D1345260

BRITISH MEDICAL ASSOCIATION

0772382

Urological Pathology

Urological Pathology

Mahul B. Amin, MD
Professor and Chairman
Department of Pathology and Laboratory Medicine
Cedars-Sinai Medical Center
Los Angeles, California

David J. Grignon, MD
Centennial Professor
Department of Pathology and Laboratory Medicine
Indiana University School of Medicine
Indianapolis, Indiana

John R. Srigley, MD, FRCPC, FRCPath, FRCPA(Hon)
Professor and Chief
Department of Pathology and Molecular Medicine, McMaster University and
Program of Laboratory Medicine and Genetics, Trillium Health Partners
Mississauga, Ontario, Canada

John N. Eble, MD, FRCPA
Nordschow Professor and Chairman
Department of Pathology and Laboratory Medicine
Indiana University School of Medicine
Indianapolis, Indiana

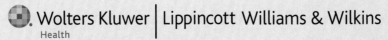
. Wolters Kluwer | Lippincott Williams & Wilkins
Health

Philadelphia • Baltimore • New York • London
Buenos Aires • Hong Kong • Sydney • Tokyo

Acquisitions Editor: Ryan Shaw
Product Manager: Kate Marshall
Production Product Manager: Priscilla Crater
Senior Manufacturing Coordinator: Beth Welsh
Marketing Manager: Dan Dressler
Designer: Joan Wendt
Production Service: SPi Global

Printed in China

Library of Congress Cataloging-in-Publication Data
Urological pathology (2014)
   Urological pathology / [edited by] Mahul B. Amin, John Eble. — First edition.
      p. ; cm.
   Includes bibliographical references and index.
   ISBN 978-0-7817-8281-4
  I. Amin, Mahul B., editor of compilation. II. Eble, John N., editor of compilation. III. Title.
  [DNLM: 1. Male Urogenital Diseases—pathology. 2. Urologic Diseases. WJ 140]
  RC900.9
  616.6'07—dc23

2013022749

Care has been taken to confirm the accuracy of the information presented and to describe generally accepted practices. However, the authors, editors, and publisher are not responsible for errors or omissions or for any consequences from application of the information in this book and make no warranty, expressed or implied, with respect to the currency, completeness, or accuracy of the contents of the publication. Application of the information in a particular situation remains the professional responsibility of the practitioner.

The authors, editors, and publisher have exerted every effort to ensure that drug selection and dosage set forth in this text are in accordance with current recommendations and practice at the time of publication. However, in view of ongoing research, changes in government regulations, and the constant flow of information relating to drug therapy and drug reactions, the reader is urged to check the package insert for each drug for any change in indications and dosage and for added warnings and precautions. This is particularly important when the recommended agent is a new or infrequently employed drug.

Some drugs and medical devices presented in the publication have Food and Drug Administration (FDA) clearance for limited use in restricted research settings. It is the responsibility of the health care provider to ascertain the FDA status of each drug or device planned for use in their clinical practice.

To purchase additional copies of this book, call our customer service department at (800) 638-3030 or fax orders to (301) 223-2320. International customers should call (301) 223-2300.

Visit Lippincott Williams & Wilkins on the Internet: at LWW.com. Lippincott Williams & Wilkins customer service representatives are available from 8:30 am to 6 pm, EST.

10 9 8 7 6 5 4 3 2 1

Preface

In *Urological Pathology*, we have aimed to bring to the practicing surgical pathologists, subspecialized urologic pathologists, and students of urologic diseases (pathology and urology residents and fellows) a comprehensive and authoritative textbook on urologic diseases. With increasing subspecialization, there is a need for surgical pathologists to have a practical resource for day-to-day management of diagnosis, reporting, and consultation on urologic diseases.

While the book aims to be all-encompassing in its coverage from etiology to clinical management, we will have succeeded if the book becomes the easy-to-navigate, yet definitive, expert resource on urologic surgical pathology kept by your microscope. Accordingly, we have focused on diagnostic morphologic criteria, differential diagnoses, pitfalls, and ancillary diagnostic tests (primarily immunohistochemistry and molecular markers only as appropriate). We have presented a broad panorama of morphologic images to compliment the diagnostic approach and the pearls highlighted in the text material and embellished this further by numerous tables and summary boxes.

This new monograph shares the title *Urological Pathology* with two other important works in the field. Herbut's *Urological Pathology* (1952) was the first comprehensive textbook on the subject. It was a monumental work comprising 1,222 pages and 522 figures. Murphy's *Urological Pathology* (first edition 1989; second edition 1997) was also an authoritative and highly respected textbook of urologic pathology.

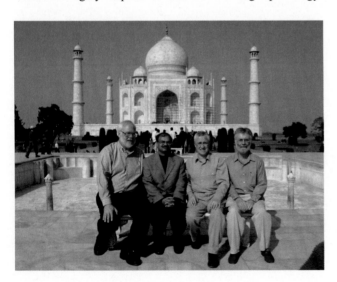

The new *Urological Pathology* is a completely new book that builds on the foundation of excellence established by these historic books and other important works in urologic pathology to provide the reader with an encyclopedic reference source on the diagnostic and prognostic assessments which are the foundation for the therapeutic decisions that follow.

The seed of this book was first planted in January 2003 while we, the editors, were on a trip to India. After delivering a 3-day national course on urologic pathology, we traveled to the Taj Mahal. Inspired by the stunning form, beauty, and timelessness of this historic monument designed and constructed because of the passion of Emperor Shah Jehan, we conceived the idea to make a major contribution (albeit on a more humble and smaller scale) to the discipline about which we are passionate. Consequently, over the past decade as we first conceptualized and then implemented the planning, authoring, and editing process, we referred to *Urological Pathology* fondly as the "Taj book."

The backbone of this book is the distinguished panel of authors of the 14 chapters, which comprise it. In creating this panel, we wanted to combine the wisdom of senior experts who have done much to make the field what it is today, with innovative ideas and passionate energy of the new generation of expert urologic pathologists whose recent work contributes to moving the field forward. We are deeply indebted to these colleagues for their generous gifts of time, enormous efforts, and incredible patience throughout this long project. We are also grateful to our clinician and scientific colleagues—urologists, oncologists and radiation oncologists who constantly seek our partnership in managing their patients, and to the many pathologists around the world who share their difficult cases with us since these cases serve as a nidus for further educational and research efforts.

In closing, we would like to dedicate this book, with the deepest of admiration, to some giants in the field who have passed away in the past decade: Dr. Robert Scully, Dr. F. K. Mostofi, Dr. Leopold Koss, and Dr. Donald Gleason. Their pioneering work laid the foundation for the establishment of the subspecialty of urologic pathology.

Mahul B. Amin
David J. Grignon
John R. Srigley
John N. Eble

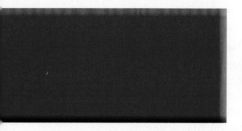

Contributors

Ferran Algaba, MD, PhD
Head Pathology Section in Fundació
  Puigvert
Autonomous University of Barcelona
Barcelona, Spain

Mahul B. Amin, MD
Professor and Chairman
Department of Pathology and
  Laboratory Medicine
Cedars-Sinai Medical Center
Los Angeles, California

Alberto G. Ayala, MD
Deputy Chair and Professor of
  Pathology
The Methodist Hospital
Weill Medical College of Cornell
  University
Ashbel-Smith Professor Emeritus of
  Pathology
The University of Texas MD Anderson
  Cancer Center
Houston, Texas

Fadi Brimo, MD, FRCPC
Assistant Professor of Pathology
McGill University
Pathologist
Department of Pathology
Montreal General Hospital
Montreal, Quebec, Canada

Antonio L. Cubilla, MD
Professor
Institute of Pathology and Investigation
National University of Asunción
Asunción, Paraguay

Brett Delahunt, ONZM, MD, FRCPA,
  FRCPath, FRSNZ
Professor of Pathology and Molecular
  Medicine
Wellington School of Medicine and
  Health Sciences
University of Otago
Wellington, New Zealand

Ronald A. DeLellis, MD
Professor
Department of Pathology and
  Laboratory Medicine
Alpert Medical School of Brown
  University
Rhode Island Hospital
Providence, Rhode Island

Mukul K. Divatia, MD
Resident
Department of Pathology and Genomic
  Medicine
The Methodist Hospital
Weill Medical College of Cornell
  University
Houston, Texas

John N. Eble, MD, FRCPA
Nordschow Professor and Chairman
Department of Pathology and
  Laboratory Medicine
Indiana University School of Medicine
Indianapolis, Indiana

Jonathan I. Epstein, MD
Professor of Pathology, Urology, and
  Oncology
Director of Surgical Pathology
The Reinhard Professor of Urological
  Pathology
The Johns Hopkins Medical
  Institutions
Baltimore, Maryland

David J. Grignon, MD
Centennial Professor
Department of Pathology and
  Laboratory Medicine
Indiana University School of Medicine
Indianapolis, Indiana

Peter A. Humphrey, MD, PhD
Ladenson Professor of Pathology and
  Immunology
Chief of Anatomic and Molecular
  Pathology
Department of Pathology and
  Immunology
Washington University School of
  Medicine
St. Louis, Missouri

Cristina Magi-Galluzzi, MD, PhD
Assistant Professor of Pathology
Lerner College of Medicine
Case Western Reserve University
Director of Genitourinary Pathology
Department of Pathology
Cleveland Clinic
Cleveland, Ohio

Shamlal Mangray, MBBS
Director, Pediatric and Autopsy
  Pathology
Lifespan Academic Medical Center
Associate Professor (Clinical)
Department of Pathology and
  Laboratory Medicine
Alpert Medical School of Brown
  University
Providence, Rhode Island

Jesse K. McKenney, MD
Head, Surgical Pathology
Robert J. Tomsich Pathology &
  Laboratory Medicine Institute
Cleveland Clinic
Cleveland, Ohio

Helen Michael, MD
Professor of Pathology and Laboratory
  Medicine
Indiana University School of Medicine
Chief of Laboratory Service
IU Health North Hospital
Indianapolis, Indiana

Esther Oliva, MD
Department of Pathology
Professor
Harvard Medical School
Pathologist
Massachusetts General Hospital
Boston, Massachusetts

Gladell P. Paner, MD
Assistant Professor
Department of Pathology
Section of Urology, Department of
  Surgery
University of Chicago
Chicago, Illinois

Victor E. Reuter, MD
Professor of Pathology and Laboratory
  Medicine
Weill Medical College of Cornell
  University
Attending Pathologist and
  Vice-Chairman
Memorial Sloan-Kettering Cancer
  Center
New York, New York

Jae Y. Ro, MD, PhD
Professor and Director of Surgical
  Pathology
The Methodist Hospital
Weill Medical College of Cornell
  University
Adjunct Professor
The University of Texas MD Anderson
  Cancer Center
Houston, Texas

Hemamali Samaratunga, MBBS,
  LRCP MRCS, FRCPA
Associate Professor
Aquesta Pathology
University of Queensland
Brisbane, Queensland, Australia

John R. Srigley, MD, FRCPC,
  FRCPath, FRCPA(Hon)
Professor
Department of Pathology and
  Molecular Medicine, McMaster
  University
Hamilton, Ontario, Canada
Chief and Medical Director
Program of Laboratory Medicine and
  Genetics, Trillium Health Partners
Mississauga, Ontario, Canada

Satish K. Tickoo, MD
Attending Pathologist
Memorial Sloan-Kettering Cancer
  Center
New York, New York

Elsa F. Velazquez, MD
Dermatopathologist
Miraca Life Sciences
Assistant Professor of Dermatology
Tufts Medical Center
Boston, Massachusetts

Mark A. Weiss, MD
Medical Director
Pathology Services
The Urology Group
Cincinnati, Ohio

Robert H. Young, MD, FRCPath
Professor of Pathology
James Homer Wright Pathology
  Laboratories
Massachusetts General Hospital
Robert E. Scully Professor of
  Pathology
Harvard Medical School
Boston, Massachusetts

Contents

Nonneoplastic Diseases of the Kidney

DAVID J. GRIGNON and MARK A. WEISS

The surgical pathologist is called on to examine kidneys removed for a wide range of nonneoplastic conditions. This chapter is not meant as a comprehensive review of nonneoplastic kidney diseases purposely excludes those conditions that are generally considered within the area of "medical kidney diseases" that pathologists are exposed to primarily through renal biopsy. For the purposes of this chapter all transplantation-related nephropathology including resection of allografts is excluded. For those diseases that are associated with renal neoplasia, the detailed discussion of the tumors is covered in Chapter 2.

EMBRYOLOGY

A detailed discussion of the embryologic development of the kidney is beyond the scope and purpose of this chapter as are the many advances in our understanding of the molecular aspects of embryogenesis. The reader is referred to more comprehensive sources if required.[1-4] The following discussion will focus on those aspects of embryology relevant to understanding the pathologic conditions covered in this chapter.

The kidney develops from the mesoderm and forms through three successive stages: the pronephros, mesonephros, and metanephros. Each of these overlaps with the preceding step as development progresses.

Pronephros

The pronephros forms from the most caudal end of the nephrogenic cord and is short-lived, appearing at the end of the 3rd week of gestation and disappearing by day 25. The pronephric ducts are the only part that persist and are incorporated into the mesonephros.

Mesonephros

The mesonephros develops from the midportion of the nephrogenic cord beginning on day 24 and results in the formation of the urogenital ridge. A series of glomeruli, each with a tubule and a capillary, form with a connection to the developing aorta. These tubules join an excretory duct, the mesonephric (Wolffian) duct. The mesonephros is a temporary functional excretory organ. These structures successively involute and by the end of the first trimester have disappeared.

Metanephros

The permanent kidney develops from the metanephros that first appears in the 5th week and becomes functional in the 9th week (Fig. 1-1). The metanephric mesenchyme, formed from the caudal end of the nephrogenic tube, gives rise to the kidney parenchyma with the ureteric bud being the origin of the collecting ducts, calyces, renal pelvis, and ureter.

Collecting System Formation

The ureteric bud develops as an outgrowth from the mesonephric duct. Signaling pathways critical to ureteric bud induction and development include GDNF and GFRα1. The *WT1* gene is involved in inducing GDNF expression. Defects in restrictive signaling pathways such as Spry-1 allow for multiple ureteric buds to form and may be related to duplicate ureters.[4] As the growing ureteric bud comes in contact with the metanephric mesenchyme it undergoes a series of dichotomous branchings. The *Wnt-11* and *GREM1* genes are among the most important in this process. The tip of the bud is known as the ampulla as is the tip of each subsequent branch as it develops. The first three to six of these give rise to the renal pelvis and major calyces (Fig. 1-2). BMP-4 is a key factor present in the metanephric mesenchyme controlling this process. Abnormalities in BMP-4 have been related to a wide range of anomalies including renal hypoplasia/dysplasia, hydroureter, megaureter, ectopic ureter, ureteral duplication, and ureteropelvic obstruction.[4] These eventually coalesce to form the structure as we see it

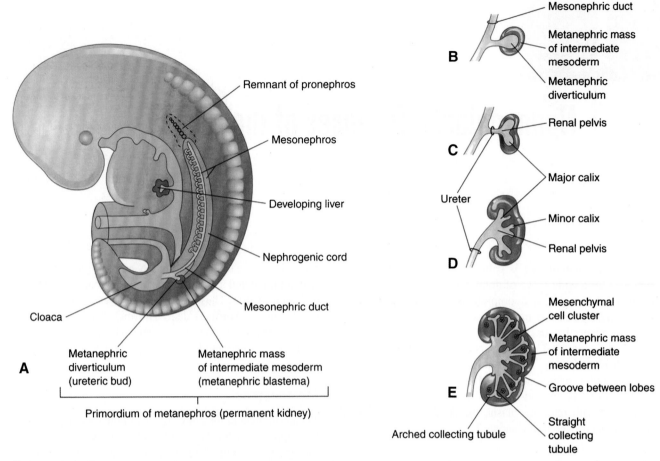

FIGURE 1-1 ■ Embryologic development of the kidney. **A:** Sketch of a lateral view of a 5-week embryo showing the primordium of the metanephros. **B–E:** Sketches showing successive stages in the development of the metanephric diverticulum or ureteric bud (5th to 8th weeks). Note the development of the ureter, renal pelvis, calices, and collecting ducts. (From Moore KL, Presaud TVN. *The Developing Human: Clinically Oriented Embryology*. 7th ed. Philadelphia, PA: Saunders; 2003, with permission.)

at birth. The continued branching and growth result in the formation of the minor calyces and ever-increasing numbers of collecting ducts (Fig. 1-3).

Nephron Formation

The nephrons develop from condensations in the metanephric mesenchyme with a condensation related to each

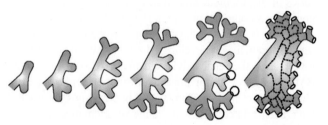

FIGURE 1-2 ■ Development of the renal pelvis. Diagram showing branching of the ureteral bud. (Reprinted from Mills SE. *Histology for Pathologists*. 3rd ed. Philadelphia, PA: Lippincott Williams & Wilkins; 2008. Modified from Potter EL. *Normal and Abnormal Development of the Kidney*. Chicago, IL: Year Book; 1972, with permission.)

tip of the branching ureteric bud ampullae (Fig. 1-4). The condensation forms an S-shaped structure (the nephrogenic vesicle) with a space that becomes continuous with the lumen of the growing collecting tubule. The nephrogenic vesicle elongates with one end forming the proximal tubule and the loop of Henle. The initial period of nephron formation ends after the 14th week of gestation. The nephrons from this initial period are localized to the corticomedullary junction. In the second period of nephrogenesis, additional glomeruli develop as arcades from the no longer branching ampullae of the ureteric bud. In the third period of nephrogenesis, between weeks 22 and 36, the ampullae grow peripherally to the outermost part of the cortex giving rise to another four to seven nephrons. The last nephrons formed are located in the subcapsular region. It is estimated that there are between 0.7 and 1.5 million glomeruli per kidney.

After 36 weeks, the ampullae regress and disappear with no additional nephrons being formed. During this last part of fetal development, the tubules lengthen and become more tortuous.

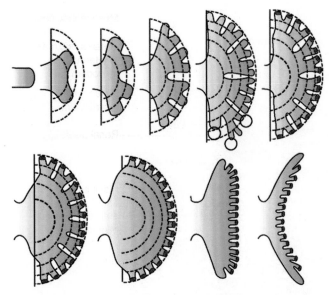

FIGURE 1-3 ■ Development of renal calyces and papillae. Diagram showing coalescence of the third to fifth generation of branches of the primordial calyx with inward prolapse of the renal papilla. (Reprinted from Mills SE. *Histology for Pathologists*. 3rd ed. Philadelphia, PA: Lippincott Williams & Wilkins; 2008. Modified from Potter EL. *Normal and Abnormal Development of the Kidney*. Chicago, IL: Year Book; 1972, with permission.)

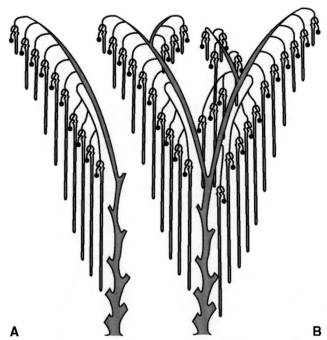

A   **B**

FIGURE 1-4 ■ Arrangement of nephrons at birth as revealed by microdissection. **A:** Usual pattern. **B:** Possible variations. (Reprinted from Mills SE. *Histology for Pathologists*. 3rd ed. Philadelphia, PA: Lippincott Williams & Wilkins; 2008. Modified from Potter EL. *Normal and Abnormal Development of the Kidney*. Chicago, IL: Year Book; 1972, with permission.)

ANATOMY AND HISTOLOGY

In this section, the anatomy and histology of the kidney relevant to the types of specimens encountered by the surgical pathologist will be reviewed. Detailed descriptions of the anatomy and histology of the kidney are available in more comprehensive references.[5,6]

Gross Anatomy

The kidneys are paired organs located in the retroperitoneum. The superior poles are usually located at the level of T12/L1 with the lower poles at L3, although the upper and lower extremes can range from T11 to L5. The right kidney is usually 1 to 2 cm lower than the left. The kidneys are related to the diaphragm at the superior posterior aspect, the psoas muscle posteriorly and the quadratus lumborum and aponeurosis of the transversus abdominus muscle laterally. Anteriorly the right kidney is juxtaposed to the liver, right colonic flexure, descending part of the duodenum, and the small intestine. On the left, the anterior surface relates to the stomach, spleen, pancreas, left colonic flexure, descending colon, and jejunum. Both superior poles are intimately related to the adrenal glands. They are surrounded by fat within Gerota fascia (Fig. 1-5). Gerota fascia is a thin fibromembranous structure that is in continuity with the transversalis fascia; it surrounds the perirenal adipose tissue superiorly, laterally, and medially but does not cover the hilar or inferior boundaries.

In newborns, the kidneys weigh between 13 and 44 g; they increase in size with age reaching 115 to 166 g in adult females and 125 to 170 g in adult males.[7] The increase in weight is related to increased tubular and interstitial tissues; the number of glomeruli remains constant. With advancing age, the kidneys begin to decrease in weight due primarily to cortical atrophy. The average adult kidney measures 11 to 12 cm in length, 5 to 7 cm in width, and 2.5 to 3 cm in thickness. The kidneys are surrounded by a well-developed fibrous capsule that can be readily stripped from the cortical surface; the capsule covers the outer convexities of the kidney but is not well-developed in the hilar region where the vascular and collecting system structures enter the renal parenchyma (Fig. 1-6). In fact, there is no capsule covering the renal cortical tissue of the columns of Bertin where the columns come in contact with the renal sinus adipose tissue. This has been shown to represent an important site of tumor extension beyond the renal parenchyma (Fig. 1-7).[8,9]

In some adults, the kidney retains the prominent fetal lobulations that are evident at birth (Fig. 1-8). In most kidneys, however, these largely disappear with the exception of two grooves extending from the hilum dividing the kidney into three poorly defined regions: a middle zone and the upper and lower poles. The cut surface reveals a continuous layer of pale tan cortex, measuring about 1 cm in thickness and making up the entire outer aspect of the renal

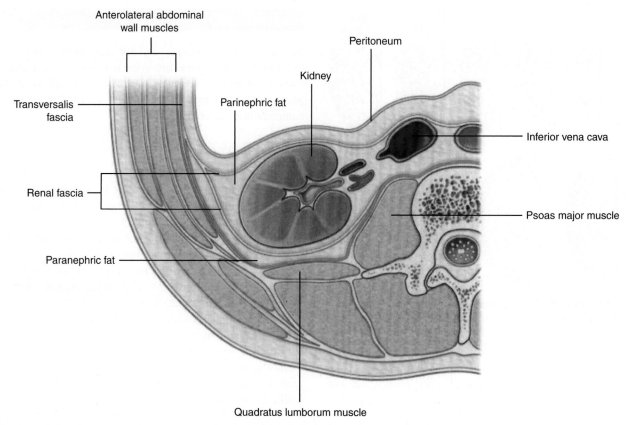

Anterolateral abdominal wall muscles

Peritoneum

Kidney

Transversalis fascia

Parinephric fat

Inferior vena cava

Renal fascia

Psoas major muscle

Paranephric fat

Quadratus lumborum muscle

FIGURE 1-5 ■ Kidney anatomy. Cross section of kidney at the level of renal hilum showing relationship to fat and renal (Gerota) fascia. (From Drake RL, Vogl AW, Mitchell AWM. *Gray's Anatomy for Students*. 2nd ed. Philadelphia, PA: Churchill Livingstone; 2010:357, with permission.)

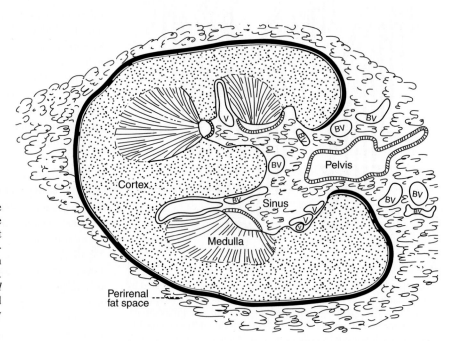

FIGURE 1-6 ■ Kidney anatomy. Line drawing of cross section of kidney at the level of the renal hilum illustrating the extent of the renal capsule (*thick line*) and in particular its absence in the renal sinus area. (From Murphy WM, Beckwith JB, Farrow GM. *Tumors of the Kidney, Bladder and Related Urinary Structures, AFIP Fascicle*. 3rd series. Washington, DC: American Registry of Pathology; 1994, with permission.)

Cortex

Medulla

Sinus

Pelvis

BV

V

Perirenal fat space

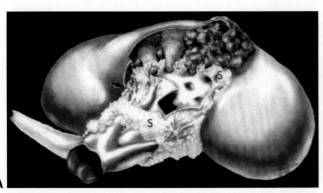
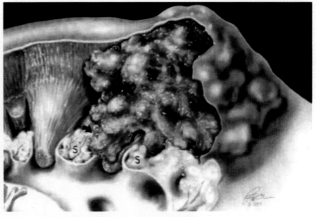

A   B

FIGURE 1-7 ■ Renal sinus and tumor invasion **(A,B)**. Drawing illustrating the propensity of tumors to infiltrate into the renal sinus soft tissue at a location lacking a renal capsule (*arrow*, **B**). (From Bonsib SM, Gibson D, Mhoon M, et al. Renal sinus involvement in renal cell carcinomas. *Am J Surg Pathol* 2000;24:452, with permission.)

parenchyma (Fig. 1-9). Cortical tissue extending from the outer aspect to the renal sinus (columns of Bertin) separates individual medullary pyramids and their draining calyces. The medulla is a darker red brown than the cortex and has a striated appearance. It can be divided into an outer or peripheral zone and an inner zone or papillae. A single unit of a pyramid with its associated cortex is the equivalent of a unipapillary kidney. In humans, the fusion of these individual units results in a multipapillary type of kidney.

Vascular Structure

The arterial supply to each kidney originates from the aorta with a main renal artery. In most kidneys, the renal artery divides into anterior and posterior divisions that pass anterior and posterior to the renal pelvis. Within the hilum, these further divide into variable numbers of segmental branches (most often the anterior division divides into four segmental branches while the posterior division continues as a single segmental branch). The main renal artery also gives rise to the suprarenal artery supplying the adrenal gland and a ureteric artery supplying the ureter. Deviation from this pattern is, however, common.

Within the renal sinus, each segmental artery gives rise to multiple lobar arteries (the vessels that typically enter the parenchyma) that then give rise to the interlobar then the arcuate arteries, followed by the interlobular arteries and finally the arterioles.[10] These are all end arteries and so occlusion leads to downstream infarction. The efferent arterioles form a complex capillary network that supplies the cortical tubules and the juxtamedullary glomeruli. The medulla derives its blood supply mainly from the efferent arterioles of the juxtamedullary glomeruli.

The venous return largely parallels the vascular supply with interlobular, arcuate, and interlobar veins paired with their corresponding artery. In contrast to the arterial system, the venous system includes a complex network of anastomoses. The interlobar veins join to form the main renal vein that passes anterior to the renal pelvis.

Lymphatic System

The major lymphatic drainage system follows the vascular system.[11] The lymphatics begin at the level of the interlobular arteries. No lymphatic channels are present in the area of the glomeruli and associated tubules. The main lymphatics drain into the hilar and periaortic lymph nodes. A second

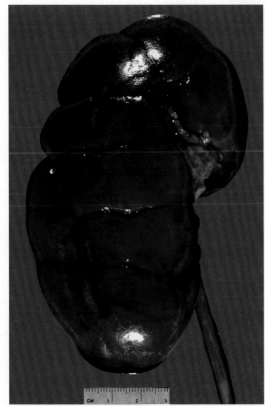

FIGURE 1-8 ■ Kidney with prominent fetal lobulations. Kidney from a 37-year-old woman with prominent grooves highlighting the normal fetal lobulations that usually disappear with maturity.

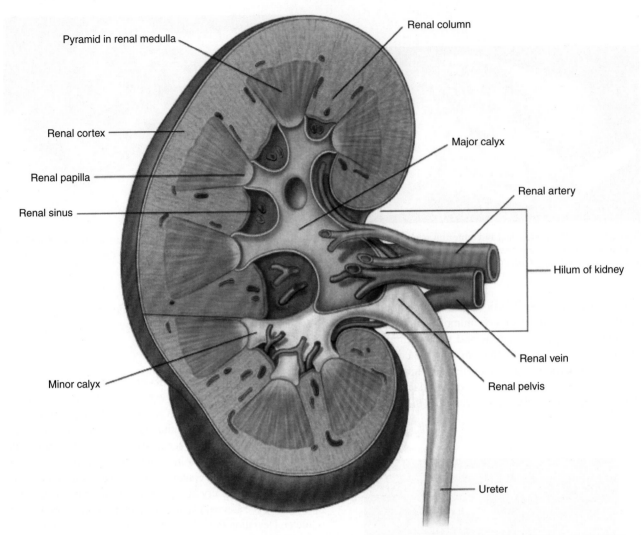

Pyramid in renal medulla

Renal column

Renal cortex

Renal papilla

Renal sinus

Major calyx

Renal artery

Hilum of kidney

Renal vein

Minor calyx

Renal pelvis

Ureter

FIGURE 1-9 ■ Kidney anatomy. Line drawing of the cut surface of the kidney. (From Drake RL, Vogl AW, Mitchell AWM. *Gray's Anatomy for Students*. 2nd ed. Philadelphia, PA: Churchill Livingstone; 2010:358, with permission.)

lymphatic system present within the renal capsule drains the outermost portion of the cortex and eventually communicates with the major lymphatic system in the hilar region.

Nerve Supply

The nerve supply of the kidney is sympathetic in type and is derived from the celiac plexus and then branches to the renal plexus via the splanchnic nerves. The nerve fibers originating in the renal plexus follow the arterial supply to the cortical region and innervate the juxtaglomerular apparatus and the renal vasculature. Nerve endings also interact with tubules, particularly the thick part of the ascending loop of Henle. Sensory fibers in the kidney follow the sympathetic nerves to the T10–T11 region.

Microscopic Anatomy

The renal cortex is covered by the renal capsule which is composed of dense fibrous connective tissue (Fig. 1-10). In the cortex of the kidney, the components are arranged in two distinct

patterns defined by the cortical labyrinth and the medullary rays. The major components of the cortical labyrinth are the glomeruli and the proximal tubules, but this area also includes distal convoluted tubules, connecting tubules, and the most proximal portions of the collecting ducts (Fig. 1-11). The medullary rays contain collecting ducts, and the proximal and distal straight tubules. The outer medulla contains the straight portion of the proximal tubules, the thin descending limb of the loop of Henle, and the thin and thick ascending limb of the loop of Henle as well as portions of the collecting ducts. The inner medulla (papilla) includes the thin descending and ascending limbs of the loop of Henle and the collecting ducts (Fig. 1-12).

Glomerulus

The normal glomerulus is about 200 μm in diameter. It consists of the glomerular tuft that is suspended in Bowman space, a fluid-filled space that empties into the proximal convoluted tubule (Fig. 1-13). The glomerular tuft consists of a complex capillary network supported by the glomerular

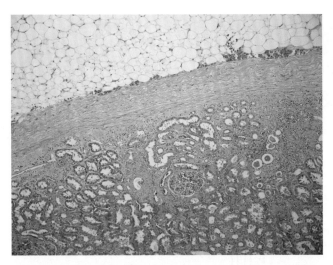

FIGURE 1-10 ■ Renal capsule. External surface of the kidney illustrating a well-defined fibrous capsule covering the surface of the renal cortex and separating the parenchyma from the perinephric fat.

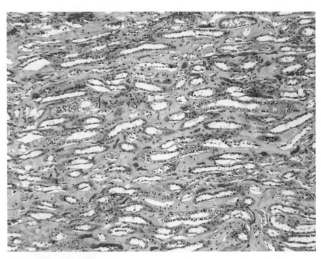

FIGURE 1-12 ■ Renal medulla. Normal renal medulla with distal tubules and collecting ducts.

mesangium and fed by the afferent arteriole and drained by an efferent arteriole. The glomerular tuft contains three types of cells: endothelial, mesangial, and epithelial (podocytes) cells. The glomerular visceral epithelial cells (podocytes) transition into the parietal epithelial cells that line Bowman space. These squamous-like cells form a complete layer on the inner surface of Bowman capsule.

The juxtaglomerular apparatus is located at the vascular pole of the glomerulus. This structure is composed of specialized epithelial cells, vascular smooth muscle cells, the macula densa of the distal tubule, and specialized cells of the extraglomerular mesangium (lacis cells). This complex structure is responsible for regulating glomerular hemodynamics.

Proximal Tubule

The proximal tubule originates at the urinary end of the glomerulus and includes both a proximal convoluted and a distal straight portion. The lining cells are cuboidal to columnar

with densely eosinophilic cytoplasm. Ultrastructural examination shows that the cells contain abundant mitochondria and have a prominent brush border.

Loop of Henle

The loop of Henle consists of a descending thin limb, an ascending thin limb, and an ascending thick limb. At the beginning of the descending thin limb, the proximal tubular cells change to a flattened inconspicuous squamous-like epithelium. In general, the cells throughout the thin limbs of the loop of Henle have nuclei that bulge into the tubular lumens and a surface that contains few to no microvilli. The thick ascending limb of the loop of Henle is considered to be part of the distal tubule.

Distal Tubule

The distal tubule includes three distinct components; the thick ascending limb, the distal convoluted tubule, and the macula densa. In the medullary portion of the thick ascending limb, the lining consists of low cuboidal cells with eosinophilic cytoplasm and apically located nuclei. These cells have no brush border. The cells of the cortical segment are shorter but otherwise similar. In the distal convoluted tubule, the cells are also cuboidal with pale eosinophilic cytoplasm and closely packed nuclei. They have short microvilli along the surface. At the junction with the connecting tubule the cells are intermingled with the connecting tubule and intercalated cells.

Collecting Duct

The collecting ducts begin in the cortex and make up much of the medullary rays as they descend and then pass into the medulla and finally terminate in the papilla. The collecting ducts are lined by two types of cells: the principal cells

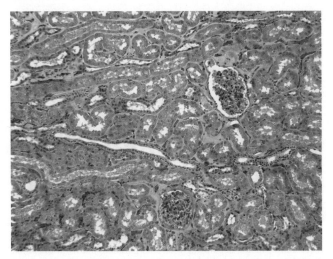

FIGURE 1-11 ■ Renal cortex. Normal renal cortex containing glomeruli and tubules of the proximal and distal nephron.

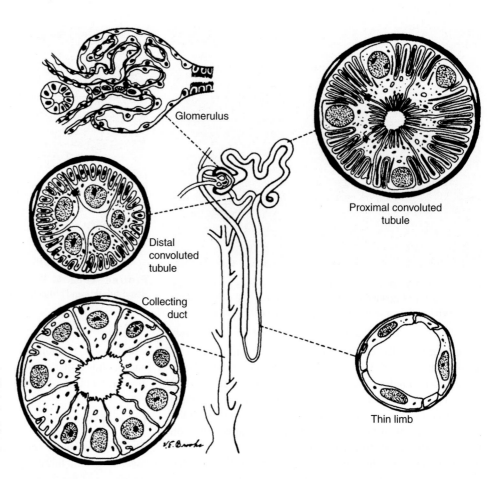

FIGURE 1-13 ■ Normal histology of the nephron. Line drawing illustrating the various components of the nephron from the glomerulus to the collecting ducts. (From Bennington JL, Kradjian R. *Renal Carcinoma*. Philadelphia, PA: WB Saunders; 1967, with permission.)

and the intercalated cells. The intercalated cells are largely restricted to the cortical and outer medullary segments of the collecting ducts. By light microscopy, both the principal cells and intercalated cells are cuboidal with pale cytoplasm and centrally located nuclei. The principal cells tend to get taller in the more distal portion of the collecting duct with the cells being columnar in the distal collecting ducts (ducts of Bellini).

Interstitium

The interstitium of the kidney includes a mixture of cells and stromal matrix. The predominant cell type within the interstitium is the fibroblast. The fibroblasts have specialized functions in different areas of the kidney. The medullary interstitial cell is a specialized lipid-laden fibroblast. These cells are involved in control of blood flow and produce prostanoids that have an antihypertensive effect.[12] Other cells normally present are dendritic cells, macrophages, and lymphocytes. The matrix includes many substances including types I, II, and VI collagen, fibronectin, and sulfated and nonsulfated glycosaminoglycans.

Renal Sinus

The junction between the renal cortex and the renal sinus fat is not well-defined by a fibrous capsule (Fig. 1-14).

Often there is a loose hypocellular connective tissue between the renal parenchymal tissue and the adipose tissue within the sinus. The sinus contains an abundance of thin-walled vascular and lymphatic channels embedded within the fat.

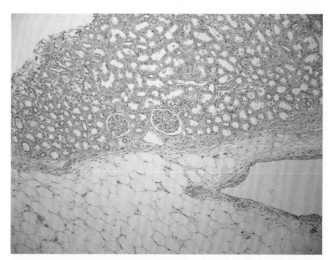

FIGURE 1-14 ■ Renal sinus. In the area of the renal sinus there is no capsule separating the renal parenchyma from the sinus fat. Note tubular epithelium immediately adjacent to fat cells.

CONGENITAL ANOMALIES

Congenital anomalies involving the kidney and urinary tract have become known under the general label "congenital abnormalities of the kidney and urinary tract" or CAKUT.[13] The use of this broad umbrella recognizes that in many cases multiple anomalies are present and further that single gene mutations can give rise to diverse abnormalities.[14] The frequency is 3 to 6 per 1,000 births, and they are a significant cause of morbidity and mortality in the 1st year.[15] Congenital anomalies are responsible for an estimated 50% of cases of end-stage renal failure in childhood and continue to be responsible for a small percentage in the 20- to 30-year-old age group.[16,17]

Renal Agenesis and Hypoplasia

Renal Agenesis

Clinical Features

Renal agenesis refers to the complete absence of one or rarely both kidneys.[1,18,19] This can occur sporadically or in the setting of a large number of syndromes (Table 1-1).[20] The majority of patients with renal agenesis have other abnormalities involving the genitourinary tract.[20] In males, the most common organs involved are the epididymis, vas deferens, and seminal vesicle, with seminal vesicle cysts being among the more frequent. The association of unilateral renal agenesis with seminal vesicle cysts is known as Zinner syndrome.[21] In females, the fallopian tube, uterus, and vagina can all have associated abnormalities. Patients with unilateral agenesis may be asymptomatic and the abnormality found incidentally even in adulthood.[22] In other cases, it is symptoms related to an associated anomaly that bring the patient to medical attention. It is recommended that close evaluation of patients be undertaken when absence of a kidney is discovered incidentally.[23]

Bilateral renal agenesis (Potter syndrome) occurs in 0.1 of 1,000 births and is incompatible with life.[1,14] The typical manifestation is severe oligohydramnios. Oligohydramnios, irrespective of cause, results in a characteristic phenotype that includes Potter facies; positional deformities of the hips, knees, and feet; and hypoplastic lungs (Fig. 1-15A and B). Infants with Potter syndrome are either stillborn or die shortly after birth due to respiratory failure.

Table 1-1 ■ SYNDROMES ASSOCIATED WITH RENAL AGENESIS

Trisomy 13
Trisomy 18
Müllerian aplasia syndrome
Fraser syndrome
William syndrome
Cloacal exstrophy
Sirenomelia
Hereditary renal dysplasia
VATER syndrome
Many others

Pathology

The apparent absence of a kidney does not always indicate renal agenesis and ultimately the diagnosis of true renal agenesis requires confirmation of the absence of the kidney at autopsy or surgery. In unilateral agenesis, the remaining kidney may be significantly enlarged and hyperplastic.

Renal Hypoplasia

Clinical Features

Renal hypoplasia is defined by the presence of kidneys that are significantly smaller than normal. The kidneys are normally differentiated and should be distinguished from abnormal small kidneys. The condition can result from deficient metanephric induction, metanephric blastema, or postnatal renal growth.[24,25] Bernstein and Gilbert-Barness[26] have recognized three distinct categories of renal hypoplasia: oligonephric hypoplasia, simple hypoplasia, and unirenicular hypoplasia. Simple hypoplasia is rare and usually bilateral.[26,27] Clinical diagnosis is based on the identification of a significant reduction in kidney size (more than 2 standard deviations), no evidence of scarring by dimercaptosuccinic acid scan, and compensatory hyperplasia of the contralateral kidney.[14] Confirmation does require pathologic evaluation to exclude dysplasia.

Oligonephric hypoplasia (oligomeganephronia) is characterized by severe polyuria and polydipsia developing before the age of 2 years. This is associated with dehydration, anorexia, failure to thrive, and growth retardation. The condition progresses to renal failure before the age of 20 years and patients do well with renal transplantation. Mutations in the *PAX2* gene have been described in some cases of oligonephric hypoplasia.[28]

Segmental hypoplasia (Ask-Upmark kidney) is now considered to be an acquired condition and is discussed later in this chapter.

Pathology

Gross Features. Both kidneys are affected except in cases associated with contralateral agenesis or dysplasia. They are smaller than normal with a mean weight of 20 g (Fig. 1-16).[24,26] The lobes and the number of pyramids are usually reduced in number and the pelvis and calyces are normally formed.

Microscopic Features. In simple hypoplasia, there may be reduced numbers of glomeruli, but the kidneys are otherwise morphologically normal. In oligonephric hypoplasia, there are reduced numbers of markedly enlarged glomeruli (Fig. 1-17). Tubules are also enlarged and dilated with the formation of small cysts. The finding of any dysplastic changes excludes the diagnosis.

Abnormalities in Form and Position

Rotation Abnormality

Clinical Features

During development, the kidneys move from the pelvis into the abdomen and as part of that transition the kidneys rotate from an anterior-facing renal pelvis to the normal medial

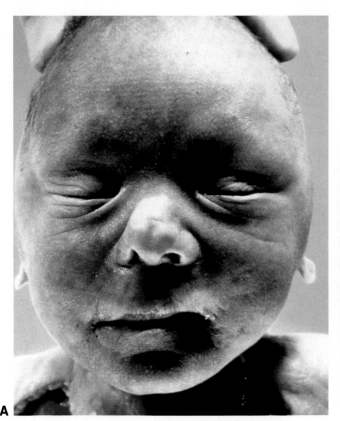

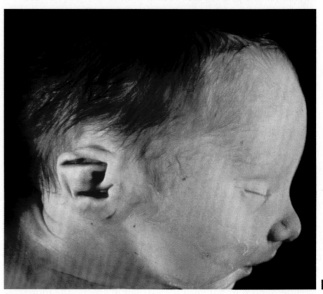

A   **B**

FIGURE 1-15 ■ Potter syndrome. Infant born with bilateral renal agenesis. Characteristic features of the face include **(A)** the widely spaced eyes, flattened nose, prominent inner canthic folds, and the receding chin; **(B)** the lateral view highlights the flattened nose, receding chin, and the low set ears with little cartilage.

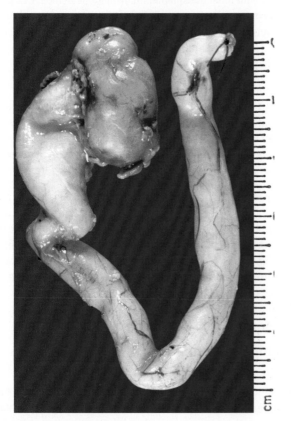

orientation. This rotation can be disrupted with the renal pelvis remaining oriented to the anterior or less frequently over rotation results in a more posterior orientation. These abnormalities may have no clinical consequences and might be identified incidentally.[22] In others, the abnormal position of the renal pelvis and ureter may result in obstruction and the associated complications including hydronephrosis, obstructive nephropathy, and lithiasis.

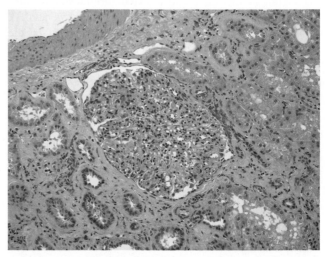

FIGURE 1-16 ■ Renal hypoplasia. The kidney is small but largely retains a normal reniform shape.

FIGURE 1-17 ■ Oligomeganephronia. Enlarged glomeruli in the setting of renal hypoplasia.

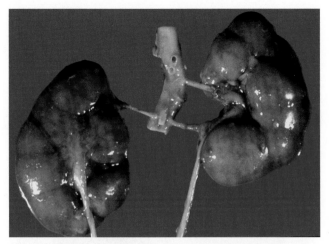

FIGURE 1-18 ■ Malrotation. The right kidney is abnormally rotated, resulting in a flattened, disc shape. Note also the aberrant renal arteries.

Pathology

Malrotated kidneys are often abnormal in shape. Most characteristic is a flattened or discoid shape (Fig. 1-18). Microscopically the kidney is normal. Secondary changes related to obstruction and its consequences may be seen.

Horseshoe Kidney

Clinical Features

Renal fusion refers to the joining of the two kidneys to form a single structure. The most common expression of renal fusion is the horseshoe kidney due to fusion of the lower poles of the two developing kidneys. This anomaly, which is more common in males, occurs in 1:350 to 1:2,000 births.[29,30] These are essentially all ectopic in location; the majority located anterior to the aorta and vena cava with others located posterior to the great vessels. The pelves face anterior. In many cases, there are additional abnormalities. Many of these remain asymptomatic unless complicated by nephrolithiasis and/or obstruction with its associated complications.[31] Renal cell carcinoma develops in horseshoe kidneys in a frequency similar to normally located, nonfused kidneys.[32,33] There is an apparent unusually high frequency of renal carcinoid tumors in horseshoe kidneys.[34,35] Squamous cell carcinoma has also been described in association with nephrolithiasis.[36]

Pathology

The kidneys are typically fused at the lower pole and may or may not be associated with other abnormalities (Figs. 1-19 and 1-20). The amount of renal parenchyma in the isthmus is variable. The arterial supply is often anomalous. Abnormalities of the ureteral location are also common. The renal parenchyma is normal. Secondary changes resulting from obstruction and its complications may be present.

Malposition (Renal Ectopia)

Clinical Features

Ectopic location of the kidney is a relatively common congenital anomaly with an estimated prevalence of 1:1,000.

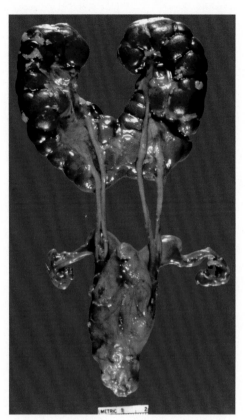

FIGURE 1-19 ■ Horseshoe kidney. In this example, there is a fairly large isthmus at the lower poles, bilateral bifid ureters, and prominent fetal lobulations.

The kidney can be located in the thorax but is more often located inferiorly in the pelvis. When the kidney is on the same side as the ureter and blood supply, the ectopy is termed simple; when located on the opposite side it is referred to as crossed. In crossed ectopy, fusion is also often present. Ectopy is frequently associated with other congenital

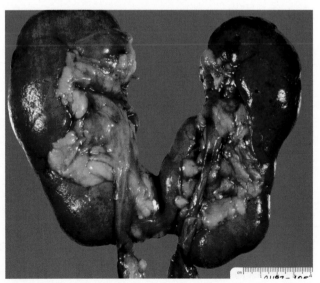

FIGURE 1-20 ■ Horseshoe kidney. In this case the isthmus joins the lower pole of the right with the lower midportion on the left.

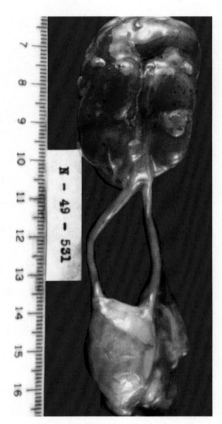

FIGURE 1-21 ■ Crossed fused ectopia. There is a fused single kidney with two ureters.

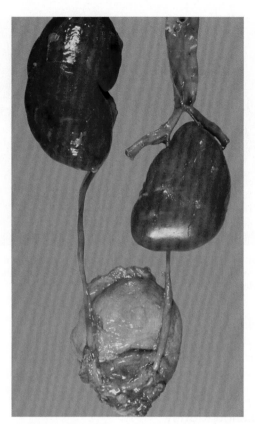

FIGURE 1-22 ■ Ectopia. The right kidney is located in the pelvis at the bifurcation of the aorta. There is also malrotation with the kidney having a disc-like shape.

anomalies, including anomalies of the cardiovascular and central nervous systems. The malposition is typically associated with aberrant vascular and ureteral locations resulting in obstructive phenomena. Many ectopic kidneys are dysplastic. If undetected in childhood, these may present in adulthood with pain, hematuria, recurrent infections, lithiasis, and obstruction. Treatment depends on the specific type of ectopy and its clinical associations.

Pathology
Ectopic kidneys are often abnormally shaped with a disc-like appearance frequent in pelvic kidneys (Figs. 1-21 and 1-22). The gross appearance reflects other associated abnormalities. A wide range of microscopic features can range from essentially normal to dysplastic.

CYSTIC DISEASES

Cystic diseases of the kidney have long been considered among the most difficult to understand categories of kidney pathology that the surgical (or autopsy) pathologist is called upon to resolve. The past decade has seen remarkable growth in the understanding of the genetics and pathogenesis of this diverse group of conditions.[37] These have been classified in a variety of ways over the years. Table 1-2 outlines the diseases discussed in this section organized by whether they are known to be inherited, acquired, or uncertain.

Cysts in Hereditary Syndromes

Autosomal Recessive (Infantile) Polycystic Disease

Genetics
Autosomal recessive polycystic kidney disease is present in 1 per 6,000 to 1 per 14,000 live births.[38,39] It is inherited as an autosomal recessive defect, and the genetic defect has been

Table 1-2 ■ CYSTIC DISEASES OF THE KIDNEY
Inherited disorders
Autosomal recessive (infantile) polycystic kidney disease
Autosomal dominant (adult) polycystic kidney disease
Nephronophthisis
Medullary cystic kidney disease
von Hippel-Lindau disease
Tuberous sclerosis
Primarily nonhereditary disorders
Multicystic renal dysplasia
Glomerulocystic disease
Medullary sponge kidney
Simple cyst
Acquired cystic kidney disease
Segmental cystic disease
Cyst-like lesions
Pyelocalyceal diverticulum (cyst)
Perinephric pseudocyst

localized to the *PKHD1* (polycystic kidney and hepatic disease) gene on chromosome 6.[40] This gene codes for the fibrocystin/polyductin protein.[41] The protein is localized to the primary cilium within renal epithelial cells of the collecting ducts. It is critical to ciliary function and within the cilium is primarily found in the basal body.[42]

Clinical Features

The clinical expression of the disorder is considered to represent a continuous spectrum; however, for practical purposes two general categories of expression predominate.[43,44] In the more common pattern, the presentation is with marked abdominal distension caused by gross renal enlargement at birth (Fig. 1-23). This may lead to intrapartum dystocia manifest as Potter syndrome.[1] These infants usually die shortly after birth secondary to pulmonary insufficiency; therapy is generally supportive only.[45] In individuals presenting later in childhood, the picture is dominated by both the renal disease and the associated hepatic fibrosis. Renal involvement is variable with about one-half retaining renal function and the remainder progressing to renal failure.[38] Hypertension may be severe and lead to heart failure. Hepatic fibrosis manifests predominantly as portal hypertension with bleeding esophageal varices being a common and frequently fatal complication[46]; liver function usually remains normal. Other associations include cholangitis and hypersplenism. Treatment in these patients may include renal transplantation and surgical shunting procedures for the portal hypertension.[47] Recent clinical experience has demonstrated significant improvement in survival for these patients. Perinatal mortality is in the 30% to 50% range; for patients who survive past 30 days, a 5-year survival rate of up to 87% has been reported.[48]

Pathology

Gross Features. The kidneys are bilaterally grossly enlarged weighing up to 10 times normal in patients with severe disease (Fig. 1-24). A normal reniform shape is maintained. The cortical surface is smooth with numerous small cysts (1 to 2 mm). The cut surface reveals radially arranged cylindrical cysts replacing the cortex and medulla with loss of definition of the corticomedullary junction (Fig. 1-25). In those individuals surviving into childhood, the findings are much more variable. The cysts tend to be fewer, more haphazardly distributed, and larger; the kidneys may be normal or enlarged.[46]

Microscopic Features. The pathogenesis of cyst formation is believed to be related to abnormal ciliary function.[41] The cysts in the cortex are elongate and fusiform with a cuboidal epithelial lining (Fig. 1-26). In the medulla, the shape of the cysts is more variable. The cysts originate from collecting ducts with the proximal tubules and glomeruli being spared. In patients diagnosed at an older age, the cysts tend to be much less uniform in appearance. Dysplastic elements such as immature tubules and cartilage are not found.

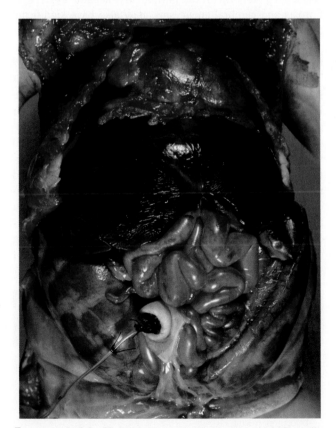

FIGURE 1-23 ■ Autosomal recessive polycystic kidney disease. In situ photograph of a neonate at autopsy. The markedly enlarged kidneys can be seen filling the abdomen and pelvis. Note the marked displacement of the liver upward resulting in severe compromise of the chest cavity. The lungs were severely hypoplastic.

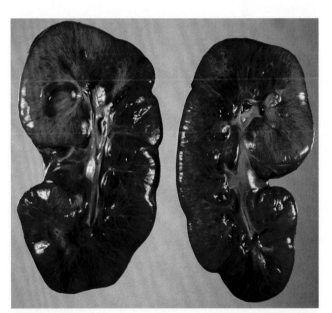

FIGURE 1-24 ■ Autosomal recessive polycystic kidney disease. Bilateral kidneys at autopsy showing markedly enlarged kidneys with normal reniform appearance. The long tubular cysts can be appreciated in this photograph to result in a radiating pattern outward toward the cortical surface (see Fig. 1-25).

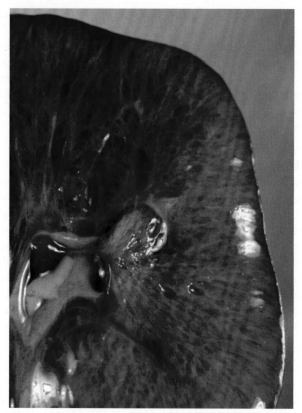

Figure 1-25 ■ Autosomal recessive polycystic kidney disease. Close-up view of the cut surface of the kidney illustrating the elongated fusiform cysts involving the cortex and medulla.

Autosomal Dominant (Adult) Polycystic Kidney Disease

Genetics

Adult or autosomal dominant polycystic disease is among the most common inherited disorders with about 1 in 600 to 1 in 1,000 persons being affected.[49,50] The defective gene

in 85% to 90% of cases has been localized to the short arm of chromosome 16 (*PKD1*, 16p13.3).[51] The remaining cases are related to the *PKD2* gene at 4q13-23 with evidence that a third gene *PKD3* may also be involved.[51] The *PKD1* and *PKD2* genes encode for the polycystin 1 and polycystin 2 proteins, respectively. These proteins localize to the primary cilia of renal epithelial cells.[52] The *TSC1* gene is located near the *PKD1* gene, and in some patients both genes are affected resulting in kidneys with overlapping features of tuberous sclerosis and autosomal dominant polycystic kidney disease.[53]

Clinical Features

There is a very high rate of penetrance, and most affected individuals will show some signs of the disease.[54] Autosomal dominant polycystic kidney disease is the most common inherited cause of end-stage renal disease in the United States.[55] The majority of cases present in the third or fourth decades with development in infancy or childhood infrequent. Ultrasound abnormalities are detectable in 85% of patients by age 25.[56] In children, the kidneys are of normal size.[57] Most patients present with abdominal pain and palpably enlarged kidneys; gross or microscopic hematuria and hypertension may also be present. In symptomatic patients, renal failure ensues on average 10 years after presentation. Associated abnormalities, particularly hepatic cysts with fibrosis and cerebral aneurysms, may also have significant clinical impact (Table 1-3).[58–62]

Treatment is symptomatic with dialysis or transplantation required in about one-half of affected patients.[55,56,63] The most common renal complications (excluding end-stage renal disease) are pain, hematuria, and infection. Hypertension develops in almost all patients and is a major part of the management required. In general, the native kidneys are not resected as even limited function is considered valuable.[64] The most common indications for native nephrectomy are recurrent infection, pain, persistent hematuria, and recurrent nephrolithiasis. Renal calculi complicate the condition in up to 35% of patients. For those with large calculi that fail medical management, open surgery or percutaneous nephrolithotomy may be necessary.[65,66] Understanding of the genetics of this disorder has identified a number of

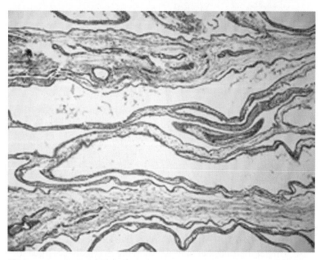

Figure 1-26 ■ Autosomal recessive polycystic kidney disease. The elongated, saccular cysts are lined by a flattened to cuboidal epithelium.

Table 1-3 ■ EXTRARENAL MANIFESTATIONS OF AUTOSOMAL DOMINANT POLYCYSTIC KIDNEY DISEASE (APPROXIMATE FREQUENCY)
Hepatic cysts (>90%)
Seminal tract cysts (40%)
Bronchiectasis (35%)
Pericardial effusion (35%)
Mitral valve prolapse (25%)
Abdominal hernia (10%)
Intracranial aneurysms (8%)
Arachnoid membrane cysts (8%)
Spinal meningeal cysts (<2%)
Pancreatic cysts (10%)

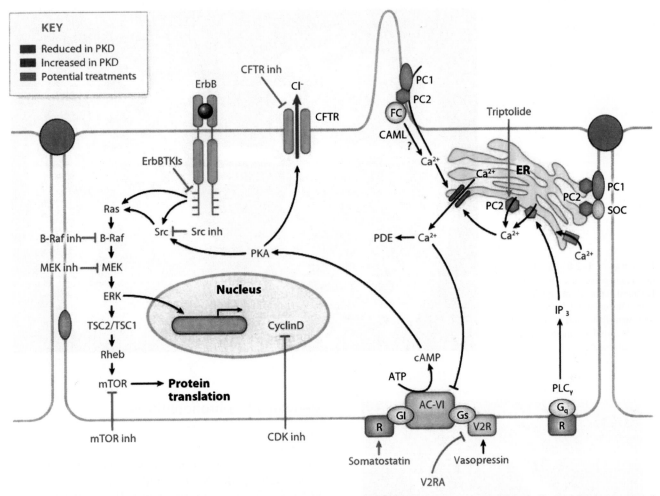

FIGURE 1-27 ■ Autosomal dominant polycystic kidney disease. Cellular changes with polycystic kidney disease. Components and pathways that are down-regulated and up-regulated are indicated. Potential treatments that target these defective pathways are shown in *red*. (From Harris PC, Torres VE. Polycystic kidney disease. *Annu Rev Med* 2009;60:325, with permission.)

molecular pathways that are potential targets for therapy[67,68] (Fig. 1-27). In transplanted patients, the major causes of death are cardiovascular disease, infection, malignancies, and cerebrovascular causes.[55]

The association with malignant tumors is controversial.[69] It has been estimated that the number of cases of renal cell carcinoma in patients with autosomal dominant polycystic kidney disease is no more than could be expected by chance.[68] Other observations such as a higher incidence of multifocal and bilateral tumors in these patients indicate an increased risk of tumor development.[70] The frequent development of epithelial proliferations including papillary adenomas in these cysts also would support the latter point of view.[71]

Pathology
Gross Features. Involved kidneys are diffusely enlarged, weighing on average 5 to 10 times the normal[72] (Fig. 1-28). There is diffuse involvement of the kidney parenchyma by unilocular cysts with the normal reniform shape of the kidney

being generally maintained (Fig. 1-29). The cysts range from less than a millimeter to several centimeters. Most contain translucent clear to straw-colored fluid, but hemorrhagic fluid and blood clots may be present. The amount of intervening stroma depends on the degree of advancement of the process.

Microscopic Features. The diagnosis of autosomal dominant polycystic kidney disease requires the demonstration of normal renal elements in the septa between the cysts (Fig. 1-30). These elements may be distorted by secondary changes related to compression or pyelonephritis. The cysts affect any part of the nephron from the glomerulus to the distal collecting ducts.[54] The cysts are lined by flattened to cuboidal epithelial cells. In over 90% of kidneys, areas of epithelial hyperplasia can be identified within the cysts ranging from increased numbers of cell layers to papillary proliferations (Fig. 1-31A and B).[71] In some cases, the papillary proliferations can become more prominent and complex (Fig. 1-32).

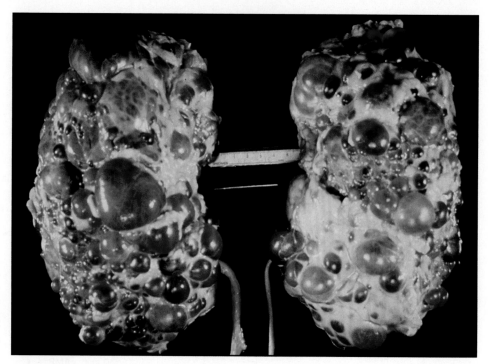

FIGURE 1-28 ■ Autosomal dominant polycystic kidney disease. Bilateral nephrectomy specimen with markedly enlarged kidneys, normal reniform shape, and the external surface distorted by innumerable cysts of variable size.

Medullary Nephronophthisis

Genetics

Nephronophthisis refers to multiple disease complexes having essentially identical pathologic findings and mutations involving the *NPHP* family of genes (*NPHP1* to *NPHP9*).[73–77] These are also referred to as the juvenile, infantile, and adolescent forms. They are autosomal recessive inherited disorders.[74,78] The pure renal juvenile form is related to a gene *NPHP1* on chromosome 2q13[79] with an infantile form related to *NPHP2* and an adolescent form to

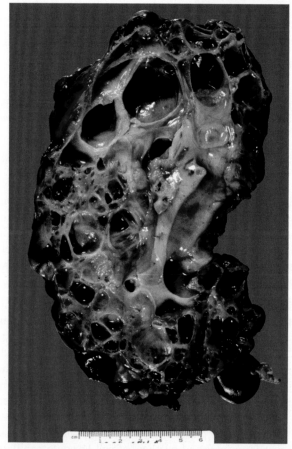

FIGURE 1-29 ■ Autosomal dominant polycystic kidney disease. Cut surface of a kidney with innumerable cysts replacing the entire kidney. In this 57-year-old patient there is no grossly visible normal parenchyma.

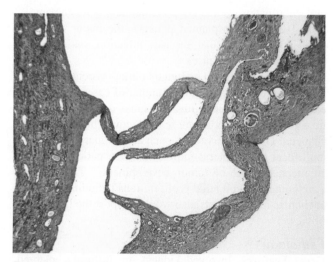

FIGURE 1-30 ■ Autosomal dominant polycystic kidney disease. Several cysts with varying amounts of stroma containing residual renal parenchyma. In the wider septa residual normal epithelial elements are apparent.

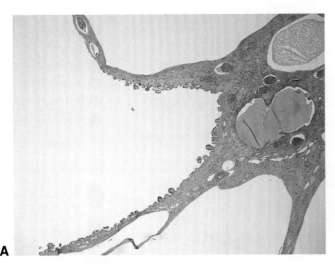

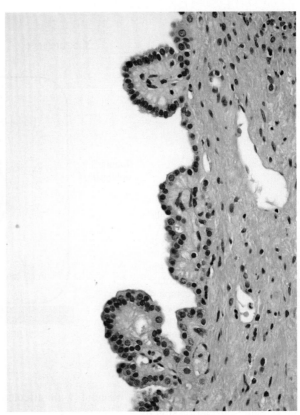

FIGURE 1-31 ■ **A,B:** Autosomal dominant polycystic kidney disease. The photomicrograph shows several cysts with varying amounts of stroma and residual parenchyma between them. In one of the cysts, there are multiple small papillae protruding into the lumen. These are a relatively common finding and are covered by cuboidal epithelium without cytologic atypia.

NPHP3. The *NPHP3* gene has been implicated in a small subset of patients with the infantile form.[76] The NPHP genes code for a series of proteins known as nephrocystins that are expressed in primary cilia or centrosomes of renal epithelial cells (Fig. 1-33).[75,80] It has been suggested that this group of diseases is best classed as "ciliopathies."[81] Cysts presumably develop due to altered signaling pathways resulting in cell polarity and tissue maintenance abnormalities.[80]

Clinical Features

The incidence varies geographically with approximately 1 in 50,000 to 1 in 100,000 births affected in North America.[75] The presentation is dependent on the type. Both sexes are affected equally. The juvenile form is most common and is estimated to be responsible for 5% to 10% of cases of end-stage renal failure in children.[75] Most patients present between 4 and 6 years of age with polyuria and polydipsia related to a decrease in urinary concentrating ability and loss of sodium conservation. The diagnosis is confirmed by radiologic studies with renal parenchymal hyperechogenicity and loss of corticomedullary differentiation. Development of small medullary cysts occurs later. End-stage renal disease develops in the early teens but can occur later. In 10% to 20% of patients, there are extrarenal manifestations with ocular, neurologic, liver, and musculoskeletal being most frequent (Table 1-4).[74,75] The adolescent form is associated with the development of end-stage renal disease at an older age (mean 19 years vs. 13 years for the juvenile form). The infantile form progresses to end-stage renal disease much more rapidly, usually by 2 years of age. Clinically severe hypertension is common.

Treatment is supportive with most patients developing end-stage renal disease requiring dialysis or transplantation within 5 to 10 years of diagnosis.[82] The disease does not recur after transplantation.[83]

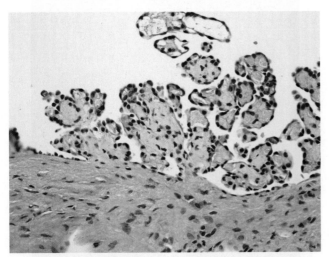

FIGURE 1-32 ■ Autosomal dominant polycystic kidney disease. Infrequently the papillae become more complex but retain the very bland cytologic features. The nature of these proliferations is unknown, but there is no evidence to suggest they have any clinical significance.

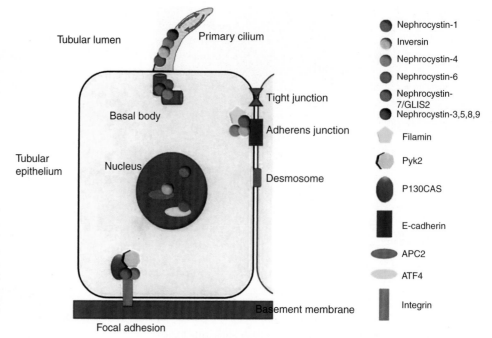

Tubular lumen

Primary cilium

Basal body

Tight junction

Adherens junction

Tubular epithelium

Nucleus

Desmosome

Basement membrane

Focal adhesion

Nephrocystin-1
Inversin
Nephrocystin-4
Nephrocystin-6
Nephrocystin-7/GLIS2
Nephrocystin-3,5,8,9
Filamin
Pyk2
P130CAS
E-cadherin
APC2
ATF4
Integrin

FIGURE 1-33 ■ Nephronophthisis. Schematic representation of a tubular epithelial cell and the subcellular localization of the nephrocystin proteins. Most of the nephrocystin proteins interact with one another forming a nephrocystin complex. (From Salomon R, Saunier S, Niaudet P. Nephronophthisis. *Pediatr Nephrol* 2009;24:2338, with permission.)

Pathology

Gross Features. The process is bilateral with affected kidneys being normal or slightly smaller than normal with thinning of both the cortex and the medulla.[84] Cysts are multiple, <2 cm in size, and are concentrated at the corticomedullary junction but may involve the medulla and pyramids (Fig. 1-34).[85] In the infantile form the kidneys can be enlarged mimicking autosomal recessive polycystic kidney disease. In some cases no cysts are recognizable grossly.

Microscopic Features. The cysts derive from the loop of Henle, distal convoluted tubules, and collecting ducts and are lined by a flattened to squamous type of epithelium.[86,87] The remainder of the parenchyma shows diffuse interstitial

Table 1-4 ■ EXTRARENAL MANIFESTATIONS OF NEPHRONOPHTHISIS
Ocular
Retinitis pigmentosa
Coloboma
Isolated oculomotor apraxia
Nystagmus
Ptosis
Neurologic
Mental retardation
Cerebellar ataxia
Hypopituitarism
Liver
Fibrosis
Biliary duct proliferation
Skeletal
Short ribs
Phalangeal cone-shaped epiphyses
Postaxial polydactyly
Skeletal dysplasia
Other
Situs inversus
Cardiac malformations
Ectodermal dysplasia

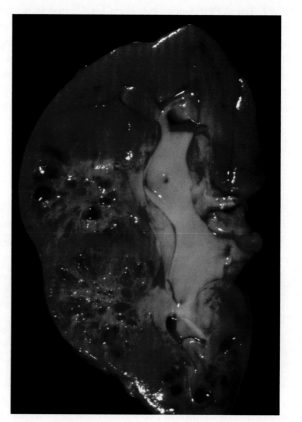

FIGURE 1-34 ■ Nephronophthisis. Kidney from a patient with juvenile nephronophthisis showing multiple small cysts within the renal medullary pyramids.

fibrosis, tubular basement membrane thickening, atrophic dilated tubules, periglomerular fibrosis, and numerous sclerotic glomeruli resulting in features similar to that found in chronic pyelonephritis. The dilated tubules contain Tamm-Horsfall protein. Ultrastructurally the tubular basement membranes show patchy basement membrane thickening with duplication alternating with areas of splitting and thinning. The basement membrane changes are seen in the juvenile and adolescent but not the infantile forms.[75]

Medullary Cystic Disease

Genetics
This is inherited as an autosomal dominant disease that includes two and possibly a third gene. Medullary cystic disease was first linked to a gene on chromosome 1q21-q23 that is now known as the medullary cystic kidney disease 1 gene (*MCKD1*); however, the specific gene involved has not yet been identified.[88] A second gene, *MCKD2*, has been localized to chromosome 16p12.[89] This is also the site of mutation in familial juvenile hyperuricemic nephropathy and some cases of glomerulocystic disease. The *MCKD2* gene codes for the protein uromodulin (Tamm-Horsfall protein). The specific type of mutation of the uromodulin gene has a modest effect on kidney survival.[90] A third possible gene at 1q41 has been proposed.[91]

Clinical Features
Medullary cystic disease and nephronophthisis have similar clinical features. Patients present with polydipsia and polyuria, have cysts at the corticomedullary junction and in the medulla, and ultimately can develop end-stage renal disease. The mean age for the development of end-stage renal failure (type 1, 62 years; type 2, 32 years) is older than for nephronophthisis.[74] The clinical features are quite variable. There is a known association with hyperuricemia and gout.[92,93] The cysts are often clinically undetectable and are bilateral in a minority of patients.

Pathology
Gross Features. There is considerable overlap in the pathologic features of medullary cystic disease and nephronophthisis. The kidneys are normal to slightly small with cysts localized to the corticomedullary junction and the medulla (Fig. 1-35). The cysts tend to be smaller than in nephronophthisis.

Microscopic Features. The findings are similar to nephronophthisis described above including the characteristic basement membrane changes. In type 2 medullary cystic kidney disease, immunohistochemistry for thrombomodulin demonstrates abnormal dense deposits in the renal tubular epithelial cells.[94] Because of the association with hyperuricemia, changes of gouty nephropathy might also be present.

von Hippel-Lindau Disease

Genetics
von Hippel-Lindau disease is inherited as an autosomal dominant genetic disorder due to a defect in the von

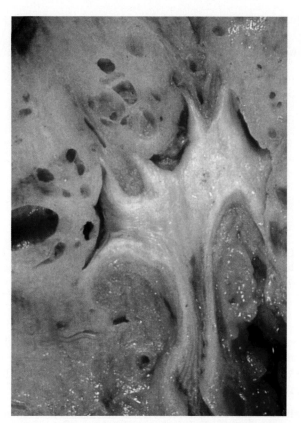

FIGURE 1-35 ■ Medullary cystic disease. Kidney showing multiple cysts within the renal medullary areas.

Hippel-Lindau gene (*VHL*) located at 3p25-p26.[95,96] It occurs in one of every 30,000 to 50,000 live births.[97] Different types of mutations have been identified with specific patterns of expression.[98] Truncating mutations are associated with all the typical features of the disease except the development of pheochromocytoma (type 1). In contrast, missense mutations result in a high risk for the development of pheochromocytoma (type 2).[99]

Clinical Features
Renal cysts are detected in up to 75% of affected individuals.[97,100] In addition to renal tumors, patients also develop tumors of the adrenal gland (pheochromocytoma), pancreas (islet cell tumors, serous cystic tumors), central nervous system (hemangioblastoma), petrous bone (endolymphatic sac tumors),[101] and retina (angioma). Males and females can have papillary cystadenoma of the epididymis and the broad ligament, respectively (Table 1-5). Renal cell carcinoma develops in about 50% of patients with many having multiple bilateral tumors.[97,102,103]

Pathology
Gross Features. The kidneys are generally normal in size unless involved by large tumors. Several lesions occur in the kidney including benign cysts, cysts with intracystic tumor formation, adenomas, and renal cell carcinoma (Fig. 1-36).[100,104] The cysts can be unilateral or bilateral and are variable in size but are generally small (<5 cm). Larger

Table 1-5 ■ EXTRARENAL MANIFESTATIONS OF VON HIPPEL-LINDAU DISEASE
Cerebellar hemangioblastoma
Retinal hemangioblastoma
Spinal hemangioma
Ependymoma
Endolymphatic tumor of the inner ear
Pancreatic cysts
Pancreatic serous cystadenoma
Pancreatic islet cell tumors
Hepatic cysts
Hepatic adenoma
Splenic cysts
Splenic angioma
Epididymal papillary cystadenoma
Broad ligament papillary cystadenoma
Café au lait spots (skin)
Syringobulbia
Syringomyelia

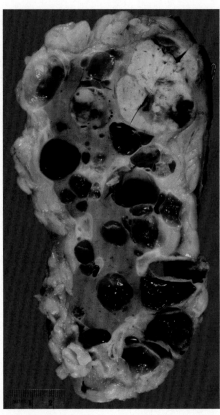

FIGURE 1-37 ■ von Hippel-Lindau disease. Cut surface of a nephrectomy specimen illustrating multiple cysts with the development of tumors evident within several of the cysts.

cysts can be multilocular. Tumors are typically multifocal with a variegated appearance (Fig. 1-37). In a study of 33 kidneys from 23 patients with von Hippel-Lindau disease, 190 solid lesions were identified.[105]

Microscopic Features. The cysts are lined by an attenuated epithelium or cuboidal to columnar cells with clear to eosinophilic cytoplasm (Figs. 1-38 and 1-39). These may show stratification, and even solid nodules of clear cell renal cell carcinoma can be found inside the cysts.[106] In 138 cystic lesions examined microscopically by Paraf et al.,[105] 103 (75%) were simple cysts, 20 (14%) were atypical with a multilayered clear cell epithelium, and 15 (11%) were cystic clear cell renal cell carcinomas. Hemorrhage into the cysts is common, and hemosiderin-laden macrophages can be present in the cyst lumen or surrounding fibrous tissue. The clear cells lining the cysts have an immunohistochemical expression

profile similar to that of clear cell renal cell carcinoma. In a study of grossly normal renal parenchyma, Walther et al.[107] found numerous microscopic abnormalities ranging from cysts to tumors. Based on these findings, the authors estimated that the average kidney in von Hippel-Lindau disease contains approximately 1,000 small cysts and 600 small tumors.[107] The parenchyma can contain microscopic foci of

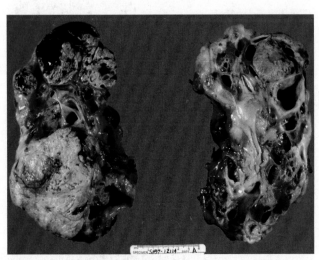

FIGURE 1-36 ■ von Hippel-Lindau disease. Bilateral nephrectomy from a young woman showing multiple variably sized cysts and multiple clear cell renal cell carcinomas.

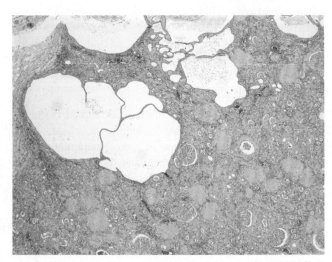

FIGURE 1-38 ■ von Hippel-Lindau disease. Multiple variably sized cysts lined by flattened epithelium. There are changes secondary to chronic pyelonephritis in the background.

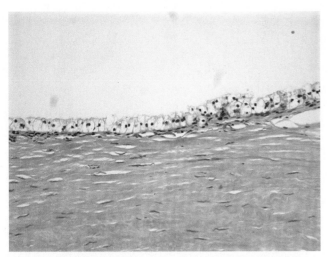

Figure 1-39 ■ von Hippel-Lindau disease. Example of a cyst lined by clear cells with morphologic features typical of the cells of clear cell renal cell carcinoma.

Table 1-6 ■ MANIFESTATIONS OF TUBEROUS SCLEROSIS COMPLEX
Major features
Renal angiomyolipoma
Lymphangioleiomyomatosis
Facial angiofibroma
Ungula and periungual fibroma
Hypomelanotic macules
Shagreen patches
Retinal hamartoma and astrocytoma
Cortical tubers
Subendymal nodules and giant cell astrocytoma
Cardiac rhabdomyoma
Minor features
Renal cysts
Hamartomatous rectal polyp
Bone cysts
Cerebral white matter migration lines
Gingival fibroma
Enamel dental pits
Retinal achromic patches
Confetti skin lesions

clear cell proliferation, and individual abnormal clear cells can be present within tubules (Fig. 1-40). These also have an immunohistochemical profile similar to that of clear cell renal cell carcinoma.

Tuberous Sclerosis

Genetics

The tuberous sclerosis complex is an autosomal dominant inherited disorder with a high (95%) degree of penetrance.[108] The prevalence is estimated at 1:11,000 births.[109] The disease is due to germline mutations of the *TSC1* (9q34) or *TSC2* (16p13.3) genes.[110,111] The disease manifestations tend to be less severe in the *TSC1*-related cases.[112] The protein products of the *TSC1* and *TSC2* genes are hamartin and tuberin, respectively. The adult polycystic kidney disease gene *PKD1*

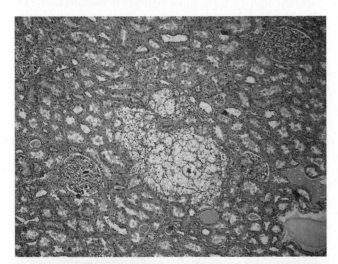

Figure 1-40 ■ von Hippel-Lindau disease. Tiny focus of clear cell renal cell carcinoma. Note the edge of a small cyst in the right lower corner that is lined by clear cells similar to those illustrated in Figure 1-39.

is located in the immediate vicinity of the *TSC2* gene and in some patients both genes are affected resulting in features of both conditions being found in the same kidney (*TSC2/ADPKD1* contiguous gene syndrome).[53] The TSC1 and TSC2 proteins have a critical role in cell proliferation and death through mTOR-dependent and mTOR-independent signaling pathways.[113]

Clinical Features

Tuberous sclerosis is a complex disease characterized by multiple manifestations involving multiple organs.[114,115] Currently the diagnosis of tuberous sclerosis is defined by a combination of major and minor features (Table 1-6).[116] The diagnosis requires two or more distinct lesions rather than multiple single lesions in one organ. Although the clinical picture is often dominated by neurologic complications such as mental retardation and seizures, the renal lesions are significant. The combination of cysts and angiomyolipomas may reduce the functional renal mass and result in renal failure. In the *TSC2/ADPKD1* contiguous gene syndrome, severe cystic kidney disease may be present at birth.[117] Second, angiomyolipomas can become large and can be complicated by retroperitoneal hemorrhage. Finally these patients have a significantly increased risk for the development of renal cell carcinoma at a young age including in children.[118] Targeted therapies hold promise in the treatment of the associated neurodevelopmental disorders, angiomyolipoma, and other manifestations of this disease.[119–121]

Pathology

Gross Features. Indications for nephrectomy in patients with tuberous sclerosis are usually an enlarging angiomyolipoma or the presence of a solid tumor suspicious for renal cell carcinoma. The combination of characteristic cysts and angiomyolipomas is typical of this inherited disorder

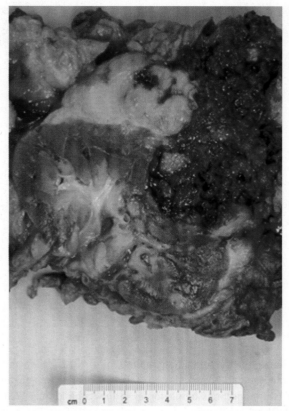

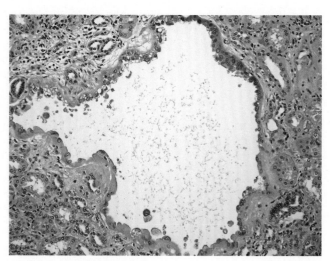

Figure 1-42 ■ Tuberous sclerosis. Cyst lined by cells with moderate to abundant amphophilic cytoplasm.

Figure 1-41 ■ Tuberous sclerosis. Nephrectomy specimen with multiple angiomyolipomas (small yellow nodules). The large tumor is an epithelioid angiomyolipoma with rupture and a retroperitoneal hemorrhage.

(Fig. 1-41).[122,123] In one study, 80% of children with tuberous sclerosis developed renal lesions by age 10 with angiomyolipomas (75%) being more common than cysts (17%).[124] Approximately 50% of patients develop renal cysts. The cysts are generally small and can be located in the cortex and medulla. There may only be a few cysts or they can be sufficiently numerous to produce a sponge-like appearance. The tumors range from a few millimeters to several centimeters and have a variable appearance depending on the proportion of the components; hemorrhage is common.

Microscopic Features. The cysts are characteristically lined by tall cells with granular eosinophilic cytoplasm and large nuclei resembling proximal tubular epithelial cells (Figs. 1-42 and 1-43). Pseudostratification and papillary tufting can be present (Fig. 1-44).[125] Cysts involving the glomeruli are also a characteristic feature. The cysts can contain eosinophilic secretions. In the absence of grossly visible tumors, there are frequently microscopic angiomyolipomas (Figs. 1-45 and 1-46). The pathology of the tumors in tuberous sclerosis is covered in detail in Chapter 2.

Multicystic Renal Dysplasia

Although the pathogenesis continues to be the subject of debate, it is generally accepted that most cases of renal

dysplasia are related to urinary tract obstruction or urinary reflux during kidney development.[24,26] Multicystic dysplastic kidneys are also a feature of many genetic disorders (Table 1-7).[14,52]

Clinical Features

Renal dysplasia is defined by the presence of abnormal renal organization with abnormal differentiation of metanephric elements. An associated urinary tract anomaly is identifiable in up to 90% of affected individuals; among the most frequent are ureteral atresia and urethral valves. In dysplasia related to reflux, the changes can be focal and the kidney can retain some level of function; otherwise, dysplastic kidneys are characteristically nonfunctional.

Multicystic dysplastic kidneys present as a flank mass in newborns and the diagnosis can be confirmed by ultrasound.[57,126] In up to 40% of affected patients, there are contralateral urinary tract abnormalities.[127] Nephrectomy has

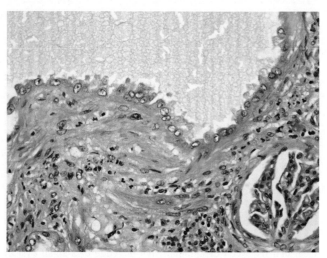

Figure 1-43 ■ Tuberous sclerosis. High-power photomicrograph of the lining epithelium in a cyst.

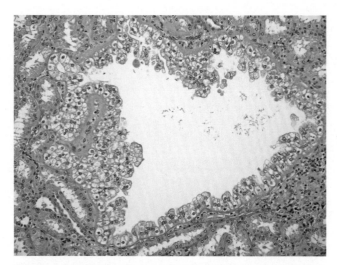

FIGURE 1-44 ■ Tuberous sclerosis. In this cyst the lining epithelium is pseudostratified and shows cytoplasmic clearing.

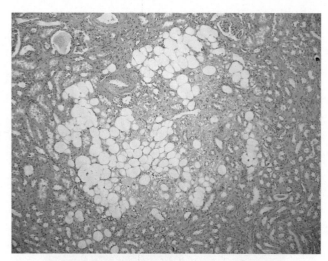

FIGURE 1-46 ■ Tuberous sclerosis. A small intraparenchymal angiomyolipoma with fat and smooth muscle.

been the standard therapy, but conservative treatment with careful monitoring for possible tumor development is an alternative.[128] Nephroblastoma and renal cell carcinoma arising in dysplastic kidneys are described.[129,130] Intrauterine diagnosis with subsequent treatment prior to birth has been tried with varied success.

Pathology

Gross Features. Most dysplastic kidneys are small, abnormally shaped, and have multiple cysts (Figs. 1-47 and 1-48).[131] In other cases, the dysplastic kidney consists of only a small nodule of rudimentary metanephric tissue. The cysts in dysplastic kidneys communicate,[132] and their size and location may correlate with the level of the obstruction.[133] Dysplasia can be segmental or focal.[134,135]

Microscopic Features. The histologic hallmarks of dysplastic kidneys are lobar disorganization, primitive ducts, and metaplastic cartilage[136] (Fig. 1-49). There is only primitive

development of the renal medulla. Collecting ducts are surrounded by a thick fibromuscular collar and may become cystic (Fig. 1-50). Small nests of hyaline cartilage are found in the cortex but not in all cases (Fig. 1-51). Nodules of renal blastema may be present (Fig. 1-52).[129,131] The presence of keratinizing squamous epithelium has been described (Fig. 1-53).[137,138]

Glomerulocystic Disease

Glomerular cysts are defined by dilation of Bowman space to two or three times the normal size. Glomerulocystic kidney

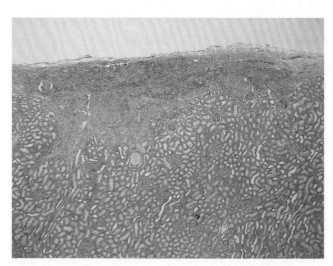

FIGURE 1-45 ■ Tuberous sclerosis. A small subcapsular angiomyolipoma that is composed entirely of smooth muscle.

Table 1-7 ■ MALFORMATION SYNDROMES ASSOCIATED WITH RENAL DYSPLASIA	
Syndrome	**Gene(s)**
Alagille syndrome	*JAG1, NOTCH2*
Bardet-Biedl syndrome	*BBS1–BBS11*
Branchiootorenal syndrome	*EYA1, SIX1, SIX2*
Di George syndrome	Del. 22q11
Hypothyroidism, sensorial deafness, renal anomalies	*GATA3*
Fraser syndrome	*FRAS1, FREM2*
Kallmann syndrome	*KALL1, FGFR1*
Renal cysts and diabetes syndrome	*TCTF2*
Simpson-Golabi-Behmel syndrome	*GPC3*
Smith-Lemli-Opitz syndrome	*DHCR7*
Townes-Brocks syndrome	*SALL1*
Cornelia de Lange syndrome	*NIPBL*
Zellweger syndrome	*PEX* family
Pallister-Hall syndrome	*GLI3*
Beckwith-Wiedemann syndrome	p57(KIP2)
Meckel-Gruber syndrome	Unknown

Adapted from Sanna-Cherchi S, Caridi G, Weng PL, et al. Genetic approaches to human renal agenesis/hypoplasia and dysplasia. *Pediatr Nephrol* 2007;22:1675–1684.

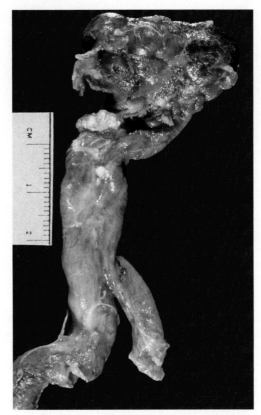

FIGURE 1-47 ■ Multicystic dysplasia. The kidney consists of a small irregularly, somewhat reniform shaped piece of soft tissue. The cysts are not grossly visible on the surface. There is an associated bifid hydroureter.

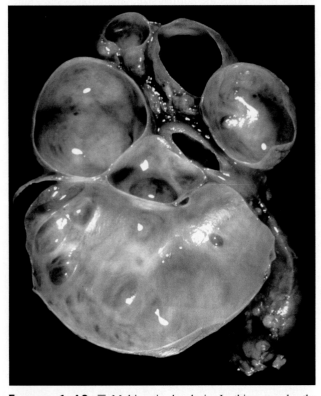

FIGURE 1-48 ■ Multicystic dysplasia. In this example, the residual kidney is almost entirely cystic with little solid tissue.

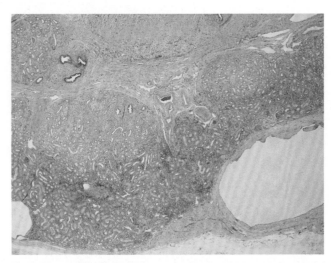

FIGURE 1-49 ■ Multicystic dysplasia. This is an example of segmental cystic dysplasia with preserved renal parenchyma, cysts, and immature stroma with entrapped tubules.

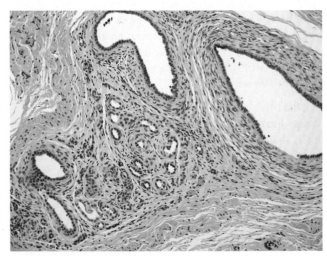

FIGURE 1-50 ■ Multicystic dysplasia. Small tubules are surrounded by a cuff of immature stroma.

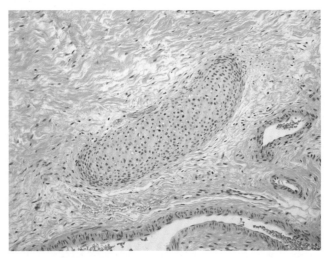

FIGURE 1-51 ■ Multicystic dysplasia. There is a nest of cartilage within loose fibrous connective tissue.

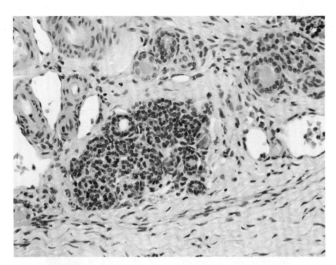

FIGURE 1-52 ■ Multicystic dysplasia. In this example, there is a nephrogenic rest with adjacent tubules and loose fibrous connective tissue.

disease as an entity is reserved for inherited types of the disease. The major form is inherited as an autosomal dominant condition. The subtypes include (i) autosomal dominant glomerulocystic kidney disease related to uromodulin gene (*UMOD*) mutations, (ii) familial hypoplastic glomerulocystic kidney disease due to mutations in the *TCF2* gene (hepatocyte nuclear factor 1β), and (iii) other genetic causes.[139] Glomerular cysts occur in a wide range of other conditions including autosomal dominant polycystic kidney disease, autosomal recessive kidney disease, numerous syndromes, and urinary obstruction with or without dysplasia (Table 1-8).[139]

Clinical Features

The clinical significance is dependent on the underlying etiology. Diagnosis is made by radiology examination. In the fetus and neonate, differentiation from other cystic diseases may not be possible.[140] In the inherited types, the disease may present early or late. In early onset, renal insufficiency

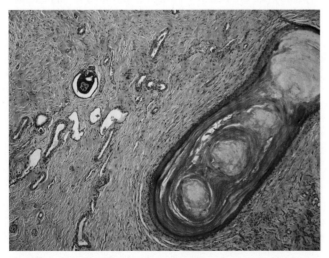

FIGURE 1-53 ■ Multicystic dysplasia. In this unusual case, the lining of a cyst shows keratinizing squamous metaplasia.

Table 1-8 ■ CONDITIONS WITH GLOMERULAR CYSTS

Glomerular cystic kidney diseases (inherited)
  Autosomal dominant glomerulocystic kidney disease
  Familial hypoplastic glomerulocystic kidney disease
  Other inherited variants
Other inherited conditions and syndromes
  Autosomal dominant polycystic kidney disease
  Autosomal recessive polycystic kidney disease
  Tuberous sclerosis
  von Hippel-Lindau disease
  Familial juvenile nephronophthisis
  Congenital nephrotic syndrome of the Finnish type
  Many others
Glomerular cysts in dysplastic kidneys
  Renal dysplasia associated with congenital obstruction
  Zellweger syndrome
  Meckel syndrome
  Many others
Miscellaneous other conditions
  Hemolytic uremic syndrome
  Systemic lupus erythematous
  Sjögren syndrome
  And many others

Adapted from Lennerz JK, Spence DC, Iskandar SS, et al. Glomerulocystic kidney: one hundred-year perspective. *Arch Pathol Lab Med* 2010;134:583–605.

develops in infants. Progression to end-stage renal disease occurs over a highly variable period of time. In more aggressive cases, renal failure can occur within 3 years of diagnosis.[139] In adults, the disease is usually asymptomatic and an infrequent cause of end-stage renal disease.

Pathology

Gross Features. In cases associated with autosomal dominant or autosomal recessive kidney disease, the gross features are those of the associated condition. In the inherited forms, the kidneys may be enlarged with variable numbers of small cysts (1 to 3 mm) grossly visible.

Microscopic Features. By definition the glomerular space is two to three times the normal size. The cysts are variable in size. In even large cysts, small residual glomerular tufts may be identifiable (Fig. 1-54). In cases related to other disorders, the histopathology of that condition is present (Table 1-8).

Medullary Sponge Kidney

The etiology of medullary sponge kidney is unknown.[74] The *GDNF* gene has been implicated as having a role.[141] There is no evidence that it is an inherited condition although the hypothesis that papillary duct ectasia is a congenital anomaly is favored.[52] It has been described in association with Marfan syndrome, Ehlers-Danlos syndrome, and Caroli disease.

Clinical Features

Medullary sponge kidney is a sporadic condition found in 1:5,000 live births.[142] Males and females are affected equally,

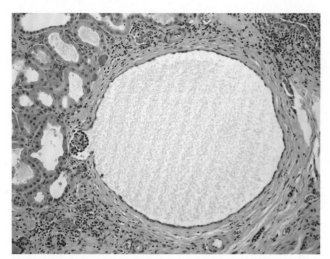

FIGURE 1-54 ■ Glomerulocystic disease. An example of a glomerular cyst in a case of adult polycystic kidney disease.

and it is seen in association with hemihypertrophy in about 10% of cases.[143] The condition is usually asymptomatic and is discovered incidentally in children or in patients in their third or fourth decades presenting with renal lithiasis[144,145]; the latter occurs in about 50% of patients.[146] Diagnosis is usually made by computed tomographic urography.[147] These patients rarely progress to chronic renal failure but complications such as recurring urolithiasis, pyelonephritis, and septicemia may cause significant clinical problems.[148] Treatment is generally directed at the complications.

Pathology

Gross Features. The kidneys are normal or slightly enlarged in most cases. The cysts are small (<5 mm) and localized to the medullary pyramids and papillary tips (Fig. 1-55).[145] Small calculi are often present within the cysts.[149]

Microscopic Features. The cysts derive from the collecting ducts; in addition to cysts, ectatic ducts in the papillae are also present. The cysts are lined by urothelial, columnar, or squamous epithelium.[143,149] Interstitial fibrosis and inflammation are present, and features resembling dysplasia including cartilage can be found.[143]

Simple Cysts

The cysts are believed to develop from diverticula that are thought to arise in the distal convoluted or collecting tubules.[150] These increase in frequency with advancing age, correlating with the increasing occurrence of cysts.[151]

Clinical Features

Simple renal cysts have an increasing prevalence with advancing age and are found in up to 50% of kidneys at autopsy.[151,152] Simple cysts can be single or multiple and are often unilateral. These are usually asymptomatic and their major significance lies in differentiating them from renal neoplasms.[84] In most instances, this is accomplished

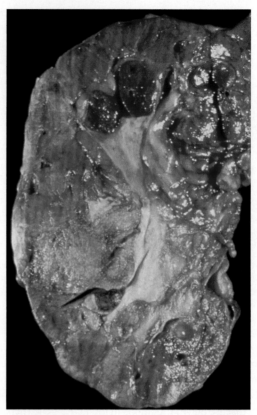

FIGURE 1-55 ■ Medullary sponge kidney. The kidney shows several small cysts that include several at the corticomedullary junction.

by radiologic evaluation but some cases are aspirated and others require surgical exploration. Symptomatic cysts have been managed by multiple approaches including percutaneous aspiration, sclerotherapy, cyst decortication, cystectomy, and cystoretroperitoneal shunt.[153–155]

Pathology

Gross Features. The cysts may be solitary or multiple and typically are unilocular although a multilocular appearance can be seen (Fig. 1-56A and B). Most are under 5 cm, but much larger cysts have been described. The fluid is under tension and is straw-colored. Cysts can be hemorrhagic or may become infected (Fig. 1-57). The inner lining is most often smooth and glistening; a shaggy, irregular surface and/ or a thick wall should heighten suspicions of a malignant tumor.

Microscopic Features. The cysts are lined by a flattened single-layered epithelium that can be difficult to demonstrate in larger lesions (Fig. 1-58). There may be associated atrophy of adjacent renal parenchyma with fibrosis, but in general the kidney is not diseased other than age-related changes. The lack of renal disease is helpful in distinguishing this from acquired cystic kidney disease. Cases complicated by hemorrhage or infection can have a thickened wall with hemosiderin-laden macrophages and a mixed inflammatory infiltrate (Fig. 1-59).

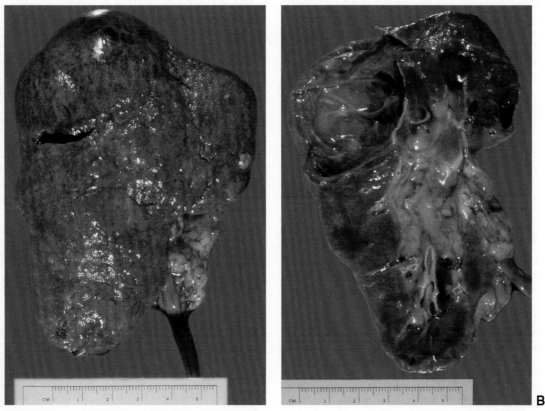

FIGURE 1-56 ■ Cortical cyst. A large, intact benign cortical cyst can be seen bulging from the external surface of the kidney **(A)**. The opened cyst shows a thin translucent lining **(B)**.

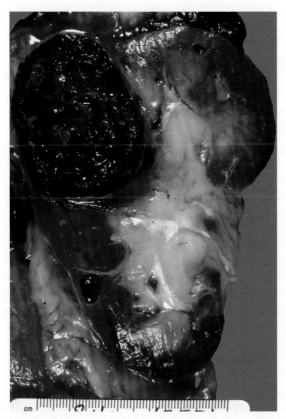

FIGURE 1-57 ■ Cortical cyst. This is an example of a benign cortical cyst complicated by intracystic hemorrhage.

Acquired Cystic Disease

Acquired cystic disease is a well-described complication of hemodialysis and peritoneal dialysis but can also occur in patients with prolonged azotemia without dialysis.[156–159] It can develop on a background of any chronic renal disease and is seen in up to 50% of all patients on hemodialysis.[160] The incidence increases with increasing time on dialysis.[161]

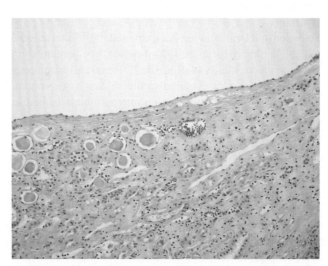

FIGURE 1-58 ■ Cortical cyst. The lining of an uncomplicated cyst has a flattened epithelium and a thin wall of connective tissue.

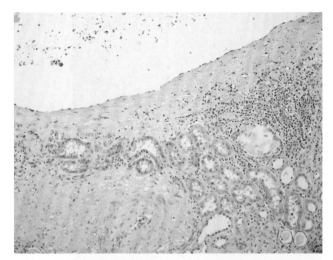

FIGURE 1-59 ■ Cortical cyst. The wall of this cortical cyst is thickened with dense fibrous tissue, and there is an associated chronic inflammatory infiltrate.

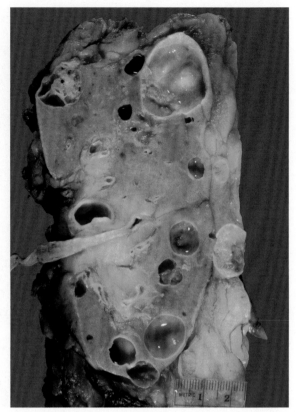

FIGURE 1-60 ■ Acquired cystic disease. The cut surface of this relatively normal sized kidney shows multiple cysts. The cysts are varied in size and in one a multilocular architecture is present (*upper left*). Histologically this was a clear cell papillary renal cell carcinoma.

The pathogenesis remains unknown with many theories having been presented over the years.[157]

Clinical Features

The diagnosis requires the demonstration of a minimum of five renal cysts in each kidney of patients with end-stage renal disease.[159] Most patients have no symptoms directly related to the development of acquired cystic disease. If symptoms do develop, they usually relate to bleeding resulting in gross or microscopic hematuria and rarely significant retroperitoneal, subcapsular, or intrarenal hemorrhage.[162] Of most importance is the association with the development of renal cell carcinoma.[156] Chronic dialysis and acquired cystic disease are associated with an estimated 10- and 50-fold increased risk of renal cell carcinoma, respectively.[156,163–165] Acquired cystic disease does not require specific treatment. Most authors advocate periodic imaging studies with computed tomography to evaluate for the development of carcinoma. In the past, nephrectomy has been recommended if a tumor larger than 3 cm develops[84]; more recently, early detection and treatment has been stressed.[166,167] Interestingly, transplantation reduces the risk of tumor development even with the native kidneys left in situ.[157] Renal cell carcinoma can also develop in acquired cystic disease occurring in allografts.[168] Surgical intervention may also be indicated in some cases complicated by hemorrhage.

Pathology

Gross Features. In most cases, the kidneys are smaller than normal although there is a wide variation in size (Figs. 1-60 and 1-61). In rare cases, the kidney can be enlarged.[169] The number of cysts is highly variable, and a minimum of five is recommended as a diagnostic criterion to separate this from simple cysts.[159] The cysts can occur anywhere but are predominantly cortical. Size ranges from a few millimeters to several centimeters; however, most are small (2 mm or less).[169] The cysts contain translucent fluid, but hemorrhage may be seen. In 15% of kidneys, single or multiple grossly visible tumor nodules are present and in 5% these are more than several centimeters in size (Fig. 1-61). Such lesions should be well-sampled for histologic evaluation, particularly any hemorrhagic or yellow tumors that are more likely to represent clear cell carcinoma.

Microscopic Features. The cysts can arise from any part of the tubular structure including proximal and distal tubules and collecting ducts (Fig. 1-62).[170] The kidney parenchyma shows changes of end-stage renal disease with interstitial fibrosis, sclerotic glomeruli, and atrophic tubules. In patients on dialysis, calcium oxalate crystal deposition is present in most cases (Fig. 1-63). The cysts are lined by a single-layered cuboidal to columnar epithelium that can show a range of hyperplastic changes up to and including formation of adenomas and carcinomas[169,171,172] (Figs. 1-64 and 1-65). Atypical epithelial proliferations within cysts have been shown to have cytogenetic abnormalities including gains in chromosomes 7, 12, 17, 20, and Y, supporting the hypothesis that these represent the precursor of at least some of the tumors that develop in these kidneys.[173] Papillary adenomas are a frequent finding in the renal parenchyma (Fig. 1-66). Tumors may develop within the cysts or in the adjacent parenchyma.[172] The pathology of neoplasms developing in this setting is described in detail in Chapter 2.

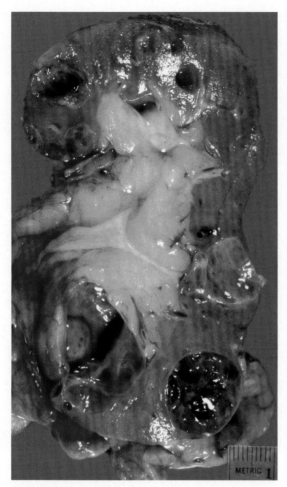

FIGURE 1-61 ■ Acquired cystic disease. In this example the kidney is small and contains multiple cysts. There is a hemorrhagic tumor arising within a cyst in the lower pole. Histologically the tumor was an acquired cystic disease–associated renal cell carcinoma.

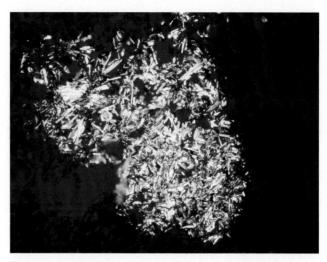

FIGURE 1-63 ■ Acquired cystic disease. Calcium oxalate crystals as seen with polarized light.

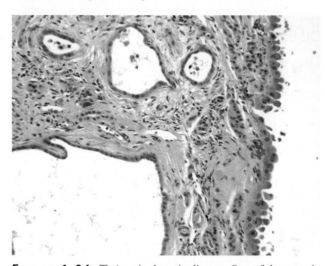

FIGURE 1-64 ■ Acquired cystic disease. One of the cysts in this photomicrograph is lined by cells with moderate amphophilic cytoplasm and large nuclei that contain prominent nucleoli.

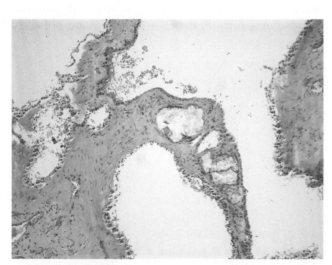

FIGURE 1-62 ■ Acquired cystic disease. Several cysts in this image are lined by a single- to multilayered cuboidal epithelium. There is fibrotic stroma between the cysts that contains several calcium oxalate crystal deposits.

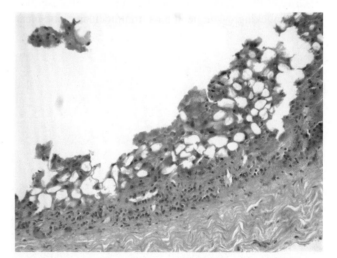

FIGURE 1-65 ■ Acquired cystic disease. An example of a cyst lined by a pseudostratified epithelium. The cells have abundant eosinophilic cytoplasm and cytoplasmic vacuoles producing a sieve-like appearance.

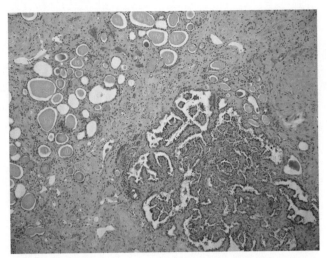

FIGURE 1-66 ■ Acquired cystic disease. Papillary adenoma developing in a kidney with acquired cystic disease.

Other Cystic Diseases

There are numerous other conditions that may include the presence of cysts in the kidney.[52] Cystic neoplasms are described in detail in Chapter 2. There are a few lesions that occasionally present as renal masses and that can cause diagnostic difficulty and warrant brief discussions.

Segmental Cystic Disease

Unilateral and partial renal involvement by multiple cysts has been reported under a variety of terms including unilateral polycystic kidney disease, localized cystic disease, and segmental cystic disease.[174,175] The lesion is not inherited and is unrelated to adult polycystic kidney disease. The etiopathogenesis is unknown. It can be symptomatic with hematuria, flank pain, and an abdominal mass but often is discovered incidentally. The complex cystic renal mass can mimic a renal tumor on imaging studies.

Grossly these can appear as a relatively circumscribed mass mimicking cystic nephroma, multilocular cystic clear

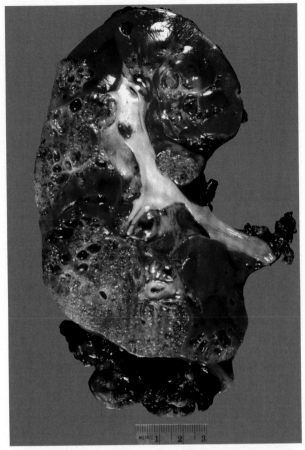

FIGURE 1-67 ■ Segmental cystic disease. The cut surface of the kidney shows three or four relatively discrete areas with extensive cyst formation that are separated from each other by normal appearing parenchyma.

cell renal cell carcinoma, or tubulocystic carcinoma (Fig. 1-67). Because these represent multiple cysts that are closely packed, the septa between the cysts contain normal elements of the nephron including tubules and glomeruli (Fig. 1-68A and B). Recognition of this feature is the key

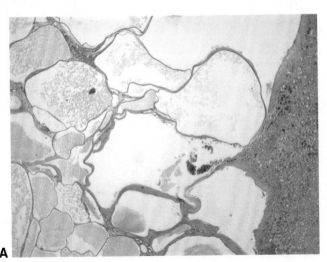
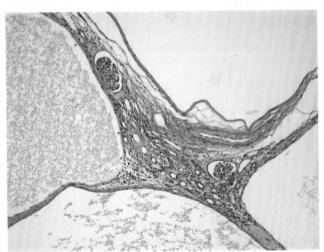

FIGURE 1-68 ■ Segmental cystic disease. The cysts are separated from each other by fibrous septa that in many locations contain normal tissues including glomeruli and tubules (**A** and **B**).

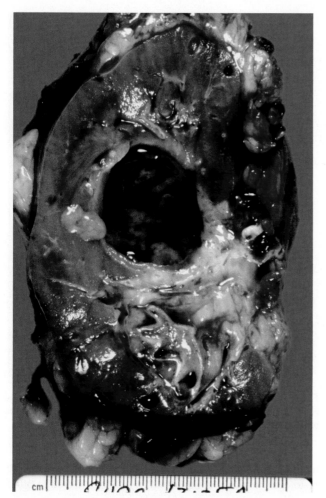

FIGURE 1-69 ■ Pyelocalyceal pseudocyst. There is a cystic structure in the renal sinus area that is lined by a fibrous wall. Microscopically there was no epithelial lining.

to reaching a correct diagnosis. The possibility of segmental cystic renal dysplasia should also be considered as it can present in adult patients.[134]

Pyelocalyceal Diverticula

These lesions are typically seen in children and present as filling defects in the pelvis or calyces on excretory urography or as cysts on imaging studies.[176] They normally communicate with the renal pelvis or calyx and are lined by urothelium. Squamous metaplasia can occur, and there can be associated calcification. The connection to the pelvis or calyx can be lost, and the lesion can present as a cystic mass.[177] Particularly in the rare adult patient, this can mimic a neoplasm and the lesion may be resected with that as the clinical diagnosis.

Perinephric Pseudocyst

Perinephric pseudocyst is usually the consequence of extravasated urine into the perinephric fat with subsequent secondary reactive changes.[178] These can also develop following perinephric hemorrhage. They may present as mass lesions and in some instances clinically appear to be renal parenchymal in origin. When these occur in the subepithelial tissue of the renal pelvis the term Antopol-Goldman lesion has been applied (Fig. 1-69).[179] The pseudocyst is lined by fibrous connective tissue with varying degrees of inflammation. Calcification can be present. In cases related to hemorrhage, hemosiderin-laden macrophages are present. In some hemorrhage-related pseudocysts, spherical laminated structures known as Liesegang rings are found (Fig. 1-70A and B); these can be seen in aspirates of fluid from the pseudocyst.[180,181] Liesegang rings have been mistaken in the past for parasitic organisms.[180]

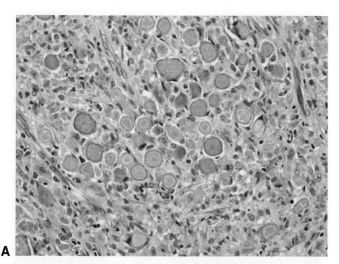
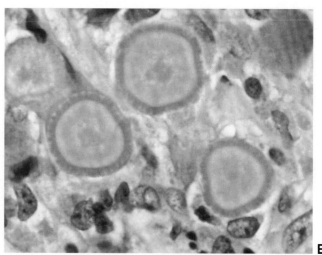

FIGURE 1-70 ■ Liesegang rings. The contents of a perinephric pseudocyst include numerous round structures with a thick outer wall and a laminated internal structure (**A** and **B**).

RENAL VASCULAR DISEASES

Involvement of the renal vasculature by pathologic conditions are important clinically particularly the role of arterial diseases as a cause of hypertension. Occasionally these lead to surgical intervention and so it is important for surgical pathologists to have knowledge of those processes that may require their assessment.

Arterial Diseases

Renal Artery Stenosis

Clinical Features
Renal artery stenosis is an important cause of systemic hypertension (2% to 5%). The vast majority of cases of renal artery stenosis are related to two conditions: atherosclerosis and fibromuscular dysplasia (Table 1-9). Atherosclerotic renal artery stenosis accounts for about two-thirds of cases and is most common in middle-aged to elderly men. It is usually seen in the presence of significant atherosclerosis of other major arteries and often with a background of essential hypertension. In about one-third of cases, both renal arteries are involved and if severe can lead to renal failure.[182]

Fibromuscular dysplasia is the most common cause of renal artery stenosis in children.[183,184] Overall, however, the disease is most common in young to middle-aged women.[185,186] The pathogenesis of this condition is unknown. The proximal renal arteries are most commonly involved, but the renal artery can be involved elsewhere as can other muscular arteries.[187] A "string of beads" appearance due to multiple stenoses is the most characteristic radiologic feature (Fig. 1-71).[188] Treatment with percutaneous transluminal renal angioplasty produces good long-term results in over 60% of patients.[187] In pediatric patients, a surgical approach is also frequently employed.[184]

Pathology
In atherosclerotic renal artery stenosis, the plaque is most often located at the ostium or proximal renal artery. The degree of luminal narrowing is variable. Other features of complex atherosclerotic plaques are present. The ipsilateral kidney shows generalized or localized ischemic changes depending on the site of the renal artery lesion (Fig. 1-72). With chronic ischemia the atrophic tubules typically have thickened basement

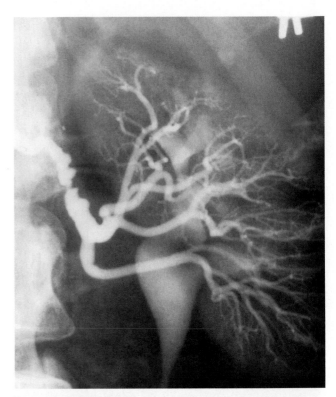

FIGURE 1-71 ■ Fibromuscular dysplasia. Renal artery arteriogram demonstrating multiple points of stenosis along the main renal artery resulting in the "string of beads" appearance.

membranes. There is variable fibrosis in the interstitium. The histologic picture is complicated by changes related to other conditions such as long-standing hypertension.

A number of discrete histologic patterns have been described in fibromuscular dysplasia. Harrison and McCormack[189] classified the lesions of fibromuscular dysplasia into three major

Table 1-9 ■ CAUSES OF RENAL ARTERY STENOSIS
Atherosclerosis
Renal artery dysplasia
Renal artery dissection
Renal artery aneurysm
Arteritis (Takayasu and others)
Arteriovenous fistula
External compression
Trauma
Others

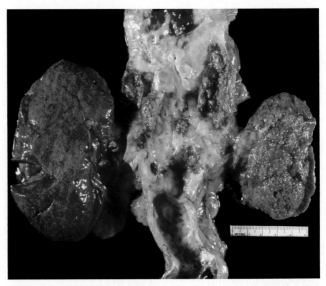

FIGURE 1-72 ■ Renal artery stenosis. Severe complicated atherosclerosis resulting in stenosis of the left renal artery and atrophy of the left kidney.

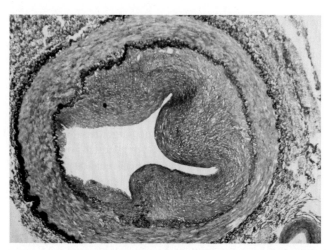

FIGURE 1-73 ■ Fibromuscular dysplasia. Section of renal artery with eccentric intimal fibroplasia producing renal artery stenosis.

categories based on the most prominent site of the fibroplasias: intimal, medial, and adventitial. The medial group was further classified into four subtypes: medial hyperplasia, medial fibroplasias with aneurysms, perimedial fibroplasias, and medial dissection (discussed later). Intimal fibroplasia is rare and is characterized by the accumulation of loose, moderately cellular connective tissue on the luminal side of the internal elastic lamina (Fig. 1-73). Medial hyperplasia accounts for 5% to 15% of cases with a proliferation of the smooth muscle cells of the media resulting in luminal narrowing. Medial fibroplasia with aneurysms is the most common pattern (60% to 70% of cases) and is often bilateral. The media shows alternating areas of smooth muscle loss with and without replacement by fibrous tissue. This results in the formation of ridges (corresponding to the fibrous tissue) and troughs or aneurysms (corresponding to areas of muscle loss). Perimedial fibroplasia (15% to 25% of cases) has dense collagen replacing the outer one-third of the media. Periarterial (adventitial) fibroplasia is rare (<1% of cases) and has dense collagen deposition in the adventitia and extending into the surrounding fibroadipose tissue.

Renal Artery Aneurysm

Clinical Features
Renal artery aneurysms are distinctly uncommon with a reported incidence of 0.01% to 0.1%.[190] They occur more commonly in men. Symptomatic presentation includes hypertension, hematuria, and flank pain.[190,191] The vast majority involve the extrarenal portions of the renal artery and its major branches. They can be associated with fibromuscular dysplasia. Most are small and the risk of rupture is low. There is considered to be an increase risk of rupture in pregnancy.[192,193]

Pathology
Renal artery aneurysms have been divided into three general categories: saccular, fusiform, and dissecting (discussed below). Saccular aneurysms typically have changes of atherosclerosis but are believed to be congenital in origin. Fusiform aneurysms most often develop distal to a site of

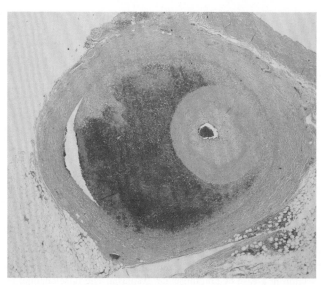

FIGURE 1-74 ■ Renal artery dissection. Renal artery dissection in a case of fibromuscular dysplasia.

stenosis such as fibromuscular dysplasia. Intrarenal aneurysms are usually secondary to other processes such as trauma and so generally represent false aneurysms.

Renal Artery Dissection

Clinical Features
Dissection of the renal artery is uncommon.[194] In many cases, the dissection is due to extension of an aortic dissection. Primary dissection of the renal artery is most often related to traumatic injury with catheterization being the most important cause. Dissection is also a significant complication of fibromuscular dysplasia.[195] Presentation is somewhat dependent on the pathogenesis but almost always has severe flank pain and hypertension. Secondary thrombosis of the renal artery can occur.

Pathology
There is accumulation of blood in the media resulting in a false lumen (Fig. 1-74). The dissection can be localized or can extend along the renal artery branches. In cases with fibromuscular dysplasia, the features of the underlying disease are evident (Fig. 1-75). Secondary changes in the kidney include acute renal infarction or more chronic ischemic changes.

Renal Arteriovenous Anastomosis

Clinical Features
Connections between the renal arterial and venous systems can be congenital or acquired.[196,197] Congenital lesions (arteriovenous malformations) are rare and most often involve vessels in the renal pelvicalyceal mucosa or the medulla. Acquired lesions are most often the result of surgery or traumatic injury. Cases have also been reported following renal biopsy.[198] Symptoms include hypertension, hematuria, and renal failure.

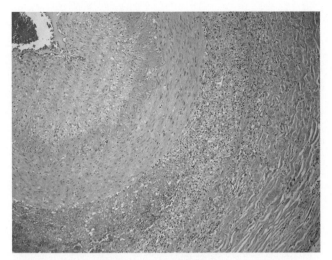

FIGURE 1-75 ■ Renal artery dissection. Renal artery dissection in a case of fibromuscular dysplasia. The false channel is located in the outer aspect of the media.

Pathology

Pathologic findings are dependent on the etiology of the lesion.

Renal Vein Thrombosis

Clinical Features

Renal vein thrombosis occurs over a wide age range and has a long list of etiologies.[199–201] Pathogenic mechanisms include hypovolemia (important in infants), primary renal disease (nephrotic syndrome in adults with hypercoagulable state), extrinsic compression, intravascular growth of tumor (renal cell carcinoma), systemic diseases associated with hypercoagulable states, extension of inferior vena caval thrombosis, and trauma.[199] With acute thrombosis there is flank pain, hematuria (gross or microscopic), and abdominal mass (in infants due to enlarged kidney). Gradual occlusion can be clinically asymptomatic. Diagnosis is generally radiologic with computed tomographic angiography being considered the most reliable.[200] Treatment depends on the acuity and underlying etiology.

Pathology

Changes in the kidney depend on the acuity of the process and any underlying disease process. Acute renal vein thrombosis results in a swollen kidney due to marked vascular congestion. There is interstitial edema. Renal venous thrombosis involves smaller venous channels within the renal parenchyma. Renal infarction is uncommon due to the presence of collateral circulation.

Renal Infarction

Clinical Features

Renal infarction most often is the result of embolic events but can also occur with acute occlusion of the renal artery or its branches for other reasons such as renal artery dissection, renal artery thrombosis, and traumatic injury to the renal artery.[202] Emboli are most often related to complicated atherosclerosis but can also originate in cardiac thrombi and be secondary to an intra-arterial procedure.[203] Infectious emboli are most often related to infective endocarditis.[204] Renal infarction is an infrequent complication of fibromuscular dysplasia.[205] Finally renal infarction has been well-described in association with cocaine abuse.[206]

Clinical presentation is dependent on the etiology. Smaller emboli are generally asymptomatic; larger renal infarcts can present with flank pain, hematuria, or hypertension. Chronic, bilateral emboli may result in sufficient renal damage to lead to renal failure. Embolization of the renal artery may also be performed for a therapeutic reason, most often for tumor infarction prior to nephrectomy.[207]

Pathology

Acute infarcts are initially red but rapidly become pale gray or yellow with a hyperemic border and are usually limited to the cortex (Fig. 1-76). They have a pyramidal shape with the base at the cortical surface. Over time, the infarct becomes fibrotic and results in a depressed scar on the cortical surface. With infectious emboli there may be liquefactive necrosis and abscess formation.

The acute infarct is characterized by coagulative necrosis with a hemorrhagic border that often contains a zone of acute inflammation. Infectious infarcts may have associated necrosis with abscess formation; the associated microorganism may be demonstrable. Embolic material may be evident in the affected vessels. With healing the tubules remain identifiable with ghost outlines of the structure but without viable cells. There is variable fibrosis, and hemosiderin-laden macrophages are present.

Other Vascular Diseases

The major renal vessels can also be involved in a wide range of vascular diseases. Among the better described are

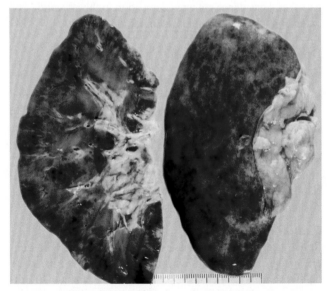

FIGURE 1-76 ■ Renal infarction. There is diffuse renal ischemia with patchy areas of infarction.

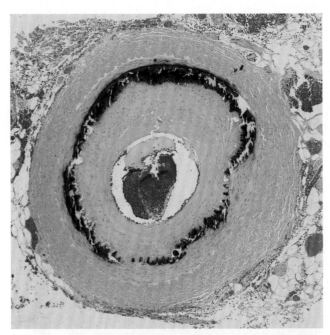

FIGURE 1-77 ■ Mönckeberg calcification. There is circumferential deposition of calcium within the media of the renal artery.

Takayasu disease[208] and polyarteritis nodosa[209]; however, many other systemic vasculitides can have renal vascular involvement.[209,210] Mönckeberg calcification can involve the renal arteries (Fig. 1-77). Patients with prior radiation treatment to the abdomen may develop renal artery stenosis related to muscle loss and fibrosis in the renal artery.

RENAL INFECTION

Renal infections are an important cause of morbidity and mortality throughout life. The kidney can become infected through a variety of routes but most common are retrograde spread from a lower urinary tract infection or blood-borne in a septic patient.[211] In this section, we will review the most common and important infectious processes that involve the kidney.

Bacterial Infection

The most common form of renal involvement is pyelonephritis, which is best defined as a nonspecific bacterial infection of the kidney that affects the parenchyma, calyces, and pelvis. It occurs in two forms, acute and chronic, and may be found with or without obstruction to the urinary tract.

Infecting organisms reach the kidney from the lower urinary tract by an ascending route. In patients without obstruction, vesicoureteral reflux is the mechanism responsible for parenchymal damage in a substantial number of cases. The term reflux nephropathy has largely replaced chronic nonobstructive pyelonephritis to describe the kidney with discrete, focal scars in a lobar distribution.[212]

Reflux, however, is not an invariable prerequisite for the development of renal scars. Scar formation can follow febrile urinary tract infections in the apparent absence of reflux,[213–215] particularly when P-fimbriated strains of *Escherichia coli* are involved. In addition, studies using dimercaptosuccinic acid scans have verified the presence of acute pyelonephritic lesions in the absence of reflux, followed at a later time by the development of discrete scars.[216,217]

Another pattern of renal infection is caused by blood-borne invasion by certain organisms, such as *Staphylococcus aureus*, which have the ability to localize, proliferate, and incite an acute inflammatory reaction in an unobstructed kidney. The infection consists of vast numbers of minute abscesses situated mainly in the cortex with no or only trivial pelvicalyceal inflammatory changes and should be termed diffuse suppurative nephritis rather than pyelonephritis.

Acute Pyelonephritis

Etiopathogenesis

Most infections of the urinary tract are caused by Gram-negative enteric organisms. *Escherichia coli* is the most common, particularly in first or uncomplicated infections.[218–220] Other organisms, such as *Klebsiella* sp., *Proteus* sp.,[221] *Pseudomonas* sp., *Enterobacter* sp., *Serratia* sp., *Morganella morganii*, and rarely *Haemophilus influenzae*,[222] are found mainly in complicated cases in which instrumentation, or an indwelling catheter, has been used,[221,223] and in patients with anatomic abnormalities, stone, or immunosuppression.[224]

The virulence of infecting organisms is a main factor in determining the occurrence of urinary tract infection. Virulence factors for *E. coli* include O serotype,[213,225–227] K antigens (capsular polysaccharides),[226,228] and H (flagellar) antigens, which relate to adherence properties and *P. fimbriae*.[226]

While Gram-positive bacteria adhere more frequently via extracellular polysaccharides, adhesion occurs via fimbriae in the case of Gram-negative bacteria. This adhesion is affected by the interaction between receptors on the epithelial cell surface and fimbriae or pili found on the surface of the infecting organism. *P. fimbriae* appear to be the most important with regard to urinary tract infections, especially with regard to renal involvement, and the class II-tip adhesin is associated with pyelonephritis.[224,229] Many novel and putative virulence factors in uropathogenic *E. coli* have been reported.[230]

Clinical Features

An acute onset of fever, chills, lumbar tenderness, and pain is the classic presentation of acute pyelonephritis in the adult.[231] Dysuria and frequency reflect lower urinary tract infections. Acute renal failure has been noted occasionally.[232] Blood cultures are positive in about a quarter or more of the cases of severe uncomplicated and complicated pyelonephritis.[233] The urine contains pus cells, pus cell casts, and organisms in excess of 100,000 cfu/mL. Hematuria and proteinuria are variable. Initial symptoms in infants and young children consist of fever, vague abdominal complaints, and vomiting. In neonates, the only symptom may be failure to thrive.

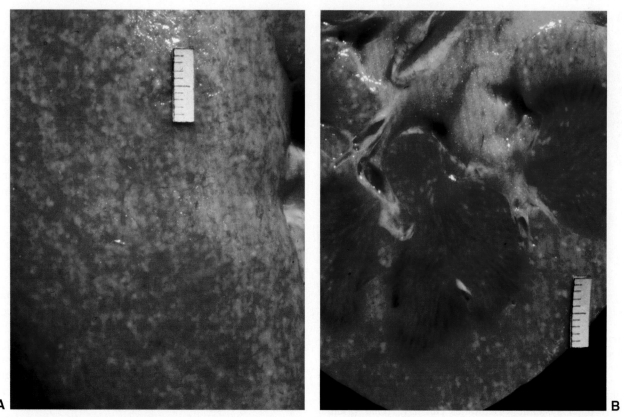

FIGURE 1-78 ■ Acute pyelonephritis. The kidney is swollen, and the cortical surface has a mottled appearance with pale yellow nodules and hyperemic areas **(A)**. The cut surface shows numerous small yellow lesions corresponding to microabscesses **(B)**.

It is often impossible to distinguish between acute pyelonephritis and lower urinary tract infections on purely clinical grounds. Various imaging techniques add precision to the diagnosis. The most reliable results have come from dimercaptosuccinic acid scintigraphy.[234]

Pathology

Gross Features. With obstructive acute pyelonephritis, the cortex has several swollen, whitish areas of acute infection. Scattered, small, discrete, whitish-yellow abscesses with a hemorrhagic rim, which may measure up to several millimeters in diameter, are noticeable on the subcapsular surface and are indicative of a secondary blood-borne infection (Fig. 1-78A and B). Intrarenal reflux caused by obstruction can cause diffuse cortical swelling and pallor.

The underlying medulla has characteristic straight, whitish-yellow streaks that correspond to collecting ducts filled with pus. Mucosal surfaces of the renal pelvis and calyces are often congested with thickening of the pelvic wall. Obstruction causes pelvicalyceal dilation, and with severe obstruction, the renal parenchyma may be thinned with blunted papillae and the pelvis filled with pus—pyonephrosis (Fig. 1-79). Severe, often terminal, acute renal infections accompanying obstruction and diabetes may be complicated by papillary necrosis (Fig. 1-80). Perinephric abscess, that is, a collection of pus in the space between the kidney and Gerota fascia, is often associated with nephrolithiasis (Fig. 1-81).[235]

Microscopic Features. Histologic findings in areas of acute infection are similar in the obstructive and nonobstructive types. The acute inflammatory process extensively destroys tubules (Fig. 1-82). Glomeruli and blood vessels are resistant to damage. Initially the interstitial inflammatory exudate consists of neutrophils. Chronic inflammatory cells, such as macrophages, lymphocytes, and plasma cells, appear within a few days of the start of infection.[236] Acute inflammatory changes are seen in relation to the pelvicalyceal epithelium.

Emphysematous Pyelonephritis

This rare, severe suppurative infection of the kidney is found predominantly in diabetics with or without urinary tract obstruction. This is associated with gas formation in the collecting system (emphysematous pyelitis), parenchyma, and sometimes in the perirenal tissue. Women are affected more often than men, with a mean age in the sixth decade. Bilateral emphysematous pyelonephritis is rare.[237–239]

Clinicopathologic features suggest a blood-borne infection. Four factors that may be involved include gas-forming bacteria, high tissue glucose level, impaired tissue perfusion, and a defective immune response.[240] *Escherichia coli* is the most common organism encountered, but *Klebsiella pneumoniae*, *Enterobacter* sp., and *Proteus mirabilis*, as well as

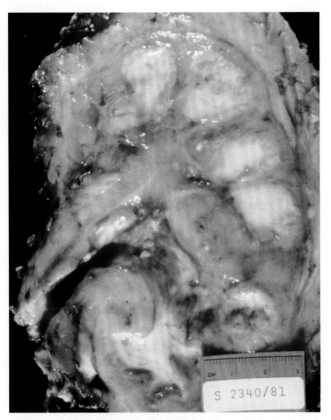

FIGURE 1-79 ■ Pyonephrosis. Acute pyelonephritis with accumulation of pus in the collecting system.

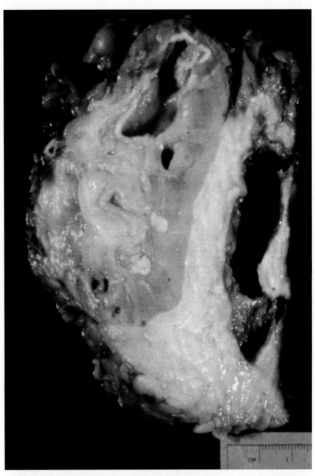

FIGURE 1-81 ■ Perinephric abscess. There is a large perinephric abscess adjacent to a kidney affected by a mixture of acute and xanthogranulomatous pyelonephritis. Note the pale yellow plaques characteristic of the latter process.

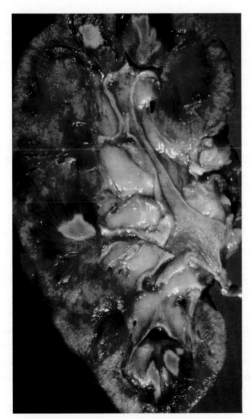

FIGURE 1-80 ■ Papillary necrosis. Multiple foci of papillary necrosis complicating acute pyelonephritis in a diabetic patient. There is a hyperemic zone surrounding the pale ischemic areas within the renal papillae.

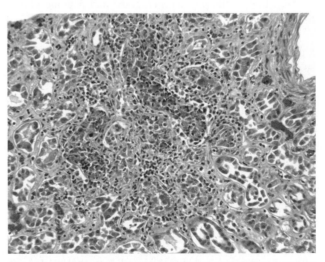

FIGURE 1-82 ■ Acute pyelonephritis. A small focus of acute inflammation with tubule destruction.

certain fungi (*Candida* sp., *Cryptococcus neoformans*), have also been described.[239]

Clinical Features

Nonspecific clinical features include chills, fever, flank pain, nausea, vomiting, abdominal pain and tenderness, and pyuria. Acute renal failure, thrombocytopenia, disturbance of consciousness, and shock can be the initial presentation and are risk factors for poor outcome and mortality.[240]

Diagnosis can be made by various imaging techniques.[241] However, a computerized tomographic scan not only confirms the diagnosis but also provides information useful for classifying the extent of intra- and extrarenal disease, which has both prognostic and therapeutic importance.[240]

Emphysematous pyelonephritis has a high mortality rate when treated with antibiotics alone.[242] Prognosis is improved considerably by prompt treatment with a combination of antibiotics and surgical intervention in the form of drainage or nephrectomy.[238–241,243,244]

Pathology

Renal lesions have included parenchymal abscesses and areas of infarction, with gas formation in necrotic areas, papillary necrosis and vascular thromboses.[239,240,242] Obstruction has been recorded in 40% of cases.

Diffuse Suppurative Nephritis

This type of renal lesion is caused by blood-borne infections. Its prototype is the lesion caused by *S. aureus*, which can localize to the kidney in the absence of obstruction. It may also be seen with *E. coli* bacteremia, but only when there is obstruction to urinary outflow.[245]

Staphylococci cause renal infection because of several microbial factors: bacterial surface receptors that recognize fibrinogen; fibronectin, vitronectin, and laminin permit bacterial adherence to endothelial cells[246] and extracellular matrix[247]; release of exotoxins,[248] including pore-forming protein[249]; various enzymes that interfere with the structure and function of the plasma membrane and degrade elastic tissue; and toxins that may function as super antigens.[250]

Other infective agents that are able to colonize a healthy kidney following bloodstream invasion include *Actinomyces* sp., yeasts, filamentous fungi, *Mycobacterium tuberculosis*, and *Brucella* sp.

Clinical Features

In patients with staphylococcal septicemia, the source of infection is often nosocomial, and *S. aureus* is the most common agent. Immunosuppressed patients are particularly vulnerable.[251] Patients present with fever, lumbar pain, symptoms of lower urinary tract infection, and renal insufficiency or renal failure.[252]

Pathology

Gross Features. With *S. aureus* infection, both kidneys are affected and are enlarged to an equal degree. With *E. coli*, only the obstructed kidney is involved. The subcapsular surface is studded with a vast number of whitish-yellow abscesses, often with red rims. The abscesses vary from pin head in size up to 5 mm in diameter and are usually discrete, but can occasionally be confluent. The cut surface of the renal cortex bulges because of interstitial edema and contains a myriad of small abscesses that predominate in the outer part; some are rounded, but others are wedge-shaped with the apex pointing inward.

Microscopic Features. The abscesses consist of large numbers of neutrophils in the interstitium, with extensive destruction of tubules. Glomeruli, arteries, and arterioles are usually undamaged, although glomerular microabscess may very rarely be seen. Organisms are readily evident. In contrast to acute pyelonephritis, there are no, or only a few, inflammatory cells beneath the pelvicalyceal epithelium.

Chronic Obstructive Pyelonephritis

The parameters that are required for renal parenchymal scarring to develop following urinary tract infection remain elusive. Persistence of uropathic bacteria in the kidney and genetic variability in the function of the host immune system may both be risk factors.

Clinical Features

The clinical presentation depends on whether chronic pyelonephritis is bilateral or unilateral and whether these are associated urinary tract abnormalities. In general, patients with bilateral chronic pyelonephritis develop slowly progressive renal insufficiency. The clinical course may be insidious or punctuated by recurrent attacks of acute pyelonephritis with back pain, fever, pyuria, and bacteriuria. In late stages of chronic pyelonephritis, bacteriuria may be absent.

Renal insufficiency principally affects tubular function, resulting in decreased concentrating power, nocturia, polyuria, and tubular acidosis. Blood urea nitrogen and phosphate levels are elevated. Mild to moderate proteinuria may occur. Terminal uremia is often associated with hypertension.

Pathology

Gross Features. Chronic pyelonephritis reduces renal size and causes irregular scarring, which is asymmetric in bilateral disease. With the renal capsule stripped, coarse, depressed scars are evident on the cortical surface (Fig. 1-83). The scars are larger and flatter than those caused by infarction. Intervening parenchyma is granular if hypertensive nephrosclerosis is present.

The characteristic changes of chronic pyelonephritis are evident on cut section of the kidney and consist of a coarse, discrete corticomedullary scar overlying a blunted or deformed calyx (Fig. 1-84). Pelvic mucosa is generally thickened and finely granular and may be hemorrhagic or covered by exudate.

In advanced stages of chronic pyelonephritis, the kidneys are markedly contracted, and the renal capsule is typically thickened, fibrotic, and difficult to strip from the capsular

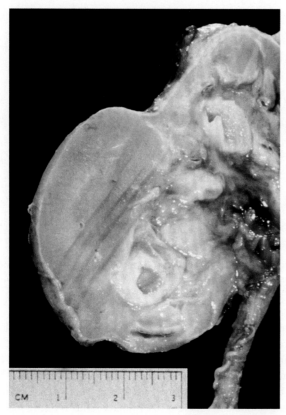

FIGURE 1-83 ■ Chronic pyelonephritis. There is a large area of scarring with relatively normal appearing adjacent renal parenchyma.

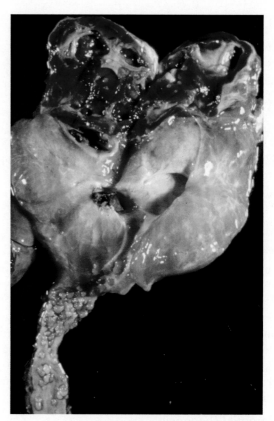

FIGURE 1-85 ■ Chronic pyelonephritis. An unusual example of segmental fibrolipomatous replacement of the lower pole of the kidney. Note also the presence of florid ureteritis cystica.

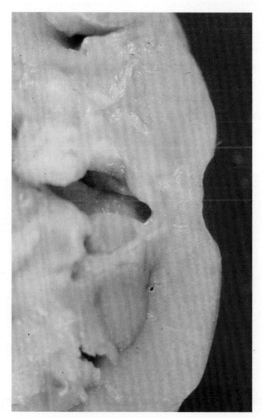

FIGURE 1-84 ■ Chronic pyelonephritis. There is an area of cortical loss resulting in a depressed scar with an underlying dilated calyx.

surface. In rare cases, chronically inflamed hilar and perirenal fat becomes fibrotic and merges with scarred renal parenchyma, leading to an appearance of diffuse or segmental fibrolipomatous replacement (Fig. 1-85).

Microscopic Features. The changes are predominately tubulointerstitial. The degree of chronic interstitial inflammation varies. In areas of preserved parenchyma, an infiltrate of lymphocytes, plasma cells, and occasional eosinophils is more likely to be prominent (Fig. 1-86). Peritubular polypoid projections of lymphocytes in the cortex are a useful indicator of infection. Cortical interstitial fibrosis may vary from fine to dense. There is a marked loss of tubular mass or prominence of atrophic tubules with flattened epithelium and thickened tubular basement membranes. Zones of atrophic tubules, which may be dilated, frequently contain waxy casts, so-called thyroidization (Fig. 1-87). These changes extend to the outer medulla, which generally has fine fibrosis. The dilated, deformed calyces are chronically inflamed and fibrotic. Pelvic mucosa is also thickened, fibrotic, and chronically inflamed.

Glomeruli within scarred zones may show variable changes, including thickening of Bowman capsule with concentric periglomerular fibrosis, ischemic collapse with collagen internal to Bowman capsule, and global hyalinization merging into the surrounding interstitium (Fig. 1-88). Compensatory hyperplasia of uninvolved

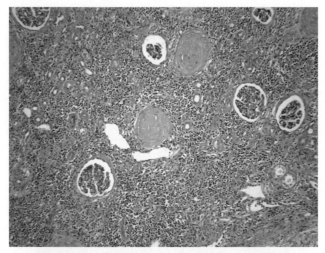

FIGURE 1-86 ■ Chronic pyelonephritis. There is a polymorphous chronic interstitial inflammatory infiltrate with glomerulosclerosis. Note the periglomerular fibrosis in the more intact glomeruli.

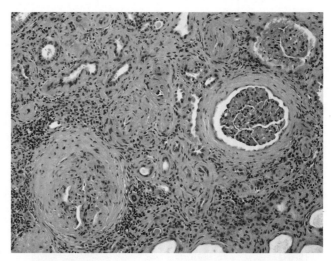

FIGURE 1-88 ■ Chronic pyelonephritis. Photomicrograph illustrating periglomerular fibrosis and thickening of Bowman capsule with eventual glomerular fibrosis.

glomeruli is often present (Fig. 1-89). Arteries within pyelonephritis scars may be normal or may show medial thickening and intimal fibrosis. The vascular fibrosis, as well as arteriolar thickening and hyalinization, are more prominent in cases complicated by hypertension.

Differential Diagnosis

The cortical tubulointerstitial changes are not diagnostic of chronic pyelonephritis. A similar histologic picture can result from a wide variety of factors, including ischemia, simple obstruction, drug reactions, irradiation, and changes secondary to papillary necrosis.

Reflux Nephropathy

Nonobstructing reversal of urine flow into the ureter, renal pelvis, and calyces may cause dilatation and damage the renal parenchyma both by increased fluid pressure and by contamination by pathogenic organisms present in the bladder urine. The combination of vesicoureteral reflux and renal scarring comprises reflux nephropathy, which replaces the term atrophic or chronic nonobstructive pyelonephritis.[253,254]

Urine reflux can be congenital (primary) or acquired and unilateral or bilateral (Table 1-10). Primary reflux is due to incompetence of the vesicoureteric junction at the point of the ureteral orifice. There is evidence that this is in part a heritable condition and multiple genes have been implicated.[255] Secondary vesicoureteral reflux in children can be the result of congenital anomalies associated with incompetent vesicoureteric junction, for example, duplicate ureters or pelvic (horseshoe) kidney.

Clinical and animal studies have confirmed that renal scarring develops in the areas where intrarenal reflux occurs. The role of superimposed urinary tract infection on the pathogenesis of vesicoureteral reflux scarring continues to be debated.

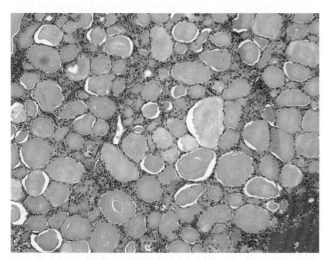

FIGURE 1-87 ■ Chronic pyelonephritis. Atrophic tubules are filled with proteinaceous secretions producing so-called thyroidization.

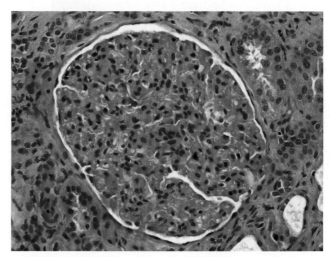

FIGURE 1-89 ■ Chromic pyelonephritis. Compensatory glomerular hyperplasia in a case of chronic pyelonephritis.

Table 1-10 ■ CAUSES OF OBSTRUCTIVE NEPHROPATHY

Hydronephrosis only
   Ureteropelvic junction obstruction
     With crossing blood vessels
     Without crossing blood vessels
   Nephrolithiasis
     Staghorn calculus
   Tumors and tumor-like conditions of renal pelvis
     Fibroepithelial polyp
     Urothelial neoplasms
     Other
Hydronephrosis and hydroureter
   Nephrolithiasis
   Ureteral valves
   Tumors and tumor-like conditions of ureter
     Fibroepithelial polyp
     Urothelial neoplasms
     Other
   Congenital anomalies of ureters
   Pregnancy
   Ureteritis
   Incompetent vesicoureteral junction
   Bladder neoplasms
   Bladder outlet obstruction
   Neurogenic bladder
   Posterior urethral valves

The presence of two types of papillae, simple and compound, explains the focal scarring in reflux nephropathy.[256] Simple papillae, located mainly in the midzone of the kidney, have slit-like collecting duct orifices that are forced closed by back pressure of urine. Compound papillae, which are situated at the poles, have larger, round openings that make them more vulnerable to reflux.

Clinical Features

Age and presence of urinary tract infection determine the clinical presentation.[257,258] Congenital reflux in infants and young children may be asymptomatic or present with nonspecific lower urinary tract symptoms, including dysuria, flank pain, and tenderness or fever.

The diagnosis of reflux nephropathy is heavily dependent on imaging studies. Ultrasound and voiding cystourethrography are the primary tests to establish the diagnosis of vesicoureteral junction reflux. Excretory urography (IVP) evaluates involvement of the upper urinary tract and is particularly suited for children with febrile urinary tract infections. The presence of one or more scars, defined as focal thinning of the renal cortex often overlying a dilated calyx, is dependent on the severity of reflux. There are five grades of reflux (I to V). High-grade reflux (grade V), often referred to as the "back-pressure type," is most frequently the type associated with cortical scars.

Patients with vesicoureteral reflux occasionally develop significant glomerular proteinuria, including the nephrotic syndrome, and prove to have secondary (hyperfiltration) focal segmental glomerulosclerosis caused by reflux. The

role of reflux in glomerulosclerosis has been well documented.[259] In one study, focal segmental glomerulosclerosis occurred in 20% of pediatric nephrectomy specimens from patients with vesicoureteral reflux.[259] It has been associated with a poor prognosis.[260]

Reflux nephropathy is reportedly responsible for 5% to 40% of end-stage renal disease in children under 16 years of age and 5% to 20% of end-stage renal disease in adults <50 years of age.[261] Progressive kidney disease is predictable based on type of scars and clinical presentation in childhood.[258] Adults with extensive scarring in childhood and/or hypertension have a worse prognosis. In high-grade reflux (grade V), medical management has been less successful than surgery[262]; however, the literature is unclear whether surgery prevents end-stage renal disease in severe cases.[263] A literature review has substantiated that very severe congenital reflux is progressive, and is often associated with other urogenital abnormalities.[264] Unilateral and mild or moderate vesicoureteral reflux in children is rather regressive instead of progressive.

Pathology

Gross Features. The appearance of reflux nephropathy consists of coarse renal scars surrounded by bulging parenchyma and overlying a dilated calyx. One or more scars may be present particularly at the poles (Fig. 1-90). Reflux-associated scars may show disproportionate centrilobar atrophy.[265]

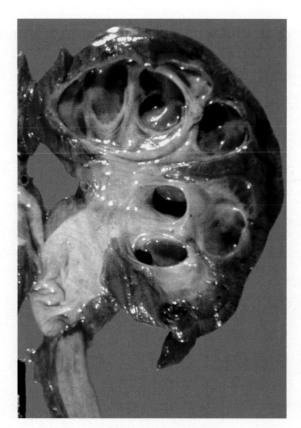

FIGURE 1-90 ■ Reflux nephropathy. There is marked hydronephrosis and loss of renal mass due to ureteropelvic obstruction.

Microscopic Features. In primary and secondary reflux nephropathy, the histology is similar and consists of linear interstitial scars with atrophic tubules and obsolescent glomeruli. In proteinuric patients with hyperfiltration focal segmental glomerulosclerosis, sclerotic glomeruli within preserved parenchyma have prominent hypertrophy.[265] Marked compensatory lengthening of glomerular capillaries secondary to hyperfiltration, tuft adhesions to Bowman capsule, and podocyte detachment are primarily found in patients with poor prognosis.[260]

Ask-Upmark Kidney

The Ask-Upmark kidney is characterized by the presence of segmental atrophy, which most investigators consider secondary to parenchymal pressure due to reflux of urine and infection.[266] Others favor an ischemic etiology related to a vascular anomaly.[267] The Ask-Upmark kidney may be unilateral or bilateral, is found both in children and in adults, and occurs predominantly in females.[266–269]

Clinical Features

Severe hypertension, which may be the presenting symptom, is seen in most children and 60% of adults. Other symptoms include recurrent urinary tract infection, proteinuria, or decreased renal function. In some patients, the hypertension is renin dependent. Nephrectomy typically cures the hypertension.

Pathology

Gross Features. The affected kidney is reduced in size with one or more sharply separated hypoplastic segments characterized by narrow cortical grooves or depressions overlying extremely thinned parenchyma and elongated or dilated calyces (Fig. 1-91A and B).[266]

Microscopic Features. The thin segment contains atrophic tubules with thyroidization, crowded thick-walled vessels, and no glomeruli. Absence of glomeruli is characteristic and contrasts with sclerotic glomeruli seen in other types of cortical atrophy, as well as the cortical scars of reflux nephropathy and chronic obstructive pyelonephritis.

Tuberculosis

The most common form of extrapulmonary tuberculosis is genitourinary disease, accounting for approximately 25% of nonpulmonary cases (range 14% to 41%).[270] In Western countries, the prevalence of renal involvement among patients with tuberculosis is around 5%,[270,271] and in African countries, the prevalence of renal tuberculosis is higher at 9.5% if diagnosed by using urine Ziehl-Nielsen stains and 14% if a combination of urine stains, sterile pyuria, and tissue histology are used.[271] Males are affected twice as often as females, and the disease most often occurs between the ages of 15 and 60 years.

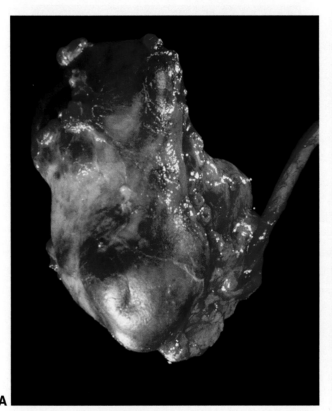

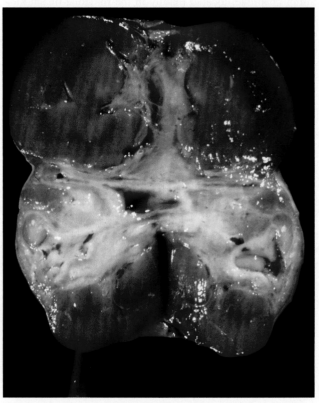

A   B

FIGURE 1-91 ■ Ask-Upmark kidney. From the external surface there is a centrally located depressed groove **(A)**. The cut surface highlights the underlying scar **(B)**.

Transplantation is a risk factor for the development of tuberculosis,[270] and immunosuppressed patients are more vulnerable to infection by mycobacteria.[270–273] Approximately 10% of all cases of tuberculosis worldwide have been HIV related, but the occurrence of the disease is as high as 60% in certain regions in sub-Saharan Africa.[270]

Clinical Features

Renal involvement may result from hematogenous dissemination of a primary tuberculous infection, from an active pulmonary lesion, or from reactivation of a healed tuberculous lesion. There are two main types of renal tuberculosis: miliary (disseminated infection) and cavitary (localized urinary tract infection). Important risk factors for renal tuberculosis in developed countries include transplantation, immunosuppression, and HIV infection. It is estimated that 10% of all cases of tuberculosis worldwide are related to HIV infection. In these patients, involvement of the kidney is often subclinical and only recognized at autopsy.

Miliary tuberculosis of the kidneys is often clinically silent[274] and overshadowed by clinical manifestations of the systemic infection.[275] With renal cavitary tuberculosis, a high proportion of men have associated genital tuberculosis, particularly affecting the epididymis and, less frequently, the prostate. Most of the symptoms from the cavitary, or so-called caseous, form of renal tuberculosis result from involvement of the lower urinary tract,[276] particularly the urinary bladder, and manifest as frequency, dysuria, and hematuria; sterile pyuria is commonly found.[275,276] Infection confined to the kidney is usually clinically silent.[274] Because involvement is usually unilateral, renal function is typically well preserved.[275] When renal failure occurs in patients with pulmonary or disseminated tuberculosis the kidney may show tuberculous interstitial nephritis. Tuberculosis is recognized to be an uncommon cause of end-stage renal disease. In developed countries the frequency is estimated at <1% of cases.[270]

The diagnosis of renal tuberculosis requires a positive culture for mycobacteria; culture of the first-voided urine specimen, obtained for 3 to 5 consecutive days, has been recommended.[277] More sensitive methodologies including urine polymerase chain reaction (PCR) for mycobacteria may improve the diagnostic accuracy.

Pathology

Gross Features. Kidneys with miliary tuberculosis have 1- to 3-mm nodules (i.e., tubercles), which occur more often in the cortex than in the medulla. In patients dying of pulmonary tuberculosis, renal tubercles are found in >60% of autopsy cases.[278] With cavitary tuberculosis, kidneys may be enlarged or decreased in size with irregular scarring on the subcapsular surface (Fig. 1-92). On cut section, pelvicalyceal dilatation or deformity and pelvi-ureteric constriction may occur with parenchymal atrophy and foci of calcification. The lesion often begins in the medulla with caseation necrosis of the papilla. Ureteral involvement can cause segmental strictures. A combination of caseation necrosis of the

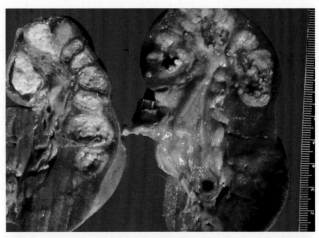

FIGURE 1-92 ■ Tuberculosis. There is marked cortical thinning in the upper pole with associated calyceal dilatation and areas of caseous necrosis.

pelvicalyceal system with ureteral stenosis leads to tuberculous pyonephrosis. "Cement," "putty," or "chalk" kidney describes replacement of renal parenchyma by caseous material, leaving rims of fibrous tissue that give the organ a loculated appearance.

Microscopic Features. The early tubercle is a granuloma that consists of epithelioid histiocytes and neutrophils and has central caseous necrosis. Often a mononuclear cell infiltrate of lymphocytes, monocytes, and plasma cells is also present. Miliary tuberculosis is characterized by numerous well-formed granulomas. In immunosuppressed patients, the granulomas are often less well defined and caseous necrosis is frequently absent. Organisms are usually identified in such lesions with special stains. The tubercle may be contained and heal, or the infection may expand and, if in the renal medulla, may reach the renal pelvis and allow release of microorganisms into the urinary tract.

Cavitary lesions consist of large zones of typical caseous material with a peripheral granulomatous reaction (Fig. 1-93). Mycobacteria are typically found in peripheral portions of areas of caseation or cavitary lesions. Less involved surrounding renal parenchyma may show variable interstitial inflammation with lymphocytes and plasma cells. Calcific foci likely represent calcified tubercles.

Tuberculous interstitial nephritis is characterized by a diffuse chronic tubulointerstitial inflammatory infiltrate with granuloma formation.[270] Chronic tuberculosis can be associated with amyloidosis. Several types of glomerular disease have also been reported in patients with tuberculosis; however, no well-defined association exists.

Differential Diagnosis

Mycobacterial stains (acid-fast or Ziehl-Nielsen) should always be requested if granulomas are present in a biopsy or nephrectomy specimen, particularly if the patient's immune system is compromised. Although *M. tuberculosis* is the most common agent, other mycobacteria, such as *M. bovis, M.*

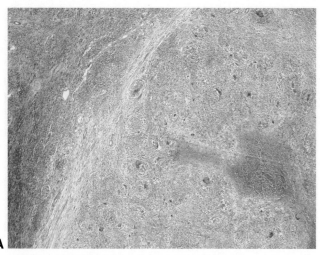
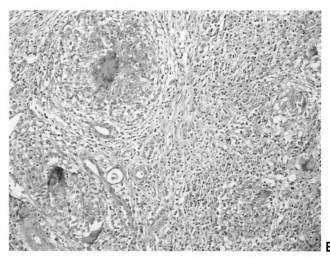

FIGURE 1-93 ■ Tuberculosis. Large confluent granulomas with numerous giant cells and necrosis (**A**). Higher-power photomicrograph with granulomas and Langhans giant cells **(B)**.

kansasii, and *M. avium intracellulare*, can cause renal infection.[279] In immunocompromised patients, including HIV-related cases, atypical mycobacteriosis can occur, including infections with *M. avium intracellulare*, which does not form typical granulomas but has abundant mycobacteria present in foamy macrophages. Fungal involvement of the kidney can also result in miliary patterns of involvement and single or multiple large cavitary lesions. Sarcoidosis can also involve the kidney with a granulomatous interstitial nephritis (Fig. 1-94).[280] The granulomas are well formed and are noncaseating. There is an associated acute and/or chronic inflammatory infiltrate with interstitial fibrosis.

Fungal Infection

Although some fungi, such as *Candida* and *Torulopsis*, may infect the lower urinary tract and involve the kidneys through the ascending route, primary infections of the kidney by fungi are rare (Table 1-11). More often, renal infections result from systemic fungal sepsis. The source may be nosocomial,[281] and almost invariably the infection occurs in immunocompromised patients, particularly those receiving chemotherapy for malignancies.[282]

Candidiasis

Clinical Features
Most renal infections by *Candida albicans* are opportunistic and result from hematogenous dissemination. Neonates,[283] granulocytopenic patients,[282,284] and immunosuppressed patients[282,285] are at risk and the source of infection is often nosocomial. In two series of systemic candidiasis, renal involvement was reported to be 52%[285] and 82%.[284]

Presenting symptoms are those of severe renal infection, with hypotension, progressive loss of renal function, and acute renal failure. Fungus balls may develop in the pelvis or calyces, and their passage may result in ureteral colic or bilateral obstruction with anuria.[286,287] Systemic candidiasis has a fatality rate of 70% to 79%.[288,289]

Pathology
The kidneys may show little or no inflammatory response, or there may be extensive necrosis, miliary abscesses, and papillary

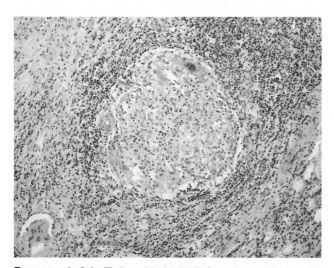

FIGURE 1-94 ■ Sarcoidosis. Well-formed granuloma with associated chronic inflammation.

Table 1-11 ■ IMPORTANT FUNGAL INFECTION OF THE KIDNEY
Candidiasis
Torulopsis
Aspergillosis
Cryptococcosis
Histoplasmosis
Blastomycosis
Coccidioidomycosis
Paracoccidioidomycosis
Mucormycosis

necrosis.[283,288] Compared with other fungi, invasion of blood vessels by *Candida* is less common, and cortical infarction is rare.[288] In tissue sections, pseudohyphae and 2 to 4 μm in diameter, rounded yeast forms are readily identified with periodic acid–Schiff (PAS) or Grocott methenamine silver (GMS) stains.

Torulopsis

Clinical Features

Torulopsis glabrata, an opportunistic yeast-like fungus, is the second most common fungal pathogen of the urinary tract.[288] The kidneys can be the site of a primary infection through the ascending route[290,291] but are usually part of disseminated infections. *Torulopsis* is an important cause of nosocomial infection.[281] Presenting symptoms are comparable to those caused by *C. albicans*. The outcome of patients with torulopsosis is poor.[292]

Pathology

Nearly one-half of patients with disseminated infection have renal involvement that is often microscopic. In severe cases, miliary or extensive abscess formation, papillary necrosis, and perinephric abscess formation have been described.[290,292–294] *Torulopsis glabrata* are demonstrable in tissue sections by GMS stain as 2- to 4-μm, budding, round to oval, nonencapsulated yeast-like organisms.

Aspergillosis

Clinical Features

Aspergillus fumigatus is the most common pathogen among the various species of aspergilli. Renal aspergillosis is frequently the result of hematogenous dissemination, usually from an invasive bronchial infection, necrotizing pneumonia, or infarct by aspergilli, particularly in immunosuppressed[282] or diabetic patients.[295,296]

Renal involvement occurs in 30% to 40% of patients who die of disseminated aspergillosis.[288] Symptoms may be comparable to acute pyelonephritis. The urinary tract may be obstructed by growth of mycelium, and fungus balls may be passed into the urine.[295]

Pathology

Multiple small abscesses, a few millimeters in diameter, are most commonly seen. However, extensive abscess formation with vascular invasion, thrombosis, and infarction also occurs and is more common in the medulla than in the cortex (Fig. 1-95).[297] The fungus takes the form of branching septate hyphae 3 to 5 μm wide that can be demonstrated within abscesses (Fig. 1-96A and B) and infarcts with PAS or GMS stain (Fig. 1-97).

Cryptococcosis

Clinical Features

Cryptococcus neoformans is a yeast-like fungus encountered in avian habitats, particularly those contaminated with pigeon droppings. The host portal of entry is the respiratory tract, and pulmonary infection is common, particularly in immunosuppressed patients.[282,298] Hematogenous dissemination

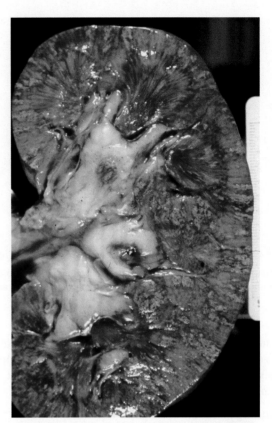

FIGURE 1-95 ■ Aspergillosis. Acute pyelonephritis due to *Aspergillus* with numerous small abscesses and pyonephrosis.

results in renal involvement, which may be clinically silent or manifest with costovertebral angle tenderness, pyuria, and gross hematuria. Renal involvement is found in about 50% of patients who die of disseminated cryptococcosis.[288]

Pathology

Small parenchymal abscesses or granulomas with central necrosis can involve the cortex and medulla, and papillary necrosis may occasionally be found.[288,299,300] Despite causing extensive tubular destruction, the organism may elicit little inflammatory reaction.

Cryptococci can be identified in tissue sections as spherical structures, 4 to 20 μm, with a polysaccharide capsule. The capsule is distinctive and stains intensely with mucicarmine, Alcian blue, and the PAS stains. Yeast forms can be recognized in the urinary sediment by negative staining with India ink.[300]

Histoplasmosis

Clinical Features

Histoplasma capsulatum is endemic in South and Central America and in the Ohio River and Mississippi River valleys in the United States.[288] Infection is caused by inhalation of dust particles containing conidia forms from soil contaminated with bird or bat droppings containing the fungus. The initial presentation resembles pulmonary tuberculosis. Disseminated histoplasmosis may result from a primary infection or from a reactivated healed lesion during

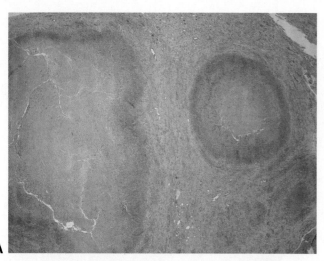
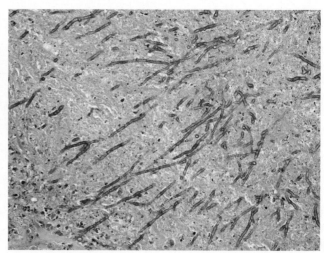

A

B

FIGURE 1-96 ■ Aspergillosis. Acute pyelonephritis due to *Aspergillus* with large granulomas having central necrosis (**A**). On higher magnification the organisms can be seen on the hematoxylin and eosin–stained section (**B**).

immunosuppression.[282] The kidneys are involved in about 40% of the patients with progressive disseminated histoplasmosis.[301] Renal involvement is usually clinically silent, and compromise of renal function is uncommon.[301]

Pathology

Grossly, the lesions range from one or more firm or soft, usually well-circumscribed nodules to diffuse inflammation and necrosis involving most of the kidney; papillary necrosis may occur.[301,302] Microscopically, small aggregates of yeast-laden macrophages may be present in all renal compartments, usually associated with granulomas at various stages and focal necrosis.[301] Macrophages contain numerous round or oval 2- to 4-μm-diameter yeast forms, usually identified with the GMS stain. At later stages dense collagenized nodules remain (Fig. 1-98).

Blastomycosis

Clinical Features

Northern American blastomycosis, caused by *Blastomyces dermatitidis*, is endemic in the Ohio River and Mississippi River valleys and the southeastern United States.[288] The fungus is a saprophytic budding yeast found in soils. Blastomycosis is prevalent among immunosuppressed patients.[282] It is four times more frequent in males than in females and occurs mainly between the ages of 30 and 50 years.[288] It is primarily a pulmonary infection.

Renal involvement, which is estimated to occur in 25% of systemic infections, is usually clinical silent, although renal insufficiency may occur in severe infections.[303] Blastomycosis tends to recur in 10% to 15% of patients and has a mortality rate of 90%.[304]

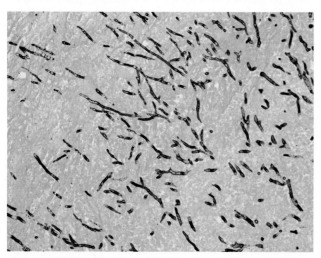

FIGURE 1-97 ■ Aspergillosis. The GMS stain highlights the branching hyphae.

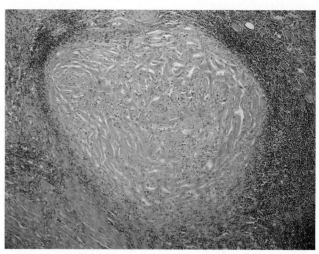

FIGURE 1-98 ■ Histoplasmosis. Old histoplasma granuloma with dense fibrotic center and surrounding chromic inflammatory infiltrate.

Pathology

Involvement is often bilateral and varies from small circumscribed nodules to diffuse inflammation and necrosis involving the whole kidney.[288] The cortex is more affected than the medulla, and extension of the infection through the renal capsule results in perinephric abscesses and discharging sinuses. Granulomatous and suppurative lesions are seen microscopically, with microabscess formation and epithelioid and giant cell granulomas that may have caseation resembling tuberculosis. Detection of *B. dermatitidis* in either type of lesion is facilitated with the GMS stain. The yeast is double contoured, 8 to 15 μm in diameter, and has broad-based branching daughter cells.

Coccidioidomycosis

Clinical Features

Coccidioides immitis, which is endemic in the southwest and western United States, exist in nature in a mycelial form.[305] Inhalation of arthrospores, the infective form, results in asymptomatic pulmonary infection in about 90% of patients. Progressive pulmonary infections are rare, and systemic dissemination in <1% of cases usually affects immunosuppressed[282,306] and diabetic patients or pregnant women.[307–309] The kidneys are involved in one-third of patients who die of disseminated disease.[288]

Pathology

Minute granulomas and multiple abscesses are present grossly. The granulomas show caseous or suppurative necrosis. *Coccidioides immitis* organisms are easily found in active lesions within macrophages or giant cells as thick-walled spherules, about 100 μm in diameter, containing endospores that are 2 to 5 μm in diameter.[288]

Paracoccidioidomycosis

Clinical Features

Paracoccidioidomycosis (i.e., South American blastomycosis), caused by *Paracoccidioides brasiliensis*, is a chronic pulmonary disease endemic in Mexico and Central America. Pulmonary infection, caused by inhalation of spores, tends to be progressive and followed by dissemination.[310] Progression and dissemination are associated with depressed cell-mediated responses.[311,312] The kidneys are involved in 10% to 15% of cases.

Pathology

Typical lesions consist of cortical and medullary miliary granulomas, a few millimeters in size, and often having necrotic centers.[288] Microorganisms, which are found in areas of inflammation, at the periphery of necrotic granulomas and within giant cells, are easily identified with the GMS stain. Nonbudding forms, between 5 and 30 μm in diameter, predominate. However, multiple buds from a single cell, up to 60 μm in diameter and resembling the pilot's wheel of a ship, are diagnostic.[288]

Mucormycosis

Clinical Features

Mucormycosis (i.e., zygomycosis) is an opportunistic pulmonary and upper respiratory tract infection caused by fungi of the order Mucorales, whose most common pathogen is *Rhizopus oryzae*. Disseminated infection occurs in immunocompromised,[282,298,313–315] diabetic and AIDS patients.[316] *Rhizopus oryzae* frequently invades blood vessels and disseminates through the hematogenous route. Involvement of the urinary tract may be clinically silent or manifest by signs or symptoms of renal infarction, including flank pain, gross hematuria, and acute renal failure.[252,288,317] Renal involvement occurs in 50% of patients dying of disseminated mucormycosis[288] and may be unilateral[316] or bilateral.[318]

Pathology

Segmental or subtotal renal infarction results from vascular thromboses. Microscopically, there is suppurative, necrotizing inflammation with thrombosis of interlobar and arcuate arteries. Granulomatous inflammation and Langhans-type giant cells are seen. Fungi can be identified with the GMS stain in areas of acute inflammation or infarction and consist of broad, nonseptate hyphae that have right-angle branching.

Parasitic Infection

Renal lesions associated with parasitic infection are quite variable. Malaria, for example, which is caused by *Plasmodium*, can lead to acute renal failure due to acute tubular necrosis, a tubulointerstitial nephritis, or chronic glomerular disease with hematuria and proteinuria or the nephrotic syndrome (quartan malarial nephropathy).[319,320] *Schistosoma mansoni* infection results in glomerulonephritis manifested by proteinuria or the nephrotic syndrome.[321] Other parasites may directly invade the kidney.

Schistosomiasis

The interstitial inflammatory response occurring in schistosomal nephropathy is most commonly nonspecific and consists of an infiltrate of mononuclear cells and interstitial fibrosis associated with obstructive uropathy.[322] Localization of ova to the kidney produces a granulomatous reaction. Ova can be easily identified in tissues; those of *S. mansoni* and *S. japonicum* are acid-fast, while those of *S. haematobium* are not.

Filariasis

Microfilaria may cause granulomatous inflammation in glomeruli[323] and the interstitium. Severe tubulointerstitial mononuclear cell infiltration with lymphocytes, plasma cells, and eosinophils, independent of granulomas, has also been described.[324]

Microsporidiosis

Microsporidia are obligate intracellular protozoa belonging to the genus *Encephalitozoon*. The organism typically infects patients with AIDS. *Encephalitozoon cuniculi*, the prototypic species, targets the kidney with involvement of macrophages, epithelium, and endothelium.[325] It has been reported to produce a necrotizing infection with microabscess-like foci that is concentrated in the distal nephron, especially the medulla.[326] Spore-laden macrophages, cellular debris and free spores, as well as sloughed epithelial cells, are present in tubular lumens.

Organisms can be identified in hematoxylin and eosin sections as oval to slightly elongated, 1- to 2-mm spores having a blue-staining outline and either a central blue band or a dense blue pole opposite a clear polar vacuole. Gram stain, polarization, and fluorescence chitin stains enhance spore detection.

Amoebiasis

Amoebiasis is a protozoal infection caused by *Entamoeba histolytica*. Renal involvement is very rare; however, with invasive infections, the kidney is the fifth most common site of abscess localization.[327] Trophozoites can be found within foci of liquefaction necrosis and abscess formation.

Hydatidosis

Unilocular hydatid disease is caused by the larval form of *Echinococcus granulosus*. Renal involvement, which occurs in 2% to 4% of all cases,[328] is usually part of disseminated disease. The most common symptoms are palpable mass, flank pain, hematuria, malaise, and fever. The passage of typical grape-like daughter cysts in the urine (hydatiduria) is a pathognomonic sign but occurs in only 5% to 25% of cases.[328]

Hydatid cysts of the kidney are usually cortical and solitary[329] and can range from a few millimeters to several centimeters in size (Fig. 1-99). A fibrous reaction usually surrounds the cyst, while atrophy and pressure necrosis occur more peripherally.[329]

Viral Infection

Glomerulonephritis may be produced by hepatitis B or C infection and arteritis by hepatitis B infection. HIV-associated nephropathy is characterized by a collapsing, rapidly progressive form of focal segmental glomerulosclerosis and interstitial nephritis with large tubular casts and numerous endothelial tuboreticular inclusions.[330-333] Hantavirus infection produces hemorrhagic fever with renal syndrome[334]; renal biopsy findings are most commonly acute interstitial nephritis with dominant lymphocytic inflammation accompanied by acute interstitial hemorrhagic and tubular necrosis.[335,336] Viral inclusions are not present. Polyoma virus and cytomegalovirus (CMV) cause an acute interstitial nephritis with characteristic viral inclusions.

Polyoma Virus

BK virus, a small nonenveloped DNA virus, is a member of the polyoma subgroup of papovaviruses. Hematogenous spread of a primary infection, which is most often a

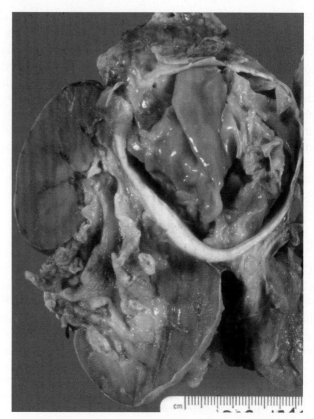

FIGURE 1-99 ■ Echinococcal cyst. A large echinococcal cyst in the kidney with the characteristic thick wall.

childhood pulmonary infection, carries BK virus to the kidney and urothelium where the virus enters latency. Organ transplant patients, HIV-infected patients, and patients with hematologic malignancies are at significant risk for reactivation of BK virus infection. An increased risk for virus replication and shedding in the urine may also occur in diabetic patients, pregnant women, and the elderly.

Clinical Features

Renal and urinary tract findings in BK virus reactivation infection include asymptomatic hematuria, hemorrhagic and nonhemorrhagic cystitis, ureteral stenosis, and renal allograft dysfunction with BK nephropathy. Reactivation BK virus infection occurs in 10% to 60% of renal transplants, and 1% to 5% of renal allografts develop BK nephropathy.[337-339] Diagnosis can be made using PCR to detect the virus in the plasma.[340]

Pathology

Histologic features include intranuclear inclusions, tubular necrosis, and interstitial inflammation, which is generally mild and has inconspicuous tubulitis.[341,342] Four different varieties of intranuclear inclusions can be seen in any part of the nephron.[341] Type 1 inclusions are the classical basophilic inclusions having an amorphous ground glass appearance with peripheral chromatin rimming (Fig. 1-100); these can be found in the renal pelvic urothelium. Type 2 inclusions are eosinophilic and granular with an incomplete

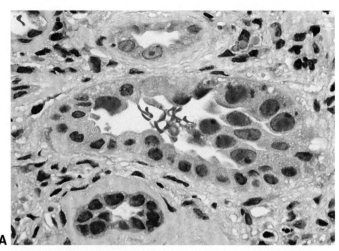 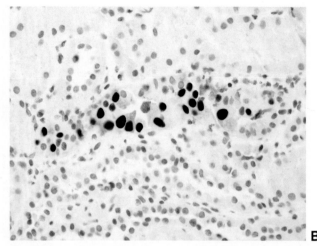

A **B**

FIGURE 1-100 ■ BK virus nephropathy. Granular amphophilic intranuclear inclusions in tubular epithelial cells (A). Positive immunoreactivity for BK virus (B).

surrounding halo. Type 3 inclusions are finely granular and lack a halo. Type 4 inclusions have a markedly enlarged nucleus with clumped, irregular chromatin and prominent nucleoli.

BK-infected cells with targetoid inclusions can be distinguished from CMV by the lack of cytomegaly and absence of cytoplasmic inclusions. The inclusions of adenovirus are more irregularly smudged than the basophilic inclusions of BK virus. BK virus inclusions lack the multinucleation and molding of herpes virus.

Urine cytology is a sensitive method for identifying urinary tract BK virus infection with nearly 100% sensitivity.[337,343] The specificity, however, is low with a <20% positive predictive value for BK nephropathy.[338] The productively infected inclusion-bearing cell in urine cytology is called the "decoy cell" because the nuclear enlargement and hyperchromasia mimics urothelial carcinoma. These degenerated cells, however, are normal or slightly increased in size, have an enlarged, rounded nucleus with a single, large, homogenous inclusion that has a smudgy appearance or a central, coarse and loose, fishnet pattern (Fig. 1-101).

Cytomegalovirus

Clinical Features
Between 20% and 60% of renal transplant recipients may suffer from CMV disease with clinical signs of fever, leukopenia, and organ dysfunction.[344] The CMV infection may be a primary infection, a reactivation infection, or a reinfection. Significant risk factors for primary CMV infection are receipt of a seropositive donor allograft by a seronegative recipient, level of immunosuppression, recipient age, and type of induction therapy.[345,346] Children are at the highest risk for primary infection. In intrauterine CMV infections the kidneys are frequently involved.[347] Management and prevention of CMV infection is a critical component of the care of renal transplant patients.[348,349] Current diagnosis and

monitoring is based on detection of the DNA virus using molecular methods.[350]

Pathology
Direct viral infection of the kidney results in CMV inclusions in glomerular and peritubular endothelial cells as well as in tubular epithelial cells (Fig. 1-102).[347,351] Large intranuclear inclusions with halos and eosinophilic cytoplasmic inclusions are characteristic and associated with cytomegaly. Immunohistochemical staining can increase the rate of detection of CMV in renal biopsy specimens.[352]

Adenovirus

Clinical Features
Adenovirus infection of the kidney occurs almost exclusively in immunocompromised patients, most often following bone marrow transplantation.[353,354] The most common

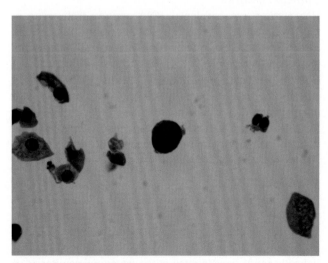

FIGURE 1-101 ■ "Decoy cell." BK virus–infected cell in urine with enlarged rounded nucleus with a smudgy granular nuclear inclusion.

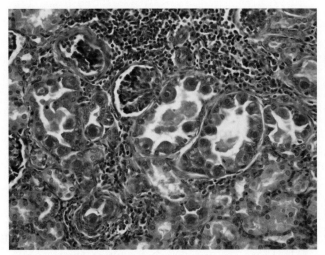

Figure 1-102 ■ Cytomegalovirus. Typical large intranuclear and intracytoplasmic eosinophilic inclusions in renal tubular cells.

serotype identified has been adenovirus type 11. The patients have gross or microscopic hematuria and can develop acute renal failure.

Pathology

The kidneys are enlarged and the cut surface has raised whitish-yellow streaks. Involvement can be unilateral or bilateral. Microscopically there is necrotizing tubulointerstitial nephritis. There is sloughing of tubular epithelial cells into the tubular lumens. The interstitium is edematous with hemorrhage. The degree of inflammatory cell infiltration is dependent on the degree of immunosuppression. Nuclear inclusions are large and basophilic, filling the nucleus. In degenerating cells, the nuclei have a smudged appearance. Inclusions are best demonstrated in the distal tubular epithelium.

Hantavirus

Clinical Features

Hantaviruses are enveloped RNA viruses that occur in rodents. Infection of humans results in two patterns of disease: hemorrhagic fever with renal syndrome and Hantavirus pulmonary syndrome.[355–357] These occur most frequently in China, Korea, and South America. Cases have been described in the southwestern United States. Hemorrhagic fever with renal syndrome is characterized clinically by an influenza-like febrile illness with hemorrhagic manifestations and renal failure. The severity is variable depending on the specific Hantavirus type. Approximately 7% of cases are fatal.

Pathology

Involvement of the kidney manifests as an acute tubulointerstitial nephritis.[335,336,358] There is interstitial edema and hemorrhage with a variable mononuclear infiltrate. The capillaries are dilated and congested. The virus targets endothelial cells and is concentrated in the interstitial capillaries of the medulla. Diagnostic features can be seen in renal biopsy if the sample includes tissue from the medulla.

HYDRONEPHROSIS AND OBSTRUCTIVE NEPHROPATHY

Hydronephrosis is dilatation of the renal pelvis irrespective of the pathogenesis. If the obstruction is below the level of the ureteropelvic junction, it is accompanied by hydroureter above the level of the obstruction. Defects involving the normal peristalsis in the pelvis and ureter can lead to a functional obstruction.[359] The consequence of chronic obstruction on the kidney is known as obstructive nephropathy. Extensive studies of ureteral obstruction in animal models have demonstrated complex mechanisms that lead to the morphologic changes observed.[360] The renal changes are similar irrespective of the etiology. Table 1-10 provides a list of the common causes of obstructive nephropathy by level of obstruction. Numerous genetic mutations have been linked to urinary tract obstruction.[359] In this section, further discussion will be restricted to ureteropelvic junction obstruction.

Ureteropelvic Junction Obstruction

Ureteropelvic junction obstruction occurs in an estimated 1:500 neonates. In this population the most common cause is anomalous vasculature with the renal vessels crossing anterior to the ureter.[361] In patients without crossing vessels the etiology remains uncertain. It is believed that defects in BMP-4 signaling may be important in the pathogenesis of ureteral smooth muscle abnormalities.[4,362] There is also evidence that abnormal function of calcineurin interferes with normal development of the renal pelvis.[363]

Clinical Features

Most patients with significant congenital ureteropelvic junction obstruction are diagnosed in utero by ultrasound. It is more common in boys than in girls and most often affects the left side. Symptoms include hematuria and flank pain. Obstruction is bilateral in up to 30% of cases. With early treatment renal function can be largely preserved. Open pyelotomy is the most commonly used treatment when surgical intervention is required.[364–366]

Pathology

Gross Features. In early lesions, dilatation of the renal pelvis only occurs followed by dilatation of the renal calyces and blunting of the renal papillae. Eventually the kidney becomes a single dilated structure with only a thin rim of surrounding atrophic renal parenchyma. Obstruction is often complicated by episodes of infection and so obstructive nephropathy often shows areas of cortical scarring as well as cortical thinning (Fig. 1-90). The term chronic obstructive pyelonephritis has been used to describe this pattern. With congenital obstruction the kidney shows cystic dysplasia.

Microscopic Features. Pyeloplasty specimens reveal five major histologic findings: normal tissue, chronic inflammation, smooth muscle hypertrophy (with or without

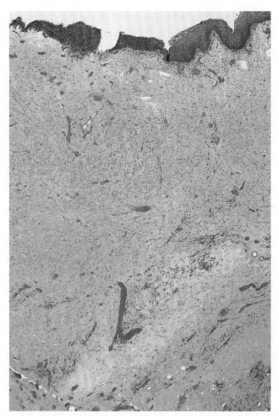

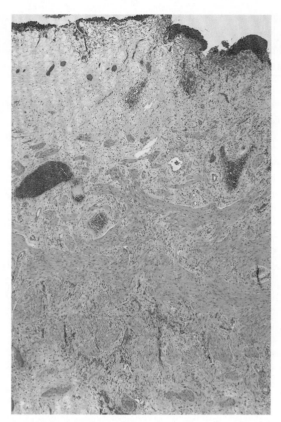

FIGURE 1-103 ■ Ureteropelvic junction obstruction. In this example of congenital ureteropelvic junction obstruction, there is no well-defined muscularis propria. Scattered individual smooth muscle cells are embedded in a fibrous stroma.

FIGURE 1-104 ■ Ureteropelvic junction obstruction. In contrast, in this case of congenital ureteropelvic junction obstruction, there is thickening and disorganization of the muscularis propria.

disorganization), fibrosis, and smooth muscle atrophy (Figs. 1-103 and 1-104).[361,367] Studies of the smooth muscle have demonstrated increased expression of SM1 and SM2 in congenital ureteropelvic junction obstruction.[368] An increased density of Cajal-like cells has also been observed.[369] In patients with crossing blood vessels, the specimens show normal histology significantly more often.[361,367] The pathology of other causes of ureteropelvic junction obstruction listed in Table 1-12 are covered elsewhere and will not be detailed here.

The earliest histologic finding in the kidney is renal tubular dilatation. This is followed by tubular atrophy and tubular basement membrane thickening. Tubular lumens contain hyaline casts. The interstitium becomes fibrotic and glomerulosclerosis begins to develop. Tamm-Horsfall protein can accumulate within the tubular lumens or can be seen within the interstitium. Tamm-Horsfall protein has a glassy pale eosinophilic to basophilic appearance on hematoxylin and eosin sections and stains strongly with PAS. The stroma can demonstrate expression of estrogen and progesterone receptors in these cases.[370] There is almost always chronic inflammation. The glomeruli can appear crowded due to the tubular atrophy and can have small glomerular tufts with dilatation of the urinary space.[169] The picture is complicated by changes related to repeated bouts of pyelonephritis.

Nephrolithiasis

Nephrolithiasis is an extremely common condition with an estimated 7% of women and 13% of men suffering from at least one event in their lives.[371,372] In the United States, kidney stones are most common in Caucasians followed by Hispanics, Asians, and African Americans.[373] They most commonly initially occur in the fourth to sixth decades and are distinctly uncommon before the age of 20.[374] There is geographic variability with the highest incidence in areas with hot, dry, or arid climates. Occupational risk seems to be most related to the degree of heat exposure and dehydration, paralleling the climate effect.

Table 1-12 ■ CAUSES OF URETEROPELVIC JUNCTION OBSTRUCTION
Congenital ureteropelvic junction obstruction
Ureteral valves
Nephrolithiasis
Fibroepithelial polyp
Other tumors
Endometriosis
Recurrent infections
Extrinsic compression
Aberrant blood vessels
Others

Table 1-13 ■ GENETIC DISORDERS ASSOCIATED WITH HYPERCALCIURIA

Disease	Inheritance	Gene
Bartter-like syndrome type 4	AD	CASR
Distal renal tubular acidosis	AD	SLC4A1
Absorptive hypercalciuria	AD	SAC
Antenatal Bartter syndrome type 1	AR	SLC12A1
Antenatal Bartter syndrome type 2	AR	KCNJ1
Bartter syndrome type 3 (classic)	AR	CLCNKB
Familial hypomagnesemia with hypercalciuria and nephrocalcinosis	AR	CLDN16
Distal renal tubular acidosis	AR	ATP6V1B1
Distal renal tubular acidosis	AR	ATPV0A4
Dent disease (X-linked hypophosphatemic rickets)	XL	CLCN5
Lowe syndrome (oculocerebrorenal syndrome)	XL	OCRL

AD, autosomal dominant; AR, autosomal recessive; XL, X-linked.

Nephrolithiasis has a broad range of pathogenic mechanisms.[375] These can be classified in a variety of ways. In this section, we will focus on the major stone types and on the major mechanisms associated with the formation of those stones. Calcium-based stones, either the oxalate or the phosphate type, are by far the most common type of stone in North America accounting for over 70% of cases. This is followed by struvite, uric acid, and cystine stones in descending order.

Calcium-based Stones

Calcium-based stones can be calcium phosphate, calcium oxalate, or a combination of the two. By far the most common etiology of idiopathic nephrolithiasis is idiopathic hypercalciuria.[376] There is often a family history[377,378] however, the genetics of this condition remain poorly understood.[379,380] Hypercalciuria can also be secondary to a specific etiology such as hyperparathyroidism.[381] There are a number of genetic diseases associated with hypercalciuria including mutations of the chloride channel gene, *CLCN5*, located on the short arm of the X chromosome,[382] Dents disease,[383] Bartter syndrome,[384] infantile hypophosphatasia,[385] and renal tubular acidosis (Table 1-13).[379]

A second major factor in the development of calcium stones is hyperoxaluria. Oxalate is not metabolized by humans and must be excreted in the urine. The number of patients with calcium oxalate stones with increased oxalate in the urine has been reported to be between 5% and 50%.[375,386] Hyperoxaluria can be primary or secondary. Primary hyperoxaluria is caused by deficiencies in the enzymes alanine

glyoxylate aminotransferase (type 1) or glyoxylate reductase (type 2). Both are inherited as autosomal recessive conditions with type 1 accounting for 70% to 80% of cases.[387,388] Secondary hyperoxaluria is most often due to hyperabsorption of oxalate in the gastrointestinal tract. This can occur in a wide range of conditions including Crohn disease and celiac sprue.[389] Increased consumption of oxalate-rich or oxalate precursor–rich foods is an important contributing factor. These include chocolate from the cacao tree, spinach, rhubarb, and tea.[375] There is also evidence that calcium oxalate stone formers have decreased *Oxalobacter formigenes* in their intestinal flora.[375,390]

Randall plaques,[391] composed principally of carbapatite, develop primarily in the basement membrane of the descending thin limb of Henle loop. These are found more often in the papillae of stone formers.[392] Their role in the pathogenesis of stone formation remains a debated issue.[375]

Other causes of calcium stones include hypocitraturia, renal tubular acidosis, and hyperuricosuria.

Clinical Features

These stones are more common in men than in women. Diagnosis is usually made at the time of the first episode of renal colic. Many small stones may pass spontaneously without an episode of colic. Larger stones lead to painful episodes when they impact in the excretory system. The most common sites of impact are within a renal calyx, at the ureteropelvic junction, at the pelvic brim, within the posterior pelvis, or at the ureterovesical junction. Congenital anomalies can be associated with other favored locations. Some large stones remain in the renal pelvis and grow there (see "Struvite Stone" discussion below).

The primary hyperoxalurias are responsible for the most severe forms of calcium stone disease although there is remarkable heterogeneity to the clinical manifestations.[388] These patients usually present prior to 10 years of age.

Treatment includes removal of the stones when they become impacted using a variety of methods. More important is identification of the etiology and therapy aimed at prevention of further stone formation. For idiopathic hypercalciuria, the primary treatment is to reduce the saturation of calcium in the urine. The most common approaches are increased fluid intake and in many patients the use of thiazide diuretics.[393,394] Other specific causes of hypercalciuria such as hyperparathyroidism require treatment of the cause of that condition.

Primary hyperoxaluria is an important cause of renal failure in children if not diagnosed early. Renal failure also leads to deposits of oxalate crystals in many other sites including the myocardium. Treatment of primary hyperoxaluria is dependent on the type and on the specific mutation responsible. Initial management is based on maintaining a high daily fluid intake. Many patients with type 1 disease respond to pyridoxine therapy. Alkali citrate treatment is also successful in some. For those not responsive to these approaches, combined liver and renal transplantation is the preferred treatment.[388]

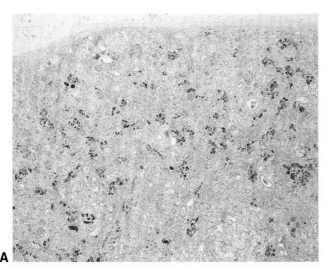
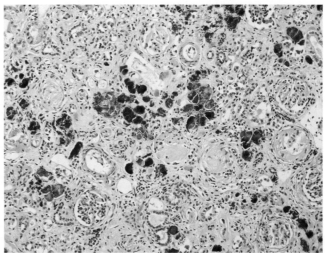

FIGURE 1-105 ■ Hypophosphatasia. In this 2-year-old patient with infantile hypophosphatasia, there is extensive tubular and interstitial calcium deposition (**A** and **B**).

Pathology

For the most part the pathology of nephrolithiasis is not specific to the type of stone but is secondary to the effects of obstruction. Pathologic features of obstructive nephropathy are covered elsewhere in this chapter and will not be further discussed here. With hypercalciuria of any cause, deposits of calcium within the distal tubules, collecting ducts, and interstitium can be seen and is referred to as nephrocalcinosis (Fig. 1-105A and B). The kidney in primary hyperoxaluria, particularly the type 1 form, shows severe nephrocalcinosis with calcium oxalate crystals deposited in the tubular epithelial cell cytoplasm, the tubular lumens, and the interstitium. Deposits of calcium crystals in the interstitium and tubular basement membranes in the papillary tips are referred to as Randall plaques. There is progressive interstitial fibrosis and inflammation.

Struvite (Infection) Stones

Calculi composed of ammonium phosphate (struvite), often in combination with carbonate apatite, are variably referred to as struvite, triple phosphate, or urease stones (Fig. 1-106). Because they characteristically develop in the setting of infection with urease-producing microorganisms (most often *Proteus* species), these are also often referred to as infection stones. Many patients have other conditions associated with stone formation.[395] Once established, these stones grow and branch forming the characteristic "staghorn calculus."[396]

Clinical Features

Struvite stones are more common in patients with a predisposition to upper tract infection such as obstructive nephropathy, vesicoureteral reflux, and neurogenic bladder. Treatment is difficult as the microorganisms are integrated into the stone material making eradication of the infection difficult if not impossible. Percutaneous nephrolithotomy is considered the best option for most patients with staghorn calculi.[396]

Pathology

Struvite stones, in particular staghorn calculi, are associated with a wide range of pathologic changes related to the effects of obstruction and infection. Changes of acute and chronic pyelonephritis are present. A particular pattern of inflammation, xanthogranulomatous pyelonephritis, is considered characteristic of staghorn calculi (Fig. 1-107). This is discussed in detail in the following section.

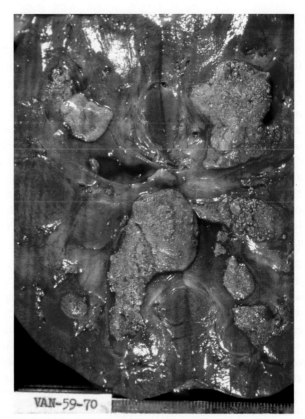

FIGURE 1-106 ■ Struvite stones. Multiple variably sized stones within the renal calyces and renal pelvis.

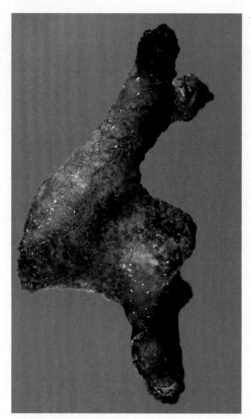

FIGURE 1-107 ■ Struvite stone. Typical staghorn calculus removed from the renal pelvis and calyces.

Uric Acid Stones

Uric acid stones account for about 5% to 10% of stones in North America. There is a higher rate among patients with gout.[375,397] In most patients, the cause is idiopathic. Inborn errors of purine and pyrimidine metabolism account for a small percentage of cases.[398] The combination of a high concentration of uric acid in low-volume urine with a low pH is most conducive to stone formation. In a small percentage of patients, conditions associated with the overproduction of uric acid are primarily responsible. A high percentage of patients with idiopathic uric acid stones have the metabolic syndrome that is associated with increased risk for type 2 diabetes mellitus and atherosclerotic coronary artery disease.[399]

Clinical Features

Gout is a general term for symptomatic disease related to the deposition of uric acid in tissues. In the kidney, this most often manifests as uric acid stones that present with episodic renal colic. An acute form related to a sudden, overwhelming excess of uric acid can lead to diffuse crystal deposition in renal tubules leading to acute renal failure. This is most often seen at the start of chemotherapy in patients with malignant lymphoma or hematopoietic malignancies. Patients with long-standing hyperuricosuria can develop interstitial crystal deposits with associated secondary changes, referred to as gouty nephropathy.

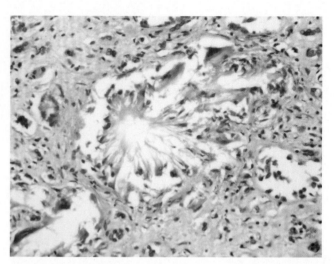

FIGURE 1-108 ■ Uric acid nephropathy. Deposit of uric acid crystals in the renal medulla.

Treatment is aimed at reducing the concentration of uric acid in the urine and inhibiting crystal precipitation. This includes increased fluid intake, alkalinization of the urine, reduced dietary intake, and treatment with allopurinol.

Pathology

In patients with gouty nephropathy, gouty tophi with needle-shaped crystals and an inflammatory reaction that includes foreign body type giant cells can be seen within the kidney interstitium (Fig. 1-108). In acute uric acid nephropathy, there is deposition of uric acid crystals within tubules in the medulla.

Cystine Stones

Cystinuria refers to the excessive secretion of cystine in the urine. This occurs in a variety of inherited conditions that can be autosomal recessive (type 1) or incomplete recessive (types 2 and 3). The defects involve a family of solute carrier genes[398] resulting in hypersecretion of cystine.

Clinical Features

The clinical features are variable depending on the mutation present. In general these patients first develop stones in the second or third decade. Stones range from small calculi to staghorn calculi. Cystine stones are often resistant to extracorporeal shock-wave lithotripsy. Treatment is aimed at reducing the concentration of cystine in the urine by increased fluid intake, reduced sodium in the diet, increasing the alkalinity of the urine, and low-protein diets.[398,400]

Pathology

Cystine crystal deposits can be seen within tubular lumens as well as in the interstitium. The crystals are hexagonal in shape. Long-term renal damage in these patients is not related to severe nephrocalcinosis but more to repeated episodes of urinary tract obstruction and infection.[398]

Other Stones

There are other rare stones that can develop. There is a rare autosomal recessive disorder that results in xanthinuria and the formation of xanthine stones.[398,401] Matrix stones are stones with little or no mineral content formed of mucopolysaccharides and mucosubstances.[402] These develop most often in the setting of infection. There are also selected medications such as ephedrine that in certain circumstances can lead to stone formation.[403]

Nephrocalcinosis

Nephrocalcinosis refers to renal parenchymal calcium deposits and is distinct from nephrolithiasis although the two do frequently coexist. Nephrocalcinosis is best considered a tubulointerstitial disorder characterized by tubular calcifications with associated tubular atrophy and interstitial fibrosis. Any condition leading to hypercalcemia or hypercalciuria can result in nephrocalcinosis. A number of other specific associations have been described including AIDS, primary hyperaldosteronism, cystic fibrosis, and Sjögren syndrome.[404–407] Several drugs have also been associated with the development of nephrocalcinosis.[408]

Clinical Features

The clinical presentation may be dominated by the underlying disease process. Nephrocalcinosis can be diagnosed by radiography, ultrasound, and computed tomography.[409] In many cases nephrocalcinosis is not clinically significant. With more diffuse tubular calcium deposition renal impairment occurs. In young children nephrocalcinosis can be associated with failure to thrive and psychomotor delay.[405] Impaired renal function can be reversed by treatment of the underlying cause.

Pathology

Grossly the calcium deposits may appear as white streaks or small granular deposits. Calcium deposition occurs throughout the nephron. There is deposition in the tubular basement membranes resulting in a purplish tinge most readily appreciated in the proximal tubules. Microconcretions are also found within tubular lumens. These are most prominent and numerous in the collecting ducts. Both small and large calcifications are present within the interstitium (Fig. 1-109). Glomeruli are infrequently involved.[410] The distribution of the calcium deposition is variable, however, and certain patterns are seen in some specific underlying condition. Secondary effects are tubular atrophy and interstitial fibrosis. The latter results in wedge-shaped scars. At later stages of the disease there is glomerulosclerosis and vascular changes occur.

Inflammatory Pseudotumors

Certain inflammatory processes involving the kidney can simulate neoplasms clinically and pathologically. Xanthogranulomatous pyelonephritis can be mistaken for renal cell carcinoma, and inflammatory pseudotumor has been mistaken for renal sarcoma or sarcomatoid carcinoma.

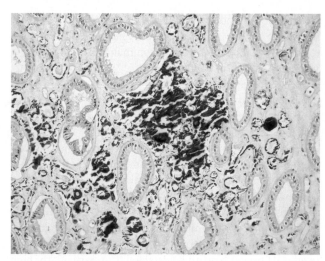

FIGURE 1-109 ■ Nephrocalcinosis. Interstitial calcium deposits in a renal papilla.

Xanthogranulomatous Pyelonephritis

Xanthogranulomatous pyelonephritis is a relatively uncommon inflammatory disease of the kidney.[411–414] However, it is a frequent histologic variant of surgically managed pyelonephritis, corresponding to almost 20% of such cases.[415]

The two most common factors predisposing to the development of xanthogranulomatous pyelonephritis are obstruction and infection. Calculi have been reported as a cause of obstruction in up to 78% of cases[413] and are frequently of the large staghorn type. Less common causes of obstruction include renal pelvic urothelial neoplasms, congenital ureteropelvic junction obstruction, tumors of the ureter and postirradiation stricture. In some cases, no cause for the obstruction is apparent.[413]

Escherichia coli and *Proteus* species are the most commonly implicated organisms. However, many other organisms have been cultured from the urine, including *Klebsiella* species, *Pseudomonas* species, and *Enterococcus faecalis*. The urine is sterile in an appreciable number of cases.[413]

Xanthogranulomatous pyelonephritis probably assumes its appearance because of massive parenchymal necrosis and interference with urinary drainage with resulting accumulation of foam cells. Ultrastructural studies of the lipid-laden macrophages, which are typically PAS-negative or only weakly positive, have demonstrated intracellular bacteria.[416]

Clinical Features

Xanthogranulomatous pyelonephritis may occur at any age. In adults, females are afflicted more often than males (4:1 ratio) and the peak incidence is in the fifth and sixth decades.[415] Appreciable numbers have been recorded in childhood[417,418] and even in infancy.[419] Of the more than 400 cases published by 1996, approximately one-fourth occurred in children.[420]

In general, xanthogranulomatous pyelonephritis is a unilateral disease, and both kidneys are involved with equal frequency[412,413]; occasionally, it is bilateral.[413,421] Usually the whole kidney is involved (the generalized form), but restricted focal forms are not uncommon and are found both in adults[413,422] and in children.[417,420,423,424]

Symptoms are frequently nonspecific and include various combinations of malaise, weight loss, fever, leukocytosis, pyuria, and hematuria. Flank tenderness and an ill-defined, palpable flank mass are common.

Increasingly sensitive radiologic investigations (ultrasonography, four-phase computed tomography, and magnetic resonance imaging) in combination with clinical suspicion have made the preoperative diagnosis of xanthogranulomatous pyelonephritis possible.[418] Renal enlargement, presence of stones or tumors in the renal pelvis, infected areas, and spread of infection to perinephric (stage II) and paranephric (stage III) tissues may all be detected.[418] A particularly high degree of diagnostic precision has been achieved with computed tomography.[425]

Nephrectomy, with or without adjunctive antibiotic therapy, has been the treatment of choice for xanthogranulomatous pyelonephritis and is considered curative. Segmental resection has been shown to be curative in the focal form.[422] There are rare reports of successful treatment of focal xanthogranulomatous pyelonephritis with antibiotics only.

Pathology

Gross Features. The kidney with diffuse xanthogranulomatous pyelonephritis is enlarged and frequently has prominent perirenal fibrosis and adhesions. The dilated pelvis frequently contains a staghorn calculus in addition to necrotic material and pus (Fig. 1-110). Calyces are dilated, papillae are lost, and there may be considerable cortical thinning. Expanded calyces are lined by a yellowish zone that is friable on the inner aspect (Fig. 1-111). The parenchyma contains similar foci of yellowish material, while the rest of it is brownish and firm due to fibrosis and cellular infiltration. In some cases a more discrete mass mimicking a tumor can be seen.

Microscopic Features. The yellow areas correspond to numerous large, finely granular foam cells, which contain lipid (neutral fat and cholesterol ester)[426] (Fig. 1-112). On the inside of the yellow zone, nearest the calyx, there is necrotic debris with many neutrophils. Foci of calcification are not uncommon. In the outer parts of the yellow zone are mononuclear inflammatory cells, plasma cells, eosinophils, and fibroblasts. Multinucleate giant cells may be present (Fig. 1-113). The spindle cell proliferation can be quite exuberant with fascicles of myofibroblasts with reactive nuclear atypia and mitotic activity (Fig. 1-114). The fascicles may be poorly formed or relatively well-defined (Fig. 1-115). Even in relatively pure spindle cell areas, occasional foamy macrophages can usually be identified. The outer cortex shows changes of chronic pyelonephritis with interstitial fibrosis, chronic inflammation, and variable tubular atrophy and/or dilation. Areas of necrosis are common (Fig. 1-116). The inflammatory process extends out into the perinephric soft

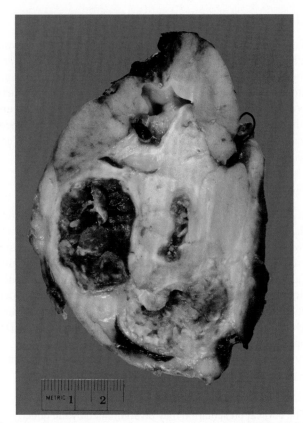

FIGURE 1-110 ■ Xanthogranulomatous pyelonephritis. Multiple and in areas confluent bright yellow plaques within the renal parenchyma, around the renal calyces, and in areas of perinephric fibrosis. Fragments of renal calculi remain in the calyces.

tissues and when combined with a mass-like lesion simulates extension of a tumor beyond the confines of the kidney.

Differential Diagnosis

The focal variant may be grossly mistaken for a tumor. These localized areas of involvement show pathologic features identical to those described for the generalized form and are often related to a stone that has formed either in a single dilated calyx or in the ureter in the case of a duplicated collecting system.[422] The foamy macrophages of xanthogranulomatous pyelonephritis can generally be distinguished from the clear cells of renal cell carcinoma by their lack of nuclear atypia and clear rather than foamy cytoplasm. The associated zonal inflammatory infiltrate and absence of a rich capillary vascular network further support a diagnosis of xanthogranulomatous pyelonephritis. Xanthogranulomatous pyelonephritis is distinguished from malakoplakia by the absence of Michaelis-Gutmann bodies and the more polymorphous nature of the inflammatory infiltrate.

Malakoplakia

Malakoplakia is an unusual inflammatory condition that is well known to urologists, who are familiar with the characteristic small, discrete, yellowish-brown plaques or nodules seen on the bladder mucosa during cystoscopy. Similar nodules

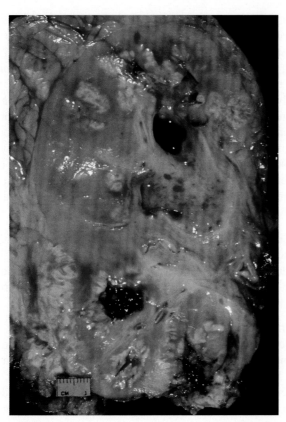

FIGURE 1-111 ■ Xanthogranulomatous pyelonephritis. Multiple variably sized yellow plaques throughout the renal parenchyma and around the renal calyces are present.

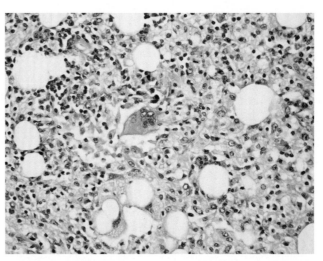

FIGURE 1-113 ■ Xanthogranulomatous pyelonephritis. A multinucleated giant cell with a mixed chronic inflammatory infiltrate in the perinephric fat.

are found less frequently in the ureter and renal pelvis and occasionally in the renal parenchyma, where they are much larger and may extensively involve the entire organ.[427,428]

While it is accepted that malakoplakia is of infective origin, it is not clear why it should take on its unique appearance. The macrophages with PAS-positive granules and the Michaelis-Gutmann bodies have been studied extensively

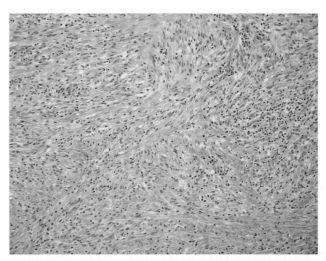

FIGURE 1-114 ■ Xanthogranulomatous pyelonephritis. An area of spindle cell proliferation with the formation of fascicles. Note the chronic inflammatory infiltrate in the background.

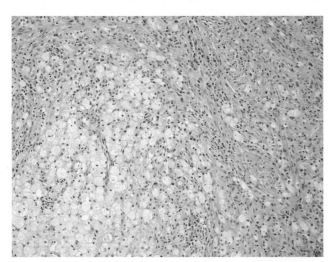

FIGURE 1-112 ■ Xanthogranulomatous pyelonephritis. A polymorphous inflammatory infiltrate that in this area includes large numbers of foamy histiocytes.

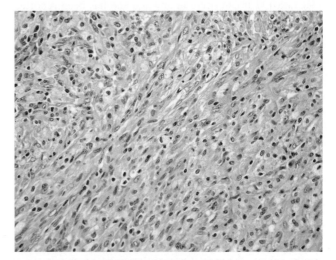

FIGURE 1-115 ■ Xanthogranulomatous pyelonephritis. A less well-defined area of spindle cell proliferation; note the presence of a few foamy histiocytes.

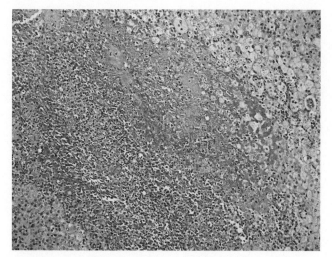

FIGURE 1-116 ■ Xanthogranulomatous pyelonephritis. An area of necrosis with surrounding foamy histiocytes.

with the electron microscope both in renal and in nonrenal cases with more or less consistent findings.[429–431] The PAS-positive granules in the macrophages correspond to phagolysosomes, which contain complex membranous whorls related to degraded bacteria. It is believed that the Michaelis-Gutmann body is formed by aggregation of crystals upon a nidus of bacterial breakdown products contained in phagolysosomes.

The frequent association of malakoplakia with various abnormalities of the immune system or with the administration of immunosuppressive agents[432] has led to the idea that there are deficiencies in the ability of leukocytes to dispose of bacteria.[433] McClure[434] concluded, however, that while a small number of patients with extensive malakoplakia may have defective monocyte bacterial function, most patients with the localized form do not.

Clinical Features

Renal malakoplakia affects females more often than males (3:1 ratio).[435] It can occur at any age and has been reported in an 8-week-old infant.[435,436] The mean age for women is 45 years, and the peak incidence for men is in the sixth decade.[435] Malakoplakia often affects both kidneys, and it has assumed a bilateral form in 33%[435] to 50% of cases.[437]

Symptoms of renal malakoplakia are generally related to urinary tract infection and include flank pain, fever and rigors; signs of perinephric abscess may be noted. Because bilateral involvement is not uncommon, renal failure may be present in a significant number of cases.[435,438,439] It is a rare cause of acute renal failure.[440] Cases presenting as an isolated renal mass are described.[441] Culture of the urine reveals *E. coli* in most cases.

Renal malakoplakia has been associated with a substantial mortality rate (70%) and poor recovery of renal function.[440] However, early diagnosis by renal biopsy, with prompt and prolonged use of appropriate antibiotics, significantly reduces the mortality rate. It can be accurately diagnosed by either open or needle biopsy.[435]

Pathology

Gross Features. The kidney may show the effects of obstruction caused by foci of ureteric malakoplakia, including pelvicalyceal dilation with pus in the pelvis and thinning of the renal parenchyma. Calculi are seldom noted in the pelvis and calyces. Perinephric abscess is not uncommon.[435] Parenchymal involvement consists of yellowish or tan nodules of variable size, which may remain discrete, coalesce to involve much of the kidney, or undergo suppuration with abscess formation. A mass lesion simulating a tumor can occur.[428] The diffuse variant of malakoplakia is much more common than the focal form. Yellow areas lining a dilated calyx are sometimes present.

Microscopic Features. The lesions of renal and urinary bladder malakoplakia are identical (see Chapter 5). In the kidney, the component structures of the kidney, particularly the tubules, are severely damaged, and changes of obstructive atrophy may be present.

Differential Diagnosis

The renal parenchymal changes of malakoplakia are accompanied by an interstitial collagenous reaction, which may be fine or coarse with a superficial resemblance to a connective tissue neoplasm. Unless Michaelis-Gutmann bodies are diligently sought, the diagnosis of malakoplakia may be overlooked.

Malakoplakia shares overlapping gross and microscopic features with xanthogranulomatous pyelonephritis.[429,430] It has been speculated that the formation of the Michaelis-Gutmann body is related to the rate of which a nidus is cleared from a focus of infection and that malakoplakia might simply represent a xanthogranulomatous reaction in which bacterial degradation is abnormal.

Megalocytic interstitial nephritis is a rare condition with many of the features of malakoplakia.[429] It may involve the kidney diffusely, with multiple grayish foci of various sizes[442] or appear as a solitary cortical nodule[443] resembling a tumor. Microscopically, there are large numbers of polygonal cells with coarsely granular eosinophilic cytoplasm. The granules are strongly PAS-positive. The absence of Michaelis-Gutmann bodies in megalocytic interstitial nephritis has been emphasized by some authors, who regard it as a prediagnostic phase of malakoplakia.[430]

Sarcoidosis

Clinical Features

Sarcoidosis is a systemic disease that can involve the kidneys. Most often renal involvement results in granulomatous tubulointerstitial nephritis. It has been estimated that approximately 1.5% of patients with sarcoidosis have renal involvement.[280] In rare cases the involvement results in formation of a mass lesion that mimics a renal tumor.[280,444] Patients present with acute renal failure with proteinuria and/or microscopic hematuria. Most patients respond to therapy with only a small percentage going on to the end-stage renal disease.

Pathology

In most cases there is a granulomatous interstitial nephritis. The granulomas are well-formed and noncaseating (Fig. 1-94). In one series, renal biopsies did not show granulomas in 10 of 47 cases. There is associated acute and chronic inflammation with tubular atrophy and interstitial fibrosis. Interstitial calcifications are present in 15% of cases.

Amyloidosis

Clinical Features

The kidney is one of the most important involved organs in patients with systemic amyloidosis.[445] In general renal amyloidosis is considered one of the medical diseases of the kidney and it is beyond the scope of this chapter to cover the topic. Amyloid deposition results in enlarged kidneys in a minority of patients. There are cases of amyloid deposition that result in the formation of mass lesions that raise the possibility of a tumor (so-called amyloidoma). These occur most often in the brain and soft tissue but have been described in many other locations.[446,447] These can form with or without systemic amyloidosis.

Pathology

The kidney in amyloidosis can be enlarged with a pale waxy appearance to the cut surface. Amyloid deposition occurs throughout the kidney with the glomerular mesangium being most prominent followed by the interstitium and the renal vasculature. Amyloidomas are formed by large deposits of amyloid having the typical histologic and ultrastructural features of amyloid.[448]

Inflammatory Myofibroblastic Tumor

Inflammatory myofibroblastic tumor (IMT), also termed plasma cell granuloma, inflammatory pseudotumor, and pseudosarcomatous fibromyxoid tumor, has been identified at multiple extrapulmonary sites.[449,450] In the genitourinary tract, the urinary bladder is the most common site of occurrence.[451,452] There have been <50 reported cases of IMT of the kidney, renal pelvis, and ureter.[453–460]

Etiopathogenesis

The pathogenesis of IMT remains uncertain. Clonal abnormalities have recently been identified, supporting the neoplastic nature of the myofibroblastic proliferation in many IMTs. Studies have demonstrated clonal abnormalities of the short arm of chromosome 2 in the region of p21-p23, the site of the anaplastic lymphoma kinase (ALK) gene that codes for tyrosine kinase inhibitor.[461,462] ALK abnormalities have been reported in 37% to 60% cases studies by immunohistochemistry and fluorescence in situ hybridization. It has been observed that ALK-negative cases tend to occur in older patients and ALK-positive cases in younger patients (children and young adults).[462,463] In a study of IMT of the urinary bladder, this age-associated occurrence of ALK-rearrangement positive tumors was not observed; however, a statistically significant gender predilection for

ALK-rearrangement-positive IMT in females versus ALK-rearrangement-negative tumors in males was identified.[464]

Clinical Features

Mean age of patients at presentation is the fifth to sixth decade (range 3 to 76 years). Childhood cases are distinctly uncommon.[455,456] There is a slight male predilection (1.5:1). The majority of tumors are discovered incidentally.[458] Less commonly, patients present with flank pain, painless gross hematuria, or ureteropelvic junction stenosis with hydronephrosis. Examples of bilateral renal infiltration with diffuse enlargement and asymptomatic renal failure have been reported.[459,465] Tumors are principally related to the renal parenchyma (56%) but also occur in the renal pelvis and adjacent soft tissue (38%) and immediate perirenal soft tissue (6%).[457]

Clinically, IMT mimics malignancy, and surgical excision remains the cornerstone of management. These tumors, however, generally behave in an indolent manner. Local recurrence and malignant transformation have been reported in a small subset of patients, particularly in those cases in which complete surgical excision was not possible.[449,450] No recurrences or metastases have been reported in IMTs arising in the urinary bladder[449,466] or kidney.[458] Resolution of the lesion with steroid therapy has been reported.[465]

Pathology

Gross Features. IMTs are nonencapsulated and completely or partially circumscribed, and can measure up to 14 cm in maximum dimension. Tumors consist primarily of firm white-tan tissue with no evidence of hemorrhage or necrosis (Fig. 1-117), or they have a myxoid "gelatinous" appearance with areas of hemorrhage (Fig. 1-118). Cystic change can be present.[467]

Microscopic Features. Three histologic patterns can be identified, with one pattern predominating in the majority of tumors: (i) loosely organized spindle cells admixed with small blood vessels and inflammatory cells, in a myxoid background (Fig. 1-119), (ii) spindle cell proliferation admixed with variable amounts of dense collagen, lymphoid aggregates often forming follicles, and plasma cells (Fig. 1-120), and (iii) hypocellular fibrous tissue with dense "keloid-like" fibrosis and sparse inflammatory cells (Fig. 1-121).

The spindle cell proliferation typically consists of relatively uniform cells with no nuclear atypia and rare mitoses (Fig. 1-122). A predominance of foamy histiocytes (plasma cell granuloma) and focal osseous metaplasia can occur. Rarely, there is prominent nuclear atypia with round cell change and/or ganglion-like cells with atypical nuclei.

Immunohistochemical Features. There is strong diffuse immunoreactivity for vimentin (Fig. 1-123A); smooth muscle actin and muscle-specific actin (HHF-35) are positive in the majority of cases (focal to diffuse) (Fig. 1-123B). A renal pelvic IMT occurring in a 3-year-old girl was positive for ALK-1.[455] However, in the renal IMTs reported by Kapusta et al., ALK-1 was negative in all cases tested (Fig. 1-123C), as were desmin, CD34, and pancytokeratins[458] (Fig. 1-123D). In contrast, cytokeratin expression is frequently identified in

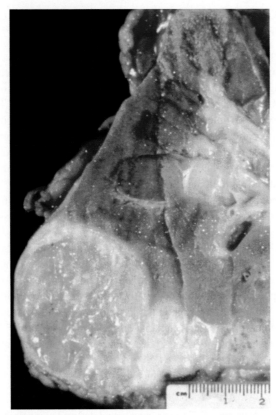

FIGURE 1-117 ■ Inflammatory myofibroblastic tumor. The tumor is well-circumscribed with an apparent fibrous capsule.

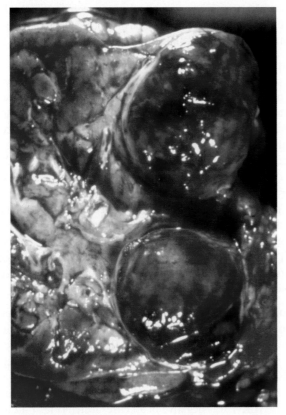

FIGURE 1-118 ■ Inflammatory myofibroblastic tumor. The mass is well-circumscribed and has a thin capsule and a glistening, gelatinous cut surface.

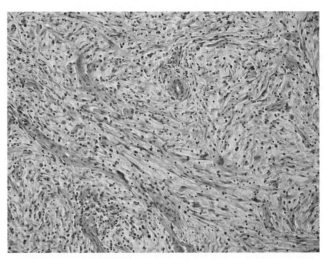

FIGURE 1-119 ■ Inflammatory myofibroblastic tumor. A myxoid pattern with elongated spindle-shaped cells and an inflammatory infiltrate in the background.

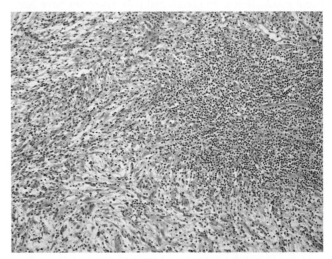

FIGURE 1-120 ■ Inflammatory myofibroblastic tumor. A myxoid lesion with an abundant chronic inflammatory infiltrate that includes large numbers of plasma cells.

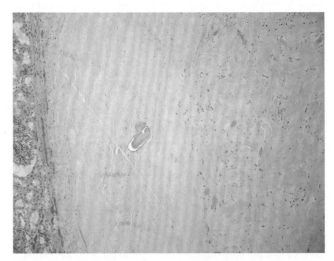

FIGURE 1-121 ■ Inflammatory myofibroblastic tumor. A case with a hypocellular keloid-like pattern containing a few scattered inflammatory cells; note the entrapped atrophic tubule.

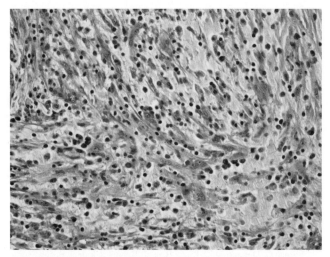

FIGURE 1-122 ■ Inflammatory myofibroblastic tumor. The spindle-shaped cells have abundant eosinophilic cytoplasm and large, uniform fusiform nuclei. There is no significant cytologic atypia.

bladder IMTs, with over 60% of tumors staining for cytokeratin AE1/AE3.[451,461,468] The spindle cells show myofibroblastic differentiation by ultrastructural examination.

Differential Diagnosis

Both leiomyosarcoma and sarcomatoid renal cell carcinoma can generally be distinguished from IMT by their infiltrative growth pattern, overt cellular pleomorphism, and high mitotic rate. Nonetheless, misdiagnosis can occur.[469] Immunohistochemistry can assist in the differential diagnosis with myxoid leiomyosarcoma expressing muscle markers including desmin and only weakly or not expressing cytokeratins. Solitary fibrous tumor, which can involve the renal capsule[470] or be intrarenal,[471] has histologic features similar to IMT. Immunohistochemistry is critical to making the correct diagnosis: solitary fibrous tumor is strongly and diffusely CD34 positive with heterogeneous staining for bcl-2 and CD99; smooth muscle actin, desmin, and keratin (AE1/AE3 and CAM 5.2) are negative.

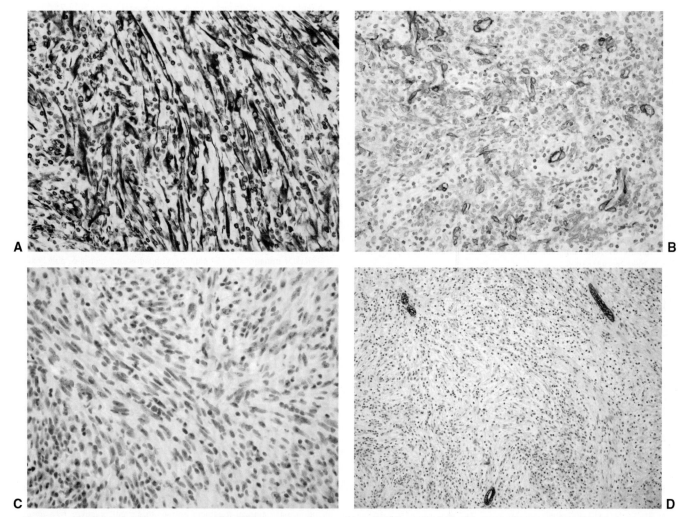

FIGURE 1-123 ■ Inflammatory myofibroblastic tumor. Immunohistochemistry results in this example revealed positive immunoreactivity for vimentin **(A)** and muscle-specific actin **(B)** with an absence of immunoreactivity for ALK **(C)** and pancytokeratin (AE1/AE3, **D**).

REFERENCES

1. Potter E. *Normal and Abnormal Development of the Kidney*. Chicago, IL: Year Book Medical Publishers; 1972.
2. Moore K, Persaud T. *The Developing Human: Clinically Oriented Embryology*. Philadelphia, PA: WB Saunders; 2003.
3. Woolf A, Jenkins D. Development of the kidney. In: Jennette J, Olson J, Schwartz M, et al., eds. *Heptinstall's Pathology of the Kidney*. 6th ed. Philadelphia, PA: Lippincott Williams & Wilkins; 2007:71.
4. Shapiro E. Clinical implications of genitourinary embryology. *Curr Opin Urol* 2009;19:427–433.
5. Bonsib S. Renal anatomy and histology. In: Jennette J, Olson J, DSchwartz M, et al., eds. *Heptinstall's Pathology of the Kidney*. 6th ed. Philadelphia, PA: Lippincott Williams & Wilkins; 2007:1.
6. Clapp W, Croker B. Kidney. In: Mills S, ed. *Histology for Pathologists*. 3rd ed. Philadelphia, PA: Lippincott Williams & Wilkins; 2007:839–907.
7. Kasiske BL, Umen AJ. The influence of age, sex, race, and body habitus on kidney weight in humans. *Arch Pathol Lab Med* 1986;110:55–60.
8. Bonsib SM, Gibson D, Mhoon M, et al. Renal sinus involvement in renal cell carcinomas. *Am J Surg Pathol* 2000;24:451–458.
9. Bonsib SM. The renal sinus is the principal invasive pathway: a prospective study of 100 renal cell carcinomas. *Am J Surg Pathol* 2004;28:1594–1600.
10. Hodson CJ. The renal parenchyma and its blood supply. *Curr Probl Diagn Radiol* 1978;7:1–32.
11. Clark RL, Cuttino JT Jr. Microradiographic studies of renal lymphatics. *Radiology* 1977;124:307–311.
12. Hao CM, Breyer MD. Physiologic and pathophysiologic roles of lipid mediators in the kidney. *Kidney Int* 2007;71:1105–1115.
13. Pope JC IV, Brock JW III, Adams MC, et al. How they begin and how they end: classic and new theories for the development and deterioration of congenital anomalies of the kidney and urinary tract, CAKUT. *J Am Soc Nephrol* 1999;10:2018–2028.
14. Sanna-Cherchi S, Caridi G, Weng PL, et al. Genetic approaches to human renal agenesis/hypoplasia and dysplasia. *Pediatr Nephrol* 2007;22:1675–1684.
15. Schulman J, Edmonds LD, McClearn AB, et al. Surveillance for and comparison of birth defect prevalences in two geographic areas—United States, 1983-88. *MMWR Morb Mortal Wkly Rep CDC Surveill Summ* 1993;42:1–7.
16. Neild GH. What do we know about chronic renal failure in young adults? I. Primary renal disease. *Pediatr Nephrol* 2009;24:1913–1919.
17. Neild GH. What do we know about chronic renal failure in young adults? II. Adult outcome of pediatric renal disease. *Pediatr Nephrol* 2009;24:1921–1928.
18. Emanuel B, Nachman R, Aronson N, et al. Congenital solitary kidney: a review of 74 cases. *J Urol* 1974;111:394–397.
19. Parikh CR, McCall D, Engelman C, et al. Congenital renal agenesis: case-control analysis of birth characteristics. *Am J Kidney Dis* 2002;39:689–694.
20. Kerecuk L, Schreuder MF, Woolf AS. Renal tract malformations: perspectives for nephrologists. *Nat Clin Pract Nephrol* 2008;4:312–325.
21. Pereira BJ, Sousa L, Azinhais P, et al. Zinner's syndrome: an up-to-date review of the literature based on a clinical case. *Andrologia* 2009;41:322–330.
22. Singer A, Simmons MZ, Maldjian PD. Spectrum of congenital renal anomalies presenting in adulthood. *Clin Imaging* 2008;32:183–191.
23. Calisti A, Perrotta ML, Oriolo L, et al. The risk of associated urological abnormalities in children with pre and postnatal occasional diagnosis of solitary, small or ectopic kidney: is a complete urological screening always necessary? *World J Urol* 2008;26:281–284.
24. Bernstein J. Developmental abnormalities of the renal parenchyma—hypoplasia and dysplasia. *Pathol Annu* 1968;3:213.
25. Foster SV, Hawkins EP. Deficient metanephric blastema—a cause of oligomeganephronia? *Pediatr Pathol* 1994;14:935–943.
26. Bernstein J, Gilbert-Barness E. Congenital malformations of the kidney. In: Tosher C, Brenner B, eds. *Renal Pathology with Clinical and Functional Correlations*. 2nd ed. Philadelphia, PA: Lippincott-Raven; 1994:1355–1386.
27. Smith SJ, Cass AS, Aliabadi H, et al. Unipapillary kidney: a case report and literature review. *Urol Radiol* 1984;6:43–47.
28. Salomon R, Tellier AL, Attie-Bitach T, et al. PAX2 mutations in oligomeganephronia. *Kidney Int* 2001;59:457–462.
29. Boatman DL, Kolln CP, Flocks RH. Congenital anomalies associated with horseshoe kidney. *J Urol* 1972;107:205–207.
30. Glodny B, Petersen J, Hofmann KJ, et al. Kidney fusion anomalies revisited: clinical and radiological analysis of 209 cases of crossed fused ectopia and horseshoe kidney. *BJU Int* 2009;103:224–235.
31. Viola D, Anagnostou T, Thompson TJ, et al. Sixteen years of experience with stone management in horseshoe kidneys. *Urol Int* 2007;78:214–218.
32. Fazio L, Razvi H, Chin JL. Malignancy in horseshoe kidneys: review and discussion of surgical implications. *Can J Urol* 2003;10:1899–1904.
33. Stimac G, Dimanovski J, Ruzic B, et al. Tumors in kidney fusion anomalies—report of five cases and review of the literature. *Scand J Urol Nephrol* 2004;38:485–489.
34. Hansel DE, Epstein JI, Berbescu E, et al. Renal carcinoid tumor: a clinicopathologic study of 21 cases. *Am J Surg Pathol* 2007;31:1539–1544.
35. Anand A, Seth A, Singh MK, et al. Neuroendocrine tumor in horseshoe kidney. *Indian J Pathol Microbiol* 2010;53:195–197.
36. Imbriaco M, Iodice D, Erra P, et al. Squamous cell carcinoma within a horseshoe kidney with associated renal stones detected by computed tomography and magnetic resonance imaging. *Urology* 2011;78:54–55.
37. Deltas C, Papagregoriou G. Cystic diseases of the kidney: molecular biology and genetics. *Arch Pathol Lab Med* 2010;134:569–582.
38. Cole BR, Conley SB, Stapleton FB. Polycystic kidney disease in the first year of life. *J Pediatr* 1987;111:693–699.
39. Cole B. Autosomal recessive polycystic kidney disease. In: Gardner KJ, Bernstein J, eds. *The Cystic Kidney*. Boston, MA: Kluwer Academic Publishers; 1990:327–350.
40. Mucher G, Becker J, Knapp M, et al. Fine mapping of the autosomal recessive polycystic kidney disease locus (PKHD1) and the genes MUT, RDS, CSNK2 beta, and GSTA1 at 6p21.1-p12. *Genomics* 1998;48:40–45.
41. Al-Bhalal L, Akhtar M. Molecular basis of autosomal recessive polycystic kidney disease (ARPKD). *Adv Anat Pathol* 2008;15:54–58.
42. Wang S, Luo Y, Wilson PD, et al. The autosomal recessive polycystic kidney disease protein is localized to primary cilia, with concentration in the basal body area. *J Am Soc Nephrol* 2004;15:592–602.
43. Blyth H, Ockenden BG. Polycystic disease of kidney and liver presenting in childhood. *J Med Genet* 1971;8:257–284.
44. Bergmann C, Senderek J, Windelen E, et al. Clinical consequences of PKHD1 mutations in 164 patients with autosomal-recessive polycystic kidney disease (ARPKD). *Kidney Int* 2005;67:829–848.
45. Kaariainen H, Koskimies O, Norio R. Dominant and recessive polycystic kidney disease in children: evaluation of clinical features and laboratory data. *Pediatr Nephrol* 1988;2:296–302.
46. Lieberman E, Salinas-Madrigal L, Gwinn JL, et al. Infantile polycystic disease of the kidneys and liver: clinical, pathological and radiological correlations and comparison with congenital hepatic fibrosis. *Medicine* 1971;50:277–318.
47. Alvarez F, Bernard O, Brunelle F, et al. Congenital hepatic fibrosis in children. *J Pediatr* 1981;99:370–375.
48. Guay-Woodford LM, Desmond RA. Autosomal recessive polycystic kidney disease: the clinical experience in North America. *Pediatrics* 2003;111:1072–1080.
49. Iglesias CG, Torres VE, Offord KP, et al. Epidemiology of adult polycystic kidney disease, Olmsted County, Minnesota: 1935–1980. *Am J Kidney Dis* 1983;2:630–639.
50. Badani KK, Hemal AK, Menon M. Autosomal dominant polycystic kidney disease and pain—a review of the disease from aetiology, evaluation, past surgical treatment options to current practice. *J Postgrad Med* 2004;50:222–226.

51. Kimberling WJ, Pieke-Dahl SA, Kumar S. The genetics of cystic diseases of the kidney. *Semin Nephrol* 1991;11:596–606.

52. Bisceglia M, Galliani CA, Senger C, et al. Renal cystic diseases: a review. *Adv Anat Pathol* 2006;13:26–56.

53. Bisceglia M, Galliani C, Carosi I, et al. Tuberous sclerosis complex with polycystic kidney disease of the adult type: the TSC2/ADPKD1 contiguous gene syndrome. *Int J Surg Pathol* 2008;16:375–385.

54. Dalgaard O. Bilateral polycystic disease of the kidney: a follow up of two hundred eighty four patients and their families. *Dan Med Bull* 1957;4:128–133.

55. Alam A, Perrone RD. Management of ESRD in patients with autosomal dominant polycystic kidney disease. *Adv Chronic Kidney Dis* 2010;17:164–172.

56. Churchill DN, Bear JC, Morgan J, et al. Prognosis of adult onset polycystic kidney disease re-evaluated. *Kidney Int* 1984;26:190–193.

57. Vester U, Kranz B, Hoyer PF. The diagnostic value of ultrasound in cystic kidney diseases. *Pediatr Nephrol* 2010;25:231–240.

58. Levey AS, Pauker SG, Kassirer JP. Occult intracranial aneurysms in polycystic kidney disease. When is cerebral arteriography indicated? *N Engl J Med* 1983;308:986–994.

59. Leier CV, Baker PB, Kilman JW, et al. Cardiovascular abnormalities associated with adult polycystic kidney disease. *Ann Intern Med* 1984;100:683–688.

60. Grunfeld JP, Albouze G, Jungers P, et al. Liver changes and complications in adult polycystic kidney disease. *Adv Nephrol Necker Hosp* 1985;14:1–20.

61. Cobben JM, Breuning MH, Schoots C, et al. Congenital hepatic fibrosis in autosomal-dominant polycystic kidney disease. *Kidney Int* 1990;38:880–885.

62. Pirson Y. Extrarenal manifestations of autosomal dominant polycystic kidney disease. *Adv Chronic Kidney Dis* 2010;17:173–180.

63. Grantham JJ, Mulamalla S, Swenson-Fields KI. Why kidneys fail in autosomal dominant polycystic kidney disease. *Nat Rev Nephrol* 2011;7:556–566.

64. Kirkman MA, van Dellen D, Mehra S, et al. Native nephrectomy for autosomal dominant polycystic kidney disease: before or after kidney transplantation? *BJU Int* 2011;108:590–594.

65. Umbreit EC, Childs MA, Patterson DE, et al. Percutaneous nephrolithotomy for large or multiple upper tract calculi and autosomal dominant polycystic kidney disease. *J Urol* 2010;183:183–187.

66. Mufti UB, Nalagatla SK. Nephrolithiasis in autosomal dominant polycystic kidney disease. *J Endourol* 2010;24:1557–1561.

67. Harris PC, Torres VE. Polycystic kidney disease. *Annu Rev Med* 2009; 60:321–337.

68. Torres V, Holley K, Offord K. General features of autosomal dominant kidney disease A: epidemiology. In: Grantham J, Gardner K, eds. *Problems in Diagnosis and Management of Polycystic Kidney Disease: Proceedings of the First International Workshop on Polycystic Kidney Disease.* Kansas City, MO: PKR Foundation; 1985:49–69.

69. Nishimura H, Ubara Y, Nakamura M, et al. Renal cell carcinoma in autosomal dominant polycystic kidney disease. *Am J Kidney Dis* 2009; 54:165–168.

70. Ng RC, Suki WN. Renal cell carcinoma occurring in a polycystic kidney of a transplant recipient. *J Urol* 1980;124:710–712.

71. Gregoire JR, Torres VE, Holley KE, et al. Renal epithelial hyperplastic and neoplastic proliferation in autosomal dominant polycystic kidney disease. *Am J Kidney Dis* 1987;9:27–38.

72. Franz KA, Reubi FC. Rate of functional deterioration in polycystic kidney disease. *Kidney Int* 1983;23:526–529.

73. Strauss MB. Clinical and pathological aspects of cystic disease of the renal medulla. An analysis of eighteen cases. *Ann Intern Med* 1962;57:373–381.

74. Hildebrandt F, Omram H. New insights: nephronophthisis-medullary cystic kidney disease. *Pediatr Nephrol* 2001;16:168–176.

75. Salomon R, Saunier S, Niaudet P. Nephronophthisis. *Pediatr Nephrol* 2009;24:2333–2344.

76. Tory K, Rousset-Rouviere C, Gubler M-C, et al. Mutations of NPHP2 and NPHP3 in infantile nephronophthisis. *Kidney Int* 2009;75:839–847.

77. Simms RJ, Hynes AM, Eley L, et al. Nephronophthisis: a genetically diverse ciliopathy. *Int J Nephrol* 2011;2011:527137.

78. Hildebrandt F, Otto E. Molecular genetics of nephronophthisis and medullary cystic kidney disease. *J Am Soc Nephrol* 2000;11:1753–1761.

79. Hildebrandt F, Otto E, Rensing C, et al. A novel gene encoding an SH3 domain protein is mutated in nephronophthisis type 1. *Nat Genet* 1997;17:149–153.

80. Hildebrandt F, Attanasio M, Otto E. Nephronophthisis: disease mechanisms of a ciliopathy. *J Am Soc Nephrol* 2009;20:23–35.

81. Fliegauf M, Benzing T, Omran H. When cilia go bad: cilia defects and ciliopathies. *Nat Rev Mol Cell Biol* 2007;8:880–893.

82. Gretz N, Scharer K, Waldherr R, et al. Rate of deterioration of renal function in juvenile nephronophthisis. *Pediatr Nephrol* 1989;3:56–60.

83. Hamiwka LA, Midgley JP, Wade AW, et al. Outcomes of kidney transplantation in children with nephronophthisis: an analysis of the North American Pediatric Renal Trials and Collaborative Studies (NAPRTCS) registry. *Pediatr Transplant* 2008;12:878–882.

84. Welling L, Grantham J. Cystic and development diseases of the kidney. In: Brenner B, Rector FJ, eds. *The Kidney.* 3rd ed. Philadelphia, PA: WB Saunders; 1986:1341–1376.

85. Zollinger HU, Mihatsch MJ, Edefonti A, et al. Nephronophthisis (medullary cystic disease of the kidney). A study using electron microscopy, immunofluorescence, and a review of the morphological findings. *Helv Paediatr Acta* 1980;35:509–530.

86. Sherman FE, Studnicki FM, Fetterman G. Renal lesions of familial juvenile nephronophthisis examined by microdissection. *Am J Clin Pathol* 1971;55:391–400.

87. Pascal RR. Medullary cystic disease of the kidney: study of a case with scanning and transmission electron microscopy and light microscopy. *Am J Clin Pathol* 1973;59:659–665.

88. Wolf MTF, Mucha BE, Hennies HC, et al. Medullary cystic kidney disease type 1: mutational analysis in 37 genes based on haplotype sharing. *Hum Genet* 2006;119:649–658.

89. Scolari F, Puzzer D, Amoroso A, et al. Identification of a new locus for medullary cystic disease, on chromosome 16p12. *Am J Hum Genet* 1999;64:1655–1660.

90. Bollee G, Dahan K, Flamant M, et al. Phenotype and outcome in hereditary tubulointerstitial nephritis secondary to UMOD mutations. *Clin J Am Soc Nephrol* 2011;6:2429–2438.

91. Hodanova K, Majewski J, Kublova M, et al. Mapping of a new candidate locus for uromodulin-associated kidney disease (UAKD) to chromosome 1q41. *Kidney Int* 2005;68:1472–1482.

92. Stavrou C, Koptides M, Tombazos C, et al. Autosomal-dominant medullary cystic kidney disease type 1: clinical and molecular findings in six large Cypriot families. [Erratum appears in *Kidney Int* 2002;62:1920]. *Kidney Int* 2002;62:1385–1394.

93. Kiser RL, Wolf MTF, Martin JL, et al. Medullary cystic kidney disease type 1 in a large Native-American kindred. *Am J Kidney Dis* 2004; 44:611–617.

94. Bleyer AJ, Hart TC, Willingham MC, et al. Clinico-pathologic findings in medullary cystic kidney disease type 2. *Pediatr Nephrol* 2005; 20:824–827.

95. Latif F, Tory K, Gnarra J, et al. Identification of the von Hippel-Lindau disease tumor suppressor gene. *Science* 1993;260:1317–1320.

96. Maher ER, Neumann HP, Richard S. von Hippel-Lindau disease: a clinical and scientific review. *Eur J Hum Genet* 2011;19:617–623.

97. Chauveau D, Duvic C, Chretien Y, et al. Renal involvement in von Hippel-Lindau disease. *Kidney Int* 1996;50:944–951.

98. Gallou C, Chauveau D, Richard S, et al. Genotype-phenotype correlation in von Hippel-Lindau families with renal lesions. [Erratum appears in *Hum Mutat* 2004;24:435–436]. *Hum Mutat* 2004;24:215–224.

99. Nielsen SM, Rubinstein WS, Thull DL, et al. Genotype-phenotype correlations of pheochromocytoma in two large von Hippel-Lindau (VHL) type 2A kindreds with different missense mutations. *Am J Med Genet A* 2011;155A:168–173.

100. Solomon D, Schwartz A. Renal pathology in von Hippel-Lindau disease. *Hum Pathol* 1988;19:1072–1079.

101. Bell D, Gidley P, Levine N, et al. Endolymphatic sac tumor (aggressive papillary tumor of middle ear and temporal bone): sine qua non radiology-pathology and the University of Texas MD Anderson Cancer Center experience. *Ann Diagn Pathol* 2011;15:117–123.

102. Poston CD, Jaffe GS, Lubensky IA, et al. Characterization of the renal pathology of a familial form of renal cell carcinoma associated with von Hippel-Lindau disease: clinical and molecular genetic implications. *J Urol* 1995;153:22–26.

103. Meister M, Choyke P, Anderson C, et al. Radiological evaluation, management, and surveillance of renal masses in von Hippel-Lindau disease. *Clin Radiol* 2009;64:589–600.

104. Loughlin KR, Gittes RF. Urological management of patients with von Hippel-Lindau's disease. *J Urol* 1986;136:789–791.

105. Paraf F, Chauveau D, Chretien Y, et al. Renal lesions in von Hippel-Lindau disease: immunohistochemical expression of nephron differentiation molecules, adhesion molecules and apoptosis proteins. *Histopathology* 2000;36:457–465.

106. Christenson PJ, Craig JP, Bibro MC, et al. Cysts containing renal cell carcinoma in von Hippel-Lindau disease. *J Urol* 1982;128:798–800.

107. Walther MM, Lubensky IA, Venzon D, et al. Prevalence of microscopic lesions in grossly normal renal parenchyma from patients with von Hippel-Lindau disease, sporadic renal cell carcinoma and no renal disease: clinical implications. *J Urol* 1995;154:2010–2014.

108. Henske EP. Tuberous sclerosis and the kidney: from mesenchyme to epithelium, and beyond. *Pediatr Nephrol* 2005;20:854–857.

109. O'Callaghan FJ, Shiell AW, Osborne JP, et al. Prevalence of tuberous sclerosis estimated by capture-recapture analysis. *Lancet* 1998;351:1490.

110. van Slegtenhorst M, de Hoogt R, Hermans C, et al. Identification of the tuberous sclerosis gene TSC1 on chromosome 9q34. *Science* 1997;277:805–808.

111. European Chromosome 16 Tuberous Sclerosis Consortium. Identification and characterization of the tuberous sclerosis gene on chromosome 16. *Cell* 1993;75:1305–1315.

112. Dabora SL, Jozwiak S, Franz DN, et al. Mutational analysis in a cohort of 224 tuberous sclerosis patients indicates increased severity of TSC2, compared with TSC1, disease in multiple organs. *Am J Hum Genet* 2001;68:64–80.

113. Tomasoni R, Mondino A. The tuberous sclerosis complex: balancing proliferation and survival. *Biochem Soc Trans* 2011;39:466–471.

114. Franz DN, Bissler JJ, McCormack FX. Tuberous sclerosis complex: neurological, renal and pulmonary manifestations. *Neuropediatrics* 2010;41:199–208.

115. Borkowska J, Schwartz RA, Kotulska K, et al. Tuberous sclerosis complex: tumors and tumorigenesis. *Int J Dermatol* 2011;50:13–20.

116. Roach ES, Gomez MR, Northrup H. Tuberous sclerosis complex consensus conference: revised clinical diagnostic criteria. *J Child Neurol* 1998;13:624–628.

117. Brook-Carter PT, Peral B, Ward CJ, et al. Deletion of the TSC2 and PKD1 genes associated with severe infantile polycystic kidney disease—a contiguous gene syndrome. *Nat Genet* 1994;8:328–332.

118. Al-Saleem T, Wessner LL, Scheithauer BW, et al. Malignant tumors of the kidney, brain, and soft tissues in children and young adults with the tuberous sclerosis complex. *Cancer* 1998;83:2208–2216.

119. de Vries PJ. Targeted treatments for cognitive and neurodevelopmental disorders in tuberous sclerosis complex. *Neurotherapeutics* 2010;7:275–282.

120. Lam C, Bouffet E, Tabori U, et al. Rapamycin (sirolimus) in tuberous sclerosis associated pediatric central nervous system tumors. *Pediatr Blood Cancer* 2010;54:476–479.

121. Dabora SL, Franz DN, Ashwal S, et al. Multicenter phase 2 trial of sirolimus for tuberous sclerosis: kidney angiomyolipomas and other tumors regress and VEGF-D levels decrease. *PLoS One* 2011;6:e23379.

122. Yu DT, Sheth KJ. Cystic renal involvement in tuberous sclerosis. *Clin Pediatr (Phila)* 1985;24:36–39.

123. Stillwell TJ, Gomez MR, Kelalis PP. Renal lesions in tuberous sclerosis. *J Urol* 1987;138:477–481.

124. Ewalt DH, Sheffield E, Sparagana SP, et al. Renal lesion growth in children with tuberous sclerosis complex. *J Urol* 1998;160:141–145.

125. Bernstein J, Robbins TO, Kissane JM. The renal lesions of tuberous sclerosis. *Semin Diagn Pathol* 1986;3:97–105.

126. Stuck KJ, Koff SA, Silver TM. Ultrasonic features of multicystic dysplastic kidney: expanded diagnostic criteria. *Radiology* 1982;143:217–221.

127. Kleiner B, Filly RA, Mack L, et al. Multicystic dysplastic kidney: observations of contralateral disease in the fetal population. *Radiology* 1986;161:27–29.

128. Lennert T, Tetzner M, Er M, et al. Multicystic renal dysplasia: nephrectomy versus conservative treatment. *Contrib Nephrol* 1988;67:183–187.

129. Dimmick JE, Johnson HW, Coleman GU, et al. Wilms tumorlet, nodular renal blastema and multicystic renal dysplasia. *J Urol* 1989;142:484–485; discussion 489.

130. Birken G, King D, Vane D, et al. Renal cell carcinoma arising in a multicystic dysplastic kidney. *J Pediatr Surg* 1985;20:619–621.

131. Vellios F, Garrett RA. Congenital unilateral multicystic disease of the kidney. A clinical and anatomic study of seven cases. *Am J Clin Pathol* 1961;35:244–254.

132. Saxton HM, Golding SJ, Chantler C, et al. Diagnostic puncture in renal cystic dysplasia (multicystic kidney). Evidence on the aetiology of the cysts. *Br J Radiol* 1981;54:555–561.

133. Sanders RC, Nussbaum AR, Solez K. Renal dysplasia: sonographic findings. *Radiology* 1988;167:623–626.

134. Suzuki K, Kurokawa S, Muraishi O, et al. Segmental multicystic dysplastic kidney in an adult woman. *Urol Int* 2001;66:51–54.

135. Iscaife A, Barbosa M, Ortiz V, et al. Segmental multicystic dysplastic kidney: a rare situation. *J Pediatr Urol* 2011;7:491–494.

136. Bernstein J. The morphogenesis of renal parenchymal maldevelopment (renal dysplasia). *Pediatr Clin North Am* 1971;18:395–407.

137. Chan JK, Saw D, Myint A, et al. Squamous cysts in renal dysplasia. *Arch Pathol Lab Med* 1986;110:148–149.

138. Fan R, Grignon DJ, Cheng L. Squamous cysts arising from segmental renal dysplasia. *Pediatr Nephrol* 2011;26:1893–1896.

139. Lennerz JK, Spence DC, Iskandar SS, et al. Glomerulocystic kidney: one hundred-year perspective. *Arch Pathol Lab Med* 2010;134:583–605.

140. Chaumoitre K, Brun M, Cassart M, et al. Differential diagnosis of fetal hyperechogenic cystic kidneys unrelated to renal tract anomalies: a multicenter study. *Ultrasound Obstet Gynecol* 2006;28:911–917.

141. Torregrossa R, Anglani F, Fabris A, et al. Identification of GDNF gene sequence variations in patients with medullary sponge kidney disease. *Clin J Am Soc Nephrol* 2010;5:1205–1210.

142. Kuiper JJ. Medullary sponge kidney. *Perspect Nephrol Hypertens* 1976;4:151–171.

143. Harrison AR, Rose GA. Medullary sponge kidney. *Urol Res* 1979;7:197–207.

144. Patriquin HB, O'Regan S. Medullary sponge kidney in childhood. *AJR Am J Roentgenol* 1985;145:315–319.

145. Forster JA, Taylor J, Browning AJ, et al. A review of the natural progression of medullary sponge kidney and a novel grading system based on intravenous urography findings. *Urol Int* 2007;78:264–269.

146. O'Neill M, Breslau NA, Pak CY. Metabolic evaluation of nephrolithiasis in patients with medullary sponge kidney. *JAMA* 1981;245:1233–1236.

147. Maw AM, Megibow AJ, Grasso M, et al. Diagnosis of medullary sponge kidney by computed tomographic urography. *Am J Kidney Dis* 2007;50:146–150.

148. MacDougall JA, Prout WG. Medullary sponge kidney. Clinical appraisal and report of twelve cases. *Br J Surg* 1968;55:130–133.

149. Ekstrom T, Engfeldt B, Lagergren C. *Medullary Sponge Kidney: A Roentgenologic, Clinical, Histopathologic and Biophysical Study.* Stockholm, Sweden: Almqvist & Wiksell; 1959.

150. Baert L, Steg A. Is the diverticulum of the distal and collecting tubules a preliminary stage of the simple cyst in the adult? *J Urol* 1977;118:707–710.

151. Tada S, Yamagishi J, Kobayashi H, et al. The incidence of simple renal cyst by computed tomography. *Clin Radiol* 1983;34:437–439.

152. Steinhardt GF, Slovis TL, Perlmutter AD. Simple renal cysts in infants. *Radiology* 1985;155:349–350.

153. Ham WS, Lee JH, Kim WT, et al. Comparison of multiple session 99% ethanol and single session OK-432 sclerotherapy for the treatment of simple renal cysts. *J Urol* 2008;180:2552–2556.

154. Thwaini A, Shergill IS, Arya M, et al. Long-term follow-up after retroperitoneal laparoscopic decortication of symptomatic renal cysts. *Urol Int* 2007;79:352–355.

155. Rane A. Laparoscopic management of symptomatic simple renal cysts. *Int Urol Nephrol* 2004;36:5–9.

156. Ishikawa I, Saito Y, Shikura N, et al. Ten-year prospective study on the development of renal cell carcinoma in dialysis patients. *Am J Kidney Dis* 1990;16:452–458.

157. Ishikawa I. Acquired cystic disease: mechanisms and manifestations. *Semin Nephrol* 1991;11:671–684.

158. Ishikawa I. Uremic acquired renal cystic disease. Natural history and complications. *Nephron* 1991;58:257–267.

159. Matson MA, Cohen EP. Acquired cystic kidney disease: occurrence, prevalence, and renal cancers. *Medicine* 1990;69:217–226.

160. Leichter HE, Dietrich R, Salusky IB, et al. Acquired cystic kidney disease in children undergoing long-term dialysis. *Pediatr Nephrol* 1988;2:8–11.

161. Frifelt JJ, Larsen C, Elle B, et al. Multicystic transformation of the kidneys in dialysis patients. *Scand J Urol Nephrol* 1989;23:51–54.

162. Moore AE, Kujubu DA. Spontaneous retroperitoneal hemorrhage due to acquired cystic kidney disease. *Hemodial Int* 2007;11:S38–S40.

163. Ishikawa I, Kovacs G. High incidence of papillary renal cell tumours in patients on chronic haemodialysis. *Histopathology* 1993;22:135–139.

164. Matas AJ, Simmons RL, Kjellstrand CM, et al. Increased incidence of malignancy during chronic renal failure. *Lancet* 1975;1:883–886.

165. Lakey W, Leieskovsky G. Tumors of the kidney. In: Karaffin L, Kendallo A, eds. *Urology*. Hagerstown, MD: Harper & Row; 1996:1–46.

166. Filocamo MT, Zanazzi M, Li Marzi V, et al. Renal cell carcinoma of native kidney after renal transplantation: clinical relevance of early detection. *Transplant Proc* 2009;41:4197–4201.

167. Klatte T, Seitz C, Waldert M, et al. Features and outcomes of renal cell carcinoma of native kidneys in renal transplant recipients. *BJU Int* 2010;105:1260–1265.

168. Williams JC, Merguerian PA, Schned AR, et al. Acquired renal cystic disease and renal cell carcinoma in an allograft kidney. *J Urol* 1995;153:395–396.

169. Truong LD, Shen SS, Park M-H, et al. Diagnosing nonneoplastic lesions in nephrectomy specimens. *Arch Pathol Lab Med* 2009;133:189–200.

170. Vandeursen H, Van Damme B, Baert J, et al. Acquired cystic disease of the kidney analyzed by microdissection. *J Urol* 1991;146:1168–1172.

171. Hughson MD, Hennigar GR, McManus JF. Atypical cysts, acquired renal cystic disease, and renal cell tumors in end stage dialysis kidneys. *Lab Invest* 1980;42:475–480.

172. Tickoo SK, dePeralta-Venturina MN, Harik LR, et al. Spectrum of epithelial neoplasms in end-stage renal disease: an experience from 66 tumor-bearing kidneys with emphasis on histologic patterns distinct from those in sporadic adult renal neoplasia. *Am J Surg Pathol* 2006;30:141–153.

173. Cheuk W, Lo ESF, Chan AKC, et al. Atypical epithelial proliferations in acquired renal cystic disease harbor cytogenetic aberrations. *Hum Pathol* 2002;33:761–765.

174. Hwang DY, Ahn C, Lee JG, et al. Unilateral renal cystic disease in adults. *Nephrol Dial Transplant* 1999;14:1999–2003.

175. Slywotzky CM, Bosniak MA. Localized cystic disease of the kidney. *AJR Am J Roentgenol* 2001;176:843–849.

176. Casale P, Grady RW, Feng WC, et al. The pediatric caliceal diverticulum: diagnosis and laparoscopic management. *J Endourol* 2004;18:668–671.

177. Mosli H, MacDonald P, Schillinger J. Caliceal diverticula developing into simple renal cyst. *J Urol* 1986;136:658–661.

178. Healy ME, Teng SS, Moss AA. Uriniferous pseudocyst: computed tomographic findings. *Radiology* 1984;153:757–762.

179. Eccher A, Brunelli M, Gobbo S, et al. Subepithelial pelvic hematoma (Antopol—Goldman lesion) simulating renal neoplasm: report of a case and review of the literature. *Int J Surg Pathol* 2009;17:264–267.

180. Sneige N, Dekmezian RH, Silva EG, et al. Pseudoparasitic Liesegang structures in perirenal hemorrhagic cysts. *Am J Clin Pathol* 1988;89:148–153.

181. Raso DS, Greene WB, Finley JL, et al. Morphology and pathogenesis of Liesegang rings in cyst aspirates: report of two cases with ancillary studies. *Diagn Cytopathol* 1998;19:116–119.

182. Sinclair AM, Isles CG, Brown I, et al. Secondary hypertension in a blood pressure clinic. *Arch Intern Med* 1987;147:1289–1293.

183. Ingelfinger JR. Renovascular disease in children. *Kidney Int* 1993;43:493–505.

184. Stanley JC, Criado E, Upchurch GR Jr, et al. Pediatric renovascular hypertension: 132 primary and 30 secondary operations in 97 children. *J Vasc Surg* 2006;44:1219–1228.

185. Slovut DP, Olin JW. Fibromuscular dysplasia. *N Engl J Med* 2004;350:1862–1871.

186. Olin JW, Sealove BA. Diagnosis, management, and future developments of fibromuscular dysplasia. *J Vasc Surg* 2011;53:826–836.e1.

187. Luscher TF, Keller HM, Imhof HG, et al. Fibromuscular hyperplasia: extension of the disease and therapeutic outcome. Results of the University Hospital Zurich Cooperative Study on Fibromuscular Hyperplasia. *Nephron* 1986;44:109–114.

188. Das CJ, Neyaz Z, Thapa P, et al. Fibromuscular dysplasia of the renal arteries: a radiological review. *Int Urol Nephrol* 2007;39:233–238.

189. Harrison EG Jr, McCormack LJ. Pathologic classification of renal arterial disease in renovascular hypertension. *Mayo Clin Proc* 1971;46:161–167.

190. Bulbul MA, Farrow GA. Renal artery aneurysms. *Urology* 1992;40:124–126.

191. Kalko Y, Ugurlucan M, Basaran M, et al. Visceral artery aneurysms. *Heart Surg Forum* 2007;10:E24–E29.

192. Browne RFJ, Riordan EO, Roberts JA, et al. Renal artery aneurysms: diagnosis and surveillance with 3D contrast-enhanced magnetic resonance angiography. *Eur Radiol* 2004;14:1807–1812.

193. Soliman KB, Shawky Y, Abbas MM, et al. Ruptured renal artery aneurysm during pregnancy, a clinical dilemma. *BMC Urol* 2006;6:22.

194. Stawicki SP, Rosenfeld JC, Weger N, et al. Spontaneous renal artery dissection: three cases and clinical algorithms. *J Hum Hypertens* 2006;20:710–718.

195. Doody O, Adam WR, Foley PT, et al. Fibromuscular dysplasia presenting with bilateral renal infarction. *Cardiovasc Intervent Radiol* 2009;32:329–332.

196. Kopchick JH, Bourne NK, Fine SW, et al. Congenital renal arteriovenous malformations. *Urology* 1981;17:13–17.

197. Smaldone MC, Stein RJ, Cho J-S, et al. Giant idiopathic renal arteriovenous fistula requiring urgent nephrectomy. *Urology* 2007;69:576.e1–576.e3.

198. Lang EK, Earhart V, Atug F, et al. Slow progressive loss of renal function due to arteriovenous fistula caused by renal biopsy. *J Urol* 2007;177:735.

199. Witz M, Korzets Z. Renal vein occlusion: diagnosis and treatment. *Isr Med Assoc J* 2007;9:402–405.

200. Asghar M, Ahmed K, Shah SS, et al. Renal vein thrombosis. *Eur J Vasc Endovasc Surg* 2007;34:217–223.

201. Lau KK, Stoffman JM, Williams S, et al. Neonatal renal vein thrombosis: review of the English-language literature between 1992 and 2006. *Pediatrics* 2007;120:e1278–e1284.

202. Gasparini M, Hofmann R, Stoller M. Renal artery embolism: clinical features and therapeutic options. *J Urol* 1992;147:567–572.

203. Meyrier A. Cholesterol crystal embolism: diagnosis and treatment. *Kidney Int* 2006;69:1308–1312.

204. Zakaria R, Forsyth V, Rosenbaum T. A rare case of renal infarction caused by infective endocarditis. *Nat Rev Urol* 2009;6:568–572.

205. Van den Driessche A, Van Hul E, Ichiche M, et al. Fibromuscular dysplasia presenting as a renal infarction: a case report. *J Med Case Rep* 2010;4:199.

206. Hoefsloot W, de Vries RA, Bruijnen R, et al. Renal infarction after cocaine abuse: a case report and review. *Clin Nephrol* 2009;72:234–236.

207. Schwartz MJ, Smith EB, Trost DW, et al. Renal artery embolization: clinical indications and experience from over 100 cases. *BJU Int* 2007;99:881–886.

208. Hall S, Barr W, Lie JT, et al. Takayasu arteritis. A study of 32 North American patients. *Medicine* 1985;64:89–99.

209. Cakar N, Ozcakar ZB, Soy D, et al. Renal involvement in childhood vasculitis. *Nephron* 2008;108:c202–c206.

210. Samarkos M, Loizou S, Vaiopoulos G, et al. The clinical spectrum of primary renal vasculitis. *Semin Arthritis Rheum* 2005;35:95–111.

211. Weiss M, Liapis H, Tomaszewski J, et al. Pyelonephritis and other infections, reflux nephropathy, hydronephrosis and nephrolithiasis. In: Jennette J, Olson J, Schwartz M, et al., eds. *Heptinstall's Pathology of the Kidney*. 6th ed. Philadelphia, PA: Lippincott Williams & Wilkins; 2007:991–1082.

212. Bailey RR. The relationship of vesico-ureteric reflux to urinary tract infection and chronic pyelonephritis-reflux nephropathy. *Clin Nephrol* 1973;1:132–141.

213. Lomberg H, Hanson LA, Jacobsson B, et al. Correlation of P blood group, vesicoureteral reflux, and bacterial attachment in patients with recurrent pyelonephritis. *N Engl J Med* 1983;308:1189–1192.

214. Meyrier A, Condamin MC, Fernet M, et al. Frequency of development of early cortical scarring in acute primary pyelonephritis. *Kidney Int* 1989;35:696–703.

215. Winberg J, Bollgren I, Kallenius G, et al. Clinical pyelonephritis and focal renal scarring. A selected review of pathogenesis, prevention, and prognosis. *Pediatr Clin North Am* 1982;29:801–814.

216. Benador D, Benador N, Slosman DO, et al. Cortical scintigraphy in the evaluation of renal parenchymal changes in children with pyelonephritis. *J Pediatr* 1994;124:17–20.

217. Majd M, Rushton HG, Jantausch B, et al. Relationship among vesicoureteral reflux, P-fimbriated *Escherichia coli*, and acute pyelonephritis in children with febrile urinary tract infection. *J Pediatr* 1991;119:578–585.

218. Bergstrom T, Lincoln K, Redin B, et al. Studies of urinary tract infections in infancy and childhood. X. Short or long-term treatment in girls with first or second-time urinary tract infections uncomplicated by obstructive urological abnormalities. *Acta Paediatr Scand* 1968;57:186–194.

219. Freedman L. Prolonged observations on a group of patients with acute urinary tract infections. In: Quinn E, Kass E, eds. *Henry Ford Hospital Symposium on Biology of Pyelonephritis*. Detroit, MI: Little Brown; 1960:345.

220. Winberg J, Andersen HJ, Bergstrom T, et al. Epidemiology of symptomatic urinary tract infection in childhood. *Acta Paediatr Scand Suppl* 1974;252:1–20.

221. Coker C, Poore CA, Li X, et al. Pathogenesis of *Proteus mirabilis* urinary tract infection. *Microbes Infect* 2000;2:1497–1505.

222. Demetrios P, Constantine B, Demetrios S, et al. *Haemophilus influenzae* acute pyelonephritis in the elderly. *Int Urol Nephrol* 2002;34:23–24.

223. Kunin C. *Detection, Prevention, and Management of Urinary Tract Infections*. 4th ed. Philadelphia, PA: Lea & Febiger; 1987.

224. Roberts JA. Tropism in bacterial infections: urinary tract infections. *J Urol* 1996;156:1552–1559.

225. Vosti KL, Goldberg LM, Monto AS, et al. Host-parasite interaction in patients with infections due to *Escherichia coli*. I. The serogrouping of *E. coli* from intestinal and extraintestinal sources. *J Clin Invest* 1964;43:2377–2385.

226. Johnson JR. Virulence factors in *Escherichia coli* urinary tract infection. *Clin Microbiol Rev* 1991;4:80–128.

227. Vaisanen V, Elo J, Tallgren LG, et al. Mannose-resistant haemagglutination and P antigen recognition are characteristic of *Escherichia coli* causing primary pyelonephritis. *Lancet* 1981;2:1366–1369.

228. Svanborg C, Godaly G. Bacterial virulence in urinary tract infection. *Infect Dis Clin North Am* 1997;11:513–529.

229. Svanborg C, Agace W, Hedges S, et al. Bacterial adherence and mucosal cytokine production. *Ann N Y Acad Sci* 1994;730:162–181.

230. Kanamaru S, Kurazono H, Ishitoya S, et al. Distribution and genetic association of putative uropathogenic virulence factors iroN, iha, kpsMT, ompT and usp in *Escherichia coli* isolated from urinary tract infections in Japan. *J Urol* 2003;170:2490–2493.

231. Roberts JA. Management of pyelonephritis and upper urinary tract infections. *Urol Clin North Am* 1999;26:753–763.

232. Kooman JP, Barendregt JN, van der Sande FM, et al. Acute pyelonephritis: a cause of acute renal failure? *Neth J Med* 2000;57:185–189.

233. Nickel JC. The management of acute pyelonephritis in adults. *Can J Urol* 2001;8:29–38.

234. Goldraich NP, Goldraich IH. Update on dimercaptosuccinic acid renal scanning in children with urinary tract infection. *Pediatr Nephrol* 1995;9:221–226.

235. Truesdale BH, Rous SN, Nelson RP. Perinephric abscess: a review of 26 cases. *J Urol* 1977;118:910–911.

236. Heptinstall RH. Experimental pyelonephritis. Bacteriological and morphological studies on the ascending route of infection in the rat. *Nephron* 1964;204:73–92.

237. Pontin AR, Barnes RD, Joffe J, et al. Emphysematous pyelonephritis in diabetic patients. *Br J Urol* 1995;75:71–74.

238. Lowe BA, Poage MD. Bilateral emphysematous pyelonephritis. *Urology* 1991;37:229–232.

239. Michaeli J, Mogle P, Perlberg S, et al. Emphysematous pyelonephritis. *J Urol* 1984;131:203–208.

240. Huang JJ, Tseng CC. Emphysematous pyelonephritis: clinicoradiological classification, management, prognosis, and pathogenesis. *Arch Intern Med* 2000;160:797–805.

241. Pontin AR, Barnes RD. Current management of emphysematous pyelonephritis. *Nat Rev Urol* 2009;6:272–279.

242. Evanoff GV, Thompson CS, Foley R, et al. Spectrum of gas within the kidney. Emphysematous pyelonephritis and emphysematous pyelitis. *Am J Med* 1987;83:149–154.

243. Mokabberi R, Ravakhah K. Emphysematous urinary tract infections: diagnosis, treatment and survival (case review series). *Am J Med Sci* 2007;333:111–116.

244. Yao J, Gutierrez OM, Reiser J. Emphysematous pyelonephritis. *Kidney Int* 2007;71:462–465.

245. Mallory G, Crane A, Edward J. Pathology of acute and of healed experimental pyelonephritis. *Arch Pathol* 1940;30:330.

246. Cheung AL, Krishnan M, Jaffe EA, et al. Fibrinogen acts as a bridging molecule in the adherence of *Staphylococcus aureus* to cultured human endothelial cells. *J Clin Invest* 1991;87:2236–2245.

247. Lopes JD, dos Reis M, Brentani RR. Presence of laminin receptors in *Staphylococcus aureus*. *Science* 1985;229:275–277.

248. Iandolo JJ. Genetic analysis of extracellular toxins of *Staphylococcus aureus*. *Annu Rev Microbiol* 1989;43:375–402.

249. Bhakdi S, Tranum-Jensen J. Alpha-toxin of *Staphylococcus aureus*. *Microbiol Rev* 1991;55:733–751.

250. Swaminathan S, Furey W, Pletcher J, et al. Crystal structure of staphylococcal enterotoxin B, a superantigen. *Nature* 1992;359:801–806.

251. Scroggs MW, Wolfe JA, Bollinger RR, et al. Causes of death in renal transplant recipients. A review of autopsy findings from 1966 through 1985. *Arch Pathol Lab Med* 1987;111:983–987.

252. Wiecek A, Zeier M, Ritz E. Role of infection in the genesis of acute renal failure. *Nephrol Dial Transplant* 1994;9:40–44.

253. Dillon MJ, Goonasekera CD. Reflux nephropathy. *J Am Soc Nephrol* 1998;9:2377–2383.

254. Mattoo TK. Vesicoureteral reflux and reflux nephropathy. *Adv Chronic Kidney Dis* 2011;18:348–354.

255. Murawski IJ, Watt CL, Gupta IR. Vesico-ureteric reflux: using mouse models to understand a common congenital urinary tract defect. *Pediatr Nephrol* 2011;26:1513–1522.

256. Ransley PG, Risdon RA. Renal papillae and intrarenal reflux in the pig. *Lancet* 1974;2:1114.

257. Woodard JR, Holden S. The prognostic significance of fever in childhood urinary infections: observations in 350 consecutive patients. *Clin Pediatr* 1976;15:1051–1054.

258. Smellie JM, Prescod NP, Shaw PJ, et al. Childhood reflux and urinary infection: a follow-up of 10-41 years in 226 adults. *Pediatr Nephrol* 1998;12:727–736.

259. Hinchliffe SA, Kreczy A, Ciftci AO, et al. Focal and segmental glomerulosclerosis in children with reflux nephropathy. *Pediatr Pathol* 1994;14:327–338.

260. Tada M, Jimi S, Hisano S, et al. Histopathological evidence of poor prognosis in patients with vesicoureteral reflux. *Pediatr Nephrol* 2001;16:482–487.

261. Ataei N, Madani A, Esfahani ST, et al. Screening for vesicoureteral reflux and renal scars in siblings of children with known reflux. *Pediatr Nephrol* 2004;19:1127–1131.

262. Austin JC, Cooper CS. Vesicoureteral reflux: surgical approaches. *Urol Clin North Am* 2004;31:543–557.

263. Fanos V, Cataldi L. Antibiotics or surgery for vesicoureteric reflux in children. *Lancet* 2004;364:1720–1722.

264. O'Donnell B. Reflections on reflux. *J Urol* 2004;172:1635–1636.

265. Bathena D, Holland N, Weiss J. Morphology of course renal scars in reflux associated nephropathy in man. In: Hodson J, Kincaid-Smith P, eds. *Reflux Nephropathy*. New York: Mason Publishing USA Inc.; 1979.

266. Arant BS Jr, Sotelo-Avila C, Bernstein J. Segmental "hypoplasia" of the kidney (Ask-Upmark). *J Pediatr* 1979;95:931–939.

267. Marwali MR, Rossi NF. Ask-Upmark kidney associated with renal and extrarenal arterial aneurysms. *Am J Kidney Dis* 1999;33:e4.

268. Babin J, Sackett M, Delage C, et al. The Ask-Upmark kidney: a curable cause of hypertension in young patients. *J Hum Hypertens* 2005;19:315–316.

269. Shindo S, Bernstein J, Arant BS Jr. Evolution of renal segmental atrophy (Ask-Upmark kidney) in children with vesicoureteric reflux: radiographic and morphologic studies. *J Pediatr* 1983;102:847–854.

270. Eastwood JB, Corbishley CM, Grange JM. Tuberculosis and the kidney. *J Am Soc Nephrol* 2001;12:1307–1314.

271. Chijioke A. Current views on epidemiology of renal tuberculosis. *West Afr J Med* 2001;20:217–219.

272. Spence RK, Dafoe DC, Rabin G, et al. Mycobacterial infections in renal allograft recipients. *Arch Surg* 1983;118:356–359.

273. Lenk S, Oesterwitz H, Scholz D. Tuberculosis in cadaveric renal allograft recipients. Report of 4 cases and review of the literature. *Eur Urol* 1988;14:484–486.

274. Benn JJ, Scoble JE, Thomas AC, et al. Cryptogenic tuberculosis as a preventable cause of end-stage renal failure. *Am J Nephrol* 1988;8:306–308.

275. Simon HB, Weinstein AJ, Pasternak MS, et al. Genitourinary tuberculosis. Clinical features in a general hospital population. *Am J Med* 1977;63:410–420.

276. Alvarez S, McCabe WR. Extrapulmonary tuberculosis revisited: a review of experience at Boston City and other hospitals. *Medicine* 1984;63:25–55.

277. Weinberg AC, Boyd SD. Short-course chemotherapy and role of surgery in adult and pediatric genitourinary tuberculosis. *Urology* 1988;31:95–102.

278. Medlar E. Cases of renal infection in pulmonary tuberculosis: evidence of healed tuberculous lesions. *Am J Pathol* 1926;2:401.

279. Grange JM, Yates MD. Survey of mycobacteria isolated from urine and the genitourinary tract in south-east England from 1980 to 1989. *Br J Urol* 1992;69:640–646.

280. Mahevas M, Lescure FX, Boffa J-J, et al. Renal sarcoidosis: clinical, laboratory, and histologic presentation and outcome in 47 patients. *Medicine* 2009;88:98–106.

281. Taylor GD, Buchanan-Chell M, Kirkland T, et al. Trends and sources of nosocomial fungaemia. *Mycoses* 1994;37:187–190.

282. Samonis G, Bafaloukos D. Fungal infections in cancer patients: an escalating problem. *In Vivo* 1992;6:183–193.

283. Tomashefski JF Jr, Abramowsky CR. *Candida*-associated renal papillary necrosis. *Am J Clin Pathol* 1981;75:190–194.

284. Myerowitz RL, Pazin GJ, Allen CM. Disseminated candidiasis. Changes in incidence, underlying diseases, and pathology. *Am J Clin Pathol* 1977;68:29–38.

285. Hughes WT. Systemic candidiasis: a study of 109 fatal cases. *Pediatr Infect Dis* 1982;1:11–18.

286. Biggers R, Edwards J. Anuria secondary to bilateral ureteropelvic fungus balls. *Urology* 1980;15:161–163.

287. Eckstein CW, Kass EJ. Anuria in a newborn secondary to bilateral ureteropelvic fungus balls. *J Urol* 1982;127:109–110.

288. Sinniah R, Churg J, Sobin L. *Renal Disease: Classification and Atlas of Infectious and Tropical Diseases*. Chicago, IL: ASCP Press; 1988.

289. Rantala A. Postoperative candidiasis. *Ann Chir Gynaecol* 1993;205:1–52.

290. Khauli RB, Kalash S, Young JD Jr. *Torulopsis glabrata* perinephric abscess. *J Urol* 1983;130:968–970.

291. Kauffman CA, Tan JS. *Torulopsis glabrata* renal infection. *Am J Med* 1974;57:217–224.

292. Berkowitz ID, Robboy SJ, Karchmer AW, et al. *Torulopsis glabrata* fungemia—a clinical pathological study. *Medicine* 1979;58:430–440.

293. Vordermark JS II, Modarelli RO, Buck AS. Torulopsis pyelonephritis associated with papillary necrosis: a case report. *J Urol* 1980;123:96–97.

294. High KP, Quagliarello VJ. Yeast perinephric abscess: report of a case and review. *Clin Infect Dis* 1992;15:128–133.

295. Flechner SM, McAninch JW. Aspergillosis of the urinary tract: ascending route of infection and evolving patterns of disease. *J Urol* 1981;125:598–601.

296. Warshawsky AB, Keiller D, Gittes RF. Bilateral renal aspergillosis. *J Urol* 1975;113:8–11.

297. Barnes PD, Marr KA. Aspergillosis: spectrum of disease, diagnosis, and treatment. *Infect Dis Clin North Am* 2006;20:545–561.

298. Reis MA, Costa RS, Ferraz AS. Causes of death in renal transplant recipients: a study of 102 autopsies from 1968 to 1991. *J R Soc Med* 1995;88:24–27.

299. Salyer WR, Salyer DC. Involvement of the kidney and prostate in cryptococcosis. *J Urol* 1973;109:695–698.

300. Randall RE Jr, Stacy WK, Toone EC, et al. Cryptococcal pyelonephritis. *N Engl J Med* 1968;279:60–65.

301. Goodwin RA Jr, Shapiro JL, Thurman GH, et al. Disseminated histoplasmosis: clinical and pathologic correlations. *Medicine* 1980;59:1–33.

302. Superdock KR, Dummer JS, Koch MO, et al. Disseminated histoplasmosis presenting as urinary tract obstruction in a renal transplant recipient. *Am J Kidney Dis* 1994;23:600–604.

303. Kaplan W, Clifford MK. Blastomycosis. I. A review of 198 collected cases in Veterans Administration Hospitals. *Am Rev Respir Dis* 1964;89:659–672.

304. Eickenberg HU, Amin M, Lich R Jr. Blastomycosis of the genitourinary tract. *J Urol* 1975;113:650–652.

305. Ampel NM. Coccidioidomycosis: a review of recent advances. *Clin Chest Med* 2009;30:241–251.

306. Ampel NM, Dols CL, Galgiani JN. Coccidioidomycosis during human immunodeficiency virus infection: results of a prospective study in a coccidioidal endemic area. *Am J Med* 1993;94:235–240.

307. Barbee RA, Hicks MJ, Grosso D, et al. The maternal immune response in coccidioidomycosis. Is pregnancy a risk factor for serious infection? *Chest* 1991;100:709–715.

308. Peterson CM, Schuppert K, Kelly PC, et al. Coccidioidomycosis and pregnancy. *Obstet Gynecol Surv* 1993;48:149–156.

309. Spinello IM, Johnson RH, Baqi S. Coccidioidomycosis and pregnancy: a review. *Ann N Y Acad Sci* 2007;1111:358–364.

310. Ferreira MS. Paracoccidioidomycosis. *Paediatr Respir Rev* 2009;10:161–165.

311. Brummer E, Castaneda E, Restrepo A. Paracoccidioidomycosis: an update. *Clin Microbiol Rev* 1993;6:89–117.

312. Shikanai-Yasuda MA, Conceicao YMT, Kono A, et al. Neoplasia and paracoccidioidomycosis. *Mycopathologia* 2008;165:303–312.

313. Levy E, Bia MJ. Isolated renal mucormycosis: case report and review. *J Am Soc Nephrol* 1995;5:2014–2019.

314. Morrison VA, McGlave PB. Mucormycosis in the BMT population. *Bone Marrow Transplant* 1993;11:383–388.

315. Spellberg B, Walsh TJ, Kontoyiannis DP, et al. Recent advances in the management of mucormycosis: from bench to bedside. *Clin Infect Dis* 2009;48:1743–1751.

316. Vesa J, Bielsa O, Arango O, et al. Massive renal infarction due to mucormycosis in an AIDS patient. *Infection* 1992;20:234–236.

317. Yu J, Li RY. Primary renal zygomycosis due to *Rhizopus oryzae*. *Med Mycol* 2006;44:461–466.

318. Dansky AS, Lynne CM, Politano VA. Disseminated mucormycosis with renal involvement. *J Urol* 1978;119:275–277.

319. Barsoum RS. Malarial nephropathies. *Nephrol Dial Transplant* 1998;13:1588–1597.

320. Barsoum RS. Malarial acute renal failure. *J Am Soc Nephrol* 2000; 11:2147–2154.

321. Barsoum RS. Schistosomal glomerulopathies. *Kidney Int* 1993;44:1–12.

322. Barsoum RS. Schistosomiasis and the kidney. *Semin Nephrol* 2003;23:34–41.

323. Date A, Gunasekaran V, Kirubakaran MG, et al. Acute eosinophilic glomerulonephritis with Bancroftian filariasis. *Postgrad Med J* 1979; 55:905–907.

324. Sitprija V, Boonpucknavig V. Renal involvement in parasitic disease. In: Tisher C, Brennan B, eds. *Renal Pathology with Clinical and Functional Considerations*. Philadelphia, PA: JB Lippincott; 1994:626.

325. Didier ES. Microsporidiosis: an emerging and opportunistic infection in humans and animals. *Acta Trop* 2005;94:61–76.

326. Mertens RB, Didier ES, Fishbein MC, et al. *Encephalitozoon cuniculi* microsporidiosis: infection of the brain, heart, kidneys, trachea, adrenal glands, and urinary bladder in a patient with AIDS. *Mod Pathol* 1997;10:68–77.

327. Guvel S, Kilinc F, Kayaselcuk F, et al. Emphysematous pyelonephritis and renal amoebiasis in a patient with diabetes mellitus. *Int J Urol* 2003;10:404–406.

328. Gogus C, Safak M, Baltaci S, et al. Isolated renal hydatidosis: experience with 20 cases. *J Urol* 2003;169:186–189.

329. Diamond HM, Lyon ES, Hui NT, et al. Echinococcal disease of the kidney. *J Urol* 1976;115:742–744.

330. D'Agati V, Suh JI, Carbone L, et al. Pathology of HIV-associated nephropathy: a detailed morphologic and comparative study. *Kidney Int* 1989;35:1358–1370.

331. Cohen AH, Nast CC. HIV-associated nephropathy. A unique combined glomerular, tubular, and interstitial lesion. *Mod Pathol* 1988;1:87–97.

332. Atta MG. Diagnosis and natural history of HIV-associated nephropathy. *Adv Chronic Kidney Dis* 2010;17:52–58.

333. Kaufman L, Collins SE, Klotman PE. The pathogenesis of HIV-associated nephropathy. *Adv Chronic Kidney Dis* 2010;17:36–43.

334. Peters CJ, Simpson GL, Levy H. Spectrum of Hantavirus infection: hemorrhagic fever with renal syndrome and Hantavirus pulmonary syndrome. *Annu Rev Med* 1999;50:531–545.

335. Bren AF, Pavlovcic SK, Koselj M, et al. Acute renal failure due to hemorrhagic fever with renal syndrome. *Ren Fail* 1996;18:635–638.

336. Mustonen J, Helin H, Pietila K, et al. Renal biopsy findings and clinicopathologic correlations in nephropathia epidemica. *Clin Nephrol* 1994;41:121–126.

337. Hirsch HH, Knowles W, Dickenmann M, et al. Prospective study of polyomavirus type BK replication and nephropathy in renal-transplant recipients. *N Engl J Med* 2002;347:488–496.

338. Nickeleit V, Hirsch HH, Binet IF, et al. Polyomavirus infection of renal allograft recipients: from latent infection to manifest disease. *J Am Soc Nephrol* 1999;10:1080–1089.

339. Blanckaert K, De Vriese AS. Current recommendations for diagnosis and management of polyoma BK virus nephropathy in renal transplant recipients. *Nephrol Dial Transplant* 2006;21:3364–3367.

340. Nickeleit V, Klimkait T, Binet IF, et al. Testing for polyomavirus type BK DNA in plasma to identify renal-allograft recipients with viral nephropathy. *N Engl J Med* 2000;342:1309–1315.

341. Nickeleit V, Hirsch HH, Zeiler M, et al. BK-virus nephropathy in renal transplants-tubular necrosis, MHC-class II expression and rejection in a puzzling game. *Nephrol Dial Transplant* 2000;15:324–332.

342. Randhawa PS, Finkelstein S, Scantlebury V, et al. Human polyoma virus-associated interstitial nephritis in the allograft kidney. *Transplantation* 1999;67:103–109.

343. Boldorini R, Brustia M, Veggiani C, et al. Periodic assessment of urine and serum by cytology and molecular biology as a diagnostic tool for BK virus nephropathy in renal transplant patients. *Acta Cytol* 2005;49:235–243.

344. Hibberd PL, Tolkoff-Rubin NE, Cosimi AB, et al. Symptomatic cytomegalovirus disease in the cytomegalovirus antibody seropositive renal transplant recipient treated with OKT3. *Transplantation* 1992;53:68–72.

345. Farrugia E, Schwab TR. Management and prevention of cytomegalovirus infection after renal transplantation. *Mayo Clin Proc* 1992;67:879–890.

346. Kanter J, Pallardo L, Gavela E, et al. Cytomegalovirus infection renal transplant recipients: risk factors and outcome. *Transplant Proc* 2009;41:2156–2158.

347. Gabrielli L, Bonasoni MP, Lazzarotto T, et al. Histological findings in foetuses congenitally infected by cytomegalovirus. *J Clin Virol* 2009;46(suppl 4):S16–S21.

348. Taherimahmoudi M, Ahmadi H, Baradaran N, et al. Cytomegalovirus infection and disease following renal transplantation: preliminary report of incidence and potential risk factors. *Transplant Proc* 2009;41:2841–2844.

349. Valenzuela M, Ortiz AM, Troncoso P, et al. Strategies for prevention of cytomegalovirus infection in renal transplant patients. *Transplant Proc* 2009;41:2673–2675.

350. Drew WL. Laboratory diagnosis of cytomegalovirus infection and disease in immunocompromised patients. *Curr Opin Infect Dis* 2007;20:408–411.

351. Payton D, Thorner P, Eddy A, et al. Demonstration by light microscopy of cytomegalovirus on a renal biopsy of a renal allograft recipient: confirmation by immunohistochemistry and in situ hybridization. *Nephron* 1987;47:205–208.

352. Sachdeva MUS, Nada R, Jha V, et al. Viral infections of renal allografts—an immunohistochemical and ultrastructural study. *Indian J Pathol Microbiol* 2004;47:189–194.

353. Ito M, Hirabayashi N, Uno Y, et al. Necrotizing tubulointerstitial nephritis associated with adenovirus infection. *Hum Pathol* 1991;22: 1225–1231.

354. Mazoyer E, Daugas E, Verine J, et al. A case report of adenovirus-related acute interstitial nephritis in a patient with AIDS. *Am J Kidney Dis* 2008;51:121–126.

355. Lordemann AG, Hjelle B, Theegarten D, et al. Young man with kidney failure and hemorrhagic interstitial nephritis. *Am J Kidney Dis* 2009;54:1162–1166.

356. Lednicky JA. Hantaviruses. a short review. *Arch Pathol Lab Med* 2003;127:30–35.

357. Jonsson CB, Figueiredo LTM, Vapalahti O. A global perspective on Hantavirus ecology, epidemiology, and disease. *Clin Microbiol Rev* 2010;23:412–441.

358. Ferluga D, Vizjak A. Hantavirus nephropathy. *J Am Soc Nephrol* 2008;19:1653–1658.

359. Chen F. Genetic and developmental basis for urinary tract obstruction. *Pediatr Nephrol* 2009;24:1621–1632.

360. Chevalier RL, Forbes MS, Thornhill BA. Ureteral obstruction as a model of renal interstitial fibrosis and obstructive nephropathy. *Kidney Int* 2009;75:1145–1152.

361. Richstone L, Seideman CA, Reggio E, et al. Pathologic findings in patients with ureteropelvic junction obstruction and crossing vessels. *Urology* 2009;73:716–719.

362. Wang GJ, Brenner-Anantharam A, Vaughan ED, et al. Antagonism of BMP4 signaling disrupts smooth muscle investment of the ureter and ureteropelvic junction. *J Urol* 2009;181:401–407.

363. Chang C-P, McDill BW, Neilson JR, et al. Calcineurin is required in urinary tract mesenchyme for the development of the pyeloureteral peristaltic machinery. *J Clin Invest* 2004;113:1051–1058.

364. Williams B, Tareen B, Resnick MI. Pathophysiology and treatment of ureteropelvic junction obstruction. *Curr Urol Rep* 2007;8:111–117.

365. Herndon CD, Kitchens DM. The management of ureteropelvic junction obstruction presenting with prenatal hydronephrosis. *ScientificWorld Journal* 2009;9:400–403.

366. Heinlen JE, Manatt CS, Bright BC, et al. Operative versus nonoperative management of ureteropelvic junction obstruction in children. *Urology* 2009;73:521–525.

367. Zhang PL, Peters CA, Rosen S. Ureteropelvic junction obstruction: morphological and clinical studies. *Pediatr Nephrol* 2000;14:820–826.

368. Hosgor M, Karaca I, Ulukus C, et al. Structural changes of smooth muscle in congenital ureteropelvic junction obstruction. *J Pediatr Surg* 2005;40:1632–1636.

369. Koleda P, Apoznanski W, Wozniak Z, et al. Changes in interstitial cell of Cajal-like cells density in congenital ureteropelvic junction obstruction. *Int Urol Nephrol* 2012;44:7–12.

370. Tickoo SK, Gopalan A, Tu JJ, et al. Estrogen and progesterone-receptor-positive stroma as a non-tumorous proliferation in kidneys: a possible metaplastic response to obstruction. *Mod Pathol* 2008;21: 60–65.

371. Stamatelou KK, Francis ME, Jones CA, et al. Time trends in reported prevalence of kidney stones in the United States: 1976-1994. *Kidney Int* 2003;63:1817–1823.

372. Cupisti A. Update on nephrolithiasis: beyond symptomatic urinary tract obstruction. *J Nephrol* 2011;24:S25–S29.

373. Soucie JM, Thun MJ, Coates RJ, et al. Demographic and geographic variability of kidney stones in the United States. *Kidney Int* 1994;46:893–899.

374. Pearle MS, Calhoun EA, Curhan GC; Urologic Diseases of America Project. Urologic diseases in America project: urolithiasis. *J Urol* 2005;173:848–857.

375. Sakhaee K. Recent advances in the pathophysiology of nephrolithiasis. *Kidney Int* 2009;75:585–595.

376. Parks JH, Coe FL. Pathogenesis and treatment of calcium stones. *Semin Nephrol* 1996;16:398–411.

377. Pak CY, Britton F, Peterson R, et al. Ambulatory evaluation of nephrolithiasis. Classification, clinical presentation and diagnostic criteria. *Am J Med* 1980;69:19–30.

378. Levy FL, Adams-Huet B, Pak CY. Ambulatory evaluation of nephrolithiasis: an update of a 1980 protocol. *Am J Med* 1995;98:50–59.

379. Devuyst O, Pirson Y. Genetics of hypercalciuric stone forming diseases. *Kidney Int* 2007;72:1065–1072.

380. Srivastava T, Schwaderer A. Diagnosis and management of hypercalciuria in children. *Curr Opin Pediatr* 2009;21:214–219.

381. Berger AD, Wu W, Eisner BH, et al. Patients with primary hyperparathyroidism—why do some form stones? *J Urol* 2009;181:2141–2145.

382. Lloyd SE, Pearce SH, Fisher SE, et al. A common molecular basis for three inherited kidney stone diseases. *Nature* 1996;379:445–449.

383. Scheinman SJ. X-linked hypercalciuric nephrolithiasis: clinical syndromes and chloride channel mutations. *Kidney Int* 1998;53:3–17.

384. Chadha V, Alon US. Hereditary renal tubular disorders. *Semin Nephrol* 2009;29:399–341.

385. Deeb AA, Bruce SN, Morris AA, et al. Infantile hypophosphatasia: disappointing results of treatment. *Acta Paediatr* 2000;89:730–733.

386. Asplin J, Favus M, Coe F. Nephrolithiasis. In: Brenner B, ed. *Brenner and Rector's the Kidney*. 5th ed. Philadelphia, PA: WB Saunders; 1996:1983.

387. Danpure CJ. Primary hyperoxaluria: from gene defects to designer drugs? *Nephrol Dial Transplant* 2005;20:1525–1529.

388. Hoppe B, Beck BB, Milliner DS. The primary hyperoxalurias. *Kidney Int* 2009;75:1264–1271.

389. Vella M, Karydi M, Coraci G, et al. Pathophysiology and clinical aspects of urinary lithiasis. *Urol Int* 2007;79:26–31.

390. Kaufman DW, Kelly JP, Curhan GC, et al. *Oxalobacter formigenes* may reduce the risk of calcium oxalate kidney stones. *J Am Soc Nephrol* 2008;19:1197–1203.

391. Randall A. Papillary pathology as a precursor of primary renal calculus. *J Urol* 1940;44:580.

392. Low RK, Stoller ML. Endoscopic mapping of renal papillae for Randall's plaques in patients with urinary stone disease. *J Urol* 1997;158:2062–2064.

393. Borghi L, Schianchi T, Meschi T, et al. Comparison of two diets for the prevention of recurrent stones in idiopathic hypercalciuria. *N Engl J Med* 2002;346:77–84.

394. Lewandowski S, Rodgers AL. Idiopathic calcium oxalate urolithiasis: risk factors and conservative treatment. *Clin Chim Acta* 2004;345:17–34.

395. Smith LH. The pathophysiology and medical treatment of urolithiasis. *Semin Nephrol* 1990;10:31–52.

396. Healy KA, Ogan K. Pathophysiology and management of infectious staghorn calculi. *Urol Clin North Am* 2007;34:363–374.

397. Miller NL, Evan AP, Lingeman JE. Pathogenesis of renal calculi. *Urol Clin North Am* 2007;34:295–313.

398. Cochat P, Pichault V, Bacchetta J, et al. Nephrolithiasis related to inborn metabolic diseases. *Pediatr Nephrol* 2010;25:415–424.

399. Eckel RH, Alberti KGMM, Grundy SM, et al. The metabolic syndrome. *Lancet* 2010;375:181–183.

400. Mattoo A, Goldfarb DS. Cystinuria. *Semin Nephrol* 2008;28:181–191.

401. Pais VM Jr, Lowe G, Lallas CD, et al. Xanthine urolithiasis. *Urology* 2006;67:1084.e9–e11.

402. Bani-Hani AH, Segura JW, Leroy AJ. Urinary matrix calculi: our experience at a single institution. *J Urol* 2005;173:120–123.

403. Bennett S, Hoffman N, Monga M. Ephedrine- and guaifenesin-induced nephrolithiasis. *J Altern Complement Med* 2004;10:967–969.

404. Katz SM, Krueger LJ, Falkner B. Microscopic nephrocalcinosis in cystic fibrosis. *N Engl J Med* 1988;319:263–266.

405. Ammenti A, Pelizzoni A, Cecconi M, et al. Nephrocalcinosis in children: a retrospective multi-centre study. *Acta Paediatr* 2009;98:1628–1631.

406. Mocan H, Yildiran A, Camlibel T, et al. Microscopic nephrocalcinosis and hypercalciuria in nephrotic syndrome. *Hum Pathol* 2000;31: 1363–1367.

407. Rajput R, Sehgal A, Jain D, et al. Nephrocalcinosis: a rare presenting manifestation of primary Sjogren's syndrome. *Mod Rheumatol* 2012;22:479–482.

408. Markowitz GS, Nasr SH, Klein P, et al. Renal failure due to acute nephrocalcinosis following oral sodium phosphate bowel cleansing. *Hum Pathol* 2004;35:675–684.

409. Semins MJ, Lang E, Matlaga BR. Nephrocalcinosis. *J Urol* 2009; 182:2910–2911.

410. Henegar JR, Coleman JP, Cespedes J, et al. Glomerular calcification in hypercalcemic nephropathy. *Arch Pathol Lab Med* 2003;127:E80–E85.

411. Chuang CK, Lai MK, Chang PL, et al. Xanthogranulomatous pyelonephritis: experience in 36 cases. *J Urol* 1992;147:333–336.

412. Rosi P, Selli C, Carini M, et al. Xanthogranulomatous pyelonephritis: clinical experience with 62 cases. *Eur Urol* 1986;12:96–100.

413. Parsons MA, Harris SC, Longstaff AJ, et al. Xanthogranulomatous pyelonephritis: a pathological, clinical and aetiological analysis of 87 cases. *Diagn Histopathol* 1983;6:203–219.

414. Li L, Parwani AV. Xanthogranulomatous pyelonephritis. *Arch Pathol Lab Med* 2011;135:671–674.

415. Korkes F, Favoretto RL, Broglio M, et al. Xanthogranulomatous pyelonephritis: clinical experience with 41 cases. *Urology* 2008;71: 178–180.

416. Khalyl-Mawad J, Greco MA, Schinella RA. Ultrastructural demonstration of intracellular bacteria in xanthogranulomatous pyelonephritis. *Hum Pathol* 1982;13:41–47.

417. Hammadeh MY, Nicholls G, Calder CJ, et al. Xanthogranulomatous pyelonephritis in childhood: pre-operative diagnosis is possible. *Br J Urol* 1994;73:83–86.

418. Zugor V, Schott GE, Labanaris AP. Xanthogranulomatous pyelonephritis in childhood: a critical analysis of 10 cases and of the literature. *Urology* 2007;70:157–160.

419. Clapton WK, Boucaut HA, Dewan PA, et al. Clinicopathological features of xanthogranulomatous pyelonephritis in infancy. *Pathology* 1993;25:110–113.

420. Gregg CR, Rogers TE, Munford RS. Xanthogranulomatous pyelonephritis. *Curr Clin Top Infect Dis* 1999;19:287–304.

421. Husain I, Pingle A, Kazi T. Bilateral diffuse xanthogranulomatous pyelonephritis. *Br J Urol* 1979;51:162–163.

422. Elder JS, Marshall FF. Focal xanthogranulomatous pyelonephritis in adulthood. *Johns Hopkins Med J* 1980;146:141–147.

423. Watson AR, Marsden HB, Lendon M, et al. Renal pseudotumours caused by xanthogranulomatous pyelonephritis. *Arch Dis Child* 1982;57:635–637.

424. Bingol-Kologlu M, Ciftci AO, Senocak ME, et al. Xanthogranulomatous pyelonephritis in children: diagnostic and therapeutic aspects. *Eur J Pediatr Surg* 2002;12:42–48.

425. Zorzos I, Moutzouris V, Korakianitis G, et al. Analysis of 39 cases of xanthogranulomatous pyelonephritis with emphasis on CT findings. *Scand J Urol Nephrol* 2003;37:342–347.

426. Saeed SM, Fine G. Xanthogranulomatous pyelonephritis. *Am J Clin Pathol* 1963;39:616–625.

427. Kobayashi A, Utsunomiya Y, Kono M, et al. Malakoplakia of the kidney. *Am J Kidney Dis* 2008;51:326–330.

428. Trillo A, Lorentz WB, Whitley NO. Malakoplakia of kidney simulating renal neoplasm. *Urology* 1977;10:472–477.

429. Kelly DR, Murad TM. Megalocytic interstitial nephritis, xanthogranulomatous pyelonephritis, and malakoplakia. An ultrastructural comparison. *Am J Clin Pathol* 1981;75:333–344.

430. Esparza AR, McKay DB, Cronan JJ, et al. Renal parenchymal malakoplakia. Histologic spectrum and its relationship to megalocytic interstitial nephritis and xanthogranulomatous pyelonephritis. *Am J Surg Pathol* 1989;13:225–236.

431. Lou TY, Teplitz C. Malakoplakia: pathogenesis and ultrastructural morphogenesis. A problem of altered macrophage (phagolysosomal) response. *Hum Pathol* 1974;5:191–207.

432. Stanton MJ, Maxted W. Malakoplakia: a study of the literature and current concepts of pathogenesis, diagnosis and treatment. *J Urol* 1981;125:139–146.

433. Biggar WD, Crawford L, Cardella C, et al. Malakoplakia and immunosuppressive therapy. Reversal of clinical and leukocyte abnormalities after withdrawal of prednisone and azathioprine. *Am J Pathol* 1985;119:5–11.

434. McClure J. Malakoplakia. *J Pathol* 1983;140:275–330.

435. Dobyan DC, Truong LD, Eknoyan G. Renal malacoplakia reappraised. *Am J Kidney Dis* 1993;22:243–252.

436. Saleem MA, Milford DV, Raafat F, et al. Renal parenchymal malakoplakia—a case report and review of the literature. *Pediatr Nephrol* 1993;7:256–258.

437. Hartman DS, Davis CJ Jr, Lichtenstein JE, et al. Renal parenchymal malacoplakia. *Radiology* 1980;136:33–42.

438. Cadnapaphornchai P, Rosenberg BF, Taher S, et al. Renal parenchymal malakoplakia an unusual cause of renal failure. *N Engl J Med* 1978;299:1110–1113.

439. Mokrzycki MH, Yamase H, Kohn OF. Renal malacoplakia with papillary necrosis and renal failure. *Am J Kidney Dis* 1992;19:587–591.

440. Tam VKK, Kung WH, Li R, et al. Renal parenchymal malacoplakia: a rare cause of ARF with a review of recent literature. *Am J Kidney Dis* 2003;41:E13–E17.

441. Wielenberg AJ, Demos TC, Rangachari B, et al. Malacoplakia presenting as a solitary renal mass. *AJR Am J Roentgenol* 2004;183:1703–1705.

442. Ravel R. Megalocytic interstitial nephritis. An entity probably related to malakoplakia. *Am J Clin Pathol* 1967;47:781–789.

443. Jander HP, Pujara S, Murad TM. Tumefactive megalocytic interstitial nephritis. *Radiology* 1978;129:635–636.

444. Mizunoe S, Yamasaki T, Tokimatsu I, et al. Sarcoidosis associated with renal masses on computed tomography. *Intern Med* 2006;45:279–282.

445. Dember LM. Amyloidosis-associated kidney disease. *J Am Soc Nephrol* 2006;17:3458–3471.

446. Gandhi D, Wee R, Goyal M. CT and MR imaging of intracerebral amyloidoma: case report and review of the literature. *Am J Neuroradiol* 2003;24:519–522.

447. Yang MC, Blutreich A, Das K. Nodular pulmonary amyloidosis with an unusual protein composition diagnosed by fine-needle aspiration biopsy: a case report. *Diagn Cytopathol* 2009;37:286–289.

448. Garcia CA, Abell-Aleff PC, Gamb SI, et al. Ultrastructural analysis of amyloidoma. *Ultrastruct Pathol* 2009;33:123–127.

449. Coffin CM, Watterson J, Priest JR, et al. Extrapulmonary inflammatory myofibroblastic tumor (inflammatory pseudotumor). A clinicopathologic and immunohistochemical study of 84 cases. *Am J Surg Pathol* 1995;19:859–872.

450. Coffin CM, Humphrey PA, Dehner LP. Extrapulmonary inflammatory myofibroblastic tumor: a clinical and pathological survey. *Semin Diagn Pathol* 1998;15:85–101.

451. Harik LR, Merino C, Coindre J-M, et al. Pseudosarcomatous myofibroblastic proliferations of the bladder: a clinicopathologic study of 42 cases. *Am J Surg Pathol* 2006;30:787–794.

452. Young RH. Tumor-like lesions of the urinary bladder. *Mod Pathol* 2009;22:S37–S52.

453. Horn LC, Reuter S, Biesold M. Inflammatory pseudotumor of the ureter and the urinary bladder. *Pathol Res Pract* 1997;193:607–612.

454. Harper L, Michel J-L, Riviere J-P, et al. Inflammatory pseudotumor of the ureter. *J Pediatr Surg* 2005;40:597–599.

455. Ho P-H, Chen S-Y, Hsueh C, et al. Inflammatory myofibroblastic tumor of renal pelvis presenting with prolonged fever and abdominal pain in children: report of 1 case and review of literature. *J Pediatr Surg* 2005;40:e35–e37.

456. Boo Y-J, Kim J, Kim J-H, et al. Inflammatory myofibroblastic tumor of the kidney in a child: report of a case. *Surg Today* 2006;36:710–713.

457. Larbcharoensub N, Chobpradit N, Kijvikai K, et al. Primary renal inflammatory myofibroblastic tumor. *Urol Int* 2006;76:94–96.

458. Kapusta LR, Weiss MA, Ramsay J, et al. Inflammatory myofibroblastic tumors of the kidney: a clinicopathologic and immunohistochemical study of 12 cases. *Am J Surg Pathol* 2003;27:658–666.

459. Li JY, Yong TY, Coleman M, et al. Bilateral renal inflammatory pseudotumour effectively treated with corticosteroid. *Clin Exp Nephrol* 2010;14:190–198.

460. Gupta P, Dhingra KK, Singhal S, et al. Inflammatory myofibroblastic tumour of the kidney with a papillary adenoma. *Pathology* 2010;42:193–196.

461. Coffin CM, Patel A, Perkins S, et al. ALK1 and p80 expression and chromosomal rearrangements involving 2p23 in inflammatory myofibroblastic tumor. *Mod Pathol* 2001;14:569–576.

462. Lawrence B, Perez-Atayde A, Hibbard MK, et al. TPM3-ALK and TPM4-ALK oncogenes in inflammatory myofibroblastic tumors. *Am J Pathol* 2000;157:377–384.

463. Cook JR, Dehner LP, Collins MH, et al. Anaplastic lymphoma kinase (ALK) expression in the inflammatory myofibroblastic tumor: a comparative immunohistochemical study. *Am J Surg Pathol* 2001;25:1364–1371.

464. Sukov WR, Cheville JC, Carlson AW, et al. Utility of ALK-1 protein expression and ALK rearrangements in distinguishing inflammatory myofibroblastic tumor from malignant spindle cell lesions of the urinary bladder. *Mod Pathol* 2007;20:592–603.

465. Williams ME, Longmaid HE, Trey G, et al. Renal failure resulting from infiltration by inflammatory myofibroblastic tumor responsive to corticosteroid therapy. *Am J Kidney Dis* 1998;31:E5.

466. Hojo H, Newton WA Jr, Hamoudi AB, et al. Pseudosarcomatous myofibroblastic tumor of the urinary bladder in children: a study of 11 cases with review of the literature. An Intergroup Rhabdomyosarcoma Study. *Am J Surg Pathol* 1995;19:1224–1236.

467. Hori J-I, Komiyama M. A case of inflammatory myofibroblastic tumor of the kidney with cystic change. *Jpn J Clin Oncol* 2009;39:410.

468. Montgomery EA, Shuster DD, Burkart AL, et al. Inflammatory myofibroblastic tumors of the urinary tract: a clinicopathologic study of 46 cases, including a malignant example inflammatory fibrosarcoma and a subset associated with high-grade urothelial carcinoma. *Am J Surg Pathol* 2006;30:1502–1512.

469. Ryu KH, Im CM, Kim MK, et al. Inflammatory myofibroblastic tumor of the kidney misdiagnosed as renal cell carcinoma. *J Korean Med Sci* 2010;25:330–332.

470. Gelb AB, Simmons ML, Weidner N. Solitary fibrous tumor involving the renal capsule. *Am J Surg Pathol* 1996;20:1288–1295.

471. Magro G, Cavallaro V, Torrisi A, et al. Intrarenal solitary fibrous tumor of the kidney report of a case with emphasis on the differential diagnosis in the wide spectrum of monomorphous spindle cell tumors of the kidney. *Pathol Res Pract* 2002;198:37–43.

Tumors of the Kidney

BRETT DELAHUNT, DAVID J. GRIGNON, and JOHN N. EBLE

CLASSIFICATION

The classification of tumors of the kidney has changed a great deal in the past three decades. The modern era of classification of epithelial tumors began in 1986 with the Mainz classification that was based on cytoplasmic staining characteristics and ultrastructural features.[1] This was followed by proposals based on the emerging recognition of the cytogenetic characteristics of these tumors[2] that expanded our understanding of this group of tumors. These led to classification schemes proposed at meetings held in Heidelberg[3] in 1996 and at the Mayo Clinic[4] in 1997 that formed the basis for the World Health Organization classification that subsequently gained near-uniform acceptance.[5,6] In 2012, the International Society of Urologic Pathology (ISUP) held a consensus conference to review and update the 2004 WHO classification. The recommendations of this group are included in the following discussions. The past few years have also seen changes in the classification of mesenchymal tumors of the kidney. This system is summarized in Table 2-1 and forms the basis for the following discussions.[7] Readers interested in a more detailed discussion of the history of the classification of renal cell carcinoma (RCC) are referred to the review by Delahunt and Eble.[8] Urothelial neoplasms of the renal pelvis are discussed in Chapter 4.

EPITHELIAL TUMORS—BENIGN

Papillary Adenoma

Introduction

Renal adenoma was first utilized as a diagnostic category for renal neoplasia in the classification proposed by Sturm in 1875. In this and subsequent classifications, it was noted that adenomas could be solitary or multiple and may show transformation into malignant tumors. In later studies, adenomas were distinguished from carcinomas on the basis of size, circumscription, and absence of metastases, and both papillary and alveolar forms were described.[9] A number of authors noted difficulties in distinguishing between adenoma and their malignant counterparts, and in some series giant forms were diagnosed on the basis of low-grade nuclear pleomorphism and lack of metastases.

In 1938, Bell proposed a classification of renal neoplasia based upon the findings of 30,000 autopsies and defined renal adenoma as tumors <3 cm in diameter. He further differentiated between these and multiple adenomas associated with atherosclerotic kidneys, for which he claimed there was no evidence of malignant potential.[10] Bell expanded his series in 1950, noting that tumors <3 cm in diameter rarely formed metastases. Somewhat paradoxically, he also noted that all solid adenomas appeared to be small carcinomas.[11]

Several studies investigated the importance of tumor size in differentiating renal adenoma and carcinoma, with metastasis being demonstrated in primary tumors as small as 9 mm in diameter. In the Mainz classification published in 1986, renal adenomas were defined as low-grade tumors <1 cm in diameter.[1] In this classification adenomas were not identified on the basis of morphology, implying that all small, well-differentiated, renal cortical tumors were benign.

Autopsy data have shown that localized papillary renal epithelial neoplasms <5 mm in diameter occur in up to 37% of adults.[12] From this, it was concluded that almost all small papillary neoplasms exhibit benign behavior and are probably incapable of progression without some transforming event. Based upon these observations, it has been proposed that the term papillary adenoma be confined to low-grade tumors of papillary or tubular architecture, measuring <5 mm in maximum diameter.[9] This recommendation was endorsed by the Heidelberg and Rochester consensus conferences and the workgroup that established the 2004 WHO classification of tumors of the kidney.[5] Small epithelial tumors other than these papillary ones should be classified as carcinomas regardless of size.

Epidemiology and Clinical Features

In several studies, small renal epithelial tumors were found in the renal cortex of 4% to 37% of autopsy patients.[12] Where

Table 2-1 ■ THE INTERNATIONAL SOCIETY OF UROLOGICAL PATHOLOGY VANCOUVER CLASSIFICATION OF RENAL NEOPLASIA

Renal cell tumors
  Papillary adenoma
  Oncocytoma
  Clear cell renal cell carcinoma
    Multilocular clear cell renal cell neoplasm of low
      malignant potential
  Papillary renal cell carcinoma
  Chromophobe renal cell carcinoma
    Hybrid oncocytic chromophobe tumor
  Carcinoma of the collecting ducts of Bellini
  Renal medullary carcinoma
  MiT family translocation renal cell carcinoma
    Xp11 translocation renal cell carcinoma
    t(6;11) renal cell carcinoma
  Carcinoma associated with neuroblastoma
  Mucinous tubular and spindle cell carcinoma
  Tubulocystic renal cell carcinoma
  Acquired cystic disease–associated renal cell
    carcinoma
  Clear cell papillary renal cell carcinoma
  Hereditary leiomyomatosis-associated renal cell
    carcinoma
  Renal cell carcinoma, unclassified
Metanephric tumors
  Metanephric adenoma
  Metanephric adenofibroma
  Metanephric stromal tumors
Nephroblastic tumors
  Nephrogenic rests
  Nephroblastoma
Mesenchymal tumors
Occurring mainly in children
  Clear cell sarcoma
  Rhabdoid tumor
  Congenital mesoblastic nephroma
  Ossifying renal tumor of infants

Occurring mainly in adults
  Leiomyosarcoma (including renal vein)
  Angiosarcoma
  Rhabdomyosarcoma
  Malignant fibrous histiocytoma
  Hemangiopericytoma
  Osteosarcoma
  Synovial sarcoma
  Angiomyolipoma
    Epithelioid angiomyolipoma
  Leiomyoma
  Hemangioma
  Lymphangioma
  Juxtaglomerular cell tumor
  Renomedullary interstitial cell tumor
  Schwannoma
  Solitary fibrous tumor
Mixed mesenchymal and epithelial tumors
  Cystic nephroma/mixed epithelial and stromal tumor
Neuroendocrine tumors
  Carcinoid (low-grade neuroendocrine tumor)
  Neuroendocrine carcinoma (high-grade neuroendocrine
    tumor)
  Primitive neuroectodermal tumor
  Neuroblastoma
  Pheochromocytoma
Hematopoietic and lymphoid tumors
  Lymphoma
  Leukemia
  Plasmacytoma
Germ cell tumors
  Teratoma
  Choriocarcinoma
Metastatic tumors
Other tumors

Modified from Srigley JR, Delahunt B, Eble JN, et al. Vancouver classification of renal neoplasia. *Am J Surg Pathol* 2013; In press.

detailed sectioning of the kidney was undertaken, these were detected in 10% of individuals aged 21 to 40 years and 40% of those aged 70 to 90 years. Papillary adenomas occur more frequently in sclerotic kidneys associated with renal vascular disease, and their occurrence has been positively correlated with chronic tobacco use.[13,14] Papillary adenomas are more commonly seen in patients on long-term hemodialysis and have been reported in 33% of patients with acquired cystic renal disease.[15] In a more recent series, renal adenomas were found in 14% of patients undergoing transplantation for end-stage renal disease, with increased occurrence independently associated with male sex, older age, and longer dialysis duration.[16] Papillary adenomas have been reported in kidneys bearing RCCs.[17]

Virtually all papillary adenomas are clinically silent and are detected in kidneys removed for other reasons. The use of high-definition modern imaging techniques does allow for the detection of papillary adenomas in vivo.

Pathology

Gross Features

Papillary adenomas are usually confined to the renal cortex and are often subcapsular in distribution. On sectioning they are gray or tan or yellow, and larger adenomas are often wedge shaped, with the base adjacent to the cortical surface.[9] In some instances, numerous papillary adenomas may be present in the same kidney, and the term renal adenomatosis is applied.

Microscopic Features

Papillary adenomas show a papillary, tubular, or tubulopapillary architecture.[9] Tumor cells have basophilic to eosinophilic cytoplasm, and either a type 1 or type 2 morphology (Figs. 2-1 through 2-4), as described for papillary RCC, may be present. Similarly, cytoplasmic clearing can be present, and this should not lead to a diagnosis of clear

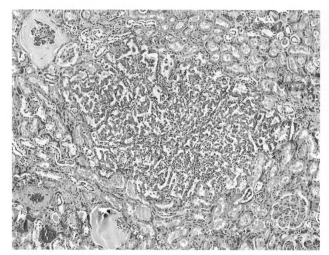

FIGURE 2-1 ■ Papillary adenoma type 1 arising in the renal cortex.

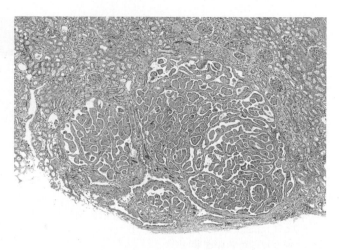

FIGURE 2-3 ■ Papillary adenoma type 2 arising in the renal cortex just beneath the renal capsule. The branching pattern of the papillae is simpler than that of papillary adenoma type 1.

cell RCC. The nuclei are round to oval with stippled to clumped chromatin. Nuclear grooves are often seen. There is minimal nuclear pleomorphism, nucleoli are inconspicuous, and mitotic figures are rarely identified. Aggregates of foamy macrophages and psammoma bodies may be present in papillary adenomas; however, necrosis and hemorrhage are rare. Small papillary adenomas are usually not encapsulated and blend with adjacent benign tubular epithelium. Larger adenomas may be enclosed by a partial or fully investing thin connective tissue capsule.[18] In rare instances, adenomatous proliferation is confined to the Bowman capsule, and this is most commonly seen in individuals with hepatic malignancy.[19]

Ancillary and Special Studies
Most adenomas show positive expression of epithelial membrane antigen, cytokeratin 7, low molecular weight cytokeratin, and high molecular weight cytokeratin. There is usually positive expression for alpha-methylacyl-CoA-racemase

(AMACR) and peanut agglutinin, while NSE and α-1-antitrypsin are occasionally positive.[20,21]

Genetics
Papillary adenomas may be either diploid or aneuploid[22] and frequently show trisomy 7 and 17.[23] The common genetic abnormalities and frequent presence in end-stage kidneys have led to the hypothesis that these are the precursor lesions for papillary carcinoma.[24] In parallel with the immunohistochemical phenotype of these tumors, ultrastructural studies show adenomas to have features of either proximal or distal convoluted tubules.[25]

Differential Diagnosis

Papillary adenoma should be differentiated from papillary RCC. The presence of significant nuclear pleomorphism, infiltration of adjacent renal tissue, and tumor size >5 mm excludes a diagnosis of papillary adenoma.

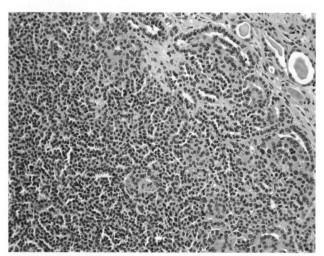

FIGURE 2-2 ■ Papillary adenoma type 1 growing with closely packed papillae giving an appearance of solidity.

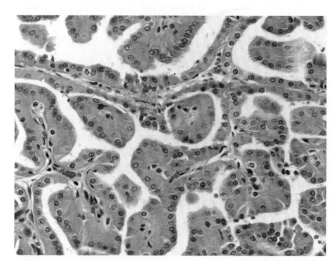

FIGURE 2-4 ■ Papillary adenoma type 2 showing pseudostratification of nuclei and voluminous eosinophilic cytoplasm.

Prognosis and Treatment

Papillary adenomas are benign tumors, although in kidneys with papillary adenomatosis there may be coexisting papillary RCC. Papillary adenoma detected incidentally on imaging studies should show no significant growth when followed serially. These tumors are of some importance if detected in kidneys intended for transplantation. Current protocols indicate that the presence of renal adenoma in a donor kidney is not a contraindication for renal transplantation.

Renal Oncocytoma

Introduction

Renal oncocytoma was firmly established as a distinct category of renal neoplasia by Klein and Valensi in 1976,[26] although the potential for malignant behavior by these tumors continued to be debated.[27] The detailed study of large series of oncocytoma has subsequently confirmed the benign nature of these tumors.

Epidemiology

In large series, patient ages range from 24 to 91 years (mean 65 to 73 years), although multiple and bilateral oncocytic neoplasms have been reported in a 10-year-old male.[28–33]

In a population-based study, the age standardized incidence of oncocytoma was 0.3 per 100,000, with a male-to-female ratio of 1.7:1.[30] In this series, oncocytomas constituted 5.5% of renal epithelial neoplasms (excluding renal adenomas), and in a separate study, the proportion of oncocytomas within a cohort of 1,043 renal tumors increased with increasing decade of life.[34]

Clinical Features

Approximately 80% of oncocytomas are asymptomatic and are diagnosed as an incidental finding in patients undergoing investigation for unrelated disease or at autopsy. For symptomatic tumors, hematuria (32%), abdominal flank pain (29%), and weight loss (10%) are the most common presenting features.[30] Occasionally, oncocytoma presents as an abdominal mass, and rarely the tumor has been associated with hypertension or erythrocytosis.

Radiologic features of oncocytoma are the presence of a central stellate scar, a "spoke-wheel" pattern of peripheral arteries with the absence of intraneoplastic vascular disarray, an homogeneous capillary phase on renography, and the presence of a so-called lucent rim. While these features are frequently seen in oncocytoma, they may also be seen in other types of renal neoplasia.

Pathology

Gross Features

Oncocytomas are highly variable in size ranging up to 26 cm in maximum extent, with mean diameters of 4.4 to 5.5 cm being reported.[29–31,35] Tumors discovered incidentally

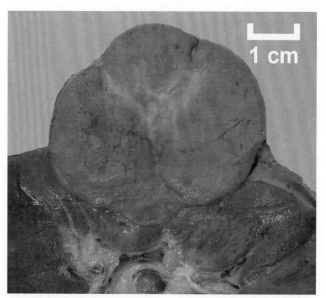

FIGURE 2-5 ■ Renal oncocytoma. This formalin-fixed specimen shows the characteristic brown color and the central zone of edematous stroma that is common in oncocytomas.

or at autopsy are often smaller, with a mean diameter of 3.8 cm.[30] On sectioning, oncocytomas are usually well circumscribed with a pushing rather than an infiltrative margin (Fig. 2-5). In most cases, a tumor capsule is not visible. Infrequently, the tumor extends into perirenal fat, and macroscopic extension of tumor into vessels is seen rarely.[29,33,36] In such cases, the diagnosis of oncocytoma should be made with caution. The cut surface of the tumor has a characteristic mahogany brown color with a homogenous consistency. In larger tumors, there is frequently a central zone of whitish, often myxoid stroma, which is usually irregular and stellate, being described as a central stellate scar. Bands of connective tissue may extend from this central scar to the periphery of the tumor, resulting in superficial bosselation. Foci of confluent hemorrhage are frequently present usually at the periphery of the tumor. Extensive necrosis is not a feature of oncocytoma, although areas of cystic degeneration may be present.

Microscopic Features

Oncocytomas may show a variable morphology. The predominant pattern is growth as tightly packed nests producing a sheet-like arrangement of the cells with inconspicuous blood vessels (Fig. 2-6). A common and more characteristic pattern is islands composed of oncocytoma cells within loose edematous connective tissue (Fig. 2-7). Less frequently, cysts ranging from microscopic up to a few millimeters in diameter are present. Rarely, groups of tumor cells contain hyaline deposits of type IV collagen resulting in a cylindromatous appearance (Fig. 2-8).[37]

Oncocytoma cells have moderate to abundant intensely finely granular eosinophilic cytoplasm. The nuclei are usually ovoid to round with stippled chromatin, and binucleate cells are often present. Nucleoli are frequent but are small to

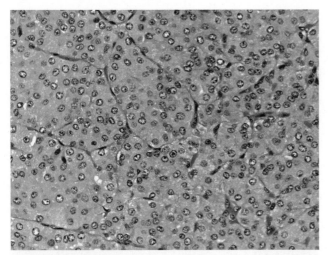

FIGURE 2-6 ■ Renal oncocytoma. This is the compact growth pattern in which sheets of oncocytoma cells are divided into nests by delicate blood vessels. The nuclei are nearly spherical, and many contain visible nucleoli.

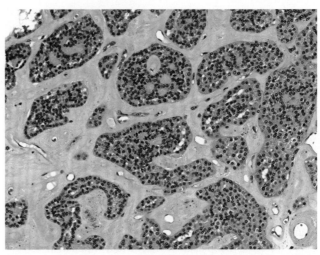

FIGURE 2-8 ■ Renal oncocytoma. The tumor is growing in nests with type IV collagen deposition producing a cylindromatous pattern.

inconspicuous. Cells showing moderate to marked nuclear pleomorphism are frequently seen in oncocytoma and are degenerative in nature, not being associated with prominent nucleoli or mitotic activity (Fig. 2-9). Focally, aggregates of tumor cells may have scanty cytoplasm (so-called oncoblasts) giving rise to apparent increased cellularity that blends with more typical oncocytes. Extracellular hyalinization, predominantly involving the walls of small vessels, is frequently seen in oncocytoma. Very occasionally, foci of dystrophic calcification or ossification may be present within the stroma. In 5% of cases, extension of tumor into small vessels may be seen, while 10% of tumors have microscopic extension into perirenal fat (Fig. 2-10). In neither instance does this appear to have any prognostic significance. Detailed comparison of oncocytomas with and without vascular infiltration show identical morphologic, genetic, and immunohistochemical features.[36]

Ancillary and Special Studies

The immunohistochemical phenotype of oncocytoma varies somewhat between studies. CD15, CD117, E-cadherin, claudin 7, claudin 8, S-100A1 protein, pancytokeratin, low molecular weight cytokeratin, *Ron* protooncogene, BCL2, antimitochondrial antibody, and EMA immunostaining are usually positive.[38–45] Tumors show only occasional positivity for CD10, RCC antigen, caveolin-1, parvalbumin, and AMACR.[43,45–47] Cytokeratin 7 expression has been reported in up to 100% of cases in some series with expression having a characteristic pattern of strongly positive single cells or small groups of cells in areas of compact growth and in many of the cells within areas of edematous stroma (Fig. 2-11A and B).[45] Cytokeratin 8, 18, and 20 also show focal positive expression, which is usually dot-like or perinuclear.[48,49] In areas of compact growth the oncocytic cells give negative reactions for vimentin, but within areas of edematous

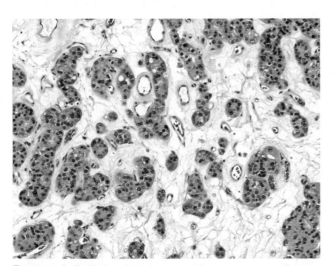

FIGURE 2-7 ■ Renal oncocytoma. The oncocytoma cells grow as islands in a background of edematous stroma.

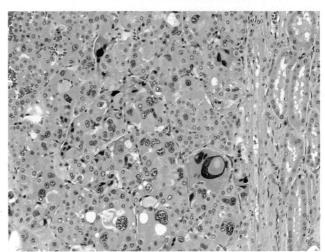

FIGURE 2-9 ■ Renal oncocytoma showing a focus of cells in which the nuclei vary widely in size and shape.

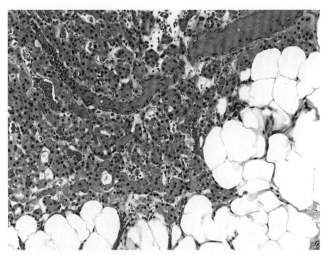

FIGURE 2-10 ■ Renal oncocytoma invading the perinephric fat.

stroma many of the cells give positive reactions (Fig. 2-11C and D). The tumor cells are generally negative with the Hale colloidal iron stain. Some authors will accept staining with Hale colloidal iron in oncocytoma when it is limited to the luminal aspect of cells in areas with tubule formation.[50] It is not uncommon to find hemosiderin pigment in oncocytoma that will react positively with the Hale colloidal iron.

Electron microscopy shows the cells of oncocytoma to have abundant mitochondria while other organelles are scanty (Fig. 2-12). Surface microvilli are sparse, and completely formed brush borders are not usually present. Lipid vacuoles and glycogen are rarely seen. The microvesicles of chromophobe RCC are not seen in oncocytomas.

Genetics

A variety of genetic abnormalities are associated with renal oncocytoma and three characteristic mutational patterns are

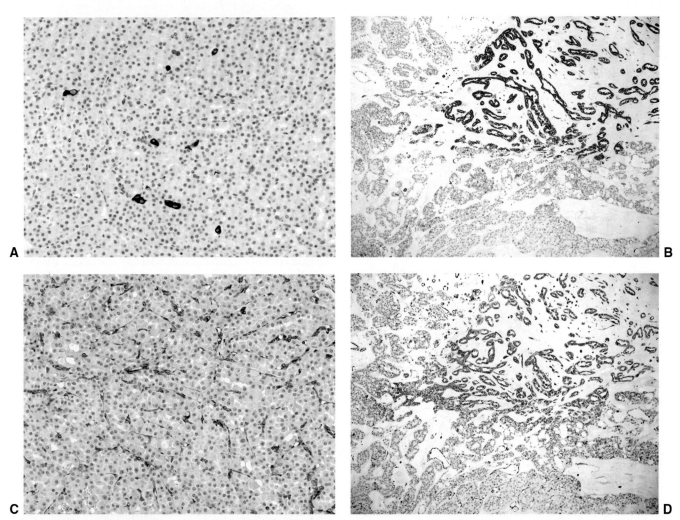

FIGURE 2-11 ■ **A:** Renal oncocytoma. Immunohistochemistry for cytokeratin 7 decorates a few scattered cells and small groups of cells in an area of compact growth similar to that seen in Figure 2-6. **B:** Immunohistochemistry for cytokeratin 7 stains most of the oncocytoma cells in an area where the growth is narrow islands in edematous stroma. In the rest of the photograph, the reaction is the same as is shown in **(A)**. **C:** Immunohistochemistry for vimentin decorates only blood vessels in an area of compact growth similar to that seen in Figure 2-6. **D:** Immunohistochemistry for vimentin stains most of the oncocytoma cells in an area where the growth is narrow islands in edematous stroma. In the rest of the photograph, the reaction is the same as is shown in **(A)**.

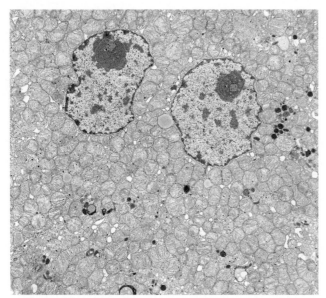

FIGURE 2-12 ■ Renal oncocytoma. Electron microscopy shows the cytoplasm of the oncocytoma cells to be filled with mitochondria.

recognized. The most common abnormality is loss of the whole of chromosome 1 or part of its short or long arm, and loss of chromosome Y.[51–53] Rearrangements of 11q13, especially the translocation t(5;11) (q35;q13), and chromosome 14 deletions are also seen.[53–55] Oncocytomas often show mosaicism, and in some tumors there is evidence of microsatellite instability.[56] Fluorescence in situ hybridization (FISH) analysis has been shown to differentiate oncocytoma from chromophobe RCCs, with the loss of two or more of chromosomes 1, 2, 6, 10, and 17 favoring a diagnosis of chromophobe RCC.[57]

Oncocytosis

Oncocytomas are usually solitary; however, multifocal or bilateral tumors are seen in 5% of cases. In rare instances, numerous tumors of varying size may be present in both kidneys, and the terms oncocytosis and oncocytomatosis have been applied (Fig. 2-13).[58,59] In cases of renal oncocytosis, not only are tumors resembling oncocytomas present but coexisting tumors resembling chromophobe RCC and unique tumors that look like mixtures of oncocytoma and chromophobe RCC are often present (Figs. 2-14, 2-15A and B). A hallmark of oncocytosis is the presence of numerous minute patches of oncocytic cells throughout the renal cortex (Fig. 2-16). The classification of these tumors remains uncertain; in the current ISUP classification, these are placed as a variant of chromophobe RCC.[7] Genetic studies have demonstrated the absence of the characteristic findings of both chromophobe RCC and of renal oncocytoma, and some authors have suggested the designation renal cell neoplasm of oncocytosis to reflect their unique characteristics.[60] This is the term we are currently using for these tumors. Little is known of the behavior of these tumors though to date metastases have not been described.[59,60]

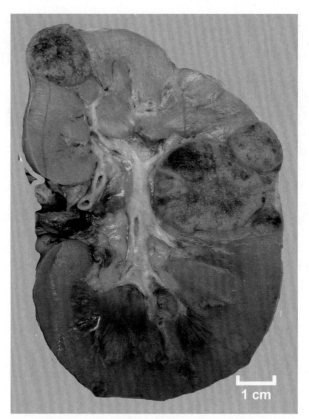

FIGURE 2-13 ■ Oncocytosis. This gross photograph shows multiple yellow to brown tumors of varying size.

Differential Diagnosis

Oncocytomas must be differentiated from other renal tumors that can have eosinophilic cytoplasm (Box 2-1). This includes variants of clear cell RCC with granular eosinophilic cytoplasm. The presence of clear cells (other than in edematous or fibrotic areas) or a papillary architecture excludes a diagnosis of oncocytoma. Other features indicative of malignancy

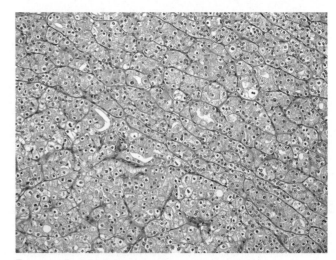

FIGURE 2-14 ■ Oncocytosis. Sections from this macroscopically visible tumor closely resemble renal oncocytoma or the eosinophilic variant of chromophobe renal cell carcinoma.

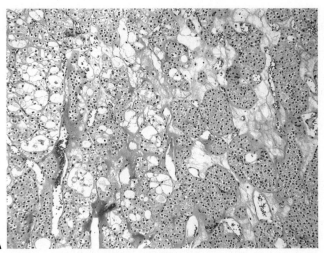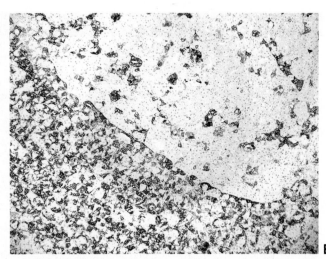

FIGURE 2-15 ■ **A:** Oncocytosis. This tumor shows areas resembling chromophobe renal cell carcinoma and areas resembling oncocytoma. Some have called these "hybrid" tumors. **B:** Immunohistochemistry for cytokeratin 7 shows areas with positive reactions similar to oncocytoma and others with positive reactions similar to chromophobe renal cell carcinoma.

that are not seen in oncocytoma are extensive perirenal fat or vascular invasion by tumor, confluent tumor necrosis, and any more than very occasional or atypical mitotic figures.

The principal differential diagnosis is the eosinophilic variant of chromophobe RCC (see Table 2-2). Oncocytomas rarely consist of diffuse sheets of cells, and neither perinuclear halos nor typical chromophobe cells are seen. The presence of wrinkled nuclei or basophilic intracytoplasmic inclusions is also suggestive of chromophobe RCC. Hale colloidal iron staining can be useful: oncocytomas give diffusely negative reactions. Immunohistochemical expression does assist in differentiating between those two tumor types. While there is some overlap in cytokeratin 7, cytokeratin 20, and CD15 expression, it has been proposed that in combination this panel has diagnostic utility. In particular, it has been shown that the

oncocytoma-specific immunoprofile of scattered strongly cytokeratin 7–positive cells or occasionally completely negative staining for cytokeratin 7 correctly classified 90% of cases of oncocytoma and all cases of chromophobe RCC.[43] Usually chromophobe RCC shows diffuse positivity for cytokeratin 7, with membrane-like expression at the cell margin.

Tumors described under the term oncocytic papillary RCC should present little diagnostic difficulty as anything more than minute and focal papillary projections within neoplastic tubules excludes a diagnosis of oncocytoma. In some areas, so-called oncocytic papillary RCC may have a solid oncocytoma-like growth pattern; however, unlike oncocytoma, these areas are usually positive for AMACR, EMA, vimentin, and CD10.[61]

Prognosis and Treatment

It is now accepted that oncocytomas are benign tumors. When correctly characterized, no case of oncocytoma has been shown to develop metastases.

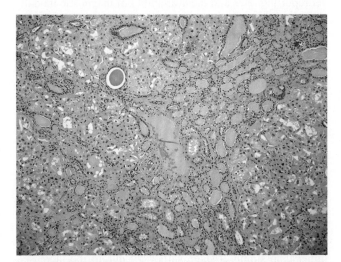

FIGURE 2-16 ■ Oncocytosis. In kidneys from patients with oncocytosis, there are numerous microscopic lesions composed of cells with eosinophilic cytoplasm identical to those of the renal tumors of oncocytosis.

Box 2-1 ● TUMORS THAT CAN HAVE PINK CYTOPLASM
• Oncocytoma
• Chromophobe renal cell carcinoma
• Clear cell renal cell carcinoma
• Papillary adenoma
• Papillary renal cell carcinoma
• Collecting duct carcinoma
• Medullary carcinoma
• Translocation-associated renal cell carcinoma
• Acquired cystic disease–associated renal cell carcinoma
• Renal cell carcinoma of hereditary leiomyomatosis and renal cell carcinoma syndrome
• Epithelioid angiomyolipoma
• Unclassified renal cell carcinoma

Table 2-2 ■ PATHOLOGIC FEATURES OF ONCOCYTOMA VERSUS CHROMOPHOBE CARCINOMA

Feature	Oncocytoma	Chromophobe Carcinoma—Eosinophilic type
Gross appearance	"Mahogany" brown +/− central scar	Pale tan-brown +/− zones of necrosis
Architecture	Closely packed nests (periphery) and nests in loose hypocellular stroma No trabeculae/sheets Tubule formation frequent	Closely packed nests and occasional streaming of cells in edematous myxoid stroma +/− broad trabeculae/sheets +/− tubule formation
Nuclear features	Uniform, round Degenerative pleomorphism	Uniform, round +/− raisinoid Pleomorphism only in high grade
Mitoses	None to very rare	Occasional
Cytoplasm	Granular, acidophilic Clearing can be seen	Granular, acidophilic with perinuclear halos Plant-like cells focally in some
Hales colloidal iron	Negative except at luminal surface in tubular areas	Strongly positive, diffuse
Cytokeratin	Positive CK7—isolated strongly positive cells (except in atrophic areas)	Positive CK7—diffuse, strongly positive in most
RCC antigen	Negative	50% positive (in some reports)
Vimentin	Negative (except atrophic areas)	Negative
Ultrastructure	Numerous mitochondria with lamellar cristae No microvesicles	Numerous mitochondria with tubulovesicular cristae Interspersed microvesicles

EPITHELIAL TUMORS—MALIGNANT

Clear Cell Renal Cell Carcinoma

Introduction

Clear cell RCC is the most common form of renal malignancy, comprising 70% of tumors in reported series. Although the morphology of these tumors was clearly described in early series, their relationship to the other subtypes of RCC remained uncertain. In 1855, Robin correctly speculated that these tumors were of renal tubular origin; however, this observation was overshadowed by the theory of Grawitz that clear cell (alveolar) RCC was of intrarenal adrenal rest origin.[8] Such was the influence of Grawitz that the term hypernephroma was adopted for these tumors, and this gained widespread currency. Despite ongoing debate as to the tissue of origin for clear cell RCC, it was not until 1959, when ultrastructural studies confirmed that tumor cells resembled proximal convoluted tubules epithelium,[62] that the question was finally settled.

Prior to the formulation of the Mainz classification in 1986, RCCs were classified according to morphologic features and as recently as 1998, the World Health Organization classification of renal tumors included clear cell RCC and granular cell RCC as separate categories of renal parenchymal malignancy. It is now clear that granular cell carcinoma, rather than being a separate diagnostic entity, consists of a variety of tumor types including clear cell RCC, chromophobe RCC, and collecting duct carcinoma. It is acknowledged that clear cell RCCs may have a granular and eosinophilic cytoplasm, and for this reason the term conventional RCC was proposed for these tumors at both the Heidelberg and Rochester Consensus Conferences.[3,4]

Despite this morphologic variability, clear cell RCC typically exhibit a characteristic vascular pattern and on genetic studies, almost always show mutation in chromosome 3p.[63,64]

Epidemiology

Although much of the epidemiologic data for RCC relate to mixed series of tumors, the majority of these tumors are the clear cell subtype. RCC accounts for 2% of all new cancer diagnoses worldwide and 3% in the United States of America.[65,66] There is a marked variation in the incidence of RCC internationally, and this is probably a reflection of cancer reporting rates and the availability of diagnostic modalities. It may also be influenced by differences in both risk factors and population genetics. The annual incidence of RCC in the United States has been increasing with tumors of the kidney and ureter accounting for an estimated 64,770 new cases and 13,570 cancer deaths in 2012.[67] This is not simply a reflection of population change but is the result of the increased use of axial imaging, as the age-adjusted incidence per 100,000 population has increased from 6.2 in 1972 to 9.6 in 1998.[68]

The increased utilization of imaging has resulted in the detection of small tumors as incidental findings, with the incidence of small asymptomatic tumors increasing from 15% to 60% in some series.[69] There is also a reported increase in the numbers of advanced-stage, symptomatic tumors, thus reflecting a true increase in tumor incidence, rather than simply a stage shift,[68,70,71] due to the increased detection of small malignancies.

Incidence rates also vary among ethnic groups and according to gender. In the United States of America, the highest incidence is seen in black males (11.5 per 100,000 population). This is slightly higher than that for white non-Hispanic (10.0/100,000 population) and white Hispanics (9.7 per 100,000 population), while that for those of Asian or Pacific Island descent is lower at 4.7 per 100,000 population. In these groups, the male-to-female ratio is relatively stable at 1.9 to 2.1 to 1.[72]

Metastatic disease is seen in approximately 25% to 30% of patients who present with RCC, and while incidence data have been derived by mathematical manipulation of tumor incidence figures, clinical data regarding the true prevalence of metastatic disease are not available.[73]

Localized (asymptomatic) tumors are associated with increased survival rates when compared to those who present with symptomatic disease. Of 4,000 cases of renal carcinoma treated surgically between 1983 and 1999, the disease-free survival for incidentally detected tumor was 73%, while that for symptomatic patients was 59%.[74] Over a 30-year period, disease-free survivals for all stages have increased with a reported doubling of survival rates between 1963–1973 and 1982–1992.[75] While this improvement in survival is largely due to the detection of tumors at a lower stage, survival rates have increased for all stages of renal carcinoma, suggesting an improvement in the management of tumors showing regional and metastatic spread.[76]

In large studies where cases were divided according to histologic subtype, the proportion of clear cell RCCs in each series ranged from 63% to 92% of tumors.[77–83] Patients ranged in age from 2 to 96 years with mean ages ranging from 56 to 64 years. There was a male predominance in all series, with the male-to-female ratio ranging from 1.1:1 to 2.8:1.

Pathogenesis

The major subtypes of RCC are associated with one or more specific genetic mutations, and a family history is associated with an increased risk for tumor development. In two studies, tumor in a first-degree relative was associated with a 1.6- and 2.5-fold risk of developing cancer,[84,85] while the risk to siblings was found to be 4% in an additional series.[86] Despite this, familial RCC syndromes account for only 4% of RCCs, and the majority of tumors occur sporadically (Table 2-3).[87,88]

A variety of risk factors for the development of RCC have been identified, and of these, the association with smoking and obesity are the most reproducible. The risk for developing renal carcinoma is increased 1.54 fold in males and 1.22 in females for those who smoke cigarettes. There is a significant dose-dependent effect for males, with a risk of 1.6× for those who smoke <10 cigarettes per day compared to 2.03× for those who smoke >20 cigarettes per day. The risk was found to decrease by 15% to 30%, 10 to 15 years after cessation of smoking.[89]

Obesity is a risk factor for RCC for both males and females, with the risk increasing by 24% for males and 34% for females for each 5 kg/m^3 increase in body mass index.[90] The role of nutrition in the development of RCC is less certain although consumption of meat, milk, margarine, oils, and butter is associated with greater risk, while consumption of vegetables and fruits has a protective effect.[69] There is also an association with physical activity, with lower risk among those who undertake recreational or occupational-related exercise.[91,92]

Diabetes mellitus, long-term dialysis, and hypertension have been shown to be associated with an increased risk for RCC[93,94]; however, this may be a function of associated obesity or the development of renal scarring. Although experimental animal studies have linked diuretics to the development of renal carcinoma, it is likely that hypertension itself, rather than its treatment, is a risk factor, with a relative risk of up to 2.0 being reported.[65]

RCC is probably not associated with aspirin or acetaminophen usage or alcohol consumption, although alcohol has been shown to have a preventative effect in some studies.[95,96]

Table 2-3 ■ HEREDITARY RENAL CELL CARCINOMA SYNDROMES

Syndrome	Genetics	Kidney Pathology
Von Hippel Lindau	*VHL* gene (3p25-26)	Cysts Clear cell RCC
Tuberous sclerosis	*TSC1* (9q34) *TSC2* (16p13)	Cysts Angiomyolipoma Clear cell RCC Papillary RCC Chromophobe RCC
Birt-Hogg-Dubé	*FLCN* (17p11.2)	BHD-associated RCC (so-called hybrid tumor) Clear cell RCC Papillary RCC
Hereditary leiomyomatosis and RCC	*FH* (1q42-43)	HLRCC-associated papillary RCC
Hereditary papillary RCC	*MET* (7q31)	Papillary RCC (type 1), Papillary adenoma
Chromosome 3 translocation	Unknown	Clear cell RCC
Hereditary paraganglioma	*SDHB* (1p36) *SDHC* (1q21) *SDHD* (11q23)	SDHB-associated RCC Clear cell RCC

RCC, renal cell carcinoma.

The role of occupation as a causative factor for RCC is debated. While most studies fail to demonstrate that occupation is a risk factor for RCC, in some reports, asbestos and trichloroethylene exposure has been implicated in tumor development.[97,98] In other studies, occupations associated with exposure to industrial toxins, such as oil refinery workers, firefighters, painters, printers, and metal workers, have been shown to have an increased risk for renal carcinoma; however, results appear inconsistent.[72,99]

Clinical Features

Increasing numbers of RCCs are found in asymptomatic patients, being detected as incidental findings during investigations for unrelated disease.[69] In large series of RCCs, with cases divided according to tumor subtype, 25% to 85% of patients with clear cell RCCs were asymptomatic at the time of diagnosis.[77,78,81,82]

Symptoms from RCC result from local tumor effects or from metastatic disease. The classic renal cancer triad of abdominal mass, flank pain, and hematuria, indicative of extrarenal extension of tumor and involvement of the renal outflow tract, is uncommon. In contemporary series, this is reported in <10% to 20% of mixed (predominantly clear cell) subtypes of RCC.[100,101]

Nonspecific systemic signs and symptoms, usually indicative of metastatic disease, are seen in 30% of patients. In descending order of frequency fatigue, weight loss, fever, nausea, and vomiting are most commonly encountered.[100] Rarer presenting features include night sweats, acute varicocele resulting from obstruction of the ipsilateral spermatic vein, and pathologic fracture.

RCC is unusual in that 10% to 40% of patients may develop a paraneoplastic syndrome (Table 2-4). These result from elaboration of tumor-related proteins or as a result of an immune response to tumor and in the case of RCC involve virtually all organ systems.[102] Hypertension is twice

as common in patients with RCC and is probably multifactorial in origin. Postulated mechanisms include renin hypersecretion, renal outflow tract obstruction, and tumor-related polycythemia.[102] Polycythemia results from the production of erythropoietin by tumor cells, which has been demonstrated in up to two-thirds of cases. Hepatic abnormalities, consisting of elevated alkaline phosphatase, transaminases, bilirubin, and gamma globulin are seen in approximately two-thirds of patients with RCC. Known as Stauffer syndrome, this is associated with the histologic features of hepatitis and usually resolves following tumor resection. The mechanism leading to these abnormalities of hepatic function is unknown, and this may be a cytokine effect or the result of the release of tumor-related hepatotoxins.[102] Hypercalcemia is the most common form of paraneoplastic syndrome associated with RCC and is usually indicative of advanced disease with 50% of patients having bony metastases.[103] In the absence of metastases, it is thought that tumor-related hypercalcemia results from elaboration of parathormone-related peptide. A wide variety of endocrine abnormalities are seen in association with RCC, and many of these are the result of release of hormones and hormone-like proteins by tumor cells. Similarly elevated glucagon or insulin may be present, and it is thought that this leads to the tumor-related abnormalities of glucose metabolism that are associated with this tumor type.[104] Anemia is frequently seen in patients with RCC.

Inflammation, occurring as a response to localized or metastatic tumor, results in increased circulating cytokines and other inflammatory mediators. The association between chronic inflammation and the development of amyloidosis is well recognized, and it is likely that this also has an important role in the pathogenesis of paraneoplastic neuropathy, myopathy, vasculitis, and nephropathy,[102] all of which are recognized in patients with RCC.

Pathology

Gross Features

Clear cell RCCs are typically solid globular masses that, when large, often deform the surface of the kidney (Fig. 2-17). Clear cell RCC is very prone to forming cysts and may be extensively cystic (Fig. 2-18). On sectioning, these tumors are frequently variegated with most tumors containing bright yellow areas reflecting the high lipid content of tumor cells. Foci of necrosis and recent and old hemorrhage are common, and these appear as red to tan-brown areas, while edematous stroma is white to gray. Cystic degeneration may be seen associated with areas of necrosis. Dystrophic calcification is seen in up to 15% of cases, and occasionally, there may be foci of intratumoral ossification. Firm white areas within tumors may indicate the presence of sarcomatoid carcinoma (Fig. 2-19).

When small, tumors are usually well circumscribed, confined to the renal cortex, and show an expansive, rather than an infiltrative growth pattern. There is often an investing

---

Table 2-4 ■ PARANEOPLASTIC SYNDROMES ASSOCIATED WITH RENAL CELL CARCINOMA

- Hypertension
- Polycythemia
- Hepatic dysfunction (Stauffer syndrome)
- Hypercalcemia
- Galactorrhea
- Cushing syndrome
- Hyperglycemia/hypoglycemia
- Amyloidosis
- Anemia
- Neuropathy
- Myopathy
- Vasculitis
- Coagulopathy
- Nephropathy (light chain nephropathy/membranous glomerulonephritis)
- Proteinopathy (prostaglandin, fibroblast growth factor, α-fetoprotein)

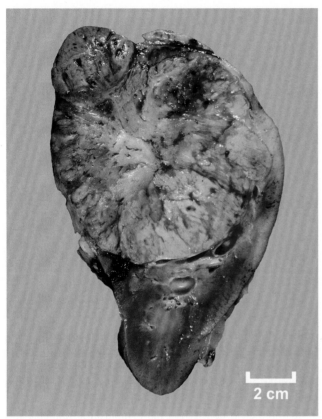

FIGURE 2-17 ■ Clear cell renal cell carcinoma. This gross photograph shows the typical variegated appearance with yellow-to-orange parenchyma with central areas of pale stroma, and foci of hemorrhage and necrosis. A few small cysts also are present.

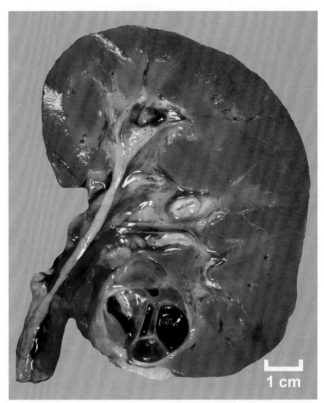

FIGURE 2-18 ■ Clear cell renal cell carcinoma. This gross photograph shows an extensively cystic tumor in the lower pole.

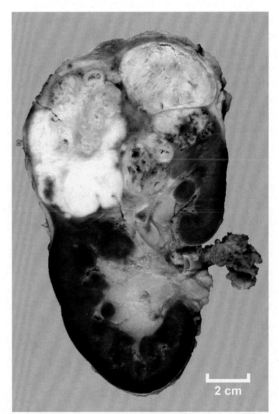

FIGURE 2-19 ■ Clear cell renal cell carcinoma. While the pale gray tissue at the superior end of the tumor is necrosis, the paler nearly white tissue is an area of sarcomatoid change.

pseudocapsule, which may be attenuated in some areas. Larger tumors are more frequently infiltrative and investing pseudocapsules, overgrown by tumor, may be represented by persistent fibrous bands within aggregates of malignant tissue.

Larger tumors often show a pronounced nodularity. Intrarenal metastatic spread may also occur, although in sporadic clear cell RCC true multifocality is uncommon. Larger peripheral tumors usually show expansion of the renal capsule, and this may adhere to adjacent perirenal fibroadipose tissue in the absence of direct infiltration. Tumor may also extend into the renal hilum and renal pelvis. Clear cell RCC often invades the renal venous system, occasionally filling the renal vein and extending into the vena cava or even the right atrium.

Microscopic Features

Clear cell RCC predominantly exhibits an alveolar architecture (Fig. 2-20), although microcystic, tubular, and pseudopapillary areas may also be seen (Fig. 2-21). These tumors consist of nests of cells, often with inconspicuous lumens containing eosinophilic proteinaceous fluid and freshly extravasated erythrocytes. Where the lumens are larger, the alveoli take on the appearance of compressed tubules. Often there is also cyst formation, usually with intraluminal exudate. Occasionally, cysts are traversed by trabeculae of fibrovascular tissue lined by tumor cells.

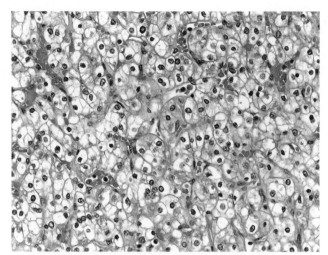

FIGURE 2-20 ■ Clear cell renal cell carcinoma. This photomicrograph shows the characteristic architecture of alveolar nests of carcinoma cells surrounded by extremely delicate blood vessels.

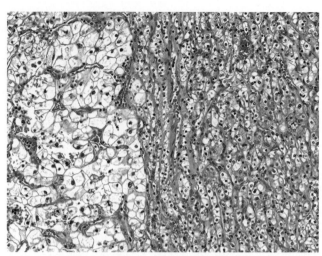

FIGURE 2-22 ■ Clear cell renal cell carcinoma with zones composed of large cells and of smaller cells.

A feature of clear cell RCC is the presence of a network of fine vessels that surround tumor nests. These are thin walled and of a uniformly small caliber. This vascular pattern is not seen in other subtypes of RCC and is of considerable diagnostic utility.

Occasionally an apparent papillary architecture may be present focally. On careful inspection there is cellular degeneration with formation of pseudopapillary structures. Very rarely true papillae are found; however, many if not all of these tumors would now be classified as clear cell papillary RCC or translocation carcinoma.

The cells of clear cell RCC have moderate to abundant, pale to clear cytoplasm. The clarity of the cytoplasm is the result of tissue processing, which causes the dissolution of cytoplasmic lipids and cholesterol. In unfixed tissues, lipid stains reveal intracytoplasmic lipid, while in fixed tissues periodic acid–Schiff staining shows the presence of

intracytoplasmic glycogen. Although the cytoplasmic volume of clear cell RCC is variable, it is typical that the cells in one area of a tumor are similar in size (Fig. 2-22). Cell borders are usually clearly visible, although they lack the prominence associated with chromophobe RCC.

In some clear cell RCCs, the cytoplasm is granular and eosinophilic. This is a feature more commonly seen in carcinomas exhibiting higher degrees of nuclear pleomorphism. Occasionally, the cytoplasm may contain numerous eosinophilic inclusions, and rarely granular melanin-like inclusions may also be seen. In some tumors there are hyaline eosinophilic globules that may occupy much of the cytoplasm of individual cells. When present, the globules may also be seen in the tumor interstitium, and these show positive staining with periodic acid–Schiff. Mucin is very rarely found in tumors with clear cytoplasm. This is not a feature of clear cell RCC, and mucin-containing clear cell tumors are more appropriately categorized as RCC, unclassified.

The nuclei of clear cell RCC show varying degrees of pleomorphism. Well-differentiated tumors have ovoid to round nuclei with inconspicuous basophilic nucleoli. More pleomorphic nuclei are larger and angulated, with granular chromatin and a prominent eosinophilic nucleolus. Tumor giant cells are frequently present in poorly differentiated tumors.

The presence of cells with a rhabdoid (Fig. 2-23) or sarcomatoid morphology is indicative of high-grade disease and results from the metaplasia of malignant epithelial cells. Rhabdoid differentiation is seen in 4% of clear cell RCC and is characterized by the presence of cells with abundant granular and eosinophilic cytoplasm, and a large eccentric irregular nucleus with a prominent eosinophilic nucleolus.[105,106] Rhabdoid differentiation is usually focal and even if extensive, areas of typical clear cell RCC are usually found, although this may require extensive sampling of the tumor.

Sarcomatoid differentiation is seen in approximately 5% of clear cell RCCs.[107] These tumors have a sarcoma-like

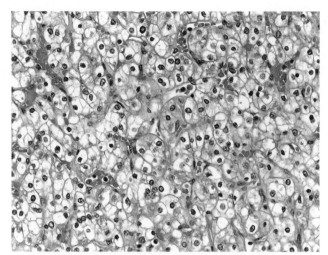

FIGURE 2-21 ■ Clear cell renal cell carcinoma with blood-filled microscopic cysts.

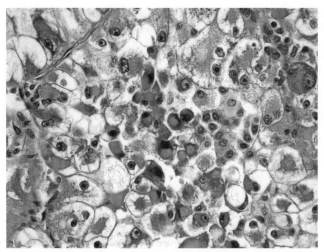

FIGURE 2-23 ■ Clear cell renal cell carcinoma with rhabdoid morphology.

spindle cell morphology, which may overgrow and replace the epithelial component of the tumor. In approximately 25% of these cases, areas of tumor showing rhabdoid and sarcomatoid differentiation may coexist. Clear cell RCC usually contains scattered lymphocytes and plasma cells, and in rare cases, there may be a pronounced lymphoid infiltrate. Granulomatous inflammation can rarely be present.

Ancillary and Special Studies
Numerous antibody markers have been investigated for clear cell RCC. These tumors typically coexpress vimentin and cytokeratin AE1/AE3. Low molecular weight cytokeratins (CK8, CK18, and CK9), EMA, CD10, and RCC antibody are also frequently positive.[49,108–112] There is strong expression of carbonic anhydrase IX, usually with a membrane pattern.[113–115] Well over 90% of tumors are strongly positive for PAX8 and to a lesser extent PAX2.[116,117] MUC-1 expression is seen in 84% of tumors and varies according to the degree of nuclear pleomorphism. High-grade tumors show diffuse membranous staining, while in low-grade tumors, membranous staining is predominantly apical.[118]

E-cadherin, CD117 (c-kit), S-100 protein, placental alkaline phosphatase, and AMACR are occasionally expressed in clear cell RCC, while staining for high molecular weight cytokeratin (CK14 and 34βE12), cytokeratin 7, cytokeratin 20, and parvalbumin is usually negative.[6,118–121]

Electron microscopy shows the cells of clear cell RCC to have abundant cytoplasmic glycogen and lipid. Two types of hyaline globules may be present within the cytoplasm. These both consist of concentric membranes, one with central lipid and the other with peripheral peroxisomes and endoplasmic reticulum. There is a prominent basal lamina, and desmosomes and junctional complexes are frequently seen. Numerous microvilli 1,000 to 2,120 nm in length are present on the luminal surface of the cell. Clear cell RCC cells with granular cytoplasm contain increased numbers of mitochondria.[122,123]

Genetics
Clear cell RCC typically shows loss of chromosome 3p, which has been demonstrated in 75% to 100% of cases.[124–126] The von Hippel-Lindau tumor suppressor gene (*VHL*) is sited at 3p25 and in clear cell RCC inactivation occurs by deletion, mutation, or hypermethylation. *VHL* regulates hypoxia-inducible factor-α, which promotes vascular and somatic growth factors.[127] The gene also regulates the mammalian target of rapamycin (mTOR) pathway leading to tumor cell growth and survival. Chromosome 3p harbors two additional tumor suppressor genes, *FHIT* at 3p14.2 and *RASSF1A* at 3p21, and possibly a further tumor suppressor gene at 3p12.[126,127] Additional mutations may be present in clear cell RCC, with loss of heterozygosity at 6q, 8p, 9q, and 14q being most frequently seen.[128,129] In addition to these, mutations at 5q, 9q, 10q, 13p, and 17p have also been reported.[130,131]

Differential Diagnosis

The diagnosis of clear cell RCC is usually not a difficult one to make; however, there is potential for these tumors to be confused with other primary renal tumors that have clear cytoplasm (Box 2-2).

Clear cell RCC must be differentiated from translocation carcinoma. Both tumor subtypes usually contain clear cells, although the presence of cells with voluminous cytoplasm, eosinophilic hyaline (basement membrane) nodules, and psammoma bodies favors a diagnosis of translocation carcinoma. A well-defined papillary component is often present in translocation carcinoma and its presence excludes clear cell RCC. Routine immunohistochemistry can be helpful with carbonic anhydrase IX almost always strongly positive in clear cell RCC and negative or weak in translocation carcinoma. Positive reactivity for cathepsin K supports translocation carcinoma but negative reactivity is not helpful. Melanocytic markers HMB-45 and melan-A are positive in some translocation carcinomas, especially those with t(6;11), and are negative in clear cell RCC. Positive immunoreactivity for the TFE3 protein is usually diagnostic (Table 2-5).

Multilocular cystic clear cell RCC is differentiated by its architecture and the presence of well-differentiated clear cells with small round nuclei within septal walls. These tumors may contain foci resembling clear cell RCC; however, if these are visible macroscopically, a diagnosis of clear cell RCC is more appropriate. Clear cell papillary RCC is usually low grade and unlike clear cell RCC has a

---

Box 2-2 ● KIDNEY TUMORS THAT CAN HAVE CLEAR CYTOPLASM

- Clear cell renal cell carcinoma
- Clear cell papillary renal cell carcinoma
- Translocation-associated renal cell carcinoma
- Chromophobe renal carcinoma
- Papillary renal cell carcinoma

Table 2-5 ■ IMMUNOHISTOCHEMISTRY OF CLEAR CELL TUMORS

Marker	Clear Cell	Clear Cell Papillary	Translocation Associated	Chromophobe	Epithelioid Angiomyolipoma	Adrenal Cortical Tumors
CA IX	Strong, diffuse, membranous	Positive, cup-like	Weak and focal or negative	Negative (<10% weak)	Negative	Positive (3%–50%)
CK7	Negative	Positive	Negative	Strong, diffuse, membrane-like	Negative	Negative
CD117	Negative	Negative	Negative	Positive, membranous	Negative	Negative
CD10	Strong, membranous	Negative or focal	Positive	Negative	Negative	Negative
Cathepsin-K	Negative	Negative	50% positive	Negative	Positive	Negative
PAX8	Positive	Positive	50% Positive	Positive	Negative	Negative
HMB-45	Negative	Negative	Positive in some	Negative	Positive	Negative
Melan-A	Negative	Negative	Positive in some	Negative	Positive	Negative
Vimentin	Positive	Positive	Variable	Negative	Positive	Positive
EMA	Positive	Positive	Negative or weak	Positive	Negative	Negative
Inhibin	Negative (<10% positive)	Negative	Negative	Negative	Negative	Positive

papillary architecture (typically short stubby papillae) and is cytokeratin 7 positive and CD10 negative (or only focally positive on the luminal surface). Chromophobe RCC can occasionally mimic clear cell RCC, particularly in limited biopsy samples. The strong positive reactivity for cytokeratin 7 and lack of carbonic anhydrase IX and CD10 reactivity readily differentiates between the two. Infrequently epithelioid angiomyolipoma can include a population of polygonal cells with pale to clear cytoplasm. These tumors do not express epithelial markers but do express muscle and melanocytic markers.

Tumors showing extensive sarcomatoid differentiation may mimic one of several types of renal sarcoma. Unlike true sarcomas, sarcomatoid tumors often have foci of parent carcinoma, while electron microscopy and immunohistochemistry usually confirm the epithelial nature of the tumor. In adults, infiltrative urothelial carcinomas of the renal pelvis may be confused with clear cell RCC. The correct diagnosis may further be complicated if the urothelial carcinoma shows sarcomatoid differentiation. In some cases, extensive sampling may reveal areas of typical urothelial carcinoma, while identification of foci of carcinoma in situ within the epithelium of the renal pelvis is particularly helpful. Urothelial carcinomas may be differentiated from clear cell RCC through positive expression of high molecular weight cytokeratin, p63, GATA3, and carcinoembryonic antigen.

A number of benign conditions may resemble clear cell RCC. Xanthogranulomatous pyelonephritis is often symptomatic with clinical features that may mimic malignancy. The gross appearances may also cause confusion as there is often a tumor-like mass that is yellow and appears to infiltrate into perirenal fat. The renal outflow tract is almost always obstructed, usually by a calculus or deformity of the pelvi-ureteric junction.[132] Microscopically, xanthogranulomatous

pyelonephritis consists of sheets of foamy macrophages, which may resemble the clear cells of RCC.[133] The cytoplasm of the tumor cells is, however, not foamy, and most importantly, the typical vascular network of clear cell RCC is not seen. Malakoplakia may also resemble renal carcinoma[134] although the diffusely granular cytoplasm, the presence of Michaelis-Guttmann bodies, and the absence of both nuclear pleomorphism and the vascular network of clear cell RCC are usually diagnostic.

Extrarenal metastases of clear cell RCC may present difficulties in diagnosis. PAX8 is presently considered the most sensitive and specific marker for the renal tubular origin of a metastasis. A limited number of other tumors do express PAX8, and other markers may be necessary if any of these are in the differential diagnosis (Box 2-3). Coexpression of pancytokeratin and vimentin, as well as the presence of intracytoplasmic glycogen is suggestive of a renal primary, and on electron microscopy, luminal or intercellular dense arrays of microvilli are a confirming feature.[135]

RCC infiltrating the adrenal gland may be differentiated from adrenal cortical carcinoma through staining for epithelial membrane antigen or cytokeratin as these are negative or only weakly positive in adrenal carcinoma.[136] Metastases to the thyroid may be correctly differentiated from primary clear cell carcinoma by negative staining for thyroglobulin

Box 2-3 ● TUMORS THAT EXPRESS PAX8

- Renal cell carcinoma (all types)
- Thyroid tumors
- Müllerian tumors
- Wolffian duct lesions
- Thymic neoplasms

and transcription terminator factor 1 (TTF1), while metastases to the ovary are CA-125 negative and usually retain the immunohistochemical phenotype typical of renal convoluted tubules.

Hemangioblastoma of the central nervous system, which can be associated with VHL disease, can resemble clear cell RCC. A positive immunohistochemical reaction for epithelial membrane antigen is normally diagnostic as this is not seen in hemangioblastoma.[137]

Prognosis and Predictive Factors

Staging

Of all the prognostic parameters investigated for clear cell RCC, tumor stage most consistently predicts outcome in individual cases.[138] In the TNM staging system, intrarenal tumors are categorized according to size, and in numerous studies investigating a variety of size cut points, maximum tumor diameter has been shown to be of prognostic significance.[78,79,139–142] By treating size as a continuous variable, it has been shown that the probability of death increases by a factor of 3.5× for each doubling of tumor size.[143]

Tumors showing regional spread are categorized as pT3 in the TNM system, and it is recognized that this pT category is associated with a variable outcome.[138] Infiltration of renal sinus fat is associated with increased risk of metastatic disease.[144] It has also been shown that this has a less favorable outcome when compared to patients with infiltration of the perirenal fat. This finding has been recently challenged as similar rates of survival were reported for patients with perirenal and renal sinus fat invasion.[145] Macroscopic invasion of the renal vein is associated with a worse prognosis when compared to patients with organ-confined disease.[146]

Invasion of the adrenal gland is an important prognostic marker and is associated with a poor outcome. Direct extension of tumor to the adrenal has a 5-year survival of 20%, which is similar to that for pT4 tumors.[146,147] Somewhat surprisingly, metastatic spread of tumor to the adrenal gland appears to have a better outcome as patients with solitary adrenal metastases have 5- and 10-year survival rates of 61% and 31%, respectively. This compares with rates of 19% and 16% for patients with combined adrenal and extra-adrenal metastatic spread of tumor.[148]

Multicenter studies have suggested that a modification of pT3 and pT4 criteria may improve the predictive value of tumor staging. In this modification, cases were grouped according to the presence of tumor in renal vein or infradiaphragmatic vena cava or perirenal fat invasion (group 1), perirenal fat invasion with either renal vein or infradiaphragmatic vena cava thrombus or adrenal gland invasion (group 2), and adrenal involvement with renal vein or infradiaphragmatic vena cava thrombus, supradiaphragmatic vena cava thrombus, or Gerota fascia invasion (group 3) with the 5-year survival for each group being 61%, 35%, and 13%, respectively.[149]

There are limited studies that investigate the prognostic significance of microvascular invasion of the renal vein, although this has been shown to correlate with outcome, independent of pT category and tumor grade.[150,151] Intrarenal microvascular invasion has also been shown to correlate with both the development of metastases and survival, independent of pT1-pT3 category and grade.[152]

Spread of tumor to the regional lymph nodes has prognostic significance independent of pT category, with 5-year survivals for patients with N0 and N+ being 74% and 10%, respectively.[153] A 5-year survival rate of 52% for N+ tumors with no evidence of extrarenal metastases has also been reported, and this was significantly higher than the 7% observed for patients with metastatic spread of tumor.[154]

Grading

Grading of RCC in general is discussed later in the chapter, but Fuhrman grading of clear cell RCC has been shown to have a significant association with outcome on univariate analysis[78,79,155]; however, this was lost on multivariate analysis in one series where N category was found to be the only parameter to retain prognostic significance.[79] In some instances, a significant association with survival was seen only when two or more grades were grouped together.[138] Fuhrman grading has also been correlated with pT staging categories, when grading was grouped into two categories (G1 + G2 vs. G3 + G4).[156] Many pathologists base their Fuhrman grading on nucleolar prominence alone, and in support of this, nucleolar prominence has been correlated with tumor stage.[157] In a mixed series of RCC, in which 74% of cases were clear cell RCCs, the percentage of high-grade carcinoma (Fuhrman grades 3 and 4) was highly correlated with metastasis-free interval, overall survival, and cancer-specific survival.[158]

Other Morphologic Features

Sarcomatoid differentiation of clear cell RCC is an important prognostic indicator with reported disease-specific survival at 2, 3, and 5 years of 29% to 37%, 19% to 32%, and 1% to 22%, respectively.[107,159–162] The prognosis of sarcomatoid RCC is also stage dependent with a reported median survival for localized disease of 17 months. For patients with regional or distant metastases, the survival was 8 and 7 months, respectively.[161] The proportion of tumor showing sarcomatoid morphology is, at best, of limited significance as the survival difference of patients with tumors ≤50% and >50% sarcomatoid component has been shown to be only weakly significant.[161]

Patients with tumors containing foci of rhabdoid differentiation are twice as likely to present with extrarenal metastases, and in one series, 71% of patients developed metastases, with a mean follow-up of 5 months. Within 2 years, 43% of patients had died, with a mean survival interval of 8 months.[163]

The presence of microscopic tumor necrosis within clear cell RCC has been correlated with survival on univariate analysis.[78,79,164] The significance of this as an independent marker of prognosis is uncertain as, on multivariate analysis that included stage and grade, the presence of necrosis has been shown to have both a significant and insignificant association with survival.[79,164]

Mitotic rates in most clear cell RCCs are too low to provide discriminative prognostic information; however, in some series, markers of cell proliferation have been correlated with survival. Nuclear staining by Ki-67, which is expressed in actively cycling cells, has been correlated with outcome on univariate and multivariate analysis.[158,165–167] Similarly, numbers of silver-staining nucleolar organizer regions, which are most visible during interphase of the cell cycle, have been significantly associated with survival for clear cell RCC.[165] Other markers of cell cycle activity ($p27^{Kip1}$, $p21^{waf1/cip1}$) have also been correlated with either survival or other prognostic markers.[168,169]

Other histologic features that have been shown to have prognostic significance for clear cell RCC are tumor vascularity[170–172] and immunohistochemical detection of caveolin-1, CD-44S,[173] human kallikrein,[174] hypoxia-inducible factor-1-alpha,[175] matrix metalloprotease inducer,[176] MUC-1,[177] and osteopontin.[178]

Multiple genetic mutations have been demonstrated for clear cell RCC, and specific mutations have been correlated with aggressive disease. Loss of heterozygosity at 14q correlates with advanced tumor stage and poor survival.[129,179] Similarly loss of chromosome 9p is associated with advanced-stage, high-grade tumors and decreased survival.[180,181]

Clear cell RCCs that are detected as an incidental finding have a favorable prognosis while anemia, hypercalcemia, and systemic symptoms such as fever and weight loss are usually indicative of extrarenal spread or metastatic disease.[182]

In an attempt to stratify outcome for patients with clear cell RCC, several prognostic nomograms have been proposed. The Memorial Sloan-Kettering Cancer Center prognostic nomogram for RCC was established in 2001. This contained a category for histologic type that included the three main types of RCC.[183] In 2005, the nomogram was refined to focus on clear cell RCC.[184] The revised nomogram was based upon tumor size, TNM 2000 pT category, Fuhrman grade, presence of necrosis, presence of microvascular invasion, and presence of systematic symptoms, although on multivariate analysis, only Fuhrman grade and the presence of microvascular invasion were found to retain a significant relationship with survival. In a separate study, the nomogram was found to have poor predictive accuracy.[185] While the nomogram contains several dependent and possibly insignificant variables, there is also a likelihood that a number of the tumors utilized to define it were understaged, as many of the cases were accessioned prior to the recognition of renal sinus invasion as an important prognostic indicator. A similar predictive scoring system, designated the SSIGN (stage, size, grade, necrosis) score, has been proposed by a group from the Mayo Clinic (Table 2-6).[186,187] A dynamic prediction model has now been incorporated into this scoring system (D-SSIGN). This dynamic model is aimed to provide more accurate assessment of distant postoperative survival, as it has been shown that cancer-specific survival increases with increasing postoperative disease-free interval (Table 2-7).[187]

Table 2-6 ■ SSIGN SCORE ALGORITHM FOR PREDICTING OUTCOME IN RENAL CELL CARCINOMA

Feature	Score
Primary tumor classification:	
pT1	0
pT2	1
pT31	2
pT3b	2
pT3c	2
pT4	0
Regional lymph node involvement:	
pNx	0
pN0	0
pN1	2
pN2	2
Distant metastases	
pM0	0
pM1	4
Primary tumor size (cm):	
<5	0
5 or greater	2
Nuclear grade:	
1	0
2	0
3	1
4	3
Coagulative tumor necrosis:	
Absent	0
Present	2

Modified from Frank I, Blute ML, Cheville JC, et al. An outcome prediction model for patients with clear cell renal cell carcinoma treated with radical nephrectomy based on tumor stage, size, grade and necrosis: the SSIGN score. *J Urol* 2002;168:2395–2400.

Table 2-7 ■ FIVE AND TEN-YEAR CANCER-SPECIFIC SURVIVAL ACCORDING TO SSIGN SCORE AT SURGERY

Score	Cancer-specific Survival	
	Five years	Ten years
0–1	98.6	95.1
2	94.9	87.0
3	88.9	77.6
4	82.3	70.4
5	69.6	58.5
6	67.2	50.4
7	44.9	27.2
8+	17.6	13.3

Modified from Thompson RH, Leibovich BC, Lohse CM, et al. Dynamic outcome prediction in patients with clear cell renal cell carcinoma treated with radical nephrectomy: the D-SSIGN score. *J Urol* 2007;177:477–480.

Treatment

Surgery is the only curative treatment for clear cell RCC. For small lesions, nephron-sparing partial nephrectomy is the treatment of choice while larger or locally advanced tumors are managed by radical nephrectomy. The latter involves removing the entire kidney with the perirenal fat and Gerota fascia.[101] Although this surgery includes the adrenal gland, many surgeons now leave the adrenal gland behind.

Numerous studies have demonstrated that partial nephrectomy has an equivalent outcome to radical nephrectomy.[188–190] There are recent data showing that outcome is better for patients treated by partial versus radical nephrectomy.[190] Partial nephrectomy has led to an increased utilization of frozen sections in RCC surgery principally for margin control.[191] Several studies have however demonstrated that positive surgical margins at surgery do not correlate with a higher rate of local recurrence or with outcome.[192,193] Laparoscopic approaches are commonly used currently for both radical and partial nephrectomy procedures with excellent results.[194,195] This can result in morcellated specimens making pathologic staging and histologic typing challenging but possible in most cases.[196]

Ablation procedures including cryoablation and radio frequency ablation to treat small renal tumors have become increasingly popular with early results indicating equivalent cancer control to surgical approaches in selected patients.[197–199] Surveillance is another treatment option in selected patients that is gaining interest though only limited long-term outcome data are available.[189,200] The latter two approaches have resulted in an increasing role for needle biopsy of renal masses.[201,202]

Spread of tumor into the renal vein, inferior vena cava, and even the right atrium is not infrequent in patients with RCC. For these patients, surgical resection remains a valid treatment option. Numerous studies have demonstrated the potential curability of such advanced disease.

Regional lymphadenectomy has not been routinely performed at the time of nephrectomy. There has been a phase III clinical trial evaluating the role for lymphadenectomy that demonstrated no survival advantage gained by the performance of a lymph node dissection although it did provide for more accurate staging.[203] In that study, lymph node metastases were identified in 4% of patients, a substantially lower percentage than had been reported in the older literature.

Adjuvant therapy is of limited efficacy for metastatic disease. High-dose interleukin 2 is not associated with improved survival despite an increase in the rate of initial durable remissions, while interferon has a proven, but limited effect.[204] More recently, a variety of targeted therapies have been developed that affect the gene products of the hypoxia-inducible factor pathway, which include transforming growth factor, platelet-derived growth factor, and vascular endothelial growth factor.[205] Agents currently available for clinical use include bevacizumab (antivascular endothelial growth factor), sunitinib (antivascular endothelial growth factor receptor and platelet-derived growth factor receptor-β), sorafenib (antivascular endothelial growth factor receptor, anti-Rafkinase), and temsirolimus (mTOR inhibitor). These inhibitors all show efficacy in promoting tumor shrinkage and delaying progression of metastatic disease and have shown promise in improving outcome over traditional biologic therapies.[206,207] In selected patients, resection of metastases may be beneficial.[208,209]

Multilocular Cystic Renal Cell Carcinoma

Introduction

Clear cell RCCs frequently contain cysts, and these are usually degenerative in nature. In up to 5% of clear cell RCCs, cyst formation is pronounced, with flattened septa lined by cells with clear cytoplasm and minimal nuclear pleomorphism.[210] In early studies, these tumors were considered to be cystic lymphangioma[211]; however, these tumors are now recognized to be a distinctive subtype of renal epithelial neoplasia.[212]

Epidemiology and Clinical Features

Multilocular cystic RCC has been reported in patients aged from 8 to 80 years.[213,214] The mean age at presentation for 208 cases published between 1928 and 2009 was 52 years.[212–217] In more recent series, this is somewhat lower at 46 years, which reflects the influence of improved imaging modalities. The mean age at diagnosis for females is slightly younger than that for males. Tumors are more commonly seen in males, with a male-to-female ratio of 2:1. No predisposing risk factors have been reported.

In recent series, multilocular cystic RCC has been diagnosed incidentally in up to 90% cases, including two cases diagnosed during pregnancy.[216,217] For symptomatic patients, presenting features are flank or abdominal pain, hematuria, and abdominal mass.

As with cystic nephroma and mixed epithelial stromal tumor of kidney, multilocular cystic RCCs show Bosniak type II or III features.[218] Hypodense cystic areas with focal hyperdense hemorrhage or gelatinous fluid are usually seen on CT imaging, and utilizing strict criteria, these tumors may be differentiated from cystic clear cell RCC.[219] Rarely, dystrophic calcification is present within the septa.

Pathology

Gross Features
Tumors range in size up to 14 cm in maximum diameter,[212] with a mean diameter of 4 to 7 cm.[214] Tumors are encapsulated and consist of cysts of variable size containing serous, gelatinous, or hemorrhagic fluid (Fig. 2-24). The cyst walls are thin, and neither expansive nodules nor solid areas of growth are present. Foci of calcification may be seen. Occasionally tumors are bilateral or multifocal.[214]

Microscopic Features
Cysts are usually lined by a single layer of cuboidal to flat tumor cells, although in areas the epithelial lining of the cyst wall may be absent. Focally, several layers of lining cells may

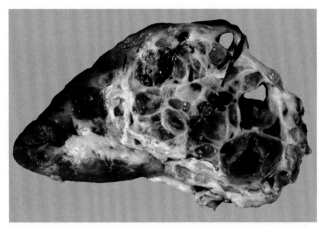

FIGURE 2-24 ■ Multilocular cystic renal cell carcinoma. The tumor is entirely cystic without solid nodules of expansile growth.

be present, and these occasionally form small papillary projections. The tumor cells have clear cytoplasm, and there is a low grade of nuclear pleomorphism. Nuclei often have dense chromatin, and although most tumors are Fuhrman nuclear grade 1, occasional tumors may show grade 2 features.

The cyst walls are composed of fibrous tissue that may be densely collagenous. Dystrophic calcification may also be seen, and rarely there may be osseous metaplasia. Nests and individual tumor cells are typically seen within cyst walls, and not infrequently microscopic aggregates of clear cells may be present (Fig. 2-25).

Ancillary and Special Studies

The immunohistochemical profile is similar to that of clear cell RCC with strong membrane expression of carbonic anhydrase IX and EMA. CD10 is negative in a small percentage, and a few cases do show weak expression of cytokeratin 7.[220] Tumor cells frequently show positive expression of the proximal nephron markers peanut agglutinin and MUC-1, while distal nephron markers LeuM1 and LTA are negative.[221] Tumor cells also show positivity with Cam 5.2 and

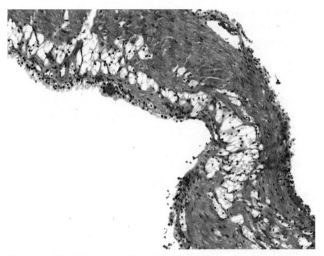

FIGURE 2-25 ■ Multilocular cystic clear cell renal cell carcinoma. The carcinoma cells are embedded in the stroma of a septum.

pancytokeratin. This latter feature may be used to confirm the epithelial nature of clear cells within cyst walls, as these may resemble histiocytes. Ultrastructurally, multilocular cystic RCC is similar to clear cell RCC. In a single study, these tumors have been shown to harbor *VHL* gene mutations.[222]

Differential Diagnosis

Multilocular cystic RCC must be differentiated from other tumors that can have a complex cystic gross appearance (Box 2-4). This includes cystic nephroma, tubulocystic renal carcinoma, clear cell papillary RCC, and localized cystic disease. The cysts of cystic nephroma are lined by a largely flattened to attenuated epithelium that typically has hobnail cells at least focally. The epithelial cells are never seen within the cyst septa. Additionally, the stroma of cystic nephroma often has areas that resemble ovarian stroma. In tubulocystic carcinoma, the spaces range from small round tubules to large cystic spaces. The cells are usually cuboidal with amphophilic cytoplasm and apocrine-like blebs on the surface. Cytoplasmic clearing is not a feature, and clear cells are not present within the septa. Clear cell papillary RCC is almost always partially solid and cystic, but the solid component can be quite minor. Recognition of small blunt papillae, aggregates of small tubules within the wall, cells with prominent subnuclear vacuoles, or a smooth muscle-containing stroma should suggest this possibility. Demonstration of strong reactivity for CK7 and negative or at most focal weak CD10 reactivity can confirm the diagnosis. Localized (segmental) cystic disease shows variably sized cysts with normal structures including glomeruli identifiable between the cystic spaces.

Multilocular cystic clear cell RCC must also be distinguished from usual clear cell RCC with prominent cystic change. Some series of multilocular clear cell RCC have included cystic tumors with solid areas. Utilizing the criteria recommended in the 2004 WHO classification, no solid areas of tumor should be visible macroscopically, and there should be no evidence of tumor infiltration or necrosis.

Prognosis and Treatment

For those reported cases that conform to the diagnostic criteria of the 2004 WHO Classification, there have been no reports of tumor recurrence or metastasis.[212,214] Because of this, the term "multilocular clear cell renal cell neoplasm of low malignant potential" was proposed in the ISUP classification of renal tumors.[7] In one case where tumor was enucleated from a donor kidney prior to transplantation, no recurrence occurred after 10 years' follow-up.[223] When feasible, nephron-sparing partial nephrectomy is the treatment of choice.[215,219,224]

Papillary Renal Cell Carcinoma

Introduction

Renal parenchymal tumors with a papillary morphology were described in the earliest reports of renal malignancy and were included in the first case series of renal tumors reported by Rayer in 1842.[225] In subsequent studies, the biologic behavior of tumors with a papillary architecture was debated with some preferring to consider localized tumors, even of large dimensions, to be adenomas.[9]

In 1976, the clinical and pathological features of papillary RCC were described in detail by Mancilla-Jimenez et al.[226] Papillary RCC was first recognized as a distinct form of renal parenchymal neoplasia in 1986, with the publication of the Mainz classification of renal tumors.[1] In this classification, papillary RCCs were termed chromophilic cell carcinoma on the basis of widespread cytoplasmic basophilia. It was also noted that a proportion of papillary carcinomas exhibited varying degrees of cytoplasmic eosinophilia, due to increased numbers of mitochondria, and the term chromophilic cell carcinoma, oncocytic-like was proposed.

Subsequent studies have confirmed that papillary RCC has distinctive clinical, histologic, and genetic features.[227,228] Papillary RCC was accepted as a tumor type in the classifications proposed by the Heidelberg and Rochester consensus conferences.[3,4] More recently, two specific variants of papillary RCC, designated type 1 and type 2, have been recognized, and these were included in the 2004 edition of the World Health Organization Classification of renal neoplasia.[5] The 2012 ISUP classification similarly recommends classifying papillary RCC into types 1 and 2.[7]

Epidemiology

Papillary RCC is the second most frequently encountered subtype of renal parenchymal malignancy. There is some variation in the proportion of papillary RCCs in contemporary series of renal epithelial neoplasia published subsequent to the Heidelberg and Rochester consensus conferences. In these series, the proportion of papillary RCC ranged from 6% to 19% of cases.[77–83,164] Of interest, lower proportions of papillary RCC were reported from large case series not subject to central histologic review.[80,83] These would seem to underestimate the true proportion of papillary RCC in these series, as review of cases accessioned before 1997 in one series showed that 2% of papillary RCC had been incorrectly classified as other tumor subtypes.[82]

There is a male predominance (1.2:1), and in larger series patients' ages ranged from 15 to 97 years, with mean ages ranging from 59 to 63 years.[77,81–83,229] Papillary RCC has also been reported in pediatric patients, and in this age group these tumors are more frequently encountered when compared to adult series.[230]

While the great majority of papillary RCCs occur sporadically, several familial renal cancer syndromes are associated with this tumor type (Table 2-3). These syndromes are detailed in a separate section on familial renal neoplasia.

Clinical Features

The clinical presentation of papillary RCC is not specific to this particular type of RCC, being similar to other forms of renal parenchymal malignancy. In earlier studies, hematuria was a common presenting feature, with abdominal pain and the detection of an abdominal mass being less frequently seen.[226] Tumors are detected as incidental findings in approximately 20% of cases, and the classic triad of hematuria, abdominal mass, and abdominal pain is observed in approximately 5% to 10% of cases, a finding similar to clear cell RCC. Spontaneous hemorrhage, which is rarely seen in clear cell RCC, was found to be a presenting feature for 8% of papillary RCC.[231]

In more recent series, where tumors were divided according to type, papillary RCCs were asymptomatic in up to half of cases.[77,78,81] In particular, it has been noted that these tumors are less likely to be symptomatic, but more likely to be multifocal and exhibit necrosis, than clear cell RCC and chromophobe RCC.[78]

Papillary renal cell carcinoma is more frequently associated with end-stage renal failure than clear cell renal cell carcinoma, and in these cases, multifocality is more common.[232]

Many of the studies on paraneoplastic syndromes associated with renal cell carcinoma do not divide tumors according to subtype.[102] While it is likely that a number of syndromes reported in these series are associated with papillary renal cell carcinoma, hypercalcemia, hypophosphatemia, and reversible hypertension have been specifically associated with this type.[226]

Renal arteriography shows papillary renal cell carcinoma to be either avascular or markedly hypovascular, a feature less commonly seen in clear cell renal cell carcinoma.[226] Tumor calcification is present in approximately one-third of cases. On ultrasound, these tumors show no evidence of neovascularity and are echo free at low gain. T1-weighted images of papillary renal cell carcinoma and clear cell renal cell carcinoma are similar on magnetic resonance imaging, while T2-weighted images of papillary tumors are hypodense. Pre- and postcontrast computerized tomography demonstrates a significantly lesser enhancement for type 1 papillary renal cell carcinoma when compared to type 2 tumors,[233] which reflects the apparent increased vascularity of type 2 tumors. Type 1 tumors have also been shown to have more distinct margins and a more homogeneous density than type 2 tumors.

Pathology

Gross Features

Papillary renal cell carcinomas are usually well circumscribed and vary in color from pale white or yellow to dark

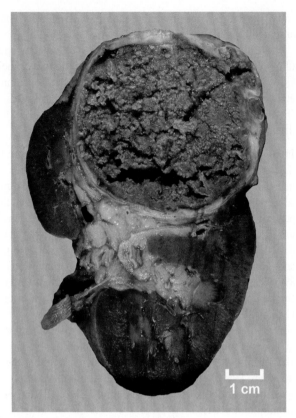

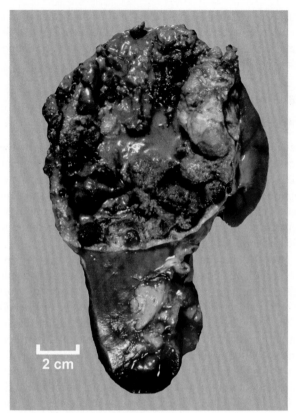

FIGURE 2-26 ■ Papillary renal cell carcinoma. The carcinoma is encased in a thick pseudocapsule. Its friable parenchyma reflects the papillary architecture of the neoplasm.

FIGURE 2-27 ■ Papillary renal cell carcinoma. This large tumor has undergone extensive hemorrhagic necrosis. In such cases, often the only place diagnosable carcinoma is found is embedded in the thick pseudocapsule.

brown, this being a reflection of the degree of hemorrhage, necrosis, and macrophage accumulation present within individual tumors (Fig. 2-26). Tumors may be solitary or multifocal, with multifocality being more frequently seen in larger tumors and those associated with familial neoplasia. Larger tumors often show cystic degeneration, necrosis, and intratumoral hemorrhage, and these features occur more frequently in papillary renal cell carcinoma than in clear cell renal cell carcinoma (Fig. 2-27).[226] In particular, necrosis has been reported in 39% to 52% of cases,[78,164,234] and this accounts for the hypovascularity that is recognized as a radiographic feature of these tumors.[235] There is frequently a prominent investing pseudocapsule, which is most commonly present in larger and well-circumscribed tumors.[226,236,237] Intratumoral calcification is present in approximately one-third of cases,[235] and rarely ossification may be present.[226] Papillary renal cell carcinomas are more frequently associated with renal scarring than clear cell renal cell carcinomas, and in these kidneys multifocal tumors are more frequently present.

Microscopic Features

A papillary or tubulopapillary architecture is present in more than 90% of cases. Solid-appearing areas, resulting from compressive growth of both tubules and papillae, may also be seen.[226,237] Tumor papillae have delicate fibrovascular cores covered by a single layer of neoplastic epithelial cells

that vary in size and morphology. In some tumors papillae are short and blunt and resemble glomeruli, while in other tumors, papillae may show complex branching or form long parallel arrays. Infrequently small amounts of mucin are found. The papillary cores contain variable amounts of fibrous tissue and may be expanded by edema or foamy macrophages. Foci of dystrophic calcification and psammoma bodies may also be seen, both in papillae and adjacent desmoplastic stroma,[119,237] and the presence of calcium oxalate crystals has also been reported.[238] In those tumors where a tubular architecture predominates, the tubules are composed of cells of similar morphology to those lining tumor papillae. In scarred kidneys, epithelial-lined cystic structures may be present with luminal papillae, and renal adenomas are also frequently seen.

Two separate types of papillary renal cell carcinoma have been identified on the basis of histological features.[237,239] Type 1 tumors are characterized by papillary cores covered by tumor cells with nuclei aligned in a linear fashion parallel to the basement membrane (Fig. 2-28). In these tumors the nuclei are usually small with mild to moderate nuclear pleomorphism and inconspicuous nucleoli. Tumor cell cytoplasm is usually pale and inconspicuous. Papillae are often short and blunt and frequently have edematous cores (Fig. 2-29), often containing psammoma bodies, and aggregates of foamy macrophages. Occasionally the cells

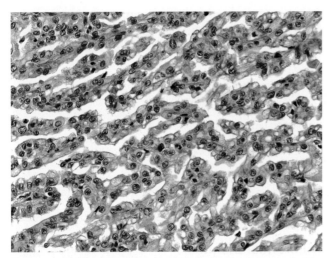

FIGURE 2-28 ■ Papillary renal cell carcinoma, type 1. The cytoplasm is pale, and the nuclei are small with inconspicuous nucleoli.

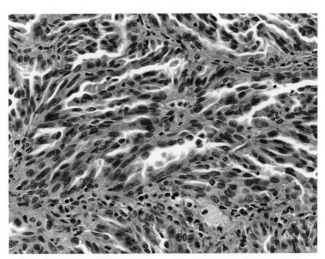

FIGURE 2-30 ■ Papillary renal cell carcinoma, type 1. Some of the carcinoma cells have become elongate and spindle shaped.

become elongate and spindle-shaped (Fig. 2-30). Type 2 papillary renal cell carcinomas differ from type 1 tumors by the presence of pseudostratification of tumor nuclei. The cells are usually larger with prominent eosinophilic cytoplasm and large nuclei with more prominent nucleoli (Fig. 2-31). Psammoma bodies and foamy macrophages are less frequently seen. In both type 1 and type 2, the papillae may become very crowded and growth may appear solid (Fig. 2-32). Classification of a papillary renal cell carcinoma as a type 1 or type 2 tumor should primarily be based on the presence or absence of pseudostratification of tumor nuclei. This is of some importance as occasionally there is overlap in the other morphologic features between the two tumor types. In particular, type 1 tumors may have voluminous cytoplasm, while type 2 tumors may have only scanty amounts of cytoplasm and small nuclei.

Fine needle aspirates of papillary renal cell carcinoma usually show a variety of distinctive features and

a definitive diagnosis is often possible.[240] Aspirates have abundant papillary clusters with fibrovascular cores, nuclei are of varying size, and nuclear grooves are often seen. Histiocytes, hemosiderin granules—often within tumor cytoplasm—and psammoma bodies are also frequently present.

Ancillary and Special Studies

Papillary renal cell carcinomas show positive immunohistochemical reactions for cytokeratin AE1/AE3, Cam 5.2, CK 19, Callus, EMA, CD10, CD15, AMACR, vimentin, and RCC antigen; tumors are also frequently positive for S100 protein.[108,119,237,239,241–244] Carbonic anhydrase IX is expressed in approximately 50% of cases but without the striking membrane pattern of clear cell renal cell carcinoma. Well over 90% of cases are PAX8 positive.[245] Type 1 and type 2 papillary renal cell carcinomas do show somewhat differing

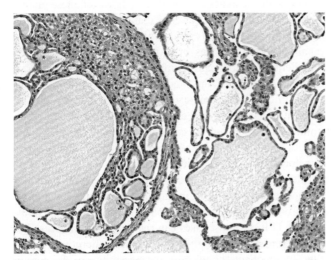

FIGURE 2-29 ■ Papillary renal cell carcinoma, type 1. The papillary cores are edematous and could be mistaken for cysts or glands.

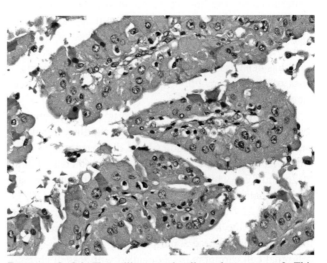

FIGURE 2-31 ■ Papillary renal cell carcinoma, type 2. This photomicrograph shows the nuclear pseudostratification, voluminous cytoplasm, and prominent nucleoli, which are typical of papillary renal cell carcinoma type 2.

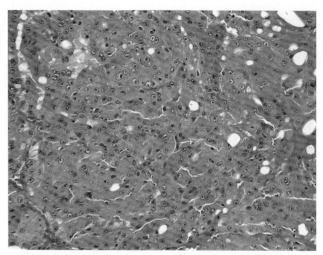

FIGURE **2-32** ■ Papillary renal cell carcinoma type 2. In some areas, the papillae may grow so closely together that the tumor appears solid.

immunohistochemical staining patterns. Type 1 tumors more frequently express cytokeratin 7, vimentin, and MUC1, while cytokeratin 20 and E-cadherin staining is more frequently seen in type 2 tumors.[49,110,239,246]

The ultrastructural features of papillary renal cell carcinoma are similar to those of clear cell renal cell carcinoma, although cilia numbers have been shown to be higher in papillary renal cell carcinoma.[247] Tumors with eosinophilic cytoplasm contain increased numbers of mitochondria.[122]

Genetics

It has been demonstrated that the characteristic genetic changes associated with papillary renal cell carcinoma are trisomy and tetrasomy 7, trisomy 17, and loss of the Y chromosome. It has been suggested that the presence of other genetic changes, especially trisomy 12, 16, and 20, are associated with malignancy.[248] This is somewhat contradicted by the finding of trisomy of chromosomes 7, 12, 16, 17, and 20 and loss of Y in papillary adenomas.[23] In higher-stage tumors, trisomy 8 and loss of chromosome 7 have been noted,[249] while loss of heterozygosity at 9p13 has been associated with shorter survival intervals.[250] Loss of 1p, 4q, 6q, 9p, 13q, Xp, and Xq has also been reported.[251]

More recent studies have focused upon the genetic differences between type 1 and type 2 papillary renal cell carcinoma and several studies have disclosed a significant difference in genotype. Type 1 tumors show increased gains of 7p and 17p, while type 2 tumors more frequently have allelic imbalance of chromosomes 1p, 3p, 5, 6, 8, 9p, 10, 11, 15, 18, and 22.[45,251–254] It has also been noted that tumors with mutations of the *c-met* gene, situated at 7q31, were more likely to exhibit a type 1 morphology.[255,256] Although clear cell renal cell carcinoma is associated with loss in chromosome 3p, this mutation has also been noted in some papillary renal cell carcinomas, including loss of heterozygosity at both the *VHL* and *FHIT* loci.[126,257,258]

Box 2-5 ● KIDNEY TUMORS THAT CAN HAVE PAPILLARY ARCHITECTURE

- Papillary adenoma
- Papillary renal cell carcinoma
- Clear cell papillary renal cell carcinoma
- Translocation-associated renal cell carcinoma
- Hereditary leiomyomatosis and renal cell carcinoma syndrome tumors
- Collecting duct carcinoma
- Medullary carcinoma
- Mucinous tubular and spindle cell carcinoma
- Acquired cystic disease–associated renal cell carcinoma
- Unclassified renal cell carcinoma

Differential Diagnosis

The differential diagnosis of papillary renal cell carcinoma is extensive and somewhat dependent on the age of the patient (Box 2-5). In the pediatric age group, Wilms tumor with epithelial predominance may show a resemblance to papillary renal cell carcinoma,[259] although blastema or differentiated stroma is usually revealed by thorough sampling. The nuclear features are also helpful as these are spheroidal in renal cell carcinoma, while in Wilms tumors the nuclei are elongate with tapered ends.

In adult patients clear cell renal cell carcinoma, clear cell papillary renal cell carcinoma, translocation-associated carcinoma, renal cell carcinoma of the hereditary leiomyomatosis and renal cell carcinoma syndrome, collecting duct carcinoma, medullary carcinoma, mucinous tubular and spindle cell carcinoma, and acquired cystic disease–associated renal cell carcinoma all can at least focally mimic papillary renal cell carcinoma. In most cases, these can be distinguished based on routine histology; however, limited samples as in needle biopsies can create challenging differential diagnoses. Immunohistochemistry can be helpful in certain cases (Table 2-8). Papillary renal cell carcinoma may show degeneration with apparent clearing of cells; however, these tumors lack the typical water clear cells that are diffusely present in clear cell papillary renal cell carcinoma.[260] Clear cell papillary renal cell carcinoma has small blunt papillae, not the more well-defined and delicate papillae of most papillary renal cell carcinomas. Further, the moderate to abundant clear cytoplasm in clear cell papillary renal cell carcinoma would be unusual in papillary renal cell carcinoma. In problem cases, immunohistochemistry for carbonic anhydrase IX, CD10, and AMACR will distinguish between the two (see Table 2-8). In translocation-associated carcinoma, the papillary architecture is often focal with solid and alveolar architectures predominating, features not seen in papillary renal cell carcinoma. Weak or absent reactivity for epithelial markers and expression of TFE3 in most cases can resolve problem cases. The presence of a solid or infiltrative tubular pattern with a papillary component should raise the possibility of the hereditary leiomyomatosis and renal cell carcinoma syndrome. The nucleolar features of the latter are characteristic but

Table 2-8 ■ IMMUNOHISTOCHEMISTRY IN TUMORS WITH PAPILLARY ARCHITECTURE				
Marker	Papillary	Clear Cell Papillary	Translocation Associated	Collecting Duct
CA IX	Weak—50%	Strong, membranous	Focal or negative	Negative
Cytokeratin 7	Positive (type1 > type2)	Strong, diffuse	Negative	Positive
CK 34βE12	<25% positive	Negative	Negative	Positive (approximately 50%)
Pan cytokeratin	Positive	Positive	Negative or focal	Positive
CD10	Positive	Negative or focal	Positive	approximately 25% positive
AMACR	Positive	Negative	Positive	Negative or weak
Cathepsin K	Negative	Negative	Positive (60%–80%)	Negative
TFE3/TFEB	Negative	Negative	Positive	Negative
INI1	Positive	Positive	Positive	Negative (15%)

not specific. Both collecting duct carcinoma and medullary carcinoma can focally have papillary architecture. The presence of a high-grade infiltrative component, stromal desmoplasia, and multiple histologic patterns would suggest one of these two possibilities. Collecting duct carcinoma is usually but not always negative for CD10 and AMACR, and expression of high molecular weight cytokeratin (34βE12) is present in about half of the cases. Medullary carcinoma has a similar immunohistochemical profile to collecting duct carcinoma but in addition shows loss of INI1 expression. Mucinous tubular and spindle renal cell carcinoma may have compact tubules, although the presence of extracellular mucin and spindle cells showing bland nuclear morphology is diagnostic. Care should be taken not to misinterpret mucinous tubular and spindle cell carcinoma as papillary renal cell carcinoma with sarcomatoid differentiation. Immunohistochemistry is generally not helpful as these have a similar profile to papillary renal cell carcinoma. Papillary renal cell carcinoma has been found in association with mucinous tubular and spindle cell carcinoma and tubulocystic carcinoma, and some studies have suggested that these three tumor types are related.[261–264] Acquired cystic disease–associated renal cell carcinoma usually has a range of morphologies including solid and sheet-like, alveolar and micro and macrocystic, features not present in papillary renal cell carcinoma. Prominent cytoplasmic vacuoles and a sieve-like pattern would favor acquired cystic disease–associated renal cell carcinoma. Immunohistochemistry is generally not helpful.

Prognosis and Predictive Factors

Staging

In early series of papillary renal cell carcinoma, it was noted that these tumors were more likely to be organ confined than clear cell renal cell carcinoma,[265] and a reported median survival of 13 years for these tumors was longer than the 6 years for nonpapillary (predominantly clear cell renal cell carcinoma) tumors.[226] In recent series, papillary renal cell carcinoma has been shown to be smaller[80,229] and more likely to be localized to the kidney at the time of diagnosis than clear cell renal cell carcinoma.[77,80,236,266] The reported 5-year survival for all stages

of papillary cell renal cell carcinoma ranges from 66% to 90%, which compares to 55% to 81% for clear cell renal cell carcinoma.[80,236,266] The survival difference between these two tumor types has been shown to be significant.[81,82] Stage at diagnosis has prognostic significance and tumor size has been correlated with outcome, specifically; 1997 tumor stage (pT1 vs. pT2 vs. pT3 vs. p T4) and the presence of metastatic disease have been significantly associated with survival.[78,108] When survival was analyzed according to stage, organ-confined papillary renal cell carcinoma was found to have a significantly improved 5-year survival rate, when compared to clear cell renal cell carcinoma (63% vs. 50%), while the 5-year survival rates for patients with metastatic disease was similar.[80]

Grading

The various grading classifications proposed following analysis of a series of mixed subtypes of renal cell carcinoma are largely unproven for papillary renal cell carcinoma. Especially in North America, the Fuhrman grading classification is in widespread usage for the various subtypes of renal cell carcinoma, although validating data are limited. Fuhrman grading has been shown to predict outcome on univariate analysis in eight studies of papillary renal cell carcinoma, although in three of these grading categories were grouped for analytical purposes.[78,79,155,267–271] In four of eight studies that investigated the prognostic significance of grading using multivariate analysis, grading was significantly associated with outcome[267–269,271] while in the remaining four[78,79,239,270] it was not. Analysis of the relationship of each of the defining criteria of the Fuhrman grading classification with outcome, showed a significant association with nucleolar prominence (determined from the high power field in the tumor showing the greatest degree of nuclear pleomorphism), but not for nuclear size or nuclear pleomorphism.[272] In view of these findings, it has been recommended that, for papillary renal cell carcinoma, Fuhrman nucleolar criteria should be used for assigning grades 1 to 3. In practice most pathologists do rely on nucleolar size (± nuclear chromatin granularity) alone to define grade 1 to 3 tumors,[6,273] and this is reflected in the reporting recommendations of the Association of Directors of Anatomic and Surgical Pathology.[274] Assignment of Grade 4 using the criteria of the

Fuhrman classification requires the presence of marked nuclear pleomorphism, tumor giant cells, or sarcomatoid differentiation. Sarcomatoid change occurs in 5% of papillary renal cell carcinomas and is seen in both type 1 and type 2 tumors.[236]

Other Features

Sarcomatoid change is infrequent but when present has been correlated with poor prognosis independent of tumor stage and grade for these tumors.[78,164,268]

The presence of venous tumor thrombosis has been shown to have independent prognostic significance,[268] while tumor necrosis, which has prognostic significance for clear cell renal cell carcinoma, does not correlate with survival.[78,164] Markers of cell proliferation (silver-staining nucleolar organizer region score and Ki-67 index) have also been correlated with outcome for papillary renal cell carcinoma.[239,275,276]

Prognostic studies relating to genetic status are limited. Hypoploidy has been associated with an adverse outcome as has allelic loss on chromosome 9p13.[250,277]

Division of papillary renal cell carcinomas according to type 1 and type 2 morphology appears to have prognostic significance. Type 2 tumors are larger and more frequently of higher stage than type 1 tumors.[237,256,278–280] Typing of these tumors has been shown to correlate with outcome on univariate analysis[164,239,246,250,256,267,276,279–282] although this was retained on multivariate analysis that included tumor stage in only three studies.[239,279,280]

Prognosis and Treatment

Patients with papillary renal cell carcinoma are more likely to have other primary visceral malignancies than are patients with clear cell renal cell carcinoma, with colonic, prostatic, and bladder cancers predominating.[283,284] Overall the prognosis is considered to be better than for clear cell renal cell carcinoma.[77,78] The management of papillary renal cell carcinoma is similar to that of clear cell renal cell carcinoma and is primarily surgical. Systemic therapy for these tumors has limited efficacy.[285]

Chromophobe Renal Cell Carcinoma

Introduction

Chromophobe renal cell carcinoma was recognized as a distinct form of renal parenchymal neoplasia by Wolfgang Thoenes et al. in 1985.[286] It was soon recognized that many of these tumors contain both chromophobe and eosinophilic cell types in varying proportions and sometimes the eosinophilic cells greatly predominated or were even the exclusive cell type.[287] Immunohistochemical studies have suggested that chromophobe renal cell carcinomas are derived from intercalated cells of the collecting duct.[1]

Epidemiology

In large registries from multiple locations, the proportion of chromophobe renal cell carcinoma within mixed series of renal cell carcinoma is approximately 4%.[77,78,80–83,288–290] Chromophobe renal cell carcinoma occurs almost exclusively in adults with reported mean ages from several series being approximately 58 years.[77,78,80–83,290,291] Chromophobe renal cell carcinoma is very rare in children.[230] There is a slight male predominance with the reported male-to-female ratio ranging from 1:1 to 1.6:1.[77,78,288]

Clinical Features

In recent series, the majority of patients were asymptomatic, with the tumors discovered as incidental findings.[288,291–293] In common with other renal neoplasms, when symptomatic, the most common presenting features are flank pain, hematuria, weight loss, or flank mass.[292] The radiological findings for chromophobe renal cell carcinoma are nonspecific. Tumors are usually hypodense and well circumscribed. Laboratory tests are usually noncontributory, although rare instances of anemia have been reported.[292]

Pathology

Gross Features

In large series, chromophobe renal cell carcinomas were unilateral and ranged in size from 1.5 to 25 cm, with mean diameters ranging from 5.4 to 9 cm (Fig. 2-33).[77,78,288,291,292] Chromophobe renal cell carcinoma is typically unifocal although multifocality occurs occasionally.[77,291]

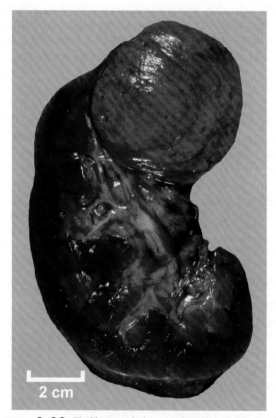

FIGURE 2-33 ■ Chromophobe renal cell carcinoma. This gross photograph shows a relatively homogeneous tumor with a brownish color.

The tumors are well circumscribed, and a prominent pseudocapsule may be present. The cut surface of chromophobe renal cell carcinoma in the unfixed state is beige, light brown, or tan, while after formalin fixation the tumors are gray to white. The eosinophilic variant tumors are darker brown than the classic type, more closely mimicking oncocytoma. Chromophobe renal cell carcinomas are usually solid, and there may be a central zone of edematous stroma similar to that sometimes seen in oncocytomas. Rarely, small cysts may be present; however, visible cysts are not typical of chromophobe renal cell carcinoma, and the tumors do not show the variegation typical of clear cell renal cell carcinoma.[287,291–293]

Microscopic Features

Histologically, chromophobe renal cell carcinoma most frequently consists of sheets or broad trabeculae of cells, although occasionally areas with small cysts are present.[287,291–293] The archetypal chromophobe cell varies in size from small to quite large and has pale-staining flocculent cytoplasm and a prominent cell membrane (Fig. 2-34). The nucleus is central or slightly eccentric, usually with a mild degree of nuclear pleomorphism, although occasionally large, but regular, nuclei may be present. Sometimes the nuclei show fixation artifact and have a wrinkled contour. Small nucleoli are usually visible. Often there is an area of cytoplasmic clearing around the nucleus forming a pronounced perinuclear halo. Intracytoplasmic basophilic inclusions may also be present. Tumor cells often show dyscohesion, and although this is a processing artifact, this feature can be diagnostically helpful. The cytoplasm of the tumor cells contains mucopolysaccharide, and this stains diffusely and strongly with Hale colloidal iron stain.[50] Most chromophobe renal cell carcinomas also contain some cells with eosinophilic cytoplasm. These cells are usually smaller than the average chromophobe cell, and because of the cytoplasmic staining, the perinuclear halos are more prominent. In about 10% of chromophobe renal

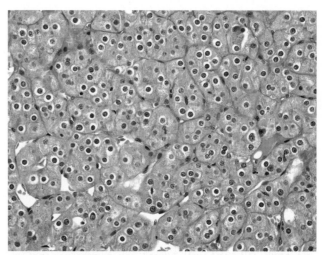

FIGURE 2-35 ■ Chromophobe renal cell carcinoma. This eosinophilic variant of chromophobe renal cell carcinoma resembles the compact growth pattern of renal oncocytoma.

cell carcinomas, these eosinophilic cells predominate to the extent that the tumor resembles an oncocytoma and these tumors are designated as the eosinophilic variant of chromophobe renal cell carcinoma (Fig. 2-35).[287,288,293]

The sheets of neoplastic cells are a random mosaic of large, medium, and small cells. In some tumors, large balloon-like chromophobe cells surround some of the blood vessels (Fig. 2-36). While there are thin-walled vessels and delicate fibrous septa, a striking feature is the presence of thick-walled hyalinized vessels of fairly small caliber. While occasional psammoma bodies may be present, a distinctive common finding is the presence of scattered small irregular aggregates of fine calcific granules.

Rarely, chromophobe renal cell carcinomas show atypical features. Focally, the tumors may exhibit microcystic change with associated lipochrome pigmentation.[294] Neuroendocrine differentiation has been reported.[295] Tumors may also show

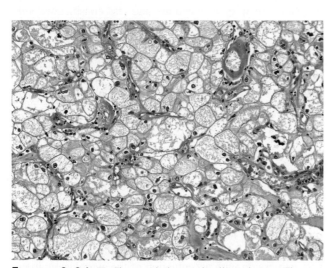

FIGURE 2-34 ■ Chromophobe renal cell carcinoma. The random mosaic-like mixture of large and small cells, thick-walled vasculature, and coarsely granular cytoplasm are typical features.

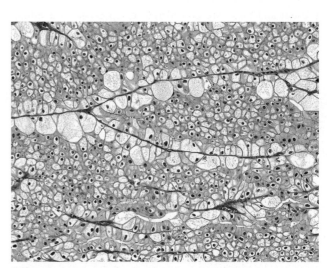

FIGURE 2-36 ■ Chromophobe renal cell carcinoma. The large cells surround the blood vessels.

extensive calcification and even osseous metaplasia.[296,297] Chromophobe renal cell carcinoma undergoes sarcomatoid change at about the same frequency as clear cell and papillary renal cell carcinoma: 4% to 8%. There may be some ethnic or geographic variability in this since the prevalence of sarcomatoid change was higher in a series from Saudi Arabia.[298] Rarely in sarcomatoid tumors, squamous, rhabdomyosarcomatous, osteosarcomatous, or chondrosarcomatous differentiation have been reported.[299–302] Rhabdoid morphology has also been reported.[303]

Chromophobe renal cell carcinoma has distinctive cytologic features and may be diagnosed by fine needle aspiration. In cytological preparations the carcinoma cells are arranged in small clusters and as single cells. The cells in the smears show the mosaic-like pattern of large and medium and small cells and well-defined cell membranes that are seen in paraffin sections. In Diff-Quik-stained smears, perinuclear halos can be seen in some cells.[304,305]

Ancillary and Special Studies

Immunohistochemical staining of chromophobe renal cell carcinoma is diffusely positive for EMA, CK7, CK14, parvalbumin, MUC-1, E-cadherin, and c-kit (CD117).[43,111,306–309] The CK7 staining is cytoplasmic with accentuation at the cell membranes. Focal positivity has been reported for CD10, AMACR, CD82, caveolin-1, beta defensin, and kidney-specific cadherin.[43,47,307,310–313] There is no or only focal weak expression of carbonic anhydrase IX.[113–115] Claudin-7 shows diffuse expression, while claudin-8 staining is negative. There is negative or at best focal expression of high molecular weight cytokeratin, vimentin, S100A1 protein, and RCC antigen.[45,307–309,314,315]

Electron microscopic examination of chromophobe renal cell carcinoma shows the presence of numerous pleomorphic, round to elongate microvesicles within the cytoplasm, ranging in size from 130 to 550 μM.[316,317] It has been suggested that these microvesicles are of mitochondrial origin.[293] Large vacuoles containing microvesicles are often present and these are considered to represent intracellular degradation.[318] Cell boundaries are prominent due to the presence of short microvilli, and occasional aggregates of dense core granules and cytokeratin microfilaments have been reported.[287,316] The eosinophilic variant of chromophobe renal cell carcinoma has been shown to contain greater numbers of mitochondria. These mitochondria are abnormal, often with tubulovesicular cristae, and in both types of chromophobe renal cell carcinoma budding from the mitochondrial membrane has been observed, which may be the mechanism of microvesicle formation. In the eosinophilic variant of the tumor, fewer intracytoplasmic microvesicles are seen.[287,293,317]

It has been noted that microvesicles are disrupted by alcohol and xylene, and are not usually visible in paraffin-embedded tissue processed for electron microscopy. It is considered that the disruption of these vesicles during processing releases the mucopolysaccharides that stain positively with Hales colloid iron. Although most difficult cases are generally resolved by light microscopy and immunohistochemistry, in the past, it has been recommended that tissue be retained for ultrastructural studies in cases of potential diagnostic difficulty.[319]

Genetics

Cytogenetic and molecular studies on chromophobe renal cell carcinoma show widespread loss of chromosomes and chromosomal regions, with monosomy of chromosomes 1, 2, 6, 10, 13, 17, and 21 being most frequently observed.[320] While this pattern is also seen in metastatic chromophobe renal cell carcinoma, sarcomatoid transformation of the tumors is associated with additional mutations, resulting in multiple gains of chromosomes 1, 2, 6, 10, and 17.[321]

The genetic profile of chromophobe renal cell carcinoma differs from that of oncocytoma, and FISH studies have been used to differentiate between these two tumor types.[57] While 91% of chromophobe renal cell carcinomas showed multiple losses among chromosomes 1, 2, 6, 10 and 17, 92% of oncocytomas showed no chromosomal losses or losses involving only one of these five chromosomes.

Differential Diagnosis

The cellular morphology of typical chromophobe renal cell carcinoma, coupled with sheet-like growth pattern and hyalinized vasculature, is usually diagnostic. Eosinophilic chromophobe renal cell carcinoma can be more problematic and in particular may mimic both oncocytoma and clear cell renal cell carcinoma with granular cytoplasm (see Table 2-2).

Unlike oncocytoma, chromophobe renal cell carcinoma has wrinkled nuclei although these are often few in the eosinophilic variant. Prominent perinuclear halos is a feature often seen and can be particularly prominent in the eosinophilic variant, a feature that is usually only focally seen in oncocytoma. The cell nests are more variable in size in oncocytoma, and separation by loose edematous stroma is characteristic of oncocytoma and less conspicuous with chromophobe carcinoma. Evidence of significant infiltration into perirenal fat with a desmoplastic stromal response is also indicative of carcinoma. Colloidal iron staining may be helpful in differentiating these two tumor types. In chromophobe renal cell carcinoma, staining is usually diffuse within the cytoplasm (Fig. 2-37A). Oncocytoma may also show positive staining, which has been reported in up to 84% of cases. This is, however, often focal and weak, and may be confined to the luminal aspect of the cell.[294]

Immunohistochemical stains are often of utility in differentiating eosinophilic chromophobe renal cell carcinoma from oncocytoma. There is an extensive literature promoting many markers as being helpful in this distinction, but for the most part, these have not stood the test of time. One marker that has proven useful is cytokeratin 7 that usually shows diffuse expression with accentuation of the cytoplasmic membrane in chromophobe renal cell carcinoma (Fig. 2-37B). In contrast, oncocytomas may be negative, but more often

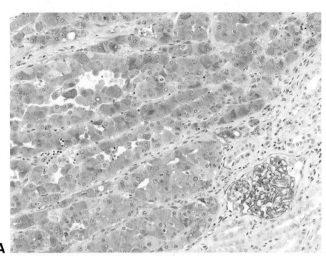
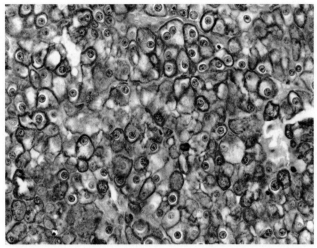

FIGURE 2-37 ■ **A:** Chromophobe renal cell carcinoma. The colloidal iron stain makes the entire cytoplasm of nearly all of the neoplastic cells blue. The nearby glomerulus and epithelium lining nonneoplastic tubules are useful positive and negative controls by which to evaluate the success of the staining procedure. **B:** Immunohistochemistry for cytokeratin 7 shows a positive reaction the cytoplasm of nearly all of the neoplastic cells. The reaction is heightened at the plasma membrane and rarefied around the nucleus.

individual cells or groups of cells are positive. Both tumors express CD117 with a membranous pattern and are negative for CD10 and vimentin.

While morphology assessment usually permits differentiation of chromophobe renal cell carcinoma from clear cell renal cell carcinoma, some cases may be problematic. The strong positive reactivity for cytokeratin 7 and lack of carbonic anhydrase IX and CD10 reactivity readily differentiates between the two.[109,307–309,314]

Prognosis and Predictive Factors

Staging

Chromophobe renal cell carcinoma has a more favorable outcome than clear cell renal cell carcinoma with 5-year survival probability rates of 80% to 100% being reported.[77,81,82,287,290,322–324] These tumors are more likely to be organ confined than other types of renal cell carcinoma at diagnosis, but have also been reported as being of larger size at presentation.[77,287] Up to 97% of tumors are localized to the kidney at diagnosis, and in larger series, the distribution of pT1, pT2, and pT3 tumors was 36% to 67%, 21% to 48%, and 11% to 29%, respectively.[78,83,288] There are limited data relating stage to outcome, and it has been shown that there was no significant survival difference between pT1 + pT2 and pT3 + pT4 tumors. The presence of lymph node metastases (pN1) was, however, significantly associated with outcome (Fig. 2-38). The presence of necrosis on histologic examination has also been correlated with survival.[78]

Extrarenal metastatic disease is a poor prognostic feature, with a reported median survival of 0.6 years.[325] In view of this, it is of significance that these tumors may metastasize at intervals >5 years after primary treatment, with pulmonary metastases 10 years after diagnosis being noted.

Grading

There are few validation studies for grading of chromophobe renal cell carcinoma due to the small number of cases available for study. Some studies have reported Fuhrman grading to correlate significantly with outcome[290,326] while others have not.[327] Using modified Fuhrman criteria that focused upon nuclear shape and nucleolar size, combined grades 1 and 2 tumors were shown to have significantly better survival, when compared to grade 3 and grade 4 tumors on univariate analysis.[78]

When each of the three components of the Fuhrman grading system was tested independently, it was shown that none of these correlated with outcome.[327] It was also shown that chromophobe nuclei are usually too small to satisfy Fuhrman grade 3 nuclear size criteria. Further, these tumors frequently

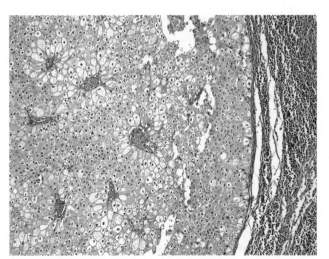

FIGURE 2-38 ■ Chromophobe renal cell carcinoma metastatic to lymph node.

have a small nucleolus, which does not accord with the degree of nuclear pleomorphism these tumors usually exhibit, which may account for the wide variation in patient numbers assigned to each grade in various reported series. In view of these findings, it has been recommended that Fuhrman grading is inappropriate for chromophobe renal carcinoma.

Alternate grading schemes for chromophobe renal cell carcinoma have been proposed but have not been validated.[328] In the absence of a reproducible and proven grading system for these tumors, the ISUP has recommended against grading chromophobe renal cell carcinoma.[329]

Other Features

Sarcomatoid dedifferentiation of chromophobe renal cell carcinoma has a poor prognosis, with a reported 24-month survival rate of 25%.[325] This is comparable to sarcomatoid dedifferentiation of other subtypes of renal parenchymal neoplasia, where 24-month survival rate was found to be 29%.

Prognosis and Treatment

The management of chromophobe renal cell carcinoma is similar to that of clear cell renal cell carcinoma and is primarily surgical. For patients with metastatic disease, there are limited data regarding the efficacy of adjuvant therapy. In a small study, a response was noted in 3 of 12 patients treated with tyrosine kinase inhibitors, with a progression-free interval of 11 months.[330]

Collecting Duct Carcinoma

Introduction

While the first report of what is now recognized as collecting duct carcinoma was published in 1949,[331] it was not until 1976 that it was suggested that tumors with atypical changes in the collecting duct epithelium were of collecting duct origin.[226] In 1986, these tumors were recognized as a distinctive form of renal cell carcinoma.[332]

Epidemiology and Clinical Features

Collecting duct carcinoma constitutes <1% of renal malignancies.[333–336] These tumors occur within a wide patient age range with pediatric examples being recognized. They are most commonly seen in patients in their fourth to seventh decades (mean 55 years), with a male predominance of approximately 2:1.[335–345]

Patients with collecting duct carcinoma often present with advanced-stage disease. These tumors are often symptomatic at diagnosis with typical presenting features being hematuria, abdominal mass, intermittent flank or back pain, fatigue, pyrexia, and weight loss. In <25% of cases, the tumor is discovered as an incidental finding.[338,339,342] The frequency of symptoms at presentation reflects the rapid growth of the tumors and early metastatic spread, with one-third to one-half of patients having clinical evidence of metastases at the time of diagnosis.[343,345,346]

Pathology

Gross Features

While the collecting ducts are present in the cortex and the medulla, the gross pathologic finding of a tumor arising in the medulla, where most other components of the renal tubular system are absent, is an important aid to the diagnosis.[337] Unfortunately, precise localization to the medulla is only possible with small tumors, and many tumors are too large at the time of resection for the specific site of origin within the kidney to be recognizable.[337] Typically, collecting duct carcinomas are white to gray, with infiltrative borders and have a firm consistency on sectioning (Fig. 2-39). Confluent central necrosis of the tumor is common; however, hemorrhage is not usually seen macroscopically. These tumors may extend into the renal pelvis and on imaging studies, may mimic pelvic urothelial carcinoma.[337]

Microscopic Features

Characteristically, these are histopathologically distinctive carcinomas with features that may resemble a mixture of both adenocarcinoma and urothelial carcinoma.[335,347,348] Microscopic examination shows highly irregular tubules and duct-like structures, nests, and cords of cells in an abundant loose, slightly basophilic desmoplastic stroma, often containing a diffuse chronic active inflammatory cell infiltrate (Fig. 2-40).[337,349] The carcinoma cells lining the lumens have small or moderate amounts of pale to eosinophilic cytoplasm

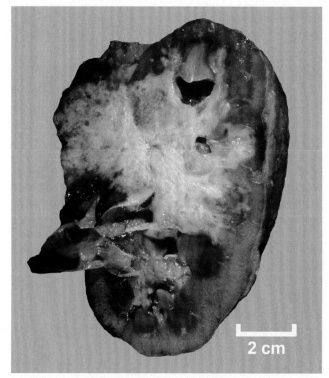

FIGURE 2-39 ■ Collecting duct carcinoma. This gross photograph shows a highly infiltrative carcinoma central in the kidney, which invades the collecting system and perinephric fat while causing early hydronephrosis.

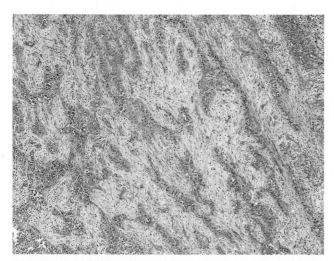

FIGURE 2-40 ■ Collecting duct carcinoma. Irregular, even jagged, cords of carcinoma cells in a background of desmoplasia with inflammation is the typical architecture of collecting duct carcinoma.

and nuclei that are pleomorphic, and have thick nuclear membranes. Prominent nucleoli are commonly seen and mitotic figures are frequently present. An especially useful feature, rarely found in renal cell carcinoma and not found in urothelial carcinoma, is the hobnail appearance sometimes present in the cells lining duct lumens. Some of the reported cases have a different pattern, consisting of papillary fronds covered by cells with small amounts of cytoplasm, similar to the basophilic cell type of renal cell carcinoma.[338,343,349] Atypical epithelium in the medullary tubules adjacent to the carcinoma has been seen in some cases.[338,347,348] Occasional foci of spindle cells may be present; however, if this is more than a rare occurrence, the tumor should be considered to be a sarcomatoid carcinoma arising in a collecting duct carcinoma. Tumor architecture may be recapitulated in extrarenal metastases.

Extracellular and intracellular mucin may be seen in collecting duct carcinoma, and histochemically this may be either neutral or acidic.[350]

Ancillary and Special Studies

The immunohistochemical expression of collecting duct carcinoma reflects its origin from the collecting duct of the distal nephron.[337,351–353] These tumors stain strongly for cytokeratin 19, lectins (*Ulex europaeus* agglutinin-1, peanut lectin), e-cadherin, c-kit, and low molecular weight cytokeratins. Expression of high molecular weight cytokeratin (34βE12) is seen in up to 50% of cases.[345,352,354] The tumors express PAX2 and PAX8.[345,354] Vimentin reactivity is variable and usually weakly to moderately positive. There is also variable expression of Leu M1 and EMA. Expression of antigens associated with convoluted tubules (CD10, RCC antigen, and AMACR) is usually but not always negative. Expression of p63 has been reported to be positive in some cases, but this was in a series that included tumors with a minor urothelial carcinoma component in the collecting duct category.[354]

Genetics

Genetic studies on collecting duct carcinoma to date have been inconclusive and only limited studies have been published. In three cases, there was monosomy of chromosomes 1, 6, 14, 15, and 22, with loss of chromosomes 4 and 18 in two patients.[340] Some question has, however, been raised regarding the diagnosis of some of these cases.[341] In a further study, these tumors have shown trisomy for chromosomes 4, 7, 8, 17, and 20, and loss of chromosomes 14, 18, and 22.[342] Loss of heterozygosity for 8p and 13q has also been shown in collecting duct carcinoma.[355]

Differential Diagnosis

Awareness of the features of collecting duct carcinoma should establish the diagnosis in most cases. The differential diagnosis includes urothelial carcinoma with glandular differentiation, renal medullary carcinoma, high-grade papillary renal cell carcinoma, renal cell carcinoma of the hereditary leiomyomatosis and renal cell carcinoma syndrome, and metastatic carcinoma (see Table 2-8).

High-grade upper tract urothelial carcinoma may mimic the architecture of collecting duct carcinoma and is the most problematic differential diagnosis. In such cases, the presence of atypical cells within the distal collecting ducts may represent direct extension of pelvic urothelial carcinoma. The presence of an identifiable urothelial component including urothelial carcinoma in situ within the renal pelvis indicates a diagnosis of urothelial carcinoma. PAX8 is positive in most collecting duct carcinomas and is negative in most but not all urothelial carcinomas of upper tract origin. PAX2 is less specific as it is expressed in 20% of upper tract urothelial carcinomas. Urothelial carcinomas are often positive for cytokeratin 20 and low molecular weight cytokeratins, and negative for vimentin. *Ulex europaeus* agglutinin-1 expression is considered typical for collecting duct carcinoma; however, this has also been demonstrated for high-grade urothelial carcinoma.[356]

Renal medullary carcinoma may mimic collecting duct carcinoma although it usually exhibits a sheet-like, yolk sac-like, or nested growth pattern. The presence of rhabdoid cells and a heavy neutrophilic infiltrate would favor medullary carcinoma. Medullary carcinoma also shows loss of INI1 expression though this has also been reported in a small percentage of collecting duct carcinomas. Patients with renal medullary carcinoma are usually <20 years of age and have sickle cell trait. High-grade papillary renal cell carcinoma with a tubulopapillary growth pattern may also resemble collecting duct carcinoma. Papillary renal cell carcinoma is usually positive for CD10, RCC antigen, and AMACR and is negative for high molecular weight cytokeratin (34βE12), *Ulex europaeus* agglutinin-1, and peanut lectin. Metastatic tumor is often multifocal and may show geographic necrosis. A previous history of extrarenal malignancy and appropriate clinical and immunohistochemical investigations are usually diagnostic.

Prognosis and Treatment

Survival data from case reports and small case series show collecting duct carcinoma to be associated with a poor prognosis.[343] Up to 40% of patients with collecting duct carcinoma have clinical evidence of metastatic disease at diagnosis, and most patients die within 1 to 3 years. The largest tumor series reported to date consists of a nationwide survey from Japan.[357] In this series of 81 confirmed cases, 65% of patients were symptomatic at diagnosis, 44% had lymph node metastases, and 32% had remote metastases. The 1-, 3-, and 10-year disease-specific survival of patients in this series was 69%, 45%, and 14%, respectively.

Treatment of these tumors has been similar to the treatment for other renal cell carcinomas but with the more frequent use of chemotherapy including gemcitabine and cisplatin. Reports of response to multiple agent protocols including tyrosine kinase inhibitors have appeared in the literature,[358] although most studies have shown limited response to targeted therapies.

Renal Medullary Carcinoma

Introduction

Renal medullary carcinoma was initially recognized from retrospective analysis of a series of renal carcinomas in younger patients, collected by the Armed Forces Institute of Pathology.[359] In this series, all patients were black and had sickled erythrocytes on histologic examination. Since this original case study in 1995, nearly 200 cases of renal medullary carcinoma have been reported.[345,360–372]

Epidemiology and Clinical Features

The overwhelming majority of reported cases of renal medullary carcinoma have been in African Americans with a smaller proportion in those of Hispanic or Brazilian origin.[362] These tumors are rarely seen in Caucasians with fewer than 10 cases reported.

Almost all patients have sickle cell trait or hemoglobin SC disease. The tumor has been reported in one patient with a normal blood profile.[362] The patients' ages at diagnosis have ranged from 5 to 69 years with a mean of 19 years. There is a male predominance with a male to female ratio of 2:1, although for patients <10 years of age, the ratio is 5:1.[362]

Virtually all patients are symptomatic at diagnosis with hematuria and flank or abdominal pain predominating. Other common presenting symptoms are abdominal mass, dysuria, and weight loss.

Pathology

Gross Features

Renal medullary carcinomas are usually poorly circumscribed ranging in size from 4 to 12 cm (mean 7 cm). Greater than 75% of tumors occur in the right kidney, and on sectioning, the tumor is frequently tan or gray-white and often shows extensive necrosis and hemorrhage.

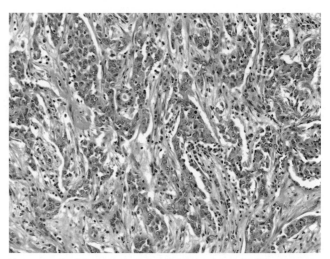

FIGURE 2-41 ■ Renal medullary carcinoma. Like collecting duct carcinoma, renal medullary carcinoma often consists of cords of carcinoma cells embedded in an inflamed desmoplastic stroma.

Microscopic Features

Renal medullary carcinomas are composed of cells exhibiting marked nuclear pleomorphism, prominent nucleoli, and eosinophilic cytoplasm. Mitotic figures are common. The tumors usually consist of infiltrating sheets with poorly formed vacuoles. The tumor may also form cords, nests, microcysts, and tubular structures (Fig. 2-41). Sharply defined round empty spaces within cords or nests are common and when numerous can impart a lacey appearance (Fig. 2-42). Pyknotic cells are sometimes seen within these holes, so it appears that they arise through a mechanism of individual cell necrosis. Carcinoma cells with rhabdoid morphology may be prominent (Fig. 2-43). There is usually a pronounced desmoplastic reaction with an associated chronic active inflammatory cell infiltrate. Areas of necrosis are often present. There is sometimes a conspicuous retraction artifact between the carcinoma and the surrounding

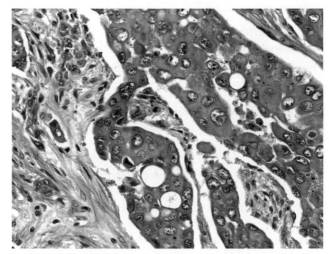

FIGURE 2-42 ■ Renal medullary carcinoma often shows sharp-edged holes in the cords and sometimes a retraction artifact at the border with the stroma.

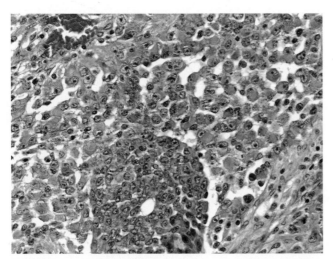

FIGURE 2-43 ■ Renal medullary carcinoma. Rhabdoid morphology is commonly found in medullary carcinoma and can be prominent.

stroma. Sickle cell erythrocytes are a frequent finding within the tumor and renal tissue.

Ancillary and Special Studies

The immunohistochemical expression profile of medullary carcinoma has been reported from several studies.[343,360,361,367,372] Medullary carcinomas frequently show diffuse positive reactions for cytokeratin AE1/AE3, low molecular weight cytokeratin, epithelial membrane antigen, vimentin, HIF, and VEGF. There is variable expression of cytokeratin 7, high molecular weight cytokeratin, CEA, *Ulex europaeus*, agglutinin-1, and TP53. Immunohistochemical reactions for HER2 (ERBB2) are negative. Immunohistochemistry with antibody to OCT4 is strongly positive in about 50% of cases.[373] *SMARCB1* is very frequently lost in medullary carcinoma of the kidney and can be detected by loss of INI1 expression immunohistochemically.[372]

Electron microscopic findings are inconsistent. In some studies tumor cells have been shown to contain vesicles lined by long microvilli and prominent desmosomes, and condensed fibrillary electron-dense deposits have also been identified. Intracytoplasmic glycogen or lipids is not a feature of these tumors.[360,361]

Genetics

Genetic studies on renal medullary carcinoma are, to date, limited. The most common genetic abnormality is inactivation of the *SMARCB1* gene.[374] In one case loss of chromosome 22 has been noted, and in three cases FISH analysis showed amplification of the *ABL* gene, with no evidence of *BCR-ABL* translocation. Gene expression profiling has shown 487 genes to be expressed differently from that of other types of renal tumor, with expression most closely resembling that of urothelial carcinoma.[361]

Differential Diagnosis

The main differential diagnosis for renal medullary carcinoma is high-grade invasive urothelial carcinoma and collecting duct carcinoma. Clinical evidence of sickle cell trait and young age at presentation are seen with renal medullary carcinoma, while the presence of in situ urothelial carcinoma and cytokeratin 20 positivity favors urothelial carcinoma.

The infiltrative components of medullary carcinoma may form tubules resembling collecting duct carcinoma and this has been considered to be evidence that these two tumor types are related. Sickle cell trait is not associated with collecting duct carcinoma. The immunohistochemical profile of medullary carcinoma and collecting duct carcinoma has significant overlap limiting its value.[345] Loss of INI1 expression would favor medullary carcinoma but can be seen in a small number of cases of collecting duct carcinoma. Loss of INI1 expression is also characteristic of rhabdoid tumor of the kidney, and the presence of rhabdoid-like cells in medullary carcinoma could lead to misdiagnosis. The presence of other patterns in medullary carcinoma should lead to the correct diagnosis. Collecting duct carcinoma is usually positive for high molecular weight cytokeratin and *Ulex europaeus* agglutinin-1 and negative for CEA.

Prognosis and Treatment

These tumors have a poor prognosis with 95% of patients having metastatic disease at the time of diagnosis.[359–362,367,369] In one series, survival ranged from 1 day to 68 weeks with a mean interval of 18 weeks. Three patients with organ-confined disease at presentation were alive at 9 months, 2 years, and 8 years postnephrectomy.[362,367] These are generally treated as other renal carcinomas with no specific treatment of demonstrated efficacy.

Translocation Carcinomas

Introduction

In recent years, a number of carcinomas showing distinctive features have been described, and in 1996, tumors of this type were characterized as showing Xp11.2 translocation.[375,376] Since then, a family of renal carcinomas, which contains a variety of translocations involving Xp11.2, has been identified. All of these translocations have resulted in gene fusions involving *TFE3*,[377] and this family of carcinomas was classified as Xp11 translocation carcinomas in the 2004 WHO Classification. Subsequently, carcinomas with a t(6;11) translocation, producing a fusion with *TFEB* transcription factor gene, have been identified.[378] *TFEB* and *TFE3* are members of the *MITF/TFE* family of transcription factors and the tumors have a number of morphologic features in common. For this reason, it has been suggested that this group of tumors be designated *MITF/TFE* family translocation carcinomas.[377]

Epidemiology and Clinical Features

While carcinomas make up <5% of renal tumors in children, more than a third of pediatric renal carcinomas are translocation carcinomas.[230] These tumors also occur in adults, and in a recent large series of cases the mean patient age was 25 years. There is a female predominance with a female-to-male ratio of 2.5:1.[379] In adult series, approximately 1% of tumors are translocation carcinomas and an association with previous chemotherapy has been noted.[380]

A melanotic variant of Xp11 translocation carcinomas has been recently reported.[381] Although the two genetically confirmed cases in this study were reported in children, 19 additional suggestive cases collected from the literature included tumors in adults, with patient ages ranging from 3 to 71 years.

The typical presenting features of hematuria, flank pain, or abdominal pain are the most common presenting features for translocation carcinomas. As is common for other forms of renal cell neoplasia, approximately one-third of tumors are detected as incidental findings following imaging studies. In some series almost half the patients presented with visceral or lymph node metastases.[379]

Pathology

Gross Findings

Translocation carcinomas are frequently large tumors at diagnosis, and recorded cases have ranged up to 20 cm in diameter, with the mean diameter of reported cases being approximately 7 cm.[377,379]

The cut surface of the tumors is similar to clear cell renal cell carcinoma usually being solid yellow-tan. Foci of hemorrhage and necrosis are common, and occasionally focal cystic degeneration is present. In early reports, it was noted that carcinomas with fusion of *PRCC-TFE3* had a pronounced fibrous pseudocapsule[382] with intramural dystrophic calcification. Melanotic translocation cancers showing varying degrees of dark pigmentation on gross examination have been reported (Fig. 2-44).[381]

Microscopic Features

Translocation carcinomas may exhibit a variety of morphologic patterns, most frequently being papillary, solid, alveolar, or nested. A useful diagnostic feature is the presence

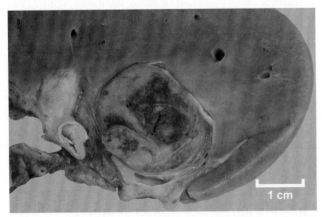

FIGURE 2-44 ■ Translocation carcinoma. This melanotic Xp11 translocation cancer shows areas of brown color corresponding to melanin pigment.

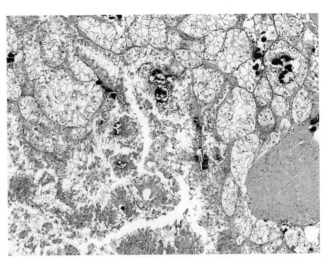

FIGURE 2-45 ■ Translocation carcinoma. Papillae and alveoli populated by large cells with clear or eosinophilic cytoplasm are typical, as are the psammoma bodies and large calcifications.

of papillae covered by clear cells with voluminous cytoplasm, although eosinophilic tumor cells may also be present (Fig. 2-45).

The nuclei may show some variability in size and are generally large with a prominent eosinophilic nucleolus. Eosinophilic hyaline droplets, psammoma bodies, and large calcifications may also be present. Focal necrosis is a common feature, and rarely there may be a lymphocytic infiltrate or aggregates of foamy macrophages.[377,378,382,383]

Subtle morphologic variations have been described in some of the carcinomas showing Xp11 translocations. Tumors with the *ASPL-TFE3* fusion are predominantly nested with pseudopapillary architecture, and foam cells are not a feature, although psammoma bodies may be present.[383] Carcinomas with the *PRCC-TFE3* fusion usually show a papillary or alveolar architecture. Foam cells and more rarely psammoma bodies may be seen, and there is often focal tumor necrosis.[377,382]

TFEB translocation carcinomas were originally described as showing a biphasic growth pattern with sheets of large cells having abundant eosinophilic cytoplasm and aggregates of small cells, which focally form rosette-like structures that surround eosinophilic hyaline nodules of basement membrane-like material (Fig. 2-46).[378] It is now recognized that this architecture may also be present in *TFE3* tumors.[380]

The melanotic variant of Xp11 translocation carcinoma consists of nests and sheets of epithelioid cells, with clear to finely granular cytoplasm and varying amounts of cytoplasmic pigmentation showing positive staining for melanin (Fig. 2-47). The nuclei are rather spherical with inconspicuous nucleoli.[381]

Ancillary and Special Studies

These tumors are typically positive for CD10, AMACR, E-cadherin, and RCC antigen, and are negative for EMA and cytokeratin 7. There is variable vimentin expression, and other cytokeratins are either negative or weakly positive.[377,379]

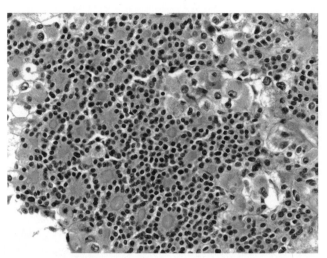

FIGURE 2-46 ■ Translocation carcinoma. Small cells with deeply basophilic nuclei forming rosette-like structures are typical of those with *TFEB* mutation.

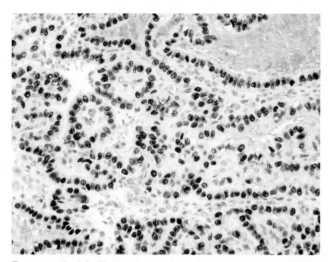

FIGURE 2-48 ■ Translocation carcinoma. Antibody to TFE3 gives a strongly positive reaction in the nuclei of most of the neoplastic cells.

Carbonic anhydrase IX is expressed in about 50% of cases as is PAX8. Melanocytic markers (melan-A, HMB45) are positive in a few TFE3-associated tumors and are more often expressed by TFEB-associated tumors. Cathepsin K immunostaining is positive in up to 50% of cases. Specific staining for TFE3 protein shows nuclear positivity in >80% of TFE3 translocation carcinomas (Fig. 2-48),[377,379,384] while a positive nuclear immunohistochemical reaction for TFEB protein is a feature of tumors showing this translocation.[385] The cores of the rosette-like structures contain collagen type IV (Fig. 2-49A and B). Melanotic translocation cancers show positive immunohistochemical reactions for TFE3 protein, and limited studies have shown these tumors to also be positive for HMB45 and melan-A. They are rarely positive for S-100 protein, and negative for cytokeratins, EMA, CD10, and RCC antigen.[381]

Ultrastructural studies of most TFE3 carcinomas show features similar to clear cell renal cell carcinoma. ASPL-TFE3

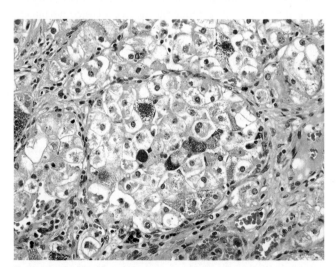

FIGURE 2-47 ■ Melanotic Xp11 cancer. Polygonal epithelioid cells form nests. Some of the cells contain melanin pigment.

tumors usually contain membrane-bound granules and rhomboid crystals within the cytoplasm.[383] Ultrastructurally, the melanotic translocation tumors contain type 2 and type 3 premelanosomes, with no evidence of epithelial or muscle differentiation.

Genetics

FISH and PCR studies show the presence of translocations typical of this tumor group. Melanotic translocation carcinomas have been shown to exhibit *TFE3* gene fusion. FISH analysis has demonstrated both balanced and unbalanced *TFE3* gene rearrangement, while *ASPL* was not the fusion partner.[381]

Differential Diagnosis

Translocation carcinoma must be differentiated from clear cell renal cell carcinoma, clear cell papillary renal cell carcinoma, and papillary renal cell carcinoma, especially for pediatric cases. The histologic features of the tumor are often characteristic, while staining for transcription factors, or molecular or genetic studies are usually diagnostic (see Tables 2-5 and 2-8). With the ever-expanding morphologic spectrum for translocation carcinoma, we include this entity in the differential diagnosis of the majority of unclassified renal cell carcinomas.

Prognosis and Treatment

TFE3 tumors show a high proportion of lymph node or visceral metastases. Despite this it appears that translocation carcinomas have an indolent clinical course, with late recurrences more than three decades after nephrectomy being reported.[377,379,386,387] Although limited numbers of cases have been studied, the tumor-related death rate in one series was 14% over a follow-up interval of 11 to 81 months. A repeat study has provided further evidence that high-stage TFE3 tumors have a prolonged disease-free interval over a mean follow-up period of 6 years.[388] Although tumor-related deaths have been reported

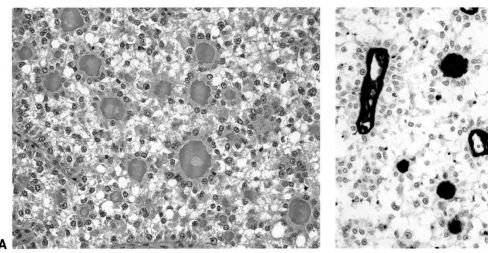

FIGURE 2-49 ■ **A:** Translocation carcinoma. At higher magnification, the rosette-like structures are seen to contain acellular eosinophilic deposits surrounded by a wreath of cells with eosinophilic cytoplasm and with the nuclei close to the basement membrane. **B:** Immunohistochemistry demonstrates the presence of collagen IV in the central eosinophilic nodules.

for TFEB and melanocytic TFE3 carcinomas, there are insufficient cases with follow-up to provide an accurate assessment of the prognosis associated with those tumors.[379,381]

Postneuroblastoma Carcinoma

Epidemiology and Clinical Features

Medeiros et al. published an account of four survivors of neuroblastoma who had histologically distinctive renal tumors and suggested that they constituted a distinct clinicopathologic entity; subsequently, another series of similar tumors in neuroblastoma survivors was published.[389,390] Postneuroblastoma renal cell carcinoma was included as a distinctive entity in the 2004 World Health Organization consensus conference on the classification of renal neoplasms.[5] Details of more than 20 cases of postneuroblastoma renal cell carcinoma have been reported.[390,391]

The tumors occurred in patients who were diagnosed with neuroblastoma within the first 2 years of life (mean age 13 months). The patients' ages at the time of diagnosis of renal carcinoma ranged from 3 to 36 years (mean 20 years) with a slight female predominance (60%). The shortest interval between the diagnosis of neuroblastoma and subsequent renal carcinoma was 3 years, while the longest interval was 35 years. In two cases, patients developed second renal carcinomas, each 2 years after the diagnosis of the first renal tumor.[389] Pooled data from the Childhood Cancer Survivor Study showed that survivors of neuroblastoma had a 329-fold increased risk of developing renal carcinoma.[392]

Although the majority of neuroblastoma survivors with renal cell carcinoma had received radiation or chemotherapy, two patients received no adjuvant therapy for their neuroblastomas.[389,390] There is also evidence that the development of these renal carcinomas is not confined to patients with neuroblastoma as a similar tumor was noted in a child who had received chemotherapy for cardiac leiomyosarcoma.[393]

Presenting features for postneuroblastoma carcinoma are varied. The majority of patients were asymptomatic while abdominal and back pain, abdominal mass, and hypertension have been reported.[391,394]

Pathology

Gross Features

Limited gross findings have been reported. Tumors were bilateral and multifocal in four cases and ranged in size from 3.5 to 8 cm. Two tumors showed involvement of the renal capsule, renal vessels, and renal sinus lymphatic vessels.[389,391]

Microscopic Features

Postneuroblastoma carcinoma consists of cells frequently showing abundant eosinophilic cytoplasm reminiscent of oncocytoma. Solid and papillary growth patterns may be present. Aggregates of foamy macrophage and psammoma bodies are occasionally seen. The nuclei of tumor cells are often irregular with a moderate degree of pleomorphism. Nucleoli are readily seen, and mitoses are often present but not plentiful. One tumor was reported as showing high nuclear grade and with extensive parenchymal infiltration.[389]

Ancillary and Special Studies

Studies of the immunohistochemical phenotype of these tumors are limited. Tumors reported to date showed positivity for cytokeratin (CAM 5.2), EMA, and vimentin. There was less frequent positivity for CK19 and CK20, while stains for CK7, S-100 protein, and HMB45 were negative.[389]

To date, no ultrastructural or genetic studies have been reported.

Differential Diagnosis

Although postneuroblastoma carcinoma has a characteristic morphology, the tumors show some resemblance to oncocytoma, chromophobe renal cell carcinoma, and type 2 papillary renal cell carcinoma. Papillary growth is not seen in oncocytoma and the presence of aggregates of foamy macrophages are not features of either oncocytoma or chromophobe renal cell carcinoma. Postneuroblastoma carcinoma lacks perinuclear halos associated with classic chromophobe cells.

While postneuroblastoma carcinoma may contain papillary areas, unlike type 2 papillary renal cell carcinoma, areas showing a solid or compacted nested pattern are usually present. The clinical features of postneuroblastoma, even in the absence of a confirmed past history of neuroblastoma, may also assist in diagnosis as these tumors occur in younger patients.

Prognosis and Treatment

Data are too limited to allow specific comment on specific prognostic factors for this tumor type. Of 14 cases for which follow-up was available, two patients died of tumor-related causes, two were alive with active disease, and seven were alive and well 12 months to 8 years following diagnosis of their renal tumors.[389,394] There is no specific treatment for these rare tumors.

Mucinous Tubular and Spindle Cell Carcinoma

Introduction

Histologically, distinctive renal neoplasms composed of cuboidal and spindle cells with mucinous extracellular matrix have been described in reports of single cases and in small series since 1998. In early reports, these tumors were known by a variety of terms that include low-grade collecting carcinoma,[395] low-grade tubular mucinous renal neoplasm,[396] and spindle and cuboidal renal cell carcinoma.[397] In these studies, emphasis was placed on the apparent low nuclear grade of these tumors, despite the presence of a spindle cell morphology. At the World Health Organization consensus conference in December 2002, the diagnostic phrase "mucinous tubular and spindle cell carcinoma" was adopted[5] reflecting the histologic features of these tumors.

Epidemiology and Clinical Features

Approximately 100 cases of mucinous tubular and spindle cell carcinoma have been reported to date, including several large series having typical and atypical morphology.[398–400] The mean age at presentation is approximately 50 years. The tumors are more common in females with a female-to-male ratio of 4:1. In one series, more than four cases was associated with nephrolithiasis.[397] Despite a wide range of reported tumor sizes, most tumors are asymptomatic at presentation and are discovered as incidental findings.

Pathology

Gross Features

Tumors range in size up to 18 cm in diameter and are usually well circumscribed. The cut surface is usually tan-brown to pink although in some studies cut surfaces has been described

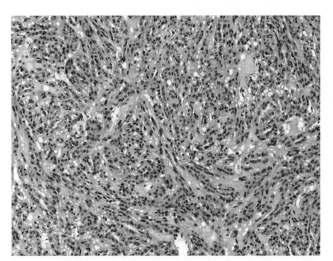

FIGURE 2-50 ■ Mucinous tubular and spindle cell carcinoma. Strands of spindle cells form tubules with narrow lumens in a background of extracellular mucinous material.

as gray to white, tan, and yellow to pinkish. Tumors are often cortical, being localized to the kidney, although localized medullary tumors have also been described. Macroscopic necrosis and hemorrhage has rarely been reported, and most tumors have a homogeneous appearance.

Microscopic Features

Mucinous tubular and spindle cell carcinoma usually has a characteristic morphology and is readily recognizable. The tumors consist of cuboidal cells arranged in long cords and tubules set in a loose and often myxoid or basophilic mucinous stroma (Fig. 2-50). In some areas, the cords appear collapsed, and here the tumor has a spindle cell appearance. The spindle cell component of the tumor may form sheets and the tumor may resemble a leiomyoma. The nuclei are usually spherical to ovoid and are of low nuclear grade, with a few small chromatin clumps and small nucleoli. Mitotic figures are rarely seen. Occasionally, tumor nuclei may show focal high nuclear grade, and recently tumors with sarcomatoid change have been reported.[401–403]

The mucinous background material may dominate focally and the epithelial elements form small cords in lakes of mucin (Fig. 2-51). This mucin reacts strongly with alcian blue and may be weakly positive for mucicarmine. Plasma cells, mast cells, clusters of foamy histiocytes, and psammoma bodies are occasionally present (Fig. 2-52).[396,404] Atypical forms of mucinous tubular and spindle cell carcinoma have recently been described.[400] In these tumors there were focal papillae, absence of mucinous stromal material, clear cells, oncocytes, and cellular vacuolation. Areas of neuroendocrine differentiation in mucinous tubular and spindle carcinoma have also been described, and this has been confirmed by ultrastructural studies.[405]

Ancillary and Special Studies

The immunohistochemical phenotype of mucinous tubular and spindle cell carcinoma varies between series. Tumors are usually positive for low molecular weight cytokeratin

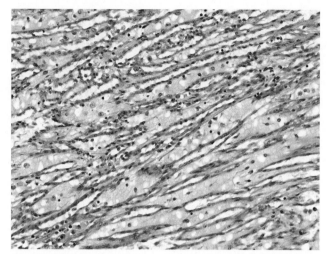

FIGURE 2-51 ■ Mucinous tubular and spindle cell carcinoma. Parallel arrays of elongate cells form long tubules with empty-looking lumens in a background of extracellular mucinous material.

(CAM 5.2), cytokeratin 7, and AMACR, and are usually negative for high molecular weight cytokeratin (CK 20 and 34βE12), CD10, RCC antigen, and *Ulex europaeus* agglutinin-1. There is variable expression for CD15.[261,398–398,403,405,406] In foci showing neuroendocrine differentiation, cells are positive for synaptophysin, chromogranin, and neuron-specific enolase.[405]

Genetics

It has been suggested that mucinous tubular and spindle cell carcinomas are related to papillary renal cell carcinomas on the basis of an overlap in immunohistochemical expression.[261,399] In spite of this, the typical genetic features of papillary renal cell carcinoma were not demonstrated in the largest genetic study to be undertaken to date.[407] Extensive losses of chromosomes have been shown in genetic studies, including loss of chromosomes 1, 4, 6, 8, 9, 13, 14, 15, 18, and 22.[396–398,407,408]

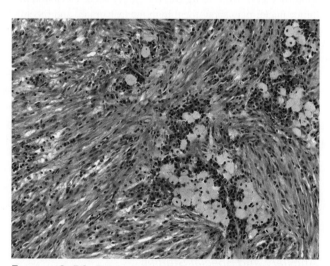

FIGURE 2-52 ■ Mucinous tubular and spindle cell carcinoma. In some tumors, there are areas consisting of sheets of spindle cells without lumens or mucin. Infiltrates of foamy macrophages and plasma cells are common in these tumors.

Differential Diagnosis

Mucinous tubular and spindle cell carcinomas are usually readily recognizable and the major differential diagnosis is type 1 papillary renal cell carcinoma. This is compounded by an overlap of immunohistochemical expression and the recent description of five cases of papillary renal cell carcinoma with low-grade spindle cell foci.[409] These spindle cell papillary renal cell carcinomas usually show typical papillary areas, at least focally, and unlike mucinous tubular and spindle cell carcinomas exhibit a male predominance. Additionally, mucinous tubular and spindle cell carcinomas are usually CD10 negative and genetic studies may also assist in differentiating between these two tumor types.

It is likely that in the past these tumors have been misdiagnosed as renal cell carcinoma showing sarcomatoid features; however, the presence of bland nuclear features and a low mitotic rate should exclude this extreme form of tumor differentiation. In mucin-poor tumors, where the spindle cell component predominates, there is some resemblance to tumors of smooth muscle origin. In such cases, negative staining for smooth muscle markers and cytokeratin positivity will lead to the correct diagnosis.

Prognosis and Treatment

In earlier studies, these tumors were considered to follow a benign course, and the vast majority of cases reported to date have behaved in a low-grade fashion. Regional lymph node involvement has been described in a few cases, and in one patient multiple intra-abdominal recurrences were seen.[396,397] Metastases have been reported in two out of five cases where the tumor showed sarcomatoid differentiation.[401–403,410] Metastases to the liver and retroperitoneal lymph nodes have also been seen in a single tumor that showed typical features of mucinous tubular and spindle cell carcinoma. There is no specific treatment for these tumors.

Tubulocystic Renal Carcinoma

Introduction

Tubulocystic carcinoma is a recently recognized form of renal neoplasia that was not included in the 2004 World Health Organization classification. The tumor was first described by Masson as "Bellinian epithelioma" in 1970 and was classified as a low-grade collecting duct carcinoma in Series III Armed Forces Institute of Pathology fascicle on tumors of the kidney.[411] In 2004, the term tubulocystic carcinoma was proposed by an international collaborative group, and to date three series have detailed the features of 55 tumors.[412–414]

Epidemiology and Clinical Features

Tubulocystic carcinoma shows a strong gender association with the male to female ratio being 7:1. Age at diagnosis is similar to other forms of adult renal cell carcinoma with ages ranging from 30 to 94 years.[412–414]

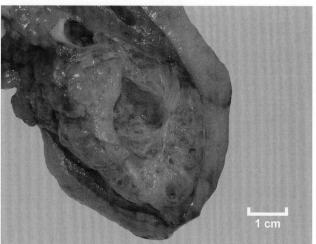

FIGURE 2-53 ■ Tubulocystic renal carcinoma. The tumor is composed of small and medium-sized cysts that contain clear fluid.

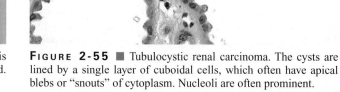

FIGURE 2-55 ■ Tubulocystic renal carcinoma. The cysts are lined by a single layer of cuboidal cells, which often have apical blebs or "snouts" of cytoplasm. Nucleoli are often prominent.

Patients are often asymptomatic at diagnosis although abdominal pain and distension, and hematuria have been reported. Tumors are more frequently left sided and radiologically often have the appearances of a cystic lesion.[413,414]

Pathology

Gross Features

Tubulocystic carcinoma is usually well circumscribed within an investing pseudocapsule, although multifocal examples have been reported. Tumors range in size from 0.5 to 17 cm (mean 4 cm) and have a white to gray spongy cut surface, which has been described as resembling cut bubble wrap (Fig. 2-53).[413]

Microscopic Features

Tubulocystic carcinoma consists of cysts and tubules within a bland connective tissue stroma (Fig. 2-54). The stroma can be relatively inconspicuous; however, the amount of stroma may vary within different parts of individual tumors. The

cysts are lined by cuboidal cells, which often have a hobnail appearance (Fig. 2-55). There is usually a moderate to marked degree of nuclear pleomorphism, and frequently a conspicuous nucleolus is present. Solid areas or desmoplastic stroma is not a feature of tubulocystic carcinoma. The tumors may occasionally contain foci of clear cells or papillae, and the coexistence of renal adenomas or papillary renal cell carcinomas has been reported.[414]

Ancillary and Special Studies

Immunohistochemistry usually shows positive reactions for cytokeratins 8, 18, and 19, CD10, AMACR, and parvalbumin, while cytokeratin 7 expression is usually focal.[412–414]

Electron microscopy shows the neoplastic cells to resemble the epithelium of the proximal convoluted tubule with abundant microvilli. Cells reminiscent of the intercalated cells of collecting ducts, with short scanty microvilli and complex cytoplasmic interdigitation are also seen.

Genetics

Gene expression studies show some similarity between tubulocystic carcinoma and papillary renal cell carcinoma and this is supported by the finding of trisomy 7 and 17 in tubulocystic carcinoma.[262,415]

Differential Diagnosis

Tumors that have a cystic growth pattern feature in the differential diagnosis for tubulocystic carcinoma (see Box 2-4). The lining cells of cystic nephroma often have a hobnail appearance and are often of low nuclear grade. The stroma in cystic nephroma is often cellular and may resemble ovarian stroma. Mixed epithelial and stromal tumor of kidney shows a more diverse morphology and usually has solid and cellular stroma. Multilocular cystic clear cell renal cell carcinoma is composed of clear cells, rather than cells with eosinophilic or amphophilic cytoplasm. These are of low nuclear grade and tumor cells are present within cyst walls.

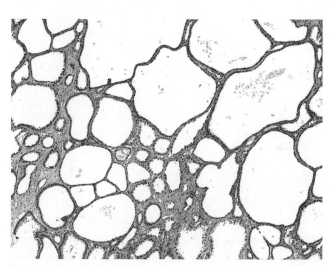

FIGURE 2-54 ■ Tubulocystic renal carcinoma. Microscopic and larger cysts of generally spherical shape are separated by thin septa.

Prognosis and Treatment

The biologic behavior of tubulocystic carcinoma is not fully established. In two recent studies follow-up was available for 30 out of 44 cases and this ranged from 1 to 104 months (mean 56 months).[413,414] Thirty-three tumors were staging category pT1 at diagnosis while three patients were pT3. One patient developed a local recurrence, while two developed metastases. A further patient developed metastases from a coexisting papillary renal cell carcinoma, while the remaining patients were either free of tumor or had died of unrelated causes. It is of interest that both patients who developed metastatic disease had focal cytoplasmic clearing of tumor cells in the primary malignancy. A single tubulocystic carcinoma with sarcomatoid change has been reported.[416] This patient developed metastases to bone and peritoneum. There is no specific treatment for tubulocystic carcinoma.

Clear Cell Papillary Renal Cell Carcinoma

Introduction

In 2006, Tickoo et al.[232] discovered a tumor with papillary architecture and abundant clear cytoplasm in a population of patients with end-stage renal disease and applied the name clear cell papillary renal cell carcinoma to them. In 2008, Gobbo et al.[260] reported examples from patients with normal renal function. Subsequently, studies reporting approximately 100 more cases have been published, clarifying aspects of the clinical, morphologic, immunophenotypic, and genetic features of these neoplasms.[417–421]

Epidemiology and Clinical Features

A little <100 cases of clear cell papillary renal cell carcinoma have been reported to date. For cases for which data were available, there was a male predominance (male-to-female ratio of 2-4:1) and all have been found in adults ranging in age from the third to tenth decades, with a mean age of approximately 60 years. The majority of patients have had normal renal function.

Pathology

Gross Features

Clear cell papillary renal cell carcinomas are usually of small size at presentation, with reported sizes ranging up to 8.5 cm in maximum diameter. The majority of tumors are cystic, with the cysts often containing serosanguinous fluid (Fig. 2-56). There is often a thick fibrous pseudocapsule, and sometimes the largest cysts are at the periphery of the tumor adjacent to the pseudocapsule (Fig. 2-57).

Microscopic Features

An acinar or glandular architecture usually predominates in these tumors. Papillae are present in approximately 80% of cases, although they often constitute only a minor component.[417] The papillae usually differ in architecture from those of papillary renal cell carcinoma types 1 and 2, and from the

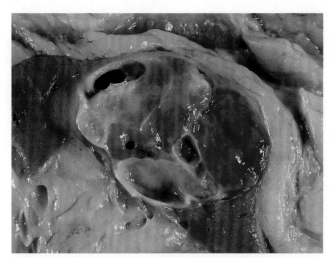

FIGURE 2-56 ■ Clear cell papillary renal cell carcinoma. The tumor is solid and cystic and surrounded by a pseudocapsule.

papillae of translocation carcinomas. The papillae are less complex, and the cores are thicker and the stroma within them often is cellular (Fig. 2-58). Additionally, sometimes stubby secondary papillae branch off the primary papillae. This architecture is distinctive, and when present, is strong evidence that the tumor is a clear cell papillary renal cell carcinoma. Nests of cells with clear cytoplasm and delicate vasculature closely resembling ordinary clear cell renal cell carcinoma (Fig. 2-59) are common and in a needle biopsy could easily be diagnosed as ordinary clear cell renal cell carcinoma. The cytoplasm is abundant and usually very clear. On papillae, it is sometimes so voluminous that the apical cytoplasm of the cells on one papilla touches that of the cells on an opposite papilla, creating a broad clear band between the wide cores. Uncommonly, the cytoplasm is weakly eosinophilic. The nuclei of the epithelial cells show

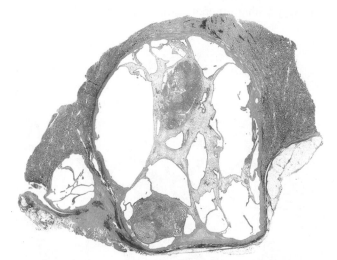

FIGURE 2-57 ■ Clear cell papillary renal cell carcinoma. There are multiple cysts and solid nodules. The cysts often are not spherical, and the solid nodules tend to be located away from the periphery of the mass.

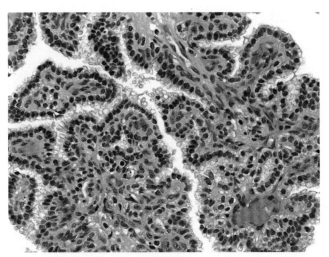

FIGURE 2-58 ■ Clear cell papillary renal cell carcinoma. When present, a highly specific feature is the peculiar papillary architecture with thick and cellular stromal cores and bulbous ends. The clear cytoplasm of the epithelial cells is sometimes so voluminous as to abut the cytoplasm of the cells on the opposite papilla.

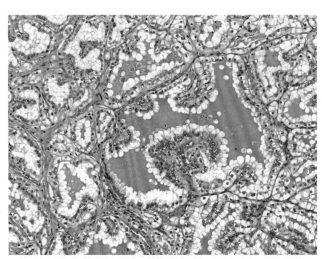

FIGURE 2-59 ■ Clear cell papillary renal cell carcinoma. Small cysts lined by clear cells resemble clear cell renal cell carcinoma. However, the small papillae and vascular architecture differ from clear cell renal cell carcinoma.

little pleomorphism and mitotic figures are difficult to find. It is common for the nuclei to be high in the cytoplasm, away from the basement membrane resulting in a pattern that has been likened to secretory phase endometrium. Psammoma bodies and foamy macrophages are not found in these tumors. The stroma of the papillary stalks and between the epithelial elements is more abundant and more cellular than is expected in an ordinary clear cell renal cell carcinoma, and this can be a helpful clue to the nature of the tumor. The cells are mostly nondescript spindle cells but sometimes show smooth muscle differentiation.

Ancillary and Special Studies

The epithelial elements usually show an immunophenotypic profile that distinguishes them from papillary renal cell carcinoma and clear cell renal cell carcinoma. A diffuse and strongly positive reaction with antibody to cytokeratin 7 is typical (Fig. 2-60A), while reactions for alpha-methylacyl CoA racemase and CD10 are consistently negative. Less helpful, but occasionally useful are the positive reactions for carbonic anhydrase IX (Fig. 2-60B) and vimentin and negative reactions for TFE3, which are typical of clear cell papillary renal cell carcinoma.

Genetics

While genetic studies on these tumors are limited it is becoming clear that they lack the gains of chromosomes 7 and 17 typical of papillary renal cell carcinomas, nor do they have the mutations in the *VHL* gene or losses in chromosome 3p25 that are characteristic of clear cell renal cell carcinomas.[260,422]

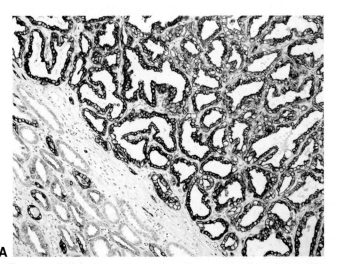

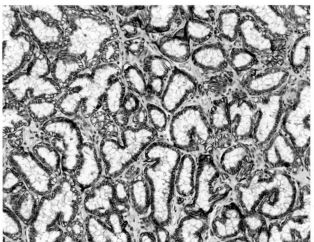

FIGURE 2-60 ■ **A:** Clear cell papillary renal cell carcinoma. The neoplastic cells react strongly positively with antibody to cytokeratin 7. **B:** The neoplastic cells react strongly positively with antibody to carbonic anhydrase IX.

Prognosis and Treatment

Although the diagnosis of carcinoma is applied to them, all tumors described to date were localized to the kidney at the time of diagnosis and no recurrence or metastasis has been reported.[417–419]

Acquired Cystic Disease–Associated Renal Cell Carcinoma

Epidemiology and Clinical Features

There is an increased prevalence of renal cell carcinoma in patients with end-stage renal disease. From 852 patients studied prospectively from 1994 to 2000, 19 had clinical evidence of renal neoplasia.[423] Seventeen of these patients underwent nephrectomy, with fourteen being subsequently diagnosed with renal cell carcinoma, giving a prevalence of 2%. This compared with a renal cancer incidence of 0.04% for the general population. The incidence of neoplasia appears to be further increased in patients with acquired cystic disease, which is usually associated with dialysis.[423] In a multinational study of 831 patients, there was an increased risk factor for renal neoplasia of 3.6 in patients who were on maintenance dialysis.[93]

The spectrum of renal tumors associated with end-stage renal disease is wide, and in single cases and small series, clear cell renal cell carcinomas, papillary renal cell carcinomas, chromophobe renal cell carcinoma, collecting duct carcinoma, tubulocystic carcinoma, clear cell papillary renal cell carcinoma, angiomyolipoma, oncocytoma, and mixed epithelial and stromal tumor have been reported.[232,424,425] In up to 70% of cases, more than one tumor was present in a single kidney.[426] In a detailed study of 66 tumor-bearing kidneys from patients with end-stage renal disease, a wide variety of renal neoplasia was noted.[232] In total, 261 tumors were examined with 55% of kidneys containing >1 tumor in each kidney ranging from 0.6 to 8.5 cm (mean 3.0 cm, median 2.6 cm). Of the recognized types of renal cell carcinoma, papillary renal cell carcinomas were most frequently encountered (18%), whereas 23% were clear cell renal cell carcinoma or chromophobe renal carcinoma. Sarcomatoid differentiation has been reported in association with these tumors.[427]

The majority of tumors associated with end-stage renal disease are discovered incidentally, either through imaging studies or the examination of nephrectomy specimens. Very occasionally hematuria is a presenting feature.[423,424,426]

Additional to sporadically occurring forms of renal neoplasia, a novel tumor type associated with end-stage renal failure has been described.[232] Designated acquired cystic disease–associated renal cell carcinoma, these tumors are seen in 46% of kidneys with acquired cystic disease.

Pathology

Gross Features

These tumors are usually well circumscribed and where large, show pseudoencapsulation, often with dystrophic

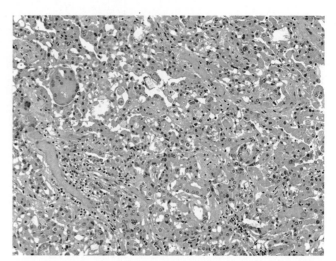

FIGURE 2-61 ■ Acquired cystic disease–associated renal cell carcinoma. In this area, the neoplastic cells grow as sheets of cells with abundant eosinophilic cytoplasm. There are urate crystals in the extracellular compartment and some of these have attracted multinucleated phagocytes.

calcification. The tumors can be seen partially filling cysts. In cases of acquired cystic disease, cysts containing apparent hemorrhage or blood clot should be sampled as this may rather be an acquired cystic disease–associated renal cell carcinoma.

Microscopic Features

Microscopically, there are a variety of architectural patterns ranging from solid (Fig. 2-61) and acinar to cystic and papillary. Frequently the presence of irregular lumens gives the tumor a cribriform or sieve-like appearance (Fig. 2-62). In 67% of reported cases, the tumor appeared to arise in a cyst.

The tumor cells contain bulky eosinophilic cytoplasm with a rounded nucleus and large nucleolus. Occasional cells have vacuolated cytoplasm, and focally clear cells

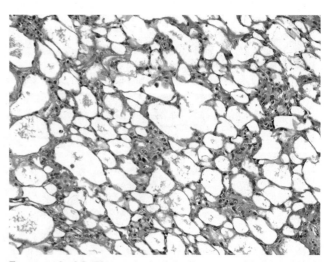

FIGURE 2-62 ■ Acquired cystic disease–associated renal cell carcinoma. The cribriform pattern of empty spaces is a characteristic feature of these tumors.

are present. Oxalate crystals are present in the majority of tumors (Fig. 2-61), and calcium aggregates, rarely forming psammoma bodies, are also seen.

Ancillary and Special Studies

These tumors are positive for vinculin and AMACR on immunohistochemical examination, and in a proportion of cases show variable and predominantly focal staining for cytokeratin 7 and parvalbumin. These tumors have also been shown to have positive immunohistochemical reactions for cytokeratin AE1/AE3, RCC antigen and CD10, and variable expression for vimentin and CAM 5.2. Staining for EMA and high molecular weight cytokeratin is negative.[428,429]

Genetics

Genetic studies on the various types of renal cell carcinoma associated with end-stage kidneys are limited; however, clear cell renal cell carcinomas arising in these kidneys have shown *VHL* gene mutations.[428,430] Genetic analysis of acquired cystic disease–associated renal cell carcinoma shows gains of chromosomes 7 and 17.[431] FISH analysis has also shown gains of chromosomes 1, 2, 3, 6, 16, and Y in several cases, with additional gains of chromosomes 1, 5, 11, 12, and X being occasionally seen.[429] Mutations of the *VHL* gene have not been identified in these tumors.[432]

Differential Diagnosis

The presence of papillary architecture may suggest the possibility of papillary renal cell carcinoma; however, the solid areas with the sieve-like architecture would not be compatible with that diagnosis. The presence of solid and papillary architectures could also suggest collecting duct carcinoma or renal cell carcinoma associated with the hereditary leiomyomatosis and renal cell carcinoma syndrome. In collecting duct carcinoma, the tumor has a more infiltrative growth pattern with stromal desmoplasia. The latter is also a feature of tumors in the hereditary leiomyomatosis and renal cell carcinoma syndrome.

Prognosis and Treatment

Outcome data for acquired cystic disease–associated renal cell carcinoma are limited with one death from metastatic disease, 34 months following diagnosis, being reported. In two other cases, regional lymph node metastases were seen.[232] Treatment is as for other renal cell carcinomas.

Thyroid-Like Follicular Renal Cell Carcinoma

Epidemiology and Clinical Features

Recently, a few cases of a primary renal tumor resembling follicular carcinoma of the thyroid have been reported arising in the kidney.[433–437] The tumors reported to date were from seven women and four men with an age range of 29 to 83 years (median 41 years) and almost half of the patients were in the age range of 29 to 35 years. All tumors were incidental findings, and three patients had a history of unrelated malignancy (breast and colonic carcinoma, Hodgkin disease).

Pathology

Gross Features

Tumors ranged in size from 2 to 12 cm (median 4 cm) and were tan on cut surface. One tumor invaded perirenal fat.[437]

Microscopic Features

Thyroid like follicular renal cell carcinoma has a follicular architecture with varying proportions of large and small follicles (Fig. 2-63). The follicles are lined by cuboidal to columnar cells showing low-grade nuclear pleomorphism with eosinophilic to amphophilic cytoplasm. Pseudoinclusions and nuclear grooves may be present, and follicles frequently contain colloid-like proteinaceous fluid. No areas of papillary architecture or clear cells have been reported.

Ancillary and Special Studies

Immunohistochemical studies are somewhat limited. All reported cases were negative for TTF1 and thyroglobulin. All of the six tumors studied by Amin et al.[433] were negative for PAX2, while the tumor reported by Dhillon et al.[436] was positive for PAX2 and PAX8.

Genetics

Genetic studies have shown gains of 8q24, 12, and 16 and loss of 1p36.3 and 9q21.33 for one tumor.[433] Gene expression profiling of three cases showed widespread underexpression or overexpression, particularly involving chromosomes 1, 2, 3, 5, 6, 10, 11, 16, and 17.[435]

Differential Diagnosis

Metastasis from primary thyroid follicular carcinoma is the principal differential diagnosis for thyroid-like follicular renal cell carcinoma. A positive reaction for TTF1 or thyroglobulin strongly supports that diagnosis.

Prognosis and Treatment

Follow-up data are limited. One patient had metastases to regional lymph nodes and another had metastases to regional

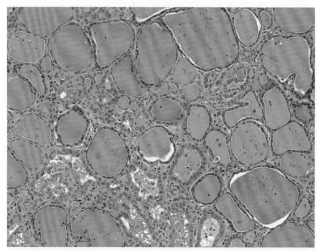

FIGURE 2-63 ■ Thyroid-like follicular renal cell carcinoma. These carcinomas form structures closely resembling colloid-filled thyroid follicles.

lymph nodes and lungs. Treatment would be as for other types of renal cell carcinoma.

Renal Angiomyoadenomatous Tumor

In 2000, Michal et al.[438] reported a case of a renal tumor characterized by a mixture of epithelial elements comprised of nests and tubules of cells with clear cytoplasm embedded in a stroma containing abundant smooth muscle. A subsequent report by Kuhn et al.[439] described five similar tumors with an epithelial component the authors considered to represent clear cell renal cell carcinoma associated with smooth muscle stroma and an angiomatous vascular proliferation. The tumors occurred over a wide age range with a predominance of females. Further studies to evaluate the epithelial component identified *VHL* gene and 3p abnormalities in some cases[440] while others found no *VHL* gene abnormalities[441] and some have identified monosomies of chromosomes 1, 11, and 16.[442] Others have reported that some clear cell renal cell carcinomas, confirmed to have *VHL* gene mutations, can have smooth muscle stroma mimicking renal angiomyoadenomatous tumors.[443] Further, the morphologic features and immunohistochemical profile of these tumors have suggested that some of these tumors may represent examples of clear cell papillary renal cell carcinoma. The current ISUP classification has followed the latter approach.[7] It can be concluded that tumors reported under this designation likely represent more than one entity and it remains to be determined if a specific tumor type unrelated to clear cell renal cell carcinoma and clear cell papillary renal cell carcinoma will emerge from the group. To date, these tumors have behaved in a benign fashion.

The cases reported to date in this category have mostly been small and relatively circumscribed. The tumors have been solid and firm and gray-white with the largest measuring 8.5 cm (Fig. 2-64). Many have had infiltrative borders histologically, particularly at the periphery with extension

FIGURE 2-65 ■ Renal angiomyoadenomatous tumor. Tendrils of the smooth muscle of the tumor extend into the perirenal fat.

of fibromuscular tissue into the perinephric fat (Fig. 2-65). The epithelial component has mostly formed small glandular or branching tubular structures lined by cells with small basally located hyperchromatic nuclei and moderate amounts of clear cytoplasm. Apocrine-like snouting of the clear cytoplasm can be prominent. In other areas, there are nests of cells with abundant clear cytoplasm and apically located nuclei with a sinusoidal vascular network resembling clear cell renal cell carcinoma (Fig. 2-66). The stroma has a leiomyomatous appearance with bundles of smooth muscle cells interspersed between the epithelial nests (Fig. 2-67). In some areas, there is a proliferation of small vascular spaces within the leiomyomatous stroma producing an angioleiomyoma-like appearance (Fig. 2-66). Immunohistochemical studies have demonstrated consistent reactivity for cytokeratin 7 (and other cytokeratins) in the epithelial cells. CD10 reactivity has been variable but generally has been negative. Carbonic anhydrase IX has

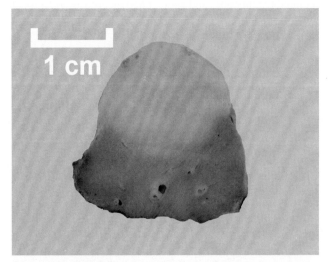

FIGURE 2-64 ■ Renal angiomyoadenomatous tumor. In this formalin-fixed specimen the tumor is off-white and homogeneous, and the border with the nonneoplastic renal parenchyma is fuzzy.

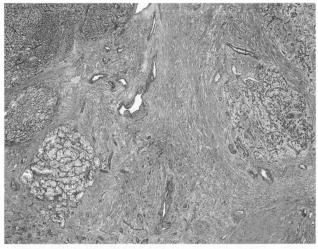

FIGURE 2-66 ■ Renal angiomyoadenomatous tumor. Nests of epithelial cells with clear cytoplasm resembling clear cell renal cell carcinoma (**left**) and angioma-like vascular proliferations (**right**) are embedded in abundant smooth muscle stroma.

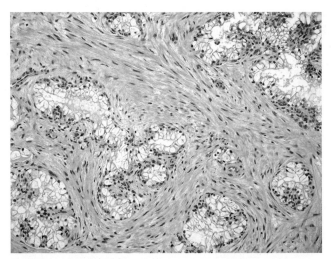

FIGURE 2-67 ■ Renal angiomyoadenomatous tumor. At higher magnification, the resemblance to clear cell renal cell carcinoma is striking.

been positive. The stroma stains positively for smooth muscle markers and is negative for melanocytic markers. The immunohistochemical profile closely resembles that found in clear cell papillary renal cell carcinoma.

Renal Cell Carcinoma, Unclassified

This category was established as part of the Heidelberg and Rochester classifications in order to accomodate tumors with features that differ from the recognized tumor groups. Approximately 4% to 5% of renal neoplasms cannot be assigned into the recognized categories of the 2004 World Health Organization renal tumor classification.[5] It is from this group of tumors that a number of new forms of renal neoplasia have emerged.

Renal cell carcinoma unclassified is not a definitive diagnosis and tumors so classified have a varying prognosis. There are no specific diagnostic features, although for the present, tumors that are apparent composites of recognized types, tumors showing mixtures of epithelial and stromal elements, and tumors with unrecognized cell types should be assigned into this category. It is also recommended in the Heidelberg, Rochester, and 2004 World Health Organization classifications that sarcomatoid carcinoma without recognizable epithelial components be placed into this category.

Grading of Renal Cell Carcinoma

A grading classification for renal malignancies, based upon the degree of cellular differentiation, was first proposed by Hand and Broders in 1932.[444] This was superseded by a composite grading system proposed by Griffiths and Thackray in 1949.[445] Since the publication of this classification seven further composite classifications have been proposed, each focusing upon a variety of morphologic and architectural features (Table 2-9).[153,446-451] A recurring feature of these various grading systems is that they fail to

Table 2-9 ■ GRADING CLASSIFICATIONS FOR RENAL CELL CARCINOMA BASED UPON A VARIETY OF MORPHOLOGIC PARAMETERS

Authors	No. of Cases	Treatment	Five-year Survivals (%) According to Grade				Significance	Classification Criteria
			1	2	3	4		
Griffiths and Thackray[445]	42	S	72	32	28	—	NT	Cell morphology, architecture, mitotic rate, nuclear pleomorphism
Riches[446]	76	S	71	39	25	—	NT	Architecture, nuclear hyperchromasia, mitoses
Arner et al.[447]	172	S	93	63	41	7	0.05 (grade 1 vs. 2+3)	Architecture, cell type
Hermanek et al.[448]	188	S	10	51	39	—	1 vs. 3 "significant" 2 vs. 3 "significant"	Cell type and architecture
Boxer et al.[449]	96	S	61	36	14	—	Significant	"Overall microscopic appearance"
Hop and van der Werf Messing[450]	162	S/SR	68	57	39	—	0.01	"Degree of differentiation"
McNichols et al.[451]	486	S	63	49	27	15	<0.05–<0.001	Tumor architecture, nuclear pleomorphism, mitotic rate, necrosis
Selli et al.[153]	115	S	93	81	55	33	0.001 (grade 1 + 2 vs. 4)	Nuclear features, tubular pattern

S, nephrectomy; R, radiotherapy; N, no treatment; NT, not tested.

Table 2-10 ■ NUCLEAR GRADING CLASSIFICATIONS FOR RENAL CELL CARCINOMA

Authors	No. of Cases	Treatment	Five-Year Survivals (%) According to Grade				Significance (P)	Classification Criteria and Comment
			1	2	3	4		
Myers et al.[452]	508	S	67	56	33	28	NT	
Skinner et al.[453]	272	S	75	65	56	26	0.001	
Syrjänen and Hjelt[454]	121	S	87	69	45	28	<0.025	Only grade 2 vs. grade 3 significant
Boxer et al.[449]	96	S	50	32	25	-	<0.01	
Lieber et al.[455]	88	S	87	57	26	26	0.0001	Grades 3 and 4 combined
Fuhrman et al.[456]	103	S/R/C/N	64	34	31	10	<0.005	
Kloppel et al.[457]	135	S	81	54	22	0	Significant	3-year survivals
Delahunt and Nacey[458]	102	S	51	36	0	—	1 vs. 2 0.02 2 vs. 3 <.001	
Störkel et al.[459]	431	S	92	60	−33	-	<0.001	Thoenes et al (1986) criteria
Onodera et al.[460]	116	S	96	87	20	—	1 vs. 3 0.0001 2 vs. 3 0.0001	Japanese classification system
Lohse et al.[155]	1733	S	93	86	50	19	1 vs. 3 and 1 vs. 4 <0.001	Clear cell RCC
	222	S	100	96	72	24	1 + 2 vs. 3 and 1 + 2 vs. 4 <0.001	Papillary RCC
	87	S						Chromophobe RCC
			100	98	78	25 (2.5y)	1 + 2 vs. 3 0.2 1+2 vs. 4 <0.001	

S, nephrectomy; R, radiotherapy; C, chemotherapy; N, no treatment; NT, not tested.

stratify each of the component grading parameters according to their prognostic significance. This implies that each parameter should be given equal weighting for grading purposes, which is an assumption that has not been validated. A further difficulty is that for many of the classifications the defining criteria are, at best, limited, which serves to promote intraobserver variability. A grading system based upon nuclear anaplasia was proposed by Myers et al.[452] in 1968, although no strict defining criteria were provided. This concept was refined by Skinner et al.[453] who demonstrated a significant difference in survivals for their four-tier grading system. Since the publication of the Skinner classification several additional grading systems have been proposed (Table 2-10).[155,449,454–460] Somewhat surprisingly,

of these grading systems, only one provides criteria as to the area of the tumor that should be assessed. Of the various nuclear grading systems proposed, that of Fuhrman et al.[456] has gained widespread acceptance in clinical practice (Table 2-11 and Figs. 2-68 to 2-71). While features of more than one grade are frequently present in a single tumor (Fig. 2-72), the grade assignment is driven by the worst area. Fuhrman grading has been validated in a number of studies, although often significant differences between grades are achieved only when grades are grouped together for analytical purposes.

Despite the extensive usage of the Fuhrman grading system, there are a number of methodologic problems. In particular, the validity of the grading system, especially for

Table 2-11 ■ DEFINING FEATURES OF THE FUHRMAN GRADING CLASSIFICATION

	Nuclear Diameter	Nuclear Shape	Nucleoli
Grade 1	Small (approximately 10 μm)	Round, uniform	Absent, inconspicuous
Grade 2	Larger (approximately 15 μm)	Irregularities in outline	Visible at 400×
Grade 3	Even larger (approximately 20 μm)	Obvious irregular outline	Prominent at 100×
Grade 4	As for grade 3 with bizarre often multilobed nuclei ± spindle cells		

Fuhrman SA, Lasky LC, Limas C. Prognostic significance of morphologic parameters in renal cell carcinoma. *Am J Surg Pathol* 1982;6:655–663.

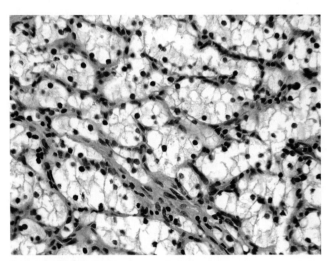

FIGURE 2-68 ■ Nuclear grade 1.

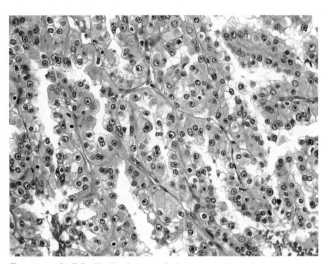

FIGURE 2-70 ■ Nuclear grade 3.

subtypes of renal cell carcinoma other than clear cell renal cell carcinoma, has been questioned. As originally defined, the system is based upon the simultaneous evaluation of three features. This implies that each of these parameters parallels one another incrementally and provides independent survival information, which has been shown not to be the case for both papillary renal cell carcinomas and chromophobe renal cell carcinomas.[272,327] The study by Fuhrman et al., which was based upon a mixed tumor series, provides no advice as to whether grading should be based upon the highest grade present or the predominant grade of the whole tumor. Further, there is no guidance as to which component of the grading system should be given priority for grading purposes, in the case of discordance between parameters. It is likely that these issues contribute to the, at best, moderate interobserver variability that has been reported for Fuhrman grading of renal cell carcinomas.[461,462] The Rochester workgroup on the grading of renal cell carcinoma noted that at present there is no ideal grading system for these tumors. They recommended that this should be reproducible and

be based upon nuclear features and that a three-tier system would seem most appropriate.[463]

It has been noted that some pathologists overcome these problems by confining grading to nucleolar prominence alone or in combination with nuclear granularity,[6] and this is endorsed by the Association of Directors of Anatomical and Surgical Pathology.[274] Anecdotally, it would appear that this practice is widespread, and although it is often referred to as Fuhrman grading, a more appropriate designation would seem to be nucleolar grading. This was confirmed in the survey done as part of the 2012 International Society of Urological Pathology consensus meeting on renal cell carcinoma.[329] A revision of the Fuhrman system was formally adopted by The International Society of Urological Pathology in 2012 (Table 2-12).[329] This system is recommended for use in clear cell and papillary renal cell carcinoma.

A novel grading system that encompasses the ISUP grading scheme and incorporates the presence or absence of microscopic coagulative necrosis (Fig. 2-73) and specifically the presence of rhabdoid or sarcomatoid features has been

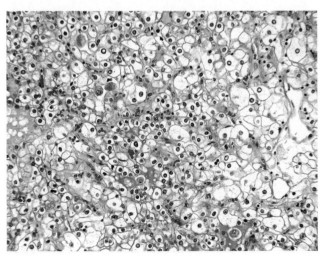

FIGURE 2-69 ■ Nuclear grade 2.

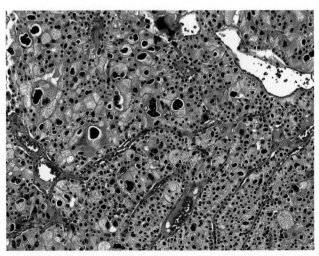

FIGURE 2-71 ■ Nuclear grade 4.

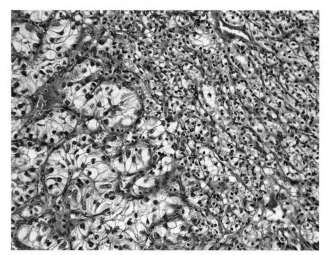

FIGURE 2-72 ■ Areas of different nuclear grade often are present in the same tumor. Grade is assigned according to the worst grade present.

FIGURE 2-73 ■ The presence of coagulative necrosis is a nonnuclear adverse prognostic finding.

proposed. This scheme results in 9-grade categories and in the initial report demonstrated a strong correlation with outcome for clear cell renal cell carcinoma.[464]

The prognostic significance of grading for renal cell carcinoma is discussed in each section relating to specific tumor subtypes.

Sarcomatoid and Rhabdoid Change

Sarcomatoid Change

Sarcomatoid change (Fig. 2-74) may be found in association with each of the main subtypes of renal cell carcinoma[107] and in the Fuhrman grading classification sarcomatoid morphology is considered a feature of grade 4 malignancy. The genetic changes that are associated with the development of a sarcomatoid phenotype are uncertain. Multiple losses of chromosomes 4q, 6q, 6p, 9, 13q, 14, and 17p and gains of chromosomes 5, 12, and 20 have been reported,[465,466] while gains of chromosomes 1, 2, 6, 10, and 17 have been demonstrated in sarcomatoid chromophobe renal cell carcinoma.[321] There is evidence that typical carcinomas evolve into sarcomatoid carcinomas through a number of mutational steps, as collagen expression of tumor cell cytoplasm and interstitium differs as tumors evolve from epithelial cells showing early spindle cell change to fully developed sarcomatoid carcinoma.[467] This reinforces the recommendation that early spindle cell change should not be classified as sarcomatoid carcinoma.[161]

The age distribution of patients with sarcomatoid renal cell carcinoma reported in large case series ranges from 29 to 81 years, with median ages ranging from 56 to 61 years. Presenting symptoms are similar to those of renal epithelial malignancies although sarcomatoid carcinomas are often of advanced stage at the time of diagnosis.[159,161,468–471]

On gross examination, sarcomatoid carcinomas are solid and gray or white with a firm to hard consistency upon sectioning. Cystic areas and a gross appearance similar to clear

Table 2-12 ■ THE INTERNATIONAL SOCIETY OF UROLOGICAL PATHOLOGY GRADING SYSTEM FOR RENAL CELL CARCINOMA	
Grade 1	Inconspicuous or absent nucleoli at 400× magnification
Grade 2	Nucleoli distinctly visible at 400× but inconspicuous at 100× magnification
Grade 3	Nucleoli distinctly visible at 100× magnification
Grade 4	Presence of rhabdoid or sarcomatoid differentiation; presence of tumor giant cells or cells showing extreme nuclear pleomorphism with clumping of chromatin

Delahunt B, Cheville JC, Martignoni G, et al. The International Society of Urological Pathology (ISUP) grading system for renal cell carcinoma and other prognostic parameters. *Am J Surg Pathol.* In press 2013.

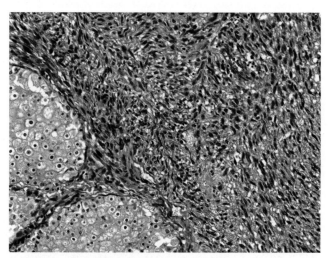

FIGURE 2-74 ■ The presence of sarcomatoid change is a nonnuclear adverse prognostic finding.

cell renal cell carcinoma may also be seen. Histologically, these tumors consist of spindle cells arranged into sheets, and occasionally a storiform architecture may be present. Rarely, there may be osteoclast-like giant cells and foci of rhabdomyomatous differentiation.

The immunohistochemical profile of these tumors provides evidence of their pathogenesis, as the majority express a variety of epithelial markers. Pancytokeratin is usually positive, at least focally, while positive expression of cytokeratins 8 and 18, CAM 5.2, and PKK1 is occasionally seen.[472] The sarcomatoid component also expressed PAX8 in 69% of cases in one series.[473] Vimentin positivity has been reported in 33% to 100% of cases,[298,472] and rarely there is actin positivity.[472] Ultrastructural studies of sarcomatoid renal cell carcinoma almost always show the presence of desmosomes, although these may be infrequent. Peripheral and intraluminal microvilli, intracytoplasmic glycogen, and lipid may also be seen. These tumors must be differentiated from a variety of renal sarcomas, with the correct diagnosis being dependent on the identification of epithelial components within the tumor, or epithelial features as demonstrated by immunohistochemistry or electron microscopy. In the 2004 edition of the World Health Organization classification of renal tumors, it is recommended that sarcomatoid carcinomas should be classified according to the morphology of the parent tumor. If the carcinoma has been completely replaced by sarcomatoid tumor, then the tumor should be classified as renal cell carcinoma, unclassified.

Because of the aggressive nature of these tumors, clinical studies have evaluated the use of combination therapies that have included chemotherapeutic agents (gemcitabine, doxorubicin), biologic agents (interferon), and targeted therapies (tyrosine kinase inhibitors, bevacizumab). To date, no optimal approach has emerged.[474]

Rhabdoid Change

As for sarcomatoid carcinoma, rhabdoid change (Fig. 2-75) has been recognized for all major subtypes of renal cell carcinoma.[105,106,163] These high-grade tumors are characterized by the presence of cells with a large irregular nucleus, with a prominent nucleolus and abundant eosinophilic cytoplasm. The proportion of rhabdoid cells within renal cell carcinoma ranges from 1% to 90%; however, this does not influence the poor prognosis associated with tumors showing this morphology. For clear cell renal cell carcinoma showing rhabdoid differentiation, a mean survival interval of 8 months has been reported.[163]

FAMILIAL RENAL CELL CARCINOMA SYNDROMES

Birt-Hogg-Dubé Syndrome

Introduction

The Birt-Hogg-Dubé syndrome was first described in 1977 in a family with multiple benign hair follicle hamartomas, trichodiscomas, and acrochordons of the face, neck, and upper torso.[475] Since this original description, a variety of extracutaneous lesions have been associated with this syndrome, including a number of renal tumors (Table 2-13).[476]

Genetics

The syndrome is caused by mutations in the *folliculin* gene (HUGO-approved gene symbol: *FLCN*), which has been mapped to chromosome 17p11.2 and consists of 14 exons.[477,478] An alias for this gene that was used in the past is *BHD*. The gene encodes the protein folliculin, which is involved in both the AMPK and MTOR signaling pathways.[479] In a large series of cases a *FLCN* mutation rate of 88% was observed and 23 separate germline mutations were demonstrated,[478] with the most frequent mutation being found on exon 11. A total of 84 *FLCN* variants have been described to date.[480] Mutations of the *FLCN* gene are infrequent in sporadic kidney tumors including chromophobe renal cell carcinoma and oncocytoma.[481]

Renal Tumors

Renal tumors are seen in 34% to 49% of affected families and 10% to 34% of affected individuals, although earlier studies indicated a much lesser frequency of renal neoplasia.[478,482,483]

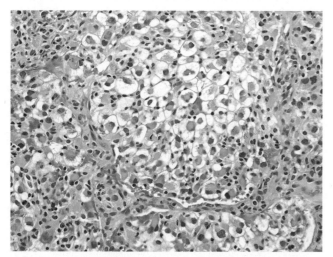

FIGURE 2-75 ■ The presence of rhabdoid change is a nonnuclear adverse prognostic finding.

Table 2-13 ■ CUTANEOUS AND EXTRACUTANEOUS MANIFESTATIONS OF THE BIRT-HOGG-DUBÉ SYNDROME
• Benign skin tumors
∘ Fibrofolliculoma
∘ Trichodiscoma
∘ Acrochordon (fibroepithelial polyp or skin tag)
• Pulmonary cysts/pneumothorax
• Oncocytoma
• Chromophobe renal cell carcinoma
• Papillary renal cell carcinoma
• Clear cell renal cell carcinoma

The mean age of presentation for renal tumors associated with the Birt-Hogg-Dubé syndrome is 50 years; however, malignant renal tumors have been detected in individuals in the third and fourth decade.[484] Over 85% to 90% of the tumors described in these patients have morphologically resembled oncocytoma and chromophobe renal cell carcinoma with many having overlapping features of the two.[476,478,484,485] The latter have been referred to as "hybrid" tumors to reflect this feature. It is difficult from the literature to determine what percentage of tumors in these patients are true oncocytomas and chromophobe renal cell carcinomas versus the so-called hybrid tumors. Recent molecular and genetic data suggest that these represent a unique tumor type unrelated to either oncocytoma or chromophobe renal cell carcinoma.[486] Hierarchical clustering shows that although similar to oncocytoma and chromophobe renal cell carcinoma, Birt-Hogg-Dubé tumors cluster into a distinct group.[486] These tumors also lack the genetic abnormalities typically associated with oncocytoma and chromophobe renal cell carcinoma.[486] Papillary renal cell carcinomas and clear cell renal cell carcinomas are less commonly seen with the latter accounting for 7% to 9% of tumors.[476,482] Renal cysts, unrelated to coexisting renal tumors, have also been reported.[476,478,484,485]

The patients who do develop renal tumors typically have multiple bilateral tumors. In one series, tumors were bilateral in 56% of patients and multiple in 65% with the number of tumors ranging from 1 to 22 (mean 7).[482] The tumors are solid with varied color ranging from brown to tan to yellow depending on the histologic type. Hemorrhage and necrosis are not a feature except in clear cell renal cell carcinomas. The most common histology is the so-called "hybrid" tumor. These are better referred to as the renal tumor of Birt-Hogg-Dubé syndrome. The tumors are composed of a mixture of cells having eosinophilic to pale to clear cytoplasm arranged in variably sized solid nests (Fig. 2-76). The eosinophilic cells resemble those of oncocytoma and the large pale cells

those of chromophobe renal cell carcinoma. The clear cells can resemble the cells of clear cell renal cell carcinoma and some authors have described such tumors as "hybrid clear cell–chromophobe renal cell carcinoma."[483] Nuclei are generally round and uniform, but some nuclear irregularity can be present. Examination of renal parenchyma not grossly involved by tumors shows numerous tiny nodules of pink (oncocytic) cells in the majority of cases.

In patients with bilateral renal tumors (synchronous or asynchronous) and a diagnosis of oncocytoma or chromophobe renal cell carcinoma in one or more of these, the possibility of Birt-Hogg-Dubé syndrome should be considered and clinical information sought. In one study that evaluated patients with bilateral kidney tumors and a diagnosis of oncocytoma or oncocytic neoplasm, 23 of 46 patients were found to have Birt-Hogg-Dubé syndrome.[487]

Prognosis and Treatment

Although there are no formal follow-up guidelines, regular imaging studies for the early detection of renal neoplasia are recommended. Where tumors larger than 3 cm are present, nephron-sparing surgery is the treatment of choice.[484,487] In one study of 23 patients, one patient developed metastases from a clear cell renal cell carcinoma; no cases of metastases occurred from the "oncocytic" tumors in the series.[487] In another series, 34 of 124 (10%) affected patients developed renal tumors and 2 of the 124 (2%) died of metastatic renal cell carcinoma (both with clear cell renal cell carcinoma).[482] The malignant potential of the non–clear cell tumors of the Birt-Hogg-Dubé syndrome remains uncertain, but it would seem to be at most limited malignant potential.[482]

von Hippel-Lindau Disease

Introduction

VHL disease is an autosomal dominant inherited disorder with a high degree of penetrance. The ocular changes of VHL disease were described by von Hippel in 1895, while the association with spinocerebral abnormalities, pancreatic and renal cysts, and renal neoplasia was reported by Lindau in 1926.[488] The full spectrum of the syndrome (Table 2-14) was fully described in 1964.[489] VHL disease has a prevalence

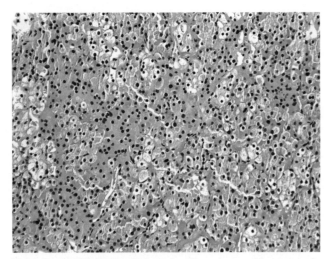

FIGURE 2-76 ■ Familial renal cell carcinoma. The tumors in Birt-Hogg-Dubé syndrome are composed of cells with eosinophilic and pale cytoplasm growing in sheets.

Table 2-14 ■ LESIONS ASSOCIATED WITH VHL DISEASE
• Renal cysts
• Clear cell renal cell carcinoma
• Pheochromocytoma
• Retinal, central nervous system angioma
• Retinal, central nervous system hemangiocytoma
• Pancreatic cysts
• Islet cell tumors
• Papillary cystadenoma, epididymis/broad ligament
• Endolymphatic sac tumor, inner ear

of approximately 1 in 36,000 and the clinical manifestations have been grouped into four clinical phenotypes. Type 1 disease is associated with a low to zero risk of pheochromocytoma, while in type 2 disease there is a high risk of pheochromocytoma. Type 2 disease is further subdivided into type 2a—occurrence of hemangioblastoma and pancreatic involvement; type 2b—occurrence of hemangioblastoma, pancreatic involvement, and high risk of clear cell renal cell carcinoma; and type 2c—predominance of pheochromocytoma, with a low risk of hemangioblastoma and pancreatic and renal cancer.[490]

Genetics

VHL disease results from germline mutation or deletion of the *von Hippel-Lindau tumor suppressor, E3 ubiquitin protein ligase* (*VHL*) gene located at 3p25.3 that is detectable in close to 100% of affected individuals. The *VHL* gene product binds to elongins that in turn bind hypoxia-inducible factor α. *VHL* gene mutation results in the accumulation of hypoxia-inducible factor α leading to up-regulation of mediators of angiogenesis and cell proliferation such as VEGF, TGFα, PDGFβ, and erythropoietin.[491–494] The wide spectrum of VHL disease results from the wide variety of mutations associated with the syndrome, with more than 300 mutations involving the three exons of the *VHL* gene being described.[490]

Renal Pathology

The renal pathology in these patients is dominated by the development of cysts and clear cell renal cell carcinomas. Both are multiple and bilateral. The cysts are described in detail in Chapter 1, but one characteristic is that they are often lined by a single layer of cuboidal cells with clear cytoplasm resembling the cells of clear cell renal cell carcinoma. It has been suggested that even a double layer of such cells indicates malignant transformation or at least a premalignant change.[495]

Renal cell carcinoma develops in 24% to 45% of VHL disease patients.[496] It occurs at a younger age (mean 39 years) than sporadic clear cell renal cell carcinoma and is often bilateral. The tumors are essentially all of the clear cell type. Some of the tumors closely resemble clear cell papillary renal cell carcinoma, and immunohistochemistry may be needed to reach the correct diagnosis. The tumors may be solid and cystic, and are often associated with renal cysts. In many cases, the tumors appear to arise within preexisting cysts. Numerous cysts and tumors, in the order of several hundreds, may be present in each kidney.[497] Careful examination of uninvolved renal parenchyma can identify individual cells or groups of cells (Fig. 2-77) with the morphologic features of clear cell renal cell carcinoma within individual tubules.

Prognosis and Treatment

VHL gene mutations are detected by screening of at-risk individuals. Annual renal imaging is recommended in order to detect the development of occult renal malignancy and for

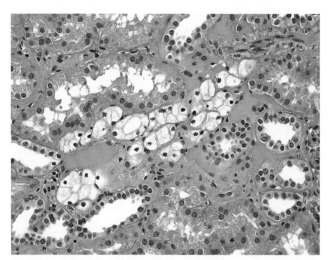

FIGURE 2-77 ■ Familial renal cell carcinoma. In von Hippel-Lindau disease, the tumors closely resemble sporadic clear cell renal cell carcinoma and small nests of these may be found throughout the kidney.

monitoring tumor size. Treatment is focused on both preserving renal function and preventing metastatic disease. A "3 cm rule" has been employed with observation until a tumor reaches >3 cm in diameter, at which time surgical intervention utilizing a nephron-sparing approach is recommended with removal of the larger tumor as well as other clinically evident tumors in the involved kidney.[498] In one series, none of the patients managed with this approach developed metastases.[499] Enucleative procedures that do not remove a rim of normal parenchyma are also being applied in these cases to further minimize the loss of renal parenchyma.[500] Close follow-up is mandatory as partial nephrectomy has been associated with a 75% risk of recurrence, within the ipsilateral or contralateral kidney.[501] Despite these approaches, metastatic renal cell carcinoma remains a significant cause of death in these patients. Targeted systemic therapies aimed at different points in the HIF pathways have shown significant potential in the treatment of metastatic clear cell renal cell carcinoma with several drugs currently being FDA approved.[207] Several of these are also being evaluated for postoperative adjuvant treatment of patients with high-risk tumors.[326] A role for these drugs as neoadjuvant treatment in these patients has not yet been demonstrated.

Tuberous sclerosis

Introduction

Tuberous sclerosis is an autosomal dominant inherited disorder associated with a high degree of penetrance and the development of a wide variety of benign tumors and tumor-like conditions affecting multiple organs. The syndrome was first recognized in 1880, although descriptions of cerebral sclerosis date back to 1862.[502] The prevalence is estimated at 1:11,000 live births.[503] The current diagnostic guidelines for recognizing this disorder, presented in Table 2-15, highlight the diversity of the manifestations of the disease.[504] In the

Table 2-15 ■ DIAGNOSTIC CRITERIA FOR TUBEROUS SCLEROSIS

Major features
- Facial angiofibromas or forehead plaque
- Nontraumatic ungual or periungual fibroma
- Hypomelanotic macules (more than three)
- Shagreen patch (connective tissue nevus)
- Cortical tuber
- Subependymal nodule
- Subependymal giant cell astrocytoma
- Multiple retinal nodular hamartomas
- Cardiac rhabdomyoma (single or multiple)
- Lymphangiomyomatosis *or* renal angiomyolipoma

Minor features
- Multiple randomly distributed pits in dental enamel
- Hamartomatous rectal polyps
- Bone cysts
- Cerebral white matter "migration tracts"
- Gingival fibromas
- Nonrenal hamartoma
- Retinal achromic patch
- "Confetti" skin lesions
- Multiple renal cysts

Definite Tuberous Sclerosis Complex: Either two major features or one major feature plus two minor features.
Probable Tuberous Sclerosis Complex: One major feature plus one minor feature.
Suspect Tuberous Sclerosis Complex: Either one major feature or two or more minor features.

pediatric age group, renal cystic disease was the presenting problem in 3 of 125 children.[505] In adults who have not yet come to clinical attention, renal tumors can be the first clinical manifestation in some cases.

Genetics

The tuberous sclerosis syndrome results from a germline mutation in one of two genes, *tuberous sclerosis 1* (*TSC1*) at 9q34 and *tuberous sclerosis 2* (*TSC2*) at 16p13.3. These mutations occur with an equal frequency. *TSC1* and *TSC2*, respectively, encode the proteins hamartin and tuberin. Hamartin has a cell adhesion function, while tuberin is a GTPase activating protein that is involved in the MTOR cell signaling pathway, which controls nutrient-stimulated cell growth.[506,507] Hamartin and tuberin function as a complex, and mutations in either *TSC1* or *TSC2* will lead to similar phenotypic changes resulting from uncontrolled cell growth signaling. Although hamartin and tuberin act as a complex, more severe manifestations are seen in individuals with *TSC2* mutations. *TSC2* is also active in VEGF expression and thus interacts with the *VHL* pathway. At 16p13.3 *TSC2* is adjacent to the gene *polycystic kidney disease 1 (autosomal dominant)* (*PKD1*), which is involved in autosomal dominant polycystic disease, and renal cysts are seen in tuberous sclerosis, where mutations involve both *TSC2* and *PKD1* (referred to as the *TSC2/PKD1* contiguous gene syndrome).[508] These patients develop severe renal cystic disease that can be present at birth.

Renal Pathology

Angiomyolipomas are the renal tumors most commonly seen in patients with tuberous sclerosis. It is important to remember however, that more than 50% of angiomyolipomas diagnosed clinically are sporadic. The demographics of angiomyolipoma associated with tuberous sclerosis differ from those of sporadic tumors. With tuberous sclerosis, there is a roughly equal gender distribution, which differs from sporadic angiomyolipoma that has a female predominance.[509,510]

Angiomyolipoma of the kidney is seen in 75% to 80% of affected individuals by the second decade and is typically bilateral and multifocal. The histologic features of syndrome-related angiomyolipoma are similar to that of sporadic tumors with varying proportions of smooth muscle, mature adipose tissue, and blood vessels with thickened walls.[510,511] There are no apparent differences in the frequency of smooth muscle– or fat-predominant angiomyolipoma between sporadic and tuberous sclerosis–associated angiomyolipoma.[511] The presence of multifocality (Fig. 2-78), particularly if more than two tumors are present, should suggest the possibility of tuberous sclerosis complex. The unusual occurrence of intraglomerular angiomyolipoma (Fig. 2-79) is also described in tuberous sclerosis. Involvement of the renal parenchyma can be so extensive as to result in renal failure. Epithelioid angiomyolipoma, with the potential to show locally infiltrative growth and the development of metastasis, may also occur in tuberous sclerosis.[512]

Single or multiple cysts is also a frequent feature in the kidney of tuberous sclerosis patients and these generally develop at an earlier age than angiomyolipoma. Renal cysts are found in approximately 50% of patients. The pathology of the renal cysts in tuberous sclerosis is covered in detail in Chapter 1.

Renal cell carcinoma has been reported to develop in 1% to 4% of patients with tuberous sclerosis.[513] Most of these have been reported as clear cell renal cell carcinomas, but

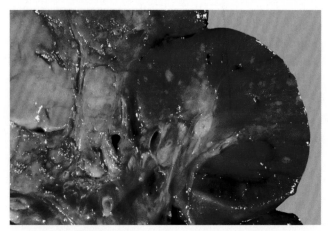

FIGURE 2-78 ■ Familial renal neoplasia. In addition to the large angiomyolipoma seen at the left, this kidney from a patient with tuberous sclerosis shows multiple small yellow spots which also are angiomyolipomas.

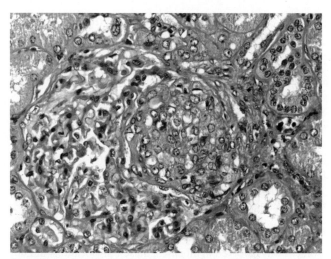

FIGURE 2-79 ■ Familial renal neoplasia. An intraglomerular angiomyolipoma is seen in this section from the kidney of a patient with tuberous sclerosis.

chromophobe renal cell carcinoma and papillary renal cell carcinoma are also described. It has, however, been suggested that many of the renal cancers reported in tuberous sclerosis are, in reality, epithelioid angiomyolipoma.[512] A meta-analysis of published cases of tuberous sclerosis provides evidence that the occurrence of most types of renal parenchymal neoplasia was not increased in tuberous sclerosis, while there did appear to be an increased incidence of oncocytoma.[514] Despite this, an increase in renal carcinoma has been reported in individuals with *TSC1* mutations, and in tuberous sclerosis it has been noted that cancers may be bilateral and multifocal with a younger age at presentation.[515]

Prognosis and Treatment

The management of renal tumors associated with tuberous sclerosis is dependent on the type of tumor present. Renal-sparing surgery with close monitoring is preferable for renal cell carcinoma in order to preserve renal function. The management of angiomyolipoma is dependent on the size of the tumor with larger masses considered at higher risk for rupture more often treated surgically. Currently targeted therapies have shown promise in the management of the neurologic disorders and for angiomyolipoma.[516] Several reports have documented inhibition of growth and reduction in the size of angiomyolipoma when treated with MTOR inhibitors.[519]

Hereditary Leiomyomatosis and Renal Cell Carcinoma Syndrome

Introduction

In 2001, Launonen et al.[518] described the clinical, histopathologic, and molecular features of a novel autosomal dominant hereditary syndrome characterized by a predisposition to uterine leiomyoma and papillary renal cell carcinomas. In addition to uterine leiomyomas these patients develop uterine leiomyosarcomas and cutaneous leiomyomas. Adrenal lesions (massive macronodular cortical disease and nodular hyperplasia) and ovarian steroid cell tumors also have been reported.[519,520]

The cutaneous and uterine leiomyomas usually present between the ages of 20 and 30 years. Cutaneous leiomyomas are found in over 80% of families when evaluated by dermatologists.[521] Renal cell carcinoma develops in 20% to 34% of families with mutations and in 2% to 21% of affected individuals.[521–524]

Genetics

Genetic studies show germline missense mutations, truncation, or whole gene deletions at 1q42.2-42.3. This region contains the 10 exons that encode for fumarate hydratase. This enzyme is essential for the conversion of fumarate to malate, and loss of function leads to up-regulation of hypoxia-inducible factor.[522–524]

Renal Tumors

Renal tumors associated with the hereditary leiomyomatosis and renal cell carcinoma syndrome develop at a younger age than sporadic renal tumors, with a mean age of 36 to 39 years (range 17 to 75 years) at presentation. There is an equal gender distribution.[525] Early reports indicated that renal tumors associated with the syndrome were type 2 papillary renal cell carcinomas.[526] Subsequent detailed studies have shown papillary tumors to predominate often combined with solid, cystic, or tubular architectures (Figs. 2-80 and 2-81). The latter areas are typically infiltrative with stromal desmoplasia and can resemble collecting duct carcinoma, and several tumors in these patients have been reported under that diagnosis. These renal tumors are characterized by cytoplasmic

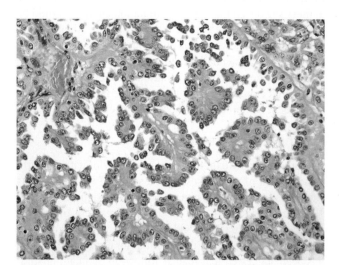

FIGURE 2-80 ■ Familial renal cell carcinoma. In hereditary leiomyomatosis and renal cell carcinoma syndrome the renal carcinomas have varied architectures. Here the structure is simple papillae covered by a single layer of cells with eosinophilic cytoplasm. The nucleoli are prominent.

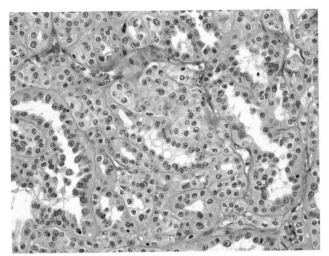

FIGURE 2-81 ■ Familial renal cell carcinoma. In hereditary leiomyomatosis and renal cell carcinoma syndrome the renal carcinomas also grow in solid and glandular patterns composed of cells with eosinophilic cytoplasm and prominent nucleoli.

eosinophilia, although occasional foci of cells with clear cytoplasm may also be seen. The tumor cells typically have pleomorphic nuclei with prominent eosinophilic or orangiophilic nucleoli and perinucleolar chromatin clearing.[525] Similar nuclear features are present in the uterine leiomyomas of these patients.[527] These tumors show negative expression of *Ulex europaeus* hemagglutinin-1 lectin, cytokeratin 7, cytokeratin 20, high molecular weight cytokeratin, and TFE-3. The clear cell areas seen in some tumors are positive for CD10.[525] These are now considered to represent a distinct type of renal cell carcinoma unique to this syndrome.

These patients can present with renal cell carcinoma without documentation of uterine or cutaneous leiomyomas. In one analysis of sporadic type 2 papillary renal cell carcinomas, *FH* gene mutations were found in 2 of 18 cases. These authors suggested that *FH* gene mutation analysis should be considered in patients under 40 years of age when a renal cell carcinoma shows features described above.[521] We concur with this recommendation and raise the possibility of this syndrome whenever the combination of a well-defined papillary architecture is mixed with a solid or infiltrative tubular component combined with the typical nuclear features.

Prognosis and Treatment

Tumors frequently exhibit aggressive behavior with the early development of metastases; in one series 17 out of 21 cases showed extrarenal extension at the time of diagnosis and 9 of 19 patients presented with metastatic disease.[523] In another series, 20 of 27 patients with renal cell carcinoma died of their tumor.[521] In view of the potential for early metastases, it has been suggested that regular follow-up by imaging studies of small tumors is appropriate.[523] Treatment is primarily surgical with some early reports indicating a possible role for tyrosine kinase inhibitors or similar drugs in metastatic disease.[521]

Clear Cell Renal Cell Carcinoma with Translocation of Chromosome 3

In 1979, hereditary clear cell renal cell carcinoma with the constitutional balanced translocation t(3;8) (p14;q24) was reported in a single family.[528] This translocation involved the tumor suppressor gene *FHIT* at 3p14, which is frequently deleted in sporadic clear cell renal cell carcinomas.[529]

Since the initial report, further instances of hereditary and sporadic clear cell renal cell carcinomas have been associated with 13 different constitutional translocations: t(3;8) (p14;q24), t(2;3)(q35;q21), t(3;6)(q12;q15), t(2;3)(q33;q21), t(1;3)(q32;qq13.3), t(3;8)(p13;q24), t(3;12)(q13.2;q24.1), t(3;6)(p13;q25.1), t(3;4)(p13;p16), t(3;15)(p11;q21), t(3;6) (q22;q16.2), and t(3;4)(q21;q31).[530–532] Although chromosome 3 was involved in all cases, these translocations did not involve the *VHL* gene at 3p25-26. Annual renal cancer screening is not recommended in these patients unless there is also a personal family history of clear cell renal cell carcinoma.[532]

Familial chromosome 3 translocation renal cell carcinomas are always of the clear cell type and are usually bilateral and multifocal. In the family with the t(3;8) translocation, carcinomas of the thyroid were also seen.[528]

Familial Clear Cell Renal Cell Carcinoma

Familial clear cell renal cell carcinoma is defined by the development of clear cell renal cell carcinoma in two or more family members with no evidence of a hereditary renal cell carcinoma syndrome or with constitutional chromosome 3 translocations.[533] Two kindreds of nine individuals with clear cell renal cell carcinoma, in the absence of *VHL* mutations, were described in 1997.[534] In this series, tumors were unilateral and in eight of nine cases, were in individuals aged >50 years. In a subsequent study of 25 cases from nine families, tumors were found to be more frequently bilateral with an earlier age at onset (mean 47.1 years) than sporadic tumors.[535] The tumors in these families are typical clear cell renal cell carcinomas without histologic features to distinguish them from sporadic cases.

A larger analysis of 145 cases from 60 families showed 2 to 5 family members to have renal tumors.[533] The gender distribution was similar to sporadic clear cell renal cell carcinoma (M:F, 1.8:1), although patients were younger with a mean age of 53 years at diagnosis. Multiple tumors were seen at diagnosis or subsequently developed in 10% of cases. Segregation analysis was most consistent with autosomal dominant inheritance. In contrast, a study of familial renal cell carcinoma in Sweden concluded that recessive genes might be important for these cases.[536] Based upon these data, it was recommended that annual renal imaging be undertaken on affected individuals and family members from the age of 30 years. In families where onset was earlier than 30 years, it was further recommended that earlier surveillance should be offered. A small percentage of patients presenting with apparent familial clear cell renal cell carcinoma will be found to harbor *FLCN* gene mutations and may represent cases of Birt-Hogg-Dubé syndrome without other features of the disease leading to the recommendation that these patients also be offered genetic testing.[533] Karyotyping for a possible chromosome 3 translocation is also recommended in such patients.[513]

Hereditary Papillary Renal Cell Carcinoma

Introduction

The occurrence of an inherited predisposition for papillary renal cell carcinoma was first described in 1994.[537] This is a rare disease with autosomal dominant inheritance and a high degree of penetrance.

Genetics

Hereditary papillary renal cell carcinoma is associated with germline mutation of the *met protooncogene (hepatocyte growth factor receptor)* gene (HUGO-approved gene symbol: *MET*) 7q31-34 that encodes the hepatocyte growth factor receptor leading to an increase of function.[538] This mutation is also occasionally seen in sporadic papillary renal cell carcinoma exhibiting a type 1 morphology.[255] Trisomy of chromosome 7 is frequently present in the tumors of hereditary papillary renal cell carcinoma; however, trisomy 17 is not a feature.[539]

Renal Tumors

The majority of tumors present in the fifth or sixth decade,[540] although in one series, a subset of tumors presenting as early as the second and third decades was reported.[541] The tumors are often occult with patients presenting late already having numerous and bilateral tumors. Radiologically the tumors are hypovascular and enhance poorly on CT scans. This can result in the number of tumors present being underappreciated in imaging studies.

In this syndrome, numerous bilateral tumors of varying size may be present with up to 3,400 papillary neoplasms being noted in some kidneys.[542] These are of type 1 morphology and almost always have a low histologic grade (Fuhrman grade 1 or 2).[542] In the series reported by Lubensky et al.,[255] 105 of 113 (93%) tumors examined were nuclear grade 1 or 2. The tumor cells are predominantly small with scant cytoplasm but eosinophilic cells and cells with cytoplasmic clearing can be present. The latter contain glycogen and lipid but in contrast to clear cell renal cell carcinoma are seen covering delicate papillae. Foamy macrophages and psammomatous calcification are common. The grossly uninvolved parenchyma typically shows numerous papillary adenomas, but these may not always be found, particularly when limited tissue is available for examination as in partial nephrectomy specimens. There are no specific features in individual tumors that allow for the distinction of sporadic from hereditary papillary renal cell carcinoma. No other forms of renal neoplasia have been seen in this syndrome, although a single report of cases associated with urothelial neoplasia has been described.[543]

Prognosis and Treatment

As many of these tumors are diagnosed in older patients, their occurrence may appear sporadic, and it has been recommended that any family with two or more individuals diagnosed with papillary renal cell carcinoma should be referred for genetic evaluation. Germline *MET* mutational analysis is also recommended for patients with bilateral, multifocal papillary renal cell carcinoma.[513] Where feasible, nephron-sparing partial nephrectomy is treatment of choice for tumors >3 cm in diameter with small tumors managed by observation.[544] Preservation of renal parenchyma is a major goal in managing these patients.[513] Although the majority of tumors are indolent, some can be aggressive and metastasize, the latter reported in 12% of patients in one study.[255] Systemic therapies targeting the MTOR pathway or the hepatocyte growth factor receptor are actively being studied for these patients.[513]

Succinate Dehydrogenase B Mutation–Associated Renal Cell Carcinoma

There have been a few examples of renal tumors developing in patients with *succinate dehydrogenase B* gene (HUGO-approved gene symbol: *SDHB*) mutations.[545–548] Isolated cases in patients with succinate dehydrogenase C and D mutations are also reported. These patients also develop pheochromocytoma, paraganglioma, and type 2 gastrointestinal stromal tumors. In a study of 358 patients from 160 kindreds, 12 patients developed renal tumors and the risk of developing a renal tumor by age 70 was estimated at 14% for those with *SDHB* mutation and 8% with *SDHD* mutations.[546] Patients reported to date have ranged from 15 to 62 years (mean and median, 37 years) with males and females affected. Bilaterality and multifocality are common. In the largest series to date, 5 of 21 patients (14, 6, and 1 each with *SDHB*, *SDHC*, and *SDHD* mutations, respectively) died of their disease.[548] Malignant behavior has also been reported in two cases with sarcomatoid morphology.

The pathology of these tumors is not well defined. Tumors have ranged from 1.8 to 11.0 cm. They have been solid or solid and cystic. The tumors have been well circumscribed and unencapsulated. The most characteristic histologic feature is a tumor composed of cuboidal or polygonal cells with moderate amounts of vacuolated eosinophilic cytoplasm arranged in small nests. The vacuoles contain pale eosinophilic fluid-like material. Ultrastructural examination has shown giant mitochondria in these tumors. Normal tubules or glomeruli are often entrapped in the tumor at the edges. Other patterns described include papillary and sarcomatoid. In one group of patients with *SDHC* mutations, the tumors were morphologically similar to clear cell renal cell carcinoma.[548] Diagnosis requires demonstration of the mutation or loss of succinate dehydrogenase expression by immunohistochemistry. Because of the limited experience with these tumors, they are not formally included in the current ISUP classification.[7]

ALK-Translocation Renal Cell Carcinoma

In 2011, there were two cases reported of renal cell carcinomas found to have a t(2;10)(p23:q22) translocation involving the *anaplastic lymphoma receptor tyrosine kinase* gene (HUGO-approved gene symbol: *ALK*).[549,550] Both were in patients with sickle cell trait, and one was considered a renal medullary carcinoma. The tumors were composed of polygonal to spindle-shaped cells with eosinophilic cytoplasm and intracytoplasmic vacuoles representing intracytoplasmic lumens. In a subsequent study, 355 renal cell carcinomas were screened for *ALK* translocations, and 2 cases were identified.[551] These occurred in two females (ages 36 and 53 years) without sickle cell trait. Both cases had papillary morphology and were considered by the authors to be renal cell carcinoma, unclassified. In another survey of 534 cases of renal cell carcinoma, *ALK* gene rearrangements were identified in only 2 cases.[552] Both patients were male (ages 59 and 61) and had tumors with papillary architecture. Of interest, there was an increase in *ALK* copy number in 8% of papillary renal cell carcinomas and 17% of clear cell renal cell carcinomas in that study. It remains unclear whether the tumors with *ALK* rearrangements represent a specific tumor type or not. The current ISUP classification does not recognize these as a distinct entity.[7]

METANEPHRIC TUMORS

Metanephric Adenoma

Epidemiology

First described in 1980, under the name néphrome néphronogène (nephronogenic nephroma), the term "metanephric adenoma" was introduced in 1979.[553,554] Although more than 100 cases of metanephric adenoma have been reported,[555] this underestimates the true incidence of these tumors in clinical practice. The patients have ranged in age from young children to the elderly,[556] and in various series the median age at presentation was around 50 years, with many cases occurring in the fifth to sixth decades.[556–559] Two-thirds of the cases of metanephric adenoma have been female. In rare cases, coexistent renal cell carcinoma was found in patients with metanephric adenoma. Metanephric adenoma is the most common epithelial neoplasm found in the kidneys of children.[230]

Pathogenesis

Although initially considered to be derived from persistent blastema, it has also been suggested that metanephric adenoma represents maturation of Wilms tumor. This is supported by the immunophenotype seen in metanephric adenoma, which parallels that seen in differentiated Wilms tumor and nephrogenic rests.[560]

Clinical Features

Metanephric adenomas are frequently discovered as incidental findings, while other presenting features are hematuria,

pyrexia, abdominal mass, and flank pain.[556,557,560] About 10% of the patients are polycythemic.[556,559] This appears to be due to tumor-derived erythropoietin and cytokines, and the polycythemia has usually disappeared after resection of the tumor.[561]

Imaging studies frequently show calcifications within the tumors, while enhanced computed tomography shows that the tumors often exhibit low attenuation.[559]

Pathology

Gross Features

Metanephric adenomas vary widely in size. Most tumors are between 3 and 6 cm in diameter, although ones as large as 15 cm in diameter have been described.[556] Metanephric adenomas are well circumscribed, and although a thin partial pseudocapsule may be rarely seen, metanephric adenoma usually directly abuts against normal renal tissue. Multifocality is rare,[562] and all tumors reported have been unilateral. On sectioning, metanephric adenomas are solid and tan to gray, and may be soft or firm (Fig. 2-82). Hemorrhage and focal necrosis may be present, especially in larger tumors. Cystic degeneration is seen in 10% of metanephric adenomas, and in one case, the tumor was entirely cystic.[556] Calcification is often seen macroscopically and may be extensive.

Microscopic Features

Histologically, metanephric adenoma is typically highly cellular and composed of tightly packed small, uniform, round

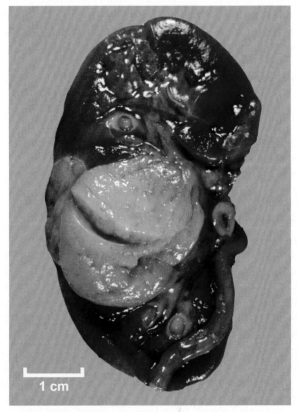

FIGURE 2-82 ■ Metanephric adenoma. The tumor is fleshy, solid, and bulges above the cut surface.

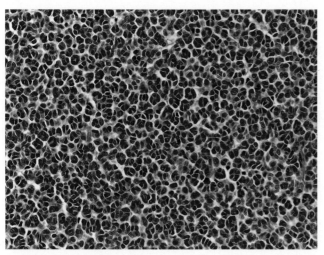

FIGURE 2-83 ■ Metanephric adenoma. The most common architecture is a dense growth of small cells with darkly basophilic nuclei arranged in clusters around small or pinpoint lumens and with inconspicuous stroma.

acini (Fig. 2-83). Since the acini and their lumens are so small, at low magnification this pattern may be mistaken for a solid sheet of cells. Long branching and angulated tubular structures also are common. The stroma ranges from inconspicuous to a loose edematous stroma to a sclerotic stroma (Fig. 2-84). Hyalinized scar, microcyst formation, or focal osseous metaplasia of the stroma is present in 10% to 20% of tumors.[556] Approximately 50% of metanephric adenomas contain papillary structures, often consisting of short blunt papillae reminiscent of immature glomeruli, growing into minute spaces. In most of these, no blood vessel is visible. Psammoma bodies are common and may be numerous and there may be dystrophic calcification in hyalinized areas. The junction with the kidney is usually abrupt and lacks a pseudocapsule. The cells of metanephric adenoma have small, uniform nuclei with absent or inconspicuous nucleoli. The nuclei are only slightly larger than lymphocytes

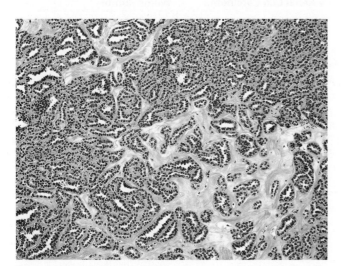

FIGURE 2-84 ■ Metanephric adenoma. Occasionally the cells form tubules or the stroma becomes sclerotic and wider.

and are round or oval and have delicate chromatin. The cytoplasm is scant and pale or light pink. Mitotic figures are absent or rare.

Ancillary and Special Studies

Immunohistochemistry shows that metanephric adenoma usually shows diffusely positive nuclear staining for WT1 (Fig. 2-85A). Staining for CD57 (Fig. 2-85B) is also frequently is positive. Negative reactions for desmin, AMACR, and epithelial membrane antigen are typical. Staining for S100 protein has been found to be strongly positive in the great majority of metanephric adenomas but this may depend upon the antibody that is used.[558] Cytokeratin 7 may be negative (Fig. 2-85C) or focally positive, with expression usually present in elongate tubules.[555,560] Positive staining for cytokeratin AE1/AE3, CAM 5.2, CK 18, and vimentin has also been reported.[558,560,562]

Genetics

In most studies metanephric adenoma has shown a normal genotype or no consistent abnormality.[563–565] In particular, it has been demonstrated that these tumors lack gains of chromosomes 7 and 17, and loss of Y, typical of papillary renal cell carcinoma, nor the pattern of chromosomal gains and losses frequently present in Wilms tumors.[566,567] In two cases, abnormalities of chromosome 2 were noted.[568,569] The V600E mutation of *BRAF* is present in approximately 90% of metanephric adenomas.[570]

Differential Diagnosis

At first inspection, metanephric adenoma brings Wilms tumor to mind because of the dense array of small blue cells and epithelial differentiation. However, the nuclei of metanephric adenoma are smaller and lack the elongation and tapered ends often present in the nuclei of epithelial cells in Wilms tumor. Further, mitotic figures are rare in metanephric adenoma and blastema is not present. Wilms tumor shows similar positive immunohistochemical reactions for α-methylacyl CoA racemase, WT1, and CK 7 to those of metanephric adenoma; however, reactions for CD57 and S100 are usually negative (Table 2-16).[555,558]

The other major consideration is type 1 papillary renal cell carcinoma because of the small cytoplasmic volume, papillary structures, and psammoma bodies. However, most metanephric adenomas are composed mainly of arrays of fairly uniform structures resembling renal tubules in cross section. This architecture is not typical of papillary renal cell carcinoma. Additionally, metanephric adenomas often have long pointed, branching channels lined by epithelial cells. These are not found in papillary renal cell carcinoma, nor in Wilms tumor. The edema of papillary cores and collections of stromal foam cells, which are common in papillary renal cell carcinoma, are not typical of metanephric adenoma. Unlike metanephric adenoma, immunohistochemistry usually shows that type 1 papillary renal cell carcinoma is negative for CD57 and WT1, and positive for CK 7 and α-methylacyl CoA racemase.[555,560]

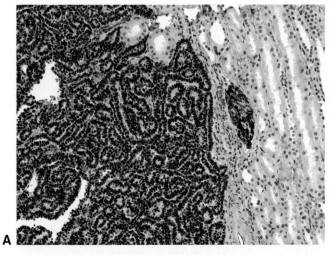

A

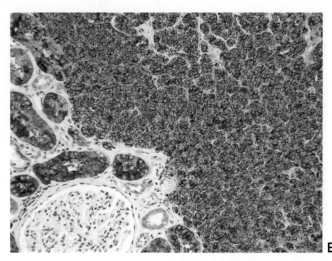

B

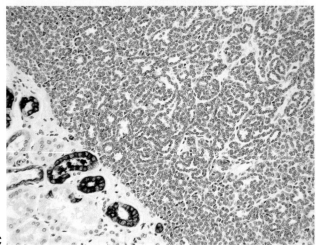

C

FIGURE 2-85 ■ **A:** Metanephric adenoma. Immunohistochemistry with antibody to WT1 usually gives a strongly positive reaction in the nuclei of nearly all of the neoplastic cells. **B:** The reaction for CD57 is often strongly positive in the cytoplasm of the metanephric adenoma cells. **C:** The reaction with antibody to cytokeratin 7 is typically negative in the neoplastic cells.

Table 2-16 ■ METANEPHRIC ADENOMA—DIFFERENTIAL DIAGNOSIS

Feature	Metanephric Adenoma	Papillary Renal Cell Carcinoma	Wilms' Tumor
Age	All ages	Middle to older age	Children
Sex (F:M)	2:1	1:3-4	1:1
Clinical	Incidental Polycythemia	Hematuria, flank pain, abdominal mass, incidental	Palpable mass Congenital anomalies
Gross	Single, circumscribed Nodular, gray-tan	Multiple in 50% Thick capsule, red–brown	Nodular, bulging Soft, gray–white
Microscopic	Most not encapsulated Closely packed tubules Small cells with little cytoplasm	Majority have capsule Tubulopapillary Basophil/eosinophil cells Foamy histiocytes	Triphasic–epithelial, mesenchymal and blastema
Special studies	Keratin + (CK 7 –/+) Vimentin + WT1 ++ EMA neg (or weak +) CD57+ S100+ Racemase (AMACR) +/– No glycogen	Keratin + (CK 7 ++) Vimentin +/– WT1 negative EMA +++ CD57 uncertain S100 negative Racemase (AMACR) ++ Glycogen +/–	Epithelium: Keratin +, Vimentin negative WT1 ++ EMA +/– CD57 + in tubules

Cyclin-dependent kinase inhibitor 2A (CDKN2A), also known as p16, can be detected immunohistochemically in most metanephric adenomas with a positive nuclear reaction in 5% to 60% of cells (median = 25%).[570]

Prognosis and Treatment

Metanephric adenoma appears to be a benign tumor. Metanephric adenoma within a regional lymph node has been described, and this was interpreted as passive seeding rather than metastatic spread.[571]

Metanephric Adenofibroma

Epidemiology and Clinical Features

In 1992, Hennigar and Beckwith described five cases of a composite neoplasm in which an epithelial component identical to metanephric adenoma was combined with a proliferation of spindle cells.[572] They proposed the name nephrogenic adenofibroma for this tumor; however, the term metanephric adenofibroma was later adopted to emphasize the close relationship of these tumors to metanephric adenoma.

The ages of the patients with metanephric adenofibroma range from 13 months to 36 years (median 4 years). Metanephric adenofibroma may also occur in association with Wilms tumor and renal cell carcinoma. Patients in the former group are younger than those with pure metanephric adenofibroma (range 5 to 33 months, median 9 months), while the latter are older (range 3 to 30 years, median 11 years). One patient with composite Wilms tumor with metanephric adenoma had a sibling with clear cell sarcoma of kidney.[572,573] While the number of reported cases is small, there does not appear to be any gender predominance.

While a significant proportion of tumors are incidental findings, other presenting features are hematuria, hypertension, urinary tract infection, and diarrhea.[572–574] Similar to metanephric adenoma, polycythemia appears to occur in about 10% of patients.[573]

Pathology

Gross Features

Metanephric adenofibromas are typically solitary firm bosselated masses without capsules and with indistinct borders. Most metanephric adenofibromas have been small (median diameter = 4 cm), but a few have been larger than 10 cm.[573,575] The tumors are yellow-tan on cut surface and may occasionally be papillary or cystic.[573]

Microscopic Features

Metanephric adenofibroma is a composite tumor in which nests of epithelial elements, identical in morphology to metanephric adenoma, are embedded in spindle cell stroma. As for metanephric adenomas, the epithelial component consists of small acini, tubules, and papillary structures, usually with psammoma bodies. Mitotic figures are usually absent or rare, although occasional metanephric adenofibroma have

>5 mitotic figures/20 HPF. The stromal cells are fibroblast-like with pale eosinophilic cytoplasm, oval or fusiform nuclei, and inconspicuous nucleoli.[572] Variable amounts of hyalinization and myxoid change are present and occasional glial-like areas may be seen.[573] The stroma may show a concentric pattern around entrapped tubules and angiodysplastic vessels. The relative proportion of the spindle cell and epithelial components varies and cases with minute epithelial foci have been described.[576] The border of the tumor with the kidney is typically irregular and the stromal component may entrap renal structures as it advances.

Reported cases of composite metanephric adenofibroma and renal cell carcinoma contain nodules of papillary or solid carcinomas within typical metanephric adenofibroma stroma. In composite metanephric adenofibroma with Wilms tumor the malignant component is epithelial predominant, without blastema.[572,573]

Ancillary and Special Studies

The stromal component is positive for CD34 in 80% of the tumors tested. Reactions for muscle-specific actin and desmin have been negative. The epithelial component is usually negative or very focally positive for CK7. CK7 is diffusely positive, however, in the carcinomatous component of composite metanephric adenofibroma with renal cell carcinoma.[573]

Genetics

In one case of metanephric adenofibroma, trisomy of chromosome 11 was demonstrated.[573]

Differential Diagnosis

Metanephric adenofibroma has a characteristic appearance and typical cases should not present diagnostic difficulty. In those tumors that are stromal predominant, extensive sampling should be undertaken as the epithelial component may be inconspicuous.

Prognosis and Treatment

Follow-up studies to date are limited. No recurrence of classic metanephric adenofibroma has been reported, even for cases that showed extension into the renal sinus. In a case reported as composite metanephric adenofibroma with carcinoma, metastatic spread of papillary carcinoma to regional lymph nodes was seen, although no follow-up details were available.[573]

Metanephric Stromal Tumor

Epidemiology and Clinical Features

Metanephric stromal tumors are benign neoplasms composed of stromal elements identical to the stroma of metanephric adenofibroma. It has been suggested that these tumors are related to Wilms tumor and may represent maturation of intralobar nephrogenic nests.

Metanephric stromal tumors are rare; fewer than 50 cases have been reported. The majority of tumors were described in patients aged 11 years or younger, with a mean age at presentation of 2 years,[555,577] although tumors in patients aged 15, 72, and 74 years have been reported.[578,579] There is no gender predisposition.

The majority of cases have presented as an abdominal mass, while other presenting features have been hypertension, hematuria, and abdominal pain.[577–579] A single example has occurred in a patient with neurofibromatosis type 1 syndrome.[580] Unlike metanephric adenoma, metanephric stromal tumor does not appear to be associated with erythrocytosis.

Pathology

Gross Features

Metanephric stromal tumor is typically lobulated and may be multifocal. When small, the tumors usually appear to be centered on the renal medulla. The mean diameter of reported tumors is 5 cm, although occasional giant tumors up to 4 kg have been seen.[577,579] Metanephric stromal tumor usually has a tan cut surface, and more than 50% contain smooth-walled cysts.

Microscopic Features

These tumors are composed of spindle cells with pale eosinophilic cytoplasm. Often times the tumors contain areas of high cellularity and other areas with less cellularity. Focally, the stroma shows concentric growth around entrapped tubules and vascular spaces. Vessels often show angiodysplasia, while there may also be hyperplasia of juxtaglomerular cells in entrapped glomeruli. These changes are histologically very similar to changes seen in the kidneys of patients with the neurofibromatosis type 1 syndrome.[580] Islands of cartilage and glial nodules are present in 20% of cases.[555] The edge of the tumor abuts upon the renal parenchyma without forming a pseudocapsule, and usually shows early intrarenal extension to surround tubules adjacent to the tumor interface.

Ancillary and Special Studies

Metanephric stromal tumors show variable immunohistochemical expression, although most are focally positive for CD34 and are negative for cytokeratins, desmin, and S-100 protein.

Differential Diagnosis

These tumors should be differentiated from congenital mesoblastic nephroma and clear cell sarcoma. Metanephric stromal tumor does not show the degree of tubular entrapment characteristic of mesoblastic nephroma, while a concentric growth pattern, glial differentiation, and positive immunohistochemical reactions for CD34 are not found in cellular mesoblastic nephroma. Clear cell sarcoma has a typical branching vascular pattern not seen in metanephric stromal tumor, which unlike clear cell sarcoma, often has heterotopic glia or cartilage.

Prognosis and Treatment

All but one of the tumors reported to date have shown a benign course with no evidence of metastatic spread. A single instance of recurrence in the scrotum with infiltration of the epididymis has been reported.[581] Lack of spread to other sites and substantial follow-up led the authors of that report to speculate that this was not blood or lymphatic metastasis, but perhaps migration down the processus vaginalis.

Metanephric Adenosarcoma

A single case of metanephric adenosarcoma has been reported in a 21-year-old woman.[582] This tumor was 10 cm in diameter and was solid and cystic, with areas of hemorrhage. Histologically, the tumor had an epithelial component typical of metanephric adenoma and a malignant spindle cell stroma. The epithelium was positive for cytokeratin AE1/AE3, while the stroma was positive for vimentin, CD34, and CD117. FISH studies showed monosomy of chromosome X. The stromal component of the tumor had spread to lymph nodes at the time of diagnosis, and the patient died within 5 weeks.

NEPHROBLASTIC TUMORS

Wilms Tumor (Nephroblastoma)

Introduction

Wilms tumor constitutes more than 90% of renal tumors of childhood.[583] Even in the first 6 months of life, Wilms tumor is the predominant renal neoplasm.[584] The origin of Wilms tumors was obscure for many years, but today nephrogenic rests are recognized as the precursors of Wilms tumors. Aggregates of cells resembling blastema have been found in pediatric autopsies and in kidneys resected from patients with Wilms tumors for decades.[585] Bove and McAdams[586] studied 69 kidneys resected for Wilms tumors and observed microscopic nodules of blastemal cells in a third of the cases. Based on these observations, they proposed a classification based on histologic features, including categories of nodular renal blastema, metanephric hamartoma, and others. Subsequently, Beckwith et al.[587] proposed a new classification based on the extensive case material of the National Wilms' Tumor Study Pathology Center (NWTS). The following discussion is based on that work: Nephrogenic rests are foci of persistent nephrogenic cells resembling those of the developing kidney. These are divided into two categories: perilobar nephrogenic rests, which are located at the periphery of the renal lobes (the cortical surfaces, the centers of the columns of Bertin, and the tissue abutting the renal sinus) (Fig. 2-86) and intralobar nephrogenic rests, which are located in the cortex or medulla within the renal lobe. In addition to the location, perilobar nephrogenic rests differ from intralobar nephrogenic rests in having well-defined smooth borders, predominance of blastema, and are often numerous or diffuse. Intralobar nephrogenic rests usually are single and mingle irregularly with renal parenchyma; stroma is usually the predominant element. Nephrogenic rests are subclassified histologically as dormant or nascent; maturing, sclerosing, and obsolescent; hyperplastic; and neoplastic.

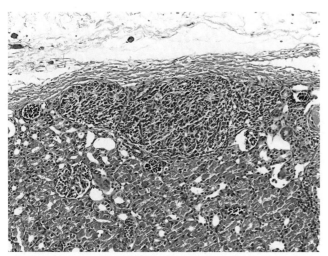

FIGURE 2-86 ■ Perilobar nephrogenic rest composed of blastema.

Tissue resembling nephrogenic rests is occasionally found outside the kidney in teratomas or in soft tissue of the pelvis or inguinal canal.[588]

Perilobar nephrogenic rests are present in approximately 1% of infants younger than 3 months, a frequency two orders of magnitude greater than that of Wilms tumor (1 per 10,000), while intralobar nephrogenic rests are almost never seen except with Wilms tumor. Nephrogenic rests are extremely rare in adults.[589] Rarely, perilobar nephrogenic rest tissue may make up the entirety or a large part of the cortex of one or both kidneys, a condition called hyperplastic perilobar nephroblastomatosis (Fig. 2-87).[590] In patients with unilateral Wilms tumor, the NWTS found that perilobar and intralobar nephrogenic rests occur approximately equally frequently and are present in 41% of cases. However, nephrogenic rests are present in more than 95% of patients with

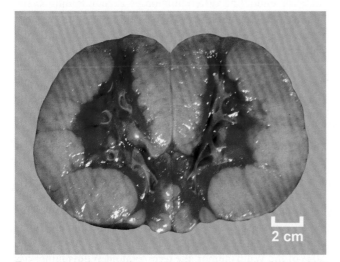

FIGURE 2-87 ■ Diffuse nephroblastomatosis in which the kidney is entirely replaced by nephrogenic rest tissue so that, while a reniform contour is retained, the distinction between cortex and medulla is no longer visible.

synchronous or metachronous bilateral Wilms tumor. Thus, careful examination of the grossly uninvolved renal tissue is important in cases of Wilms tumor, for the presence of nephrogenic rests indicates a greater probability of synchronous or metachronous bilaterality.[591]

Epidemiology and Clinical Features

Wilms tumor occurs most frequently in children 2 to 4 years old (median ages for boys and girls, respectively, are 37 and 43 months)[592] and is relatively uncommon in the first 6 months of life and in children older than 6 years.[593] Wilms tumor is rare in the neonatal period.[594] While in children aged 10 to 16 years, Wilms tumor remains the predominant renal tumor,[595] the prevalence of renal carcinomas quickly overtakes it and in the age range 11 to 20 years, Wilms tumors account for only 30% of renal tumors.[596] The incidence of Wilms tumors is about the same worldwide.[597] There is a slight preponderance of girls.[592] Wilms tumor is bilateral in 4.4% of cases,[598] and patients with bilateral tumors average more than a year younger than patients with unilateral tumors.[592] Associations with congenital anomalies, including cryptorchidism, hypospadias, other genital anomalies, hemihypertrophy, and aniridia are recognized.[599] As many as 5% of patients with Beckwith-Wiedemann syndrome develop Wilms tumor.[600] Patients with the Drash syndrome also have an increased risk of developing Wilms tumor.[601] A variety of other malformations are less frequently associated with Wilms tumor.[593,602] Prenatal and environmental risk factors for Wilms tumor include high birth weight, preterm birth, and maternal exposure to pesticides.[603] Uncommonly, Wilms tumor has a familial association.[592] Wilms tumors are rare in adults and the stage at presentation and frequency of anaplasia are higher than in children and response to therapy correspondingly less.[604,605]

Most children present with a painless abdominal mass, but a third present with pain, anorexia, vomiting, or malaise. Hypertension is the most common paraneoplastic manifestation but erythrocytosis, hypercalcemia, Cushing syndrome, and acquired von Willebrand disease also occur.[606,607] Wilms tumor is rare in adults, and most cases are in young adults (median age approximately 24 years).[608] Unfavorable histology occurs in 10% of adult cases and 5-year survival is more than 80%.[608]

Pathology

Gross Features

Wilms tumors usually are large, more than 5 cm in diameter, and a third or more are larger than 10 cm.[593] Often the specimen weighs more than 500 g. The cut surface is typically solid, soft, and gray or pink resembling brain tissue (Fig. 2-88). Foci of hemorrhage and necrosis are often present and cysts are common. Rarely, Wilms tumor is extensively cystic. The tumor usually is enclosed by a prominent pseudocapsule composed of compressed renal and perirenal tissues, giving an appearance of circumscription and even

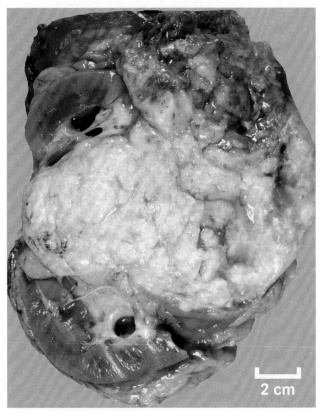

FIGURE 2-88 ■ Wilms tumor is often a large multilobular tumor with areas of necrosis.

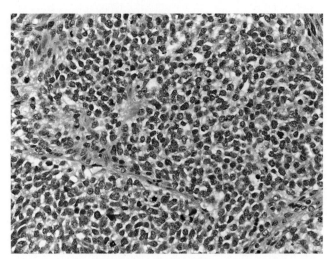

FIGURE 2-90 ■ Wilms tumor. Blastema with mitotic figures.

true encapsulation. Polypoid growth in the renal pelvic cavity, mimicking sarcoma botryoides, is a feature associated with extensive skeletal muscle differentiation[609–611] and may be mistaken for rhabdomyosarcoma.

Microscopic Features

Wilms tumor is typically composed of a variable mixture of blastema, epithelium, and stroma (Fig. 2-89), although in some tumors only one or two components are present.

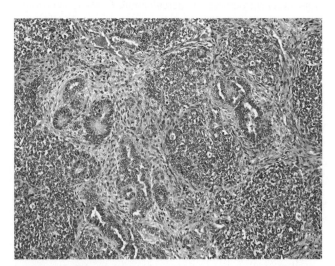

FIGURE 2-89 ■ Wilms tumor showing a mixture of blastema, stroma, and epithelial elements.

Blastema consists of sheets or randomly arranged densely packed small cells with darkly staining nuclei, frequent mitotic figures, and inconspicuous cytoplasm (Fig. 2-90), resembling other "small blue cell tumors" of childhood. Blastema is commonly arranged in three patterns, serpentine, nodular, and diffuse. Serpentine and nodular are most common and diagnostically helpful, consisting of anastomosing serpiginous or spheroidal aggregates of blastema that are sharply circumscribed from the surrounding stromal elements. When blastema is the predominant (>66%) element, the tumors are called blastemal predominant Wilms tumors and there is some evidence that this morphologic variant has adverse prognostic significance with a 5-year survival of only 65%.[612]

The epithelial component usually consists of small tubules or cysts lined by primitive columnar or cuboidal cells. The epithelium of Wilms tumor may also form structures resembling glomeruli, or may display mucinous, squamous, neural,[613] or endocrine differentiation.[259] Predominantly cystic Wilms tumor containing blastema and other Wilms tumor tissues in their septa are designated cystic partially differentiated nephroblastoma.[614,615]

The stroma of Wilms tumor may differentiate along the lines of almost any type of soft tissue. Loose myxoid and fibroblastic spindle cell stroma are most common, but smooth muscle, skeletal muscle (Fig. 2-91), fat, cartilage, bone, and neural components also are present in some tumors.[259] Uncommonly, differentiation toward skeletal muscle is diffuse and predominant (>50%) and the diagnosis of fetal rhabdomyomatous nephroblastoma is indicated.[609,610] The importance of recognizing fetal rhabdomyomatous nephroblastoma lies in its relative resistance to chemotherapy.[616–618] When complex combinations of differentiated heterologous epithelium and stroma are present and make up more than 50% of the Wilms tumor, the term teratoid Wilms tumor has been applied.[618–620]

Wilms tumor that has been treated with chemotherapy before nephrectomy poses additional diagnostic challenges.[621]

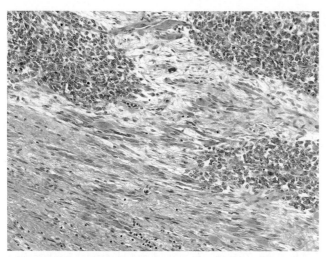

FIGURE 2-91 ■ Wilms tumor. Skeletal muscle differentiation in the stroma.

If the tumor is completely necrotic, ghostly contours of tumor elements can be seen. Nephrogenic rests are strong evidence that the necrotic tumor was a Wilms tumor, and the presence of the necrosis is supportive of the diagnosis since other types of renal neoplasia usually do not respond so completely to the chemotherapy given preoperatively. Distinction of hypocellular Wilms stroma from chemotherapy-induced changes can be difficult. The presence of rhabdomyoblasts would indicate that it is Wilms stroma and the presence of foamy macrophages would support the conclusion that it is chemotherapy effect. Estimation of the proportion of residual blastema is done semiquantitatively and so is subjective. Recognition of focal versus diffuse anaplasia can be made difficult by low mitotic rate and the consequent difficulty in finding enlarged atypical anaplastic mitotic figures.

Ancillary and Special Studies

Immunohistochemistry is of some help in making the diagnosis of Wilms tumor. Positive nuclear reactions for WT1 are typical (approximately 90%) in blastema and primitive epithelial elements, but stroma and more differentiated epithelial elements usually give weak or negative reactions.[622] PAX2 is demonstrable in nearly 100% of samples of Wilms' epithelium and blastema but only about 25% of examples of Wilms stroma, while cellular congenital mesoblastic nephroma, clear cell sarcoma, rhabdoid tumor, PNET/ Ewings sarcoma, and neuroblastoma give negative results.[623] CD56 is frequently positive in Wilms tumors (approximately 96%), mainly in the epithelial and blastemal elements, while it is negative in metanephric adenomas.[622,624] Gene expression studies show some promise as aids to diagnosis.[625]

Evidence is emerging that positive immunohistochemical reactions for TP53 are predictive of unfavorable stage and poorer survival.[626]

Genetics

Detection of deletions in 11p13 in patients with the Wilms tumor with aniridia, genitourinary anomalies, and mental retardation syndrome (WAGR syndrome) led to the identification of the *Wilms tumor 1* gene (HUGO-approved gene symbol *WT1*) that encodes a transcription factor. In these cases, *WT1* is inactivated, suggesting that it is a tumor suppressor gene. *WT1* also is inactivated in nephrogenic rests.[627] Mutations in *WT1* are detected in only about 20% of Wilms tumors, so there are more genes implicated in the genesis of Wilms tumors.[628] The *family with sequence 123B* gene (HUGO-approved gene symbol *FAM123B*) on Xq11.1 (also known as WTX for Wilms tumor on the X chromosome) plays a role in regulating the Wnt pathway and is mutated in about 20% of Wilms tumors. Mutations in *FAM123B* have been found in nephrogenic rests, suggesting that they occur early in carcinogenesis.[629] The *catenin (cadherin-associated protein) beta 1, 88 kDa* gene (HUGO-approved gene symbol *CTNNB1*) on 3p21 also codes for a protein regulating the Wnt pathway and is mutated in about 15% of Wilms tumors.[630] The gene *tumor protein 53* (HUGO-approved gene symbol *TP53*) on 17p13.1 is a tumor suppressor gene that is mutated in about 5% of Wilms tumors and is associated with anaplasia in Wilms tumors. Loss of heterozygosity or loss of imprinting on 11p15, a region in which genes for somatic overgrowth Beckwith-Wiedeman syndrome reside, occurs in many Wilms tumors and in nephrogenic rests.[631,632] Monosomy of chromosome 22 is common in Wilms tumor and has been found in hyperplastic and adenomatous nephrogenic rests.[633] Gene expression profiling has shown promise as means of stratifying patients with Wilms tumors with distinct differences in their pathologic and clinical features.[634,635]

Differential Diagnosis

Fetal rhabdomyomatous nephroblastoma has a favorable prognosis and should not be misinterpreted as rhabdomyosarcoma. This tumor contains extensive areas of relatively mature skeletal muscle but lacks the malignant small cells and rhabdomyoblasts found in rhabdomyosarcoma.

Monophasic epithelial Wilms tumor can be difficult to distinguish from renal cell carcinoma, especially in adolescents and adults. Recognition of the nuclear characteristics typical of the epithelium of Wilms tumor is often helpful. The epithelial nuclei in Wilms tumor are often elongate or ovoid with molded, sometimes wedged, shapes that differ from those of renal cell carcinoma that are usually nearly spherical. The distinction of Wilms tumor from rhabdoid tumor and clear cell sarcoma is discussed below.

Prognosis and Predictive Factors

In the 1930s, the mortality for children with Wilms tumors was approximately 70%. Today, approximately 80% of patients are cured by the initial therapy, and about half of those who relapse are cured by salvage therapy. In the United States and Canada, patients are treated with protocols developed by the National Wilms Tumor Study Group in which primary nephrectomy and pathologic diagnosis are used while in Europe the protocols developed by the

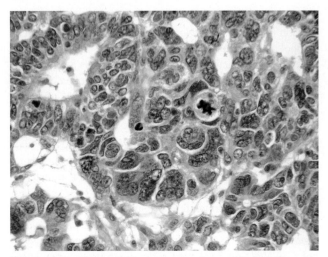

FIGURE 2-92 ■ Wilms tumor showing anaplasia with markedly enlarged and pleomorphic nuclei and a very large atypical mitotic figure.

International Society of Pediatric Oncology (SIOP) call for initial treatment with neoadjuvant chemotherapy.[636] Overall survival is similar with either protocol and is now 90%.[583,637] The co-operative groups are presently focusing on the development of protocols, which maintain the high rate of survival while reducing late effects of treatment.[638–640]

Based on the results of the NWTS, Wilms tumor is divided into categories of favorable and unfavorable histology, depending on the absence or presence of anaplasia (Fig. 2-92). Among patients with favorable histology, those with predominance of epithelial or stromal elements after preoperative chemotherapy in SIOP protocols appear to have a better prognosis than those with large amounts of blastema.[641] Anaplasia is found in approximately 11% of cases of Wilms tumor.[642] It is rare in patients younger than 1 year, and more than 80% of patients with anaplasia are older than two.[643] Early in the NWTS, the presence of anaplasia was found to be predictive of treatment failure and death.[644] However, anaplasia in a stage 1 Wilms tumor and anaplasia limited to discrete foci within a primary tumor have little or no adverse prognostic significance.[645,646] Anaplasia has been defined by the NWTS as the combination of cells with very large hyperchromatic nuclei and multipolar mitotic figures. Correct recognition of anaplasia demands good histologic preparations, including proper fixation, sectioning, and staining. The enlarged nuclei must be at least three times as large as typical blastemal nuclei in both axes, and the hyperchromasia must be obvious. In addition to the enlarged nuclei, hyperdiploid mitotic figures must be present. Several points should be borne in mind when evaluating a Wilms tumor for anaplasia. First, enlarged nuclei in skeletal muscle fibers in the stroma of Wilms tumors are not evidence of anaplasia. Second, the criteria for abnormal hyperdiploid mitotic figures are quite strict, demanding not only structural abnormalities but also enlargement of the mitotic figure as evidence of hyperploidy. Occasionally, mitotic figures of

normal ploidy appear multipolar due to artifact, but these are much smaller than the hyperploid mitotic figures of anaplasia; comparison with the normal-sized mitotic figures in blastema elsewhere in the tumor facilitates this determination. In NWTS 5, 11% of the patients had anaplastic histology and even the patients in stage I had dramatically poorer 4-year survival rates than those with favorable histology.[642] Lymph node dissection is recommended for patients with stage II anaplastic Wilms tumors.[647]

The effects of preoperative chemotherapy are often dramatic, and it has been suggested that these tumors be classified as completely necrotic tumors when after adequate sampling <1% of the tumor is seen to be viable. Tumors with greater proportions of viable tissue may be classified as intermediate tumors if <66% of the remaining viable tumor is blastema. Tumors are considered blastemal predominant if at least 66% of the remaining viable tumor is blastema. The last category is anaplastic tumors, and these must meet the criteria for focal or diffuse anaplasia. It is estimated that about 10% of the tumors will be completely necrotic tumors, 10% will be blastemal predominant tumors, 10% will be anaplastic tumors, and the majority will be intermediate tumors.[648]

Some genetic abnormalities have prognostic significance. Mutation of *WT1* and loss of heterozygosity at 11p15 are predictive of relapse in very low risk Wilms' tumors treated with surgery alone.[649] Loss of heterozygosity at 1p and at 16q also indicate increased risk for relapse.[650] More complex gene expression profiles also appear predictive for relapse.[651]

Both the Children's Oncology Group in the United States and the SIOP have established staging schemes for Wilms tumor and other pediatric renal malignancies (Table 2-17). The two systems are largely similar. In order to accurately stage the tumors, most sections should be taken at the periphery and selected to show the relationship between the tumor and the renal capsule, renal parenchyma, and renal sinus. Sections showing the juxtaposition of the tumor pseudocapsule and renal capsule facilitate evaluation of spread outside the kidney. The kidney is a concave organ and the renal sinus is within the contour of the kidney and its interface with the renal parenchyma is irregular and follows along the vessels. Lymph nodes containing small aggregates of metastatic Wilms tumor cells in the subcapsular sinuses that are not recognized at the original institution are a common cause for upstaging upon central pathology review.[648] Biopsy of the tumors has been recommended to discover anaplasia and guide therapy.[652] The College of American Pathologists has developed a synoptic report that is recommended for use with pediatric tumors (Table 2-18).

Cystic Partially Differentiated Nephroblastoma

Introduction

Joshi et al.[614] introduced the concept of cystic partially differentiated nephroblastoma in 1977 with a report of 3 new

Table 2-17 ■ STAGING SYSTEM FOR RENAL TUMORS OF CHILDHOOD

Stage I
  Tumor is limited to the kidney or surrounded by a fibrous capsule (pseudocapsule)
  Tumor can protrude into the renal pelvis or ureter
  Intrarenal vessel involvement can be present
Stage II
  Viable tumor penetrates into perirenal fat but not to surgical resection margin
  Viable tumor infiltrates the soft tissue of the renal sinus
  Viable tumor infiltrates blood or lymphatic channels outside of kidney but is completely resected
  Viable tumor infiltrates the renal pelvis or ureter wall
  Viable tumor infiltrates adjacent organs or vena cava but is completely resected
Stage III
  Viable or nonviable tumor extends beyond the resection margins
  Any abdominal lymph nodes are involved
  Tumor rupture before or intraoperatively (irrespective of other criteria)
  Tumor has penetrated through the peritoneal surface
  Tumor implants are present on the peritoneal surface
  Tumor thrombi are present at resection margins of vessels or ureter (or removed piecemeal by surgeon)
  Tumor has been surgically biopsied (wedge biopsy) prior to preoperative chemotherapy or surgery
Stage IV
  Hematogenous metastases (lung, liver, bone, brain, etc.) or lymph node metastases outside the abdominal–pelvic region
Stage V
  Bilateral renal tumors at diagnosis (each side substaged as above)

cases and a review of 10 cases from the literature, proposing it as a variant of Wilms' tumor curable by surgery. Additional reports followed,[615,653] and in 1989 Joshi and Beckwith[654] proposed terminology and criteria for the diagnosis that were later modified by Bonsib and Eble.[212]

Epidemiology and Clinical Features

Cystic partially differentiated nephroblastoma is rare. Only 21 patients received that diagnosis among the 5,100 patients enrolled in the National Wilms' Tumor Study from 1981 through 2000.[655] Similarly, in Europe the SIOP studies from 1993 to 2004 found only 7 cases of cystic partially differentiated nephroblastoma among 1,245 children who were enrolled.[656] In these populations, 22 of the children were boys and 6 were girls. The mean age at diagnosis in the NWTS was 15 months and in the SIOP population 11 months. In the NWTS group, the ages ranged from 5 months to 44 months and five patients were 24 months old or older. One patient had bilateral cystic partially differentiated nephroblastomas.

Pathology

Gross Features

Cystic partially differentiated nephroblastomas are well-circumscribed encapsulated tumors composed entirely of cysts of various sizes. The presence of one or more solid nodules indicates that the tumor is an extensively cystic Wilms tumor and precludes the diagnosis of cystic partially differentiated nephroblastoma. In 1990, Joshi and Beckwith[657] recognized that cystic partially differentiated nephroblastomas occasionally have papillary or nodular structures protruding into the lumens from the walls of some of the cysts and designated this as a papillonodular variant of cystic partially differentiated nephroblastoma.[657] Subsequently, another case was reported, illustrating the capability of magnetic resonance imaging to discern the papillonodular architecture preoperatively.[658]

Microscopic Features

The cysts are mostly lined by flattened, cuboidal, or hobnail epithelium. Occasionally, some of the lining epithelium may consist of immature-looking cells with dark nuclei or of cells containing mucin.[654] The septa contain variable amounts and combinations of Wilms' tumor tissues such as tubules, blunt papillae in small cysts reminiscent of glomeruli, blastema, and immature mesenchyme. Stroma with skeletal muscle or cartilaginous differentiation is occasionally seen.[659] In the papillonodular variant, the sorts of tissue seen in the septa are also found in the papillae or nodule protruding into the lumens.

Ancillary and Special Studies

Ancillary and special studies play little role in establishing the diagnosis of cystic partially differentiated nephroblastoma.

Differential Diagnosis

Cystic partially differentiated nephroblastoma grossly resembles cystic nephroma. Whether tumors with this gross appearance in which Wilms' tumor elements, such as blastema, Wilms' tumor epithelium, or stroma with skeletal muscle differentiation are not found should be considered extreme examples of cystic partially differentiated nephroblastoma or diagnosed as cystic nephroma is unclear and controversial. A review of the literature shows that patients with tumors considered to be cystic nephroma in children had a predominance of boys, while adult patients with cystic nephroma are mainly women, so if a second type of tumor with this gross appearance arises in children it is a different tumor than what is diagnosed as cystic nephroma in adults.[660] Since the elements typical of Wilms tumor may be inconspicuous, cystic renal tumors in children should be sampled extensively before cystic partially differentiated nephroblastoma is excluded. A weakness of studies based upon specimens referred to a central laboratory[654] is variable and sometimes inadequate sampling performed at the referring institutions.

Cystic Wilms tumors may grossly and radiographically resemble cystic partially differentiated nephroblastoma. Thorough dissection of the specimen, looking for expansile

Table 2-18 ■ COLLEGE OF AMERICAN PATHOLOGISTS RECOMMENDED CANCER CASE SUMMARY FOR PEDIATRIC RENAL TUMORS (2012)

Procedure

___ Partial nephrectomy
___ Radical nephrectomy
___ Bilateral partial nephrectomies
___ Other (specify): _____
___ Not specified

Specimen Size

Kidney dimensions: ___ x ___ x ___ cm
Weight: ___ g

Specimen Laterality

___ Right
___ Left
___ Not specified

+Tumor Site(s) (select all that apply)

+___ Upper pole
+___ Middle
+___ Lower pole
+___ Other (specify): _____
+___ Not specified

Tumor Size

Greatest dimension: ___ cm
+Additional dimensions: ___ x ___ cm
___ Cannot be determined (provide Comment)
For specimens with multiple tumors, specify greatest
  dimension of each additional tumor
Greatest dimension tumor #2: ___ cm Etc.

Tumor Focality

___ Unifocal
___ Multifocal
Number of tumors in specimens (specify): _____
___ Indeterminate
___ Cannot be assessed

Macroscopic Extent of Tumor

Gerota fascia
___ Gerota fascia intact
___ Gerota fascia disrupted
___ Indeterminate
___ Cannot be assessed
Renal Sinus
___ Renal sinus involvement by tumor not identified
___ Tumor minimally extends into renal sinus soft
  tissue
___ Tumor extensively involves renal sinus soft
  tissue
___ Tumor involves lymph–vascular spaces in the renal
  sinus
Renal Vein
___ Renal vein invasion present
___ Renal vein invasion not identified
___ Indeterminate
___ Cannot be assessed

Adjacent Organ Involvement
___ Tumor extension into adjacent organ present (specify
  organ): _____
___ Tumor extension into adjacent organ not identified

Histologic type (select all that apply)

___ Wilms' tumor, favorable histology
___ Wilms' tumor, focal anaplasia
___ Wilms' tumor, diffuse anaplasia
___ Congenital mesoblastic nephroma, classical
___ Congenital mesoblastic nephroma, cellular
___ Congenital mesoblastic nephroma, mixed
___ Clear cell sarcoma
___ Rhabdoid tumor
___ Other (specify): _____
___ Malignant neoplasm, type indeterminate

+Nephrogenic Rests (select all that apply)

+___ Nephrogenic rests not identified
+___ Nephrogenic rests present
    +___ Nephrogenic rests, intralobar
    +___ Nephrogenic rests, perilobar
        +___ Diffuse, hyperplastic
        +___ Multifocal
        +___ Focal
    +___ Nephrogenic rests, unclassified
+___ Cannot be assessed

Margins (select all that apply)

___ Cannot be assessed
___ Margin involvement by tumor not identified
  Distance of tumor from closest margin: ___ mm or ___ cm
  Specify margin: _____
___ Margin(s) involved by tumor
    ___ Gerota fascia
    ___ Renal vein
    ___ Inferior vena cava
    ___ Ureter
    ___ Other (specify): _____

Lymph Nodes

___ Regional lymph node metastasis not identified
___ Regional lymph node metastasis present (specify site, if
  known): _____
___ No nodes submitted or found
Number of lymph nodes examined
Specify: ___
___ Number of lymph nodes cannot be determined
  (explain): _____
Number of lymph nodes involved
Specify: ___
___ Number cannot be determined (explain): _____

Distant Metastasis

___ Not applicable
___ Distant metastasis present
  +Specify site(s) if known: _____

Stage—see Table 2.17
+ Data elements preceded by this symbol are not required. However, these elements may be clinically important but are not yet validated or regularly used in patient management.
Reproduced from Hill DA, Amin MB, Bowen J, et al. Protocol for the examination of specimens from pediatric patients with Wilms tumors. In: Washington K, ed. *Reporting on Cancer Specimens. Case Summaries and Background Documentation.* Northfield, IL: College of American Pathologists; 2012, with permission.

solid nodules, must be performed and none found, before a diagnosis of cystic partially differentiated nephroblastoma can be made.

Prognosis and Treatment

Cystic partially differentiated nephroblastoma is almost always cured by nephrectomy or partial nephrectomy.[656,661] Recurrence has been reported in less than a handful of cases.[654,662] For stage I patients, chemotherapy may do more harm than good and the role of chemotherapy in the treatment of patients with cystic partially differentiated nephroblastoma is very limited.[648,655]

MESENCHYMAL TUMORS—OCCURRING MAINLY IN CHILDREN

Congenital Mesoblastic Nephroma

Introduction

Congenital mesoblastic nephroma is a mesenchymal neoplasm that occurs in infants and accounts for approximately 3% to 4% of renal tumors of childhood.[663] While these tumors were first recognized in 1966[664] and have been described under several names, the terminology "congenital mesoblastic nephroma" that was coined by Bolande[665] in 1967 is now standard. Based upon morphology and genetics, congenital mesoblastic nephromas are classified as classic, cellular, or, occasionally, mixed. The classic type makes up about 30% of cases, the cellular type about 50%, and a mixture of the two in about 20%.

Epidemiology and Clinical Features

Although comprising <3% of primary renal tumors in children, mesoblastic nephroma is the predominant renal neoplasm in the first 3 months of life, and is uncommon after 6 months.[594,666] The median age at presentation is 2 months or less.[663] That a tumor is present is recognized before birth in more than 10% of cases.[663] Only 10% of cases are diagnosed in the 2nd year and in patients older than 24 months, the diagnosis should be regarded with suspicion. Polyhydramnios and prematurity are associated with this tumor.[667,668] An abdominal mass is almost always the presenting finding, and with the widespread use of prenatal ultrasonography, the tumors are frequently recognized before birth. A few congenital mesoblastic nephromas have been reported in patients with Beckwith-Wiedemann syndrome. Some patients have been hypercalcemic, and this has been attributed to paraneoplastic production of prostaglandin E. Hyper-reninism, apparently caused by secretion by juxtaglomerular cells entrapped within the tumor, is fairly common.

Pathology

Gross Features

Congenital mesoblastic nephroma is usually large relative to the infant's kidney. Prenatal ultrasonographic examinations

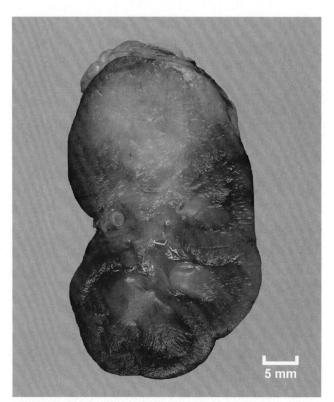

FIGURE 2-93 ■ Congenital mesoblastic nephroma. At its periphery, this solid off-white fleshy tumor infiltrates the renal parenchyma.

have revealed some smaller ones. Externally, the surface of the tumor and kidney is smooth, and the renal capsule and calyceal systems are stretched over the tumor. The surface may be bosselated. The cut surface resembles that of a leiomyoma: firm, whorled or trabeculated, and light colored (Fig. 2-93).[669] Renal vein invasion also occurs occasionally.[669] Cysts, hemorrhage, and necrosis are present in some tumors, particularly those that are cellular on microscopic examination.[669] The tumor is unencapsulated, typically interdigitates with the surrounding kidney, and may extend into surrounding tissues, particularly in the renal sinus. The medial margin of the nephrectomy specimen must be carefully examined to establish that it is free of neoplasm.

Microscopic Features

The classical pattern of congenital mesoblastic nephroma described by Bolande[670] is a moderately cellular proliferation of thick interlacing bundles of spindle cells with elongate nuclei that usually infiltrate renal and perirenal tissues (Fig. 2-94). Entrapment of glomeruli and renal tubules is common. The spindle cells resemble smooth muscle cells or myofibroblasts (Fig. 2-95). Mitotic figures are usually in the range of 0 to 1 per 10 high power fields.[669] Islands of cartilage and foci of extramedullary hematopoiesis are present in some tumors.

Cellular congenital mesoblastic nephroma was recognized later.[671] It consists of a densely cellular proliferation of polygonal cells (Fig. 2-96) with mitotic figures in the range of 8 to 30 per 10 high power fields, and often pushing borders.

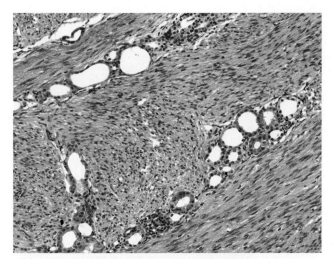

FIGURE 2-94 ■ Congenital mesoblastic nephroma. The classic form is highly infiltrative and entraps tubules and glomeruli.

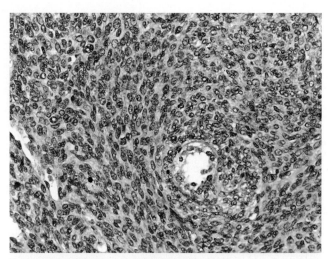

FIGURE 2-96 ■ Congenital mesoblastic nephroma. The cellular form consists of short spindle cells which are densely packed. A few mitotic figures are visible.

Moderate nuclear pleomorphism may be present. Cysts are common in this pattern. Prominent nucleoli and foci of necrosis may be present. Mixed congenital mesoblastic nephromas usually are composed of nodules of cellular congenital mesoblastic nephroma arising within sheets of classic congenital mesoblastic nephroma. This appearance suggests that cellular congenital mesoblastic nephroma might sometimes arise from classic congenital mesoblastic nephroma.

Ancillary and Special Studies

Both classic and cellular types give positive immunohistochemical reactions for vimentin, desmin, actin, and fibronectin. They are typically unreactive with antibodies to laminin, cytokeratins, and S-100 protein. Positive reactions with antibodies to WT1 have been reported but this appears at best to be an inconsistent finding. Nestin can be detected in almost all congenital mesoblastic nephromas.[672]

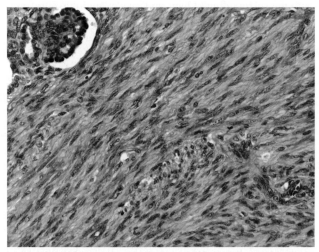

FIGURE 2-95 ■ Congenital mesoblastic nephroma. The tumor consists of elongate spindle cells resembling smooth muscle cells or myofibroblasts.

Genetics

Cellular congenital mesoblastic nephromas typically have a translocation [t(12;15)(p13;q25)] that results in the fusion of the gene *ets variant 6* (HUGO-approved gene symbol *ETV6*) on chromosome 12p13 with the gene *neurotrophic tyrosine kinase, receptor, type 3* (HUGO-approved gene symbol *NTRK3*) on chromosome 15q24-q25.[673–675] This mutation is also found in infantile fibrosarcoma arising in other parts of the body, and cellular congenital mesoblastic nephroma and infantile fibrosarcoma are very similar in histologic appearance. Classic congenital mesoblastic nephromas lack this gene fusion, as does infantile fibromatosis, which they closely resemble. For classic congenital mesoblastic nephroma, no consistent genetic abnormalities have been discovered.[676] Detection of the gene fusion in paraffin-embedded tissue is possible and can be of diagnostic assistance.[677] Gene expression profiling shows promise for aiding in the diagnosis of congenital mesoblastic nephroma.[625]

The few examples of "mixed" congenital mesoblastic nephroma that have been tested have been found to contain the fusion.[674,675]

Differential Diagnosis

Congenital mesoblastic nephroma usually is easily diagnosed when the histology and patient age are considered. Wilms tumor with stromal predominance may be confused with congenital mesoblastic nephroma, particularly Wilms tumor, which has been treated preoperatively and contains much spindle cell stroma. This problem can usually be resolved by the identification of blastema, which is not found in mesoblastic nephroma. Skeletal muscle differentiation is not found in congenital mesoblastic nephroma. Also, Wilms tumor usually has sharply circumscribed borders, whereas those of mesoblastic nephroma often are infiltrative. Age assists in making the correct diagnosis, and bilaterality favors Wilms tumor.

The differential diagnosis with clear cell sarcoma is important. Some laboratory findings (hypercalcemia, hyperreninism) weigh in favor of congenital mesoblastic nephroma, while the detection of metastases (particularly to bone) weighs in favor of clear cell sarcoma. Microscopically, the presence of cartilage is evidence in favor of congenital mesoblastic nephroma, while the presence of any of the variant patterns recognized in clear cell sarcoma weighs against congenital mesoblastic nephroma. A high mitotic rate weighs in favor of congenital mesoblastic nephroma, as does the presence of extensive infiltration at the periphery of the tumor. Extensive sclerosis weighs in favor of clear cell sarcoma. Immunohistochemically, a positive reaction for actin or desmin is evidence for congenital mesoblastic nephroma.

Although both occur in the same age group, congenital mesoblastic nephroma, even the cellular variant, and rhabdoid tumor are usually easily distinguished. In cases of congenital mesoblastic nephroma with exceptionally prominent nucleoli, immunohistochemistry for actin is expected to be positive, while rhabdoid tumors may react positively with antibodies to cytokeratins and epithelial membrane antigen.

Prognosis and Treatment

The vast majority of patients are cured by surgical resection, with 5-year overall survival of approximately 95%.[585,678–680] Local recurrences or metastases, or both, have occurred in approximately 7% of cases, principally in patients older than 3 months at presentation.[681,682] Mesoblastic nephroma has infiltrative borders, which the surgical pathologist must study carefully because the risk of recurrence appears to be dependent upon the completeness of the resection.[683,684] Metastasis is rare.[685] The principal risk factors for recurrence or metastasis appear to be cellular morphology, stage III (NWTS staging system) or greater, and vascular invasion.[686]

Clear Cell Sarcoma of Kidney

Epidemiology and Clinical Features

Originally called "bone-metastasizing renal tumor of childhood" by Marsden and Lawler,[687] clear cell sarcoma[688] is a highly malignant neoplasm resistant to conventional therapy for Wilms' tumor, but often responsive to doxorubicin-containing regimens. Thus, it is of considerable therapeutic importance that clear cell sarcoma be correctly diagnosed.

Occurring in the same general age range as Wilms tumor, clear cell sarcoma constitutes approximately 6% of pediatric renal tumors.[689] Most are diagnosed in patients between 12 and 36 months of age.[690] Approximately 66% of the patients are male. In a review of 351 cases from the NWTS, only one clear cell sarcoma was associated with a perilobar nephrogenic rest and none was associated with an intralobar nephrogenic rest.[690] No association with developmental syndromes nor any familial predisposition has been discovered. The propensity for metastasis to bone is marked; it is at least ten times more likely to metastasize to bone than other pediatric renal cancers.

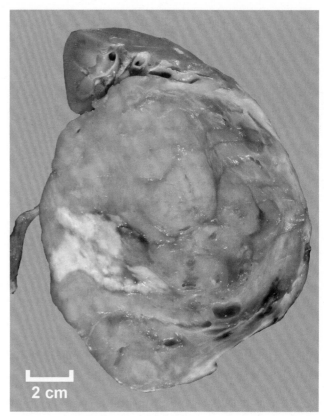

FIGURE 2-97 ■ Clear cell sarcoma of kidney. The tumor is unifocal and contains a few cysts and an area of necrosis.

Pathology

Gross Features

The appearance of the cut surfaces of this tumor is variable: it may be homogeneous, gray and lobular or variegated, including firm gray whorled tissue and light pink soft areas (Fig. 2-97).[691] Cysts ranging from a few millimeters to centimeters in diameter are present in nearly all tumors and may be so extensive as to bring cystic nephroma to mind.[690] Foci of necrosis and hemorrhage are present in more than 70% of tumors.[690] Often, the tumor weighs more than 500 g.[691] Bilaterality has not been reported.[690]

Microscopic Features

At low magnification, clear cell sarcoma of kidney usually consists of a monotonous sheet of cells with lightly staining cytoplasm. At higher magnification, it is apparent that the cells are arranged in cords separated by septa composed of spindle cells with dark nuclei and a distinctive branching pattern of small blood vessels (Fig. 2-98).[692] The cells in the cords have pale or vacuolated cytoplasm and indistinct borders. Despite the name, the cytoplasm of clear cell sarcoma is usually much less clear than that of clear cell renal cell carcinoma and cytoplasmic clarity should not be relied upon to establish the diagnosis. The nuclei contain finely dispersed chromatin and the nucleoli are small. These nuclear characteristics are helpful in distinguishing clear cell sarcoma from rhabdoid tumor. A characteristic feature is the

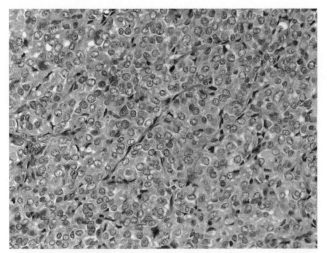

FIGURE 2-98 ■ Clear cell sarcoma of kidney. The tumor consists of cord cells with pale cytoplasm and nuclei with open chromatin and inconspicuous nucleoli and septal cells that are spindle shaped and have darkly basophilic nuclei. The septal cells form a network about the cord cells.

infiltrative border between the clear cell sarcoma and the surrounding renal parenchyma; renal tubules are frequently seen surrounded by the sarcoma.[691] While more than 90% of tumors are composed either predominantly or secondarily of the classical pattern described above, a majority also contain one or more variant patterns.[690,693] These confusing variations on the classical appearance include myxoid pattern, which is present in 50% of tumors (Fig. 2-99), sclerosing pattern (present in 35% of tumors), cellular pattern (present in 25% of tumors), palisading pattern (present in 11% of tumors), spindle cell pattern (present in 7% of tumors), storiform pattern (present in 4% of tumors), and anaplastic pattern (present in 3% of tumors).[690] The tumor should be sampled generously to find areas in which the septal vascular pattern and finely dispersed chromatin and small nucleoli in the nuclei of the cord cells indicate the correct diagnosis.

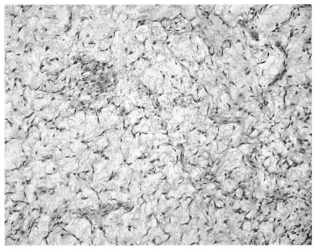

FIGURE 2-99 ■ Clear cell sarcoma of kidney. In this myxoid variant, the characteristic architecture of cords and septa is obscured.

Ancillary and Special Studies

Clear cell sarcomas react immunohistochemically with few antibodies. Reactions for vimentin can be elicited in essentially all tumors. Weak staining for actin is found in less than half of tumors but desmin is not detectable. Markers for epithelial differentiation (AE1/3, CAM 5.2, epithelial membrane antigen) are not detectable. Results with antibodies to S100 protein, synaptophysin, glial fibrillary acidic protein, leukocyte-common antigen, neuron-specific enolase, carcinoembryonic antigen, CD34, and factor 8 were negative.[690]

Genetics

The genetics of clear cell sarcoma of the kidney include translocation (10;17) and deletions in 14q.[694] The translocation (10;17) results in rearrangement of *YWHAE* on chromosome 17 and *FAM22* on chromosome 10 and fusing the two genes.[695,696] Gene expression profile studies indicate that genes for neural markers, in the Sonic hedgehog pathway and in the phosphoinositide-3-kinase/AKT pathway, are likely to be important in the development of clear cell sarcoma of kidney.[697]

Differential Diagnosis

In distinguishing clear cell sarcoma of kidney from Wilms tumor, some pertinent negatives are important: blastema is not found in clear cell sarcoma; nonrenal elements such as cartilage or muscle are not found in clear cell sarcoma; clear cell sarcoma is unilateral and unicentric, and sclerotic stroma is uncommon in Wilms tumor before therapy. The distinctive vascular pattern of clear cell sarcoma is often helpful in distinguishing it from Wilms tumor. The border with the kidney is usually infiltrative while the border of Wilms tumor is typically "pushing." Exceptionally, clear cell sarcoma of kidney may contain foci in which the cells have prominent nucleoli, similar to those of rhabdoid tumor of kidney; other areas with patterns typical of clear cell sarcoma usually will clarify the diagnosis.

Prognosis and Treatment

The most important factors for survival are treatment with doxorubicin, stage (NWTS 5 definitions), age at presentation, and tumor necrosis, but tumor necrosis was not significant when relapse-free survival was the end point.[690] Today, the overall survival rate for stage 1 patients is close to 100%.[698]

By far the most common site of metastases at presentation is to lymph nodes (present in almost 30% of cases), while the most common sites of recurrence are bone, lung, abdominal and retroperitoneal spaces, and brain.[690,699] Twenty percent or more of metastases appear 3 years or more after original presentation and some as long as 10 years later.

Rhabdoid Tumor of Kidney

Epidemiology and Clinical Features

Rhabdoid tumor of the kidney was first recognized by Beckwith and Palmer in 1978, when it was considered a possible rhabdomyosarcoma-like manifestation of Wilms tumor.[688] Shortly thereafter, it was recognized as an entity independent of Wilms tumor, and the name "rhabdoid tumor of the kidney" was applied.[700]

Patients with rhabdoid tumors of the kidney made up only 1.5% of 9,232 patients with renal tumors registered in the National Wilms Tumor Study between 1969 and 2002.[701] The patients usually are very young at the time of diagnosis (NWTS median age 11 months and SIOP median age 13 months) and rare after 3 years.[701,702] The oldest patient with rhabdoid tumor of kidney reported by the NWTS and SIOP was 9 years old.[701,702] There is a 1.4:1 predominance of boys over girls.[701] Associations with atypical teratoid/rhabdoid tumors of the central nervous system[703] in 10% to 15% of patients and paraneoplastic hypercalcemia[704,705] are recognized.

Pathology

Gross Features

Rhabdoid tumor lacks the appearance of encapsulation often seen in cases of Wilms tumor or clear cell sarcoma. The tumors usually are located medially in the kidney, and the renal sinus and pelvis are almost always infiltrated.[706] They are typically yellow-gray or light tan easily fragmented tumors with indistinct borders (Fig. 2-100). Necrosis and hemorrhage are common.

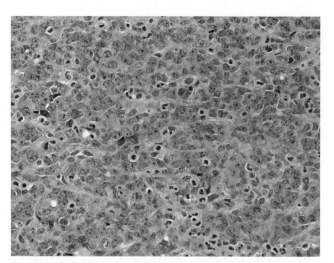

Figure 2-101 ■ Rhabdoid tumor of kidney. The tumor grows as infiltrative sheets of undifferentiated malignant cells with prominent nucleoli.

Microscopic Features

Rhabdoid tumor of kidney is typically diffuse and monotonous, consisting of medium or large polygonal cells with abundant eosinophilic cytoplasm and round nuclei with thick nuclear membranes and large nucleoli (Fig. 2-101). It is the resemblance of the cytoplasm of these cells to differentiating rhabdomyoblasts that gave the tumor its name (Fig. 2-102).[688] However, the resemblance to skeletal muscle is merely superficial, and if definite evidence of differentiation toward skeletal muscle is present, the tumor is not a rhabdoid tumor. Often, the cytoplasm contains a large eosinophilic globular inclusion that displaces the nucleus. Electron microscopy has shown that these consist of aggregates of whorled filaments.[707] As more cases have accrued to the NWTS, a wide range of patterns has been appreciated, including sclerosing, epithelioid, spindle cell, lymphomatoid, vascular, pseudopapillary, and cystic.[706] Typically, these patterns are mixed with

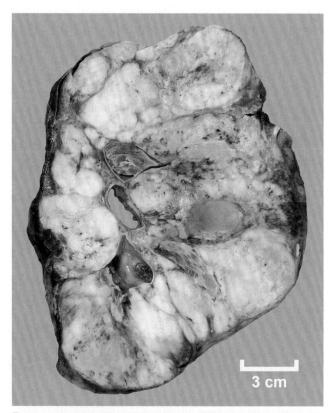

Figure 2-100 ■ Rhabdoid tumor of kidney. This bulky multilobular tumor has replaced the kidney except for part of the collecting system and shows foci of hemorrhage and necrosis.

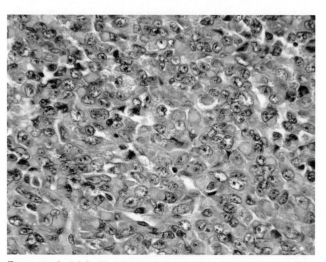

Figure 2-102 ■ Rhabdoid tumor of kidney. The eosinophilic globules that displace the nuclei bring rhabdomyoblasts to mind and are the reason for the name of this tumor.

the common pattern and with each other. The characteristic nuclear features of large centrally placed nucleoli and thick nuclear membranes are usually retained.

Ancillary and Special Studies

Immunohistochemistry shows a negative reaction for SMARCB1/INI1 in 98% or more of rhabdoid tumors.[708] Expression of epithelial, neural, and mesenchymal markers, including cytokeratins and epithelial membrane antigen, S100 protein, neuron-specific enolase, synaptophysin, glial fibrillary acidic protein, vimentin, smooth muscle–specific actin, desmin, and CD99 have been reported.[708,709]

Genetics

Rhabdoid tumor of kidney has, in common with rhabdoid tumors at other sites, mutation or deletion of the gene *SWI/SNF-related, matrix-associated, actin-dependent regulator of chromatin, subfamily b, member 1* (HUGO-approved gene symbol *SMARCB1*).[710] This gene has also been called *INI1* and *SNF5*. *SMARCB1* codes for a protein with a role in transcriptional regulation. Further genetic studies have identified additional genes that are mutated in rhabdoid tumor of the kidney.[711] The rhabdoid tumor predisposition syndrome is a familial transmission of mutations in *SMARCB1*, which leads to the development of rhabdoid tumor of kidney, atypical teratoid/rhabdoid tumor, choroid plexus carcinoma, medulloblastoma, and extrarenal rhabdoid tumor.[712,713] Rhabdoid tumors of the kidney often express a variety of stem cell factors, such as glypican3 and SALL4.[714,715]

Differential Diagnosis

A wide variety of renal and extrarenal tumors may mimic rhabdoid tumor in routine sections. The NWTS has been receiving cases of Wilms tumor, congenital mesoblastic nephroma, renal cell carcinoma, urothelial carcinoma, collecting duct carcinoma, oncocytoma, rhabdomyosarcoma, neuroendocrine carcinoma, and lymphoma that have been confused with rhabdoid tumor of kidney.[716] Filamentous cytoplasmic inclusions or conspicuous macronucleoli are the misleading features in most cases. Conventional light microscopy is able to clarify most cases, but electron microscopy and immunohistochemistry are sometimes necessary to show the characteristic features of the mimics and exclude rhabdoid tumor. Occasionally, blastemal cells contain inclusions suggestive of rhabdoid tumor, but the presence of characteristic aggregates of blastema, such as nodules or serpentine groupings, clarifies the diagnosis. Immunohistochemistry for SMARCB1 (INI1) was found to be negative in 100% of 44 rhabdoid tumors (29 renal) and positive in 100% of 45 varied soft tissue tumors in children, correlating with the mutation or deletion of *SMARCB1* that is typical of rhabdoid tumors.[717,718]

Prognosis and Treatment

Rhabdoid tumor of the kidney is a highly aggressive cancer that presents with advanced stage in two-thirds or more of cases and has a 5-year survival of approximately 25% in the largest series.[701,702,719] Age at diagnosis is a significant prognostic factor with younger children doing worse than ones older than 2 years.[701] High stage at presentation and the presence of an atypical teratoid–rhabdoid tumor of the central nervous system also diminish the outlook

Ossifying Renal Tumor of Infancy

Epidemiology and Clinical Features

Ossifying renal tumor of infancy was first recognized by Caillet, Massot, and Taillard in 1966.[720] Up to the present, 19 cases have been reported.[721–733]

This rare tumor of uncertain histogenesis has been reported only in 13 boys and 4 girls, and hematuria has been the presenting symptom in all but 2 cases. Radiography often reveals a calcified mass in the renal collecting system or pelvis, and these tumors have been mistaken clinically for staghorn calculi. All of the tumors were resected, and no case of recurrence or of metastasis has been reported.

Pathology

Gross Features

Grossly, the tumor typically projects into the lumen of the renal pelvis. Some are densely calcified and very hard. The margins with the underlying medullary tissue are ill defined.

Microscopic Features

Microscopically, the bulk of the tumor often consists of an osteoid core associated with variable numbers of osteoblasts. In older patients, these cores often appear more mature with increased calcification and decreased numbers of osteoblasts. The osteoblasts blend into a population of round to oval cells and spindle cells. The spindle cell elements resemble intralobar nephrogenic rests. Immunohistochemistry and electron microscopy disclose cells with epithelial differentiation among these.[725] Mitotic figures are uncommon. Osteoclasts and cartilaginous tissues are absent.

Differential Diagnosis

The principal differential diagnostic consideration preoperatively often is a calculus. Congenital mesoblastic nephroma rarely may exhibit ossification.[734] Sotelo-Avila et al.[725] were struck by the resemblance to intralobar nephrogenic rests, while Seixas-Mikelus and colleagues were impressed by the resemblance of the spindle cell areas to congenital mesoblastic nephroma. The relationship of ossifying renal tumor infancy to other renal neoplasms remains obscure.

Prognosis and Treatment

In the few cases that have been reported, neither recurrence nor metastasis has been identified, so it appears that complete resection is curative and nephron-sparing surgical procedures can be used.[730]

Anaplastic Sarcoma of the Kidney

Anaplastic sarcoma of the kidney has been described from a series of 20 cases collected through the NWTS, the SIOP, and the United Kingdom Children's Cancer Study Group.[735] The patients ranged in age from 10 months to 41 years (median = 5 years) and there was a slight female predominance. Grossly, anaplastic sarcomas are solid tumors, about 50% with a cystic component and are frequently large at diagnosis, ranging from 4 to 21 cm in maximum extent, with a median of 13 cm.

Histologically, these tumors are characterized by the presence of spindle cells growing in fascicles and round or oval mesenchymal cells with a myxoid stroma. Cartilaginous differentiation was present in 75% of the tumors. Pleomorphic giant cells, rhabdomyoblast-like cells, and dystrophic calcification may also be present. A few of the tumors contained areas composed of small blastema-like cells. A third of the tumors contained epithelium-lined cysts. The immunohistochemical investigation was limited; however, reactions with antibodies to desmin and vimentin were usually positive while reactions with antibodies to WT1, CD34, CD56, CD99, and CAM 5.2 were negative in almost all of the tumors. Genetic investigations have been limited and have failed to detect either the *SYT1-SSX* or *ETV6-NTRK3* fusion transcripts. Cytogenetic analysis of a single tumor detected cytogenetic abnormalities of unclear significance.[736]

Follow-up details for these tumors are limited. Half of the patients showed extrarenal extension or metastases at diagnosis. Following nephrectomy and postoperative adjunct chemotherapy, 10 patients were free of disease, while 3 patients had died of tumor after follow-up intervals of 1.5 to 14 years.

MESENCHYMAL TUMORS—OCCURRING MAINLY IN ADULTS

Renomedullary Interstitial Cell Tumor

Epidemiology and Clinical Features

Renomedullary interstitial cell tumor originates from renomedullary interstitial cells. These cells contain vasoactive substances such as prostaglandins, important in the regulation of blood pressure. It is uncertain if these are true neoplasms, and it has been suggested that they are hyperplastic nodules that develop in response to hypertension. In contradiction of this, no convincing correlation has been demonstrated between hypertension, cardiac weight, and the incidence of these tumors in autopsy studies.[737,738]

These tumors are commonly found in adults, and in a large autopsy series 50% of patients had at least one tumor, while 57% of patients with renomedullary interstitial cell tumors had multiple lesions. These tumors are rarely seen in childhood and there is slight female predominance.[14,739] While most are found at autopsy or as incidental findings in nephrectomy specimens removed for cancers, they occasionally are found in needle biopsies.[740]

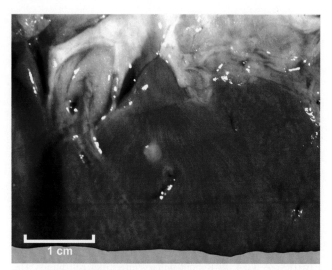

FIGURE 2-103 ■ Renomedullary interstitial cell tumor forms a small white nodule within a medullary pyramid.

Most renomedullary cell tumors are asymptomatic and remain undetected during life; however, if carefully searched for, these tumors are frequently seen in nephrectomy specimens. Rarely renomedullary tumors are symptomatic, with flank pain originating from obstruction of renal outflow.[741]

Pathology

Gross Features

The tumors are white well-circumscribed nodules within the renal medulla and are usually <0.5 cm in diameter (Fig. 2-103). Occasionally, renomedullary interstitial cell tumors are pedunculated, protruding into the lumen of the renal pelvis, and it is these forms that may result in urinary tract obstruction.[741,742]

Microscopic Features

Renomedullary interstitial cell tumors consist of small stellate cells within a loose faintly basophilic stroma (Fig. 2-104).[738,741] The stroma often has an interlacing pattern and may entrap medullary tubules at the edge of the lesion. Sections stained with Masson trichrome stain usually show little collagen within the lesions. In a minority of tumors, irregularly shaped densely eosinophilic deposits are present that resemble amyloid (Fig. 2-105).[744]

Ancillary and Special Studies

One immunohistochemical study found α-smooth muscle actin and CD35 in many of the spindle cells.[742] Electron microscopy confirms medullary interstitial cells to be the cell of origin for these tumors with the presence of cytoplasmic electron-dense lipid droplets.[738]

Differential Diagnosis

Renomedullary interstitial cell tumors have been described as fibromas on morphologic grounds; however, they are collagen poor.

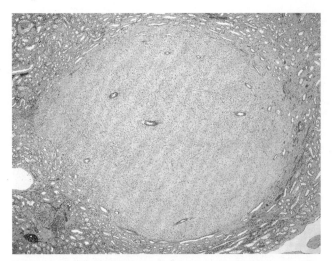

FIGURE 2-104 ■ Renomedullary interstitial cell tumor. The tumor is moderately to sparsely cellular and composed of bland spindle cells. A few medullary tubules are embedded within it.

Prognosis and Treatment

These are benign tumors. The rare pedunculated tumors that occasionally cause outflow obstruction may require surgical intervention.[744]

Juxtaglomerular Cell Tumor

Epidemiology and Clinical Features

A renin-secreting renal tumor was first reported in 1967,[745] and in 1968, the term juxtaglomerular cell tumor was coined.[746] It is now recognized that these tumors are derived from the smooth muscle cell of the glomerular afferent arteriole.[747]

Fewer than 100 cases have been reported and most patients have been young adults and adolescents, averaging 27 years of age.[748,749] Many of the patients at the time of resection have been hypertensive for years before surgery with the average age of onset of hypertension being 22 years. The tumor is found predominantly in females, with a female-to-male ratio of 2:1.

Virtually all patients with juxtaglomerular cell tumors are hypertensive, although a single case of a normotensive patient has been reported.[750] In one series, seven tumors were detected in 30,000 newly diagnosed hypertensive patients.[751] Elevation of plasma renin is typical of these patients, and selective catheterization of the renal veins has been advocated as an important guide to treatment.[752] In some patients, the clinical features of uncontrolled severe hypertension may be seen.[753]

Pathology

Gross Features

Most lesions have been smaller than 3 cm at diagnosis and some have not been visible when the renal capsule was stripped. For this reason, when a juxtaglomerular cell tumor is suspected, the specimen must be carefully dissected and all abnormal foci submitted for microscopic examination. These tumors are sharply circumscribed and composed of rubbery white or gray tissue with a capsule of variable thickness. Occasionally, tumors contain small cyst-like smooth-walled cavities or areas of hemorrhage.[754]

Microscopic Features

Juxtaglomerular cell tumors show variable histologic patterns. A common pattern is one of irregular trabeculae of polygonal cells in a loose myxoid stroma (Fig. 2-106). Tubules and cysts are often present. Sheets of tumor cells and papillary structures may also be seen (Figs. 2-107 and 2-108).[755,756] Tumor cells are amphophilic and may show a mild degree of nuclear pleomorphism. There is frequently prominent vascularity, and a lymphocytic infiltrate and mast cells may be conspicuous. Vascular invasion has been reported.[753,757]

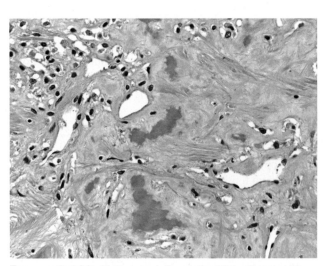

FIGURE 2-105 ■ Renomedullary interstitial cell tumor. These lesions occasionally contain deposits resembling amyloid.

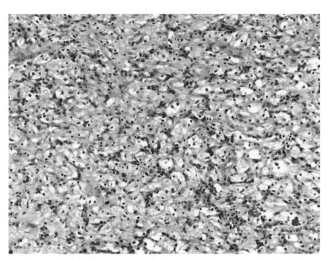

FIGURE 2-106 ■ Juxtaglomerular cell tumor. A complex vascular network invests cells with pale or clear cytoplasm and centrally located small darkly staining nuclei.

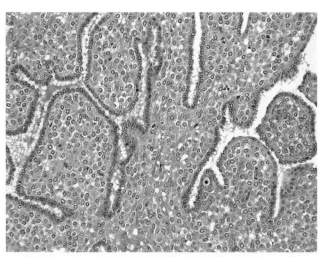

FIGURE 2-107 ■ Juxtaglomerular cell tumor. Sheets of polygonal epithelioid cells surround complex channels lined by epithelial cells that have evolved from entrapped renal tubules.

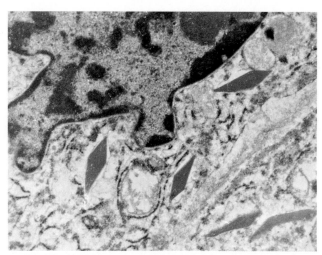

FIGURE 2-109 ■ Juxtaglomerular cell tumor. Electron microscopy shows intracytoplasmic rhomboid renin granules.

Ancillary and Special Studies

Modified Bowie stain may reveal intracytoplasmic granules. Immunohistochemistry for renin shows a positive reaction in the cytoplasm. Tumor cells are also positive for vimentin, actin, calponin, CD34, and CD117, and are negative for cytokeratins.[754–756]

Electron microscopy is helpful in demonstrating typical globular and rhomboid granules (Fig. 2-109) and smooth muscle myofilaments of juxtaglomerular cell tumors.[758] Expression of angiotensin II type 1 receptor has been detected in these tumors.[759] In other studies tumor cells have been shown to exhibit monosomy of chromosomes 6, 9, 11, 15, 21, and X on FISH, gains of chromosome 10.[747,760] Losses of chromosomes 9 and 11 are the genetic abnormalities that have been observed most frequently.

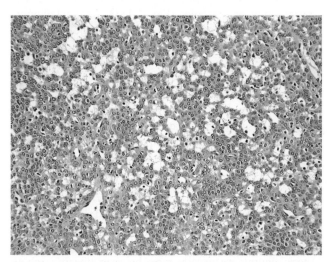

FIGURE 2-108 ■ Juxtaglomerular cell tumor. Sheets of polygonal epithelioid cells are punctuated by small spaces filled with edema fluid.

Differential Diagnosis

The association of the tumor with severe hypertension, especially in younger patients means that the nature of the tumor is often suspected preoperatively. The gross finding of a small pale-colored rubbery tumor narrows the differential diagnosis, and the histologic appearance is distinctive. The presence of renin also differentiates these tumors from renal solitary fibrous tumors. Although renin has rarely been found in renal cell carcinoma and nephroblastoma, these rarely cause diagnostic confusion.[761,762]

Prognosis and Treatment

Virtually all juxtaglomerular cell tumors appear to have been cured by resection although the reported follow-up has often been short. A single case of juxtaglomerular cell tumor metastasizing to the lung 6 years postnephrectomy has been reported.[755]

Angiomyolipoma

Introduction

Angiomyolipoma is a benign neoplasm that consists of varying proportions of smooth muscle cells, mature adipose tissue, and atypical thick-walled vessels. The existence of these tumors has been recognized for more than a century with the term angiomyolipoma being used by Paul Grawitz in 1900.[763] In early studies, angiomyolipoma was classified as a hamartoma and was noted to occur both sporadically and as part of the tuberous sclerosis complex.[764] The observation that angiomyolipomas have nonrandom inactivation of the X chromosome led to the conclusion that these tumors were clonal and neoplastic in origin.[765]

The observations that angiomyolipomas contained cells that showed positive expression of the melanoma-marker

HMB-45 and that cells showing similar features were present in clear cell tumor of the lung (sugar tumor) led to the suggestion that these tumors were related. In these tumors the HMB-45 positive cells were all shown to have a characteristic appearance, being epithelioid with a clear to acidophilic cytoplasm and a perivascular distribution.[766] It was subsequently shown that these tumors stained positively for other melanoma markers and on electron microscopy contained electron dense granules, resembling melanosomes.[767] Similar features were found in hepatic angiomyolipomas,[768] and it was suggested that all these tumors were derived from perivascular epithelioid cells that can differentiate to form fat and smooth muscle cells, as well as eosinophilic and clear epithelioid cells.[769,770] This family of tumors has now been expanded to include not only lymphangiomyomatosis, which is itself associated with renal angiomyolipoma, but also a wide variety of soft tissue, abdominal, gynecologic, subcutaneous, and bone tumors.[771]

Epidemiology

Angiomyolipomas are common; 24 cases were detected in 18,000 clinically normal individuals undergoing routine health screening in Japan[772] and 9 were found in 10,000 volunteers in Germany.[773] In both of these studies, angiomyolipomas were as numerous as renal cell carcinomas. In a series of 3,512 autopsies, 4% of the 108 renal tumors present were angiomyolipomas.[774] Pain is the presenting symptom in 50% of cases, hematuria in about 25%, and the tumor is an incidental finding in about 25%.[775]

In an unselected series of 194 cases of angiomyolipoma, 8% of tumors were found in patients with tuberous sclerosis.[776] Earlier studies had shown that in large surgical series sporadic angiomyolipomas were four times more common than tumors associated with tuberous sclerosis.[777] These analyses probably underestimate the true incidence of tuberous sclerosis-related tumors due to a potential failure to recognize individuals with the syndrome. It is also likely that the number of patients with tuberous sclerosis is under-represented in surgical studies as these patients are more likely to be treated conservatively in order to preserve renal function. For individuals diagnosed with tuberous sclerosis, renal angiomyolipomas are detected in approximately 50% of cases.[778,779]

Among patients with sporadic angiomyolipoma, women predominate over men with a ratio of 4-4.5 to 1.[776,777] In patients with tuberous sclerosis, an equal gender distribution occurs.[776,779] The age at presentation for patients with sporadic angiomyolipoma ranges from 17 to 80 years, with a mean age of 45 years. This contrasts to a range of 0 to 80 years, and a mean age of 30 years, for tumors diagnosed in association with tuberous sclerosis.[775]

Clinical Features

Small angiomyolipomas are usually detected incidentally through imaging studies. Larger tumors are frequently associated with intratumoral hemorrhage and 80% of tumors >4 cm in maximum diameter are symptomatic. The most common presenting symptom is abdominal or flank pain with hematuria and abdominal mass being less frequently seen.[780] Fever, hypertension, and visceral compressive symptoms are unusual presenting features.[781] The size of angiomyolipomas may increase during pregnancy, and pregnancy-associated tumor rupture has been reported.[782] Rapid tumor growth was also noted in an adolescent female treated with hormones for menorrhagia.[783]

In patients with tuberous sclerosis, multiple tumors are common, being reported from 87% of cases, and in 71% of these patients bilateral tumors were seen.[778] Sporadically arising angiomyolipomas are more likely to be symptomatic at diagnosis and in a series of 60 cases, 50% presented with abdominal pain and 22% with hematuria, while 28% were asymptomatic.[775]

The presence of fat in angiomyolipoma is an important diagnostic feature and these tumors are usually readily diagnosed by ultrasound or computerized tomography.[784] These tumors must be differentiated from other fat-containing renal tumors and in particular may be mistaken for clear cell renal cell carcinoma.[785]

Pathology

Gross Features

On gross examination, angiomyolipomas are usually circumscribed with rounded contours. They are found within either the renal cortex or medulla and may also appear to arise from the renal capsule. There is usually no evidence of pseudocapsule. In approximately 30% of surgical specimens, multiple tumors are present.[511] Angiomyolipomas vary in size with median diameters of 7 to 9 cm being reported from larger series.[511,786] Occasionally they may be large, ranging up to 25 to 30 cm in diameter.[787] The cut surface is yellow to tan and has a soft to firm consistency dependent on the proportion of fat present. Larger tumors may show extensive hemorrhage, which may involve the whole of the tumor (Fig. 2-110). Angiomyolipomas in which smooth muscle predominates are pale gray or tan color (Fig. 2-111). Angiomyolipoma may erode through the renal capsule and bulge into perirenal fat.[777] Angiomyolipoma may also extend into intrarenal veins or into the renal vein, and rarely extension to the vena cava and right atrium has been reported.[777] When examining specimens containing renal angiomyolipomas it is important to very carefully examine the renal parenchyma and to submit for microscopic examination any small lesions since the presence of multiple angiomyolipomas is a strong indicator that the patient may have tuberous sclerosis.[788]

Microscopic Features

Angiomyolipoma typically contains varying proportions of smooth muscle, adipose tissue, and blood vessels (Fig. 2-112). Cells of the smooth muscle component of the tumor range from spindle shaped to round (Fig. 2-113). Mitotic figures are usually rare; however, focally smooth muscle cells may show nucleomegaly and hyperchromasia, occasionally with prominent nucleoli (Fig. 2-114).

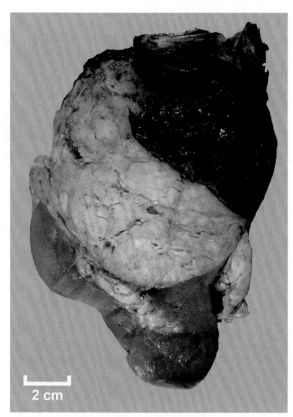

FIGURE 2-110 ■ Angiomyolipoma. This large fatty angiomyolipoma has ruptured and formed a perirenal retroperitoneal hematoma. The yellow color of the tumor indicates its fat content.

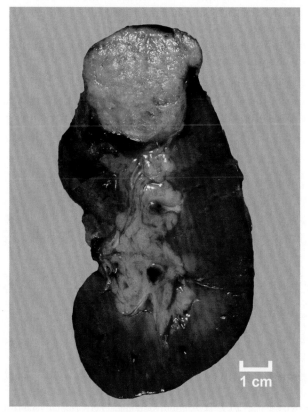

FIGURE 2-111 ■ Angiomyolipoma. The pale gray color of this angiomyolipoma indicates a high content of smooth muscle.

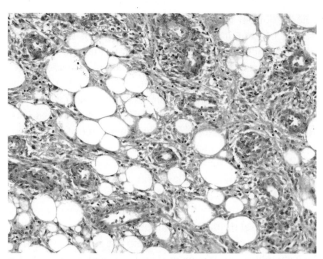

FIGURE 2-112 ■ Angiomyolipoma. Thick-walled blood vessels, fat, and spindle-shaped smooth muscle.

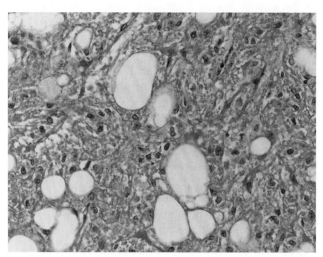

FIGURE 2-113 ■ Angiomyolipoma. Smooth muscle cells with polygonal contours: epithelioid smooth muscle.

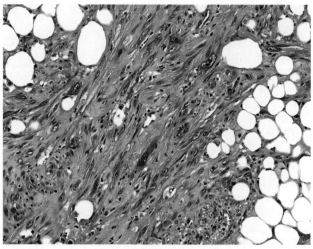

FIGURE 2-114 ■ Angiomyolipoma. The smooth muscle cells may have striking nuclear pleomorphism.

The cytoplasm of the smooth muscle cells may contain a variety of granules. These are frequently positive for periodic acid-Schiff and are not resistant to diastase digestion. Diastase resistant granules and crystalloid structures have also been reported. In rare instances the spindle cells may contain granular brown pigment. This has the histochemical features of melanin and may be quite extensive, at least focally, within a tumor.[789] The fat component of angiomyolipoma consists of mature fat cells of normal appearance. Rarely, there are foci of fat cells with cytoplasm containing multiple lipid vacuoles, bringing lipoblasts to mind (Fig. 2-115). However, these have the nuclei of typical adipocytes. The vascular component of the tumor consists mainly of blood vessels with thick walls and small lumens. Although elastin fibers may be present within the muscle wall, they lack the elastic arrangement seen in normal arteries. These vessels are often grouped into clusters with radial collarettes of smooth muscle. Lymphatic differentiation has been demonstrated throughout these tumors and is most pronounced in the smooth muscle component, where lymphatics may aggregate to form a labyrinth-like pattern (Fig. 2-116).[790]

The proportion of each of the components of the tumor may vary widely. In a series of 184 tumors, 83% had a triphasic morphology, while 13% had ≥95% smooth muscle component and 5% had ≥95% fat component.[786] Fat-predominant tumors may resemble renal lipoma, while in smooth muscle predominant tumors, fat may form small islands or be absent altogether. In these instances, the presence of thick-walled vessels may be an important key to the diagnosis. Occasionally angiomyolipomas contain areas in which there is marked perivascular sclerosis, imparting a trabecular or sclerosing appearance (Fig. 2-117).[791] Usually, the cells between the trabeculae are polygonal or round smooth muscle cells.

Coalescence of separate tumor nodules in multifocal disease may give the appearance of invasion, although angiomyolipoma does not infiltrate into the kidney and usually has a smooth contour. Very rarely, angiomyolipoma may contain

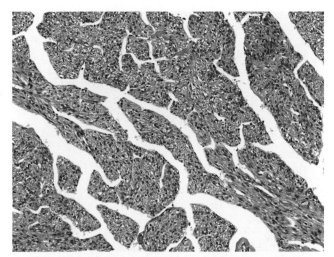

FIGURE 2-116 ■ Angiomyolipoma. Lymphangioleiomyoma-like vessels are present in some angiomyolipomas.

cysts or even have a predominantly cystic appearance grossly, with cysts measuring up to 6 cm in diameter.[792–794] The cystic areas are lined by cuboidal to hobnail epithelial cells, which may be ciliated. The cysts are thought to be entrapped renal tubules that have become dilated.

A variety of renal tumors have been reported to coexist with angiomyolipoma. Clear cell renal cell carcinoma, papillary renal cell carcinoma, and chromophobe renal cell carcinoma have been reported. Coexisting carcinomas may be ipsilateral, contralateral, or bilateral, while multiple papillary adenomas may also be present. Renal cell carcinoma is a recognized feature of tuberous sclerosis, and these patients often present with renal malignancy at younger age than patients with sporadic tumors.[795–797]

Ancillary and Special Studies

Angiomyolipomas give positive immunohistochemical reactions for HMB-45, with staining most frequently seen

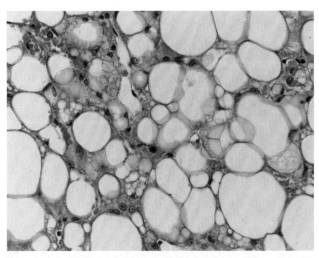

FIGURE 2-115 ■ Angiomyolipoma. A focus of fat cells with bubbly cytoplasm reminiscent of lipoblasts.

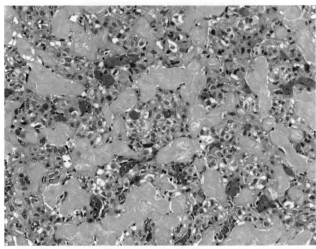

FIGURE 2-117 ■ Angiomyolipoma. Perivascular sclerosis imparts a trabecular architecture.

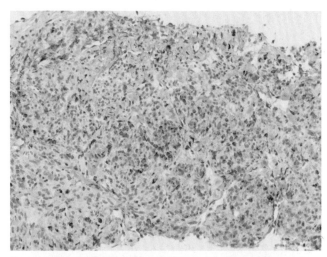

Figure 2-118 ■ Angiomyolipoma. Immunohistochemistry with HMB45 gives a positive reaction in some of the cells of a needle biopsy of a smooth muscle-predominant tumor.

in polygonal and perivascular muscle cells.[798–800] Melan-A also is frequently detected, and almost all angiomyolipomas are positive for HMB-45 (Fig. 2-118) or melan-A or both. Cathepsin K also is expressed in almost all angiomyolipomas.[801] Other melanocyte markers such as microophthalmia transcription factor, and tyrosinase are less frequently positive and less useful. Smooth muscle actin, muscle-specific actin, and vimentin are also frequently positive.[802,803] Angiomyolipomas also express hormone receptors. Immunohistochemistry is very frequently positive for estrogen receptor β (100%) and androgen receptor (80%).[804] Staining is variable for estrogen receptor α (30%) and progesterone receptor (38%).[804] Stains for epithelial markers are negative, except for the epithelial cells lining the cysts in angiomyolipoma with epithelial cysts.[792,794,805]

Genetics
Tuberous sclerosis is associated with mutations of the *TSC1* gene on chromosome 9q34 and *TSC2* gene on chromosome 16p13. Mutations of the *TSC2* gene may also be seen in sporadic angiomyolipoma.[806]

Differential Diagnosis

Tumors showing a predominance of smooth muscle or fat may be mistaken for renal leiomyoma or lipoma. Smooth muscle predominant tumors may also be mistaken for leiomyosarcoma and sarcomatoid renal cell carcinoma. Angiomyolipoma with epithelial cysts may mimic mixed epithelial and stromal tumor of kidney, although the clinical features of these tumors differ. Unlike angiomyolipoma, mixed epithelial and stromal tumors do not express melanocytic markers.[792]

The smooth muscle character of the spindle cells of angiomyolipoma is confirmed by electron microscopy. These cells contain glycogen, and the presence of lipid in some cells suggests a transition between smooth muscle cells and adipocytes. Crystalloids may also be seen. Interstitial collagen

bundles are usually present between smooth muscle cells and vascular spaces, and occasional premelanosomes have been identified.[800,807,808]

Prognosis and Predictive Factors

Angiomyolipomas are benign tumors, although in two cases leiomyosarcoma developed, causing death.[809,810] Angiomyolipoma may occasionally show regional extension to the abdominal wall and pelvis,[811,812] and tumor deposits may be found within regional lymph nodes (Fig. 2-119) and the spleen; however, these features are not indicative of malignancy.[813–815] Despite the benign nature of angiomyolipoma, larger tumors are more frequently associated with spontaneous or trauma-related hemorrhage. The likelihood of hemorrhage is dependent on tumor size, being more common in tumors >4 to 6 cm in diameter.[780] Angiomyolipomas appear more likely to undergo hemorrhage during pregnancy.[782] Hemorrhage may be intrarenal, but massive retroperitoneal hemorrhage may also occur and this is known as Wunderlich syndrome. Patients with angiomyolipoma are at increased risk of developing renal cell carcinoma and pulmonary lymphangiomyomatosis, although this is more frequently associated with tuberous sclerosis.

Treatment

Many patients with small asymptomatic angiomyolipomas require no treatment and are followed with periodic ultrasound examinations to assess the size of the tumor. A variety of treatments are available for renal angiomyolipoma. Nephrectomy is the standard treatment for large tumors, while for smaller tumors nephron-sparing partial nephrectomy often is appropriate.[816] Tumors may also be treated by selective arterial embolization[781] or laparoscopic cryoablation.[817] It is recommended that tumors >8 cm be managed surgically due to the high risk of spontaneous hemorrhage. It has also been

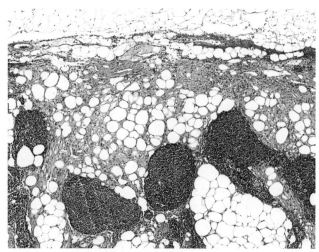

Figure 2-119 ■ Angiomyolipoma. Angiomyolipoma sometimes is found in lymph nodes draining a kidney with an angiomyolipoma.

recommended that all patients with symptomatic tumors or asymptomatic tumors ≥4 cm should be considered for treatment as these tumors are at greater risk of rupture or hemorrhage.[781] Most recently, treatment with mTOR inhibitors has been found to reduce the size of angiomyolipomas.[818,819]

Epithelioid Angiomyolipoma

Epidemiology and Clinical Features

The term "epithelioid angiomyolipoma" was coined in 1996 in a report of a case with distinctive morphology and, ultimately, fatal outcome.[820] Epithelioid angiomyolipoma is now established as a distinctive form of renal neoplasia occurring both sporadically and in association with tuberous sclerosis.

The clinical and pathologic features of nearly 100 cases of epithelioid angiomyolipoma have been described in case reports and more recently in larger studies.[512,791,821,822] There is a female predominance, with a male-to-female ratio of 1:6.5.[776] Patients ranged in age from 6 to 81 years with a mean age of 44 years, and in a mixed series of angiomyolipoma, <10% of tumors were epithelioid angiomyolipomas.[776] These tumors occur both sporadically and as part of the tuberous sclerosis complex, which in one series constituted 27% of cases.[776]

Approximately 50% of patients with epithelioid angiomyolipoma are asymptomatic, with tumors discovered as an incidental finding or as a result of investigations in individuals with known tuberous sclerosis. The most common presenting features are hemorrhage, abdominal or flank pain, and renal mass. Nonspecific systemic symptoms may also be presenting features, with fatigue, weight loss, edema, nausea, recurrent urinary tract infection, night sweats, fever, and anorexia being reported.[821] Imaging studies of epithelioid angiomyolipoma are often nonspecific. As these tumors are always fat poor, they lack the typical radiologic feature of angiomyolipoma and may be mistaken for renal cell carcinoma.[823]

Pathology

Gross Features

Epithelioid angiomyolipomas are usually well circumscribed and are, on average, larger than typical angiomyolipoma at diagnosis. Mean diameters of 8 cm have been reported from larger series, and a tumor weighing 7.1 kg was found at autopsy of a patient with tuberous sclerosis.[776,824]

The cut surface of the tumor is tan, gray, pink, or yellow and may be variegated, with macroscopic areas of hemorrhage and necrosis being frequently seen (Fig. 2-120).[823] The tumor may distort the renal capsule, extend into perirenal fat, and infiltrate adjacent organs. Occasionally tumor extends into the renal vein or vena cava. Tumor may be present in regional lymph nodes; however, as is the case for typical angiomyolipoma, this does not necessarily indicate metastatic spread of malignant disease.[825] When examining specimens containing renal angiomyolipomas, it is important to very carefully examine the renal parenchyma and to submit for microscopic examination any small lesions since the

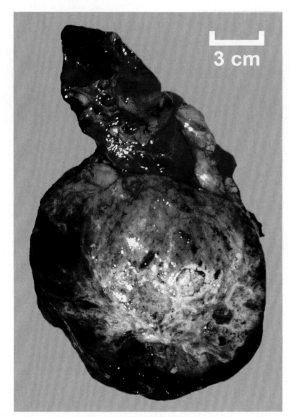

FIGURE 2-120 ■ Epithelioid angiomyolipoma. The tumor resembles a carcinoma and lacks the yellow color imparted by fat cells.

presence of multiple angiomyolipomas is a strong indicator that the patient may have tuberous sclerosis.[788]

Microscopic Features

Epithelioid angiomyolipoma is characterized by the presence of polygonal cells and short spindle-shaped cells of variable size (Fig. 2-121).[823,826] The larger epithelioid cells show

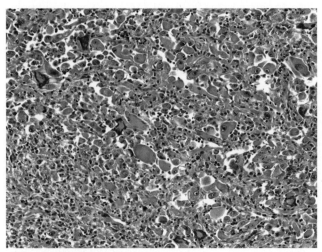

FIGURE 2-121 ■ Epithelioid angiomyolipoma. A mixture of stubby spindle cells and large mononuclear and multinuclear cells makes up the tumor.

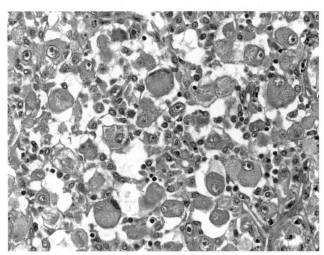

FIGURE 2-122 ■ Epithelioid angiomyolipoma. Large ganglion-like mononuclear cells are a hallmark of epithelioid angiomyolipoma.

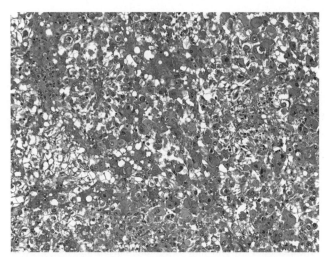

FIGURE 2-124 ■ Epithelioid angiomyolipoma. Diffuse hemorrhage and edema between the cells resembling degeneration in a high-grade carcinoma.

nuclear atypia with a prominent nucleolus and may resemble ganglion cells (Fig. 2-122). The cytoplasm is abundant and deeply eosinophilic, and large multinucleate cells, often with peripheral nuclei, may be present. Smaller epithelioid cells are relatively uniform in size with a moderate amount of pale cytoplasm and, at most, focal nuclear atypia. Adipose tissue is usually absent and when present, forms inconspicuous nests. The large vessels characteristic of typical angiomyolipoma are rarely seen. The growth pattern may be sheets, or less frequently, a carcinoma-like pattern composed of nests surrounded by vascular septa.[827] Within the sheets, areas of edema in which the individual cells are separated by edema fluid are common. Puddles of hemorrhage may give the illusion of cyst formation (Fig. 2-123). Diffuse hemorrhage and edema may resemble degeneration in high-grade carcinoma (Fig. 2-124) Tumor necrosis is present in approximately one-quarter of cases, and this may be extensive. Mitotic activity

is visible in 50% of tumors, with mitotic rates ranging from 1 to 10 mitotic figures/10 high-power fields. Invasion of intrarenal vessels or the renal vein may be present.[825] Epithelioid angiomyolipoma may coexist with areas of tumor showing the features of typical angiomyolipoma, and this may constitute up to 95% of the tumor.[825]

Ancillary and Special Studies
HMB45 and Melan-A are each positive in 80% to 90% of tumors, and one or the other is positive in nearly 100%. Cathepsin K is also detectable in nearly all epithelioid angiomyolipomas.[801] A positive reactivity for smooth muscle-specific actin is found in about 90% of tumors. Reactions with antibodies to markers of epithelial differentiation are typically negative.[776,821,823] Staining for estrogen receptor is variable, being present in up to 50% of cases.[828]

Electron microscopy of these tumors shows an absence of epithelial features, while glycogen is present. Membrane-bound granules and premelanosome-like structures may also be seen.[823]

Genetics
Genetic studies on epithelioid angiomyolipoma are limited; however, loss of heterozygosity at the *TSC2* locus on chromosome 16p has been seen in one case. Diffuse immunoreactivity for TP53 has also been demonstrated, although no mutation has been detected in the *TP53* gene.[823,824]

Differential Diagnosis

These tumors may be mistaken for renal cell carcinoma and sarcomatoid carcinoma. Epithelioid angiomyolipoma should be considered in any tumor containing poorly cohesive polygonal cells with eosinophilic cytoplasm. In such instances, positive immunoreactivity for HMB-45, melan-A, or cathepsin K, along with smooth muscle-specific actin, and negative reactions for markers of epithelial differentiation are diagnostic.

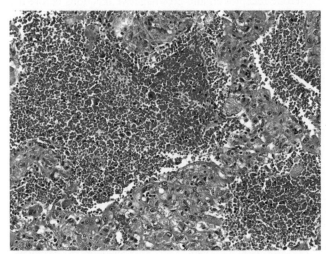

FIGURE 2-123 ■ Epithelioid angiomyolipoma. Puddles of blood resemble blood-filled cysts and heighten the resemblance to carcinoma.

Prognosis and Treatment

Epithelioid angiomyolipoma has malignant potential. In a review of published cases, metastatic spread to lymph nodes, liver, lung, or spleen was reported for 30% of patients.[829] In a separate series, 36% of tumors either recurred or metastasized over a mean follow-up interval of 52 months.[825] In contrast to this, no malignant behavior was observed in a further series of 15 cases after a mean follow-up interval of 5 years.[776]

In an analysis of features predictive of subsequent clinical behavior, it was suggested that the presence of ≥70% atypical epithelioid cells, ≥2 mitotic figures per 10 high-power fields, atypical mitotic figures, and necrosis was of prognostic significance, and that if three or more of these were identified then there was an increased risk of malignancy.[825] Another study found that large size, carcinoma-like growth pattern, invasion of perinephric fat or renal vein, and necrosis were associated with malignant behavior.[827]

Epithelioid angiomyolipoma is often larger than typical angiomyolipoma at diagnosis. Surgical management is the usual treatment for epithelioid angiomyolipoma and is often undertaken in the mistaken belief that the tumor is a renal cell carcinoma. Tumor metastases have been reported to respond to doxorubicin and possibly to dacarbazine, ifosfamide, cyclophosphamide, and cisplatin.[822]

Desmoplastic Small Round Cell Tumor

Epidemiology and Clinical Features

Eight cases of desmoplastic small round cell tumor of the kidney have been reported.[830–835] The patient initially reported by Egloff et al.[831] was also reported in two other papers.[833,836] The adult was a 41-year-old man, while the children were five girls and two boys aged from 7 to 14 years (median = 8 years).

Pathology

Grossly the tumors were solid and involved renal cortex, medulla, and renal sinus. The cut surfaces were white or tan, and foci of necrosis and hemorrhage are present. The microscopic features of the tumor are typical for desmoplastic small round cell tumor, consisting of small cells with hyperchromatic nuclei and scanty cytoplasm. Mitotic figures are commonly seen. Foci of necrosis are common and scattered areas of dystrophic calcification often present. Focal desmoplasia was seen in only one tumor.

All tumors reacted positively with antibodies to vimentin and desmin, with the staining for desmin being dot-like and near the nucleus. Some tumors also showed positive expression of neuron-specific enolase, smooth muscle and muscle-specific actin, WT1, CD56, and FLI1. The majority of tumors also showed, at least, focal expression of CAM5.2, pancytokeratin, EMA, and CD99. Electron microscopy of two cases showed intermediate junctions, thickened basal lamina, and aggregates of intermediate filaments. All cases studied showed *EWS-WT1* gene fusion [t(11;22)(p13;q12)] characteristic of desmoplastic small round cell tumor.[830,833]

Prognosis and Treatment

Of the pediatric patients, two had recurrences post surgery, and following chemotherapy these and two other patients were disease free over a follow-up period of 22 to 44 months. The adult patient had been recurrence free for 18 months following nephrectomy.

MISCELLANEOUS MESENCHYMAL NEOPLASMS

Lipoma

Epidemiology and Clinical Features

Renal lipomas are rare with fewer than two dozen cases reported in the literature.[837–841] Most of the reports are from the era before immunohistochemistry was available, and even recent reports include no more than minimal immunohistochemical evidence that the tumors are not angiomyolipomas with great predominance of fat. Renal lipoma usually presents with flank or abdominal pain and rarely with hematuria. These are benign tumors and are cured by surgical removal.

Pathology

The gross specimen consists of yellow fat-forming lobules, often with an investing capsule of varying thickness. Tumors vary in size ranging up to 14 cm in maximum diameter, and in larger tumors there may be areas of necrosis and hemorrhage.

The histologic features are those of mature adipose tissue without nuclear atypia. The differential diagnosis includes angiomyolipoma, retroperitoneal lipoma, and liposarcoma. Before a renal tumor can be accepted as a lipoma rather than an angiomyolipoma, it must be extensively sampled, and a thorough immunohistochemical investigation must be done. A battery of antibodies to HMB45, melan-A, cathepsin K, smooth muscle actin, desmin, estrogen receptor, and progesterone receptor should give negative reactions before the diagnosis of lipoma is made. Retroperitoneal lipomas show no vascular attachment to the kidney, while liposarcoma may be excluded on morphologic grounds. A single case of lipoblastoma of the kidney has been recorded in a 2-year-old male and a hibernoma in the kidney of a 51-year-old woman.[842,843] Renal replacement lipomatosis is a nonneoplastic condition in which the renal parenchyma atrophies and renal sinus fat expands to replace it.[844,845] Renal replacement lipomatosis is discussed in more detail in Chapter 1 on nonneoplastic diseases of the kidney.

Leiomyoma

Epidemiology and Clinical Features

Renal leiomyomas are benign smooth muscle tumors similar in morphology to those occurring in other parts of the body. Renal leiomyomas are very rare. Smooth muscle–predominant angiomyolipomas are much more common, so one must be skeptical of any report that does not present convincing immunohistochemical evidence that the tumor is not an angiomyolipoma. However, there are a few reports of well-investigated leiomyomas of the renal parenchyma.[846–849] Leiomyomas have been reported to arise from the renal capsule, and a few of these reports have presented immunohistochemical evidence that they were not angiomyolipomas.[850] Leiomyomas arising from the renal pelvis and renal vein where angiomyolipomas are not a significant consideration have also been reported.[851,852] Renal leiomyoma has been reported in immunodeficient patients and, as with leiomyoma in other organs in this group of patients, is thought to be induced by Epstein-Barr virus (EBV).[853]

Most tumors are discovered clinically as incidental findings following imaging studies. Rarely renal leiomyomas are symptomatic with abdominal mass, hematuria, and flank pain being reported.[846] These are benign tumors and are cured by surgical resection.

Pathology

As in other sites, renal leiomyomas are well-circumscribed solid rubbery masses with a whorled cut surface. Occasionally, cystic areas are present. Histologically, renal leiomyoma consists of bundles of smooth muscle fibers without nuclear pleomorphism. Degenerative changes and dystrophic calcification may be present, and larger tumors may show areas of hyalinization. The findings of necrosis, nuclear atypia, or more rarely atypical mitotic figures suggest a diagnosis of renal leiomyosarcoma. Immunohistochemical expression reflects the smooth muscle nature of these tumors, with positive staining for smooth muscle actin and desmin.

Differential Diagnosis

The principal differential diagnostic consideration is angiomyolipoma with predominance of smooth muscle. Before a diagnosis of renal leiomyoma can be rendered, the tumor must be extensively sampled to search for fat and the abnormal blood vessels often found in angiomyolipomas. The presence of multiple tumors favors a diagnosis of angiomyolipoma. A battery of antibodies to HMB45, melan-A, and cathepsin K should give negative reactions before the diagnosis of renal leiomyoma is made.

Hemangioma

Epidemiology and Clinical Features

Hemangiomas of the kidney have been found in a wide age range of patients although tumors most commonly occur in adults.[854–856] Solitary lesions are more frequent, but in more than 10% of cases, tumors are multiple and bilaterality has been reported. Hemangiomas may be associated with the Klippel-Trenaunay and Sturge-Weber syndromes.[857] Many hemangiomas are asymptomatic and are found only at autopsy. In symptomatic patients, recurrent hematuria is the usual complaint, frequently associated with anemia.[856]

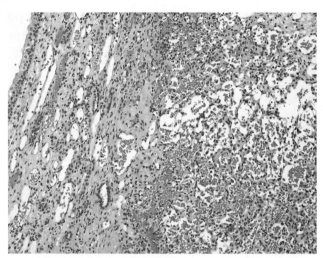

FIGURE 2-125 ■ Hemangioma. This lesion is in a medullary pyramid near the urothelial mucosa.

Pathology

Most tumors are <1 cm in diameter at presentation and are often difficult to detect with the naked eye. Larger lesions, up to 18 cm in diameter, have been reported, and these have a spongy reddish appearance. While hemangiomas may arise anywhere in the kidney, the medulla and papilla are the sites of the majority of symptomatic lesions (Fig. 2-125).

Microscopically, these lesions are composed of vascular spaces of variable size, some of which may have smooth muscle and elastic tissue in their walls. As for hemangioma of soft tissue, capillary and cavernous types are recognized[854,856] and thrombosis and organization are common. Recently, a variant of renal hemangioma composed of densely packed capillary vessels with foci of an anastomosing sinusoid-like pattern has been given the name "anastomosing hemangioma."[855,858] These lesions often have endothelium with a hobnail appearance and zones of sclerosis between the small vessels. Extramedullary hematopoiesis is sometimes present. While hemangiomas often have irregular borders and merge with the surrounding renal parenchyma, the lack of nuclear atypia and mitotic figures should make recognition of their benign nature straightforward in most cases. The lobulated architecture of anastomosing hemangiomas is also helpful in the differential with angiosarcoma. These tumors are distinguished from angiosarcoma using the same criteria applied to soft tissue tumors.

Hemangioblastoma

Epidemiology and Clinical Features

Hemangioblastoma is most common in the cerebellum and other central nervous system sites. While most of these tumors occur sporadically about 25% occur in patients with VHL disease, in whom, the differential diagnosis with clear cell renal cell carcinoma metastatic to the central nervous system must be considered. A handful of cases of primary renal hemangioblastoma have been reported.[137,859–863] The patients were three females and four males with ages ranging from 16 to 71 years (median = 58 years). None of the patients had VHL disease. No patient suffered recurrence or metastasis and were well with follow-up ranging from 5 to 108 months.

Presenting symptoms included hematuria, polycythemia, and back pain, but in half the cases, the tumors were incidental findings.

Pathology

Grossly the tumors were well circumscribed, and ranged from 12 to 68 mm in diameter. The cut surfaces of the tumors were gray or brown, and in one case tumor cavitation was present.

Histologically, these tumors show features similar to hemangioblastoma of the central nervous system and to clear cell renal cell carcinoma, with sheets of polygonal cells having bulky eosinophilic cytoplasm and an associated prominent arborizing vascular network. Intracytoplasmic eosinophilic globules were present in one case.

Differential Diagnosis

The main differential diagnostic consideration is with clear cell renal cell carcinoma. The main obstacle to making the diagnosis is having a sufficiently low threshold of suspicion. Once hemangioblastoma is under consideration, negative immunohistochemical reactions with antibodies to PAX2 and PAX8, along with a positive reaction with antibody to inhibin-α, will confirm that the tumor is a hemangioblastoma, since 95% to 100% of hemangioblastoma will give negative nuclear reactions for PAX2 and PAX8, while 90% of hemangioblastomas will give diffusely positive cytoplasmic reactions for inhibin-α.[864]

Glomus Tumor

Epidemiology and Clinical Features

A few cases of primary renal glomus tumor and a further case of glomus tumor arising in the renal pelvis have been reported.[865–869] There has been a predominance of males, and the patients' ages have ranged from 17 to 81 years. The single instance of glomus tumor of the renal pelvis was in a 53-year-old female.

Pathology

Gross Features

Most of the tumors were incidental findings and ranged in size up to 7 cm in maximum diameter. Tumors of renal origin were usually situated peripherally with distortion, but not infiltration of the renal capsule. The tumors were well circumscribed, and the cut surface had a solid or gelatinous consistency. The tumors were gray-white to brown, and in one tumor, foci of hemorrhage were seen.

Microscopic Features

Microscopically these tumors show a variety of histologic features. The neoplastic cells are usually small, round to oval, with a scanty to moderate amount of eosinophilic to amphophilic cytoplasm (Fig. 2-126A). The stromal architecture is variable, and in one tumor, classified as a solid glomus tumor, tumor cells formed sheets and nests within a myxoid and delicate fibrovascular stroma. Two tumors were classified as glomangioma having peripheral slit-like vascular spaces, with a central myxoid stroma interspersed with hyalinized areas and telangiectatic vessels. In the remaining two cases, tumor cells were round to fusiform with some degree of nuclear pleomorphism. In some areas, there was vascular proliferation with condensation of adjacent tumor cells at the vascular margin. In some areas short fascicles of smooth muscle were seen.

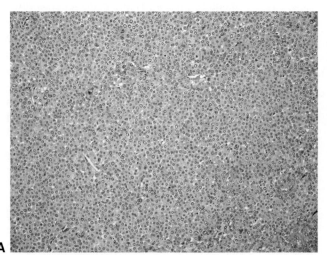 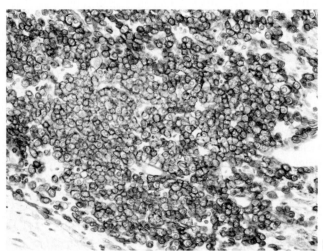

FIGURE 2-126 ■ **A:** Glomus tumor. The sheets of polygonal cells bring carcinoma or juxtaglomerular cell tumor to mind. **B:** Immunohistochemistry for laminin shows a positive reaction in the cytoplasm.

Ancillary and Special Studies

Tumors showed strongly positive cytoplasmic immunohistochemical reactions for common and smooth muscle actin, while laminin expression was pericellular (Fig. 2-126B) and there was focal expression of CD34. Epithelial markers were usually negative. In one tumor, there was positivity for NSE, S-100 protein, cytokeratin, and desmin, and on the basis of this immunoprofile, the diagnosis of glomangioma has been questioned.[868]

Prognosis and Treatment

Although malignant behavior is well recognized in nonrenal glomus tumors, most that have originated in the kidney have, to date, followed a benign course. A single case of malignant behavior in a renal glomus tumor has been reported.[870]

Lymphangioma

Epidemiology and Clinical Features

Renal lymphangioma occurs in both adults and children.[871,872] These tumors may arise in the renal parenchyma or be associated with the renal capsule or renal sinus.[873–875] Tumors may be unilateral or bilateral, while those associated with inflammation are often peripelvic. Abdominal mass is the most frequent presenting feature although abdominal pain, hematuria, or hypertension has been reported. Lesions within the renal sinus may infiltrate the renal medulla, leading to urinary obstruction.[876]

Pathology

Grossly these tumors are solitary encapsulated masses of small cysts containing clear fluid (Fig. 2-127). Occasionally, tumors are localized to the subcapsular cortex or may diffusely involve the kidney. Histologically, lymphangiomas consist of spaces lined by bland endothelial cells with fibrous septa that may contain smooth muscle. Clinically, the differential diagnosis includes a wide variety of cystic diseases of the kidney while pathologically the major differential diagnosis is cystic nephroma. Lymphangioma does not have the ovarian-like stroma typical of cystic nephroma and positive immunohistochemistry for Factor VIII, CD31, and for podoplanin in the cells lining the spaces is diagnostic.

VHL gene mutation and abnormalities of chromosomes 7 and X have been described in association with lymphangioma. In some cases, coexistent angiomas in other organs have been noted.[871,874] To date, no instance of malignant transformation of these tumors has been reported.

Schwannoma

Schwannomas originating from the Schwann cell of the peripheral nerve sheath are rarely encountered in the kidney. There is an equal gender distribution and patients ranged in age from 14 to 89 years.[877,878] Presenting symptoms are variable with flank pain, abdominal mass, fever, and anemia predominating. The majority of schwannomas occur within

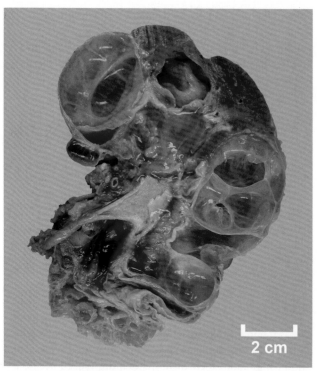

FIGURE 2-127 ■ Lymphangioma. The cystically dilated lymphatic could be mistaken for cystic nephroma, multilocular cystic renal cell carcinoma, or cystic partially differentiated nephroblastoma.

the renal sinus. Tumors have been reported arising from the renal parenchyma and renal capsule. Often the schwannomas are large. Histologically, these tumors resemble typical peripheral nerve schwannoma with absence of cellular atypia and at most, rare mitotic figures. Cellular variants have also been described.[879] Renal schwannomas have a benign clinical course with reported follow-up of up to 60 months.[879]

Solitary Fibrous Tumor

Epidemiology and Clinical Features

Solitary fibrous tumor is a spindle cell neoplasm that has been reported from many sites, including the kidney, and is most common in the pleura. The tumors that have previously been diagnosed under the name "hemangiopericytoma" are presently considered to be solitary fibrous tumors. The histogenesis of solitary fibrous tumor is unknown.

Fewer than 100 cases of renal solitary fibrous tumor have been reported.[880] There is an equal gender distribution, and patients range in age from early childhood to the ninth decade of life, with a mean age of 51 years.[880,881] These tumors are often discovered incidentally or may be associated with flank pain, abdominal mass, or hematuria.[881]

Pathology

Gross Features

Renal solitary fibrous tumors range in size from 2 to 25 cm (mean 9 cm). More than two-thirds arise in the renal parenchyma, but some are attributed to the renal capsule and renal sinus. They are usually well circumscribed with a gray to tan cut surface. Tumors are usually solitary although a single patient with bilateral tumors has been seen. In one of the two malignant solitary fibrous tumors reported to date, there was gross necrosis with extension of the tumor into Gerota fascia and adipose tissue of the ureter and renal hilum.[881]

Microscopic Features

Solitary fibrous tumors consist of spindle cells exhibiting minimal nuclear pleomorphism. The tumor may show a storiform or fascicular architecture with intervening hypocellular collagenous areas. Dilated blood vessels, occasionally with a hemangiopericytoma pattern, may also be present.[882,883] In those cases showing malignant transformation, areas of typical morphology sharply abut upon sheets of plump spindle cells with moderate to marked nuclear pleomorphism. In those areas the mitotic rate ranged from 2 to 6 mitotic figures per 10 HPF.[881,884]

Differential Diagnosis

The differential diagnosis includes sarcomatoid carcinoma and spindle cell neoplasms of smooth muscle and neural origin. Immunohistochemistry is helpful, indeed necessary, to support the diagnosis. Strong, diffusely positive reactions for CD34, BCL2, and CD99 are common in solitary fibrous tumors. Most sarcomatoid carcinomas give positive reactions with antibodies to cytokeratins (AE1/AE3 most frequently), and smooth muscle tumors and neural tumors with antibodies to smooth muscle actin and S100, respectively.

Prognosis and Treatment

All but one of the reported cases of renal solitary fibrous tumor have behaved in a benign manner with follow-up ranging from 2 to 89 months. In one case, there was sarcomatoid differentiation with extrarenal spread at the time of diagnosis and the patient developed pulmonary metastases 4 months later.[881]

Liposarcoma

Epidemiology and Clinical Features

Liposarcoma of renal origin is rare, with most liposarcomas involving the kidney being perirenal in origin (Box 2-6).[885,886] Several cases of liposarcoma arising from the renal sinus have also been reported,[887] while a single case of renal liposarcoma has been reported in association with end-stage kidney disease.[426] These tumors are most commonly found in patients in their fifth to sixth decade, with the oldest patient being in the ninth decade.[887]

Box 2-6 ● PRIMARY RENAL SARCOMA DIAGNOSTIC CRITERIA

- No history of sarcoma elsewhere
- Gross appearance compatible with renal parenchymal origin
- Sarcomatoid renal cell carcinoma excluded

Pathology

Liposarcoma localized to the kidney is usually yellow, lobulated, and well circumscribed. Larger tumors are more likely perirenal in origin. These tumors show the range of histologic patterns seen elsewhere in the body, although in one series 80% were found to be myxoid.[888] The most important differential diagnosis is angiomyolipoma, and well-differentiated liposarcomas should be widely sampled to search for smooth muscle and abnormal blood vessels. A battery of antibodies to HMB45, melan-A, cathepsin K, smooth muscle actin, desmin, estrogen receptor, and progesterone receptor should give negative reactions before the diagnosis of liposarcoma is made.

Prognosis and Treatment

Renal vein infiltration has been reported for perirenal liposarcoma, and in general those tumors have a poor prognosis. The most important indicator of outcome for renal liposarcoma, as for other renal sarcomas, is completeness of surgical excision.[887]

Leiomyosarcoma

Epidemiology and Clinical Features

Leiomyosarcoma is the most frequently encountered soft tissue sarcoma of the genitourinary tract and constitutes 0.1% of invasive renal tumors and about 50% of primary renal sarcomas.[889,890] Approximately 125 renal leiomyosarcomas have been reported, with most patients being aged >40 years.[890] The peak incidence of the tumors is in the fifth to sixth decade, although tumors have been recorded in childhood and extreme old age. There is a slight female predominance.[890] Presenting features are often abdominal pain or mass, while fever and hematuria may also be present.

Pathology

Gross Features

Renal leiomyosarcoma is often of large dimension at diagnosis with a mean tumor size of 13 cm being reported. These tumors frequently occur in the renal sinus, arising from the renal vasculature or the wall of the renal pelvis (Fig. 2-128). Tumors may also arise from the renal capsule, and only 30% of leiomyosarcomas are intrarenal. The cut surface is usually gray-white, firm, and solid with whorled cut surface. They are often well circumscribed and may have a pseudocapsule. Foci of necrosis and hemorrhage are frequently seen and there may be cystic degeneration. Perineural infiltration is also a frequent finding.[888]

Microscopic Features

Histologically, leiomyosarcoma consists of sheets and fascicles of spindle cells. There is often pronounced nuclear pleomorphism, and mitotic rates ranging from 0 to 50 per 10 high-power fields (mean 11/10 high-power fields) have been reported.[890] Occasionally, the tumor may show a myxoid morphology and microscopic necrosis, and intrarenal vascular infiltration is also frequently seen.[891]

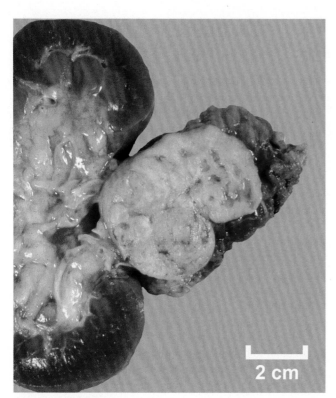

FIGURE 2-128 ■ Leiomyosarcoma. This leiomyosarcoma has arisen in the renal vein.

Differential Diagnosis

The differential diagnosis is mainly angiomyolipoma, but renal leiomyoma and sarcomatoid renal cell carcinoma may also deserve consideration. There are no strict criteria to differentiate between benign and malignant renal smooth muscle tumors. Tumors that are large with nuclear pleomorphism, frequent mitotic figures, and geographic necrosis may be confidently diagnosed as malignant; however, metastases have been reported in tumors showing few mitotic figures.[892,893] Further, nuclear atypia is fairly common in angiomyolipomas, and a few mitotic figures are seen occasionally in the smooth muscle component of angiomyolipomas. Tumors should be extensively sampled to search for fat and the abnormal blood vessels that would indicate that the tumor is smooth muscle-predominant angiomyolipoma. A battery of antibodies to HMB45, melan-A, cathepsin K, estrogen receptor, and progesterone receptor should give negative reactions before the diagnosis of leiomyosarcoma is made. Sarcomatoid renal cell carcinoma may be problematic, although extensive sampling often reveals an epithelial element, and epithelial immunohistochemical markers are often positive, albeit focally. Antibody to cytokeratin (AE1/AE3) is the one most frequently positive. The sarcomatoid component will also express PAX8 in over 50% of cases.[473]

Prognosis and Treatment

Renal leiomyosarcoma has a poor prognosis, and outcome does not appear to correlate with histologic features.

Metastases are frequently present at diagnosis, and the reported 5-year survival rate is approximately 30%, with median survival intervals of 12 to 18 months.[890,894] Treatment is primarily surgical with adjuvant chemotherapy used in selected cases.[889]

Rhabdomyosarcoma

Epidemiology and Clinical Features

Rhabdomyosarcomas of the kidney are rare tumors with an equal gender distribution and affecting patients from early childhood to the eighth decade of life.[895,896]

Pathology

Grossly, these tumors were large and pale gray. In some cases, the tumor has extended into the renal pelvis in a botryoid architecture.[897–899] Histologically, the tumors have been either embryonal rhabdomyosarcoma or pleomorphic rhabdomyosarcoma.[896,900]

As rhabdomyosarcomas are rare, the differential diagnosis is of considerable importance. In children, Wilms tumors may contain elements of skeletal muscle, and the existence of rhabdomyosarcoma distinct from Wilms tumor in children is important. The variant of Wilms tumor called fetal rhabdomyomatous nephroblastoma may have a botryoid architecture.[609] Extensive sampling to search for the blastema and epithelial elements that would indicate that the tumor is a Wilms tumor must be done if the tumor is in a child. A positive nuclear immunohistochemical reaction for WT1 would also indicate that the tumor is not a rhabdomyosarcoma but rather a Wilms tumor.

Angiosarcoma

Epidemiology and Clinical Features

Renal angiosarcomas are rare, fewer than 50 having been reported. These are tumors of adults, and there is a predominance of males over females of approximately 10:1.[901] Unlike angiosarcomas of other organs, no predisposing factors or associations with carcinogenic compounds have been determined for angiosarcomas originating in the renal parenchyma.[902]

Presenting features are weight loss, pyrexia, tiredness, hematuria, and abdominal mass.[901] In addition to angiosarcomas, hemangioendotheliomas (vascular tumors of borderline malignancy) have arisen in the kidney.[903,904]

Pathology

Grossly renal angiosarcomas often involve much of the kidney and are usually ill defined, variegated, and hemorrhagic and may be multifocal. Microscopically, there is varying cellularity with interdigitating vascular spaces. Nuclear pleomorphism and a high mitotic rate are typical.[905] Angiosarcomas show positive expression of CD31, CD34, and factor VIII.[906] Electron microscopy usually shows Weibel-Palade bodies, tight junctions, and neolumina-containing red blood cells. No consistent genetic abnormality has been reported.[902] Renal angiosarcoma has a poor prognosis with a mean survival of 7 months.[901] Metastases to the lungs, bone, and liver are common, and most patients have metastatic disease at presentation. Treatment is generally as for other sarcomas.

Osteosarcoma

Epidemiology and Clinical Features

Primary renal osteosarcoma is rarely seen, with fewer than two dozen cases reported in the literature.[907] These tumors occur in elderly patients, with most in the eighth decade. Abdominal mass is the most common presenting feature and rarely retroperitoneal hemorrhage may occur. Dense calcification is often visible on imaging studies.

Pathology

Grossly the tumors are frequently large, gray-brown and often have hard, bony foci. The histologic features are typical of osteosarcoma with osteoblast-like tumor cells and osteoid. Chondromatous differentiation may also be seen.

Osteosarcoma-like areas occurring in sarcomatoid renal cell carcinoma are probably more common than primary renal osteosarcoma. Tumors must be sampled carefully to exclude coexisting epithelial or sarcomatoid elements, and immunohistochemistry may be helpful. Osteosarcoma metastatic to the kidney must also be excluded. Most renal osteosarcomas show extensive extrarenal extension at diagnosis, and most patients die of metastatic disease within a few months.

Synovial Sarcoma

Epidemiology and Clinical Features

In 2000, a series of spindle cell tumors previously designated "embryonal sarcoma of kidney" were shown to have the *SS18-SSX1* or *SS18-SSX2* gene fusions typical of synovial sarcoma, and primary renal synovial sarcoma was recognized.[908] Approximately 40 cases of synovial sarcoma have been reported,[908–915] with patients' ages ranging from 15 to 61 years. The majority of patients were in the fourth or fifth decades at presentation, and there is an equal gender distribution.

Renal mass and abdominal or flank pain are the most frequently reported presenting features of synovial sarcoma, while hypertension and hematuria have also been described. These tumors may, on occasion, be differentiated from renal cell carcinoma clinically by the detection of cystic spaces within the tumor on ultrasonography or other imaging studies.

Pathology

Gross Features

Synovial sarcoma is frequently large when diagnosed, ranging up to 20 cm in diameter. The tumors are soft and rubbery or solid, and usually show either focal or diffuse necrosis and

hemorrhage. Smooth-walled cysts are frequently present, and occasionally they predominate to the point that the tumors resemble cystic nephroma.

Microscopic Features

Renal synovial sarcoma usually shows a monophasic morphology consisting of spindle cells with ovoid to elongate nuclei and scanty cytoplasm. Nucleoli are not prominent. Nuclei frequently overlap and mitotic figures are common. The nuclei contain clumped chromatin. Pronounced nuclear pleomorphism is uncommon. The tumor cells form intersecting fascicles and sheets, and abut directly against or infiltrate adjacent renal tissue, without pseudocapsule formation. Biphasic tumors showing rhabdoid morphology, at least focally, have been described. The rhabdoid component consists of cells with abundant eosinophilic cytoplasm, eccentric nuclei, and prominent nucleoli.[912,914] In these tumors, more typical areas of spindle cell morphology are usually present.

The majority of tumors contain epithelial-lined cysts of varying size (Fig. 2-129). The cysts are lined by a single layer of cuboidal to hobnail cells with eosinophilic cytoplasm and ovoid nuclei. On occasion the cysts may predominate, and in some areas these tumors may resemble cystic nephroma.

Ancillary and Special Studies

Variable expression of BCL2, EMA, CD99, CD56, and CD34 has been described, while cytokeratins are rarely positive. The spindle cells frequently express vimentin and calponin. Expression of desmin, smooth muscle actin, or S-100 protein is not seen. Cyst-lining epithelial cells show positivity for cytokeratins

Genetics

Synovial sarcoma shows the reciprocal translocation t(X;18) (p11.2;q11.2). This results in fusion of the *SS18* gene on chromosome 18 to one of the *SSX* genes on chromosome X.[908] There are five genes in the *SSX* gene family, although the *SS18-SSX* gene fusions seen in synovial sarcoma involve

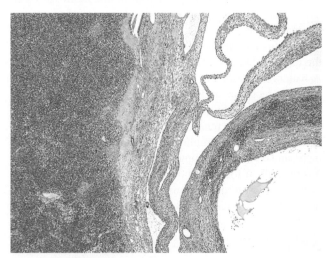

FIGURE 2-129 ■ Synovial sarcoma. Renal synovial sarcomas are sometimes markedly cystic.

only *SSX1* and *SSX2*.[911] The *SYT-SSX* fusion gene transcript is detectable in both fresh and paraffin-embedded tissue by RT-PCR and if present is diagnostic for synovial sarcoma. Most renal synovial sarcomas are of the monophasic type and this has been associated with the *SS18-SSX1* translocation. Interestingly, both spindle cell and tumors with rhabdoid elements have been found to have *SYT-SSX2* fusion transcripts.[908,912]

Differential Diagnosis

Synovial sarcomas should be differentiated from other primary renal spindle cell neoplasms. The major differential diagnosis is sarcomatoid carcinoma where the sarcomatoid component has overgrown the original epithelial neoplasm. Sarcomatoid carcinoma will often retain expression of cytokeratins, at least focally, and expression of PAX8 is present in the majority. Desmosomes may be identified by electron microscopy.

Blastema-predominant Wilms tumors may superficially resemble synovial sarcoma. Careful sampling will usually reveal the epithelial components of Wilms' tumor, while stromal differentiation should also exclude synovial sarcoma. Renal primitive neuroectodermal tumor may also cause diagnostic difficulty although positive expression of FLI1 and neuroendocrine markers is usually helpful. Clear cell sarcoma of kidney and cellular mesoblastic nephroma occur in younger patients, although in some instances these tumors, as well as other primary sarcomas of the kidney, can only be differentiated through genetic studies for the translocations typical of synovial sarcoma.

Prognosis and Treatment

Follow-up studies of renal synovial sarcoma show a high incidence of postoperative metastases. It has been suggested that monophasic synovial sarcomas have a more favorable prognosis than biphasic tumors, although this is debated.[910,911]

MIXED MESENCHYMAL AND EPITHELIAL TUMORS

Cystic Nephroma

Introduction

Cystic nephroma was first described by Walter Edmunds in 1892.[916] During the last 100 years, many terms have been applied to this lesion, reflecting diverse views on its pathogenesis. Although Edmunds regarded cystic nephroma as a neoplasm, some have considered it to be a developmental lesion. Osathanondh and Potter[917] considered multilocular cysts to be a form of renal dysplasia, an opinion shared by Tang et al.,[918] who, based upon their ultrastructural observations, concluded that cystic nephroma results from segmental maldevelopment of the ureteric bud. Coming full circle, Joshi and Beckwith[654] revived the notion that cystic nephroma is a neoplasm. They suggested that it is closely related in

pathogenesis to nephroblastoma, possibly being an extremely differentiated cystic partially differentiated nephroblastoma, a view shared by Hartman et al.[919] Progressive enlargement when followed without resection, a property suggestive of a neoplastic process, has twice been reported in detail.

Diagnostic criteria for cystic nephroma were first formulated by Powell et al.,[920] in 1951. These criteria subsequently were reformulated by Boggs and Kimmelstiel and later by Eble and Bonsib.[212,921]

Many pathologists believe that cystic nephroma and mixed epithelial stromal tumor are part of the spectrum of a single tumor.[922,923] This is the approach taken in the current International Society of Urological Pathology classification.[7] We are not convinced of this and continue to use these diagnoses separately.

Epidemiology and Clinical Features

Cystic nephroma often is found incidentally by radiologic examinations for other conditions[925] but may present as a palpable mass in the flank[916,925] or with pain or hematuria. Rarely, cystic nephroma is bilateral.[926–930] Delahunt et al.,[931] reported a familial cluster of cystic nephroma in association with pleuropulmonary blastoma (Box 2-7). Data on age and gender are available for almost 200 cases of cystic nephroma. The data are not from population-based series but instead reflect the consultation referral patterns of cystic kidney lesions to William Beaumont Hospital,[932] kidney tumors to the Armed Forces Institute of Pathology,[933] and pediatric kidney tumors to the NWTS.[654] The review of Castillo et al.[934] is a collection of reported cases from around the world. It is apparent from these studies that most lesions occur in children younger than 4 years and in that population, males predominate in a ratio of approximately 2:1. Cystic nephroma is exceptional from age 5 to age 30, accounting for merely 5% of the total. Above age 30, there is another group of patients whose ages range into old age. In this adult population, women predominate over men by approximately 8:1. Most authors believe that cystic nephroma in the pediatric age group and in adults represent two different and unrelated entities.

Pathology

Gross Features

Cystic nephromas are typically round expansile masses that are well demarcated from the surrounding kidney by a thick fibrous pseudocapsule, (Fig. 2-130) which may occasionally

---

Box 2-7 ● PLEUROPULMONARY BLASTOMA AND CYSTIC NEPHROMA

- Familial association first described in 1993
- Cystic nephroma in 6% of patients and families with pleuropulmonary blastoma
- Associated with pediatric cystic nephroma
- Mutation of *DICER1* gene implicated

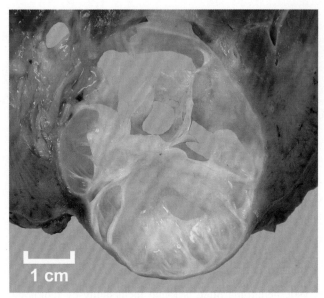

FIGURE 2-130 ■ Cystic nephroma. The tumor is entirely cystic and separated from the renal parenchyma by a fibrous pseudocapsule.

contain a few tubules and glomeruli, indicating its origin from compression of the adjacent renal tissue. The tumors vary widely in size (averaging 9 cm in diameter in a large series).[933]

The location within the kidney is variable: cystic nephroma commonly herniates into the renal pelvis[933,935] or renal sinus[936] or may bulge from the renal cortex. Rarely, the tumor may be predominantly in the renal sinus with only tenuous connection to the renal parenchyma.[933,937] The tumor is completely cystic and there are no solid nodules. The cysts contain clear or hemorrhagic fluid with chemical properties similar to serum[938] and range in size from microscopic to 5 cm or greater. The septa are thin (typically <5 mm), translucent, and uniform. Necrosis and hemorrhage are rare except when the tumor has herniated into the renal pelvis. The septa may become focally calcified.[939]

Microscopic Features
Cystic nephromas are simple structures (Fig. 2-131). The cysts are lined by a single layer of flattened, cuboidal, or hobnail epithelium. Occasionally the lining cells have pale or clear cytoplasm. Mitotic figures are not visible or are very rare. Many tumors have areas of cystic surface that lack epithelium.

The septa are thin and correspond to the outlines of the cysts, without expansile nodules. The septal stroma consists of fibrous tissue that varies from myxoid to collagenous (Fig. 2-132). Sometimes it is cellular and the cells have a wavy appearance that brings ovarian stroma to mind.[933,940] Skeletal muscle and fat are not present in the septa.[654,933,934] Smooth muscle differentiation is usually no greater than subtle in hematoxylin and eosin-stained sections. The septa of cystic nephroma often contain small cysts lined by bland cuboidal epithelial cells resembling renal tubules cut in cross section.

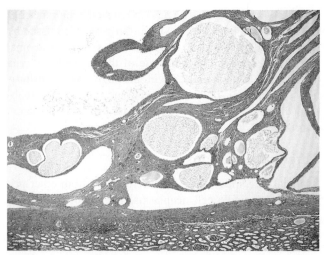

FIGURE 2-131 ■ Cystic nephroma. The septa often contain small cysts.

A few cystic nephromas have been examined by fine needle aspiration cytology.[924,941–943] The cytologic findings have included papillary clusters and small sheets of cohesive epithelial cells with vacuolated or scant cytoplasm. There has often been a high nuclear/cytoplasmic ratio and the nuclei have often had irregular contours and prominent nucleoli. The background has been proteinaceous or inflammatory without necrosis. Hughes et al.[924] emphasized the difficulty in distinguishing these findings from those of cystic renal cell carcinoma.

Ancillary and Special Studies
The epithelium lining the cysts typically gives a nicely positive immunohistochemical reaction with antibodies to cytokeratins (CAM 5.2, AE1/AE3, and cytokeratin 19).[944] A positive reaction with antibody to smooth muscle–specific actin is very common in the septal stromal cells, but positive

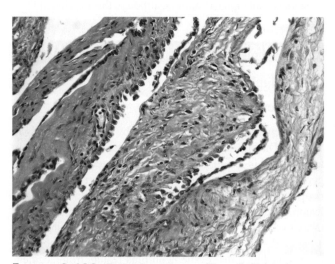

FIGURE 2-132 ■ Cystic nephroma. The cells lining the cysts may be flattened, may be cuboidal, or may have a hobnail appearance. The septa are composed of spindle cells and are often densely collagenized.

reactions for desmin are much less frequent.[944] Positive reactions for estrogen receptor and progesterone receptor are found in the stroma of about 50% of cystic nephromas.[944]

Ultrastructural studies by Coleman[945] showed that the lining cells have short microvilli, and Tang et al.[918] concluded that they closely resemble the epithelium of the collecting tubules. Shimokama and Watanabe[925] used scanning electron microcopy to demonstrate long cilia and variable numbers of microvilli on the surfaces of the epithelial cells.

Differential Diagnosis

Tumors with the gross and microscopic appearances of cystic nephroma found in young children have historically been called cystic nephroma by pediatric pathologists, surgeons, and oncologists. Almost all of these tumors have occurred in children younger than 48 months, and in this population, the ratio of boys to girls is about 2:1. An alternative that we prefer is to consider these tumors in this population to be cystic partially differentiated nephroblastomas in which the component of recognizable Wilms' tumor elements is very small or absent.

Tubulocystic renal cell carcinoma is a potential differential diagnostic consideration. Grossly, the cysts in cystic nephroma tend to be, on average, much larger than the cysts of tubulocystic renal cell carcinoma and more variable in size. The septa of cystic nephroma usually are thicker and stiffer than the septa of tubulocystic renal cell carcinoma. Microscopically, the cells lining the cysts of tubulocystic renal cell carcinoma have more prominent nucleoli, a greater tendency to form apocrine-like cytoplasmic "snouts," and are much less likely to become flattened and inconspicuous than the cells lining the cysts of cystic nephroma.

The poorly defined and rare entity known as "segmental cystic dysplasia" of the kidney also comes up in the differential diagnosis of small lesions.[946] If the lesion is an expansile roughly spherical lesion with a pseudocapsule, it should be diagnosed as a cystic nephroma. Occasionally, the collision of a few simple cysts in the renal cortex will raise the possibility of an early cystic nephroma. If any glomeruli are present in the septa it is easy to recognize that the lesion is merely a collision of simple cysts.

Prognosis and Treatment

Nephrectomy and partial nephrectomy are curative, but incomplete excision with a nephron-sparing procedure such as partial nephrectomy has occasionally been followed by local recurrence.[927,933] There are a few old reports of sarcoma arising in cystic nephroma, but these probably were examples of renal synovial sarcoma.[933]

Mixed Epithelial and Stromal Tumor

Introduction

Early reports of mixed epithelial and mesenchymal tumors in adults applied the terms "cystic hamartoma of the renal pelvis"[947] and "adult mesoblastic nephroma."[948] Mixed epithelial and stromal tumor is the name now used for these tumors.[5,6] This tumor is unrelated to congenital mesoblastic nephroma, and that term should not be used for these tumors.[949] Because of the consistent expression of estrogen and progesterone receptors in the spindle cells, the possibility of a hormonal influence in the development of these neoplasms has been raised.[950,951]

Epidemiology and Clinical Features

Mixed epithelial and stromal tumors are much more common in women than in men (4-5:1) and occur over a broad age range[950,951] including a few in prepubertal children.[952] Mixed epithelial and stromal tumors have been described in the hyperparathyroidism–jaw tumor syndrome related to germline mutations in the *cell division cycle 73* gene (HUGO-approved gene symbol: *CDC73*), previously known as *HRPT2* gene (Box 2-8).[88,953] Some studies have found an association with estrogen therapy, but the clinical information has been very sketchy for most reported cases.[950,954] Presenting complaints have been similar to other renal neoplasms. Radiologically, mixed epithelial and stromal tumors are complex solid and cystic lesions that are classified as Bosniak category 3 or 4.[955,956] Whether the epithelial component represents an intrinsic part of the tumor or entrapped tubules has been debated.[954] Genetic analysis using microdissection of the epithelial and mesenchymal components demonstrated nonrandom X chromosome inactivation in both components suggesting that both are neoplastic and of a common origin.[957]

Pathology

Gross Features

Mixed epithelial and stromal tumors are typically solid with some cysts (Fig. 2-133). The proportions of solid and cystic tissue are variable, but predominantly cystic ones are a small minority. Some tumors have been well circumscribed and others infiltrative. Some have been very small incidental findings in kidneys removed for other reasons.[958] Occasionally, they grow into the lumen of the renal pelvis and even into the ureter as a polypoid mass. A peculiar feature is the development of domed nodules that protrude into the lumens of large cysts or the renal pelvis (Fig. 2-134).

> **Box 2-8 ● FEATURES OF THE HYPERPARATHYROIDISM–JAW TUMOR SYNDROME**
>
> - Parathyroid adenoma or carcinoma with hyperparathyroidism
> - Fibro-osseous lesions of mandible and maxilla
> - Renal pathology includes (not well characterized)
>   - Mixed epithelial and stromal tumor
>   - Adult Wilms tumor
>   - Papillary renal cell carcinoma
>   - Cysts

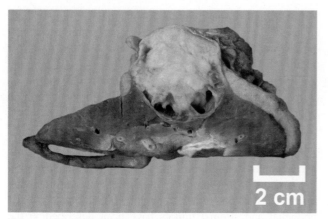

FIGURE 2-133 ■ Mixed epithelial and stromal tumor showing the typical solid and cystic gross appearance.

Microscopic Features

Mixed epithelial and stromal tumors often are remarkably complex mixtures of stromal and epithelial elements (Fig. 2-135). The epithelial components are frequently strikingly heterogeneous ranging from simple ducts to complex branching glandular formations to florid complex papillary structures to microscopic cysts and larger cysts (Figs. 2-136 and 2-137). In some there are spatulate papillae resembling those seen in mammary phyllodes tumors. The epithelial cells range from flattened to cuboidal to columnar with clear to eosinophilic cytoplasm. Urothelium is present occasionally. Ciliated and mucin-secreting cells sometimes are present. Cervical glandular and intestinal-type epithelium with Paneth-like cells have been reported.[959] A single tumor containing elements resembling a mucinous borderline tumor has been reported.[960] The mesenchymal component ranges from hypocellular and fibrotic to more cellular fibroblastic and myofibroblastic foci to more cellular spindle cell stroma. Smooth muscle differentiation often is evident in hematoxylin and eosin-stained sections, particularly at the periphery

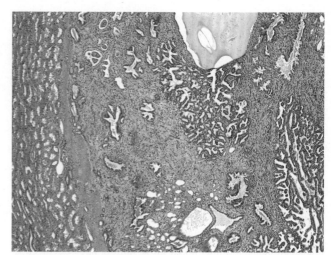

FIGURE 2-135 ■ Mixed epithelial and stromal tumor showing a complex mixture of epithelial structures in a background of spindle cells with smooth muscle differentiation.

of the tumor. Patches of closely spaced thick-walled blood vessels are sometimes present. Fat is occasionally present and may predominate.[961]

Ancillary and Special Studies

The spindle cells of the stroma express vimentin, actin, and desmin.[950,951,954] In most cases, the stromal but not the epithelial cells express estrogen and progesterone receptors (Fig. 2-138).[950,951,954] Estrogen and progesterone receptor expression is also found in the stroma of cystic nephroma and angiomyolipoma, as well as in reactive renal stroma, so their finding is not of great diagnostic utility.[962] The spindle cells are consistently found to be negative for angiomyolipoma markers HMB45 and melan-A. The epithelial cells show expression of renal tubular antigens including PAX2 and PAX8.[963] Ultrastructural studies have shown smooth muscle differentiation in the stromal cells.[954]

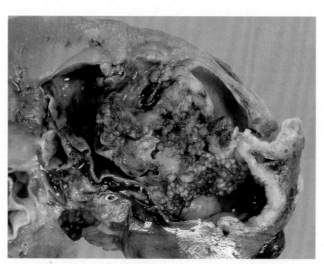

FIGURE 2-134 ■ Mixed epithelial and stromal tumor showing smooth-surfaced mural nodules on the inner surface of a large cyst.

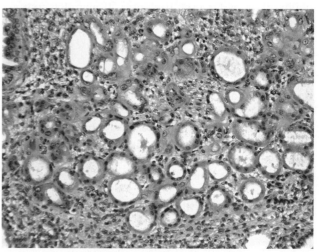

FIGURE 2-136 ■ Mixed epithelial and stromal tumor. Clusters of small cysts closely resembling nephrogenic adenoma are one of the most common epithelial elements in these tumors.

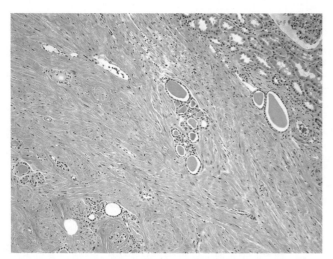

FIGURE 2-137 ■ Mixed epithelial and stromal tumor. Small cysts containing brightly eosinophilic proteinaceous fluid are a very common epithelial element. The lumens range greatly in size, down to pinpoint or smaller. The stroma here consists of smooth muscle and fibrous tissue.

Differential Diagnosis

The differential diagnosis includes other tumors that can have a mixture of epithelial and mesenchymal elements including cystic nephroma, angiomyolipoma with entrapped cysts, nephroblastoma, synovial sarcoma, and sarcomatoid carcinoma. The last three have histologic features of malignancy that exclude them. Cystic nephromas are simple cystic structures without solid areas, and their epithelial cells lack the heterogeneity of mixed epithelial and stromal tumor. Angiomyolipoma with entrapped cysts has the characteristic thick-walled blood vessels and fat; if the latter are not present, positive immunohistochemical reactions for melan-A, HMB45, or cathepsin K will confirm the diagnosis of angiomyolipoma. Nephroblastoma is recognized by a blastema

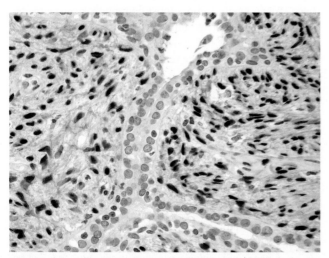

FIGURE 2-138 ■ Mixed epithelial and stromal tumor. Immunohistochemistry with antibody to progesterone receptor is frequently positive in the nuclei of the stromal cells.

component; in the absence of blastema, the epithelial component of nephroblastoma is malignant with cytologic atypia and mitotic activity.

Prognosis and Treatment

To date, the almost all of the reported cases appear to have been cured by surgical resection. A few cases have been described that may represent mixed epithelial and stromal tumor with sarcomatous or carcinomatous change in the mesenchymal component.[964–969] In these tumors, the malignant component appears to have been an obvious and substantial part of the tumor.

NEUROENDOCRINE TUMORS

Carcinoid Tumor

Epidemiology and Clinical Features

Well-differentiated neuroendocrine tumors, similar to carcinoids of the respiratory and gastrointestinal tracts, occur in the kidney. To date, fewer than 100 cases have been reported with the largest series consisting of 21 patients.[970] There is an even gender distribution, and tumors most frequently occur between the third and sixth decade, with a mean age at presentation of approximately 50 years.[970,971] There is an association with horseshoe kidney.[972] Tumors have also been seen in association with polycystic kidney.[973]

Most carcinoids are asymptomatic and are discovered incidentally. Other presenting features are abdominal mass, back or flank pain, anemia, hematuria, or fever. The carcinoid syndrome is rarely seen although other hormonal effects, such as Cushing syndrome, have been reported.[970–974]

Pathology

Gross Features

The majority of tumors are intrarenal and may extend beyond the renal capsule, while tumors may also arise from the renal pelvis.[975] These tumors are rarely small at diagnosis with 70% being >4 cm.[976] Carcinoids have a typically tan-brown cut surface and are usually solid with, at least, focal pseudoencapsulation. Occasionally, tumors may contain foci of hemorrhage or cystic degeneration.[971]

Microscopic Features

Histologically, renal carcinoids resemble carcinoids found in other organs and may form sheets, trabeculae, ribbons, and glands (Fig. 2-139A).[970,971] The nuclei are ovoid to elongate with finely stippled chromatin and an inconspicuous nucleolus. Mitotic activity is usually <2/10 HPF. Foci of tumor necrosis are rare.

Ancillary and Special Studies

Most tumors are argentaffin and argyrophil negative.[975] Immunohistochemistry for synaptophysin and chromogranin is positive in 90% or more of renal carcinoids

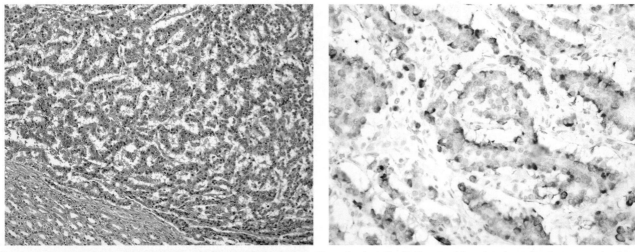

FIGURE 2-139 ■ **A:** Carcinoid showing characteristic ribbons of neoplastic cells. **B:** Immunohistochemistry for chromogranin gives a positive reaction in the cytoplasm of the carcinoid cells.

(Fig. 2-139B).[971,977] Cytokeratin CAM 5.2 and vimentin are usually positive. Importantly for the differential diagnosis with primitive neuroectodermal tumor, a strong membranous reaction for CD99 is found in approximately 85% of renal carcinoids.[977] At least focal positivity for cytokeratin 7 and 20, and prostate-specific acid phosphatase have also been reported in occasional cases.[970,978] PAX2 and PAX8 were not detected in any of nine renal carcinoids studied.[977] Ultrastructural examination shows typical membrane-bound neurosecretory granules.[970]

A few genetic studies have been undertaken, and abnormalities of chromosomes 3 and 13 have been reported.[979,980]

Differential Diagnosis

The differential diagnosis is other renal neuroendocrine tumors, although carcinoids showing a typical morphology should present little diagnostic difficulty. Small cell carcinoma, neuroblastoma, and primitive neuroectodermal tumor usually demonstrate significant mitotic activity. Small cell carcinoma often has little cytoplasm and prominent nuclear molding, while neuroblastoma has a typical stroma, and primitive neuroectodermal tumor is CD99 positive.

Prognosis and Treatment

Approximately 50% of patients, and 60% of patients with tumors >4 cm in diameter, have metastases at presentation. An age of >40 years at diagnosis, the presence of solid tumor, extrarenal spread, and a mitotic rate >1/10 HPF have been shown to be associated with an adverse prognosis.[976] Despite the high incidence of metastasis at presentation, patients with renal carcinoid have a protracted clinical course. In the largest reported series, only one patient with both liver and bone metastasis had died of disease, while 47% were alive without active disease and one had died of other causes, in follow-up periods ranging from 1 to 5 years.

Neuroendocrine Carcinoma

Epidemiology and Clinical Features

To date, fewer than 100 cases of neuroendocrine carcinoma of the kidney have been described.[981] Most are small cell carcinomas, with or without urothelial elements, that may also show foci of squamous or glandular differentiation.[982,983] Large cell neuroendocrine carcinoma of the kidney is much rarer.[984] Median age at diagnosis is 60 years, and presenting features are frequently flank pain and hematuria.[971,982,985,986] Renal neuroendocrine carcinoma has a poor prognosis. Metastases at presentation are frequent, and survival beyond a few months is uncommon.[982]

Pathology

Renal neuroendocrine carcinomas are usually irregular and large, and are tan-gray with extensive necrosis and hemorrhage. When small, tumors most commonly occur adjacent to the renal pelvis or within the renal sinus, which supports the suggestion that the majority of these tumors originate from the urothelium of the renal pelvis or calyces.

Microscopic Features

Histologically, these tumors show features similar to small cell carcinoma of the lung with round to oval cells containing scanty cytoplasm and exhibiting varying degrees of nuclear molding. Immunohistochemistry for pancytokeratin shows dot-like expression in the vast majority of these tumors.[982] Immunohistochemical reactions for synaptophysin and chromogranin are positive in 50% to 75% of renal neuroendocrine carcinomas.[982] CD56, Leu 7, and neuron-specific enolase are variable.[971,981,986] Ultrastructurally these tumors contain dense-core neurosecretory granules.[985] Genetic studies have been undertaken in a few cases, and these show multiple chromosome gains, loss of *TP53,* and amplification of the *MYC* gene.[981]

The differential diagnosis includes urothelial carcinoma with small cell differentiation of the renal pelvis and metastatic tumor, with lung being the most likely primary site. The presence of an identifiable urothelial component would be consistent with renal pelvis origin. The possibility of metastasis requires exclusion by clinical history.

Primitive Neuroectodermal Tumor or Ewing Sarcoma

Epidemiology and Clinical Features

The Ewing family of tumors is a group of tumors composed of small cells, which includes Ewing sarcoma of bone, extraskeletal Ewing sarcoma, Askin tumor, and primitive neuroectodermal tumor. Although renal primitive neuroectodermal tumors are uncommon, 79 cases were reported from the NWTS in 2001, 11 from a multicenter collaboration in 2002, and 16 from a single center in 2008.[987–989] Many of those referred to the NWTS were referred because monophasic blastemal Wilms tumor was suspected.[987]

The first case of renal primitive neuroectodermal tumor was reported in a 2-year-old male in 1975.[990] The age at presentation has ranged from <1 year to 75 years (with the majority of patients in the range of 16 to 25 years), and there is an equal gender distribution.[987,988] Primitive neuroectodermal tumors in children are much rarer than in adults.[991,992]

The presentation of these tumors is nonspecific, with abdominal flank pain being most common and hematuria, night sweats, abdominal mass, and metastatic disease less frequent.[988,993,994]

Pathology

Gross Features

Primitive neuroectodermal tumors are frequently large at presentation, and in one series ranged from 8 to 16 cm (median 11 cm) in diameter.[988] The tumors are usually poorly circumscribed, solid, and lobulated, being tan to yellow on cut surface and frequently with necrosis and hemorrhage. In occasional cases, cysts are present.

Microscopic Features

Renal primitive neuroectodermal tumor is similar histologically to its extrarenal and skeletal counterparts. The tumors are composed of sheets of small cells with scanty cytoplasm that may occasionally appear clear.[988] Where present, cells with clear cytoplasm usually show positive staining with periodic acid–Schiff, which is abolished by diastase digestion. The nuclei are vesicular; nucleoli are inconspicuous, and mitotic figures are common. Occasionally there are rosettes. The tumor usually infiltrates adjacent renal tissue, and extrarenal extension and invasion of the renal vein are common.

Ancillary and Special Studies

CD99 is expressed in more than 90% of renal primitive neuroectodermal tumors, and the CD99 staining is typically membranous.[995] About two-thirds of these tumors give a positive nuclear reaction for FLI1.[995] Positive reactions for cytokeratin are seen in <10% of these tumors.[995] In the few cases studied, expression of synaptophysin was reported.[987,996] Approximately 25% of renal primitive neuroectodermal tumors show positive nuclear reactions for WT1[987,988,995] and are rarely positive for CD31.

Electron microscopy usually demonstrates neural features with cytoplasmic processes containing microtubules and dense core granules. In some tumors, cells show epithelioid features, and intracytoplasmic glycogen may be present.[987]

Genetics

The vast majority of these tumors contain translocations involving the *EWSR1* gene on chromosome 22. Most frequently, the translocation fuses *EWSR1* with *FLI1* on chromosome 11. In a minority of these tumors *EWSR1/FLI1* fusion transcripts, representing the molecular equivalent of t(11;22), are demonstrable by RT-PCR.[995,997] *FLI1* is a member of the E26 transformation-specific family of genes and occasionally *EWSR1* is fused to other members of this family: *ERG*, *ETV*, or *FEV*. Rarely, *FUS* on chromosome 16 can substitute for *EWSR1*, and an *FUS/ERG* fusion has been reported in a renal primitive neuroectodermal tumor.[998]

Differential Diagnosis

Primitive neuroectodermal tumor must be differentiated from blastema-predominant Wilms tumor. Wilms tumor typically has overlapping nuclei and may show focal epithelial differentiation. The detection of CD99, vimentin, and FLI1 in primitive neuroectodermal tumor combined with a negative reaction for WT1 is useful diagnostically, although very occasionally Wilms tumor may give a positive reaction for CD99.[988]

Prognosis and Treatment

Most tumors are high stage at presentation[987] with extrarenal infiltration and renal vein invasion. Common metastatic sites are bone and lung. In one series, 4/14 patients died of disease with follow-up to 35 months, while in another series 5/8 patients had died with a median follow-up of 17 months.[987,988] With aggressive chemotherapy and radiotherapy, a 5-year survival of 40% to 50% has been achieved.[98,999]

Neuroblastoma

Epidemiology and Clinical Features

Primary adrenal and retroperitoneal neuroblastoma may infiltrate the kidney; however, in such instances imaging studies usually permit identification of the primary tumor site.[1000] Rarely neuroblastoma may originate in the kidney, and this can result in diagnostic difficulty especially with core biopsies. At the time of presentation, Wilms tumor is important in the differential diagnosis.[1001] Constitutional symptoms or intratumoral calcification are preoperative findings that favor neuroblastoma over Wilms tumor and suggest laboratory measurement of urinary catecholamines.[1002]

Pathology

Renal neuroblastomas are often large firm tumors with a yellow-red cut surface and areas of hemorrhage.[1000] Some are within the renal parenchyma[1001] while others arise within the renal sinus, not involving the adrenal gland.[1003] Histologically, renal neuroblastoma consists of small round cells with nuclei showing a salt and pepper chromatin pattern. Homer-Wright rosettes may be present. Although stroma-poor tumors may resemble nephroblastoma, intratumoral calcification, vascular encasement on imaging, and elevated urinary catecholamines are indicative of neuroblastoma.[1002] The presence of epithelial elements or positive nuclear immunohistochemical reactions for WT1 are diagnostic of nephroblastoma.[1004]

Pheochromocytoma or Paraganglioma

Rare cases of intrarenal pheochromocytoma or paraganglioma have been reported. These range in size from 2.5 to 20 cm and may present as abdominal pain or mass, or hypertension.[1005,1006] Tumors may be intrarenal or may originate from the renal sinus. Grossly these tumors are yellow-brown to tan and frequently appear cystic.[1005,1007] Microscopically, renal pheochromocytoma resembles similar tumors found within the adrenal and elsewhere, and have an identical immunohistochemical expression pattern.

Renal pheochromocytoma mimics renal cell carcinoma clinically and grossly, and may cause diagnostic difficulty microscopically, although immunohistochemistry is usually helpful.[1008] These tumors are usually benign, although in one case metastatic spread occurred 13 years after diagnosis.[1009]

HEMATOPOIETIC AND LYMPHOID TUMORS

Lymphoma

Epidemiology and Clinical Features

Malignant lymphoma involving the kidney is either primary or secondary disease. A diagnosis of primary renal lymphoma is usually restricted to those cases with localized renal disease, although the term has also been used to include those with renal involvement as the presenting feature.[1010] There is some debate as to whether primary lymphoma occurs in the absence of occult disseminated disease, as in most cases extranodal lymphoma developed shortly after diagnosis.[1011,1012] Despite this, cases of primary renal lymphoma without progression or with no evidence of lymphadenopathy at surgery have been reported.[1013] Secondary renal lymphoma, the involvement of the kidney as an extranodal manifestation of systemic disease, is more frequently encountered.

Primary renal lymphomas are seen in 3% of patients presenting with renal masses and account for 0.7% of extranodal lymphomas,[1010,1011,1014] with bilateral disease being present in 43% of cases.[1015] There is a male predominance, and patients range in age from 20 to 82 years, with most patients presenting in the eighth decade.[1011,1014,1015]

Secondary involvement of the kidney in systemic lymphoma is seen commonly in advanced disease and is identified in 30% to 50% of cases at autopsy.[1013,1015] In addition to renal involvement by both non-Hodgkin and Hodgkin lymphoma, infiltration of the kidney has also been reported in intravascular malignant lymphomatosis and EBV-associated posttransplant lymphoproliferative disease.[1016]

There are reports of renal cell carcinoma and lymphoma developing in the same patient.[1017,1018] This appears to be a late treatment effect and is seen more frequently with non-Hodgkin rather than Hodgkin lymphoma.

Diagnostic criteria for primary renal lymphoma are (1) renal failure as an initial presenting feature, (2) enlargement of the kidneys without obstruction or other organ or nodal involvement, (3) absence of other causes of renal failure, (4) diagnosis made by renal biopsy, and (5) rapid improvement of renal function after therapy.[1015]

A variety of signs and symptoms have been reported in association with primary renal lymphoma including abdominal mass, weight loss, back and flank pain, hematuria, anorexia, and acute renal failure.[1011,1014,1015] These features are nonspecific, and in many of the cases, a primary epithelial malignancy was suspected, with definitive diagnosis being made following nephrectomy.[1011,1014] Similarly, the clinical features of secondary renal lymphoma are nonspecific although surprisingly the majority of patients are free of renal symptoms at the time of diagnosis.[1011] Patients with HIV-related acquired immunodeficiency syndrome show a predisposition to immunoblastic and Burkett subtypes of non-Hodgkin lymphoma.

Pathology

Gross Features

The macroscopic appearance of renal lymphoma is variable, and several patterns have been described. Tumors may form solitary or multiple masses (Fig. 2-140), or show infiltration from contiguous retroperitoneal disease or diffuse infiltration, and these patterns are reflected in reported radiologic findings. With localized disease, the tumors usually form soft, fleshy or firm, white to gray nodules, which are typically visible on the cortical surface of the kidney. Localized tumors frequently arise in the renal sinus and expand to surround and infiltrate hilar structures.[468,1011,1019] In advanced disease, tumor may extend to encase the adrenal gland, ureter, renal artery, or renal vein, and this may be associated with hydronephrosis. On rare occasions, tumor occlusion or thrombosis of major renal arteries or veins may be seen, and clinically renal lymphoma may mimic renal cell carcinoma with renal vein or vena cava involvement.

Less frequently lymphoma diffusely infiltrates the kidney. Here there is expansion of the renal volume, while the renal cortex and medulla are pale, with obliteration of the corticomedullary junction.[468]

Microscopic Features

The microscopic features of renal lymphoma vary according to the type of lymphoma. Where the lymphoma consists of

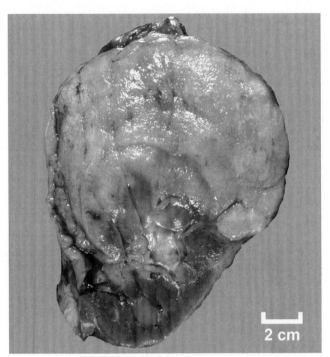

FIGURE 2-140 ■ Lymphoma forming a discrete large fleshy mass.

discrete nodules, there are sheets of tumor cells with effacement of renal architecture. At the periphery of the nodules there is often interstitial infiltration with adjacent fibrosis and relative sparing of glomeruli and tubules.[1013] In cases where there is a diffuse infiltrate of lymphoma cells, there is infiltration of the renal interstitium (Fig. 2-141) and again, relative sparing of glomeruli and tubules is commonly seen.[1013]

All morphologic varieties of lymphoma have been reported, with diffuse large B-cell lymphomas being more commonly seen than small cell lymphomas. Hodgkin lymphoma is unusual, while rare examples of low-grade mucosa-associated lymphoid tissue lymphomas have been descri bed.[468,1011,1013,1014,1020] As with all cases of lymphoma, panels of

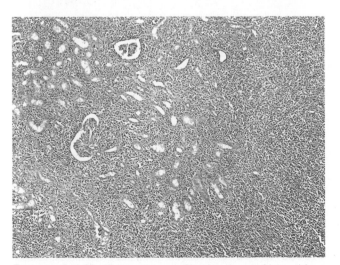

FIGURE 2-141 ■ Lymphoma infiltrating the renal interstitium.

immunohistochemical stains, supported, where appropriate, by flow cytometry and genetic studies, are necessary for definitive diagnosis.

In cases of intravascular malignant lymphomatosis neoplastic cells are seen within glomerular capillaries. Tumor cells are also marginated in interstitial capillaries, with early infiltration into the interstitium.[1016,1021]

Posttransplant lymphoproliferative disease, resulting from an uncontrolled proliferation of EBV-transformed B cells, is associated with a spectrum of lymphoproliferative lesions, including B-cell lymphoma. This is characterized by expansile nodules of atypical EBV-infected B cells with foci of serpiginous necrosis. Hemorrhage, infarction, vasculitis, tubulitis, and interstitial infiltrates are also frequently present.

Lymphoma has been associated with paraneoplastic glomerulopathy. With non-Hodgkin lymphoma, minimal change disease and amyloidosis may be seen. Glomerular lesions have been reported in association with non-Hodgkin lymphoma; however, these are rarely seen, and the wide variety of glomerulopathies reported has led to the suggestion that any association is coincidental.[1015]

Differential Diagnosis

Renal lymphoma frequently mimics renal carcinoma both clinically and on imaging studies. In these cases, the correct diagnosis may be suspected if there is involvement of perirenal structures or the renal hilum.

Prognosis and Treatment

Although remissions with up to 147 months follow-up have been recorded for primary renal lymphoma, progressive disease is frequently seen with median survivals of 5.5 to 34 months.[1022] Secondary renal lymphoma is usually associated with advanced disease and has a poor prognosis.

Plasmacytoma

Epidemiology and Clinical Features

Extraosseus plasmacytoma originating in the kidney is rare, with most instances being a manifestation of systemic disease. In multiple myeloma, extramedullary lesions are present in 76% of cases, with the organs most commonly involved being, in descending order of frequency, the liver, spleen, lymph nodes, and kidney. In some instances, plasmacytoma detected on imaging is considered to be renal cell carcinoma or urothelial carcinoma of the renal pelvis, and in such cases the correct diagnosis is only made following nephrectomy.[1023]

Fewer than 20 cases of renal plasmacytoma have been reported.[1024–1026] There is a 3:1 male predominance, and most patients present in the sixth decade.[1023] Presenting features include abdominal mass, hematuria, weight loss, and renal failure, while some tumors are detected as an incidental finding following investigations of unrelated conditions.[1023,1025]

Pathology

On macroscopic examination plasmacytoma usually forms a well-circumscribed lobulated mass, which has been reported to be up to 21 cm in maximum extent. Tumor may also involve the renal pelvis, adjacent soft tissue, and lymph nodes.[1023,1027] The cut surface of the tumor ranges from light gray to tan, and foci of hemorrhage may be present.

Microscopically, the tumors consist of plasma cells forming sheets, cords, and follicles, and occasionally a hyaline interstitial matrix may be present.[1023] The plasma cells are usually well differentiated although anaplastic plasmacytoma, with irregular nuclei, prominent nucleoli, and appreciable mitotic activity, has been described.[1024]

Leukemia

Epidemiology and Clinical Features

Leukemic involvement of the kidneys is infrequently encountered. From a series of 423 pediatric patients, 12 cases with renal involvement were detected by computerized tomography. It is, however, likely that the true incidence was underestimated in this study as not all patients underwent imaging studies.[1028] In this series, patients ranged in age from 7 months to 21 years, and the histologic diagnosis was acute lymphoblastic leukemia, acute myelogenous leukemia, or juvenile myelomonocytic leukemia. In all cases, there were additional sites of extramedullary disease. Unilateral or bilateral renal enlargement and focal renal parenchymal abnormalities were commonly seen, although renal dysfunction was present in only two patients. This contrasts to other reports where recent-onset renal failure has been shown to be associated with leukemic involvement of the kidneys.[1029,1030] Bilateral nephromegaly is a rare presentation.[1031]

Myeloid sarcoma, previously known as chloroma and granulocytic sarcoma, has, in rare instances, been reported from the kidney.[1032,1033] Most tumors were found in autopsy studies, and multiple extrarenal leukemic masses were usually present. Clinical evidence of renal impairment is uncommon, with acute renal failure being seen in only five cases to date.[1034]

Pathology

Histologically these tumors consist of primitive granulocytic precursor cells. Eosinophilic myelocytes may resemble lymphoma and it has been shown that an immunohistochemical panel of CD20, CD43, C68, and M10 will identify 96% of cases.[1035] CD33 immunoreactivity has also been reported.[1033]

Myeloid sarcoma usually develops in patients with known leukemia or myeloproliferative disorder.[1034,1036] When tumor occurs in isolation, most patients develop leukemia within 2 years.

Germ Cell Tumors

Several instances of primary renal teratoma have been reported. The majority of these tumors have been diagnosed in children, and most have had benign histologic features.[1037–1040] In rare instances, renal teratoma contained carcinoid tumor,[1041–1043] and in one case yolk sac tumor was present.[1044] Tumors involved either the renal parenchyma or renal hilum and in two cases were associated with cystic renal dysplasia.[1039]. Occasional cases of apparently primary renal choriocarcinoma have also been described.[1045]

The pathogenesis of renal germ cell tumors is uncertain. Poorly differentiated urothelial carcinomas may show syncytiotrophoblastic differentiation and express the β subunit of human chorionic gonadotropin,[1046] while nephroblastoma may show teratoma-like differentiation.[1047]

Metastases

In autopsy studies, the kidneys are involved by metastases in up to 7% of patients dying of cancer with lung being the most common site of origin (Figs. 2-142 and 2-143).[1048,1049] Infrequently tumors present with renal metastasis as the primary manifestation. In one study of patients with known nonrenal malignancy, 21 of 36 renal masses (58%) were metastases.[1050] In some cases, surgical resection of metastatic kidney lesions is indicated for intractable hematuria. Metastases can be single or multiple; in some cases only microscopic involvement, limited to glomeruli, is present.[1051] In the latter instance, presentation with proteinuria or acute renal failure may result.[1052] Of note, renal cell carcinoma is the most common "host" of tumor-to-tumor metastasis.[1053,1054]

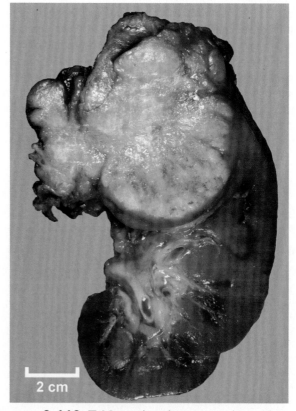

FIGURE 2-142 ■ Metastatic pulmonary carcinoma forms a large renal mass.

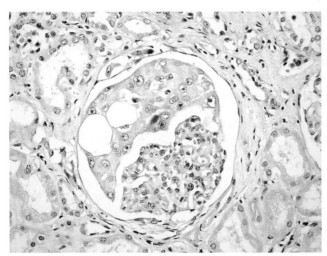

FIGURE 2-143 ■ Metastatic squamous cell carcinoma in a glomerulus.

Primary lesions detailed in this chapter are identifiable when the cytologic, clinical, and radiologic data are evaluated together. The cytologic diagnosis must adequately explain the clinical and radiologic information. If not, consideration of metastatic disease must be made. Individuals with known extrarenal primaries should have their previous tissues reviewed. Subsequent ancillary studies to resolve diagnostic dilemmas can then be intelligently selected.

Staging of Renal Cell Carcinoma

Of the many prognostic indicators investigated for renal cell carcinoma, it is recognized that tumor staging is the most powerful predictor of outcome in individual cases.[138] The earliest formalized staging system for renal cell carcinoma was proposed by Flocks and Kadesky in 1958, who devised a staging classification that focused upon local (intrarenal) spread, regional extension, and metastatic disease.[1055] This staging system was refined by Robson in 1963 and 1969 with expansion of the categories of extrarenal regional tumor extension (Table 2-19).[1056,1057] This staging system was widely adopted and in some centers remains in use today.

Table 2-19 ■ ROBSON STAGING CLASSIFICATION FOR RENAL CELL CARCINOMA	
Stage	**Features (5 year survival)**
1	Confined to kidney (66%)
2	Confined to Gerota fascia (64%)
3a	Gross renal vein invasion (42%)
3b	Lymph node invasion (42%)
3c	Combined 3a and 3b
4a	Adjacent organs involved
4b	Distant metastases (11%)

From Robson CJ. Radical nephrectomy for renal cell carcinoma. *J Urol* 1963;89:37–42.

In 1977, the Union Internationale Contre le Cancer (UICC) and the American Joint Committee for Cancer Staging and End Results Reporting (AJCC) proposed the TNM staging system for renal cell carcinoma.[1058] The first edition of the TNM classification for renal tumors was overly complex and contained a number of categories with unproven prognostic significance. As a consequence of this, the staging categories in the second edition published in 1983 were simplified.[1059] Subsequent editions continued to make revisions to the various categories (Table 2-20).[1060–1063] The current 2010 AJCC/TNM classification is presented in Table 2-21.[1064]

In the 1977 and 1983 TNM classifications, the first two staging categories were based upon tumor size (small vs. large), although no defining dimensions were identified.[1058,1059] This meant that assignment of pT1 and pT2 categories was left to the subjective assessment of the reporting pathologist. In the 1988 revision the cut point between pT1 and pT2 was set at 2.5 cm as it was considered that tumors smaller than this were unlikely to be associated with occult metastases.[1060] It was subsequently noted, however, that this cut point lacked discrimination, as only 1% to 8% of tumors in various series were <2.5 cm in diameter.[164] This was addressed in the 1997 revision of the staging system, with the cut point being raised to 7 cm.[1062] In follow-up studies, this cut point was found not to adequately stratify metastasizing and nonmetastasizing tumors, and in 2002 the pT1 category was subdivided into pT1a and pT1b with a cut point at 4.0 cm (Figs. 2-144 and 2-145).[1063] In the current edition (2010), an additional cut point was placed at 10 cm dividing the pT2 category into two subcategories (pT2a for tumors >7 and ≤10 cm and pT2b for tumors >10 cm) (Fig. 2-146).[1064]

The question of size and where to place specific cut points has been extensively studied over the past several decades and these have been consistent in finding a correlation between tumor size and prognosis. What has been inconsistent is the identified optimal cut points to be used to gain the maximum prognostic information from tumor size. The previous paragraph highlights the changes that have occurred over the evolution of the TNM staging system. There are data in the literature supporting cut points at 4.0, 4.5, 5.0, 5.5, 6.5, 7.5, and 10.0 cm.[139–142,156,1065]

Tumors showing regional spread beyond the confines of the kidney have, in all editions of the TNM classification, been assigned to the pT3 category. In the 1977 classification this incorporated a wide variety of features, but in the subsequent editions of the classification this category was simplified to include direct infiltration of perinephric tissues or the adrenal gland. In more recent studies, it was shown that infiltration of tumor into the renal sinus was of prognostic significance[1066] and this was included as a feature of the pT3a category in the 2002 edition of the TNM staging classification.

In the current staging system, invasion of the perinephric fat is staged as pT3a (Fig. 2-147). Tumors in the kidney frequently bulge beyond the contours of the kidney and into the perinephric fat. These tumors are often covered by

Table 2-20 ■ EVOLUTION OF THE UICC/AJCC PRIMARY TUMOR STAGING CATEGORY FOR RENAL CELL CARCINOMA

TNM (First Edition)[1058] T—Primary Tumor	TNM (Third Edition)[1060] T—Primary Tumor	TNM (Fifth Edition)[1062] T—Primary Tumor	TNM (Sixth Edition)[1063] T—Primary Tumor
T1 Intrarenal (small)	T1 ≤ 2.5cm, limited to kidney	T1 ≤ 7cm, limited to kidney	T1a ≤ 4 cm T1b > 4–≤7 cm
T2 Intrarenal (large)	T2 > 2.5cm, limited to kidney	T2 > 7cm, limited to kidney	T2 > 7 cm
T3a Confined to perinephric tissues	T3a Invades adrenal gland or perinephric tissues, but not beyond Gerota's fascia	T3a Invades adrenal gland or perinephric tissues but not beyond Gerota's fascia	T3a Invades adrenal gland, perirenal tissues including renal sinus (peripelvic) fat
T3b Involves renal vein	T3b Grossly into renal vein or vena cava	T3b Grossly into renal vein or vena cava below diaphragm	T3b into renal vein, including segmental (muscle containing) branches or cava below diaphragm
T3c Involves renal vein and infradiaphragmatic vena cava		T3c Grossly into vena cava above diaphragm	T3c vena cava above diaphragm
T4a Invasion of adjacent structures	T4 Invades beyond Gerota's fascia	T4 Invades beyond Gerota's fascia	T4 Invades beyond Gerota's fascia.
T4b Supradiaphragmatic vena cava infiltration			

Data from American Joint Committee for Cancer Staging and End Results Reporting. *Staging of Cancer at Genitourinary Sites: Kidney, Bladder, Prostate, and Testes. Manual for Staging of Cancer 1977.* 1st ed. Chicago, IL: American Joint Committee; 1977:109–130; American Joint Committee on Cancer. Kidney. In: Beahrs OH, Henson DE, Hutter RVP, et al., eds. *Manual for Staging of Cancer.* 3rd ed. Philadelphia, PA: J.B. Lippincott Co.; 1988:199–201; American Joint Committee on Cancer. Kidney. In: Fleming ID, Cooper JS, Henson DE, et al., eds. *AJCC Cancer Staging Manual.* 5th ed. Philadelphia, PA: Lippincott-Raven; 1997:231–234; American Joint Committee on Cancer. Kidney. In: Greene FL, Page DL, Fleming ID, et al., eds. *AJCC Cancer Staging Handbook.* 6th ed. New York: Springer-Verlag; 2002:323–328.

a thin capsule or pseudocapsule and are still considered to be confined to the kidney (pT1 or pT2) (Fig. 2-148). The diagnosis of perinephric fat invasion requires histologic confirmation of tumor invading the adipose tissue. Extension of the tumor into the perinephric tissue as irregular tongues, with or without associated desmoplasia, is also considered diagnostic of perinephric fat invasion (Fig. 2-149).[1067]

Perhaps no specific feature of staging has generated as much interest in the last decade as the renal sinus.[1068] The anatomy in this region is complex and includes the rich vascular and lymphatic networks feeding and draining the kidney as well as the collecting system including the renal pelvis and ureteropelvic junction. Further, the renal parenchyma is not separated from the adjacent soft tissue by a defined capsule as elsewhere.[1066] It has also been demonstrated that invasion of the renal sinus is a more common pathway out of the kidney than the perinephric fat (Fig. 2-150).[1069] and that invasion of the renal sinus is frequently associated with involvement of lymphatic spaces.[1070]

It has been noted that large intrarenal (pT2) tumors have similar outcomes to tumors directly invading into the renal sinus (pT3a).[1071] Renal sinus invasion has been validated as a prognostic indicator for renal cell carcinoma and has been correlated with tumor size, being seen in 97% of clear cell renal cell carcinomas >7 cm in diameter.[144] This would indicate that tumor size predicts renal sinus invasion, and for this reason it is surprising that tumors >7 cm in diameter were classified as pT2a or pT2b in the seventh edition of the TNM classification. As these tumors are almost always likely to

show renal sinus invasion, it would seem appropriate that large tumors be reassigned into the pT3a category. Since such a change was not made in the 2010 staging system, it is important for pathologists to understand this relationship and carefully assess the renal sinus prior to accepting a renal cell carcinoma, in particular a clear cell renal cell carcinoma, as being pT2. In one interesting study, resection specimens from 33 patients with pT1 tumors who had died of their disease were compared with a matched group of 33 patients not dying of renal cell carcinoma. The gross specimens were reexamined and an additional 10 sections submitted from the renal sinus; renal sinus invasion was demonstrated in 42% of the patients who died of disease compared to 6% of those who did not.[1072] There are also data that indicate that renal sinus invasion is associated with a worse outcome than perinephric fat invasion.[1073]

The current AJCC/TNM staging manual uses "renal sinus fat" to define pT3a disease; however, the histology of the renal sinus is such that tumor that clearly is outside of the kidney in this region does not necessarily involve fat. The ISUP consensus recommendations included a statement that a tumor should be considered to involve the renal sinus (pT3a) if it involved any renal sinus structures including the fat, the loose connective tissue, or endothelial-lined spaces of any size (Fig. 2-150).[1067]

As noted above, involvement of the large vascular structures (renal vein and vena cava) draining the kidney has been included in the definition of regional spread (Fig. 2-151). In the 1977 edition, involvement of the renal

Table 2-21 ■ THE 2010 UICC/AJCC/TNM STAGING CLASSIFICATION FOR RENAL CELL CARCINOMA

Pathologic staging (pTNM)
TNM descriptors (required only if applicable) (select all that apply)
- m (multiple primary tumors) (see template page V)
- y (post neoadjuvant treatment)

Primary tumor (pT)
- pTX: Primary tumor cannot be assessed
- pT0: No evidence of primary tumor
- pT1: Tumor 7 cm or less in greatest dimension, limited to the kidney
- pT1a: Tumor 4 cm or less in greatest dimension, limited to the kidney
- pT1b: Tumor more than 4 cm but no more than 7 cm in greatest dimension, limited to the kidney
- pT2: Tumor more than 7 cm in greatest dimension, limited to the kidney
- pT2a: Tumor more than 7 cm but ≤10 cm in greatest dimension, limited to kidney
- pT2b: Tumor more than 10 cm, limited to the kidney
- pT3: Tumor extends into major veins or perinephric tissues but not into the ipsilateral adrenal gland and not beyond Gerota fascia
- pT3a: Tumor grossly extends into the renal vein or its segmental (muscle containing) branches, or tumor invades perirenal and/or renal sinus fat but not beyond Gerota fascia.
- pT3b: Tumor grossly extends into the vena cava below the diaphragm.
- pT3c: Tumor grossly extends into vena cava above diaphragm or invades the wall of the vena cava
- pT4: Tumor invades beyond Gerota fascia (including contiguous extension into the ipsilateral adrenal gland)

Regional lymph nodes (pN)
- pNX: Regional lymph nodes cannot be assessed.
- pN0: No regional lymph node metastasis
- pN1: Metastasis in regional lymph node(s)
  Specify: Number examined____
      Number positive____

Distant metastasis (cM or pM)
- cM0: No distant metastasis
- cM1: Distant metastasis (proved by clinical means)
- pM1: Distant metastasis (proven by microscopic exam of specimen)

Stage groups

Stage groups			
• Stage I	T1	N0	M0
• Stage II	T2	N0	M0
• Stage III	T1 or T2	N1	M0
	T3	N0 or N1	M0
• Stage IV	T4	Any N	M0
	Any T	Any N	M1

From American Joint Committee on Cancer. Kidney. In: Edge SB, Byrd DR, Compton CC, et al., eds. *AJCC Staging Manual.* 7th ed. New York: Springer; 2009:479–489, with permission.

vein or vena cava below the diaphragm were considered pT3, but the presence of tumor within the vena cava above the diaphragm was placed in the pT4 group. This feature was omitted from the 1988 edition of the classification but was included in the pT3 category as pT3c in the 1997 and 2002 classifications. There is some debate as to the prognostic significance of the level of tumor thrombus within the renal vein and vena cava. The 2004 Mayo Clinic classification defines five levels of venous involvement dependent on the position of tumor thrombus.[1074] In subsequent studies, conflicting results as to the prognostic significance of this classification have been reported, with some studies validating the classification,[1075,1076] while others have shown that the level of tumor thrombosis, beyond the renal vein, does not influence survival.[1077–1081] In a large multi-institutional series of 1,215 patients with venous extension undergoing radical nephrectomy with thrombectomy, the 5-year cancer-specific survival was 43% with renal vein invasion, 37% with vena cava involvement below the diaphragm, and 22% with vena cava involvement above the diaphragm.[1082]

The current AJCC/TNM classification has further modified the approach to vascular invasion with renal vein involvement considered pT3a, vena cava below the diaphragm pT3b, and above the diaphragm as pT3c. An additional feature is that tumor invasion of the vena cava wall at any level is placed in the pT3c category. The definition of renal vein involvement (pT3a) is "tumor grossly extends into the renal vein or its segmental (muscle containing) branches." At the time of gross dissection, the renal vein and a few of its major branches are typically opened and examined, but all segmental (muscle containing) branches are unlikely to be evaluated. In sections taken from the renal sinus, it is not uncommon to find tumor in venous branches (2 to 3 mm or more in diameter) that have a muscular wall and where no tumor was recognized grossly but presumably could have been if the vessel had been examined grossly. The ISUP recommendation is to consider this as meeting the criteria for inclusion in the

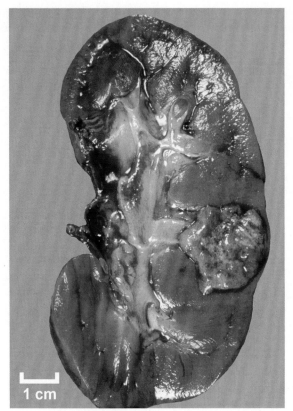

FIGURE 2-144 ■ Stage pT1a: A carcinoma within the renal capsule and smaller than 4 cm.

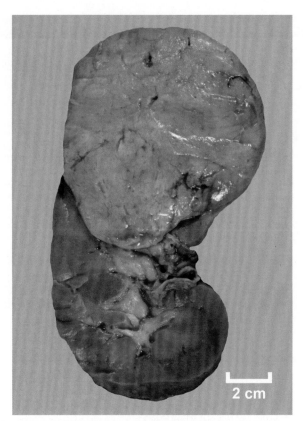

FIGURE 2-146 ■ Stage pT2a: A carcinoma within the renal capsule larger than 7 cm and smaller than 10 cm.

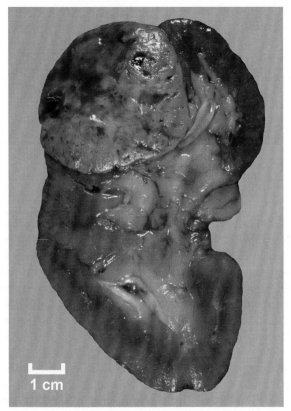

FIGURE 2-145 ■ Stage pT1b: A carcinoma within the renal capsule larger than 4 cm and smaller than 7 cm.

pT3a category.[1067] Microscopic lymph–vascular invasion has repeatedly been shown to have prognostic significance[151,1083] but is not included in the pT3a category except when found in the renal sinus.

The pT4 category of the TNM classification focuses upon extension of the tumor beyond the confines of regional boundaries. Direct invasion of the adrenal gland is reported to be present in 0.8% to 2.5% of radical nephrectomy specimens (Fig. 2-152).[208,1084] A major change incorporated into

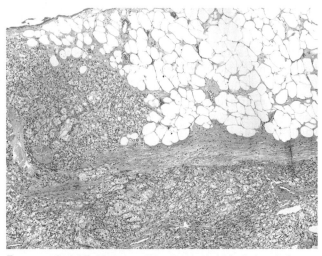

FIGURE 2-147 ■ Stage pT3a: Perinephric fat is invaded.

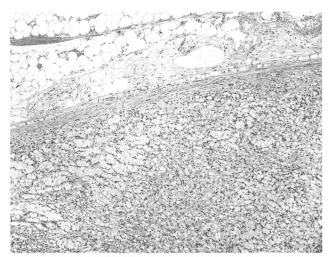

FIGURE 2-148 ■ Stage pT2: The tumor remains confined within the kidney by an attenuated renal capsule.

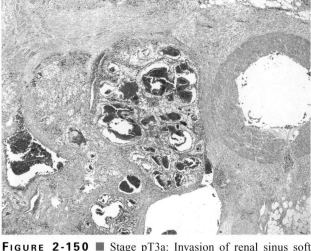

FIGURE 2-150 ■ Stage pT3a: Invasion of renal sinus soft tissue.

the 2010 AJCC/TNM classification was the reassignment of direct invasion of the ipsilateral adrenal gland from the pT3a category of earlier classifications to pT4. This change was based on studies demonstrating that these tumors had a much poorer prognosis than pT3a tumors and more in keeping with other tumors that had been included in the pT4 category in the 2002 classification.[208,1084,1085]

Infiltration of lymph nodes by renal cell carcinoma was considered to be local invasion in the Robson staging system, but was reclassified as a separate feature—the N-category—in the AJCC/TNM classification. In 1977, a series of complex N categories was proposed being N0—no nodal involvement, N1—single ipsilateral involvement, N2—tumor within multiple regional, contralateral nodes or within nodes bilaterally, N3—fixed regional nodes, and N4—involvement of juxtaregional lymph nodes. In the 1988 edition of the classification, nodal infiltration by tumor was

redefined, with criteria being based upon the size of tumor-positive nodes. In this classification a single node ≤2 cm in diameter was classified as N1, while involvement of a single lymph node >2 to <5 cm in diameter was classified as N2, and the involvement of multiple nodes <5 cm in diameter as N3. This was simplified in the 1997 edition of the classification, with tumors divided according to the presence

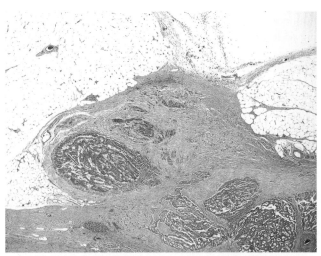

FIGURE 2-149 ■ Stage pT3a: Although surrounded by a desmoplastic pseudocapsule, the carcinoma has invaded perirenal fat.

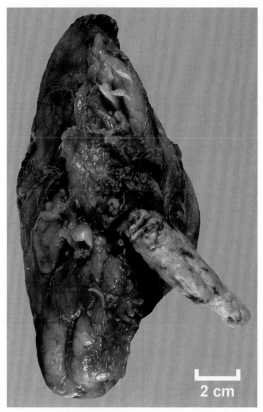

FIGURE 2-151 ■ Stage pT3a: The renal vein is filled with carcinoma.

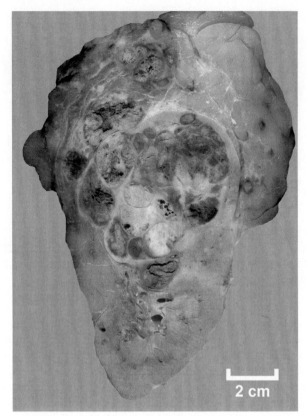

FIGURE 2-152 ■ Stage 4: The adrenal is invaded by carcinoma.

of metastases in a single regional lymph node (N1) or in multiple nodes (N2), and these criteria were retained in the 2002 edition of the classification. The current (2010) edition further simplifies the nodal classification into a single category pN1 that includes any regional lymph node metastasis (includes para-aortic, periaortic, or any retroperitoneal lymph nodes not otherwise specified).

The presence of lymph node metastases is associated with a poor prognosis for renal cell carcinoma. In patients undergoing routine lymph node dissection at the time of nephrectomy, metastases are identified in 11% to 14.6% of cases.[1086,1087] In one study, lymph node dissection was restricted to patients considered at high risk for metastases (based on intraoperative examination and frozen section to evaluate pathologic stage, nuclear grade 3 or 4, sarcomatoid component, and tumor necrosis); using this approach the lymph nodes were positive in 38% of cases.[1088] In a series of 1,260 patients undergoing lymphadenectomy at the time of nephrectomy, the 5-year cancer-specific survival was 83.8% for pN0 versus 38.4% for pN1 patients.[1086] The risk of mortality has been reported to be higher with increasing numbers of involved lymph nodes.[1089] In particular, a significant difference in outcome was noted when nodes were divided at a cut point of ≤4 and >4 involved nodes.[78] It has also been shown that the number of positive nodes increases with the number of nodes sampled.[77,1087] In one study it was recommended that >12 nodes be sampled for staging purposes,[77] and according to another report, 90% of pN1 cases

would be correctly staged if at least 15 lymph nodes were examined.[1087]

In the first edition of the TNM staging system, distant metastases were recorded as MX (not assessed), M0 (no known metastases), or M1 (distant metastases present) with a "+" added to indicate pathologic confirmation.[1058] This has essentially remained unchanged over the first six editions. The current TNM system made one significant change in the pM category with ipsilateral adrenal metastases now recognized as pM1. The other change of note is the elimination of pMX as a category (for all tumor sites). In the current system the two available categories for reporting pM are either pM1 or pM not applicable.

The presence of distant metastases portends a poor prognosis for renal cell carcinoma.[1090–1092] The median survival for patients with metastatic clear cell renal cell carcinoma is approximately 1 year with a 5-year cancer-specific survival of 15%.[1090] In an algorithm for predicting outcome for patients with metastatic clear cell renal cell carcinoma, features associated with a worse prognosis included constitutional symptoms at the time of diagnosis (+2 points), bone metastases (+2), liver metastases (+4), multiple metastases (+2), metastases within 2 years of nephrectomy (+3), presence of a tumor thrombus (+3), primary tumor nuclear grade of 4 (+3), and the presence of coagulative tumor necrosis (+2). The most favorable feature was complete resection of the metastases (−5).[1090]

The AJCC/TNM staging system, in its current form, provides powerful prognostic information.[1091–1093] Most data that have been generated have not been type specific but have included all types of renal cell carcinoma. In previous sections of the chapter covering specific types of renal cell carcinoma, staging data specific to the histologic type are discussed where available, and the reader is referred to those sections for further information on the impact of stage on outcomes of specific types of renal cell carcinoma. Despite the established validity of the AJCC/TNM staging system as an important prognostic indicator, this staging classification continues to evolve, and it is anticipated that large-scale multicenter studies will allow further refinement of its defining features.

Specimen Handling and Reporting

Introduction

The treatment of renal cell carcinoma for patients with localized disease remains largely surgical although, as discussed elsewhere, the use of ablative therapies and to a lesser extent observational protocols are becoming increasingly popular. Both partial and radical nephrectomy is widely used and the handling of these specimens will be the focus of this section. Proper handling of the specimen is critical for the determination of pathologic stage, surgical margin status, histologic classification, and tumor grading. A number of guidelines for the gross dissection, sampling, and reporting of the findings have been published.[274,1094–1096] Most recently, the International Society of Urological Pathology has issued consensus guidelines on the handling and reporting of renal cell carcinoma–containing specimens, and this section largely reflects those recommendations.[1067]

Radical Nephrectomy

The majority of radical nephrectomy specimens are received in the laboratory either fresh or in a formalin-filled container and in the latter are often in a relatively unfixed state. Specimens can be dissected fresh and this is generally preferred; if the institutional policy is to allow the specimen to fix overnight, it should be initially dissected upon arrival in the laboratory. There is usually a significant covering of fat that acts as a barrier to penetration by fixatives into the renal tissue, and sectioning is necessary to allow optimal fixation. It is also often easier to identify the renal artery and vein and the ureter in the unfixed state.

The specimen should be oriented using the ureter and adrenal gland as the principal landmarks. The ureter extends inferiorly from the renal sinus along the medial border of the specimen. It is also possible to identify the laterality of the specimen from the position of the ureter if it is a short segment, as this normally lies posterior to the renal artery and vein. Further, the anterior surface of the kidney is usually smoother than the posterior surface. In addition to the descending path of the ureter, the position of the adrenal gland, when removed as part of the radical nephrectomy procedure will provide absolute confirmation as to the identification of the upper pole of the kidney. Many surgeons do not however remove the adrenal gland routinely when performing a radical nephrectomy. Overall dimensions of the specimen should be recorded; weighing the entire specimen has little value. After further dissection, the size of the kidney should be measured, and if the perinephric fat is removed then the weight of the kidney without the fat can be recorded.

Areas that are suspicious for tumor extending to the surgical excision margin should be inked prior to dissection. Examination of the external surface can reveal roughened or disrupted areas that may represent sites of adhesion due to invasive tumor. It is unnecessary to ink the whole specimen as in most cases tumor will be contained by the perirenal fat within Gerota fascia and excessive inking makes the specimen difficult to handle. The ink also has the potential to spread to nonsurgical margins, causing confusion on examination of the histologic sections. Excessive ink will often obscure the hilar structures.

It is helpful to have an idea of the position of the tumor before commencing dissection, as this will permit sectioning through its maximum dimension. This can often be determined by palpation of the specimen. Accurate determination of the maximum dimension of the tumor is required for the assignment of the pT1-pT2 staging categories according to the staging criteria of the UICC/ AJCC TNM classification.[1064] The maximum dimension of

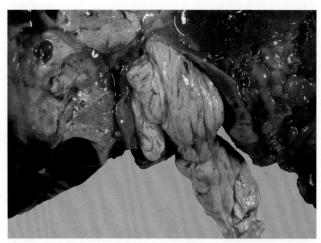

FIGURE 2-153 ■ Renal vein contains carcinoma but the margin is clear.

the tumor is based on the main tumor mass and includes tumor that has extended beyond the kidney. Special care to identify the maximum dimension of the tumor should be taken when it is around the key sizes of 4, 7, and 10 cm. If a tumor thrombus is visible, its dimensions should be recorded but are not included in the determination of the main tumor dimensions.

In the majority of specimens, the initial section is made along the long axis of the kidney. Prior to making this first section, the renal vein and ureter should be identified and opened. Careful examination of the renal vein and its major branches is important as the AJCC/TNM definition of renal vein invasion is "tumor grossly extends into the renal vein or its segmental (muscle containing) branches."[1064] If no tumor is evident, the renal vein margin is submitted for histologic evaluation (often in the same cassette with the ureter and renal artery margins). If possible tumor thrombus is identified, at least one section is submitted to confirm the nature of the thrombus; further, areas of adherence to the vein wall should be looked for and specifically sampled to evaluate for possible invasion of the vein wall (Figs. 2-153 and 2-154). The renal vein margin should also be submitted (Fig. 2-155).

The initial section may be taken from the hilar aspect or from the lateral aspect of the specimen. From the hilar aspect the section can be placed just anterior to the renal pelvis or can be made using probes in either the collecting system or the venous system as a guide. When beginning laterally, the incision is generally started at roughly the middle of the kidney and angled to exit through the renal hilum slightly off center. In either case additional parallel sections are made to more completely assess the hilar structures and the relationship of the tumor to the renal sinus. The sectioning can be adjusted based on the gross evaluation of the specimen.

The perinephric fat lies between the renal capsule and Gerota fascia. Documentation of invasion of the perirenal

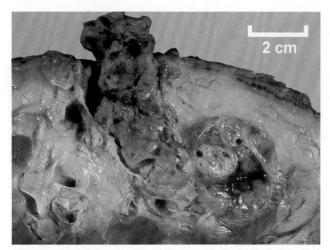

FIGURE 2-154 ■ Renal vein is invaded at the margin, so the margin is compromised.

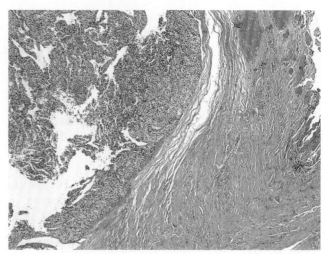

FIGURE 2-155 ■ This section of renal vein shows carcinoma at the margin.

fat is one feature that places a tumor in the pT3a category and has significant prognostic implications. Many renal cell carcinomas grossly distort the external surface of the kidney and bulge into the perinephric fat (Fig. 2-146). This does not make the tumor pT3a, which requires histologic documentation of tumor invading beyond the kidney and into the perirenal tissue. Evaluation for possible sites of perirenal fat invasion is best done by making multiple perpendicular cuts of the interface between the tumor and the perinephric fat. Careful examination for small nodules of tumor in the perinephric fat or areas of adhesion or fibrosis along the interface will direct the sampling. If tumor is grossly apparent in the fat, a single section for documentation is sufficient. In the absence of obvious invasion, areas suspicious for invasion should have more sections submitted. If there is no gross evidence of invasion, a single section of the interface is sufficient.

The initial section will usually clarify the position and extent of the tumor in relation to the surface of the kidney. If

desired, the fat can then be stripped off the surface of kidney except where it is overlying the tumor, and around to the renal sinus leaving the renal capsule intact. This approach results in an easier specimen to handle and allows for more accurate determination of the kidney dimensions and the weight of the kidney.

The careful examination of the renal hilar area is also critical to accurate staging of renal cell carcinoma. The studies of the renal sinus by Bonsib[144,1069] have clearly demonstrated the high frequency of renal sinus invasion, particularly in tumors larger than 7 cm. For cases with obvious invasion of the renal sinus, a single section for confirmation is sufficient. For those tumors that encroach on the renal sinus, even with a pushing border, it is recommended that a minimum of three sections of the interface between the tumor and the renal sinus be submitted (Fig. 2-156A and B). For clear cell renal cell carcinomas larger than 7 cm, submission of additional

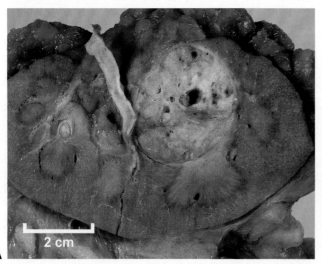

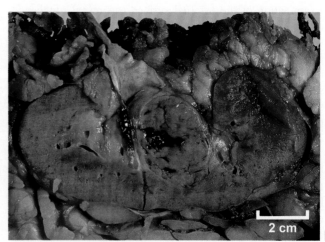

FIGURE 2-156 ■ **A:** Microscopic invasion of renal sinus soft tissue was found in this specimen. **B:** Although essentially identical to the specimen in A, thorough sampling found no invasion of renal sinus soft tissue in this specimen.

blocks should be considered if the initial sections do not show renal sinus invasion. For tumors that do not encroach on the sinus, a single section of the renal sinus should be submitted.

The tumor should be cut at 3 to 5 mm intervals, either in sections parallel to the initial incision or at right angles to the longitudinal cut that bisects the kidney; areas of the tumor that show differing gross appearances should be identified for histologic examination. The interface between the tumor and the kidney should also be examined and at least one sample taken for histology. For small (<4 cm) tumors, a minimum of three sections of tumor should be submitted. The necessary sections of tumor with perirenal fat, tumor with renal sinus, and tumor with normal parenchyma will largely meet this number, but in most cases at least one or two further sections will be needed to include varying gross appearances. Any fleshy, gray-white areas must be sampled as this often indicates a sarcomatoid component (Fig. 2-19). For tumors 4 cm or larger, the tumor sampling should include at least one section per centimeter.

For situations with multiple tumors, the greatest dimension should be recorded for those smaller than the main tumor mass; if there are innumerable tumors, this can be presented as a range of sizes. Although many would suggest sampling all discrete tumors, for cases with numerous lesions this may be impractical. In those situations at least the five largest lesions should be evaluated histologically.

Finally, the entire kidney is cut at 5 mm intervals at right angles to the sagittal bisecting cut and any abnormal tissue is sampled. Sections of apparently normal renal tissue should also be taken including adjacent to the tumor and at least one section remote from the tumor.[1094,1095]

Lymph nodes can be identified in some radical nephrectomy specimens. There are few published data on the frequency of finding lymph nodes but most estimate it to be in 10% to 20% of specimens. These are almost invariably found in the hilar area, so this region should be carefully dissected for possible lymph nodes. It is not necessary to dissect all of the perirenal adipose tissue for lymph nodes as for practical purposes lymph nodes are not present in this tissue.

The adrenal gland should be identified and sectioned at 3-mm intervals. Any nodules identified should be sampled. If there is gross evidence of tumor involving the adrenal gland, then the stage assignment is dependent on whether it is direct invasion of the gland (pT4) or a metastasis from the tumor (pM1). This is best determined by the gross examination, and sections should be selected to document the gross impression.

Partial Nephrectomy

The overall dimensions of the specimen should be recorded. Partial nephrectomy specimens may include overlying fat (Fig. 2-157) or may include only a small thin rim of

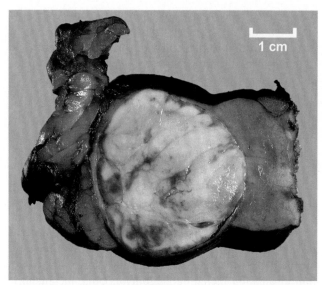

FIGURE 2-157 ■ Perirenal fat is adherent to the capsule in this partial nephrectomy specimen.

renal parenchyma (Fig. 2-158). Examination of the surgical margin for involvement by tumor is important for partial nephrectomy specimens. All surgical margins should be inked and following sectioning, the distance from the tumor to the margin recorded. A generous number of sections should be taken perpendicular to the inked margin, especially for margins closest to the tumor. Similarly, the cortical surface should be examined in detail for evidence of infiltration of perirenal fat. The proximity of tumor to the surgical margin does not appear to influence outcome, as long as there is no tumor directly at the site of surgical

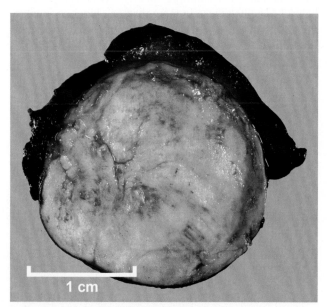

FIGURE 2-158 ■ The tumor in this partial nephrectomy specimen is covered only by the renal capsule.

resection.[1097] There is also considerable literature that indicates that the presence of a positive surgical margin is associated with a low risk of tumor recurrence, and so in most instances, the urologist will not go back and perform a radical nephrectomy but rather will follow the patient with imaging studies.[192,193]

Renal Biopsy

The European Association of Urology considers needle biopsy to always be indicated (1) before ablative therapy, (2) before systemic therapy if no prior histologic diagnosis is available, and (3) when a surveillance strategy is considered.[1098] Contemporary series have reported that needle core biopsies are adequate for definitive diagnosis in 78% to 91% of cases.[1099–1101] Needle biopsy allows for the diagnosis of benign masses that may not require resection or ablation including angiomyolipoma, metanephric adenoma, benign cysts, and oncocytoma. Rendering a definitive diagnosis of oncocytoma on needle biopsy is controversial, but pathologists in institutions where considerable experience has been gained in these specimens have been willing to commit to the diagnosis.[1100] In cases of renal cell carcinoma, the tumor is correctly classified in a high percentage of cases. Accuracy evaluated by comparing biopsy and resection specimens has been very high with reported results up to 100%. Nonetheless, the interpretation of thin needle biopsies of renal masses can be challenging. Immunohistochemical studies are helpful and in our hands are utilized more often to aid in diagnosis and classification in biopsies than in resections.[1102]

These specimens may contain relatively little tumor, and proper classification more often requires immunohistochemistry than when the whole tumor is available for examination. When multiple cores are obtained, it can be helpful to embed these in more than one block to increase the ability to utilize multiple immunohistochemical stains if required.

Morcellated Kidneys

Laparoscopic radical nephrectomy with specimen morcellation is a novel surgical approach that is used for tumors in selected patients. Following morcellation, the kidney is received in numerous fragments, with at least one dimension being <10 to 12 mm in length. It has been estimated that for initial sampling of morcellated kidneys, 5% of the total specimens should be sampled.[1103] It has also been shown that for diagnostic purposes, further sampling may be required in up to 25% of cases. While histologic diagnosis of the tumor is possible for morcellated nephrectomy specimens, it is not usually possible to assign a pT staging category.[196,1103,1104] There may also be difficulties in identifying resection margins, although marking of the specimen with methylene blue or India ink prior to piecemeal extraction has been suggested.[1105]

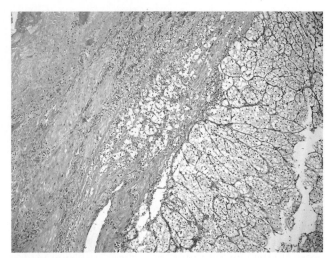

FIGURE 2-159 ■ The carcinoma invades the wall of the vena cava.

Vena Cava Thrombus Specimens

In patients with tumor extension into the vena cava the tumor thrombus is often removed at the time of nephrectomy and is submitted as a separate specimen. Involvement of the vena cava below the diaphragm is staged as pT3b unless the tumor "invades the wall," which would result in staging it as pT3c.[1064] For this reason, sections of these thrombi need to be submitted to look for evidence that the thrombus was invading the caval wall rather than being "free-floating" within the lumen (Fig. 2-159).

Specimen Reporting

Detailed guidelines for the reporting of the gross and microscopic features of kidneys removed for renal cell carcinoma have been published periodically.[274,1096] These recommendations are frequently in narrative form; however, there is now an impetus for reporting in a synoptic format. An appropriate template for this has been published by both the College of American Pathologists and the Royal College of Pathologists of Australasia.[274] The salient features that should be reported for needle biopsies and for radical and partial nephrectomy specimens using the guidelines of the College of American Pathologists are shown in Table 2-22.

The importance of careful examination of nonneoplastic renal tissue for host-related and incidental findings has recently been emphasized.[1106] In these kidneys, vascular disease is the most common abnormality followed by diabetic nephropathy (Fig. 2-160).[1107,1108] Importantly, the identification of unsuspected conditions may influence the subsequent clinical course and influence treatment. In one report of 110 patients undergoing radical nephrectomy[91] or partial nephrectomy,[19] follow-up demonstrated significantly higher serum creatinine levels 6 months after surgery in patients

Table 2-22 ■ COLLEGE OF AMERICAN PATHOLOGISTS RECOMMENDED CANCER CASE SUMMARY (2012)

Procedure

_____ Partial nephrectomy

_____ Radical nephrectomy

_____ Other (specify) _____

_____ Not specified

Specimen Laterality

_____ Right

_____ Left

_____ Not specified

+Tumor site (select all that apply)

+_____ Upper pole

+_____ Middle

+_____ Lower pole

+_____ Other (specify) _____

+_____ Not specified

Tumor size (largest tumor if multiple)

Greatest dimension: _____ cm

+Additional dimensions: _____x_____ cm

_____ Cannot be determined (see Comment)

Tumor Focality

_____ Unifocal

_____ Multifocal

Macroscopic Extent of Tumor (select all that apply)

_____ Tumor limited to kidney

_____ Tumor extension into perinephric tissues

_____ Tumor extension into renal sinus

_____ Tumor extension beyond Gerota fascia

_____ Tumor extension into major veins

_____ Tumor extension into pelvicalyceal system

_____ Tumor extension into adrenal gland

　　　_____ Direct invasion (T4)

　　　_____ Noncontiguous (M1)

Histologic type

_____ Clear cell renal cell carcinoma

_____ Multilocular cystic clear cell renal cell carcinoma

_____ Papillary renal cell carcinoma

_____ Chromophobe renal cell carcinoma

_____ Carcinoma of the collecting ducts of Bellini

_____ Renal medullary carcinoma

_____ Translocation carcinoma (Xp11 or others)

_____ Carcinoma associated with neuroblastoma

_____ Mucinous tubular and spindle cell carcinoma

_____ Tubulocystic carcinoma

_____ Renal cell carcinoma, unclassified

_____ Other (specify) _____

Sarcomatoid Features

_____ Not identified

_____ Present

　　　Specify percentage _____ %

+Tumor Necrosis (any amount)

_____ Not identified

_____ Present

Histologic Grade (Fuhrman nuclear grade)

_____ Not applicable

_____ GX: cannot be determined

_____ G1

_____ G2

_____ G3

_____ G4

_____ Other (specify): _____

Microscopic Tumor Extension (select all that apply)

_____ Tumor limited to kidney

_____ Tumor extension into perinephric tissues

_____ Tumor extension into renal sinus

_____ Tumor extension beyond Gerota fascia

_____ Tumor extension into major veins (renal vein or its segmental [muscle containing] branches

_____ Tumor extension into pelvicalyceal system

_____ Tumor extension into adrenal gland

　　　_____ Direct invasion (T4)

　　　_____ Noncontiguous (M1)

_____ Tumor extension into other organ(s)/structures(s) (specify): _____

Margins (select all that apply)

_____ Cannot be assessed

_____ Margins uninvolved by invasive carcinoma

_____ Margin(s) involved by invasive carcinoma

　　　_____ Renal parenchymal margin (partial nephrectomy only)

　　　_____ Renal capsular margin (partial nephrectomy only)

　　　_____ Perinephric fat margin

　　　_____ Gerota fascial margin

　　　_____ Renal vein margin

　　　_____ Ureteral margin

　　　_____ Other (specify): _____

+Lymphvascular Invasion

+_____ Not identified

+_____ Present

+_____ Indeterminate

Pathologic Staging (TNM)

Pathologic Findings in Nonneoplastic Kidney (select all that apply)

_____ Insufficient tissue (partial nephrectomy with <5 mm of adjacent nonneoplastic kidney)

_____ Significant pathologic alterations

　　　_____ None identified

　　　_____ Glomerular disease (specify type): _____

　　　_____ Tubulointerstitial disease (specify type): _____

　　　_____ Vascular disease (specify type): _____

　　　_____ Other (specify): _____

+Other Tumors and/or Tumor-like Conditions (select all that apply)

+_____ Cyst(s) (specify type): _____

+_____ Tubular (papillary) adenoma(s): _____

+_____ Other (specify): _____

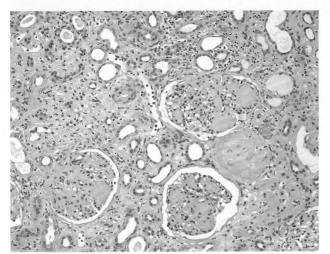

FIGURE 2-160 ■ Diabetic glomerulosclerosis (Kimmelstiel-Wilson nodules).

with vascular scarring or diabetic glomerulosclerosis (moderate and nodular).[1107]

REFERENCES

1. Thoenes W, Störkel S, Rumpelt H-J. Histopathology and classification of renal cell tumors (adenomas, oncocytomas and carcinomas) the basic cytological and histopathological elements and their use for diagnostics. *Pathol Res Pract* 1986;181:125–143.
2. Kovacs G. Molecular differential pathology of renal cell tumours. *Histopathology* 1993;22:1–8.
3. Kovacs G, Akhtar M, Beckwith JB, et al. The Heidelberg classification of renal cell tumours. *J Pathol* 1997;183:131–133.
4. Störkel S, Eble JN, Adlakha K, et al. Classification of renal cell carcinoma, workgroup 1. *Cancer* 1997;80:987–989.
5. World Health Organization Classification of Tumours. *Pathology and Genetics of Tumours of the Urinary System and Male Genital Organs.* Lyon, France: IARC Press; 2004.
6. Murphy WM, Grignon DJ, Perlman EJ. *AFIP Atlas of Tumor Pathology, Fourth Series, Fascicle 1, Tumors of the Kidney, Bladder, and Related Urinary Structures.* Washington, DC: American Registry of Pathology; 2004.
7. Srigley JR, Delahunt B, Eble JN, et al. Vancouver classification of renal neoplasia. *Am J Surg Pathol* 2013; In press.
8. Delahunt B, Eble JN. History of the development of the classification of renal cell neoplasia. *Clin Lab Med* 2005;25:231–246.
9. Delahunt B, Eble JN. Papillary adenoma of the kidney: an evolving concept. *J Urol Pathol* 1997;7:99–112.
10. Bell ET. A classification of renal tumors with observations on the frequency of the various types. *J Urol* 1938;39:238–243.
11. Bell ET. *Renal Diseases.* 2 ed. Philadelphia, PA: Lea and Febiger; 1950.
12. Grignon DJ, Eble JN. Papillary and metanephric adenomas of the kidney. *Semin Diagn Pathol* 1998;15:41–53.
13. Budin RE, McDonnell PJ. Renal cell neoplasms, their relationship to arteriolonephrosclerosis. *Arch Pathol Lab Med* 1984;108:138–140.
14. Xipell JM. The incidence of benign renal nodules (a clinicopathologic study). *J Urol* 1971;106:503–506.
15. Hughson MD, Buchwald D, Fox M. Renal neoplasia and acquired cystic kidney disease in patients receiving long-term dialysis. *Arch Pathol Lab Med* 1986;110:592–601.
16. Denton MD, Magee CC, Ovuworie C, et al. Prevalence of renal cell carcinoma in patients with ESRD pre-transplantation: a pathologic analysis. *Kidney Int* 2002;61:2201–2209.
17. Cheng WS, Farrow GM, Zincke H. The incidence of multicentricity in renal cell carcinoma. *J Urol* 1991;146:1221–1223.
18. Reese AJM, Winstanley DP. The small tumor-like lesions of the kidney. *Br J Cancer* 1958;12:507–516.
19. Reidbord HE. Metaplasia of the parietal layer of Bowman's capsule. *Am J Clin Pathol* 1968;50:240–242.
20. Cohen C, McCue PA, DeRose PB. Immunohistochemistry of renal adenomas and carcinomas. *J Urol Pathol* 1995;3:61–71.
21. Hiasa Y, Kitamura M, Nakaoka S, et al. Antigen immunohistochemistry of renal cell adenomas in autopsy cases: relevance to histogenesis. *Oncology* 1995;52:97–105.
22. Farnsworth WV, DeRose PB, Cohen C. DNA image cytometric analysis of paraffin-embedded sections of small renal cortical neoplasms. *Cytometry* 1994;18:223–227.
23. Brunelli M, Eble JN, Zhang S, et al. Gains of chromosomes 7, 17, 12, 16, and 20 and loss of Y occur early in the evolution of papillary renal cell neoplasia: a fluorescence in situ hybridization study. *Mod Pathol* 2003;16:1053–1059.
24. Ishikawa I, Kovacs G. High incidence of papillary renal cell tumours in patients on chronic haemodialysis. *Histopathology* 1993;22:135–139.
25. Holm-Nielsen P, Olsen TS. Ultrastructure of renal adenoma. *Ultrastruct Pathol* 1988;12:27–39.
26. Klein MJ, Valensi QJ. Proximal tubular adenomas of kidney with so-called oncocytic features, a clinicopathologic study of 13 cases of a rarely reported neoplasm. *Cancer* 1976;38:906–914.
27. Lieber MM, Tomera KM, Farrow GM. Renal oncocytoma. *J Urol* 1981;125:481–485.
28. Ramaekers FCS, Beck HLM, Feitz WFJ, et al. Application of antibodies to intermediate filament proteins as tissue-specific probes in the flow cytometric analysis of complex tumors. *Anal Quant Cytol Histol* 1986;8:271–280.
29. Perez-Ordonez B, Hamed G, Campbell S, et al. Renal oncocytoma: a clinicopathologic study of 70 cases. *Am J Surg Pathol* 1997;21:871–883.
30. Gudbjartsson T, Hardarson S, Petursdottir V, et al. Renal oncocytoma: a clinicopathological analysis of 45 consecutive cases. *BJU Int* 2005;96:1275–1279.
31. Morra MN, Das S. Renal oncocytoma: a review of histogenesis, histopathology, diagnosis, and treatment. *J Urol* 1993;150:295–302.
32. Dechet CB, Bostwick DG, Blute ML, et al. Renal oncocytoma: multifocality, bilaterality, metachronous tumor development and coexistent renal cell carcinoma. *J Urol* 1999;162:40–42.
33. Trpkov K, Yilmaz A, Uzer D, et al. Renal oncocytoma revisited: a clinicopathological study of 109 cases with emphasis on problematic diagnostic features. *Histopathology* 2010;57:893–906.
34. Skolarus TA, Serrano MF, Berger DA, et al. The distribution of histological subtypes of renal tumors by decade of life using the 2004 WHO classification. *J Urol* 2008;179:439–444.
35. Amin MB, Crotty TB, Tickoo SK, et al. Renal oncocytoma: a reappraisal of morphologic features with clinicopathologic findings in 80 cases. *Am J Surg Pathol* 1997;21:1–12.
36. Hes O, Michal M, Sima R, et al. Renal oncocytoma with and without intravascular extension into the branches of the renal vein have the same morphological, immunohistochemical and genetic features. *Virchows Arch* 2008;452:285–293.
37. Kragel PJ, Williams J, Emory TS, et al. Renal oncocytoma with cylindromatous changes: pathologic features and histogenetic significance. *Mod Pathol* 1990;3:277–281.
38. Lechpammer M, Resnick MB, Sabo E, et al. The diagnostic and prognostic utility of claudin expression in renal cell neoplasms. *Mod Pathol* 2008;21:1320–1329.
39. Lin F, Yang W, Betten M, et al.; The French Kidney Cancer Study Group. Expression of S-100 protein in renal cell neoplasms. *Hum Pathol* 2006;37:462–470.
40. Mai KT, Teo I, Belanger EC, et al. Progesterone receptor reactivity in renal oncocytoma and chromophobe renal cell carcinoma. *Histopathology* 2008;52:277–282.

41. Cossu Rocca P, Brunelli M, Gobbo S, et al. Diagnostic utility of S100A1 expression in renal cell neoplasms: an immunohistochemical and quantitative RT-PCR study. *Mod Pathol* 2007;20:722–728.

42. Abrahams NA, MacLennan GT, Khoury JD, et al. Chromophobe renal cell carcinoma: a comparative study of histological, immunohistochemical and ultrastructural features using high throughput tissue microarray. *Histopathology* 2004;45:593–602.

43. Garcia E, Li M. Caveolin-1 immunohistochemical analysis in differentiating chromophobe renal cell carcinoma from renal oncocytoma. *Am J Clin Pathol* 2006;125:392–398.

44. Rampino T, Gregorini M, Soccio G, et al. The Ron proto-oncogene product is a phenotypic marker of renal oncocytoma. *Am J Surg Pathol* 2003;27:779–785.

45. Zhou M, Roma A, Magi-Galluzzi C. The usefulness of immunohistochemical markers in the differential diagnosis of renal neoplasms. *Clin Lab Med* 2005;25:247–257.

46. Molinié V, Balaton A, Rotman S, et al. Alpha-methyl CoA racemase expression in renal cell carcinomas. *Hum Pathol* 2006;37:698–703.

47. Martignoni G, Pea M, Chilosi M, et al. Parvalbumin is constantly expressed in chromophobe renal carcinoma. *Mod Pathol* 2001;14:760–767.

48. Stopyra GA, Warhol MJ, Multhaupt HAB. Cytokeratin 20 immunoreactivity in renal oncocytomas. *J Histochem Cytochem* 2001;49:919–920.

49. Langner C, Wegscheider BJ, Ratschek M, et al. Keratin immunohistochemistry in renal cell carcinoma subtypes and renal oncocytomas: a systematic analysis of 233 tumors. *Virchows Arch* 2004;444:127–134.

50. Tickoo SK, Amin MB, Zarbo RJ. Colloidal iron staining in renal epithelial neoplasms including chromophobe renal cell carcinoma: emphasis on technique and patterns of staining. *Am J Surg Pathol* 1998;22:419–424.

51. Lindgren V, Paner GP, Omeroglu A, et al. Cytogenetic analysis of a series of 13 renal oncocytomas. *J Urol* 2004;171:602–604.

52. Paner GP, Lindgren V, Jacobson K, et al. High incidence of chromosome 1 abnormalities in a series of 27 renal oncocytomas, cytogenetic and fluorescence in situ hybridization studies. *Arch Pathol Lab Med* 2007;131:81–85.

53. Füzesi L, Frank D, Nguyen C, et al. Losses of 1p and chromosome 14 in renal oncocytomas. *Cancer Genet Cytogenet* 2005;160:120–125.

54. Füzesi L, Gunawan B, Braun S, et al. Renal oncocytoma with a translocation t(9;11)(p23;q13). *J Urol* 1994;152:471–472.

55. Füzesi L, Gunawan B, Braun S, et al. Cytogenetic analysis of 11 renal oncocytomas: further evidence of structural rearrangements of 11q13 as a characteristic chomosomal anomaly. *Cancer Genet Cytogenet* 1998;107:1–6.

56. Thrash-Bingham CA, Salazar H, Freed JJ, et al. Genomic alterations and instabilities in renal cell carcinomas and their relationship to tumor pathology. *Cancer Res* 1995;55:6189–6195.

57. Brunelli M, Delahunt B, Gobbo S, et al. Diagnostic usefulness of fluorescent cytogenetics in differentiating chromophobe renal cell carcinoma from renal oncocytoma, a validation study combining metaphase and interphase analyses. *Am J Clin Pathol* 2010;133:116–126.

58. Warfel KA, Eble JN. Renal oncocytomatosis. *J Urol* 1982;127:1179–1180.

59. Tickoo SK, Reuter VE, Amin MB, et al. Renal oncocytosis: a morphologic study of fourteen cases. *Am J Surg Pathol* 1999;23:1094–1101.

60. Gobbo S, Eble JN, Delahunt B, et al. Renal cell neoplasms of oncocytosis have distinct morphologic, immunohistochemical, and cytogenetic profiles. *Am J Surg Pathol* 2010;34:620–626.

61. Hes O, Brunelli M, Michal M, et al. Oncocytic papillary renal cell carcinoma: a clinicopathologic, immunohistochemical, ultrastructural, and interphase cytogenetic study of 12 cases. *Ann Diagn Pathol* 2006;10:133–139.

62. Oberling C, Rivière M, Hagueneau F. Ultrastructure of the clear cells in renal carcinomas and its importance for the demonstration of their renal origin. *Nature* 1960;186:402–403.

63. Zbar B, Brauch H, Talmadge C, et al. Loss of alleles of loci on the short arm of chromosome 3 in renal cell carcinoma. *Nature* 1987;327:721–724.

64. Presti JC Jr, Rao PH, Chen Q, et al. Histopathological, cytogenetic, and molecular characterization of renal cortical tumors. *Cancer Res* 1991;51:1544–1552.

65. McLaughlin JK, Lipworth L, Tarone RE. Epidemiologic aspects of renal cell carcinoma. *Semin Oncol* 2006;33:527–533.

66. DeCastro GJ, McKiernan JM. Epidemiology, clinical staging, and presentation of renal cell carcinoma. *Urol Clin North Am* 2008;35:581–592.

67. Siegel R, Naishadham D, Jemal A. Cancer statistics, 2012. *CA Cancer J Clin* 2012;62:10–29.

68. Hock LM, Lynch J, Balaji KC. Increasing incidence of all stages of kidney cancer in the last 2 decades in the United States: an analysis of surveillance, epidemiology and end results program data. *J Urol* 2002;167:57–60.

69. Lindblad P. Epidemiology of renal cell carcinoma. *Scand J Surg* 2004;93:88–96.

70. Mevorach RA, Segal AJ, Tersegno ME, et al. Renal cell carcinoma: incidental diagnosis and natural history: review of 235 cases. *Urology* 1992;39:519–522.

71. Chow WH, Devesa SS, Warren JL, et al. Rising incidence of renal cell cancer in the United States. *JAMA* 1999;281:1628–1631.

72. Chow W-H, Dong LM, Devesa SS. Epidemiology and risk factors for kidney cancer. *Nat Rev Urol* 2010;7:245–257.

73. Gupta K, Miller JD, Li JZ, et al. Epidemiologic and socioeconomic burden of metastatic renal cell carcinoma (mRCC): a literature review. *Cancer Treat Rev* 2008;34:193–205.

74. Patard J-J, Rodriguez A, Rioux-Leclercq N, Guillé F, et al. Prognostic significance of the mode of detection in renal tumours. *BJU Int* 2002;90:358–363.

75. Pantuck AJ, Zisman A, Belldegrun AS. The changing natural history of renal cell carcinoma. *J Urol* 2001;166:1611–1623.

76. Chow W-H, Devesa SS. Contemporary epidemiology of renal cell cancer. *Cancer J* 2008;14:288–301.

77. Amin MB, Amin MB, Tamboli P, et al. Prognostic impact of histologic subtyping of adult renal epithelial neoplasms, an experience of 405 cases. *Am J Surg Pathol* 2002;26:281–291.

78. Cheville JC, Lohse CM, Zincke H, et al. Comparisons of outcome and prognostic features among histologic subtypes of renal cell carcinoma. *Am J Surg Pathol* 2003;27:612–624.

79. Kim H, Cho NH, Kim D, et al.; Genitourinary Pathology Study Group of the Korean Society of Pathologists. Renal cell carcinoma in South Korea: a multicenter study. *Hum Pathol* 2004;35:1556–1563.

80. Patard J-J, Leray E, Rioux-Leclercq N, et al. Prognostic value of histologic subtypes of renal cell carcinoma: a multicenter experience. *J Clin Oncol* 2005;23:2763–2771.

81. Gudbjartsson T, Hardarson S, Petursdottir V, et al. Histological subtyping and nuclear grading of renal cell carcinoma and their implications for survival: a retrospective nation-wide study of 629 patients. *Eur Urol* 2005;48:593–600.

82. Ficarra V, Martignoni G, Galfano A, et al. Prognostic role of the histologic subtypes of renal cell carcinoma after slide revision. *Eur Urol* 2006;50:786–794.

83. Capitanio U, Cloutier V, Zini L, et al. A critical assessment of the prognostic value of clear cell, papillary, and chromophobe histological subtypes in renal cell carcinoma: a population-based study. *BJU Int* 2009;103:1496–1500.

84. Schlehofer B, Pommer W, Mellemgaard A, et al. International renal-cell-cancer study. VI. The role of medical and family history. *Int J Cancer* 1996;66:723–726.

85. Gago-Dominguez M, Yuan J-M, Castelao JE, et al. Family history and risk of renal cell carcinoma. *Cancer Epidemiol Biomarkers Prev* 2001;10:1001–1004.

86. Czene K, Hemminki K. Kidney cancer in the Swedish Family Cancer Database: familial risks and second primary malignancies. *Kidney Int* 2002;61:1806–1813.

87. Cohen D, Zhou M. Molecular genetics of familial renal cell carcinoma syndromes. *Clin Lab Med* 2005;25:259–277.

88. Przybycin CG, Magi-Galluzzi C, McKenney JK. Hereditary syndromes with associated renal neoplasia: a practical guide to histologic recognition in renal tumor resection specimens. *Adv Anat Pathol* 2013;20: 245–263.

89. Hunt JD, van der Hel OL, McMillan GP, et al. Renal cell carcinoma in relation to cigarette smoking: meta-analysis of 24 studies. *Int J Cancer* 2005;114:101–108.

90. Renehan AG, Tyson M, Egger M, et al. Body-mass index and incidence of cancer: a systematic review and meta-analysis of prospective observational studies. *Lancet* 2008;371:569–578.

91. Menezes RJ, Tomlinson G, Kreiger N. Physical activity and risk of renal cell cancer. *Int J Cancer* 2003;107:642–646.

92. Lindblad P, Wolk A, Bergström R, et al. The role of obesity and weight fluctuations in the etiology of renal cell cancer: a population-based case-control study. *Cancer Epidemiol Biomarkers Prev* 1994;3:631–639.

93. Stewart JH, Buccianti G, Agodoa L, et al. Cancers of the kidney and urinary tract in patients on dialysis for end-stage renal disease: analysis of data from the United States, Europe, and Australia and New Zealand. *J Am Soc Nephrol* 2003;14:197–207.

94. Chow W-H, Gridley G, Fraumeni JF Jr, et al. Obesity, hypertension, and the risk of kidney cancer in men. *N Engl J Med* 2000;343:1305–1311.

95. McCredie M, Pommer W, McLaughlin JK, et al. International renal-cell cancer study. II. Analgesics. *Int J Cancer* 1995;60:345–349.

96. Wolk A, Lindblad P, Adami H-O. Nutrition and renal cell cancer. *Cancer Causes Control* 1996;7:5–18.

97. Mandel JS, McLaughlin JK, Schlehofer B, et al. International renal-cell cancer study. IV. occupation. *Int J Cancer* 1995;61:601–605.

98. Raaschou-Nielsen O, Hansen J, McLaughlin JK, et al. Cancer risk among workers at Danish companies using trichloroethylene: a cohort study. *Am J Epidemiol* 2003;158:1182–1192.

99. Delahunt B, Bethwaite PB, Nacey JN. Occupational risk for renal cell carcinoma. A case-control study based on the New Zealand Cancer Registry. *Br J Urol* 1995;75:578–582.

100. Gibbons RP, Montie JE, Correa RJ Jr, et al. Manifestations of renal cell carcinoma. *Urology* 1976;8:201–206.

101. Sokoloff MH, DeKernion JB, Figlin RA, et al. Current management of renal cell carcinoma. *CA Cancer J Clin* 1996;46:284–302.

102. Palapattu GS, Kristo B, Rajfer J. Paraneoplastic syndromes in urologic malignancy: the many faces of renal cell carcinoma. *Rev Urol* 2002;4:163–170.

103. Chasan SA, Pothel LR, Huben RP. Management and prognostic significance of hypercalcemia in renal cell carcinoma. *Urology* 1989;33:167–170.

104. Pavelic K, Popovic M. Insulin and glucagon secretion by renal adenocarcinoma. *Cancer* 1981;48:98–100.

105. Gökden N, Nappi O, Swanson PE, et al. Renal cell carcinoma with rhabdoid features. *Am J Surg Pathol* 2000;24:1329–1338.

106. Kuroiwa K, Kinoshita Y, Shiratsuchi H, et al. Renal cell carcinoma with rhabdoid features; an aggressive neoplasm. *Histopathology* 2002;41:538–548.

107. Delahunt B. Sarcomatoid renal carcinoma: the final common dedifferentiation pathway of renal epithelial malignancies. *Pathology* 1999;31:185–190.

108. Avery AK, Beckstead J, Renshaw AA, et al. Use of antibodies to RCC and CD10 in the differential diagnosis of renal neoplasms. *Am J Surg Pathol* 2000;24:203–210.

109. Young AN, Amin MB, Moreno CS, et al. Expression profiling of renal epithelial neoplasms: a method for tumor classification and discovery of diagnostic molecular markers. *Am J Pathol* 2001;158:1639–1651.

110. Kim M-K, Kim S. Immunohistochemical profile of common epithelial neoplasms arising in the kidney. *Appl Immunohistochem Mol Morphol* 2002;10:332–338.

111. Petit A, Castillo M, Santos M, et al. KIT expression in chromophobe renal cell carcinoma, comparative immunohistochemical analysis of KIT expression different renal cell neoplasms. *Am J Surg Pathol* 2004;28:676–678.

112. Pan CC, Chen PC, Chiang H. Overexpression of KIT (CD117) in chromophobe renal cell carcinoma and renal oncocytoma. *Am J Clin Pathol* 2004;121:878–883.

113. Al-Ahmadie HA, Alden D, Qiu L, et al. Carbonic anhydrase IX expression in clear cell renal cell carcinoma, an immunohistochemical study comparing 2 antibodies. *Am J Surg Pathol* 2008;32: 377–382.

114. Gupta R, Balzer B, Picken M, et al. Diagnostic implications of transcription factor Pax 2 protein and transmembrane enzyme complex carbonic anhydrase IX immunoreactivity in adult renal epithelial neoplasms. *Am J Surg Pathol* 2009;33:241–247.

115. Genega EM, Ghebremichael M, Najarian R, et al. Carbonic anhydrase IX expression in renal neoplasms, correlation with tumor type and grade. *Am J Clin Pathol* 2010;134:873–879.

116. Ozcan A, Zhai Q, Javed R, et al. PAX-2 is a helpful marker for diagnosing metastatic renal cell carcinoma, comparison with the renal cell marker antigen and kidney-specific cadherin. *Arch Pathol Lab Med* 2010;134:1121–1129.

117. Truong LD, Shen SS. Immunohistochemical diagnosis of renal neoplasms. *Arch Pathol Lab Med* 2011;135:92–109.

118. Langner C, Ratschek M, Rehak P, et al. Expression of MUC1 (EMA) and E-cadherin in renal cell carcinoma: a systematic immunohistochemical analysis of 188 cases. *Mod Pathol* 2004;17:180–188.

119. Renshaw AA, Corless CL. Papillary renal cell carcinoma, histology and immunohistochemistry. *Am J Surg Pathol* 1995;19:842–849.

120. Wu SL, Kothari P, Wheeler TM, et al. Cytokeratins 7 and 20 immunoreactivity in chromophobe renal cell carcinomas and renal oncocytomas. *Mod Pathol* 2002;15:712–717.

121. Yamazaki K, Sakamoto M, Ohta T, et al. Overexpression of KIT in chromophobe renal cell carcinoma. *Oncogene* 2003;22:847–852.

122. Krishnan B, Truong LD. Renal epithelial neoplasms: the diagnostic implications of electron microscopic study of 55 cases. *Hum Pathol* 2002;33:68–79.

123. Mackay B, Ordóñez NG, Khoursand J, et al. The ultrastructure and immunocytochemistry of renal cell carcinoma. *Ultrastruct Pathol* 1987;11:483–502.

124. Bernués M, Casadevall C, Miró R, et al. Analysis of 3p allelic losses in renal cell carcinomas: comparison with cytogenetic results. *Cancer Genet Cytogenet* 1998;107:121–124.

125. Kaelin WG Jr. The von Hippel-Lindau tumor suppressor gene and kidney cancer. *Clin Cancer Res* 2004;10:6290s–6295s.

126. Velickovic M, Delahunt B, Störkel S, et al. *VHL* and *FHIT* locus loss of heterozygosity is common in all renal cancer morphotypes but differs in pattern and prognostic significance. *Cancer Res* 2001;61: 4815–4819.

127. Klatte T, Pantuck AJ. Molecular biology of renal cortical tumors. *Urol Clin North Am* 2008;35:573–580.

128. Thrash-Bingham CA, Greenberg RE, Howard S, et al. Comprehensive allelotyping of human renal cell carcinomas using microsatellite DNA probes. *Proc Natl Acad Sci U S A* 1995;92:2854–2858.

129. Mitsumori K, Kittleson JM, Itoh N, et al. Chromosome 14q LOH in localized clear cell renal cell carcinoma. *J Pathol* 2002;198:110–114.

130. Morita R, Saito S, Ishikawa J, et al. Common regions of deletion on chromosomes 5q, 6q, and 10q in renal cell carcinoma. *Cancer Res* 1991;51:5817–5820.

131. Velickovic M, Delahunt B, McIver B, et al. Intragenic *PTEN/MMAC1* loss of heterozygosity in conventional (clear-cell) renal cell carcinoma is associated with poor patient prognosis. *Mod Pathol* 2002;15: 479–485.

132. Chuang C-K, Lai M-K, Chang P-L, et al. Xanthogranulomatous pyelonephritis: experience in 36 cases. *J Urol* 1992;147:333–336.

133. Parsons MA, Harris SC, Longstaff AJ, et al. Xanthogranulomatous pyelonephritis: a pathological, clinical and aetiological analysis of 87 cases. *Diagn Histopathol* 1983;6:203–219.

134. Esparza AR, McKay DB, Cronan JJ, et al. Renal parenchymal malakoplakia, histologic spectrum and its relationship to megalocytic interstitial nephritis and xanthogranulomatous pyelonephritis. *Am J Surg Pathol* 1989;13:225–236.

135. Taxy JB. Renal adenocarcinoma presenting as a solitary metastasis: contribution of electron microscopy to diagnosis. *Cancer* 1981;48:2056–2062.

136. Wick MR, Cherwitz DL, McGlennen RC, et al. Adrenocortical carcinoma, an immunohistochemical comparison with renal cell carcinoma. *Am J Pathol* 1986;122:343–352.

137. Ip Y-T, Yuan J-Q, Cheung H, et al. Sporadic hemangioblastoma of the kidney: an underrecognized pseudomalignant tumor? *Am J Surg Pathol* 2010;34:1695–1700.

138. Delahunt B. Advances and controversies in grading and staging of renal cell carcinoma. *Mod Pathol* 2009;22:S24–S36.

139. Hafez KS, Fergany AF, Novick AC. Nephron sparing surgery for localized renal cell carcinoma: impact of tumor size on patient survival, tumor recurrence and TNM staging. *J Urol* 1999;162:1930–1933.

140. Kinouchi T, Saiki S, Meguro N, et al. Impact of tumor size on the clinical outcomes of patients with Robson stage I renal cell carcinoma. *Cancer* 1999;85:689–695.

141. Gettman MT, Blute ML, Spotts B, et al. Pathologic staging of renal cell carcinoma: significance of tumor classification with the 1997 TNM staging system. *Cancer* 2001;91:354–361.

142. Zisman A, Pantuck AJ, Chao D, et al. Reevaluation of the 1997 TNM classification for renal cell carcinoma: T1 and T2 cutoff point at 4.5 rather than 7 cm. better correlates with clinical outcome. *J Urol* 2001;166:54–58.

143. Delahunt B, Kittelson JM, McCredie MRE, et al. Prognostic importance of tumor size for localized conventional (clear cell) renal cell carcinoma, assessment of TNM T1 and T2 tumor categories and comparison with other prognostic parameters. *Cancer* 2002;94:658–664.

144. Bonsib SM. T2 clear cell renal cell carcinoma is a rare entity: a study of 120 clear cell renal cell carcinomas. *J Urol* 2005;174:1199–1202.

145. Margulis V, Tamboli P, Matin SF, et al. Location of extrarenal extension does not impact survival of patients with pT3a renal cell carcinoma. *J Urol* 2007;178:1878–1882.

146. Ficarra V, Novara G, Iafrate M, et al. Proposal for reclassification of the TNM staging system in patients with locally advanced (pT3-4) renal cell carcinoma according to the cancer-related outcome. *Eur Urol* 2007;51:722–731.

147. Thompson RH, Cheville JC, Lohse CM, et al. Reclassification of patients with pT3 and pT4 renal cell carcinoma improves prognostic accuracy. *Cancer* 2006;104:53–60.

148. Siemer S, Lehmann J, Kamradt J, et al. Adrenal metastases in 1635 patients with renal cell carcinoma: outcome and indication for adrenalectomy. *J Urol* 2004;171:2155–2159.

149. Ficarra V, Galfano A, Guillé F, et al. A new staging system for locally advanced (pT3-4) renal cell carcinoma: a multicenter European study including 2,000 patients. *J Urol* 2007;178:418–424.

150. van Poppel H, Vandendriessche H, Boel K, et al. Microscopic vascular invasion is the most relevant prognosticator after radical nephrectomy for clinically nonmetastatic renal cell carcinoma. *J Urol* 1997;158:45–49.

151. Gonçalves PD, Srougi M, Dall'Oglio MF, et al. Low clinical stage renal cell carcinoma: relevance of microvascular invasion as a prognostic factor. *J Urol* 2004;172:470–474.

152. Kroeger N, Rampersaud EN, Patard J-J, et al. Prognostic value of microvascular invasion in predicting the cancer specific survival and risk of metastatic disease in renal cell carcinoma: a multicenter investigation. *J Urol* 2012;187:418–423.

153. Selli C, Hinshaw WM, Woodard BH, et al. Stratification of risk factors in renal cell carcinoma. *Cancer* 1983;52:899–903.

154. Giuliani L, Giberti C, Martorana G, et al. Radical extensive surgery for renal cell carcinoma: long-term results and prognostic factors. *J Urol* 1990;143:468–474.

155. Lohse CM, Blute ML, Zincke H, et al. Comparison of standardized and nonstandardized nuclear grade of renal cell carcinoma to predict outcome among 2,042 patients. *Am J Clin Pathol* 2002;118:877–886.

156. Cheville JC, Blute ML, Zincke H, et al. Stage pT1 conventional (clear cell) renal cell carcinoma: pathological features associated with cancer specific survival. *J Urol* 2001;166:453–456.

157. Helpap B, Knüpffer J, Essmann S. Nucleolar grading of renal cancer, correlation of frequency and localization of nucleoli to histologic and cytologic grading and stage of renal cell carcinomas. *Mod Pathol* 1990;3:671–678.

158. Serrano MF, Katz M, Yan Y, et al. Percentage of high-grade carcinoma as a prognostic indicator in patients with renal cell carcinoma. *Cancer* 2008;113:477–483.

159. Tomera KM, Farrow GM, Lieber MM. Sarcomatoid renal carcinoma. *J Urol* 1983;130:657–659.

160. Cangiano T, Liao J, Naitoh J, et al. Sarcomatoid renal cell carcinoma: biologic behavior, prognosis, and response to combined surgical resection and immunotherapy. *J Clin Oncol* 1999;17:523–528.

161. Ro JY, Ayala AG, Sella A, et al. Sarcomatoid renal cell carcinoma: a clinicopathologic study of 42 cases. *Cancer* 1987;59:516–526.

162. Cheville JC, Lohse CM, Zincke H, et al. Sarcomatoid renal cell carcinoma, an examination of underlying histologic subtype and an analysis of associations with patient outcome. *Am J Surg Pathol* 2004;28:435–441.

163. Leroy X, Zini L, Buob D, et al. Renal cell carcinoma with rhabdoid features, an aggressive neoplasm with overexpression of p53. *Arch Pathol Lab Med* 2007;131:102–106.

164. Moch H, Gasser T, Amin MB, et al. Prognostic utility of the recently recommended histologic classification and revised TNM staging system for renal cell carcinoma, a Swiss experience with 588 tumors. *Cancer* 2000;89:604–614.

165. Cheville JC, Zincke H, Lohse CM, et al. pT1 clear cell renal cell carcinoma: a study of the association between MIB-1 proliferative activity and pathologic features and cancer specific survival. *Cancer* 2002;94:2180–2184.

166. Moch H, Sauter G, Buchholz N, et al. Epidermal growth factor receptor expression is accociated with rapid tumor cell proliferation in renal cell carcinoma. *Hum Pathol* 1997;28:1255–1259.

167. Kankuri M, Söderström K-O, Pelliniemi T-T, et al. The association of immunoreactive p53 and Ki-67 with T-stage, grade, occurrence of metastases and survival in renal cell carcinoma. *Anticancer Res* 2006;26:3825–3834.

168. Migita T, Oda Y, Naito S, et al. Low expression of p27^{Kip1} is associated with tumor size and poor prognosis in patients with renal cell carcinoma. *Cancer* 2002;94:973–979.

169. Weiss RH, Borowsky AD, Seligson D, et al. p21 is a prognostic marker for renal cell carcinoma: implications for novel therapeutic approaches. *J Urol* 2007;177:63–69.

170. Fukata S, Inoue K, Kamada M, et al. Levels of angiogenesis and expression of angiogenesis-related genes are prognostic for organ-specific metastasis of renal cell carcinoma. *Cancer* 2005;105:931–942.

171. Delahunt B, Bethwaite PB, Thornton A. Prognostic significance of microscopic vascularity for clear cell renal cell carcinoma. *Br J Urol* 1997;80:401–404.

172. Yoshino S, Kato M, Okada K. Evaluation of the prognostic significance of microvessel count and tumor size in renal cell carcinoma. *Int J Urol* 1998;5:119–123.

173. Gilcrease MZ, Guzman-Paz M, Niehans G, et al. Correlation of CD44S expression in renal clear cell carcinomas with subsequent tumor progression or recurrence. *Cancer* 1999;86:2320–2326.

174. Petraki CD, Gregorakis AK, Vaslamatzis MM, et al. Prognostic implications of the immunohistochemical expression of human kallikreins 5, 6, 10 and 11 in renal cell carcinoma. *Tumour Biol* 2006;27:1–7.

175. Lidgren A, Hedberg Y, Grankvist K, et al. The expression of hypoxia-inducible factor 1α is a favorable independent prognostic factor in renal cell carcinoma. *Clin Cancer Res* 2005;11:1129–1135.

176. Jin J-S, Hsieh D-S, Lin Y-F, et al. Increasing expression of extracellular matrix metalloprotease inducer in renal cell carcinoma: tissue microarray analysis of immunostaining score with clinicopathological parameters. *Int J Urol* 2006;13:573–580.

177. Leroy X, Zerimech F, Zini L, et al. MUC1 expression is correlated with nuclear grade and tumor progression in pT1 renal clear cell carcinoma. *Am J Clin Pathol* 2002;118:47–51.

178. Matusan K, Dordevic G, Stipic D, et al. Osteopontin expression correlates with prognostic variables and survival in clear cell renal cell carcinoma. *J Surg Oncol* 2006;94:323–331.

179. Wu S-Q, Hafez GR, Xing W, et al. The correlation between the loss of chromosome 14q with histologic tumor grade, pathologic stage, and outcome of patients with nonpapillary renal cell carcinoma. *Cancer* 1996;77:1154–1160.

180. Moch H, Presti JC Jr, Sauter G, et al. Genetic aberrations detected by comparative genomic hybridization are associated with clinical outcome in renal cell carcinoma. *Cancer Res* 1996;56:27–30.

181. Kinoshita H, Yamada H, Ogawa O, et al. Contribution of chromosome 9p21-22 deletion to the progression of huan renal cell carcinoma. *Jpn J Cancer Res* 1995;86:795–799.

182. Furniss D, Harnden P, Ali N, et al.; National Cancer Research Institute Renal Clinical Studies Group. Prognostic factors for renal cell carcinoma. *Cancer Treat Rev* 2008;34:407–426.

183. Kattan MW, Reuter V, Motzer RJ, et al. A postoperative prognostic nomogram for renal cell carcinoma. *J Urol* 2001;166:63–67.

184. Sorbellini M, Kattan MW, Snyder ME, et al. A postoperative prognostic nomogram predicting recurrence for patients with conventional clear cell renal cell carcinoma. *J Urol* 2005;173:48–51.

185. Hupertan V, Roupret M, Poisson J-F, et al. Low predictive accuracy of the Kattan postoperative nomogram for renal cell carcinoma recurrence in a population of French patients. *Cancer* 2006;107:2604–2608.

186. Frank I, Blute ML, Cheville JC, et al. An outcome prediction model for patients with clear cell renal cell carcinoma treated with radical nephrectomy based on tumor stage, size, grade and necrosis: the SSIGN score. *J Urol* 2002;168:2395–2400.

187. Thompson RH, Leibovich BC, Lohse CM, et al. Dynamic outcome prediction in patients with clear cell renal cell carcinoma treated with radical nephrectomy: the D-SSIGN score. *J Urol* 2007;177:477–480.

188. Kim SP, Thompson RH, Boorjian SA, et al. Comparative effectiveness for survival and renal function of partial and radical nephrectomy for localized renal tumors: a systematic review and meta-analysis. *J Urol* 2012;188:51–57.

189. Kim SP, Thompson RH. Approach to the small renal mass: to treat or not to treat. *Urol Clin North Am* 2012;39:171–179.

190. Tan H-J, Norton EC, Ye Z, et al. Long-term survival following partial vs radical nephrectomy among older patients with early-stage kidney cancer. *JAMA* 2012;307:1629–1635.

191. Miller DC, Shah RB, Bruhn A, et al.; The Urologic Diseases in America Project. Trends in the use of gross and frozen section pathological consultations during partial or radical nephrectomy for renal cell carcinoma. *J Urol* 2008;179:461–467.

192. Yossepowitch O, Thompson AD, Leibovich BC, et al. Positive surgical margins at partial nephrectomy: predictors and oncological outcomes. *J Urol* 2008;179:2158–2163.

193. Bensalah K, Pantuck AJ, Rioux-Leclercq N, et al. Positive surgical margin appears to have negligible impact on survival of renal cell carcinomas treated by nephron-sparing surgery. *Eur Urol* 2010;57:466–471.

194. Pierorazio PM, Patel HD, Feng T, et al. Robotic-assisted versus traditional laparoscopic partial nephrectomy: comparison of outcomes and evaluation of learning curve. *Urology* 2011;78:813–819.

195. Pierorazio PM, Hyams ES, Lin BM, et al. Laparoscopic radical nephrectomy for large renal masses: critical assessment of perioperative and oncologic outcomes of stage T2a and T2b tumors. *Urology* 2012;79:570–576.

196. Landman J, Lento P, Hassen W, et al. Feasibility of pathological evaluation of morcellated kidneys after radical nephrectomy. *J Urol* 2000;164:2086–2089.

197. Venkatesan AM, Wood BJ, Gervais DA. Percutaneous ablation in the kidney. *Radiology* 2011;261:375–391.

198. Best SL, Park SK, Yaacoub RF, et al. Long-term outcomes of renal tumor radio frequency ablation stratified by tumor diameter: size matters. *J Urol* 2012;187:1183–1189.

199. Olweny EO, Park SK, Tan YK, et al. Radiofrequency ablation versus partial nephrectomy in patients with solitary clinical T1a renal cell carcinoma: comparable oncologic outcomes at a minimum of 5 years of follow-up. *Eur Urol* 2012;61:1156–1161.

200. Jewett MAS, Mattar K, Basiuk J, et al. Active surveillance of small renal masses: progression patterns of early stage kidney cancer. *Eur Urol* 2011;60:39–44.

201. Lane BR, Samplaski MK, Herts BR, et al. Renal mass biopsy—a renaissance? *J Urol* 2008;179:20–27.

202. Volpe A, Cadeddu JA, Cestari A, et al. Contemporary management of small renal masses. *Eur Urol* 2011;60:501–515.

203. Blom JHM, van Poppel H, Maréchal JM, et al.; EORTC Genitourinary Tract Cancer Group. Radical nephrectomy with and without lymph-node dissection: final results of European Organization for Research and Treatment of Cancer EORTC randomized phase 3 trial 30881. *Eur Urol* 2009;55:28–34.

204. Sun M, Lughezzani G, Perrotte P, et al. Treatment of metastatic renal cell carcinoma. *Nat Rev Urol* 2010;7:327–338.

205. Kaelin WG Jr. Treatment of kidney cancer, insights provided by the VHL tumor-suppressor protein. *Cancer* 2009;115(10 suppl):2262–2272.

206. Escudier B, Szczylik C, Porta C, et al. Treatment selection in metastatic renal cell carcinoma: expert consensus. *Nat Rev Clin Oncol* 2012;9:327–337.

207. Singer EA, Gupta GN, Srinivasan R. Targeted therapeutic strategies for the management of renal cell carcinoma. *Curr Opin Oncol* 2012;24:284–290.

208. Antonelli A, Cozzoli A, Simeone C, et al. Surgical treatment of adrenal metastasis from renal cell carcinoma: a single-centre experience of 45 patients. *BJU Int* 2006;97:505–508.

209. Antonelli A, Arrighi N, Corti S, et al. Surgical treatment of atypical metastasis from renal cell carcinoma (RCC). *BJU Int* 2012;110:E559–E563.

210. Murad T, Komaiko W, Oyasu R, et al. Multilocular cystic renal cell carcinoma. *Am J Clin Pathol* 1991;95:633–637.

211. Perlmann S. Über einen Fall von Lymphangioma cysticum der Niere. *Virchows Arch Pathol Anat Physiol Klin Med* 1928;268:524–535.

212. Eble JN, Bonsib SM. Extensively cystic renal neoplasms: cystic nephroma, cystic partially differentiated nephroblastoma, multilocular cystic renal cell carcinoma, and cystic hamartoma of renal pelvis. *Semin Diagn Pathol* 1998;15:2–20.

213. Menon P, Rao KLN, Saxena AK, et al. Multilocular cystic renal cell carcinoma in a child. *J Pediatr Surg* 2004;39:e14–e16.

214. Suzigan S, López Beltrán A, Montironi R, et al. Multilocular cystic renal cell carcinoma, a report of 45 cases of a kidney tumor of low malignant potential. *Am J Clin Pathol* 2006;125:217–222.

215. Nassir A, Jollimore J, Gupta R, et al. Multilocular cystic renal cell carcinoma: a series of 12 cases and review of the literature. *Urology* 2002;60:421–427.

216. Gong K, Zhang N, He Z, et al. Multilocular cystic renal cell carcinoma: an experience of clinical management for 31 cases. *J Cancer Res Clin Oncol* 2008;134:433–437.

217. Radopoulos D, Dimitriadis G, Gologinas P, et al. Solitary multilocular cystic renal cell carcinoma in adults: diagnostic problems, pathological features and treatment. *Scand J Urol Nephrol* 2009;43:84–87.

218. Hora M, Hes O, Michal M, et al. Extensively cystic renal neoplasms in adults (Bosniak classification II or III)—possible "common" histological diagnoses: multilocular cystic renal cell carcinoma, cystic nephroma, and mixed epithelial and stromal tumor. *Int Urol Nephrol* 2005;37:743–750.

219. Aubert S, Zini L, Delomez J, et al. Cystic renal cell carcinomas in adults. Is preoperative recognition of multilocular cystic renal cell carcinoma possible? *J Urol* 2005;174:2115–2119.

220. Williamson SR, Halat S, Eble JN, et al. Multilocular cystic renal cell carcinoma similarities and differences in immunoprofile with clear cell renal cell carcinoma. *Am J Surg Pathol* 2012;36:1425–1433.

221. Imura J, Ichikawa K, Takeda J, et al. Multilocular cystic renal cell carcinoma: a clinicopathological, immuno- and lectin histochemical study of nine cases. *APMIS* 2004;112:183–191.

222. Halat S, Eble JN, Grignon DJ, et al. Multilocular cystic renal cell carcinoma is a subtype of clear cell renal cell carcinoma. *Mod Pathol* 2010;23:931–936.

223. Weiss S II, Hafez RG, Uehling DT. Multilocular cystic renal cell carcinoma: implications for nephron sparing surgery. *Urology* 1998; 51:635–637.

224. Han K-R, Janzen NK, McWhorter VC, et al. Cystic renal cell carcinoma: biology and clinical behavior. *Urol Oncol* 2004;22:410–414.

225. Delahunt B, Thornton A. Renal cell carcinoma, a historical perspective. *J Urol Pathol* 1996;4:31–49.

226. Mancilla-Jimenez R, Stanley RJ, Blath RA. Papillary renal cell carcinoma, a clinical, radiologic, and pathologic study of 34 cases. *Cancer* 1976;38:2469–2480.

227. Mydlo JH, Bard RH. Analysis of papillary renal adenocarcinoma. *Urology* 1987;30:529–534.

228. Kovacs G. Papillary renal cell carcinoma, a morphologic and cytogenetic study of 11 cases. *Am J Pathol* 1989;134:27–34.

229. Schrader AJ, Rauer-Bruening S, Olbert PJ, et al. Incidence and long-term prognosis of papillary renal cell carcinoma. *J Cancer Res Clin Oncol* 2009;135:799–805.

230. Bruder E, Passera O, Harms D, et al. Morphologic and molecular characterization of renal cell carcinoma in children and young adults. *Am J Surg Pathol* 2004;28:1117–1132.

231. Hora M, Hes O, Klecka J, et al. Rupture of papillary renal cell carcinoma. *Scand J Urol Nephrol* 2004;38:481–484.

232. Tickoo SK, dePeralta-Venturina MN, Harik LR, et al. Spectrum of epithelial neoplasms in end-stage renal disease: an experience from 66 tumor-bearing kidneys with emphasis on histologic patterns distinct from those in sporadic adult renal neoplasia. *Am J Surg Pathol* 2006;30:141–153.

233. Mydlo JH, Weinstein R, Misseri R, et al. Radiologic, pathologic and molecular attributes of two types of papillary renal adenocarcinomas. *Scand J Urol Nephrol* 2001;35:262–269.

234. Delahunt B, Bethwaite PB, Nacey JN. Outcome prediction for renal cell carcinoma: evaluation of prognostic factors for tumours divided according to histological subtype. *Pathology* 2007;39:459–465.

235. Bard RH, Lord B, Fromowitz F. Papillary adenocarcinoma of kidney, II. Radiographic and biologic characteristics. *Urology* 1982;19: 16–20.

236. Amin MB, Corless CL, Renshaw AA, et al. Papillary (chromophil) renal cell carcinoma: histomorphologic characteristics and evaluation of conventional pathologic prognostic parameters in 62 cases. *Am J Surg Pathol* 1997;21:621–635.

237. Delahunt B, Eble JN. Papillary renal cell carcinoma: a clinicopathologic and immunohistochemical study of 105 tumors. *Mod Pathol* 1997;10:537–544.

238. Dry SM, Renshaw AA. Extensive calcium oxalate crystal deposition in papillary renal cell carcinoma: report of two cases. *Arch Pathol Lab Med* 1998;122:260–261.

239. Delahunt B, Eble JN, McCredie MRE, et al. Morphologic typing of papillary renal cell carcinoma: comparison of growth kinetics and patient survival in 66 cases. *Hum Pathol* 2001;32:590–595.

240. Dekmezian R, Sneige N, Shabb N. Papillary renal-cell carcinoma: fine-needle aspiration of 15 cases. *Diagn Cytopathol* 1991;7:198–203.

241. Ordóñez NG. The diagnostic utility of immunohistochemistry in distinguishing between mesothelioma and renal cell carcinoma: a comparative study. *Hum Pathol* 2004;35:697–710.

242. Gatalica Z, Kovatich A, Miettinen M. Consistent expression of cytokeratin 7 in papillary renal-cell carcinoma. An immunohistochemical study in formalin-fixed, paraffin-embedded tissues. *J Urol Pathol* 1995;3:205–211.

243. Tretiakova MS, Sahoo S, Takahashi M, et al. Expression of alpha-methylacyl-CoA racemase in papillary renal cell carcinoma. *Am J Surg Pathol* 2004;28:69–76.

244. Medeiros LJ, Michie SA, Johnson DE, et al. An immunoperoxidase study of renal cell carcinomas: correlation with nuclear grade, cell type, and histologic pattern. *Hum Pathol* 1988;19:980–987.

245. Hu Y, Hartmann A, Stoehr C, et al. PAX8 is expressed in the majority of renal epithelial neoplasms: an immunohistochemical study of 223 cases using a mouse monoclonal antibody. *J Clin Pathol* 2012;65: 254–256.

246. Leroy X, Zini L, Leteurtre E, et al. Morphologic subtyping of papillary renal cell carcinoma: correlation with prognosis and differential expression of MUC1 between the two subtypes. *Mod Pathol* 2002;15:1126–1130.

247. Schraml P, Frew IJ, Thoma CR, et al. Sporadic clear cell renal cell carcinoma but not the papillary type is characterized by severely reduced frequency of primary cilia. *Mod Pathol* 2009;22:31–36.

248. Kovacs G, Fuzesi L, Emanuel A, et al. Cytogenetics of papillary renal cell tumors. *Genes Chromosomes Cancer* 1991;3:249–255.

249. Kattar MM, Grignon DJ, Wallis T, et al. Clinicopathologic and interphase cytogenetic analysis of papillary (chromophilic) renal cell carcinoma. *Mod Pathol* 1997;10:1143–1150.

250. Schraml P, Müller D, Bednar R, et al. Allelic loss at the D9S171 locus on chromosome 9p13 is associated with progression of papillary renal cell carcinoma. *J Pathol* 2000;190:457–461.

251. Jiang F, Richter J, Schraml P, et al. Chromosomal imbalances in papillary renal cell carcinoma: genetic differences between histologic subtypes. *Am J Pathol* 1998;153:1467–1473.

252. Sanders ME, Mick R, Tomaszewski JE, et al. Unique patterns of allelic imbalance distinguish type 1 from type 2 sporadic papillary renal cell carcinoma. *Am J Pathol* 2002;161:997–1005.

253. Antonelli A, Tardanico R, Balzarini P, et al. Cytogenetic features, clinical significance and prognostic impact of type 1 and type 2 papillary renal cell carcinoma. *Cancer Genet Cytogenet* 2010;199:128–133.

254. Furge KA, Chen J, Koeman J, et al. Detection of DNA copy number changes and oncogenic signaling abnormalities from gene expression data reveals MYC activation in high-grade papillary renal cell carcinoma. *Cancer Res* 2007;67:3171–3176.

255. Lubensky IA, Schmidt L, Zhuang Z, et al. Hereditary and sporadic papillary renal carcinomas with c-met mutations share a distinct morphological phenotype. *Am J Pathol* 1999;155:517–526.

256. Klatte T, Pantuck AJ, Said JW, et al. Cytogenetic and molecular tumor profiling for type 1 and type 2 papillary renal cell carcinoma. *Clin Cancer Res* 2009;15:1162–1169.

257. Morrisey C, Martinez A, Zatyka M, et al. Epigenetic inactivation of the RASSF1A 3p21.3 tumor suppressor gene in both clear cell and papillary renal cell carcinoma. *Cancer Res* 2001;61:7277–7281.

258. Hughson MD, Dickman K, Bigler SA, et al. Clear-cell and papillary carcinoma of the kidney: an analysis of chromosome 3, 7, and 17 abnormalities by microsatellite amplification, cytogenetics, and fluorescence in situ hybridization. *Cancer Genet Cytogenet* 1998;106: 93–104.

259. Beckwith JB. Wilms' tumor and other renal tumors of childhood: a selective review from the National Wilms' Tumor Study Pathology Center. *Hum Pathol* 1983;14:481–492.

260. Gobbo S, Eble JN, Grignon DJ, et al. Clear cell papillary renal cell carcinoma, a distinct histopathologic and molecular genetic entity. *Am J Surg Pathol* 2008;32:1239–1245.

261. Paner GP, Srigley JR, Radhakrishnan A, et al. Immunohistochemical analysis of mucinous tubular and spindle cell carcinoma and papillary renal cell carcinoma of the kidney: significant immunophenotypic overlap warrants diagnostic caution. *Am J Surg Pathol* 2006;30:13–19.

262. Zhou M, Yang XJ, Lopez JI, et al. Renal tubulocystic carcinoma is closely related to papillary renal cell carcinoma: implications for pathologic classification. *Am J Surg Pathol* 2009;33:1840–1849.

263. Daniel L, Zattara-Cannoni H, Lechevallier E, et al. Association of a renal papillary carcinoma with a low grade tumour of the collecting ducts. *J Clin Pathol* 2001;54:637–639.

264. Brennan C, Srigley JR, Whelan C, et al. Type 2 and clear cell papillary renal cell carcinoma, and tubulocystic carcinoma: a unifying concept. *Anticancer Res* 2010;30:641–644.

265. Blei CL, Hartman DS, Friedman AC, et al. Papillary renal cell carcinoma: ultrasonic/pathologic correlation. *J Clin Ultrasound* 1982;10:429–434.

266. Chow GK, Myles J, Novick AC. The Cleveland Clinic experience with papillary (chromophil) renal cell carcinoma: clinical outcome with histopathological correlation. *Can J Urol* 2001;8:1223–1228.

267. Méjean A, Hopirtean V, Bazin J-P, et al. Prognostic factors for the survival of patients with papillary renal cell carcinoma: meaning of histological typing and multifocality. *J Urol* 2003;170:764–767.

268. Margulis V, Tamboli P, Matin SF, et al. Analysis of clinicopathologic predictors of oncologic outcome provides insight into the natural history of surgically managed papillary renal cell carcinoma. *Cancer* 2008;112:1480–1488.

269. Gontero P, Ceratti G, Guglielmetti S, et al. Prognostic factors in a prospective series of papillary renal cell carcinoma. *BJU Int* 2008;102:697–702.

270. Klatte T, Remzi M, Zigeuner RE, et al. Development and external validation of a nomogram predicting disease specific survival after nephrectomy for papillary renal cell carcinoma. *J Urol* 2010;184:53–58.

271. Herrmann E, Trojan L, Becker F, et al. Prognostic factors of papillary renal cell carcinoma: results from a multi-institutional series after pathologic review. *J Urol* 2010;183:460–466.

272. Sika-Paotonu D, Bethwaite PB, McCredie MRE, et al. Nucleolar grade but not Fuhrman grade is applicable to papillary renal cell carcinoma. *Am J Surg Pathol* 2006;30:1091–1096.

273. Tickoo SK, Gopalan A. Pathologic features of renal cortical tumors. *Urol Clin North Am* 2008;35:551–561.

274. Higgins JP, McKenney JK, Brooks JD, et al.; Association of Directors of Anatomic and Surgical Pathology. Recommendations for the reporting of surgically resected specimens of renal cell carcinoma. The Association of Directors of Anatomic and Surgical Pathology. *Hum Pathol* 2009;40:456–463.

275. Delahunt B. Histopathologic prognostic indicators for renal cell carcinoma. *Semin Diagn Pathol* 1998;15:68–76.

276. de Peralta-Venturina MN, Amin MB, Keoleian CM, et al. Papillary renal cell carcinoma, assessment of proliferative activity using PCNA and MIB-1 (Ki-67) and correlation with clinicopathologic findings. *Appl Immunohistochem* 1994;2:241–247.

277. Del Vecchio MT, Lazzi S, Bruni A, et al. DNA ploidy pattern in papillary renal cell carcinoma. Correlation with clinicopathologic parameters and survival. *Pathol Res Pract* 1998;194:325–333.

278. Ku JH, Moon KC, Kwak C, et al. Is there a role of the histologic subtypes of papillary renal cell carcinoma as a prognostic factor? *Jpn J Clin Oncol* 2009;39:664–670.

279. Allory Y, Ouazana D, Boucher E, et al. Papillary renal cell carcinoma, prognostic value of morphological subtypes in a clinicopathologic study of 43 cases. *Virchows Arch* 2003;442:336–342.

280. Pignot G, Elie C, Conquy S, et al. Survival analysis of 130 patients with papillary renal cell carcinoma: prognostic utility of type 1 and type 2 subclassification. *Urology* 2007;69:230–235.

281. Kuroda N, Toi M, Hiroi M, et al. Review of papillary renal cell carcinoma with focus on clinical and pathobiological aspects. *Histol Histopathol* 2003;18:487–494.

282. Yamashita S, Ioritani N, Oikawa K, et al. Morphological subtyping of papillary renal cell carcinoma: clinicopathological characteristics and prognosis. *Int J Urol* 2007;14:679–683.

283. Thompson RH, Leibovich BC, Cheville JC, et al. Second primary malignancies associated with renal cell carcinoma histological subtypes. *J Urol* 2006;176:900–904.

284. Rabbani F, Reuter VE, Katz J, et al. Second primary malignancies associated with renal cell carcinoma: influence of histologic type. *Urology* 2000;56:399–403.

285. Ronnen EA, Kondagunta GV, Ishill N, et al. Treatment outcome for metastatic papillary renal cell carcinoma patients. *Cancer* 2006;107:2617–2621.

286. Thoenes W, Störkel S, Rumpelt H-J. Human chromophobe cell renal carcinoma. *Virchows Arch B Cell Pathol Incl Mol Pathol* 1985;48:207–217.

287. Thoenes W, Störkel S, Rumpelt H-J, et al. Chromophobe cell renal carcinoma and its variants—a report on 32 cases. *J Pathol* 1988;155:277–287.

288. Cindolo L, de la Taille A, Schips L, et al. Chromophobe renal cell carcinoma: comprehensive analysis of 104 cases from multicenter European database. *Urology* 2005;65:681–686.

289. Teloken PE, Thompson RH, Tickoo SK, et al. Prognostic impact of histological subtype on surgically treated localized renal cell carcinoma. *J Urol* 2009;182:2132–2136.

290. Cheville JC, Lohse CM, Sukov WR, et al. Chromophobe renal cell carcinoma: the impact of tumor grade on outcome. *Am J Surg Pathol* 2012;36:851–856.

291. Peyromaure M, Misrai V, Thiounn N, et al. Chromophobe renal cell carcinoma, analysis of 61 cases. *Cancer* 2004;100:1406–1410.

292. Crotty TB, Farrow GM, Lieber MM. Chromophobe renal cell carcinoma: clinicopathologic features of 50 cases. *J Urol* 1995;154:964–967.

293. Akhtar M, Kardar H, Linjawi T, et al. Chromophobe cell carcinoma of the kidney. A clinicopathologic study of 21 cases. *Am J Surg Pathol* 1995;19:1245–1256.

294. Hes O, Vanecek T, Perez-Montiel DM, et al. Chromophobe renal cell carcinoma with microcystic and adenomatous arrangement and pigmentation—a diagnostic pitfall. Morphological, immunohistochemical, ultrastructural and molecular genetic report of 20 cases. *Virchows Arch* 2005;446:383–393.

295. Parada DD, Peña KBG. Chromophobe renal cell carcinoma with neuroendocrine differentiation, case report. *APMIS* 2008;116:859–865.

296. Wu SL, Fishman IJ, Shannon RL. Chromophobe renal cell carcinoma with extensive calcification and ossification. *Ann Diagn Pathol* 2002;6:244–247.

297. Kefeli M, Yildiz L, Aydin O, et al. Chromophobe renal cell carcinoma with osseous metaplasia containing fatty bone marrow element: a case report. *Pathol Res Pract* 2007;203:749–752.

298. Akhtar M, Tulbah A, Kardar AH, et al. Sarcomatoid renal cell carcinoma: the chromophobe connection. *Am J Surg Pathol* 1997;21:1188–1195.

299. Viswanathan S, Desai SB, Prabhu SR, et al. Squamous differentiation in a sarcomatoid chromophobe renal cell carcinoma, an unusual case report with review of the literature. *Arch Pathol Lab Med* 2008;132:1672–1674.

300. Mete O, Kiliçaslan I, Ozcan F, et al. Sarcomatoid chromophobe renal cell carcinoma with squamous differentiation. *Pathology* 2007;39:598–613.

301. Magro G, Lopes M, Amico P, et al. Chromophobe renal cell carcinoma with extensive rhabdomyosarcomatous component. *Virchows Arch* 2005;447:894–896.

302. Quiroga-Garza G, Khuran H, Shen S, et al. Sarcomatoid chromophobe renal cell carcinoma with heterologous sarcomatoid elements, a case report and review of the literature. *Arch Pathol Lab Med* 2009;133:1857–1860.

303. Shannon BA, Cohen RJ. Rhabdoid differentiation of chromophobe renal cell carcinoma. *Pathology* 2003;35:228–230.

304. Salamanca J, Alberti N, López-Ríos F, et al. Fine needle aspiration of chromophobe renal cell carcinoma. *Acta Cytol* 2007;51:9–15.

305. Tejerina E, González-Peramato P, Jiménez-Heffernan JA, et al. Cytological features of chromophobe renal cell carcinoma, classic type. A report of nine cases. *Cytopathology* 2009;20:44–49.

306. Mathers ME, Pollock AM, Marsh C, et al. Cytokeratin 7: a useful adjunct in the diagnosis of chromophobe renal cell carcinoma. *Histopathology* 2002;40:563–567.

307. Liu L, Qian J, Singh H, et al. Immunohistochemical analysis of chromophobe renal cell carcinoma, renal oncocytoma, and clear cell carcinoma, an optimal and practical panel for differential diagnosis. *Arch Pathol Lab Med* 2007;131:1290–1297.

308. Wang H-Y, Mills SE. KIT and RCC are useful in distinguishing chromophobe renal cell carcinoma from the granular variant of clear cell renal cell carcinoma. *Am J Surg Pathol* 2005;29:640–646.

309. Taki A, Nakatani Y, Misugi K, et al. Chromophobe renal cell carcinoma: an immunohistochemical study of 21 Japanese cases. *Mod Pathol* 1999;12:310–317.

310. Adley BP, Gupta A, Lin F, et al. Expression of kidney-specific cadherin in chromophobe renal cell carcinoma and renal oncocytoma. *Am J Clin Pathol* 2006;126:79–85.

311. Yusenko MV, Kovacs G. Identifying CD82 (KAI1) as a marker for human chromophobe renal cell carcinoma. *Histopathology* 2009;55:687–695.

312. Hornsby CD, Cohen C, Amin MB, et al. Claudin-7 immunohistochemistry in renal tumors, a candidate marker for chromophobe renal cell carcinoma identified by gene expression profiling. *Arch Pathol Lab Med* 2007;131:1541–1546.

313. Martignoni G, Pea M, Brunelli M, et al. CD10 is expressed in a subset of chromophobe renal cell carcinomas. *Mod Pathol* 2004;17:1455–1463.

314. Khoury JD, Abrahams NA, Levin HS, et al. The utility of epithelial membrane antigen and vimentin in the diagnosis of chromophobe renal cell carcinoma. *Ann Diagn Pathol* 2002;6:154–158.

315. Li G, Barthelmy A, Feng G, et al. S100A1: a powerful marker to differentiate chromophobe renal cell carcinoma from renal oncocytoma. *Histopathology* 2007;5:642–647.

316. Erlandson RA, Reuter VE. Renal tumor in a 62-year-old male. *Ultrastruct Pathol* 1988;12:561–567.

317. Montes Moreno S, Alemany Benítez I, Martínez González MA. Ultrastructural studies in a series of 18 cases of chromophobe renal cell carcinoma. *Ultrastruct Pathol* 2005;29:377–387.

318. Thoenes W, Baum H-P, Störkel S, et al. Cytoplasmic microvesicles in chromophobe cell renal carcinoma demonstrated by freeze fracture. *Virchows Arch B Cell Pathol Incl Mol Pathol* 1987;54:127–130.

319. Bonsib SM, Bray C, Timmerman TG. Renal chromophobe cell carcinoma: limitations of paraffin-embedded tissue. *Ultrastruct Pathol* 1993;17:529–536.

320. Zambrano NR, Lubensky IA, Merino MJ, et al. Histopathology and molecular genetics of renal tumors: toward unification of a classification system. *J Urol* 1999;162:1246–1258.

321. Brunelli M, Gobbo S, Cossu Rocca P, et al. Chromosomal gains in the sarcomatoid transformation of chromophobe renal cell carcinoma. *Mod Pathol* 2007;20:303–309.

322. Leibovich BC, Lohse CM, Crispen PL, et al. Histological subtype is an independent predictor of outcome for patients with renal cell carcinoma. *J Urol* 2010;183:1309–1316.

323. Onishi T, Oishi Y, Yanada S, et al. Prognostic implications of histological features in patients with chromophobe renal carcinoma. *BJU Int* 2002;90:529–532.

324. Beck SDW, Patel MI, Snyder ME, et al. Effect of papillary and chromophobe cell type on disease-free survival after nephrectomy for renal cell carcinoma. *Ann Surg Oncol* 2005;11:71–77.

325. Lohse CM, Cheville JC. A review of prognostic pathologic features and algorithms for patients treated surgically for renal cell carcinoma. *Clin Lab Med* 2005;25:433–464.

326. Amin MB, Paner GP, Alvarado-Cabrero I, et al. Chromophobe renal cell carcinoma: histomorphologic characteristics and evaluation of conventional pathologic prognostic parameters in 145 cases. *Am J Surg Pathol* 2008;32:1822–1834.

327. Delahunt B, Sika-Paotonu D, Bethwaite PB, et al. Fuhrman grading is not appropriate for chromophobe renal cell carcinoma. *Am J Surg Pathol* 2007;31:957–960.

328. Paner GP, Amin MB, Alvarado-Cabrero I, et al. A novel tumor grading scheme for chromophobe renal cell carcinoma, prognostic utility and comparison with Fuhrman nuclear grade. *Am J Surg Pathol* 2010;34:1233–1240.

329. Delahunt B, Cheville JC, Martignoni G, et al. The International Society of Urological Pathology (ISUP) grading system for renal cell carcinoma and other prognostic parameters. *Am J Surg Pathol.* In press 2013.

330. Choueiri TK, Plantade A, Elson P, et al. Efficacy of sunitinib and sorafenib in metastatic papillary and chromophobe renal cell carcinoma. *J Clin Oncol* 2012;26:127–131.

331. Foot NC, Papanicolaou GN. Early renal carcinoma in situ detected by means of smears of fixed urinary sediment. *JAMA* 1949;139:356–358.

332. Fleming S, Lewi HJE. Collecting duct carcinoma of the kidney. *Histopathology* 1986;10:1131–1141.

333. Delahunt B, Eble JN. Renal cell neoplasia. *Pathology* 2002;34:13–20.

334. Kuroda N, Toi M, Hiroi M, et al. Review of collecting duct carcinoma with focus on clinical and pathobiological aspects. *Histol Histopathol* 2002;17:1329–1334.

335. Rumpelt HJ, Störkel S, Moll R, et al. Bellini duct carcinoma: further evidence for this rare variant of renal cell carcinoma. *Histopathology* 1991;18:115–122.

336. Karakiewicz PI, Trinh Q-D, Rioux-Leclercq N, et al. Collecting duct renal cell carcinoma: a matched analysis of 41 cases. *Eur Urol* 2007;52:1140–1146.

337. Kennedy SM, Merino MJ, Linehan WM, et al. Collecting duct carcinoma of the kidney. *Hum Pathol* 1990;21:449–456.

338. Chao D, Zisman A, Pantuck AJ, et al. Collecting duct renal cell carcinoma: clinical study of a rare tumor. *J Urol* 2002;167:71–74.

339. Carter MD, Tha S, McLoughlin MG, et al. Collecting duct carcinoma of the kidney: a case report and review of the literature. *J Urol* 1992;147:1096–1098.

340. Bielsa O, Arango O, Corominas JM, et al. Collecting duct carcinoma of the kidney. *Br J Urol* 1994;74:127–128.

341. Cavazzana AO, Prayer-Galetti T, Tirabosco R, et al. Bellini duct carcinoma, a clinical and in vitro study. *Eur Urol* 1996;30:340–344.

342. Füzesi L, Cober M, Mittermayer C. Collecting duct carcinoma: cytogenetic characterization. *Histopathology* 1992;21:155–160.

343. Srigley JR, Eble JN. Collecting duct carcinoma of kidney. *Semin Diagn Pathol* 1998;15:54–67.

344. Peyromaure M, Thiounn N, Scotté F, et al. Collecting duct carcinoma of the kidney: a clinicopathologic study of 9 cases. *J Urol* 2004;170:1138–1140.

345. Gupta R, Billis A, Shah RB, et al. Carcinoma of the collecting ducts of Bellini and renal medullary carcinoma, clinicopathologic analysis of 52 cases of rare aggressive subtypes of renal cell carcinoma with a focus on their interrelationship. *Am J Surg Pathol* 2012;36:1265–1278.

346. Karakiewicz PI, Trinh Q-D, Bhojani N, et al. Renal cell carcinoma with nodal metastases in the absence of distant metastatic disease: prognostic indicators of disease-specific survival. *Eur Urol* 2007;51:1616–1624.

347. Hai MA, Diaz-Perez R. Atypical carcinoma of kidney originating from collecting duct epithelium. *Urology* 1982;19:89–92.

348. Cromie WJ, Davis CJ Jr. Atypical carcinoma of kidney possibly originating from collecting duct epithelium. *Urology* 1979;13:315–317.

349. Aizawa S, Kikuchi Y, Suzuki M, et al. Renal cell carcinoma of lower nephron origin. *Acta Pathol Jpn* 1987;37:567–574.

350. Halenda G, Sees JN Jr, Belis JA, et al. Atypical renal adenocarcinoma with features suggesting collecting duct origin and mimicking a mucinous adenocarcinoma. *Urology* 1993;41:165–168.

351. Dimopoulos MA, Logothetis CJ, Markowitz A, et al. Collecting duct carcinoma of the kidney. *Br J Urol* 1993;71:388–391.

352. Kobayashi N, Matsuzaki O, Shirai S, et al. Collecting duct carcinoma of the kidney: an immunohistochemical evaluation of the use of antibodies for differential diagnosis. *Hum Pathol* 2008;39:1350–1359.

353. McGregor DK, Khurana KK, Cao C, et al. Diagnosing primary and metastatic renal cell carcinoma: the use of the monoclonal antibody 'renal cell carcinoma marker'. *Am J Surg Pathol* 2001;25:1485–1492.

354. Albadine R, Schultz L, Illei P, et al. PAX8 (+)/p63 (-) immunostaining pattern in renal collecting duct carcinoma (CDC) a useful immuno-profile in the differential diagnosis of CDC versus urothelial carci-noma of the upper urinary tract. *Am J Surg Pathol* 2010;34:965–969.

355. Schoenberg M, Cairns P, Brooks JD, et al. Frequent loss of chromo-some arms 8p and 13q in collecting duct carcinoma (CDC) of the kidney. *Genes Chromosomes Cancer* 1995;12:76–80.

356. Orsola A, Trias I, Raventós CX, et al. Renal collecting (Bellini) duct carcinoma displays similar characteristics to upper tract urothelial car-cinoma. *Urology* 2005;65:49–54.

357. Tokuda N, Naito S, Matsuzaki O, et al. Collecting duct (Bellini duct) renal cell carcinoma: a nationwide survey in Japan. *J Urol* 2006;176:40–43.

358. Barrascout E, Beuselinck B, Ayllon J, et al. Complete remission of pulmonary metastases of Bellini duct carcinoma with cisplatin, gem-citabine and bevacizumab. *Am J Case Rep* 2012;13:1–2.

359. Davis CJ Jr, Mostofi FK, Sesterhenn IA. Renal medullary carcinoma: the seventh sickle cell nephropathy. *Am J Surg Pathol* 1995;19:1–11.

360. Swartz M, Karth J, Schneider DT, et al. Renal medullary carcinoma: clinical, pathologic, immunohistochemical, and genetic analysis with pathogenetic implications. *Urology* 2002;60:1083–1089.

361. Yang XJ, Sugimura J, Tretiakova MS, et al. Gene expression profil-ing of renal medullary carcinoma, potential clinical relevance. *Cancer* 2004;100:976–985.

362. Simpson L, He X, Pins M, et al. Renal medullary carcinoma and *ABL* gene amplification. *J Urol* 2005;173:1883–1888.

363. Sathyamoorthy K, Teo A, Atallah M. Renal medullary carcinoma in a patient with sickle-cell disease. *Nat Clin Pract Urol* 2006;3:279–283.

364. Leitão VA, da Silva W Jr, Ferreira U, et al. Renal medullary carci-noma, case report and review of the literature. *Urol Int* 2006;77:184–186.

365. Baig MA, Lin YS, Rasheed J, et al. Renal medullary carcinoma. *J Natl Med Assoc* 2006;98:1171–1174.

366. Hakimi AA, Koi PT, Milhoua PM, et al. Renal medullary carcinoma: the Bronx experience. *Urology* 2007;70:878–882.

367. Watanabe IC, Billis A, Guimarães MS, et al. Renal medullary car-cinoma: report of seven cases from Brazil. *Mod Pathol* 2008;20:914–920.

368. Cheng JX, Tretiakova M, Gong C, et al. Renal medullary carcinoma: rhabdoid features and the absence of INI1 expression as markers of aggressive behavior. *Mod Pathol* 2008;21:647–652.

369. Wartchow EP, Trost BA, Tucker JA, et al. Renal medullary carcinoma: ultrastructural studies may benefit diagnosis. *Ultrastruct Pathol* 2008;32:252–256.

370. O'Donnell PH, Jensen A, Posadas EM, et al. Renal medullary-like carcinoma in an adult without sickle cell hemoglobinopathy. *Nat Rev Urol* 2010;7:110–114.

371. Gatalica Z, Lilleberg SL, Monzon FA, et al. Renal medullary carci-nomas: histopathologic phenotype associated with diverse genotypes. *Hum Pathol* 2011;42:1979–1988.

372. Liu Q, Galli S, Srinivasan R, et al. Renal medullary carcinoma: molecular, immunophistochemistry, and morphologic correlation. *Am J Surg Pathol* 2013;37:368–374.

373. Rao P, Tannir NM, Tamboli P. Expression of OCT3/4 in renal med-ullary carcinoma represents a potential diagnostic pitfall. *Am J Surg Pathol* 2012;36:583–588.

374. Calderaro J, Moroch J, Pierron G, et al. *SMARCB1/INI1* inactivation in renal medullary carcinoma. *Histopathology* 2012;61:428–435.

375. Sidhar SK, Clark J, Gill S, et al. The t(x;1)(p11.2;q21.2) translocation in papillary renal cell carcinoma fuses a novel gene *PRCC* to the *TFE3* transcription factor gene. *Hum Mol Genet* 1996;5:1333–1338.

376. Clark J, Lu Y-J, Sidhar SK, et al. Fusion of splicing factor genes *PSF* and *NonO(p54nrb)* to the *TFE2* gene in papillary renal cell carcinoma. *Oncogene* 1999;15:2233–2239.

377. Argani P, Ladanyi M. Translocation carcinomas of the kidney. *Clin Lab Med* 2005;25:363–378.

378. Argani P, Hawkins A, Griffin CA, et al. A distinctive pediatric renal neoplasm characterized by epithelioid morphology, basement mem-brane production, focal HMB45 immunoreactivity, and t(6;11) (p21.1;q12) chromosome translocation. *Am J Pathol* 2001;158:2089–2096.

379. Camparo P, Vasiliu V, Molinié V, et al. Renal translocation carcinomas, clinicopathologic, immunohistochemical, and gene expression profil-ing analysis of 31 cases with a review of the literature. *Am J Surg Pathol* 2008;32:656–670.

380. Argani P, Laé M, Ballard ET, et al. Translocation carcinomas of the kidney following chemotherapy in childhood. *J Clin Oncol* 2006;24:1529–1534.

381. Argani P, Aulmann S, Karanjawala Z, et al. Melanotic Xp11 transloca-tion renal cancers, a distinctive neoplasm with overlapping features of PEComa, carcinoma, and melanoma. *Am J Surg Pathol* 2009;33:609–619.

382. Argani P, Antonescu CR, Couturier J, et al. *PRCC-TFE3* renal car-cinomas: morphologic, immunohistochemical, ultrastructural, and molecular analysis of an entity associated with the t(X;1)(p11.2;q21). *Am J Surg Pathol* 2002;26:1553–1566.

383. Argani P, Antonescu CR, Illei PB, et al. Primary renal neoplasms with the ASPL-TFE3 gene fusion of alveolar soft part sarcoma: a distinc-tive tumor entity previously included among renal cell carcinomas of children and adolescents. *Am J Pathol* 2001;159:179–192.

384. Argani P, Lui MY, Couturier J, et al. A novel *CLTC-TFE3* gene fusion in pediatric renal adenocarcinoma with t(X;17)(p11.2;q23). *Oncogene* 2003;22:5374–5378.

385. Argani P, Laé M, Hutchinson B, et al. Renal carcinomas with the t(6;11)(p21;q12), clinicopathologic features and demonstration of the specific *Alpha-TFEB* gene fusion by immunohistochemistry, RT-PCR, and DNA PCR. *Am J Surg Pathol* 2005;29:230–240.

386. Argani P, Ladanyi M. Distinctive neoplasms characterised by specific chromosomal translocations comprise a significant proportion of pae-diatric renal cell carcinomas. *Pathology* 2003;35:492–498.

387. Dal Cin P, Stas M, Sciot R, et al. Translocation (X;1) reveals metas-tasis 31 years after renal cell carcinoma. *Cancer Genet Cytogenet* 1998;101:58–61.

388. Geller JI, Argani P, Adeniran A, et al. Translocation renal cell carci-noma, lack of negative implications due to lymph node spread. *Cancer* 2008;112:1607–1616.

389. Medeiros LJ, Palmedo G, Krigman HR, et al. Oncocytoid renal cell carcinoma after neuroblastoma: a report of four cases of a distinct clinicopathologic entity. *Am J Surg Pathol* 1999;23:772–780.

390. Koyle MA, Hatch DA, Furness PD III, et al. Long-term urologic com-plications in survivors younger than 15 months of advanced stage abdominal neuroblastoma. *J Urol* 2001;166:1455–1458.

391. Eble JN. Mucinous tubular and spindle cell carcinoma and post-neu-roblastoma carcinoma: newly recognised entities in the renal cell car-cinoma family. *Pathology* 2003;35:499–504.

392. Bassal M, Mertens AC, Taylor L, et al. Risk of selected subsequent carcinomas in survivors of childhood cancer: a report from the Child-hood Cancer Survivor Study. *J Clin Oncol* 2006;24:476–483.

393. Dhall D, Al-Ahmadie HA, Dhall G, et al. Pediatric renal cell carci-noma with oncocytoid features occurring in a child after chemother-apy for cardiac leiomyosarcoma. *Urology* 2007;70:178.e13–178.e15.

394. Fleitz JM, Wootton-Gorges SL, Wyatt-Ashmead J, et al. Renal cell carcinoma in long-term survivors of advanced stage neuroblastoma in early childhood. *Pediatr Radiol* 2003;33:540–545.

395. MacLennan GT, Farrow GM, Bostwick DG. Low-grade collecting duct carcinoma of the kidney: report of 13 cases of low-grade muci-nous tubulocystic renal carcinoma of possible collecting duct origin. *Urology* 1997;50:679–684.

396. Rakozy C, Schmahl GE, Bogner S, et al. Low-grade tubular-mucinous renal neoplasms: morphologic, immunohistochemical, and genetic features. *Mod Pathol* 2002;15:1162–1171.

397. Hes O, Hora M, Perez-Montiel DM, et al. Spindle and cuboidal renal cell carcinoma, a tumour having frequent association with nephrolithiasis: report of 11 cases including a case with hybrid conventional renal cell carcinoma/spindle and cuboidal renal cell carcinoma components. *Histopathology* 2002;41:549–555.

398. Ferlicot S, Allory Y, Compérat E, et al. Mucinous tubular and spindle cell carcinoma, a report of 15 cases with a review of the literature. *Virchows Arch* 2005;447:978–983.

399. Shen SS, Ro JY, Tamboli P, et al. Mucinous tubular and spindle cell carcinoma of kidney is probably a variant of papillary renal cell carcinoma with spindle cell features. *Ann Diagn Pathol* 2007;11:13–21.

400. Fine SW, Argani P, DeMarzo AM, et al. Expanding the histologic spectrum of mucinous tubular and spindle cell carcinoma of the kidney. *Am J Surg Pathol* 2006;30:1554–1560.

401. Dhillon J, Amin MB, Selbs E, et al. Mucinous tubular and spindle cell carcinoma of the kidney with sarcomatoid change. *Am J Surg Pathol* 2009;33:44–49.

402. Pillay N, Ramdial PK, Cooper K. Mucinous tubular and spindle cell carcinoma with aggressive histomorphology—a sarcomatoid variant. *Hum Pathol* 2008;39:966–969.

403. Simon RA, di Sant'Agnese PA, Palapattu GS, et al. Mucinous tubular and spindle cell carcinoma of the kidney with sarcomatoid differentiation. *Int J Clin Exp Pathol* 2008;1:180–184.

404. Parwani AV, Husain AN, Epstein JI, et al. Low-grade myxoid renal epithelial neoplasms with distal nephron differentiation. *Hum Pathol* 2001;32:506–512.

405. Kuroda N, Nakamura S, Miyazaki E, et al. Low-grade tubular-mucinous renal neoplasm with neuroendocrine differentiation: a histological, immunohistochemical and ultrastructural study. *Pathol Int* 2004;54:201–207.

406. Kuehn A, Paner GP, Skinnider BF, et al. Expression analysis of kidney-specific cadherin in a wide spectrum of traditonal and newly recognzied renal epithelial neoplasms: diagnostic and histogenetic implications. *Am J Surg Pathol* 2007;31:1528–1533.

407. Cossu Rocca P, Eble JN, Delahunt B, et al. Renal mucinous tubular and spindle cell carcinoma lacks the gains of chromosomes 7 and 17 and losses of chromosome Y that are prevalent in papillary renal cell carcinoma. *Mod Pathol* 2006;19:488–493.

408. Brandal P, Lie AK, Bassarova A, et al. Genomic aberrations in mucinous tubular and spindle cell renal cell carcinomas. *Mod Pathol* 2006;19:186–194.

409. Argani P, Netto GJ, Parwani AV. Papillary renal cell carcinoma with low-grade spindle cell foci, a mimic of mucinous tubular and spindle cell carcinoma. *Am J Surg Pathol* 2008;32:1353–1359.

410. Bulimbasic S, Ljubanovic D, Sima R, et al. Aggressive high-grade mucinous tubular and spindle cell carcinoma. *Hum Pathol* 2009;40:906–907.

411. Murphy WM, Beckwith JB, Farrow GM. *Atlas of Tumor Pathology, Third Series, Fascicle 11, Tumors of the Kidney, Bladder, and Related Urinary Structures.* Washington, DC: Armed Forces Institute of Pathology; 1994.

412. Azoulay S, Vieillefond A, Paraf F, et al. Tubulocystic carcinoma of the kidney: a new entity among renal tumors. *Virchows Arch* 2007;451:905–909.

413. Yang XJ, Zhou M, Hes O, et al. Tubulocystic carcinoma of the kidney, clinicopathologic and molecular characterization. *Am J Surg Pathol* 2008;32:177–187.

414. Amin MB, MacLennan GT, Gupta R, et al. Tubulocystic carcinoma of the kidney, clinicopathologic analysis of 31 cases of a distinctive rare subtype of renal cell carcinoma. *Am J Surg Pathol* 2009;33:384–392.

415. Osunkoya AO, Young AN, Wang W, et al. Comparison of gene expression profiles in tubulocystic carcinoma and collecting duct carcinoma of the kidney. *Am J Surg Pathol* 2009;33:1103–1106.

416. Bhullar JS, Thamboo T, Esuvaranathan K. Unique case of tubulocystic carcinoma of the kidney with sarcomatoid features: a new entity. *Urology* 2012;78:1071–1072.

417. Aydin H, Chen L, Cheng L, et al. Clear cell tubulopapillary renal cell carcinoma: a study of 36 distinctive low-grade epithelial tumors of the kidney. *Am J Surg Pathol* 2010;34:1608–1621.

418. Adam J, Couturier J, Molinié V, et al. Clear-cell papillary renal cell carcinoma: 24 cases of a distinct low-grade renal tumour and a comparative genomic hybridization array study of seven cases. *Histopathology* 2011;58:1064–1071.

419. Rohan SM, Xiao Y, Liang Y, et al. Clear-cell papillary renal cell carcinoma: molecular and immunohistochemical analysis with emphasis on the *von Hippel-Lindau* gene and hypoxia-inducible factor pathway-related proteins. *Mod Pathol* 2011;24:1207–1220.

420. Bhatnagar R, Alexiev BA. Renal-cell carcinomas in end-stage kidneys: a clinicopathological study with emphasis on clear-cell papillary renal-cell carcinoma and acquired cystic disease-associated carcinoma. *Int J Surg Pathol* 2012;20:19–28.

421. Williamson SR, Eble JN, Cheng L, et al. Clear cell papillary renal cell carcinoma: differential diagnosis and extended immunohistochemical profile. *Mod Pathol* 2013;26:697–708.

422. Kuroda N, Shiotsu T, Kawada C, et al. Clear cell papillary renal cell carcinoma and clear cell renal cell carcinoma arising in acquired cystic disease of the kidney: an immunohistochemical and genetic study. *Ann Diagn Pathol* 2011;15:282–285.

423. Farivar-Mohseni H, Perlmutter AE, Wilson S, et al. Renal cell carcinoma and end stage renal disease. *J Urol* 2006;175:2018–2021.

424. Ianhez LE, Lucon M, Nahas WC, et al. Renal cell carcinoma in renal transplant patients. *Urology* 2007;69:462–464.

425. Sangoi AR, Higgins JP. Bilateral mixed epithelial stromal tumor in an end-stage renal disease patient: the first case report. *Hum Pathol* 2008;39:142–146.

426. Hora M, Reischig T, Ürge T, et al. Tumors in end-stage kidneys. *Transplant Proc* 2008;40:3354–3358.

427. Kuroda N, Tamura M, Taguchi T, et al. Sarcomatoid acquired cystic disease-associated renal cell carcinoma. *Histol Histopathol* 2008;23:1327–1331.

428. Inoue H, Nonomura N, Kojima Y, et al. Somatic mutations of the von Hippel-Lindau disease gene in renal carcinomas occurring in patients with long-term dialysis. *Nephrol Dial Transplant* 2007;22:2052–2055.

429. Pan C-C, Chen Y-J, Chang L-C, et al. Immunohistochemical and molecular genetic profiling of acquired cystic disease-associated renal cell carcinoma. *Histopathology* 2009;55:145–153.

430. Yoshida M, Yao M, Ishikawa I, et al. Somatic von Hippel-Lindau disease gene mutation in clear-cell renal carcinomas associated with end-stage renal disease/acquired cystic disease of kidney. *Genes Chromosomes Cancer* 2002;35:359–364.

431. Cheuk W, Lo ESF, Chan AKC, et al. Atypical epithelial proliferations in acquired renal cystic disease harbor cytogenetic aberrations. *Hum Pathol* 2002;33:761–765.

432. Cossu Rocca P, Eble JN, Zhang S, et al. Acquired cystic disease-associated renal tumors: an immunohistochemical and fluorescence *in situ* hybridization study. *Mod Pathol* 2006;19:780–787.

433. Jung SJ, Chung JI, Park SH, et al. Thyroid follicular carcinoma-like tumor of kidney, a case report with morphologic, immunohistochemical, and genetic analysis. *Am J Surg Pathol* 2006;30:411–415.

434. Sterlacci W, Verdorfer I, Gabriel M, et al. Thyroid follicular carcinoma-like renal tumor: a case report with morphologic, immunophenotypic, cytogenetic, and scintigraphic studies. *Virchows Arch* 2008;452:91–95.

435. Amin MB, Gupta R, Ondrej H, et al. Primary thyroid-like follicular carcinoma of the kidney, report of 6 cases of a histologically distinctive adult renal epithelial neoplasm. *Am J Surg Pathol* 2009;33:393–400.

436. Dhillon J, Tannir NM, Matin SF, et al. Thyroid-like follicular carcinoma of the kidney with metastases to the lungs and retroperitoneal lymph nodes. *Hum Pathol* 2011;42:146–150.

437. Alessandrini L, Fassan M, Gardiman MP, et al. Thyroid-like follicular carcinoma of the kidney: report of two cases with detailed immunohistochemical profile and literature review. *Virchows Arch* 2012;461:345–350.

438. Michal M, Hes O, Havlicek F. Benign renal angiomyoadenomatous tumor: a previously unreported renal tumor. *Ann Diagn Pathol* 2000;4:311–315.

439. Kuhn E, De Anda J, Manoni S, et al. Renal cell carcinoma associated with prominent angioleiomyomatous proliferation, report of five cases and review of the literature. *Am J Surg Pathol* 2006;30:1372–1381.

440. Shannon BA, Cohen RJ, Segal A, et al. Clear cell renal cell carcinoma with smooth muscle stroma. *Hum Pathol* 2009;40:425–429.

441. Michal M, Hes O, Nemcova J, et al. Renal angiomyoadenomatous tumor: morphologic, immunohistochemical, and molecular genetic study of a distinct entity. *Virchows Arch* 2009;454:89–99.

442. Kuroda N, Michal M, Hes O, et al. Renal angiomyoadenomatous tumor: fluorescence *in situ* hybridization. *Pathol Int* 2009;59:689–691.

443. Petersson F, Grossmann P, Hora M, et al. Renal cell carcinoma with areas mimicking renal angiomyoadenomatous tumor/clear cell papillary renal cell carcinoma. *Hum Pathol* 2013;44:1412–1420.

444. Hand JR, Broders AC. Carcinoma of the kidney: the degree of malignancy in relation to factors bearing on prognosis. *J Urol* 1932;28:199–216.

445. Griffiths IH, Thackray AC. Parenchymal carcinoma of the kidney. *Br J Urol* 1949;21:128–151.

446. Riches EW. Factors in the prognosis of carcinoma of the kidney. *J Urol* 1958;79:190–194.

447. Arner O, Blanck C, von Schreeb T. Renal adenocarcinoma, morphology, grading of malignancy, prognosis, a study of 197 cases. *Acta Chir Scand Suppl* 1965;346:7–51.

448. Hermanek P, Sigel A, Chlepas S. Histological grading of renal cell carcinoma. *Eur Urol* 1976;2:189–191.

449. Boxer RJ, Waisman J, Lieber MM, et al. Renal carcinoma: computer analysis of 96 patients treated by nephrectomy. *J Urol* 1979;122:598–601.

450. Hop WCJ, van der Werf-Messing BHP. Prognostic indexes for renal cell carcinoma. *Eur J Cancer* 1980;16:833–840.

451. McNichols DW, Segura JW, DeWeerd JH. Renal cell carcinoma: long-term survival and late recurrence. *J Urol* 1981;126:17–23.

452. Myers GH Jr, Fehrenbacker LG, Kelalis PP. Prognostic significance of renal vein invasion by hypernephroma. *J Urol* 1968;100:420–423.

453. Skinner DG, Colvin RB, Vermillion CD, et al. Diagnosis and management of renal cell carcinoma, a clinical and pathological study of 309 cases. *Cancer* 1971;28:1165–1177.

454. Syrjänen KJ, Hjelt L. Grading of human renal adenocarcinoma. *Scand J Urol Nephrol* 1978;12:49–55.

455. Lieber MM, Tomera FM, Taylor WF, et al. Renal adenocarcinoma in young adults: survival and variables affecting prognosis. *J Urol* 1981;125:164–168.

456. Fuhrman SA, Lasky LC, Limas C. Prognostic significance of morphologic parameters in renal cell carcinoma. *Am J Surg Pathol* 1982;6:655–663.

457. Klöppel G, Knöfel WT, Baisch H, et al. Prognosis of renal cell carcinoma related to nuclear grade, DNA content and Robson stage. *Eur Urol* 1986;12:426–431.

458. Delahunt B, Nacey JN. Renal cell carcinoma II. Histological indicators of prognosis. *Pathology* 1987;19:258–263.

459. Störkel S, Thoenes W, Jacobi GH, et al. Prognostic parameters in renal cell carcinoma—a new approach. *Eur Urol* 1989;16:416–422.

460. Onodera Y, Matsuda N, Ohta M, et al. Prognostic significance of tumor grade for renal cell carcinoma. *Int J Urol* 2000;7:4–9.

461. Al-Aynati M, Chen V, Salama S, et al. Interobserver and intraobserver variability using the Fuhrman grading system for renal cell carcinoma. *Arch Pathol Lab Med* 2003;127:593–596.

462. Lang H, Lindner V, De Fromont M, et al. Multicenter determination of optimal interobserver agreement using the Fuhrman grading system for renal cell carcinoma, assessment of 241 patients with >15-year follow-up. *Cancer* 2005;103:625–629.

463. Medeiros LJ, Jones EC, Aizawa S, et al. Grading of renal cell carcinoma, workgroup no. 2. *Cancer* 1997;80:990–991.

464. Delahunt B, McKenney JK, Lohse CM, et al. A novel grading system for clear cell renal cell carcinoma incorporating tumor necrosis. *Am J Surg Pathol* 2013;37:311–322.

465. Jiang F, Moch H, Richter J, et al. Comparative genomic hybridization reveals frequent chromosome 13q and 4q losses in renal carcinomas with sarcomatoid transformation. *J Pathol* 1998;185:382–388.

466. Dijkhuizen T, van den Berg E, van den Berg A, et al. Genetics as a diagnostic tool in sarcomatoid renal-cell cancer. *Int J Cancer* 1997;72:265–269.

467. Delahunt B, Bethwaite PB, McCredie MRE, et al. The evolution of collagen expression in sarcomatoid renal cell carcinoma. *Hum Pathol* 2007;38:1372–1377.

468. Farrow GM, Harrison EG Jr, Utz DC. Sarcomas and sarcomatoid and mixed malignant tumors of the kidney in adults—part II. *Cancer* 1968;22:551–555.

469. Bertoni F, Ferri C, Benati A, et al. Sarcomatoid carcinoma of the kidney. *J Urol* 1987;137:25–28.

470. Sella A, Logothetis CJ, Ro JY, et al. Sarcomatoid renal cell carcinoma, a treatable entity. *Cancer* 1987;60:1313–1318.

471. Oda H, Machinami R. Sarcomatoid renal cell carcinoma: a study of its proliferative activity. *Cancer* 1993;71:2292–2298.

472. DeLong W, Grignon DJ, Eberwein P, et al. Sarcomatoid renal cell carcinoma. An immunohistochemical study of 18 cases. *Arch Pathol Lab Med* 1993;117:636–640.

473. Chang A, Brimo F, Montgomery EA, et al. Use of PAX8 and GATA3 in diagnosing sarcomatoid renal cell carcinoma and sarcomatoid urothelial carcinoma. *Hum Pathol* 2013;44:1563–1568.

474. Shuch B, Bratslavsky G, Linehan WM, et al. Sarcomatoid renal cell carcinoma: a comprehensive review of the biology and current treatment strategies. *Oncologist* 2012;17:46–54.

475. Birt AR, Hogg GR, Dubé WJ. Hereditary multiple fibrofolliculomas with trichodiscomas and acrochrodons. *Arch Dermatol* 1977;113:1674–1677.

476. Pavlovich CP, Walther MM, Eyler RA, et al. Renal tumors in the Birt-Hogg-Dubé syndrome. *Am J Surg Pathol* 2002;26:1542–1552.

477. Leter EM, Koopmans AK, Gille JJP, et al. Birt-Hogg-Dubé syndrome: clinical and genetic studies of 20 families. *J Invest Dermatol* 2007;128:45–49.

478. Toro JR, Wei MH, Glenn GM, et al. *BHD* mutations, clinical and molecular genetic investigations of Birt-Hogg-Dubé syndrome: a new series of 50 families and a review of published reports. *J Med Genet* 2008;45:321–331.

479. Baba M, Hong SB, Sharma N, et al. Folliculin encoded by the *BHD* gene interacts with a binding protein, FNIP1, and AMPK, and is involved in AMPK and mTOR signaling. *Proc Natl Acad Sci U S A* 2006;103:15552–15557.

480. Wei MH, Blake PW, Shevchenko J, et al. The *folliculin* mutation database: an online database of mutations associated with Birt-Hogg-Dubé syndrome. *Hum Mutat* 2009;30:E880–E990.

481. Murakami T, Sano F, Huang Y, et al. Identification and characterization of Birt-Hogg-Dubé associated renal carcinoma. *J Pathol* 2007;211:524–531.

482. Pavlovich CP, Grubb RL III, Hurley K, et al. Evaluation and management of renal tumors in the Birt-Hogg-Dubé syndrome. *J Urol* 2005;173:1482–1486.

483. Houweling AC, Gijezen LM, Jonker MA, et al. Renal cancer and pneumothorax risk in Birt-Hogg-Dubé syndrome; an anlysis of 115 *FLCN* mutation carriers from 35 BHD families. *Br J Cancer* 2011;105:1912–1919.

484. Kluijt I, deJong D, Teertstra HJ, et al. Early onset of renal cancer in a family with Birt-Hogg-Dubé syndrome. *Clin Genet* 2009;75:537–543.

485. Fahmy W, Safwat AS, Bissada NK, et al. Multiple/bilateral renal tumors in patients with Birt-Hogg-Dubé syndrome. *Int Urol Nephrol* 2007;39:995–999.

486. Klomp JA, Petillo D, Nierni NM, et al. Hogg-Dubé renal tumors are genetically distinct from other renal neoplasias and are associated with up-regulation of mitochondrial gene expression. *BMC Med Genomics* 2010;3:59.

487. Boris RS, Benhammou J, Merino M, et al. The impact of germline BHD mutation on histological concordance and clinical treatment of patients with bilateral renal masses and known unilateral oncocytoma. *J Urol* 2011;185:2050–2055.

488. Molino D, Sepe J, Anastasio P, et al. The history of von Hippel-Lindau disease. *J Nephrol* 2006;19(suppl 10):S119–S123.

489. Melmon KL, Rosen SW. Lindau's disease, review of the literature and study of a large kindred. *Am J Med* 1964;36:595–617.

490. Ong KR, Woodward ER, Killick P, et al. Genotype-phenotype correlations in von Hippel-Lindau disease. *Hum Mutat* 2007;28:143–149.

491. Kondo K, Kaelin WG Jr. The von Hippel-Lindau tumor suppressor gene. *Exp Cell Res* 2001;264:117–125.

492. Bindra RS, Vasselli JR, Stearman R, et al. VHL-mediated hypoxia regulation of cyclin D1 in renal carcinoma cells. *Cancer Res* 2002;62: 3014–3019.

493. Kondo K, Klco J, Nakamura E, et al. Inhibition of HIF is necessary for tumor suppression by the von Hippel-Lindau protein. *Cancer Cell* 2002;1:237–246.

494. Bratslavsky G, Sudarshan S, Neckers L, et al. Pseudohypoxic pathways in renal cell carcinoma. *Clin Cancer Res* 2007;13:4667–4671.

495. Paraf F, Chauveau D, Chrétien Y, et al. Renal lesions in von Hippel-Lindau disease: immunohistochemical expression of nephron differentiation molecules, adhesion molecules and apoptosis proteins. *Histopathology* 2000;36:457–465.

496. Lonser RR, Glenn GM, Walther M, et al. von Hippel-Lindau disease. *Lancet* 2003;361:2059–2067.

497. Walther MM, Lubensky IA, Venzon D, et al. Prevalence of microscopic lesions in grossly normal renal parenchyma from patients with von Hippel-Lindau disease, sporadic renal cell carcinoma and no renal disease: clinical implications. *J Urol* 1995;154:2010–2015.

498. Duffey BG, Choyke PL, Glenn G, et al. The relationship between renal tumor size and metastases in patients with von Hippel-Lindau disease. *J Urol* 2004;172:63–65.

499. Herring JC, Enquist EG, Chernoff A, et al. Parenchymal sparing surgery in patients with hereditary renal cell carcinoma: 10-year experience. *J Urol* 2001;165:777–781.

500. Shuch B, Singer EA, Bratslavsky G. The surgical approach to multifocal renal cancers: hereditary syndromes, ipsilateral multifocality, and bilateral tumors. *Urol Clin North Am* 2012;39:133–148.

501. Malek RS, Omess PJ, Benson RC Jr, et al. Renal cell carcinoma in von Hippel-Lindau syndrome. *Am J Med* 1987;82:236–238.

502. Gomez MR. History of the tuberous sclerosis complex. *Brain Dev* 1995;17(suppl):55–57.

503. O'Callaghan FJ, Shiell AW, Osborne JP, et al. Prevalence of tuberous sclerosis estimated by capture-recapture analysis. *Lancet* 1998;351:1490.

504. Roach ES, Sparagana SP. Diagnosis of tuberous sclerosis complex. *J Child Neurol* 2004;19:643–649.

505. Yates JRW, MacLean C, Higgins JNP, et al.; The Tuberous Sclerosis 2000 Study Group. The Tuberous Sclerosis 2000 Study: presentation, initial assessments and implications for diagnosis and management. *Arch Dis Child* 2011;96:1020–1025.

506. Sancak O, Nellist M, Goedbloed M, et al. Mutational analysis of the *TSC1* and *TSC2* genes in a diagnostic setting: genotype—phenotype correlations and comparison of diagnostic DNA techniques in tuberous sclerosis complex. *Eur J Hum Genet* 2005;13:731–741.

507. Nellist M, Sancak O, Goedbloed M, et al. Functional characterization of the TSC1-TSC2 complex to assess multiple *TSC2* variants identified in single families affected by tuberous sclerosis complex. *BMC Med Genet* 2008;9:10.

508. Brook-Carter PT, Peral B, Ward CJ, et al. Deletion of the *TSC2* and *PKD1* genes associated with severe infantile polycystic kidney disease—a contiguous gene syndrome. *Nat Genet* 1994;8:328–332.

509. Steiner MS, Goldman SM, Fishman EK, et al. The natural history of renal angiomyolipoma. *J Urol* 1993;150:1782–1786.

510. Torres VE, Zincke H, King BK, et al. Renal manifestations of tuberous sclerosis complex. *Contrib Nephrol* 1997;122:64–75.

511. Lane BR, Aydin H, Danforth TL, et al. Clinical correlates of renal angiomyolipoma subtypes in 209 patients: classic, fat poor, tuberous sclerosis associated and epithelioid. *J Urol* 2008;180:836–843.

512. Pea M, Bonetti F, Martignoni G, et al. Apparent renal cell carcinomas in tuberous sclerosis are heterogeneous: the identification of malignant epithelioid angiomyolipoma. *Am J Surg Pathol* 1998;22:180–187.

513. Linehan WM, Pinto PA, Bratslavsky G, et al. Hereditary kidney cancer, unique opportunity for disease-based therapy. *Cancer* 2009;115 (10 suppl):2252–2261.

514. Tello R, Blickman JG, Buonomo C, et al. Meta analysis of the relationship between tuberous sclerosis complex and renal cell carcinoma. *Eur J Radiol* 1998;27:131–138.

515. Torres VE, Bjornsson J, Zincke H. Inherited renal neoplasms. *J Nephrol* 1998;11:229–238.

516. Kohrman MH. Emerging treatments in the management of tuberous sclerosis complex. *Pediatr Neurol* 2012;46:267–275.

517. Dabora SL, Franz DN, Ashwal S, et al. Multicenter phase 2 trial of sirolimus for tuberous sclerosis: kidney angiomyolipomas and other tumors regress and VEGF-D levels decrease. *PLoS One* 2011;6: e23379.

518. Launonen V, Vierimaa O, Kiuru M, et al. Inherited susceptibility to uterine leiomyomas and renal cell cancer. *Proc Natl Acad Sci U S A* 2001;98:3387–3392.

519. Arora R, Eble JN, Pierce HH, et al. Bilateral ovarian steroid cell tumours and massive macronodular adrenocortical disease in a patient with hereditary leiomyomatosis and renal cell cancer syndrome. *Pathology* 2012;44:360–363.

520. Shuch B, Ricketts CJ, Vocke CD, et al. Adrenal nodular hyperplasia in hereditary leiomyomatosis and renal cell cancer. *J Urol* 2013; 189:430–435.

521. Gardie B, Remenieras A, Kattygnarath D, et al.; French National Cancer Institute "Inherited predisposition to kidney cancer" Network. Novel FH mutations in families with hereditary leiomyomatosis and renal cell carcinomaHLRCC) and patients with isolated type 2 papillary renal cell carcinoma. *J Med Genet* 2011;48:226–234.

522. Alam NA, Rowan AJ, Wortham NC, et al. Genetic and functional analyses of *FH* mutations in multiple cutaneous and uterine leiomyomatosis, hereditary leiomyomatosis and renal cancer, and fumarate hydratase deficiency. *Hum Mol Genet* 2003;12:1241–1252.

523. Grubb RL III, Franks ME, Toro J, et al. Hereditary leiomyomatosis and renal cell cancer: a syndrome associated with an aggressive form of inherited renal cancer. *J Urol* 2007;177:2074–2080.

524. Stewart L, Glenn GM, Stratton P, et al. Association of germline mutations in the fumarate hydratase gene and uterine fibroids in women with hereditary leiomyomatosis and renal cell cancer. *Arch Dermatol* 2008;144:1584–1592.

525. Merino MJ, Torres-Cabala C, Pinto P, et al. The morphologic spectrum of kidney tumors in hereditary leiomyomatosis and renal carcinoma (HLRCC) syndrome. *Am J Surg Pathol* 2007;31:1578–1585.

526. Kiuru M, Launonen V, Hietala M, et al. Familial cutaneous leiomyomatosis is a two-hit condition associated with renal cell cancer of characteristic histopathology. *Am J Pathol* 2001;159:825–829.

527. Sanz-Ortega J, Vocke C, Stratton P, et al. Morphologic and molecular characteristics of uterine leiomyomas in hereditary leiomyomatosis and renal cancer (HLRCC) syndrome. *Am J Surg Pathol* 2013;37: 74–80.

528. Cohen AJ, Li FP, Berg S, et al. Hereditary renal-cell carcinoma associated with a chromosomal translocation. *N Engl J Med* 1979;301:592–595.

529. Velickovic M, Delahunt B, Grebe SKG. Loss of heterozygosity at 3p14.2 in clear cell renal cell carcinoma is an early event and is highly localized to the *FHIT* gene locus. *Cancer Res* 1999;59:1323–1326.

530. van Kessel AG, Wijnhoven M, Bodmer D, et al. Renal cell cancer: chromosome 3 translocations as risk factors. *J Natl Cancer Inst* 1999;91:1159–1160.

531. Kuiper RP, Vreede L, Venkatachalam R, et al. The tumor suppressor gene *FBXW7* is disrupted by a constitutional t(3;4)(q21;q31) in a patient with renal cell cancer. *Cancer Genet Cytogenet* 2009;195: 105–111.

532. Woodward ER, Skytte A-B, Cruger DG, et al. Population-based survey of cancer risks in chromsome 3 translocation carriers. *Genes Chromosomes Cancer* 2010;49:52–58.

533. Woodward ER, Ricketts C, Killick P, et al. Familial non-VHL clear cell (conventional) renal cell carcinoma: clinical features,

segregation analysis, and mutation analysis of *FLCN. Clin Cancer Res* 2008;14:5925–5930.

534. Teh BT, Giraud S, Sari NF, et al. Familial non-VHL non-papillary clear-cell renal cancer. *Lancet* 1997;349:848–849.

535. Woodward ER, Clifford SC, Astuti D, et al. Familial clear cell renal cell carcinoma (FCRC): clinical features and mutation analysis of the *VHL, MET* and *CUL2* candidate genes. *J Med Genet* 2000;37:348–353.

536. Liu H, Sundquist J, Hemminki K. Familial renal cell carcinoma from the Swedish Family-Cancer Database. *Eur Urol* 2011;60:987–993.

537. Zbar B, Tory K, Merino M, et al. Hereditary papillary renal cell carcinoma. *J Urol* 1994;151:561–566.

538. Schmidt L, Duh F-M, Chen F, et al. Germline and somatic mutations in the tyrosine kinase domain of the *MET* proto-oncogene in papillary renal carcinomas. *Nat Genet* 1997;16:68–73.

539. Zhuang Z, Park W-S, Pack S, et al. Trisomy 7-harbouring non-random duplication of the mutant *MET* allele in hereditary papillary renal carcinomas. *Nat Genet* 1998;20:66–69.

540. Zbar B, Glenn G, Lubensky I, et al. Hereditary papillary renal cell carcinoma: clinical studies in 10 families. *J Urol* 1995;153:907–912.

541. Schmidt LS, Nickerson ML, Angeloni D, et al. Early onset hereditary papillary renal carcinoma: germline missense mutations in the tyrosine kinase domain of the *MET* proto-oncogene. *J Urol* 2004;172:1256–1261.

542. Ornstein DK, Lubensky IA, Venzon D, et al. Prevalence of microscopic tumors in normal appearing renal parenchyma of patients with hereditary papillary renal cancer. *J Urol* 2000;163:431–433.

543. Czene K, Hemminki K. Familial papillary renal cell tumors and subsequent cancers: a nationwide epidemiological study from Sweden. *J Urol* 2003;169:1271–1275.

544. Walther MM, Choyke PL, Weiss G, et al. Parenchymal sparing surgery in patients with hereditary renal cell carcinoma. *J Urol* 1995;153:913–916.

545. Henderson A, Douglas F, Perros P, et al. SDHB-associated renal oncocytoma suggests a broadening of the renal phenotype in hereditary paragangliomatosis. *Fam Cancer* 2009;8:257–260.

546. Ricketts CJ, Forman JR, Rattenberry E, et al. Tumor risks and genotype-phenotype-proteotype analysis in 358 patients with germline mutations in *SDHB* and *SDHD. Hum Mutat* 2010;31:41–51.

547. Gill AJ, Pachter NS, Chou A, et al. Renal tumors associated with germline SDHB mutation show distinctive morphology. *Am J Surg Pathol* 2011;35:1578–1585.

548. Ricketts CJ, Shuch B, Vocke CD, et al. Succinate dehydrogenase kidney cancer; an aggressive example of the Warburg effect in cancer. *J Urol* 2012;188:2063–2071.

549. Debelenko LV, Raimondi SC, Daw N, et al. Renal cell carcinoma with novel *VCL-ALK* fusion: new representative of ALK-associated tumor spectrum. *Mod Pathol* 2011;24:430–442.

550. Mariño-Enríquez A, Ou W-B, Weldon CB, et al. *ALK* rearrangement in sickle cell trait-associated renal medullary carcinoma. *Genes Chromosomes Cancer* 2011;50:146–153.

551. Sugawara E, Togashi Y, Kuroda N, et al. Identification of anaplastic lymphoma kinase fusions in renal cancer, large-scale immunohistochemical screening by the intercalated antibody-enhanced polymer method. *Cancer* 2012;118:4427–4436.

552. Sukov WR, Hodge JC, Lohse CM, et al. *ALK* alterations in adult renal cell carcinoma: frequency, clinicopathologic features and outcome in a large series of consecutively treated patients. *Mod Pathol* 2012;25:1516–1525.

553. Pagès A, Granier M. Le néphrome néphronogène. *Arch Anat Cytol Pathol* 1980;28:99–103.

554. Bove KE, Bhathena D, Wyatt RJ, et al. Diffuse metanephric adenoma after in utero aspirin intoxication. *Arch Pathol Lab Med* 1979;103:187–190.

555. Argani P. Metanephric neoplasms: the hyperdifferentiated, benign end of the Wilms tumor spectrum? *Clin Lab Med* 2005;25:379–392.

556. Davis CJ Jr, Barton JH, Sesterhenn IA, et al. Metanephric adenoma, clinicopathological study of fifty patients. *Am J Surg Pathol* 1995;19:1101–1114.

557. Jones EC, Pins M, Dickersin GR, et al. Metanephric adenoma of the kidney, a clinicopathological, immunohistochemical, flow cytometric, cytogenetic, and electron microscopic study of seven cases. *Am J Surg Pathol* 1995;19:615–626.

558. Azabdaftari G, Alroy J, Banner BF, et al. S100 protein expression distinguishes metanephric adenomas from other renal neoplasms. *Pathol Res Pract* 2008;204:719–723.

559. Bastide C, Rambeaud JJ, Bach AM, et al. Metanephric adenoma of the kidney: clinical and radiological study of nine cases. *BJU Int* 2009;103:1544–1548.

560. Muir TE, Cheville JC, Lager DJ. Metanephric adenoma, nephrogenic rests, and Wilms' tumor: a histologic and immunophenotypic comparison. *Am J Surg Pathol* 2001;25:1290–1296.

561. Yoshioka K, Miyakawa A, Ohno Y, et al. Production of erythropoietin and multiple cytokines by metanephric adenoma results in erythrocytosis. *Pathol Int* 2007;57:529–536.

562. Kohashi K, Oda Y, Nakamori M, et al. Multifocal metanephric adenoma in childhood. *Pathol Int* 2009;59:49–52.

563. Granter SR, Fletcher JA, Renshaw AA. Cytologic and cytogenetic analysis of metanephric adenoma of the kidney, a report of two cases. *Am J Clin Pathol* 1997;108:544–549.

564. Gatalica Z, Grujic S, Kovatich A, et al. Metanephric adenoma: histology, immunophenotype, cytogenetics, ultrastructure. *Mod Pathol* 1996;9:329–333.

565. Szponar A, Yusenko MV, Kovacs G. High-resolution array CGH of metanephric adenomas: lack of DNA copy number changes. *Histopathology* 2010;56:212–216.

566. Brunelli M, Eble JN, Zhang S, et al. Metanephric adenoma lacks the gains of chromosomes 7 and 17 and loss of Y that are typical of papillary renal cell carcinoma and papillary adenoma. *Mod Pathol* 2003;16:1060–1063.

567. Pan C-C, Epstein JI. Detection of chromosome copy number alterations in metanephric adenomas by array comparative genomic hybridization. *Mod Pathol* 2010;23:1634–1640.

568. Pesti T, Sükösd F, Jones EC, et al. Mapping a tumor suppressor gene to chromosome 2p13 in metanephric adenoma by microsatellite allelotyping. *Hum Pathol* 2001;32:101–104.

569. Stumm M, Koch A, Wieacker PF, et al. Partial monosomy 2p as the single chromosomal anomaly in a case of renal metanephric adenoma. *Cancer Genet Cytogenet* 1999;115:82–85.

570. Choueiri TK, Cheville J, Palescandolo E, et al. *BRAF* mutations in metanephric adenoma of the kidney. *Eur Urol* 2012;62:917–922.

571. Paner GP, Turk TM, Clark JI, et al. Passive seeding in metanephric adenoma, a review of pseudometastatic lesions in perinephric lymph nodes. *Arch Pathol Lab Med* 2005;129:1317–1321.

572. Hennigar RA, Beckwith JB. Nephrogenic adenofibroma, a novel kidney tumor of young people. *Am J Surg Pathol* 1992;16:325–334.

573. Arroyo MR, Green DM, Perlman EJ, et al. The spectrum of metanephric adenofibroma and related lesions, clinicopathologic study of 25 cases from the National Wilms Tumors Study Group Pathology Center. *Am J Surg Pathol* 2001;25:433–444.

574. Bigg SW, Bari WA. Nephrogenic adenofibroma: an unusual renal tumor. *J Urol* 1997;157:1835–1836.

575. Piotrowski Z, Canter DJ, Kutikov A, et al. Metanephric adenofibroma: robotic partial nephrectomy of a large Wilms' tumor variant. *Can J Urol* 2010;17:5309–5312.

576. Shek TWH, Luk ISC, Peh WCG, et al. Metanephric adenofibroma: report of a case and review of the literature. *Am J Surg Pathol* 1999;23:727–733.

577. Argani P, Beckwith JB. Metanephric stromal tumor, report of 31 cases of a distinctive pediatric renal neoplasm. *Am J Surg Pathol* 2000;24:917–926.

578. Palese MA, Ferrer F, Perlman E, et al. Metanephric stromal tumor: a rare benign pediatric renal mass. *Urology* 2001;58:462xv–462xvii.

579. Amat Villegas C, Gómez-Dorronsoro ML, Caballero Martínez MC, et al. Tumor del estroma metanéfrico: presentación de dos casos en adultos y revisión de la literatura. *Arch Esp Urol* 2006;59:88–90.

580. McDonald OG, Rodriguez R, Bergner A, et al. Metanephric stromal tumor arising in a patient with the neurofibromatosis type I syndrome. *Int J Surg Pathol* 2011;5:667–671.

581. De Pasquale MD, Diomedi-Camassei F, Serra A, et al. Recurrent metanephric stromal tumor in an infant. *Urology* 2011;78:1411–1413.

582. Picken MM, Curry JL, Lindgren V, et al. Metanephric adenosarcoma in a young adult: morphologic, immunophenotypic, ultrastructural, and fluorescence in situ hybridization analyses, a case report and review of the literature. *Am J Surg Pathol* 2001;25:1451–1457.

583. Pastore G, Znaor A, Spreafico F, et al. Malignant renal tumours incidence and survival in European children (1978-1997): report from the Automated Childhood Cancer Information System Project. *Eur J Cancer* 2006;42:2103–2114.

584. van den Heuvel-Eibrink MM, Grundy P, Graf N, et al. Characteristics and survival of 750 children diagnosed with a renal tumor in the first seven months of life: a collaborative study by the SIOP/GPOH/SFOP, NWTSG, and UKCCSG Wilms tumor study groups. *Pediatr Blood Cancer* 2008;50:1130–1134.

585. Bove KE, Koffler H, McAdams AJ. Nodular renal blastema, definition and possible significance. *Cancer* 1969;24:323–332.

586. Bove KE, McAdams AJ. The nephroblastomatosis complex and its relationship to Wilms' tumor: a clinicopathologic treatise. *Perspect Pediatr Pathol* 1976;3:185–223.

587. Beckwith JB, Kiviat NB, Bonadio JF. Nephrogenic rests, nephroblastomatosis, and the pathogenesis of Wilms' tumor. *Pediatr Pathol* 1990; 10:1–36.

588. Coli A, Angrisani B, Chiarello G, et al. Ectopic immature renal tissue: clues for diagnosis and management. *Int J Clin Exp Pathol* 2012;5:977–981.

589. Scharfenberg JC, Beckman EN. Persistent renal blastema in an adult. *Hum Pathol* 1984;15:791–793.

590. Perlman EJ, Faria P, Soares A, et al. Hyperplastic perilobar nephroblastomatosis: long-term survival of 52 patients. *Pediatr Blood Cancer* 2006;46:203–221.

591. Breslow NE, Beckwith JB, Perlman EJ, et al. Age distributions, birth weights, nephrogenic rests, and heterogeneity in the pathogenesis of Wilms tumor. *Pediatr Blood Cancer* 2006;47:260–267.

592. Breslow N, Beckwith JB, Ciol M, et al. Age distribution of Wilms' tumor: report from the National Wilms' Tumor Study. *Cancer Res* 1988; 48:1653–1657.

593. Lemerle J, Tournade M-F, Gerard-Marchant R, et al. Wilms' tumor: Natural history and prognostic factors, a retrospective study of 248 cases treated at the Institut Gustave-Roussy 1952–1967. *Cancer* 1976;37:2557–2566.

594. Hrabovsky EE, Othersen HB Jr, deLorimier A, et al. Wilms' tumor in the neonate: a report from the National Wilms' Tumor Study. *J Pediatr Surg* 1986;21:385–387.

595. Popov SD, Sebire NJ, Vujanić GM. Renal tumors in children aged 10-16 years: a report from the United Kingdom Children's Cancer and Leukaemia Group. *Pediatr Dev Pathol* 2011;14:189–193.

596. Grabowski J, Silberstein J, Saltzstein SL, et al. Renal tumors in the second decade of life: results from the California Cancer Registry. *J Pediatr Surg* 2009;44:1148–1151.

597. Innis MD. Nephroblastoma: index cancer of childhood. *Med J Aust* 1973;2:322–323.

598. Blute ML, Kelalis PP, Offord KP, et al. Bilateral Wilms tumor. *J Urol* 1987;138:968–973.

599. Breslow NE, Beckwith JB. Epidemiological features of Wilms' tumor: results of the National Wilms' Tumor Study. *J Natl Cancer Inst* 1982;68: 429–436.

600. Sotelo-Avila C, Gonzalez-Crussi F, Fowler JW. Complete and incomplete forms of Beckwith-Wiedemann syndrome: their oncogenic potential. *J Pediatr* 1980;96:47–50.

601. Heppe RK, Koyle MA, Beckwith JB. Nephrogenic rests in Wilms tumor patients with Drash syndrome. *J Urol* 1991;145:1225–1228.

602. Miller RW, Fraumeni JF Jr, Manning MD. Association of Wilms's tumor with aniridia, hemihypertrophy and other congenital malformations. *N Engl J Med* 1964;270:922–927.

603. Chu A, Heck JE, Ribeiro KB, et al. Wilms' tumour: a systematic review of risk factors and meta-analysis. *Paediatr Perinat Epidemiol* 2011;24:449–469.

604. Huser J, Grignon DJ, Ro JY, et al. Adult Wilms' tumor: a clinicopathologic study of 11 cases. *Mod Pathol* 1990;3:321–326.

605. Arrigo S, Beckwith JB, Sharples K, et al. Better survival after combined modality care for adults with Wilms' tumor, a report from the National Wilms' Tumor Study. *Cancer* 1990;66:827–830.

606. Coppes MJ. Serum biological markers and paraneoplastic syndromes in Wilms tumor. *Med Pediatr Oncol* 1993;21:213–221.

607. Segers H, van der Heyden JC, van den Akker ELT, et al. Cushing syndrome as a presenting symptom of renal tumors in children. *Pediatr Blood Cancer* 2009;53:211–213.

608. Segers H, van den Heuvel-Eibrink MM, Pritchard-Jones K, et al.; SIOP-RTSG, COG-Renal Tumour Committee. Management of adults with Wilms' tumor: recommendations based on international consensus. *Expert Rev Anticancer Ther* 2011;11:1105–1113.

609. Eble JN. Fetal rhabdomyomatous nephroblastoma. *J Urol* 1983;130: 541–543.

610. Gonzalez-Crussi F, Hsueh W, Ugarte N. Rhabdomyogenesis in renal neoplasia of childhood. *Am J Surg Pathol* 1981;5:525–532.

611. Losty P, Kierce B. Botryoid Wilms' tumour—an unusual variant. *Br J Urol* 1993;72:251–252.

612. Kinoshita Y, Suminoe A, Inada H, et al. The prognostic significance of blastemal predominant histology in initally resected Wilms' tumors: a report from the Study Group for Pediatric Solid Tumors in the Kyushi Area, Japan. *J Pediatr Surg* 2012;47:2205–2209.

613. Grimes MM, Wolff M, Wolff JA, et al. Ganglion cells in metastatic Wilms' tumor, review of a histogenetic controversy. *Am J Surg Pathol* 1982;6:565–571.

614. Joshi VV, Banerjee AK, Yadav K, et al. Cystic partially differentiated nephroblastoma, a clinicopathologic entity in the spectrum of infantile renal neoplasia. *Cancer* 1977;40:789–795.

615. Joshi VV. Cystic partially differentiated nephroblastoma: an entity in the spectrum of infantile renal neoplasia. *Perspect Pediatr Pathol* 1979;5:217–235.

616. Maes P, Delemarre J, de Kraker J, et al. Fetal rhabdomyomatous nephroblastoma: a tumour of good prognosis but resistant to chemotherapy. *Eur J Cancer* 1999;35:1356–1360.

617. Pollono D, Drut R, Tomarchio S, et al. Fetal rhabdomyomatous nephroblastoma: report of 14 cases confirming chemotherapy resistance. *J Pediatr Hematol Oncol* 2003;25:640–643.

618. Nayak A, Iyer VK, Agarwal S, et al. Fine needle aspiration cytology of fetal rhabdomyomatous and teratoid Wilms tumor. *Acta Cytol* 2010;54:563–568.

619. Magee JF, Ansari S, McFadden DE, et al. Teratoid Wilms' tumour: a report of two cases. *Histopathology* 1992;20:427–431.

620. Treetipsatit J, Raveesunthornkiet M, Ruangtrakool R, et al. Teratoid Wilms' tumor: case report of a rare variant that can mimic aggressive biology during chemotherapy. *J Pediatr Surg* 2011;46:E1–E6.

621. Vujanić GM, Sandstedt B. The pathology of Wilms' tumour (nephroblastoma): the International Society of Paediatric Oncology approach. *J Clin Pathol* 2010;63:102–109.

622. Bisceglia M, Ragazzi M, Galliani CA, et al. TTF-1 expression in nephroblastoma. *Am J Surg Pathol* 2009;33:454–461.

623. Davis JL, Matsumura L, Weeks DA, et al. PAX2 expression in Wilms tumor and other childhood neoplasms. *Am J Surg Pathol* 2011; 35:1186–1194.

624. Vasei M, Moch H, Mousavi A, et al. Immunohistochemical profiling of Wilms tumor, a tissue microarray study. *Appl Immunohistochem Mol Morphol* 2008;16:128–134.

625. Huang C-C, Cutcliffe C, Coffin C, et al. Classification of malignant pediatric renal tumors by gene expression. *Pediatr Blood Cancer* 2006;46:728–738.

626. Franken J, Lerut E, van Poppel H, et al. p53 immunohistochemistry in Wilms' tumor: a prognostic tool in the detection of tumor aggressiveness. *J Urol* 2013;189:664–670.

627. Park S, Bernard A, Bove KE, et al. Inactivation of *WT1* in nephrogenic rests, genetic precursors to Wilms' tumour. *Nat Genet* 1994;5: 363–367.

628. Huff V. Wilms' tumours: about tumour suppressor genes, an oncogene and a chameleon gene. *Nat Rev Cancer* 2011;11:111–121.

629. Fukuzawa R, Holman SK, Chow CW, et al. *WTX* mutations can occur both early and late in the pathogenesis of Wilms tumour. *J Med Genet* 2010;47:791–794.

630. Cardoso LC, De Souza KR, De O Reis AH, et al. *WT1*, *WTX* and *CTNNB1* mutation analysis in 43 patients with sporadic Wilms' tumor. *Oncol Rep* 2013;29:315–320.

631. Fukuzawa R, Anaka MR, Heathcott RW, et al. Wilms tumour histology is determined by distinct types of precursor lesions and not epigenetic changes. *J Pathol* 2008;215:377–387.

632. Vuononvirta R, Sebire NJ, Dallosso AR, et al. Perilobar nephrogenic rests are nonobligate molecular genetic precursor lesions of insulin-like growth factor-II-associated Wilms tumors. *Clin Cancer Res* 2008; 14:7635–7644.

633. MdZin R, Phillips M, Edwards C, et al. Perilobar nephrogenic rests and chromosome 22. *Pediatr Dev Pathol* 2011;14:485–492.

634. Gadd S, Huff V, Huang C-C, et al. Clinically relevant subsets identified by gene expression patterns support a revised ontogenic model of Wilms tumor: a Children's Oncology Group study. *Neoplasia* 2012;14: 742–756.

635. Royer-Pokora B. Genetics of pediatric renal tumors. *Pediatr Nephrol* 2013;28:13–23.

636. Sonn G, Shortliffe LMD. Management of Wilms tumor: current standard of care. *Nat Clin Pract Urol* 2008;5:551–560.

637. Sayed HAR, Ali AM, Hamza HM, et al. Long-term follow-up of infantile Wilms tumor treated according to International Society of Pediatric Oncology protocol: seven years' follow-up. *Urology* 2011;77:446–451.

638. Ko EY, Ritchey ML. Current Management of Wilms' tumor in children. *J Pediatr Urol* 2009;5:56–65.

639. Cotton CA, Peterson S, Norkool PA, et al. Early and late mortality after diagnosis of Wilms tumor. *J Clin Oncol* 2009;27:1304–1309.

640. Green DM. The evolution of treatment for Wilms tumor. *J Pediatr Surg* 2013;48:14–19.

641. Verschuur AC, Vujanić GM, van Tinteren H, et al. Stromal and epithelial predominant Wilms tumours have an excellent outcome: the SIOP 93 01 experience. *Pediatr Blood Cancer* 2010;55:233–238.

642. Dome JS, Cotton CA, Perlman EJ, et al. Treatment of anaplastic histology Wilms' tumor: results from the fifth National Wilms' Tumor Study. *J Clin Oncol* 2006;24:2352–2358.

643. Bonadio JF, Storer B, Norkool P, et al. Anaplastic Wilms' tumor: clinical and pathologic studies. *J Clin Oncol* 1985;3:513–520.

644. Breslow NE, Palmer NF, Hill LR, et al. Wilms' tumor: prognostic factors for patients without metastases at diagnosis, results of the National Wilms' Tumor Study. *Cancer* 1978;41:1577–1589.

645. Beckwith JB, Zuppan CW, Browning NG, et al. Histological analysis of aggressiveness and responsiveness in Wilms' tumor. *Med Pediatr Oncol* 1996;27:422–428.

646. Beckwith B. Focal versus diffuse anaplasia in nephroblastoma. *Arch Anat Cytol Pathol* 1996;44:53.

647. Kieran K, Anderson JR, Dome JS, et al. Lymph node involvement in Wilms tumor: results from National Wilms Tumor Studies 4 and 5. *J Pediatr Surg* 2012;47:700–706.

648. Perlman EJ. Pediatric renal tumors: practical updates for the pathologist. *Pediatr Dev Pathol* 2005;8:320–338.

649. Perlman EJ, Grundy PE, Anderson JR, et al. WT1 mutation and 11P15 loss of heterozygosity predict relapse in very low-risk Wilms tumors treated with surgery alone: a Children's Oncology Group study. *J Clin Oncol* 2011;29:698–703.

650. Geller JI. Genetic stratification of Wilms tumor, is *WT1* analysis ready for prime time? *Cancer* 2008;113:893–896.

651. Sredni ST, Gadd S, Huang C-C, et al. Subsets of very low risk Wilms tumor show distinctive gene expression, histologic, and clinical features. *Clin Cancer Res* 2009;15:6800–6809.

652. Hamilton TE, Green DM, Perlman EJ, et al. Bilateral Wilms' tumor with anaplasia: lessons from the National Wilms' Tumor study. *J Pediatr Surg* 2006;41:1641–1644.

653. Andrews MJ Jr, Askin FB, Fried FA, et al. Cystic partially differentiated nephroblastoma and polycystic Wilms tumor: a spectrum of related clinical and pathologic entities. *J Urol* 1983;129: 577–580.

654. Joshi VV, Beckwith JB. Multilocular cyst of the kidney (cystic nephroma) and cystic, partially differentiated nephroblastoma, terminology and criteria for diagnosis. *Cancer* 1989;64:466–479.

655. Blakely ML, Shamberger RC, Norkool P, et al. Outcome of children with cystic partially differentiated nephoblastoma treated with or without chemotherapy. *J Pediatr Surg* 2003;38:897–900.

656. Luithle T, Szavay P, Furtwängler R, et al. Treatment of cystic nephroma and cystic partially differentiated nephroblastoma—a report from the SIOP/GPOH Study Group. *J Urol* 2007;177:294–296.

657. Joshi VV, Beckwith JB. Pathologic delineation of the papillonodular type of cystic partially differentiated nephroblastoma, a review of 11 cases. *Cancer* 1990;66:1568–1577.

658. Shiraishi A, Kuwatsuru R, Kurosaki Y, et al. Papillonodular type of cystic partially differentiated nephroblastoma: a case report. *Radiat Med* 2001;19:313–316.

659. Raut WK, Gadkari RU, Bobhate SK. Cystic partially differentiated nephroblastoma with skeletal muscle differentiation: a case report. *Indian J Cancer* 1998;35:129–131.

660. Eble JN. Cystic nephroma and cystic partially differentiated nephroblastoma: two entities or one? *Adv Anat Pathol* 1994;1:99–102.

661. Rajangam K, Narasimhan KL, Trehan A, et al. Partial nephrectomy in cystic partially differentiated nephroblastoma. *J Pediatr Surg* 2000;35: 510–512.

662. Baker JM, Viero S, Kim PC, et al. Stage III cystic partially differentiated nephroblastoma recurring after nephrectomy and chemotherapy. *Pediatr Blood Cancer* 2008;50:129–131.

663. England RJ, Haider N, Vujanić GM, et al. Mesoblastic nephroma: a report of the United Kingdom Children's Cancer and Leukemia Group (CCLG). *Pediatr Blood Cancer* 2011;56:744–748.

664. Kay S, Pratt CB, Salzberg AM. Hamartoma (leiomyomatous type) of the kidney. *Cancer* 1966;19:1825–1832.

665. Bolande RP, Brough AJ, Izant RJ Jr. Congenital mesoblastic nephroma of infancy, a report of eight cases and the relationship to Wilms' tumor. *Pediatrics* 1967;40:272–278.

666. Marsden HB, Lawler W. Primary renal tumours in the first year of life. A population based review. *Virchows Arch A Pathol Anat Histopathol* 1983;399:1–9.

667. Blank E, Neerhout RC, Burry KA. Congenital mesoblastic nephroma and polyhydramnios. *JAMA* 1978;240:1504–1505.

668. Favara BE, Johnson W, Ito J. Renal tumors in the neonatal period. *Cancer* 1968;22:845–855.

669. Pettinato G, Manivel JC, Wick MR, et al. Classical and cellular (atypical) congenital mesoblastic nephroma: a clinicopathologic, ultrastructural, immunohistochemical, and flow cytometric study. *Hum Pathol* 1989;20:682–690.

670. Bolande RP. Congenital mesoblastic nephroma of infancy. *Perspect Pediatr Pathol* 1973;1:227–250.

671. Beckwith JB. Mesenchymal renal neoplasms in infancy revisited. *J Pediatr Surg* 1974;9:803–805.

672. Murphy AJ, Viero S, Ho M, et al. Diagnostic utility of nestin expression in pediatric tumors in the region of the kidney. *Appl Immunohistochem Mol Morphol* 2009;17:517–523.

673. Takahashi T, Habuchi T, Kakehi Y, et al. Clonal and chronological genetic analysis of multifocal cancers of the bladder and upper urinary tract. *Cancer Res* 1998;58:5835–5841.

674. Knezevich S, Garnett MJ, Pysher TJ, et al. ETV6-NTRK3 gene fusions and trisomy 11 establish a histogenetic link between mesoblastic nephroma and congenital fibrosarcoma. *Cancer Res* 1998;58:5046–5048.

675. Rubin BP, Chen C-J, Morgan TW, et al. Congenital mesoblastic nephroma t(12;15) is associated with ETV6-NTRK3 gene fusion;

cytogenetic and molecular relationship to congenital (infantile) fibrosarcoma. *Am J Pathol* 1998;153:1451–1458.

676. Anderson J, Gibson S, Sebire NJ. Expression of ETV6-NTRK in classical, cellular and mixed subtypes of congenital mesoblastic nephroma. *Histopathology* 2006;48:748–753.

677. Argani P, Fritsch M, Kadkol SS, et al. Detection of the ETV6-NTRK3 chimeric RNA of infantile fibrosarcoma/cellular congenital mesoblastic nephroma in paraffin-embedded tissue: application to challenging pediatric renal stromal tumors. *Mod Pathol* 2000;13:29–36.

678. Howell CG, Othersen HB, Kiviat NE, et al. Therapy and outcome in 51 children with mesoblastic nephroma: a report of the National Wilms' Tumor Study. *J Pediatr Surg* 1982;17:826–131.

679. Chan HSL, Cheng M-Y, Mancer K, et al. Congenital mesoblastic nephroma: a clinicoradiologic study of 17 cases representing the pathologic spectrum of the disease. *J Pediatr* 1987;111:64–70.

680. Sandstedt B, Delemarre JFM, Krul EJ, et al. Mesoblastic nephromas: a study of 29 tumours from the SIOP nephroblastoma file. *Histopathology* 1985;9:741–750.

681. Joshi VV, Kasznica J, Walters TR. Atypical mesoblastic nephroma. Pathologic characterization of a potentially aggressive variant of conventional congenital mesoblastic nephroma. *Arch Pathol Lab Med* 1986;110:100–106.

682. Gonzalez-Crussi F, Sotelo-Avila C, Kidd JM. Malignant mesenchymal nephroma of infancy, report of a case with pulmonary metastases. *Am J Surg Pathol* 1980;4:185–190.

683. Beckwith JB, Weeks DA. Congenital mesoblastic nephroma, when should we worry? *Arch Pathol Lab Med* 1986;110:98–99.

684. Gormley TS, Skoog SJ, Jones RV, et al. Cellular congenital mesoblastic nephroma: what are the options. *J Urol* 1989;142:479–483.

685. Heidelberger KP, Ritchey ML, Dauser RC, et al. Congenital mesoblastic nephroma metastatic to the brain. *Cancer* 1993;72:2499–2502.

686. Furtwaengler R, Reinhard H, Leuschner I, et al. Mesoblastic nephroma—a report from the Gesellschaft fur Pädiatrische Onkologie und Hämatologie (GPOH). *Cancer* 2006;106:2275–2283.

687. Marsden HB, Lawler W. Bone-metastasizing renal tumour of childhood. *Br J Cancer* 1978;38:437–441.

688. Beckwith JB, Palmer NF. Histopathology and prognosis of Wilms tumor, results from the First National Wilms' Tumor Study. *Cancer* 1978;41:1937–1948.

689. Mierau GW, Weeks DA, Beckwith JB. Anaplastic Wilms' tumor and other clinically aggressive childhood renal neoplasms: ultrastructural and immunocytochemical features. *Ultrastruct Pathol* 1989;13:225–248.

690. Argani P, Perlman EJ, Breslow NE, et al. Clear cell sarcoma of the kidney, a review of 351 cases from the National Wilms Tumor Study Group Pathology Center. *Am J Surg Pathol* 2000;24:4–18.

691. Sotelo-Avila C, Gonzalez-Crussi F, Sadowinski S, et al. Clear cell sarcoma of the kidney: a clinicopathologic study of 21 patients with long-term follow-up evaluation. *Hum Pathol* 1986;16:1219–1230.

692. Marsden HB, Lawler W. Bone metastasizing renal tumour of childhood, histopathological and clinical review of 38 cases. *Virchows Arch A Pathol Anat Histol* 1980;387:341–351.

693. Balarezo FS, Joshi VV. Clear cell sarcoma of the pediatric kidney: detailed description and analysis of variant histologic patterns of a tumor with many faces. *Adv Anat Pathol* 2000;8:98–108.

694. Brownlee NA, Perkins LA, Stewart W, et al. Recurring translocation (10;17) and deletion (14q) in clear cell sarcoma of the kidney. *Arch Pathol Lab Med* 2007;131:446–451.

695. O'Meara E, Stack D, Lee C-H, et al. Characterization of the chromosomal translocation t(10;17)(q22;p13) in clear cell sarcoma of kidney. *J Pathol* 2012;227:72–80.

696. Fehr A, Hansson MC, Kindblom L-G, et al. *YWHAE-FAM22* gene fusion in clear cell sarcoma of the kidney. *J Pathol* 2012;227:e5–e7.

697. Cutcliffe C, Kersey D, Huang C-C, et al. Clear cell sarcoma of the kidney: up-regulation of neural markers with activation of the sonic hedgehog and Akt pathways. *Clin Cancer Res* 2005;11:7986–7994.

698. Kalapurakal JA, Perlman EJ, Seibel NL, et al. Outcomes of patients with revised stage I clear cell sarcoma of kidney treated in National Wilms Tumor Studies 1-5. *Int J Radiat Oncol Biol Phys* 2013;85:428–431.

699. Gooskens SLM, Furtwängler R, Vujanić GM, et al. Clear cell sarcoma of the kidney: a review. *Eur J Cancer* 2012;28:2219–2226.

700. Palmer NF, Sutow W. Clinical aspects of the rhabdoid tumor of the kidney: a report of the National Wilms' Tumor Study Group. *Med Pediatr Oncol* 1983;11:242–245.

701. Tomlinson GE, Breslow NE, Dome J, et al. Rhabdoid tumor of the kidney in the National Wilms' Tumor Study: age at diagnosis as a prognostic factor. *J Clin Oncol* 2005;23:7641–7645.

702. van den Heuvel-Eibrink MM, van Tinteren H, Rehorst H, et al. Malignant rhabdoid tumours of the kidney (MRTKs), registered on recent SIOP protocols from 1993 to 2005: a report of the SIOP Renal Tumour Study Group. *Pediatr Blood Cancer* 2011;56:733–737.

703. Bonnin JM, Rubinstein LJ, Palmer NF, et al. The association of embryonal tumors originating in the kidney and in the brain, a report of seven cases. *Cancer* 1984;54:2137–2146.

704. Rousseau-Merck MF, Boccon-Gibod L, Nogues C, et al. An original hypercalcemic infantile renal tumor without bone metastasis: heterotransplantation to nude mice, report of two cases. *Cancer* 1982;50:85–93.

705. Mayes LC, Kasselberg AG, Roloff JS, et al. Hypercalcemia associated with immunoreactive parathyroid hormone in a malignant rhabdoid tumor of the kidney (rhabdoid Wilms' tumor). *Cancer* 1984;54:882–884.

706. Weeks DA, Beckwith JB, Mierau GW, et al. Rhabdoid tumor of kidney, a report of 111 cases from the National Wilms' Tumor Study Pathology Center. *Am J Surg Pathol* 1989;13:439–458.

707. Haas JE, Palmer NF, Weinberg AG, et al. Ultrastructure of malignant rhabdoid tumor of the kidney, a distinctive renal tumor of children. *Hum Pathol* 1981;12:646–657.

708. Hollman TJ, Hornick JL. INI1-deficient tumors: diagnostic features and molecular genetics. *Am J Surg Pathol* 2011;35:e47–e63.

709. Machado I, Noguera R, Santonja N, et al. Immunohistochemical study as a tool in differential diagnosis of pediatric malignant rhabdoid tumor. *Appl Immunohistochem Mol Morphol* 2010;18:150–158.

710. Biegel JA, Zhou J, Rorke LB, et al. Germ-line and acquired mutations of *INI1* in atypical teratoid and rhabdoid tumors. *Cancer Res* 1999;59:74–79.

711. Gadd S, Sredni ST, Huang C-C, et al. Rhabdoid tumor: gene expression clues to pathogenesis and potential therapeutic targets. *Lab Invest* 2010;90:724–738.

712. Lee H-Y, Yoon C-S, Sevenet N, et al. Rhabdoid tumor of the kidney is a component of the rhabdoid predisposition syndrome. *Pediatr Dev Pathol* 2002;5:395–399.

713. Roberts CWM, Biegel JA. The role of SMARCB1/INI1 in development of rhabdoid tumor. *Cancer Biol Ther* 2009;8:412–416.

714. Venneti S, Le P, Martinez D, et al. Malignant rhabdoid tumors express stem cell factors, which relate to the expression of EZH2 and Id proteins. *Am J Surg Pathol* 2011;35:1463–1472.

715. Deisch J, Raisanen J, Rakheja D. Immunohistochemical expression of embryonic stem cell markers in malignant rhabdoid tumors. *Pediatr Dev Pathol* 2011;14:353–359.

716. Weeks DA, Beckwith JB, Mierau GW, et al. Renal neoplasms mimicking rhabdoid tumor of kidney, a report from the National Wilms' Tumor Study Pathology Center. *Am J Surg Pathol* 1991;15:1042–1054.

717. Hoot AC, Russo P, Judkins AR, et al. Immunohistochemical analysis of hSNF5/INI1 distinguishes renal extra-renal malignant rhabdoid tumors from other pediatric soft tissue tumors. *Am J Surg Pathol* 2004;28:1485–1491.

718. Wu X, Dagar V, Algar E, et al. Rhabdoid tumour: a malignancy of early childhood with variable primary site, histology and clinical behaviour. *Pathology* 2008;40:664–670.

719. Reinhard H, Reinert J, Beier R, et al. Rhabdoid tumors in children: prognostic factors in 70 patients diagnosed in Germany. *Oncol Rep* 2008;19:819–823.

720. Küss MR. Un cas de néphroblastome calcifié simulant un calcul. *J Urol Nephrol* 1966;73:653–655.

721. Chatten J, Cromie WJ, Duckett JW. Ossifying tumor of infantile kidney, report of two cases. *Cancer* 1980;45:609–612.

722. Jerkins GR, Callihan TR. Ossifying renal tumor of infancy. *J Urol* 1986;135:120–121.

723. Middlebrook PF, Jimenez CL, Schillinger JF. Ossifying renal tumor of infancy: a case report. *J Urol* 1992;147:1337–1339.

724. Steffens J, Kraus J, Misho B, et al. Ossifying renal tumor of infancy. *J Urol* 1993;149:1080–1081.

725. Sotelo-Avila C, Beckwith JB, Johnson JE. Ossifying renal tumor of infancy: a clinicopathologic study of nine cases. *Pediatr Pathol* 1995;15:745–762.

726. Charles AK, Berry PJ, Joyce MRL, et al. Ossifying renal tumor of infancy. *Pediatr Pathol Lab Med* 1997;17:332–334.

727. Ito J, Shinohara N, Koyanagi T, et al. Ossifying renal tumor of infancy: the first Japanese case with long-term follow-up. *Pathol Int* 1998;48:151–159.

728. Vazquez JL, Barnewolt CE, Shamberger RC, et al. Ossifying renal tumor of infancy presenting as a palpable abdominal mass. *Pediatr Radiol* 1998;28:454–457.

729. El-Husseini TK, Egail SA, Al-Orf AM, et al. Ossifying renal tumor of infancy. *Saudi Med J* 2005;26:1978–1979.

730. Schelling J, Schröder A, Stein R, et al. Ossifying renal tumor of infancy. *J Pediatr Urol* 2007;3:258–261.

731. Seixas-Mikelus SA, Khan A, Williot PE, et al. Three-month-old boy with juvenile granulosa cell tumor of testis and ossifying renal tumor of infancy. *Urology* 2009;74:311–313.

732. Höglund HHE, Kellner MW, Körber F, et al. Ossifying renal tumor of infancy (ORTI)—a rare diagnosis. *Klin Padiatr* 2011;223:178–179.

733. Liu J, Guzman MA, Pawel BR, et al. Clonal trisomy 4 cells detected in the ossifying renal tumor of infancy: study of 3 cases. *Mod Pathol* 2013;26:275–281.

734. Fernbach SK, Schlesinger AE, Gonzalez-Crussi F. Calcification and ossification in a congenital mesoblastic nephroma. *Urol Radiol* 1985;7: 165–167.

735. Vujanić GM, Kelsey A, Perlman EJ, et al. Anaplastic sarcoma of the kidney, a clinicopathologic study of 20 cases of a new entity with polyphenotypic features. *Am J Surg Pathol* 2007;31:1459–1468.

736. Gomi K, Hamanoue S, Tanaka M, et al. Anaplastic sarcoma of the kidney with chromosomal abnormality: first report on cytogenetic findings. *Hum Pathol* 2010;41:1495–1499.

737. Stuart R, Salyer WR, Salyer DC, et al. Renomedullary interstitial cell lesions and hypertension. *Hum Pathol* 1976;7:327–332.

738. Lerman RJ, Pitcock JA, Stephenson P, et al. Renomedullary interstitial cell tumor (formerly fibroma of the renal medulla). *Hum Pathol* 1972;3:559–568.

739. Agras K, Tuncel A, Aslan Y, et al. Adolescent renomedullary interstitial cell tumor: a case report. *Tumori* 2005;91:555–557.

740. Horita Y, Tadokoro M, Taura K, et al. Incidental detection of renomedullary interstitial cell tumour in a renal biopsy specimen. *Nephrol Dial Transplant* 2004;19:1007–1008.

741. Glover SD, Buck AC. Renal medullary fibroma: a case report. *J Urol* 1982;127:758–760.

742. Kuroda N, Toi M, Miyazaki E, et al. Participation of α-smooth muscle actin-positive cells in renomedullary interstitial cell tumors. *Oncol Rep* 2002;9:745–750.

743. Zimmermann A, Luscieti P, Flury B, et al. Amyloid-containing renal interstitial cell nodules (RICNs) associated with chronic arterial hypertension in older age groups. *Am J Pathol* 1981;105:288–294.

744. Faris G, Nashashibi M, Friedman B, et al. Urosepsis as a presenting symptom of renomedullary interstitial cell tumor causing renal obstruction. *Isr Med Assoc J* 2009;11:509–510.

745. Robertson PW, Klidjian A, Harding LK, et al. Hypertension due to a renin-secreting renal tumour. *Am J Med* 1967;43:963–976.

746. Kihara I, Kitamura S, Hoshino T, et al. A hitherto unreported vascular tumor of the kidney: a proposal of "juxtaglomerular cell tumor". *Acta Pathol Jpn* 1968;18:197–206.

747. Capovilla M, Couturier J, Molinié V, et al. Loss of chromosomes 9 and 11 may be recurrent chromosome imbalances in juxtaglomerular cell tumors. *Hum Pathol* 2008;39:459–462.

748. Capovilla M, Couturier J, Molinié V, et al. Tumeur à rénine du rein: à propos de deux cas, avec analyse génomique. *Ann Pathol* 2008;28:474–476.

749. Remynse LC, Begun FP, Jacobs SC, et al. Juxtaglomerular cell tumor with elevation of serum erythropoietin. *J Urol* 1989;142:1560–1562.

750. Hayami S, Sasagawa I, Suzuki H, et al. Juxtaglomerular cell tumor without hypertension. *Scand J Urol Nephrol* 1998;32:231–233.

751. Corvol P, Pinet F, Galen FX, et al. Seven lessons from seven renin secreting tumors. *Kidney Int Suppl* 1988;34(Suppl 25):S-38–S-44.

752. Valdés G, Lopez JM, Martinez P, et al. Renin-secreting tumor, case report. *Hypertension* 1980;2:714–718.

753. Beaudoin J, Périgny M, Têtu B, et al. A patient with a juxtaglomerular cell tumor with histological vascular invasion. *Nature Clin Pract Nephrol* 2008;4:458–462.

754. Kim HJ, Kim CH, Choi YJ, et al. Juxtaglomerular cell tumor of kidney with CD34 and CD117 immunoreactivity: report of 5 cases. *Arch Pathol Lab Med* 2006;130:707–711.

755. Duan X, Bruneval P, Hammadeh R, et al. Metastatic juxtaglomerular cell tumor in a 52-year-old man. *Am J Surg Pathol* 2004;28: 1098–1102.

756. Martin SA, Mynderse LA, Lager DJ, et al. Juxtaglomerular cell tumor, a clinicopathologic study of four cases and review of the literature. *Am J Clin Pathol* 2001;116:854–863.

757. Kuroda N, Gotoda H, Ohe C, et al. Review of juxtaglomerular cell tumor with focus on pathobiological aspect. *Diagn Pathol* 2011;6:80.

758. Lindop GBM, Stewart JA, Downie TT. The immunocytochemical demonstration of renin in a juxtaglomerular cell tumour by light and electron microscopy. *Histopathology* 1983;7:421–431.

759. Tanabe A, Naruse M, Naruse K, et al. Angiotensin II type 1 receptor expression in two cases of juxtaglomerular cell tumor: correlation to negative feedback of renin secretion by angiotensin II. *Horm Metab Res* 1999;31:429–434.

760. Shao L, Manalang M, Cooley L. Juxtaglomerular cell tumor in an 8-year-old girl. *Pediatr Blood Cancer* 2008;50:406–409.

761. Steffens J, Bock R, Braedel HU, et al. Renin-producing renal cell carcinoma. *Eur Urol* 1990;18:56–60.

762. Lindop GBM, Fleming S, Gibson AAM. Immunocytochemical localisation of renin in nephroblastoma. *J Clin Pathol* 1984;37:738–742.

763. Grawitz P. Demonstration eines grossen Angio-Myo-Lipoms der Niere. *Dtsch Med Wochenschr* 1900;26:290.

764. Moolten SE. Hamartial nature of the tuberous sclerosis complex and its bearing on the tumor problem. Report of a case with tumor anomaly of the kidney and adenoma sebaceum. *Arch Intern Med* 1942;69:589–623.

765. Green AJ, Sepp T, Yates JRW. Clonality of tuberous sclerosis hamartomas shown by non-random X-chromosome inactivation. *Hum Genet* 1996;97:240–243.

766. Bonetti F, Pea M, Martignoni G, et al. The perivascular epithelioid cell and related lesions. *Adv Anat Pathol* 1997;4:343–358.

767. Weeks DA, Chase DR, Malott RL, et al. HMB-45 staining in angiomyolipoma, cardiac rhabdomyoma, other mesenchymal processes, and tuberous sclerosis-associated brain lesions. *Int J Surg Pathol* 1994;1:191–197.

768. Weeks DA, Malott RL, Arnesen M, et al. Hepatic angiomyolipoma with striated granules and positivity with melanoma-specific antibody (HMB-45): a report of two cases. *Ultrastruct Pathol* 1991;15:563–571.

769. Bonetti F, Pea M, Martignoni G, et al. Clear cell ("sugar") tumor of the lung is a lesion strictly related to angiomyolipoma—the concept of a family of lesions characterized by the presence of the perivascular epithelioid cells (PEC). *Pathology* 1994;26:230–236.

770. Zamboni G, Pea M, Martignoni G, et al. Clear cell "sugar" tumor of the pancreas, a novel member of the family of lesions characterized by the presence of perivascular epithelioid cells. *Am J Surg Pathol* 1996;20:722–730.

771. Folpe AL, Mentzel T, Lehr HA, et al. Perivascular epithelioid cell neoplasms of soft tissue and gynecologic origin. *Am J Surg Pathol* 2005;29:1558–1575.

772. Fujii Y, Ajima J, Oka K, et al. Benign renal tumors detected among healthy adults by abdominal ultrasonography. *Eur Urol* 1995;27:124–127.

773. Filipas D, Spix C, Schulz-Lampel D, et al. Screening for renal cell carcinoma using ultrasonography: a feasibility study. *BJU Int* 2003;91:595–599.

774. Kozlowska J, Okoń K. Renal tumors in postmortem material. *Pol J Pathol* 2008;59:21–25.

775. Seyam RM, Bissada NK, Kattan SA, et al. Changing trends in presentation, diagnosis, and management of renal angiomyolipoma: comparison of sporadic and tuberous sclerosis complex-associated forms. *Urology* 2008;72:1077–1082.

776. Aydin H, Magi-Galluzzi C, Lane BR, et al. Renal angiomyolipoma clinicopathologic study of 194 cases with emphasis on the epithelioid histology and tuberous sclerosis association. *Am J Surg Pathol* 2009;33:289–297.

777. Eble JN. Angiomyolipoma of kidney. *Semin Diagn Pathol* 1998;15:21–40.

778. Stillwell TJ, Gomez MR, Kelalis PP. Renal lesions in tuberous sclerosis. *J Urol* 1987;138:477–481.

779. Cook JA, Oliver K, Mueller RF, et al. A cross sectional study of renal involvement in tuberous sclerosis. *J Med Genet* 1996;33:480–484.

780. Oesterling JE, Fishman EK, Goldman SM, et al. The management of renal angiomyolipoma. *J Urol* 1986;135:1121–1124.

781. Sooriakumaran P, Gibbs P, Coughlin G, et al. Angiomyolipomata: challenges, solutions, and future prospects based on over 100 cases treated. *BJU Int* 2009;105:101–106.

782. Forsnes EV, Eggleston MK, Burtman M. Placental abruption and spontaneous rupture of renal angiomyolipoma in a pregnant woman with tuberous sclerosis. *Obstet Gynecol* 1996;88:725.

783. Gould Rothberg BE, Grooms MC, Dharnidharka VR. Rapid growth of a kidney angiomyolipoma after initiation of oral contraceptive therapy. *Obstet Gynecol* 2006;108:734–736.

784. Halpenny D, Snow A, McNeill G, et al. The radiological diagnosis and treatment of renal angiomyolipoma—current status. *Clin Radiol* 2010;65:99–108.

785. Morrison ID, Reznek RH, Webb JAW. Case report: renal adenocarcinoma with ultrasonographic appearances suggestive of angiomyolipoma. *Clin Radiol* 1995;50:659–661.

786. Price EB Jr, Mostofi FK. Symptomatic angiomyolipoma of the kidney. *Cancer* 1965;18:761–774.

787. Sola JE, Pierre-Jerome F, Sitzmann JV, et al. Multifocal angiomyolipoma in a patient with tuberous sclerosis. *Clin Imaging* 1996;20:99–102.

788. Roach ES, Gomez MR, Northrup H. Tuberous sclerosis complex consensus conference: revised clinical diagnostic criteria. *J Child Neurol* 1998;13:624–628.

789. Fukunaga M, Harada T. Pigmented perivascular epithelioid cell tumor of the kidney. *Arch Pathol Lab Med* 2009;133:1981–1984.

790. Bonsib SM, Moghadamfalahi M, Bhalodia A. Lymphatic differentiation in renal angiomyolipomas. *Hum Pathol* 2009;40:374–380.

791. Matsuyama A, Hisaoka M, Ichikawa K, et al. Sclerosing variant of epithelioid angiomyolipoma. *Pathol Int* 2008;58:306–310.

792. Fine SW, Reuter VE, Epstein JI, et al. Angiomyolipoma with epithelial cysts (AMLEC): a distinct cystic variant of angiomyolipoma. *Am J Surg Pathol* 2006;30:593–599.

793. Davis CJ, Barton JH, Sesterhenn IA. Cystic angiomyolipoma of the kidney, a clinicopathologic description of 11 cases. *Mod Pathol* 2006;19:669–674.

794. Mikami S, Oya M, Mukai M. Angiomyolipoma with epithelial cysts of the kidney in a man. *Pathol Int* 2008;58:664–647.

795. Gutierrez OH, Burgener FA, Schwartz S. Coincidental renal cell carcinoma and renal angiomyolipoma in tuberous sclerosis. *AJR Am J Roentgenol* 1979;132:848–850.

796. Huang J-K, Ho DM, Wang J-H, et al. Coincidental angiomyolipoma and renal cell carcinoma—report of 1 case and review of the literature. *J Urol* 1988;140:1516–1518.

797. Ohigashi T, Iigaya T, Hata M. Coincidental renal cell carcinoma and renal angiomyolipomas in tuberous sclerosis. *Urol Int* 1991;47:160–163.

798. Ashfaq R, Weinberg AG, Albores-Saavedra J. Renal angiomyolipoma and HMB-45 reactivity. *Cancer* 1993;71:3091–3097.

799. Abdulla M, Bui HX, del Rosario AD, et al. Renal angiomyolipoma, DNA content and immunohistochemical study of classic and multicentric variants. *Arch Pathol Lab Med* 1994;118:735–739.

800. Kaiserling E, Kröber S, Xiao J-C, et al. Angiomyolipoma of the kidney. Immunoreactivity with HMB-45. Light- and electron-microscopic findings. *Histopathology* 1994;25:41–48.

801. Martignoni G, Bonetti F, Chilosi M, et al. Cathepsin K expression in the spectrum of perivascular epthelioid cell (PEC) lesions of the kidney. *Mod Pathol* 2012;25:100–111.

802. L'Hostis H, Deminière C, Ferriere J-M, et al. Renal angiomyolipoma: a clinicopathologic, immunohistochemical, and follow-up study of 46 cases. *Am J Surg Pathol* 1999;23:1011–1020.

803. Glenthøj A, Partoft S. Ultrasound-guided percutaneous aspiration of renal angiomyolipoma. Report of two cases diagnosed by cytology. *Acta Cytol* 1984;28:265–268.

804. Boorjian SA, Sheinin Y, Crispen PL, et al. Hormone receptor expression in renal angiomyolipoma: clinicopathologic correlation. *Urology* 2008;72:927–932.

805. Rosenkrantz AB, Hecht EM, Taneja SS, et al. Angiomyolipoma with epithelial cysts: mimic of renal cell carcinoma. *Clin Imaging* 2010;34:65–68.

806. Henske EP, Neumann HPH, Scheithauer BW, et al. Loss of heterozygosity in the tuberous sclerosis (TSC2) region of chromosome band 16p13 occurs in sporadic as well as TSC-associated renal angiomyoplipomas. *Genes Chromosomes Cancer* 1995;13:295–298.

807. Perez-Atayde AR, Iwaya S, Lack EE. Angiomyolipomas and polycystic renal disease in tuberous sclerosis, ultrastructural observations. *Urology* 1981;18:607–610.

808. Holm-Nielsen P, Sørensen FB. Renal angiomyolipoma: an ultrastructural investigation of three cases with histogenetic considerations. *APMIS Suppl* 1988;4:37–47.

809. Ferry JA, Malt RA, Young RH. Renal angiomyolipoma with sarcomatous transformation and pulmonary metastases. *Am J Surg Pathol* 1991;15:1083–1088.

810. Lowe BA, Brewer J, Houghton DC, et al. Malignant transformation of angiomyolipoma. *J Urol* 1992;147:1356–1358.

811. Farrow GM, Harrison EG Jr, Utz DC, et al. Renal angiomyolipoma, a clinicopathologic study of 32 cases. *Cancer* 1968;22:564–570.

812. Kragel PJ, Toker C. Infiltrating recurrent renal angiomyolipoma with fatal outcome. *J Urol* 1985;133:90–91.

813. Taylor RS, Joseph DB, Kohaut EC, et al. Renal angiomyolipoma associated with lymph node involvement and renal cell carcinoma in patients with tuberous sclerosis. *J Urol* 1989;141:930–932.

814. Ro JY, Ayala AG, El-Naggar A, et al. Angiomyolipoma of kidney with lymph node involvement, DNA flow cytometric analysis. *Arch Pathol Lab Med* 1990;114:65–67.

815. Hulbert JC, Graf R. Involvement of the spleen by renal angiomyolipoma: metastasis or multicentricity. *J Urol* 1983;130:328–329.

816. Boorjian SA, Frank I, Inman B, et al. The role of partial nephrectomy for the management of sporadic renal angiomyolipoma. *Urology* 2011;70:1064–1068.

817. Byrd GF, Lawatsch EJ, Mesrobian H-G, et al. Laparoscopic cryoablation of renal angiomyolipoma. *J Urol* 2006;176:1512–1516.

818. Davies DM, de Vries PJ, Johnson SR, et al. Sirolimus therapy for angiomyolipoma in tuberous sclerosis and sporadic lymphangioleiomyomatosis; a phase 2 trial. *Clin Cancer Res* 2011;17:4071–4081.

819. Franz DN. Everolimus: an mTOR inhibitor for the treatment of tuberous sclerosis. *Expert Rev Anticancer Ther* 2011;11:1181–1192.

820. Mai KT, Perkins DG, Collins JP. Epithelioid variant of renal angiomyolipoma. *Histopathology* 1996;28:277–280.

821. Cibas ES, Goss GA, Kulke MH, et al. Malignant epithelioid angiomyolipoma ('sarcoma ex angiomyolipoma') of the kidney: a case report and review of the literature. *Am J Surg Pathol* 2001;25:121–126.

822. Park HK, Zhang S, Wong MKK, et al. Clinical presentation of epithelioid angiomyolipoma. *Int J Urol* 2007;14:21–25.

823. Martignoni G, Pea M, Bonetti F, et al. Carcinoma-like monotypic epithelioid angiomyolipoma, in patients without evidence of tuberous sclerosis, a clinicopathologic and genetic study. *Am J Surg Pathol* 1998;22:663–672.

824. Sato K, Ueda Y, Tachibana H, et al. Malignant epithelioid angiomyolipoma of the kidney in a patient with tuberous sclerosis: an autopsy case report with *p53* gene mutation analysis. *Pathol Res Pract* 2008;204:771–777.

825. Brimo F, Robinson B, Guo C, et al. Renal epithelioid angiomyolipoma with atypia: a series of 40 cases with emphasis on clinicopathologic prognostic indicators of malignancy. *Am J Surg Pathol* 2010;34: 715–722.

826. Eble JN, Amin MB, Young RH. Epithelioid angiomyolipoma of the kidney, a report of five cases with a prominent and diagnostically confusing epithelioid smooth muscle component. *Am J Surg Pathol* 1997;21:1123–1130.

827. Nese N, Martignoni G, Fletcher CD, et al. Pure epithelioid PEComas (so-called epithelioid angiomyolipoma) of the kidney: a clinicopathologic study of 41 cases: detailed assessment of morphology and risk stratification. *Am J Surg Pathol* 2011;35:161–176.

828. Cho NH, Shim HS, Choi YD, et al. Estrogen receptor is significantly associated with the epithelioid variants of renal angiomyolipoma: a clinicopathological and immunohistochemical study of 67 cases. *Pathol Int* 2004;54:510–515.

829. Ooi SM, Vivian JB, Cohen RJ. The use of the Ki-67 marker in the pathological diagnosis of the epithelioid variant of renal angiomyolipoma. *Int Urol Nephrol* 2009;41:559–565.

830. Su M-C, Jeng Y-M, Chu Y-C. Desmoplastic small round cell tumor of the kidney. *Am J Surg Pathol* 2004;28:1379–1383.

831. Egloff AM, Lee EY, Dillon JE, et al. Desmoplastic small round cell tumor of the kidney in a pediatric patient: sonographic and multiphase CT findings. *AJR Am J Roentgenol* 2005;185:1347–1349.

832. Collardeau-Frachon S, Ranchère-Vince D, Delattre O, et al. Primary desmoplastic small round cell tumor of the kidney: a case report in a 14-year-old girl with molecular confirmation. *Pediatr Dev Pathol* 2007;10:320–324.

833. Wang LL, Perlman EJ, Vujanić GM, et al. Desmoplastic small round cell tumor of the kidney in childhood. *Am J Surg Pathol* 2007;31: 576–584.

834. Cardoso da Silva R, Medeiros Filho P, Chioato L, et al. Desmoplastic small round cell tumor of the kidney mimicking Wilms tumor, a case report and review of the literature. *Appl Immunohistochem Mol Morphol* 2009;17:557–562.

835. Janssens E, Desprechins B, Ernst C, et al. Desmoplastic small round cell tumor of the kidney. *JBR-BTR* 2009;92:60.

836. Eaton SH, Cendron M. Primary desmoplastic small round cell tumor of the kidney in a 7-year-old girl. *J Pediatr Urol* 2006;2:52–54.

837. Dineen MK, Venable DD, Misra RP. Pure intrarenal lipoma—report of a case and review of the literature. *J Urol* 1984;132:104–107.

838. Safak M, Baltaci S, Akyar S, et al. Intrarenal lipoma: report of a case. *Urol Int* 1989;44:113–115.

839. Ke HL, Hsiao HL, Guh JY, et al. Primary intrarenal lipoma: a case report. *Kaohsiung J Med Sci* 2005;21:383–386.

840. Chiang I-C, Jang M-Y, Tsai K-B, et al. Huge renal lipoma with prominent hypervascular non-adipose elements. *Br J Radiol* 2006;79: e148–e151.

841. Liu X, Wu X, He D, et al. The first case of renal lipoma in a child. *J Pediatr Surg* 2011;46:1281–1283.

842. Kucera A, Snajdauf J, Vyhnánek M, et al. Lipoblastoma in children: an analysis of 5 case. *Acta Chir Belg* 2008;108:580–582.

843. Delsignore A, Ranzoni S, Arancio M, et al. Kidney hibernoma: case report and literature review. *Arch Ital Urol Androl* 2010;82:189–191.

844. Shah VB, Rupani AB, Deokar MS, et al. Idiopathic renal replacement lipomatosis; a case report and review of literature. *Indian J Pathol Microbiol* 2009;52:552–553.

845. Romero FR, Pilati R, Caboclo MFSF, et al. Renal replacement lipomatosis and xanthogranulomatous pyelonephritis: differential diagnosis. *Rev Assoc Med Brasil* 2011;57:262–265.

846. Shum CF, Yip SKH, Tan PH. Symptomatic renal leiomyoma: report of two cases. *Pathology* 2006;38:454–456.

847. Kuroda N, Inoue Y, Taguchi T, et al. Renal leiomyoma: an immunohistochemical, ultrastructural and comparative genomic hybridization study. *Histol Histopathol* 2007;22:883–888.

848. Terad T. Leiomyoma of the kidney parenchyma. *Pathol Int* 2011;61: 495–497.

849. Mashali N, Awad AT, Trevisan G, et al. Renal leiomyoma. *Pathologica* 2011;105:22–24.

850. Hogan A, Smyth GK, D'Arcy C, et al. Renal capsular leiomyoma. *Urology* 2008;71:1226.e1–1226.e3.

851. Gómez Pérez L, Budía Alba A, Delgado Oliva FJ, et al. Leiomioma de pelvis renal. *Actas Urol Esp* 2006;30:641–643.

852. Zelić M, Uravić M, Petrosić N, et al. Leiomyoma of the left renal vein, a report of a case. *Acta Chir Belg* 2009;109:782–784.

853. Dionne JM, Carter JE, Matsell D, et al. Renal leiomyoma associated with Epstein-Barr virus in a pediatric transplant patient. *Am J Kidney Dis* 2005;46:351–355.

854. Brown JG, Folpe AL, Rao P, et al. Primary vascular tumors and tumor-like lesions of the kidney: a clinicopathologic analysis of 25 cases. *Am J Surg Pathol* 2010;34:942–949.

855. Kryvenko ON, Gupta NS, Meier FA, et al. Anastomosing hemangioma of the genitourinary system: eight cases in the kidney and ovary with immunohistochemical and ultrastructural analysis. *Am J Clin Pathol* 2011;136:450–457.

856. Zhao X, Zhang J, Zhong Z, et al. Large renal cavernous hemangioma with renal vein thrombosis: case report and review of the literature. *Urology* 2009;73:443.e1–443.e3.

857. Schofield D, Zaatari GS, Gay BB. Klippel-Trenaunay and Sturge-Weber syndromes with renal hemangioma and double inferior vena cava. *J Urol* 1986;136:442–445.

858. Montgomery E, Epstein JI. Anastomosing hemangioma of the genitourinary tract, a lesion mimicking angiosarcoma. *Am J Surg Pathol* 2009;33:1364–1369.

859. Faraji H, Nguyen BN, Mai KT. Renal epithelioid angiomyolipoma: a study of six cases and a meta-analytic study. Development of criteria for screening the entity with prognostic significance. *Histopathology* 2009;55:525–534.

860. Verine J, Sandid W, Miquel C, et al. Sporadic hemangioblastoma of the kidney: an underrecognized pseudomalignant tumor? *Am J Surg Pathol* 2011;35:623–624.

861. Liu Y, Qiu X-S, Wang E-H. Sporadic hemangioblastoma of the kidney: a rare renal tumor. *Diagn Pathol* 2012;7:49.

862. Wang CC, Wang S-M, Liau J-Y. Sporadic hemangioblastoma of the kidney in a 29-year-old man. *Int J Surg Pathol* 2012;20:519–522.

863. Yin W-H, Li J, Chan JKC. Sporadic hemangioblastoma of the kidney with rhabdoid features and focal CD10 expression: report of a case and literature review. *Diagn Pathol* 2012;7:39.

864. Carney EM, Banerjee P, Ellis CL, et al. PAX2(-)/PAX8(-)/inhibin A(+) immunoprofile in hemangioblastoma: a helpful combination in the differential diagnosis with metastatic clear cell renal cell carcinoma to the central nervous system. *Am J Surg Pathol* 2011;35:262–267.

865. Billard F, Dumollard JM, Cucherousset J, et al. Deux tumeurs vasculaires bénignes de la capsule du rein. *Ann Pathol* 1991;11:266–270.

866. Siddiqui NH, Rogalska A, Basil IS. Glomangiomyoma (glomus tumor) of the kidney. *Arch Pathol Lab Med* 2005;129:1172–1174.

867. Herawi M, Parwani AV, Edlow D, et al. Glomus tumor of renal pelvis: a case report and review of the literature. *Hum Pathol* 2005;36:299–302.

868. Al-Ahmadie HA, Yilmaz A, Olgac S, et al. Glomus tumor of the kidney, a report of 3 cases involving renal parenchyma and review of the literature. *Am J Surg Pathol* 2007;31:585–591.

869. Nuwayhid Z, Rodriguez MM, Prescott A, et al. Renal glomus tumor in an adolescent: a conservative approach. *J Pediatr Surg* 2010;45: E23–E26.

870. Lamba G, Rafiyath SM, Kaur H, et al. Malignant glomus tumor of kidney: the first reported case and review of the literature. *Hum Pathol* 2011;42:1200–1203.

871. Caduff RF, Schwöbel MG, Willi UV, et al. Lymphangioma of the right kidney in an infant boy. *Pediatr Pathol Lab Med* 1997;17:631–637.

872. Honma I, Takagi Y, Shigyo M, et al. Lymphangioma of the kidney. *Int J Urol* 2002;9:178–182.

873. Nakai Y, Namba Y, Sugao H. Renal lymphangioma. *J Urol* 1999;162: 484–485.

874. Zapzalka DM, Krishnamurti L, Manivel JC, et al. Lymphangioma of the renal capsule. *J Urol* 2002;168:220.

875. Mahdavi R, Khooei A, Asadi L. Hygroma renalis: an extremely rare renal lesion. *Urol J* 2007;4:118–120.

876. Pickering SP, Fletcher BD, Bryan PJ, et al. Renal lymphangioma: a cause of neonatal nephromegaly. *Pediatr Radiol* 1984;14:445–448.

877. Gobbo S, Eble JN, Huang J, et al. Schwannoma of the kidney. *Mod Pathol* 2008;21:779–783.

878. Hung S-F, Chung S-D, Lai M-K, et al. Renal schwannoma: case report and literature review. *Urology* 2008;72:716.e3–716.e6.

879. Alvarado-Cabrero I, Folpe AL, Srigley JR, et al. Intrarenal schwannoma: a report of four cases including three cellular variants. *Mod Pathol* 2000;13:851–856.

880. Hirano D, Mashiko A, Murata Y, et al. A case of solitary fibrous tumor of the kidney: an immunohistochemical and ultrastructural study with a review of the literature. *Med Mol Morphol* 2009;42:239–244.

881. Fine SW, McCarthy DM, Chan TY, et al. Malignant solitary fibrous tumor of the kidney, report of a case and comprehensive review of the literature. *Arch Pathol Lab Med* 2006;130:857–861.

882. Wang J, Arber DA, Frankel K, et al. Large solitary fibrous tumor of the kidney: report of two cases and review of the literature. *Am J Surg Pathol* 2001;25:1194–1199.

883. Magro G, Cavallaro V, Torrisi A, et al. Intrarenal solitary fibrous tumor of the kidney, report of a case with emphasis on the differential diagnosis in the wide spectrum of monomorphous spindle cell tumors of the kidney. *Pathol Res Pract* 2002;198:37–43.

884. Hsieh T-Y, ChangChien Y-C, Chen W-H, et al. *De novo* malignant solitary fibrous tumor of the kidney. *Diagn Pathol* 2011;6:96.

885. Mayes DC, Fechner RE, Gillenwater JY. Renal liposarcoma. *Am J Surg Pathol* 1990;14:268–273.

886. Cano JY, D'Altorio RA. Renal liposarcoma: case report. *J Urol* 1976;115:747–749.

887. Matsushita M, Ito A, Ishidoya S, et al. Intravenous extended liposarcoma arising from renal sinus. *Int J Urol* 2007;14:769–770.

888. Farrow GM, Harrison EG Jr, Utz DC, et al. Sarcomas and sarcomatoid and mixed malignant tumors of the kidney in adults—part I. *Cancer* 1968;22:545–550.

889. Dotan ZA, Tal R, Golijanin D, et al. Adult genitourinary sarcoma: the 25-year Memorial Sloan-Kettering experience. *J Urol* 2006;176: 2033–2039.

890. Miller JS, Zhou M, Brimo F, et al. Primary leiomyosarcoma of the kidney: a clinicopathologic study of 27 cases. *Am J Surg Pathol* 2010; 34:238–242.

891. Yokose T, Fukuda H, Ogiwara A, et al. Myxoid leiomyosarcoma of the kidney accompanying ipsilateral ureteral transitional cell carcinoma. A case report with cytological, immunohistochemical and ultrastructural study. *Acta Pathol Jpn* 1991;41:694–700.

892. Krech RH, Loy V, Dieckmann K-P, et al. Leiomyosarcoma of the kidney: immunohistological and ultrastructural findings with special emphasis on the growth fraction. *Br J Urol* 1989;63:132–134.

893. Grignon DJ, Ayala AG, Ro JY, et al. Primary sarcomas of the kidney, a clinicopathologic and DNA flow cytometric study of 17 cases. *Cancer* 1990;65:1611–1618.

894. Deyrup AT, Montgomery E, Fisher C. Leiomyosarcoma of the kidney, a clinicopathologic study. *Am J Surg Pathol* 2004;28:178–182.

895. Grignon DJ, McIsaac GP, Armstrong RF, et al. Primary rhabdomyosarcoma of the kidney, a light microscopic, immunohistochemical, and electron microscopic study. *Cancer* 1988;62:2027–2032.

896. Raney B, Anderson J, Arndt C, et al.; Soft-tissue Sarcoma Committee of the Children's Oncology Group. Primary renal sarcomas in the Intergroup Rhabdomyosarcoma Study Group (IRSG) experience, 1972–2005: a report from the Children's Oncology Group. *Pediatr Blood Cancer* 2008;51:339–343.

897. Kren L, Goncharuk VN, Votava M, et al. Botryoid-type of embryonal rhabdomyosarcoma of renal pelvis in an adult, a case report and review of the literature. *Cesk Patol* 2003;39:31–35.

898. Tsai W-C, Lee S-S, Cheng M-F, et al. Botryoid-type rhabdomyosarcoma of the renal pelvis in an adult, a rare case report and review of the literature. *Urol Int* 2006;77:89–91.

899. Sola JE, Cova D, Casillas J, et al. Primary renal botryoid rhabdomyosarcoma: diagnosis and outcome. *J Pediatr Surg* 2007;42:E17–E20.

900. Dalfior D, Eccher A, Gobbo S, et al. Primary pleomorphic rhabdomyosarcoma of the kidney in an adult. *Ann Diagn Pathol* 2008;12:301–303.

901. Zenico T, Saccomani M, Salomone U, et al. Primary renal angiosarcoma: case report and review of world literature. *Tumori* 2011;97: e6–e9.

902. Cerilli LA, Huffman HT, Anand A. Primary renal angiosarcoma: a case report with immunohistochemical, ultrastructural, and cytogenetic features and review of the literature. *Arch Pathol Lab Med* 1998;122:929–935.

903. Indolfi P, Donofrio V, Fusco C, et al. Kaposiform hemangioendothelioma of the kidney: an unusual presentation of a rare vascular neoplasm. *J Pediatr Hematol Oncol* 2010;32:e195–e198.

904. Shin DH, Chen M, Niemeier LA. Primary epithelioid hemangioendothelioma of the kidney and penis. *Can J Urol* 2010;17:5480–5482.

905. Lee TY, Lawen J, Gupta R. Renal angiosarcoma: a case report and literature review. *Can J Urol* 2007;14:3471–3476.

906. Singh C, Xie L, Schmechel SC, et al. Epithelioid angiosarcoma of the kidney: a diagnostic dilemma in fine-needle aspiration cytology. *Diagn Cytopathol* 2012;40(suppl 2):E131–E139.

907. Cioppa T, Marrelli D, Neri A, et al. Primary osteosarcoma of the kidney with retroperitoneal hemorrhage. Case report and review of the literature. *Tumori* 2007;93:213–216.

908. Argani P, Faria PA, Epstein JI, et al. Primary renal synovial sarcoma: molecular and morphologic delineation of an entity previously included among embryonal sarcomas of the kidney. *Am J Surg Pathol* 2000;24:1087–1096.

909. Divetia M, Karpate A, Basak R, et al. Synovial sarcoma of the kidney. *Ann Diagn Pathol* 2008;12:333–339.

910. Perlmutter AE, Saunders SE, Zaslau S, et al. Primary synovial sarcoma of the kidney. *Int J Urol* 2005;12:760–762.

911. Kim D-H, Sohn JH, Lee MC, et al. Primary synovial sarcoma of the kidney. *Am J Surg Pathol* 2000;24:1097–1104.

912. Jun S-Y, Choi J, Kang GH, et al. Synovial sarcoma of the kidney with rhabdoid features, report of three cases. *Am J Surg Pathol* 2004;28:634–637.

913. Shao L, Hill DA, Perlman EJ. Expression of WT-1, Bcl-2, and CD34 by primary renal spindle cell tumors in children. *Pediatr Dev Pathol* 2004;7:577–582.

914. Paláu MA, Pham TT, Barnard N, et al. Primary synovial sarcoma of the kidney with rhabdoid features. *Int J Surg Pathol* 2007;15: 421–428.

915. Gabilondo F, Rodríguez F, Mohar A, et al. Primary synovial sarcoma of the kidney: corroboration with in situ polymerase chain reaction. *Ann Diagn Pathol* 2008;12:134–137.

916. Edmunds W. Cystic adenoma of kidney. *Trans Path Soc London* 1892;43:89–90.

917. Osathanondh V, Potter EL. Pathogenesis of polycystic kidneys. Historical survey. *Arch Pathol* 1964;77:459–465.

918. Tang TT, Harb JM, Oechler HW, et al. Multilocular renal cyst: electron microscopic evidence of pathogenesis. *Am J Pediatr Hematol Oncol* 1984;6:27–32.

919. Hartman DS, Davis CJ Jr, Johns T, et al. Cystic renal cell carcinoma. *Urology* 1986;28:145–153.

920. Powell T, Shackman R, Johnson HD. Multilocular cysts of the kidney. *Br J Urol* 1951;23:142–152.

921. Boggs LK, Kimmelstiel P. Benign multilocular cystic nephroma: report of two cases of so-called multilocular cyst of the kidney. *J Urol* 1956;76:530–541.

922. Turbiner J, Amin MB, Humphrey PA, et al. Cystic nephroma and mixed epithelial and stromal tumor of kidney: a detailed clinicopathological analysis of 34 cases and proposal for renal epithelial and stromal tumor (REST) as a unifying term. *Am J Surg Pathol* 2007; 31:489–500.

923. Zhou M, Kort E, Hoekstra P, et al. Adult cystic nephroma and mixed epithelial and stromal tumor of the kidney are the same disease entity, molecular and histologic evidence. *Am J Surg Pathol* 2009;33:72–80.

924. Hughes JH, Niemann TH, Thomas PA. Multicystic nephroma: report of a case with fine-needle aspiration findings. *Diagn Cytopathol* 1996; 14:60–63.

925. Shimokama T, Watanabe T. Multilocular renal cyst, scanning and transmission electron microscopic observations. *Pathol Res Pract* 1989; 184:255–259.

926. Chatten J, Bishop HC. Bilateral multilocular cysts of the kidneys. *J Pediatr Surg* 1977;12:749–750.

927. Geller RA, Pataki KI, Finegold RA. Bilateral multilocular renal cysts with recurrence. *J Urol* 1979;121:808–810.

928. Ferrer FA, McKenna PH. Partial nephrectomy in a metachronous multilocular cyst of the kidney (cystic nephroma). *J Urol* 1994;151: 1358–1360.

929. Yamamoto H, Maruyama T, Kuwae H, et al. Bilateral multilocular cystic renal cell carcinoma: a case report. *Acta Urol Jpn* 1996;42:513–516.

930. Cheng EY, Cohn RA, Palmer LS, et al. A rare case of bilateral multilocular renal cysts. *J Urol* 1997;157:1861–1862.

931. Delahunt B, Thomson KJ, Ferguson AF, et al. Familial cystic nephroma and pleuropulmonary blastoma. *Cancer* 1993;71:1338–1342.

932. Kajani N, Rosenberg BF, Bernstein J. Multilocular cystic nephroma. *J Urol Pathol* 1993;1:33–42.

933. Madewell JE, Goldman SM, Davis CJ Jr, et al. Multilocular cystic nephroma: a radiographic-pathologic correlation of 58 patients. *Radiology* 1983;146:309–321.

934. Castillo OA, Boyle ET Jr, Kramer SA. Multilocular cysts of kidney, a study of 29 patients and review of the literature. *Urology* 1991; 37:156–162.

935. Gibson TE. Multilocular cyst of the kidney: case report. *Trans Am Assoc Genitourin Surg* 1961;53:53–59.

936. Kettritz U, Semelka RC, Siegelman ES, et al. Multilocular cystic nephroma: MR imaging appearance with current techniques, including gadolinium enhancement. *J Magn Reson Imaging* 1996;6:145–148.

937. Gibbons AB, Waisman J, Fligiel S. Multilocular cyst of renal hilum. *Urology* 1983;22:306–308.

938. Abt AB, Demers LM, Shochat SJ. Cystic nephroma: an ultrastructural and biochemical study. *J Urol* 1979;122:539–541.

939. Brown RC, Cornell SH, Culp DA. Multilocular renal cyst with diffuse calcification simulating renal-cell carcinoma. *Radiology* 1970;95: 411–412.

940. Steele R, Daroca PJ, Hill S, et al. Multilocular renal cyst (cystic nephroma) with müllerian-like stroma. *Urology* 1994;43:549–553.

941. Drut R. Cystic nephroma: cytologic findings in fine-needle aspiration cytology. *Diagn Cytopathol* 1992;8:593–595.

942. Clark SP, Kung ITM, Tang SK. Fine-needle aspiration of cystic nephroma (multilocular cyst of the kidney). *Diagn Cytopathol* 1992;8: 349–351.

943. Morgan C, Greenberg ML. Multilocular renal cyst: a diagnostic pitfall on fine-needle aspiration cytology: case report. *Diagn Cytopathol* 1995;13:66–70.

944. Mukhopadhyay S, Valente AL, de la Roza G. Cystic nephroma, a histologic and immunohistochemical study of 10 cases. *Arch Pathol Lab Med* 2004;128:1404–1411.

945. Coleman M. Multilocular renal cyst, case report, ultrastructure and review of the literature. *Virchows Arch A Pathol Anat Histol* 1980; 387:207–219.

946. Ding Y, Chen L, Deng F-M, et al. Localized cystic disease of the kidney, distinction from cystic neoplasms and hereditary polycystic disorders. *Am J Surg Pathol* 2013;37:506–513.

947. Pawade J, Soosay GN, Delprado W, et al. Cystic hamartoma of the renal pelvis. *Am J Surg Pathol* 1993;17:1169–1175.

948. Truong LD, Williams R, Ngo T, et al. Adult mesoblastic nephroma; expansion of the morphologic spectrum and review of the literature. *Am J Surg Pathol* 1998;22:827–839.

949. Pierson CR, Schober MS, Wallis T, et al. Mixed epithelial and stromal tumor of the kidney lacks the genetic alterations of cellular congenital mesoblastic nephroma. *Hum Pathol* 2001;32:513–520.

950. Adsay NV, Eble JN, Srigley JR, et al. Mixed epithelial and stromal tumor of the kidney. *Am J Surg Pathol* 2000;24:958–970.

951. Michal M, Hes O, Bisceglia M, et al. Mixed epithelial and stromal tumors of the kidney. A report of 22 cases. *Virchows Arch* 2004; 445:359–367.

952. Teklali Y, Piolat C, Durand C, et al. Mixed epithelial and stromal renal tumour in a 12-year-old boy. *J Pediatr Urol* 2010;6:320–323.

953. Tan MH, Teh BT. Renal neoplasia in the parathyroidism-jaw tumor syndrome. *Curr Mol Med* 2004;4:895–897.

954. Antic T, Perry KT, Harrison K, et al. Mixed epithelial and stromal tumor of the kidney and cystic nephroma share overlapping features, reappraisal of 15 lesions. *Arch Pathol Lab Med* 2006;130:80–85.

955. Sahni VA, Mortele KJ, Glickman J, et al. Mixed epithelial and stromal tumour of the kidney: imaging features. *BJU Int* 2009;105:932–939.

956. Chu LC, Hruban RH, Horton KM, et al. Mixed epithelial and stromal tumor of the kidney: radiologic-pathologic correlation. *Radiographics* 2010;30:1541–1551.

957. Kum JB, Grignon DJ, Wang M, et al. Mixed epithelial and stromal tumors of the kidney: evidence for a single cell of origin with capacity for epithelial and stromal differentiation. *Am J Surg Pathol* 2011;35:1114–1122.

958. Parikh P, Chan TY, Epstein JI, et al. Incidental stromal-predominant mixed epithelial-stromal tumors of the kidney, a mimic of intraparenchymal renal leiomyoma. *Arch Pathol Lab Med* 2005;129:910–914.

959. Yang Y, Hes O, Zhang L, et al. Mixed epithelial and stromal tumor of the kidney with cervical and intestinal differentiation. *Virchows Arch* 2005;447:669–671.

960. Chu PG, Lau SK, Weiss LM, et al. Intestinal type of mucinous borderline tumor arising from mixed epithelial and stromal tumor of kidney. *Virchows Arch* 2009;455:389–394.

961. Sireci AN, Rodriguez R, Swierczynski SL, et al. Fat-predominant mixed epithelial and stromal tumor (MEST): report of a unique case mimicking angiomyolipoma. *Int J Surg Pathol* 2008;16:73–77.

962. Tickoo SK, Gopalan A, Tu JJ, et al. Estrogen and progesterone receptor-positive stroma as a non-tumerous proliferation in kidneys: a possible meataplstic response to obstructioin. *Mod Pathol* 2008;21: 60–65.

963. Karafin M, Parwani AV, Netto GJ, et al. Diffuse expression of PAX2 and PAX8 in the cystic epithelium of mixed epithelial stromal tumor, angiomyolipoma with epithelial cysts, and primary renal synovial sarcoma: evidence supporting renal tubular differentiation. *Am J Surg Pathol* 2011;35:1264–1273.

964. Svec A, Hes O, Michal M, et al. Malignant mixed epithelial and stromal tumor of the kidney. *Virchows Arch* 2001;439:700–702.

965. Nakagawa T, Kanai Y, Fujimoto H, et al. Malignant mixed epithelial and stromal tumor of the kidney: a report of the first two cases with a fatal clinical outcome. *Histopathology* 2004;44:302–304.

966. Jung SJ, Shen SS, Tran T, et al. Mixed epithelial and stromal tumor of kidney with malignant transformation: report of two cases and review of literature. *Hum Pathol* 2008;39:463–468.

967. Kuroda N, Sakaida N, Kinoshita H, et al. Carcinosarcoma arising in mixed epithelial and stromal tumor of the kidney. *APMIS* 2008;116:1013–1015.

968. Menéndez CL, Rodríguez Villar D, et al. A new case of malignant mixed epithelial and stromal tumor of the kidney with rhabdomyosarcomatous transformation. *Anal Quant Cytol Histol* 2012;34: 331–334.

969. Suzuki T, Hiragata S, Hosaka K, et al. Malignant mixed epithelial and stromal tumor of the kidney: report of the first male case. *Int J Urol* 2013;20:448–450.

970. Hansel DE, Epstein JI, Berbescu E, et al. Renal carcinoid tumor: a clinicopathologic study of 21 cases. *Am J Surg Pathol* 2007;31: 1539–1544.

971. Lane BR, Chery F, Jour G, et al. Renal neuroendocrine tumours: a clinicopathological study. *BJU Int* 2007;100:1030–1035.

972. Krishnan B, Truong LD, Saleh G, et al. Horseshoe kidney is associated with an increased relative risk of primary renal carcinoid tumor. *J Urol* 1997;157:2059–2066.

973. Shibata R, Okita H, Shimoda M, et al. Primary carcinoid tumor in a polycystic kidney. *Pathol Int* 2003;53:317–322.

974. Hannah J, Lippe B, Lai-Goldman M, et al. Oncocytic carcinoid of the kidney associated with periodic Cushing's syndrome. *Cancer* 1988;61:2136–2140.

975. Kuroda N, Katto K, Tamura M, et al. Carcinoid tumor of the renal pelvis: consideration on the histogenesis. *Pathol Int* 2008;58:51–54.

976. Romero FR, Rais-Bahrami S, Permpongkosol S, et al. Primary carcinoid tumors of the kidney. *J Urol* 2006;176:2359–2366.

977. Jeung JA, Cao D, Selli BW, et al. Primary renal carcinoid tumors: clinicopathologic features of 9 cases with emphasis on novel immunohistochemical findings. *Hum Pathol* 2011;42:1554–1561.

978. Raslan WF, Ro JY, Ordonez NG, et al. Primary carcinoid of the kidney. Immunohistochemical and ultrastructural studies of five patients. *Cancer* 1993;72:2660–2666.

979. El-Naggar AK, Troncoso P, Ordonez NG. Primary renal carcinoid tumor with molecular abnormality characteristic of conventional renal cell neoplasms. *Diagn Mol Pathol* 1995;4:48–53.

980. van den Berg E, Gouw ASH, Oosterhuis JW, et al. Carcinoid in a horseshoe kidney. Morphology, immunohistochemistry, and cytogenetics. *Cancer Genet Cytogenet* 1995;84:95–98.

981. La Rosa S, Bernasconi B, Micello D, et al. Primary small cell neuroendocrine carcinoma of the kidney: morphological, immunohistochemical, ultrastructural, and cytogenetic study of a case and review of the literature. *Endocr Pathol* 2009;20:24–34.

982. Si Q, Dancer J, Stanton ML, et al. Small cell carcinoma of the kidney: a clinicopathologic study of 14 cases. *Hum Pathol* 2011;42: 1792–1798.

983. Masuda T, Oikawa H, Yashima A, et al. Renal small cell carcinoma (neuroendocrine carcinoma) without features of transitional cell carcinoma. *Pathol Int* 1998;48:412–415.

984. Dundr P, Pesl M, Povýsil C, et al. Primary large cell neuroendocrine carcinoma of the kidney. *Pathol Oncol Res* 2010;16:139–142.

985. Capella C, Eusebi V, Rosai J. Primary oat cell carcinoma of the kidney. *Am J Surg Pathol* 1984;8:855–861.

986. Morgan KG, Banerjee SS, Eyden BP, et al. Primary small cell neuroendocrine carcinoma of the kidney. *Ultrastruct Pathol* 1996;20: 141–144.

987. Parham DM, Roloson GJ, Feely M, et al. Primary malignant neuroepithelial tumors of the kidney: a clinicopathologic analysis of 146 adult and pediatric cases from the National Wilms' Tumor Study Group Pathology Center. *Am J Surg Pathol* 2001;25:133–146.

988. Jimenez RE, Folpe AL, Lapham RL, et al. Primary Ewing's sarcoma/primitive neuroectodermal tumor of the kidney, a clinicopathologic and immunohistochemical analysis of 11 cases. *Am J Surg Pathol* 2002;26:320–327.

989. Thyavihally YB, Tongaonkar HB, Gupta S, et al. Primitive neuroectodermal tumor of the kidney: a single institute series of 16 patients. *Urology* 2008;71:292–296.

990. Seemayer TA, Thelmo WL, Bolande RP, et al. Peripheral neuroectodermal tumors. *Perspect Pediatr Pathol* 1975;2:151–172.

991. Citak EC, Oguz A, Karadeniz C, et al. Primitive neuroectodermal tumor of the kidney in a child. *Pediatr Hematol Oncol* 2009;26: 481–486.

992. Asiri M, Al-Sayyad A. Renal primitive neuroectodermal tumour in childhood. *Can Urol Assoc J* 2010;4:E158–E160.

993. Karnes RJ, Gettman MT, Anderson PM, et al. Primitive neuroectodermal tumor (extraskeletal Ewing's sarcoma) of the kidney with vena caval tumor thrombus. *J Urol* 2000;164:772.

994. Rodriguez-Galindo C, Marina NM, Fletcher BD, et al. Is primitive neuroectodermal tumor of the kidney a distinct entity? *Cancer* 1997;79:2243–2250.

995. Ellison DA, Parham DM, Bridge J, et al. Immunohistochemistry of primary malignant neuroepithelial tumors of the kidney: a potential source of confusion? A study of 30 cases from the National Wilms Tumor Study Pathology Center. *Hum Pathol* 2007;38:205–211.

996. Ranadive NU, Urmi C, Kumar M. Primary primitive neuroectodermal tumor (PNET) of the kidney: a case report. *Arch Esp Urol* 1999;52:190–192.

997. Takeuchi T, Iwasaki H, Ohjimi Y, et al. Renal primitive neuroectodermal tumor: a morphologic, cytogenetic, and molecular analysis with the establishment of two cultured cell lines. *Diagn Mol Pathol* 1997;6:309–317.

998. Berg T, Kalsaas A-H, Buechner J, et al. Ewing sarcoma—peripheral neuroectodermal tumor of the kidney with a *FUS-ERG* fusion transcript. *Cancer Genet Cytogenet* 2009;194:53–57.

999. Bartholomew T, Parwani A. Renal primitive neuroectodermal tumors. *Arch Pathol Lab Med* 2012;136:686–690.

1000. Gohji K, Nakanishi T, Hara I, et al. Two cases of primary neuroblastoma of the kidney in adults. *J Urol* 1987;137:966–968.

1001. Sellaturay SV, Arya M, Banisadr S, et al. Primary intrarenal neuroblastoma: a rare, aggressive tumour of childhood mimicking Wilms' tumour. *J Pediatr Urol* 2006;2:522–524.

1002. Dickson PV, Sims TL, Streck CJ, et al. Avoiding misdiagnosing neuroblastoma as Wilms tumor. *J Pediatr Surg* 2008;43:1159–1163.

1003. Fan R. Primary renal neuroblastoma—a clinical pathologic study of 8 cases. *Am J Surg Pathol* 2012;36:94–100.

1004. Sebire NJ, Vujanic GM. Paediatric renal tumours: recent developments, new entities and pathological features. *Histopathology* 2009; 54:516–528.

1005. Simon H, Carlson DH, Hanelin J, et al. Intrarenal pheochromocytoma: report of a case. *J Urol* 1979;121:805–807.

1006. Pengelly CDR. Phaeochromocytoma within the renal capsule. *Br Med J* 1959;2:477–478.

1007. Preger L, Gardner RE, Kawala BO, et al. Intrarenal pheochromocytoma, preoperative angiographic diagnosis. *Urology* 1976;8: 194–196.

1008. Takahashi M, Yang XJ, McWhinney S, et al. cDNA microarray analysis assists in diagnosis of malignant intrarenal pheochromocytoma originally masquerading as a renal cell carcinoma. *J Med Genet* 2005;42:e48.

1009. Lagacé R, Tremblay M. Non-chromaffin paraganglioma of the kidney with distant metastases. *Can Med Assoc J* 1968;99:1095–1098.

1010. Dimopoulos MA, Moulopoulos LA, Constantinides C, et al. Primary renal lymphoma: a clinical and radiological study. *J Urol* 1996;155: 1865–1867.

1011. Ferry JA, Harris NL, Papanicolaou N, et al. Lymphoma of the kidney, a report of 11 cases. *Am J Surg Pathol* 1995;19:134–144.

1012. Ferry JA, Young RH. Malignant lymphoma of the genitourinary tract. *Curr Diagn Pathol* 1997;4:145–169.

1013. Osborne BM, Brenner M, Weitzner S, et al. Malignant lymphoma presenting as a renal mass: four cases. *Am J Surg Pathol* 1987;11:375–382.

1014. Harris GJ, Lager DJ. Primary renal lymphoma. *J Surg Oncol* 1991;46: 273–277.

1015. Da'as N, Polliack A, Cohen Y, et al. Kidney involvement and renal manifestations in non-Hodgkin's lymphoma and lymphocytic leukemia: a retrospective study of 700 patients. *Eur J Haematol* 2001;67: 158–164.

1016. D'Agati V, Sablay LB, Knowles DM, et al. Angiotropic large cell lymphoma (intravascular malignant lymphomatosis) of the kidney: presentation as minimal change disease. *Hum Pathol* 1989;20:263–268.

1017. Nishikubo CY, Kunkel LA, Figlin R, et al. An association between renal cell carcinoma and lymphoid malignancies, a case series of eight patients. *Cancer* 1996;78:2421–2426.

1018. Kunthur A, Wiernik PH, Dutcher JP. Renal parenchymal tumors and lymphoma in the same patient: case series and review of the literature. *Am J Hematol* 2006;81:271–280.

1019. Kuo C-C, Li W-Y, Huang C-C, et al. Primary renal lymphoma. *Br J Haematol* 2008;144:628.

1020. Qiu L, Unger PD, Dillon RW, et al. Low-grade mucosa-associated lymphoid tissue lymphoma involving the kidney, report of 3 cases and review of the literature. *Arch Pathol Lab Med* 2006;130:86–89.

1021. Wang BY, Strauchen JA, Rabinowitz D, et al. Renal cell carcinoma with intravascular lymphomatosis, a case report of unusual collision tumors with review of the literature. *Arch Pathol Lab Med* 2001;125:1239–1241.

1022. Kose F, Sakalli H, Mertsoylu H, et al. Primary renal lymphoma: report of four cases. *Onkologie* 2009;32:200–202.

1023. Igel TC, Engen DE, Banks PM, et al. Renal plasmacytoma: Mayo Clinic experience and review of the literature. *Urology* 1991;37:385–389.

1024. Fan F, Deauna-Limayo D, Thrasher JB, et al. Anaplastic plasmacytoma of the kidney. *Histopathology* 2005;47:432–433.

1025. Yazici S, Inci K, Dikmen A, et al. Port site and local recurrence of incidental solitary renal plasmacytoma after retroperitoneoscopic radical nephrectomy. *Urology* 2009;73:210.e15–210.e17.

1026. Mongha R, Narayan S, Dutta A, et al. Plasmacytoma of the kidney. *Saudi J Kidney Dis Transpl* 2010;21:931–934.

1027. Kandel LB, Harrison LH, Woodruff RD, et al. Renal plasmacytoma: a case report and summary of reported cases. *J Urol* 1984;132:1167–1169.

1028. Hilmes MA, Dillman JR, Mody RJ, et al. Pediatric renal leukemia: spectrum of CT imaging findings. *Pediatr Radiol* 2008;38:424–430.

1029. Sato A, Imaizumi M, Chikaoka S, et al. Acute renal failure due to leukemic cell infiltration followed by relapse at multiple extramedullary sites in a child with acute lymphoblastic leukemia. *Leuk Lymphoma* 2004;45:825–828.

1030. Sharma A, Gupta R, Rizvi Y, et al. Acute renal failure in a patient with acute lymphoblastic leukemia: a rare cause. *Saudi J Kidney Dis Transpl* 2013;24:93–96.

1031. Akbayram S, Akgun C, Peker E, et al. T-cell lymphoblastic leukemia as a rare cause of bilateral nephromegaly. *J Emerg Med* 2012;43:e65–e66.

1032. Bagg MD, Wettlaufer JN, Willadsen DS, et al. Granulocytic sarcoma presenting as a diffuse renal mass before hematological manifestations of acute myelogenous leukemia. *J Urol* 1994;152:2092–2093.

1033. Park H-J, Jeong D-H, Song H-G, et al. Myeloid sarcoma of both kidneys, the brain, and multiple bones in a nonleukemic child. *Yonsei Med J* 2003;44:740–743.

1034. Usmani SZ, Shahid Z, Saleh H, et al. Myeloid sarcoma presenting with acute renal failure and bilateral ureteral obstruction: a case report and review of the literature. *Am J Med Sci* 2007;334:136–138.

1035. Traweek ST, Arber DA, Rappaport H, et al. Extramedullary myeloid cell tumors, an immunohistochemical and morphologic study of 28 cases. *Am J Surg Pathol* 1993;17:1011–1019.

1036. Jeong SH, Han JH, Jeong SY, et al. A case of donor-derived granulocytic sarcoma after allogeneic hematopoietic stem cell transportation. *Korean J Hematol* 2010;45:70–72.

1037. Dehner LP. Intrarenal teratoma occurring in infancy: report of a case with discussion of extragonadal germ cell tumors in infancy. *J Pediatr Surg* 1973;8:369–378.

1038. Aubert J, Casamayou J, Denis P, et al. Intrarenal teratoma in a newborn child. *Eur Urol* 1978;4:306–308.

1039. Otani M, Tsujimoto S, Miura M, et al. Intrarenal mature cystic teratoma associated with renal dysplasia: case report and literature review. *Pathol Int* 2001;560:564.

1040. Aaronson IA, Sinclair-Smith C. Multiple cystic teratomas of the kidney. *Arch Pathol Lab Med* 1980;104:614.

1041. Yoo J, Park S, Lee HJ, et al. Primary carcinoid tumor arising in a mature teratoma of the kidney, a case report and review of the literature. *Arch Pathol Lab Med* 2002;126:979–981.

1042. Kojiro M, Ohishi H, Isobe H. Carcinoid tumor occurring in cystic teratoma of the kidney, a case report. *Cancer* 1976;38:1636–1640.

1043. Fetissof F, Benatre A, Dubois MP, et al. Carcinoid tumor occurring in a teratoid malformation of the kidney, an immunohistochemical study. *Cancer* 1984;54:2305–2308.

1044. Liu Y-C, Wang J-S, Chen C-J, et al. Intrarenal mixed germ cell tumor. *J Urol* 2000;164:2020–2021.

1045. Mihatsch MJ, Bleisch A, Six P, et al. Primary choriocarcinoma of the kidney in a 49-year-old woman. *J Urol* 1972;108:537–539.

1046. Grammatico D, Grignon DJ, Eberwein P, et al. Transitional cell carcinoma of the renal pelvis with choriocarcinomatous differentiation: immunohistochemical and immunoelectron microscopic assessment of human chorionic gonadotropin production by transitional cell carcinoma of the urinary bladder. *Cancer* 1993;71:1835–1841.

1047. Fernandes ET, Parham DM, Ribeiro RC, et al. Teratoid Wilms' tumor: the St. Jude experience. *J Pediatr Surg* 1988;23:1131–1134.

1048. Wagle DG, Moore RH, Murphy GP. Secondary carcinomas of the kidney. *J Urol* 1975;114:30–32.

1049. Bracken RB, Chica G, Johnson DE, et al. Secondary renal neoplasms: an autopsy study. *South Med J* 1979;72:806–807.

1050. Patel U, Ramachandran N, Halls J, et al. Synchronous renal masses in patients with a nonrenal malignancy: incidence of metastasis to the kidney versus primary renal neoplasia and differentiating features on CT. *AJR Am J Roentgenol* 2011;197:W680–W686.

1051. Perl SI, Yong JC, Higgins SG. Tumor crescents from intraglomerular metastases. *Clin Nephrol* 1987;27:260–262.

1052. Belghiti D, Hirbec G, Bernaudin JF, et al. Intraglomerular metastases, report of two cases. *Cancer* 1984;54:2309–2312.

1053. Shin T, Kan T, Sato F, et al. Tumor-to-tumor metastasis to chromophobe renal cell carcinoma: a first report. *Case Rep Urol* 2011;2011:520839.

1054. Aggarwal N, Amin RM, Parwani AV. Tumor-to-tumor metastasis: case report of a pulmonary adenocarcinoma metastatic to a clear cell renal cell carcinoma. *Pathol Res Pract* 2012;208:50–52.

1055. Flocks RH, Kadesky MC. Malignant neoplasms of the kidney: an analysis of 353 patients followed five years or more. *J Urol* 1958;79:196–201.

1056. Robson CJ. Radical nephrectomy for renal cell carcinoma. *J Urol* 1963;89:37–42.

1057. Robson CJ, Churchill BM, Anderson W. The results of radical nephrectomy for renal cell carcinoma. *J Urol* 1969;101:297–301.

1058. American Joint Committee for Cancer Staging and End Results Reporting. *Staging of Cancer at Genitourinary Sites: Kidney, Bladder, Prostate, and Testes. Manual for Staging of Cancer 1977*. 1st ed. Chicago, IL: American Joint Committee; 1977:109–130.

1059. American Joint Committee on Cancer. Kidney. In: Beahrs OH, Myers MH, eds. *Manual for Staging of Cancer*. 2nd ed. Philadelphia, PA: J.B. Lippincott Co.; 1983:177–180.

1060. American Joint Committee on Cancer. Kidney. In: Beahrs OH, Henson DE, Hutter RVP, et al., eds. *Manual for Staging of Cancer*. 3rd ed. Philadelphia, PA: J.B. Lippincott Co.; 1988:199–201.

1061. American Joint Committee on Cancer. Kidney. In: Beahrs OH, Henson DE, Hutter RVP, et al., eds. *Manual for Staging of Cancer*. 4th ed. Philadelphia, PA: J.B. Lippincott Co.; 1992:201–204.

1062. American Joint Committee on Cancer. Kidney (sarcomas and adenomas are not included). In: Fleming ID, Cooper JS, Henson DE, et al., eds. *AJCC Cancer Staging Manual*. 5th ed. Philadelphia, PA: Lippincott-Raven; 1997:231–234.

1063. American Joint Committee on Cancer. Kidney (sarcomas and adenomas are not included). In: Greene FL, Page DL, Fleming ID, et al., eds. *AJCC Cancer Staging Handbook*. 6th ed. New York: Springer-Verlag; 2002:355–360.

1064. American Joint Committee on Cancer. Kidney. In: Edge SB, Byrd DR, Compton CC, et al., eds. *AJCC Staging Manual*. 7th ed. New York: Springer; 2010:479–489.

1065. Guinan P, Saffrin R, Stuhldreher D, et al. Renal cell carcinoma: comparison of the TNM and Robson stage groupings. *J Surg Oncol* 1995;59:186–189.

1066. Bonsib SM, Gibson D, Mhoon M, et al. Renal sinus involvement in renal cell carcinomas. *Am J Surg Pathol* 2000;24:451–458.

1067. Trpkov K, Grignon DJ, Bonsib SM, et al. Handling and staging of renal cell carcinoma: the International Society of Urological Pathology (ISUP) consensus conference recommendations. *Am J Surg Pathol*. In press 2013.

1068. Grignon D, Paner GP. Renal cell carcinoma and the renal sinus. *Adv Anat Pathol* 2007;14:63–68.

1069. Bonsib SM. The renal sinus is the principal invasive pathway, a prospective study of 100 renal cell carcinomas. *Am J Surg Pathol* 2004;28:1594–1600.

1070. Bonsib SM. Renal lymphatics, and lymphatic involvement in sinus vein invasive (pT3b) clear cell renal cell carcinoma: a study of 40 cases. *Mod Pathol* 2006;19:746–753.

1071. Gofrit ON, Shapiro A, Pizov G, et al. Does stage T3a renal cell carcinoma embrace a homogeneous group of patients? *J Urol* 2007;177:1682–1686.

1072. Thompson RH, Blute ML, Krambeck AE, et al. Patients with pT1 renal cell carcinoma who die from disease after nephrectomy may have unrecognized renal sinus fat invasion. *Am J Surg Pathol* 2007;31:1089–1093.

1073. Thompson RH, Leibovich BC, Cheville JC, et al. Is renal sinus fat invasion the same as perinephric fat invasion for pT3a renal cell carcinoma? *J Urol* 2005;174:1218–1221.

1074. Blute ML, Leibovich BC, Lohse CM, et al. The Mayo Clinic experience with surgical management, complications and outcome for patients with renal cell carcinoma and venous tumor thrombus. *BJU Int* 2004;94:33–41.

1075. Klaver S, Joniau S, Suy R, et al. Analysis of renal cell carcinoma with subdiaphragmatic macroscopic venous invasion. *BJU Int* 2007;101:444–449.

1076. Haferkamp A, Bastian PJ, Jakobi H, et al. Renal cell carcinoma with tumor thrombus extension into the vena cava: prospective long-term followup. *J Urol* 2007;177:1703–1708.

1077. Klatte T, Pantuck AJ, Riggs SB, et al. Prognostic factors for renal cell carcinoma with tumor thrombus extension. *J Urol* 2007;178:1189–1195.

1078. Lambert EH, Pierorazio PM, Shabsigh A, et al. Prognostic risk stratification and clinical outcomes in patients undergoing surgical treatment for renal cell carcinoma with vascular tumor thrombus. *Urology* 2007;69:1054–1058.

1079. Moinzadeh A, Libertino JA. Prognostic significance of tumor thrombus level in patients with renal cell carcinoma and venous tumor thrombus extension. Is all T3b the same? *J Urol* 2004;171:598–601.

1080. Leibovich BC, Cheville JC, Lohse CM, et al. Cancer specific survival for patients with pT3 renal cell carcinoma—can the 2002 primary tumor classfication be improved? *J Urol* 2005;173:716–719.

1081. Terakawa T, Miyake H, Takenaka A, et al. Clinical outcome of surgical management for patients with renal cell carcinoma involving the inferior vena cava. *Int J Urol* 2011;14:781–784.

1082. Martínez-Salamanca JI, Huang WC, Millán I, et al.; International Renal Cell Carcinoma-Venous Thrombus Consortium. Prognostic impact of the 2009 UICC/AJCC TNM staging system for renal cell carcinoma with venous extension. *Eur Urol* 2011;59:120–127.

1083. Katz MD, Serrano MF, Humphrey PA, et al. The role of lymphovascular space invasion in renal cell carcinoma as a prognostic marker of survival after curative resection. *Urol Oncol* 2011;29:738–744.

1084. Han KR, Bui MH, Pantuck AJ, et al. TNM T3a renal cell carcinoma: adrenal gland involvement is not the same as renal fat invasion. *J Urol* 2003;169:899–903.

1085. Thompson RH, Leibovich BC, Cheville JC, et al. Should direct ipsilateral adrenal invasion from renal cell carcinoma be classified as pT3a? *J Urol* 2005;173:918–921.

1086. Sun M, Bianchi M, Hansen J, et al. Nodal involvement at nephrectomy is associated with worse survival: a stage-for-stage and grade-for-grade analysis. *Int J Urol* 2013;20:372–380.

1087. Capitanio U, Suardi N, Matloob R, et al. Staging lymphadenectomy in renal cell carcinoma must be extended: a sensitivity curve analysis. *BJU Int* 2012;111:412–418.

1088. Crispen PL, Breau RH, Allmer C, et al. Lymph node dissection at the time of radical nephrectomy for high-risk clear cell renal cell carcinoma: indications and recommendations for surgical templates. *Eur Urol* 2011;59:18–23.

1089. Joslyn SA, Sirintrapun SJ, Konety BR. Impact of lymphadenectomy and nodal burden in renal cell carcinoma: retrospective analysis of the National Surveillance, Epidemiology, and End Results database. *Urology* 2005;65:675–680.

1090. Leibovich BC, Cheville JC, Lohse CM, et al. A scoring algorithm to predict survival for patients with metastatic clear cell renal cell carcinoma: a stratification tool for prospective clinical trials. *J Urol* 2005;174:1759–1763.

1091. Novara G, Ficarra V, Antonelli A, et al.; Members of the SATURN Project-LUNA Foundation. Validation of the 2009 TNM version in a large multi-institutional cohort of patients treated for renal cell carcinoma: are further improvements needed? *Eur Urol* 2010;58:588–595.

1092. Veeratterapillay R, Simren R, El-Sherif A, et al. Accuracy of the revised 2010 TNM classification in predicting the prognosis of patients treated for renal cancer in the north east of England. *J Clin Pathol* 2012;65:367–371.

1093. Kim SP, Alt AL, Weight CJ, et al. Independent validation of the 2010 American Joint Committee on Cancer TNM classification for renal carcinoma: results from a large, single institution cohort. *J Urol* 2011;185:2035–2039.

1094. Eble JN. Recommendations for examining and reporting tumor-bearing kidney specimens from adults. *Semin Diagn Pathol* 1998;15:77–82.

1095. Che M, Grignon DJ. Handling and reporting of tumor-containing kidney specimens. *Clin Lab Med* 2005;25:417–432.

1096. Srigley JR, Amin MB, Delahunt B, et al.; Members of the Cancer Committee CoAP. Protocol for the examination of specimens from patients with invasive carcinoma of renal tubular origin. *Arch Pathol Lab Med* 2010;134:e25–e30.

1097. Castilla EA, Liou LS, Abrahams NA, et al. Prognostic importance of resection margin width after nephron-sparing surgery for renal cell carcinoma. *Urology* 2002;60:993–997.

1098. Ljungberg B, Cowan NC, Hanbury DC, et al. EAU guidelines on renal cell carcinoma: the 2010 update. *Eur Urol* 2010;58:398–406.

1099. Somani BK, Nabi G, Thorpe P, et al.; Aberdeen Academic and Clinical Urological Surgeons (ABACUS) Group. Image-guided biopsy-diagnosed renal cell carcinoma: critical appraisal of technique and long-term follow-up. *Eur Urol* 2007;51:1289–1297.

1100. Shannon BA, Cohen RJ, de Bruto H, et al. The value of preoperative needle core biopsy for diagnosing benign lesions among small, incidentally detected renal masses. *J Urol* 2008;180:1257–1261.

1101. Volpe A, Mattar K, Finelli A, et al. Contemporary results of percutaneous biopsy of 100 small renal masses: a single center experience. *J Urol* 2008;180:2333–2337.

1102. Al-Ahmadie HA, Alden D, Fine SW, et al. Role of immunohistochemistry in the evaluation of needle core biopsies in adult renal cortical tumors: an ex vivo study. *Am J Surg Pathol* 2011;35:949–961.

1103. Rabban JT, Meng MV, Yeh B, et al. Kidney morcellation in laparoscopic nephrectomy of tumor: recommendations for specimen sampling and pathologic tumor staging. *Am J Surg Pathol* 2001;25:1158–1166.

1104. Wu SD, Lesani A, Zhao LC, et al. A multi-institutional study on the safety and efficacy of specimen morcellation after laparoscopic radical nephrectomy for clinical stage T1 or T2 renal cell carcinoma. *J Endourol* 2009;23:1513–1518.

1105. Meng MV, Koppie TM, Duh Q-Y, et al. Novel method of assessing surgical margin status in laparoscopic specimens. *Urology* 2001;58:677–682.

1106. Bonsib SM, Pei Y. The non-neoplastic kidney in tumor nephrectomy specimens, what can it show and what is important? *Adv Anat Pathol* 2010;17:235–250.

1107. Bijol V, Mendez GP, Hurwitz S, et al. Evaluation of the nonneoplastic pathology in tumor nephrectomy specimens, predicting the risk of progressive renal failure. *Am J Surg Pathol* 2006;30:575–584.

1108. Henriksen KJ, Meehan SM, Chang A. Non-neoplastic renal diseases are often unrecognized in adult tumor nephrectomy specimens. *Am J Surg Pathol* 2007;31:1703–1708.

Pathology of the Adrenal Gland

SHAMLAL MANGRAY and RONALD A. DeLELLIS

Although considerably less common than diseases of the kidney, urinary bladder, and prostate, disorders of the adrenal glands form a significant proportion of the material submitted for pathologic examination to surgical pathologists. Adrenal diseases may be nonfunctional or may be associated with a complex array of clinical syndromes resulting from abnormalities in the production and secretion of steroid hormones or catecholamines. As with other endocrine diseases, the same clinical syndromes can develop as a consequence of diverse pathophysiologic mechanisms. It is essential, therefore, that the pathologist is familiar with basic pathophysiologic concepts of adrenal disorders and with appropriate ancillary techniques that aid in the differential diagnosis of specific disorders.

The role of the surgical pathologist and cytopathologist has been further complicated by the detection of a variety of mass lesions by ultrasonography, computed tomography (CT), magnetic resonance imaging (MRI), or positron emission tomography (PET) in the workup of patients for reasons other than expected adrenal pathology. The presence of incidental lesions of varying sizes (incidentalomas) has been demonstrated in up to 5% of individuals subjected to abdominal CT studies.[1] By far the majority are of cortical origin and a subset of these lesions are subjected to needle core biopsy or fine needle aspiration biopsy, which frequently pose considerable diagnostic challenges.

The purpose of this chapter is to provide an overview of the pathology of the adrenal glands, including the use of immunohistochemical and molecular approaches for the differential diagnosis and prognostic assessment of a wide range of neoplastic and nonneoplastic lesions.

EMBRYOLOGY OF THE ADRENAL GLANDS

The adrenal cortex is first recognizable at 5 to 6 weeks of gestation (9-mm embryo stage) as a proliferation of cells from the peritoneum at the base of the dorsal mesentery close to the cranial aspect of the mesonephros.[2] By 8 weeks, the cortical cells separate from the mesothelium and are enveloped by a fibrous capsule. By the second trimester, the cortex includes a broad inner zone composed of large eosinophilic cells referred to as the provisional zone or fetal cortex and an outer zone that is destined to become the adult cortex (Fig. 3-1). Dehydroepiandrosterone sulfate is the major steroid product of the fetal cortex, while cortisol, aldosterone, and sex steroids are the main products of the adult cortex. Relative to total body weight, the weight of the adrenals is maximal at the 4th week of development. At birth, the fetal cortex occupies about 75% of the cortical volume, but shortly thereafter it begins to undergo involution, which is associated with an approximate 50% reduction in glandular weight.[3] At birth, the adrenal glands together weigh close to 10 g (Table 3-1). Further involution of the fetal cortex and proliferation of the permanent cortex toward the center of the gland occur simultaneously. As a result the fetal cortex accounts for approximately 20% of the cortical volume by the 12th postgestational week.

The neural crest–derived intra-adrenal (adrenal medulla) and extra-adrenal paraganglia and the sympathetic nervous system are intimately associated during embryonic development. In the 14-mm embryo, the cortical anlage is invaded on its medial aspect by primitive sympathetic cells and nerve fibers that originate from the contiguous prevertebral and paravertebral sympathetic tissue. Some primitive sympathetic cells, however, may penetrate the anlage without associated nerve fibers.[4,5] They are first apparent as nodular aggregates in the cortex (Fig. 3-2), where they may form rosettes or pseudorosettes. Mature medullary (chromaffin) cells are identifiable among the primitive sympathetic cells between the 27- and 33-mm stages and gradually increase in number. Nodules of primitive sympathetic cells peak in number and size between 17 and 20 weeks and then decline. Groups of these cells may, however, persist until birth and may also be apparent in early infancy (see "Neuroblastoma"). As the medullary chromaffin cells reach their maximum volume, there is a progressive involution of extra-adrenal chromaffin cells. However, the formation of the adrenal medulla is not completed until the 3rd year of life.

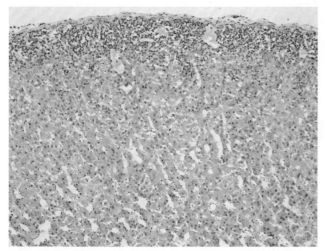

FIGURE 3-1 ■ Adrenal cortex of a 16-week fetus demonstrating the broad inner zone of eosinophilic cells (provisional zone or fetal cortex) and the thin outer zone that will form the adult cortex.

FIGURE 3-2 ■ Groups of primitive sympathetic cells forming neuroblastic nodules within the fetal cortex in the adrenal gland of a 16-week fetus (same specimen as Fig. 3-1).

NORMAL ANATOMY AND PHYSIOLOGY OF THE ADRENAL CORTEX AND MEDULLA

The adrenal glands are present on the superior surfaces of the kidneys. There is considerable variation in reported adrenal weights in different published series (Table 3-1). In adults who have died suddenly, the average adrenal weight is between 4 and 5 g and measures $5 \times 3 \times 1$ cm in the normal adult. However, greater weights occur in hospitalized patients dying after prolonged illnesses, presumably as a result of

Table 3-1 ■ AVERAGE COMBINED WEIGHTS OF ADRENAL GLAND FROM SERIES OF AUTOPSY PATIENTS*

| Age | Combined Weight | |
	Mean (grams)	Range (grams)
Fetal (Wk)		
30–33	2.3	1.6–3.2
33–38	4.4	3.1–5.8
38–41	6.2	2.0–10.5
Infants and Toddlers (Wk)		
0–1	6.3	3.8–8.8
1–3	4.4	3.1–5.8
3–9	2.4	1.8–3.0
9–14	2.0	1.2–2.6
14–32	2.3	1.6–3.2
32–78	2.5	1.6–4.0
Children and Adults (Y)		
1.5–4	4.0	0–8.0
4–8	4.1	2.3–5.8
8–14	6.2	3.5–9.0
14–18	8.8	6.0–11.2
18–25	8.0	5.6–9.8
25–35	9.0	6.2–11.4

*Derived from Figure 9-1 in Lack EE. *AFIP Atlas of Tumor Pathology (series 4) Tumors of the Adrenal Gland and Extraadrenal Paraganglia.*

prolonged stimulation of the glands by adrenocorticotropin during stress.[6,7] The right gland has a pyramidal shape, while the left gland has a crescentic shape. Each gland has a tripartite structure consisting of head (medial), body (middle), and tail (lateral) portions.[8,9] The central vein emerges from the gland at the junction of the head and body of the gland. Within the gland itself, the muscle bundles of the central vein are eccentric and are oriented toward the medulla.

In the fresh state, the outer cortex is bright yellow, while the inner cortical zone is brown to tan. The cortex measures approximately 1 mm in thickness in adults and constitutes approximately 90% of the total glandular weight. Cortical extrusions, which are characterized by the presence of nodular groups of cortical cells that extend into the periadrenal fat, are common. They are attached to the adjacent cortex by a small pedicle and are surrounded by a fibrous capsule; however, they may be completely separated from the gland in some instances.

The zones of the cortex include glomerulosa, fasciculata, and reticularis[6,10] (Fig. 3-3). The glomerulosa, which is composed of relatively small lipid-poor cells that synthesize mineralocorticoids, accounts for 15% of the cortical volume. The glomerulosa layer is often incomplete so the fasciculata may abut the capsule of the gland directly. The fasciculata, on the other hand, is composed of columns of lipid-rich cells, which synthesize both glucocorticoids and sex steroids and occupy 70% to 80% of the cortical volume. Stimulation of the adrenal by adrenocorticotropic hormone (ACTH) during times of stress leads to depletion of lipid stores from the fasciculata.[6] As a result, the cells of this layer become compact and eosinophilic.[11] In some patients, the solid cords of the outer cortex are replaced by tubular structures lined by lipid-depleted cells. Proteinaceous material and degenerated cells may also be present within the tubular structures. In some patients dying from infections, chronic renal failure, and overexposure to cold, cells within the zona fasciculata may have intracytoplasmic vacuoles.[11] The lipid content becomes replenished (lipid reversion)

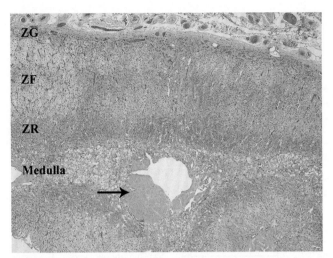

Figure 3-3 ■ Histology of the normal adrenal gland. The three cortical zones (ZG, zona glomerulosa; ZF, zona fasciculata; ZR, zona reticularis), and medulla (MED) are demonstrated. There is slight nodularity of the cortex as occurs in normal adults. Also demonstrated is the eccentric smooth muscle wall of the central vein (*arrow*).

during the process of recovery. The remainder of the cortex is composed of the reticularis, which is capable of synthesis of both glucocorticoids and sex steroids. The cells of the reticularis have eosinophilic cytoplasm, scanty lipid

vacuoles, and prominent deposits of lipochrome pigment, which are responsible for the brown color of the reticularis. Ultrastructurally, the cells of the glomerulosa contain lamelliform mitochondria while tubulovesicular mitochondria predominate in the fasciculata and reticularis. The intermediate filaments of cortical cells include vimentin and variable amounts of low-molecular-weight cytokeratins.[12] Cortical cells are also positive for calretinin, inhibin A, melan-A, and synaptophysin.[13–16]

Focal aggregates of lymphocytes are an incidental finding in the adrenal cortices of normal adults, and increase in frequency with the age of the patient.[17] Most of the lymphocytes are of T lineage.[18]

Cholesterol, which is derived from circulating low-density lipoproteins, is the precursor of all steroid hormones. Following internalization into the cortical cells, the lipoproteins are hydrolyzed with the production of cholesterol esters, which yield cholesterol and free fatty acids.[19,20] There are four cytochrome P-450 enzymes that are involved in the biosynthesis of adrenal steroids (P-450$_{scc}$, P-450$_{c17}$, P-450$_{c21}$, P-450$_{c11}$). The enzyme 3β-hydroxysteroid dehydrogenase does not belong to the P-450 cytochrome family (Fig. 3-4). The synthesis and secretion of glucocorticoids, 18-hydroxysteroids, and androgens are regulated by a complex set of control mechanisms. Hypothalamic corticotropin-releasing hormone

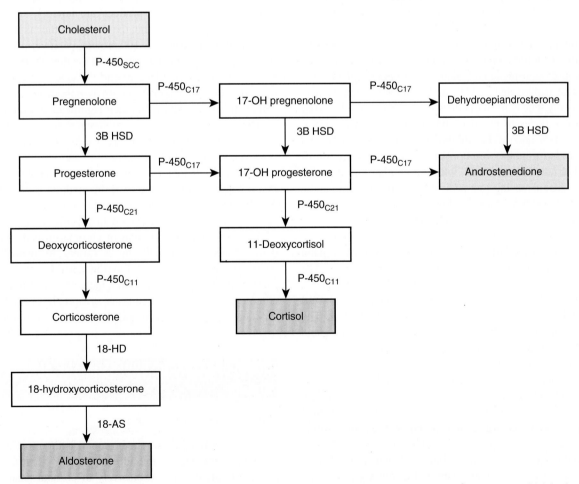

Figure 3-4 ■ Biosynthesis of adrenal steroid hormones. 18-AS, 18-aldehyde synthetase; 3B HSD, 3-β hydroxysteroid dehydrogenase; 18 HD, 18 hydroxylase.

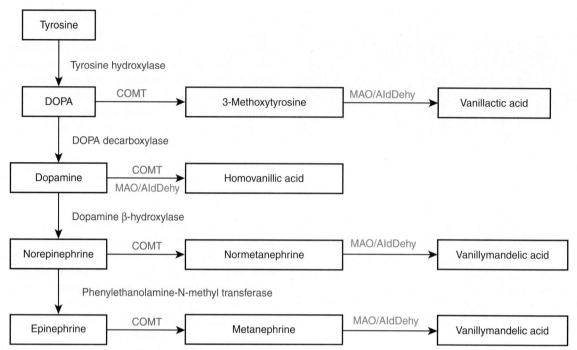

FIGURE 3-5 ■ Catecholamine biosynthesis and metabolism. COMT, catecholamine-*O*-methyl transferase; DOPA, 3,4-dihydroxyphenylalanine; MAO/AldDehy, monoamine oxidase and aldehyde dehydrogenase.

(CRH), a 41-amino-acid polypeptide, reaches the anterior pituitary gland via the hypophyseal portal system, where it stimulates the release of ACTH.[20]

In the adrenal cortex, ACTH stimulates cortical cells by activation of intracytoplasmic cyclases that form cyclic adenosine monophosphate and guanosine monophosphate from adenosine triphosphate (ATP) and guanosine triphosphate, respectively. The control of cortisol synthesis is mediated by a complex series of positive and negative feedback loops. Both cortisol and ACTH inhibit the release of CRH, and cortisol also inhibits secretion of ACTH. The secretion of ACTH is normally episodic, with the number and duration of episodes increasing to a peak in the early morning and a nadir in the evening, resulting in the characteristic circadian rhythm of cortisol secretion.[20] The secretion of aldosterone is regulated primarily by the renin–angiotensin system.[20–22]

The adrenal medulla occupies 8% to 10% of each gland volume in adults and has an average weight of 0.4 g.[7] The major portion of the medulla lies within the head of the gland, while the body of the gland contains medullary (chromaffin) cells within its crest and usually within one alar region.[8] The average corticomedullary ratio is 5:1 in the head of the gland and 14.7:1 in the body. The tail of the adrenal does not normally contain medullary tissue.

Medullary (chromaffin) cells are arranged in small nests and cords that are separated by a rich capillary network. A few medullary cells, particularly those found in the juxtacortical regions, may have enlarged and hyperchromatic nuclei, which increase in number with age[23] in addition to periodic acid-Schiff (PAS) positive hyaline globules.[24] At the ultrastructural level, the most characteristic feature of medullary cells is the presence of membrane-bound secretory granules in which catecholamines and other products are stored.[25,26] A few ganglion cells are present within the medulla either as single cells or as small-cell clusters. S-100 protein–positive sustentacular cells are present at the peripheries of the medullary cords and nests and are also evident around the ganglion cells. There may also be small collections of lymphocytes and plasma cells within the medulla, but their significance is unknown.

The precursor of the catecholamines is tyrosine, which is converted sequentially to 3, 4-dihydroxyphenylalanine (DOPA), dopamine, norepinephrine, and epinephrine by a series of well-characterized enzymatic steps (Fig. 3-5).[27] The major catecholamine product of the medulla is epinephrine, which affects the activities of a wide variety of cells and tissues following its interactions with specific receptors.

The catecholamine content of chromaffin cells has been demonstrated traditionally by a variety of histochemical techniques including the chromaffin reaction.[28–31] In current surgical pathology practice, immunohistochemical stains for chromogranins, chromomembrins, synaptophysin, and regulatory peptides are most commonly utilized for this purpose.[32–35]

NONNEOPLASTIC DISORDERS OF THE ADRENAL GLAND

Developmental Disorders

Accessory adrenal tissue (heterotopia) is the most common congenital anomaly of the adrenal gland.[36] Most accessory adrenal tissue consists exclusively of cortical tissue, but a few examples, particularly those in the region of the celiac ganglion, may also contain medullary tissue.[37] Based on autopsy studies accessory adrenal tissue is most frequently found in the retroperitoneal space (32%) along the celiac axis, the upper pole of the kidney just beneath the renal capsule (0.1% to 6%), the broad ligament (23%), adnexa of the testes (7.5%), and along the course of the spermatic cord (3.8% to 9.3%).[11] Less common sites include the pancreas, spleen, liver, lung placenta, and brain. In surgical pathology series, the most commonly encountered site is in inguinal hernia sacs. One percent of hernia sacs have been reported to contain accessory adrenal tissue.[38] Accessory adrenals may undergo hyperplasia in response to increased levels of ACTH and may serve as the site of origin of cortical neoplasms.[23,39,40] True heterotopic adrenal glands may be fused with the liver or kidney and are typically surrounded by a common connective tissue capsule.[41,42] In such cases, a concern for a metastatic renal cell carcinoma (RCC) or other clear-cell tumors may arise.

Adrenal union (fusion) and adhesion are rare anomalies that are distinguished by the presence (adrenal union) or absence (adhesion) of a connective tissue capsule. Fusion is occasionally associated with midline congenital defects, including spinal dysraphism, indeterminate visceral situs, and the Cornelia de Lange syndrome. Fusion of the adrenal glands can occur in patients with bilateral renal agenesis.[43]

Aplasia of the adrenal glands has been reported in association with anencephaly, but in most instances, the glands are markedly hypoplastic rather than completely absent.[44] In approximately 10% of patients with unilateral renal agenesis, the ipsilateral adrenal gland is also absent. There are four main types of congenital adrenal hypoplasia (OMIM #300200): sporadic with hypopituitarism, autosomal recessive, X-linked cytomegalic type with hypogonadotrophic hypogonadism, and the form associated with glycerol kinase deficiency.[44,45] The majority of patients present early in childhood and most typically in infancy; however, occasional individuals with mild forms of these disorders may present as adults. Patients commonly have signs and symptoms of adrenal insufficiency, but other clinical manifestations include hearing loss, coal black pigmentation of the skin, hypogonadism, and precocious puberty.[45]

In primary hypoplasia, the adult cortex is markedly hypoplastic, but the fetal zone is retained and often has cytomegalic features. This disorder has an X-linked pattern of inheritance and has been associated with mutations or deletions of the *DAX-1* gene (Xp21).[37,46,47] The miniature adult type of hypoplasia may appear sporadically or as an inherited abnormality with an autosomal recessive pattern of inheritance. Despite their small size, the adrenals have a normal architecture.

The differential diagnosis of primary hypoplasia includes disorders in which adrenal insufficiency precedes other manifestations. For example, if hypoadrenalism occurs prior to neurologic manifestations, patients with adrenoleukodystrophy will present with clinical symptomology simulating that of primary adrenal hypoplasia. Chronic maternal exogenous glucocorticoid administration induces secondary hypoplasia of the adrenal glands in the newborn. In such instances the adrenal glands are small for age, have decreased fetal zone volume, and contain cells with decreased lipid and scattered cytomegalic features.

Adrenal Cytomegaly and Beckwith-Wiedemann Syndrome

Adrenal cytomegaly is characterized by the presence of collections of markedly enlarged (up to 150 μm) eosinophilic cortical cells containing hyperchromatic and pleomorphic nuclei (Fig. 3-6), with occasional nuclear cytoplasmic pseudoinclusions within the fetal cortex. Cytomegaly may be seen in neonates but is more common in premature infants (3% to 7%) and is also relatively common in infants with Rh incompatibility.[17] In Beckwith-Wiedemann syndrome, cytomegaly usually affects most of the cells of the fetal cortex and both adrenal glands are typically hyperplastic.[11,37,48] Characteristic features of Beckwith-Wiedemann syndrome include macroglossia, prenatal and postnatal overgrowth (gigantism/hemihypertrophy), abdominal wall defects (exomphalos), and pancreatic islet cell hyperplasia leading to hypoglycemia (Table 3-1).

The adrenal glands in Beckwith-Wiedemann syndrome are enlarged and the combined weight of both glands may be as high as 16 g. Because of the cortical hyperplasia the external aspects of the glands appear cerebriform as a result of the presence redundant folds and nodules.[11] Microscopic sections demonstrate collections of cells similar to those seen in isolated adrenal cytomegaly, but they are present in greater numbers. The enlarged cells may raise a concern for an infectious etiology, such as cytomegalovirus (CMV) infection, but the cells lack the characteristic eosinophilic nuclear inclusions, perinuclear halos, and granular cytoplasmic inclusions.

Hemorrhagic adrenal cortical macrocysts may also be found.[49,50] Patients with Beckwith-Wiedemann syndrome

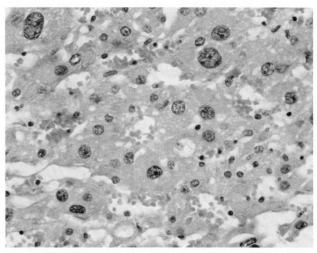

FIGURE 3-6 ■ Focal cytomegaly of cells of the fetal cortex from a newborn.

are predisposed to the development of a variety of malignant tumors including Wilms tumor, adrenal cortical carcinoma, neuroblastoma (NB), hepatoblastoma, and pancreaticoblastoma. However, the hyperplastic cortical cells in this syndrome do not represent a preneoplastic lesion.[43,50] Adrenal cortical adenomas and ganglioneuromas have also been reported in affected patients.[49] Autosomal dominant inheritance is well established in Beckwith-Wiedemann syndrome, but approximately 85% of cases are actually sporadic. The molecular basis of this syndrome is complex and involves downregulation of imprinted genes within the chromosome 11p15 region (Table 3-2). Other syndromes that predispose to adrenal tumors are discussed in subsequent sections.

Metabolic Disorders

Storage Diseases

Adrenoleukodystrophy (Addison-Schilder disease; OMIM 300100) is a rare, X-linked recessive disorder characterized by progressive demyelination of the central and peripheral nervous system and by adrenal cortical insufficiency.[51,52] In the classic form, the disorder is characterized by early behavioral manifestations including inattention, hyperactivity, and emotional lability becoming apparent through school difficulties. Subsequently there are visual symptoms, auditory processing difficulties, and motor incoordination. Once the neurologic manifestations appear, progression of the illness

Table 3-2 ■ SYNDROMES ASSOCIATED WITH ADRENAL TUMORS

Syndrome	Gene	Chromosome Locus	Adrenal Tumor	Extra-Adrenal Features
Beckwith-Wiedemann (OMIM: 130650)	CDKN1/NSD1, KCNQ1, KCNQ1OT1 (domain 2); IGF2 and H19 (domain 1)	11p15.5	Cortical carcinoma, cortical adenoma, neuroblastoma, ganglioneuroma	Exomphalos, macroglossia, pancreatic islet cell hyperplasia, gigantism/hemihypertrophy, Wilms tumor, hepatoblastoma, pancreaticoblastoma
Li-Fraumeni syndrome (OMIM:151623)	TP53	17p13.1	Cortical carcinoma	Other neoplasms/cancers
Carney complex (OMIM:160980)	PRKAR1A	17q23-q24	PPNAD	Lentigines and other pigmented skin lesions, myxomas, LCCST of testis, pituitary adenoma.
MEN 1 (Wermer syndrome) (OMIM:131100)	MEN1	11q13	Cortical adenoma	Endocrine lesions of parathyroid, pituitary, pancreas, GI tract lesions, skin lesions
MEN 2A (Sipple syndrome) (OMIM:171400)	RET (exon 10, 11)	10q11.2	Pheochromocytoma	MTC, primary hyperparathyroidism (hyperplasia)
MEN 2B (OMIM:162300)	RET (exon 16)	10q11.2	Pheochromocytoma	MTC, mucosal neuromas, ganglioneuromatosis of intestine, marfanoid habitus, corneal nerve lesions
von Hippel-Lindau disease (OMIM:193300)	VHL	3p26-p35	Pheochromocytoma	Retinal and cranial hemangioblastoma, RCC, cysts of multiple, organs, pancreatic endocrine tumors, ELST of ear
Familial pheochromocytoma-paraganglioma (OMIM:115310)	SDHD, SDHC, SDHB	1p36.1-p35	Pheochromocytoma	Paraganglioma of abdomen, thorax, head, and neck
Neurofibromatosis type 1 (OMIM:162200)	NF1	17q11.2	Pheochromocytoma	Café au lait macules, neurofibromas or plexiform neurofibroma, optic glioma, axillary or inguinal freckling, Lisch nodules, osseous lesions

ELST, endolymphatic sac tumor; GI, gastrointestinal; LCCST, large cell calcifying Sertoli cell tumor; MEN, multiple endocrine neoplasia; MTC, medullary thyroid carcinoma; PPNAD, primary pigmented nodular adrenocortical disease.

is tragically rapid and the child is often in a vegetative state within 1 to 2 years. According to Moser et al.[53] there are seven phenotypes that include the childhood cerebral form, adrenomyeloneuropathy, adult cerebral, adolescent, adrenal insufficiency without neurologic disease, asymptomatic, and heterozygotes. Clinical manifestations can, therefore, vary widely even within the same family.

The disorder is caused by mutations of the gene on chromosome Xq28 encoding an ATP-binding transporter ALDP—adrenoleukodystrophy protein that is localized in the peroxisomal membrane. The mutations result in the defective oxidation of very long fatty acids[54] and the diagnosis can be established by the presence of hexacosanoate and other long-chain fatty acids in cultured skin fibroblasts.[55]

The adrenal glands in this disorder are grossly atrophic with weights ranging from 1 to 2 g or less, with ballooning and striation of the cells of the inner zona fasciculata and zona reticularis. Groups of ballooned cells form nodules that may undergo degenerative changes with the formation of large cortical vacuoles. The medulla is usually normal. Ultrastructurally, there is proliferation of smooth endoplasmic reticulum and the presence of lamellar inclusions with a trilaminar structure.[51] An adult variant with an onset in the second or third decades is known as adrenomyeloneuropathy, a condition that can be associated with unexplained adrenal insufficiency in the absence of neurologic manifestations at first clinical presentation.[56] Cortical cells typically appear ballooned and contain linear lamellar inclusions.[55,56] A third form of the disease has been reported in women who are carriers of the abnormal gene.

The presence of primary adrenal insufficiency and atrophic adrenal glands may raise the possibility of autoimmune adrenalitis. However, in autoimmune adrenalitis the adrenal glands have a chronic inflammatory infiltrate (see section on "Primary Hypofunction") and the degenerative changes in the cortical cells described above are lacking. Additionally, correlation with the clinical presentation and autoimmune serology will assist in making the distinction.

Wolman disease (primary familial xanthomatosis) is a rare lipid storage disorder caused by an autosomal recessive deficiency of lysosomal acid lipase.[57] The disease is characterized by the accumulation of triglycerides and cholesterol esters in a variety of tissues including the liver, spleen, and adrenal glands. Most of the affected individuals die by the age of 6 months. Typically, the adrenal glands are markedly enlarged even though they often retain their normal configurations. The glands often demonstrate multiple foci of calcification in association with necrosis and fibrosis, and vacuolated zona reticularis cells.[57] Other storage diseases (e.g., Niemann-Pick disease) may also result in adrenal enlargement and hypofunction.

Congenital Adrenal Hyperplasia (Congenital Adrenogenital Syndrome)

Congenital adrenal hyperplasia encompasses a spectrum of abnormalities that result from autosomal recessive enzymatic defects in adrenal steroid biosynthesis.[58]

This group of disorders is caused by deficient activity of one of the following enzymes: 21-hydroxylase (P-450$_{c21}$), 11β-hydroxylase (P-450$_{c11}$), 3β-hydroxysteroid dehydrogenase, 17-hydroxylase/17,20-lyase (P-450$_{c17}$), and 20,22 desmolase (P-450$_{scc}$). Approximately 95% of cases of congenital adrenal hyperplasia are due to 21-hydroxylase deficiency (OMIM +201910) in which there are four clinically recognized forms: salt wasting (approximately 65%), simple virilizing (approximately 30%), nonclassic (also referred to as attenuated or acquired), and cryptic.[59] The worldwide incidence of classic 21-hydroxylase deficiency is 1 in 14,500 births, with a heterozygote frequency of approximately 1 in 60. Affected children have evidence of glucocorticoid deficiency, aldosterone deficiency with salt wasting, and excess adrenal androgen production resulting in virilization. Excess adrenal androgen production is a consequence of the accumulation of 17-hydroxypregnenolone, which is subsequently metabolized to androgenic steroids. Nonclassic (cryptic) 21-hydroxylase deficiency has a frequency of 1 in 100 in certain parts of the United States and is one of the most common autosomal recessive disorders. Affected individuals have mild degrees of cortisol deficiency, normal aldosterone production, and excess production of adrenal androgens. This form of 21-hydroxylase deficiency is most often diagnosed in childhood or early adulthood. A small proportion of individuals with 21-hydroxylase deficiency may have no apparent symptoms.

Masculinization of females in utero usually occurs while males generally appear normal at birth. Postnatally, untreated males as well as females may manifest rapid growth, penile or clitoral enlargement, precocious adrenarche, and early epiphyseal closure with resultant short stature. A mild form of late-onset adrenal hyperplasia due to 21-hydroxylase deficiency can occur in adults and is characterized by hirsutism as the only manifestation in the most attenuated form. The detailed biochemical, genetic, and molecular features of these disorders are discussed elsewhere.[58–62] Prenatal screening of amniotic fluid and neonatal screening by blood spot for elevated upstream hormones is available. Confirmation by testing for mutation of the underling *CYP21* gene is then performed.[59]

Deficiency of 11β-hydroxylase (P-450$_{c11}$; OMIM #202010) accounts for approximately 5% of all cases of congenital adrenal hyperplasia and is associated with increased production of androgens and deoxycorticosterone.[60–62] As a result, affected patients typically exhibit signs of hyperandrogenism and hypertension. Deficiency of 17α-hydroxylase (OMIM #202110) is responsible for approximately 1% of cases. External genitalia are female in both sexes. Increased levels of deoxycorticosterone are responsible for the hypertension seen in these patients. In 3β-hydroxysteroid dehydrogenase deficiency (OMIM #201810), there is deficiency of all steroid hormones including androstenedione. As a result virilization is less developed, but salt loss is a prominent feature. The adrenal glands are similar to those of the normal fetus.[63]

Adrenal hyperplasia in the congenital adrenogenital syndromes result from inadequate production of glucocorticoids, leading to stimulation of the cortex by increased pituitary ACTH production. The adrenal glands become markedly enlarged (up to 15 g) with a characteristic cerebriform appearance and a tan-brown color due to lipid depletion of cortical cells.[43] This contrasts with ACTH pituitary–dependent adrenocortical hyperplasia in which there is an outer yellow and inner tan-brown appearance as a result of hyperplasia of the fasciculata (see Hyperfunctional States). In paraneoplastic ACTH-dependent adrenocortical hyperplasia, the adrenal glands are usually larger than those seen in congenital adrenal hyperplasia, but they typically appear tan-brown as well because of lipid depletion. In patients with 20,22-desmolase (P-450$_{scc}$) deficiency, also referred to congenital lipoid hyperplasia, the adrenal glands are pale yellow or white and are characterized on microscopic examination by vacuolated cells, occasionally with formation of cholesterol clefts and an accompanying giant-cell reaction. These disorders are usually treated by replacement of the deficient steroid hormone and surgical correction of ambiguous genitalia or hypospadias.

Rarely, adrenal cortical adenomas and carcinomas may develop, in the setting of congenital adrenal hyperplasia.[64,65] Testicular tumors can also arise in affected patients. The testicular lesions are not autonomous neoplasms, since they are dependent on the presence of elevated levels of ACTH for their maintenance.[66] They are commonly bilateral and are most typically located in the hilar regions of the testes. The cell of origin is unknown, but the component cells of these lesions contain abundant amounts of eosinophilic cytoplasm, which lack crystalloids of Reinke. In the series reported by Rutgers et al.,[66] the diagnosis of congenital adrenal hyperplasia was made only after the appearance of testicular tumors in 18% of the cases.

Hypofunctional States

Primary Hypofunction

Autoimmune Adrenalitis

Autoimmune adrenalitis is responsible for approximately 75% of cases of the inflammatory conditions affecting the adrenal glands in North America and Western Europe, followed by infection and a variety of other conditions (Box 3-1). In idiopathic (autoimmune) Addison disease (chronic adrenocortical insufficiency), the glands are markedly atrophic and the residual cortical tissue is infiltrated by lymphocytes and plasma cells. The presence of a few aggregates of lymphocytes in the adrenal cortex should not be considered evidence of adrenalitis. All layers of the cortex are involved in autoimmune adrenalitis, but the medulla is unaffected. Typically, the capsules of the glands are fibrotic. Both humoral and cell-mediated immune mechanisms have been implicated in the development of autoimmune adrenal hypofunction. Autoantibodies to cortical cells are present in 50% of all patients and in more than 70% of women with newly diagnosed disease. The major targets for autoantibody

---

Box 3-1 ● HYPOFUNCTION AND HYPERFUNCTION OF THE ADRENAL GLAND

Primary Adrenal Insufficiency
Congenital adrenal hypoplasia
Autoimmune adrenalitis
Polyglandular autoimmune syndrome
Infections
    Bacterial
    Fungal
    Viral (CMV, HIV, HSV)
Drugs
Radiation
Metabolic (adrenoleukodystrophy, amyloidosis, Wolman disease)
Neoplastic (metastatic tumor)
Miscellaneous (Adrenal hemorrhage and necrosis, adrenal cysts)

Secondary and Tertiary Adrenal Insufficiency
Pituitary or hypothalamic dysfunction

Primary Hyperfunction (glucocorticoid, mineralocorticoid or sex hormone overproduction)
Primary hyperplasia
Macronodular hyperplasia
Primary pigmented adrenocortical disease
Tumors (adenoma, carcinoma)

Secondary Hyperfunction
Cushing disease (pituitary tumor; primarily hypercortisolism)
Ectopic ACTH syndrome (primarily hypercortisolism)
Ectopic CRH syndrome (primarily hypercortisolism)
Renal artery stenosis (hyperaldosteronism)
Juxtaglomerular cell tumor (hyperaldosteronism)

---

reactivity are the adrenal cytochrome P-450 enzymes.[67] Affected patients can also have antibodies to gonadal, gastric parietal, and thyroid follicular cells.

Adrenocortical hypofunction may be associated with hypofunction of other endocrine glands.[68] The type I polyglandular autoimmune syndrome is associated with mucocutaneous candidiasis, alopecia, hypoparathyroidism, adrenal insufficiency, autoimmune thyroiditis, and diabetes mellitus. This form of the disease has also been termed autoimmune polyendocrinopathy–candidiasis–ectodermal dystrophy (APECED). Mutations in the *APECED* or autoimmune regulatory gene (*21q22.3*) have been implicated in the development of this syndrome.[69,70] The type II polyglandular autoimmune syndrome is characterized by adrenal insufficiency, autoimmune thyroiditis, and insulin-dependent diabetes mellitus. The type I syndrome is inherited as an autosomal recessive trait, while the pattern of inheritance of the type II syndrome is usually dominant.

Infectious Disorders

Infectious disorders including tuberculosis and fungal diseases (histoplasmosis, North and South American blastomycosis, coccidiomycosis, cryptococcosis) can affect both the cortical and medullary regions of the adrenal glands. Although tuberculosis is now a rare cause of adrenal insufficiency in the United States and Western Europe, it is a common cause in parts of the world where tuberculosis is endemic. In contrast to the shrunken appearance of the adrenal glands in idiopathic Addison disease, the glands in mycobacterial infection are typically enlarged and necrotic. Infection with *Mycobacterium avium intracellulare* is typically associated with the presence of confluent masses of histiocytes containing acid-fast organisms.

CMV has been identified in the adrenal glands of a large proportion of patients dying of the acquired immunodeficiency syndrome.[71] Adrenal cortical necrosis associated with CMV infection can be severe enough to result in acute adrenal insufficiency in some instances. Both herpes simplex and varicella zoster may also involve the adrenal glands and may lead to adrenal cortical insufficiency when they are associated with extensive cortical necrosis.

Amyloidosis

Rarely, amyloid deposition can result in cortical hypofunction.[72] Typically, adrenal involvement is associated with extensive systemic amyloid disease of the AA type. The adrenal glands may have a normal shape and size or may be enlarged. In severe cases, the glands are pale tan to yellow. Amyloid deposits typically affect the fasciculata and reticularis zones and are present between the cortical cells and capillary endothelium. The cortical cells ultimately become atrophic as a result of the progressive deposition of intercellular amyloid. In patients with AL disease, the amyloid deposits are usually vascular in distribution.

Adrenal Hemorrhage

Adrenal hemorrhage may develop in a segmental fashion or may involve the entire adrenal (Fig. 3-7).[73] This syndrome may be seen in association with sepsis and shock due to meningococcal infection or infection with other bacteria, including *Haemophilus influenzae*, *Streptococcus pneumoniae*, and *Pseudomonas aeruginosa* (Waterhouse-Friderichsen syndrome). Typically, the glands are enlarged and hemorrhagic, with necrosis of both cortical and medullary tissue. Adrenal

hemorrhage in the Waterhouse-Friderichsen syndrome is regarded as the consequence rather than the cause of shock. Anticoagulant therapy has also been associated with adrenal hemorrhage. Corticomedullary necrosis of milder degrees can occur in association with hypotension and shock.[74] In patients with segmental lesions, examination of the capsular vessels and sinusoids often reveals evidence of thrombus formation. Affected cortical areas show a pattern of ischemic necrosis that ultimately heals by the process of fibrosis.

Miscellaneous Causes of Hypofunction

Adrenal hypofunction may result from bilateral involvement by tumor, most commonly metastatic carcinoma. Typically, clinically apparent hypofunction occurs when more than 95% of the glands are replaced by tumor. A rare case of hypofunction has been reported secondary to involvement by Erdheim-Chester disease, a non-Langerhans histiocytosis that typically involves bone, but in which extraskeletal manifestations are present in up to 50% of cases. In this condition, there is diffuse enlargement of the adrenal gland secondary to infiltration by foamy histiocytes.[75]

In patients with acquired immune deficiency syndrome (AIDS), involvement of the adrenals by opportunistic infections or neoplasms such as Kaposi sarcoma can lead to significant glucocorticoid insufficiency. However, most AIDS patients also have decreased adrenal reserves characterized by a defect in the production of 17-deoxycorticosteroid by the zona fasciculata. This is associated with morphologic changes of lipid depletion as described earlier in stress-related changes of the adrenal gland. Also, peripheral resistance to glucocorticoids related to decreased affinity for type II glucocorticoid receptors has been reported in a subset of patients with AIDS.[17]

Drugs such as 12-methylbenzathracene and hexadimethane can cause direct necrosis of the cortex. Ketoconazole, etomidate, cyanoketone, and trilostane have inhibitory effects on adrenal steroidogenesis while rifampicin and dilantin can lead to increased breakdown of glucocorticoids.[17]

Patients with increased iron stores can have excess deposition of iron in the adrenal cortex, particularly the zona glomerulosa. High-dose radiation to the abdomen, pelvis, or lumbar regions for treatment of malignancies can lead to fibrosis of the adrenal glands. While the adrenal cortex is relatively resistant to radiation compared to other endocrine organs, fibrosis of the inner cortex, particularly the zone reticularis along with reduction in the zona fasciculata, can occur.[17]

Secondary Hypofunction

Adrenocortical atrophy may be found in association with lesions primarily affecting the pituitary or hypothalamus, leading to diminished secretion of ACTH.[6] The administration of exogenous corticosteroids will produce similar changes as a result of suppression of endogenous ACTH. The adrenal glands in secondary hypofunctional states are considerably smaller than normal, although the overall

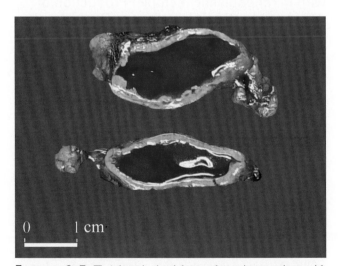

FIGURE 3-7 ■ Adrenal gland hemorrhage in a patient with cholangiocarcinoma. There was no evidence of metastatic disease.

configurations of the glands are retained. Typically, the cortex is bright yellow owing to lipid accumulation in the cortical cells, the capsule is fibrotic, and the medulla is unaffected. The zona glomerulosa is usually of normal thickness in these cases.

Hyperfunctional States

Adrenocortical Hyperplasia

Hyperplasia of the adrenal cortex, which represents an increased cortical mass resulting from stimulation of the cortex by ACTH derived from the pituitary gland or from a variety of extrapituitary sources, can be associated with a wide variety of clinical syndromes. Cortical hyperplasia can also selectively involve the zona glomerulosa in patients with idiopathic hyperaldosteronism.

Pituitary/Hypothalamic-based Hyperplasia (Cushing Disease)

Hyperplasia may be the result of stimulation of the adrenal glands by ACTH-producing pituitary adenomas or of hypothalamic stimulation of the pituitary ACTH cells by CRH.[76,77] Basophilic pituitary adenomas were originally described in association with hypercortisolism by Harvey Cushing in 1932, and this association has been termed Cushing disease or ACTH-dependent Cushing syndrome. Immunohistochemical studies have shown that ACTH-producing pituitary adenomas are considerably more common than had been recognized on light microscopy alone, and many of them have been classified as microadenomas measuring considerably <1 cm.

Adrenocortical hyperplasia in patients with ACTH-dependent Cushing syndrome can be either diffuse or nodular and combinations of diffuse and nodular hyperplasia are common. In diffuse hyperplasia, gland weights may be increased minimally.[6] In more advanced cases, the combined average weight is considerably in excess of normal with combined weights of >25 g. The glands have rounded contours rather than the sharp outlines typical of normal glands. The inner portion of the cortex is widened and often appears pale brown or tan. The outer layers of the cortex are typically yellow. On microscopy, the inner brown zone corresponds to lipid-depleted cells of the fasciculata, whereas the cells of the outer cortex are more characteristically vacuolated.[78] The glomerulosa in adults with Cushing disease is often difficult to identify, but in children the glomerulosa may also appear slightly hyperplastic.[79]

In some cases, the cortex may appear nodular with individual nodules measuring <0.5 or 1.0 cm in diameter, depending on varying criteria used by different authors.[43] This type of change is classified as "diffuse and micronodular hyperplasia." If the nodules exceed 1 cm in diameter, the hyperplasia is defined as "diffuse and macronodular type."

In diffuse and nodular (micro- or macro-)hyperplasia, multiple cortical nodules are present in association with a

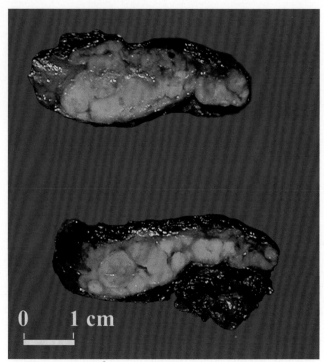

FIGURE 3-8 ■ Diffuse and nodular adrenocortical hyperplasia. Adrenal gland from a patient with pituitary-dependent Cushing syndrome (Courtesy Dr. A. Mc Nicol, Glasgow, Scotland, UK.).

diffusely hyperplastic cortex (Figs. 3-8 and 3-9). Formation of nodules is often asymmetric. While one adrenal gland may show diffuse and nodular cortical hyperplasia, the contralateral adrenal gland may appear diffusely hyperplastic. Most often, the nodules are composed of admixtures of clear- and compact-type cells. In contrast to the atrophic cortex adjacent to a functioning adenoma, the cortex between or adjacent to the nodules in nodular hyperplasia is diffusely hyperplastic.

Adrenocortical Hyperplasia Associated with Paraneoplastic (Ectopic) Production of Adrenocorticotropic Hormone or Corticotropin-releasing Hormone

Hyperplasia can be found in association with a variety of neoplasms producing ACTH, CRH, or both ACTH and CRH.[77,80,81] In most series, bronchial carcinoids and small-cell carcinomas are responsible for the paraneoplastic production of these hormones. Other tumors associated with the paraneoplastic ACTH syndrome include pancreatic endocrine neoplasms, medullary thyroid carcinoma, thymic carcinoids, and pheochromocytomas. In patients with the paraneoplastic ACTH syndrome, the adrenals are usually larger (average combined weight of 20 to 30 g) than those seen in association with hyperplasia stemming from pituitary ACTH overproduction. The cortex is diffusely hyperplastic and appears tan-brown throughout its width. On microscopy, there is evidence of diffuse hyperplasia of the fasciculata cells, which are characterized by

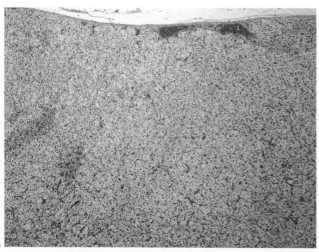
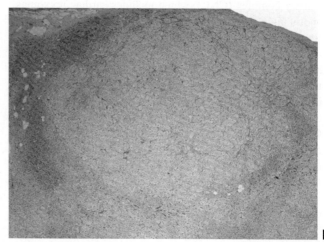

FIGURE 3-9 ■ Diffuse and nodular adrenocortical hyperplasia. Histologic section of diffuse **(A)** and nodular hyperplasia **(B)** from a patient with Cushing syndrome. There is predominantly hyperplasia of the vacuolated fasciculata.

a compact or lipid-depleted appearance.[82] Foci of nuclear enlargement and hyperchromasia of reticularis cells may be noted, and these features may be particularly striking adjacent to metastatic foci in the glands.[23] Both bronchial carcinoids and small-cell bronchogenic carcinomas may also produce CRH.

Macronodular Hyperplasia (Massive Macronodular Adrenocortical Disease)

In macronodular hyperplasia with marked adrenal enlargement, the adrenal glands may together weigh up to 180 g, and individual nodules may measure up to 4.0 cm in diameter.[37,83,84] Nodules are composed of clear cells, compact cells, or admixtures of these cell types. Macronodular hyperplasia is ACTH-independent, and this entity can involve a single gland in some instances.[85] The cortex between the nodules is often atrophic, as might be expected in an ACTH-independent process. This entity, which has also been referred to as massive macronodular adrenocortical disease, has a bimodal age distribution. A small proportion of patients may present during the 1st year of life with association with the McCune-Albright syndrome. Most of the patients present clinically in the fifth decade with a male to female ratio of 1:1. Rare examples of familial massive macronodular adrenocortical disease have also been reported. This disorder has been associated with aberrant (ectopic) expression and regulation of various G-protein-coupled receptors.[86] These lesions are treated by bilateral adrenalectomy.[17]

Primary Pigmented Nodular Adrenocortical Disease—Microadenomatous Hyperplasia of the Adrenal Gland

Primary pigmented nodular adrenocortical disease (PPNAD) is a rare disorder, which is seen in association with ACTH-independent Cushing syndrome and treated by bilateral adrenalectomy. Morphologically, PPNAD is characterized

by the presence of multiple pigmented nodules of cortical cells with intervening atrophic cortical tissue.[87–90] The glands may be either smaller than normal or enlarged (range 0.9 to 13.4 g).[17] Individual nodules, which can vary in color from gray to black, typically measure from 1 to 3 mm in diameter, although larger nodules measuring up to 3 cm in diameter may also be evident.[43] The nodules are composed of large, granular eosinophilic cells that often contain hyperchromatic nuclei with prominent nucleoli (Fig. 3-10). Because of the atypical nuclear features, this entity had been referred to previously as micronodular dysplasia. The black color is due to the presence of lipochrome pigment. The presence of pigmented nodules might raise the possibility of metastatic melanoma, but this will be readily excluded on careful examination and review of the clinical data.

Primary pigmented adrenal cortical disease may occur sporadically or in a familial form that can be associated with

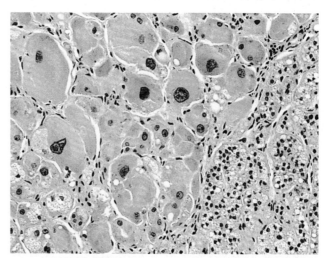

FIGURE 3-10 ■ Primary pigmented nodular adrenocortical disease (PPNAD). The nodule is composed of large cells with hyperchromatic nuclei. In this photomicrograph pigment is absent.

Carney complex (CNC), which includes cardiac myxomas, spotty pigmentation, neurofibromatosis, testicular Leydig or Sertoli cell tumors, mammary myxoid fibroadenomas, and cerebral hemangiomas.[89,91] The Carney complex may occur sporadically or may be inherited as an autosomal dominant trait. The gene encoding the protein kinase A type Iα regulatory subunit PRKAR1A has been mapped to 17q22-q24 and loss of heterozygosity (LOH) studies from patients with CNC have revealed mutations in this gene in approximately 50% of affected individuals. No mutations have been found on 2p16. Studies of sporadic and isolated cases of (CNC) have also revealed inactivating mutations of *PRKAR1A*. The wild-type alleles could be inactivated by somatic mutations consistent with the hypothesis that the gene belongs to the tumor suppressor class.[92,93] Some studies have suggested that PPNAD may have an autoimmune etiology.[94]

Howath et al. reported mutations in the gene encoding phosphodiesterase 11A4 (*PDE11A4*) in cases of PPNAD and other forms of micronodular adrenocortical hyperplasia. LOH and other analyses showed susceptible genes at the 2q31-2q25 locus.[95] *PDE*s regulate cyclic nucleotide levels. The same group subsequently reported that missense mutations of *PDE11A* were frequently present in patients from the general population with adrenal cortical hyperplasia and adenoma, resulting in speculation that *PDE11A* genetic defects may be associated with adrenal pathology in a wider clinical spectrum.[96]

Adrenocortical Hyperplasia Associated with Hyperaldosteronism

Primary hyperaldosteronism is characterized by the excessive secretion of aldosterone from the adrenal glands and is associated with suppression of plasma renin activity with resultant hypokalemia and hypertension. At least six subtypes of primary hyperaldosteronism have been recognized, including aldosterone-producing adenoma, idiopathic hyperaldosteronism, primary adrenal hyperplasia, aldosterone-producing adrenal cortical carcinoma, aldosterone-producing ovarian tumor, and familial hyperaldosteronism (FH).[97] FH is subdivided into two groups: FH-I (glucocorticoid-remediable hyperaldosteronism) and FH-II (aldosterone-producing adenoma and idiopathic hyperaldosteronism).

In approximately 40% of cases of primary hyperaldosteronism, the only apparent adrenal abnormality is hyperplasia of the zona glomerulosa with or without the formation of micronodules.[9,43,98,99] Generally, biochemical abnormalities in patients with hyperplasia are less severe than in those with adenomas. On histologic examination, hyperplasia of the glomerulosa is characterized by thickening of this cell layer, with extensions of the glomerulosa extending toward the fasciculata (Fig. 3-11). Micronodules, when present, are usually composed of clear fasciculata-type cells[9,23] and are thought to be a consequence of the associated hypertension. In about 10% of cases, it may not be possible to distinguish a micronodule from a true adenoma associated with aldosterone production.

ADRENAL NEOPLASMS

A host of syndromes predispose to adrenocortical or adrenomedullary tumors. In addition to the previously discussed (CNC) and Beckwith-Wiedemann syndrome, other disorders associated with adrenal tumors include Li-Fraumeni syndrome, multiple endocrine neoplasia (MEN) types 1, 2A, and 2B, familial pheochromocytoma–paraganglioma, neurofibromatosis type 1, and von Hippel-Lindau disease (Table 3-2). Unlike Beckwith-Wiedemann syndrome, which predisposes to both cortical and medullary tumors, the other syndromes give rise to either cortical or medullary tumors. While Beckwith-Wiedemann syndrome presents early in infancy and childhood, the manifestations of the other syndromes usually occur later in life; however, features of MEN2B, which include oral, ocular, and gastrointestinal ganglioneuromatosis associated with a Marfanoid habitus, may present at birth.

Adrenal medullary hyperplasia, although viewed as a nonneoplastic lesion, is seen in patients with inherited syndromes that predispose to the development of pheochromocytoma. This change has been reported in association with MEN2A and 2B and von Hippel-Lindau disease, but rare examples have been reported without an apparent associated familial syndrome. This topic is further discussed in "Pheochromocytoma."

ADRENOCORTICAL NEOPLASMS

Adrenocortical Adenomas

Adrenocortical adenomas represent a heterogeneous group of benign neoplasms that can differentiate toward any of the cortical layers.[43,100] Most adenomas are nonfunctional. In order of decreasing frequency, functional adenomas can be associated with the production of mineralocorticoids (Conn syndrome), glucocorticoids (Cushing syndrome), or sex steroids (adrenogenital syndrome). Mixed syndromes can also occur.

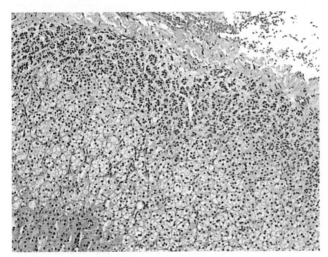

FIGURE 3-11 ■ Hyperplasia of the zona glomerulosa in a patient with primary hyperaldosteronism.

Nonfunctional Adrenocortical Adenomas and Cortical Nodules

Epidemiology and Etiopathogenesis

The classification of nonfunctional cortical nodes is controversial. While some studies refer to them as cortical adenomas, others classify them as hyperplastic nodules. In this chapter, the terms "nonfunctional adenoma" and "hyperplastic nodule" will be used interchangeably.

Adrenocortical nodules occur commonly in patients without clinical or biochemical evidence of steroid hormone hypersecretion,[43] and they are detected frequently by abdominal imaging techniques. A significant proportion of these lesions occur as "incidentalomas." Autopsy studies have revealed cortical nodules in approximately 25% of individuals without evidence of biochemical abnormalities. They occur frequently in the adrenals of elderly individuals and in patients with essential hypertension or diabetes mellitus. Most nodules represent foci of compensatory cortical hyperplasia that have developed in response to focal atrophy of the cortex induced by narrowing of adrenal capsular arterioles.[101] Nonfunctional cortical nodules may be particularly prominent in patients with aldosterone-secreting adenomas, presumably as a result of the associated hypertension.

Gross Pathology

Although cortical nodules are commonly multicentric and bilateral, dominant nodules measuring up to 2 to 3 cm in diameter or larger may be present. The smaller nodules are often nonencapsulated, whereas the larger single nodules may be surrounded by a fibrous pseudocapsule. The nodules are generally bright yellow with foci of brownish discoloration (Fig. 3-12A). Those arising in the zona reticularis are more homogeneously brown or black.

Microscopic Features

Adenomas have pushing borders with a pseudocapsule derived from compression of the adjacent cortex or expansion of the adrenal capsule.[11] They can be composed of small nests,

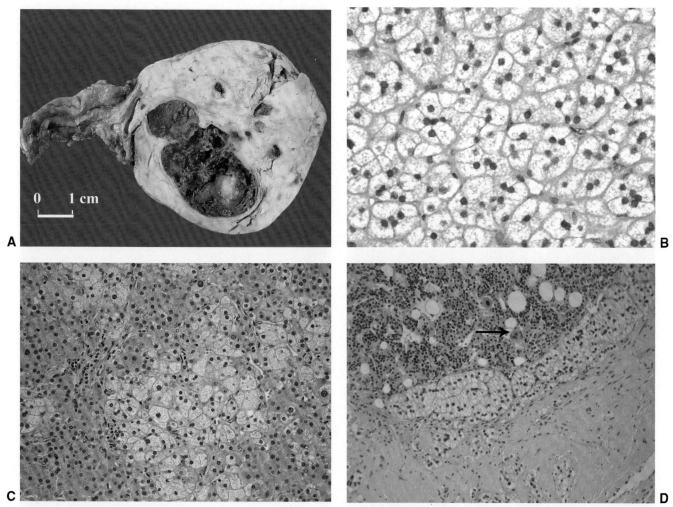

FIGURE 3-12 ■ Nonfunctional adrenocortical adenoma. The cut surface is *bright yellow* with central hemorrhage and fibrosis **(A)** (Courtesy of Dr. A. Matoso, Providence, RI). The tumor is composed predominantly of clear cells that resemble normal cells of the fasciculata **(B)**, but compact cells are also present **(C)**. Myelolipomatous change was present in a section from the central hemorrhagic area **(D,** *arrow* megakaryocyte).

cords, or alveolar arrangements of vacuolated (clear) cells that most closely resemble those of the normal fasciculata (Fig. 3-12B). Variable numbers of compact-type cells are also present (Fig. 3-12C). Black adenomas are composed exclusively of lipochrome-rich compact cells.[6] The nuclear/cytoplasmic ratio is generally low, although a few single cells and small groups of cells may have enlarged and hyperchromatic nuclei. Typically, the nuclei are vesicular with small, distinct nucleoli and little or no mitotic activity. In fine-needle aspiration biopsy specimens, the cells are round to polyhedral with round nuclei and foamy cytoplasm. Numerous naked nuclei in a background of granular to foamy material may be prominent.

Foci of myelolipomatous change, calcification, or ossification may be evident within the nodules, particularly the larger ones (Fig. 3-12D). In contrast to functional adenomas associated with glucocorticoid production, the cortex adjacent to nonfunctional nodules is of normal thickness.

Adenomas Producing Cushing Syndrome

Epidemiology and Etiopathogenesis

Functional adenomas associated with Cushing syndrome occur more commonly in females than in males and are typically unilateral and unicentric. X-chromosome inactivation analyses have shown that some adenomas are clonal while others are polyclonal. Monoclonal adenomas are larger than polyclonal lesions and have a higher prevalence of nuclear pleomorphism.[102] This heterogeneity may reflect different pathogenetic mechanisms or different stages of a common multistep process.

Gross Pathology

The tumors are typically unilateral and present as sharply circumscribed masses that usually weigh <50 g and measure 3 to 3.5 cm in average diameter. Larger tumors should be examined with particular care to rule out malignancy.[9,23,37] On cross section, adenomas vary from yellow to brown, and occasional examples of heavily pigmented (black) adenomas associated with Cushing syndrome have been reported (Fig. 3-13A). Necrosis is rare, but cystic change is relatively common, particularly in larger tumors.

Microscopic Features

The microscopic features are similar to those of nonfunctional adenomas.[11] Adenomas are most often composed of small nests, cords, or alveolar arrangements of vacuolated (clear) cells that resemble those of the normal fasciculata. Generally, adenoma cells are somewhat larger than normal cortical cells. Variable numbers of lipochrome-rich compact-type cells are also evident[6] and predominate in cases of black adenomas (Fig. 3-13B). Foci of spindle-cell growth may be present in some cases, and some adenomas may exhibit considerable fibrosis or myxoid change. The nuclear/cytoplasmic ratio is generally low, although a few single cells and small groups of cells may have enlarged hyperchromatic nuclei. Typically, the nuclei are vesicular with small, distinct nucleoli. Mitotic activity is rare. In fine needle aspiration biopsy specimens, the cells are round to polyhedral with round nuclei and foamy cytoplasm. Numerous naked nuclei in a background of granular to foamy material may

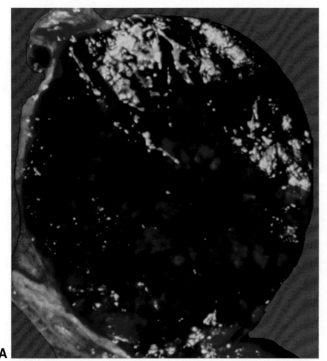
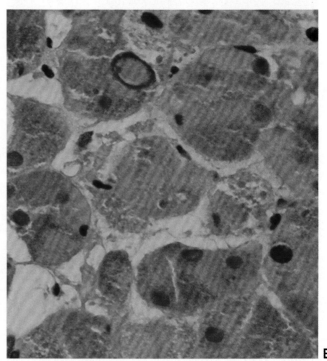

FIGURE 3-13 ■ Pigmented (*black*) adenoma associated with Cushing syndrome **(A)**. The tumor is composed predominantly of compact cells containing abundant lipochrome pigment **(B)**.

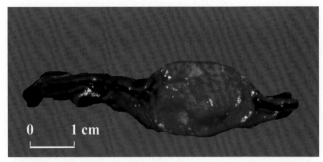

FIGURE 3-14 ■ Adrenocortical adenoma associated with Conn syndrome. This tumor has a *yellow-brown* color or *orange* cut surface rather than a *bright yellow* appearance that is more characteristic.

be prominent. Foci of myelolipomatous change or calcification may be seen, particularly in larger adenomas.[23] On ultrastructural examination, adenoma cells most closely resemble the cells of the normal fasciculata or reticularis.[6]

Adenomas Producing Conn Syndrome

Epidemiology and Clinical Features

Initial studies suggested that cortical adenomas were responsible for Conn syndrome in up to 90% of cases; however, more recent analyses indicate that adenomas are present in a considerably smaller proportion of cases. As in cases of hyperplasia of the zona glomerulosa, these patients present with symptoms and signs of hypokalemia and hypertension.

Gross Pathology

Most adenomas associated with hyperaldosteronism measure <2 cm in diameter and are round to ovoid in configuration.[103] They are usually unilateral, bright yellow in color and are demarcated from the adjacent cortex by a fibrous pseudocapsule. Occasional cases have a yellow brown or orange appearance (Fig. 3-14).

Microscopic Features

The tumor cells, which are usually arranged in small nests and cords, can resemble cells of the glomerulosa, fasciculata, or reticularis or combine the features of both glomerulosa and fasciculata cells (hybrid cells)[23,103] (Fig. 3-15A). Some of the tumors may be highly pigmented.[104] In patients treated with spironolactone, occasional cells may contain lamellar eosinophilic inclusions (spironolactone bodies) measuring up to 10 µm in diameter. They are often demarcated from the adjacent cytoplasm by a clear halo (Fig. 3-15B). Ultrastructurally, spironolactone bodies resemble myelin figures.

Although most of the tumor cells have relatively small vesicular nuclei and small but distinct nucleoli, some tumors exhibit considerable variation in nuclear size and shape. At the ultrastructural level, the mitochondria manifest tubular or vesicular cristae, although some may have lamelliform cristae typical of the zona glomerulosa. The fasciculata adjacent to aldosterone-secreting adenomas is of normal thickness. Hyperplasia of the zona glomerulosa may be present, however, in association with these tumors.[103]

Adenomas Producing Adrenogenital Syndromes

Epidemiology and Clinical Features

Benign adrenocortical tumors may be associated with syndromes of virilization or feminization, but the presence of a pure adrenogenital syndrome, particularly feminization, should suggest the possibility of malignancy. Some authors, in fact, consider all feminizing cortical neoplasms as being potentially malignant.

Gross and Microscopic Pathology

Virilizing adenomas are generally larger than those found in the context of pure Cushing syndrome, and a few adenomas associated with adrenogenital syndromes have

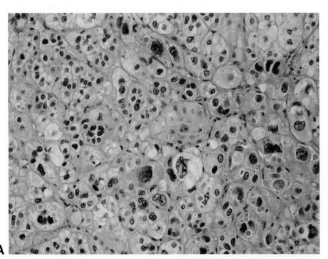 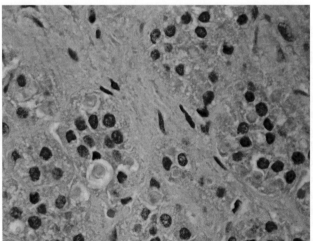

FIGURE 3-15 ■ Adrenocortical adenoma associated with Conn syndrome. The tumor is composed of an admixture of fasciculata- and glomerulosa-type cells. Cells with enlarged, hyperchromatic nuclei are evident **(A)**. Spironolactone bodies that have a typical lamellar appearance are prominent in this section **(B)**.

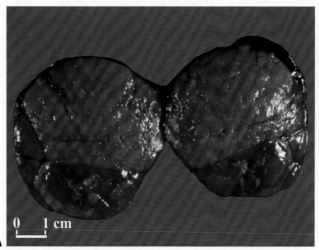
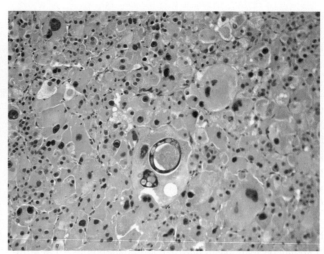

FIGURE 3-16 ■ Adrenocortical adenoma associated with virilizing syndrome. This tumor from a 2-year-old girl has a *brown* cut surface **(A)**. The neoplastic cells are eosinophilic and granular with focal nuclear enlargement and hyperchromasia **(B)**. Nuclear pseudoinclusions are also present.

weighed up to 500 g.[9,23,43] Similar to tumors associated with glucocorticoid overproduction, virilizing adenomas are sharply circumscribed or encapsulated; however, they tend to be red-brown rather than yellow on cross section[23] (Fig 3.16A). Smaller tumors have an alveolar pattern of growth, whereas larger tumors tend to have more solid or diffuse growth patterns. Although most tumor cells have a low nuclear/cytoplasmic ratio, single cells and small-cell groups may exhibit considerable nuclear enlargement and hyperchromasia. The cytoplasm is usually eosinophilic and granular (Fig. 3.16B). Rare virilizing tumors contain Reinke crystalloids and have been termed Leydig cell adenomas similar to their testicular counterparts.[105,106] On ultrastructural examination, the mitochondria are of the tubulolamellar type. Sex steroid–producing adenomas are not associated with atrophy of the adjacent cortex or the contralateral adrenal gland.

Oncocytic Adrenocortical Tumors

Epidemiology and Clinical Features

Tumors with oncocytic features develop rarely as primary adrenocortical neoplasms. While some behave as benign neoplasms (oncocytomas), others may be malignant, as discussed in the section on adrenocortical carcinomas. Most oncocytomas are nonfunctional,[107–109a] but up to a quarter of tumors may be associated with virilization[109–110] or Cushing syndrome.[109a,111] A case of a giant oncocytoma arising in retroperitoneal accessory adrenal tissue has been described.[112]

Gross and Microscopic Features

Typically, adrenal cortical oncocytomas are dark brown, similar to oncocytomas at other sites. Reported cases have ranged

in size from 8 g to over 500 g. They have abundant granular eosinophilic cytoplasm (Fig. 3-17), which corresponds to the presence of numerous mitochondria with both lamellar and tubulovesicular cristae and small, electron-dense inclusions.[113] However, smaller eosinophilic cells (small oncocytes), may be present and may be quite frequent in some cases.[109a] The nuclei are enlarged, irregularly shaped, and vesicular with coarse chromatin and prominent nucleoli. Nuclear psuedoinclusions may be seen. Mitotic activity is minimal to absent and there is no evidence of necrosis. The cells have a tendency to be arranged in diffuse sheets, but variable trabecular, alveolar, and microcystic architecture can be seen.

Bisceglia et al.[113a] suggested that oncocytic adrenocortical tumors be classified as pure when the tumor was composed of 90% oncocytic cells and mixed when the

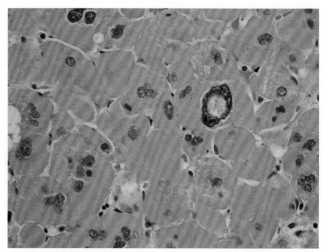

FIGURE 3-17 ■ Adrenocortical oncocytoma. The cells contain densely granular eosinophilic cytoplasm and pleomorphic nuclei with a pseudoinclusion.

tumors were composed of 50% to 90% oncocytic cells. Subsequently, Duregon et al.[113b] classified oncocytic adrenocortical tumors as being pure, mixed, having focal oncocytic features, or being conventional adrenocortical tumors when the oncocytic cells constituted >90%, 50% to 90%, 10% to 49%, and <10% of the tumor cells, respectively (Box 3-2). Because of variations in sampling with fine needle or core biopsies it is appropriate to render a diagnosis of "adrenocortical neoplasm with oncocytic features" in such samples.

Recognition of adrenocortical oncocytoma and distinction from conventional adrenocortical carcinoma is an important one since these tumors have many of the features that would fulfill criteria for malignancy in conventional adrenocortical neoplasms. Therefore, the criteria for malignancy in oncocytic adrenocortical tumors are different (Box 3-2) and are fully discussed in "Adrenocortical Carcinomas."

Although the granular cell variants of conventional RCC and chromophobe RCC tend to have eosinophilic cytoplasm, adrenocortical oncocytic neoplasms generally tend to have more voluminous cytoplasm that demonstrate diffuse strong positive granular cytoplasmic staining with the antimitochondrial antibody mES-13.[109,109a] Immunohistochemical staining with markers for adrenocortical tumors and RCC will assist in the diagnosis. Melan-A-positive staining of neoplastic cells is the most sensitive adrenocortical marker.[109,109a] As noted in a subsequent section, pheochromocytomas rarely have oncocytic cytoplasm (oncocytic pheochromocytoma), but staining with antibodies to chromogranin will assist in establishing the diagnosis of pheochromocytoma. Interestingly, like oncocytic neoplasms of other organs,

9 of 12 tumors classified by Duregon et al.[113b] as oncocytic adrenal adenomas were shown to have the 4,977-bp mitochondrial DNA "common deletion" by real-time polymerase chain reaction (PCR) and fluorescent in situ hybridization (FISH). However, this finding was not entirely specific since it was demonstrated in some normal adrenocortical cells and some examples of conventional adrenocortical adenomas.[113b]

Adrenocortical Carcinomas

Epidemiology and Etiopathogenesis

Adrenocortical carcinomas account for 0.05% to 0.2% of all malignancies and have an incidence of approximately one to two cases per million population per year. They have a bimodal age distribution with a small peak occurring in the first two decades and a larger peak in the fifth decade.[114] Adrenocortical carcinomas develop somewhat more commonly in women than in men in most large clinical series, although some studies have demonstrated a slight male predominance. They occur in approximately 1% of patients with the Li-Fraumeni syndrome, with most affected individuals harboring p53 mutations at chromosome locus 17p13. These tumors, in fact, may be the only manifestation of this disorder in childhood.[115] The frequency of cortical malignancies is also increased in patients with the Beckwith-Wiedemann syndrome (Table 3-2) and congenital adrenal hyperplasia.

Gene expression profiling studies have demonstrated that the most significantly upregulated genes in carcinomas include ubiquitin-specific protease 4 (*USP4*) and ubiquitin degradation 1-like (*UFD1L*). Additional upregulated genes include members of the insulin-like growth factor (IGF) family such as *IGF2, IGF2R, IGFBP3,* and *IGFBP6*.[116] Giordano et al. also demonstrated increased expression of IGF2 in adrenal cortical carcinomas.[117] Downregulated genes in carcinomas include the chemokine (C-X-C motif) ligand 10 (*CXCL10*), the retinoic acid receptor responder 2, the aldehyde dehydrogenase family member A1 (*ALD1f1A1*), cytochrome b reductase 1, and glutathione S-transferase A4.[117]

Similar patterns of gene expression occur in pediatric adrenal cortical tumors with a consistent marked decrease in the expression of all histocompatibility class II genes in carcinomas as compared to adenomas.[118] These results parallel the observations by Marx et al.[119] that pre- and postnatal adrenals do not express major histocompatibility complex class II antigens in contrast to adult adrenals, which express these antigens.

Clinical Features

Some patients may present with abdominal pain, and up to 30% may have a palpable abdominal mass. The tumors may be associated with Cushing syndrome or evidence of sex steroid overproduction, and mixed syndromes are more common than in patients with cortical adenomas. In exceptional circumstances, mineralocorticoid production may be

---

Box 3-2 ● ONCOCYTIC ADRENOCORTICAL TUMORS (OACTS)

Classification of OACT

Pure OACT	>90% oncocytic cells
Mixed OACT	50%–90% oncocytic cells
Focal OACT	10%–49% oncocytic cells
Conventional adrenocortical tumors	<10% oncocytic cells

Clinical Behavior

Malignant OACT	Any major criteria
Borderline OACT	One to four minor criteria
Benign OACT	Absence of major or minor criteria

Major Criteria

>5 mitoses per 50 HPFs
Atypical mitoses
Venous invasion

Minor Criteria

Size >10 cm or >200 g
Microscopic necrosis
Capsular invasion
Sinusoidal invasion

present. A significant proportion of cortical carcinomas (up to 75% in some series) may be unassociated with syndromes of hormone overproduction.[120] In some instances, patients may show signs of hypoglycemia due to the production of IGFs by the tumor or hypercalcemia due to the production of parathyroid hormone–related peptide.

Gross Pathology

Adrenocortical carcinomas generally weigh more than 100 g in adults, and most often, tumor weight is in excess of 750 g.[9,121–124] Rarely, however, tumors weighing <50 g will metastasize, while a small proportion of tumors weighing more than 1,000 g will not.[43] It should be remembered, however, that benign tumors associated with sex steroid overproduction, however, can weigh considerably more than 100 g. Tumor weight is a useful predictor of malignancy in children. Tumors weighing more than 500 g in a series of 23 cases reported by Cagle et al.[125] were malignant, whereas only a single tumor weighing <500 g pursued a malignant course.

Many cortical malignancies have a multinodular appearance with individual nodules varying from pink to yellow-tan, depending on their lipid content. Carcinomas associated with feminization or virilization tend to be red-brown, while those associated with Cushing syndrome are more often yellow-tan. Rare cases may have a myxoid appearance. Foci of necrosis,

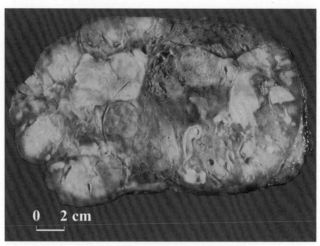

FIGURE 3-18 ■ Adrenocortical carcinoma. The cut surface of this large tumor shows prominent necrosis.

cystic change, hemorrhage, and calcification are common, particularly in large tumors (Fig. 3-18). The larger tumors often invade contiguous structures, including the kidney and liver.

Microscopic Features

Adrenocortical carcinomas have diverse architectural patterns, including alveolar (Fig. 3-19), trabecular, or solid patterns of growth, and many tumors exhibit admixtures

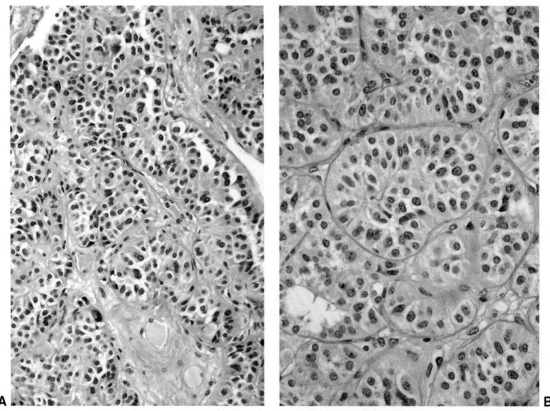

FIGURE 3-19 ■ Adrenocortical carcinoma. The tumor has an alveolar pattern of growth (**A**, low power; **B**, high power).

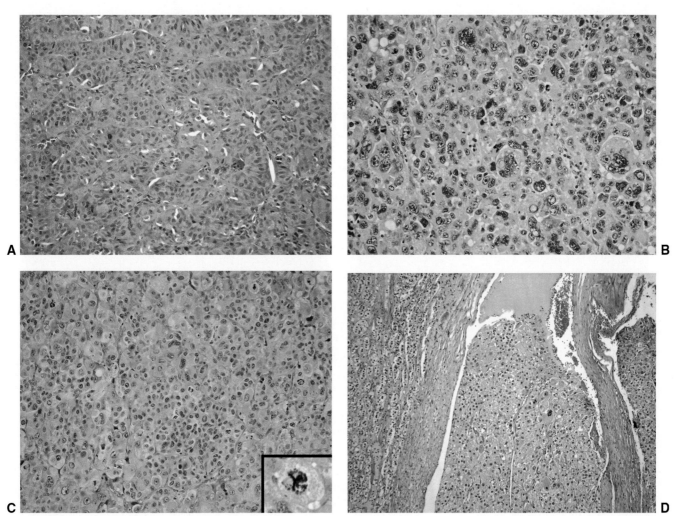

FIGURE 3-20 ■ Adrenocortical carcinoma. Trabecular growth pattern **(A)**, nuclear pleomorphism **(B)**, prominent mitotic activity **(C, inset** atypical mitotic figure), and vascular space invasion **(D)** are demonstrated.

of these patterns.[23,37,43] Many tumors are composed of widened trabeculae separated by endothelium-lined sinusoidal channels (Fig. 3-20A) in contrast to the thin cell cords characteristic of adenomas. Necrosis, particularly in large tumors, may be extensive (Fig. 3-21A). Foci of myxoid change, pseudoglandular patterns, and spindle-cell growth may be prominent in some cases.[126] Depending on their lipid content, the cytoplasm may vary from vacuolated to eosinophilic. Some tumors may have eosinophilic globular inclusions resembling those seen in pheochromocytomas. Rare cases may exhibit adenosquamous differentiation.[127] There may be considerable variation in the appearance of the nuclei. In some instances, they may appear relatively small and uniform, while in others they may exhibit marked pleomorphism (Fig. 3-20B), coarse chromatin, and multiple enlarged nucleoli. Mitotic activity, including atypical forms (Fig. 3-20C), is often prominent. Nuclear pseudoinclusions may be particularly striking in some cortical carcinomas.

Some adrenocortical carcinomas are composed of oncocytic cells.[109,128–130] While some of these tumors may be associated

with Cushing syndrome or feminization,[109] others may be nonfunctional. Hoang et al.[129] concluded that large tumor size, extracapsular extension, vascular invasion, necrosis, and metastasis are features of malignancy in these tumors, while mitotic rate was less than 1 per 10 high-power fields (HPFs).[129] Cytologic atypia and mitotic rate, therefore, were not reliable criteria for the prediction of biologic behavior of these neoplasms according to this study.[129] On the other hand, Bisceglia et al.[109] have also reviewed the criteria for the distinction of benign and malignant adrenal oncocytic tumors.[109] According to these authors, major criteria for malignancy included high mitotic rate, atypical mitoses, and venous invasion while minor criteria included large tumor size, necrosis, capsular invasion, and sinusoidal invasion (Box 3-2, section on Oncocytic Adrenocortical Tumors). The presence of one major criterion was sufficient for the diagnosis of malignancy while one to four minor criteria were sufficient for a diagnosis of tumors of uncertain malignant potential. The absence of all criteria indicated benignancy.

Rarely, adrenocortical carcinomas may contain sarcomatous foci (carcinosarcoma). In the case reported by

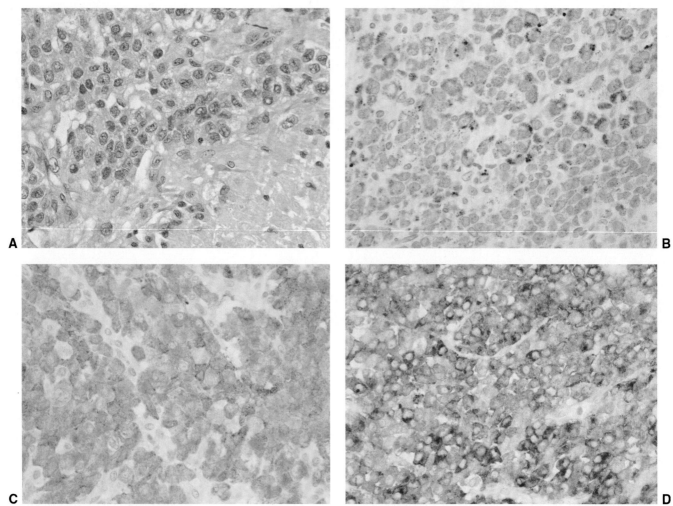

FIGURE 3-21 ■ Adrenocortical carcinoma. There was extensive necrosis of this tumor and viable tumor cells have high nuclear to cytoplasmic ratio (**A**, hematoxylin–eosin section; necrosis in right lower aspect). Neoplastic cells stain positively with antibodies to melan-A (**B**), inhibin (**C**), and synaptophysin (**D**).

Fischler et al.,[131] the sarcomatous component had features of rhabdomyosarcoma and stained positively for muscle-specific actin and desmin. Although this tumor was associated with virilization, the case reported by Decorato et al.[132] was nonfunctional. Recently, Thway et al.[132a] reported an example of oncocytic adrenocortical carcinosarcoma in a 45-year-old man with pleomorphic rhabdomyosarcoma that metastasized to the mesentery, hilar lymph nodes, lungs, and brain over the 11-month terminal course from diagnosis.

In fine needle aspiration biopsy samples, cortical carcinomas generally contain single cells and poorly cohesive cell clusters in a necrotic background. Although there may be considerable nuclear atypia and mitotic activity, some cortical carcinomas appear deceptively bland.[126] According to Ren et al.[133] common cytologic features include hypercellularity, necrosis, nuclear pleomorphism, mitotic figures, and prominent nucleoli. Twenty percent of their cases exhibited all five features while necrosis and/or mitoses were found in every case.

Differential Diagnosis and Ancillary Studies

Adrenocortical carcinomas must be distinguished from cortical adenomas and a variety of secondary tumors involving the adrenal gland, including RCC, hepatocellular carcinoma (HCC), metastatic carcinoma, and liposarcoma. Immunohistochemistry may be of particular value in discriminating these tumors,[12,134–139] (Table 3-3; Box 3-3). The most commonly utilized immunohistochemical antibodies for adrenal cortical tumors are those that react with melan-A, calretinin, and inhibin A (Fig. 3-21) and synaptophysin. The monoclonal antibody A103, which reacts with melan-A, an antigen recognized by cytotoxic T cells and expressed in melanocytes, has also been used for the identification of adrenocortical and other steroid hormone–producing tumors.[14] With the exception of melanoma, the only tumors that are reactive with A103 are adrenocortical adenomas and carcinomas, testicular Leydig cell tumors, and ovarian Sertoli-Leydig cell tumors. Antibodies to inhibin A also provide an additional useful approach for the identification of steroid-producing

Table 3-3 ■ DIFFERENTIAL DIAGNOSIS OF ADRENOCORTICAL CARCINOMA

Tumor	Limited Panel of Antibodies										Other Antibodies
	CK	VIM	Mel-A	INH	CAL	SYN	CHR	S-100	EMA	pCEA	
Cortical carcinoma	+/−	+	+	+	+	+/−	−	−	−	−	D2-40+, SF-1+
Pheochromocytoma	−	+/−	−	−	−	+	+	−	−	−	
Hepatocellular carcinoma	+	+/−	−	−	−	−	−	−	+/−	+	AFP+, Hep+, CD10+ (pCEA pattern)
Renal cell carcinoma	+	+	−	−/+	−/+	−	−	+/−	+	−	RCC+, CD10+
Metastatic NSCLCA	+	+/−	−	−	−	−	−	−	+	+	TTF-1+, CK7+, SP-A+
Metastatic BrCA	+	+/−	−	−	−	−	−	−/+	+	+	GCDFP-15+, MMG+
Metastatic CRCA	+	+/−	−	−	−	−	−	−	+/−	+	CK20+, CDX2+
Metastatic melanoma	−	+	+	−	−	−	−	+	−	−	HMB-45+, MITF+
Liposarcoma	−/+	+	−	−	−	−	−	+	−	−	CDK4+, MDM2+

AFP, alpha fetoprotein; BrCA, breast carcinoma; CAL, calretinin; CDK-4, cyclin dependent kinase 4; CDX2, caudal type homeobox 2; CK, cytokeratin; CHR, chromogranin; CRCA, colorectal carcinoma; EMA, epithelial membrane antigen; GCDFP, gross cystic disease fluid fluid protein; Hep, hepatocyte; HMB-45, human melanoma black 45; INH, inhibin; MDM2, mouse double minute 2; Mel-A, melan A; MITF, microphthalmic transcription factor; MMG, mammoglobin; NSCLCA, non-small cell lung carcinoma; pCEA, polyclonal carcinoembryonic antigen; RCC, renal cell carcinoma antigen; SF-1, steroidogenic factor 1; SP-A, surfactant protein A; SYN, synaptophysin; TTF-1, thyroid transcription factor 1; VIM, vimentin.

cells. Renshaw and Granter[15] have demonstrated that inhibin A and A103 are both useful for the identification of adrenal cortical neoplasms and that A103 is marginally more specific and inhibin A slightly more sensitive. Calretinin is also expressed in adrenal cortical neoplasms and is a useful adjunct in cases where stains for inhibin A are negative. Jorda et al.[13] demonstrated that almost 75% of cortical neoplasms were positive for inhibin A; however, when calretinin was added, the numbers of tumors staining positively for the two markers increased to 94% (31/33 cases).

There are considerable differences in the reported incidences of keratin positivity in cortical carcinomas, depending on the specificities of the antibodies and the types of tissue preparation (Table 3-3). With microwave retrieval methods, cytokeratin immunoreactivity is present focally in up to 60% of adrenal cortical neoplasms.[140,141] Interestingly, all four of the oncocytic carcinomas reported by Hoang et al.[129] were positive for cytokeratins using AE1/AE3 and CAM 5.2 antibodies. Epithelial membrane antigen is consistently negative in adrenocortical neoplasms.[134,136,142] Vimentin is evident in most cortical carcinomas following microwave-induced

Box 3-3 ● IMMUNOPROFILE OF ADRENOCORTICAL LESIONS

Positive
Melan-A
Calretinin
Inhibin
SF-1
Synaptophysin
AE1/AE3 keratin

Negative
HMB-45
Chromogranin
Epithelial membrane antigen

antigen retrieval. Some cortical carcinomas may, therefore, exhibit a vimentin-positive, cytokeratin-negative phenotype while others may coexpress cytokeratins and vimentin.[131]

Some adrenocortical carcinomas exhibit evidence of neuroendocrine differentiation, as is manifest by the presence of immunoreactivity for synaptophysin (Fig. 3-21D), neurofilament proteins, and neuron-specific enolase.[143,144] In contrast to pheochromocytomas, however, cortical carcinomas are negative for the chromogranin/secretogranin proteins. Ultrastructural analysis of cortical carcinomas with neuroendocrine differentiation showed clusters of membrane-bound secretory granules that measured 150 to 300 nm in diameter resembling neurosecretory granules. The tumor cells also contained synaptophysin messenger RNA.[144] Several other approaches have been used for the identification of adrenocortical neoplasms, including antibodies reactive with steroidogenic enzymes and transcription factors that regulate the expression of these genes.[145,146] Schröder et al.[16] have developed a monoclonal antibody (D11) that is reactive with normal and neoplastic cortical cells but nonreactive with normal adrenal medullary cells and pheochromocytomas. This antibody recognizes several 59-kD proteins that are capable of binding apolipoprotein E. The D11 antibody, however, is not specific for steroid hormone–producing cells, since it is also present in several other tumor types, including HCC, RCC, and some cases of bronchogenic carcinoma.[147] Browning et al.[148] reported that D2-40, a marker that is commonly used to highlight lymphatic endothelial cells, was highly specific and sensitive for differentiating adrenal cortical tumors from both metastatic RCCs and pheochromocytomas. In this series, D2-40 was strongly and diffusely positive in the cells of the neoplastic and nonneoplastic adrenal cortex, but was negative in 13 cases of clear-cell renal carcinomas and in normal and neoplastic medullary cells. Sangoi and McKenney[149] reported that a commercially available nuclear antibody to steroidogenic factor-1 (SF-1) was helpful in eliminating interpretative issues of artifactual or background reactivity to distinguish adrenocortical lesions from pheochromocytoma when used in conjunction with chromogranin and either calretinin or inhibin. However, in the vast majority of cases of pheochromocytoma, positive staining for chromogranin will be diagnostic. Sbiera et al.[150] also reported high sensitivity and specificity of SF-1 in distinguishing the adrenocortical origin of tumors from nonsteroidogenic tumors.

Ultrastructurally, the mitochondria of cortical carcinomas may be round, ovoid, or elongated. Silva et al.[151] have found isolated mitochondria with tubular cristae in virtually every case, but tumors containing a predominance of tubular mitochondria were found in only about half of the cases. Abundant smooth endoplasmic reticulum is present in approximately 10% of cases.[151]

Criteria for Malignancy

The distinction between benign and malignant cortical tumors is occasionally challenging, and different authors have used a variety of parameters to differentiate these groups of neoplasms.[121,123,152–158] Hough et al.[123] found that the presence of necrosis (larger than 2 HPFs in diameter) and broad fibrous bands were the most useful histologic discriminants. In addition, a diffuse pattern of growth, nuclear hyperchromasia, and vascular invasion were also helpful in making the distinction between benign and malignant cortical neoplasms.

Weiss[121] proposed a system for the distinction of benign and malignant tumors based on the following nine parameters (Table 3-4): high nuclear grade (Fuhrman grade 3 or 4); >5 mitoses per 50 HPF; atypical mitoses (Fig. 3-20C); diffuse patterns of growth; necrosis; invasion of venous (Fig. 3-20D), sinusoidal, or capsular structures; and clear cells comprising <25% of the tumor.[121,158] In a series of 43 cases, Weiss[121] found

that tumors with fewer than two of these features never metastasized, while those with more than four almost invariably recurred or metastasized. Subsequently, Weiss et al.[159] lowered the threshold for malignancy from four to three parameters. Aubert et al.[160] confirmed the value of the Weiss system, but have proposed a modification based on the most reproducible criteria, including mitotic rate (>5 per 50 HPF), cytoplasmic features (<25% clear cells), abnormal mitoses, necrosis, and capsular invasion. The first two features were assigned values of 2 while the remainder was assigned values of 1. According to this system, each tumor could be given a score of 0 to 7 and the threshold for malignancy remained a score of 3 or more.

Volante et al.[160a] proposed an algorithm in which disruption of the reticulin network combined with any one of the three criteria: mitotic rate >5 per 50 HPFs, necrosis, or vascular space invasion for the diagnosis of adrenocortical carcinomas. According to the authors, tumors classified as adrenocortical carcinomas and adenomas by the Weiss system were similarly classified with 100% sensitivity and specificity using this alternative approach. Disruption of the reticulin network was assessed by silver histochemical staining and basal lamina was assessed using immunohistochemical antibodies to laminin and collagen type IV. Disruption of the reticulin/basal lamina network was defined by loss of continuity of the reticular fibers or basal membrane network in 1 HPF ($400\times = 0.2$ mm^2) extended to at least one-third of the lesion. The authors suggest that this method was easier to use and more practical. More recently, Duregon et al.[113b] also applied this algorithm to their series of oncocytic adrenocortical tumors and found that there tended to be a more heterogenous pattern of reticulin framework and that disruption was more likely to occur in nononcocytic areas, thus posing additional challenges. However, they concluded that its applicability was justified because it avoided undestimation of malignancy in this group of tumors.

In the study of myxoid adrenocortical tumors by Papotti et al.,[161] 8 of 10 cases with myxoid areas that ranged from 5% to 90% fulfilled Weiss' criteria for malignancy (score > 3), but 2 cases with 90% myxoid areas had a Weiss score of 1. In one of the latter tumors that measured 5 cm and weighed 55 g, there was local and peritoneal recurrence at 60 months after resection and the patient eventually died of disease at 68 months. The other patient with a 20-g tumor had no evidence of disease at 9 months of follow-up. In their study they also cited four other cases with conventional features of adrenocortical carcinoma with focal myxoid degenerative changes. The authors concluded that myxoid adrenocortical tumors represent a rare but histologically and phenotypically distinct entity exhibiting malignant behavior.[161]

The issue of malignancy is even more complicated in the pediatric population in which the criteria of Weiss are less predictive of an aggressive course. Cagle et al.[125] found tumor weight >500 g to be the most useful determinant in predicting malignant behavior. Even tumors with evidence of vascular invasion failed to pursue an aggressive course. Wieneke et al recently more reported their experience with

Table 3-4 ■ CRITERIA FOR THE DIAGNOSIS OF ADRENOCORTICAL CARCINOMA

Histologic Features	Weiss (121,159)	Aubert et al. (160) Modification of Weiss System
Nuclear grade (Fuhrmann grade 3 or 4)	1	N/A
Necrosis	1	1
Diffuse architecture (>30% of tumor)	1	N/A
Capsular invasion	1	1
Atypical mitoses	1	1
Sinusoidal invasion	1	N/A
Venous invasion	1	N/A
Mitoses (>5/50 HPF)	1	2
Clear cells (<25%)	1	2
Threshold for malignancy	**>3**	**≥3**

83 cortical neoplasms in patients <20 years of age. Twenty-three of seventy-four cases with a malignant histology based on adaptation of Weiss' criteria had a clinically malignant course.[162] From their analysis, features associated with an increased probability of malignant behavior included tumor weight >400 g, size >10.5 cm, vena cava invasion, capsular and/or vascular invasion, extension into periadrenal soft tissue, confluent necrosis, severe nuclear atypia, >15 mitoses per 20 HPFs, and the presence of atypical mitotic figures. Of these, vena cava invasion, necrosis, and mitotic activity independently predicted malignant behavior in multivariate analyses. Because of the added uncertainty in pediatric tumors, Dehner has suggested labeling tumors fulfilling Weiss' criteria as "atypical adenomas."[163]

Unlike pediatric cases where it is recommended that a diagnosis of "atypical adenoma" should be rendered instead of carcinoma despite the presence of criteria for malignancy, in adults the presence of a single worrisome feature including weight >200 g, prominent diffuse growth pattern, conspicuous mitotic activity or necrosis is sufficient cause for rendering a diagnosis of "atypical adenoma" or "adrenocortical neoplasm of uncertain malignant potential."

Prognostic Factors, Treatment, and Outcome

There are no generally accepted criteria for the grading of cortical carcinomas. In an analysis of 42 carcinomas, the only parameter that had a strong statistical association with patient outcome was mitotic rate.[159] Patients with tumors containing more than 20 mitoses per 50 HPFs had a mean survival of 14 months while tumors with fewer than 20 mitoses had a mean survival of 58 months. Atypical mitoses, capsular invasion, tumor weight in excess of 250 g, and size in excess of 10 cm each had a marginal association with survival. Other features including nuclear grade, presence of necrosis, venous or sinusoidal invasion, character of the tumor cell cytoplasm, or architectural pattern had no impact on survival.

Based on multivariate analysis, Volante et al.[160a] also stratified adrenocortical carcinomas in their proposed algorithm into low-, intermediate- and high-risk groups: low risk, stage 1 to 2 and mitosis ≤9 per 50 HPF; intermediate risk, stage 1 to 2 and >9 mitoses per 50 HPF or stage 3 to 4 and ≤9 mitoses per 50 HPFs; high risk, stage 3 to 4 and >9 mitoses per 50 HPF. Mean disease-free survivals were reported to be 61.9, 17.3, and 12.2 months in the low-, intermediate-, and high-risk groups, respectively.

Other approaches for predicting outcome include DNA content, MIB-1 labeling index, and p53 status.[154–156] Early studies indicated that carcinomas were aneuploid and adenomas diploid, but subsequent analyses demonstrated aneuploidy in some adenomas and diploidy in some carcinomas.[157,158] Vargas et al.[164] demonstrated that the mean proliferative fraction, as determined by counting the proportion of MIB-1-positive cells was 1.49% in adenomas, 20.8%

in carcinomas, and 16.6% in recurrent or metastatic tumors. None of the 20 benign lesions had a MIB-1 score that exceeded 8%, while only one of 20 malignancies had a score of <8%. Forty-five percent of the carcinomas were positive for p53, while none of the 20 adenomas was p53-positive. Aubert et al.[160] also observed a statistically significant difference in MIB-1 labeling indices between benign (2.4 ± 1.3%) and malignant (21.2 ± 18.44%) tumors.

Comparative genomic hybridization studies have revealed that genetic alterations are more common in malignant than in benign cortical tumors while they occur rarely in hyperplastic lesions. Losses of 1p21-p31, 2q, 3p, 3q, 6q, 9p, and 11q14-qter and gains of 5q12, 9q32-qter, 12q, and 20q were the most frequent abnormalities present in carcinomas. Gains in 17q, 17p, and 9q32-qter were most frequent abnormalities in adenomas while gains in two of six cases of cortical hyperplasia involved 17 or 17q.[165] Several groups have demonstrated LOH of 11q13 in a significant proportion of adrenal cortical carcinomas; however, none of the tumors demonstrated a mutation in the MEN1 gene.[166,167] LOH of 17p13 and 11p15 have been demonstrated in approximately 80% of cortical carcinomas. Gicquel et al.[168] have further demonstrated that 17p13 LOH and histologic grade were independently associated with tumor recurrence. Sbiera et al.[150a] reported strong SF-1 protein expression correlating with poor clinical outcome in adrenocortical carcinomas independent of stage of tumor.

Didolkar et al.[120] have studied the natural history of a large series of patients with adrenocortical carcinoma. The mean duration of symptoms in patients with or without hormonal manifestations was 6 months. Fifty-two percent had distant metastases at the time of diagnosis, 41% had locally advanced disease, and 7% had tumor confined to the adrenal gland. The overall median survival was 14 months, and the 5-year survival rate was 24%. The median survival of patients with functional tumors was somewhat longer than that of those patients with nonfunctional tumors. The most common sites of metastasis were the lungs, followed by retroperitoneal lymph nodes, liver, and bone. While acknowledging the low numbers and limited follow-up, Duregon et al.[113b] have suggested that pure oncocytic adrenocortical carcinomas tended to have a more indolent course. The staging of adrenocortical carcinoma is summarized in Table 3-5.[169]

In view of the improvements in sensitivity of imaging modalities, the question arises as to whether there have been improvements in the diagnosis of adrenocortical carcinoma at earlier stages with resultant improved survival. Paton et al.[170] recently analyzed data from the Surveillance, Epidemiology and End results database for the period 1988 through 2002. Of 602 tumors, 3% were <5 cm and localized (stage I), 36% were >5 cm and localized (stage II), and 20.3% invaded adjacent structures (stage III). There were distant metastases (stage IV) in 31.4% of cases and stage was unknown in 8.8%. While 5-year survivals were better in localized disease (62%) compared to 7% in advanced

Table 3-5 ■ PATHOLOGIC STAGING OF ADRENOCORTICAL CARCINOMA

Definitions of TNM

Primary Tumor (T)

TX:	Primary tumor cannot be assessed
T0:	No evidence of primary tumor
T1:	Tumor 5 cm or less in greatest dimension, no extra-adrenal extension
T2:	Tumor >5 cm, no extra-adrenal extension
T3:	Tumor of any size with local invasion, but not invasion of adjacent organs*
T4:	Tumor of any size with invasion of adjacent organs*

Regional Lymph Nodes (N)

Nx:	Regional lymph nodes cannot be assessed
N0:	No regional node metastasis
N1:	Metastasis in regional lymph node(s)

Distant Metastases (M)

M0:	No distant metastases
M1:	Distant metastases

Anatomic Stage/Prognostic Groups

Stage I:	T1	N0	M0
Stage II:	T2	N0	M0
Stage III:	T1	N1	N0
	T2	N1	M0
	T3	N0	M0
Stage IV:	T3	N1	M0
	T4	N0	M0
	T4	N1	M0
	Any T	Any N	M1

From Edge et al (eds). *Adrenal Gland Staging, AJCC Cancer Staging Manual.* 7th ed. New York, NY: Springer; 2009:515–520.
*Adjacent organs include kidney, diaphragm, great vessels, pancreas, spleen, and liver.

disease, tumor stage and survival did not improve over the 15-year study period.

Handling and Reporting of Adrenalectomy Specimens for Adrenocortical Lesions

Knowledge of the clinical, radiologic, and endocrinologic findings of patients is essential for appropriate assessment of adrenalectomy specimens. Subsequent handling and processing of the resected specimens are dictated by the presence or absence of a mass lesion. If the adrenals have been resected for bilateral adrenocortical hyperplasia, the periadrenal adipose tissue should be dissected from the glands in order to determine accurate glandular weights. Multiple cross sections should be prepared at 0.2- to 0.3-cm intervals from the head to tail regions of the glands in order to determine the thickness of the cortical layer and the presence or absence of small nodules or other lesions. Intraoperative gross examination of the resected specimen and review of radiologic findings in the contralateral adrenal are of value in the distinction of adenoma and nodular hyperplasia. Gross photographs

should be taken to document the presence of any abnormalities. Representative sections from the head, body, and tail regions in addition to sections from any focal lesions will provide adequate histologic sampling. Frozen section examination is generally not indicated although there may be some exceptional situations in which frozen sections may be necessary.

Adrenals resected for relatively small mass lesions measuring <2 cm should be weighed and measured following dissection of periadrenal adipose tissue. For these cases, the lesions with the adjacent adrenal gland should be sectioned at 0.3- to 0.5-cm intervals with at least three sections selected for histologic examination. Sections should include the capsule of the lesion. Additional sections of the adjacent cortex should be obtained in order to assess the presence of associated cortical abnormalities.

Larger adrenal resection samples with surrounding adipose tissue should be measured, weighed, and inked prior to sectioning at 0.5- to 1-cm intervals. Gross photographs are of value for documenting the appearance of the tumor and the presence or absence of areas of invasive growth.

If there is a suspicion of malignancy, the periadrenal soft tissues should be left in continuity with the tumor in order to assess the presence or absence of capsular invasion and periadrenal soft tissue involvement. In general, one section for each centimeter of the largest tumor diameter will provide adequate sampling. Sections should include areas of differing consistencies, hemorrhage, and necrosis in addition to the surrounding capsule and periadrenal soft tissue in areas that are grossly suspicious for invasion. Although occasional adrenocortical tumors may be relatively small (<50 g), the utility of frozen sections to distinguish adenomas from small cortical carcinomas is negligible. This distinction should be based on the assessment of permanent sections. However, frozen section examination is of value in determining the status of the margins intraoperatively.

Although there are no strict guidelines at present, it may be of value to collect fresh tumor samples in culture medium for possible cytogenetic studies and to obtain snap-frozen samples for possible molecular studies.

Features that need to be reported in cases of adrenocortical carcinoma are summarized in Box 3-4.[171] Pathologic stage (Table 3-5) is reported in the final diagnosis only in cases that fulfill criteria for malignancy. In cases diagnosed as "atypical adenoma" or "adrenocortical neoplasm of uncertain malignant potential" a comment with pertinent negatives that are usually included in the assessment of malignancy will address the relevant findings.

Box 3-4 ● REPORTING OF ADRENAL GLAND SPECIMENS (MODIFIED FROM CAP CHECKLIST)

Macroscopic
Manner received (unfixed versus fixed)
Procedure type (biopsy, partial or total adrenalectomy)
Specimen laterality
Specimen integrity (intact versus fragmented)
Specimen size (dimensions in centimeters) and weight (grams)
Tumor size (greatest dimension and additional dimensions in centimeters)
Tumor descriptors (cut surface appearance with associated hemorrhage, necrosis, presence of invasion into capsule, vessels or extra-adrenal tissue)

Microscopic
Histologic type (adrenocortical carcinoma)
Microscopic tumor extension (capsular invasion, extension into extra-adrenal soft tissue, extension into adjacent viscera)
Margin status (Involved versus uninvolved with distance from nearest margin)
Lymphatic/sinusoidal or venous involvement (small and large vessel)
Perineural invasion
Lymph node involvement (size of tumor deposit with or without extranodal extension)
Treatment effect (when applicable)
Pathologic stage (pTNM)

MEDULLARY NEOPLASMS

Pheochromocytoma

Epidemiology and Etiopathogenesis

Pheochromocytomas (intra-adrenal paragangliomas) occur in 0.005% to 0.1% of unselected autopsies.[172,173] Their average annual incidence is eight per million person-years in the United States, and they are responsible for <0.1% of cases of hypertension. The term "pheochromocytoma" was introduced by Pick in 1912 to express the fact that the tumors darkened after exposure to potassium dichromate.[174,175] By definition pheochromocytomas are tumors of the adrenal medulla, but tumors of similar morphology and function may also develop in a variety of extra-adrenal sites. While the extra-adrenal tumors have also been referred to as pheochromocytomas by some authors, the preferred terminology for such neoplasms is extra-adrenal paraganglioma with a designation indicating their sympathetic (predominantly abdominal) or parasympathetic (predominantly head and neck) origins.

Most pheochromocytomas are sporadic (nonfamilial). Although previous studies indicated that approximately 10% of tumors were familial, more recent analyses indicate that a considerably higher proportion have a heritable basis. This distinction is of particular importance since most familial tumors are bilateral and multicentric while most sporadic tumors are unilateral. Familial pheochromocytomas are found in 30% to 50% of patients with types 2A and 2B MEN syndromes, 10% to 20% of patients with von Hippel-Lindau (VHL) disease, and 1% to 5% of patients with von Recklinghausen disease.[176] Familial paragangliomas and pheochromocytomas also occur in patients with germ line mutations of succinate dehydrogenase (*SDH*) subunits B, C, D, and AF2,[177–177b] the kinesin family member 1B (*KIF1B*), transmembrane protein 127 (*TMEM127*), and the *MYC*-associated factor X (*MAX*) genes.[177a–177e]

Although generations of medical students have been taught the 10% rule of pheochromocytomas (10% hereditary, 10% bilateral/multifocal, 10% pediatric, 10% extra-adrenal, 10% malignant), recent studies indicate that this axiom represents an oversimplification. In fact, up to 25% of these tumors are heritable and significantly more than 10% occur in the pediatric population and are multifocal, consistent with a familial origin. Moreover, considerably <10% of adrenal primaries are malignant while more than 10% of retroperitoneal paragangliomas pursue an aggressive course.[178]

Germ line mutations in the *RET* protooncogene, a member of the transmembrane protein kinase family, are responsible for MEN 2A and 2B. The mutations, which typically affect exons 10, 11, and 16, convert this protooncogene into a dominant activating oncogene. From the description of an 18-year-old woman with bilateral adrenal tumors (originally diagnosed as sarcoma and angiosarcoma) in 1886 and the presence of a germ line mutation of the *RET* gene in her living relatives, Neumann et al.[179] have concluded that this represents the first description of pheochromocytoma in a patient with MEN 2. Approximately 10% of sporadic pheochromocytomas harbor somatic mutations involving the *RET* protooncogene.[180] LOH surrounding the neurofibromatosis I (*NFI*) locus and loss of neurofibromin expression are evident in pheochromocytomas from patients with neurofibromatosis.[181] These findings support the view that mutations of the neurofibromin gene contribute to the development of pheochromocytomas in patients with von Recklinghausen disease. The VHL gene, located on chromosome 3p25, encodes a protein that operates by a mechanism involving transcription elongation that is mediated by interactions with elongation factors B and C. This raises the possibility that the disease may control oncogenes that are regulated at the level of elongation, such as c-*myc*, n-*myc*, l-*myc*, and c-*fos*.[182] In VHL-associated pheochromocytomas, the VHL protein often harbors a missense mutation at codon 238. In VHL families without pheochromocytomas, the mutation is more often a nonsense codon, frame shift, or deletion.[183]

Nearly 25% of patients with apparent sporadic pheochromocytomas have germ line mutations of one of the pheochromocytoma susceptibility genes including *VHL* (45%), *RET* gene (19.6%), *SDHD* (16.6%), and *SDHB* (18.2%).[184] Interestingly, only 32% of patients who were positive for mutations had multifocal tumors, while 35% of patients presented after the age of 30 and 17% after the age of 40. Most true sporadic pheochromocytomas become clinically evident in the fourth to fifth decades.

Gill et al.[184a] have reported the utility of immunohistochemical staining with the antibody to the SDHB protein for triaging genetic testing of *SDHB*, *SDHC*, and *SDHD* in paraganglioma–pheochromocytoma syndromes from a series of cases with known *SDH* gene mutation status. According to these authors, all 12 *SDH*-mutated tumors in their series showed weak diffuse positive or negative staining with this antibody while 9 of 10 tumors with known mutations of *VHL, RET*, and *NF1* and 34 of 36 tumors without germ line mutations showed strong positive staining. There was weak positive or negative staining of one tumor with *VHL* mutation and two tumors without germ line mutation. They reasoned that since *SDH* mutations are virtually always germ line, this immunohistochemical method is useful for screening cases for *SDH* gene mutations.

Comparative genomic hybridization studies have revealed that gene copy alterations in pheochromocytomas and paragangliomas are common. Loss of 1p has been observed in more than 80% of these tumors.[185] The minimal region of loss was 1cen-p31. Additional losses have involved 3q22-q25, 11p, 3p13-p14, 4q, 2q, and 11q22-23 while gains were found on 19p, 19q, 17q24-qter, 11cen-q13, and 16p. Dannenberg et al.[186] reported similar findings and have further demonstrated that losses of 6q and 17p may play an important role in the progression to malignancy. Petri et al.[187] have demonstrated that although there is frequent loss of the *TP53* locus on 17p, the *TP53* gene does not appear to play a major role in pheochromocytoma tumorigenesis.

Interestingly, deletions of 1p have also been demonstrated in NBs and adrenal cortical carcinomas, as discussed in the respective sections.

Clinical Features

The clinical manifestations of pheochromocytoma are protean but are generally dominated by signs and symptoms of catecholamine hypersecretion or by the complications of hypertension. Common symptoms include headache, diaphoresis, palpitations, anxiety, chest pain, and weight loss. In most series, hypertension, which may be sustained or paroxysmal, is the most common sign at presentation. A few patients with pheochromocytomas are normotensive, and a few may even be hypotensive. Tachycardia, postural hypotension, and a hypermetabolic state are also common. Most pheochromocytomas produce a combination of norepinephrine and epinephrine, with a predominance of norepinephrine. Tumors producing epinephrine exclusively may be associated with hypotension. The diagnosis depends on the presence of increased urinary and plasma levels of catecholamines and their metabolites. Preoperative localization of pheochromocytomas is accomplished most effectively with CT or MRI.

The syndrome of pseudopheochromocytoma is more of clinical dilemma rather than one for the surgical pathologist. The term "pseudopheochromocytoma" was used initially for patients with paroxysmal hypertension without biochemical or imaging evidence of pheochromocytoma. However, the syndrome has been expanded to include conditions with symptoms of excess catecholamines, without the presence of pheochromocytoma or adrenal lesions that may mimic pheochromocytoma on imaging studies. Underlying conditions include hyperadrenergic essential hypertension, anxiety disorder, obstructive sleep apnea, toxic effect of drugs, and metabolic disorders.[188,189]

Pheochromocytomas are rare in childhood, but they are more likely to be bilateral and multicentric than those in adults.[190] Approximately 90% of affected children have sustained hypertension; polydipsia, polyuria, and convulsions are considerably more common than in adults. In addition, the rate of metachronous or synchronous extra-adrenal paragangliomas is considerably higher in children than in adults.[172] The high rate of bilaterality and multicentricity suggests that many of these cases may represent unrecognized examples of familial pheochromocytomas.

Gross Features

In patients with nonfamilial forms of pheochromocytoma, the right adrenal gland is somewhat more commonly involved than the left. Most nonfamilial tumors are unilateral and sharply circumscribed solid masses with fibrous pseudocapsules. In most surgical series, the tumors measure 3 to 5 cm with tumor weights ranging from 70 to 150 g.[23] Size and weight variations may be considerable, and even very small tumors can be associated with signs and symptoms of catecholamine hypersecretion. The tumors vary

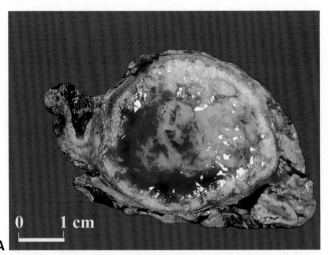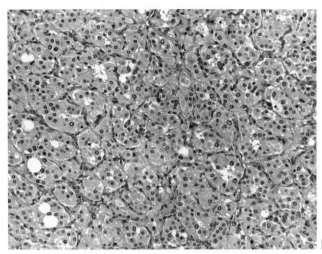

A   **B**

FIGURE 3-22 ■ Pheochromocytoma. This tumor has a gray-white fleshy appearance and hemorrhage **(A)**. This histologic section shows an alveolar pattern of growth of eosinophilic neoplastic cells and a capillary-rich framework producing the characteristic "Zellballen" appearance **(B)**.

in color from gray-white to pink-tan, with foci of congestion (Fig. 3-22A). Larger tumors can contain central areas of fibrosis. Occasionally, very large pheochromocytomas undergo cystic degeneration, and they may be difficult to distinguish from nonneoplastic adrenal cysts. Familial pheochromocytomas are typically bilateral and multicentric and the adjacent medulla may appear hyperplastic grossly.[191–193] Large tumor masses in patients with familial pheochromocytomas most likely develop as a result of the confluence of multiple small tumor nodules.

Microscopic Features and Ancillary Studies

The tumors are composed of intermediate to large polygonal cells that may be arranged in alveolar, trabecular, or solid patterns. Most pheochromocytomas exhibit admixtures of these growth patterns. In tumors with alveolar arrangements, the groups of tumor cells are surrounded by a capillary-rich framework that results in a characteristic "Zellballen" appearance (Fig. 3-21B). In some instances, the capillary channels are prominent enough to result in an angiomatous appearance. Some tumor cells may be arranged in a glandular or acinar pattern. In patients with familial pheochromocytomas, the adjacent medulla is often hyperplastic.

The cytoplasm may be acidophilic, amphophilic, or basophilic and typically has a finely granular texture. A few pheochromocytomas contain abundant cytoplasmic vacuoles resulting from lipid degeneration, and tumors with these features may be particularly difficult to distinguish from adrenocortical tumors. In some instances, however, extensive cytoplasmic vacuolation is the result of fixation artifacts. Rarely, pheochromocytomas may show oncocytic features.[194] Periodic acid–Schiff–positive eosinophilic globules are evident in a high proportion of cases (Fig. 3-23). The globules are most likely derived from the membrane components of secretory granules.

Although most pheochromocytomas are composed of intermediate- to large-sized polygonal cells, some tumors may be composed of spindle cells (Fig. 3-24) or relatively small cells resembling pheochromoblasts. Moreover, very large cells resembling ganglion cells may also be evident in some cases. In addition to chromaffin cells, pheochromocytomas also contain a population of sustentacular cells, which are difficult to recognize in hematoxylin and eosin–stained preparations; however, they can be demonstrated selectively with antibodies to S-100 protein. Typically, the sustentacular cells are present at the peripheries of the cell nests.

The nuclei are round to ovoid, with coarsely clumped chromatin and a single prominent nucleolus. Nuclear pseudoinclusions may be particularly prominent in some tumors. However, similar pseudoinclusions can also be a feature of adrenal cortical tumors. Nuclear pleomorphism and hyperchromasia may be particularly prominent in some

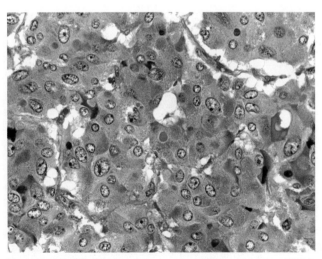

FIGURE 3-23 ■ Pheochromocytoma. The cytoplasm in this case is amphophilic and cytoplasmic globules are present centrally.

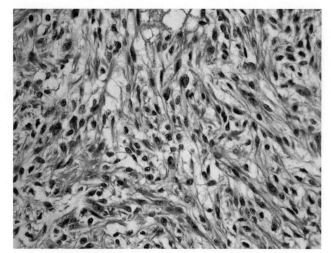

FIGURE 3-24 ■ Pheochromocytoma. Neoplastic spindle cells were prominent in this tumor.

pheochromocytomas, but this finding does not correlate with malignant behavior. Benign pheochromocytomas can occasionally contain mitotic figures. Thirty-five percent of benign tumors compared with 65% of malignant tumors contain mitoses.[195] Mitotic counts in the malignant tumors were slightly higher (3 per 30 HPF) than in the benign tumors, (1 per 30 HPF); however, these differences were not statistically significant.

Large tumors frequently display areas of hemorrhage and may show necrosis. The stroma may have areas of myxoid change with foci of lymphocytic infiltration. Amyloid deposits may be present in a small number of cases.[196] Foci of capsular and venous invasion may also be evident, but these features do not correlate with malignant behavior. Brown fat has been reported in the retroperitoneum surrounding pheochromocytomas; however, this change is not specific.[197]

The diagnosis of an adrenal tumor as a pheochromocytoma depends in part on the ability to determine its catecholamine

content by biochemical or histochemical methods. The chromaffin reaction is an insensitive procedure for the demonstration of catecholamines since some tumors that contain catecholamines, as determined by biochemical analysis, have shown negative results with the standard chromaffin reaction. Catecholamine-synthesizing enzymes, including tyrosine hydroxylase, dopamine beta-hydroxylase, and phenylethanolamine N-methyltransferase, may also be demonstrated in pheochromocytomas using immunohistochemical procedures.[31] These tumors are usually positive for vimentin and neurofilament proteins and negative for cytokeratins. However, focal cytokeratin immunoreactivity (AE1/AE3 and CK1) can occur.[198] Pheochromocytomas exhibit positivity for chromogranin proteins (Fig. 3-25A) and synaptophysin (Box 3-5), but synaptophysin is also present in a large proportion of adrenal cortical tumors. The S-100 protein is restricted to the sustentacular cells and is particularly evident in those areas with a "Zellballen" pattern (Fig. 3-25B). Pheochromocytomas may also contain a large array of regulatory peptide products, including leu- and met-enkephalin, endorphins, ACTH, somatostatin, and calcitonin.[33,199] The overproduction of these substances may give rise, in rare cases, to syndromes of hormone excess, including Cushing syndrome.[200] Ultrastructurally, pheochromocytomas contain variable numbers of membrane-bound, dense-core, secretory-type granules.[201–203]

Criteria for Malignancy in Pheochromocytoma and Outcome

The diagnosis of malignancy in pheochromocytomas is particularly challenging. Differences in criteria have resulted in considerable variation in the reported rates of malignancy, which have ranged from 2.4% to 14%. With the exception of the presence of lymph node or distant metastases, there are no absolute criteria that distinguish benign from malignant pheochromocytomas. Capsular invasion, even when it

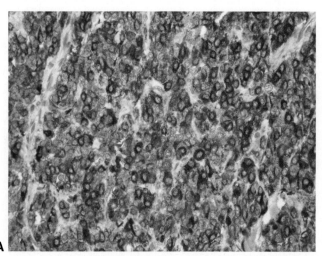

A

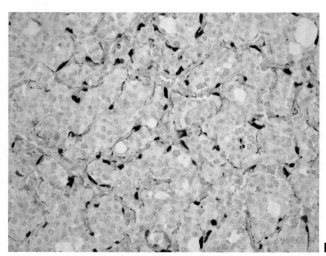

B

FIGURE 3-25 ■ Pheochromocytoma. The tumor cells in this focus are small and stained with antibodies to chromogranin A **(A)**. Antibodies to the S-100 protein stain the sustentacular cells at the peripheries of the tumor cells in this section from another tumor **(B)**.

Box 3-5 ● IMMUNOPROFILE OF PHEOCHROMOCYTOMA

Positive
Synaptophysin
Chromogranin

Negative
Melan-A
Calretinin
Inhibin
SF-1
Cytokeratin

is extensive, is a poor predictor of metastatic behavior, while the absence of invasion does not preclude the development of metastases. In a study of adrenal and extra-adrenal sympathoadrenal paragangliomas, Linnoila et al.[195] noted the following features more frequently in malignant tumors: male predominance, extra-adrenal location, greater tumor weight (mean of 383 g for malignant vs. 73 g for benign tumors), confluent tumor necrosis, and the presence of vascular invasion and/or extensive local invasion. Hyaline globules were found in 59% of benign and 32% of malignant tumors. Logistic regression analysis of 16 nonhistologic and histologic parameters revealed that four were most predictive of malignancy: extra-adrenal location, coarse nodularity of the primary tumor, confluent tumor necrosis, and absence of cytoplasmic hyaline globules. Although most malignant tumors had two or three of these features, most benign tumors had only one or none.

In a series from the Armed Forces Institute of Pathology, Thompson[198] was unable to demonstrate a statistically significant difference in weight between benign and malignant pheochromocytomas. He developed a system for the assessment of malignancy of pheochromocytomas (PASS, *P*heochromocytomas of the *A*drenal gland *S*caled *S*core). In this system, each of the following features was assigned a value of 1: vascular invasion, capsular invasion, profound nuclear pleomorphism, and hyperchromasia. Features assigned a value of 2 included periadrenal adipose tissue invasion, large tumor nests or diffuse growth pattern, focal or confluent necrosis, high cellularity, tumor cell spindling, cellular monotony, mitotic figures in excess of 3 per 10 HPFs, and atypical mitoses. Among 50 tumors that were classified as histologically malignant and assigned a PASS ≥ 4, metastases developed in 33 patients, while 17 were free of metastases. Patients with tumors with a PASS ≤ 3 remained free of metastases with a mean follow-up of 14.1 years.

Wu et al.[204] reviewed the reproducibility of the PASS on a cohort of 57 pheochromocytomas from a single institution as assessed by five pathologists with at least 10 years' experience in endocrine pathology from different institutions. The authors found significant interobserver and intraobserver disagreement in assignment of PASS as a result of variable interpretations of the histologic parameters. They concluded that PASS required further refinement and validation and concluded that it could not be used for clinical prognostication.[204]

Other parameters have also been used for the assessment of malignancy. Clarke et al.[205] reported that a cutoff value of MIB-1 of >3% yielded a specificity of 100% and a sensitivity of 50% for predicting malignancy. The value of S-100 protein for the distinction of benign and malignant pheochromocytomas has been controversial. In general, those tumors with a "Zellballen" pattern show well-developed staining in the sustentacular cells present at the peripheries of cell nests. Tumors with a large nesting or diffuse growth pattern, on the other hand, may be devoid of S-100-positive sustentacular cells. Most malignant pheochromocytomas demonstrated a decreased number of sustentacular cells, which undoubtedly reflects the diffuse growth pattern so commonly seen in these tumors. It should be noted that abundant S-100 positivity may be present in sustentacular cells in metastatic tumors, particularly those with a well-developed "Zellballen" pattern.

Cytomorphometry has been used in the differential diagnosis of malignant and benign pheochromocytomas. In a study reported by Lewis,[206] benign pheochromocytomas had a mode corresponding to a diploid (2n) DNA content and a wide range of values with nuclei measuring up to 40n. Malignant pheochromocytomas, on the other hand, had a hyperdiploid or triploid mode with a smaller range of values.

Recent interest has been focused on the vascular patterns of pheochromocytomas.[207] Malignant tumors have an abnormal vascular architecture with an irregular pattern of large vascular volumes flattened between tumor nodules. Benign pheochromocytomas exhibit a regular pattern of short, straight capillaries.[208] Correlative molecular studies have shown an increase of EPAS1 (a hypoxia-inducible transcription factor), VEGF (vascular endothelial growth factor), and ETB (endothelin receptor, type B) of 4.5-, 3.5-, and 10-fold, respectively, in malignant versus benign pheochromocytomas. Expression of stromal tenascin has also been suggested as a marker to distinguish benign (predominantly negative) from malignant (strongly positive) pheochromocytomas.[209]

Gene expression profiling studies of malignant pheochromocytomas have revealed consistent downregulation of genes involved in catecholamine metabolism (fumaryl acetate hydrolase and monoamine oxidase), peptide processing (glutaminyl-peptide cyclotransferase, peptidylglycine alpha-amidating monooxygenase), and hormone secretion (synaptophysin-like 3 and secretogranin II) while expression of astrotactin and plexin C1, which are involved in cell adhesion, are also downregulated in these tumors.[210,211]

Malignant pheochromocytomas are generally slowly growing neoplasms with 5-year survival rates in the range of 40% to 50%. The most common sites of metastatic spread include lymph nodes, bone, and liver. In assessing lymph node metastases, all efforts should be directed to distinguishing concurrent extra-adrenal paragangliomas that compress adjacent lymph nodes from true nodal metastases.

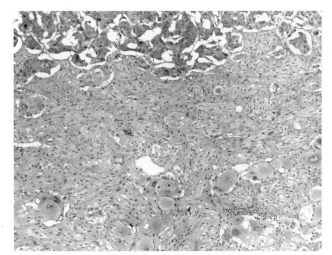

FIGURE 3-26 ■ Composite tumor (pheochromocytoma and ganglioneuroma) of the adrenal medulla. The pheochromocytoma component at the top of the field demonstrates a typical "Zellballen" arrangement while the ganglioneuroma contains mature ganglion cells in a Schwannian-dominant stroma (lower field).

Composite Pheochromocytoma

The terms composite pheochromocytoma and compound tumor of the adrenal medulla have been used to describe tumors containing pheochromocytoma together with foci of NB, ganglioneuroblastoma, ganglioneuroma, or malignant peripheral nerve sheath tumor (Fig. 3-26).[43] Composite pheochromocytomas are rare tumors that make up <3% of sympathoadrenal pheochromocytomas. Rarely, they may be associated with neurofibromatosis type I[212] or MEN 2A or MEN 2B. The predominant component of the tumor is usually pheochromocytoma. The possibility of differentiation along more than one cell line has been supported by studies that have shown that normal and neoplastic chromaffin cells are capable of differentiation into ganglion cells under the influence of nerve growth factor.[213] It has been suggested that the sustentacular cells of pheochromocytomas could serve as the progenitors of the malignant peripheral nerve sheath component of some composite pheochromocytomas. Many

of the reported composite tumors have been associated with signs and symptoms typical of pheochromocytomas, and some have been found in the context of the Verner-Morrison syndrome of watery diarrhea and hypokalemia. A unique case of composite pheochromocytoma consisting of typical pheochromocytoma and neuroendocrine carcinoma has been reported.[214]

Adrenal Medullary Hyperplasia

Although adrenal medullary hyperplasia is classified as a nonneoplastic lesion, it is discussed in this section because of its relationship to pheochromocytoma. Diffuse and nodular hyperplasia of the medulla has been recognized only relatively recently as a distinct clinical and pathologic entity[193,208,215] (Fig. 3-27). This change has been reported in association with MEN 2A and MEN 2B and von Hippel-Lindau disease and has also been noted in a few patients without an apparent familial syndrome. Of the four patients with nonfamilial hyperplasia reported by Rudy et al.,[216] three underwent unilateral adrenalectomy, and one had bilateral adrenalectomy. In this series, the hyperplasia was diffuse in three cases and diffuse and nodular in the fourth. The diagnosis of adrenal medullary hyperplasia should be made with considerable care. In the context of cortical atrophy, for example, the medulla may appear more prominent than usual. The diagnosis of medullary hyperplasia should be made only on the basis of increased medullary volume, as determined morphometrically. Other findings suggestive of medullary hyperplasia include the presence of medullary tissue in both alar regions of the gland and extension of the medulla into the tail region. Naeye[217] has suggested that adrenal medullary hyperplasia may also be found in victims of the sudden infant death syndrome.

Molecular studies of microdissected nodules in patients with MEN 2A-associated nodular adrenal medullary hyperplasia have shown that this disorder is a multifocal monoclonal proliferation. Interestingly, the same X chromosome is inactivated in individual nodules from the same patient. This observation has suggested an early clonal expansion of adrenal medullary precursors in these patients.[218]

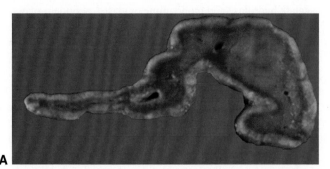
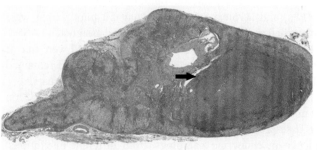

A   B

FIGURE 3-27 ■ Diffuse and nodular medullary hyperplasia. Adrenal gland resected from a patient with type 2A multiple endocrine neoplasm (MEN 2A). In addition to the diffuse hyperplasia of the medulla, there is focal nodule formation **(A)**. Histologic section from another MEN 2A patient highlights the nodular (*arrow*) and diffuse hyperplasia **(B)**.

Handling of Adrenalectomy Specimens for Pheochromocytoma

Pheochromocytomas should be handled in a manner similar to cortical neoplasms. Historically, suspected cases were fixed in chromate-containing fixatives to demonstrate a positive chromaffin reaction, but in the era of immunohistochemistry all cases are fixed in formalin. For cases of suspected adrenal medullary hyperplasia, periadrenal fat should be dissected from the glands and sections should be prepared at 0.2- to 0.3-cm intervals. These glands should be submitted in their entireties for histologic examination and evaluation of medullary volume.

Neuroblastic Tumors

Epidemiology and Etiopathogenesis

Neuroblastic tumors are embryonic neoplasms of the adrenal medulla and sympathetic nervous system. They are the second most common solid neoplasms in childhood after central nervous system tumors and account for approximately 15% of all neoplasms in children 4 years and younger (mean age, 21 months).[219] Neuroblastoma (NB), ganglioneuroblastoma, and ganglioneuroma constitute the main categories of neuroblastic tumors and are conceptually regarded as a continuum from the most immature to the most mature forms of neuroblastic tumors. The epidemiologic and clinical characteristics of these tumors are largely related to NB, which account for the majority of these neoplasms.

The vast majority occur sporadically, although cases of familial NB have been recorded.[220] Activating mutations of the anaplastic lymphoma kinase (*ALK*) oncogene have been shown to account for the vast majority of familial NBs.[221] NBs may be found in association with the Beckwith-Wiedemann syndrome, von Recklinghausen disease, Hirschsprung disease, opsoclonus/myoclonus, heterochromia iridis, watery diarrhea, or Cushing syndrome.[43] Children with sporadic or familial NB in conjunction with congenital central hypoventilation syndrome, Hirschsprung disease, or both have been demonstrated to have loss of function mutations in the homeobox gene *PHOX2B*.[221] Rare examples of NBs have been reported in adults.[222–224]

The ratio of adrenal to extra-adrenal primary sites is approximately 1.5 to 2:1. The remaining tumors may develop within the head and neck region, mediastinum or pelvic area. In approximately 10% of cases, it may not possible to establish the primary site of origin with certainty.

The concept of in situ NBs was introduced by Beckwith and Perrin[225] for neuroblastomatous foci confined to the adrenals of newborns. At the microscopic level, these lesions are composed of clusters of immature neuroblasts ranging in size from 0.7 to 9.5 mm, with frequent foci of cystic change. In different autopsy series, the incidence ranges from 0.4% to 2.5%, which is considerably higher than that of clinically apparent NBs, suggesting that a substantial number of cases undergo spontaneous regression, degeneration, or

maturation. The distinction between in situ NBs and nodules of normal developing neuroblasts is difficult. Neuroblastic nodules measuring more than 2 mm in diameter are considered to represent latent NBs by Bolande,[226] while smaller lesions are thought to be an integral part of adrenal morphogenesis.[227]

Clinical Features

NBs/neuroblastic tumors most often come to clinical attention as abdominal masses. Increased levels of catecholamines and their metabolites are found in most patients with NBs; however, hypertension is present only rarely in affected patients and cardiogenic shock has been reported.[228] In advanced-stage tumors, increased catecholamine and a positive bone marrow biopsy are employed rather than a biopsy of the primary tumor. Mass screening with analysis of urinary catecholamines in infants has been successful in detecting occult cases of NB both in Japan and in other countries,[229] but subsequent studies have reported little or no survival advantage from detection of occult cases in infants.[230–232]

Classification of Neuroblastic Tumors

Several classification and grading schemes have been proposed to correlate morphologic features with prognosis.[233–236] The current system is a consensus classification developed by member pathologists of the International Neuroblastoma Pathology Committee (INPC) by applying criteria from previous schemes to neuroblastic tumors from the Children's Cancer Group registry. The resulting classification system is largely based on the Shimada classification, but also draws from traditional and other recent schemes.[237,238] It is though to be the most reproducible, biologically relevant, and prognostically significant system. Neuroblastic tumors are divided into four major categories (Table 3-6): NB (Schwannian stroma–poor neuroblastic tumor); ganglioneuroblastoma, intermixed (Schwannian stroma–rich neuroblastic tumor); ganglioneuroblastoma (Schwannian stroma–dominant neuroblastic tumor); and the composite neuroblastic tumor ganglioneuroma, nodular (composite Schwannian stroma–rich/stroma–dominant and stroma–poor neuroblastic tumor).[237]

Neuroblastoma (Schwannian Stroma–poor Neuroblastic Tumor)

Gross and Microscopic Features

NBs vary in size from those measuring <1 cm in diameter to those that may fill the abdomen or thorax. They are generally soft and white to gray-pink[23,43,239] (Fig. 3-28). However, more differentiated tumors may have a yellow-tan appearance and firmer consistency similar to ganglioneuroma. Larger tumors tend to undergo hemorrhage, necrosis, cyst formation, and calcification (Fig. 3-29), but these features can also be seen in small tumors. Adrenal primaries tend to

Table 3-6 ■ CLASSIFICATION OF NEUROBLASTIC TUMORS (NTs)

International Neuroblastoma Pathology Committee (Shimada et al.[237])

Neuroblastoma (Schwannian stroma-poor NT)	
Undifferentiated	Absence of neuropil and <5% ganglionic differentiation*
Poorly differentiated	Neuropil present and <5% ganglionic differentiation
Differentiating	Neuropil present, >5% ganglionic differentiation and <50% Schwannian stroma
Ganglioneuroblastoma, intermixed (Schwannian stroma–rich NT)	Nests of neuroblasts and neuropil intermixed with ganglion cells and >50% Schwannian stroma
Ganglioneuroma (Schwannian stroma–dominant NT)	
Maturing	Mature ganglion cells and Schwannian stroma with intermixed individual neuroblasts without formation of nests of neuroblasts
Mature	Mature ganglion cells and Schwannian stroma without neuroblasts
Ganglioneuroblastoma, nodular composite Schwannian stroma–rich/stroma–dominant and stroma–poor neuroblastic tumor)	Composite tumor of neuroblastoma nodule in a background of either ganglioneuroblastoma, intermixed, or ganglioneuroma

Shimada[235]	Joshi[236]
Stroma-poor NT	**Neuroblastoma**
Undifferentiated	*Undifferentiated*
	Poorly differentiated
Differentiated	*Differentiated*
Stroma-rich NT, intermixed	**Ganglioneuroblastoma (intermixed)**
Stroma-rich NT, well differentiated	**Ganglioneuroblastoma (borderline)**
Ganglioneuroma	**Ganglioneuroma**
Stroma-rich NT, nodular	**Ganglioneuroblastoma (nodular)**

*Ganglionic differentiation refers to synchronous enlargement of nucleus and cell body such that the diameter of the cell is twice that of the nucleus.

grow toward the midline and can extend to the contralateral side. Large, right-sided tumors can invade the liver directly, whereas large, left-sided tumors can invade the pancreatic parenchyma.

NBs are composed of sheets of small cells with hyperchromatic nuclei and scanty cytoplasm. A lobular appearance is common because of the presence of thin fibrovascular septa between groups of tumor cells (Figs. 3-30A and 3-31A). Most cases have a finely fibrillary matrix (neuropil) between the tumor cells that corresponds to unmyelinated axons at the ultrastructural level[240] (Figs. 3-31 and 3-32). Homer-Wright pseudorosettes are found in about 30% of cases.[23] They are characterized by one to two layers of neuroblasts arranged around a central space filled with neuropil (Fig. 3-31B). In the presence of hemorrhage, pseudorosettes or nests of cells may assume a papillary configuration resembling Schiller-Duvall bodies of yolk sac tumors.

In the INPC classification,[237] undifferentiated NB lacks neuropil and is characterized by the presence of small- to medium-sized cells with scant cytoplasm and indistinct cytoplasmic borders. Nuclei are round to ovoid with "salt and pepper" chromatin and indistinct nucleoli (Fig. 3-30B). Areas of coagulative necrosis should not be mistaken for neuropil. Occasional cells with vesicular nuclei and prominent nucleoli apparently differentiating toward immature ganglion cells provide a useful clue for distinguishing these tumors from other small blue cell tumors, including Ewing sarcoma/primitive neuroectodermal tumor (EWS/PNET), rhabdomyosarcoma, desmoplastic small round cell tumor, blastemal Wilms tumor, and lymphoma. Immunohistochemical and molecular genetic studies are critical in arriving at the

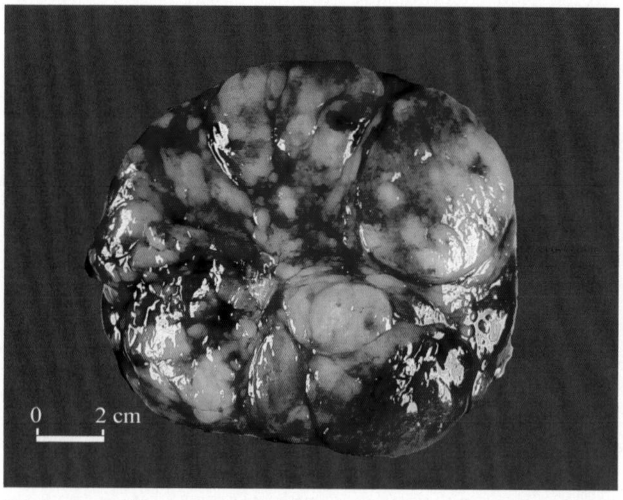

FIGURE 3-28 ■ Neuroblastoma. The tumor has a lobular gray-pink fleshy appearance.

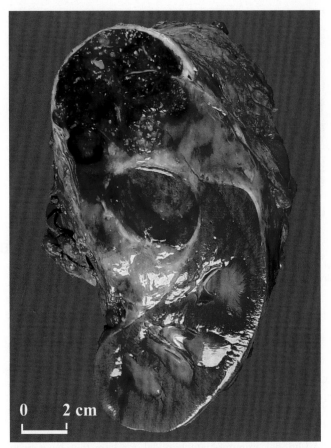

FIGURE 3-29 ■ NB with attached kidney, resected after chemotherapy. The upper part of the lesion contains calcification (*white* stippling) and is composed of viable poorly differentiated tumor. The lower part of the tumor including, involvement of the renal hilum, is fibrous and myxoid corresponding to chemotherapy response with maturation.

correct diagnosis (Table 3-7). Most neoplastic cells are undifferentiated, but cells with evidence of ganglionic differentiation (differentiating neuroblasts) are usually present. By definition, differentiating neuroblasts account for <5% of the neoplastic cells.[237] Differentiation is manifested by synchronous differentiation of the nucleus (enlarged eccentric nucleus, vesicular chromatin, single prominent nucleolus) and cytoplasm that may appear eosinophilic or amphophilic. A cell diameter at least twice the nuclear diameter is required for categorization of ganglionic differentiation.

Poorly differentiated NB contains a neuropil background (Fig. 3-31) and <5% of neuroblasts with evidence of ganglionic differentiation. Pleomorphic cells containing large nuclei and prominent nucleoli may be present. These pleomorphic cells may be present and may occasionally have rhabdoid features. These cells should not be mistaken for cells showing ganglionic differentiation when grading NBs. Both undifferentiated and poorly differentiated NBs contain no or minimal ganglioneuromatous stroma.

Differentiating NBs are characterized by the presence of more than 5% of cells showing evidence of ganglionic differentiation. Usually, differentiating NBs contain more abundant neuropil than poorly differentiated NBs although the most critical feature of the differentiating tumors is the proportion of differentiating neuroblasts (Fig. 3-32). Both ganglionic differentiation and Schwannian stromal formation, which are frequently present at the periphery of the tumor, may be prominent in differentiating NBs. However, these features should comprise <50% of the tumor in contrast to ganglioneuroblastoma, intermixed in which they represent more than 50% of the tumor.[237] Also, the distinction of differentiating NBs from nodular ganglioneuroblastoma may at times be difficult.

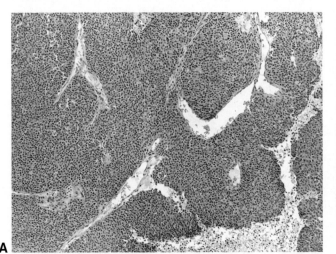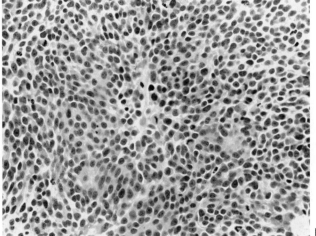

FIGURE 3-30 ■ NB, undifferentiated. This section demonstrates a typical lobular appearance and an area of coagulative necrosis in the lower field **(A)**. There is absence of neuropil and the coagulative necrosis should not be mistaken for neuropil. At high power mitoses and karyorrhexis are evident as well as occasional cells with prominent nucleoli suggesting an attempt at ganglionic differentiation **(B)**.

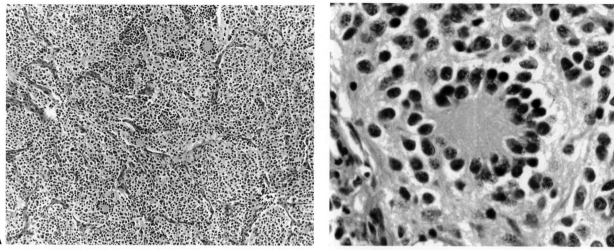

FIGURE 3-31 ■ NB, poorly differentiated. A lobular growth pattern and neuropil including Homer-Wright pseudorosettes are present on low power **(A)**. The pseudorosette is composed of two layers of neuroblasts arranged around central neuropil **(B)**.

Generally, the transitional zone between the NB and ganglio-neuroblastomatous component is poorly defined in the differentiating NBs. Although not included in the International Neuroblastoma Pathology Committee classification, it should be noted that a large cell variant of neuroblastoma with an aggressive clinical behavior has been reported.[241]

Ancillary Studies

Ultrastructural examination of NBs has been largely supplanted by immunohistochemistry and molecular genetic studies since undifferentiated tumors that pose the most difficulty on H&E sections cannot be reliably distinguished from other small blue cell tumors by electron microscopy.

NBs most commonly express neurofilament proteins,[242–246] which may be helpful in making the distinction from other small round blue cell tumors of infancy and childhood. However, neurofilament proteins can be present in other small round blue cell tumors, including rhabdomyosarcoma[247] (Table 3-6). The most commonly utilized antibodies are chromogranin and synaptophysin, which demonstrate positive cytoplasmic staining[32,248,249] (Fig. 3-33A). Neuron-specific enolase (NSE) is present in virtually all NB but is also positive in an array of nonneuroblastic tumors.[35] Additional immunohistochemical markers that have been reported to be positive in NBs include CD57 (leu-7),[250] ganglioside D2,[251] protein gene product 9.5[249] (Fig. 3-33B), microtubule (MAP-1, MAP-2), and tau proteins,[246,252] and certain epitopes detectable with NB-directed monoclonal antibodies, including UJ13A[253,254] and HSAN 1.2.[255,256] Antibodies to neural adhesion molecule (NCAM/CD56), a family of cell surface glycoproteins involved in direct cell to cell adhesion, frequently react with NB.[257–259] NB84, a monoclonal antibody raised against NB cells, recognizes a large

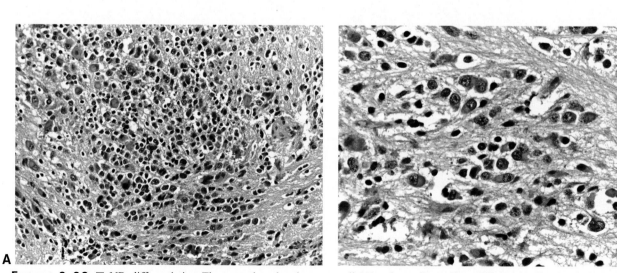

FIGURE 3-32 ■ NB, differentiating. The tumor has abundant neuropil **(A)** and ganglion cells at different levels of maturity **(B)**.

Table 3-7 ■ IMMUNOHISTOCHEMICAL AND GENETIC MARKERS OF SMALL BLUE CELL TUMORS IN THE DIFFERENTIAL DIAGNOSIS OF NEUROBLASTOMA

Neoplasm	Immunohistochemical Profile	Genetics
Neuroblastoma	CHR+, SYN+, CD99–, WT-1–, CK–, DES–, MYOG–, CD45+	MYCN amplification, 1p deletion and 17q gain (these are not specific for neuroblastoma but have prognostic significance)
EWS/PNET	CD99+, SYN–/+, CHR–, DES–, MYOG–, CD45–, CK–	t(11;22)(q24;q12) EWS/FLI-1 t(21;22)(q22;q12) EWS/ERG t(7;22)(p22;q12) EWS/ETV1 t(17;22)(q12;q12) EWS/E1AF
Rhabdomyosarcoma	DES+, MYOG+, CD99–/+, SYN–/+, CK–, WT-1–	**Alveolar RMS** t(2;13)(q35-37;q14) PAX3/FKHR t(1;13)(p36;q14) PAX7/FKHR PAX3/FKHR translocation reported to be associated with decreased survival compared to no translocation or PAX7/FKHR translocation MYCN amplification may be associated with a worse prognosis **Embryonal** Allelic loss of 11p15; extra 2, 8, 13 Rearrangement of 2, 8, 13, 1p11-1q11, 12q13
Wilms (blastemal)	WT-1+ (both N- and C-terminal abs), CK+/–, DES+/–, CD99–/+, CHR–, SYN–, MYOG–	No consistent cytogenetic/genetic abnormality in sporadic cases
Desmoplastic small round cell tumor	DES+, CK+, WT-1+ (C-terminal ab), CD99–/+, SYN–/+, MYOG–, CHR–, CD45–	t(11;22)(p13;q12) EWS/WT1
Lymphoblastic lymphoma	CD45+ (rare cases negative), TdT+, CD99–/+, CK–, MYOG–, CHR–, SYN–	T-cell β, γ, immunoglobulin heavy or light chain gene rearrangement

CHR, chromogranin; CK, cytokeratin; DES, desmin; EWS/PNET, Ewing sarcoma/primitive neuroectodermal tumor; MYOG, myogenin; SYN, synaptophysin; TdT, terminal deoxynucleotidyl transferase; WT, Wilms tumor.

proportion of NBs as well as EWS/PNETs and desmoplastic small round cell tumors.[260] Additionally, cases of rhabdomyosarcomas, lymphoblastic lymphomas rhabdomyosarcomas, and small-cell osteosarcomas have been reported to be positive for NB84.[261] Immunohistochemical staining with S-100 protein highlights cells in the Schwannian stroma, but the neuroblasts are negative. Membranous staining with CD99 (detectable by monoclonal antibodies HBA-71, 12E7, and O13), which is typically seen in the EWS/PNET tumor group of tumors, is negative in NBs.[262]

A number of genetic and molecular features are seen in NBs including MYCN gene amplification, chromosome 1p loss, and 17q gain. These parameters along with other genetic features are discussed in detail in "Prognosis of Neuroblastic Tumors."

Spread and Metastases

NBs can metastasize widely through both lymphatic and vascular routes.[23] Common sites of spread include bone marrow (78%), bone (69%), lymph nodes (42%), and liver (20%) while pulmonary and brain metastases are uncommon. Pulmonary metastases have been reported in 3% of cases

in one study, and are usually associated with widespread disease and unfavorable histology with poor outcome.[263] In these cases, the metastatic nodules tend to be small when present, NB is considered less likely to be the primary than other small round cell tumors such as EWS/PNET. Skin (2%) and testes (2%) may also be involved. Spontaneous regression is well documented. Increasing evidence suggests that genetic prerequisites that are involved include an intact chromosome 1 short arm, lack of *MYCN* amplification, and near triploidy.[237]

Differential Diagnosis

Distinguishing undifferentiated and poorly differentiated NBs from other small round blue cell tumors (Table 3-7) is challenging on routine hematoxylin and eosin–stained sections, particularly in small biopsy samples. Distinction from EWS/PNET poses the most difficulty. Both tumors can have a lobular growth pattern and may contain Homer-Wright pseudorosettes, but EWS/PNET lacks the neuropil background of poorly differentiated NB. While both tumors react with antibodies to NSE and synaptophysin, EWS/PNET is almost never positive for chromogranin and CD99

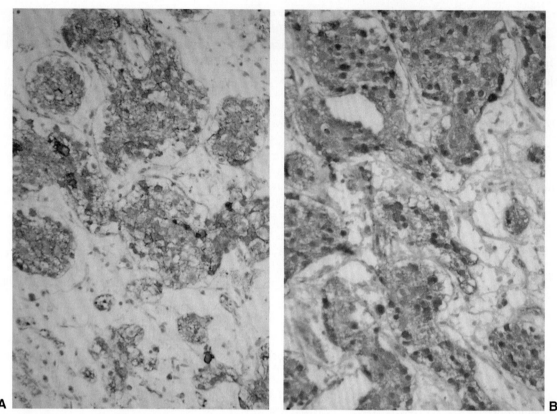

FIGURE 3-33 ■ NB, poorly differentiated. Immunohistochemical stains show positive granular cytoplasmic staining of neuroblasts with chromogranin (**A**) and protein gene product 9.5 (**B**).

is positive in EWS/PNET but negative in NB. Molecular genetic studies are useful adjuncts in making the distinction (Table 3-7), but Burchill et al.[264] reported that 2 of 12 cases of typical NB had the *EWS/FLI-1* fusion transcript by reverse transcriptase-PCR. In the cases described, serum and urinary markers as well as histologic features were consistent with NB. Immunohistochemical staining of both tumors revealed positivity for NB84, PGP 9.5, and NSE, while CD99 was negative. These observations underscore the need for detailed clinical–pathologic correlation in arriving at a diagnosis, particularly when faced with limited material in biopsy samples. Since NB is much more common than EWS/PNET in children under 5 years of age, and a significant proportion have metastatic disease, NB needs to be excluded when the latter diagnosis is being considered.[265]

Rhabdomyosarcoma, particularly embryonal rhabdomyosarcoma, occurs in the same age group as NB, but the presence of rhabdomyoblasts and strap cells usually helps in making the distinction. However, as discussed, undifferentiated or poorly differentiated NB may have pleomorphic cells with rhabdoid features, but immunohistochemistry will permit their specific identification. Similarly, Wilms tumor occurs in the same age group. Triphasic or epithelial tumors pose less of a diagnostic problem, but blastemal Wilms is more likely to be mistaken for NB on routine sections. This is complicated by small biopsy specimens from

large tumors that may show extension between the adrenal gland and kidney. Serum and urinary catecholamines and immunohistochemistry (Table 3-7) are key elements the distinction.

Lymphoblastic lymphoma is another important differential diagnosis when there is bulky disease of the retroperitoneum. The distinction is particularly difficult on small biopsies in which neuropil is not apparent. CD45 can be negative in a subset of these tumors,[266] so stains for terminal deoxynucleotidyl transferase and T and B lymphocytes may be necessary for conclusive exclusion.

A less common newly recognized entity first described in childhood is the *Nu*clear protein in *t*estis (NUT) midline carcinoma. These tumors most commonly occur in the head and neck and mediastinum, but have also been reported in the abdomen. A large proportion of cases have features of poorly differentiated carcinoma including small-cell morphology, but some may have more pleomorphic cells or even squamous differentiation. French et al.[267] have characterized the specific translocation t(15,19) resulting in the *BRD4-NUT* oncogene seen in these tumors and their group have developed an immunohistochemical antibody for paraffin-embedded sections.[268] This antibody along with positive keratin and CD34 staining will assist in distinguishing NUT midline carcinoma from NB.

Metastatic medulloblastoma may enter the differential diagnosis since medulloblastoma can metastasize to bone as is the case with NB and NB may rarely metastasize to the brain. Since there is wide histologic and immunohistochemical overlap with these tumors, correlation with imaging studies for a primary site and biochemistry will assist in making the distinction. It should be noted that the peak incidence of medulloblastomas is in a slightly older age group of 5 to 10 years compared to NB (under 5 years). In terms of bone lesions, small-cell osteogenic sarcoma may enter the differential diagnosis, but again these tumors will follow the age range for conventional osteogenic sarcomas, have imaging characteristics of osteogenic sarcoma, and contain osteoid with lack of expression of neuroendocrine markers and absence of the typical biochemical findings.

As noted earlier, NB rarely occurs in older patients. Therefore, the possibility of metastatic carcinoid tumor or small-cell carcinoma will enter the differential diagnosis. In such instances the lack of neuropil will be helpful, but immunohistochemical staining for keratin and thyroid transcription factor 1 (TTF-1) in the case of lung primaries will be useful in the immunohistochemical workup.

Ganglioneuroblastoma, Intermixed (Schwannian Stroma–rich Neuroblastic Tumor)

Ganglioneuroblastoma, intermixed, can have the same gross appearance as NB or ganglioneuroma depending on the extent of differentiation. It is characterized by the random intermingling of neuroblastic nests within the stroma-rich (ganglioneuromatous) component (Fig. 3-34). The neuroblasts are usually in various stages of differentiation, with differentiating neuroblasts and ganglion cells present within ample neuropil. Ganglioneuroblastoma, intermixed, is distinguished from ganglioneuroblastoma, nodular, by the lack of a macroscopically distinct hemorrhagic nodule, and, microscopically, the interface between the stroma-poor and stroma-rich components is infiltrative rather than pushing (see section on "Ganglioneuroblastoma, nodular"). Differentiation from

differentiating NB is based on the extent of the ganglioneuromatous component, which should exceed 50% of the total volume in microscopic field(s) from representative section(s) of the tumor in the case of ganglioneuroblastoma, intermixed.[237]

Ganglioneuroma (Schwannian Stroma–dominant Neuroblastic Tumor)

In the INPC classification ganglioneuroma is subdivided into ganglioneuroma, maturing, and ganglioneuroma, mature, subtypes.[237,238] The ganglioneuroma, maturing, subtype was previously classified as "stroma-rich, well differentiated neuroblastic tumor" in the original Shimada classification.[235] It is composed predominantly of ganglioneuromatous stroma with a minor component of scattered, evenly or unevenly distributed collections of differentiating neuroblasts and/or maturing ganglion cells in addition to fully mature ganglion cells. Separation from ganglioneuroblastoma, intermixed, is based on the fact that neuroblastomatous foci do not form distinct microscopic nests, but instead individual neuroblasts merge into the ganglioneuromatous stroma.

Ganglioneuroma, mature, subtype is the prototypic ganglioneuroma of traditional classification schemes. Less than 30% of these tumors occur in the adrenal glands where they are most commonly asymptomatic.[269,270] The remainder develop in the posterior compartment of the mediastinum, retroperitoneum, and other sites. Rarely, they are associated with hypertension, watery diarrhea, and hypokalemia, or masculinization.[271] Adrenal ganglioneuromas (ganglioneuroma, mature, subtype) are generally smaller than those in the mediastinum or retroperitoneum. They are sharply circumscribed but do not have a true capsule (Fig. 3-35). The cut surface is gray to tan, and the consistency varies from soft and gelatinous to firm and whorled with an appearance similar to that of a leiomyoma. Microscopically, ganglioneuroma, mature, subtype contains varying numbers of mature ganglion cells and Schwann cells together with variable amounts of collagen[272]

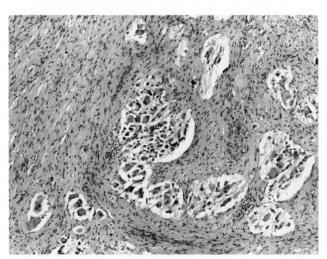

FIGURE 3-34 ■ Ganglioneuroblastoma, intermixed. The nests of neuroblasts and ganglion cells within neuropil are intermixed with the spindle-cell Schwannian stroma.

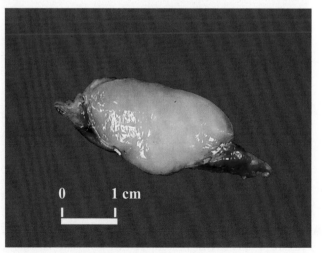

FIGURE 3-35 ■ Ganglioneuroma. The tumor is sharply circumscribed but not encapsulated and has a myxoid glistening cut surface because of the rich Schwann cell stroma.

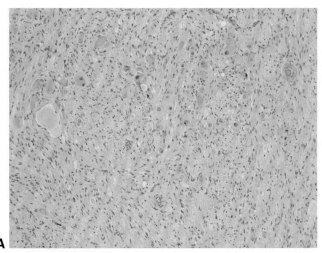

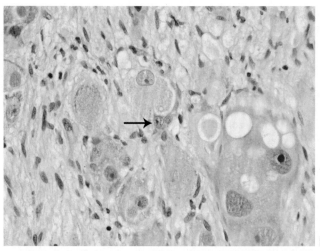

FIGURE 3-36 ■ Ganglioneuroma. Mature ganglion cells are surrounded by a Schwann cell–rich stroma on low power **(A)**. Individual neuroblasts (*arrow*) are present among the mature ganglion cells (**B**, high power) resulting in the case being classified as the maturing subtype of ganglioneuroma.

(Fig. 3-36). Multinucleated ganglion cells may also be present. The Schwann cells and collagen are often arranged in interlacing bundles. Ganglion cells may be distributed diffusely throughout the tumor or arranged in small clusters. Fully mature ganglion cells are usually surrounded by satellite cells. Complete maturation requires the absence of neuroblasts. Because lymphocytes are commonly present within these tumors, immunohistochemical staining with CD45 may be necessary in some instances to exclude the presence of a neuroblastic component. Surgical excision of ganglioneuroma, mature and maturing, subtypes is usually curative. Very rarely, ganglioneuroma, mature, may transform into malignant peripheral nerve sheath tumors either spontaneously or following irradiation for NB or ganglioneuroblastoma.[43]

Ganglioneuroblastoma, Nodular (Composite Schwannian Stroma–Rich/Stroma-dominant, and Stroma-poor Neuroblastic Tumor)

While the other neuroblastic tumors form a spectrum from the immature stroma-poor NB to the mature stroma-dominant ganglioneuroma, ganglioneuroblastoma, nodular (ganglioneuroblastoma, nodular) is a composite tumor composed of a NB component in a background of ganglioneuroma or ganglioneuroblastoma, intermixed. The classic adrenal ganglioneuroblastoma, nodular, is characterized by a gross appearance in which a frequently hemorrhagic and soft NB nodule (Fig. 3-37) is present in a firm tan-pink whorled or myxomatous cut surface of ganglioneuroma or

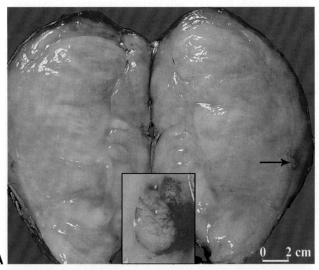

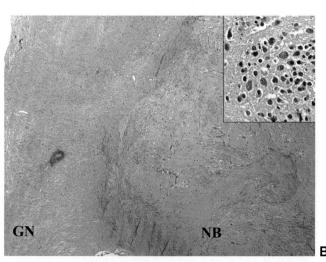

FIGURE 3-37 ■ Ganglioneuroblastoma, nodular (composite Schwannian stroma–rich/stroma–dominant and stroma–poor neuroblastic tumor). This very large tumor is predominantly ganglioneuroma **(A)** with a fibrous and myxoid cut surface, but a small *white* hemorrhagic nodule of NB (*arrow* and **inset**) was found. The circumscribed interface between ganglioneuroma (GN) and neuroblastoma (NB, **inset**) is demonstrated on this histologic section **(B)**.

ganglioneuroblastoma, intermixed. Microscopically, there is usually an abrupt demarcation of the neuroblastic (stroma-poor) component from the stroma-rich (ganglioneuroblastoma, intermixed) or stroma-dominant (ganglioneuroma) component. Neuroblastic nodules therefore have pushing borders and may even have a fibrous pseudocapsule. These nodules probably develop as a consequence of evolution of one or more aggressive clones within the tumor. This may be the result of newly acquired genetic alterations or the persistence of two or more genetically and biologically different clones.[237]

The stroma-rich/stroma-dominant component is often located at the periphery, but there is variability in the proportion of both components. Rarely the neuroblastic component may dominate the tumor with the stroma-rich/stroma-dominant component being in the periphery. Therefore, examination of the periphery of these tumors is essential for accurate classification since the category of ganglioneuroblastoma, nodular, is grouped in the unfavorable histology group of neuroblastic tumors. The proportion of stroma-rich/stroma-dominant tissue is not critical for the diagnosis. In variants of ganglioneuroblastoma nodular there are multiple nodules of NB rather than a single nodule, or ganglioneuroblastoma, intermixed, or ganglioneuroma constitute the primary adrenal tumor, but NB is found in sections from a metastatic site, either regional lymph node or distant metastasis.

Problematic Cases of Histologic Classification and Grading

Categorization of a neuroblastic tumor may be hampered by small biopsies in which clear distinction of NB, ganglioneuroblastoma, nodular, ganglioneuroblastoma, intermixed, and ganglioneuroma is not possible. In these instances, a diagnosis of "neuroblastic tumor unclassifiable" is appropriate, and a multidisciplinary discussion is useful in determining the adequacy of the biopsy. A diagnosis of NB, not otherwise specified (NOS), is appropriate where there is poor quality of sections, extensive hemorrhage, cystic degeneration, necrosis, crush artifact, and/or diffuse calcification. These factors may also impede evaluation of neuroblastic differentiation, mitosis karyorrhexis index (MKI), and mitotic rate. Similarly, a diagnosis of ganglioneuroblastoma, NOS, is appropriate when extensive calcification may obscure a stroma-poor nodule.[237]

Posttherapeutic Specimens

Posttherapeutic resection specimens are difficult to assess. There is usually extensive fibrosis and calcification of specimens from the abdomen or retroperitoneum complicating the assessment of margins and the presence of residual tumor. Microscopically, necrotic foci, fibrosis, chronic inflammation, and calcification are commonly seen. In residual foci of tumor, both features of differentiation and nuclear enlargement may be seen. Grading of these tumors with stratification into favorable or unfavorable categories is not performed.[237]

Specimen Handling and Reporting

The surgical pathologist must be involved in evaluating neuroblastic tumors immediately after surgery so that fresh tissue can be appropriately submitted for genetic and biologic markers. Specimen dimensions and weight are obtained. Although accurate staging of NBs can be quite problematic by gross examination, careful examination of all specimens for the presence or absence of a capsule and the adequacy of margins is mandatory. Specimens should be sectioned at 1.0- to 1.5-cm intervals such that the relationships to identifiable structures are maintained. Fresh tissue should be submitted in culture medium for conventional cytogenetics. Snap-frozen fresh tissue and touch/squash preparations (fixed in acetone or ethanol for 10 to 15 minutes) should be prepared for molecular genetic studies. Tissue fixed in glutaraldehyde is used for ultrastructural examination as needed. Representative sections from all heterogeneous-appearing areas must be submitted making sure to demonstrate the interface between these areas (to facilitate making the diagnosis of nodular ganglioneuroblastoma), as well as those areas between tumor and recognizable normal/anatomic structures. In resection specimens, sections to delineate margins are necessary. A photograph, photocopy, or diagram clearly demonstrating a map of the sections should be made.[237,273] By and large the same general principle of submitting one section for each centimeter of tumor applies. Using this principle, along with the sections as indicated above, the number of sections is usually twice the maximum dimension of the tumor.

The final report should include the following information: site and weight, a specific and descriptive diagnosis based on the INPC classification, and the stage. The results of DNA content studies and the presence or absence of *MYCN* amplification when available, together with cytogenetic results, should be included in the final report.

Prognosis of Neuroblastic Tumors

The prognosis of neuroblastic tumors is determined by multiple variables, including age, histopathologic features, and stage, as well as series molecular, genetic, and biologic parameters. Age at diagnosis is an important independent prognostic factor with outcome being inversely related to age at diagnosis.[274] In the past, the cutoff age of 1 year was used for risk stratification for treatment purposes compared to the 18 months used in the age-linked histologic grading. However, more recently the latter cutoff is now also being used for treatment stratification based on the International Neuroblastoma Risk Group (INRG) Classification System in an effort to standardize risk stratification across the globe.[274a]

MKI was adopted by the INPC over mitotic rate expressed per 10 HPFs and presence of calcification for stratifying NBs into different prognostic groups.[272,275] The number of cells undergoing mitosis and karyorrhexis is expressed as a percentage of 5,000 cells and is assessed on high power (400X). MKI is designated as low, intermediate, or high

Table 3-8 ■ AGE-LINKED PROGNOSTIC EFFECTS USING THE INPC CLASSIFICATION

Grade	MKI	Age (Y)		
		<1.5	1.5–5	≥5
Undifferentiated	Low	○	○	○
	Intermediate	○	○	○
	High	○	○	○
Poorly differentiated	Low	●	○	○
	Intermediate	●	○	○
	High	○	○	○
Differentiating	Low	●	●	○
	Intermediate	●	○	○
	High	○	○	○

●, good (favorable histology); ○, poor (unfavorable histology).
MKI, mitosis karyorrhexis index.

based on counts of <100 (<2%), 100 to 200 (2% to 4%), and more than 200 (>4%) mitotic and karyorrhectic cells, respectively.[235] There may be variability in the MKI in different fields of a section or variability between sections, but the overall MKI is the average determined by assessing all sections. Of note, MKI should not be assessed adjacent to areas of necrosis. MKI can be assessed in metastatic tumor. The MKI along with age and grade of NB is used to assign NBs into favorable and unfavorable histology categories similar to the original Shimada classification[235,276] (Table 3-8). Ganglioneuroblastoma, intermixed, and ganglioneuroma were classified as favorable histology neuroblastic tumors (100% 5-year overall survival). Ganglioneuroblastoma, nodular, is classified as unfavorable histology (5-year overall survival 59.1%),[276] but Umehara et al.[277] reported prognostic subsets of ganglioneuroblastoma, nodular, based on the grade of the NB component using the same parameters as those used for favorable and unfavorable histology in NBs. Favorable and unfavorable subsets, with 5-year overall survivals of 95% and 40.7%, respectively, were defined.

Tumor stage is clearly an important independent prognostic indicator. The staging system employed based on the degree of surgical resection is the International Neuroblastoma Staging System (INSS)[278,279] (Table 3-9). Stage 4S is considered essentially localized disease (stage 1 and 2) with limited distant spread. In the revised INSS, stage 4S is restricted to patients younger than 1 year of age. There

Table 3-9 ■ INTERNATIONAL NEUROBLASTOMA STAGING SYSTEM AND INTERNATIONAL NEUROBLASTOMA RISK GROUP STAGING SYSTEM

INSS Stage	Definition
1	Localized tumor with gross excision, with or without microscopic residual disease, representative ipsilateral lymph nodes negative for tumor microscopically.
	Nodes attached to and removed with primary tumor may be positive; includes grossly resectable tumor arising in the midline from pelvic ganglia or organ of Zuckerkandl
2A	Localized tumor with incomplete gross excision; representative ipsilateral nonadherent lymph nodes negative for tumor microscopically.
	Includes a midline tumor that extends beyond one side of the vertebral column and is unresectable
2B	Localized tumor with or without gross excision, with ipsilateral nonadherent lymph nodes positive for tumor. Enlarged contralateral lymph nodes must be negative microscopically.
	Includes a midline tumor that extends beyond one side of the vertebral column, is unresectable with positive ipsilateral lymph node involvement (on side of extension); a thoracic tumor with malignant unilateral pleural effusion
3	Unresectable unilateral tumor infiltrating across the midline with or without regional lymph node involvement; or localized unilateral tumor with contralateral regional lymph node involvement.
	Includes midline tumor with bilateral extension by infiltration (unresectable) or by lymph node involvement; a tumor of any size with malignant ascites or peritoneal implants
4	Any primary tumor with dissemination to distant lymph nodes, bone, bone marrow, liver, skin, and/or other organs (except as defined for 4S)
4S	Localized primary tumor (stage 1, 2A, or 2B) with dissemination limited to skin, liver, and/or bone marrow (limited to infants <1 y of age)
	Marrow involvement should be minimal (<10% of total nucleated cells identified as malignant on biopsy or aspirate); more extensive involvement should be considered stage 4

INRGSS Stage	Description
L1	Localized tumor without involvement of image-defined vital structures and confined to one body compartment
L2	Locoregional tumor with one or more image-defined risk factors
M	Distant metastatic disease (except stage MS)
MS*	Metastatic disease in children younger than 18 mo with metastases confined to skin, liver, and/or bone marrow

INSS, International Neuroblastoma Staging System; INRGSS, International Neuroblastoma Risk Group Staging System.
Note: Midline is defined as the vertebral column with the vertebral body margin as the limit.
Multifocal primary tumors should be staged according to the greatest extent of disease and followed by the subscript letter M in the INSS. Similarly, multifocal primary tumors in the INRG staging are staged on the basis of the greatest extent of disease.
*MS in the INRGSS uses an upper limit of 18 mo compared to that of 12 mo in the INSS.

Table 3-10 ■ PROGNOSTIC SUBSETS OF NEUROBLASTOMA BASED ON CLINICAL AND BIOLOGIC PARAMETERS

Prognostic Feature	Low-Risk Tumors	Intermediate-Risk Tumors	High-Risk Tumors
Age	<1 y	>1 y	1–5 y
Stage (INSS)	1, 2, 4S	3, 4	3, 4
MYCN	1 copy	1 copy	Amplified
DNA ploidy	Hyperdiploid or near triploid	Near diploid or near tetraploid	Near diploid or near tetraploid
TRK-A/C expression	High	Low or absent	Low or absent
TRK-B expression	Truncated	Low or absent	High
Chromosome 1p36	Usually intact	Usually intact	Usually intact
Chromosome 17q gain	Absent	Present	High
Clinical course	Very good response to therapy with 5-y survival 95%	Initial response to therapy, but tends to relapse with 5-y survival 40%–50%	Rapidly progressive disease in spite of therapy with 5-y survival 25%

Modified from Brodeur GM. Neuroblastoma: biological insights into a clinical enigma. *Nat Rev* 2003;3:203–216.

are no significant differences in 4-year overall survival rates for patients younger than 1 year of age with stage 1, 2A, 2B, 3, or 4S disease (98.5% survival) compared to those with stage 4 disease (73.1% survival).[280] Similarly, patients older than 1 year of age with stage 1, 2A, 2B, or 3 disease had similar 4-year overall survival rates as compared to stage 4 disease in which survival was 48.5%.

Although stage 4 cases are usually associated with progressive disease and a poor outcome, a series of chronic NB in children diagnosed with stage 4 NB in the first decade of life who had metastatic disease for 5 years or more from diagnosis has been reported.[281] This represents indolent or smoldering NB, a concept traditionally restricted to adolescents and adults. This phenomenon may be attributed to the expanding repertoire of chemotherapeutic modalities, including biologic therapies currently in use.

It is important to recognize that the INRG has devised a staging system (Table 3-9) that is based on imaging rather than the extent of surgical resection.[281a] This system allows for preoperative treatment stratification and facilitates comparison of clinical trials across continents. However, it should be pointed out that in a report from the INRG that demonstrated age, stage, MYCN status, and time from diagnosis to first relapse were predictive of overall survival,[281b] it was the INSS stage that was used rather than the INRG staging system. This reflects the retrospective nature of the study in which the database relies on the INSS.

Serum ferritin and lactate dehydrogenase have been reported to be useful prognostic markers for NB at diagnosis, but lack sensitivity and specificity to monitor disease activity.[279] Serum levels of NSE also reflect the extent of disease in patients with these tumors.[282] NSE, chromogranin (CGA), and GD2 (tumor-associated ganglioside) are more specific but not as sensitive as serum ferritin levels. Catecholamine levels have also been associated with prognosis.[283]

Several genetic and molecular features have been proposed as prognostic indicators in neuroblastic tumors, including

MYCN amplification, chromosome 1p deletion, ploidy, and gains in chromosome 17q (Table 3-10). *MCYN* amplification (>10 copies of *MYCN*) and ploidy are used routinely for stratification into treatment groups by the Children's Oncology Group. *MYCN* amplification is present in 25% to 30% of NBs with advanced-stage disease and is associated with rapid tumor progression and poor clinical outcome.[284–286] *MYCN* amplification is used as a determinant in applying more aggressive treatment protocols for stage 1, 2, and 4S tumors (similar to more advanced-stage tumors). *MYCN* amplification is present almost exclusively in NBs, with a smaller proportion in the ganglioneuroblastoma, nodular, category and none in ganglioneuroblastoma, intermixed, and ganglioneuroma categories.[287] Five-year overall survival rates for favorable histology-nonamplified and -amplified tumors are 99% and 50%, respectively, while corresponding survival rates for unfavorable histology-nonamplified and -amplified tumors are 47.1% and 23%, respectively. Kobayashi et al.[288] have suggested that the presence of enlarged and prominent nucleoli may be indicative of the presence of *MYCN* amplification in NB. Detection of *MYCN* amplification can be determined with Southern blot, FISH, and PCR. Recently, Thorner et al.[289] employed chromogenic in situ hybridization (CISH) for determining *MYCN* gene copy number in routine tissue sections. Therefore, although routinely determined on frozen tissue for biology protocol, *MYCN* amplification can be assessed from paraffin-embedded tissue by FISH and CISH.

Ambros et al.[290] attempted to correlate morphologic features of NB, independent of age, that might be able to identify clinically favorable and unfavorable groups. Prominent nucleoli in undifferentiated and poorly differentiated neuroblasts, cellularity, and nuclear size appeared to have clinical significance. Indeed, more recently Suganuma et al.[290a] assessed discordance between histology and *MYCN* amplification (phenotype–genotype discordance) and identified two prognostic groups; presence of prominent nucleoli (bull's eye) and tumors with "conventional" stippled (salt-and-pepper) chromatin pattern. The group with prominent nucleoli had a worse prognosis. Immunohistochemical expression of the N-myc protein was positive in the majority of the former tumors while it was negative in the latter cases. By and large the morphology and biology of NBs are rather homogenous. However, Sano et al.[291] reported a case in a 12-month-old child in which two distinct histologic and biologic clones could be distinguished. Both were poorly differentiated but one clone had a high MKI falling into an unfavorable histology and the other a low MKI and so favorable histology. *MYCN* was amplified in the unfavorable histology clone and nonamplified in the favorable histology clone. Metastasis to lymph nodes contained the former clone. Because of these findings they considered this to be a composite NB.

Deletion of chromosome 1p is the most characteristic cytogenetic abnormality described in NBs and has been identified in 30% to 50% of cases.[292] While there has been some debate as to whether 1p loss has independent prognostic value, multivariate analysis has suggested that it is associated with decreased event-free survival.[293] FISH studies have demonstrated unbalanced translocations involving 17q resulting in gains of 17q. Such unbalanced partial 17q gain is significantly associated with well-established indicators of clinical risk in NB including advanced stage and older age.[294] Interestingly, *MYCN* amplification almost never occurs in the absence of 1p allele loss, 17q gain, or both.

Tumors with a near-diploid karyotype have a poorer prognosis than those with a hyperdiploid or triploid karyotype,[285] and *MYCN* amplification is significantly more frequent in diploid than in hyperdiploid tumors.[292] Furthermore, chromosome 1p abnormalities, double minutes, and heterogenous staining regions appear to be more prevalent in diploid and tetraploid tumors (Table 3-10).

Other prognostic factors reported are expression of the tyrosine kinase receptor for nerve growth factor (*Trk-A, Trk-B and Trk-C*) (Table 3-10), CD44 expression, *HRAS* expression, LOH of chromosome 11q23 (in stage 4 NBs), deletions in the region of chromosome 9p22-p24, LOH of chromosome 14q, expression of the multidrug resistance genes (*MDR1*) or multidrug resistance-related protein (MRP), telomerase activity, partial genetic instability, *bcl-2* overexpression, and allelic imbalances of chromosomes 8q, 10p11, 12q24, and 19q13 and proliferation index assessed by immunohistochemical staining.[292–302]

High level of apoptosis and low AKT activation has been reported in mass screening NBs that tend to be associated with spontaneous regression compared to classical NBs.[302a] Interestingly, the expression of CD133, a cell membrane protein thought to be a marker of cancer stem cells in a host of tumors, has recently been shown by the same group to be present in just over a third of primary NBs and associated with poor outcome via chemoresistance mediated by the AKT pathway.[302b] Upregulation of carbonic anhydrase IX (hypoxia induced enzyme) and hypoxia-inducible factor 1α have been reported to be associated with adverse clinicopathologic and biologic factors by Dungwa et al.[302c,d] using immunohistochemistry and enzyme-linked immunosorbent assays. This group also reported that upregulation of the endothelial marker LYVE-1 assessed by the density of immunohistochemical staining and presence of lymphatic invasion correlated with adverse prognostic factors and lymph node metastases.[302e] They further performed expression analysis of the lymphangiogenic growth factors VEGF-C and VEGF-D, and their receptor VEGFR-3 in prechemotherapy biopsies from NBs and ganglioneuroblastomas. Increased VEGFR-3 lymphovascular receptor (VEGFR-3v), VEGF-D expression, and lymphovascular invasion were found to be associated with advanced clinical stage and high-risk disease.[302f] Duijkers et al.[302g] reported that high ALK immunohistochemical expression in NBs and ganglioneuroblastomas was a predictor of poor outcome.

Gene expression profiling has been used to predict behavior of NBs. Wei et al.[303] identified 19 predictor genes and reported that they were able to predict outcome for 98% of patients in the study group of 56 pretreatment samples from 49 NB patients. Along with *MYCN*, four other genes were upregulated in the poor outcome group (*DLK1, PRSS3, ARC,* and *SLIT3*) and three were downregulated (*CNR1, ROBO2,* and *BTBD3*). *DLK1*, a transmembrane protein that activates the Notch signaling pathway and has also been shown to inhibit neuronal differentiation, ranked highest. Of interest, one of the genes *ARH1*, which is downregulated in the poor prognostic group, maps to chromosome 1p31 and lies in close proximity to the 1p36 region, deletion of which has already been noted to be associated with high-risk NBs. Asgharzadeh et al.[304] determined the gene expression profiles of 102 untreated primary NBs without *MYCN* amplification but having metastatic disease. In their analysis, two subgroups of patients older than 12 months that were classified as having clinically high-risk disease were identified: a low-risk group with progression-free survival (PFS) of 79% and a high-risk group with a PFS of 16%. The *TrkB* gene was found to be the most statistically significant gene associated with risk of progression in the 55 candidate genes studied. More recently the role of miRNA profiling for risk stratification has been investigated. In the largest study, DePreter et al.[303a] reported that this modality enabled stratification into high- and low-risk groups from both fresh and archived paraffin-embedded tissue.

In summary, a wide array of biologic parameters, using different modalities, has been reported to influence prognosis of NBs. However, the INRG Biology Committee Biology Committee has recommended obligatory testing of *MYCN*, 11q23, and ploidy status for stratification into risk treatment groups.[303b]

OTHER ADRENAL MASS LESIONS

Abdominal imaging techniques, including ultrasound, CT, and MRI, have markedly increased the rate of discovery of nonfunctional adrenal mass lesions.[305–309] These are detected in approximately 5% of normal individuals and their prevalence

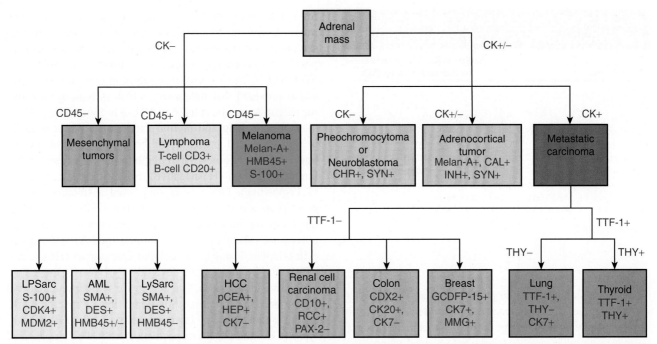

FIGURE 3-38 ■ Algorithm for immunohistochemical workup of adrenal tumor on needle biopsy. AML, angiomyolipoma; CAL, calretinin; CHR, chromogranin; CK, cytokeratin; DES, desmin; GCDFP, gross cystic disease fluid protein; HEP, hepatocyte; INH, inhibin; LySarc, leiomyosarcoma; MMG, mammoglobin; pCEA, polyclonal CEA; RCC, renal cell carcinoma; SMA, smooth muscle actin; THY, thyroglobulin; TTF-1, thyroid transcrption factor 1.

increases with the age of the population. As a group, these lesions have been referred to as "incidentalomas," and the differential diagnosis includes primary cortical and medullary tumors, metastatic tumors, cysts, myelolipomas, hyperplastic lesions, lymphoid hyperplasia, and periadrenal lesions.

According to the National Institutes of Health guidelines,[310,311] all patients with incidentalomas should have a 1-mg dexamethasone suppression test and measurement of plasma-free metanephrines. In addition, patients with hypertension should have measurements of serum potassium and plasma aldosterone concentration–plasma renin activity ratio. The presence of a homogeneous mass with a low attenuation (<10 Hounsfield units) on CT most likely represents a lipid-rich cortical adenoma. Patients with tumors >6 cm are usually treated surgically while those with tumors <4 cm are generally monitored. In those patients with tumors between 4 and 6 cm, criteria in addition to size should be considered in the decision to monitor or proceed with adrenalectomy. In general, surgery should be considered for all patients with functional adrenocortical tumors that are clinically apparent while all patients with pheochromocytomas should undergo surgery.

Fine-needle aspiration and core biopsies are important approaches for the differential diagnosis of adrenal mass lesions.[312] These procedures are typically performed when adrenal lesions cannot be accurately characterized by ultrasound, CT, MR imaging, or PET scanning. However, the interpretation of adrenal masses on core needle or fine-needle aspiration biopsies is a challenging process. Foremost is the determination of whether the biopsy is lesional. In the case of benign adrenocortical nodules or tumors, the lesions

may recapitulate the histology of the normal adrenal cortex, precluding a definite diagnosis of neoplasia on biopsy. As noted in the section on adrenocortical carcinomas, the diagnosis of adrenocortical carcinoma can be difficult even in resection specimens. Because of variability in a neoplasm, the area sampled may only permit a diagnosis of "consistent with adrenocortical neoplasm," to be rendered. Clearly, in functional tumors, differentiation from metastatic tumors or extension from adjacent structures is aided by biochemical studies when available. However, since the majority of cases that are encountered on needle biopsies are nonfunctional tumors, an immunohistochemical approach (Fig. 3-38) is most often used in conjunction with the cytologic features.

Metastatic Tumors

Secondary involvement of the adrenal glands has been reported in almost 30% of patients with metastatic tumors of diverse sites of origin[23] with bilateral involvement in almost 50%. The high frequency of adrenal metastases is most likely a result of the rich sinusoidal blood supply of the glands. In most series, from the United States and Western Europe, primary tumors of the lung and breast account for 60% of the cases (Box 3-6), followed by primary tumors of the gastrointestinal tract, kidney, and skin (melanoma). Adrenocortical carcinomas may also occasionally metastasize to the contralateral adrenal gland. Patients with metastatic carcinoma involving one or both adrenal glands may be seen initially for diagnosis of an intra-adrenal mass, and in such cases the primary tumor may not be evident until the time of autopsy. Although adrenal

Box 3-6 ● METASTATIC CARCINOMAS TO
ADRENAL GLAND (AUTOPSY BASED STUDIES)*

Carcinoma	Cases with Metastases to Adrenal Gland (%)
Breast	53.9
Lung	35.6
Kidney	24
Stomach	21
Pancreas	19
Ovary	17
Colon	14.4

*From Lack EE. AFIP Atlas of Tumor Pathology (series 4). *Tumors of the Adrenal Gland and Extra-Adrenal Paraganglia.* Washington, DC: American Registry of Pathology and Armed Forces Institute of Pathology; 2007.

insufficiency is uncommon in patients with adrenal metastasis, mild degrees of insufficiency may be evident.[313] Clinically significant adrenal hemorrhage secondary to adrenal metastases may occur but is rare.[314] Metastases to cortical adenomas[315] and pheochromocytomas[316] have been reported.

Grossly, metastases appear as multiple or single firm masses that replace all or part of the glands (Fig. 3-39A). Larger metastases are often necrotic and hemorrhagic, and may therefore simulate adrenocortical carcinomas. The microscopic appearances of metastatic lesions differ according to their sites of origin. While most such lesions are recognizable as metastases, their distinction from primary adrenal tumors may be difficult. Generally, however, metastatic carcinomas can be distinguished from other tumor types on the basis of immunohistochemistry (Fig. 3-38).

Metastatic carcinomas are positive for broad-spectrum cytokeratins while adrenocortical tumors may be positive or negative. Most melanomas and sarcomas are negative for cytokeratins; however, some sarcomas (e.g., synovial sarcoma, epithelioid variants of leiomyosarcoma, and liposarcoma) and occasional melanomas may be cytokeratin-positive. Accordingly, melan-A, inhibin, calretinin, and SF-1 will be most useful in establishing an adrenocortical origin provided that melanoma, which is typically positive for melan-A, can be ruled out. TTF-1 is commonly positive in metastatic lung and thyroid carcinomas, but is negative in non-small-cell primaries of breast, the gastrointestinal tract, liver, and kidney. Thyroglobulin (THY) is used to differentiate lung (THY-negative) from thyroid carcinomas (THY-positive). Other commonly used antibodies include gross cystic disease fluid protein 15 (GCDFP-15) and mammoglobin for breast; CDX2 for gastrointestinal primaries; polyclonal carcinoembryonic antigen (pCEA) and hepatocyte (HepPar-1) for hepatocellular carcinomas (HCC); and CD10, RCC antigen, and PAX-2[141,317,318] for RCCs. CD45 is positive in and is used to screen for lymphoreticular and hematopoietic neoplasms. Additional lineage specific markers are used for further classification into T-cell or B-cell subtypes (CD3 and CD20, respectively). It must be emphasized that the algorithmic approach, summarized in Figure 3-38, is a simplification, since sensitivity and specificity of the different immunohistochemical markers vary, so that despite adequate material on a biopsy, one neoplasm can only be favored over another, without a definitive diagnosis in some cases.

Malignant Lymphoma and Leukemia

Secondary involvement of the adrenal glands occurs in up to 25% of patients with disseminated malignant lymphoma studied at autopsy.[43] Both Hodgkin disease and non-Hodgkin lymphomas have been reported, with a higher frequency for non-Hodgkin lymphomas. Adrenal insufficiency as a result of leukemic or lymphomatous involvement is rare and most likely to occur in patients with high-grade tumors.[319,320]

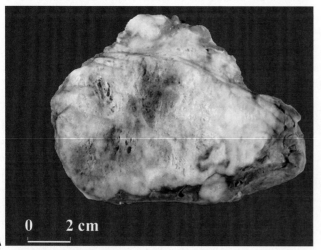

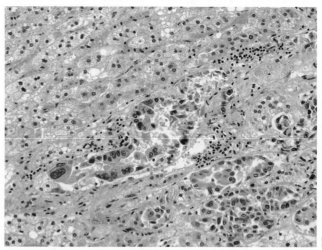

A   **B**

FIGURE 3-39 ■ Adrenal gland involved by metastatic carcinoma. The adrenal gland from an autopsy case in which there was a large lung primary. Grossly, the metastatic tumor is relatively circumscribed, but also infiltrates the periadrenal fat (**A,** courtesy of Dr. K. Singh, Providence, RI). The histologic section demonstrates an adenocarcinoma adjacent to adrenocortical cells (**B**).

Adrenal involvement can be unilateral or bilateral, and tumors can range in size from those of microscopic dimensions to those that replace the adrenal and adjacent structures (Fig. 3-40A and B). The gross appearance can be identical to that of adrenocortical carcinomas. Histologic characteristics vary according to the type of lymphoma. These tumors can be distinguished from other tumor types on the basis of positive staining for CD45 and other markers of lymphoid differentiation. Very rare examples of primary lymphomas of the adrenal glands have also been reported.[319–322] Virtually all of the primary adrenal lymphomas have been of the non-Hodgkin large-cell type (Fig. 3-40C), including the large-cell angiotrophic variant.[320] Leukemic involvement of the kidney is typically identified as an incidental finding at autopsy.

Myelolipoma

The myelolipoma is a benign tumor-like lesion of the adrenal gland composed of mature adipose tissue admixed with hematopoietic cells. Lesions of identical morphology may develop in a variety of extra-adrenal sites, particularly the retroperitoneum. Foci of myelolipomatous change may be found in cortical tumors and within otherwise normal adrenal glands.[23,323] As a result, it has been debatable as to whether myelolipomas are true neoplasms or represent a reactive process. However, Bishop et al.[324] demonstrated nonrandom X-chromosome inactivation in the hematopoietic elements and fat in 8 of 11 myelolipomas from female patients in support of a clonal origin of these lesions and hence neoplastic nature.

The mean age at diagnosis is approximately 50 years, and most patients are asymptomatic. Sometimes, however, patients have evidence of flank pain with or without a palpable mass or hematuria. Myelolipomas are unilateral non-encapsulated but circumscribed lesions that are bright yellow with foci of tan-brown discoloration[43] (Fig. 3-41A). They vary considerably in size, from those that are of microscopic

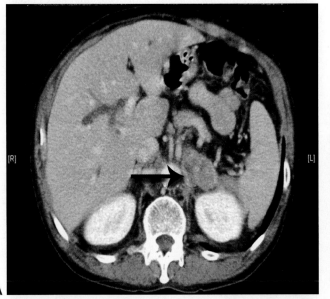

A

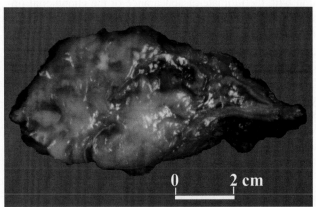

B

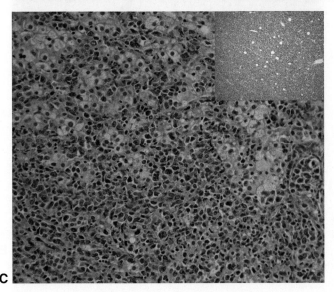

C

FIGURE 3-40 ■ Adrenal lymphoma. CT image of the abdomen demonstrates effacement of the left adrenal gland by tumor (**A; arrow**) without evidence of retroperitoneal lymph node enlargement. The gross image of the gland demonstrates involvement by a grey "fish flesh" tumor with *white* areas corresponding to foci of necrosis (**B**). The H&E section demonstrates infiltration by large neoplastic cells with high nuclear to cytoplasmic ratio in the lower filed and adrnocotical cells in the upper field (**C**). The neoplastic cells are diffusely positive for CD20 (**inset**), confirming the diagnosis of diffuse large B-cell non-Hodgkin lymphoma.

dimensions to those that fill the abdomen. At the microscopic level, the lesions are composed of mature adipose tissue with scattered islands of hematopoietic cells[325] (Fig. 3-41B). Areas of necrosis, hemorrhage, cyst formation, and calcification or ossification may also be evident, particularly in larger lesions.

Cysts and Pseudocysts

Although adrenal cysts are uncommon, their rate of detection as a result of CT and MRI scanning has increased dramatically. Most adrenal cysts are unilateral, and occur more frequently in females than in males. Symptomatic cysts may be associated with flank pain or gastrointestinal complaints. Adrenal cysts may be divided into four major categories, including epithelial cysts, parasitic cysts, endothelial (vascular) cysts, and pseudocysts.[43,326] The term pseudocyst describes a lesion that lacks recognizable endothelial or epithelial cells. Typically, pseudocysts are unilocular. Pseudocysts range in size from 1.8 to 10 cm, but lesions of considerably larger size have been reported. The cysts usually contain hemorrhagic fibrinous material while the wall is composed of dense fibrous tissue with areas of calcification and granulation tissue. Many adrenal pseudocysts probably develop as lymphangioendothelial cysts that undergo episodes of hemorrhage, fibrosis, and hemosiderin deposition with the ultimate disappearance of the endothelial lining.[327] This conclusion is based on the occasional presence of residual lining cells that are positive for factor VIII–related antigen. Occasionally, abundant elastic tissue may be present within the cyst wall, further suggesting a vascular origin.

True vascular cysts are typically multilocular and are most likely related to preexisting adrenal hemorrhage with subsequent organization and endothelialization or to benign vascular lesions. They are lined by flattened endothelial cells. True epithelial cysts include retention cysts, some of which are of mesothelial origin, embryonal cysts, and cystic neoplasms. As noted in the other sections, any adrenal neoplasm may contain foci of cystic change. Rarely such cystic change may involve a neoplasm almost entirely so that on imaging studies they simulate a cyst or pseudocyst, but on pathologic examination residual mural tumor nodules are present. Erickson et al.[328] reported 2 adrenal cortical carcinomas, 2 adrenal cortical adenomas, and 2 pheochromocytomas associated with 6 of 32 pseudocysts from the archives of the Mayo Clinic over a 25-year period.[328] An additional case of pheochromocytoma was associated with an endothelial cyst. Parasitic cysts are the least common adrenal cysts and are most often due to echinococcal infection.

Adenomatoid Tumor

Adenomatoid tumors occur most commonly in the genital tract, but similar lesions may rarely arise within the adrenal gland. They are generally small, with infiltrative margins, and may appear solid or cystic with occasional cases having a papillary architecture.[329] Adenomatoid tumors are composed of nests and cords of epithelioid cells forming glands and tubules (Fig. 3-42). The epithelioid cells may have a flattened appearance resembling endothelial cells; however, the tumor cells are positive for cytokeratins and are characterized by the presence of desmosomes and microvilli, consistent with mesothelial origin.[330,331] Moreover, the cells are positive for calretinin.[332]

Mesenchymal Tumors

Both benign and malignant mesenchymal tumors may occur as primary adrenal tumors and include hemangiomas, lipomas, leiomyomas, osteomas, neurofibromas, angiomyolipomas, and schwannomas (neurilemomas).[23,43,72,333] Among

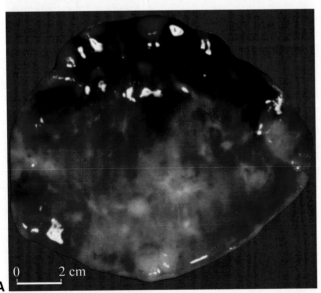

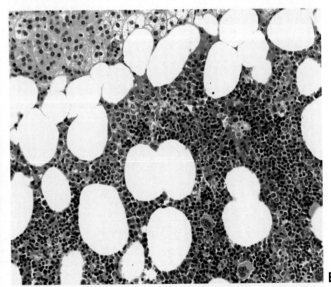

FIGURE 3-41 ■ Adrenal myelolipoma. The cut surface this tumor has a mottled *yellow brown* appearance (**A**). Histologic section demonstrates islands of hematopoietic tissue scattered among the fat cells (**B**).

the benign tumors, cavernous hemangiomas are the most common and are usually detected as incidental findings at surgery or autopsy. Most hemangiomas are solitary and unilateral (Fig. 3-43). Hemangiomas should be distinguished from adrenal cortical adenomas with degenerative changes and secondary vascular proliferation. The gross and histologic features of adrenal neurofibromas and schwannomas are identical to those of similar tumors found at other sites. Of note, Lau et al.[333a] reported two cases of primary adrenal schwannomas that were over 9 cm in size, one of which had a cellular morphology. Leiomyomas are rare and most

likely originate from smooth muscle cells of the central vein. Solitary fibrous tumor and calcifying fibrous tumor/pseudotumor have also been reported within the adrenal gland[334–336].

Although primary adrenal sarcomas have been reported, it must be remembered that a primary retroperitoneal sarcomas growing around the adrenal gland may simulate an adrenal primary on imaging studies. Angiosarcomas arising within the adrenal gland are extremely rare. In a series of 10 angiosarcomas reported by Wenig and Heffess,[337] the tumors ranged in size from 6 to 10 cm and were composed

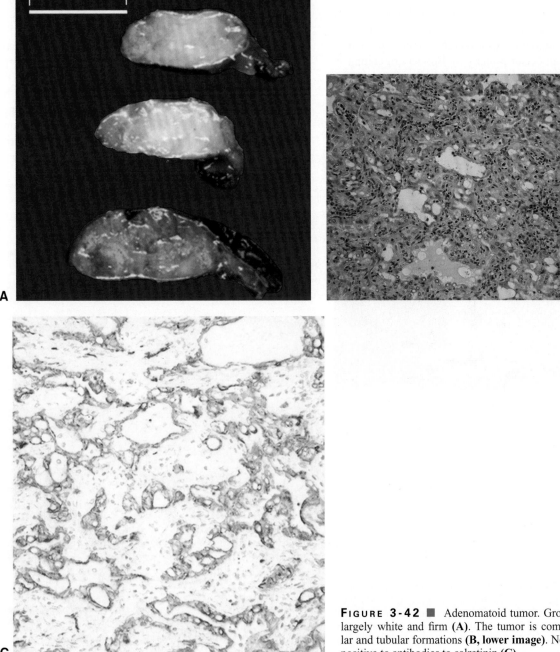

FIGURE 3-42 ■ Adenomatoid tumor. Grossly, the tumor is largely white and firm **(A)**. The tumor is composed of glandular and tubular formations **(B, lower image)**. Neoplastic cells are positive to antibodies to calretinin **(C)**.

of spindle-shaped and/or epithelioid cells. A vascular origin was confirmed by the finding of positive staining for factor VIII–related antigen and CD34. Epithelioid angiosarcomas may show focal keratin immunoreactivity, similar to epithelioid angiosarcomas occurring at other sites. Rarely, extensive hemorrhagic infarction of an adrenal adenoma with the formation of pseudovascular spaces lined by large, atypical fibroblasts may mimic a primary adrenal angiosarcoma.[338] Leiomyosarcomas, including cases of pleomorphic leiomyosarcoma of the adrenal gland with osteoclast-like giant cells, and malignant peripheral nerve sheath tumors rarely may develop as primary adrenal gland malignancies.[339–341]

Other Tumors and Tumor-like Lesions

Primary adrenal melanomas are rare and controversial tumors with approximately 10 well documented cases reported in the literature. Considerably more common is the presence of an occult primary melanoma originating in the skin, mucous membranes, or eyes with metastasis to the adrenal gland.[342,343] Dao et al.[343] have proposed that adrenal melanomas can arise from pheochromocytomas, which produce melanin rather than catecholamines. Moreover, they suggest that these tumors should be classified as malignant melanotic pheochromocytomas. It should be remembered, however, that some pheochromocytomas, similar to other neuroectodermal tumors, may contain melanin pigment. Typically, pheochromocytomas are positive for synaptophysin and chromogranin while melanomas are positive for S-100 protein, tyrosinase, melan-A, and HMB-45. Of particular interest has been the observation that approximately one-third of nonmelanotic pheochromocytomas exhibit positivity for the melanoma-specific antibody HMB-45.[344]

Angiomyolipoma may be primary within the adrenal gland[333] or may arise from the upper pole of adjacent kidney such that its exact origin may not be discernible on imaging studies. Since these lesions can be dominated by HMB-45-positive epithelioid cells, distinction from melanoma is made by absent staining with melan-A.

Ovarian thecal metaplasia refers to a focal subcapsular proliferation of spindle cells that resemble ovarian stroma.[345] This is an uncommon lesion that has been reported in <5% of women undergoing adrenalectomy for metastatic breast carcinoma. A similar lesion may occur in men but is exceptionally uncommon. The spindle cells may be surrounded by a collagenous matrix, and groups of cortical cells may be admixed with the spindle cells. Very rarely, gross enlargement of the adrenals may result from similar proliferations of spindle cells.[346] Granulosa cell and Leydig cell tumors have also been reported within the adrenal glands.[347,348]

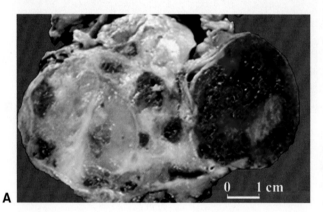

A

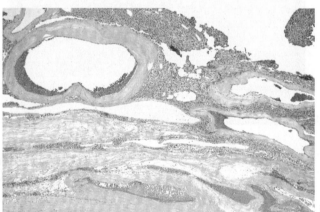

B

C

FIGURE 3-43 ■ Adrenocortical hemangioma. This tumor is composed of a large area of sclerosis on the left (**A**, Courtesy of Dr. W. Greaves, Providence, R.I.). Histologic sections demonstrate different caliber vessels intermixed with adrenal cortical tissue and cavernous spaces with some vessels having sclerosed walls (**B**). High-power demonstrates normal appearing endothelial cells of the vessels (**C**).

Dysembryonic neoplasms and adrenocortical blastomas are exceptionally uncommon. Santonja et al.[349] have reported a single case of a primary adrenal tumor in a 4-year-old boy with features of Wilms tumor. The tumor was composed of blastemal nodules, primitive tubules, glomeruloid structures, and areas resembling sclerotic nephrogenic rests. Molberg et al.[350] have reported a malignant virilizing adrenocortical tumor in a 21-month-old child with elevated alpha fetoprotein levels. The neoplasm was composed of immature epithelial and mesenchymal elements including slit-like spaces lined by primitive epithelial cells. They felt the histologic features were reminiscent of the embryonic adrenal cortex so they used the term "adrenocortical blastoma."[350]

Mixed corticomedullary tumors composed of admixtures of cortical and medullary cells are exceptionally rare and <20 cases have been reported.[351,352] While some of these cases most likely represent collision tumors, others have been characterized by intimate admixtures of cortical and medullary cells. A recent example has been reported to demonstrate features of malignancy.[352]

Sustentaculoma is a distinctive neoplasm of the adrenal medulla reported by Lau et al.[353] that pursued a benign course on limited follow-up. The authors described a well circumscribed tumor characterized by ill-defined, irregular nests of spindle cells with eosinophilic cytoplasm and elongated nuclei having tiny nucleoli. There was an accompanying lymphoplasmacytic inflammatory infiltrate. Immunohistochemical staining demonstrated positive staining with antibodies to S-100 protein and CD56, but distinction from a spindle-cell pheochromocytoma was aided by negative staining with antibodies to synaptophysin and chromogranin. Dendritic cell markers and melanoma-associated antigens were also negative. On ultrastructural examination, the lesional cells were devoid of secretory granules and basal lamina. The latter feature was used to distinguish the lesion from a schwannoma.

REFERENCES

1. Young WF. The incidentally discovered adrenal mass. *N Engl J Med* 2007;356:601–610.
2. Seron-Ferre M, Jaffee RB. The fetal adrenal gland. *Annu Rev Physiol* 1981;43:141–162.
3. Beck K, Tygstrup I, Nerup J. The involution of the fetal adrenal cortex: a light microscopic study. *Acta Pathol Microbiol Scand* 1969;76:391–400.
4. Coupland RE. The development and fate of catecholamine secreting endocrine cells. In: Parvez H, Parez S. *Biogenic Amines in Development.* Amsterdam: Elsevier/North Holland; 1980:3–28.
5. Tischler AS. Paraganglia. In: Sternberg SS, ed. *Histology for Pathologists.* 2nd ed. Philadelphia, PA: Lippincott-Raven Publishers; 1997.
6. Symington T. The adrenal cortex. In: Bloodworth JMB Jr, ed. *Endocrine Pathology General and Surgical.* Baltimore, MD: Williams & Wilkins; 1982:419–472.
7. Quinan C, Berger AA. Observations on human adrenals with especial reference to the relative weight of the normal medulla. *Ann Intern Med* 1933;6:1180–1192.
8. Dobbie JW, Symington T. The human adrenal gland with special reference to the vasculature. *J Endocrinol* 1966;34:479–489.
9. Neville AM, O'Hare MJ. Aspects of structure, function and pathology. In: James VHT, ed. *The Adrenal Gland.* New York, NY: Raven Press; 1979:165.
10. Motto P, Muto M, Fujita T. Three dimensional organization of mammalian adrenal cortex. *Cell Tissue Res* 1979;196:23–38.
11. Lack EE. AFIP Atlas of Tumor Pathology (series 4). *Tumors of the Adrenal Gland and Extra-Adrenal Paraganglia.* Washington, DC: American Registry of Pathology and Armed Forces Institute of Pathology; 2007.
12. Miettinen M, Lehto VP, Virtanen I. Immunofluorescence microscopic evaluation of the intermediate filament expression of the adrenal cortex and medulla and their tumors. *Am J Pathol* 1985;118:360–366.
13. Jorda M, De MB, Nadji M. Calretinin and inhibin A are useful in separating adrenal cortical neoplasms from pheochromocytomas. *Appl Immunohistochem Mol Morph* 2002;10:67–70.
14. Busam KJ, Iversen K, Coplan KA, et al. Immunoreactivity for A103, an antibody to Melan-A (Mart-1), in adrenocortical and other steroid tumors. *Am J Surg Pathol* 1998;22:57–63.
15. Renshaw AA, Granter SR. A comparison of A103 and inhibin reactivity in adrenal cortical tumors: distinction from hepatocellular carcinoma and renal tumors. *Mod Pathol* 1998;11:1160–1164.
16. Schröder S, Padberg BC, Achilles E, et al. Immunohistochemistry in adrenocortical tumors: a clinicomorphological study of 72 neoplasms. *Virchows Arch A Pathol Anat Histopathol* 1992;420:65–70.
17. Lloyd RV, Douglas BR, Young WF. *Atlas of Non Tumor Pathology. Endocrine Disease.* Washington, DC: American Registry of Pathology & AFIP; 2002.
18. Hayashi Y, Hiyoshi T, Takemura T, et al. Focal lymphocytic infiltration in the adrenal cortex of the elderly: immunohistological analysis of infiltrating lymphocytes. *Clin Exp Immunol* 1998;77:101–105.
19. Boggaram V, Funkenstein B, Waterman MR, et al. Lipoproteins and the regulation of adrenal steroidogenesis. *Endocr Res* 1985;10:387–409.
20. Bondy P. Disorders of the adrenal cortex. In: Wilson JD, Foster DW, eds. *Williams' Textbook of Endocrinology.* Philadelphia, PA: WB Saunders; 1985:816–891.
21. Carey RM, Sen S, Dolan LM, et al. Idiopathic hyperaldosteronism: a possible role for aldosterone stimulation factor. *N Engl J Med* 1984; 311:94–100.
22. Sen S, Bumpus FM, Oberfield S, et al. Development and preliminary application of a new assay for aldosterone stimulation factor. *Hypertension* 1983;5(suppl 1):127–131.
23. Page DL, DeLellis RA, Hough AJ. Tumors of the adrenal. *Atlas of Tumor Pathology.* 2nd series, fascicle 23. Washington, DC: Armed Forces Institute of Pathology; 1985.
24. Dekker A, Oehrle JS. Hyaline globules of the adrenal medulla of man. *Arch Pathol* 1971;91:353–364.
25. Grynszpan-Winograd O. Ultrastructure of the chromaffin cell. In: Greep RO, Astwood EB, eds. *Handbook of Physiology.* Washington, DC: American Physiological Society; 1975:295–308.
26. Fawcett DW, Long JA, Jones AL. The ultrastructure of endocrine glands. *Recent Prog Horm Res* 1969;25:315–380.
27. Winkler H, Smith AD. The chromaffin granule and the storage of catecholamines. In: Greep RO, Astwood EB, eds. *Endocrinology.* Washington, DC: American Physiological Society; 1975:321–339.
28. Sherwin RP. The adrenal medulla paraganglia and related tissues. In: Bloodworth JMB, ed. *Endocrine Pathology.* Baltimore, MD: Williams & Wilkins; 1968:256–315.
29. DeLaTorre JC, Surgeon JW. A methodological approach to rapid and sensitive monoamine histofluorescence using a modified glyoxylic acid technique. *Histochemistry* 1976;45:81–99.
30. Falck B, Owman C. A detailed methodological description of the fluorescence method for the cellular demonstration of biogenic monoamines. *Acta Univ Lund* (Sect II) 1965;2:523.
31. Lloyd RV, Sisson JC, Shapiro B, et al. Immunohistochemical localization of epinephrine, norepinephrine, catecholamine synthesizing enzymes and chromogranin in neuroendocrine cells and tumors. *Am J Pathol* 1986;125:45–54.
32. Gould VE, Lee I, Wiedemann B, et al. Synaptophysin: a novel marker for neurons, certain neuroendocrine cells and their neoplasms. *Hum Pathol* 1986;17:979–983.
33. Hassoun J, Monges G, Giraud P, et al. Immunohistochemical study of pheochromocytomas: an investigation of methionine enkephalin,

vasoactive intestinal peptide, somatostatin corticotropin, β-endorphin and calcitonin in 16 tumors. *Am J Pathol* 1984;114:56–63.

34. Lloyd RV, Blaivas M, Wilson BS. Distribution of chromogranin and S-100-protein in normal and abnormal adrenal medullary tissues. *Arch Pathol Lab Med* 1985;109:633–635.

35. Schmechel D. Gamma subunit of the glycolytic enzyme enolase: non-specific or neuron specific? *Lab Invest* 1985;52:239–242.

36. Gutowski T, Gray GF. Ectopic adrenal in inguinal hernia sacs. *J Urol* 1979;121:353–354.

37. Lack EE. *Pathology of the Adrenal Glands*. New York, NY: Churchill Livingstone; 1990.

38. MacLennan A. On the presence of adrenal rests in hernial sac walls. *Surg Gynecol Obstet* 1919;29:387.

39. Burke EF, Gilbert E, Uehling DT. Adrenal rest tumors of the testes. *J Urol* 1973;109:649–652.

40. Johnson RE, Scheithauer B. Massive hyperplasia of testicular adrenal rests in a patient with Nelson's syndrome. *Am J Clin Pathol* 1982; 77:501–507.

41. Dolan MF, Janouski NA. Adrenohepatic union. *Arch Pathol* 1968;86:22.

42. O'Crowley CR, Martland HS. Adrenal heterotopia, rests and the so-called Grawitz tumor. *J Urol* 1943;50:576.

43. Lack EE. *Tumors of the Adrenal Gland and Extra-Adrenal Paraganglia*. Washington, DC: Armed Forces Institute of Pathology; 1997.

44. Benirschke K. Adrenals in anencephaly and hydrocephaly. *Obstet Gynecol* 1956;8:442.

45. McKusick VA, et al. Adrenal hypoplasia, congenital. www.ncbi.nlm.nih.gov/omim/300200

46. Wise JE, Matalon R, Morgan AM, et al. Phenotypic features of patients with congenital adrenal hypoplasia and glycerol kinase deficiency. *Am J Dis Child* 1987;141:744–747.

47. Burris TP, Guo W, McCabe ER. The gene responsible for congenital adrenal hypoplasia DAX-1, encodes a nuclear hormone receptor that defines a new class within the superfamily. *Recent Prog Horm Res* 1996;54:241.

48. Oppenheimer EH. Adrenal cytomegaly: studies by light and electron microscopy in Beckwith's syndrome. *Arch Pathol* 1970;90:57–64.

49. McCawley RG, Beckwith JB, Elias ER, et al. Benign hemorrhagic macrocysts in Beckwith-Wiedemann syndrome. *AJR* 1991;157:549–552.

50. Cohen MM Jr. Beckwith-Wiedemann syndrome: historical clinicopathological and etiopathogenetic perspectves. *Pediatr Dev Pathol* 2005;8:287–304.

51. Ghatak NR, Nochlin D, Peris M. Morphology and distribution of cytoplasmic inclusions in adrenoleukodystrophy. *J Neurol Sci* 1981;50:391.

52. McKusick VA, et al. Adrenoleukodystrophy. www.ncbi.nlm.nih.gov/omim/300100

53. Moser HW, Loes DJ, Melhem ER, et al. X-linked adrenoleukodystrophy: overview and prognosis as a function of age and brain magnetic resonance imaging abnormality: a study involving 372 patients. *Neuropediatrics* 2000;31:227–239.

54. Cartier N, Lopez J, Moullier P, et al. Retroviral-mediated gene transfer connects very long chain fatty acid metabolism in adrenoleukodystrophy fibroblasts. *Proc Natl Acad Sci U S A* 1995;92:1674.

55. Powers JM, Schaumberg HH, Johnson AB, et al. A correlative study of the adrenal cortex in adrenoleukodystrophy: evidence for a fatal intoxication with very long chain saturated fatty acids. *Invest Cell Pathol* 1980;3:3–53.

56. Schaumberg HH, Powers JM, Raine CS. Adrenomyeloneuropathy: a probable variant of adrenoleukodystrophy. II. General pathologic, neuropathologic and biochemical aspects. *Neurology* 1977;27:11–14.

57. Wolman M, Sterk VV, Gratt S, et al. Primary familial xanthomatosis with involvement and calcification of adrenal. Report of two more cases in siblings of a previously described infant. *Pediatrics* 1961;28:742–757.

58. White PC, New MI, Dupont D. Congenital adrenal hyperplasia. *N Engl J Med* 1987;316:1519–1524, 1580–1586.

59. McKusick VA, et al. Adrenal hyperplasia, congenital, due to 21-hydroxylase deficiency. www.ncbi.nlm.nih.gov/omim/201910

60. Hughes I. Congenital adrenal hyperplasia: phenotype and genotypes. *J Pediatr Endocrinol Metab* 2002;15(suppl 15):1529–1340.

61. Peter M. Congenital adrenal hyperplasia: 11 beta-hydroxylase deficiency. *Semin Reprod Med* 2002;20:249–254.

62. Auchus RJ. The genetics, pathophysiology and management of deficiencies of P450$_{c17}$. *Endocrinol Metab Clin North Am* 2001;30:101–119.

63. McKusick VA, et al. 3-beta hydroxysteroid dehydrogenase II: HSD3B2. www.ncbi.nlm.nih.gov/omim/201810

64. Daeschner GL. Adrenal cortical adenoma arising in a girl with congenital adrenogenital syndrome. *Pediatr Pathol* 1965;36:140–142.

65. Jaursch-Hancke C, Allollio B, Meltzer U, et al. Adrenal cortical carcinoma in patients with untreated congenital adrenal hyperplasia. *Acta Endocrinol* 1988;117:146–147.

66. Rutgers JL, Young RH, Scully RE. The testicular tumor of the adrenogenital syndrome: a report of 6 cases and review of the literature on testicular masses in patients with adrenocortical disorders. *Am J Surg Pathol* 1988;12:503–513.

67. Weetman AP. Autoimmunity to steroid producing cells and familial polyendocrinopathy. *Ballieres Clin Endocrinol Metab* 1995;9:157–174.

68. Neufeld M, MacLaren NK, Blizzard RM. Two types of autoimmune Addison's disease associated with different polyglandular autoimmune syndromes. *Medicine* 1981;60:355–362.

69. Wang CY, Davoodi-Semiromi A, Huang W, et al. Characterization of mutations in patients with autoimmune polyglandular syndrome type I (APSI). *Hum Genet* 1998;103:681–685.

70. Ahonen P. Autoimmune polyendocrinopathy—candidiasis ectodermal dystrophy (APECED): autosomal recessive inheritance. *Clin Genet* 1985;27:535–542.

71. Grinspoon SK, Bilezikian JP. HIV disease and the endocrine system. *N Engl J Med* 1992;327:1360–1365.

72. Wenig BM, Heffess CS, Adair CF. *Atlas of Endocrine Pathology*. Philadelphia, PA: WB Saunders; 1997.

73. Friderichsen C. Waterhouse-Friderichsen syndrome. *Acta Endocrinol* 1955;18:482–492.

74. Kuhajda FP, Hutchins GM. Adrenal corticomedullary junction necrosis: a morphological marker for hypotension. *Am Heart J* 1979;98:294–297.

75. Haroche J, Amoura Z, Toouraine P, et al. Bilateral adrenal infiltration in Erdheim-Chester disease. Report of seven cases and literature review. *J Clin End Metab* 2007;92:2007–2012.

76. Burch C. Cushing's disease: a review. *Arch Intern Med* 1985;145: 1106–1111.

77. Upton GV, Amatruda TT. Evidence for the presence of tumor peptide with corticotropin-releasing factor like activity in the ectopic ACTH syndrome. *N Engl J Med* 1971;285:419–424.

78. Reibord H, Fisher ER. Electron microscopic study of adrenal cortical hyperplasia in Cushing's syndrome. *Arch Pathol* 1968;86:419–426.

79. Neville AM, Symington T. Bilateral adrenal cortical hyperplasia in children with Cushing's syndrome. *J Pathol* 1972;107:95–106.

80. Carey RM, Varma SK, Drake CR, et al. Ectopic secretion of corticotropin releasing factor as a cause of Cushing's syndrome: a clinical, morphological and biochemical study. *N Engl J Med* 1984;311:13–20.

81. Zarate A, Kovacs K, Flores M, et al. ACTH and CRF-producing bronchial carcinoid associated with Cushing's syndrome. *Clin Endocrinol (Oxf)* 1986;24:523.

82. Neville AM, Symington T. The pathology of the adrenal in Cushing's syndrome. *J Pathol Bacteriol* 1967;93:19–35.

83. Hidai H, Fuji H, Otsuka K, et al. Cushing's syndrome due to huge adrenocortical multinodular hyperplasia. *Endocrinol Jpn* 1975;22:555–560.

84. Neville AM. The nodular adrenal. *Invest Cell Pathol* 1978;1:99–111.

85. Josse RG, Bear R, Kovacs K, Higgins HP. Cushing's syndrome due to unilateral nodular adrenal hyperplasia: a new pathophysiologic entity? *Acta Endocrinol* 1980;93:495–504.

86. Bourdeau I, Stratakis CA. Cyclic AMP dependent signaling aberrations in macronodular adrenal disease. *Ann N Y Acad Sci* 2002;968:240–255.

87. Meador CK, Bowdoin B, Owen WC, et al. Primary adrenocortical nodular dysplasia: a rare cause of Cushing's syndrome. *J Clin Endocrinol Metab* 1967;27:1255–1263.

88. Hasleton PS, Ali HH, Anfield C, et al. Micronodular adrenal disease: a light and electron microscopic study. *J Clin Pathol* 1982;35:1078–1085.

89. Schweizer-Cagianut M, Froesch ER, Hedinger C. Familial Cushing's syndrome with primary adrenocortical microadenomatosis (primary adrenocortical nodular dysplasia). *Acta Endocrinol* 1980;94:529–535.

90. Shenoy BV, Carpenter PC, Carney JA. Bilateral primary pigmented nodular adrenocortical disease: rare cause of the Cushing syndrome. *Am J Surg Pathol* 1984;8:335–344.

91. Carney JA, Young WF. Primary pigmented nodular adrenal cortical disease and its associated conditions. *Endocrinologist* 1992;2:6–21.

92. Groussin L, Jullian E, Perlemoine K, et al. Mutations of the PRKAR1A gene in Cushing's syndrome due to sporadic primary pigmented nodular adrenal cortical disease. *J Clin Endocrinol Metab* 2002;87:4324–4329.

93. Stratakis CA. Mutations of the gene encoding the protein kinase A type Iα regulatory subunit (PRKAR1A) in patients with the "complex of spotty skin pigmentation, myxomas, endocrine overactivity and schwannomas" (Carney complex). *Ann N Y Acad Sci* 2002;968:3–21.

94. Wulffraat NM, Drexhage HA, Wiersinga WM, et al. Immunoglobulins of patients with Cushing's syndrome due to pigmented adrenocortical micronodular dysplasia stimulate in vitro steroidogenesis. *J Clin Endocrinol Metab* 1988;66:601.

95. Howarth A, Boikos S, Giatzakis C, et al. A genome wide scan identifies mutations in the gene encoding phosphodiesterase 11A4 (PDE11A) in individuals with adrenocortical hyperplasia. *Nat Genet* 2006;38:794–800.

96. Howath A, Giatzakas C, Robinson-White A, et al. Adrenal hyperplasia and adenomas are associated with inhhibition of phosphodiesterase 11A in carriers of PDE11A sequence variants that are frequent in the population. *Cancer Res* 2006;66:1157-S.

97. Young WF. Pheochromocytoma and primary aldosteronism: diagnostic approaches. *Endocrinol Metab Clin North Am* 1997;26:801–827.

98. Bravo EL, Tarazi RC, Dustan HP, et al. The changing clinical spectrum of primary aldosteronism. *Am J Med* 1983;74:641–651.

99. Conn JW, Knopf RF, Nesbit RM. Clinical characteristic of primary aldosteronism from an analysis of 145 cases. *Am J Surg* 1964;107:159.

100. Bertagna C, Orth DN. Clinical and laboratory findings and results of therapy in 58 patients with adrenocortical tumors admitted to a single medical center (1951–1978). *Am J Med* 1981;71:855–875.

101. Dobbie JM. Adrenal cortical nodular hyperplasia: the aging adrenal. *J Pathol* 1969;99:1–18.

102. Gicquel C, Leblond-Francillard M, Bertagna X, et al. Clonal analysis of human adrenal cortical carcinomas and secreting adenomas. *Clin Endocrinol (Oxf)* 1994;40:465–477.

103. Neville AM, Symington T. Pathology of primary aldosteronism. *Cancer* 1966;19:1854–1868.

104. Caplan RH, Virata RL. Functional black adenoma of the adrenal cortex: a rare cause of primary aldosteronism. *Am J Clin Pathol* 1974;62:97–103.

105. Pollock WJ, McConnell CF, Hilton C, et al. Virilizing Leydig cell adenoma of the adrenal gland. *Am J Surg Pathol* 1986;10:816–822.

106. Ryan JJ, Rezkalla MA, Rizk SN, et al. Testosterone-secreting adrenal adenoma that contained crystalloids of Reinke in an adult female patient. *Mayo Clinic Proc* 1995;70:380–383.

107. Sasano H, Szuki T, Sano T, et al. Adrenocortical oncocytoma: a true nonfunctioning adrenal cortical tumor. *Am J Surg Pathol* 1991;15:949–956.

108. Lin BT, Bonsib SM, Mierau GW, et al. Oncocytic adrenocortical neoplasms: a report of seven cases and review of the literature *Am J Surg Pathol* 1998;22:603–614.

109. Bisceglia M. Ludovico O, Di Mattia A, et al. Adrenocortical oncocytic tumors: report of 10 cases and review of the literature. *Int J Surg Pathol* 2004;12:231–243.

109a. Wong DD, Spagnolo DV, Bisceglia M, et al. Oncocytic adrenocortical neoplasms—a clinicopathologic study of 13 new cases emphasizing the importance of their recognition. *Hum Pathol* 2011;42:489–499.

110. Erlandson RA, Reuter VE. Oncocytic adrenal cortical adenoma. *Ultrastruct Pathol* 1991;15:539–547.

111. Xiao GQ, Pertsemlidis DS, Unger PD. Functioning adrenocortical oncocytoma: a case report and review of the literature. *Ann Diagn Pathol* 2005;9:295–297.

112. Corsi A, Riminucci M, Petrozza V, et al. Incidentally detected giant oncocytoma arising in retroperitoneal heterotopic adrenal tissue. *Arch Pathol Lab Med* 2002;126:1118–1122.

113. El-Naggar AK, Evans DB, Mackay B. Oncocytic adrenal cortical carcinoma. *Ultrastruct Pathol* 1991;15:549–556.

113a. Bisceglia M, Ben-Dor D, Pasquinelli G. Oncocytic adrenocortical tumors. *Pathol Case Rev* 2005;10:228–242.

113b. Duregon E, Volante M, Cappia S, et al. Oncocytic adrenal cortical tumors: diagnostic algorithm and mitochondrial DNA profile in 27 cases. *Am J Surg Pathol* 2011;35:1882–1893.

114. Correa P, Chen VW. Endocrine gland cancer. *Cancer* 1995;75:338–352.

115. Sameshima Y, Tsunematsu Y, Watanabe S, et al. Detection of novel germline p53 mutations in diverse cancer prone families identified by selecting patients with childhood adrenocortical carcinoma. *J Natl Cancer Inst* 1992;84:703–710.

116. Velazquez-Fernandez D, Laurell C, Geli J, et al. Expression profiling of adrenocortical neoplasms suggests a molecular signature of malignancy. *Surgery* 2005;138:1087–1094.

117. Giordano TJ, Thomas DG, Kuiche R, et al. Distinct transcriptional profiles of adrenocortical tumors uncovered by microarray analysis. *Am J Pathol* 2003;162:521–531.

118. West AN, Neale GA, Pounds S, et al. Gene expression profiling of childhood adrenocortical tumors. *Cancer Res* 2007;67:600–608.

119. Marx C, Bornstein SR, Wolkersdorfer GW, et al. Relevence of major histocompatibility complex class II expression as a hallmark for the cellular differentiation in the human adrenal cortex. *J Clin Endocrinol Metab* 1997;82:2136–2140.

120. Didolkar MD, Bescher RA, Elias EG, et al. Natural history of adrenal cortical carcinoma: a clinicopathologic study of 42 patients. *Cancer* 1981;47:2153–2161.

121. Weiss LM. Comparative histological study of 43 metastasizing and nonmetastasizing adrenocortical tumors. *Am J Surg Pathol* 1984;8:163–169.

122. Hutter AM, Kayhoe DE. Adrenal cortical carcinoma: clinical features of 138 patients. *Am J Med* 1966;41:572–592.

123. Hough AJ, Hollifield JW, Page DL, et al. Prognostic factors in adrenal cortical tumors: a mathematical analysis of clinical and morphologic data. *Am J Clin Pathol* 1979;72:390–399.

124. Hajjar RA, Hickey RC, Samaan NA. Adrenal cortical carcinoma: a study of 32 patients. *Cancer* 1975;35:549–554.

125. Cagle PT, Hough A, Pysher J, et al. Comparison of adrenal cortical tumors in children and adults. *Cancer* 1986;57:2235–2237.

126. Brown FM, Gaffey TA, Wold LE, et al. Myxoid neoplasms of the adrenal cortex: a rare histologic variant. *Am J Surg Pathol* 2000;24:396–401.

127. Drachenberg CB, Lee HK, Gann DS, et al. Adrenal cortical carcinoma with adenosquamous differentiation. Report of a case with immunohistochemical and ultrastructural studies. *Arch Pathol Lab Med* 1995;119:260–265.

128. Alexander A, Paulose KP. Oncocytic variant of adrenal carcinoma presenting as Cushing's syndrome. *J Assoc Physicians India* 1998;46:235–237.

129. Hoang MP, Ayala AG, Albores-Saavedra J. Oncocytic adrenal cortical carcinoma: a morphologic immunohistochemical and ultrastructural study of four cases. *Mod Pathol* 2002;15:973–978.

130. Song SY, Park S, Kim SR, et al. Oncocytic adrenocortical carcinomas: a pathological and immunohistochemical study of four cases in comparison with conventional adrenocortical carcinomas. *Pathol Int* 2004;54:603–610.

131. Fischler DF, Nunez C, Levin HS, et al. Adrenal carcinosarcoma presenting in a woman with clinical signs of virilization: a case report with immunohistochemical and ultrastructural findings. *Am J Surg Pathol* 1992;16:626–631.

132. Decorato JW, Gruber H, Petti M, et al. Adrenal carcinosarcoma. *J Surg Oncol* 1990;45:134–136.

132a. Thway K, Olmos D, Shah C, et al. Oncocytic adrenal cortical carcinosarcoma with pleomorphic rhabdomyosarcomatous metastases. *Am J Surg Pathol* 2012;36:470–477.

133. Ren R, Guo M, Sneige N, et al. Fine-needle aspiration of adrenal cortical carcinoma: cytologic spectrum and diagnostic challenges. *Am J Clin Pathol* 2006;126:389–398.

134. Gaffey MJ, Traweek ST, Mills S, et al. Cytokeratin expression in adrenal cortical neoplasia: an immunohistochemical and biochemical study with implications for the differential diagnosis of adrenocortical, hepatocellular and renal cell carcinoma. *Hum Pathol* 1992;23:144–153.

135. Wick Mr, Cherwitz DL, McGlennen RC, et al. Adrenal cortical carcinoma: an immunohistochemical comparison with renal cell carcinoma. *Am J Pathol* 1986;122:343–352.

136. Cote RJ, Cardon Cardo C, Reuter VE, et al. Immunopathology of adrenal and renal cortical tumors: coordinated changes in antigen expression is associated with neoplastic conversion in the adrenal cortex. *Am J Pathol* 1990;136:1077–1084.

137. Binh MB, Sastre-Garau X, Guillou L, et al. MDM2 and CDK4 immunostaining are useful adjuncts in diagnosing well-differentiated and dedifferentiated liposarcoma subtypes: a comparative analysis of 559 soft tissue neoplasms with genetic data. *Am J Surg Pathol* 2005;29:1340–1347.

138. Binh MB, Sastre-Garau X, Guillou L, et al. Reproducibility of MDM2 and CDK4 staining in soft tissue tumors. *Am J Clin Pathol* 2006;125:693–697.

139. Huang HY, Antonescu CR. Epithelioid variant of pleomorphic liposarcoma: a comparative immunohistochemical and ultrastructural analysis of six cases with emphasis on overlapping features with epithelial malignancies. *Ultrastruct Pathol* 2002;26:299–308.

140. Delellis RA, Shin SJ, Treaba DO. Immunohistochemistry of endocrine tumors. In: Dabbs DJ, ed. *Diagnostic Immunohistochemistry. Theranostic and Genomic Applications.* Philadelphia, PA: Saunders; 2010:291–339.

141. Shin SJ, Hoda RS, Ying L, et al. Diagnostic utility of the monoclonal antibody A103 in fine needle aspiration biopsies of the adrenal. *Am J Clin Pathol* 2002;10:295–302.

142. Pan CC, Chen PC, Tsay SH, et al. Differential immunoprofiles of hepatocellular carcinoma, renal cell carcinoma and adrenocortical carcinoma: a systemic immunohistochemical survey using tissue array technique. *Appl Immunohistochem Mol Morphol* 2005;13:347–352.

143. Miettinen M. Neuroendocrine differentiation in adrenal cortical carcinoma: new immunohistochemical findings supported by electron microscopy. *Lab Invest* 1992;66:169–174.

144. Komminoth P, Roth J, Schröder S, et al. Overlapping expression of immunohistochemical markers and synaptophysin mRNA in pheochromocytomas and adrenocortical carcinomas: implications for the differential diagnosis of adrenal gland tumors. *Lab Invest* 1995;72:424–431.

145. Sasano H, Suzuki T, Nagura H, et al. Steroidogenesis in human adrenocortical carcinoma: biochemical activities, immunohistochemistry and in situ hybridization of steroidogenic enzymes and histopathologic study in 9 cases. *Hum Pathol* 1993;24:397–404.

146. Sasano H, Shizawa S, Suzuki T, et al. Transcription factor adrenal 4 binding protein is a marker of adrenocortical malignancy. *Hum Pathol* 1995;26:1154–1156.

147. Tartour E, Caillou B, Tennenbaum F, et al. Immunohistochemical staining of adrenocortical carcinoma: prediction value of the D11 antibody. *Cancer* 1993;72:3296–3303.

148. Browning L, Bailey D, Parlcer A. D2-40 is a sensitive and specific marker in differentiating primary adrenal cortical tumors from both metastatic clear cell reneal cell carcinoma and pheochromocytoma. *J Clin Pathol* 2008;61:293–296.

149. Sangoi AR, McKenney JK. A tissue microarray-based comparative analysis of novel and traditional immunohistochemical markers in the distinction between adrenal cortical lesions and pheochromocytoma. *Am J Surg Pathol* 2010;34:423–432.

150. Sbiera S, Schull S, Assie G, et al. High diagnostic and prognostic value of steroidogenic factor-1 expression in adrenal tumors. *J Clin Endocrinol Metab* 2010;95:E161–E171.

151. Silva EG, Mackay B, Samaan NA, et al. Adrenal cortical carcinomas: an ultrastructural study of 22 cases. *Ultrastruct Pathol* 1982;3:1–7.

152. King DR, Lack EE. Adrenal cortical carcinoma. *Cancer* 1979;44:239–244.

153. Van Slooten H, Schaberg A, Smeenk D, et al. Morphological characteristics of benign and malignant adrenal cortical tumors. *Cancer* 1985;55:766–773.

154. Amberson JB, Vaughn ED, Gray G, et al. Flow cytometric analysis of nuclear DNA from adrenal cortical neoplams. *Cancer* 1987;59:2091–2095.

155. Bowlby LS, DeBault LE, Abraham SR. Flow cytometric analysis of adrenal cortical tumor DNA: relationship between cellular DNA and histopathologic classification. *Cancer* 1986;58:1499–1505.

156. Taylor SR, Roederer M, Murphy RF. Flow cytometric DNA analysis of adrenal cortical tumors in children. *Cancer* 1987;59:2059–2063.

157. Cibas ES, Medeiros LJ, Weinberg ES, et al. Cellular DNA profiles of benign and malignant adrenal cortical tumors. *Am J Surg Pathol* 1990;14:948–955.

158. Medeiros LJ, Weiss LM. New developments in the pathological diagnosis of adrenal cortical neoplasms. *Am J Clin Pathol* 1992;97:73–83.

159. Weiss LM, Medeiros LJ, Vickery AL Jr. Pathologic features of prognostic significance in adrenocortical carcinoma. *Am J Surg Pathol* 1989;13:202–206.

160. Aubert S, Wacrenier A, Leroy X, et al. Weiss system revisited. A clinicopathologic and immunohistochemical study of 49 adrenocortical tumors. *Am J Surg Pathol* 2002;26:1612–1619.

160a. Volante M, Bollito E, Sperone P, et al. Clinicopathologic study of a series of 92 adrenocortical carcinomas: from a simplified algorithm to prognostic stratification. *Histopathology* 2009;55:535–543.

161. Papotti M, Volante M, Duregon E, et al. Adrenocortical tumors with myxoid features: a distinct morphologic and phenotypical variant exhibiting malignant behavior. *Am J Surg Pathol* 2010;34:973–983.

162. Wieneke JA, Thompson LDR, Heffess CS. Adrenal cortical neoplasms in the pediatric population. A clinicopathologic and immunophenotypic analysis of 83 patients. *Am J Surg Pathol* 2003;27:867–881.

163. Dehner LP. Pediatric adrenocortical neoplasms. On the road to some clarity. *Am J Surg Pathol* 2003;27:1005–1007.

164. Vargas MP, Vargas HI, Kleiner DE, et al. Adrenocortical neoplasms: role of prognostic markers MIB-1, p53, and RB. *Am J Surg Pathol* 1997;21:556–562.

165. Zhao J, Speel EMJ, Muletta-Feurer S, et al. Analysis of genomic alterations in sporadic adrenal cortical lesions. Gain of chromosome 17 is an early event in adrenocortical tumorigenesis. *Am J Pathol* 1999;155:1039–1045.

166. Heppner C, Reincke M, Agarwal SK, et al. MEN1 gene analysis in sporadic adrenocortical neoplasms. *J Clin Endocrinol Metab* 1999;84:216–219.

167. Gortz B, Roth J, Speel EJ, et al. MEN1 gene mutation analysis of sporadic adrenocortical lesions. *Int J Cancer* 1999;80:373–379.

168. Gicquel C, Bertagna X, Gaston V, et al. Molecular markers and long term recurrence in a large cohort of patients with sporadic adrenocortical tumors. *Cancer Res* 2001;61:6762–6676.

169. Edge SB, Byrd DR, Carducci MA, Compton CC, eds. *AJCC Cancer Staging Manual.* 7th ed. New York, NY: Springer; 2010.

170. Paton BL, Novitsky YW, Zerey M, et al. Outcomes of adrenal cortical carcinoma in the United States. *Surgery* 2006;140:914–920.

171. Wieneke J, Amin M, Chang SS, et al. Protocol for the examination of specimens form patients with carcinoma of the adrenal gland. www.cap.org/apps/docs/committee/cancer/cancer_protocols/2009/Adrenal_09protocol.pdf

172. Manger WM, Gifford RW Jr. *Pheochromocytoma.* New York, NY: Springer-Verlag; 1977.

173. Remine WH, Chong GC, Van Heerden JA, et al. Current management of pheochromocytoma. *Ann Surg* 1974;179:741–748.

174. Manasse P. Zur Histologie und Histogenese der primaren Nierengeschwulske. *Arch Pathol Anat Klin Med* 1893;133:391–404.

175. Pick L. Das Ganglioma embryonale sympathicum. *Klin Wochenschrv* 1912;49:16–22.

176. Koch CA, Vortmeyer A, Zhuang Z, et al. New insights into the genetics of familial chromaffin cell tumors. *Ann N Y Acad Sci* 2002;970:11–28.

177. Maher ER, Eng C. The pressure rises: update on the genetics of phaeochromocytoma. *Hum Mol Genet* 2002;11:2347–2354.

177a. Welander J, Soderkvist P, Gimm O. Genetics and clinical characteristics of hereditary pheochromocytomas and paragangliomas. *Endocr Relat Cancer* 2011;18:R253–R276.

177b. Burnichon N, Briere JJ, Rosella L, et al. *SDHA* is a tumor suppressing gene causing Paraganglioma. *Hum Mol Genet* 2010;19:3011–3020.

177c. Yeh I-T, Lenci RE, Qin Y, et al. A germline mutation of the *KIF1Bβ* gene on 1p36 in a family with neural and nonneural tumors. *Hum Genet* 2008;124:279–285.

177d. Yao L, Schiavi F, Cascon A, et al. Spectrum and prevalence of *FP/TMEM 127* gene mutations in pheochromocytomas and paragangliomas. *JAMA* 2010;304:2611–2619.

177e. Comino-Mendez I, Gracia-Aznarez FJ, Schiavi F. Exome sequencing identifies *MAX* mutations as a cause of hereditary pheochromocytoma. *Nat Genet* 2008;124:279–285.

178. Dluhy RG. Pheochromocytoma—death of an axiom. *N Engl J Med* 2002;346:1486–1488.

179. Neumann HP, Vortmeyer A, Schmidt D, et al. Evidence of MEN-2 in the original description of calssic pheochromocytoma. *N Engl J Med* 2007;357:1311–1315.

180. Lindor NM, Honchel R, Khsla S, et al. Mutations in the ret proto-oncogene in sporadic pheochromocytomas. *J Clin Endocrinol Metab* 1995;80:627–629.

181. Gutmann DH, Cole JH, Stone WJ, et al. Loss of neurofibromin in adrenal gland tumors from patients with neurofibromatosis type I. *Genes Chromosomes Cancer* 1993;10:55–58.

182. Krumm A, Meulia T, Groudine M. Common mechanisms for the control of eukaryotic transcriptional elongation. *Bioassays* 1993;15:659–665.

183. Crossey PA, Richards FM, Foster K, et al. Identification of intragenic mutations in the von Hippel–Lindau disease tumor suppressor gene and correlation with disease phenotype. *Hum Mol Genet* 1994;3:1303–1308.

184. Neumann HPH, Bausch B, McWhinney S, et al. Germ-line mutations in non syndromic pheochromocytoma. *N Engl J Med* 2001;346:1459–1466.

184a. Gill AJ, Benn DE, Chou A, et al. Immunohistochemistry for SDHB traiages genetic testing of SDHB, SDHC, and SDHD in paraganglioma-pheochromocytoma syndromes. *Hum Pathol* 2010;41:805–814.

185. Edstrom E, Mahlamaki E, Nord B, et al. Comparative genomic hybridization reveals frequent losses of chromosomes 1p and 3q in pheochromocytomas and abdominal paragangliomas, suggesting a common genetic etiology. *Am J Pathol* 2000;156:651–659.

186. Dannenberg H, Speel EJM, Zhao J, et al. Losses of chromosomes 1p and 3q are early genetic events in the development of sporadic pheochromocytomas. *Am J Pathol* 2002;157:353–359.

187. Petri BJ, Speel EJ, Korpershoek E, et al. Frequent loss of 17p, but no p53 mutations or protein overexpression in benign and malignant pheochromocytomas. *Mod Pathol* 2008;21:407.

188. Mann SJ. Severe paroxysmal hypertension (pseudopheochromocytoma). Understanding the cause and treatment. *Arch Intern Med* 1999;159:670–674.

189. Hoy LJ, Emery M, Wedzicha JA, et al. Obstructive sleep apnea presenting as pseudopheochromocytoma: a case report. *J Clin Endocrinol Metab* 2004;89:2033–2038.

190. Stackpole RH, Melicow MM, Uson AC. Pheochromocytoma in children. *J Pediatr* 1953;63:315–330.

191. Atuk NO, McDonald T, Wood T, et al. Familial pheochromocytoma, hypercalcemia and von Hippel–Linden disease. *Medicine* 1979;58:209–218.

192. DeLellis RA, Dayal Y, Tischler AS, et al. Multiple endocrine neoplasia (MEN) syndromes: cellular origins and inter-relationships. *Int Rev Exp Pathol* 1986;28:163–215.

193. Carney JA, Sizemore GW, Sheps SG. Adrenal medullary disease in multiple endocrine neoplasia, type 2. *Am J Clin Pathol* 1976;66:279–290.

194. Li M, Wenig BM. Adrenal oncocytic pheochromocytoma. *Am J Surg Pathol* 2000;24:1552–1557.

195. Linnoila RI, Keiser HR, Steinberg SM, et al. Histopathology of benign versus malignant sympathoadrenal paragangliomas: clinicopathologic study of 120 cases including unusual histological features. *Hum Pathol* 1990;21:1168–1180.

196. Steinhoff MN, Wells SA, DeSchryver-Kelskemeti K. Stromal amyloid in pheochromocytomas. *Hum Pathol* 1992;23:33–36.

197. Medeiros LJ, Katsas GG, Balogh K. Brown fat and adrenal pheochromocytoma: association or coincidence? *Hum Pathol* 1985;16:580–589.

198. Thompson LDR. Pheochromocytoma of the adrenal gland scaled score (PASS) to separate benign form malignant neoplasms. A clinicopathologic and immunophenotypic study of 100 cases. *Am J Surg Pathol* 2002;26:551–556.

199. DeLellis RA, Tischler AS, Lee AK, et al. Leuenkephalin-like immunoreactivity in proliferative lesions of the human adrenal medulla and extra-adrenal paraganglia. *Am J Surg Pathol* 1983;7:29–37.

200. Berenyi MR, Singh G, Gloster ES, et al. ACTH-producing pheochromocytoma. *Arch Pathol Lab Med* 1977;101:31–35.

201. Tannenbaum M. Ultrastructural pathology of adrenal medullary tumors. In: Sommers SC, ed. New York, NY: Appleton-Century-Crofts; 1970:145–171.

202. Wantanabe H, Burnstock G, Jarrott B, et al. Mitochondrial abnormalities in human phaeochromocytoma. *Cell Tissue Res* 1976;171:281–288.

203. Yokoyama M, Takayasu H. An electron microscopic study of the human adrenal medulla and pheochromocytoma. *Urol Int* 1969;24:79–95.

204. Wu D, Tischler AS, Lioyd RV, et al. Observer variation in the application of the pheochromocytoma of the adrenal gland scaled score. *Am J Surg Pathol* 2009;33:599–608.

205. Clarke MR, Weyant RJ, Watson CG, et al. Prognostic markers in pheochromocytoma. *Hum Pathol* 1998;29:522–526.

206. Lewis PD. A cytophotometric study of benign and malignant pheochromocytomas. *Virchows Arch B [Zellpathol]* 1971;9:371–376.

207. Favier J, Plouin PF, Corvol P, et al. Angiogenesis and vascular architecture in pheochromocytomas. Distinctive traits in malignant tumors. *Am J Pathol* 2002;161:1235–1246.

208. DeLellis RA, Wolfe HJ, Gagel RF, et al. Adrenal medullary hyperplasia: a morphometric analysis in patients with familial medullary thyroid carcinoma. *Am J Pathol* 1976;83:177–196.

209. Salmenkivi K, Haglund C, Arola J, et al. Increased expression of tenascin in pheochromocytomas correlates with malignancy. *Am J Surg Pathol* 2001;25:1419–1423.

210. Thouennon E, Elkahlom AG, Guillemot J, et al. Identification of potential gene markers and insights into the pathophysiology of pheochromocytoma malignancy. *J Endocrinol Metab* 2007;92:4865–4872.

211. Brouwers FM, Elkahloun AG, Munson PJ. Gene expression profiling of benign and malignant pheochromocytoma. *Ann N Y Acad Sci* 2006;1073:541–556.

212. Kimura N, Wata nabe T, Fukase M, et al. Neurofibromin and NF1 gene analysis in composite pheochromocytoma and tumors associated with von Recklinghausen's disease. *Mod Pathol* 2002;15:183–188.

213. Tischler AS, DeLellis RA, Biales B, et al. Nerve growth factor induced neurite outgrowth from normal human chromaffin cell. *Lab Invest* 1980;43:399–409.

214. Juarez D, Brown RW, Ostrowski M, et al. Pheochromocytoma associated with neuroendocrine carcinoma. A new type of composite pheochromocytoma. *Arch Pathol Lab Med* 1999;123:1274–1279.

215. Visser JW, Axt R. Bilateral adrenal medullary hyperplasia: a clinicopathological entity. *J Clin Pathol* 1975;28:298–304.

216. Rudy FR, Bates RD, Cimorelli AJ, et al. Adrenal medullary hyperplasia: a clinicopathologic study of four cases. *Hum Pathol* 1980;11:650–657.

217. Naeye RL. Brainstem and adrenal abnormalities in the sudden infant death syndrome. *Am J Clin Pathol* 1976;66:526–530.

218. Diaz-Cano SJ, de Miguel M, Blanes A, et al. Clonal patterns in pheochromocytomas and MEN2 adrenal medullary hyperplasia: histologic and kinetic correlates. *J Pathol* 2000;192:221–228.

219. Ross JA, Severson RK, Pollock BH, et al. Childhood cancer in the United States: a geographical analysis of cases from the Pediatric Cooperative Clinical Trials Group. *Cancer* 1996;77:201–207.

220. Hardy PC, Nesbit ME Jr. Familial neuroblastoma: report of a kindred with a high incidence of familial tumors. *J Pediatr* 1973;80:74–77.

221. Maris JM. Recent advances in neuroblastoma. *N Engl J Med* 2010;362:2202–2211.

222. MacKay B, Luna MA, Butler JJ. Adult neuroblastoma. *Cancer* 1976; 37:1334–1351.

223. Allan SG, Cornbleet MA, Carmichael J, et al. Adult neuroblastoma: report of three cases and review of the literature. *Cancer* 1986;57: 2419–2421.

224. Kaye JA, Warhol NJ, Kretschmar C, et al. Neuroblastoma in adults: three case reports and review of the literature. *Cancer* 1986;58:1149–1157.

225. Beckwith JB, Perrin EV. In situ neuroblastomas: a contribution to the natural history of neural crest tumors. *Am J Pathol* 1963;43:1089–1104.

226. Bolande RP. Developmental pathology. *Am J Pathol* 1979;94:623–683.

227. Turkel SB, Itabashi HH. The natural history of neuroblastic cells in the fetal adrenal gland. *Am J Pathol* 1974;76:225–244.

228. Chauty A, Raimondo G, Vergeron H, et al. Discovery of a neuroblastoma producing cardiogenic shock in a two-month-old child. *Arch Pediatr* 2002;9:602–605.

229. Sawada T. Past and future of neuroblastoma screening in Japan. *Am J Pediatr Hematol Oncol* 1992;14:320–326.

230. Woods WG, Gao RN, Shuster JJ, et al. Screening of infants and mortality due to Neuroblastoma. *N Engl J Med* 2002;346:1041–1046.

231. Schilling FH, Spix C, Berthold F, et al. Neuroblastoma screening at one year of age. *N Engl J Med* 2002;346:1047–1053.

232. Yamato K, Ohta S, Ito E, et al. Marginal decrease in mortality and marked increase in incidence as a result of neuroblastoma screening at 6 months of age: cohort study in seven prefectures in Japan. *J Clin Oncol* 2002;20:1209–1214.

233. Beckwith JB, Martin RF. Observations on the histopathology of neuroblastomas. *J Pediatr Surg* 1968;3:106–110.

234. Hughes M, Marsden HB, Palmer MK. Histological patterns of neuroblastomas related to prognosis and clinical staging. *Cancer* 1974;34:1706–1711.

235. Shimada H, Chatten J, Newton WA, et al. Histopathologic prognostic factors in neuroblastic tumors: definition of subtypes of ganglioneuroblastoma and an age linked classification of neuroblastomas. *J Natl Cancer Inst* 1984;73:405–413.

236. Joshi VV, Cantor AB, Altshuler G, et al. Age linked prognostic categorization based on a new histologic grading system of neuroblastomas. *Cancer* 1992;69:2197–2211.

237. Shimada H, Ambros IM, Dehner LP, et al. Terminology and morphologic criteria of neuroblastic tumors. Recommendations by the International Neuroblastoma Pathology Committee. *Cancer* 1999;86: 349–363.

238. Shimada H, Ambros IM, Dehner LP, et al. The International Neuroblastoma Pathology Classification (the Shimada System). *Cancer* 1999;86:364–372.

239. Russell DS, Rubinstein LJ. *Pathology of Tumors of the Nervous System*. Baltimore, MD: Williams & Wilkins; 1971.

240. Taxy JB. Electron microscopy in the diagnosis of neuroblastoma. *Arch Pathol Lab Med* 1980;104:355–360.

241. Tornoczky T, Kalman E, Kajar PG, et al. Large cell neuroblasoma. A distinct phenotype of neuroadenoma with aggressive clinical behavior. *Cancer* 2004;100:390–397.

242. Moll R, Lee I, Gould V, et al. Immunocytochemical analysis of Ewing's tumors: patterns of expression of intermediate filaments and desmosomal proteins indicate cell type heterogeneity and pluripotential differentiation. *Am J Pathol* 1987;127:288–304.

243. Osborn M, Dirk T, Kaser H, et al. Immunohistochemical localization of neurofilaments and neuron specific enolase in 19 cases of neuroblastoma. *Am J Pathol* 1986;122:433–442.

244. Hachitanda Y, Tsuneyoshi M, Enjoji M. An ultrastructural and immunohistochemical evaluation of cytodifferentiation in neuroblastic tumors. *Mod Pathol* 1989;2:13–19.

245. Mukai M, Torikata C, Iri H, et al. Expression of neurofilament triplet proteins in human neural tumors: an immunohistochemical study of paraganglioma, ganglioneuroma, ganglioneuroblastoma and neuroblastoma. *Am J Pathol* 1985;122:28–35.

246. Molenaar WM, Baker DL, Pleasure D, et al. The neuroendocrine and neural profiles of neuroblastomas, ganglioneuroblastomas and ganglioneuromas. *Am J Pathol* 1990;136:375–382.

247. Hasegawa T, Matsumo Y, Hiroshashi S, et al. Second primary rhabdomyosarcoma in patients with bilateral retinoblastoma: a clinical and immunohistochemical study. *Am J Surg Pathol* 1998;22:1351–1360.

248. Brook FB, Raafat F, Eldeeb BB, et al. Histological and immunohistochemical investigation of neuroblastomas and correlation with prognosis. *Hum Pathol* 1988;19:879–888.

249. Wiedemann B, Franke W. Identification and localization of synaptophysin in integral membrane protein of Mr38000 characteristic of presynaptic vesicles. *Cell* 1985;41:1017–1028.

250. Wirnsberger GH, Becker H, Ziervogel K, et al. Diagnostic immunohistochemistry of neuroblastic tumors. *Am J Surg Pathol* 1992;16:49–57.

251. Sariola H, Terava H, Rapola J, et al. Cell surface ganglioside D2 in the immunohistochemical detection and differential diagnosis of neuroblastoma. *Am J Clin Pathol* 1991;96:248–252.

252. Artlieb V, Krepler R, Wiche G. Expression of microtubule associated proteins, Map-1 and Map-2, in human neuroblastomas and differential diagnosis of immature neuroblasts. *Lab Invest* 1985;53:684–691.

253. Oppedal BR, Strom-Mathiesen I, Kemshead JT, et al. Bone marrow examination in neuroblastoma patients: a morphological, immunocytochemical and immunohistochemical study. *Hum Pathol* 1989;20:800–805.

254. Reid MM, Wallis JP, McGuckin AG, et al. Routine histological compared to immunohistological examination of bone marrow trephine biopsy specimens in disseminated neuroblastoma. *J Clin Pathol* 1991;44:483–486.

255. Smith RG, Reynolds CP. Monoclonal antibody recognizing a human neuroblastoma-associated antigen. *Diagn Clin Immunol* 1987;5: 209–220.

256. Moss TJ, Reynolds CP, Sather HN, et al. Prognostic value of immunocytologic detection of bone marrow metastases in neuroblastoma. *N Engl J Med* 1991;324:219–226.

257. Shipley WR, Hammer RD, Lennington WJ, et al. Paraffin immunohistochemical detection of CD56, a useful marker for neural adhesion molecule (NCAM) in normal and neoplastic fixed tissues. *Appl Immunohistochem* 1997;5:87–93.

258. Wick MR. Immunohistology of neuroendocrine and neuroectodermal tumors. *Semin Diagn Pathol* 2000;17:194–203.

259. Phimister E, Kiely F, Kemshead JT, et al. Expression of neural adhesion molecule (NCAM) isoforms in neuroblastoma. *J Clin Pathol* 1991;44:580–585.

260. Miettinen M, Chatten J, Paetau A, et al. Monoclonal antibody NB84 in the differential diagnosis of neuroblastoma and other small round cell tumors. *Am J Surg Pathol* 1998;22:327–332.

261. Folpe AL, Patterson K, Gown AM. Antineuroblastoma antibody NB84 also identifies a significant subset of other small round blue cell tumors. *Appl Immunohistochem* 1997;5:239–245.

262. Stevenson AJ, Chatten J, Bertoni F, et al. CD99 (p30/32 mic2) neuroectodermal/Ewing's sarcoma antigen, an immunohistochemical marker: review of more than 600 tumors and the literature experience. *Appl Immunohistochem* 1994;2:231—240.

263. Kammen BF, Matthay KK, Pacham P, et al. Pulmonary metastases at diagnosis of neuroblastoma in pediatric patients: CT findings and prognosis. *AJR* 2001;176:755–759.

264. Burchill SA, Wheeldon J, Cullinane C, et al. EWS-FLI1 fusion transcripts identified in patients with typical neuroblastoma. *Eur J Cancer* 1997;33:239–243.

265. Kempson RL, Fletcher CDM, Evans HL, et al. Tumors of Soft Tissues. *Atlas of Tumor Pathology,* 3rd series, fascicle 30. Washington, DC: Armed Forces Institute of Pathology; 2001.

266. Ozdermirli M, Farnburg-Smith JC, Hartman DP. Differentiating lymphoblastic lymphoma and Ewing's sarcoma: lymphocyte markers and gene rearrangement. *Mod Pathol* 2001:1175–1182.

267. French CA, Kutol JL, Faquin WC, et al. Midline carcinoma of children and young adults with NUT rearrangement. *J Clin Oncol* 2004;22:4135–4139.

268. Haack H, Johnson LA, Fry CJ, et al. Diagnosis of NUT midline carcinoma using a NUT-specific monoclonal antibody. *Am J Surg Pathol* 2009;33:984–991.

269. Stout JP. Ganglioneuroma of the sympathetic nervous system. *Surg Gynecol Obstet* 1947;84:101–110.

270. Stowens D. Neuroblastomas and related tumors. *Arch Pathol* 1957; 63:451–459.

271. Mack E, Sarto GE, Crummy AB, et al. Virilizing adrenal ganglioneuroma. *JAMA* 1978;239:2273–2274.

272. Joshi VV, Silverman JF. Pathology of neuroblastic tumors. *Semin Diagn Pathol* 1994;11:107–117.

273. Askin FB, Perlman EJ. Neuroblastoma and peripheral neuroectodermal tumors. *Am J Clin Pathol* 1998;(suppl 1):S23–S30.

274. Evans AE, D'Angio GJ, Propert K, et al. Prognostic factors in neuroblastoma. *Cancer* 1987;59:1853–1859.

274a. Cohn SL, Pearson ADJ, London WB, et al. The International Neuroblastoma Risk Group (INRG) Classification System: An INRG task force report. *J Clin Oncol* 2009;27:289–297.

275. Chatten J, Shimada H, Sather HN, et al. Prognostic value of histopathology in advanced neuroblastoma: a report from the Children's Cancer Group. *Hum Pathol* 1988;19:1187–1198.

276. Shimada H, Umehara S, Monobe Y, et al. International neuroblastoma pathology classification for prognostic evaluation of patients with peripheral neuroblastic tumors. A report from the children's cancer group. *Cancer* 2001;92:2451–2461.

277. Umehara S, Nakagawa A, Matthay KK, et al. Histopathology defines prognostic subsets of ganglioneuroblastoma, nodular. A report from the children's cancer group. *Cancer* 2000;89:1150–1161.

278. Brodeur GM, Seeger RC, Barrett A, et al. International criteria for diagnosis, staging, and response to treatment in patients with neuroblastoma. *J Clin Oncol* 1988;6:1874–1881.

279. Brodeur GM, Pritchard J, Berthold F, et al. Revisions of the international criteria for neuroblastoma diagnosis, staging and response to treatment. *J Clin Oncol* 1993;11:1466–1477.

280. Ikeda H, Iehara T, Tsuchida Y, et al. Experience with the international neuroblastoma staging system and pathology classification. *Br J Cancer* 2002;86:1110–1116.

281. Kushner BH, Kramer K, Cheung NKV. Chronic neuroblastoma. Indolent stage 4 disease in children. *Cancer* 2002;95:1366–1375.

281a. Monclair T, Brodeur GM, Ambros PF et al. The International Neuroblastoma Risk Group (INRG) Staging System: An INRG task force report. *J Clin Oncol* 2009;27:298–303.

281b. London WB, Castel V, Monclair T, et al. Clinical and biologic features predictive of survival after relapse of neuroblastoma: A report from the International Neuroblastoma Risk Group Project. *J Clin Oncol* 2011;29:3286–3292.

282. Zeltzer PM, Marangos PA, Evans AE, Schneider AL. Serum neuron specific enolase in children with neuroblastoma: relationship to stage and disease course. *Cancer* 1986;57:1230–1234.

283. Berthold F, Hunnemann DH, Harms D, et al. Serum vanillylmandelic acid/homovanillic acid contributes to prognosis estimation in patients with localized but not with metastatic neuroblastoma. *Eur J Cancer* 1992;28A:1950.

284. Brodeur GM, Seeger RC, Schwab M, et al. Amplification of N-myc in untreated human neuroblastomas correlates with advanced stage disease. *Science* 1984;224:1121–1124.

285. Brodeur GM. Molecular pathology of human neuroblastomas. *Semin Diagn Pathol* 1994;11:125.

286. Brodeur GM. Neuroblastoma: biological insights into a clinical enigma. *Nat Rev Cancer* 2003;3:203–216.

287. Goto S, Umehara S, Gerbing RB, et al. Histopathology (international neuroblastoma pathology classification) and MYCN status in patents with peripheral neuroblastic tumors. A report from the Children's Cancer Group. *Cancer* 2001;92:2699–2708.

288. Kobayashi C, Monforte-Munoz HL, Gerlsing RB, et al. Enlarged and prominent nucleoli may be indicative of MYCN amplification. A study of neuroblastoma (Schwannian Stroma-poor), undifferentiated/poorly differentiated subtype with high mitosis-Karyorrhexis index. *Cancer* 2005;103:174–180.

289. Thorner PS, Ho M, Chilton-MacNeill S, et al. Use of chromogenic in situ hybridization to identify MYCN copy number in neuroblastoma using routine tissue sections. *Am J Surg Pathol* 2006;30:635–642.

290. Ambros IM, Hata J, Joshi VV, et al. Morphologic features of neuroblastoma (schwannian stroma-poor tumors) in clinically favorable and unfavorable groups. *Cancer* 2002;94:1574–1583.

290a. Suganuma R, Wang LL, Sano H, et al. Peripheral neuroblastic tumors with genotype-phenotype discordance: a report from the Children's Oncology Group and the International Neuroblastoma Pathology Committee. *Pediatr Blood Cancer* 2013;60:363–370.

291. Sano H, Gonzalez-gomez, Wu SQ, et al. A case of composite neuroblastoma composed of histologically and biologically distinct clones. *Ped Dev Pathol* 2007;10:229–232.

292. Bown N. Neuroblastoma tumor genetics: clinical and biological aspects. *J Clin Pathol* 2001;54:897–910.

293. Caron H, van Sluis P, de Kraker J, et al. Allelic loss of chromosome 1p as a predictor of unfavorable outcome in patients with neuroblastoma. *N Engl J Med* 1996;334:225–230.

294. Bown N, Cotterill S, Lastowska M, et al. Gain of chromosome arm 17q and adverse outcome in patients with neuroblastoma. *N Engl J Med* 1999;340:1954–1961.

295. Nakagawara A, Arima M, Azar CG, et al. Inverse relationship between trk expression and N-myc amplification in human neuroblastomas. *Cancer Res* 1992;52:1364–1368.

296. Brodeur GM, Maris JM, Yamashiro DJ, et al. Biology and genetics of human neuroblastomas. *J Pediatr Hematol Oncol* 1997;19: 93–101.

297. Mora J, Gerald WL, Qin J, Cheung NKV. Evolving significance of prognostic markers associated with treatment improvement in patients with stage 4 neuroblastoma. *Cancer* 2002;94:2756–2765.

298. Giordani L, Iolascon A, Servedio V, et al. Two regions of deletion in 9p22-p24 in neuroblastoma are frequently observed in favorable tumors. *Cancer Genet Cytogenet* 2002;135:42–47.

298a. Prognostic value of partial genetic instability in neuroblastoma with <50% neuroblastic cell content. *Histopathol* 2011;59:22–30.

299. Ramani R. Expression of bcl-2 gene product in neuroblastoma. *J Pathol* 1994;172:273–278.

300. Chan HSL, Haddad G, Thorner PS, et al. P-glycoprotein expression as a predictor of outcome in therapy for neuroblastoma. *N Engl J Med* 1991;325:1608–1614.

301. Mora J, Cheung NK, Oplanich S, et al. Novel regions of allelic imbalance identified by genome-wide analysis of neuroblastoma. *Cancer Res* 2002;62:1761–1767.

302. Krams M, Hero B, Berthold F, et al. Proliferation marker KI-S5 discriminates between favorable and adverse prognosis in advanced stages of neuroblastoma with and without MYCN amplification. *Cancer* 2002;94:854–861.

302a. Sartelet H, Ohta S, Barrette S, et al. High level of apoptosis and low AKT activation in mass screening as opposed to standard neuroblastoma. *Histopathol* 2010;56:607–616.

302b. Sartelet H, Imbriglio T, Nyalendo C, et al. CD133 expression is associated with poor outcome in neuroblastoma via chemoresistance mediated by the AKT pathway. *Histopathol* 2012;60:1144–1155.

302c. Dungwa JV, Hunt LP, Ramani P. Carbonic anhydrase IX up-regulation is associated with E-adverse clinicopathologic and biologic factors in neuroblastomas. *Hum Pathol* 2012;43:1651–1660.

302d. Dungwa JV, Hunt LP, Ramani P. HIF-1α up-regulation is associated with adverse clinicopathological and biologic factors in neuroblastomas. *Histopathol* 2012;61:417–427.

302e. Ramani P, Dungwa JV, May MT. LYVE-1 upregulation and lymphatic invasion correlate with adverse prognostic factors and lymph node metastasis in neuroblastoma. *Virchows Arch* 2012;460:183–191.

302f. Ramani P, Nash R, Radevsky L, et al. VEGF-C, VEGF-D and VEGFR-3 expression in peripheral neuroblastic tumors. *Histopathol* 2012;61(6):1006-16.

302g. Duijkers FAM, Gaal J, Meijerink JPP, et al. High anaplastic lymphoma kinase immunohistochemical staining in neuroblastoma and ganglioneuroblastoma is an independent predictor of poor outcome. *Am J Pathol* 2012;180:1223–1231.

303. Wei JS, Greer BT, Westerman F, et al. Prediction of clinical outcome using gene expression profiling and artificial neural networks for patients with neuroblastoma. *Cancer Res* 2004;64:6883–6891.

303a. DePreter K, Mestdagh P, Vermeulen J, et al. miRNA expression profiling ennables stratification in archived and fresh neuroblastoma tumor samples. *Clin Cancer Res* 2011;17:7684–7692.

303b. Ambros PF, Ambros IM, Brodeur GM, et al. International consensus for neuroblastoma molecular diagnostics: report from the International Neuroblastoma Risk Group (INRG) Biology Committee. *Br J Cancer* 2009;100:1471–1482.

304. Asgharzadeh A, Pique-Regi R, Sposto R, et al. Prognostic significance of gene expression profiles of metastatic neuroblastomas lacking gene amplification. *J Natl Cancer Inst* 2006;98:1193–1203.

305. Belldegrun A, Hussain S, Seltzer SE, et al. Incidentally discovered mass of the adrenal gland. *Surg Gynecol Obstet* 1986;163:203–208.

306. Copeland PM. The incidentally discovered adrenal mass. *Ann Intern Med* 1983;98:940–945.

307. Geelhoed GW, Druy EM. Management of the adrenal "incidentaloma." *Surgery* 1982;92:866–874.

308. Glazer HS, Weyman PJ, Sagel SS, et al. Nonfunctioning adrenal masses: incidental discovery on computed tomography. *AJR* 1982;39:81–85.

309. Katz RL, Shirkhoda A. Diagnostic approach to incidental adrenal nodules in the cancer patient. *Cancer* 1985;55:1995–2000.

310. Grumbach MM, Shaw EB, Biller BMK, et al. NIH state-of-the-science statement on management of clinically inapparent adrenal mass ("incidentaloma"). *NIH Consens State Sci Statements* 2002;19:1–25.

311. Grumbach MM, Shaw EB, Biller BMK, et al. Management of clinically inapparent adrenal mass ("incidentaloma"). *Ann Intern Med* 2003;138:424–429

312. Nosher JL, Amorosa JK, Seiman S, et al. Fine needle aspiration of the kidney and adrenal gland. *J Urol* 1982;128:895–899.

313. Redman BG, Pazdur R, Zingas AP, et al. Prospective evaluation of adrenal insufficiency in patients with adrenal metastasis. *Cancer* 1987;60:103–107.

314. Lam K-Y, Lo C-Y. Metastatic tumors of the adrenal glands: a 30 year experience in a teaching hospital. *Clin Endocrinol* 2002;56:95–101.

315. McMahon RF. Tumor-to-tumor metastasis: bladder carcinoma metastasizing to an adrenocortical adenoma. *Br J Urol* 1991;67:216

316. Lack EE. *Pathology of the Adrenal and Extra-Adrenal Paraganglia. Major Problems in Pathology.* Philadelphia, PA: WB Saunders; 1994.

317. Gokden N, Gokden M, Phan DC, et al. The utility of PAX-2 in distinguishing metastatic renal cell carcinoma from its morphologic mimics. An immunohistochemical study with comparison to renal cell carcinoma marker. *Am J Surg Pathol* 2008;32:1462–1467.

318. Gupta R, Balzer B, Picken M, et al. Diagnostic implications of transcription factor Pax 2 protein and transmembrane enzyme complex carbonic anhydrase IX immunoreactivity in adult renal epithelial neoplasms. *Am J Surg Pathol* 2009;33(2):241-7.

319. Schnitzer B, Smid D, Lloyd RV. Primary T-cell lymphoma of the adrenal glands with adrenal insufficiency. *Hum Pathol* 1986;17:634–636.

320. Chu P, Costa J, Lackman MF. Angiotropic large cell lymphoma presenting as primary adrenal insufficiency. *Hum Pathol* 1996;27:209–211.

321. Choi GH, Durishin M, Garbudawala ST, et al. Non-Hodgkin's lymphoma of the adrenal gland. *Arch Pathol Lab Med* 1990;114:883–885.

322. Donner LR, Mott FE, Tafur I. Cytokeratin positive, CD45 negative primary centroblastic lymphoma of the adrenal gland: a potential for a diagnostic pitfall. *Arch Pathol Lab Med* 2002;125:1104–1106.

323. Bennett B, McKenna TJ, Hough AJ, et al. Adrenal myelolipoma associated with Cushing's disease. *Am J Clin Pathol* 1980;73:443–447.

324. Bishop E, Eble JN, Cheng L, et al. Adrenal myelolipomas show nonrandom X- chromosome inactivation in hematopoietic elements and fat: support for a clonal origin of myelolipomas. *Am J Surg Pathol* 2006;30:838–843.

325. Selye H, Stone H. Hormonally induced transformation of adrenal into myeloid tissue. *Am J Pathol* 1950;26:211–233.

326. Foster DG. Adrenal cysts: review of the literature and report of a case. *Arch Surg* 1966;92:131–143.

327. Incze JS, Lui PS, Merriam JC, et al. Morphology and pathogenesis of adrenal cysts. *Am J Pathol* 1979;95:423–432.

328. Erickson LA, Lloyd RV, Hartman R, et al. Cystic adrenal neoplasms. *Cancer* 2004;101:1537–1544.

329. Glantz K, Wegmann W. Papillary adenomatoid tumor of the adrenal gland. *Histopathology* 2000;37:376–377.

330. Simpson PR. Adenomatoid tumor of the adrenal glands. *Arch Pathol Lab Med* 1990;114:725–727.

331. Travis WD, Lack EE, Azumi N, et al. Adenomatoid tumors of the adrenal gland with ultrastructural and immunohistochemical demonstrations of a mesothelial origin. *Arch Pathol Lab Med* 1990;114:722–727.

332. Isotalo PA, Keeney GL, Sebo TJ, et al. Adenomatoid tumor of the adrenal gland: clinicopathologic study of five cases and review of the literature. *Am J Surg Pathol* 2003;27:969–977.

333. Lam KY, Lo CY. Adrenal lipomatous tumors: a 30 year clinicopathological experience at a single institution. *J Clin Pathol* 2001;54:707–712.

333a. Lau SK, Spagnolo DV, Weiss LM. Schwannoma of the adrenal gland: report of two cases. *Am J Surg Pathol* 2006;30:630–634.

334. Prevot S, Penna CT, Imbert J-C, et al. Solitary fibrous tumor of the adrenal gland. *Mod Pathol* 1996;9:1170–1174.

335. Eftekhari F, Ater JL, Ayala AG, et al. Calcifying fibrous pseudotumor of the adrenal gland. *Br J Radiol* 2001;74:452–454.

336. Lau SK, Weiss LM. Calcifying fibrous tumor of the adrenal gland. *Hum Pathol* 2007;38:656–659.

337. Wenig B, Heffess C. Adrenal angiosarcoma; a clinicopathologic and immunocytochemical study. *Lab Invest* 1992;66:39A.

338. Granger JK, Hoan H-Y, Collins C. Massive hemorrhagic functional adrenal adenoma histologically mimicking angiosarcoma: report of a case with immunohistochemical study. *Am J Surg Pathol* 1991;15:699–704.

339. Lack EE, Graham CW, Azumi N, et al. Primary leiomyosarcoma of adrenal gland: case report with immunohistochemical and ultrastructural study. *Am J Surg Pathol* 1991;15:899.

340. Candanedo-Gonzalez FA, Chavez TV, Cerubulo-Vasquez A. Pleomorphic leiomyosarcoma of the adrenal gland with osteoclast-like giant cells. *Endocr Pathol* 2005;16:75–82.

341. Zetler PJ, Filipanko JD, Bilbey JH, et al. Primary adrenal leiomyosarcoma in a man with acquired immunodeficiency syndrome (AIDS): further evidence for an increase in smooth muscle tumors related to Epstein Barr virus infection in AIDS. *Arch Pathol Lab Med* 1995;119:1164–1167.

342. Carstens PHB, Kuhns JG, Ghazi C. Primary malignant melanomas of the lung and adrenal. *Hum Pathol* 1984;15:910–914.

343. Dao AH, Page DL, Reynold VH, et al. Primary malignant melanoma of the adrenal glands: a report of two cases and review of the literature. *Am Surg* 1990;56:199–203.

344. Unger PD, Hoffman K, Thung SN, et al. HMB-45 reactivity in adrenal pheochromocytomas. *Arch Pathol Lab Med* 1992;116:151–153.

345. Fidler WJ. Ovarian thecal metaplasia in adrenal glands. *Am J Clin Pathol* 1976;67:318–323.

346. Carney JA. Unusual tumefactive spindle cell lesions in the adrenal glands. *Hum Pathol* 1987;18:980.

347. Orselli, RC, Bassler, TJ. Theca granulosa cell tumor arising in adrenal. *Cancer* 1973;31:474

348. Pollock WJ, McConnell CF, Hilton C, Lavine RL. Virilizing Leydig cell adenoma of adrenal gland. *Am J Surg Pathol* 1986;10:816.

349. Santonja C, Diaz MA, Dehner LP. A unique dysembryonic neoplasm of the adrenal gland composed of nephrogenic rests in a child. *Am J Surg Pathol* 1996;20:118–124.

350. Molberg K, Vuitch F, Stewart D, et al. Adrenocortical blastoma. *Hum Pathol* 1992;23:1187–1190.

351. Wieneke JA, Thompson LA, Heffess CS. Corticomedullary mixed tumor of the adrenal gland. *Ann Diagn Pathol* 2001;5:304–308.

352. Turk AT, Asad H, Trapasso J, et al. Mixed corticomedullary carcinoma of the adrenal gland: a case report. *Endocr Pract* 2012;18:e37–e42.

353. Lau SK, Romansky SG, Weiss LM. Sustentaculoma: report of a distinctive neoplasm of the adrenal medulla. *Am J Surg Pathol* 2006;30:268–273.

Pathology of the Renal Pelvis and Ureter

BRETT DELAHUNT and HEMAMALI SAMARATUNGA

The renal pelvis and ureter are tubular structures that facilitate passage of the urine from the kidney to the urinary bladder. Despite their relatively simple architecture, these organs are subject to a wide variety of pathologic processes. In particular, the complex nature of nephro-ureterogenesis accounts for the observed diversity of congenital abnormalities seen at this site, which may lead to urinary reflux, urinary tract infections, and ultimately renal failure. In addition to these congenital abnormalities, chronic exposure to toxins and metabolites within the urine may promote the development of clinically important diseases such as lithiasis, and mucosal metaplasia and neoplasia. Although a number of reported pelviureteral disorders are rarely encountered in clinical practice, many of the more common conditions account for a significant morbidity and mortality in both pediatric and adult populations.

ANATOMY AND HISTOLOGY

The renal pelvis and ureter are fibromuscular tubes lined by mucosa. The ureter is 30 cm long with an average diameter of 5 mm. There are narrowings of the lumen at the ureteropelvic junction where the external and common iliac vessels cross and where the ureter enters the bladder. These are natural sites for obstruction and impaction of stones and are frequently the sites where pathology is observed.[1]

Urothelium lines the complete length of the renal pelvis and ureter and varies in thickness from two to three cells in the renal pelvis to four to six cells in the ureter. The surface of the urothelium consists of larger cells aligned parallel to the surface (umbrella cells). These have eosinophilic cytoplasm and occasional binucleate forms and mucin-filled vacuoles are seen.[2] The surface of the superficial layer is covered by an impervious trilaminar membrane, which is convoluted in the resting nondistended state.[3] Desmosomes are present between cells of the superficial layer and between superficial and intermediate cells. Beneath the superficial layer, cells are aligned perpendicular to the basement membrane, and in thickened epithelium a condensed basal cell layer may be present. Scattered glycogen-filled vacuoles are often present within

the deeper layers. It has been demonstrated that the nuclei of cells of the renal pelvic urothelium are larger than those of the bladder. As a consequence of this, caution is required in interpreting dysplasia and carcinoma in situ (CIS) in frozen sections of ureter.

The lamina propria consists of vascular fibrous tissue, which is more condensed toward the deep aspect.[1] Scattered elastin fibers are present, which cause folding of the mucosa in the resting state. Beneath the submucosa, bands of smooth muscle form the muscularis propria, which increases in thickness distally (Fig. 4-1). This is arranged into an inner longitudinal layer and an outer circular layer, although this division is not discernible within the renal pelvis and proximal ureter. The passage of urine through the renal pelvis and ureter is facilitated by peristalsis, with an action potential being propagated between myocytes by numerous close contacts or nexuses.[1] In the renal pelvis the fibers of the muscularis have a spiral arrangement, which extends into the immediate proximal ureter.[4] This spiral arrangement gives rise to a fragmented appearance to the muscularis in histologic sections, and this has been considered, erroneously, to be a diagnostic feature of ureteropelvic junction obstruction.

In the renal pelvis the muscularis propria is covered by fat, which blends into the fat of the renal hilum.[2] The adventitia of the proximal ureter consists of loose connective tissue containing collagen, fibroblasts, myocytes, and nerve fibers. This is condensed and thickened in the distal ureter to form Waldeyer fascia, which continues as the adventitia of the bladder.

EMBRYOLOGY

The urinary tract develops from intermediate mesoderm, and three separate renal structures form sequentially. Initially the transient pronephros is formed with an associated nephrogenic duct, which opens into the cloaca. With the development of this structure into the mesonephros by week 4, the nephrogenic duct forms the mesonephric duct from which the ureteric bud develops on its dorsomedial surface. The bud elongates caudally and its junction with the mesonephric

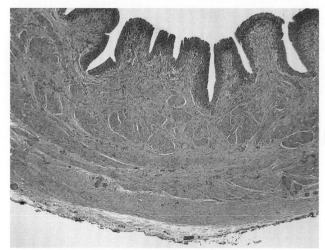

FIGURE 4-1 ■ Distal ureter showing prominence of the inner longitudinal and outer circular layers of the muscularis propria.

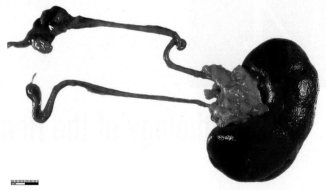

FIGURE 4-2 ■ Kidney with duplex renal pelves and ureters.

duct migrates toward the cloaca to form separate ureteric and Wolffian ducts by week 6.[5] The caudal end of the ureteric duct forms the ampulla, and this fuses with the metanephric mesenchyme. This fusion induces branching of the ampullary bud to form the renal pelvis, calyces, and collecting ducts, and also induces differentiation of metanephric mesenchyme into nephrons and supporting stroma.[6,7] By week 12 the ureteral muscularis develops, and by week 14 there is recognizable urothelium lining the upper tract.[8]

It has been claimed that the ureter becomes temporarily obliterated during week 6 and recanalization commences in the midportion and extends both proximally and distally.[9] This process of obliteration and recanalization has been questioned, and it has been suggested that this is merely a collapse of the ureteral lumen prior to the onset of urine output by the metanephros.[10] There is a further temporary obstruction of the ureter by the Chawalla membrane that forms as a thin band of epithelial cells across the ureteral orifice during week 6.[11] Persistence of luminal obliteration or of the Chawalla membrane has been implicated as a cause of ureteral valves and ureteral stenosis.

MALFORMATIONS

Agenesis, Duplication, and Ectopia

Renal agenesis and duplication, and positional abnormalities of the upper tract are the result of growth failure or abnormal branching of the ureteric duct from the mesonephric duct.

Total failure of the ureteric duct to develop results in renal agenesis. Bilateral renal agenesis is rare, with a reported incidence of 3.5/10[5] live births,[12,13] while unilateral agenesis is more frequently encountered[12] and in one series was detected in 1/1,200 of children on screening.[14] Renal agenesis may also arise when there is failure of the ureteric duct to fuse with the metanephros, and where the ureteric duct may persist to form a blind diverticulum part way along the length of the ureter.

During elongation of the ureteric duct, with associated renal ascent, splitting of the ampullary bud may occur. In cases where this splitting occurs early in nephrogenesis or if two separate ampullary buds form along the length of the mesonephric duct, then double renal pelves and ureters will form, giving rise to a duplex collecting system (Fig. 4-2). Typically the vesicoureteral orifice of the upper pole ureter in a duplex system lies medial and caudal to the lower pole orifice, although exceptions to this rule have been reported. When splitting of the ureteric duct is a late event, a bifid ureter forms with two renal pelves, which drain into separate ureters that fuse to terminate in a single vesicoureteral orifice[15,16] (Fig. 4-3). The site of the junction of bifid ureters depends on timing of the branching of the ureteric

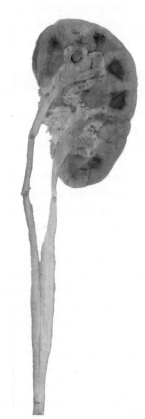

FIGURE 4-3 ■ Double renal pelves and ureters fusing superior to the vesicoureteric orifice to form a single ureter.

duct; however, in the majority of cases, this is in the lower third of the ureter and may be sited in the bladder wall.[17]

During embryogenesis the developing ureteric duct migrates distally along the mesonephric duct to fuse with the bladder, and the vesicoureteral orifice migrates to its normal trigonal position. If the ureteric duct develops in close proximity to the bladder, then migration of the vesicoureteral orifice extends beyond the trigone in both the caudal and lateral planes. Often the ectopic ureter is inserted more directly into the bladder wall with loss of the valve mechanism and resulting vesicoureteral reflux.[18] In extreme cases the ureteral orifice extends beyond the bladder, and the ureter terminates in the urethra or the genital structures that develop from the mesonephric duct.[16] In females ureteral ectopia is associated with a duplex system in 80% of cases, while in males there is usually a single renal outflow tract.[18] Further, as the ureteric duct takes its origin from the mesonephric duct, upper tract abnormalities are often associated with other malformations of the urogenital system and are found in the prune belly and VATER syndromes and trisomy 21.

Clinical features of congenital abnormalities of the upper tract are variable although there is often reflux and urinary stasis leading to urinary tract infection, lithiasis, and fistula formation. Ureteral duplications are often asymptomatic although cyclic abdominal pain may occasionally be a presenting feature.[17] Ultrasonography is valuable in the demonstration of malformations in utero and in neonates. The role of the pathologist may be to define the anatomic basis of a functional deficiency.

Ureteropelvic Junction Obstruction

Ureteropelvic Junction (UPJ) obstruction refers to the significant functional impairment of urinary flow from the renal pelvis to the ureter leading to hydronephrosis (Fig. 4-4). The majority of cases are congenital and occur in the pediatric age group. More rarely the obstruction may be secondary to postoperative or inflammatory strictures, renal stones, and urothelial neoplasms, including fibroepithelial polyps.[19,20] Rarely UPJ obstruction is associated with renal parenchymal neoplasia. There is also a reported association with congenital renal abnormalities in 15% to 20% of patients,[21] with agenesis and cystic renal dysplasia in the contralateral kidney,[22] and with vasculitis.[23] Functional obstruction has also been reported due to extrinsic compression by an aberrant lower pole vessel. This is seen in 16% to 20% of patients with UPJ obstruction with a median age of 67 months at presentation.[24] UPJ obstruction is more likely to be unilateral in adults, while pediatric cases are more frequently bilateral.

Congenital UPJ obstruction affects 13,000 newborns annually in the United States with hospitalization rates of 2.4/100,000 for patients aged ≤18 years. The highest incidence is in children <3 years of age with hospital admission rates of 9.3/100,000 being reported,[19] and in this age group there is a male predominance.[25] Ethnicity appears not to be a significant factor although slightly higher hospitalization rates for UPJ obstruction have been noted for patients of Hispanic origin.[19]

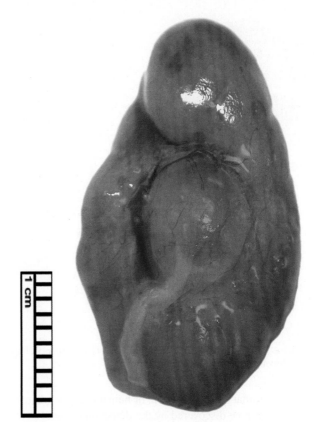

FIGURE 4-4 ■ Ureteropelvic junction obstruction. The renal pelvis is distended proximal to the UPJ obstruction.

Transport of urine from the renal papilla to the bladder is active and dependent on smooth muscle contraction, with some modulation by the autonomic nervous system.[26] In many cases of clinical UPJ obstruction, no identifiable lesion is seen and the impairment is functional.[27] Earlier studies have demonstrated abnormalities at both a cellular and ultrastructural level, and in particular increased interstitial collagen has been implicated,[28] although this is likely to be a secondary effect. Folds in the muscle or overlying mucosa, or the development of kinks or strictures that lead to reorientation of muscle bundles into a predominantly longitudinal pattern, have also been suggested as a pathogenic mechanism for UPJ obstruction.[29,30] Recent reports utilizing S100 protein, CKIT protooncogene protein (CD117), and synaptophysin immunohistochemistry suggest a defect in innervation as the cause of UPJ obstruction.[31] The UPJ is not normally innervated, and in cases of obstruction it is apparent that this segment extends for a longer distance down the proximal ureter.[32] Defective innervation is supported by a finding of increased vasoactive intestinal peptide and decreased levels of synaptophysin and nerve growth factor receptor in UPJ obstruction.[32] Transforming growth factor beta 1 (TGF-β1) has recently been shown to be increased in UPJ obstruction; however, this may be a secondary effect leading to the promotion of extracellular matrix formation and collagen synthesis.[33]

Prior to the advent of ultrasound investigations, UPJ obstruction was usually diagnosed during investigations for

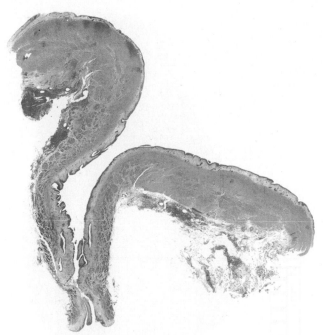

FIGURE 4-5 ■ UPJ obstruction showing a typical funnel shape with fibrosis of proximal ureter.

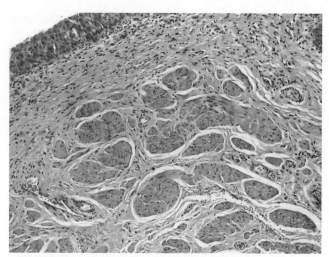

FIGURE 4-6 ■ Ureteropelvic junction obstruction. The distal renal pelvis shows marked interstitial fibrosis.

azotemia, urinary tract infection, or hematuria. The majority of cases are now discovered by the detection of renal pelvis dilatation on prenatal or perinatal ultrasound, and it is recommended that a dilatation of ≥5 mm be further investigated.[34] Asymptomatic cases of UPJ obstruction are usually treated conservatively, and in those patients with good renal function, the outcome is favorable whether the treatment is conservative or surgical. While patients with moderate impairment may benefit from pyeloplasty, those with poor function usually have minimal recovery following pyeloplasty.[27]

The gross surgical specimen in congenital UPJ obstruction is usually funnel shaped (Fig. 4-5), and thickening of the portion of the renal pelvis in the vicinity of the UPJ may be present. The histologic findings are variable and nonspecific, and occasionally no abnormality is seen. The mucosa is usually normal although projections resembling mucosal folds may be present.[35] There is occasionally hypertrophy of the smooth muscle layer[32] although this is more commonly thinned, and segmental loss of smooth muscle has also been reported.[36] Interstitial fibrosis is the most common finding although this is variable and may be associated with a mild diffuse chronic inflammatory infiltrate (Fig. 4-6). On electron microscopy, increased interstitial collagen is usually observed.

Ureteral and Paraureteral Diverticulum

Ureteral diverticula are rare and may be congenital or acquired. Symptoms are nonspecific; however, dysuria and hematuria may be presenting features.[37] Congenital diverticula are related to sites of weakness within the ureteral wall and are most commonly found adjacent to the ureteropelvic and vesicoureteral junctions. Other abnormalities of the urinary tract may be found in conjunction with congenital diverticula.[38]

Acquired diverticula are probably secondary to chronic infection or ureteral obstruction.[39,40] Occasionally multiple diverticula may be present, and it has been suggested that these are acquired, being the result of chronic infection.[41] It is recommended that treatment of small acquired diverticula should be directed toward management of the predisposing condition,[36] although larger diverticula may require surgical resection.

Histologically, congenital diverticula contain all three layers of the ureteral wall, while acquired diverticula usually have a thinned mucosal layer.[37]

Paraureteral diverticula originate within the bladder wall, adjacent to the ureteral orifice, and are due to a failure of normal muscle development or a defect in Waldeyer fascia.[42] In some cases, these can expand to involve the ureter with vesicoureteral reflux or outflow obstruction.[43] There is occasionally coexisting renal dysplasia, and an association with pelvicalyceal duplication has been reported.[44,45] Treatment is surgical and consists of diverticulectomy with or without ureteral reimplantation.[43]

Ureterocele

Ureterocele is the cystic dilatation of the distal ureter that projects into the bladder (Fig. 4-7). This most commonly occurs in Caucasian females,[46] and there is an annual hospitalization rate of $1/10^5$ in the pediatric age group, with 92% of hospital admissions being children under the age of 2 years.[47] The pathogenesis is uncertain and persistence of Chawalla membrane has been suggested, as has abnormality of the ureteral muscularis.[48] It has been estimated that there is an association with a duplex system in 95% of cases in females and 44% of cases in males.[47] Ureterocele associated with duplex ureter usually occurs in the upper pole ureter and is situated more inferiorly than ureterocele that arises from a single ureter. Previously ureteroceles arising in association with duplex ureters have been designated ectopic ureterocele; however, this term is now limited to those

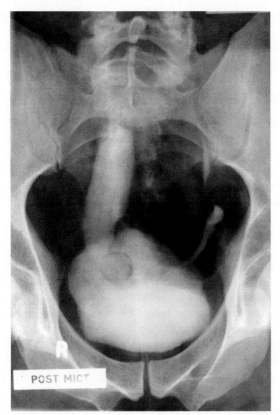

FIGURE 4-7 ■ Cystogram showing a ureterocele with typical cobra-head appearance.

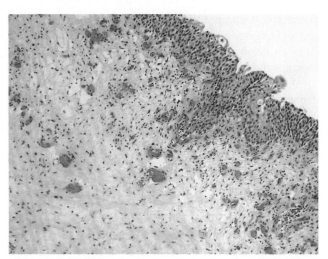

FIGURE 4-8 ■ Ureterocele. There is hyperplasia of the urothelium with edema, telangiectasia, and chronic inflammation of the grossly thickened lamina propria.

ureteroceles that extend beyond the bladder into the bladder neck or urethra.[49] If a ureterocele burrows between the bladder mucosa and muscularis to lie intramurally, the term cecoureterocele is applied.

Ureterocele is associated with dilatation of the proximal ureter and often results in reflux and hydronephrosis. Larger ureteroceles may also obstruct the contralateral ureter or the normal ipsilateral ureter in a duplex system. Obstruction of renal outflow from ureterocele may lead to cystic renal dysplasia or renal scarring, and in 10% of cases hypertension develops.[50]

The histologic features of ureterocele relate to chronicity. The surface mucosa of ureterocele originates from the bladder, while the cyst lumen is lined by ureteral mucosa[51] (Fig. 4-8). The muscularis may show hypertrophy or be attenuated and atrophic, with interstitial edema and variable interstitial fibrosis.

Treatment of ureterocele consists of early prophylactic antibiotic therapy, to minimize the effect of urinary tract infection. Endoscopic puncture may be undertaken as an emergency procedure, followed by surgical excision of the ureterocele and ureteral reconstruction.[52]

Megaureter

Megaureter is dilation of the ureter. This is considered to be primary if it is the result of a defect of intrinsic smooth muscle. It is most commonly seen in the pediatric age group and is

characterized by a ureteral diameter of >7 mm. Megaureter is not a specific diagnosis and may be associated with reflux or outflow obstruction, although a significant proportion is nonrefluxing and nonobstructed. These three categories of megaureter are further subdivided into primary and secondary groups[53] (Table 4-1). The pathogenesis of megaureter is dependent on the type; however, there is an association with abnormalities of the urinary tract, particularly cystic renal dysplasia.[54]

Refluxing Megaureter

Refluxing megaureter is characterized by retrograde flow from the bladder into the ureter. This may be unilateral or bilateral and is more common in females.[55] Primary refluxing megaureter results from abnormalities of the vesicoureteral junction, associated with loss of the valve function of the intramural ureteral segment.[54] The histologic features are

Table 4-1 ■ CLASSIFICATION OF MEGAURETER

Refluxing megaureter	Primary	- Primary refluxing megaureter
	Secondary	- Urethral obstruction - Neurogenic bladder
Obstructed megaureter	Primary	- Intrinsic obstruction (adynamic segment, ureteral stenosis)
	Secondary	- Urethral obstruction - Neurogenic bladder - Extrinsic obstruction
Non-refluxing, non-obstructed megaureter	Primary	- Non refluxing, non obstructed megaureter
	Secondary	- Polyuria - Infection

nonspecific with mural thickening, loss of smooth muscle, and an increase in interstitial connective tissue. Widespread collagen deposition is seen, and quantitative studies have shown a predominance of type III (juvenile) collagen.[56] Treatment is dependent on the severity of the reflux and degree of abnormality of the intravesical ureter. In severe cases early reimplantation is required, and in mild cases reflux may cease as the child grows. Secondary refluxing megaureter may be associated with urethral obstruction, neurogenic bladder, prune belly syndrome, and megacystis.[53,57]

Obstructed Megaureter

Primary obstructed megaureter results from the presence of an aperistaltic ureteral segment situated immediately proximal to the vesicoureteral junction[58] (Fig. 4-9). Ureteral obstruction in these cases is functional as no stricture is seen, and abnormalities of neuromuscular transmission, resulting in an adynamic segment, have been implicated. Histologic findings are nonspecific, and there is often muscle hypoplasia with disorganization of myofibrils. Increased amounts of collagen are present, and in particular, an increase in collagen types I and III has been noted.[56] Hyperplasia of the ureteral muscularis, associated with ectopic insertion,[59] as well as total loss of the muscularis,[60] have been described. Obstructed megaureter is treated by excision of the lower stenotic segment and ureteral reimplantation.[53]

Obstructed megaureter may occur secondary to urethral obstruction (Fig. 4-10), including urethral valves, neurogenic bladder, and external obstruction such as retroperitoneal fibrosis and neoplasia.[54]

Nonobstructed, Nonrefluxing Megaureter

In the majority of cases of perinatal megaureter, there is no evidence of either ureteral obstruction or reflux.

The pathogenesis of nonobstructed, nonrefluxing megaureter is unknown although abnormal ureteral compliance or persistence of fetal ureteral architecture, with transient obstruction, have been proposed.[61,62] This is confined to the distal ureter immediately proximal to the vesicoureteric junction with ureteral dilatation proximal to this,[57] and the dilated segment of the ureter is often fusiform and lacks the tortuosity associated with other forms of megaureter (Fig. 4-11). There is overlap with the histology of obstructed megaureter with interstitial fibrosis, fibrosis of the periureteral sheath, and hypoplasia of the inner (longitudinal) muscle layer being reported.[63]

Management of nonobstructed, nonrefluxing megaureter is usually expectant in the absence of urinary tract infection or loss of renal function. In severe cases, with declining renal function, ureteral reimplantation is undertaken.[57]

Secondary causes of nonobstructed, nonrefluxing megaureter may result from conditions leading to polyuria and from bacterial toxins associated with urinary tract infection.[53]

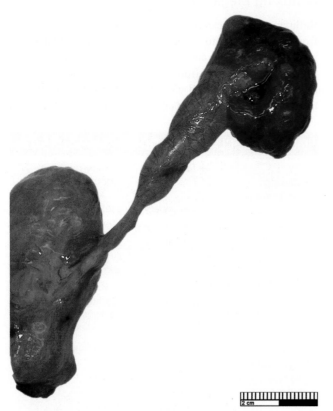

FIGURE 4-9 ■ Primary obstructed megaureter with ureter of normal caliber adjacent to the vesicoureteral junction.

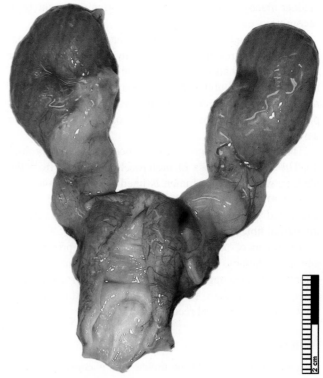

FIGURE 4-10 ■ Bilateral obstructed megaureter secondary to urethral valves.

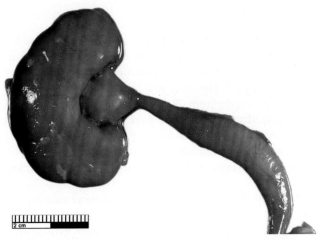

FIGURE 4-11 ■ Nonobstructed, nonrefluxing megaureter showing typical fusiform ureteral dilatation.

Ureteral Dysplasia

Rarely congenital nonrefluxing megaureter is associated with ureteral dysplasia where the muscularis has poorly formed myocytes, with absent or poor organization into muscle bundles. There is usually pronounced interstitial fibrosis with a variable infiltrate of lymphocytes and plasma cells.[64,65] On ultrastructural examination there is thinning of myofilaments, wide separation of cell membranes, a decrease in numbers of nexuses, and an increase in collagen fibers and ground substance.[65]

It has been shown that ureteral dysplasia is evident at 11 weeks' gestation, and as there is an association with urinary outflow obstruction early in nephrogenesis, cystic renal dysplasia frequently occurs.[63] The pathogenesis of ureteral dysplasia is unknown although muscle contractility studies show decreased amplitude of contractions and decreased response to adrenergic drugs.[66] On imaging there is dilatation of the involved ureteral segment, which is usually sited in the distal ureter. In severe cases interstitial fibrosis leads to ureteral obstruction, although, in most cases this obstruction is functional rather than anatomical.[67]

Treatment of ureteral dysplasia involves resection of the dysplastic segment with ureteral reimplantation.[68]

Ureteral Stricture

Ureteral stricture may be either congenital or secondary to trauma and inflammation. The pathogenesis of congenital stricture is uncertain and may be associated with failure of complete recanalization of the ureter, which undergoes temporary obliteration during fetal development.[69,70] An alternative theory is that congenital ureteral stricture is due to external compression of the ureter by fetal vessels leading to incomplete smooth muscle development.[71] This latter theory accords with the histologic findings, which consist of segmental absence of muscle and narrowing of the ureteral lumen. Congenital ureteral stricture may occur in isolation or may be a component of multiple organ syndromes.[72]

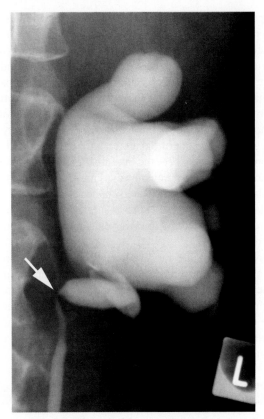

FIGURE 4-12 ■ Ascending ureteropyelogram showing stricture and medial deviation of the upper ureter (*arrow*) secondary to infiltration by retroperitoneal tumor.

There is also an association with ipsilateral and contralateral cystic renal dysplasia, solitary kidney, and blind ending of the contralateral ureter.

Secondary ureteral stricture is a recognized complication of ureteral endoscopy and pelvic surgery, with an incidence ranging from 0.5% to 3%.[73] Other secondary causes of ureteral stricture are trauma, ureteral infections, including tuberculosis and inflammation in adjacent organs, radiation, ureteral lithiasis; vasculitis and ischemia, amyloidosis, and endometriosis.[74–79]

Primary tumors of the ureter, especially urothelial carcinoma, usually present with ureteral stricture, and hydronephrosis and stricture may also be seen in association with extraureteral tumors that involve the ureter by direct infiltration or metastatic spread (Fig. 4-12).

Ureteral Valves

Ureteral valves are a rare cause of ureteral outflow obstruction with <60 cases being reported.[80] The majority of cases occur in males in the pediatric age group, with hydronephrosis being the most frequently associated finding. In many cases there is also an association with abnormalities of the kidney and ureters.[11]

The pathogenesis of ureteral valves is debated; however, it has been suggested that they represent a persistent Chawalla membrane or an exuberant form of the ureteral folds seen in normal fetal development.[11,81]

Specific criteria for the diagnosis of ureteral valves have been proposed; (i) The leaflets should be covered by mucosa and contain smooth muscle, (ii) There should be ureteral obstruction proximal to the fold but not distal to it, and (iii) There should be no other evidence of either functional or mechanical obstruction.[81] The requirement for the identification of smooth muscle in the leaflet is debated, while others require smooth muscle in the leaflet base.[11] Valves may occur throughout the length of the ureter, with 50% reported from the proximal ureter, 17% the mid ureter, and 33% the distal ureter. Histologically, ureteral valves may form leaflets or an annular ring of mucosal-covered connective tissue.

Management of valve leaflets is surgical with most treated by ureteroureterostomy, ureteropyelostomy, or longitudinal ureterotomy.[11]

Ureteral folds are rarely detected on excretory urography, and these occasionally have a corkscrew appearance.[10] These folds consist of lamina propria and smooth muscle and probably represent persistent fetal ureteral tortuosity.[10,82] Most cases of ureteral folds are not associated with outflow obstruction, although rarely hydronephrosis may be a presenting feature.[83]

INFLAMMATION AND INFECTION

Renal Pelvis and Ureteral Infection

Infection of the upper urinary tract is usually secondary to lower tract infection and may be associated with urinary tract obstruction, voiding dysfunction, and urinary tract abnormalities (ureteral duplication, megaureter, and UPJ obstruction). Other significant contributing factors include catheterization, instrumentalization, and urinary tract lithiasis, while ureteral infection may occur secondary to pyelonephritis.

The most common pathogenic bacterial organism in the urinary tract is *Escherichia coli* although *Proteus, Klebsiella, Enterococcus, Pseudomonas,* and *Serratia* are frequently encountered. Struvite lithiasis is often associated with *Proteus* and less commonly *Morganella* infection.[84]

Mycobacterium infection of the ureter (Fig. 4-13A and B) is usually secondary to renal infection and may result in the development of stricture leading to hydronephrosis. *Mycobacterium tuberculosis* is most frequently involved, although *M. avium, M. kansasii,* and *M. bovis* infections are also well described.

Upper tract fungal infections are usually associated with systemic disease or localized renal infection in an immunocompromised patient. A wide variety of fungi have been reported as renal pelvis and ureteral pathogens with *Candida* being the most commonly seen. This may form a fungal bezoar within the renal pelvis and, as is reported for *Aspergillus* and *Coccidioides,* may result in ureteral stricture formation.[85,86] There is a single case report of extragenital granuloma inguinale presenting as a soft tissue neoplasm involving the ureter.[87]

Malacoplakia

While more commonly occurring in the urinary bladder, renal parenchyma, and genital tract, occasional cases of malacoplakia of the renal pelvis and ureter (Fig. 4-13C) have been reported.[88–90] There is a female predominance with ages of patients ranging from 24 to 78 years (mean 66 years).[88,91] In the majority of cases, there were no reported preexisting conditions although an association with concurrent acute inflammation and immunosuppression has been noted,[89,92] and there is a single case report of malacoplakia in a transplant ureter.[93]

Malacoplakia of the renal pelvis and/or ureter usually presents as an exophytic tumor-like lesion on imaging and may be mistaken for urothelial carcinoma.[94] Urinary cytology has also been shown to be diagnostic in rare instances.[95] Disease may be bilateral or unilateral and is often associated with urinary obstruction and hydronephrosis.[94] Malacoplakia has also been reported as a cause of secondary UPJ obstruction.[96] On occasion inflammation may be limited to the renal pelvis or ureter; however, there is usually concurrent malacoplakia in the urinary bladder or renal parenchyma, and it has been suggested that involvement of the urinary outflow tract is a secondary feature.[97]

Grossly the lesion may be solitary or multifocal and is soft friable and exophytic ranging from white to pale yellow in color.

Histology shows typical features of malacoplakia with early lesions resembling xanthogranulomatous inflammation without Michaelis-Gutmann bodies, while later lesions may be associated with interstitial fibrosis.[92,98] On ultrastructural examination both histiocytes and urothelial cells contain cytoplasmic multilamellar bodies.[99]

Few reports have identified organisms within foci of malacoplakia although *E. coli* has been isolated,[86] and treatment usually involves either localized or radical resection with adjuvant antibiotic therapy. Occasionally antibiotic treatment alone, or in combination of ureteral stenting, is successful.[88,89,100]

Renal Pelvis and Ureter Lithiasis

Renal lithiasis is a common problem, especially in Western countries, and is increasing in frequency. Within the United States, it is estimated that 13% of males and 7% of females will be diagnosed with a renal stone and that the likelihood of recurrence is up to 50% on a 5-year follow-up.[101,102] The advent of nonsurgical treatments has led to a decline in hospitalization for renal lithiasis although in 2000, 62/100,000 population were treated as inpatients for upper tract stones in the United States, with the rates being highest for the 55- to 64-year age group.[101]

Stone composition is variable (Table 4-2) and in the majority of instances stones form as the result of metabolic disorders, dietary factors, and/or urinary tract abnormalities, although medications such as adenosine, ephedrine, indinavir, and triamterene have been implicated. There is a strong

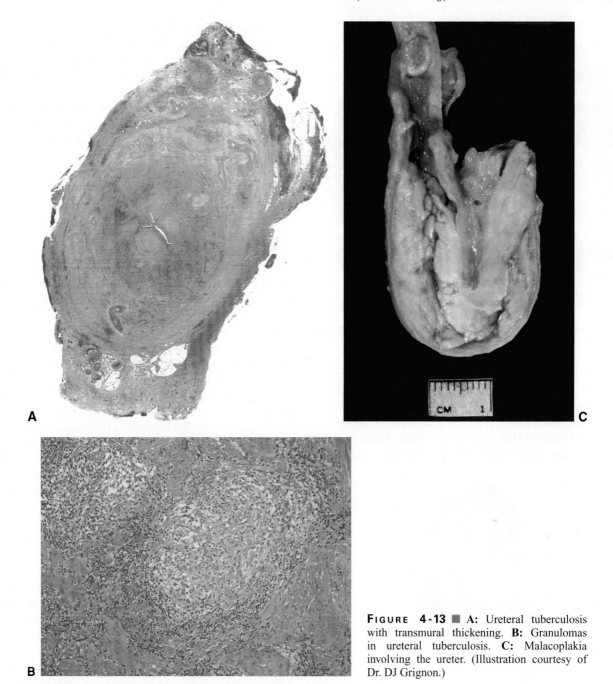

FIGURE 4-13 ■ **A:** Ureteral tuberculosis with transmural thickening. **B:** Granulomas in ureteral tuberculosis. **C:** Malacoplakia involving the ureter. (Illustration courtesy of Dr. DJ Grignon.)

Table 4-2 ■ FREQUENCY OF TYPE OF UPPER TRACT STONE

Calcium oxalate and phosphate	34%
Calcium oxalate	33%
Magnesium ammonium phosphate (struvite)	15%
Uric acid	8%
Calcium phosphate	6%
Cystine	3%
Others	1%

Adapted from Balaji KC, Menon M. Mechanism of stone formation. *Urol Clin North Am* 1997;24:1.

genetic predisposition to some forms of nephrolithiasis, and genes associated with cystinuria, hyperoxaluria, and X-linked nephrolithiasis have been identified.[103] In many cases multiple genetic loci are involved and this reflects the many and diverse causes of hypercalciuria. A separate pathogenesis is described for struvite stones, which form as a result of chronic bacterial infection of the urinary tract, with the presence of urea-splitting bacteria being necessary for the generation of inorganic carbonate and phosphate.[104]

The natural history of stones within the renal pelvis and ureter is dependent on stone type and the metabolic environment. In general terms calyceal stones are asymptomatic

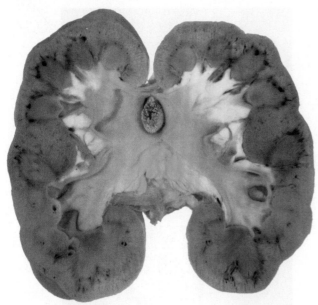

FIGURE 4-14 ■ Calcium oxalate renal stone impacted at the level of the UPJ.

when small, but if untreated, almost 50% will become symptomatic in 5 years.[105] Larger stones within the renal pelvis may present with urinary tract infection, pain, hematuria, dysuria, and obstruction, especially at the UPJ[106] (Fig. 4-14).

Ureteral stones (Fig. 4-15) are often symptomatic, and impaction, with urinary outflow obstruction, may be

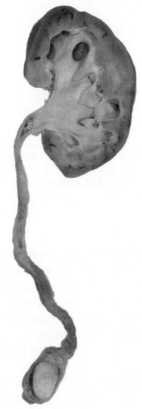

FIGURE 4-15 ■ Ureteral stone situated superior to the vesico-ureteral junction. There is dilation of the ureter and hydronephrosis.

a presenting feature. Stones >5 mm in diameter usually require intervention as they are unlikely to pass spontaneously,[105] and complications include localized mucosal ulceration and edema, leading to scarring and stricture formation, or ureteral perforation.

The pressure effect of renal stones on the mucosa of the renal pelvis is compounded by recurrent acute or chronic inflammation. This results in mucosal ulceration, reactive hyperplasia of adjacent urothelium, granulation tissue formation, and fibrosis. Chronic inflammation predisposes to reactive epithelial changes with a predominance of squamous metaplasia. Other benign mucosal changes reported from the renal pelvis in association with renal lithiasis are pyelitis follicularis, pyelitis cystica, polypoid pyelitis, xanthogranulomatous pyelitis, encrusted pyelitis, and fibroepithelial polyposis.[107] Similar changes are seen in the ureter with chronic inflammation being associated with squamous metaplasia, ureteritis follicularis, ureteritis cystica, and polypoid ureteritis.[107]

Renal lithiasis is a recognized risk factor for renal pelvic and ureteral malignancy.[108] The risk of developing malignancy is enhanced by recurrent urinary tract infections and is most commonly associated with struvite staghorn calculi. In some series the risk of malignancy increased with chronicity, while in others the risk remained stable over a 10-year follow-up.[109] Urothelial carcinoma (UC) is the tumor most frequently associated with lithiasis, although squamous cell carcinoma (SCC) occurs in 20% of cases and has been found in 2% of patients with recurrent staghorn calculi.[110] In addition to these tumors, verrucous carcinoma, sarcomatoid SCC, small cell (neuroendocrine) carcinoma, and adenocarcinoma have been reported.[111–113]

Vasculitis

Although the kidney is the most common organ to be involved in many of the forms of systemic vasculitis,[114] reports of vasculitis of the renal pelvis and ureter are rare and are usually confined to single cases. Vasculitis of the urinary outflow tract often occurs as part of multisystem disease and presents as UPJ obstruction or ureteral stenosis, which may be unilateral or bilateral, with secondary hydronephrosis.

Renal pelvic or ureteral vasculitis has been reported as part of the polyarteritis group of systemic vasculitis (classic polyarteritis nodosa,[115] polyarteritis nodosa associated with hepatitis B,[116] and acute febrile mucocutaneous lymph node syndrome),[23] as well as with Henoch-Schönlein hypersensitivity angiitis[117]. In these cases ureteral stenosis was associated with typical clinical and pathologic systemic features. Renal pelvic and ureteral vasculitis has also been noted in Churg-Strauss syndrome[118] and Wegener granulomatosis[119] in patients with established pulmonary disease. Limited Wegener granulomatosis, involving the urogenital tract, has also been associated with ureteral vasculitis.[120]

Ureteral angiitis as part of the systemic manifestation of rheumatic connective tissue disease occurs rarely and has been noted in cases of systemic sclerosis,[121] systemic lupus erythematosus,[122] and dermatomyositis.[123]

Renal Pelvis and Ureter Injury

Trauma

Renal injury occurs in up to 3% of major trauma; however, direct involvement of the renal pelvis is rare.[124] In cases of blunt or penetrating trauma to either the UPJ or renal pelvis, there is usually hematuria and urinary extravasation may occur. Rarely a urinoma may form and this can become secondarily infected.[125,126] Ureteral trauma is most frequently iatrogenic, with gynecologic procedures predominating and in those cases requiring reconstruction, outcome is predicted by the length of ureteral injury and a history of previous radiotherapy.[127] In cases of noniatrogenic ureteral injury in the United States, 81% result from gunshot wounds, while 10% are related to blunt trauma and 9% to stab wounds.[128]

Radiation

Ureteral stenosis has been reported in 0.3% of patients with a mean follow-up of 5.7 years following curative radiotherapy for gynecologic carcinomas.[129]

In the acute phase following radiotherapy, ureteral dilation occurs in two-thirds of cases, and this usually resolves over 6 months.[130] In experimental animal models asymptomatic fibrotic ureteral stenosis was observed in dogs following doses of 20 Gy, and this has been associated with increased levels of TGF-β1.[131]

High-dose radiation is associated with capillary thrombosis, and in early lesions epithelial atypia and mucosal ulceration are seen. Chronic effects consist of cytoplasmic vacuolation of epithelial cells, loss of pleating with associated telangiectasia of ureteral mucosa, submucosal chronic active inflammation and fibrosis (Fig. 4-16), ureteritis cystica, and squamous metaplasia.[129,132,133] In experimental

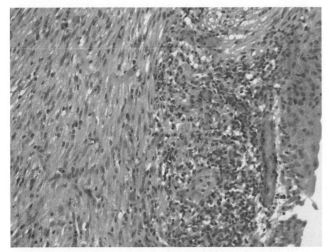

FIGURE 4-16 ■ Ureter, chronic radiation effect. There is chronic inflammation situated predominantly within the mucosa with neovascularization, telangiectasia, and submucosal fibrosis.

animal models these changes have been shown to increase in severity for the first 12 months following radiotherapy. In these studies the resulting stenosis was found to be functional as secondary hydronephrosis developed in the presence of a patent ureter.[132] Ureteral UC has been reported as a secondary effect of radiation,[134] and renal pelvis SCC has also been noted.[135]

Renal Pelvis Hemorrhage

Hemorrhage into the renal pelvis may be associated with subepithelial hematoma (Antopol-Goldman lesion).[136] Often misdiagnosed as renal pelvic neoplasia, 25 cases of subepithelial hematoma have been reported. There is a female predominance with the ages of patients ranging from 24 to 84 years.[136–138] In several cases the cause of the hematoma could not be determined, while in others it was shown to be secondary to trauma, hypertension, analgesic abuse, or coagulopathy. In five cases subepithelial hematomas were associated with congenital renal abnormalities.[136–138] Histologic findings are nonspecific and consist of subepithelial hemorrhage, which may be associated with peripelvic hemorrhage, renal cortical infarction, or hydronephrosis.[138] The majority of cases have been treated by nephrectomy or partial nephrectomy; however, once the diagnosis is established, conservative therapy is advocated.[138]

Hemorrhage into the renal pelvis, in the absence of subepithelial hematoma or neoplasia, has been associated with coumadin anticoagulant therapy[139] and has been recognized as a complication of retrograde endopyelotomy.[140]

Retroperitoneal Fibrosis (Sclerosing Retroperitoneal Fibrosis)

Retroperitoneal fibrosis is typically a diffuse fibrous process that involves the aorta, vena cava, and structures of the retroperitoneum. It may be primary or idiopathic or in approximately 25% of cases is secondary to autoimmune diseases, malignancy, trauma and surgery, chronic infection, drugs (methysergide, pergolide, ergotamine, methyldopa, hydralazine, and beta-blockers), and radiation.[141] There is a prevalence of 1 to 2 cases per 200,000 with a male predominance, and although pediatric cases are well recognized,[142] the majority of patients are 50 to 60 years of age at diagnosis.[143]

The pathogenesis of retroperitoneal fibrosis is uncertain, and the association of secondary forms of the disease with hyperimmune states suggests an autoimmune etiology. There is also a reported association with asbestosis, autoimmune thyroid disease including Riedel thyroiditis, Wegener granulomatosis, mediastinal fibrosis, polyarteritis nodosa, systemic lupus erythematosus, sclerosing cholangitis and primary biliary cirrhosis, UC, and sclerosing lymphoma.[144]

Clinical features are nonspecific and relate to the structure encased in fibrous tissue. Often there is ureteral involvement, and in neglected cases renal failure is a common complication. Laboratory results are similarly nonspecific

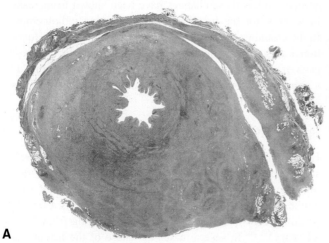
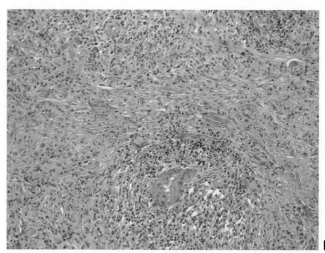

FIGURE 4-17 ■ **A:** Retroperitoneal fibrosis. The ureter is encased in a dense mat of fibrous tissue. **B:** Retroperitoneal fibrosis consisting of sheets of fibroblasts, thick-walled vessels, and a predominantly perivascular chronic inflammatory cell infiltrate.

with elevated C-reactive protein and erythrocyte sedimentation rate, as well as positive antinuclear antibodies being the most frequent findings.

Macroscopically, retroperitoneal fibrosis consists of white fibrous plaques that encase retroperitoneal structures. The fibrosis is usually diffuse; however, in occasional cases the fibrosis is confined to single organs, and localized ureteral (Fig. 4-17A) and perirenal retroperitoneal fibrosis has been reported.[145] On microscopic examination (Fig. 4-17B) the lesions consist of sheets of fibroblasts showing variable cellularity. There is frequently an associated inflammatory infiltrate consisting predominantly of lymphocytes and plasma cells. In older lesions the inflammatory cell infiltrate is less prominent, and there is hyalinization, occasionally with dystrophic calcification.[141] Vascular changes resembling vasculitis, with intramural inflammatory cells and fibrinoid necrosis, are often present.

In the majority of cases, there is both a symptomatic and clinical response to steroids with a resulting decrease in the volume of fibrous tissue.[141] Stenting of ureters is frequently necessary, and in cases refractile to steroids, surgical intervention, consisting of ureteral replacement and autotransplantation of the kidney may be required. Often the disease relapses and long-term follow-up is necessary.[143] In cases of secondary retroperitoneal fibrosis, treatment of the primary disease process may lead to a reduction in the volume of fibrous tissue.

OTHER LESIONS

Reactive Atypia Due to Chemotherapeutic Agents

Topical chemotherapeutic agents such as triethylenethiophosphoramide (thiotepa) and mitomycin C are used to treat superficial urothelial cancer of the upper tract and may produce urothelial atypia.[146,147] Reactive urothelial atypia may also be caused by chemotherapeutic agents given

systemically to treat neoplastic and nonneoplastic disorders. Among these, cyclophosphamide is known to have significant effects on urothelium and can reactivate polyoma virus infection, which morphologically can also mimic carcinoma. busulfan, adriamycin, epirubicin, ethoglucid, cisplatin, and mitoxantrone are other agents known to cause urothelial changes.[147]

Thiotepa and mitomycin C cause a pronounced necroinflammatory process and mucosal denudation accompanied by enlargement, vacuolization, and multinucleation of urothelial cells. These changes can last for several weeks after treatment.[147] Cyclophosphamide produces variable cellular and nuclear enlargement, with binucleation and multinucleation. In these cases, usually there are large, bizarre nuclei resembling those seen after radiotherapy. Nuclei are often eccentric, irregular in outline, and hyperchromatic, with coarse chromatin mimicking carcinoma cells. However, unlike carcinoma, there is loss of chromatin texture with nuclear pyknosis. Cyclophosphamide may also cause hemorrhagic pyelitis and ureteritis, in addition to cystitis. The histologic changes include vascular ectasia with severe edema and hemorrhage of the lamina propria, usually associated with necrosis of the epithelial lining, and mucosal ulceration.[148]

Reactive Atypia Due to Instrumentation, Stents, and Strictures

Biopsies from patients with stents or strictures and after instrumentation can have atypical changes mimicking urothelial CIS. In contrast to urothelial CIS, reactive atypia displays cellular and nuclear enlargement with prominent nucleoli and mitotic activity in the absence of significant pleomorphism and chromatin abnormalities. Immunohistochemistry (CK20, P53, and CD44) may be helpful however, correlation with morphology is critical due to overlap in immunoprofile in reactive versus neoplastic conditions.

Endometriosis and Müllerianosis

Endometriosis, the benign proliferation of ectopic endometrial mucosa, involves the urinary tract in 2% of reported cases.[149] In most of these instances, endometriosis is confined to the urinary bladder; however, in 16% of cases one or both ureters are also involved.[150] In most cases of urinary tract endometriosis, symptoms of dysuria, frequency, recurrent urinary tract infection, and/or renal angle pain are reported, although endometriosis confined to the ureter is asymptomatic in 60% of patients.[151]

In endometriosis diffusely spread within the pelvis and in the urinary tract, lesions are more commonly found on the left side, and it has been speculated that this is a reflection of the direction of flow of peritoneal fluid that carries regurgitated endometrial tissue to ectopic sites.[149]

In 65% of cases involving the ureters, endometriosis is superficial within the overlying peritoneal tissues, and in a further 30% of cases, the endometriotic deposits lie adjacent to the ureter. Intramural endometriosis is present in only 5% of lesions, and these are usually associated with ureteral stenosis.[150,152]

The histologic features of ureteral endometriosis are similar to those seen in other organs. Recognizable endometrial epithelium and stroma may be present, or there may be recent hemorrhage and/or aggregates of hemosiderin and hemosiderin-laden macrophages (Fig. 4-18). In the latter instance CD10 immunohistochemistry is often useful for detecting small foci of residual endometrial stroma. Rarely, Müllerianosis with endocervicosis or endosalpingiosis can be seen as ureteric lesions. In some cases there is associated endometriosis.[153]

Rarely endometrioid adenocarcinoma may arise in ureteral endometriosis, and in one reported case there was no evidence of residual endometriosis in the genital tract or elsewhere in the urinary tract.[154]

Management of endometriosis of the ureter is dependent on the site of the lesion. Peritoneal deposits are amenable to laparoscopic excision, while intramural endometriosis may require ureteral resection and anastomosis.[153,155]

Amyloidosis

Primary localized amyloidosis is rarely seen in the urinary tract with <50 reported cases involving the renal pelvis and ureter.[156–158] There is a male predominance, and patients are usually >50 years of age, with pyrexia, hematuria, and flank pain being common presenting features.[156] On imaging, ureteral stricture and hydronephrosis are frequent findings. This may be unilateral or bilateral and in most cases mimics invasive UC.[157] Although urinary cytology may provide evidence of the correct diagnosis,[157] most cases are diagnosed following surgery.

Histologically, amyloid deposits are interstitial and most commonly involve the lamina propria and muscularis. The amyloid is usually of the AL type, as demonstrated by congophilia with resistance to permanganate treatment, and on immunohistochemistry consists of lambda light chains. Rarely osseous metaplasia may occur.[159] Management usually involves surgical resection of the involved segment.

HYPERPLASIA AND METAPLASIA

Pyeloureteritis Cystica and Glandularis

Pyeloureteritis cystica is a cystic dilation of mucosal urothelial nests (Brunn nests) and is the renal pelvic and ureteral equivalent of cystitis cystica. This may be a variant of normal histology as it is present in up to 10% of normal ureters at autopsy.[160] Pyeloureteritis cystica is usually asymptomatic and is more commonly found in female patients and in the elderly. There is an association with chronic or recurrent infection (including schistosomiasis), lithiasis, and chemical irritants such as formalin instilled for treatment of cyclophosphamide-induced cystitis.[161,162] Although occasionally associated with UC and adenocarcinoma, long-term follow-up suggests that pyeloureteritis cystica has no malignant potential and represents a reactive response to chronic mucosal irritation.[161]

In both the renal pelvis and ureter, cystic lesions are either confined to the mucosa or form polyps covered by urothelium with a loose connective tissue stroma and may be visible on radiologic imaging. Intramural cysts are lined by urothelium, which, in the case of larger cysts, may become attenuated, and there is usually an associated chronic inflammatory cell infiltrate (Fig. 4-19). Transition of urothelium to mucus-secreting and columnar epithelium similar to that of the colon is known as pyeloureteritis glandularis, and this has been suggested as a precursor to adenocarcinoma.[161,163,164]

Various treatments have been recommended, and in the bladder resolution of cystitis cystica has been noted following installation of 2% silver nitrate and with long-term antibiotic treatment.[165,166]

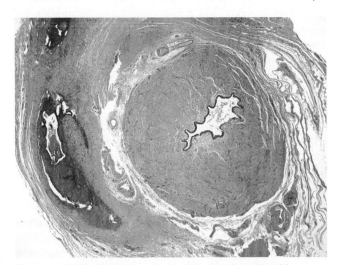

FIGURE 4-18 ■ Endometriosis within the adventitia of the ureter.

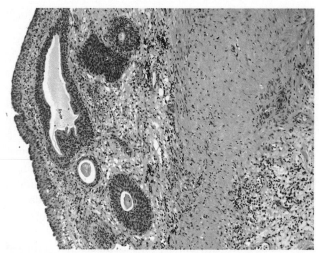

FIGURE 4-19 ■ Pyelitis cystica within the mucosa of the renal pelvis.

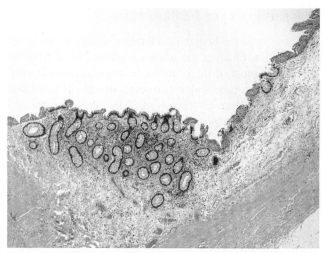

FIGURE 4-20 ■ Glandular metaplasia resembling colonic mucosa within the renal pelvis.

Pyeloureteral Urothelial Hyperplasia and Metaplasia

Irritation of the renal pelvis and ureter may result in epithelial hyperplasia or metaplasia. Hyperplasia of the surface epithelium leads to a thickened flat overgrowth of urothelium.[167] This is seen as a reactive phenomenon but is rarely present in bladders with coexisting low-grade urothelial neoplasms. In cases where irritation is chronic, squamous metaplasia of the urothelium (leukoplakia) may develop. This is most commonly associated with mechanical stimuli such as lithiasis, although an association with radiation, xanthogranulomatous pyelonephritis, and recurrent infection, including schistosomiasis, is well recognized.[132,168–170] Squamous metaplasia is more frequently seen in females, and there is a slight predominance of left-sided lesions[167]; however, unlike those seen in the bladder, pyeloureteral lesions are usually focal. There is often hyperkeratosis and in these cases the term cholesteatoma has been applied, and occasionally dystrophic calcification may also develop.[171] The underlying lamina propria usually contains a variable chronic inflammatory cell infiltrate, and foreign body–type giant cells may develop as a response to the implantation of keratin.[172] There is often atypia of metaplastic epithelial cells, and in 8% to 12% of cases there is an associated SCC.

Glandular metaplasia usually occurs within foci of pyeloureteritis cystica, with formation of colonic-type epithelium, which may contain Paneth cells and intraluminal mucin.[168] Goblet cell metaplasia and diffuse glandular metaplasia are infrequently seen (Fig. 4-20) and most commonly develop in association with lithiasis and chronic infection.[173] Glandular metaplasia may present as a polypoid or sessile mass, and on occasion colonic-type glands may be implanted within the lamina propria mimicking invasive carcinoma.[174] In such cases the benign nature of the epithelium may be determined by a uniform lack of nuclear atypia. There is, however, an association between glandular metaplasia and adenocarcinoma, and this has been reported for both pyeloureteritis glandularis and diffuse glandular metaplasia.[175]

Unusual forms of urothelial metaplasia have been reported. müllerian metaplasia has been noted in the ureter of an otherwise well 39-year-old female. This was characterized by metaplasia of surface epithelium, and additionally Müllerian epithelium–lined cysts were present within the lamina propria.[176] Osseous metaplasia within the ureter is rare and in animal models has developed in response to ischemia, necrosis, fibrosis, and trauma.[177] In single cases osseous metaplasia has been reported in association with amyloidosis and trauma and has also been observed in the ureter of a donor kidney, post-transplantation.[159,178,179] Foci of osseous metaplasia may occasionally act as a nidus for the formation of stones within the renal pelvis and ureter.[159]

Nephrogenic Adenoma

Nephrogenic adenomas are benign lesions of the urothelium and lamina propria. The majority of cases are confined to the bladder; however, in various series 11% to 31% were present in the renal pelvis and ureter, respectively.[180–182] There is a male predominance and the age of patients ranges from 9 to 75 years, which is a similar age distribution for nephrogenic adenoma of the bladder.[180] The pathogenesis is uncertain although the frequent association with coexisting chronic inflammation and stones supports the suggestion that nephrogenic adenoma is a form of urothelial metaplasia. It has also been shown that some of the lesions result from implanted renal tubular cells.[183–185]

Nephrogenic adenoma of the renal pelvis is almost always an incidental finding on histologic examination of nephrectomy specimens and has been reported in association with tuberculosis, renal calculi, calyceal diverticulum, previous surgery, and coexisting urothelial neoplasia.[180,182]

As with renal pelvic lesions, ureteral nephrogenic adenoma is also frequently diagnosed incidentally in resected nephroureterectomy specimens, although rarely cases are initially detected as an incidental finding during radiologic studies.[180] Painless hematuria may also be a presenting feature.[180,183]

Occasionally ureteral nephrogenic adenoma may lead to proximal ureteral dilatation and hydronephrosis,[180] necessitating endoscopic removal. Preexisting conditions associated with ureteral nephrogenic adenoma include neuropathic bladder, tuberculosis, and UC and cytomegalovirus infection in renal transplant patients.[180,186] The histologic features of ureteral and renal pelvic nephrogenic adenoma are similar to those of lesions found elsewhere in the urinary tract (see Chapter 5).

POLYPS, CYSTS, AND OTHER PSEUDOTUMORS

Fibroepithelial Polyps

Fibroepithelial polyps are benign mucosal lesions which rarely occur in the ureter and renal pelvis. The etiology of most fibroepithelial polyps is obscure, but many are considered to be either of congenital or inflammatory origin and are often associated with calculi.[187,188]

Polyps usually occur in young to middle-aged adults, but can also occur in children and the elderly, with a higher frequency in males. Patients present with flank pain, hematuria, or evidence of UPJ obstruction. A filling defect is usually seen on intravenous urography.[187–189]

Polyps occur most commonly in the renal pelvis, proximal ureter, or UPJ. Grossly, one or more fleshy soft polyps may be present, and most are round or bilobed and lobulated (Fig. 4-21). Histologically the polyps are characterized by exophytic projections of fibrous tissue covered by urothelium with varying degrees of inflammation[187,188] (Fig. 4-22).

Cysts

Cysts reported in the upper urinary tract include epidermoid cysts of ureter[190] and parapelvic cysts.[191]

Inflammatory Pseudotumor

Inflammatory pseudotumor, also known as pseudosarcomatous myofibroblastic proliferation, inflammatory myofibroblastic tumor, and postoperative spindle cell nodule, occurs rarely in the upper tract. In contrast to visceral and soft tissue lesions, which occur predominantly in children and young adults, inflammatory pseudotumor of the urinary tract occurs in a

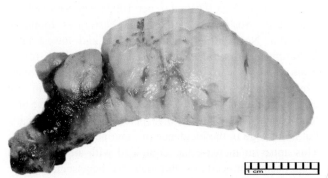

FIGURE 4-21 ■ Ureteral fibroepithelial polyp with surface lobulation.

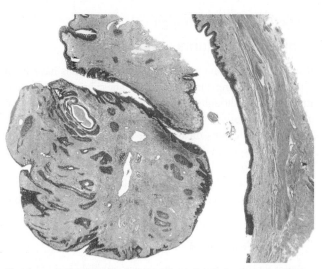

FIGURE 4-22 ■ Renal pelvis fibroepithelial polyp. The fibrous core is covered by urothelium.

wide age range, but predominantly in adults.[192,193] These lesions from elsewhere in the urinary tract have been shown to have anaplastic lymphoma kinase (*ALK*) gene alterations; however, no case reported from the ureter or renal pelvis has shown immunostaining for *ALK* rearrangements.[192,193] Although no recurrences or metastases were reported in a series of cases involving the renal pelvis,[192] one case involving the ureter and renal pelvis was associated with sarcomatoid UC.[193]

Inflammatory pseudotumor is characterized by a proliferation of spindle cells admixed with a chronic inflammatory cell infiltrate, similar to that seen in other locations. Three histologic patterns have been reported with lesions being described as myxoid vascular, compact spindle cell, and hypocellular fibrous. The spindle cells in inflammatory pseudotumor display myofibroblastic characteristics and are positive for vimentin and smooth muscle actin and variably express HHF-35, cytokeratins, desmin, and CD68.[192,193]

NEOPLASMS

The renal pelvis and ureter give rise to a variety of benign and malignant neoplasms of both epithelial and mesenchymal types. These account for about 9% of all urinary tract neoplasms[194] and 10% to 15% of renal tumors.[194,195] Carcinomas arising in this location are derived from the urothelium and are therefore similar to bladder cancers. Compared to bladder cancers, however, these tumors are less common and may be associated with several familial syndromes. Other differences include the relative inaccessibility of the renal pelvis and ureter to topical therapies and, given the anatomical differences such as thickness of the muscularis, the possibility of early metastatic spread. More than 90% of renal pelvic and ureteral carcinomas are UCs, with adenocarcinoma and SCC being more rarely encountered.[196] Similar to those of the bladder, pelviureteral tumors are more common in males and in older patients.[197]

Epithelial Tumors: Benign

Urothelial Papilloma

Rare cases of pelviureteral urothelial papillomas have been reported in children and adults.[198,199] These are usually found incidentally although some may present with hematuria, and radiologically a filling defect is usually seen. These are mostly small lesions measuring a few millimeters in diameter and being treated by fulguration are not usually sent for histopathologic evaluation.

Histologically these delicate papillary lesions have a thin fibrovascular core covered by benign urothelium of normal thickness.

Inverted Papilloma

Pelviureteral inverted papillomas are rare[200,201] and are more frequently seen in the ureter than in the renal pelvis.[202] These occur in adults and there is a male predominance. Some inverted papillomas present with gross or microscopic painless hematuria, flank pain, or colic or may be detected as a filling defect seen on intravenous urography.

Inverted papillomas of the renal pelvis and ureter are either sessile or pedunculated polyps, usually measuring <3 cm in maximum dimension and having a similar histology to those seen in the bladder.

Inverted papillomas are benign neoplasms usually treated by local excision. However, the long-term outcome is unknown. Some cases are associated with multicentricity and coexistent malignancy,[200,202] and for these reasons, long-term follow-up is recommended.

Villous Adenoma

Tumors similar in morphology to villous adenoma of the colon occur in the urinary tract, with rare examples reported in the ureter[203,204] and renal pelvis.[205,206] These tumors occur in adults with a similar incidence in males and females. There is an association with renal calculi, long-standing chronic inflammation, and intestinal metaplasia, and patients usually present with hematuria or flank pain. Abundant mucus production and mucus retention causing distension of the renal pelvis (muconephrosis) and proximal ureter may also occur.[204,206] Histologically these are papillary exophytic tumors with pointed or blunt, finger-like processes lined by pseudostratified columnar epithelium displaying variable atypia (Fig. 4-23). Most adenomas have cytoplasmic mucin and are positive for cytokeratins CK7 and CK20, while some are positive for carcinoembryonic antigen and epithelial membrane antigen (EMA). Patients without coexistent adenocarcinoma have an excellent prognosis with no recurrence being reported after local excision.[203] Given the rarity of reported cases in the upper tract, it is advisable that these patients are followed closely, even after apparent complete excision of the lesion. If the lesion is not entirely submitted for examination, a definite diagnosis of villous adenoma should not be made as there is a risk of missing deeper and occult adenocarcinoma.

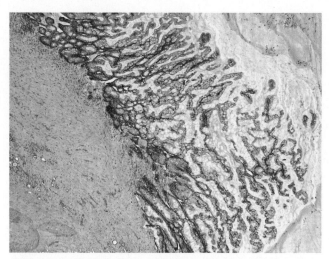

FIGURE 4-23 ■ Villous adenoma of the renal pelvis.

Pheochromocytoma

Extraadrenal pheochromocytomas or paragangliomas develop in the paraganglionic chromaffin cells of the sympathetic nervous system, and rare cases have been reported in the renal pelvis and ureter.[207] Magnetic resonance imaging is now considered preferable to computed tomography scans for the diagnosis of these lesions because of increased diagnostic accuracy and because they avoid the possible risk of a hypertensive crisis that can be precipitated by intravenous contrast medium.[207]

Epithelial Tumors: Malignant

Urothelial Carcinoma

Epidemiology

UC of the renal pelvis and ureter accounts for about 5% of all urothelial tumors of the urinary tract.[208] Two-thirds of the upper tract tumors occur in the renal pelvis, while most ureteral cancers occur in the distal ureter.[197] Pelviureteral UC is multifocal in about one-third of patients, but bilaterality is uncommon, seen in only about 3% of patients.[209] These tumors are twice as common in males as in females and twice as common in whites as in African-Americans. The mean age at presentation for UC is 65 years, and tumors are rare in those <40 years of age.[208] The incidence of tumors is 0.6 to 1.1 per 100,000 person-years[197] and varies worldwide, with the highest rates found in Australia, North America, and Europe and lowest rates in South and Central America and Africa.[210,211] In recent years, there appears to have been an increase in the incidence of UC.[207] Other studies report an increase in situ carcinoma ranging from 7.2% to 23.1% and in invasive ureteral cancers from 0.69 to 0.73 per 100,000 person-years, but no change in the incidence of renal pelvic tumors.[197,212] This apparent increase has coincided with an increase in ureteroscopic procedures, but may also be associated with increased environmental exposure to carcinogens as well as the effects of an aging population.

The incidence of UC of the upper tract after bladder cancer varies between 2% and 13.4%, with most upper tract tumors found within 3 to 6 years after the diagnosis of the bladder primary. The risk is significantly higher in patients with high-grade tumors, multifocal tumors, urothelial CIS, and urethral involvement,[213-215] and patients with CIS of the bladder and upper tract involvement show high rates of tumor bilaterality.[215]

Etiopathogenesis

Genetic Susceptibility. A familial risk has been found in some patients with upper tract UC[216,217] whose carcinomas have identical karyotypic profiles to those of bladder UC.[218,219] Rearrangements of chromosome 9 resulting in loss of material from 9p, 9q or of the entire chromosome are the most frequent alterations, seen in 50% to 75% of all patients.[218] Loss of material from chromosome arms, 1p, 8p, and 11p, with gains of chromosome 7, 1q, and 8q seem to be early changes occurring in superficial low-grade tumors, whereas loss of material from 17p, formation of isochromosome 5p, and p53 mutations are seen in more aggressive, invasive tumor phenotypes.[218,220] Mutations of *FGFR3, KRT20, UPK2, FXYD, 3 hTERT,* and *BIRC5* have also been reported.[221] Upper tract UC may also develop as a component of the hereditary nonpolyposis colorectal cancer (HNPCC) syndrome (Lynch syndrome), which is characterized by germline mutations in a number of DNA mismatch repair (MMR) genes, detectable as microsatellite instability (MSI) or loss of the respective protein by immunostaining. MSI occurs in 20% to 31% of patients with upper tract UC,[222,223] although a recent population-based study from Sweden found an incidence of only 6% in these tumors.[224] About 90% of cases show loss of MMR proteins hMSH2, hMLH1, or hMSH6, and in 7% to 33% of cases, there is alteration of coding sequence microsatellites (TGFbetaRII, Bax, hMSH3, and hMSH6).[223] These tumors have been shown to have significantly different clinical findings from sporadic upper tract UC, including a high prevalence in females and characteristic histopathologic features such as frequent papillary and inverted growth patterns. In one study, an inverted morphology of at least 20% of the tumor was found in 65.7% of microsatellite-unstable tumors, compared with only 17.5% of microsatellite-stable tumors.[225] Inverted growth in upper tract urothelial cancers may serve as a marker lesion for MSI and may assist in identifying patients who should be tested for HNPCC.[223,225] Some studies have shown a low tumor stage and grade for these tumors,[223,225] while a recent study has shown a high-grade potential similar to that in the general population with an almost equal gender ratio.[226] These occur at a younger age and are more likely to be in the ureter (Box 4-1).[226]

Tobacco Smoking. Significantly increased relative risks for development of upper tract UC are seen in smokers compared with nonsmokers.[227,228] The risk of urothelial cancer in smokers is higher in the ureter than in the renal pelvis and is higher in the renal pelvis, when compared to the urinary bladder.

Box 4-1 ● MOLECULAR ALTERATIONS, ASSOCIATIONS, AND PREDISPOSING FACTORS

Genetic susceptibility
  Deletion of part or all of chromosome 9
  Loss of 1p, 8p, and 11p
  Gains of chromosome 7, 1q, and 8q
  Loss of material from 17p, isochromosome 5p
  Mutations of *p53, FGFR3, KRT20, UPK2, FXYD3*
    and *hTERT, BIRC5*
  HNPCC syndrome
Tobacco smoking
Occupational exposures
Analgesic abuse
Balkan and endemic nephropathy
Thorotrast exposure
Chronic infection associated with staghorn calculi
Chinese herbal nephropathy
Arsenic exposure (blackfoot disease)

Occupational Exposure. There are several occupational exposures linked to renal pelvic cancers. The dry-cleaning, iron, and steel industries are reported as high-risk occupations,[229] and significantly increased risks have also been reported in the petrochemical, chemical, and plastic industries and from exposure to coal and coke, asphalt, and tar.[227,229]

Analgesic Abuse. Chronic abuse of analgesics, and especially that of phenacetin, is an established risk factor for carcinoma of the upper urinary tract.[230,231] Regular consumption of phenacetin-containing analgesics confers a 10-fold relative risk in women and four- to eightfold relative risks in men for the development of renal pelvic cancer. There also appears to be an increased risk from aspirin use among women.[232] There is a synergistic effect, when there is both analgesic abuse and tobacco smoking,[232] with a reduction in the incidence of renal pelvic cancer resulting from cessation of both risk factors.[233] A history of analgesic abuse is strongly associated with the presence and severity of diffuse renal papillary scarring with thickening of the basement membrane around subepithelial capillaries (capillary sclerosis), and this lesion confers an increased risk of UC.[234] For both phenacetin and aspirin, a dose effect has been observed as moderate consumption doubles the risk of renal pelvic cancer, and heavy consumption increases the risk to 6 to 16 times that for nonconsumers.[232] The histologic grade of the tumors also tends to rise in a dose-dependent fashion.[235] Patients with renal transplants for end-stage analgesic nephropathy also have an increased risk of upper tract UC in the transplanted kidney.[236]

Balkan Endemic Nephropathy. Balkan endemic nephropathy (BEN) is a chronic tubulointerstitial nephritis with notable concentric atrophy of the ureter and renal cortex. BEN is endemic in Bosnia, Bulgaria, Croatia, Romania, and Serbia in settlements around the South Morava River and its tributaries. There is evidence that BEN is an environmentally induced disease related to exposure to organic vegetable and/or fungal toxins, especially aristolochic acid, in patients with familial metabolic abnormalities. The disease has an insidious onset and slow progression to terminal renal failure, and patients have an increased incidence of upper tract UC.[237,238] These tumors are more likely to be low grade and bilateral when compared to those from nonendemic areas,[238] and there is an increased risk of UC after renal transplantation in these patients.[239]

Other Risk Factors. Renal pelvic carcinomas have been reported between 14 and 41 years after thorotrast pyelography.[240] There is also a well-reported association between long-standing chronic infection in the presence of staghorn (struvite) calculi and renal pelvic UC.[241,242] Chinese herb nephropathy, a chronic tubulointerstitial nephritis related to use of Chinese herbs containing aristolochic acid, is also associated with a high risk of UC, and >50% of these tumors occur in the upper tract.[243,244] An unusually high incidence of upper tract UC has been reported from endemic areas for "blackfoot disease" of southern Taiwan, due to arsenic contamination of water.[245]

Clinical Features

Gross or microscopic hematuria is the most common presenting symptom for upper tract UC, while there may also be dull flank pain, resulting from gradual onset of outflow obstruction with hydronephrotic distension. Pain may be acute and mimic renal colic due to the passage of blood clot or necrotic tumor fragments. Some patients are asymptomatic at presentation, and the tumor is diagnosed as an incidental finding on radiologic evaluation. Advanced cancers usually present with an abdominal or flank mass, weight loss, anorexia, and bone pain.[246,247]

Pathology. Diagnosis of upper tract UC is usually made with intravenous urography or retrograde pyelography by detection of a discrete filling defect. Diagnosis is confirmed by cystoscopy and ureteropyeloscopy, with biopsy, while cytologic assessment of washings and brushings from the upper tract may be useful. Only superficial biopsies are performed to avoid risk of perforation due to the thinness of the muscular walls, and therefore, biopsy samples are usually not reliable for staging purposes.[248]

Voided urine cytology is positive in 60% of renal pelvic UC and in 35% of ureteral UC.[249] There is a high positive predictive value for high-grade lesions including CIS, whereas the predictive value for low-grade lesions is <50%.[250,251] Upper tract cytology specimens can be difficult to interpret as benign cells in this location frequently have an atypical appearance, while lithiasis and inflammation may also result in a false-positive diagnosis. In cases with concurrent bladder UC, there is a possibility of contamination of the upper tract sample.

The morphologic characteristics of urothelial dysplasia and carcinoma of the upper tract are similar to those tumors found in the bladder.

Urothelial dysplasia (low-grade intraurothelial neoplasia) may not be apparent macroscopically, or there may be erythema, erosions, or rarely ulceration. Variable loss of

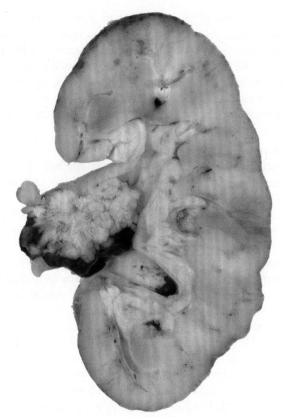

FIGURE 4-24 ■ Multifocal papillary urothelial carcinoma of the renal pelvis.

polarity and significant cytologic atypia, not severe enough to merit a diagnosis of CIS, characterize these lesions.[252,253]

CIS (high-grade intraurothelial neoplasia) is a flat lesion with nuclear anaplasia similar to high-grade UC. This lesion is frequently seen in association with invasive UC, particularly in patients with analgesic nephropathy.[252,253]

Macroscopically, noninvasive UC may be solitary or multifocal, and there is usually distension of the renal pelvis or ureter (Figs. 4-24 to 4-26). As for bladder UC, papillary

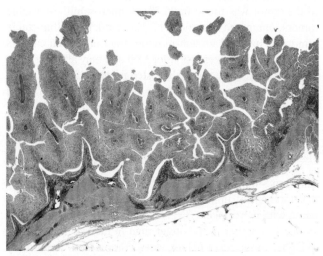

FIGURE 4-25 ■ Papillary urothelial carcinoma of the renal pelvis.

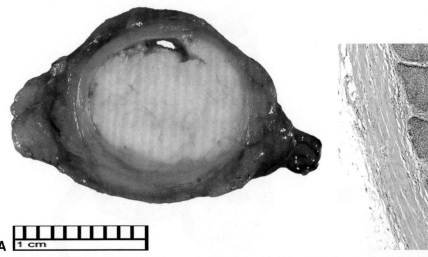
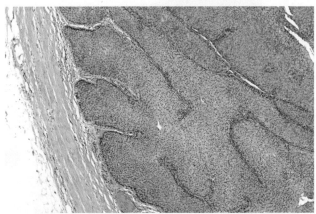

FIGURE 4-26 ■ **A:** Noninvasive urothelial carcinoma distends the lumen of the ureter. **B:** Noninvasive low-grade UC of the ureter.

noninvasive tumors are classified as papillary urothelial neoplasm of low malignant potential or papillary UC depending on the architectural abnormalities and the degree of nuclear atypia.

Invasive UC may be solitary or multifocal and are papillary, polypoid, solid nodular (Fig. 4-27), ulcerated, or diffusely infiltrative causing thickening of the renal pelvis or ureter. Infiltration of the renal medulla is preceded by in situ extension of the UC into collecting ducts (Fig. 4-28), and invasive tumors usually form a solid mass involving renal parenchyma, which may mimic a primary renal cell carcinoma (Fig. 4-29). In advanced cases the carcinoma may infiltrate diffusely and often has marked associated desmoplasia (Fig. 4-30). Ureteral tumors may be associated with ureteral obstruction and proximal hydronephroureter (Fig. 4-31).

Invasive UC is classified as low grade or high grade depending on the degree of nuclear atypia and architectural abnormality. As in the bladder, invasion is characterized by suburothelial

nests, clusters, or single cells with a stromal reaction and paradoxical differentiation. The stromal reaction can be in the form of retraction artifact, desmoplasia, inflammation, or a pseudosarcomatous reaction. Invasive carcinoma in this location may show the entire morphologic spectrum of bladder UC. Lymph node metastasis from renal pelvic UC is primarily to the renal hilar, paracaval, retrocaval, and para-aortic lymph nodes; from the upper two-thirds of the ureter to the paraaortic, retrocaval, and interaortocaval nodes; and from the lower ureter, to nodes inferior to the aortic bifurcation.[254] Metastatic spread is most commonly to the liver, lungs, and bone,[255] although rare metastatic sites include the heart, skin, and penis.[256,257]

Cytologic evaluation is not useful in distinguishing papillary from invasive UC as these have similar cytologic characteristics.

High-grade invasive UC, particularly when there is divergent differentiation, can be difficult to differentiate from other invasive carcinomas of the renal pelvis such as poorly

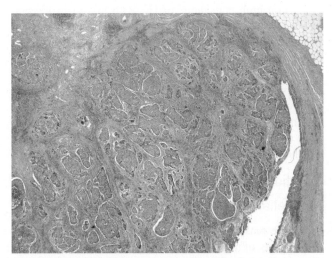

FIGURE 4-27 ■ UC of the renal pelvis showing a nodular infiltrative pattern.

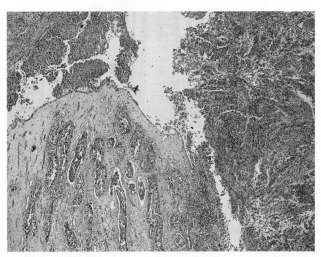

FIGURE 4-28 ■ High-grade UC of the renal pelvis with in situ extension into distal collecting ducts.

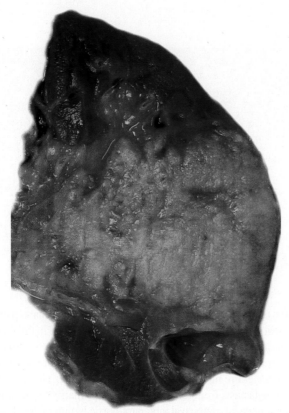

FIGURE 4-29 ■ Advanced UC of the renal pelvis with renal infiltration.

differentiated SCC and adenocarcinoma. High-grade UC invading into the renal parenchyma can mimic renal cell carcinoma, and in such instances the detection of urothelial CIS or a papillary component can be diagnostically helpful. p63 immunostaining is of value in differentiating UC from renal cell carcinoma as even in poorly differentiated tumors it is positive in 96% of upper tract UC, but not in most renal cell

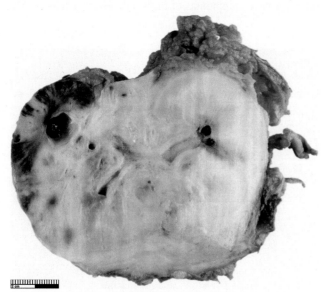

FIGURE 4-30 ■ Kidney with diffusely infiltrative desmoplastic UC.

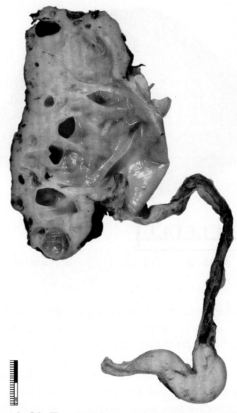

FIGURE 4-31 ■ UC of the ureter with dilatation of the proximal ureter and hydronephrosis.

carcinomas.[258,259] A PAX8+/p63− immunoprofile supports the diagnosis of collecting duct carcinoma with most UC showing an inverse pattern of staining.[259] Monoclonal antibodies against placental S100 protein (S100P) and GATA3 have also been found useful, as a high percentage of UC is positive, whereas clear cell renal cell carcinomas are negative.[260] CD10 is positive in about 50% upper tract UC, compared to 90% of renal cell carcinomas.[261]

Immunodetection of various antigens has been correlated with outcome for upper tract UC. Uroplakin III staining is found in a high percentage of UC with loss of expression associated with a poor prognosis.[262] Ki-67 overexpression is significantly correlated with tumor grade and stage and is of prognostic value, while p53, matrix metalloproteinase MMP-2, and MMP-9 are of limited value in predicting outcome.[263,364] The expression of CD44 isoforms is associated with tumor differentiation and progression; however, this is not independent of stage.[265] Alpha-methylacyl-CoA racemase (AMACR) expression may be of prognostic utility, as it is most frequent in high stage and high-grade tumors.[266]

Morphologic Variants

Urothelial Carcinoma with Mixed Differentiation

UC of the renal pelvis may display divergent differentiation, and a variety of morphologic patterns may be seen in association with UC. Mixed morphologic patterns are present in about 40% of high-grade pelvic UC[267] with the most common subtype

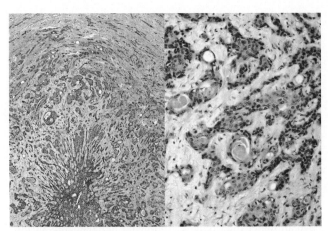

FIGURE 4-32 ■ Invasive UC of the ureter (*left*) showing focal squamous differentiation (*right*).

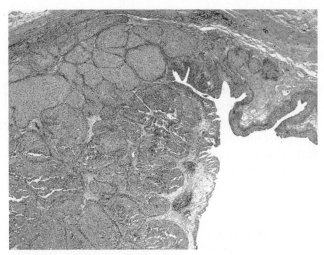

FIGURE 4-33 ■ Low-grade UC of the renal pelvis exhibiting a prominent inverted growth pattern.

being SCC (Fig. 4-32), which comprises 10% of cases.[267,268] Foci of other types of differentiation including adenocarcinoma, sarcomatoid carcinoma, small cell neuroendocrine carcinoma, micropapillary UC, and lymphoepithelioma-like carcinoma may also be present. The median survival for patients with these tumors is <3 years although a small proportion of patients, who present with renal pelvis tumor showing minimal or no infiltration of the renal parenchyma, have a more favorable prognosis following radical nephrectomy (Box 4-2).[267]

Microcystic Carcinoma

Rare cases of a deceptively bland variant of invasive UC have been reported in the renal pelvis. In these tumors, there are cysts of varying size lined by single or multiple layers of cuboidal or flattened cells, with minimal cytologic atypia.[269]

Micropapillary Urothelial Carcinoma

Micropapillary UC is found in about 3% of UC of the renal pelvis and ureter. These tumors usually present at an advanced stage with lymphovascular invasion and distant metastasis. The presence of invasive micropapillary UC, even focally, appears to indicate a poor clinical course.[270,271]

Urothelial Carcinoma with Inverted Growth Pattern

Papillary urothelial neoplasms may show an endophytic growth pattern, and this should be distinguished from true invasion[272] (Fig. 4-33). In some cases inverted carcinoma extends into the kidney along collecting ducts. These lesions have an excellent prognosis following nephrectomy.[267]

Osteoclast-rich Sarcomatoid Carcinoma

Sarcomatoid (undifferentiated) carcinoma containing osteoclastic giant cells has been reported in the renal pelvis with associated urothelial CIS and/or high-grade papillary UC. These tumors are composed of evenly spaced multinucleated giant cells on a background of ovoid or spindled mononuclear cells. Multinucleated cells have the morphologic and immunohistochemical properties of osteoclasts being positive for CD68, leukocyte common antigen, CD51, and CD54 and negative for cytokeratins and EMA. These tumors are invariably at a high stage at presentation and have a poor prognosis.[273,274]

Urothelial Carcinoma with Choriocarcinoma or Syncytiotrophoblastic Giant Cells

UC with trophoblastic differentiation occurs rarely in the renal pelvis. A close genetic relationship between these two neoplastic components has been documented, pointing to clonal evolution of UC with acquisition of trophoblastic differentiation. In these tumors HCG staining is seen within the choriocarcinoma and focally within the associated high-grade UC. Widespread hepatic and pulmonary metastases with choriocarcinomatous features have been reported with

---

Box 4-2 ● HISTOLOGIC VARIANTS OF UC SEEN IN THE UPPER TRACT

UC with squamous differentiation
UC with glandular differentiation
Microcystic urothelial carcinoma
Micropapillary urothelial carcinoma
UC with inverted growth pattern
Osteoclast-rich undifferentiated carcinoma
Urothelial carcinoma with choriocarcinoma or syncytiotrophoblastic giant cells
Sarcomatoid variant
Lipid-cell variant
Lymphoepithelioma-like carcinoma
Nested variant
Plasmacytoid variant
Signet-ring cell
Clear cell variant
UC showing rhabdoid differentiation

these tumors. In some cases there are syncytiotrophoblastic giant cells in association with invasive high-grade UC.[275,276]

Sarcomatoid Variant

Sarcomatoid carcinoma (formerly known as carcinosarcoma) is a rare aggressive malignancy composed of epithelial and stromal components. Coexisting UC is present in most cases, and some tumors display heterologous elements. These tumors often coexpress keratins, EMA, and vimentin[276] and usually present with metastatic disease or advanced involvement of renal parenchyma. The prognosis is extremely poor with most patients dying within 2 years.[277,278]

Lipid-cell Variant

Rare cases of lipid-cell variant, composed of large epithelial cells with abundant clear multivacuolated cytoplasm mimicking lipoblasts, have been reported in the renal pelvis. Tumor cells lack mucin and are strongly positive for cytokeratins 7 and 20 and EMA. High-grade UC is invariably present. These tumors exhibit aggressive behavior and have a poor prognosis.[279]

Lymphoepithelioma-like Carcinoma

Carcinoma that histologically resembles lymphoepithelioma-like carcinoma of the nasopharynx and characterized by a heavy lymphocytic or mixed inflammatory infiltrate has been reported in the upper tract. EBV-encoded RNA has not been demonstrated in these tumors, and most are at an advanced stage at presentation.[267]

Other Variants of Urothelial Carcinoma

Nested, plasmacytoid, signet-ring cell, and clear cell variants of UC, as well as tumors showing rhabdoid differentiation, rarely occur in the renal pelvis and ureter.[267,280–284]

Prognosis and Predictive Factors

Tumor stage and grade are the most significant factors predicting recurrence and survival. The pT3 stage for renal pelvic UC differs from that of the ureter based on anatomical differences and includes invasion of the renal parenchyma. Involvement of renal tubules without stromal invasion in renal pelvic tumors should not be considered pT3. Patients with pT3 tumors, who have macroscopic or extensive renal parenchymal and/or fat infiltration, appear to have a worse prognosis than those with pT3 tumors displaying only microscopic invasion of these areas.[285,286] In some studies, the prognosis of these tumors was found to be similar to pT4 cancers.[285,286] There appears to be no significant difference in the stage-specific 5-year survival for renal pelvic and ureteral UC.[197] Although upper tract tumors usually present at a higher stage than bladder UC, they have a similar behavior to bladder UC of the same stage and grade.[287] The overall 5-year disease-specific survival of patients diagnosed with an upper tract UC has improved over the last 45 years and currently is about 75%.[197,288] Actuarial 5-year disease-specific survival rates by the primary tumor stage are 95% to 100% for Ta/CIS, 85% to 92% for T1, 75% to 83%

for T2, and 40% to 60% for T3.[197,288,289] Patients with stage 4 tumors have a very poor prognosis with a median survival of 6 months.[288] The ISUP/WHO grading system for bladder UC, incorporated in the 2004 WHO classification of bladder tumors,[210,290,291] is also applied to UC of the upper tract and has prognostic significance. Other independent prognostic factors are patient age, sex, race, type of surgical procedure, tumor multifocality, and vascular invasion.[288,290]

Patients with upper tract UC are at risk of developing synchronous or metachronous tumors in other urothelial locations, including the contralateral upper tract.[292,293] Ipsilateral upper tract recurrence is common in patients managed without nephroureterectomy, and one-third of patients with UC have an upper tract relapse, following percutaneous or ureteroscopic tumor resection, or ablation. The risk of relapse is grade dependent as <20% of low grade tumors relapse, which compares with >50% of high grade tumors.[294] Between 20% and 50% of patients with upper tract carcinoma subsequently develop bladder UC,[255,295] and in particular, those with locally resected tumors require lifelong surveillance.

Treatment

Open or laparoscopic radical nephroureterectomy or distal ureterectomy for distal ureteral tumors is the standard treatment for all but the lowest risk tumors.[248,296] Endoscopic resection may be undertaken for small low-grade tumors, while BCG and interferon alpha 2B after tumor ablation have also been found effective for papillary tumors.[297] Adjuvant radiotherapy, with and without concurrent chemotherapy, after tumor resection has been found by some to be beneficial for locally advanced cancers[298]; however, others have found that these therapies do not affect the outcome of patients with advanced disease.[255] Surgery and subsequent adjuvant chemotherapy, with paclitaxel and carboplatin for locally advanced high-risk upper tract cancers, have shown a reduced risk for the development of distant metastases.[299]

Squamous Cell Carcinoma

SCC accounts for 0.5% of renal tumors and 6% to 15% of upper tract malignancies.[268,300,301]

Most SCC of the upper tract is associated with chronic infection, renal calculi of long duration, and outflow obstruction with hydronephrosis. A history of urolithiasis is found in 25% of patients with SCC of the renal pelvis,[196,301] and it is presumed that chronic irritation and inflammation promotes neoplastic transformation. A history of abuse of analgesics containing phenacetin produces a risk of SCC higher than that of UC. Occasionally SCC is related to a history of external beam radiotherapy to the abdominal or pelvic region.[268] These tumors have been associated with paraneoplastic syndromes such as hypercalcemia, leucocytosis, and thrombocytosis.[302–305]

The age distribution of patients with SCC of the upper tract is similar to that seen with UC, with a median age at presentation of 72 years.[268] These tumors are more frequent in females in contrast to UC of the upper tract and bladder. Common presenting symptoms are hematuria and flank pain. Radiologic findings are nonspecific, and solid space-occupying lesion, hydronephrosis, and calcification are common.

Typically, SCC is large and unifocal within the renal pelvis or ureter and frequently involves the kidney and perinephric tissues.

Histologically these tumors typically have a solid or mixed solid and papillary pattern, while other microscopic features are similar to SCC seen in other locations, although upper tract tumors are typically high grade.

Metastatic SCC from another location, such as lung, needs to be considered in the differential diagnosis and may require clinical investigation for exclusion. UC with squamous differentiation, rather than SCC, is diagnosed when there is any associated UC including urothelial CIS.[267] This is of little practical importance, however, as there is no significant difference in prognosis between patients with pure SCC and those with focal areas showing other histology, including UC.

Tumor stage, but not grade, appears to have strong prognostic value, as most tumors present at an advanced stage. Compared with 62% of UCs, <5% of SCCs are at stage pT2 or lower at diagnosis; however, there is no significant difference in the disease-specific 5-year survival rates between patients with SCC and UC of the same stage.[268,306] The outcome for patients with advanced upper tract SCC is poor with a mean survival in the order of a few months. Bladder SCC and metachronous contralateral upper tract tumors following surgery for an upper tract SCC are more unusual than with upper tract UC, and for this reason the value of regular cystoscopy and follow-up urography after an upper tract SCC is questionable. Vascular invasion, solid tumor growth pattern, and large tumor size have prognostic significance, and the most common metastatic sites are the regional lymph nodes, lungs, liver, and bone.

Patients with stage T1 to T2 SCC can be treated with radical surgery, and these have a good prognosis. Advanced tumors respond poorly to adjuvant or neoadjuvant chemotherapy and radiotherapy.[268]

Adenocarcinoma

Adenocarcinoma of the upper tract is rarely seen and accounts for <1% of renal pelvic tumors. Males and females are equally affected, and predisposing factors include chronic irritation, repeated infections, nephrolithiasis, pyeloureteral glandularis, and urothelial glandular (intestinal) metaplasia.[307] Typically, patients present with gross or microscopic hematuria, or flank pain.

Hydronephrosis, with distension of the renal pelvis or the involved segment of ureter, with copious thick viscid mucus, is a typical finding.[307] Adenocarcinomas, particularly those in elderly patients, may be of the intestinal type and can show tubulovillous, mucinous (Fig. 4-34), clear cell, and signet-ring cell varieties. Nonintestinal papillary adenocarcinomas account for 7% of adenocarcinomas. These occur in a much younger patient population and are characterized by the presence of psammoma bodies.[307–309]

Metastatic adenocarcinoma, collecting duct carcinoma, and UC with glandular differentiation need to be considered

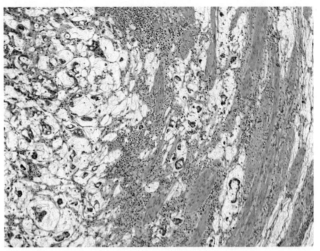

FIGURE 4-34 ■ Ureteral mucinous adenocarcinoma.

in the differential diagnosis. Nonintestinal-type adenocarcinoma, which has been postulated to be of collecting duct origin, is differentiated from Bellini duct carcinoma by its almost entirely renal pelvic location, minimal cytologic atypia, and the presence of frequent psammoma bodies. Absence of atypia and proliferation in adjacent collecting ducts are also helpful feature in differentiation.

Survival of patients with upper tract adenocarcinoma depends on histologic subtype, histology grade, and tumor stage at presentation. Tubulovillous adenocarcinomas are the most aggressive subtype of adenocarcinoma with a 5-year survival rate of <30%. In comparison, mucinous tumors have a 5-year survival rate of 67%, while that of papillary nonintestinal tumors approaches 100%.[307] Nephrectomy or nephroureterectomy is beneficial for lower-stage tumors, although most adenocarcinomas are high grade and present at a high stage[196,308] and chemotherapy and/or radiotherapy may improve short-term survival.

Small Cell Carcinoma

Primary small cell carcinoma of the renal pelvis and ureter is very rare and usually presents at an advanced stage.[196,310,311] These tumors occur in an age group similar to that of UC, with a median age at presentation of 62 years. There is a female predominance (male to female ratio 1:3.4), and the most common presenting symptoms are abdominal pain and hematuria. Distant metastases are present in 32% of patients at the time of diagnosis.[311]

Most small cell carcinomas are large at presentation and have gross and microscopic features similar to those of small cell neuroendocrine carcinomas from other locations. Neuroendocrine markers such as CD56, chromogranin A, synaptophysin, and neuron-specific enolase (NSE) are usually positive.

As with small cell neuroendocrine carcinoma in other locations, these tumors have propensity to spread via the lymphatics and blood vessels and to infiltrate to lymph nodes and distant organs, and death usually occurs within 1 year of diagnosis.[311] Surgery and systemic chemotherapy are the primary therapeutic modalities for small cell carcinomas, and the use of platinum-based chemotherapy has been shown to improve overall survival.[311]

Carcinoid Tumor

Carcinoid tumors have rarely been reported from the ureter[312] and renal pelvis.[312–314] These tumors usually occur in patients younger than 50 years of age, and males and females are equally affected. Carcinoid syndrome has not been reported in association with these tumors, and patients frequently present with lymph node metastases. Despite the presence of distant metastases, these tumors often have a prolonged clinical course.[314]

Upper tract carcinoids have morphologic features similar to those of carcinoid tumors occurring elsewhere, and cytologic examination of urine sediment may occasionally be diagnostic.[315] These tumors are positive for pancytokeratin, synaptophysin, vimentin, chromogranin, and NSE and contain dense core granules on ultrastructural examination.[313–315]

Mesenchymal Tumors: Benign

Leiomyoma

Despite being the most commonly reported benign mesenchymal neoplasms of the ureter and renal pelvis, upper tract leiomyomas are rarely seen. These tumors are usually found in adults with an average age at presentation of 44 years, although occasional cases have been reported in children.[316–318]

The clinical presentation of these tumors is variable, and although most are asymptomatic and discovered incidentally, others present with flank pain, hematuria, upper quadrant mass, outflow obstruction, or hydronephroureter.[316]

Grossly, leiomyomas are well-circumscribed whorled white tumors and may be polypoid, with histologic features similar to those of leiomyomas in other organs. Mitotic figures are rare (<2 per 10 high-power fields),[316] and occasionally tumors with cellular atypia resembling bizarre (symplastic) leiomyoma of the myometrium are seen.[319] Upper tract leiomyomas usually express one or more smooth muscle markers (desmin, muscle-specific actin; MSA and SMSA), but unlike renal capsular leiomyomas are negative for HMB 45.[320]

Hemangioma

Rare cases of sporadic hemangioma have been reported in the upper tract, in both adults and children,[321,322] while multiple renal pelvic hemangiomas may occur as part of the Klippel-Trenaunay-Weber syndrome.[323]

These tumors typically present with massive hematuria, usually necessitating nephrectomy. Renal pelvic lesions may cause UPJ obstruction and hydronephrosis, while pericalyceal hemangiomas can result in renal papillary necrosis.[324] Histologically upper tract hemangiomas can show a cavernous, capillary, or fibrous morphology.

Neurofibroma

Neurofibromas rarely occur in the renal pelvis.[325] Segmental neurofibromatosis and solitary neurofibroma involving the ureter have also been reported.[326,327] These tumors may occur sporadically or may be a manifestation of von Recklinghausen neurofibromatosis. Patients present with flank pain and a mass lesion is usually found on radiologic investigation.[327] The pathologic features of upper tract neurofibroma are similar to those seen in other locations.

Other Tumors

Hemangiomyoma of the ureter has been reported in a child.[328] Periureteric lipoma[329] and benign *schwannoma*,[330] causing extrinsic UPJ obstruction, and hibernoma[331] are also rare tumors reported in this location.

Mesenchymal Tumors: Malignant

Leiomyosarcoma

Leiomyosarcomas arising in the renal pelvis are rare. These tumors occur in adults and are more common in females. They usually present at a relatively late stage with gross hematuria,[332–334] and patient age and stage at diagnosis are the strongest predictors for survival. Overall survival for leiomyosarcoma in this location is similar to that of UC.[333]

Rhabdomyosarcoma

Rhabdomyosarcoma of the renal pelvis is extremely rare. Botryoid-type pleomorphic rhabdomyosarcoma and embryonal rhabdomyosarcoma, producing a polypoid mass attached to the renal pelvis, have been reported in adults[335] and children.[336]

Other Tumors

Rare cases of ureteral angiosarcoma have been reported, with a case described in a long-term functional renal allograft.[337,338] Botryoid nephroblastoma of the renal pelvis and ureter, with limited parenchymal involvement, occurs rarely in the pediatric age group.[339,340] These patients present with a flank mass, low-grade fever, abdominal pain, and gross hematuria. Radiology displays renal enlargement, with typically a heterogeneous mass occupying a dilated pelvical-yceal system and ureter. Malignant peripheral nerve sheath tumors rarely occur in the renal pelvis.[341] *Ewing sarcoma/primitive neuroectodermal tumor* is a highly malignant tumor and has a poor prognosis.[342] Another malignant mesenchymal tumor reported in the renal pelvis is malignant fibrous *histiocytoma*, which is an extremely aggressive neoplasm, with little response to radiotherapy and chemotherapy.[343]

Primary malignant melanoma of the renal pelvis occurs in both adults and children.[344,345] These tumors are composed of large eosinophilic cells, but are rarely of clear cell type. Melanoma in this location is more commonly metastatic and is usually part of a disseminated process.

Hematopoietic and Lymphoid Tumors

Lymphomatous involvement of the upper tract usually occurs in association with systemic disease, or renal or retroperitoneal lymphoma.[346–349] Rare cases of non-Hodgkin lymphoma involving the ureter and renal pelvis have been reported,[350] and lymphomatous infiltration of the ureter is an uncommon cause of ureteral obstruction.[351,352]

Obstructive nephropathy may result from granulocytic sarcoma (chloroma) arising within the renal pelvis.[353] Ureteral obstruction due to an isolated focus of chronic lymphocytic leukemia has also been reported.[354] In a patient with a history of leukemia, this possibility needs to be considered in the differential diagnosis of urinary obstruction, even in the absence of other evidence of active disease, as the treatment is nonsurgical.

Plasmacytoma involving the kidney and renal pelvis is a rare manifestation of extramedullary plasmacytoma. While these tumors may be part of multiple myeloma, in rare cases the neoplastic plasma cell proliferation has been confined to the renal pelvis, hilar region, and renal capsule.[355]

Secondary Tumors

The majority of ureteropelvic metastatic tumors are of nonurologic origin and occur as part of widespread dissemination. Reported metastatic tumors include testicular seminoma, colonic, rectal and gastric adenocarcinoma, pulmonary carcinoma, breast carcinoma, cutaneous melanoma, renal cell carcinoma, and tumors of pelvic organs.

STAGING

The TNM clinical classification of the American Joint Committee on Cancer (AJCC)/Union Internationale Contre Le Cancer (UICC) is the most commonly employed staging system for tumors of the renal pelvis and ureter[356] (Table 4-3).

The thickness of the suburothelial stroma and muscularis varies in the calyces, the renal pelvis, and the ureter and may cause difficulties in staging of tumors. Further, staging of large and often friable pelvicalyceal tumors can be difficult, particularly if the tumor is poorly fixed. Large papillary

Table 4-3 ■ TNM CLASSIFICATION OF CARCINOMAS OF THE RENAL PELVIS AND URETER

Primary Tumor (T)

TX	Primary tumor cannot be assessed
T0	No evidence of primary tumor
Ta	Papillary noninvasive carcinoma
Tis	Carcinoma in situ
T1	Tumor invades subepithelial connective tissue
T2	Tumor invades muscularis
T3	(Renal pelvis) Tumor invades beyond muscularis into peripelvic fat or renal parenchyma
	(Ureter) Tumor invades beyond muscularis into periureteric fat
T4	Tumor invades adjacent organs or through the kidney into perinephric fat

Regional Lymph Nodes (N)

NX	Regional lymph nodes cannot be assessed
N0	No regional lymph node metastases
N1	Metastasis in a single lymph node, 2 cm or less in greatest dimension
N2	Metastasis in a single lymph node more than 2 cm but not more than 5 cm in greatest dimension, or in multiple lymph nodes, none more than 5 cm in greatest dimension
N3	Metastasis in a lymph node more than 5 cm in greatest dimension

Distant Metastasis (M)

MX	Distant metastasis cannot be assessed
M0	No distant metastasis (no pathologic M0: use clinical M to complete stage group)
M1	Distant metastasis

Stage Grouping

Stage 0a	Ta	N0	M0
Stage 0is	Tis	N0	M0
Stage 1	T1	N0	M0
Stage 11	T2	N0	M0
Stage 111	T3	N0	M0
Stage 1V	T4	N0	M0
	Any T	N1, N2, N3	M0
	Any T	Any N	M1
Stage unknown			

tumors in this location may have a prominent endophytic growth pattern and appear to push into renal sinus fat. This raises the possibility of misinterpreting these tumors as invasive carcinomas. Pagetoid spread of UC into renal tubules may also mimic renal parenchymal invasion. It should also be noted that tubular spread of carcinoma without invasion remains an in situ process, in contrast to renal parenchymal invasion, which is classified as pT3 disease. Unlike tumor showing renal parenchymal invasion, tumor confined to the renal tubules maintains a renal tubular contour and there is no stromal reaction.[357]

SPECIMEN HANDLING

Appropriate handling and assessment of specimens is necessary for accurate diagnosis and evaluation of prognostic features and is crucial for appropriate patient management.[358] Surgical specimens must be accompanied by adequate clinical history of urologic and nonurologic disease, including information regarding previous treatment.

Biopsy

Biopsy is obtained with cold cup forceps, diathermy forceps, or small diathermy loops. These must be transferred to formalin with minimal handling. The entire biopsy specimen must be submitted for processing and multiple sectioning. Given the thinness of the wall and relative inaccessibility of the upper tract, ureteral and pelvicalyceal biopsies are typically small and superficial, sometimes displaying crush artifact. Therefore, these may be suboptimal for assessment, which may prevent definitive diagnosis. This can also prevent accurate assessment of the grade and pathologic stage of tumors from this location.

Nephro-ureterectomy

Frozen section of ureter resection margins may be requested. Longitudinal sections or a cross section of the inked ureter margin may be examined.

For nephro-ureterectomy specimens dissection is best commenced at the renal hilum following identification of the ureter, renal artery, and renal vein. The ureteral and hilar soft tissue margins are inked, and a cut, beginning in the renal pelvis, is extended to bivalve the kidney and then extended through the perinephric fat and down the ureter. The location of any tumor within the pelvicalyceal system or ureter is recorded, along with a description of the macroscopic features, dimensions, depth of invasion, involvement of renal parenchyma, renal sinus, perinephric fat, hilar lymph nodes, and blood vessels, and distance from the surgical resection margins. Photographs of the opened specimen are desirable. Tissues demonstrating the tumor and its relationship to renal parenchyma and peripelvic/periureteral soft tissue are submitted for histology. Separate sections of the resection margins (ureteral, closest hilar soft tissue, and perinephric) and representative sections of nonneoplastic kidney, renal pelvis

and ureter, renal sinus, hilar lymph nodes (if present), and hilar blood vessels are also taken.

Ureterectomy

The cut margins are inked and both ends are submitted for separate evaluation. The entire ureter is then opened, and careful inspection of the ureteral mucosa and wall is undertaken. Any tumor is identified and the distance to the resection margins is recorded along with the macroscopic level of invasion and involvement of periureteral soft tissues. Several blocks of the tumor are submitted, and these should include the closest approach to the periureteral soft tissue margin.

REPORTING

College of American Pathologists guidelines should be used in reporting (Box 4-3).

Box 4-3 ● COLLEGE OF AMERICAN PATHOLOGISTS GUIDELINES

URETER, RENAL PELVIS: Biopsy
Specimen
Specimen Laterality
Histologic Type
Associated Epithelial Lesions
Histologic Grade
Tumor Configuration
Adequacy of Material for Determining T Category
Microscopic Tumor Extension
Pathologic Staging (pTNM)
Additional Pathologic Findings

RENAL PELVIS: Resection/Nephro-ureterectomy,
    Partial or Complete
Procedure
Specimen Laterality
Tumor Size
Histologic Type
Associated Epithelial Lesions
Histologic Grade
Microscopic Tumor Extension
Tumor Configuration
Margins
Lymphovascular Invasion
Pathologic Staging (pTNM)
Additional Pathologic Findings
Pathologic Findings in Non-neoplastic Kidney

URETER: Resection
Procedure
Specimen Laterality
Tumor Size
Histologic Type
Associated Epithelial Lesions
Histologic Grade
Microscopic Tumor Extension
Tumor Configuration
Margins
Lymphovascular Invasion
Pathologic Staging (pTNM)
Additional Pathologic Findings

Biopsy

The biopsy report should record the tissues present. In case of malignancy, tumor type, and ISUP/WHO grade, the extent of invasion into the different layers and presence of vascular, lymphatic, and perineural invasion must be recorded. It is also important to report the adequacy of the specimen and the presence of any urothelial denudation.

Nephro-ureterectomy

The histologic report of nephroureterectomy specimens should contain a description of the location, size, morphologic features, grade, and stage of tumor, detailing the extent of invasion into the layers of the renal pelvic or ureteral wall. The report should also note any involvement of the renal parenchyma and renal sinus, the presence of vascular lymphatic and perineural invasion, and adequacy of resection.

Ureterectomy

The location, size, and distance to resection margins of any tumor should be recorded in addition to the histologic type, grade, and extent of invasion into the different layers. Any vascular, lymphatic, and perineural invasion should be noted along with an assessment of the completeness of resection.

REFERENCES

1. Hanna MK, Jeffs RD, Sturgess JM, et al. Ureteral structure and ultrastructure. Part 1 the normal human ureter. *J Urol* 1976;116:718.
2. Woodburne RT. The ureter, ureterovesical junction and vesical trigone. *Anat Rec* 1965;151:243.
3. Motola JA, Shahon RS, Smith AD. Anatomy of the ureter. *Urol Clin North Am* 1988;15:295.
4. Notley RG. The musculature of the human ureter. *Br J Urol* 1970;40:724.
5. Marshall FF. Embryology of the lower genitourinary tract. *Urol Clin North Am* 1978;5:3.
6. Gyllensten L. Contributions to embryology of the urinary bladder: development of definitive relations between openings of the Wolffian ducts and ureters. *Acta Anat* 1949;7:305.
7. Vainio S, Muller U. Inductive tissue interactions, cell signaling and the control of kidney organogenesis. *Cell* 1997;90:975.
8. Baker LA, Gomez RA. Embryonic development of the ureter and bladder. Acquisition of smooth muscle. *J Urol* 1998;160:545.
9. Alcarez A, Vinaita F, Tejedo-Mateu A, et al. Obstruction and recanalization of the ureter during embryonic development. *J Urol* 1991;145:410.
10. Kirks DR, Currarino G, Weinberg AG. Transverse folds in the proximal ureter: a normal variant in infants. *AJR Am J Roentgenol* 1978;130:463.
11. Rabinowitz R, Kingston TE, Wesselhoeft C, et al. Ureteral valves in children. *Urology* 1998;51:7.
12. Magee MC, Lucey DT, Fried FA. A new embryologic classification for urogynecologic malformations: the syndromes of mesonephric duct induced müllerian deformities. *J Urol* 1979;121:265.
13. Stroup NE, Edmonds L, O'Brien TR. Renal agenesis and dysgenesis: are they increasing? *Teratology* 1990;42:383.
14. Shieh CP, Hung CS, Wei CF, et al. Cystic dilatations within the pelvis in patients with ipsilateral renal agenesis or dysplasia. *J Urol* 1990;144:324.
15. Stephens FD. Anatomical vagaries of double ureters. In: Webster R, ed. *Congenital Malformations of the Rectum, Anus and Genitourinary Tracts*. Edinburgh, UK: Livingstone; 1963:171–177.
16. Fernbach SK, Feinstein KA, Spencer K, et al. Ureteral duplication and its complications. *Radiographics* 1997;17:109.
17. Lenaghan D. Bifid ureters: an anatomical physiological and clinical study. In: Webster R, ed. *Congenital Malformations of the Rectum, Anus and Genitourinary Tracts*. Edingburgh, UK: Livingstone; 1963:196–208.
18. Pope JC, Brock JW, Adams MC, et al. How they begin and how they end. Classic and new theories for the development and detection of congenital anomalies of the kidney and urinary tract, CAKUT. *J Am Soc Nephrol* 1999;10:2018.
19. Lam JS, Breda A, Schulam PG. Ureteropelvic junction obstruction. *J Urol* 2007;177:1652.
20. Karaca I, Sencan A, Mir E, et al. Ureteral fibroepithelial polyps in children. *Pediatr Surg Int* 1997;12:603.
21. Dewan PA, Penington E, Jeyaseelan D. Upper pole pelviureteric junction obstruction. *Pediatr Surg Int* 1998;13:290.
22. Aslam M, Watson AR. Unilateral multicystic dysplastic kidney: long term outcomes. *Arch Dis Child* 2006;91:820.
23. Subramaniam R, Lama T, Chong CY. Pelviureteric junction obstruction as a sequelae of Kawasaki disease. *Pediatr Surg Int* 2004;20:553.
24. Dewan PA, Ng KP, Ashwood PJ. The relationship of age to pathology in pelviureteric junction obstruction. *J Paediatr Child Health* 1998;34:384.
25. Johnston JH, Evans JP, Glassberg KI, et al. Pelvic hydronephrosis in children: a review of 219 personal cases. *J Urol* 1977;117:97.
26. Le Normand L, Buzelin J-M, Bouchot O, et al. Upper urinary tract: physiology, pathophysiology of obstructions and clinical investigations. *Ann Urol (Paris)* 2005;39:30.
27. Ylinen E, Ala-Houhala M, Wikstrom S. Outcome of patients with antenatally-detected pelviureteric junction obstruction. *Pediatr Nephrol* 2004;19:880.
28. Gosling JA, Dixon JS. Functional obstruction of the ureter and renal pelvis. A histological and electron microscopic study. *Br J Urol* 1978;50:145.
29. Starr NJ, Maizels M, Chou P, et al. Microanatomy and morphometry of the hydronephrotic obstructed renal pelvis in asymptomatic infants. *J Urol* 1992;148:519.
30. Kaneto H, Orikasa S, Chiba T, et al. Three-D muscular arrangement at the ureteropelvic junction and its changes in congenital hydronephrosis. A stero-morphometric study. *J Urol* 1991;146:909.
31. Kuvel M, Canguven O, Murtazaoglu M, et al. Distribution of Cajal like cells and innervation in intrinsic ureteropelvic junction obstruction. *Arch Ital Urol Androl* 2011;83:128–132.
32. Harish J, Joshi KLN, Rao KL, et al. Pelviureteric junction obstruction: how much is the extent of the upper ureter with defective innervation needing resection? *J Pediatr Surg* 2003;38:1194.
33. Yang Y, Zhou X, Gao H, et al. The expression of epidermal growth factor and transforming growth factor beta 1 in the stenotic tissue of urogenital pelvi-ureteric junction obstruction in children. *J Pediatr Surg* 2003;38:1656.
34. Jaswon MS, Dibble L, Puri S, et al. Prospective study of outcome in antenatally diagnosed renal pelvis dilatation. *Arch Dis Child Fetal Neonatal Ed* 1999;80:135.
35. Takeyama J, Sakai K. Mucosal abnormalities in congenital ureteropelvic junction obstruction. *Histopathology* 2007;51:716.
36. Foote JW, Blennerhassett JB, Wiglesworth FW, et al. Observations on the ureteropelvic junction. *J Urol* 1970;104:252.
37. Schoborg TW, Florence TJ. Ureteral diverticulosis. *J Urol* 1976;116:107.
38. Rank WB, Mellinger GT, Spiro E. Ureteral diverticula: etiologic consideration. *J Urol* 1906;83:566.
39. Scarcello NS, Kumar S. Multiple ureteral diverticula. *J Urol* 1971;106:36.
40. Summers JL, Keitzer WA, Hathaway TR. Multiple ureteral diverticula. Case report with a discussion of etiology. *Ohio State Med J* 1972;68:1027.
41. Lester PD, Kyaw MM. Ureteral diverticulosis. Roentgenologic manifestation of ureteritis. *Radiology* 1973;106:77.

42. Blane CE, Zerin JM, Bloom DA. Bladder diverticula in children. *Radiology* 1994;190:695.

43. Yu TJ. Extravesical diverticuloplasty for the repair of a paraureteral diverticulum and the associated refluxing ureter. *J Urol* 2002;168:1135.

44. Tokunaka S, Koyanagi T, Matsuno T, et al. Paraureteral diverticula: clinical experience with 17 cases with associated renal dysmorphism. *J Urol* 1980;124:791.

44. Atwell JD, Allen NH. The interrelationship between paraureteric diverticula, vesicoureteral reflux and duplication of the pelvicaliceal collecting system: a family study. *Br J Urol* 1980;52:269.

46. Rickwood AMK, Reiner I, Jones M, et al. Current management of duplex-system ureteroceles: experience with 41 patients. *Br J Urol* 1992;70:196.

47. Pohl HG, Joyce GF, Wise M, et al. Vesicoureteral reflux and ureteroceles. *J Urol* 2007;177:1659.

48. Tokunaka S, Gotoh T, Koyanagi T, et al. Morphological study of the ureterocele: a possible clue to its embryogenesis as evidenced by a locally arrested myogenesis. *J Urol* 1981;126:726.

49. Glassberg KI, Braren V, Duckett JW, et al. Suggested terminology for duplex systems, ectopic ureters and ureteroceles. *J Urol* 1984;132:1153.

50. Friedland GW, Cunningham J. The elusive ectopic ureterocele. *AJR Am J Roentgenol* 1972;116:792.

51. Merlini E, Lelli Chiesa P. Obstructive ureterocele – an ongoing challenge. *World J Urol* 2004;22:107.

52. Devy JB, Vandersteen DR, Morgenstern BZ, et al. Hypertension after surgical management of renal duplication associated with an upper pole ureterocele. *J Urol* 1997;158:1241.

53. King LR. Megaloureter: definition, diagnosis and management. *J Urol* 1980;123:222.

54. Berrocal T, López-Pereira P, Arjonilla A, et al. Anomalies of the distal ureter, bladder, and urethra in children: embryologic, radiologic and pathologic features. *Radiographics* 2002;22:1139.

55. Jerkins GR, Noe HN. Familial vesicoureteral reflux: a prospective study. *J Urol* 1982;128:774.

56. Lee BR, Silver RI, Partin AW, et al. A quantitative histologic analysis of collagen subtypes: the primary obstructed and refluxing megaureter of childhood. *Urology* 1998;51:820.

57. Shokeir AA, Nijman RJM. Primary megaureter: current trends in diagnosis and treatment. *BJU Int* 2000;86:861.

58. Meyer JS, Lebowitz RL. Primary megaureter in infarcts and children: a review. *Urol Radiol* 1992;14:296.

59. Dixon JS, Jen PYP, Yeung CK, et al. The vesicoureteric junction in three cases of primary obstructive megaureter associated with ectopic ureteric insertion. *Br J Urol* 1998;81:580.

60. MacKinnon KJ. Primary megaureter. *Birth Defects Orig Artic Ser* 1977;13:15.

61. Nicotina PA, Romeo C, Arena F, et al. Segmental up-regulation of transforming growth factor-beta in the pathogenesis of primary megaureter. An immunohistochemical study. *Br J Urol* 1997;80:946.

62. Baskin LS, Zderic SA, Snyder HM, et al. Primary dilated megaureter: long term follow-up. *J Urol* 1994;152:618.

63. Belman AB. Megaureter. Classification, etiology and management. *Urol Clin North Am* 1974;1:497.

64. Tokunaka S, Koyanagi T. Morphologic study of primary nonrefluxing megaureters with particular emphasis on the role of ureteral sheath and ureteral dysplasia. *J Urol* 1982;128:399.

65. Hanna MK. Ureteral structure and ultrastructure. Part V. The dysplastic ureter. *J Urol* 1979;122:796.

66. Kirpatovski VI, Mudraia IS, Pugachev AG, et al. Contractile function of ureter in its anomalies in children. *Urologila* 1999;4:12.

67. Derevianko IM, Derevianko TI. Segmentary dysplasia of the perivesical portion of the ureter. *Urol Nefrol (Mosk)* 1997;1:19.

68. Pugacher AG, Kudriavtsev IV, Pavlov AI, et al. Neuromuscular dysplasia of the ureters in children. *Urol Nefrol (Mosk)* 1993;1:16.

69. Cauchi JA, Chandran H. Congenital ureteric structures: an uncommon cause of antenatally detected hydronephrosis. *Pediatr Surg Int* 2005;21:566.

70. Ruano-Gil D, Tejedo-Mateu A. Human embryo (12 mm) with mesohydronephrosis and ureterohydronephrosis. *Acta Anat* 1975;93:135.

71. Allen TD. Congenital ureteral strictures. *J Urol* 1970;104:196.

72. Plotz FB, van Essen AJ, Bosschaart AN, et al. Cerebro-costo-mandibular syndrome. *Am J Med Genet* 1996;62:286.

73. Cholkeri-Singh A, Narepalem N, Miller CE. Laparoscopic ureteral injury and repair: case reviews and clinical update. *J Minim Invasive Gynecol* 2007;14:356.

74. Carl P, Stark L. Indications for surgical management of genitourinary tuberculosis. *World J Surg* 1997;21:505.

75. Kubo M, Taguchi K, Fujisue H, et al. Hydronephrosis as a complication of appendicitis: a case report. *Hinyokika Kiyo* 1996;42:679.

76. Tremps Velazquez E, Ramon Dalmou M, Garcia Rojo D, et al. Ureteral stenosis secondary to Churg-Strauss allergic granulomatous vasculitis. *Arch Esp Urol* 1997;50:82.

77. Awakura Y, Mizutani Y, Kakehi Y, et al. A case of localized amyloidosis of the ureter. *Hinyokika Kiyo* 1996;42:135.

78. Fernandez Gonzalez I, Serrano Pascual A, Garcia Cuerpo E, et al. Endometriosis: the cause of hematuria in the dysfunctional ureter. *Arch Esp Urol* 1997;50:881.

79. Giessing M. Transplant ureter stricture following renal transplantation: surgical options. *Transplant Proc* 2011;43:383.

80. Nonira Y, Feki W, Kallel Y, et al. Ureteric valves: a report of two cases. *Ann Chir* 2006;131:567.

81. Maizels M, Stephens FD. Valves of the ureter as a cause of primary obstruction of the ureter: embryologic and clinical aspects. *J Urol* 1980;123:742.

82. Dorph S, Horn T, Steven K. Transverse folds of the adult obstructed ureter. Case report. *Scand J Urol Nephrol* 1994;157:153.

83. Lincke P, Bassler R, Funke R. Morphology of sub-pelvic ureter folds in childhood. Pathogenesis of infantile hydronephrosis. *Pathologe* 1980;1:147.

84. Stamm WE, Hooten TM. Management of urinary tract infections in adults. *N Engl J Med* 1993;329:1328.

85. Modi P, Goel R. Synchronous endoscopic management of bilateral kidney and ureter fungal bezoar. *Urol Int* 2007;78:374.

86. Wise GJ, Talluri GS, Marella VK. Fungal infections of the genitourinary system: manifestations, diagnosis and treatment. *Urol Clin North Am* 1999;26:701.

87. Barnes R, Masood S, Lammert N, et al. Extragenital granuloma inguinale mimicking a soft-tissue neoplasm: a case report and review of the literature. *Hum Pathol* 1990;21:559.

88. Koroku M, Tanda H, Katoh S, et al. Malakoplakia of the ureter and bladder. *Hinyokika Kiyo* 2005;51:183.

89. Long JP, Althausen AF. Malacoplakia: a 25-year experience with a review of the literature. *J Urol* 1989;141:1328.

90. Sozer IT. A rare localization of malakoplakia: renal pelvis. *J Urol* 1966;95:746.

91. Chenonfi MB, Moalla R, Petrov N, et al. A triple association: renal malacoplakia, bilateral vulvar hypertrophy, upper limb algodystrophy. *Ann Urol (Paris)* 1998;32:138.

92. Kato T, Suzuki Y, Sugimura J, et al. A cases of ureterovesical malakoplakia that manifested hydronephrosis. *Hinyokika Kiyo* 2001;47:195.

93. Teahan SJ, OMalley KJ, Little DM, et al. Malacoplakia of transplant ureter resulting in an anuric renal failure. *J Urol* 1999;162:1375.

94. Suzuki K, Sotoma T, Umemiya A, et al. Ureteral malakoplakia: a case report. *Hinyokika Kiyo* 1996;42:131.

95. Tsung SH. Urinary sediment cytology: potential diagnostic tool for malakoplakia. *Urology* 1982;20:546.

96. Halpern GN, Kalles DW, Factor S, et al. Malacoplakia causing bilateral ureteropelvic junction obstruction. *Urology* 1974;3:628.

97. Joos H, Frick J. Malacoplakia of the kidney and urinary bladder. *Eur Urol* 1983;9:372.

98. Tamboli P, Ro JY, Amin MB, et al. Benign tumors and tumor-like lesions of the adult kidney. Part II: benign mesenchymal and mixed neoplasms and tumor-like lesions. *Adv Anat Pathol* 2000;7:47.

99. Breda G, Artibani W, Vancini P, et al. Ultrastructural features in a case of ureteric malakoplakia. *Eur Urol* 1977;3:132.

100. Dohle GR, Zwartendijk J, Van Krieken JH. Urogenital malakoplakia treated with fluoroquinolones. *J Urol* 1993;150:1518.

101. Pearle MS, Clahoun EA, Curhan GC, et al. Urologic diseases in America project: urolithiasis. *J Urol* 2005;173:848.

102. Balaji KC, Menon M. Mechanism of stone formation. *Urol Clin North Am* 1997;24:1.

103. Scheinman SJ. Nephrolithiasis. *Semin Nephrol* 1999;19:381.

104. Hinman F. Directional growth of renal calculi. *J Urol* 1979;121:700.

105. Segura JW, Preminger GM, Assimos DG, et al. Ureteral Stones Clinical Guidelines Panel summary report on the management of ureteral calculi. The American Urological Association. *J Urol* 1997;158:1915.

106. Glowacki LS, Becroft ML, Cook RJ, et al. The natural history of asymptomatic urolithiasis. *J Urol* 1992;147:319.

107. Ozdamar AS, Ozkurkcugil C, Gultekin Y, et al. Should we get routine urothelial biopsies in every stone surgery? *Int Urol Nephrol* 1997;29:415.

108. Yeh CC, Lin TH, Wu HC, et al. A high association of upper tract transitional cell carcinoma with non-functioning kidney caused by stone disease in Taiwan. *Urol Int* 2007;79:19.

109. Chow W-H, Lindblad P, Grindley G, et al. Risk of urinary tract cancers following kidney or ureter stones. *J Natl Cancer Inst* 1997;89:1453.

110. Shah HN, Jain P, Chibber PJ. Laparoscopic nephrectomy for giant staghorn calculus with non-functioning kidneys: is associated unsuspected urothelial carcinoma responsible for conversion? Report of 2 cases. *BMC Urol* 2006;6:1.

111. Shaeff M, Fociani P, Badenoch D, et al. Verrucous carcinoma of the renal pelvis: case, presentation and review of the literature. *Virchows Arch* 1996;428:375.

112. Kayaselcuk F, Bal N, Guvel S, et al. Carcinosarcoma and squamous cell carcinoma of the renal pelvis associated with nephrolithiasis: a case report of each tumor type. *Pathol Res Pract* 2003;199:489.

113. Kim TS, Seong PH, Ro JY. Small cell carcinoma of the ureter with squamous cell and transitional cell carcinomatous components associated with ureteral stone. *J Korean Med Sci* 2001;16:796.

114. Churg J, Churg A. Idiopathic and secondary vasculitis: a review. *Mod Pathol* 1989;2:144.

115. Melin JP, Lemaine P, Birembaut P, et al. Polyarteritis nodosa with bilateral ureteric involvement. *Nephron* 1982;32:87.

116. Casserly LF, Reddy SM, Rennke HG, et al. Reversible bilateral hydronephrosis without obstruction in hepatitis B–associated polyarteritis nodosa. *Am J Kidney Dis* 1999;34:e11.

117. de la Prada Alvarez FJ, Prados Gallardo AM, Tugores Vazquez A, et al. Schönlein-Henoch nephritis complicated with pulmonary renal syndrome. *An Med Interna* 2005;22:441.

118. Tremps Velazquez E, Ramon Dalmau M, Garcia Rojo D, et al. Ureteral stenosis secondary to Churg-Strauss allergic granulomatous vasculitis. *Arch Esp Urol* 1997;50:82.

119. Rich LM, Piering WF. Ureteral stenosis due to recurrent Wegener's granulomatosis after kidney transplantation. *J Am Soc Nephrol* 1994;4:1516.

120. Davenport A, Downey SE, Goel S, et al. Wegener's granulomatosis involving the urogenital tract. *Br J Urol* 1996;78:354.

121. Fernandez Garcia ML, de la Fuentes Buceta A, Gomez Rodriguez N, et al. Ureteral stenosis caused by systemic sclerosis. *Arch Esp Urol* 1999;52:881.

122. Benson CH, Pennebaker JB, Harisdangkul V, et al. Spontaneous ureteral rupture in a patient with systemic lupus erythematosus. *South Med J* 1983;76:1053.

123. Borrelli M, Prado MJ, Cordeiro P, et al. Ureteral necrosis in dermatomyositis. *J Urol* 1988;139:1275.

124. Santucci RA, Wessells H, Bartsch G, et al. Evaluation and management of renal injuries: consensus statement of the renal trauma subcommittee. *BJU Int* 2004;93:937.

125. Kawashima A, Sandler CM, Corl FM, et al. Imaging of renal trauma: a comprehensive review. *Radiographics* 2001;21:557.

126. Titton RL, Gervais DA, Hahn PF, et al. Urine leaks and urinomas: diagnosis and image-guided intervention. *Radiographics* 2003;23:1133.

127. Cormio L, Ruutu M, Selvaggi FP. Prognostic factors in the management of ureteric injuries. *Ann Chir Gynaecol* 1994;83:41.

128. Elliott SP, McAninch JW. Ureteral injuries: external and iatrogenic. *Urol Clin North Am* 2006;33:55.

129. Masier U, Ehrenbock PM, Hofbauer J. Late urological complications and malignancies after curative radiotherapy for gynecological carcinomas. A retrospective analysis of 10,709 patients. *J Urol* 1997;158:814.

130. Taylor JS. The behaviour of the ureters following radiotherapy and Wertheim hysterectomy. *Br J Urol* 1977;49:203.

131. Buglione M, Toninelli M, Pietta N, et al. Post-radiation pelvic disease and ureteral stenosis: pathophysiology and evolution in the patient treated for cervical carcinoma. Review of the literature and experience of the Radium Institute. *Arch Ital Urol Androl* 2002;74:6.

132. van Kampen M, Eble MJ, Krempien R, et al. Influence of irradiated volume on ureteral injury after intraoperative radiation therapy: experimental study in dogs. *Radiology* 2003;228:139.

133. Suresh UR, Smith VJ, Lupton EW, et al. Radiation disease of the urinary tract: histological features of 18 cases. *J Clin Pathol* 1993;46:228.

134. Saito M, Kondo A, Kato T, et al. Radiation-induced urothelial carcinoma. *Urol Int* 1996;56:254.

135. Weshler Z, Sulkes A, Kopolovic J. Squamous cell carcinoma of the renal pelvis as a late complication of hepatic irradiation: a case report. *J Surg Oncol* 1983;22:84.

136. Deffan P, Morel D, Basseau F, et al. Antopol-Goldman lesion: a rare course of hematuria. *Nephrol Ther* 2005;1:131.

137. Villar-Pastor CM, López-Beltrán A, Alvarez-Kindelán J, et al. Subepithelial hemorrhage of renal pelvis (Antopol-Goldman Lesion). Report of 4 cases and review of the literature. *Actas Urol Esp* 2000;24:805.

138. Iczkowski KA, Sweat SD, Bostwick DG. Subepithelial pelvic hematoma of the kidney, clinically mimicking cancer: report of six cases and review of the literature. *Urology* 1999;53:276.

139. Danaci M, Kesici GE, Kesici H, et al. Coumadin-induced renal and retroperitoneal hemorrhage. *Ren Fail* 2006;28:129.

140. Wagnor JR, D'Agostino R, Babyan RK. Renal arterioureteral hemorrhage: a complication of acucise endopyelotomy. *Urology* 1996;48:139.

141. Vaglio A, Salvarani C, Buzio C. Retroperitoneal fibrosis. *Lancet* 2006;367:241.

142. Miller OF, Smith LJ, Ferrara LJ, et al. Presentation of idiopathic retroperitoneal fibrosis in the pediatric population. *J Pediatr Surg* 2003;38:1685.

143. Li KP, Zhu J, Zhang JL, et al. Idiopathic retroperitoneal fibrosis (RPF): clinical features of 61 cases and literature review. *Clin Rheumatol* 2011;30:601.

144. Uibu T, Okso P, Auvinen A, et al. Asbestos exposure as a risk factor for retroperitoneal fibrosis. *Lancet* 2004;363:1422.

145. Triantopoulou C, Rizos S, Bourli A, et al. Localized unilateral perirenal fibrosis. CT and MRI appearances. *Eur Radiol* 2002;12:2743.

146. Bassi P, Iafrate M, Longo F, et al. Intracavitary therapy of non-invasive transitional cell carcinoma of the upper urinary tract. A review of the literature. *Urol Int* 2001;67:189.

147. Lopez-Beltran A, Luque RJ, Mazzucchelli R, et al. Changes produced in the urothelium by traditional and newer therapeutic procedures for bladder cancer. *J Clin Pathol* 2002;55:641.

148. Wong TM, Yeo W, Chan LW, et al. Hemorrhagic pyelitis, ureteritis and cystitis secondary to cyclphosphamide: case report and review of the literature. *Gynaecol Oncol* 2000;76:223.

149. Chapron C, Chopin N, Borghese B, et al. Deeply infiltrated endometriosis: pathogenetic implications of the anatomical distribution. *Hum Reprod* 2006;21:1839.

150. Frenna V, Santos L, Ohana E, et al. Laparoscopic management of ureteral endometriosis: our experience. *J Minim Invasive Gynecol* 2007;14:169.

151. Carmignani L, Vercellini P, Spinelli M, et al. Pelvic endometriosis and hydroureteronephrosis. *Fertil Steril* 2010;93:1741.

152. Chen CCG, Falcone T. Endoscopic management of endometriosis. *Minerva Ginecol* 2006;58:347.

153. Li WM, Yang SF, Lin HC, et al. Müllerianosis of ureter: a rare cause of hydronephrosis. *Urology* 2007;69:1208.e9–e11.

154. Salerno MG, Masciullo V, Naldini A, et al. Endometrioid adenocarcinoma with squamous differentiation arising from ureteral endometriosis in a patient with no history of gonadal endometriosis. *Gynecol Oncol* 2005;99:749.

155. Zugos V, Schott GE. Endometriosis involving the ureter. The Erlangen experience exemplified by two case reports. *Aktuelle Urol* 2007;38:55.

156. Merrimen JLO, Alkhudair WK, Gupta R. Localized amyloidosis of the urinary tract: case series of nine patients. *Urology* 2006;67:904.

157. Takahashi T, Miura H, Matsu-ura Y, et al. Urine cytology of localized primary amyloidosis of the ureter: a case report. *Acta Cytol* 2005;49:319.

158. Iida S, Chujyo T, Nakata Y, et al. A case of amyloidosis of the renal pelvis. *Hinyokika Kiyo* 2003;49:423.

159. Kawashima A, Alleman WG, Takahashi N, et al. Imaging evaluation of amyloidosis of the urinary tract and retroperitoneum. *Radiographics* 2011;31:1569.

160. Wiener DP, Koss LG, Sablay B, et al. The prevalence and significance of Brunn's nests, cystitis cystica and squamous metaplasia in normal bladders. *J Urol* 1979;122:317.

161. Kylye S, Sargin SY, Gunes A, et al. A rare condition: the ureteritis cystica. *Sci World J* 2004;4:175.

162. Gupta R, Kehinde EO, Sinan T, et al. Urinary schistosomiasis: urographic features and significance of drooping kidney appearance. *Int Urol Nephrol* 2001;33:461.

163. Binous MY, Chtourou M, Kbaier I, et al. Ureteritis cystica. A case report and review of the literature. *Tunis Med* 2003;81:425.

164. Ward AM. Glandular neoplasia within the urinary tract. The aetiology of adenocarcinoma of the urothelium with a review of the literature. *Virchows Arch A* 1971;352:296.

165. Kopp JH. Pyelitis, ureteritis and cystitis cystica. *J Urol* 1946;56:28.

166. del Real M, Zaboleta JS, Padial MC, et al. Cystic ureteritis: importance of chronic infection–inflammation as etiologic factor. Report of a clinical case. *Actas Urol Esp* 2000;24:496.

167. Hertle L, Androulakakis P. Keratinizing desquamative squamous metaplasia of the upper urinary tract: leukoplakia–cholesteatoma. *J Urol* 1982;127:631.

168. Blacklock ARE, Geddes JR, Black JW. Mucinous and squamous metaplasia of the renal pelvis. *J Urol* 1983;130:544.

169. Zahran MM, Kamel M, Mooro H, et al. Bilharziasis of the urinary bladder and ureter: comparative histopathologic study. *Urology* 1974;8:73.

170. Dhingra KK, Singal S, Jain S. Rare co-existence of keratinizing squamous metaplasia with xanthogranulomatous pyelonephritis. Report of a case with the role of immunocytochemistry in the differential diagnosis. *Acta Cytol* 2007;51:92.

171. Noyes WE, Palubinskas AJ. Squamous metaplasia of the renal pelvis. *Radiology* 1967;89:292.

172. Harada H, Seki T, Togashi M, et al. Squamous metaplasia mimicking papillary carcinoma in the upper urinary tract. *Hokkaido Igaku Zasshi* 2004;79:15.

173. Mather S, Singh MK, Rao SI, et al. Mucinous metaplasia of the renal pelvic epithelium in a case of recurrent urolithiasis and pyelonephritis. *Urol Int* 2004;72:355.

174. Bullock PS, Thoni DE, Murphy WM. The significance of colonic mucosal (intestinal metaplasia) involving the urinary tract. *Cancer* 1987;59:2086.

175. Richmond HG, Robb WAT. Adenocarcinoma of the ureter secondary to ureteritis cystica. *Br J Urol* 1967;39:359.

176. Nogales FF, Zuluaga A, Arrabal M, et al. Müllerianosis of the ureter: a metaplastic lesion. *J Urol* 1999;162:2090.

177. Meyer AJ, Kausch I, Behm A, et al. Bone formation in the ureter. Osseous metaplasia of an obstructed ureter. *Urologe A* 2006;45:1438.

178. Selli C, Risaliti A, De Antoni P, et al. Ureteral obstruction after kidney transplantation secondary to bone metaplasia. *Urology* 2000;56:153.

179. Willis SF, Bariol SV, Tolley DA. Bone formation in the urinary tract: case report. *J Endourol* 2005;19:878.

180. Ford TF, Watson GM, Cameron KM. Adenomatous metaplasia (nephrogenic adenoma) of the urothelium. *Br J Urol* 1985;57:427.

181. Oliva E, Young RH. Nephrogenic adenoma of the urinary tract: a review of the microscopic appearance of 80 cases with emphasis on unusual features. *Mod Pathol* 1995;8:722.

182. Martinez-Pineiro L, Hidalgo M, Picazo JM, et al. Nephrogenic adenoma of the renal pelvis. *Br J Urol* 1991;67:100.

183. Jackman SV, Moore RG, Nelson JB. Nephrogenic adenoma of the ureter: endoscopic diagnosis and management. *Urology* 1998;52:316.

184. Rehemtullah A, Oliva E. Nephrogenic adenoma: an update on an innocuous but troublesome entity. *Adv Anat Pathol* 2006;13:247.

185. Hung SY, Tseng HH, Chung HM. Nephrogenic adenoma with cytomegalovirus infection of the ureter in a renal transplant patient: presentation as ureteral obstruction. *Transpl Int* 2001;14:111.

186. Tong G-X, Melamed J, Mansukhani M. PAX2: a reliable marker for nephrogenic adenoma. *Mod Pathol* 2006;19:356.

187. Kojima Y, Lambert SM, Steixner BL, et al. Multiple metachronous fibroepithelial polyps in children. *J Urol* 2011;185:1053.

188. Bolton D, Stoller ML, Irby P. Fibroepithelial ureteral polyps and urolithiasis. *Urology* 1994;44:582.

189. Williams TR, Wagner BJ, Corse WR, et al. Fibroepithelial polyps of the urinary tract. *Abdom Imaging* 2002;27:217.

190. Ishizaki H, Iida S, Koga H, et al. Epidermoid cyst of the ureter: a case report. *Int J Urol* 2007;14:443.

191. Basiri A, Hosseini SR, Tousi VN, et al. Ureteroscopic management of symptomatic, simple parapelvic renal cyst. *J Endourol* 2010;24:537.

192. Kapusta LR, Weiss MA, Ramsay J, et al. Inflammatory myofibroblastic tumors of the kidney. *Am J Surg Pathol* 2003;27:658.

193. Montgomery EA, Shuster DD, Burkart AL, et al. Inflammatory myofibroblastic tumors of the urinary tract: a clinical pathologic study of 46 cases, including a malignant example inflammatory fibrosarcoma and a subset associated with high-grade urothelial carcinoma. *Am J Surg Pathol* 2006;30:1502.

194. Lynch CF, Cohen MB. Urinary system. *Cancer* 1995;75:316.

195. Latham HS, Kay S. Malignant tumors of the renal pelvis. *Surg Gynecol Obstet* 1974;138:613.

196. Busby JE, Brown GA, Tamboli P, et al. Upper urinary tract tumors with nontransitional histology: a single-center experience *Urology* 2006;67:518.

197. Munoz JJ, Ellison LM. Upper tract urothelial neoplasms: incidence and survival during the last 2 decades. *J Urol* 2000;164:1523.

198. Kanamori S, Okamura S, Nishimura T, et al. Papilloma of renal pelvis in childhood. *Urology* 1990;35:523.

199. Overgaard S, Thomsen NB, Olsen LH, et al. Percutaneous endoscopic management of bilateral transitional cell papillomas of the renal pelvis. *Scand J Urol Nephrol* 1990;24:157.

200. Spevack L, Herschorn S, Srigley J. Inverted papilloma of the upper urinary tract. *J Urol* 1995;153:1202.

201. Chiura AN, Wirtschafter A, Bagley DH. Upper urinary tract inverted papillomas. *Urology* 1998;52:514.

202. Kyriakos M, Royce RK. Multiple simultaneous inverted papillomas of the upper urinary tract. A case report with a review of ureteral and renal pelvic inverted papillomas. *Cancer* 1989;63:368.

203. Cheng L, Montironi R, Bostwick DG. Villous adenoma of the urinary tract. A report of 23 cases, including 8 with coexistent adenocarcinoma. *Am J Surg Pathol* 1999;23:764.

204. Shih CM, Wu SC, Lee CC, et al. Villous adenoma of the ureter with manifestations of mucus hydroureteronephrosis. *J Chin Med Assoc* 2007;70:33.

205. Bos I, Lichtenauer HP, Frontzeck M. Villoses adenom des nierenbeckens vom intestinalen typ (Intestinal type of villous adenoma of the kidney pelvis). *Pathologe* 1988;9:109.

206. Bhat S, Chandran V. Villous adenoma of the renal pelvis and ureter. *Indian J Urol* 2010;26:598.

207. Atiyeh BA, Barakat AJ, Abumrad NN. Extra-adrenal pheochromocytoma. *J Nephrol* 1997;10:25.

208. Jemal A, Tiwari RC, Murray T, et al. Cancer statistics, 2004. *CA Cancer J Clin* 2004;54:8.

209. Charbit L, Gendreau MC, Mee S, et al. Tumors of the upper urinary tract: 10 years of experience. *J Urol* 1991;146:1243.

210. Delahunt B, Amin MB, Hofstadter F. Tumours of the renal pelvis and ureter. In: Eble JN, Sauter G, Epstein JI, et al., eds. *Pathology and Genetics: Tumours of the Urinary System and Male Genital Organs. WHO Classification of Tumors.* Lyon, France: IARC Press; 2004:150–153.

211. Parkin DM, Whelan SL, Ferlay J, et al. *Cancer Incidence in Five Continents.* IARC Scientific Publications No 155. Lyon, France: IARC Press; 2003.

212. Mellemgaard A, Carstens B, Norgaard N, et al. Trends in the incidence of cancer in the kidney, pelvis, ureter and bladder in Denmark 1943–1988. *Scand J Urol Nephrol* 1993;27:327.

213. Raman JD, Messer J, Sielatycki JA, et al. Incidence and survival of patients with carcinoma of the ureter and renal pelvis in the USA, 1973–2005. *BJU Int* 2011;107:1059.

214. Takayanagi A, Masumori N, Takahashi A, et al. Upper urinary tract recurrence after radical cystectomy for bladder cancer: incidence and risk factors. *Int J Urol* 2012;19:229.

215. Sanderson KM, Cai J, Miranda G, et al. Upper tract urothelial recurrence following radical cystectomy for transitional cell carcinoma of the bladder: an analysis of 1069 patients with 10-year follow-up. *J Urol* 2007;177:2088.

216. Ross RK, Paganini-Hill A, Landolph J, et al. Analgesics, cigarette smoking, and other risk factors for cancer of the renal pelvis and ureter. *Cancer Res* 1989;49:1045.

217. Aben KK, Witjes JA, Schoenberg MP, et al. Familial aggregation of urothelial cell carcinoma. *Int J Cancer* 2002;98:274.

218. Fadl-Elmula I. Chromosomal changes in uroepithelial carcinomas. *Cell Chromosome* 2005;4:1.

219. Fadl-Elmula I, Goruňova L, Mandahl N, et al. Cytogenetic analysis of upper urinary tract transitional cell carcinomas. *Cancer Genet Cytogenet* 1999;115:123.

220. Rouprêt M, Drouin SJ, Cancel-Tassin G, et al. Genetic variability in 8q24 confers susceptibility to urothelial carcinoma of the upper urinary tract and is linked with patterns of disease aggressiveness at diagnosis. *J Urol* 2012;187:424.

221. Izquierdo L, Mengual L, Gazquez C, et al. Molecular characterization of upper urinary tract tumours. *BJU Int* 2010;106:868.

222. Blaszyk H, Wang L, Dietmaier W, et al. Upper tract urothelial carcinoma: a clinicopathologic study including microsatellite instability analysis. *Mod Pathol* 2002;15:790.

223. Hartmann A, Zanardo L, Bocker-Edmonston T, et al. Frequent microsatellite instability in sporadic tumours of the upper urinary tract. *Cancer Res* 2002;62:6796.

224. Ericson KM, Isinger AP, Isfoss BL, et al. Low frequency of defective mismatch repair in a population-based series of upper urothelial carcinoma. *BMC Cancer* 2005;5:23.

225. Hartmann A, Dietmaier W, Hofstadter F, et al. Urothelial carcinoma of the upper urinary tract: inverted growth pattern is predictive of microsatellite instability. *Hum Pathol* 2003;34:222.

226. Crockett DG, Wagner DG, Holmäng S, et al. Upper urinary tract carcinoma in Lynch syndrome cases. *J Urol* 2011;185:1627.

227. Jensen OM, Knudsen JB, McLaughlin JK, et al. The Copenhagen case-controlled study of renal pelvis and ureter cancer: role of smoking and occupational exposure. *Int J Cancer* 1988;41:557.

228. Simsir A, Sarsik B, Cureklibatir I, et al. Prognostic factors for upper urinary tract urothelial carcinomas: stage, grade, and smoking status. *Int Urol Nephrol* 2011;43:1039.

229. McCredie M, Stuart JH. Risk factors for kidney cancer in New South Wales. IV. Occupation. *Br J Ind Med* 1993;50:349.

230. Steffens J, Nagel R. Tumors of the renal pelvis and ureter: observations in 170 patients. *Br J Urol* 1988;61:277.

231. Jensen OM, Knudsen JB, Tomasson H, et al. The Copenhagen case-control study of renal pelvis and ureter cancer: role of analgesics. *Int J Cancer* 1989;44:965.

232. McCredie M, Ford JM, Taylor JS, et al. Analgesics and cancer of the renal pelvis in New South Wales. *Cancer* 1982;49:2617.

233. McCredie M, Stewart J, Smith D, et al. Observations on the effect of abolishing analgesic abuse and reducing smoking on cancers of the kidney and bladder in New South Wales, Australia, 1972–1995. *Cancer Causes Control* 1999;10:303.

234. Palvio DH, Andersen JC, Falk E. Transitional cell tumors of the renal pelvis and ureter associated with capillarosclerosis, indicating analgesic abuse. *Cancer* 1987;59:972.

235. Stuart JH, Hobbs JB, McCredie MR. Morphologic evidence that analgesic induced kidney pathology contributes to the progression of tumors of the renal pelvis. *Cancer* 1999;86:1576.

236. Thon WF, Kliem V, Truss MC, et al. Denovo urothelial carcinoma of the upper and lower urinary tract in kidney-transplant patients with end-stage analgesic nephropathy. *World J Urol* 1995;13:254.

237. Stefanovic V, Toncheva D, Atanasova S, et al. Etiology of Balkan endemic nephropathy and associated urothelial cancer. *Am J Nephrol* 2006;26:1.

238. Nikolic J, Djokic M, Ignjatovic I, et al. Upper urothelial tumors in emigrants from Balkan endemic nephropathy areas in Serbia. *Urol Int* 2006;77:240.

239. Basic-Jukic N, Hrsak-Puljic I, Kes P, et al. Renal transplantation in patients with Balkan endemic nephropathy. *Transplant Proc* 2007;39:1432.

240. Almgard LE, Ahlgren L, Boeryd B, et al. Thorotrast-induced renal tumours after retrograde pyelogram. *Eur Urol* 1977;3:69.

241. Katz R, Gofrit ON, Golijanin D, et al. Urothelial cancer of the renal pelvis in percutaneous nephrolithotomy patients. *Urol Int* 2005;75:17.

242. Raghavendran M, Rastogi A, Dubey D, et al. Stones associated renal pelvic malignancies. *Indian J Cancer* 2003;40:108.

243. Colin P, Koenig P, Ouzzane A, et al. Environmental factors involved in carcinogenesis of urothelial cell carcinomas of the upper urinary tract. *BJU Int* 2009;104:1436.

244. Chang CH, Wang YM, Yang AH, et al. Rapidly progressive interstitial renal fibrosis associated with Chinese herbal medications. *Am J Nephrol* 2001;21:441.

245. Chou YH, Huang CH. Unusual clinical presentation of upper urothelial carcinoma in Taiwan. *Cancer* 1999;85:1342.

246. Raabe NK, Fossa SI, Bjerkehagen B. Carcinoma of the renal pelvis. Experience of 80 cases. *Scand J Urol Nephrol* 1992;26:357.

247. Guinan P, Vogelzang NJ, Randazzo R, et al. Renal pelvic cancer: a review of 611 patients treated in Illinois, 1975–1985. Cancer Incidence and End Results Committee. *Urology* 1992;40:393.

248. Gilligan T, Dreicer R. The atypical urothelial cancer patient: management of bladder cancers of non-transitional cell histology and cancers of the ureters and renal pelvis. *Semin Oncol* 2007;34:145.

249. Potts SA, Thomas PA, Cohen MB, et al. Diagnostic accuracy and key cytologic features of high-grade transitional cell carcinoma in the upper urinary tract. *Mod Pathol* 1997;10:657.

250. Lomax-Smith JD, Seymour AE. Neoplasia in analgesic nephropathy. A urothelial field change. *Am J Surg Pathol* 1980;4:565.

251. Nocks BN, Heney NM, Daly JJ, et al. Transitional cell carcinoma of renal pelvis. *Urology* 1982;19:472.

252. Chow NH, Tzai TS, Cheng HL, et al. Urinary cytodiagnosis: can it have a different prognostic implication than a diagnostic test. *Urol Int* 1994;53:18.

253. Witte D, Truong LD, Ramzy I. Transitional cell carcinoma of the renal pelvis; the diagnostic role of pelvic washings. *Am J Clin Pathol* 2002;117:444.

254. Kondo T, Nakazawa H, Ito F, et al. Primary site and incidence of lymph node metastases in urothelial carcinoma of the upper urinary tract. *Urology* 2007;69:265.

255. Kirkali Z, Tuzel E. Transitional cell carcinoma of the ureter and renal pelvis. *Crit Rev Oncol Hematol* 2003;47:155.

256. Pomara G, Pastina I, Simone M, et al. Penile metastasis from primary transitional cell carcinoma of the renal pelvis: first manifestation of systemic spread. *BMC Cancer* 2004;4:90.

257. Murakami T, Komiya A, Mikata K, et al. Cardiac metastasis of renal pelvic cancer. *Int J Urol* 2007;14:240.

258. Langner C, Ratschek M, Tsybrovskyy O, et al. P63 immunoreactivity distinguishes upper urinary tract transitional-cell carcinoma and renal-cell carcinoma even in poorly differentiated tumors. *J Histochem Cytochem* 2003;51:1097.

259. Albadine R, Schultz L, Illei P, et al. PAX8 (+)/p63 (−) immunostaining pattern in renal collecting duct carcinoma (CDC): a useful immunoprofile in the differential diagnosis of CDC versus urothelial carcinoma of upper urinary tract. *Am J Surg Pathol* 2010;34:965.

260. Higgins JP, Kaygusuz G, Wang L, et al. Placental S100 (S100P) and GATA 3: markers for transitional epithelium and urothelial carcinoma discovered by complementary DNA Microarray. *Am J Surg Pathol* 2007;31:673.

261. Langner C, Ratschek M, Rehak P, et al. CD10 is a diagnostic and prognostic marker in renal malignancies. *Histopathology* 2004;45:460.

262. Ohtsuka Y, Kawakami S, Fujii Y, et al. Loss of uroplakin III expression is associated with a poor prognosis in patients with urothelial carcinoma of the upper urinary tract. *BJU Int* 2006;97:1322.

263. Kamijima S, Tobe T, Suyama T, et al. The prognostic value of p53, Ki-67 and matrix metalloproteinases MMP-2 and MMP-9 in transitional cell carcinoma of the renal pelvis and ureter. *Int J Urol* 2005;12:941.

264. Hashimoto H, Sue Y, Saga Y, et al. Roles of p53 and MDM2 in tumor proliferation and determination of the prognosis of transitional cell carcinoma of the renal pelvis and ureter. *Int J Urol* 2000;7:457.

265. Masuda M, Takano Y, Iki M, et al. Expression and prognostic value of CD44 isoforms in transitional cell carcinoma of renal pelvis and ureter. *J Urol* 1999;161:805.

266. Langner C, Rupar G, Leibl S, et al. A-methylacyl-CoA racemase (AMACR/P 504S) protein expression in urothelial carcinoma of the upper urinary tract correlates with tumour progression. *Virchows Arch* 2006;448:325.

267. Perez-Montiel D, Wakely PE, Hes O, et al. High-grade urothelial carcinoma of the renal pelvis: clinicopathologic study of 108 cases with emphasis on unusual morphologic variants. *Mod Pathol* 2006;19:494.

268. Holmang S, Lele SM, Johansson SL. Squamous cell carcinoma of the renal pelvis and ureter: incidence, symptoms, treatment and outcome. *J Urol* 2007;178:51.

269. Pacchioni D, Bosco M, Allia E. Microcystic urothelial cell carcinoma with neuroendocrine differentiation arising in renal pelvis. Report of a case. *Virchows Arch* 2009;454:223.

270. Perez-Montiel D, Hes O, Michael M, et al. Micropapillary urothelial carcinoma of the upper urinary tract: clinicopathologic study of five cases. *Am J Clin Pathol* 2006;126:86.

271. Guo CC, Tamboli P, Czerniak B. Micropapillary variant of urothelial carcinoma in the upper urinary tract: a clinicopathologic study of 11 cases. *Arch Pathol Lab Med* 2009;133:62.

272. Amin MB, Gomez JA, Young RH. Urothelial transitional cell carcinoma with endophytic growth patterns: a discussion of patterns of invasion and problems associated with assessment of invasion in 18 cases. *Am J Surg Pathol* 1997;21:1057.

273. Baydar D, Amin MB, Epstein JI. Osteoclast-rich undifferentiated carcinomas of the urinary tract. *Mod Pathol* 2006;19:161.

274. McCash SI, Unger P, Dillon R, et al. Undifferentiated carcinoma of the renal pelvis with osteoclast-like giant cells: a report of two cases. *APMIS* 2010;118:407.

276. Zettl A, Konrad MA, Polzin S, et al. Urothelial carcinoma of the renal pelvis with choriocarcinomatous features: genetic evidence of clonal evolution. *Hum Pathol* 2002;33:1234.

276. Grammatico D, Grignon DJ, Eberwein P, et al. Transitional cell carcinoma of the renal pelvis with choriocarcinomatous differentiation. Immunohistochemical and immunoelectron microscopic assessment of human chorionic gonadotropin production by transitional cell carcinoma of the urinary bladder. *Cancer* 1993;71:1835.

277. López-Beltran A, Escudero AL, Cavazzana AO, et al. Sarcomatoid transitional cell carcinoma of the renal pelvis. A report of five cases

with clinical, pathological, immunohistochemical and DNA ploidy analysis. *Pathol Res Pract* 1996;192:1218.

278. Wang X, MacLennan GT, Zhang S, et al. Sarcomatoid carcinoma of the upper urinary tract: clinical outcome and molecular characterization. *Hum Pathol* 2009;40:211.

279. Leroy X, González S, Zini L, et al. Lipid-cell variant of urothelial carcinoma: a clinical pathologic and immunohistochemical study of five cases. *Am J Surg Pathol* 2007;31:770.

280. Pusztaszeri M, Hauser J, Iselin C, et al. Urothelial carcinoma "nested variant" of renal pelvis and ureter. *Urology* 2007;69:778.

281. Parwani AV, Herawi M, Volmar K, et al. Urothelial carcinoma with rhabdoid features: report of 6 cases. *Hum Pathol* 2006;37:168.

282. Weeks DA, Beckwith JB, Mierau GW, et al. Renal neoplasms mimicking rhabdoid tumor of kidney. A report from the National Wilms' Tumor Study Pathology Center. *Am J Surg Pathol* 1991;15:1042.

283. Lau SK. Nested variant of urothelial carcinoma of the renal pelvis. *Pathol Res Pract* 2009;205:508.

284. Keck B, Giedl J, Kunath F, et al. Clinical course of plasmacytoid urothelial carcinoma of the upper urinary tract: a case report. *Urol Int* 2012;89:120–122.

285. Fujimoto H, Tobisu K, Sakamoto M, et al. Intraductal tumor involvement and renal parenchymal invasion of transitional cell carcinoma in the renal pelvis. *J Urol* 1995;153:57.

286. Yoshimura K, Arai Y, Fujimoto H, et al. Prognostic impact of extensive parenchymal invasion pattern in pT3 renal pelvic transitional cell carcinoma. *Cancer* 2002;94:3150.

287. Catto JW, Yates DR, Rehman I, et al. Behavior of urothelial carcinoma with respect to anatomical location. *J Urol* 2007;177:1715.

288. Hall MC, Womack S, Sagalowsky AI, et al. Prognostic factors, recurrence, and survival in transitional cell carcinoma of the upper urinary tract: a 30-year experience in 252 patients. *Urology* 1998;52:594.

289. Rey A, Lara PC, Redondo E, et al. Overexpression of p53 in transitional cell carcinoma of the renal pelvis and ureter. Relation to tumor proliferation and survival. *Cancer* 1997;79:2178.

290. Kim DS, Lee YH, Cho KS, et al. Lymphovascular invasion and pT stage are prognostic factors in patients treated with radical nephroureterectomy for localized upper urinary tract transitional cell carcinoma. *Urology* 2010;75:328.

291. Olgac S, Mazumdar M, Dalbagni G. Urothelial carcinoma of the renal pelvis: a clinicopathologic study of 130 cases. *Am J Surg Pathol* 2004;28:1545.

292. Holmang S, Johansson SL. Bilateral metachronous ureteral and renal pelvic carcinomas: incidence, clinical presentation, histopathology, treatment and outcome. *J Urol* 2006;175:69.

293. Holmang S, Johansson SL. Synchronous bilateral ureteral and renal pelvic carcinomas: incidence, etiology, treatment and outcome. *Cancer* 2004;101:741.

294. Chen GL, Bagley DH. Ureteroscopic surgery for upper tract transitional cell carcinoma: complications and management. *J Endourol* 2001;15:399.

295. Azémar MD, Comperat E, Richard F, et al. Bladder recurrence after surgery for upper urinary tract urothelial cell carcinoma: frequency, risk factors, and surveillance. *Urol Oncol* 2011;29:130.

296. Razdan S, Johannes J, Cox M, et al. Current practice patterns in urologic management of upper-tract transitional-cell carcinoma. *J Endourol* 2005;19:366.

297. Katz MH, Lee MW, Gupta M. Setting a new standard for topical therapy of upper-tract transitional-cell carcinoma: BCG and interferon-alpha2B. *J Endourol* 2007;21:374.

298. Czito B, Zietman A, Kaufman D, et al. Adjuvant radiotherapy with and without concurrent chemotherapy for locally advanced transitional cell carcinoma of the renal pelvis and ureter. *J Urol* 2004;172:1271.

299. Bamias A, Deliveliotis C, Fountzilas G, et al. Adjuvant chemotherapy with paclitaxel and carboplatin in patients with advanced carcinoma of the upper urinary tract: a study by the Hellenic Corporative Oncology Group. *J Clin Oncol* 2004;22:2150.

300. Rausch S, Hofmann R, von Knobloch R. Nonbilharzial squamous cell carcinoma and transitional cell carcinoma with squamous differentiation of the lower and upper urinary tract. *Urol Ann* 2012;4:14.

301. Li MK, Cheung WL. Squamous cell carcinoma of the renal pelvis. *J Urol* 1987;138:269.

302. Lee M., Sharifi R, Kurtzman NA. Humoral hypercalcaemia due to squamous cell carcinoma the renal pelvis. *Urology* 1988;32:250.

303. Diaz Gonzalez R, Barrientos A, Larrodera L, et al. Squamous cell carcinoma of the renal pelvis associated with hypercalcaemia and the presence of parathyroid hormone-like substances in the tumor. *J Urol* 1985;133:1029.

304. Morita T, Izumi T, Shinohara N, et al. Squamous cell carcinoma of the ureter with marked leucocytosis producing granulocyte colony-stimulating factor. *Urol Int* 1995;55:32.

305. Er O, Coskun HS, Altinbas M, et al. Rapidly relapsing squamous cell carcinoma of the renal pelvis associated with paraneoplastic syndromes of leucocytosis, thrombocytosis and hypercalcaemia. *Urol Int* 2001;67:175.

306. Berz D, Rizack T, Weitzen S, et al. Survival of patients with squamous cell malignancies of the upper urinary tract. *Clin Med Insights Oncol* 2012;6:11.

307. Spires SE, Banks ER, Cibull ML, et al. Adenocarcinoma of renal pelvis. *Arch Pathol Lab Med* 1993;117:1156.

308. Delahunt B, Nacey JN, Meffan PJ, et al. Signet ring cell adenocarcinoma of the ureter. *Br J Urol* 1991;68:555.

309. Shih CM, Huang CT, Chi CH, et al. CA125-producing clear cell adenocarcinoma arising from the upper ureter and renal pelvis. *J Chin Med Assoc* 2010;73:4.

310. Miller RJ, Holmäng S, Johansson SL, et al. Small cell carcinoma of the renal pelvis and ureter: clinicopathologic and immunohistochemical features. *Arch Pathol Lab Med* 2011;135:1565.

311. Majhail NS, Elson P, Bukowski RM. Therapy and outcome of small cell carcinoma of the kidney: report of two cases and a systematic review of the literature. *Cancer* 2003;97:1436.

312. Al-Ali M, Samalia KP. Genitourinary carcinoid tumors: initial report of ureteral carcinoid tumours. *J Urol* 2000;163:1864.

313. Ji X, Li W. Primary carcinoid of the renal pelvis. *J Environ Pathol Toxicol Oncol* 1994;13:269.

314. Hansel DE, Epstein JI, Berbescu E, et al. Renal carcinoid tumor. A clinicopathologic study of 21 cases. *Am J Surg Pathol* 2007;31:1539.

315. Rudrick B, Nguyen GK, Lakey WH. Carcinoid tumor of the renal pelvis: report of a case with positive urine cytology. *Diagn Cytopathol* 1995;12:360.

316. Yusim IE, Neulander EZ, Eidelberg I, et al. Leiomyoma of the genitourinary tract. *Scand J Urol Nephrol* 2001;35:295.

317. Belis JA, Post GJ, Rochman SC, et al. Genitourinary leiomyomas. *Urology* 1979;13:424.

318. Yashi M, Hashimoto S, Muraishi O, et al. Leiomyoma of the ureter. *Urol Int* 2000;64:40.

319. Kho GT, Duggan MA. Bizarre leiomyoma of the renal pelvis with ultrastructural and immunohistochemical findings. *J Urol* 1989;141:928.

320. Bonsib SM. HMB-45 reactivity in renal leiomyomas and leiomyosarcomas. *Mod Pathol* 1996;9:664.

321. Pumberger W, Gindl K, Amann G, et al. Polypoid fibro-haemangioma of the kidney in a child with gross haematuria. *Scand J Urol Nephrol* 1999;33:344.

322. Coulier B, Lefebvre Y, Petein M. Renal pelvis haemangioma demonstrated by MSCT urography with ureteral compression and 3D reconstruction. *JBR-BTR* 2005;88:187.

323. Campistol JM, Agusti C, Torras A, et al. Renal hemangioma and renal artery aneurysm in Klippel-Trenaunay syndrome. *J Urol* 1988;140:134.

324. Chabrel CM, Hickey BB, Parkinson C. Pericaliceal haemangioma-a cause of papillary necrosis? Case report and review of 7 similar vascular lesions. *Br J Urol* 1982;54:334.

325. Le Cheong L, Khan AN, Bisset RA. Sonographic features of a renal pelvic neurofibroma. *J Clin Ultrasound* 1990;18:129.

326. Gersell DJ, Fulling KH. Localized neurofibromatosis of the female genitourinary tract. *Am J Surg Pathol* 1989;13:873.

327. Varela-Duran J, Urdiales-Viedma M, Taboada-Blanco F, et al. Neurofibroma of the ureter. *J Urol* 1987;138:1425.

328. Ogata S, Mizoguchi H, Arita M, et al. A case of hemangiomyoma of the ureter in a child. *Eur Urol* 1985;11:355.

329. Smith EM, Resnick MI. Ureteropelvic junction obstruction secondary to periureteric lipoma. *J Urol* 1994;151:150.

330. Micali S, Virgili G, Vespasiani G, et al. Benign schwannoma surrounding and obstructing the ureteropelvic junction. First case report. *Eur Urol* 1997;32:121.

331. Gulmez I, Dogan A, Balkanli S, et al. The first case of periureteric hibernoma. Case report. *Scand J Urol Nephrol* 1997;31:203.

332. Kartsanis G, Douros K, Zolota V, et al. Case report: leiomyosarcoma of the renal pelvis. *Int Urol Nephrol* 2006;38:211.

333. Kendal WS. The comparative survival of renal leiomyosarcoma. *Can J Urol* 2007;14:3435.

334. Dhamne SA, Gadgil NM, Padmanabhan A. Leiomyosarcoma of the renal pelvis. *Indian J Pathol Microbiol* 2009;52:549.

335. Tsai WC, Lee SS, Cheng MF, et al. Botryoid-type pleomorphic rhabdomyosarcoma of the renal pelvis in an adult. A rare case report and review of the literature. *Urol Int* 2006;77:89–91.

336. Harbaugh JT. Botryoid sarcoma of the renal pelvis: a case report. *J Urol* 1968;100:424.

337. Coup AJ. Angiosarcoma of the ureter. *Br J Urol* 1988;62:275.

338. Askari A, Novick A, Braun W, et al. Late ureteral obstruction and hematuria from de novo angiosarcoma in a renal transplant patient. *J Urol* 1980;124:717.

339. Yanai T, Okazaki, T, Yamataka A, et al. Botryoid Wilms' tumor: a report of two cases. *Pediatr Surg Int* 2005;21:43.

340. Tu BW, Ye WJ, Li YH. Botryoid Wilms' tumor: report of two cases. *World J Pediatr* 2011;7:274.

341. Voznesensky MA, Yamase H, Taylor JA III. Malignant peripheral nerve sheath tumor of the renal pelvis. *Urol Int* 2009;83:370.

342. Song HC, Sun N, Zhang WP, et al. Primary Ewing's sarcoma/primitive neuroectodermal tumor of the urogenital tract in children. *Chin Med J (Engl)* 2012;125:932.

343. Anderson JD, Scardino P, Smith RB. Inflammatory fibrous histiocytoma presenting as a renal pelvic and bladder mass. *J Urol* 1977;118:470.

344. Ehara H, Takahashi Y, Saitoh A, et al. Clear cell melanoma the renal pelvis presenting as a primary tumor. *J Urol* 1997;157:634.

345. Frasier BL, Wachs BH, Watson LR, et al. Malignant melanoma of the renal pelvis presenting as a primary tumor. *J Urol* 1988;140:812.

346. Maeda K, Hawkins ET, Oh HK, et al. Malignant lymphoma in transplanted renal pelvis. *Arch Pathol Lab Med* 1986;110:626.

347. Bozas G, Tassidou A, Moulopoulos LA, et al. Non-Hodgkin's lymphoma of the renal pelvis. *Clin Lymphoma Myeloma* 2006;6:404.

348. Mita K, Ohnishi Y, Edahiro T, et al. Primary mucosa-associated lymphoid tissue lymphoma in the renal pelvis. *Urol Int* 2002;69:241.

349. Hara M, Satake M, Ogino H, et al. Primary ureteral mucosa-associated lymphoid tissue (MALT) lymphoma-pathological and radiological findings. *Radiat Med* 2002;20:41.

350. Boscolo-Berto R, Raduazzo DI, Vezzaro R, et al. Aggressive non-Hodgkin's lymphoma mimicking unilateral transitional cell carcinoma of renal pelvis. The risk of making a diagnostic mistake. *Arch Ital Urol Androl* 2011;83:163.

351. Al Shaibani KM, AlMeshari KA, Raza SM, et al. Early post transplant lymphoproliferative disorder presenting with ureteric obstruction in en block kidneys. *Am J Nephrol* 2000;20:142.

352. Comiter S, Glasser J, al-Askari S. Ureteral obstruction in a patient with Burkitt's lymphoma, and AIDS. *Urology* 1992;39:277.

353. Breatnach E, Stanley RJ, Carpenter JT Jr. Intrarenal chloroma causing obstructive nephropathy: CT characteristics. *J Comput Assist Tomogr* 1985;9:822.

354. Greenstein F, Novetsky AD, Kahn AI, et al. Ureteral obstruction from isolated focus of chronic lymphocytic leukaemia. *Urology* 1984;24:70.

355. Igel TC, Engen DE, Banks PM, et al. Renal plasmacytoma: Mayo Clinic experience and review of the literature. *Urology* 1991;37:385.

356. Edge SB, Byrd DR, Compton CC, et al. *American Joint Committee on Cancer (AJCC) Cancer Staging Manual.* 7th ed. Chicago, IL: Springer; 2009.

357. Gupta R, Paner GP, Amin MB. Neoplasms of the upper urinary tract. A review with focus on urothelial carcinoma of the pelvicalyceal system and aspects related to its diagnosis and reporting. *Adv Anat Pathol* 2008;15:127.

358. Lopez-Beltran A, Bassi PF, Pavone-Macaluso M, et al. Handling and pathology reporting of specimens with carcinoma of the urinary bladder, ureter, and renal pelvis. a joint proposal of the European Society of Uropathology and the Uropathology Working Group. *Virchows Arch* 2004;445:103.

Nonneoplastic Lesions of the Urinary Bladder

JESSE K. McKENNEY, JOHN N. EBLE, and ROBERT H. YOUNG

A broad spectrum of nonneoplastic lesions occurs in the urinary bladder. These range from congenital abnormalities to infectious/inflammatory conditions of only microscopic dimension to mass forming pseudotumors. As background, this chapter first presents a brief review of the embryology, normal anatomy, and histology of the urinary bladder and then details the full spectrum of nonneoplastic conditions that may be encountered in diagnostic surgical pathology practice.

NORMAL EMBRYOLOGY, ANATOMY, AND HISTOLOGY

Embryology

The urinary bladder develops during the first 12 weeks of gestation. It derives predominantly from the vesical (rostral) part of the urogenital sinus; the trigone originates from the caudal end of the mesonephric ducts. The urothelium is derived from the endoderm, while all other layers are from the splanchnic mesenchyme. The formation of the bladder and trigone is regulated by complex epithelial–mesenchymal signaling events.[1,2] Initially in development, the bladder is continuous with the allantois; however, neither the urachus nor the allantois is involved in the formation of the bladder. The allantois typically regresses to a fibrous cord in adults, contained within the urachus, which is also called the median umbilical ligament. As the bladder increases in size, the distal parts of the mesonephric ducts are incorporated into the dorsal wall forming the connective tissue of the trigone, where the developing ureters implant. The anterior bladder wall is formed with the caudal migration of the cloacal membrane. In the 7th week of gestation, the urorectal septum separates the rectum from the part of urogenital sinus that forms the dome and the posterior wall of the bladder.

Anatomy

The urinary bladder is located in the pelvis but, when filled, may extend up to the level of the umbilicus. The bladder is wider at the superior aspect and narrows toward the inferior region, creating the shape of an inverted pyramid. The anatomic regions of the bladder are the bladder neck (inferior), the dome (superior), the apex (most anterior and superior point), the fundus (posterior wall), and the trigone, the last defined as the triangular region at the base of the bladder, bounded posterolaterally by the ureteric orifices and inferiorly by the internal urethral orifice.[3,4]

In the male, the bladder is held in place at the bladder neck by the puboprostatic ligaments that attach to the prostate gland and directly in the female by the pubovesical ligament. The remainder of the bladder is surrounded by the loose fibrous connective tissue and adipose tissue of the pelvis, which allows it to expand with filling. Other points of attachment include the rectovesical ligaments that attach to the rectum and sacrum, and the median umbilical ligament that extends from the apex to the anterior abdominal wall.

In the male, the anatomic relation to surrounding structures is (a) fundus: the rectovesical septum, seminal vesicles, and vas deferens; (b) apex: median umbilical ligament; (c) superior: peritoneal surface; (d) inferolateral: space of Retzius; and (e) neck: prostate. In the female, the fundus is separated from the anterior aspect of the uterus by the vesicouterine pouch and more inferiorly by the cervix and upper vaginal wall, while the inferior surface rests on the pelvic and urogenital diaphragms. The uterus also rests on the superior surface of the bladder in the emptied state.

The ureters course obliquely through the bladder wall and are surrounded by smooth muscle and fibrous tissue called Waldeyer sheath. The ureters enter the lumen at the trigone, where their muscle fibers are admixed with the muscularis propria. The urethra begins at the neck where the walls of the bladder converge. The smooth muscle fibers of the muscularis propria and urethra intermix at the bladder neck, but the internal sphincter consists predominantly of muscularis propria.

The blood supply for urinary bladder is derived from the superior and inferior vesical arteries, which arise from the internal iliac artery. Blood drains through the vesical venous plexus, which empties into the internal iliac veins. Most of the lymphatics drain to the internal and external iliac nodes; however, the bladder neck drains to the sacral or common

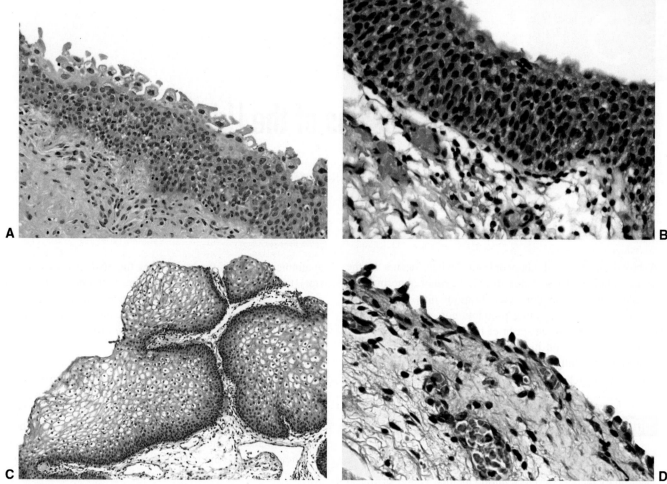

FIGURE 5-1 ■ **A:** Normal urothelium may have a prominent umbrella cell layer. These cells may have enlarged nuclei with multilobulation and cytoplasmic vacuolization. These features should not be regarded as neoplastic. **B:** In general, normal urothelium shows a streaming arrangement of the urothelial cells arranged perpendicular to the basement membrane. The urothelial cells often have nuclear grooves along the long axis of the cell. **C:** In the trigone of women, the surface lining is often composed of a glycogenated nonkeratinizing squamous epithelium. **D:** In biopsy specimens, particularly those performed with "hot" loops, denudation of the surface urothelium is not uncommon. Scattered residual benign basal cells may be present.

iliac nodes. The sympathetic nerves that innervate the bladder are derived from the T11–L2 nerve roots; these sympathetic nerves play no role in micturition. The parasympathetic nerves originate from the S2–S4 roots and travel to the bladder via the pelvic nerve and inferior hypogastric plexus. These peripheral nerves cause contraction of the muscularis propria fibers, which leads to traction of the bladder, opening of the internal sphincter, and emptying of urine into the urethra.

HISTOLOGY

Urothelium

Urothelium is a multilayered epithelium comprised of oval to fusiform cells that typically have pale nuclei containing longitudinal nuclear grooves in many of the cells. These urothelial cells mature to form very large surface cells known as "umbrella" or superficial cells.[5,6] Umbrella cells may have binucleation, prominent eosinophilic cytoplasm, and nuclear atypia characterized by nucleomegaly, nuclear multilobation,

and smudgy nuclear hyperchromasia, which should not be misconstrued to be dysplastic or preneoplastic (Fig. 5-1A). The number of cell layers varies considerably depending on distention of the bladder, but typically is three to six cell layers. The urothelial cells (previously referred to as transitional cells) typically have a somewhat linear organization streaming upward, perpendicular to the basement membrane (Fig. 5-1B). Nonkeratinizing, glycogenated squamous metaplasia is relatively common in the trigone of women and is generally considered a variation of normal histology (Fig. 5-1C).[6] In routine diagnostic biopsies, the surface urothelium may be denuded due to biopsy technique (i.e., thermal effect), but the retained basal cells that may be present are cytologically benign (Fig. 5-1D).

Heterogeneity of the thickness, the relation of the individual urothelial cells to the basement membrane, and the nuclear size of the urothelium are common, even within the same biopsy. Historically, there has been overuse of the term "mild dysplasia" for urothelium with a minimally disordered architecture and mild nuclear variation.[7]

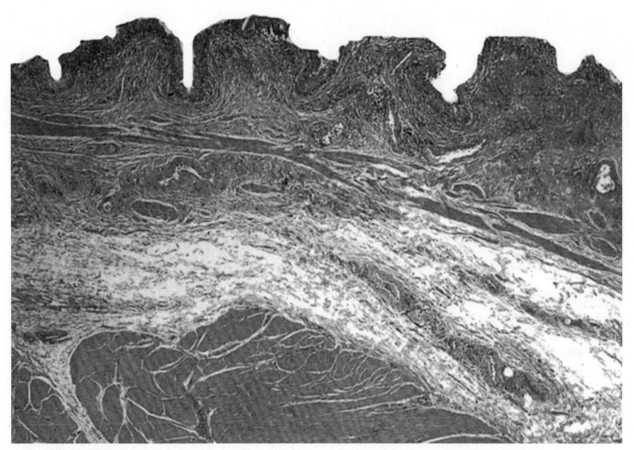

FIGURE 5-2 ■ The lamina propria is defined as the tissue between the urothelium and the muscularis propria. It often contains disorganized wispy fascicles of smooth muscle called the muscularis mucosae, as well as loose stroma and varying caliber blood vessels.

Lamina Propria

The lamina propria lies between the basement membrane of the urothelium and the muscularis propria (Fig. 5-2).[5,6] It consists predominantly of hypocellular, loosely collagenized stroma (Fig. 5-3A). Rare, scattered stromal cells that are hyperchromatic and often multinucleated are common in the lamina propria (Fig. 5-3B) (see giant-cell cystitis).[8] These atypical stromal cells may occasionally be numerous (Fig. 5-3C). In addition, prominent medium-sized blood vessels are common (Fig. 5-3D) and may be associated with smooth muscle that comprises the muscularis mucosae. Normal adipose tissue is also present within the lamina propria.[9] The thickness of the lamina propria varies; it is usually thinner in the trigone and bladder neck.

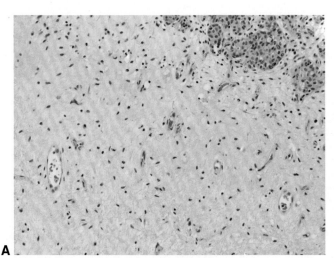
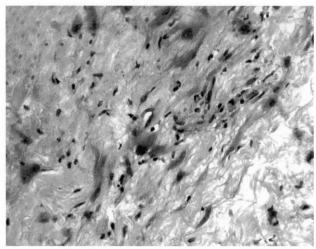

FIGURE 5-3 ■ **A:** The stroma within the lamina propria may be edematous or finely collagenized, as in this example. The majority of the stroma cells are small and inconspicuous. **B:** However, scattered stromal cells with enlarged hyperchromatic or multilobated nuclei are not uncommon, and (**C**) these stromal cells may be numerous.

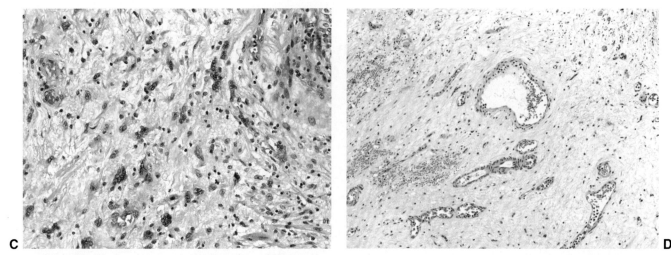

FIGURE 5-3 ■ (*Continued*) **D:** Varying caliber blood vessels set in a fine stroma are also characteristic of the lamina propria.

The muscularis mucosae is generally composed of irregular, usually isolated, thin wispy fascicles of smooth muscle within the lamina propria (Fig. 5-4A).[10] The muscularis mucosae varies considerably between individuals, but it is typically discontinuous; a continuous layer of smooth muscle layer is only rarely seen in the lamina propria. Recent detailed studies of the muscularis mucosae suggest greater heterogeneity of appearance than previously reported.[11,12] Particularly in the dome, the muscularis mucosae may be characterized by individual thick bundles of compact "hypertrophic" smooth muscle, even in women (Fig. 5-4B and C). These newly described round contoured smooth muscle bundles of the muscularis mucosae are separated by the stroma of the lamina propria, in contrast to the more typical larger aggregates of smooth muscle that comprise the muscularis propria. In men with benign prostatic hyperplasia, the muscularis mucosae may become more prominent throughout the entire bladder due to compensatory hypertrophy (Fig. 5-4D). These compensatory hypertrophic fibers are generally irregular, haphazard aggregates of smooth muscle fibers splayed in multiple direction; however, there is morphologic variation and overlap with muscularis propria may make distinction very difficult in a subset of biopsy specimens. For cancer staging purposes, we recommend defining the border between the muscularis propria and lamina propria as the line of demarcation where the dense smooth muscle bundles become organized into large aggregates (Table 5-1).

The lamina propria also contains a continuous band of ill-defined haphazardly oriented compact spindle cells that are immediately subjacent to the urothelium that has been termed the suburothelial band of myofibroblasts (Fig. 5-5). These spindle cells blend with the thin slender fascicles of the muscularis mucosae and show immunoreactivity for smooth muscle actin, but not desmin.[13]

Muscularis Propria

The muscularis propria, or detrusor muscle, consists of aggregates of large, thick, compact bundles of smooth muscle with variable amounts of interspersed collagen

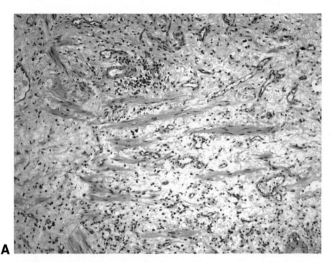

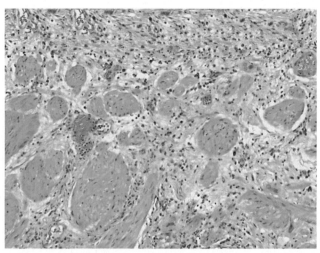

FIGURE 5-4 ■ **A:** The histology of the muscularis mucosae is classically described as disorganized wispy fascicles of smooth muscle within the lamina propria. **B:** However, recent studies have described more histologic variability. In the dome, individual rounded bundles of smooth muscle are common.

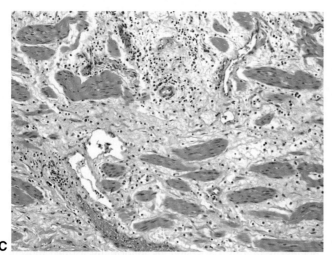

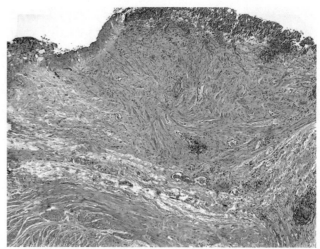

C   D

FIGURE 5-4 ■ (*Continued*) **C:** Unlike muscularis propria, these individual rounded bundles of muscularis mucosae are separated by stroma. **D:** In patients with urinary outlet obstruction, typically due to prostatic hyperplasia, the muscularis mucosae may become hypertrophic. The disarray of the smooth muscle fibers characterizes hyperplastic muscularis mucosae.

and adipose tissue (Fig. 5-6A).[5,6] Although the muscularis mucosae may have individual thick muscle bundles (i.e., hyperplastic muscularis mucosae), the muscularis propria has distinct tight aggregates of several discernable compact smooth muscle bundles that aid in their recognition (Fig. 5-6B). Because of variation in thickness of the lamina propria, the muscularis propria may be surprisingly superficial in some biopsies, particularly in the trigone (Fig. 5-6C). In this location, typical deeper muscularis propria bundles become smaller in caliber as they reach toward the surface and are found in almost a suburothelial location.

Recent studies have described distinct patterns of immunoreactivity between the muscularis mucosae and muscularis propria with the antibody to smoothelin, a monoclonal antibody to contractile smooth muscle.[13–19] Muscularis propria reportedly shows strong and diffuse immunoreactivity to smoothelin, while the muscularis mucosae is negative or have only weak, focal staining (Fig. 5-7). Some studies, however, have reported more overlap in intensity between the muscularis mucosae and muscularis propria; therefore, marked caution should be maintained while using this antibody in a diagnostic setting for the recognition of muscularis propria.[20–22]

Adventitia and Perivesical Adipose Tissue

These tissues are deep to the muscularis propria and consist of loose fibroconnective and adipose tissue with interspersed small peripheral nerves. The demarcation between the muscularis propria and perivesical fat is not well delineated, which may create problems in staging some bladder cancers that extend to this irregular border (i.e., pT2 vs. pT3 disease) (Fig. 5-8).

Paraganglia

Paraganglia may be present at any level within the bladder wall, but are more commonly deep seated (Fig. 5-9). They are generally not diagnostically important, but their existence explains the occasional occurrence of paraganglioma in the bladder. Occasionally, they may be mistaken as nests of carcinoma in resections for prostatic or urothelial carcinoma. The typically prominent nucleoli in the endocrine cell population of paraganglia may lead to the consideration of prostatic carcinoma. The presence of coarse intracytoplasmic granules or prominent interspersed capillary-sized blood vessels may aid in recognition as paraganglia. The endocrine cells of paraganglia express synaptophysin and other neuroendocrine markers, but are nonreactive for cytokeratins.

Table 5-1 ■ MUSCULARIS MUCOSAE VERSUS MUSCULARIS PROPRIA	
Muscularis Propria	**Muscularis Mucosae**
• ***Typical***: Dense compact smooth muscle bundles arranged into large solid aggregates.	• ***Typical***: Thin, irregular, wispy fascicles of smooth muscle of variable caliber.
• ***Dispersed***: In some examples, there may be dispersion of thin smooth muscle bundles from the muscularis propria into the deep lamina propria. In this setting, we use the point at which the muscle is comprised of a solid compact layer as the line of demarcation between muscularis propria and lamina propria.	• ***Dome/trigone variation***: The muscularis mucosae in the dome/trigone may consist of small individual rounded dense bundles of smooth muscle separated by stroma.
	• ***Compensatory hyperplasia***: With obstruction, the number of fascicles of muscularis mucosae may be markedly increased; however, they remain disorganized and are often splayed in multiple directions.

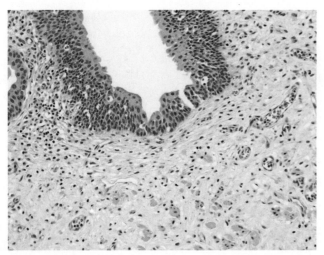

FIGURE 5-5 ■ There is a variably cellular layer of spindled myofibroblasts beneath the urothelium. These cells often show elongated nuclei and long cytoplasmic processes.

MALFORMATIONS

Agenesis and Hypoplasia

Congenital absence of the urinary bladder is extremely rare, and <70 cases are reported. By definition, the ureters empty into a structure other than the bladder such as the vagina,[23,24] uterus,[25] rectum,[26] or skin.[27] Accompanying hydronephrosis secondary to ureteral obstruction is common. In a subset of cases, a cloaca persists. Agenesis has been associated with a variety of other malformations[28] and is reportedly common in sirenomelia.[29] Agenesis is most often associated with stillbirth, but viable live births with agenesis are reported, most commonly female neonates.

Hypoplasia of the urinary bladder is defined as a small bladder with a thin wall and an abnormally formed muscularis propria. Hypoplasia is almost always found in the setting of congenital renal malformations such as bilateral renal

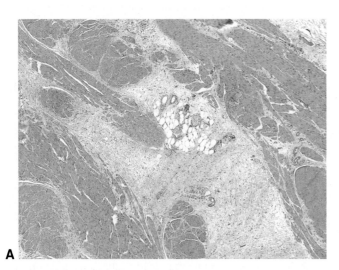

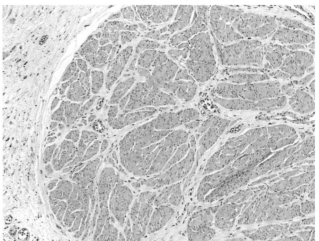

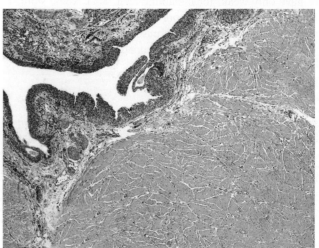

FIGURE 5-6 ■ A: Adipose tissue may be present at any level within the bladder wall. In this example, a lobule of adipose tissue is seen within the muscularis propria. B: The muscularis propria is comprised of compact well-delineated aggregates of smooth muscle. C: In some areas, such as the trigone, the muscularis propria is located very superficially.

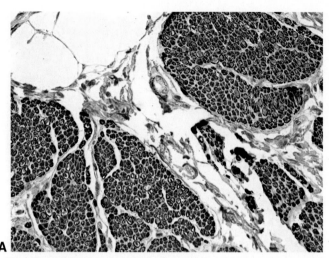

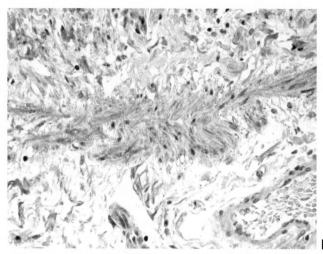

FIGURE 5-7 ■ Antismoothelin antibodies highlight the muscularis propria **(A)** with a strong and diffuse pattern of immunoreactivity. In contrast, the muscularis mucosae **(B)** are typically negative or show only weak, focal staining.

agenesis or other abnormalities that lead to an absence of urine entering the bladder (e.g., bilateral ureteral ectopia).[30] Rarely, bladder hypoplasia may be due to an absence of urine collection in the bladder due to low outlet resistance from causes such as epispadias.

Megacystis

This is defined as massive congenital dilatation of the bladder. Some authors have restricted the term to cases with thin and untrabeculated walls (i.e., functional obstruction), while others have included cases with bladder neck or urethral obstruction showing classic hypertrophy of the bladder musculature. Severe vesicoureteral reflux is common with associated hydroureter, hydronephrosis, and cystic renal dysplasia.

In rare cases, megacystitis is associated with the intestinal pseudoobstructive, autosomal recessive disorder termed megacystitis–microcolon–intestinal hypoperistalsis

syndrome. One report has suggested a loss of interstitial cells of Cajal as part of the pathogenesis,[31] but a consensus has not been reached.[32]

Duplication and Septation

Congenital division of the urinary bladder refers to the presence of more than one vesical lumen. This may result from a spectrum of abnormalities that range from complete duplication with separate bladders to the presence of an intravesical septum that divides the lumen of a single bladder. Although many patients are asymptomatic, incomplete bladder emptying may predispose to urinary tract infections. The clinical treatment is extremely variable, depending on the extent of anomalies and the presence of any functional impairment in an individual patient.[33]

Congenital division of the bladder may occur by complete or partial duplication.[34,35] In complete duplication, there are

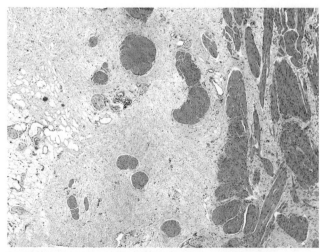

FIGURE 5-8 ■ The interface between the muscularis propria and the perivesical soft tissue is often irregular, which may cause difficulties in assessing microscopic invasion for staging purposes.

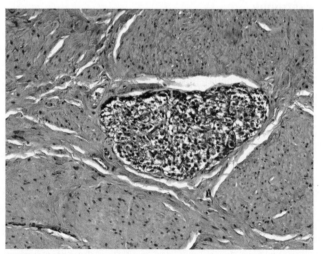

FIGURE 5-9 ■ Incidental paraganglia may rarely be found in the bladder wall. These are likely the origin of rare bladder paragangliomas.

two bladders with fully formed mucosal and muscular walls. Each side receives a single ureter and drains into separate duplicate urethras. Complete duplication is typically associated with duplication of the internal and external genital organs, hindgut, and caudal vertebral column.[36] Partial duplication, which is less common than the complete form, is defined as two bladders that share a common bladder neck and drain into a common urethra.

Septation is most commonly characterized by a complete sagittal septum that divides the bladder into two compartments. The bladder may appear grossly normal from the external surface. In contrast to partial duplication, only one side drains to the urethra. If a ureter empties into the blind-ending, obstructed side, then resultant unilateral dilatation with hydroureter, hydronephrosis, and cystic renal dysplasia are expected. Microscopically, the septum consists of two mucosal surfaces divided by fibroconnective tissue, with or without smooth muscle. Coronal septations are very rare, as are incomplete, nonobstructing septations. Finally, the "hourglass" bladder has a horizontal narrowing near the middle secondary to a horizontal band of smooth muscle, giving it its distinctive shape.

Diverticula

Bladder diverticula may be congenital or acquired. The majority occur in men >50 years of age with urinary outflow obstruction secondary to benign prostatic hyperplasia. In children, causes include localized alterations of the muscularis propria, neurogenic bladder, and a variety of syndromes including Menkes,[37] Williams,[38] prune-belly, and Ehlers-Danlos syndromes.[39] Diverticula typically occur in the region of the ureterovesical junction, likely secondary to the normal disruption of the muscularis propria by the adjoining ureter. While most diverticula are small and asymptomatic, larger lesions may cause ureteral obstruction, recurring infections, or stones. Diverticula also are at risk for the development of neoplasia secondary to urinary stasis.[40–42]

Exstrophy

Exstrophy is a congenital defect in the anterior bladder wall and ventral body wall, which results in external protrusion of exposed bladder mucosa (Fig. 5-10). At the margins of the defect, the urothelial lining is contiguous with the epidermis. With exstrophy, urine drains from the ureteric orifices onto this exposed surface of the bladder, which has a hyperemic appearance and may contain polyps.[43] The prevalence of exstrophy at birth is approximately 1 per 30,000 (ranging from 1:10,000 to 1:50,000 in published reports), and there is a male predominance up to 6:1; it is usually diagnosed with routine prenatal imaging. The recurrence risk for an individual family is approximately 1 in 100, which is approximately 500 times the expected risk. It is usually associated with other defects in the bony pelvis and external genitalia. In males, an open (epispadic) urethral plate covers the whole dorsum of the penis from the open bladder to the glandular groove. Females typically have a split clitoris next to the open urethral plate with associated narrowed vagina

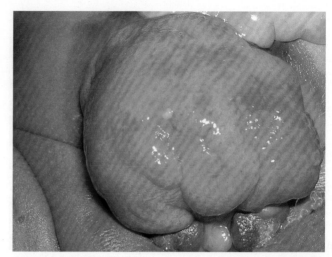

FIGURE 5-10 ■ Bladder exstrophy is clinically striking with the bladder mucosa exposed on the surface of the abdominal wall. (Courtesy: Dr. Michael Hsieh, Stanford University.)

and shortened perineum. The frequent association with epispadias has led to the use of the term exstrophy–epispadias complex. Associated bilateral inguinal hernias are also common, and spina bifida is present in 18% of cases.

The etiology of exstrophy is not fully understood. The defect in the urinary bladder and anterior body walls results from incomplete closure of the mesoderm. There are varying theories about the mechanism of this incomplete closure that include (a) overdevelopment of the cloacal membrane, (b) premature rupture of the cloacal membrane, and (c) caudal maldevelopment of the genital tubercles.[44]

Histologically, the mucosa of the extruded bladder is comprised of metaplastic epithelium with acute and chronic inflammation and ulceration. Squamous metaplasia and cystitis glandularis with intestinal metaplasia are minimal at birth, but develop with time.[45] After closure, squamous metaplasia and inflammation persist, but glandular changes become less prominent.[46] Unusual "hyperplastic"-appearing benign mucosal polyps are also commonly seen.

Patients with exstrophy have a well-described risk of developing cancer, most commonly adenocarcinoma.[47,48] Squamous cell carcinoma may also arise, and urothelial carcinoma and even rhabdomyosarcoma are rarely reported.[49–52] Although this cancer risk seems greatest in bladders without complete repair or those surgical repairs in which fecal exposure to the urothelium is present,[53] the risk following complete surgical repair is likely low, but remains uncertain.[54] These neoplasms may occur in the bladder proper or in urinary–intestinal anastomoses.

Vascular Malformations and Other Benign Vascular Abnormalities

Vascular malformations may rarely involve the urinary bladder.[55–57] Patients may present with hematuria, or the lesions may be discovered incidentally during cystoscopic evaluation. They may be small hemorrhagic submucosal lesions to large broad-based polypoid masses measuring up to 6 cm.[57]

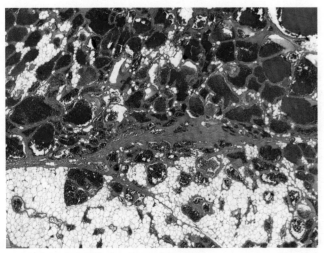

FIGURE 5-11 ■ Vascular malformations are typically comprised of dilated vascular spaces admixed with fat or normal bladder tissues.

Some are associated with syndromes such as Klippel-Trenaunay-Weber syndrome.[58,59] Preoperative imaging often suggests a vascular lesion, and in large masses Doppler flow studies may show a shunt in lesions with an arterial component. Morphologically, these lesions consist of large abnormally dilated vascular channels with varying components of arterial, venous, and lymphatic vessels (Fig. 5-11). The vessel walls vary in thickness with varying amounts of medial and elastic layers. Vascular malformations may have overlying ulceration and associated reactive urothelial atypia, including pseudosarcomatous epithelial hyperplasia.[60]

Some cases may show rather florid papillary endothelial hyperplasia, either with or without an associated vascular malformation, and this hyperplasia can mimic angiosarcoma. The overall circumscription of this endothelial hyperplasia within the confines of a vascular space and the absence of significant cytologic atypia generally allow distinction from an angiosarcoma. Papillary endothelial hyperplasia is well described in the setting of prior local radiation.[57] A component of adipose tissue is often admixed with large vascular malformations and may cause confusion with adipocytic tumors; however, the presence of the large dilated vascular channels excludes the possibility of an adipocytic tumor. Angiomyolipoma is distinguished by the presence of neoplastic cells within the walls of the vessels that have eosinophilic to clear cytoplasm and coexpress actin and HMB-45 or other melanocytic markers.[61]

Persistent Cloaca

Persistent cloaca, also called cloacogenic bladder, is defined as a retained connection between the urinary bladder, rectum, and/or vagina. The cloaca is a single embryonic canal from which the urinary, genital, and intestinal tracts arise at gestational weeks 5 to 6. Although the diagnosis has historically been restricted to females due to relatively arbitrary distinctions, many now accept that it occurs in both sexes when the diagnosis is based on contemporary embryologic criteria. The literature has referred to these abnormalities in the male

as "partial urorectal septum malformation sequence" and "cloacal dysgenesis sequence." Determining its frequency is difficult because of variable definitions employed in the literature and the exclusion of male defects. By traditional definitions based on malformations in females, it occurs in 1 per 20,000 births. In females, the defect is characterized by the terminal rectum, vagina, and urinary tracts all opening into a shared cloacal pouch. The persistent cloacal pouch is often connected to a single perineal opening, but this is occasionally absent. In males, the lumen of the rectum and urinary bladder are connected by a fistula, and the anus is imperforate. Associations with a variety of other complex malformations of the genital tract are common. Some of the associated malformations may actually be due to the resultant oligohydramnios. Persistent cloaca is presumably due to incomplete septation of the embryonic cloaca by the urorectal septum, but the underlying cause of this has not been determined and may be multifactorial.[44] Some animal models suggest the role of B-class Eph/ephrin signaling.[62] Complex surgical reconstruction is the standard treatment.[63]

INFLAMMATION AND INFECTION

Reactive Urothelial Atypia

Reactive urothelial changes, sometimes florid, may be associated with instrumentation, indwelling catheters, and any inflammatory condition. Morphologically, the reactive urothelial cells may show some degree of nucleomegaly and hyperchromasia, but the overall architecture of the urothelial cells (i.e., even spacing and alignment perpendicular to the basement membrane) is generally maintained. Intercellular edema may be conspicuous, and an associated intraurothelial inflammatory infiltrate is common.[7,64] Despite the prominence of one or multiple nucleoli and increased mitotic activity (which may be striking), the chromatin remains finely dispersed throughout the nucleus (Fig. 5-12A and B). These nuclear changes suggest urothelial carcinoma in situ (CIS), but the nuclear pleomorphism, irregular distribution of nuclear chromatin (i.e., striking nuclear hyperchromasia), and the loss of orderly alignment of the individual cells in CIS are distinctive (Table 5-2). The use of adjunctive immunohistochemistry to aid in this distinction has been studied, and a panel of antibodies to cytokeratin 20, p53, and standard isoform CD44 may be useful in some settings (Fig. 5-13).[64] CIS shows strong diffuse cytoplasmic immunoreactivity for CK20 in approximately 80% of cases, while diffuse nuclear p53 reactivity is seen in up to 57%. CD44s expression is either limited to the basal layer or absent in CIS. In contrast, reactive atypia is characterized by full-thickness membranous reactivity for CD44s with CK20 expression limited to superficial umbrella cells. p53 may show patchy nuclear staining in benign and reactive urothelium, but it does not have the intensity or the diffuse immunoreactivity pattern typical of CIS. Reactive urothelial atypia due to radiation and chemotherapy is discussed in detail below (see Box 5-1).

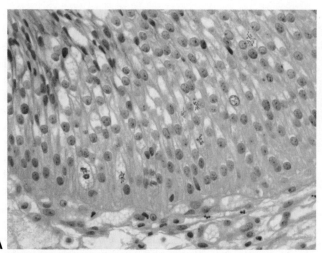
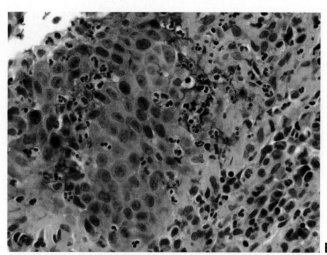

FIGURE 5-12 ■ **A:** This example of reactive urothelial atypia is associated with an indwelling catheter. Nuclear enlargement and small nucleoli are typical in reactive urothelial changes. In contrast to flat neoplasia, the nuclear contours are sharp and the chromatin remains fine and evenly distributed. Mitotic figures may be increased and may extend into the upper layers of the urothelium. **B:** In this example of reactive atypia, the nucleoli are more prominent, but the chromatin remains fine. Neutrophilic infiltrates are also common.

Papillary–Polypoid Cystitis

Papillary/polypoid cystitis is a clinically benign pattern of urothelial injury often secondary to an indwelling catheter or vesical fistula, but of diverse potential etiologies.[65–69] This lesion affects a broad age range, but the mean patient age is 49 years, and the majority of patients are male. It is relatively rare, but polypoid cystitis may be seen in up to 80% of the patients with an indwelling catheter. It may also be seen after radiation therapy. Although usually of microscopic size, grossly visible polypoid lesions may be seen. The entire bladder may be involved when a catheter has been present for a prolonged period of time, usually 6 months or more. With vesical fistula, extravesical symptoms may be initially absent in approximately half the cases, making diagnosis difficult. The cystoscopic appearance may also closely mimic a neoplasm.

Morphologically, the papillary and polypoid patterns may be intermixed, but lesions with relatively slender, nonbranching exophytic projections are termed papillary cystitis, while broad-based, edematous lesions have been termed

polypoid cystitis (Fig. 5-14A and B). Characteristically, the exophytic appearance results from edema in the lamina propria, but variable fibrosis, chronic inflammation, and associated dilated blood vessels are also present. These lesions exist along a morphologic continuum with bullous cystitis depending on the degree of edema; some authors have used the following convention: Lesions that are taller than they are wide are termed papillary/polypoid cystitis and vice versa for bullous cystitis. Older lesions tend to have less edema with more stromal fibrosis. As papillary and polypoid cystitis are usually associated with inflammation, there may be metaplastic changes in the lesional or adjacent urothelium. In both types of cystitis, the urothelium may be hyperplastic and reactive appearing, but usually is not as stratified as in a neoplasm. Some authors have suggested that the lesion described as "fibroepithelial polyp" of the bladder has many similar histologic features and may represent an end-stage phase of papillary–polypoid cystitis.

The main diagnostic consideration is a low-grade papillary urothelial neoplasm, particularly urothelial papilloma or papillary urothelial neoplasm of low malignant potential. In

Table 5-2 ■ IMMUNOPHENOTYPE OF FLAT LESIONS

	CIS	Reactive Atypia
CK20	• Strong cytoplasmic reactivity in neoplastic cell population • May be full thickness or individual cell staining depending on pattern of CIS (e.g., pagetoid CIS)	• Strong cytoplasmic reactivity in the umbrella cell layer only • Typically no staining in basal and intermediate cell population
CD44	• Strong membranous reactivity may be seen in residual basal cells, if present • Membranous reactivity may also be seen in surrounding benign cells in pagetoid CIS	• Strong membranous immunoreactivity typically seen in the full thickness of the urothelium
p53	• Strong diffuse nuclear reactivity in the neoplastic cell population (requires high threshold for positive staining)	• Various levels of patchy nuclear staining may be seen depending on individual lab

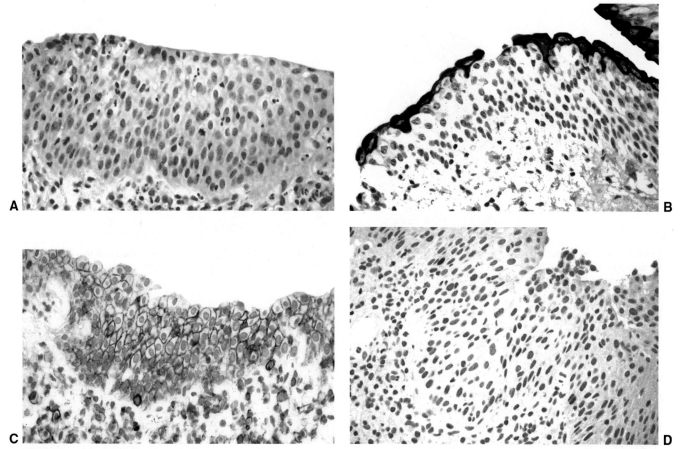

FIGURE 5-13 ■ Reactive urothelial atypia (**A**, H&E) has a characteristic immunophenotype with CK20, CD44, and p53 immunohistochemistry. CK20 (**B**) highlights the umbrella cell layer, while CD44 (**C**) shows strong membranous reactivity in the full thickness of the urothelial cells. p53 (**D**) shows weak and isolated nuclear staining, but strong and diffuse reactivity is not seen.

some cases, usually with recent catheterization, papillary/polypoid cystitis shows marked reactive epithelial changes with small, prominent nucleoli, urothelial hyperplasia, and mitotic activity mimicking a high-grade lesion.[70] In general, papillomas have more slender papillae; the papillae of papillary cystitis often have a bulbous tip with prominent stromal edema. In addition, urothelial papillomas have other features that, at least in aggregate, may aid in the distinction when

present: a very prominent umbrella cell layer or marked cytoplasmic vacuolization, a gland-in-gland pattern within the papillae, a dilated lymphatic space filling the papillae, a more complex papillary pattern with secondary and tertiary branching, and an admixed endophytic (inverted) component.[71,72] Significant cytologic atypia within a papillary lesion or the adjacent urothelium favors a diagnosis of neoplasia.

Giant-Cell Cystitis

Atypical, mononucleated or multinucleated mesenchymal cells are a relatively frequent finding in the lamina propria of the bladder (Fig. 5-15). Wells found them in one-third of cases of cystitis at autopsy and applied the term giant-cell cystitis to those cases.[8] Cells of this type are relatively common in the lamina propria of routine biopsies without significant cystitis. Their nuclei are frequently hyperchromatic and multilobated, but mitotic figures are typically absent. The cells resemble those that may be seen in various benign mesenchymal tumors and in the stroma of the female genital tract; therefore, when clustered closely, they may mimic a mesenchymal neoplasm. Similar cells may be seen in patients treated with chemotherapeutic agents and radiation.[73]

Box 5-1 ● NONNEOPLASTIC FLAT LESIONS OF URINARY BLADDER

Reactive urothelial atypia
  May have rounded nuclei with increased mitotic activity
  Retains finely dispersed nuclear chromatin
  Nuclei enlarged, but typical size is <3–4 lymphocyte nuclei
  Often associated with acute inflammation
Polyoma virus
  Urothelium may have scattered cells with hyperchromatic, smudgy chromatin.
  Can be confirmed by antibodies to polyoma virus
Flat nephrogenic adenoma
  Surface lined by a single layer of short cuboidal epithelial cells
  Express PAX8

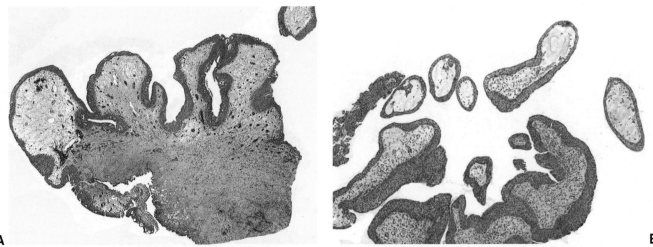

A   **B**

FIGURE 5-14 ■ **A:** In papillary/polypoid cystitis, the exophytic projections have a broad base due to underlying edema. In addition, the complex hierarchical branching of papillary neoplasia is absent. **B:** Biopsies taken near the tips of the papillary component may easily be mistaken for papillary neoplasia.

Follicular Cystitis

Follicular cystitis, which is also called cystitis follicularis or lymphofollicular cystitis, is reportedly more prevalent in children, but occurs across a wide age range and may have multiple etiologies.[74–76] It is often associated with repeated bacterial urinary tract infections and factors that contribute to prolonged infection such as paraplegia and indwelling catheters.[77] Other associations include carcinomas of the urinary bladder (with sterile urine), intravesical Bacillus Calmette-Guérin (BCG) or interferon therapy, and *Salmonella* infection.[78] Grossly, the urothelial mucosa is edematous with small pale to white nodules. Microscopically, the nodules are composed of lymphoid follicles in the lamina propria with or without germinal center formation (Fig. 5-16). When due to infection, the lymphoid follicles often disappear when abacteriuria is achieved.[74] Although rare, the main differential diagnosis is a low-grade malignant lymphoma, such as follicular lymphoma, involving the urinary bladder. Lymphoma may be excluded by a routine immunohistochemistry evaluation to distinguish reactive lymphoid from neoplastic proliferations.[79,80] Clinically, the nodular lesions seen on cystoscopy may mimic other infections such as tuberculosis, but the absence of granulomatous inflammation excludes that possibility.

Painful Bladder Syndrome or Interstitial Cystitis

Interstitial cystitis, now commonly referred to as "painful bladder syndrome," is a poorly defined chronic inflammatory process of unknown etiology that affects the urinary bladder.[81–83] The clinical symptoms include urinary frequency, urgency, nocturia, suprapubic pressure, and pain with either bladder distention or voiding. By definition, patients experience the clinical urinary symptoms despite sterile urine cultures by routine laboratory techniques. Urodynamic studies typically reveal decreased bladder filling capacity. Prior therapies with

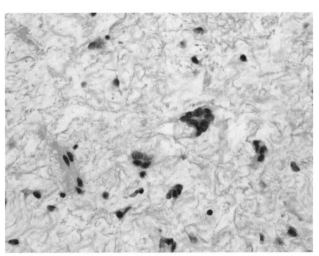

FIGURE 5-15 ■ Increased numbers of multinucleated atypical stromal cells within the lamina propria have been termed giant-cell cystitis.

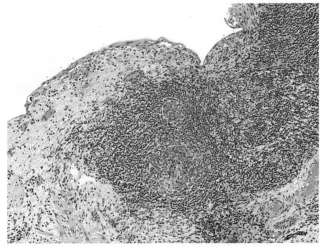

FIGURE 5-16 ■ Follicular cystitis is characterized by mature lymphocytic infiltrates with germinal center formation.

known bladder irritants, concomitant urothelial neoplasia, and infections would exclude the diagnosis of interstitial cystitis.[81] The American Urologic Association guidelines have provided the following modified definition: "An unpleasant sensation (pain, pressure, discomfort) perceived to be related to the urinary bladder, associated with lower urinary tract symptoms of more than 6 weeks duration, in the absence of infection or other identifiable causes."[83]

The reported incidence of painful bladder syndrome/interstitial cystitis varies widely, ranging from 10 to 510 per 100,000. This variation is likely due to the varied criteria that have been utilized for diagnosis between different studies. Despite being described almost 100 years ago, the disease remains a clinical and therapeutic enigma. Some research has suggested the possibility of an autoimmune disorder, but there is no general agreement about the pathophysiology of the disease.

Cystoscopic evaluation of the disease may be categorized as "nonulcer or early disease" and the classic type. The nonulcer disease is characterized by normal mucosa at initial evaluation with the development of small submucosal hemorrhagic foci, called glomerulations, and linear cracks during/after distention (Fig. 5-17). In the classic pattern, there are single or multiple patches of reddened mucosa with small blood vessels radiating from a central mucosal scar. Classically, the mucosa ruptures under hydrodistention creating oozing of blood, which is the prototypical Hunner ulcer. In well-developed cases, the entire wall may be fibrotic and contracted. The trigone, in general, is not involved.

The role of morphology in the diagnosis of interstitial cystitis remains controversial. In our opinion, the role of the surgical pathologist is twofold: (a) most importantly, to exclude other specific forms of cystitis and urothelial CIS and (b) to detail histologic features for correlation with cystoscopy. There are no pathognomonic histologic features of interstitial cystitis, but common findings include ulceration with variably admixed fibrin, erythrocytes, and inflammatory cells, especially neutrophils. Associated granulation tissue and

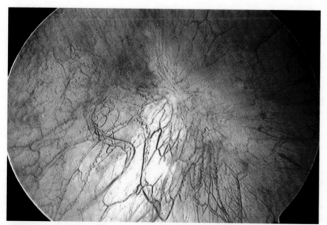

FIGURE 5-17 ■ Interstitial cystitis is often characterized cystoscopically by small foci of mucosal hemorrhage called glomerulations.

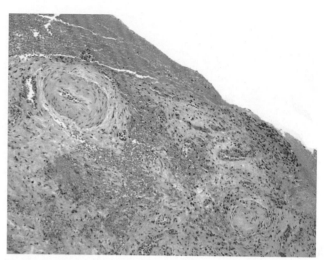

FIGURE 5-18 ■ In interstitial cystitis, variable surface erosion with hemorrhage is common.

perineural lymphocytic infiltrates are common, and urothelial denudation is frequent. Ulcers typically extend deep into the lamina propria with surrounding edema and congestion. In patients without ulcers, the morphologic changes may be subtle and include suburothelial hemorrhage, edema, and possibly mucosal tears (Fig. 5-18). In long-standing disease, fibrosis of the muscularis propria may be present. There is considerable debate regarding the utility (i.e., specificity) of mast cell counts in the distinction from other inflammatory processes. However, there are reports of increased intravesical mast cell infiltrates in patients with interstitial cystitis (Fig. 5-19A and B).[84–86] One of the major roles of biopsy evaluation is to exclude other lesions in the clinical differential diagnosis, particularly urothelial CIS. When the urothelium is extensively denuded, additional levels may be necessary to exclude this possibility. Since the morphologic features are not entirely specific, the final diagnosis of interstitial cystitis requires close clinical (i.e., history, cystoscopy, and voiding studies) and pathologic correlation.

A recent review of patient management identified >180 published treatment modalities.[82] These modalities include variations of behavioral, dietary, pharmacologic, and surgical interventions. There is general agreement on the use of some oral and intravesical agents, such as amitriptyline, hydroxyzine, and pentosan polysulfate sodium; however, there is a lack of definitive conclusions regarding optimal therapy.

Radiation and Chemotherapy Cystitis

In radiation or chemotherapy cystitis, patients often present with hematuria or voiding symptoms. Biopsy evaluation of the urothelium may show striking cytologic atypia.[73] Cytoplasmic and nuclear vacuolation, karyorrhexis, and a normal nuclear–cytoplasmic ratio are features suggestive of radiation injury (Fig. 5-20A and B). In general, robust mitotic activity is absent. These histologic and clinical changes are both time and dose dependent; however, histologic changes may be seen for years. In addition, the

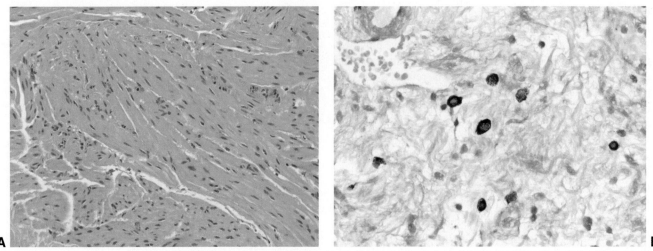

FIGURE 5-19 ■ **A:** Although its specificity has been debated, increased mast cells within the muscularis propria are reported in interstitial cystitis. **B:** The mast cells may be highlighted by a toluidine blue stain.

toxicity may be potentiated by concomitant therapy with cyclophosphamide. Radiation-induced histologic changes are similar to those seen with intravesical chemotherapy, but with intravesical chemotherapy the histologic changes are often more restricted to the superficial urothelial cell layer. Atypical mesenchymal cells similar to those seen in giant-cell cystitis are also typically present in the lamina propria (Fig. 5-21). Other characteristic changes of radiation injury including marked stromal edema or fibrosis; prominent telangiectatic change, hyalinization, and thrombosis of the vessels are also helpful. Pseudocarcinomatous hyperplasia of the epithelium (discussed later) may be striking.

In the posttherapy setting, one should have a high threshold for the diagnosis of urothelial CIS. In difficult cases with uncertainty as to the appropriate diagnosis, use of the diagnostic

term "atypia of unknown significance" is warranted. This allows repeat cystoscopy and biopsy evaluation after inflammation resides and avoids the potential overdiagnosis of reactive urothelial neoplasia.

Marked urothelial changes may be seen following radiation or chemotherapy. In general, radiation atypia is characterized by changes in the umbrella cell layer that include cytoplasmic vacuolization, nucleomegaly, and multinucleation. A reactive immunophenotype is maintained in reactive urothelial changes secondary to radiation therapy.[87] Intravesical chemotherapy with agents such as mitomycin may also cause marked epithelial atypia. There are very little data available in the diagnostic pathology literature on the specific urothelial alterations after intravesical chemotherapy,[88] but in our experience the cytoplasm of the urothelial cells becomes more

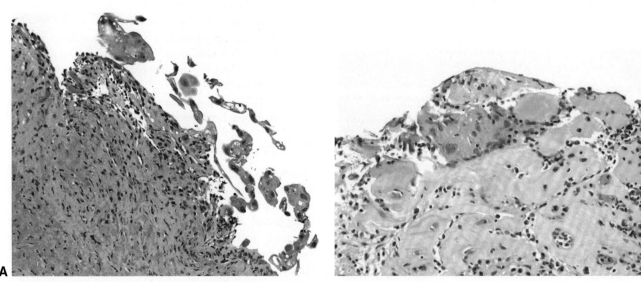

FIGURE 5-20 ■ **A:** Urothelial atypia secondary to radiation therapy is generally characterized by nuclear enlargement, prominent cytoplasmic vacuolization, and **(B)** multinucleation. The underlying tissue, including blood vessels, commonly shows hyalinization.

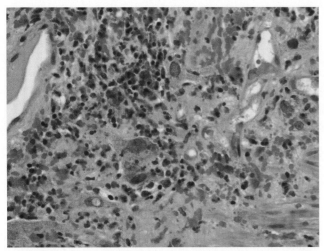

FIGURE 5-21 ■ With radiation therapy, the stromal cells of the bladder may suggest prior radiation exposure given the degree of atypia with marked variation in size.

uniformly eosinophilic, and nuclear changes similar to those seen with radiation are common (Fig. 5-22A and B).

Hemorrhagic Cystitis

Hemorrhagic cystitis is caused predominantly by chemotherapeutic agents, most commonly cyclophosphamide, methotrexate, and radiation therapy,[89] but viral etiologies are also well described (see "Viral Cystitis"). Less common causes include other chemotherapeutic agents such as busulfan and thiotepa, aniline and toluidine derivatives used in dyes and insecticides, and many other compounds.[90] The clinical presentation is typically onset of severe hematuria shortly after exposure to the inciting agent (Fig. 5-23).

Morphologically, hemorrhagic cystitis is characterized by extensive hemorrhage into the lamina propria with vascular congestion and edema. The overlying epithelium may show striking nuclear atypia similar to that seen in association with radiation or intravesical chemotherapy.

Eosinophilic Cystitis

"Eosinophilic cystitis" is a descriptive term that has been applied to mixed inflammatory infiltrates of the lamina propria rich in eosinophils (Fig. 5-19).[91,92] This type of inflammatory infiltrate is seen in a broad age range, but approximately 20% of cases occur in children. There is an equal sex distribution. Patients often present with dysuria, frequency, hematuria, and/or flank pain. Rarely, patients can present with an infiltrative mass lesion that may induce urinary obstruction. On cystoscopy, the lesions often have a polypoid appearance that may mimic polypoid cystitis or urothelial carcinoma in adults or a botryoid rhabdomyosarcoma in children.

Eosinophilic cystitis is best regarded as a pattern of inflammation associated with a variety of causes and not a single diagnostic entity; however, there are two general settings: (a) allergy related and (b) injury related. Bladder eosinophilia has been reported in association with allergic gastroenteritis, asthma, or other allergic disorders, especially in women and children.[91] This likely represents a systemic eosinophilic process that is distinct from the other nonspecific infiltrates. In adults, most commonly older males, eosinophilic infiltrates are more frequently associated with bladder injury from underlying prostatic hyperplasia, bladder carcinoma, or prior biopsy. Rarely, eosinophilic cystitis may be seen secondary to a parasitic infection.[93] The word "eosinophilic" occasionally causes some confusion with neoplastic entities in children and

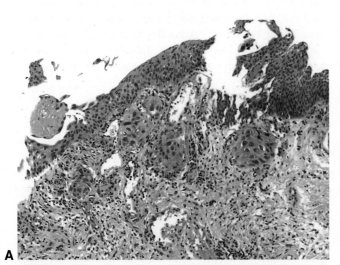

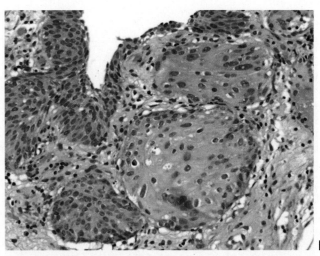

FIGURE 5-22 ■ **A:** After intravesical chemotherapy, nests of urothelial cells with atypical features may underlie a relatively normal appearing re-epithelialized urothelium. These reactive cells have enlarged nuclei and commonly have more eosinophilic cytoplasm imparting a squamoid appearance. **B:** At higher magnification, the fine chromatin of the reactive urothelial cells with enlarged nuclei can be seen. Compared to the overlying urothelium, these nests of cells with prior exposure to intravesical chemotherapy have a more pronounced cytoplasmic eosinophilia.

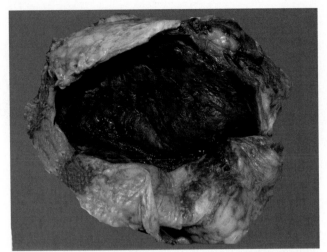

FIGURE 5-23 ■ In this postmortem bladder specimen, the diffuse mucosal hemorrhage characteristic of hemorrhagic cystitis due to prior systemic chemotherapy is seen. (Courtesy: Dr. Don Regula, Stanford University.)

young adults; however, it should be emphasized that there is no relationship to Langerhans cell histiocytosis (previously called eosinophilic granuloma).

Histologically, early lesions of eosinophilic cystitis are characterized by inflammatory infiltrates rich in eosinophils (Fig. 5-24). In some cases with extensive infiltrates, necrosis of the muscularis propria may be seen. As lesions mature, the eosinophilic infiltrate becomes less prominent with an admixture of mature lymphocytes and plasma cells.

Patient management depends on the clinical setting. With allergy-associated lesions, removal of the inciting agent may alleviate the symptoms in the bladder. In idiopathic cases, a course of antihistamines and nonsteroidal anti-inflammatory agents are often tried. Other intravesical therapies, such as mitomycin C, dimethylsulfoxide, cyclosporine A, and oral

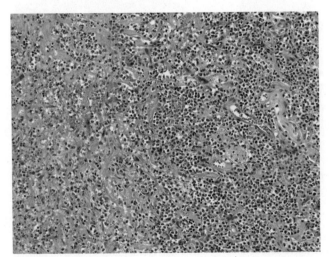

FIGURE 5-24 ■ Although nonspecific, the extensive infiltrates of eosinophils typical of eosinophilic cystitis are seen in this biopsy specimen from a bladder mass in a child.

corticosteroids, have also been utilized. In severe cases with unremitting symptoms, transurethral surgical resection and rarely cystectomy may be required.

Nonspecific Acute and Chronic Cystitis

In some patients with symptomatic inflammatory conditions of the urinary bladder, no identifiable etiology is determined after workup for an infectious etiology, and the patients do not have clinical features of interstitial cystitis. When biopsied, nonspecific histologic changes may be seen. Recent changes may include edema, hyperemia, neutrophilic infiltrate, and histiocytes. Surface ulceration as well as associated reactive urothelial atypia may also be present. Chronic changes include fibrosis and mixed chronic inflammatory infiltrates.

Bacterial Cystitis

Bacterial cystitis is typically secondary to coliform bacteria such as *Escherichia coli, Klebsiella pneumoniae,* and *Streptococcus faecalis.*[94–96] Another important cause is *Proteus mirabilis.* These infections are typically diagnosed by urine culture, so tissue biopsy plays little role in management.

Encrusted Cystitis

Encrusted cystitis refers to the deposition of inorganic salts in the bladder mucosa and is caused by urea-splitting bacteria that alkalinize the urine.[97–99] It is most common in women, and presenting symptoms are similar to other urinary tract infections. Cystoscopically, the lesions may be diffuse and have a gritty appearance. Morphologically, encrusted cystitis is characterized by a fibrinous exudate with admixed calcified, necrotic debris and inflammatory infiltrates (Fig. 5-25A and B). The main differential consideration is urothelial carcinoma associated calcification, which may be seen in areas of necrosis or prior biopsy/resection.[100] Accordingly, in a limited sample the carcinoma may be missed, and careful correlation with the cystoscopic impression is important to avoid a delay in diagnosis.

Gangrenous Cystitis

Gangrenous necrosis of the bladder is most commonly a complication of infection, but may also be due to systemic disorders (e.g., severe diabetes mellitus, metastatic carcinoma, sepsis, vascular disease) or corrosive chemical injury.[101–103] The necrosis generally begins in the mucosa and may progress to involve the entire wall to the serosa.

Emphysematous Cystitis

Emphysematous cystitis, which is more common in women than men, is defined as the presence of gas-filled vesicles that are visible by cystoscopy or gross examination.[104,105] A clinical diagnosis is typically made based on plain film and CT imaging, which show air within the wall of the

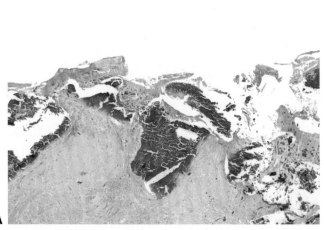

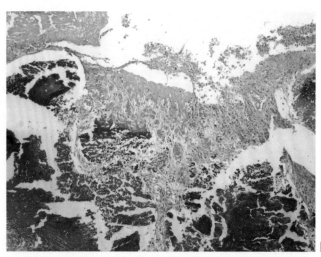

FIGURE 5-25 ■ **A:** With encrusted cystitis, surface erosions are covered by calcified debris. **B:** Associated hemorrhage, granulation tissue, and fibrin are common.

bladder. This lesion is typically associated with bacterial infections such as *E. coli* or *Aerobacter zaerogenes*. In adults, an association with diabetes/hyperglycemia is described in up to 50% of cases, but it may also be seen in association with neurogenic bladder, chronic cystitis, or immunosuppressed states.[105,106] In children, this is most commonly seen as a complication of necrotizing enterocolitis, secondary to gas extending from the bowel wall.[107] Rare cases are associated with fungal infection. Gross examination reveals easily ruptured cysts that typically range from 0.5 to 3 mm in size. Microscopically, the lamina propria contains cysts that are surrounded by a thin wall of fibrous connective tissue (Fig. 5-26). The mortality rate is approximately 7%. Patients typically receive aggressive antibiotic therapy and must undergo relief of any urinary obstruction.

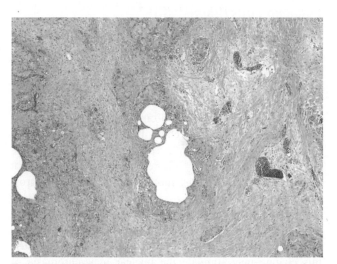

FIGURE 5-26 ■ Although not commonly seen in pathology specimens, sharply delineated cysts or spaces within resected bladder tissue are characteristic of emphysematous cystitis caused by gas-forming bacteria.

Malakoplakia

Malakoplakia is an inflammatory lesion that is caused by impaired intraphagosomal digestion resulting in histiocytic accumulation.[108–111] It occurs in a variety of anatomic locations, but is most common in the urinary bladder and typically associated with a coliform bacterial infection (e.g., *E. coli*). On gross examination the lesions in malakoplakia are often multiple and are typically soft yellow or yellow-brown plaques frequently with central umbilication and a hyperemic rim. They typically measure under 2 cm, but larger nodules are seen in approximately one-quarter of the cases, and occasionally striking papillary or polypoid tumor–like lesions are seen. Morphologically, it consists of sheets of histiocytes with granular eosinophilic cytoplasm (von Hansemann cells) and small basophilic intracytoplasmic inclusions (Michaelis-Gutmann bodies) (Fig. 5-27A).[112] The histiocytes are typically in the lamina propria with an intact, overlying urothelium. The inclusions are spherical, concentrically laminated (imparting a "bull's eye" appearance), and typically range from 5 to 8 µm in size. The inclusions contain calcium and are highlighted by a von Kossa stain (Fig. 5-27B). In late stages of malakoplakia, the picture may be complicated by extensive granulation tissue and fibrosis, and in all stages a prominent inflammatory cell infiltrate may partially obscure the nature of the process.

The main differential diagnostic consideration is a urothelial carcinoma with a sheet-like growth pattern. The small bland nuclei of the histiocytes and identification of the Michaelis-Gutmann bodies are usually sufficient for this distinction. In more difficult cases, an absence of cytokeratin immunoreactivity may be helpful.

Patients with malakoplakia typically receive antibiotics that concentrate in macrophages (e.g., quinolones or trimethoprim–sulfamethoxazole). Some cases associated with *E. coli* may require surgical debridement. Some have suggested a role for bethanechol, which may help correct

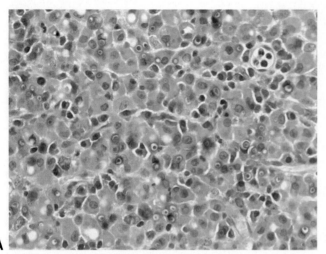
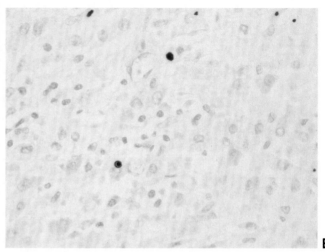

A   **B**

FIGURE 5-27 ■ **A:** This example of malakoplakia shows sheets of epithelioid histiocytes containing the characteristic targetoid intracytoplasmic inclusions (Michaelis-Gutmann bodies). **B:** These intracytoplasmic inclusions may be highlighted by von Kossa stains that highlight the phosphate associated with the calcium.

intraphagosomal digestion. Discontinuation of any immunosuppressive drugs is also warranted.

Fungal Cystitis

Fungal cystitis is uncommon. It is usually caused by *Candida albicans*, either secondary to ascending urethral infection or hematogenous spread[113,114] and is most common in debilitated patients or those on antibiotic therapy, particularly diabetic women. Cystoscopically, the lesions are typically small white mucosal plaques, but large fungal balls may rarely be seen. The fungal hyphae may be visible on routine stains, but special stains may be useful in highlighting the organisms in an acutely inflamed and ulcerated lamina propria. *Aspergillus* species and other fungal organisms have been rarely reported in the bladder.

Actinomycosis

Actinomycotic infection of the bladder is rare, but is present in 10% of women with actinomycosis of the ovary and/or fallopian tube.[115–118] Clinically, actinomycosis may present as a mass lesion that closely mimics a neoplasm secondary to direct continuity between adjacent organs. Morphologically, the bladder shows abscesses containing the classic "sulfur granule" colonies of *Actinomyces*. The individual bacteria may be highlighted by a Gram stain (Gram positive).

VIRAL CYSTITIS

Human Papillomavirus

Although more common in the urethra, condyloma acuminata may rarely involve the bladder and is morphologically identical to lesions occurring on the external genitalia, anus,

and perineum.[119–122] They are characterized by a squamous epithelial-lined papillary/polypoid growth with koilocytotic atypia (i.e., perinuclear halos, large hyperchromatic nuclei, frequent binucleation) (Fig. 5-28A and B). As in other sites, these lesions may progress to high-grade dysplasia or carcinoma.[123,124] The classic nuclear features aid in the distinction from verrucous carcinoma, papillary squamous cell carcinoma, and squamous papilloma.

Adenovirus

Adenovirus is an important cause of hemorrhagic cystitis in children, particularly types 11 and 21.[125–129] The cystitis may occur after bone marrow or solid organ transplantation in any age group or in otherwise healthy children.

Polyoma Virus (BK and JC)

Rarely, cystitis may be due to infection with BK or JC virus, human polyoma viruses. Although infection with polyoma virus is relatively common in childhood, it may become reactivated in states of relative immune deficiency. Polyoma viral infection infrequently causes clinical symptoms, except in immunocompromised patients with organ or marrow transplantation, chemotherapy, or HIV infection. Symptomatic patients may present with ureteral stenosis or interstitial nephritis.[130] Rarely, patients may present with hemorrhagic cystitis, more commonly after marrow transplantation.[131,132]

Infection may be identified in urine cytology specimens (Fig. 5-29A). Polyoma viral changes are characterized by large, homogeneous basophilic nuclear inclusions. Because this change may simulate the nuclear hyperchromasia of urothelial CIS, the infected cells are commonly referred to as "decoy cells" in the pathology literature. In bladder biopsies, similar cytologic changes may be seen in superficial

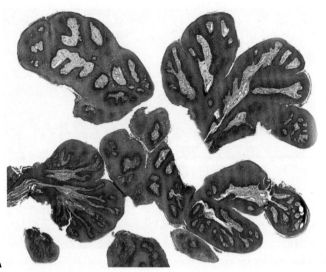
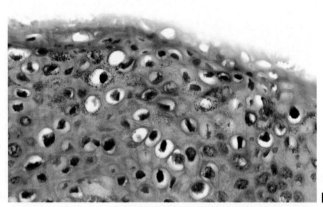

FIGURE 5-28 ■ **A:** Condyloma in the urinary tract often has an exophytic papillary appearance. **B:** The perinuclear clearing typical of HPV infection is seen in this bladder condyloma, but the cytologic features are often less pronounced than those more typically seen in the uterine cervix.

umbrella cells (Fig. 5-29B); however, urine cytology is much more sensitive for identifying infected cells .[132a] Antibodies against the LT antigen of polyoma may be used as an ancillary diagnostic test. In addition, PCR methods can be used to identify BK virus DNA in urine; however, BK viruria does not necessarily correlate with kidney or bladder damage. Treatment usually consists of intravenous antiviral therapy (e.g., cidofovir).

Other Viruses

Other viral causes of hemorrhagic cystitis include polyoma virus and herpes simplex type 2.[133] Herpes zoster may be associated with reversible voiding dysfunction, and cytomegalovirus may also rarely involve the bladder in immunocompromised patients.[134,135]

Schistosomiasis

Schistosomiasis is a waterborne trematode infection that is also known as bilharziasis.[136,137] Infection with *Schistosoma haematobium* is an important cause of bladder pathology, particularly in Africa and the eastern Mediterranean. In endemic regions, large percentages of the population are affected, particularly those with occupational exposure to infested water. The initial symptom of involvement in the genitourinary tract, which is the established phase of infection characterized by egg deposition, is typically hematuria. Diagnosis is usually by identification of eggs in the urine or by newer serologic tests.[138] The infection is a chronic process that, if untreated, may lead to hydronephrosis, pyelonephritis, and renal failure. There is a high incidence of primary bladder cancer, particularly

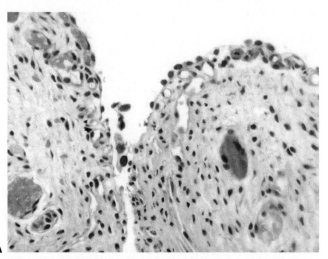
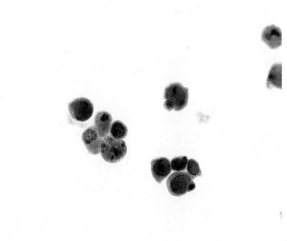

FIGURE 5-29 ■ **A:** Polyoma virus infection may be hard to recognize in biopsy samples, but the nuclei show a typical inclusion. **B:** Polyoma virus infection is more typically diagnosed in cytology preparations, where the enlarged nuclei have intracytoplasmic inclusions. These so-called "decoy" cells may mimic urothelial neoplasia.

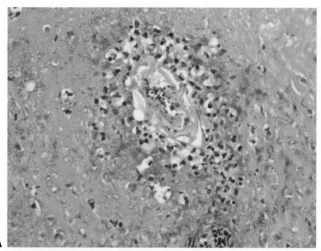
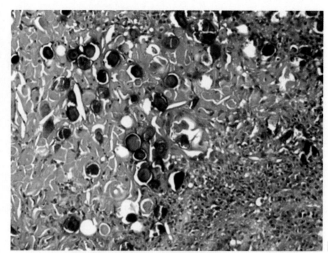

FIGURE 5-30 ■ **A:** This single egg of *Schistosoma haematobium* is surrounded by an acute inflammatory response. **B:** Over time, the eggs become calcified and may be numerous.

squamous cell carcinoma, in patients with chronic urinary schistosomiasis, which is more fully discussed in the chapter on neoplasia. Other complications include hydroureter, hydronephrosis with renal failure, and bacterial coinfection. The current treatment for *Schistosoma* infection is praziquantel.

Grossly, the bladder mucosa may show rough granular foci (i.e., sandy patches), sharp ulcerations with firm base, transverse fissures, and less commonly polyps. These features may simulate a neoplasm cystoscopically. Microscopically, numerous ova are seen with a surrounding granulomatous response, chronic inflammation, hemorrhage, and mucosal ulceration (Fig. 5-30A). The schistosomal eggs become calcified over time (Fig. 5-30B). Metaplastic urothelial changes, including keratinizing squamous metaplasia and intestinal metaplasia, are common. In long-standing

infections, considerable fibrosis may be present, and the associated complications may occur in this inactive phase when diagnosis is more difficult.

Granulomatous Cystitis

Postsurgical necrobiotic granulomas are relatively common following previous transurethral biopsies/curettings (present in 14% of patients with two surgical procedures). Histologically, they are linear or serpiginous in shape and are characterized by central granular eosinophilic material surrounded by palisading histiocytes and multinucleated giant cells (Fig. 5-31).[139] The surrounding tissue typically shows dense fibrosis and mixed chronic inflammation that may be eosinophil-rich. These lesions progress to dense fibrous scars that occasionally calcify.

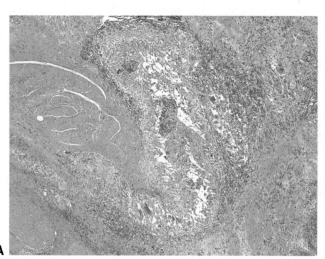
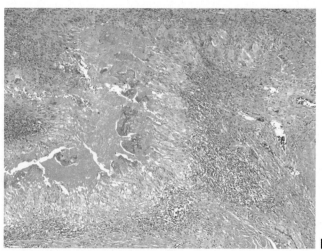

FIGURE 5-31 ■ **A:** Granulomas due to prior biopsy/curettage are fairly common in bladder follow-up biopsies or resection specimens. These postbiopsy granulomas often have a linear or serpiginous shape. **B:** They characteristically have central granular eosinophilic material surrounded by palisading histiocytes and multinucleated giant cells.

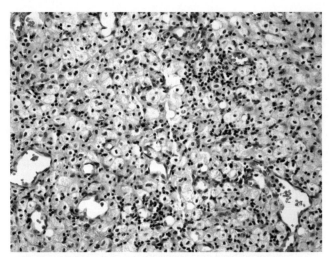

FIGURE 5-32 ■ Xanthogranulomatous inflammation is characterized by sheets of foamy histiocytes, often admixed with other inflammatory cells.

Xanthogranulomatous cystitis consists of sheets of foamy histiocytes without well-formed granulomas (Fig. 5-32).[140–142] Unlike malakoplakia, Michaelis-Gutmann bodies are not present. A similar reaction may be rarely seen in association with carcinoma of the bladder.

Granulomas are commonly associated with administration of intravesical BCG, which has become common therapy for urothelial CIS and high-grade superficial bladder cancer. BCG induces a marked inflammatory response with denudation of the urothelium; the lamina propria typically shows mixed chronic inflammation admixed with small epithelioid granulomas, typically with associated multinucleated giant cells (Fig. 5-33).[143,144] The granulomas are usually superficial with a round contour and no necrosis. Acid-fast stains are

not necessary in the proper clinical context, but they may highlight organisms.[145]

Tuberculous cystitis is most commonly caused by *Mycobacterium tuberculosis,* but *Mycobacterium bovis* may rarely be a causative agent.[146,147] It is almost always secondary to renal tuberculosis as organisms are carried to the bladder through infected urine. Because of this descending route of infection, the early lesions are generally in the region of the ureteral orifice. These lesions consist of small 1 to 3 mm tubercles that may coalesce and ulcerate. Morphologically, there is central necrosis surrounded by histiocytes with admixed multinucleated giant cells and lymphocytes. *Mycobacterium* may be demonstrated by acid-fast stains, molecular techniques, or cultures.

Other noninfectious granulomatous processes may involve the urinary bladder and include sarcoidosis, Crohn disease, rheumatoid arthritis (rheumatoid nodule), and granulomatous disease of childhood.

Calculi

Vesical calculi, which are much less common than renal calculi, occur most frequently in men with urinary outflow obstruction secondary to benign prostatic hyperplasia or in patients with neurogenic bladder.[148] Children in developing countries, mostly boys, are also prone to developing stones, likely due to low protein and fluid intake. Patients typically present with urinary frequency, urgency, and nocturia, but hematuria, dysuria, and suprapubic pain are also frequent. The diagnosis is usually confirmed by cystoscopy or radiography. The stones are most commonly composed of calcium oxalate or a mixture of calcium oxalate and calcium phosphate, but struvite stones may be found in association with *P. mirabilis* or other urease-producing bacterial infections.

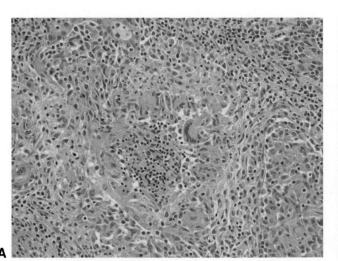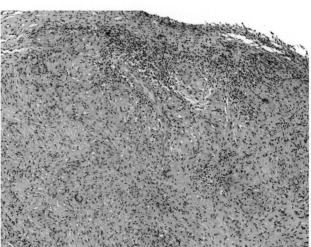

A   **B**

FIGURE 5-33 ■ **A:** Granulomas due to previous intravesical BCG therapy are typically characterized by a chronic inflammatory infiltrate admixed with small epithelioid granulomas, often with associated multinucleated giant cells. **B:** Infectious granulomas, such as this example of *M. tuberculosis* in a bladder biopsy, are often larger and more confluent. Areas of acute inflammation and caseating necrosis are common.

METAPLASIA AND HYPERPLASIA

Squamous Metaplasia

Squamous metaplasia is the replacement of urothelium by stratified squamous epithelium, which may be nonkeratinized or keratinized. The nonkeratinizing type occurs commonly in the trigone of the bladder of women (so-called pseudomembranous trigonitis) and is considered a normal variation. In women, this metaplastic process is likely hormonally regulated.[149,150] It is also rarely seen in children[151] and may be seen in association with inverted papilloma. In general, nonkeratinizing squamous metaplasia is not associated with chronic irritation and does not predispose to carcinoma.

Keratinizing squamous metaplasia, often clinically referred to as leukoplakia, is more common in men and is often associated with settings of chronic irritation such as indwelling catheters, calculi, and schistosomiasis (Fig. 5-34). Macroscopically, white plaques are often seen, and flakes of keratin may be evident. Keratinizing squamous metaplasia can be a predisposing factor to the development of squamous cell carcinoma or other complications such as bladder contracture or obstruction.[152,153] When squamous dysplasia and/or invasive squamous cell carcinoma is present, keratinizing squamous metaplasia is frequently seen in the adjacent epithelium and may help to confirm a primary squamous carcinoma.

von Brunn Nests

von Brunn nests are a normal variation of bladder histology that most commonly occurs in the trigone and may result from a prior inflammatory insult.[154] They are generally incidental microscopic findings without any associated clinical symptoms, but when florid may appear as small cysts or the mucosa may have a distinctive cobblestone appearance at cystoscopy. They are characterized by well-circumscribed,

---

Box 5-2 ● NONNEOPLASTIC ENDOPHYTIC LESIONS OF URINARY BLADDER

von Brunn nests
   Collection of rounded nests of normal urothelium in superficial lamina propria
   Have sharp line of demarcation at base
Cystitis glandularis
   Collection of rounded urothelial nests in superficial lamina propria with central lumen lined by cells with apical cytoplasm
   Also have sharp line of demarcation at base
   May have intestinal metaplasia and mucin extravasation
Nephrogenic adenoma
   The endophytic component may be complex with tubular, cystic, or solid patterns.
   Small tubules may have intraluminal blue secretions and may resemble a small capillary.
   Solid pattern resembles clear cell renal cell carcinoma.
   Express PAX8 by immunohistochemistry
Pseudocarcinomatous hyperplasia
   Most often associated with ischemia from radiation or chemotherapy
   Nests of invaginated epithelium have squamoid appearance.
   Epithelium is enmeshed with fibrin and surrounds vessels with fibrinoid change.
   Lamina propria often shows atypical cells, vascular injury, and hemorrhage.

---

evenly spaced nests of invaginated urothelium in the lamina propria (Fig. 5-35). In the bladder, the nests typically have smooth, rounded contours and are often clustered in groups, but the connection with the overlying urothelium may not be identifiable.[155] They are usually located in the superficial lamina propria, but deeper nests occur on occasion. The urothelial cells are devoid of significant cytologic atypia (see Box 5.2).

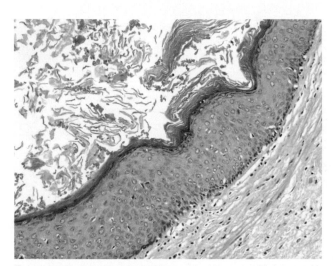

FIGURE 5-34 ■ Keratinizing squamous metaplasia may be seen in the setting of chronic bladder irritation.

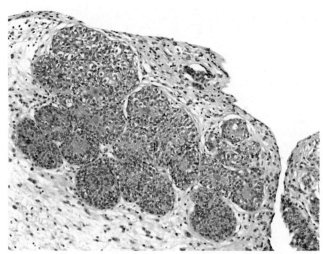

FIGURE 5-35 ■ von Brunn nests are characterized by rounded invaginations of benign urothelium. These nests are typically clustered in a lobular arrangement and extend to a uniform depth in the lamina propria.

Although there is usually a sharp line of demarcation at the base of the nests, diagnostic problems may arise in rare cases where von Brunn nests lie relatively deep in the lamina propria, as this displacement from the overlying epithelium may suggest an invasive urothelial carcinoma. Although the bland histology of the cells in von Brunn nests contrasts with the significant atypia seen in most invasive bladder cancers, the epithelium in von Brunn nests, like the surface epithelium, may exhibit hyperplasia and reactive atypia including mitotic activity. Even when invasive carcinoma has relatively bland cytologic features, the cell nests generally have a more disorderly distribution in the lamina propria and more variation in size and shape of the nests than von Brunn nests. The main differential diagnosis is a "deceptively benign" form of urothelial carcinoma such as the nested variant.[155] The most useful distinguishing feature is the extension of von Brunn nests to a uniform level within the lamina propria creating a sharp, linear border at the base that contrasts with the irregular, infiltrative base of nested carcinoma. Other subtle features of invasion may be seen in nested carcinomas such as small clusters or individual neoplastic cells with surrounding retraction artifact. The overall architectural arrangement and cytology of the neoplastic cells may also have a subtle difference when compared to von Brunn nests, but these features are not as definitive. The presence of small, irregularly sized, unevenly distributed nests creating confluent, branching patterns should serve as a clue to carefully consider the possibility of a nested carcinoma, as von Brunn nests are often clustered, evenly spaced, and round. Invasion of the muscularis propria, despite the bland nuclear features, is diagnostic of carcinoma and is the most definitive distinguishing feature. Unfortunately, the distinction of nested carcinoma from von Brunn nests may not be possible in superficial biopsies when some of the subtle clues are not present, particularly when complicated by extensive cautery artifact. In difficult cases, correlation with the clinical impression of the urologist may suggest the presence of a more aggressive lesion suggesting the need for rebiopsy.

Occasionally, urothelial CIS may extend into von Brunn nests and may mimic invasion. The relatively smooth, round contour of the nests, the absence of surrounding retraction spaces, the lobular or linear arrangement of the nests with a noninfiltrative base, and the absence of a stromal reaction should aid in that distinction.

Cystitis Glandularis and Cystitis Cystica

Although similar to von Brunn nests, the term cystitis cystica is used when the nests are cystically dilated with an inner luminal surface. When the inner adluminal cells have a columnar or cuboidal appearance with prominent apical cytoplasm, but no intestinal-type goblet cells, the term cystitis glandularis (cystitis cystica et glandularis) is used (Fig. 5-36).[156,157] Although usually a microscopic finding, cystitis cystica or glandularis is occasionally visible grossly (Fig. 5-37). At cystoscopy, it may have a cobblestone or

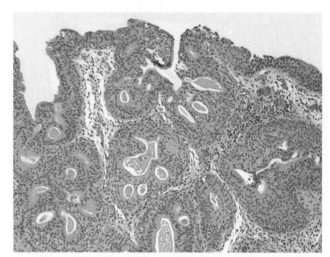

FIGURE 5-36 ■ Cystitis glandularis is similar to von Brunn nests, except that there is central lumen formation with the lining luminal cells showing abundant apical cytoplasm.

polypoid appearance. On microscopic examination the lesion usually occurs in a nonpolypoid mucosa, but occasionally an exuberant proliferation produces a papillary or polypoid lesion helping to explain the occasional case, which simulates a neoplasm at cystoscopy.

As discussed for von Brunn nests, deceptively bland patterns of urothelial carcinoma such as tubular or microcystic patterns may also be confused with cystitis glandularis cystica, and the same histologic considerations are valid here. One other differential consideration, though not as clinically relevant, is inverted papilloma. In some instances, the distinction from inverted papilloma (cystitis cystica–like pattern) may be somewhat arbitrary.[158] Inverted papillomas typically show a more anastomosing pattern of the epithelial nests and retain the peripheral palisading of cells even when central lumina are present.

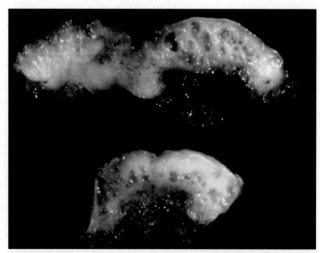

FIGURE 5-37 ■ Cystitis cystica may produce a clinically apparent polypoid lesion. In this gross specimen, the cysts underlying the surface may be seen.

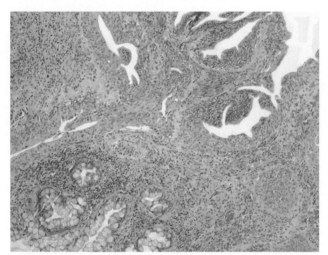

FIGURE 5-38 ■ Cystitis glandularis with intestinal metaplasia is defined by the presence of cells with abundant intracytoplasmic mucin within cystitis glandularis. Typical cystitis glandularis and von Brunn nests are commonly admixed.

Cystitis Glandularis with Intestinal Metaplasia

The presence of intestinal-type goblet cells within the nests warrants the designation cystitis glandularis with intestinal metaplasia (Fig. 5-38). Occasionally, mucinous epithelium, including that showing intestinal metaplasia, may replace the lining urothelium. This is usually associated with underlying cystitis glandularis of typical or intestinal type but may be seen on its own. In the latter situation, the lesion should be referred to as mucinous metaplasia (Fig. 5-39), if the epithelium is nonintestinal in type, or intestinal metaplasia. Worrisome-appearing, fleshy polypoid lesions may rarely be present, particularly in cases with mucin extravasation, in which the radiologic and/or cystoscopic appearance may suggest a malignant tumor.

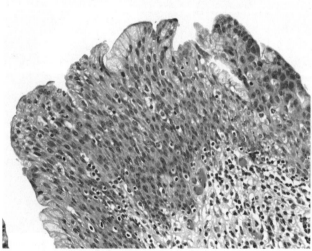

FIGURE 5-39 ■ Mucinous metaplasia may occasionally be seen within the surface urothelium, typically in association with a chronic irritative process.

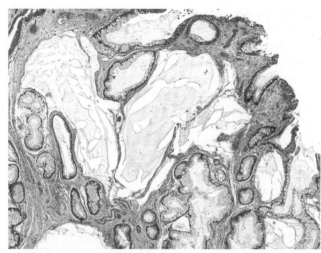

FIGURE 5-40 ■ Cystitis glandularis with intestinal metaplasia may be associated with extensive mucin extravasation in some cases. This may create a clinical mass lesion that closely mimics adenocarcinoma.

Diagnostic problems usually arise in cases of the intestinal, rather than typical, form of cystitis glandularis. Even with a very florid proliferation, the glands retain an essentially orderly arrangement and lack the irregular stromal infiltration that generally facilitates the diagnosis of adenocarcinoma. Rare examples of florid cystitis glandularis with extensive intestinal metaplasia and mucin extravasation have been reported (Fig. 5-40).[159,160] These florid metaplasias may closely mimic invasive adenocarcinoma because they fill the lamina propria and abut the muscularis propria. Adenocarcinomas typically show greater nuclear atypia with irregular tumor cell aggregates, including within mucin, and more mitotic activity. In addition, adenocarcinomas often show obvious, destructive invasion of the muscularis propria. Cystitis glandularis with intestinal metaplasia and mucin extravasation, despite the abundant extracellular mucin within the lamina propria, maintains cytologically benign-appearing epithelium. These benign glands may be intact or ruptured. When ruptured, they may closely mimic a colloid/mucinous adenocarcinoma, but there are no architecturally irregular or complex epithelial aggregates. One series of florid cystitis cystica glandularis with intestinal metaplasia reported two cases with "focal, superficial extension" into the muscularis propria, but this likely represents an irregular muscularis propria-lamina propria junction and is distinctive from the extensive, irregular invasion of the muscularis propria by cancer.[159]

Finally, it should be noted that extraordinary "borderline" cases meriting the designation "cystitis glandularis with atypia" are very rarely seen. Although rare case reports have described adenocarcinoma adjacent to cystitis glandularis, cystitis cystica and glandularis are relatively common and are not currently regarded as a precursor to vesical carcinoma. Despite this occasional association and the presence of cases in "transition" to malignancy, evidence suggests that even intestinal metaplasia is not a significant risk factor for progression to adenocarcinoma.[160,161]

Pseudocarcinomatous Hyperplasia

Rarely, patients who have received radiation or chemotherapy, and even some patients without such histories, present with an unusual benign epithelial proliferation on biopsy that can closely mimic invasive urothelial carcinoma.[60,162,163] Cystoscopy may show an ulcerated mucosa. Histologically, these epithelial proliferations are within the lamina propria and consist of small nests of urothelium with variable rounded to irregular, jagged contours creating an infiltrative appearance. The individual urothelial cells may have eosinophilic cytoplasm with a "squamoid" appearance and show some nuclear enlargement with slight variation in nuclear size, but the nuclear chromatin is bland and they do not show significant atypia. A helpful and unique feature of these lesions is that the epithelial nests wrap around blood vessels with associated fibrin and congestion (Fig. 5-41A–D). The fibrin is found both within the wall of the vessels and within the lamina propria. Associated hemorrhage, fibrosis, acute and chronic inflammation, and ulceration are also common, as well as other, radiation-induced changes such as ectatic vessels with intimal proliferation and squamous metaplasia. Rare cases without prior treatment have been thought secondary to ischemia or chronic irritation.[60]

Nephrogenic Adenoma

Nephrogenic adenoma is a benign proliferative lesion occurring in the bladder (80%), urethra (12%), or ureters (8%) that is thought to arise secondary to urothelial injury.[164–166] It is much more common in male adults (approximately 66% men) and is only rarely reported in children.[167,168] Typically, nephrogenic adenoma is an incidental histologic finding, but patients may present with hematuria or voiding symptoms. These lesions are usually small (<1 cm), but have been reported to reach sizes as large as 7 cm. At cystoscopy,

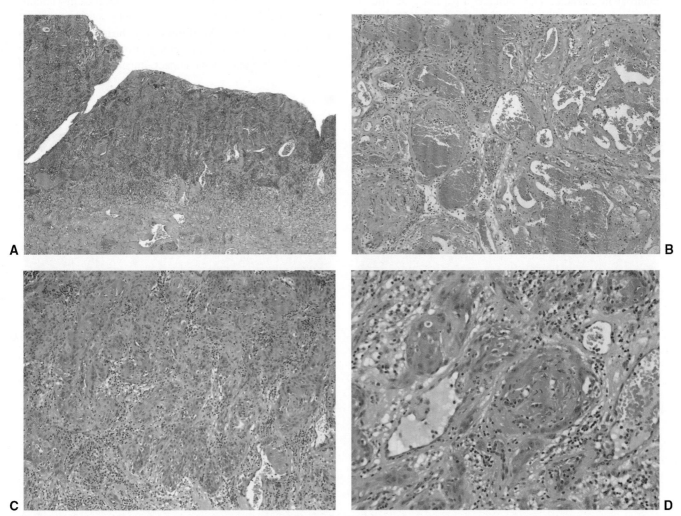

FIGURE 5-41 ■ **A:** In "pseudocarcinomatous" hyperplasia, usually due to prior radiation therapy, a florid epithelial proliferation may be seen. **B:** There is often a background of dilated vessels with fibrinoid change associated with the proliferation. **C:** The nests of epithelium often have a more pronounced cytoplasmic eosinophilia, which may create a squamoid appearance. **D:** One useful diagnostic feature is the intimate association of the epithelium with fibrin aggregates and blood vessels. Characteristically, the epithelium "wraps around" the fibrin.

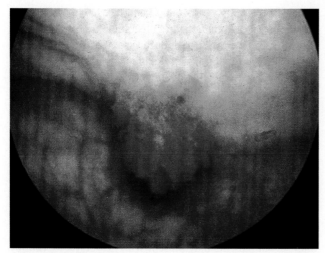

FIGURE 5-42 ■ This single hemorrhagic polypoid lesion on cystoscopy represents a nephrogenic adenoma. This may mimic a neoplastic urothelial process.

nephrogenic adenoma may simulate a papillary, sessile, or in situ carcinoma (Fig. 5-42). Approximately 55% of the lesions are papillary, 10% polypoid, and 35% sessile. They are typically single, but almost 20% are multiple; rarely there is diffuse bladder involvement.

The main importance of recognizing this lesion pathologically is its distinction from papillary urothelial bladder neoplasms, clear cell adenocarcinoma, and prostatic adenocarcinoma. Although a broad histologic spectrum has been reported for nephrogenic adenoma, there are three main growth patterns that are often intermixed and will be discussed separately: tubular, papillary or polypoid, and diffuse (Fig. 5-43A–C).[164–166,169] The individual cells also have a variable morphology; they are typically low cuboidal with scant eosinophilic cytoplasm. They frequently have prominent nucleoli, but, by definition, nephrogenic adenomas do not show marked nuclear atypia or easily identified mitotic activity. Degenerative-type atypia has been described, however, and is characterized by large cells with a hyperchromatic appearance secondary to a smudged, indistinct chromatin pattern. Some uncommon features include cytoplasmic clearing or bulbous apical nuclei producing a hobnail pattern. Recently, a distinct fibromyxoid pattern was also described.[170]

The tubular pattern is most common and consists of well-delineated tubules lined by a single layer of low columnar to cuboidal epithelium occasionally with prominent nucleoli (Fig. 5-43A). Most frequently, the individual tubules are well spaced with intervening stroma (Fig. 5-44), but the tubules may be very compact, imparting a solid, nested

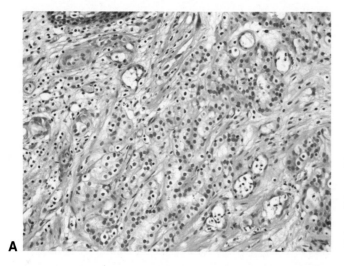

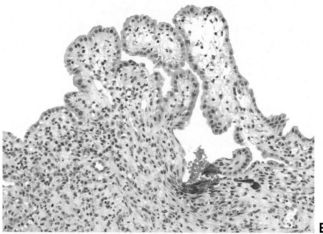

FIGURE 5-43 ■ Nephrogenic adenoma may have a **(A)** tubular, **(B)** papillary or polypoid, or **(C)** diffuse or solid architecture.

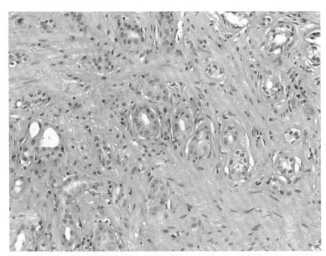

FIGURE 5-44 ■ The tubules in nephrogenic adenoma are typically separated by intervening stroma. In this example, some of the tubules have a subtle peritubular basement membrane–like material.

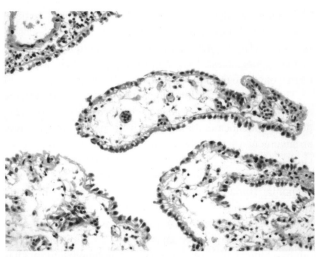

FIGURE 5-46 ■ The papillary excrescences in nephrogenic adenoma are characteristically lined by a single layer of cuboidal epithelium.

appearance focally, and some may also have a branching pattern. The tubules may also become dilated imparting a cystic appearance; in these cystic patterns, the epithelial lining is frequently flattened and attenuated. There is also variable peritubular hyalinization with a basement membrane–like appearance (Fig. 5-44), and intraluminal eosinophilic and basophilic secretions are relatively common. Small compressed tubules with only a single lining cell apparent at the periphery of the lumen may closely resemble a signet-ring cell, but this is usually present only focally (Fig. 5-45). The degenerative-appearing cells described above typically line tubules that are flattened and may resemble blood vessels.

The papillary or polypoid pattern of nephrogenic adenoma is most commonly characterized by large edematous polypoid excrescences, but a relatively simple, filiform branching pattern is also seen in a minority of cases (approximately 10%) (Fig. 5-43B). Complex epithelial budding is

rare and usually focal. The polypoid excrescences and papillae are lined by a single layer of low cuboidal cells with scant eosinophilic cytoplasm (Fig. 5-46). The cytoplasm is occasionally more prominent with an eosinophilic appearance or more cuboidal with pale cytoplasm.

The "diffuse" pattern is quite rare and is almost always admixed with other patterns of nephrogenic adenoma. It is characterized by a very compact or solid growth pattern with little to no intervening stroma (Fig. 5-43C). A cord-like growth pattern somewhat reminiscent of a carcinoid tumor has also been reported. The fibromyxoid pattern is also rare and is characterized by prominent myxoid stroma and scattered, compressed, spindled, or corded epithelial cells (Fig. 5-47).

There are rare reports of extension of nephrogenic adenoma into the superficial muscularis propria and into prostatic stroma. We would recommend extreme caution in making the diagnosis

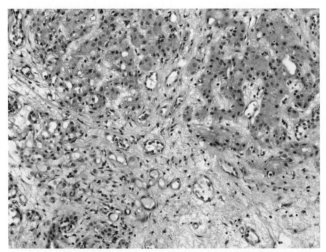

FIGURE 5-45 ■ Some foci of nephrogenic adenoma contain minute tubules with a single lining cell and intraluminal basophilic material that may mimic a signet-ring cell.

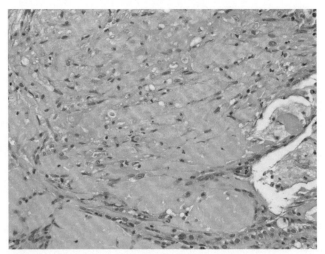

FIGURE 5-47 ■ The fibromyxoid pattern of nephrogenic adenoma is characterized by cords of epithelial cells set in a myxoid to densely collagenized background stroma.

of nephrogenic adenoma with muscularis propria involvement; a "deceptively bland" pattern of urothelial carcinoma, such as nested, tubular, or microcystic, should be carefully considered in that setting. Nested carcinomas typically show a greater degree of cytologic atypia in areas of deep invasion.

The main differential diagnostic consideration for the tubular pattern is primary adenocarcinoma or extension from prostatic adenocarcinoma. The well-spaced architectural arrangement of the tubules, the peritubular hyalinization, epithelial flattening with cystic change, and mixed papillary/polypoid patterns should aid in the diagnosis of nephrogenic adenoma. Immunohistochemistry may be misleading and can cause confusion with prostate cancer; weak cytoplasmic immunoreactivity with PSA or PSAP is reported in up to half of nephrogenic adenomas.[164–166,169] In addition, P504S (alpha-methylacyl-CoA racemase) immunoreactivity has also been documented in nephrogenic adenoma and should, therefore, not be used as a distinguishing marker for prostatic adenocarcinoma in this setting.[171] Nuclear PAX2 and PAX8 reactivity is present in nephrogenic adenoma, but has not been reported in prostatic adenocarcinoma (Fig. 5-48).[170,172,173]

The main differential diagnosis for papillary or polypoid nephrogenic adenoma is a low-grade papillary urothelial neoplasm. In general, papillary urothelial neoplasms have a stratified lining consisting of multiple cell layers. In addition, the individual neoplastic cells of urothelial tumors have more elongated cells, often with nuclear grooves. Higher-grade urothelial carcinomas have nuclear pleomorphism, nuclear hyperchromasia, and increased mitotic activity, making their distinction straightforward. Identification of a mixed tubular pattern in a nephrogenic adenoma may also be helpful in this differential diagnostic setting (see Box 5-3).

The diagnosis of clear cell adenocarcinoma of the bladder may be considered when there is a mixed papillary and tubulocystic pattern. Clear cell carcinomas, however, typically have marked nuclear pleomorphism, obviously increased

mitotic activity, more cellular stratification, and more prominent cytoplasmic clearing. Conspicuous clear cells are uncommon in nephrogenic adenoma. Some authors have suggested the utility of p53 stains in this differential setting (nuclear reactivity in adenocarcinoma), but routine morphologic features will usually suffice.[174] PAX2 and PAX8 are not useful as they are expressed in both nephrogenic adenoma and clear cell carcinoma.[172,173]

There is continuing debate regarding the etiology of nephrogenic adenoma. While there is a strong association with inflammatory insults due to a variety of factors including intravesical chemotherapy,[175,176] transurethral surgical biopsy,[177] diverticula,[178] vesical infection,[179] ibuprofen abuse,[180] and various types of cystitis, an origin from renal epithelial cells has long been postulated. The latter theory has been supported by some studies showing nephrogenic adenoma origin from donor renal tubule cells in renal transplant patients.[181]

POLYPS, CYSTS, AND OTHER PSEUDOTUMOROUS LESIONS

Fibroepithelial Polyp

These rare bladder lesions occur at all ages. They are much more common in the ureter and renal pelvis.[182–184] In children, they are the most common benign bladder lesion. Morphologically, they are characterized by large bulbous polypoid excrescences covered by urothelium (Fig. 5-49).

Box 5-3 ● NONNEOPLASTIC POLYPOID/ PAPILLARY LESIONS OF URINARY BLADDER

Papillary/polypoid cystitis
  Typically result of injury (e.g., indwelling catheter)
  Papillae have broad base, but become progressively more slender to tip.
  No complex hierarchical branching (as expected in urothelial neoplasia)
  Lining may show reactive urothelial atypia.
Nephrogenic adenoma
  Variety of architectural patterns
    Papillae lined by a single layer of cuboidal epithelial cells
    Underlying pattern in lamina propria may be solid, small tubular, or cystic.
    Tubules may be surrounded by dense basement membrane.
    Express PAX8 by immunohistochemistry
Prostatic-type polyp
  Usually <1 cm
  Lined by prostatic secretory-type cells admixed with urothelial cells
Fibroepithelial polyp
  Mostly males, first decade
  <4 cm
  Club-like projections most common pattern
  Lined by normal urothelium

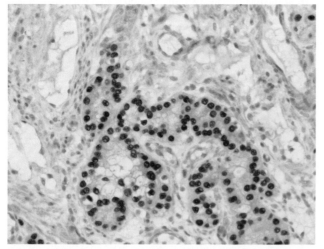

FIGURE 5-48 ■ The lesional cells in nephrogenic adenoma typically show strong nuclear reactivity with PAX2 and PAX8. To date, all evaluated prostate cancers have been negative with these markers.

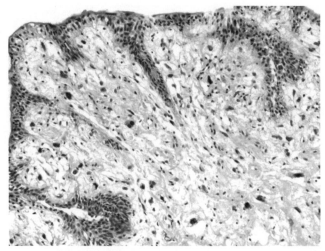

FIGURE 5-49 ■ Fibroepithelial polyps have a polypoid growth lined by benign urothelium or metaplastic squamous epithelium with underlying collagenous stroma. Similar to lesions in other anatomic locations, the stroma may contain "atypical" cells with multinucleation.

The cores show loose, edematous stroma with scattered blood vessels. One unusual case had atypical stromal cells similar to those seen in fibroepithelial polyps of the lower female genital tract, and myxoid stroma with associated cystitis cystica has been described.[184] The polypoid appearance may suggest the possible diagnosis of botryoid rhabdomyosarcoma on microscopic examination; however, the absence of a cambium layer, rhabdomyoblasts, and myogenin reactivity helps establish the diagnosis.

Prostatic-Type Polyp (Ectopic Prostate)

Ectopic prostate tissue presenting as a polypoid mass lesion in the bladder, usually the trigone, has been reported.[185] The morphologic appearance is identical to that described for

benign prostatic urethral polyps. The submucosal component consists of admixed stroma and histologically benign prostate glands. The overlying surface is often papillary with a lining consisting of prostatic secretory epithelium, urothelium, or an admixture of both (Fig. 5-50A and B). Identification of the prostatic secretory epithelial component usually allows distinction from a papillary urothelial neoplasm. Immunohistochemistry for PSA and PSAP highlights the prostatic secretory cells and is helpful in difficult cases.

Collagen Polyp or "Collagenoma"

Patients may receive collagen injections into the urethral or bladder wall as part of the management of urinary stress incontinence or in the creation of urinary pouches from intestinal segments. After therapeutic failures, surgical specimens may be received with subsequent surgical reconstruction. In these specimens, submucosal polyps have been described that result from collagen accumulation.[186] Rarely, clinically detectable mass lesions resulting from collagen accumulation are reported.[187] Histologically, the polyps or masses show a submucosal accumulation of collagen that is comprised of a dense homogeneous eosinophilic, acellular material. The material is typically positive by periodic acid–Schiff reaction and strongly positive by trichrome stain.

Tamm-Horsfall Protein

Although it is much more commonly identified in the kidney or within renal hilar lymph nodes, the accumulation of Tamm-Horsfall protein may occasionally produce a lesion in the urinary bladder.[188,189] One group has studied a series of over 250 consecutive bladder specimens and found incidental Tamm-Horsfall protein in 6.9% of cases, confirmed by the anti-THP antibody. This finding appears to be more common in cystectomy specimens. Histologically, there are two

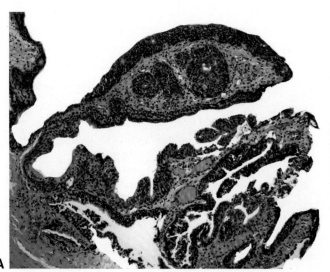
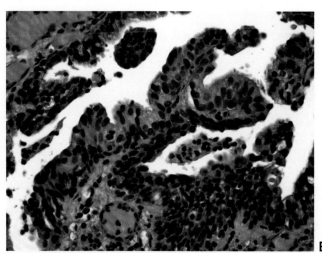

FIGURE 5-50 ■ **A:** Benign prostatic-type polyps (ectopic prostate) present as exophytic papillary projections into the bladder lumen. **B:** On high-power examination, the presence of prostate-type secretory cells admixed with the urothelium is diagnostic.

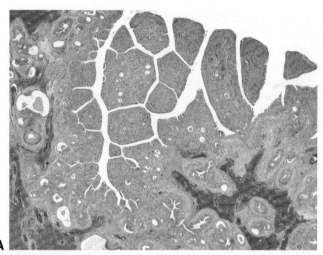
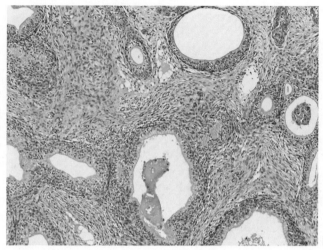

FIGURE 5-51 ■ **A:** Hamartomas of the bladder have a polypoid architecture and **(B)** consist of an admixture of epithelium resembling cystitis glandularis with a variably cellular stroma.

patterns: (a) classic large aggregates of "waxy" eosinophilic or pale extracellular material with a variable minor admixture of fibroblasts, inflammatory cells, and granulation tissue or (b) inconspicuous small, homogeneous eosinophilic "flecks" or interconnecting eosinophilic strands in areas of fibrinous exudate, necrosis, or ulcer. Aggregates of Tamm-Horsfall protein are incidental morphologic findings of no clinical significance.

Hamartoma

Hamartomas of the bladder have typically been polypoid and composed microscopically of foci resembling von Brunn nests, cystitis glandularis, or cystitis cystica dispersed irregularly in a stroma, which has varied from muscular to fibrous or edematous (Fig. 5-51A and B).[190–195] One reported case had a markedly cellular stroma, particularly around the glandular component, suggesting the possible diagnosis of

a low-grade neoplasm[190]; however, current evidence points toward a nonneoplastic nature for these rare lesions.

Amyloidosis

The bladder may be involved by amyloidosis, either as a primary process or secondarily with systemic amyloidosis.[196–199] The initial urinary presentation is hematuria, which may be severe. Although secondary amyloidosis is more prevalent, the primary form is more likely to be biopsied because associated bladder symptoms are more common. Cystoscopically, amyloid has the appearance of a neoplasm. The morphologic appearance is identical to that seen elsewhere: deposits of eosinophilic, amorphous extracellular material (Fig. 5-52A and B). The amyloid is typically present in the lamina propria, but vascular involvement is also seen. Amyloid involving blood vessels should be distinguished from the hyalinized blood vessels occasionally seen in the

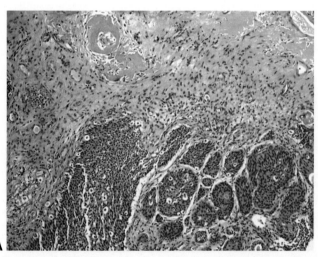
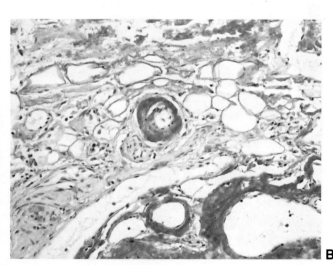

FIGURE 5-52 ■ **A:** The dense deposits of amorphous eosinophilic material characteristic of amyloid are present within the walls of multiple blood vessels in this bladder biopsy. **B:** On Congo red stain, the amyloid is brightly orangeophilic.

cores of papillary urothelial carcinomas. Congo red stains, thioflavin T fluorescence, or electron microscopy may be used for diagnostic confirmation. Primary localized amyloidosis of the bladder is usually AL type (immunoglobulin light chains).[197,200] Some studies have shown that patients with rare forms of hereditary amyloidosis, such as familial amyloidotic polyneuropathy, frequently present with lower urinary dysfunction (up to 50% of patients).[201] Therapy is usually guided by the cause of the amyloid deposition, but surgery may be required to control bleeding in severe cases.

MÜLLERIAN LESIONS

Endometriosis

Although the urinary bladder is the most common site of endometriosis in the genitourinary tract, it occurs in <2% of all patients with endometriosis. Many cases of bladder involvement are associated with prior surgery, such as cesarean section. Endometriosis may present as a mass lesion in the urinary bladder (approximately 50%) or may be an incidental microscopic finding. Rarely, bladder symptoms that exacerbate at the time of menstruation suggest the diagnosis, but otherwise there are no specific symptoms.[202] When grossly evident, there may be a hemorrhagic or blue-tinged mucosal appearance. It most commonly involves serosal surfaces, typically near the vesicouterine pouch, but implants may grow into the muscular wall producing a luminal bulge or, rarely, a polypoid mass.[203,204] Morphologically, the process is identical to that seen in other anatomic sites with admixed benign endometrial glands and stroma (Fig. 5-53).[205] There are a few case reports of vesical endometriosis occurring in men, possibly related to antiandrogen therapy for prostate cancer.[206,207] Rarely, endometriosis of the bladder may be associated with a Müllerian-type malignancy such as clear cell or endometrioid adenocarcinoma.[208–210] Patients

are typically treated with hormonal therapy, but partial cystectomy may be required.[211]

Endocervicosis

Glandular lesions characterized by a prominent component of endocervical-type epithelium involving the wall of the urinary bladder in women of reproductive age are referred to as endocervicosis.[212] Five of the initially reported patients presented with bladder symptoms. In each patient a mass that ranged from 2 to 5 cm was typically located in the posterior wall or posterior dome. Microscopic examination typically reveals extensive involvement of the bladder wall by irregularly dispersed benign-appearing or mildly atypical endocervical-type glands, some of which are cystically dilated (Fig. 5-54). In some cases the glands are associated with fibrosis, edema, or extravasated mucin in the adjacent stroma. Although primarily intramural, mucosal involvement may be seen, including even intraluminal papillae lined by endocervical-type mucinous epithelium. Rarely there is a focal endometriotic stroma indicating a relationship of this lesion to endometriosis. This and other features, such as an occasional association with a history of a cesarean section, suggest that this is a unique müllerian lesion of the bladder and represents the mucinous analogue of endometriosis. Lack of awareness of this entity may lead to a misdiagnosis of adenocarcinoma, but the absence of significant nuclear atypia or an irregular invasive pattern facilitates distinction.

Endosalpingiosis

Rarely, glands within the wall of the bladder may be lined by tubal-type epithelium including ciliated, intercalated, and peg cells (Fig. 5-55A and B).[213,214] Rarely, a striking number of glands may be present, resulting in a mass effect.

Müllerianosis

When benign intramural glandular lesions show a mixture of endocervical, tubal, and endometrial epithelium, the term müllerianosis has been applied.[214]

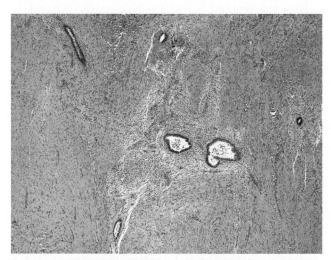

FIGURE 5-53 ■ Endometriosis of the bladder is morphologically similar to that seen in other sites. The mixed endometrial type glands and stroma may be seen within the muscularis propria.

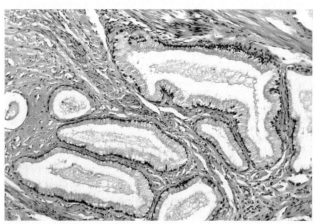

FIGURE 5-54 ■ Endocervicosis is characterized by columnar cells of endocervical mucinous type.

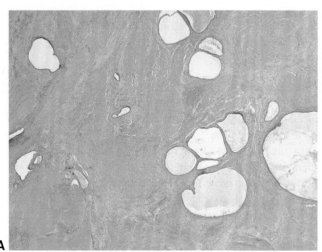
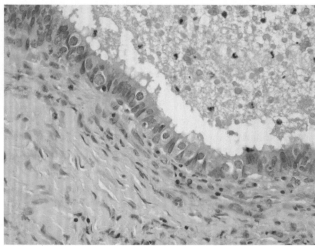

FIGURE **5-55** ■ **A:** The individual glands of endosalpingiosis may be present within the wall of the bladder. **B:** On higher-power evaluation, the tubal nature of the lining cells is seen.

Müllerian Duct Cyst

Müllerian duct cysts may occur in men and lie between the bladder and rectum; they may involve the posterior wall of the bladder.[215–217] Patients typically present with irritative bladder symptoms or identification of a midline supraprostatic mass. The cysts may be unilocular or multilocular and are lined by müllerian-type epithelium, but complete denudation of the cyst lining is not uncommon. Spermatozoa are not present within the lumen, in contrast to a seminal vesicle cyst. Rarely, a müllerian sinus may connect the posterolateral wall of the bladder to the broad ligament.

Fallopian Tube Prolapse

There is one published case in which a patient developed a vesicovaginal fistula 3 months after a total abdominal hysterectomy and was subsequently found to have a polypoid mass at the bladder base.[218] Although the gross lesion was interpreted clinically as papillary carcinoma, microscopic examination showed fragments of fallopian tube plicae.

Fistulas

Fistulous tracts between the urinary bladder and the gastrointestinal tract may occur secondary to diverticular disease, colorectal carcinoma, Crohn disease, or appendicitis.[219,220] Vesicovaginal fistulas are most commonly secondary to prior gynecologic procedures or obstetrical trauma, but other causes include high stage cervical carcinoma, radiation therapy, cerclage, and long-standing foreign body.[221,222] Clinical symptoms with well-developed fistulas include pneumaturia and fecaluria, but initial presentation may be more subtle with only vague urinary symptoms such as dysuria, urgency, and frequency. The cystoscopic appearance may closely mimic papillary urothelial neoplasia because of edema with resultant papillary/polypoid cystitis.[65]

Cystocele and Bladder Prolapse

Cystocele, also referred to as a prolapsed bladder, occurs in women, predominantly in the postmenopausal years. A cystocele is caused by weakening of the musculature between the urinary bladder and the anterior vaginal wall, allowing the bladder to bulge into the vagina. Patients typically present with urinary incontinence or dyspareunia. Cystocele is easily diagnosed by routine pelvic examination. The development of cystocele is often associated with previous vaginal childbirth, but other factors include chronic constipation and heavy lifting. The low estrogen levels after menopause also play a role in laxity of the surrounding connective tissues, which further increases the risk of cystocele development. Patients are usually treated conservatively with pessary, estrogen therapy, activity modification, and pelvic strengthening exercises; however, surgical repair may be needed for patients with severe symptoms refractory to other interventions. Surgical pathology plays little role in the diagnosis/management of cystocele because, in general, tissue is not removed during reparative procedures.

Benign Myofibroblastic Proliferations

Myofibroblastic proliferations of the urinary bladder have been described under a variety of names including postoperative spindle cell nodule, inflammatory pseudotumor, pseudosarcomatous fibromyxoid tumor, pseudosarcomatous myofibroblastic proliferation (PSMP), pseudosarcomatous spindle cell proliferation, and inflammatory myofibroblastic tumor (IMT). Although different names have been applied, these lesions are commonly divided into two categories: those with a prior history of bladder instrumentation and de novo lesions with no predisposing factors. It should be emphasized that, for practical purposes, these two lesions are morphologically indistinguishable in most cases. Although recent publications have begun to combine all myofibroblastic lesions into one category, we maintain the separation by clinical setting for this discussion.

Postoperative Spindle Cell Nodule

This designation was given by Proppe et al.[223] in 1984 to a proliferative spindle cell lesion that developed in the lower urinary tract of five men and the lower genital tract of four women. All of the lesions developed within 3 months after a surgical procedure had been performed at the same site. Two of the lesions in men were in specimens obtained by transurethral resection of the bladder both of whom had had a similar procedure performed 2 months previously. At cystoscopy, "heaped up tumor" and a "friable vegetant mass" were noted.

The low-power appearance/architectural arrangement of the cells is generally compact spindle cells, but foci may be myxoid and rarely there is a sclerotic/hyalinized appearance. The myxoid pattern has a very loose, disorganized appearance similar to that seen in nodular fasciitis. There is often an associated mixed chronic inflammatory infiltrate and an irregular network of poorly organized small blood vessels. The compact spindle cell component is more cellular with a better-developed fascicular architecture. The fascicles are not as tightly formed and do not show the precise, acute intersecting fascicles typical of a sarcoma. Cytologically, the individual cells are spindled to stellate; the ends of the cells are usually tapered with elongated cytoplasmic processes identifiable at high-power examination. The cytoplasm varies from eosinophilic to more amphophilic. The nuclei are also tapered; have bland, noncondensed chromatin; and may show prominent nucleoli (Fig. 5-56). Mitoses may be conspicuous. The lesional cells may extend into the muscularis propria, a feature that should not be regarded as an indication of malignancy (Fig. 5-57).

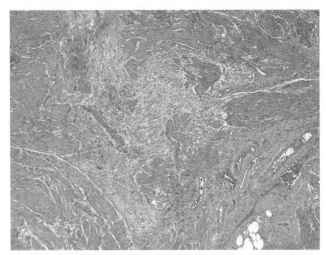

FIGURE 5-57 ■ Myofibroblastic proliferations may extend into the muscularis propria, a feature that should not be regarded as malignant.

By definition, these proliferations occur after trauma, typically following bladder instrumentation. The interval of time between the procedure and the development of a proliferation is typically a few weeks to months. Although postoperative spindle cell nodule is basically morphologically identical to nonprocedure-related myofibroblastic proliferations of the bladder, they are usually small and rarely exceed 1 cm. The differential diagnosis is discussed under PSMP, as the same issues apply to both.

Pseudosarcomatous Myofibroblastic Proliferation (Inflammatory Pseudotumor)

Individual cases of nontrauma-related, de novo myofibroblastic proliferations of the urinary bladder are indistinguishable from postoperative spindle cell nodules; however, overall they are typically more myxoid, reach a larger size (e.g., usually 2 to 8 cm, but over 30 cm reported) (Fig. 5-58), and

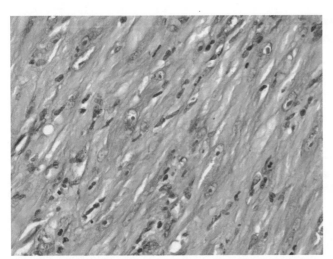

FIGURE 5-56 ■ The myofibroblastic cells show the elongated cytoplasmic processes and nuclei typical of myofibroblasts, but there may be some degree of variation in the size of the cells and nucleoli may be prominent. Despite these features, the chromatin distribution remains even.

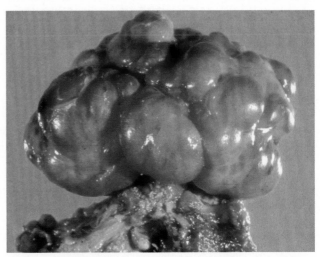

FIGURE 5-58 ■ This gross specimen from a resection of PSMP shows an exophytic mass projecting into the bladder lumen.

may have somewhat more variation in the size of the cells. By the original definition, they are not related to trauma or an overlying urothelial carcinoma. Recent studies of vesical PSMP have documented both ALK 1 (anaplastic lymphoma kinase) expression by immunohistochemistry and ALK gene rearrangements by FISH analysis, findings typical of IMT in other anatomic sites.[224–228] The reported incidence of ALK 1 expression is quite variable and ranges from 8% to 89% of cases. Freeman et al.[224] confirmed ALK gene rearrangement by FISH in four of six cases demonstrating ALK immunoreactivity. ALK expression is not entirely specific for IMT and is reported in other mesenchymal neoplasms (e.g., up to 20% of rhabdomyosarcomas).[229]

The recurrence rate for PSMP in the urinary bladder has ranged from 0% to 19%, and no metastases have been reported. One patient death has been reported from urinary obstruction due to local mass effect of an unresected vesical PSMP.[230]

There is controversy regarding diagnostic terminology for these lesions, which can be confirmed by a survey of the nomenclature employed in current textbooks. Some authors suggest that vesical myofibroblastic proliferations are distinct from IMT. Whether the presence or absence of ALK reactivity has any clinical significance or defines subsets of myofibroblastic lesions in the bladder remains to be determined. Under current clinical management standards, however, this is mostly a semantic argument because histologically benign-appearing proliferations are followed clinically after a simple excision procedure. The clinically relevant decision is their distinction from malignant spindle cell lesions (e.g., leiomyosarcoma or sarcomatoid carcinoma) in which a more radical excision procedure is indicated.

Most diagnostic difficulties are related to the morphologic overlap with leiomyosarcoma and sarcomatoid carcinoma; the distinction is based predominantly on cytologic features. Although there may be some variation in the size of nuclei in PSMP, the chromatin is evenly distributed giving the nucleus a bland cytologic appearance, often with one or more large nucleoli. Malignant lesions, in contrast, have irregular chromatin with marked hyperchromasia and may focally have obvious nuclear pleomorphism. The associated stroma and the low-power architecture of PSMP may be indistinguishable from a malignant neoplasm. Myxoid stroma is common in PSMP, but may be seen in sarcomatoid carcinoma and leiomyosarcoma.[231] Both types of malignant tumors may have areas with a loose, hypocellular arrangement or more cellular fascicles. All three lesions commonly infiltrate the muscularis propria, have increased mitotic activity, and show necrosis superficially making these unreliable distinguishing features.

Other morphologic features that are reportedly more common in malignant neoplasms include necrosis at the tumor/muscularis propria interface, acute inflammation, and lack of prominent blood vessels. Deep necrosis (at the tumor/muscularis propria interface) has been reported as a specific histologic feature of malignancy,[230] but this has been questioned in more recent series.[225]

The immunohistochemical profiles of all three lesions are compared in Table 5-3 (Fig. 5-59A–C). Carcinomas express high molecular weight cytokeratin, cytokeratin 5/6, and p63, while PSMP and leiomyosarcoma are negative.[232] Keratin expression in both PSMP and leiomyosarcoma is generally seen with only low molecular weight types. Strong and diffuse desmin and actin reactivity generally supports the diagnosis of leiomyosarcoma, as long as heterologous differentiation in a sarcomatoid carcinoma is excluded. PSMP also expresses smooth muscle actin, but does not typically express desmin.

Table 5-3 ■ IMMUNOHISTOCHEMISTRY IN SPINDLE CELL LESIONS

	Smooth Muscle	Skeletal Muscle	Myofibroblastic	Epithelial
Cytokeratin (broad spectrum)	• May be positive (cytoplasmic)	• Negative	• May be positive (cytoplasmic with membranous accentuation)	• Positive (cytoplasmic), may be focal
Cytokeratin (high molecular weight)	• Negative	• Negative	• Negative	• Positive (cytoplasmic), may be focal
Smooth muscle actin	• Positive (cytoplasmic)	• Positive (cytoplasmic)	• Positive (cytoplasmic)	• Negative
Desmin	• Positive (cytoplasmic)	• Positive (cytoplasmic)	• Typically negative	• Negative
Caldesmon	• Positive (cytoplasmic)	• Positive (cytoplasmic)	• May be positive (cytoplasmic)	• Negative
Myogenin	• Negative	• Strong nuclear immunoreactivity	• Negative	• Negative
Smoothelin	• May be positive (cytoplasmic)	• Negative	• Negative	• Negative
ALK-1	• Negative	• May be positive	• Variable immunoreactivity reported	• Negative

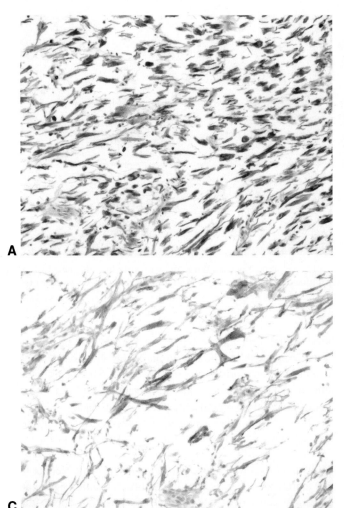

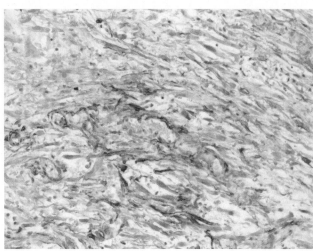

FIGURE 5-59 ■ Pseudosarcomatous myofibroblastic proliferations are often immunoreactive for **(A)** pancytokeratin, **(B)** smooth muscle actin, and **(C)** ALK-1.

NEOBLADDER

Patients undergoing radical cystectomy have varying options for urinary diversion, but one common technique is the creation of an orthotopic neobladder, which allows patients to void without the need for an external urine reservoir (i.e., continent urinary diversion).[233] In this procedure, a segment of small intestine is resected, opened, and constructed into a pouch. The ureters are connected to the superior aspect of the pouch, while the inferior aspect is connected to the urethra. The distal urethral sphincter muscles are preserved to maintain continence.

Invasive and in situ urothelial carcinoma may recur in the neobladder after surgery for urinary bladder cancer; therefore, endoscopic biopsies may be performed in some settings. For these reasons, it is important for pathologists to be aware of the spectrum of benign changes that may be seen in neobladder mucosa. Since the pouch is formed from small bowel, the mucosa is expectedly of intestinal type with goblet cells; this should not be regarded as "intestinal metaplasia." Histologic changes in the mucosa occur gradually over time, but are quite variable.[234] The intestinal villi become shorter with urine exposure and may progress to show areas with complete atrophy; however, this change is topographically uneven, and some foci may have a preserved villous architecture even after many years (Fig. 5-60A).[235–239] There is also variable increase in lamina propria lymphocytes with some lymphoid nodules and associated edema (Fig. 5-60B). Fibrosis of the submucosa has also been reported. In addition, the epithelial cells may vary with areas of increased goblet cells to foci with mainly enterocytes, especially in regions of flat mucosa. At an ultrastructural level, microvilli are also decreased.[239] There are rare reports of primary intestinal-type dysplasia and adenocarcinomas arising within a neobladder,[240] but this seems to be a rare occurrence.[236,237] In our experience, it is much more common for benign changes in a neobladder to be confused for dysplasia, than to encounter a true neoplastic precursor lesion.

URACHUS

Embryology and Anatomy

In early embryonic life, the allantois projects outward from the yolk sac into the body stalk, which is the structure that later forms the umbilical cord. The allantois originates from a portion of the yolk sac that subsequently gives rise

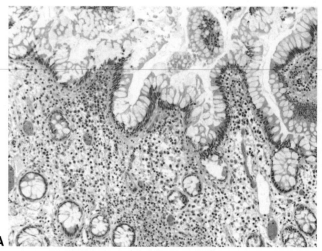
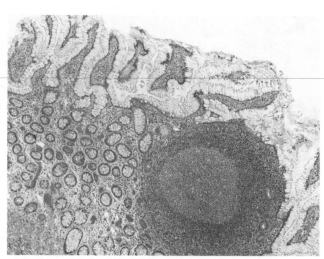

FIGURE 5-60 ■ **A:** Cystoscopic biopsies from neobladders show small bowel–type mucosa, frequently with atrophic villi. This feature varies considerably from region to region and with time. **B:** There is often a mixed chronic inflammatory infiltrate that includes well-formed lymphoid follicles.

to the cloacal portion of the hindgut. The allantois remains connected to the apex of the bladder as the urinary bladder differentiates from the cloaca.[241] The urachus is the intraabdominal structure that contains the allantois and connects the apex of the urinary bladder to the body wall at the umbilicus. The relative embryologic contributions of the allantois and the cloaca to the development of the urachus have been debated and are still not fully known.[242–244] With growth of the embryo, the urachus also grows and lengthens to maintain its connection with the bladder dome and body stalk. By the beginning of the 6th month, the urachus has become an elongate structure little more than a millimeter in diameter. At birth, the dome of the bladder and the umbilicus are in close proximity. At this developmental phase, the urachus is only 2.5 to 3 mm in length with a diameter of 1 mm throughout most of its course; however, it expands to 3 mm as it joins the bladder.[243] In comparison, the neighboring umbilical arteries are 5 to 7 mm in diameter, and the umbilical vein is 10 mm in diameter. At its superior end, the urachus commonly divides into three separate fibrous strands. Two of these fibrous strands attach to the adventitia of the umbilical arteries, but the middle one passes through the body wall into the umbilical cord. Within the cord, it breaks up into a number of fine fibrous strands, the last remnants of the allantois, about 10 mm from the surface of the body.[243]

The urachus lies in a space between the anterior abdominal wall and the peritoneum. It is bounded anteriorly and posteriorly by the umbilicovesical fascia and laterally by the two umbilical arteries, which are surrounded by umbilicovesical fascia. Inferiorly, the umbilicovesical fascial layers spread out over the surface of the dome of the bladder. These fascial planes separate a roughly pyramidal anatomic space, termed the space of Retzius, from the peritoneum and other structures. This anatomic space contains adipose tissue, which allows for filling and expansion of the bladder. As the apex of the urinary bladder descends into the pelvis with continued growth after birth, the urachus and obliterated umbilical arteries descend with it. The adventitia of the umbilical arteries is attached superiorly to the fibrous tissue, which closes the umbilical fascial tunnel, and this adventitia fans out into a complex of fibrous strands, the plexus of Luschka.

Based on the relationship of the urachus to the umbilical arteries, four anatomic variants were recognized by Hammond et al.[245] in adults and children (Fig. 5-61). In type I, the urachus is well defined and extends from the bladder to the umbilicus, separate from the umbilical arteries. The type II variant consists of union of the urachus with one of the umbilical arteries and their joint continuation to the umbilicus. When the urachus and both umbilical arteries join and continue to the umbilicus as a cord, the ligamentum commune, the variant is type III. Type IV occurs when the urachus and both umbilical arteries merge into a tangle of strands (the plexus of Luschka), which extends from the point of merging above the bladder to the umbilicus.

Hammond et al.[245] found type I in 7 of 20 adult specimens, type II in 4 of 20, type III in 4 of 20, and type IV in 5 of 20 adult specimens. In a study of 81 specimens, Blichert-Toft et al.[246] found 7 of type I (2 adults, 1 child, and 4 stillborn infants), 10 of type II, 20 of type III, and 44 of type IV. Since the bladder had not yet descended into the pelvis in the four stillborns, it would be expected that all are of type I (the fetal type). Both these classic studies demonstrate that the fetal type of anatomy may persist into adulthood, but they report different prevalence rates of that variant.

In the adult, the urachus outside the urinary bladder wall has a wide range in length with reports from 2 to 15 cm, but it most commonly ranges from 5 to 5.5 cm in length.[243,246] At its junction with the urinary bladder, the width of the urachus most often ranges from 4 to 8 mm and tapers to about 2 mm at its superior end.[246] For descriptive purposes, it is convenient to divide the urachus into three parts: supravesical, intramural, and intramucosal. When

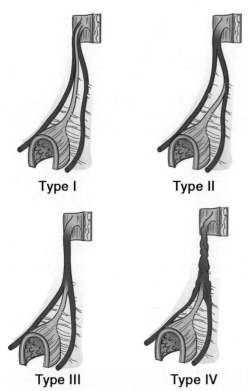

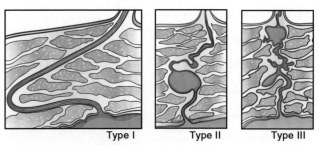

FIGURE 5-62 ■ Common patterns of the urachus within the muscularis propria of the urinary bladder. Type I: a smooth tubular canal. Type II: a canal with an irregular course and a few saccular dilatations. Type III: a canal with a markedly irregular course and multiple outpouchings and saccular dilatations.

FIGURE 5-61 ■ Common variants of urachal anatomy as described by Hammond et al. Type I: The urachus extends from the bladder to the umbilicus, separate from the umbilical arteries. This is also called the fetal type. Type II: The urachus joins with one of the umbilical arteries, and they continue together to the umbilicus. Type III: The urachus and two umbilical arteries join together above the bladder and continue together to the umbilicus. Type IV: The urachus and both umbilical arteries merge into a tangle of strands (the plexus of Luschka), which extends from the point of merging above the bladder to the umbilicus.

in most cases and that there was a small fold of mucosa, which covered the opening and prevented the efflux of urine into the urachus, which has been referred to as the "valve of Wutz." The existence of this valve has been the subject of much controversy. Begg described only one example of this structure in his series of dissections and Hammond et al. reported none.[243,245] Bucchiere[249] concluded that the valve does exist, but that it is particularly difficult to demonstrate in fixed specimens. Begg described the presence of a delicate orifice in one-third of his specimens; however, in the remaining two-thirds, microscopic sections did not demonstrate an orifice. Hammond et al.[245] reported an identifiable orifice in only 10% of their specimens.

there is no communication with the bladder lumen, only the intramural and supravesical portions are present. Tubular urachal remnants lined by epithelium are not uncommon and reportedly present within the wall of the urinary bladder in approximately one-third of the adult population. These intramural remnants are evenly distributed between men and women.[247] Schubert et al. classified the architecture of the intramural urachal canals into three types, ranging from simple tubular canals to more complex passages: Type I has a simple tubular canal, type II consists of a canal with a slightly irregular course and one or more saccular dilatations, and type III consists of a canal with a very irregular course and numerous blind outpockets and saccular dilatations (Fig. 5-62).

The mucosal portion of the urachus also has anatomic variation (Fig. 5-63). It may consist of a wide diverticular opening, a papilla, or a small opening flush with the mucosal surface. In some patients, the urachus does not open into the bladder lumen and is covered by the urinary bladder mucosa, which may be even with the adjacent mucosal surface or have a slight indentation or "dimple." Wutz[248] considered that an opening into the bladder lumen existed

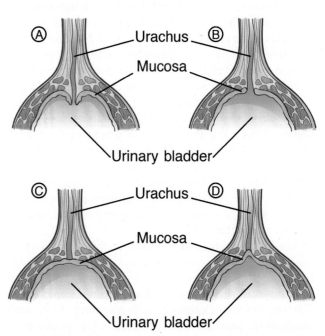

FIGURE 5-63 ■ Common patterns of the intramucosal segment of the urachus. **A:** Patent lumen with wide opening that invaginates into the bladder lumen (i.e., termination in a papilla); **(B)** patent lumen with a small smooth opening flush with the mucosal surface; **(C)** no luminal connection with smooth bladder mucosa; and **(D)** no luminal connection with small invagination of bladder mucosa (a "dimple").

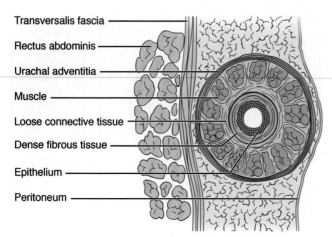

FIGURE 5-64 ■ The microscopic anatomy of the urachus.

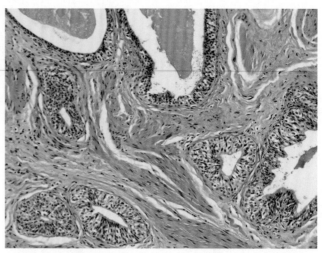

FIGURE 5-65 ■ Urachal remnants are most commonly lined by a urothelial layer.

Histology

Microscopically, the urachus consists of a central lumen surrounded by an epithelial lining, which is invested by multiple layers of connective tissue that include (from the lumen outward): (a) a subepithelial coat of dense fibrous tissue, (b) a layer of loose fibrous tissue, (c) an array of bundles of smooth muscle, and (d) an outer adventitia of connective tissue (Fig. 5-64).[243] All of these elements of the urachus are located between the transversalis fascia and the peritoneum. At least some epithelium frequently persists into adulthood.[243,246,247] It is reported that the distribution of persistent urachal epithelium varies with the anatomic type of urachus (i.e., Hammond types I to IV). Blichert-Toft et al. found that persistent epithelium was present in six of seven examples of the type I anatomic variant and that it extended at least half the distance to the umbilicus. In three cases, epithelium extended all the way to the level of the umbilicus.[246] In contrast, only 16 of 44 examples of the type IV variant (36%) had persistent epithelium. In most of those cases, the epithelium was limited to the region of the apex/dome of the urinary bladder. The normal urachus is not always a smooth tube, and it often has small buds or ramifications branching from it in the wall of the urinary bladder and in the supravesical segment.[243,247] Patients presenting with symptoms from urachal remnants typically have epithelium present, but the absence of symptoms does not necessarily correlate with an absence of epithelium.[250]

The histologic type of persistent epithelium also varies considerably. While most examples consist of urothelium (Fig. 5-65), a columnar intestinal-type lining with goblet cells may also be seen as well as squamous epithelium. The simple layer of columnar cells may rarely form small intraluminal papillary excrescences.[247] The presence of intestinal-type goblet epithelial cells in the urachus may not represent a metaplastic process given that they have been identified in the urachus of a newborn.[251] As would be expected, there are immunohistochemical staining differences in the varying types of epithelium found within the urachus. Urothelium within the urachus stains as typical urothelium, while glandular epithelium often shows an intestinal phenotype.[252]

MALFORMATIONS

Patent Urachus

The first observation of urachal disease is generally attributed to Bartolomeo Cabriolus, whose 1550 *Alphabet Anatomique* contained a description of a patient with a patent urachus. The patent urachus has been classified into five types (Fig. 5-66), which are defined as complete or incomplete. In its complete form, patent urachus is a dramatically symptomatic lesion in which urine drains from the umbilical stump or umbilicus.[241,249,253] These reviews found a preponderance of males to females (2:1) and an age range from neonatal to old age. Often, the umbilicus was swollen and inflamed. Although most of the patients had no other detectable developmental anomaly, Lattimer[254] found that 50% of the 22 children who had congenital deficiency of the abdominal musculature ("prune-belly syndrome") also had a patent urachus. The etiology of patent urachus has been debated. Based on the associations with hydronephrosis, hydroureter, and dilation of the bladder in these children, Lattimer[254] argued that elevated pressure may lead to a failure of urachal closure. Others have argued that increased pressure is not an adequate explanation and suggest failure of the urachus to develop normally, errors in timing of the developmental sequences, or malformations of the urinary bladder resulting in its apex remaining near the umbilicus.[243,255]

The incomplete forms of patent urachus, as proposed by Vaughan[256] in 1905, are umbilicourachal sinus, vesicourachal sinus or diverticulum, and the blind variant in which the urachus is closed at both ends but remains patent in between. In 1961, Hinman[257] added the alternating urachal sinus to the classification in order to account for adults without histories of urinary drainage from the umbilicus in whom urachal

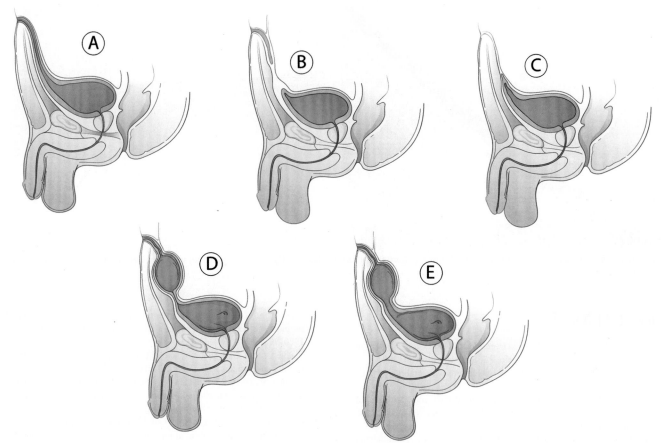

FIGURE 5-66 ■ Variants of patent urachus. **A:** Completely patent urachus. **B:** Umbilicourachal sinus. **C:** Vesicourachal sinus or vesicourachal diverticulum. **D:** Blindly patent urachus. **E:** Alternating urachal sinus.

infections drained both through the umbilicus and the bladder. He distinguished this from complete patent urachus, in which the lumen from bladder to umbilicus is patent at birth, and concluded that in the alternating sinus the lumen was a potential one in which cellular debris accumulated and formed a focus for infection.

Rarely, calculi are formed within the cavities of urachal malformations.[256,258,259] These stones are often similar in salt composition to those more commonly found in the urinary bladder.

Urachal Cysts

Urachal cysts may occur at any level in the urachus and range from small incidental findings to large symptomatic lesions. Smaller cysts commonly are lined with urothelium or cuboidal cells (Fig. 5-67A). However, columnar epithelium may also form the lining. Larger cysts are usually lined by flattened, attenuated epithelium (Fig. 5-67B).

Infections

Bacterial infections of the urachus most often occur in the presence of a urachal malformation or cyst.[260] Purulent bacterial infections are reported in association with a variety of malformations including umbilicourachal sinus, vesicourachal sinus, blind urachus or cyst, and alternating urachal sinus.[241,261–266] These infections often develop into abscesses and may drain spontaneously through the umbilicus or into the bladder. In advanced infections, rupture through the peritoneum may occur and is a serious complication. When the abscess is large and advanced, it may be difficult to determine the exact nature of the associated urachal anomaly and may clinically mimic a primary bladder cancer with extensive extravesical invasion.[267] Treatment with antibiotics followed by prompt surgical removal of the infected cyst has been shown to be effective therapy.[268] Tuberculous, echinococcal, actinomycotic, and tineal infections have been reported to involve the urachus, but these etiologies appear to be rare.[169,249,269–271] The fetal, or type I, anatomical variant of urachal structure reportedly predisposes patients to pilonidal disease and granulomas. Steck and Helwig reported that 40 of 82 patients with type I anatomic variant had chronic granulomatous omphalitis, and 13 of these 40 also had umbilical pilonidal disease. It was argued that this predisposition is due to a urachal attachment that produces umbilical dimples of greater depth than normal.[272] Xanthogranulomatous inflammation has also been reported in association with urachal malformations.[273]

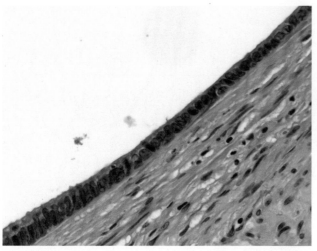
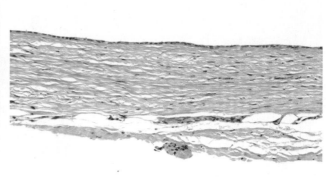

FIGURE 5-67 ■ **A:** This urachal cyst shows a cuboidal lining epithelium, **(B)** but many have an atrophic epithelial layer.

REFERENCES

1. Moore KL, Persaud TVN. *The Developing Human: Clinically Oriented Embryology*. 8th ed. Philadelphia, PA: Saunders/Elsevier; 2007.
2. Shapiro E. Clinical implications of genitourinary embryology. *Curr Opin Urol* 2009;19:427–433.
3. Brooks JD. Anatomy of the lower urinary tract and male genitalia. In: Wein AJ, et al., eds. *Campbell-Walsh Urology*. Philadelphia, PA: Saunders/Elsevier; 2007:38–77.
4. Moore KL, Dalley AF. *Clinically Oriented Anatomy*. 4th ed. Philadelphia, PA: Lippincott Williams and Wilkins; 1999.
5. Fawcett DW. *Bloom and Fawcett: A Textbook of Histology*. 11th ed. Philadelphia, PA: WB Saunders; 1986.
6. Reuter VR. Urinary bladder, ureter, and renal pelvis. In: Mills SE, ed. *Histology for Pathologists*. Philadelphia, PA: Lippincott Williams & Wilkins; 2007:909–922.
7. Epstein JI, et al. The World Health Organization/International Society of Urological Pathology consensus classification of urothelial (transitional cell) neoplasms of the urinary bladder. Bladder Consensus Conference Committee. *Am J Surg Pathol* 1998;22:1435–1448.
8. Wells HG. Giant cells in cystitis. *Arch Pathol Lab Med* 1938;26:32–43.
9. Philip AT, et al. Intravesical adipose tissue: a quantitative study of its presence and location with implications for therapy and prognosis. *Am J Surg Pathol* 2000;24:1286–1290.
10. Ro JY, Ayala AG, el-Naggar A. Muscularis mucosa of urinary bladder. Importance for staging and treatment. *Am J Surg Pathol* 1987;11:668–673.
11. Paner GP, et al. Further characterization of the muscle layers and lamina propria of the urinary bladder by systematic histologic mapping: implications for pathologic staging of invasive urothelial carcinoma. *Am J Surg Pathol* 2007;31:1420–1429.
12. Vakar-Lopez F, et al. Muscularis mucosae of the urinary bladder revisited with emphasis on its hyperplastic patterns: a study of a large series of cystectomy specimens. *Ann Diagn Pathol* 2007;11:395–401.
13. Paner GP, et al. Diagnostic utility of antibody to smoothelin in the distinction of muscularis propria from muscularis mucosae of the urinary bladder: a potential ancillary tool in the pathologic staging of invasive urothelial carcinoma. *Am J Surg Pathol* 2009;33:91–98.
14. Aneiros-Fernandez J, Nicolae A, Preda O. Smoothelin in bladder and gastrointestinal tract again. *Histopathology* 2011;58:1173.
15. Council L, Hameed O. Differential expression of immunohistochemical markers in bladder smooth muscle and myofibroblasts, and the potential utility of desmin, smoothelin, and vimentin in staging of bladder carcinoma. *Mod Pathol* 2009;22:639–650.
16. Hansel DE, et al. Limited smoothelin expression within the muscularis mucosae: validation in bladder diverticula. *Hum Pathol* 2011;42:1770–1776.
17. Maake C, et al. Expression of smoothelin in the normal and the overactive human bladder. *J Urol* 2006;175:1152–1157.
18. Montani M, Thiesler T, Kristiansen G. Smoothelin is a specific and robust marker for distinction of muscularis propria and muscularis mucosae in the gastrointestinal tract. *Histopathology* 2010;57:244–249.
19. Paner GP, et al. Diagnostic use of antibody to smoothelin in the recognition of muscularis propria in transurethral resection of urinary bladder tumor (TURBT) specimens. *Am J Surg Pathol* 2010;34:792–799.
20. Chakravarthy R, et al. In response—a modified staining protocol for smoothelin immunostaining. *Virchows Arch* 2011;459:119–120.
21. Lindh C, et al. Detection of smoothelin expression in the urinary bladder is strongly dependent on pretreatment conditions: a critical analysis with possible consequences for cancer staging. *Virchows Arch* 2011;458:665–670.
22. Miyamoto H, et al. Pitfalls in the use of smoothelin to identify muscularis propria invasion by urothelial carcinoma. *Am J Surg Pathol* 2010;34:418–422.
23. Glenn JF. Agenesis of the bladder. *J Am Med Assoc* 1959;169:2016–2018.
24. Miller HL. Agenesis of the urinary bladder and urethra. *J Urol* 1948;59:1156.
25. Kasat LS, et al. Bladder agenesis with urometrocolpos. *Pediatr Surg Int* 1999;15:415–416.
26. Weight CJ, Chand D, Ross JH. Single system ectopic ureter to rectum subtending solitary kidney and bladder agenesis in newborn male. *Urology* 2006;68:1344 e1–e3.
27. Bhagwat AD, et al. Agenesis of the urinary bladder with cutaneous ectopic ureteric orifice and multiple birth defects. *Pediatr Surg Int* 1997;12:63–65.
28. Karaguzel G, Aslan A, Melikoglu M. An uncommon association relating to cloacal maldevelopment: bladder agenesis, anorectal atresia, and absence of vulva, vagina, and uterus. *J Pediatr Surg* 1999;34:612–614.
29. Stocker JT, Heifetz SA. Sirenomelia. A morphological study of 33 cases and review of the literature. *Perspect Pediatr Pathol* 1987;10:7–50.
30. Perlmutter AD, Retik AB, Bauer SB. Anomalies of the upper urinary tract. In: Walsh PC, et al., eds. *Campbells' Urology*. Philadelphia, PA: Saunders; 1986:1665.
31. Piaseczna Piotrowska A, et al. Interstitial cells of Cajal in the human normal urinary bladder and in the bladder of patients with megacystis-microcolon intestinal hypoperistalsis syndrome. *BJU Int* 2004;94:143–146.

32. Drake M. Interstitial cells of cajal in the human normal urinary bladder and in the bladder of patients with megacystis-microcolon intestinal hypoperistalsis syndrome. *BJU Int* 2004;94:1402.

33. Gastol P, et al. Complete duplication of the bladder, urethra, vagina, and uterus in girls. *Urology* 2000;55:578–581.

34. Abrahamson J. Double bladder and related anomalies: clinical and embryological aspects and a case report. *Br J Urol* 1961;33:195.

35. Lacson A, et al. Renal system. Kidneys and urinary tract. In: Gilbert-Barnes E, ed. *Potter's Pathology of the Fetus, Infant, and Child.* Philadelphia, PA: Elsevier; 2007:1330–1344.

36. Dominguez R, et al. Caudal duplication syndrome. *Am J Dis Child* 1993;147:1048–1052.

37. Harcke HT Jr, et al. Bladder diverticula and Menkes' syndrome. *Radiology* 1977;124:459–461.

38. Morris CA, et al. Adults with Williams syndrome. *Am J Med Genet Suppl* 1990;6:102–107.

39. Breivik N, et al. Ehlers-Danlos syndrome and diverticula of the bladder. *Z Kinderchir* 1985;40:243–246.

40. Faysal MH, Freiha FS. Primary neoplasm in vesical diverticula. A report of 12 cases. *Br J Urol* 1981;53:141–143.

41. Knappenberger ST, Uson AC, Melicow MM. Primary neoplasms occurring in vesical diverticula: a report of 18 cases. *J Urol* 1960;83:153–159.

42. Thomas AA, et al. Urethral diverticula in 90 female patients: a study with emphasis on neoplastic alterations. *J Urol* 2008;180:2463–2467.

43. Ebert AK, et al. The exstrophy-epispadias complex. *Orphanet J Rare Dis* 2009;4:23.

44. Siebert JR, Kapur RP. Back and perineum. In: Gilbert-Barnes E, ed. *Potter's Pathology of the Fetus, Infant and Child.* Philadelphia, PA: Elsevier; 2007:950–951.

45. Culp DA. The Histology of the exstrophied bladder. *J Urol* 1964;91:538–548.

46. Rudin L, Tannenbaum M, Lattimer JK. Histologic analysis of the exstrophied bladder after anatomical closure. *J Urol* 1972;108:802–807.

47. Beare JB, Tormey AR Jr, Wattenberg CA. Exstrophy of the urinary bladder complicated by adenocarcinoma. *J Urol* 1956;76:583–594.

48. Mc Intosh J, Worley G Jr. Adenocarcinoma arising in exstrophy of the bladder: report of two cases and review of the literature. *J Urol* 1955;73:820–829.

49. Semerdjian HS, Texter JH Jr, Yawn DH. Rhabdomyosarcoma occurring in repaired exstrophied bladder: a case report. *J Urol* 1972;108:354–356.

50. Rieder JM, et al. Primary squamous cell carcinoma in unreconstructed exstrophic bladder. *Urology* 2006;67:199.

51. Sahai A, Rosenblatt GS, Parra RO. Squamous cell carcinoma arising in an augmented bladder in a patient with bladder exstrophy. *J Urol* 2004;172:2187–2188.

52. Vik V, Gerharz EW, Woodhouse CR. Invasive carcinoma in bladder exstrophy with transitional, squamous and mucus-producing differentiation. *Br J Urol* 1998;81:173–174.

53. Smeulders N, Woodhouse CR. Neoplasia in adult exstrophy patients. *BJU Int* 2001;87:623–628.

54. Novak TE, et al. Polyps in the exstrophic bladder. A cause for concern? *J Urol* 2005;174:1522–1526; discussion 1526.

55. Nuovo GJ, Nagler HM, Fenoglio JJ Jr. Arteriovenous malformation of the bladder presenting as gross hematuria. *Hum Pathol* 1986;17:94–97.

56. Shekarriz B, et al. Massive hematuria in adults with Klippel-Trenaunay syndrome associated with vascular malformation of the bladder. *Urol Int* 2000;64:226–228.

57. Tavora F, Montgomery E, Epstein JI. A series of vascular tumors and tumorlike lesions of the bladder. *Am J Surg Pathol* 2008;32:1213–1219.

58. Furness PD III, et al. Klippel-Trenaunay syndrome: 2 case reports and a review of genitourinary manifestations. *J Urol* 2001;166:1418–1420.

59. Husmann DA, Rathbun SR, Driscoll DJ. Klippel-Trenaunay syndrome: incidence and treatment of genitourinary sequelae. *J Urol* 2007;177:1244–1249.

60. Lane Z, Epstein JI. Pseudocarcinomatous epithelial hyperplasia in the bladder unassociated with prior irradiation or chemotherapy. *Am J Surg Pathol* 2008;32:92–97.

61. Sukov WR, et al. Perivascular epithelioid cell tumor (PEComa) of the urinary bladder: report of 3 cases and review of the literature. *Am J Surg Pathol* 2009;33:304–308.

62. Yucel S, et al. Hypospadias and anorectal malformations mediated by Eph/ephrin signaling. *J Pediatr Urol* 2007;3:354–363.

63. Matsui F, et al. Bladder function after total urogenital mobilization for persistent cloaca. *J Urol* 2009;182:2455–2459.

64. McKenney JK, et al. Discriminatory immunohistochemical staining of urothelial carcinoma in situ and non-neoplastic urothelium: an analysis of cytokeratin 20, p53, and CD44 antigens. *Am J Surg Pathol* 2001;25:1074–1078.

65. Buck EG. Polypoid cystitis mimicking transitional cell carcinoma. *J Urol* 1984;131:963.

66. Ekelund P, et al. The reversibility of catheter-associated polypoid cystitis. *J Urol* 1983;130:456–459.

67. Ekelund P, Johansson S. Polypoid cystitis: a catheter associated lesion of the human bladder. *Acta Pathol Microbiol Scand A* 1979;87A:179–184.

68. Kilic S, et al. Polypoid cystitis unrelated to indwelling catheters: a report of eight patients. *Int Urol Nephrol* 2002;34:293–297.

69. Young RH. Papillary and polypoid cystitis. A report of eight cases. *Am J Surg Pathol* 1988;12:542–546.

70. Lane Z, Epstein JI. Polypoid/papillary cystitis: a series of 41 cases misdiagnosed as papillary urothelial neoplasia. *Am J Surg Pathol* 2008;32:758–764.

71. Magi-Galluzzi C, Epstein JI. Urothelial papilloma of the bladder: a review of 34 de novo cases. *Am J Surg Pathol* 2004;28:1615–1620.

72. McKenney JK, Amin MB, Young RH. Urothelial (transitional cell) papilloma of the urinary bladder: a clinicopathologic study of 26 cases. *Mod Pathol* 2003;16:623–629.

73. Fajardo LF, Berthrong M. Radiation injury in surgical pathology. Part I. *Am J Surg Pathol* 1978;2:159–199.

74. Hansson S, et al. Follicular cystitis in girls with untreated asymptomatic or covert bacteriuria. *J Urol* 1990;143:330–332.

75. Marsh FP, Banerjee R, Panchamia P. The relationship between urinary infection, cystoscopic appearance, and pathology of the bladder in man. *J Clin Pathol* 1974;27:297–307.

76. Sarma KP. On the nature of cystitis follicularis. *J Urol* 1970;104:709–714.

77. Vaidyanathan S, et al. The method of bladder drainage in spinal cord injury patients may influence the histological changes in the mucosa of neuropathic bladder—a hypothesis. *BMC Urol* 2002;2:5.

78. Giannopoulos A, et al. The immunomodulating effect of interferon-gamma intravesical instillations in preventing bladder cancer recurrence. *Clin Cancer Res* 2003;9:5550–5558.

79. Ohsawa M, et al. Malignant lymphoma of bladder. Report of three cases and review of the literature. *Cancer* 1993;72:1969–1974.

80. Pawade J, et al. Lymphomas of mucosa-associated lymphoid tissue arising in the urinary bladder. *Histopathology* 1993;23:147–151.

81. Gillenwater JY, Wein AJ. Summary of the National Institute of Arthritis, Diabetes, Digestive and Kidney Diseases Workshop on Interstitial Cystitis, National Institutes of Health, Bethesda, Maryland, August 28-29, 1987. *J Urol* 1988;140:203–206.

82. Giannantoni A, et al. Contemporary management of the painful bladder: a systematic review. *Eur Urol* 2012;61:29–53.

83. Hanno PM, et al. AUA guideline for the diagnosis and treatment of interstitial cystitis/bladder pain syndrome. *J Urol* 2011;185:2162–2170.

84. Johansson SL, Fall M. Clinical features and spectrum of light microscopic changes in interstitial cystitis. *J Urol* 1990;143:1118–1124.

85. Kastrup J, et al. Histamine content and mast cell count of detrusor muscle in patients with interstitial cystitis and other types of chronic cystitis. *Br J Urol* 1983;55:495–500.

86. Lundeberg T, et al. Interstitial cystitis: correlation with nerve fibres, mast cells and histamine. *Br J Urol* 1993;71:427–429.

87. Oliva E, et al. Immunohistochemistry as an adjunct in the differential diagnosis of radiation-induced atypia vs. carcinoma in situ of the bladder: a study of 48 cases. *Mod Pathol* 2007;20:167A.

88. Murphy WM, Soloway MS, Crabtree WN. The morphologic effects of mitomycin C in mammalian urinary bladder. *Cancer* 1981;47:2567–2574.

89. Rubin JS, Rubin RT. Cyclophosphamide hemorrhagic cystitis. *J Urol* 1966;96:313–316.

90. deVries CR, Freiha FS. Hemorrhagic cystitis: a review. *J Urol* 1990;143:1–9.

91. Gregg JA, Utz DC. Eosinophilic cystitis associated with eosinophilic gastroenteritis. *Mayo Clin Proc* 1974;49:185–187.

92. Hellstrom HR, Davis BK, Shonnard JW. Eosinophilic cystitis. A study of 16 cases. *Am J Clin Pathol* 1979;72:777–784.

93. Oh SJ, Chi JG, Lee SE. Eosinophilic cystitis caused by vesical sparganosis: a case report. *J Urol* 1993;149:581–583.

94. Hooton TM. Pathogenesis of urinary tract infections: an update. *J Antimicrob Chemother* 2000;46:1–7.

95. Hooton TM. The current management strategies for community-acquired urinary tract infection. *Infect Dis Clin North Am* 2003;17:303–332.

96. Hooton TM, Stamm WE. Diagnosis and treatment of uncomplicated urinary tract infection. *Infect Dis Clin North Am* 1997;11:551–581.

97. Canning DA. Encrusted cystitis and pyelitis in children: an unusual condition with potentially severe consequences. *J Urol* 2005;173:237–238.

98. Giannakopoulos S, et al. Encrusted cystitis and pyelitis. *Eur Urol* 2001;39:446–448.

99. Meria P, et al. Encrusted cystitis and pyelitis. *J Urol* 1998;160:3–9.

100. Pollack HM, et al. Diagnostic considerations in urinary bladder wall calcification. *AJR Am J Roentgenol* 1981;136:791–797.

101. Ballas K, et al. Gangrenous cystitis. *Int Urogynecol J Pelvic Floor Dysfunct* 2007;18:1507–1509.

102. Devitt AT, Sethia KK. Gangrenous cystitis: case report and review of the literature. *J Urol* 1993;149:1544–1545.

103. White MD, Das AK, Kaufman RP Jr. Gangrenous cystitis in the elderly: pathogenesis and management options. *Br J Urol* 1998;82:297–299.

104. Quint HJ, et al. Emphysematous cystitis: a review of the spectrum of disease. *J Urol* 1992;147:134–137.

105. Thomas AA, et al. Emphysematous cystitis: a review of 135 cases. *BJU Int* 2007;100:17–20.

106. Dutta P, et al. Presentation and outcome of emphysematous renal tract disease in patients with diabetes mellitus. *Urol Int* 2007;78:13–22.

107. Morrison SC. Pneumatosis of the bladder wall associated with necrotizing enterocolitis. *J Clin Ultrasound* 2000;28:497–499.

108. Long JP Jr, Althausen AF. Malacoplakia: a 25-year experience with a review of the literature. *J Urol* 1989;141:1328–1331.

109. Smith BH. Malacoplakia of the urinary tract: a study of twenty-four cases. *J Urol* 1965;43:409.

110. Thorning D, Vracko R. Malakoplakia. Defect in digestion of phagocytized material due to impaired vacuolar acidification? *Arch Pathol* 1975;99:456–460.

111. Abdou NI, et al. Malakoplakia: evidence for monocyte lysosomal abnormality correctable by cholinergic agonist in vitro and in vivo. *N Engl J Med* 1977;297:1413–1419.

112. Michaelis L, Gutmann C. Ueber Einschlusse in Blasentumoren. *Z Klin Med* 1902;47:208.

113. Rohner TJ Jr, Tuliszewski RM. Fungal cystitis: awareness, diagnosis and treatment. *J Urol* 1980;124:142–144.

114. Wise GJ, Silver DA. Fungal infections of the genitourinary system. *J Urol* 1993;149:1377–1388.

115. King DT, Lam M. Actinomycosis of the urinary bladder. Association with an intrauterine contraceptive device. *JAMA* 1978;240:1512–1513.

116. Makar AP, et al. Primary actinomycosis of the urinary bladder. *Br J Urol* 1992;70:205–206.

117. Ozyurt C, et al. Actinomycosis simulating bladder tumour. *Br J Urol* 1995;76:263–264.

118. Villani U, et al. Actinomycosis of bladder and intrauterine devices. *Br J Urol* 1987;60:463–464.

119. Chrisofos M, et al. HPV 16/18-associated condyloma acuminatum of the urinary bladder: first international report and review of literature. *Int J STD AIDS* 2004;15:836–838.

120. Karim RZ, et al. Condylomata acuminata of the urinary bladder with HPV 11. *Pathology* 2005;37:176–178.

121. Kleiman H, Lancaster Y. Condyloma acuminata of the bladder. *J Urol* 1962;88:52.

122. Del Mistro A, et al. Condylomata acuminata of the urinary bladder. Natural history, viral typing, and DNA content. *Am J Surg Pathol* 1988;12:205–215.

123. Koss LG. Warty carcinoma of bladder containing HPV type 11. *Int J Surg Pathol* 2000;8:367.

124. Querci della Rovere G, et al. Development of bladder tumour containing HPV type 11 DNA after renal transplantation. *Br J Urol* 1988;62:36–38.

125. Akiyama H, et al. Adenovirus is a key pathogen in hemorrhagic cystitis associated with bone marrow transplantation. *Clin Infect Dis* 2001;32:1325–1330.

126. Hofland CA, Eron LJ, Washecka RM. Hemorrhagic adenovirus cystitis after renal transplantation. *Transplant Proc* 2004;36(10):3025–3027.

127. Keswani M, Moudgil A. Adenovirus-associated hemorrhagic cystitis in a pediatric renal transplant recipient. *Pediatr Transplant* 2007;11:568–571,

128. Miyamura K, et al. Hemorrhagic cystitis associated with urinary excretion of adenovirus type 11 following allogeneic bone marrow transplantation. *Bone Marrow Transplant* 1989;4:533–535.

129. Umekawa T, Kurita T. Acute hemorrhagic cystitis by adenovirus type 11 with and without type 37 after kidney transplantation. *Urol Int* 1996;56:114–116.

130. Meehan SM, et al. Nephron segment localization of polyoma virus large T antigen in renal allografts. *Hum Pathol* 2006;37:1400–1406.

131. Giraud G, et al. BK-viruria and haemorrhagic cystitis are more frequent in allogeneic haematopoietic stem cell transplant patients receiving full conditioning and unrelated-HLA-mismatched grafts. *Bone Marrow Transplant* 2008;41:737–742.

132. de Padua Silva L, et al. Hemorrhagic cystitis after allogeneic hematopoietic stem cell transplants is the complex result of BK virus infection, preparative regimen intensity and donor type. *Haematologica* 2010;95:1183–1190.

132a. Herawi M, Parwani AV, Chan T, et al. Polyoma virus-associated cellular changes in the urine and bladder biopsy samples: a cytohistologic correlation. *Am J Surg Pathol* 2006;30:345.

133. Childs R, et al. High incidence of adeno- and polyomavirus-induced hemorrhagic cystitis in bone marrow allotransplantation for hematological malignancy following T cell depletion and cyclosporine. *Bone Marrow Transplant* 1998;22:889–893.

134. Spach DH, et al. Cytomegalovirus-induced hemorrhagic cystitis following bone marrow transplantation. *Clin Infect Dis* 1993;16:142–144.

135. Tutuncuoglu SO, Yanovich S, Ozdemirli M. CMV-induced hemorrhagic cystitis as a complication of peripheral blood stem cell transplantation: case report. *Bone Marrow Transplant* 2005;36:265–266.

136. Ghoneim MA. Bilharziasis of the genitourinary tract. *BJU Int* 2002;89:22–30.

137. Zahran MM, et al. Bilharziasis of urinary bladder and ureter: comparative histopathologic study. *Urology* 1976;8:73–79.

138. Van Gool T, et al. Serodiagnosis of imported schistosomiasis by a combination of a commercial indirect hemagglutination test with *Schistosoma mansoni* adult worm antigens and an enzyme-linked immunosorbent assay with *S. mansoni* egg antigens. *J Clin Microbiol* 2002;40:3432–3437.

139. Eble JN, Banks ER. Post-surgical necrobiotic granulomas of urinary bladder. *Urology* 1990;35:454–457.

140. Tai HL, Chen CC, Yeh KT. Xanthogranulomatous cystitis associated with anaerobic bacterial infection. *J Urol* 1999;162:795–796.

141. Chung MK, et al. Xanthogranulomatous cystitis associated with suture material. *J Urol* 1998;159:981–982.

142. Walther M, Glenn JF, Vellios F. Xanthogranulomatous cystitis. *J Urol* 1985;134:745–746.

143. Lage JM, et al. Histological parameters and pitfalls in the interpretation of bladder biopsies in bacillus Calmette-Guerin treatment of superficial bladder cancer. *J Urol* 1986;135:916–919.

144. Rigatti P, et al. Local bacillus Calmette-Guerin therapy for superficial bladder cancer: clinical, histological and ultrastructural patterns. *Scand J Urol Nephrol* 1990;24:191–198.

145. Oates RD, et al. Granulomatous prostatitis following bacillus Calmette-Guerin immunotherapy of bladder cancer. *J Urol* 1988; 140:751–754.

146. Christensen WI. Genitourinary tuberculosis: review of 102 cases. *Medicine (Baltimore)* 1974;53:377–390.

147. Stoller JK. Late recurrence of Mycobacterium bovis genitourinary tuberculosis: case report and review of literature. *J Urol* 1985;134: 565–566.

148. Schwartz BF, Stoller ML. The vesical calculus. *Urol Clin North Am* 2000;27:333–346.

149. Pacchioni D, et al. Immunohistochemical detection of estrogen and progesterone receptors in the normal urinary bladder and in pseudomembranous trigonitis. *J Endocrinol Invest* 1992;15:719–725.

150. Stephenson TJ, et al. Pseudomembranous trigonitis of the bladder: hormonal aetiology. *J Clin Pathol* 1989;42:922–926.

151. Jurkiewicz B, et al. Bladder squamous metaplasia of the urothelium—introductory report. *Urol Int* 2006;77:46–49.

152. Khan MS, et al. Keratinising squamous metaplasia of the bladder: natural history and rationalization of management based on review of 54 years experience. *Eur Urol* 2002;42:469–474.

153. Tannenbaum M. Inflammatory proliferative lesion of urinary bladder: squamous metaplasia. *Urology* 1976;7:428–429.

154. von Brunn A. Ueber drusenahnliche bildungen in der scheimhaut des ureters und der harnblasebeim menschen. *Arch F Mikosc Anat* 1935;41:303.

155. Volmar KE, et al. Florid von Brunn nests mimicking urothelial carcinoma: a morphologic and immunohistochemical comparison to the nested variant of urothelial carcinoma. *Am J Surg Pathol* 2003; 27:1243–1252.

156. Davies G, Castro JE. Cystitis glandularis. *Urology* 1977;10:128–129.

157. Mostofi FK. Potentialities of bladder epithelium. *J Urol* 1954;71: 705–714.

158. Kunze E, Schauer A, Schmitt M. Histology and histogenesis of two different types of inverted urothelial papillomas. *Cancer* 1983; 51:348–358.

159. Jacobs LB, Brooks JD, Epstein JI. Differentiation of colonic metaplasia from adenocarcinoma of urinary bladder. *Hum Pathol* 1997;28:1152–1157.

160. Young RH, Bostwick DG. Florid cystitis glandularis of intestinal type with mucin extravasation: a mimic of adenocarcinoma. *Am J Surg Pathol* 1996;20:1462–1468.

161. Corica FA, et al. Intestinal metaplasia is not a strong risk factor for bladder cancer: study of 53 cases with long-term follow-up. *Urology* 1997;50:427–431.

162. Baker PM, Young RH. Radiation-induced pseudocarcinomatous proliferations of the urinary bladder: a report of 4 cases. *Hum Pathol* 2000;31:678–683.

163. Chan TY, Epstein JI. Radiation or chemotherapy cystitis with "pseudocarcinomatous" features. *Am J Surg Pathol* 2004;28:909–913.

164. Oliva E, Young RH. Nephrogenic adenoma of the urinary tract: a review of the microscopic appearance of 80 cases with emphasis on unusual features. *Mod Pathol* 1995;8:722–730.

165. Rutgers JL, Young RH. Nephrogenic adenoma of the urinary bladder: a comparison of its cytologic and histopathologic features in ten cases. *Diagn Cytopathol* 1988;4:210–216.

166. Young RH, Scully RE. Nephrogenic adenoma. A report of 15 cases, review of the literature, and comparison with clear cell adenocarcinoma of the urinary tract. *Am J Surg Pathol* 1986;10:268–275.

167. Crook TJ, et al. A case series of nephrogenic adenoma of the urethra and bladder in children: review of this rare diagnosis, its natural history and management, with reference to the literature. *J Pediatr Urol* 2006;2:323–328.

168. Husain AN, Armin AR, Schuster GA. Nephrogenic metaplasia of urinary tract in children: report of three cases and review of the literature. *Pediatr Pathol* 1988;8:293–300.

169. Allan CH, Epstein JI. Nephrogenic adenoma of the prostatic urethra: a mimicker of prostate adenocarcinoma. *Am J Surg Pathol* 2001;25:802–808.

170. Hansel DE, Nadasdy T, Epstein JI. Fibromyxoid nephrogenic adenoma: a newly recognized variant mimicking mucinous adenocarcinoma. *Am J Surg Pathol* 2007;31:1231–1237.

171. Skinnider BF, et al. Expression of alpha-methylacyl-CoA racemase (P504S) in nephrogenic adenoma: a significant immunohistochemical pitfall compounding the differential diagnosis with prostatic adenocarcinoma. *Am J Surg Pathol* 2004;28:701–705.

172. Tong GX, et al. PAX2: a reliable marker for nephrogenic adenoma. *Mod Pathol* 2006;19:356–363.

173. Tong GX, et al. Expression of PAX8 in nephrogenic adenoma and clear cell adenocarcinoma of the lower urinary tract: evidence of related histogenesis? *Am J Surg Pathol* 2008;32:1380–1387.

174. Gilcrease MZ, et al. Clear cell adenocarcinoma and nephrogenic adenoma of the urethra and urinary bladder: a histopathologic and immunohistochemical comparison. *Hum Pathol* 1998;29: 1451–1456.

175. Wood DP Jr, Streem SB, Levin HS. Nephrogenic adenoma in patients with transitional cell carcinoma of the bladder receiving intravesical thiotepa. *J Urol* 1988;139:130–131.

176. Stilmant MM, Siroky MB. Nephrogenic adenoma associated with intravesical bacillus Calmette-Guerin treatment: a report of 2 cases. *J Urol* 1986;135:359–361.

177. Piper NY, Thompson IM. Large nephrogenic adenoma following transurethral resection of the prostate. *J Urol* 1999;161:605.

178. Medeiros LJ, Young RH. Nephrogenic adenoma arising in urethral diverticula. A report of five cases. *Arch Pathol Lab Med* 1989;113: 125–128.

179. Hung SY, Tseng HH, Chung HM. Nephrogenic adenoma associated with cytomegalovirus infection of the ureter in a renal transplant patient: presentation as ureteral obstruction. *Transpl Int* 2001;14: 111–114.

180. Scelzi S, et al. Nephrogenic adenoma of bladder after ibuprofen abuse. *Urology* 2004;64:1030.

181. Mazal PR, et al. Derivation of nephrogenic adenomas from renal tubular cells in kidney-transplant recipients. *N Engl J Med* 2002; 347:653–659.

182. Al-Ahmadie H, et al. Giant botryoid fibroepithelial polyp of bladder with myofibroblastic stroma and cystitis cystica et glandularis. *Pediatr Dev Pathol* 2003;6:179–181.

183. Tsuzuki T, Epstein JI. Fibroepithelial polyp of the lower urinary tract in adults. *Am J Surg Pathol* 2005;29:460–466.

184. Young RH. Fibroepithelial polyp of the bladder with atypical stromal cells. *Arch Pathol Lab Med* 1986;110:241–242.

185. Remick DG Jr, Kumar NB. Benign polyps with prostatic-type epithelium of the urethra and the urinary bladder. A suggestion of histogenesis based on histologic and immunohistochemical studies. *Am J Surg Pathol* 1984;8:833–839.

186. Smith VC, Boone TB, Truong LD. Collagen polyp of the urinary tract: a report of two cases. *Mod Pathol* 1999;12:1090–1093.

187. Crites MA, Ghoniem GM. Bladder mass "collagenoma". *Int Urogynecol J* 2011;22:621–623.

188. Truong LD, Ostrowski ML, Wheeler TM. Tamm-Horsfall protein in bladder tissue. Morphologic spectrum and clinical significance. *Am J Surg Pathol* 1994;18:615–622.

189. Howie AJ. Tamm-Horsfall protein outside the kidney. *J Pathol* 1987;153:399–404.

190. Billis A, et al. Adenoma of bladder in siblings with renal dysplasia. *Urology* 1980;16:299–302.

191. Borski AA. Hamartoma of the bladder. *J Urol* 1970;104:718–719.

192. Brancatelli G, et al. Hamartoma of the urinary bladder: case report and review of the literature. *Eur Radiol* 1999;9:42–44.

193. Keating MA, et al. Hamartoma of the bladder in a 4-year-old girl with hamartomatous polyps of the gastrointestinal tract. *J Urol* 1987;138:366–369.

194. McCallion WA, Herron BM, Keane PF. Bladder hamartoma. *Br J Urol* 1993;72:382–383.

195. Williams MP, Ibrahim SK, Rickwood AM. Hamartoma of the urinary bladder in an infant with Beckwith-Wiedemann syndrome. *Br J Urol* 1990;65:106–107.

196. Livneh A, et al. Light chain amyloidosis of the urinary bladder. A site restricted deposition of an externally produced immunoglobulin. *J Clin Pathol* 2001;54:920–923.

197. Merrimen JL, Alkhudair WK, Gupta R. Localized amyloidosis of the urinary tract: case series of nine patients. *Urology* 2006;67:904–909.

198. Oka N, et al. Secondary amyloidosis of the bladder causing macroscopic hematuria. *Int J Urol* 2001;8:330–332.

199. Tirzaman O, et al. Primary localized amyloidosis of the urinary bladder: a case series of 31 patients. *Mayo Clin Proc* 2000;75:1264–1268.

200. Monge M, et al. Localized amyloidosis of the genitourinary tract: report of 5 new cases and review of the literature. *Medicine (Baltimore)* 2011;90:212–222.

201. Andrade MJ. Lower urinary tract dysfunction in familial amyloidotic polyneuropathy, Portuguese type. *Neurourol Urodyn* 2009;28:26–32.

202. Comiter CV. Endometriosis of the urinary tract. *Urol Clin North Am* 2002;29:625–635.

203. Parker RL, et al. Polypoid endometriosis: a clinicopathologic analysis of 24 cases and a review of the literature. *Am J Surg Pathol* 2004;28:285–297.

204. Wong-You-Cheong JJ, et al. From the archives of the AFIP: inflammatory and nonneoplastic bladder masses: radiologic-pathologic correlation. *Radiographics* 2006;26:1847–1868.

205. Clement PB. Lesions of the secondary mullerian system. Urinary tract endometriosis. In: Kurman RJ, ed. *Blaustein's Pathology of the Female Genital Tract*. New York, NY: Springer-Verlag; 2002:762–764.

206. Pinkert TC, Catlow CE, Straus R. Endometriosis of the urinary bladder in a man with prostatic carcinoma. *Cancer* 1979;43:1562–1567.

207. Schrodt GR, Alcorn MO, Ibanez J. Endometriosis of the male urinary system: a case report. *J Urol* 1980;124:722–723.

208. Garavan F, Grainger R, Jeffers M. Endometrioid carcinoma of the urinary bladder complicating vesical Mullerianosis: a case report and review of the literature. *Virchows Arch* 2004;444:587–589.

209. Oliva E, et al. Clear cell carcinoma of the urinary bladder: a report and comparison of four tumors of mullerian origin and nine of probable urothelial origin with discussion of histogenesis and diagnostic problems. *Am J Surg Pathol* 2002;26:190–197.

210. al-Izzi MS, et al. Malignant transformation in endometriosis of the urinary bladder. *Histopathology* 1989;14:191–198.

211. Chapron C, et al. Surgery for bladder endometriosis: long-term results and concomitant management of associated posterior deep lesions. *Hum Reprod* 2010;25:884–889.

212. Clement PB, Young RH. Endocervicosis of the urinary bladder. A report of six cases of a benign mullerian lesion that may mimic adenocarcinoma. *Am J Surg Pathol* 1992;16:533–542.

213. Edmondson JD, et al. Endosalpingiosis of bladder. *J Urol* 2002;167:1401–1402.

214. Young RH, Clement PB. Mullerianosis of the urinary bladder. *Mod Pathol* 1996;9:731–737.

215. Felderman T, et al. Mullerian duct cysts: conservative management. *Urology* 1987;29:31–34.

216. Ritchey ML, et al. Management of mullerian duct remnants in the male patient. *J Urol* 1988;140:795–799.

217. Steele AA, Byrne AJ. Paramesonephric (mullerian) sinus of urinary bladder. *Am J Surg Pathol* 1982;6:173–176.

218. Anastasiades KD, Majmudar B. Prolapse of fallopian tube into urinary bladder, mimicking bladder carcinoma. *Arch Pathol Lab Med* 1983;107:613–614.

219. Joffe N. Roentgenologic abnormalities of the urinary bladder secondary to Crohn's disease. *AJR Am J Roentgenol* 1976;127:297–302.

220. Slade N, Gaches C. Vesico-intestinal fistulae. *Br J Surg* 1972;59:593–597.

221. Bird GC. Obstetric vesico-vaginal and allied fistulae. A report on 70 cases. *J Obstet Gynaecol Br Commonw* 1967;74:749–752.

222. Zoubek J, et al. The late occurrence of urinary tract damage in patients successfully treated by radiotherapy for cervical carcinoma. *J Urol* 1989;141:1347–1349.

223. Proppe KH, Scully RE, Rosai J. Postoperative spindle cell nodules of genitourinary tract resembling sarcomas. A report of eight cases. *Am J Surg Pathol* 1984;8:101–108.

224. Freeman A, et al. Anaplastic lymphoma kinase (ALK 1) staining and molecular analysis in inflammatory myofibroblastic tumours of the bladder: a preliminary clinicopathological study of nine cases and review of the literature. *Mod Pathol* 2004;17:765–771.

225. Harik LR, et al. Pseudosarcomatous myofibroblastic proliferations of the bladder: a clinicopathologic study of 42 cases. *Am J Surg Pathol* 2006;30:787–794.

226. Hirsch MS, Dal Cin P, Fletcher CD. ALK expression in pseudosarcomatous myofibroblastic proliferations of the genitourinary tract. *Histopathology* 2006;48:569–578.

227. Montgomery EA, et al. Inflammatory myofibroblastic tumors of the urinary tract: a clinicopathologic study of 46 cases, including a malignant example inflammatory fibrosarcoma and a subset associated with high-grade urothelial carcinoma. *Am J Surg Pathol* 2006;30:1502–1512.

228. Tsuzuki T, Magi-Galluzzi C, Epstein JI. ALK-1 expression in inflammatory myofibroblastic tumor of the urinary bladder. *Am J Surg Pathol* 2004;28:1609–1614.

229. Cessna MH, et al. Expression of ALK1 and p80 in inflammatory myofibroblastic tumor and its mesenchymal mimics: a study of 135 cases. *Mod Pathol* 2002;15:931–938.

230. Iczkowski KA, et al. Inflammatory pseudotumor and sarcoma of urinary bladder: differential diagnosis and outcome in thirty-eight spindle cell neoplasms. *Mod Pathol* 2001;14:1043–1051.

231. Jones EC, Young RH. Myxoid and sclerosing sarcomatoid transitional cell carcinoma of the urinary bladder: a clinicopathologic and immunohistochemical study of 25 cases. *Mod Pathol* 1997;10:908–916.

232. Westfall DE, et al. Utility of a comprehensive immunohistochemical panel in the differential diagnosis of spindle cell lesions of the urinary bladder. *Am J Surg Pathol* 2009;33:99–105.

233. Hautmann RE, et al. The ileal neobladder: complications and functional results in 363 patients after 11 years of followup. *J Urol* 1999;161:422–427; discussion 427–428.

234. Chen KK, et al. Histopathological changes in Kock pouch. *Br J Urol* 1993;72:433–440.

235. Hockenstrom T, et al. Morphologic changes in ileal reservoir mucosa after long-term exposure to urine. A study in patients with continent urostomy (Kock pouch). *Scand J Gastroenterol* 1986;21:1224–1234.

236. Gatti R, et al. Histological adaptation of orthotopic ileal neobladder mucosa: 4-year follow-up of 30 patients. *Eur Urol* 1999;36:588–594.

237. Senkul T, et al. Histopathologic changes in the mucosa of ileal orthotopic neobladder—findings in 24 patients followed up for 5 years. *Scand J Urol Nephrol* 2003;37:202–204.

238. Kojima Y, et al. Mucosal morphological changes in the ileal neobladder. *Br J Urol* 1998;82:114–117.

239. Aragona F, et al. Structural and ultrastructural changes in ileal neobladder mucosa: a 7-year follow-up. *Br J Urol* 1998;81:55–61.

240. Robles MW, Rutgers JK, Shanberg AM. Adenocarcinoma and dysplasia in an ileal neobladder after ileocystoplasty for interstitial cystitis. *Int J Surg Pathol* 2004;12:63–65.

241. Cullen TS. *Embryology, Anatomy, and Diseases of the Umbilicus Together with Diseases of the Urachus.* Philadelphia, PA: W.B. Saunders; 1916.

242. Bauer SB, Retik AB. Urachal anomalies and related umbilical disorders. *Urol Clin North Am* 1978;5:195–211.

243. Begg RC. The urachus: its anatomy, histology, and development. *J Anat* 1930;64:170–182.

244. Trimingham HL, McDonald JR. Congenital anomalies in the region of the umbilicus. *Surg Gynecol Obstet* 1945;80:152–163.

245. Hammond G, Yglesias L, Davis JE. The urachus, its anatomy and associated fasciae. *Anat Rec* 1941;80:271–287.

246. Blichert-Toft M, Koch F, Nielsen OV. Anatomic variants of the urachus related to clinical appearance and surgical treatment. *Surg Gynecol Obstet* 1973;137:51–54.

247. Schubert GE, Pavkovic MB, Bethke-Bedurftig BA. Tubular urachal remnants in adult bladders. *J Urol* 1982;127:40–42.

248. Wutz JB. Ueber Urachus and Urachuscysten. *Arch Pathol Anat Physiol Klin Med* 1883;92:387–423.

249. Bucchiere JJ Jr. *Diseases of the Urachus.* Minneapolis, MN: University of Minnesota; 1978.

250. Copp HL, et al. Clinical presentation and urachal remnant pathology: implications for treatment. *J Urol* 2009;182:1921–1924.

251. Tyler DE. Epithelium of intestinal type in the normal urachus: a new theory of vesical embryology. *J Urol* 1964;92:505–507.

252. Paner GP, et al. Immunohistochemical analysis in a morphologic spectrum of urachal epithelial neoplasms: diagnostic implications and pitfalls. *Am J Surg Pathol* 2011;35:787–798.

253. Herbst WP. Patent urachus. *Southern Med J* 1937;30:711–719.

254. Lattimer JK. Congenital deficiency of the abdominal musculature and associated genitourinary anomalies: a report of 22 cases. *J Urol* 1958;79:343–352.

255. Schreck WR, Campbell WA III. The relation of bladder outlet obstruction to urinary-umbilical fistula. *J Urol* 1972;108:641–643.

256. Vaughan GT. Patent urachus. Review of the cases reported. Operation on a case complicated by stones in the kidneys. A note on tumors and cysts of the urachus. *Trans Am Surg Assoc* 1905;23:273–294.

257. Hinman F Jr. Urologic aspects of the alternating urachal sinus. *Am J Surg* 1961;102:339–342.

258. Nargund VH, Donaldson RA. Urachal calculi: a case report and review of the literature. *Int Urol Nephrol* 1994;26:409–411.

259. Dreyfuss ML, Fliess MM. Patent urachus with stone formation. *J Urol* 1941;47:77–81.

260. Iuchtman M, et al. Management of urachal anomalies in children and adults. *Urology* 1993;42:426–430.

261. Berman SM, et al. Urachal remnants in adults. *Urology* 1988;31:17–21.

262. Brodie N. Infected urachal cysts. *Am J Surg* 1945;69:243–248.

263. Hinman F Jr. Surgical disorders of the bladder and umbilicus of urachal origin. *Surg Gynecol Obstet* 1961;113:605–614.

264. Lees VC, Doyle PT. Urachal cyst presenting with abscess formation. *J R Soc Med* 1991;84:367–368.

265. MacMillan RW, Schullinger JN, Santulli TV. Pyourachus: an unusual surgical problem. *J Pediatr Surg* 1973;8:387–389.

266. MacNeily AE, et al. Urachal abscesses: protean manifestations, their recognition, and management. *Urology* 1992;40:530–535.

267. Chen WJ, Hsieh HH, Wan YL. Abscess of urachal remnant mimicking urinary bladder neoplasm. *Br J Urol* 1992;69:510–512.

268. Newman BM, et al. Advances in the management of infected urachal cysts. *J Pediatr Surg* 1986;21:1051–1054.

269. Micheli E, et al. Primary actinomycosis of the urachus. *BJU Int* 1999;83:144–145.

270. Nagy V, et al. Actinomycosis of the urachus persistens penetrating into the ileum. *Int Urol Nephrol* 1997;29:627–631.

271. Thompson NP, Stoker DL, Springall RG. Urachal abscess as a complication of tinea corporis. *Br J Urol* 1994;73:319.

272. Steck WD, Helwig EB. Umbilical granulomas, pilonidal disease, and the urachus. *Surg Gynecol Obstet* 1965;120:1043–1057.

273. Carrere W, et al. Urachal xanthogranulomatous disease. *Br J Urol* 1996;77:612–613.

Tumors of the Urinary Bladder

DAVID J. GRIGNON

CLASSIFICATION OF UROTHELIAL TUMORS

The last decade has seen a tremendous upheaval in this very important area that only recently seems to have settled down to a level of general concurrence.[1] For over two decades, the World Health Organization (WHO) classification and grading of urothelial neoplasms[2] dominated although several variations and different schemes were published. In the early 1990s, several factors emerged that resulted in the need to reevaluate this approach. First, the controversy of calling grade 1 papillary tumors "carcinoma" arose with several groups led by Dr. William Murphy calling all tumors in the low-grade end as papilloma.[3,4] Second, the use of intravesical therapy as a standard practice in the treatment of high-risk noninvasive papillary tumors demanded that high-risk tumors be clearly identified. Third, the WHO (1973) system was criticized for the imprecision of the published criteria (Table 6-1), leading many pathologists to essentially use this three-grade system to create five grade groups (1, 1–2, 2, 2–3, and 3), one result being that only a small percentage of cases were placed in the grade 3 group. For example, in a review of three clinical studies only 25 of 280 (8.9%) newly diagnosed noninvasive papillary tumors (pTa) were called grade 3.[5] The effect of the latter was confusion as to how to treat grade 2 Ta tumors, a category that included many high-risk patients who could benefit from intravesical therapy as well as many patients with low-risk disease for whom intravesical therapy may not be appropriate or necessary. Multiple studies have demonstrated that this group includes high-risk patients with progression to invasive carcinoma reported in up to 20% of patients and cancer-specific death in 13% to 20%.[6,7]

Recognizing the many emerging issues, in 1997 Dr. F. K. Mostofi organized a meeting of a small group of urologic pathologists, urologists, and urologic oncologists to address these concerns. This was followed by a much larger consensus conference that was held under the auspices of the International Society of Urologic Pathology (ISUP) in March of 1998. The results of this consensus were adopted by the WHO and the results published in 1998 as the WHO/ISUP consensus classification (Table 6-2).[8] Most controversial was the adoption of the term papillary urothelial neoplasm of low malignant potential. This represented a compromise term where the papilloma and carcinoma advocates could be comfortable and allowed that controversy to be brought to resolution. Most important was the adoption of the grading system that had been described by Malmström et al.[9] The value of the latter was viewed as twofold; first, the morphologic criteria for applying the scheme were well defined and, second, it appeared to place the majority of patients with high-risk disease into the high-grade category.

The publication of the 1999 WHO blue book the following year introduced a variation on this system with the splitting of the low- and high-grade categories of the 1998 WHO/ISUP classification into three groups (grades 1, 2, and 3) while retaining the papillary urothelial neoplasm of low malignant potential category.[10] This reignited the controversy with some experts urging a return to the 1973 WHO grading system.[11] Others criticized the 1998 WHO/ISUP system as simply representing a renaming of the 1973 WHO,[12] a clearly incorrect interpretation.[13] At a subsequent meeting in Ancona, Italy (2001), a modified version of the 1973 WHO was proposed.[13]

This issue became the primary focus of discussion at the WHO meetings prior to the release of the 2004 WHO classification. Following extensive debate and discussion, it was agreed overwhelmingly to essentially reproduce the 1998 WHO/ISUP classification as the 2004 WHO recommended classification scheme (Table 6-2).[14] The authors of the Fourth Series Armed Forces Institute of Pathology fascicle covering bladder neoplasia also followed this system.[15] With this consistent approach adopted by arguably the two most influential references for tumor classification and grading, work can continue on evaluating the biologic and clinical relevance and value of this system.[16]

The success of the 2004 WHO/ISUP classification in addressing the key issues outlined in the first paragraph has been stressed, in particular the reclassification of high-risk

Table 6-1 ■ 1973 WHO GRADING CRITERIA	
Grade 1	Tumors with the least degree of cellular anaplasia compatible with a diagnosis of malignancy
Grade 2	Histologic features between grades 1 and 3
Grade 3	Tumors with the most severe degrees of cellular anaplasia

From Mostofi F, Sobin L. *Histologic Typing of Urinary Bladder Tumors.* Geneva, Switzerland: World Health Organization; 1973.

grade 2 tumors (WHO 1973) into the high-grade papillary carcinoma category.[13,17,18] For example, in the study by Yin and Leong,[18] 13 of 46 WHO (1973) grade 2 tumors (28%) were placed in the WHO (2004) high-grade category resulting in 23% of all cases being considered high-grade in WHO 2004 compared to only 4% being called grade 3 in the 1973 WHO system. Similarly, Samaratunga et al.[17] reviewed 134 papillary tumors of which 6 (4%) had been reported as grade 3 (WHO, 1973); on review they considered 29 (22%) to be high grade by WHO/ISUP 1998.

This approach has been embraced by many urologic oncologists with interest in bladder cancer. It has important application in the contemporary treatment of Ta tumors. The reclassification of high-risk grade 2 tumors (WHO 1973) into the high-grade category (WHO 2004) has resulted in a large and better-defined group of patients with low-risk Ta tumors. In a series of 215 patients with low-grade (papilloma, papillary urothelial neoplasm of low malignant potential and low-grade papillary carcinoma) Ta tumors from the Memorial Sloan Kettering Cancer Center treated by transurethral resection only, progression to high-grade Ta or invasive carcinoma occurred in only 3% and 5% of patients, respectively, with

Table 6-2 ■ 2004 WHO/1998 ISUP CLASSIFICATION
• Normal
• Hyperplasias
• Flat lesions with atypia
◦ Reactive (inflammatory) atypia
◦ Atypia of unknown significance
◦ Dysplasia (low-grade intraurothelial neoplasia)
◦ CIS (high-grade intraurothelial neoplasia)
• Papillary neoplasms
◦ Papilloma
◦ Inverted papilloma
◦ Papillary urothelial neoplasm of low malignant potential
◦ Papillary carcinoma, low grade
◦ Papillary carcinoma, high grade
• Invasive neoplasms

From Epstein JI, Amin MB, Reuter VR, et al. The World Health Organization/International Society of Urological Pathology consensus classification of urothelial (transitional cell) neoplasms of the urinary bladder. Bladder Consensus Conference Committee. *Am J Surg Pathol* 1998;22:1435–1448; Eble J, Epstein J, Sauter G, et al. *World Health Organization Histologic and Genetic Typing of Tumours of the Kidney, Urinary Bladder, Prostate Gland and Testis.* Lyon, France: IARC Press; 2004.

a median follow-up of 8 years.[19] A prospective study lent further support to these findings.[20] This experience has led to the suggestion that patients with low-grade Ta tumors can be followed less frequently.[21] Similarly, Nieder and Soloway[22] recommended treating patients with papilloma and papillary urothelial neoplasm of low malignant potential by transurethral resection alone, low-grade Ta tumors by transurethral resection with a single dose of mitomycin C, and high-grade Ta tumors by transurethral resection with mitomycin C and bacillus Calmette-Guérin (BCG) immunotherapy. In December 2007, the American Urological Association (AUA) reinforced the current approach in its guidelines for the treatment of non–muscle-invasive bladder cancers by separating noninvasive papillary tumors into two groups—low grade and high grade[23]—with different treatment recommendations for each group. The use of this system has also been advocated by the European Urology Association.[24] The College of American Pathologists (CAP) utilizes WHO 2004 in its recommendations for the reporting of urothelial tumors.[25,26] Support for this system was further emphasized in the International Consultation on Bladder Cancer.[27]

EPITHELIAL TUMORS—BENIGN

Urothelial Papilloma

There has been a long-standing controversy regarding the nature of papillary lesions with minimal cytologic atypia.[28] An early definition by Mostofi restricted the term papilloma to noninvasive papillary lesions covered by urothelium that was indistinguishable from normal urothelium.[29] This definition was adopted in the WHO (1973) classification.[2] The use of this term by some experts for up to one-third of all papillary lesions was a major stimulant to the reevaluation of these lesions that began in 1997.[3,4] The current classification retains the restrictive traditional WHO criteria.[2,14,15] These tumors do harbor the *FGFR3* mutations characteristic of papillary neoplasia.[30]

Clinical Features

Lesions meeting these restricted criteria occur at a younger age than other urothelial bladder tumors and often present with only one or a few papillary processes. The mean patient age in two large series was 51 years (range, 8 to 87 years).[31,32] In one series with individual data presented, 50% of the patients were under 40 years of age.[31] They are more common in men (male:female ratio is 2.4:1).[31] There does not appear to be a predilection for a specific location in the bladder. Using the restrictive criteria recommended, these lesions account for approximately 1% of papillary tumors.[28] In patients with urothelial papilloma and no other urothelial neoplasia, the recurrence rate is <10% and there is a low risk for the subsequent development of higher-grade tumors.[28,31–34] In contemporary studies, the progression to higher-grade tumors has been low, and the subsequent development of

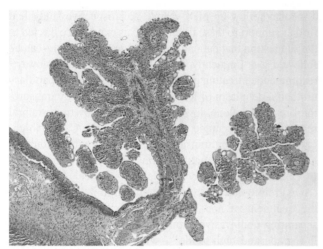

FIGURE 6-1 ■ Urothelial papilloma showing a small tumor with fine papillary fronds.

invasive disease has been reported to be <1%.[31-33] In these studies, the one case with progression was on immunosuppressive therapy following renal transplantation.

Pathology

Grossly, urothelial papilloma consists of a small lesion with a few distinct and separate fronds. Histologically, papilloma is characterized by fine papillary fronds without fusion or complexity (Fig. 6-1). There is minimal if any branching. Individual fronds are covered by an essentially normal urothelium without architectural or cytologic atypia (Fig. 6-2). The absolute number of cell layers is not a criterion for diagnosis, but the urothelium should not be obviously thickened. In some cases, the urothelium can be quite attenuated with only a couple of cell layers. As in normal urothelium, some variability in the histology is allowed. The umbrella cell layer can have enlarged nuclei and cytoplasmic vacuoles, and an apocrine-like appearance of the cytoplasm can be seen. There should be no atypia of the cells other

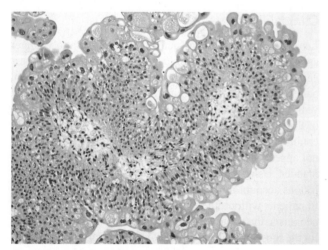

FIGURE 6-2 ■ Urothelial papilloma with the surface urothelium showing no cytologic or architectural atypia.

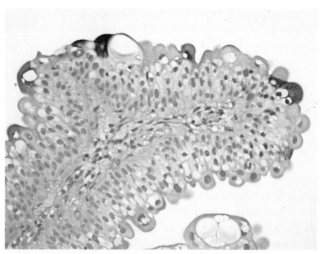

FIGURE 6-3 ■ Urothelial papilloma with immunohistochemistry for cytokeratin 20 highlighting a few umbrella cells.

than the umbrella cells. Mitoses are absent. Although immunohistochemistry is not recommended for diagnosis, similar to papillary urothelial neoplasm of low malignant potential, expression of cytokeratin 20 is limited to the umbrella cell layer (Fig. 6-3)[35] and proliferation determined by Ki-67 immunohistochemistry is low.[36]

Differential Diagnosis

The differential diagnosis includes papillary cystitis, papillary hyperplasia, and low-grade papillary urothelial carcinoma. Papillary cystitis occurs in an inflammatory background and the clinical setting—indwelling catheter, bladder stones, nonfunctioning bladder—may be helpful. The papillae are shorter and broader than typical of papillary neoplasia.[37,38] Branching of the papillae is not a feature. The stroma is inflamed and may be edematous (polypoid cystitis). The urothelium often shows a reactive type of atypia. Papillary hyperplasia has more of a pseudopapillary architecture with tenting of the urothelium characterized by a thicker stromal core at the base of the lesion that thins toward the tip of the lesion.[39] The uniformly thin fibrovascular core typical of papilloma is absent. The lesion often is associated with thickening of the urothelium of the pseudopapillary projection and the adjacent flat surface. Distinction from papillary urothelial neoplasm of low malignant potential can be difficult. The presence of complex branching, thickening of the epithelium, or increased cell density favors the diagnosis of papillary urothelial neoplasm of low malignant potential, while any fusion of the papillae, architectural disturbance, nuclear enlargement or atypia, and mitoses indicates the diagnosis of low-grade papillary carcinoma.

Inverted Urothelial Papilloma

Clinical Features

Inverted urothelial papilloma accounts for approximately 1% of urothelial neoplasms. It is a distinct clinical and pathologic entity that occurs over a wide age range but most often after the age of 50.[5,40–47] They are much more common in men than women. These develop throughout the urinary tract but are most common in the urinary bladder, in particular the trigone and bladder neck region. Cases of synchronous inverted papilloma and papillary carcinoma are well described though rare. In rare cases, they can be multifocal.[42] Inverted papilloma is treated by transurethral resection and is associated with a low risk of recurrence (<5%) that is distinctly different from low-grade papillary urothelial neoplasms.[42,43]

Genetic data have confirmed that these represent a neoplastic process with clonality demonstrated by X-linked inactivation studies.[42,48] Loss of heterozygosity studies have demonstrated that inverted urothelial papilloma does not have the typical genetic abnormalities of papillary urothelial neoplasms, supporting the concept that these are unrelated.[48] There is no association with human papilloma virus (HPV) infection.[49]

Pathology

Grossly, these lesions typically have an exophytic polypoid growth pattern and can be pedunculated (Box 6-1). Histologically, inverted urothelial papilloma consists of anastomosing trabeculae of urothelium covered by a normal or attenuated urothelium (Fig. 6-4). Multiple sites of origin from the surface urothelium are usually present. The basal

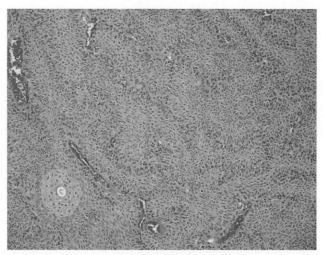

FIGURE 6-5 ■ Inverted urothelial papilloma with palisading of basilar cells and streaming of centrally located cells.

layer is often prominent with the basilar nuclei lined up perpendicular to the basement membrane. The cells in the central part of the trabeculae can be spindled with a streaming growth pattern (Fig. 6-5). In general, there is no significant nuclear pleomorphism although occasionally mild atypia can be present.[50] Mitotic figures are rare or absent. The cytoplasm can be foamy or vacuolated.[51] This can resemble the "glycogenated" squamoid morphology that can be present in some urothelial carcinomas. Squamous or glandular differentiation may be present. In many cases, glands or gland-like spaces that are lined by a cuboidal to columnar epithelium are found (Fig. 6-6). These typically do not appear to be mucin-containing cells on hematoxylin and eosin–stained sections. The lumens can contain eosinophilic secretions that can stain with mucicarmine. In transurethral resection material, the fragmentation of the lesion may result in apparent papillary structures, making diagnosis difficult. There is no stromal desmoplasia and minimal inflammation.

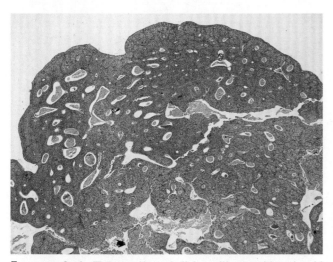

FIGURE 6-4 ■ Inverted urothelial papilloma with polypoid appearance, flattened surface epithelium, and complex trabecular architecture.

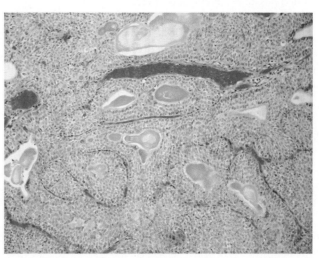

FIGURE 6-6 ■ Inverted urothelial papilloma with glandular spaces lined by columnar epithelium.

Differential Diagnosis

The major problem is the distinction from papillary carcinoma with an inverted growth pattern.[48,50,52] These carcinomas generally have larger pushing borders with more defined nested architecture rather than the complex anastomosing architecture typical of inverted papilloma. The striking peripheral palisading, maturation toward the center of the trabeculae and the spindling growth pattern are also absent.[53] In most cases, there is a greater degree of nuclear pleomorphism than is acceptable for inverted papilloma, and mitoses may be frequent. Foci of stromal invasion are often present and would exclude the diagnosis of inverted papilloma.

Florid cystitis glandularis can produce a localized polypoid lesion that can be confused with inverted papilloma. These have well-defined nests without the complex trabecular architecture of inverted papilloma. Similarly, exuberant proliferations of von Brunn nests can mimic inverted papilloma, but the nests are separated and a complex trabecular architecture is absent.[54] Finally other tumors that can have a nested architecture such as the nested variant of urothelial carcinoma, paraganglioma, and carcinoid tumor could potentially mimic inverted papilloma in small biopsy specimens.

Villous Adenoma

Clinical Features

Villous adenoma is an uncommon lesion that can arise in the urinary bladder proper or the urachus.[55–59] It is more common in men than women and occurs over a wide age range from young adults to the elderly with most found in the sixth or seventh decade. The most frequent presentation is with hematuria or irritative symptoms. Mucusuria can occur but is infrequent. Lesions in the urinary bladder most often arise in the trigone or bladder dome region. Involvement of bladder diverticula is also described.[60] Development following bladder augmentation has been reported.[61] At cystoscopy, the lesion has an exophytic appearance.

Villous adenoma is treated by transurethral resection or local resection. If the lesion is a pure villous adenoma, complete local resection is curative. There is, however, a frequent association with adenocarcinoma, and without complete resection and examination of the lesion this possibility cannot be excluded.[59] In one series, 50% of cases had either in situ adenocarcinoma (17%) or invasive adenocarcinoma (33%) associated with the villous adenoma.[59]

Pathology

Villous adenoma in the bladder is morphologically identical to that occurring in the gastrointestinal tract. There are tall villous projections covered by an intestinal-type epithelium with variable numbers of goblet cells (Fig. 6-7). The nuclei are oval to fusiform, enlarged, and frequently pseudostratified with variable degrees of atypia (Fig. 6-8). Nucleoli can be prominent. Mitoses are present but are not frequent. In

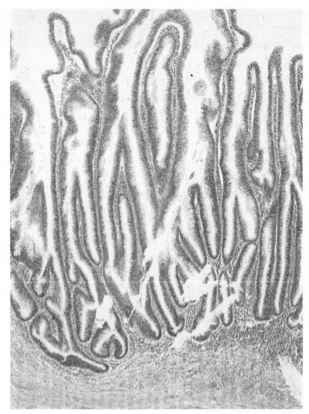

FIGURE 6-7 ■ Villous adenoma with tall villiform papillae.

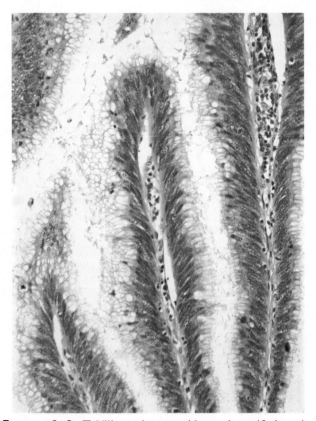

FIGURE 6-8 ■ Villous adenoma with pseudostratified mucin-secreting epithelium.

some cases the degree of atypia is sufficient to warrant the designation of adenocarcinoma in situ.[59] Cystitis glandularis can be present.[62] Acidic and neutral mucin is demonstrable in most cases.[58] The tumors have a similar immunohistochemical profile as in the gastrointestinal tract with cytokeratin 20 (100%) and carcinoembryonic antigen (CEA) positivity (89%).[58] Many also express cytokeratin 7 (56%). In one study, expression of prostate-specific membrane antigen (PSMA) was described in one case but without immunoreactivity for prostate-specific antigen (PSA) or prostate-specific acid phosphatase (PSAP).[63] There is also a single report of reactivity for PSA in a villous adenoma of the urachus.[64]

Differential Diagnosis

The major consideration is with adenocarcinoma, with either primary or secondary involvement from the gastrointestinal tract. Up to 50% of cases of villous adenoma have associated malignancy, and so, careful examination for areas of in situ and invasive adenocarcinoma is essential (Fig. 6-9). The invasive tumor typically has an enteric pattern with infiltrating glands and reactive stromal desmoplasia. The presence of glands with a wreath-like arrangement with central necrosis also indicates malignant transformation. In reporting a diagnosis of villous adenoma in biopsy or transurethral resection specimens, a note should always be added that the possibility of adenocarcinoma can only be excluded by complete resection and microscopic evaluation of the entire tumor.

Papillary urothelial carcinoma with villoglandular differentiation should also be considered in the differential diagnosis.[65] These are papillary urothelial carcinomas where the covering epithelium includes mucin-secreting cells, often with intraepithelial gland formation, mimicking an intestinal-type epithelium. This is almost always a partial change with other areas of the papillae having more a typical urothelial surface. The papillae are branching and irregular in length without the tall villous architecture of villous adenoma.

Squamous Papilloma

Clinical Features

Squamous papilloma is an uncommon lesion in the urinary bladder.[66,67] It is more common in women than men (female:male ratio of 1.5:1). They can occur over a wide age range with a mean age of 62 years (range, 28 to 82 years). There should not be a history of urogenital condylomata. They may be asymptomatic or present with hematuria. At cystoscopy, these may appear as erythematous areas, plaque-like, or as exophytic papillary lesions. In the series reported by Guo et al.,[67] one of four patients had a history of papillary urothelial neoplasia and subsequently developed additional urothelial neoplasms. Cheng et al.[66] included two patients with a history of urothelial neoplasia in their series of seven cases of squamous papilloma. Cases such as these suggest that some squamous papillomas represent low-grade papillary urothelial tumors with squamous differentiation.

Pathology

The lesion is exophytic with true papillary projections covered entirely by squamous epithelium (Fig. 6-10). The squamous epithelium is essentially normal in appearance. There is no koilocytotic atypia. These do not contain HPV DNA and are diploid.[66] There is no overexpression of p53; there is expression of epidermal growth factor receptor (EGFR).[66,67]

Differential Diagnosis

The differential diagnosis includes verrucous squamous hyperplasia, condyloma acuminatum, papillary urothelial neoplasia with squamous differentiation, and well-differentiated squamous cell carcinoma. Verrucous squamous hyperplasia is characterized by keratinizing squamous epithelium with hyperkeratosis and a spike-like proliferation rather than the well-developed papillae of squamous papilloma.[67]

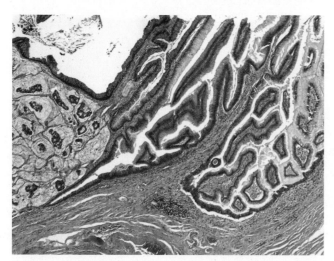

FIGURE 6-9 ■ Villous adenoma with associated mucinous adenocarcinoma.

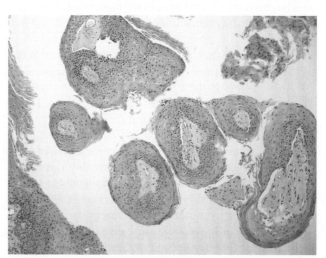

FIGURE 6-10 ■ Squamous papilloma with fine papillary structures covered by keratinizing squamous epithelium.

Condyloma acuminatum occurs in patients with genital condyloma or in patients who are immunosuppressed.[66,68] The lesions tend be more sessile with less well-defined papillae, thickened epithelium, and koilocytic atypia. The lesions contain HPV DNA and many overexpress p53.[66] In papillary urothelial neoplasia, there is often a history of prior papillary tumors, and the covering epithelium has areas more typical of urothelium. In the setting of known urothelial neoplasia, the diagnosis of squamous papilloma should be restricted to cases where the surface epithelium is uniformly benign squamous in type. Squamous cell carcinoma is typically a solid, invasive tumor. Infrequently there can be a component with papillary architecture, but the covering epithelium is neoplastic in nature and even in low-grade tumors would not have a benign appearance.

EPITHELIAL TUMORS—MALIGNANT

Urothelial Carcinoma

Epidemiology

Bladder cancer is estimated to be the ninth most common cancer worldwide (an estimated 357,000 cases in 2002) and the thirteenth most common cause of death from cancer (145,000 deaths in 2002).[69] It is the seventh most common malignancy of men and the seventeenth most common tumor in women worldwide.[70] There are significant geographic differences with an approximately 10-fold difference in incidence and death rates between countries. The highest rates of bladder cancer are found in southern European countries (Spain, Italy) and Egypt, closely followed by Israel, the United States, Denmark, and the United Kingdom. The lowest rates are in the Far East, including Japan, China, and Korea. The worldwide age-adjusted mortality rates for bladder cancer are 2 to 10 per 100,000 for males and 0.5 to 4 per 100,000 for females.[70] Overall bladder cancer is approximately four times more common in men than in women.[71] This has been largely attributed to the higher rate of smoking and more frequent occupational exposure to bladder carcinogens in men.[71]

In the United States, the most recent data estimate is that there will be 72,570 new cases of bladder cancer diagnosed in 2013, with 54,610 of these in males and 17,960 in females.[72] The estimated number of cancer deaths for 2013 is 15,210 with 10,820 and 4,390 in males and females, respectively.[72] Bladder cancer is most common in Caucasians (excluding Hispanic Caucasians). Despite the lower incidence of bladder cancer in African Americans the mortality rate is significantly higher.[73] This has been partly attributed to tumors being higher stage at diagnosis, but this is not considered to completely explain the observed differences.[73]

Bladder cancer is generally a disease of older individuals with most patients being diagnosed in the seventh decade or older. The tumor can occur in younger individuals.[74] In patients under the age of 20 years, the tumors are almost all low grade with no high-grade tumors identified in the review by Paner et al.[74] The rate of recurrence in this age group is significantly lower (3%) than would be expected for papillary tumors with progression being very rare.[74]

Etiopathogenesis

The most important risk factors for the development of bladder cancer are tobacco smoke and occupational exposure to carcinogens (Table 6-3). Tobacco smoke is estimated to be responsible for 30% to 50% of cases of bladder cancer.[75–77] Smokers have a two- to six-fold increased risk of developing bladder cancer over those who have never smoked.[75–77] Stopping smoking decreases the risk of bladder cancer development, and smoking filtered cigarettes confers a lower risk than smoking nonfiltered types. Cigarette smoke contains numerous carcinogenic compounds including 4-aminophenol (considered the most important), β-naphthylamine, benzene, cadmium, chromium, radon, vinyl chloride, nickel, and many others.[71] Changes in worldwide smoking patterns are reflected in the changing incidences in bladder cancer.

Occupational exposure to carcinogens is estimated to account for up to 20% of bladder cancer cases.[78] The best documented occupational carcinogens are β-naphthylamine, 4-aminobiphenyl, and benzidine, most often associated with textile dye and rubber industries. With the banning of these compounds in Western countries, these no longer account for a significant percentage of occupation-related bladder cancers. Increased risk for bladder cancer has been reported in a wide range of diverse industries with a varying degree of evidence. In the Western world, even for those that have been most often documented, the relative risks have been low, most often in the range of 1.1 to 1.2.[71]

Table 6-3 ■ UROTHELIAL CARCINOMA: IMPLICATED CARCINOGENIC AGENTS

Tobacco (smoking)
  4-Aminophenol
  β-Naphthylamine
  Benzene
  Others
Occupational
  Benzidine
  β-Naphthylamine
  Chlorinated aliphatic hydrocarbons
  Arylamines
  4-Aminobiphenyl
  Others
Drugs
  Phenacetin
  Cyclophosphamide
Infectious
  Schistosoma haematobium
Dietary
  Nitrites (weak evidence)
Other

There have been extensive analyses of the relationship of drinking water to bladder cancer. Many of these have focused on chlorinated water and the carcinogenic risk of chlorination by products such as trihalomethane.[79,80] In a recent review, Wu et al.[71] concluded that although exposure to chlorinated drinking water might increase the risk of bladder cancer, this is relatively small. Contamination of drinking water with arsenic has been shown to be associated with an increased risk of bladder cancer.[81] There is a dose/effect relationship, and the very low level of arsenic in drinking water in developed countries is not considered to be an important carcinogenic factor. Finally there has been interest in the volume of fluid intake based on the hypothesis that high volumes of liquid would result in dilution of excreted carcinogens and thereby reduce carcinogenic risk. To date, studies of this possible effect have not yielded consistent results.[71]

Dietary factors have been the subject of intense interest. Although studies have not been entirely consistent, the data have generally supported a protective effect for high consumption of fruit and vegetables.[82,83] It has been suggested that this is an effect of antioxidants that detoxify excreted metabolites. In one meta-analysis, diet low in fruit intake was associated with an increased risk of bladder cancer.[84] In a prospective analysis of women, however, no association between intake of fruits, vegetables, or vitamins was found.[85] In addition, there has been weak evidence linking nitrite and meat-associated nitrates with bladder cancer risk.[86] Studies of pesticides have failed to identify a relationship between pesticide exposure and bladder cancer.[87] No other dietary factors, including artificial sweeteners and coffee, have been demonstrated to have a relationship to bladder cancer development.

Infectious agents are an important contributor to bladder cancer development. In particular the strong relationship between *Schistosoma haematobium* and the development of bladder cancer is well known.[88,89] This has been most strongly related to the development of squamous cell carcinoma,[90] but other histologic types including urothelial carcinoma and adenocarcinoma are also more frequent in areas where *Schistosoma* infection is endemic. There is no evidence that viral infection plays a role in bladder cancer development.[91]

Hereditary factors are not considered to be a major contributor to bladder cancer.[92] There have been a number of reports of familial clustering of bladder cancer cases, but these have largely been isolated reports. Some of these have been associated with an early age of bladder cancer development supporting a significant hereditary component.[92] The reported higher risk in first-degree relatives of bladder cancer patients also suggests a hereditary component, but the importance relative to other environmental factors is unclear.[93,94] Urothelial cancers have been found in certain hereditary syndromes such as Costello syndrome,[95] Lynch syndrome,[96] and the Muir-Torre syndrome.[97]

Bladder cancer risk has also been associated with a number of other factors including drug exposure (cyclophosphamide, phenacetin)[98,99] and radiation therapy.[100] Despite

considerable interest, exposure to hair dyes has now largely been eliminated as a risk factor.[101] Other causes of long-standing irritation of the bladder mucosa such as chronic urinary tract infections, lithiasis, and nonfunctioning bladders of any cause have been linked to the development of bladder cancer.

Genetics

Studies of the genetics of urothelial carcinoma have led to the development of a model of tumorigenesis that includes distinct pathways for papillary and nonpapillary neoplasia (Fig. 6-11). Both pathways can result in the development of invasive high-grade urothelial carcinoma that has the capacity to metastasize and result in the death of the patient. In this section, these pathways and the relevant genetic changes are briefly reviewed.[102,103]

The major genes implicated in the transformation of normal urothelium into low-grade papillary neoplasia include *H-Ras*, *FGFR3*, *PI3K*, and 9p deletion. Abnormalities in the *H-Ras* gene are most often the result of mutations, in particular those involving codon 12.[104] These are activating mutations and are found in approximately 15% of noninvasive papillary tumors. Mutations in the fibroblast growth factor receptor-3 (*FGFR3*) gene are present in 60% to 80% of low-grade noninvasive papillary tumors.[35,105,106] The rate is much lower in high-grade invasive carcinomas and in urothelial CIS.[35] It has been reported that the absence of *FGFR3* gene mutations is a predictor of a higher likelihood of progression.[36,107] Since the *FGFR3* and *H-Ras* genes are in the same pathway, they are considered to be mutually exclusive events in bladder cancer.[108] Mutations in the *PI3-kinase* gene (*PIK3CA*) have been described in a subset of approximately 15% of low-grade papillary tumors with the highest frequency in papillary neoplasms of low malignant potential.[109] Some tumors harbor more than one of these genetic abnormalities, and it has been suggested that tumors with multiple abnormalities are associated with progression to high-grade tumors.[102]

Loss of heterozygosity studies have demonstrated abnormalities in both 9p and 9q in over 50% of bladder tumors.[103] In many tumors, there is loss of an entire copy of the chromosome. Implicated in the 9p abnormalities are the *CDKN2A* and *CDKN2B* genes, the former coding for the p16 protein.[110] Loss of heterozygosity studies has demonstrated abnormality of the *CDKN2A* gene in up to 60% of papillary tumors.[111] Mutations in the *INK4* gene and deletions of 9q (including the *PTCH*, *DBC1*, and *TSC1* genes) are frequently present in high-grade papillary tumors and are believed to be important in the progression of low- to high-grade papillary tumors.[112,113] Inactivating mutations of the TSC1 gene have been found in approximately 10% of bladder tumors.[114] Mutations of the *PTCH* gene are infrequent.

A second pathway in the development of invasive carcinoma is through urothelial CIS. The major genes implicated in this pathway are the tumor suppressor genes

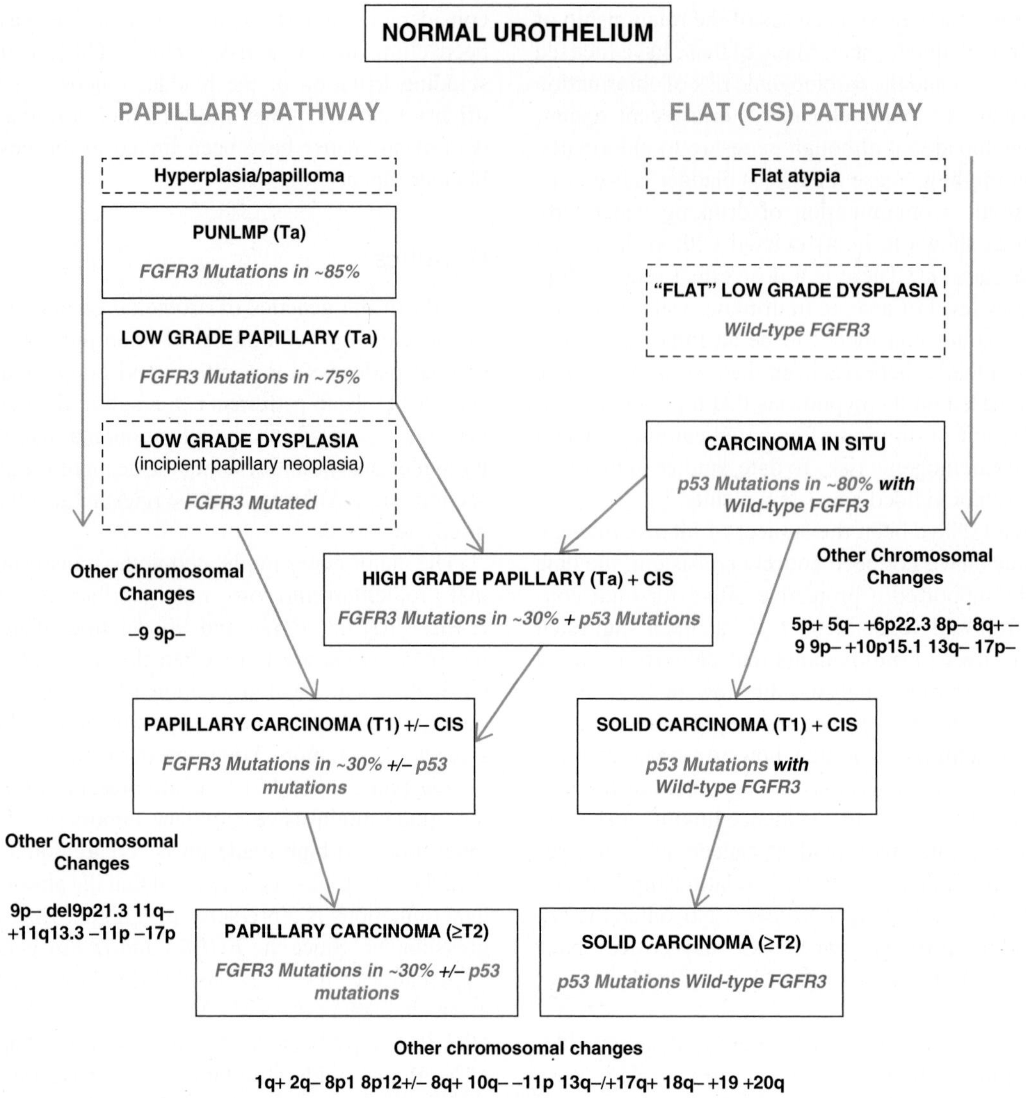

NORMAL UROTHELIUM

PAPILLARY PATHWAY

FLAT (CIS) PATHWAY

Hyperplasia/papilloma

Flat atypia

PUNLMP (Ta)

FGFR3 Mutations in ~85%

"FLAT" LOW GRADE DYSPLASIA

Wild-type FGFR3

LOW GRADE PAPILLARY (Ta)

FGFR3 Mutations in ~75%

LOW GRADE DYSPLASIA
(incipient papillary neoplasia)

FGFR3 Mutated

CARCINOMA IN SITU

*p53 Mutations in ~80% **with** Wild-type FGFR3*

Other Chromosomal Changes

–9 9p–

HIGH GRADE PAPILLARY (Ta) + CIS

FGFR3 Mutations in ~30% + p53 Mutations

Other Chromosomal Changes

5p+ 5q– +6p22.3 8p– 8q+ – 9 9p– +10p15.1 13q– 17p–

PAPILLARY CARCINOMA (T1) +/– CIS

FGFR3 Mutations in ~30% +/– p53 mutations

SOLID CARCINOMA (T1) + CIS

*p53 Mutations **with** Wild-type FGFR3*

Other Chromosomal Changes

9p– del9p21.3 11q– +11q13.3 –11p –17p

PAPILLARY CARCINOMA (≥T2)

FGFR3 Mutations in ~30% +/– p53 mutations

SOLID CARCINOMA (≥T2)

p53 Mutations Wild-type FGFR3

Other chromosomal changes

1q+ 2q– 8p1 8p12+/– 8q+ 10q– –11p 13q–/+17q+ 18q– +19 +20q

FIGURE 6-11 ■ Pathways for the development of urothelial tumors.

TP53, retinoblastoma (*RB*), and *PTEN*.[102] Both the *RB* and *TP53* genes have generated intense interest in bladder cancer. *RB* gene deletions are common in high-grade bladder tumors and have been associated with an aggressive clinical course.[115] The absence of RB protein or inactivation of RB protein affects multiple critical pathways including the E2F family of transcription factors. As in the case of *RB*, the importance of the *TP53* tumor suppressor gene has been extensively studied in bladder cancer. *TP53* mutations are present in up to 70% of urothelial carcinomas and are related to high-grade and high-stage disease and also to poor clinical outcome.[116] Studies related to loss of chromosome 9 in CIS have had variable results[103]; in one report chromosome 9 loss was significantly higher in primary CIS than in CIS associated with papillary tumors.[117] The *TP53* mutation analysis demonstrated a similar relationship suggesting that these might represent two different types of CIS.[103] *FGFR3* mutations are not present in primary CIS and are infrequent in CIS associated with papillary tumors.[106,118]

Clinical Features

The single most frequent presenting symptom of bladder cancer is painless hematuria, present in around 85% of patients. When microscopic hematuria is included, almost all patients have some degree of hematuria. Hematuria can, however, be intermittent, and so a negative examination of the urine for hematuria does not exclude a bladder tumor. In general, most urologists recommend cystoscopy for even a single episode of unexplained hematuria for patients in the right age group for bladder cancer. The latter would include any patient over the age of 60 years or younger patients with a history of smoking or exposure to other significant risk factors.

The second most common presentation is with a group of symptoms that includes urinary frequency, urgency, and irritative voiding symptoms. This group of symptoms is often indicative of an invasive carcinoma or diffuse CIS. Less frequent presentations include those related to ureteral obstruction, a pelvic mass, or obstruction of pelvic lymphatics. Least common are presentation as a metastasis of unknown origin or general cancer cachexia.

Diagnosis

Urine Markers

Ultimately the diagnosis of bladder cancer relies on direct visualization of the lesion with tissue diagnosis. Prior to tissue diagnosis, there is reliance on a series of markers evaluable in urine specimens and the use of cytology for the identification of malignant cells (Table 6-4).

The current practice of urology includes numerous tools for the diagnosis of bladder neoplasia through application to urine specimens. Some of these depend on bladder tumor antigens (BTA) and others on determination of gene expression or gene copy number. Interested readers are referred to more comprehensive reviews of these tests.[123,124,137] The role of these tests is an area of active discussion and debate in terms of both effectiveness and cost.[138–141]

Among the more commonly utilized tests are the BTA-Stat and BTA-TRAK tests that are both FDA-approved for surveillance. These detect the presence of complement factor H–related protein by immunoassay and a standard enzyme-linked immunosorbent assay (ELISA) method, respectively. These have overall sensitivities in the 17% to 89% range and specificities in the 50% to 86% range.[124,142] The sensitivity is related to tumor grade, stage, and size. Although overall sensitivity is slightly better than cytology,[123] the frequency of false-positive tests is a significant problem and has limited the value of these tests.[137]

Another popular test is NMP22, which is also FDA approved, and based on the detection of nuclear matrix proteins. Nuclear matrix protein 22 is a regulator of mitosis that is increased up to 25-fold in carcinoma cells compared to normal urothelial cells. The first NMP22 test utilized a quantitative sandwich ELISA method; the current BladderChek test is a point of care test that utilizes monoclonal antibodies. This test has reported sensitivity in the 47% to 70% range

with specificities in the 40% to 87% range depending on the clinical setting.[124,137,142] In most studies, it has fared better than cytology in terms of sensitivity but lacks the same degree of specificity.

Several other soluble and other urine markers that have been evaluated include BLCA-1, BLCA-4, HA-HAse, cytokeratins, telomerase, and survivin.[124,137,143] Although some of these appear quite promising at the time of this writing (HA-HAse, survivin), their eventual usefulness remains uncertain.

The ImmunoCyt/uCyt tests are FDA-approved and are dependent on detection of fluorescein-labeled antibodies to three proteins, M344, LDQ10, and 19A211. The M344 and LDQ10 antibodies detect mucin-like antigens present in approximately 70% of pTa and pT1 urothelial carcinomas.[144] The 19A211 antibody detects a high molecular weight form of CEA expressed in approximately 90% of pTa and pT1 tumors.[145] The test has been promulgated as an adjunct to urine cytology and is generally performed by personnel in the cytology department. Sensitivity has averaged 90% (range of 57% to 100%) and specificity 74% (range of 64% to 95%).[124] The major roles for the test have been in the detection of upper tract tumors, in the identification of high-grade lesions not visualized at cystoscopy, and in detecting recurrences.[124] The test is limited by the need for performance in a specialized laboratory with specialized equipment and a high degree of expertise. FDA approval is only for use in conjunction with cytology.

UroVysion is an FDA-approved test that has also enjoyed widespread application. Initial FDA approval was for monitoring patients with bladder cancer for recurrence and later for diagnosis of patients with hematuria suspected of having bladder cancer. This test uses fluorescence in situ hybridization to evaluate exfoliated cells in the urine for aneuploidy of chromosomes 3, 7, and 17 as well as loss of 9p21. Use of multiple markers is aimed at improving sensitivity. Studies on paraffin-embedded tissue specimens have reported the detection of abnormalities in 93% of dysplasias, 91% of CIS, and 100% of invasive carcinomas.[146] In the same study, 17% of normal urothelial samples, hyperplasia, and reactive atypia also resulted in abnormal findings.[146] In urine specimens, sensitivity has ranged from 39% to 97% (average 74%) with low sensitivity in low-grade tumors.[124,135,147] The specificity has been high with reported results in the 89% to 100% range.[124,135,148] For high-grade tumors and CIS, the sensitivity has been in the 83% to 97% range with a high degree of specificity (89% to 96%). In the majority of studies, in all clinical settings, FISH tests have outperformed cytology.[136] The suggested value for this test has been in the setting of the workup of hematuria,[148] detection of upper tract tumors, detection of tumor recurrences,[136] and in cases of atypical urine cytology specimens.[149–151] A limiting factor of this test has remained its requirement for specialized equipment, labor intensiveness requiring a high degree of expertise, and the high cost.[137]

Table 6-4 ■ URINE-BASED MARKERS FOR BLADDER CANCER

Mucin-like proteins and CEA (ImmunoCyt)[119]
Nuclear matrix protein 22 (NMP22)[120,121]
Other nuclear matrix proteins (BLCA-4)[122]
Complement factor H-related protein (BTA-stat, BTA-TRAK)[123,124]
Hyaluronic acid and hyaluronidase (HA-ase)[125]
Cytokeratins (CYFRA 21-1)[126,127]
Survivin[128,129]
Telomerase[127,130]
Fibroblast growth factor receptor-3[131]
Vascular endothelial growth factor[127,132]
DNA ploidy[133]
Microsatellites[134]
Chromosomal abnormalities (UroVysion)[135,136]

Cytology

Urine cytology has played a major role in the diagnosis and monitoring of bladder carcinoma for many years. With the increasing availability of a wide variety of alternative urine-based tests, the role of cytology as the gold standard is being challenged. Specimens available for evaluation include voided urine, urine obtained by catheter, urine obtained at cystoscopy, and bladder washings. Each of these has its own advantages and disadvantages.

The value of urine cytology is dependent on the specific situation in which it is being applied. It is particularly valuable in the diagnosis and monitoring of high-grade tumors. Although published data on sensitivity and specificity are highly variable, it is reasonable to say that urine cytology has moderate to high sensitivity for the detection of high-grade tumors and is highly specific. On the other hand, urine cytology is much less useful in the setting of low-grade disease. Here the sensitivity is much lower although the specificity is largely retained. From a clinical standpoint, this weakness is not a substantive issue as low-grade tumors are not life threatening and there is little if any value in detecting them before they are visible to the urologist.

One other limitation of urine cytology is the inability to identify the source of the malignant cells when present. Tumors in the upper urinary tracts and the urethra will shed cells into the urine. In patients without visible lesions in the urethra or urinary bladder, selective sampling from the upper tracts is used in an effort to localize the origin of the malignant cells.

Cystoscopy

Cystourethroscopy is the mainstay of bladder cancer diagnosis and for some tumors, treatment.[152] Advances in the optical technology used have resulted in significant improvement in the diagnosis of bladder neoplasia.[153] Both rigid and flexible instruments have advantages and disadvantages. The major advantages of the rigid cystourethroscope are the superior optics; the larger working channel that allows for use of a wider range of accessory instruments and increased water flow, improving visualization; and the ease of manipulation. Flexible cystourethroscopes provide greater patient comfort, more flexibility in patient positioning, and ability to inspect the bladder surface from more angles.[154] The procedure can be performed in the office setting or in endoscopic suites depending somewhat on the indication. In the outpatient setting, the procedure is well tolerated and does allow for the performance of biopsies and fulguration of small recurrent tumors.[155] Intraurethral and intravesical topical anesthesia are sufficient for control of discomfort.

The procedure allows for direct visualization of the bladder mucosa, collection of cytologic specimens, and biopsy of any abnormalities. In the evaluation of hematuria, if the source is in the urinary bladder it can usually be detected or if it is coming from the upper tracts, that can also often be determined. The published sensitivity and specificity for detecting urothelial tumors have shown considerable variation and depend on the indication. For follow-up of patients with known papillary neoplasia, sensitivity and specificity are generally in the 85% to 95% and 90% to 100% range, respectively. The sensitivity is greater for papillary than for flat lesions. Because of the latter, routine biopsy of normal-appearing mucosa has been advocated in order to enhance the detection of CIS.[156,157] In more contemporary studies, a low yield has been reported for such biopsies.[158] Recent advances in the application of photodynamic diagnosis that significantly improve the detection of CIS will also impact the routine performance of random biopsies.[153] Experienced urologists have a high degree of reliability in predicting the pathologic features of papillary tumors based on the cystoscopy findings.[159] Evaluation of the upper tracts is also possible through this procedure by the performance of retrograde pyelography, selective sampling of material from the upper tracts for cytologic examination, and direct visualization by ureteroscopy.

There have also been advances in the type of light source utilized to evaluate the bladder mucosa. White light cystoscopy has been the standard and remains most widely used. The use of fluorescein labeling with 5-aminolevulinic acid and hexaminolevulinic acid has been extensively studied and in general has resulted in significantly improved detection of CIS.[160] The sensitivity for the identification of CIS increases from 56%–68% to 92%–97%.[161] The diagnosis of papillary lesions is also improved.[162] Studies have also demonstrated an improvement in the transurethral resection of visible tumors with a decrease in residual tumor from 25%–53% to 5%–33%.[153]

This method does, however, yield a high rate of false-positive findings, particularly in the presence of inflammation.[153,163] This limits the value of this technique following BCG therapy.

More recently narrow band imaging cystoscopy has been evaluated as potentially being superior in the detection of bladder tumors.[164,165] Results have been variable, and it remains to be determined whether this or other alternatives being tested will ultimately change the standard use of white light. The application of real-time Raman spectroscopy and optical coherence tomography to enhance the prediction of tissue diagnosis are under investigation and appears promising.[153]

Biopsy and Transurethral Resection

Methods for sampling of bladder lesions include hot and cold cup biopsy, strip biopsy, and transurethral resection. Evaluation of flat lesions largely relies on the hot and cold cup biopsy methods. The cold cup biopsy does not use electrocautery, and so, thermal tissue artifacts are avoided.[166]

Transurethral resection of lesions in the bladder is performed to (i) remove the entire visible abnormality as both a diagnostic and therapeutic procedure, (ii) obtain a larger sample of a lesion than is possible by a biopsy technique, and (iii) obtain tissue deeper to the lesion to allow for staging of the tumor. The general approach to resection of a tumor (TURBT, transurethral resection of bladder tumor) is to first remove the bulk or entirety of the tumor and second to sample the base of the tumor. These may be submitted as a single specimen or as two separately designated specimens. In situations where the complete resection of the lesion is not possible or not indicated, the urologist should be removing sufficient tissue for accurate diagnosis and staging (meaning evaluation of the muscularis propria). The procedure is usually performed with an instrument that cauterizes the remaining surface as the tissue fragments are removed. Depending on instrument settings, this can result in a considerable degree of artifact that can hamper interpretation of tissue specimens removed. The degree of tissue artifact is not related to the use of unipolar or bipolar energy.[167]

Pathology

Flat Lesions

As discussed above, both our genetic understanding of urothelial carcinoma and the clinical behavior and treatment of these tumors have led to a general classification of urothelial carcinoma into flat and papillary lesions. Flat lesions refer to neoplastic transformation of the urothelium that is not associated with the formation of papillary structures. The following sections discuss the two categories of noninvasive neoplastic change of the urothelium, urothelial dysplasia and urothelial CIS. In the past, there have been many proposed classifications of flat lesions that have included multiple categories such as low-grade dysplasia, moderate dysplasia, severe dysplasia, and CIS as distinct categories. Studies of reproducibility have demonstrated the poor performance of pathologists in applying these types of schemes.[168,169] Stratification into a three-tier system (benign, dysplasia, CIS) enhances overall reproducibility particularly in the CIS category; the diagnosis of dysplasia, however, remains problematic.[168] Changes in the management of patients with flat lesions have also impacted on the value of stratification of flat lesions into multiple tiers. With the 1998 and 2004 WHO/ISUP classifications, the category of neoplastic flat lesions has been simplified into a two-tier system of low-grade (dysplasia) and high-grade lesions (CIS).[8,14]

The current classification of flat urothelial lesions also includes nonneoplastic categories of urothelial hyperplasia, reactive urothelial atypia, and a category for lesions that cannot be placed into a neoplastic or nonneoplastic category with certainty (atypia of unknown significance). Detailed discussions of specific patterns of urothelial atypia are presented in Chapter 5 and will not be repeated here. Rather, a brief review of salient morphologic features important in the distinction from urothelial dysplasia and urothelial CIS is presented.

Urothelial Hyperplasia

Historically, the term "hyperplasia" has been equated with counting cell layers and specifically considering the epithelium to be hyperplastic if there were more than seven cell layers. It is well recognized that the apparent number of cell layers in the normal urothelium is variable and dependent on the state of contraction of the bladder wall. Reactive hyperplasia can result from a wide range of causes of bladder irritation. It can also be present in the setting of known urothelial neoplasia including both flat and papillary lesions. There is no evidence to suggest that flat urothelial hyperplasia is a preneoplastic process when diagnosed in isolation of bladder neoplasia. In patients with known papillary tumors, there have been some data to indicate that flat hyperplasia in this setting contains genetic abnormalities, indicating that this may be an early manifestation of low-grade papillary neoplasia.[170] In this study, chromosome 9 abnormalities similar to those in the associated papillary tumor were present in 70% of biopsies with flat hyperplasia and in 50% with histologically normal urothelium.[170] The presence of *FGFR3* mutations has also been demonstrated in urothelial hyperplasia in the setting of papillary neoplasia.[171] These data indicate that urothelial hyperplasia may be an early manifestation of low-grade papillary neoplasms.

The current classification recognizes hyperplasia when there is a "markedly thickened mucosa without atypia." Counting cell layers is not recommended. The urothelium retains a normal architecture with the epithelial cells having elongated nuclei oriented perpendicular to the basement membrane (Fig. 6-12). The umbrella cell layer is present. The nuclei may be slightly enlarged but otherwise are cytologically normal with nuclear grooves preserved. Mitoses can be found but are largely restricted to the basal layer (Table 6-5). Hyperplasia can have a pseudopapillary architecture with some tenting of the mucosa, but these areas lack the formation of a true central fibrovascular core.

Reactive Urothelial Atypia

In the presence of acute and/or chronic inflammation, the urothelium shows a wide range of reactive changes. There

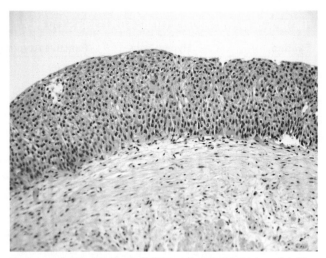

FIGURE 6-12 ■ Urothelial hyperplasia with thickened epithelium lacking any architectural or cytologic atypia.

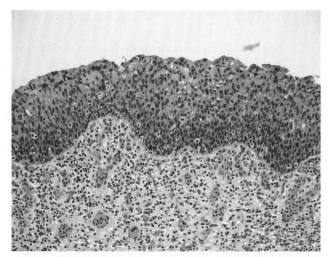

FIGURE 6-13 ■ Reactive urothelial atypia with thickened epithelium, no architectural atypia, and mildly enlarged nuclei, many containing small nucleoli.

is usually a history of instrumentation, infection, lithiasis, or some other cause of irritation. Urothelial atypia can also result from treatment with intravesical agents (thiotepa, mitomycin-C, BCG), systemic chemotherapeutic drugs (cyclophosphamide), or radiation therapy. Some patterns of atypia are associated with specific etiologies (see Chapter 5).[172] Available data in the literature indicate that reactive atypia is not associated with the subsequent development of urothelial carcinoma.[173]

In reactive atypia, the epithelium may or may not be thickened. Although a thickened epithelium is typically associated with a reactive process, CIS can also produce a thicker than normal epithelium. Nuclei are uniformly enlarged, vesicular, and may have a prominent usually centrally located nucleolus (Fig. 6-13). The degree of enlargement is, however, significantly less than is typical of CIS (Table 6-5). The nuclei often have a round shape. Mitoses can be frequent and are

located in the lower epithelial layers. The normal architecture is largely preserved though there may be some variation in nuclear orientation. The orientation can also be made unclear by the rounding of the nuclei resulting in no obvious perpendicular orientation to the basement membrane. The cytoplasm can be normal in appearance or have either increased eosinophilia or basophilia. Cytoplasmic clearing or vacuolization can be a feature (Table 6-5). Inflammation is almost always present and often obscures the epithelial stromal interface. Intraepithelial inflammatory cells are a feature of reactive atypia and are infrequently found in urothelial CIS.

Atypia of Unknown Significance

One of the gray zones in any consideration of intraepithelial lesions is between reactive atypia and true neoplastic (dysplastic) alterations. Reproducibility studies have clearly demonstrated the lack of consistency in this particular area. This category was created to include those instances where a lesion cannot be confidently placed in the reactive versus dysplastic categories.[8]

Histologically, there is usually an inflammatory background. The degree of cytologic atypia is judged to be outside of the accepted range for reactive processes although this possibility cannot be excluded. Re-evaluation after inflammation subsides may resolve the problem, particularly in the follow-up of patients with known urothelial neoplasia who have been treated with intravesical therapy. In one study, none of the 35 patients diagnosed with atypia of unknown significance developed urothelial neoplasia with a median 3.5 years of follow-up.[173]

Urothelial Dysplasia (Low-grade Intraurothelial Neoplasia)

This category also suffers from a significant problem in diagnostic reproducibility.[168,169] Previous classification schemes have included grading systems for urothelial dysplasia, but the current approach is to place neoplastic intraepithelial

Table 6-5 ■ MORPHOLOGIC FEATURES OF FLAT LESIONS

Feature	Hyperplasia	Reactive Atypia	Dysplasia	Carcinoma In Situ
Thickness	Thickened	Variable	Variable	Variable
Architecture	Normal	Normal	Mildly abnormal	Disorganized
Pagetoid spread	No	No	No	Yes
Denudation	No	Variable	Variable	Commonly present
Nuclear size	Normal or slight enlargement	Normal or slight enlargement	Enlarged	Markedly enlarged
Nuclear shape	Regular	Regular or rounded	Slight irregularities	Pleomorphic
Nuclear membrane	Smooth	Smooth	Some irregularities—notching	Irregular with thickening
Chromatin	Fine	Fine	Variable hyperchromasia	Hyperchromatic
Nucleoli	Inconspicuous	Large	Small or inconspicuous	Large, may be multiple
Mitoses	Infrequent	May be common—basal location	Infrequent	Frequent including abnormal forms
Cytoplasm	Uniform	Uniform or vacuolated	Uniform	Uniform

lesions into only two categories: urothelial dysplasia and urothelial CIS. Urothelial dysplasia has been divided into primary dysplasia for when the lesion is diagnosed de novo and secondary dysplasia when it is found in the setting of known urothelial neoplasia.[174] There is evidence, largely genetic, that it shares some abnormalities with CIS and therefore likely represents a precursor lesion.[175]

The natural history of lesions with dysplastic features of a lesser degree than the moderate to severe categories is unknown.[176] Given the difficulties with reproducibility of the diagnosis and changes in the reporting of these lesions over the past several decades, it is difficult to interpret the published data regarding the natural history of this lesion. It is most often diagnosed in the context of known urothelial neoplasia. In the latter group, urothelial dysplasia can be identified in the flat epithelium of 22% to almost 100% of cases.[177–180] Studies that have applied the 1998 WHO/ISUP criteria for primary dysplasia have indicated a 15% to 19% risk of developing cancer with a mean follow-up of 4.9 to 8.2 years.[173,181]

The limitations of diagnostic criteria and reproducibility also make it difficult to interpret published data on the genetics of urothelial dysplasia. Aberrant expression of cytokeratin 20 in the midlayers of the urothelium has been described.[182–184] Studies have also described overexpression of p53 protein and increased proliferation as indicated by the expression of Ki67.[183] Loss of CD44 expression occurs in dysplasia.[184] Studies utilizing loss of heterozygosity have demonstrated abnormalities of chromosome 9 in these lesions.[185] These findings have supported the hypothesis that urothelial dysplasia is related to CIS and does represent a neoplastic process.

Histologically, the epithelium is of variable thickness, but most often it is within the normal range. The nuclei are irregularly enlarged and tend to be more oval or rounded than normal. In general, the degree of enlargement is significantly less than in CIS. There is some degree of disruption of the normal architecture with variable degrees of loss of polarity and focal nuclear crowding (Fig. 6-14). There is mild nuclear hyperchromasia and pleomorphism but not to the degree seen in CIS. The nuclear membranes are irregularly thickened and notching and sharp angulation can be present. Nucleoli when present are small and inconspicuous. Mitoses can be present but are few and limited to the lower epithelial layers. Cytoplasmic changes may be present with increased eosinophilia. Overall, the features are those of a neoplastic atypia but fall short of the criteria for CIS outlined below. Denudation can be present but is much less frequent than in CIS.

In some instances, the features resemble those of the urothelium present in low-grade papillary carcinoma. In the setting of papillary neoplasia, this may represent the earliest indication of the development of new papillary tumors (Fig. 6-15).[185]

Carcinoma In Situ (High-grade Intraurothelial Neoplasia)

The current classification recognized the need to expand the category of CIS to include lesions that had been graded in the moderate to severe dysplasia categories in previous systems. This change reflects current practice in major institutions treating bladder cancer. It also recognizes the general trend for underdiagnosis of higher-grade lesions.[16] There is further recognition that this is the most reproducible diagnostic category.[168,169] CIS is accepted as a precursor of invasive carcinoma.

CIS is most often seen in association with high-grade papillary or invasive urothelial carcinoma. De novo CIS accounts for only 1% to 3% of newly diagnosed cases of bladder cancer.[186–188] These patients are at significant risk for the development of invasive carcinoma. In contemporary series progression to invasive carcinoma occurs in up to 25% of patients and the cancer-specific survival is in the 75% to 85% range with long-term follow-up.[189–191] The presence of

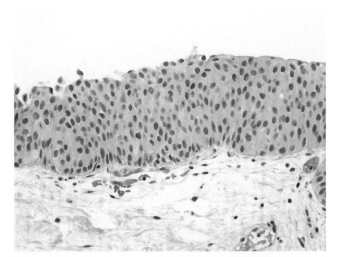

FIGURE 6-14 ■ Urothelial dysplasia with flat epithelium showing a mild degree of architectural and cytologic atypia.

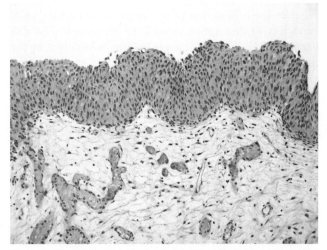

FIGURE 6-15 ■ Urothelial dysplasia with slight tenting of the surface.

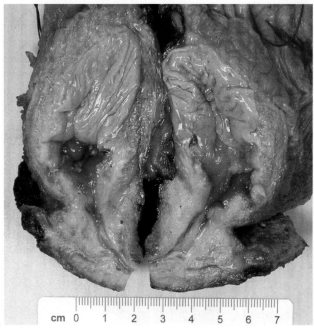

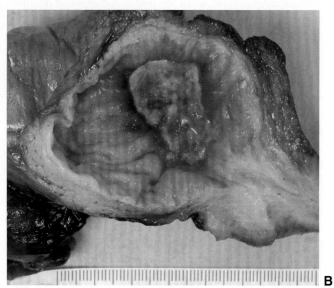

FIGURE 6-16 ■ Gross appearance of CIS localized to area around an invasive carcinoma **(A)** and more diffusely involving the mucosa **(B)**.

CIS of the bladder in patients with other urothelial tumors is also important.[192] The risk of having CIS in the upper tract is three- to four-fold higher and in the prostatic urethra is seven-fold higher than when a bladder tumor does not have associated CIS.[193,194] For patients with noninvasive papillary tumors, the presence of CIS is associated with a higher risk of recurrence and progression.[195] In cases with lamina propria invasion (T1), the presence of CIS also indicates an increased risk of progression to muscle-invasive disease and has been used as one of the indications for early cystectomy.[195,196]

Grossly, CIS most often appears as an erythematous area (Fig. 6-16). This can be focal, multifocal, or diffuse. In some cases, the mucosa has a velvety or granular character.

The histologic diagnosis of CIS fundamentally requires the recognition of cytologically malignant cells. A variety of descriptive terms have been applied to CIS (Table 6-6).[15,172,176,197] These are helpful in highlighting the morphologic variability of the lesion but have no clinical significance. Histologically, CIS is characterized by

architectural disorder with haphazard orientation of nuclei and nuclear crowding and clustering (Fig. 6-17). There is nuclear pleomorphism with significant nuclear enlargement, hyperchromasia, and single to multiple nucleoli. The atypical cells need not involve the full thickness of the epithelium, and at the minimum single malignant cells growing in a pagetoid fashion are sufficient for the diagnosis (Fig. 6-18). Individual cells tend to show marked cytologic atypia but an increased nuclear-to-cytoplasmic ratio is not a prerequisite (not present in the large cell type of CIS).

In the large cell patterns of CIS, the malignant cells have moderate to abundant cytoplasm that often has increased

Table 6-6 ■ MORPHOLOGIC PATTERNS OF UROTHELIAL CIS
• Small cell
• Large cell
• Denuding (denuding cystitis)
• Pagetoid
• Undermining
• CIS with glandular differentiation
• CIS with squamous differentiation

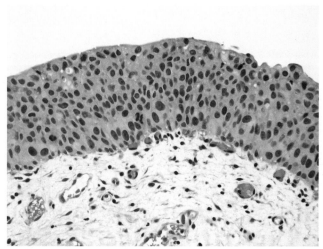

FIGURE 6-17 ■ Urothelial CIS with haphazardly arranged cells with significant nuclear pleomorphism.

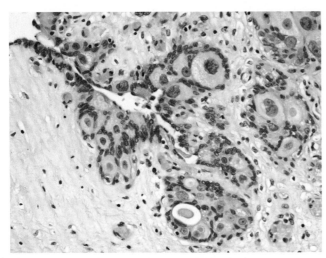

FIGURE 6-18 ■ Urothelial CIS showing pagetoid spread into von Brunn nests.

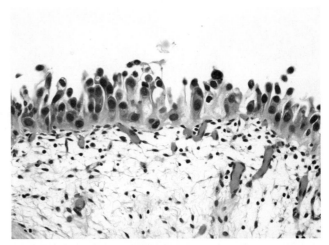

FIGURE 6-20 ■ Urothelial CIS with a denuding pattern.

eosinophilia (Fig. 6-19). These cells can have relatively uniform but markedly enlarged hyperchromatic nuclei or nuclei with a high degree of pleomorphism. The small cell pattern gets its name because the cells have scant cytoplasm that is often basophilic. This gives a similar impression to small cell carcinoma, but the nuclei are actually enlarged and typically have severe hyperchromasia. This is not considered to be related to small cell neuroendocrine carcinoma. Tumor cells in CIS are often discohesive, and in some cases, only a few isolated cells are present clinging to the basement membrane (denuding or clinging CIS) (Fig. 6-20). It has been suggested that this is related to loss of the normal polarity of MUC-1 expression.[198] The nuclei in these cases are often intensely hyperchromatic, and it is not possible to appreciate the chromatin pattern. In other cases, the surface may be completed denuded with the CIS present in von Brunn nests only (Fig. 6-21). This pattern should not be overdiagnosed as invasive carcinoma

(Fig. 6-22). There is a propensity for the malignant cells to invade the adjacent normal urothelium. This can take the form of single malignant cells resulting in a pagetoid pattern. In other cases the malignant cells burrow beneath and lift up the adjacent benign urothelium. Less frequently the malignant cells will spread within the upper level of the adjacent urothelium. Squamous and glandular differentiation can be seen in CIS (Fig. 6-23).[199] When glandular differentiation is present, the term adenocarcinoma in situ should not be used as this implies a precursor lesion of primary adenocarcinoma (see section on adenocarcinoma).

Cytologic Features

Urothelial CIS is a high-grade lesion, and urine cytology is highly sensitive for its detection. The lesion is characterized by discohesive cells, and so the tumor cells are often shed singly in the urine (Fig. 6-24). In specimens obtained at cystoscopy, more intact fragments of the epithelium are present.

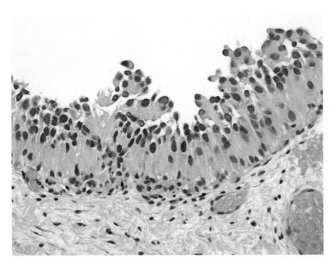

FIGURE 6-19 ■ Urothelial CIS with cells having abundant eosinophilic cytoplasm.

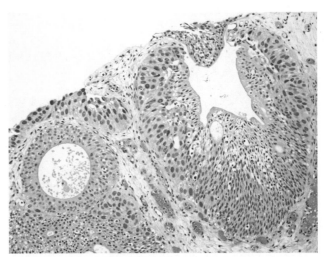

FIGURE 6-21 ■ Urothelial CIS spreading into von Brunn nest and lifting the overlying benign urothelium.

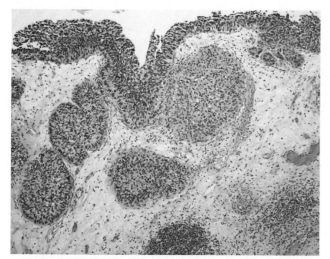

FIGURE 6-22 ■ Urothelial CIS extending into and expanding von Brunn's nests simulating an invasive tumor. There is a small focus of early invasion in the upper right.

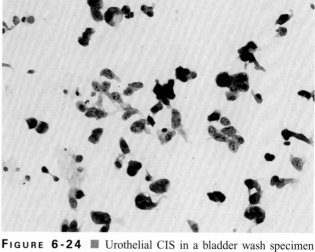

FIGURE 6-24 ■ Urothelial CIS in a bladder wash specimen with discohesive individual malignant cells.

The cells typically are enlarged and have large hyperchromatic nuclei with scant cytoplasm. The nuclear outlines are irregular, and nucleoli are prominent. As described above, there are several histologic patterns to CIS, and in some, the cells can have more abundant cytoplasm. This can result in the malignant cells having an appearance resembling squamous cell carcinoma. It is not possible to distinguish CIS reliably from invasive carcinoma. The presence of necrosis and tissue debris would indicate that invasion is likely present.

Immunohistochemistry in Flat Lesions

A variety of immunohistochemical markers have been studied as adjuncts to the diagnosis of flat lesions. The first marker used was cytokeratin 20.[182] In normal or reactive urothelium, cytokeratin 20 expression is limited to the umbrella cell layer whereas there is diffuse reactivity for cytokeratin 20 throughout the full thickness of the urothelium in the majority but not

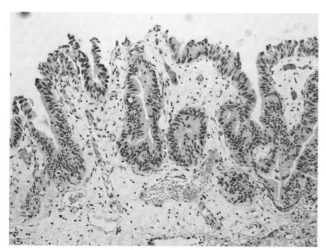

FIGURE 6-23 ■ Urothelial CIS with cells having fusiform nuclei mimicking adenocarcinoma in situ.

all cases of CIS (Fig. 6-25A and B).[182–184,200] In normal or reactive urothelium p53, protein is generally expressed by only a few cells and with weak intensity.[184] In some cases, however, 50% or more of the nuclei show variably intense immunoreactivity. Most cases of CIS show diffuse and intense nuclear expression of p53 (Fig. 6-25C).[183,184,201] However, not all cases of CIS are p53 positive, and so absence of staining for p53 does not exclude a diagnosis of CIS. Cellular proliferation is significantly higher in CIS than in reactive atypia, and so, Ki67 has been used in this distinction.[184,200] There is, however, sufficient overlap in Ki67 scores between CIS and reactive atypia to make this a difficult feature to use in individual cases.[200] CD44 is expressed in the basal cells of normal urothelium and shows more diffuse expression throughout all layers in hyperplasia and reactive atypia. In contrast, there is loss of expression of CD44 in dysplasia and CIS.[184] Other markers that have been applied to this challenge include p16 and E-cadherin, but there is less experience with these, making their routine use of limited value.[202,203] In one study, E-cadherin showed more diffuse and intense immunoreactivity in CIS than in normal epithelium[198] while in another loss of E-cadherin staining was observed in 32% of cases.[204] The RNA-binding protein IMP3 has been found to be expressed in 48% of cases of CIS compared to 13% in reactive atypia in one study.[205]

Because of the variability in results for individual markers, it has been recommended that a panel of three markers (cytokeratin 20, p53, and CD44) be applied (i) where the diagnosis of CIS is strongly favored on routine stains but the pathologist is hesitant to make a definitive diagnosis, (ii) when making a diagnosis of de novo CIS in patients without a history of urothelial neoplasia, and (iii) in cases with unusual morphologic patterns of CIS.[172]

Fluorescence in situ hybridization has also been proposed as an adjunct to histologic evaluation of flat lesions.[146] Over 90% of cases of dysplasia and CIS contain polysomies compared with 36% in hyperplasia, 26% in reactive atypia, and

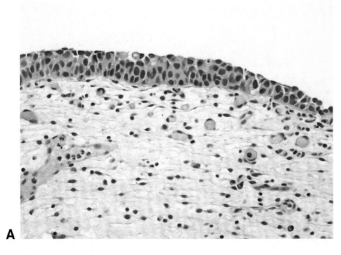

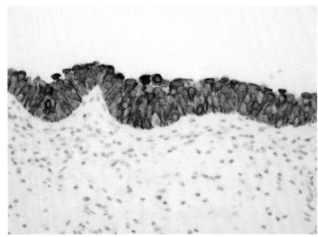

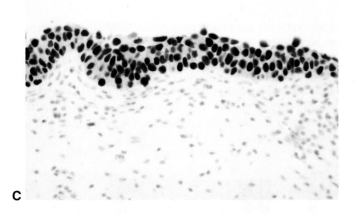

FIGURE 6-25 ■ Urothelial CIS with malignant cells forming a thin epithelium **(A)**. Immunohistochemistry shows diffuse reactivity for cytokeratin 20 **(B)** and p53 **(C)**.

30% in normal epithelium. The high frequency of abnormalities in histologically benign urothelium limits the application of this approach.

Papillary Tumors

In the majority of cases the diagnosis of a lesion as being "papillary" in the urinary bladder is straightforward and the features to be determined are related to proper classification (grading) and evaluation of stage. Occasionally there can be problems in differential diagnosis with lesions that can mimic a papillary process (polypoid or papillary cystitis, fragmented or tangentially cut flat lesions) or papillary lesions that are not strictly speaking urothelial (nephrogenic adenoma, condyloma acuminatum, etc.).[206,207]

More problematic is the concept of papillary hyperplasia and when to call a small lesion a true papillary neoplasm particularly in the setting of known papillary neoplasia. If a true papillary stalk is evident then the lesion is graded and classified into the categories described below (Fig. 6-26). A papillary stalk is defined by the presence of a central fibrovascular core in an exophytic lesion. In the presence of known neoplasia, I am quite aggressive in diagnosing a lesion as a papillary tumor (Fig. 6-27).

For cases with an undulating surface or tenting of the urothelium where no fibrovascular core is evident, the term papillary hyperplasia has been suggested (Fig. 6-28).[39] In some instances, small capillaries are present in the stroma at the base of the pseudopapillae, but these do not extend upward into the stroma. These are therefore more "pseudopapillary"

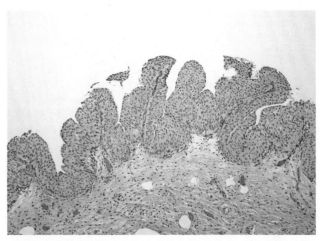

FIGURE 6-26 ■ Papillary urothelial carcinoma with short papillary fronds.

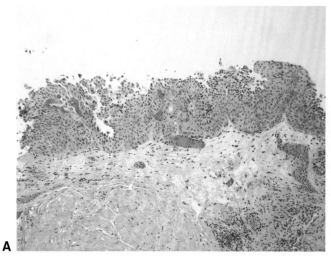

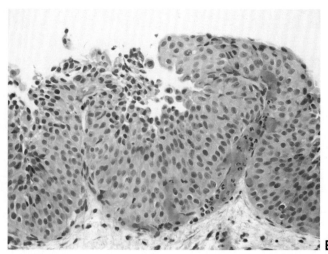

FIGURE 6-27 ■ Papillary urothelial carcinoma with early formation of identifiable papillae **(A,B)**.

than truly papillary, and that is the terminology I use in my practice. The diagnosis in specimens with a pseudopapillary architecture is dependent on evaluating the surface urothelium as a "flat" lesion; if unequivocal dysplasia or CIS is present the diagnosis should be dysplasia or CIS.

Several studies have looked at a variety of biologic markers in papillary tumors and their relationship to the three groups; for the most part these have demonstrated significant differences of the respective marker in the different categories.[18,208]

Grossly papillary tumors may be single or multiple (Fig. 6-29). In low-grade tumors, the papillary architecture can often be appreciated grossly. In some cases, the tumors cover much or all of the mucosal surface (Fig. 6-30). In high-grade carcinoma, the tumors often have a more sessile appearance (Fig. 6-31).

Histologically, papillary tumors are defined by the presence of true papillae with central fibrovascular cores

covered by the neoplastic epithelium. While the cores tend to be delicate, in some cases they can be quite thickened and hyalinized (Fig. 6-32). Infrequently the stalks are expanded by an inflammatory infiltrate (Fig. 6-33) or by collections of foamy macrophages (Fig. 6-34). The classification (grading) of papillary tumors is based on the features of the covering epithelium and is detailed in the following sections.

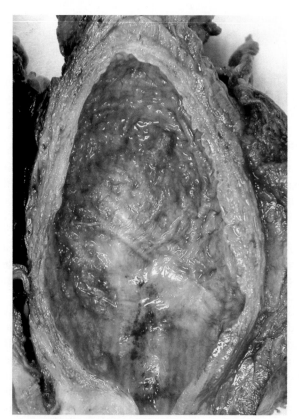

FIGURE 6-29 ■ Small, single papillary urothelial carcinoma on the posterior wall of the bladder.

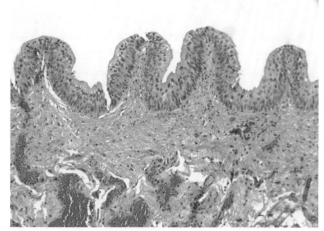

FIGURE 6-28 ■ Prominent tenting of the mucosal surface producing pseudopapillae (papillary hyperplasia).

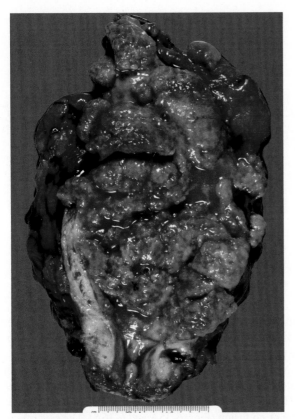

FIGURE 6-30 ■ Diffuse involvement of the bladder by noninvasive (pTa) low-grade papillary urothelial carcinoma.

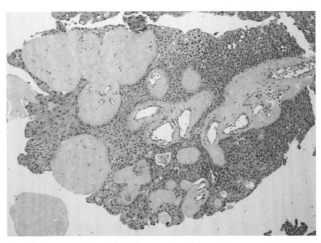

FIGURE 6-32 ■ Papillary urothelial carcinoma with hyalinization of the papillary cores.

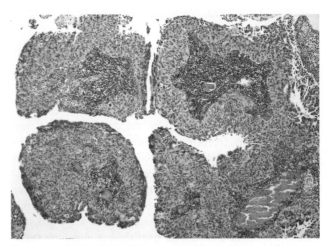

FIGURE 6-33 ■ Papillary urothelial carcinoma with intense chronic inflammatory infiltrate in the papillary cores.

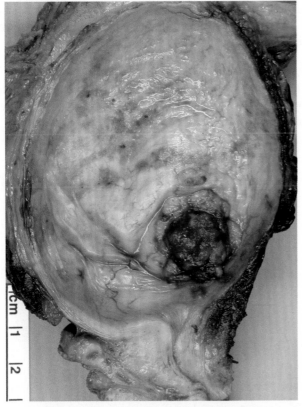

FIGURE 6-31 ■ Invasive (pT2a), high-grade papillary urothelial carcinoma.

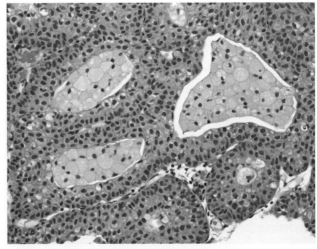

FIGURE 6-34 ■ Papillary urothelial carcinoma with foamy macrophages in the papillary cores.

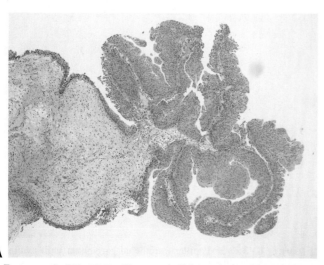

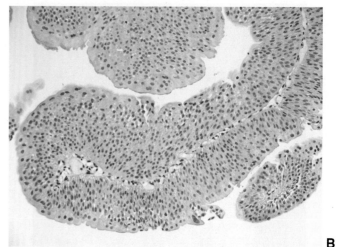

FIGURE 6-35 ■ Papillary urothelial neoplasm of low malignant potential at low **(A)** and high **(B)** magnification.

Papillary Urothelial Neoplasm of Low Malignant Potential

The creation of this category represented a compromise between the "papilloma" camp and those insisting on the use of "carcinoma" for all papillary lesions. The 1998 consensus statement acknowledged that the lower-grade papillary neoplasms were not intrinsically malignant but were associated with a significant risk for the development of new papillary tumors (recurrence). These lesions at the lower end of the spectrum were accepted as clinically significant with close clinical follow-up necessary but further intravesical therapy not indicated. These tumors have a significantly lower rate of recurrence than either low- or high-grade papillary carcinomas and have a very low rate of stage progression.[9,18,34,209–212] In a review of published studies, the mean tumor recurrence rate was found to be 36% and the stage progression rate to be 4%.[13] The largest single institution experience with 212 cases (representing 21% of the 1,006

noninvasive papillary tumors) reported a recurrence rate of 18% and progression to invasive disease in 2%.[213] None of the patients died of bladder cancer.

Morphologically, this category largely though not completely corresponds to grade 1 papillary carcinoma in the 1973 WHO system.[2] The tumor consists of delicate papillae with little or no fusion (Figs. 6-35A and 6-36A). The covering urothelium is usually but not always thickened and shows minimal if any architectural irregularity. Nuclei are normal in size to slightly enlarged and lack significant nuclear hyperchromasia or pleomorphism (Figs. 6-35B and 6-36B). The chromatin is fine, and nucleoli are inconspicuous. Mitoses are infrequent and basally located when present (Tables 6-7 and 6-8).

Papillary Urothelial Carcinoma, Low Grade

This category contains the intermediate group of lesions. In the 1973 WHO system, this would include roughly the lower one-half to two-thirds of grade 2 papillary carcinoma.[17,18]

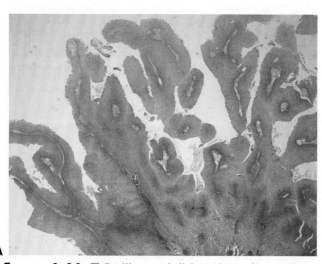

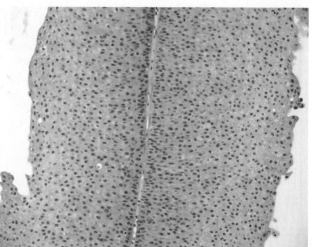

FIGURE 6-36 ■ Papillary urothelial neoplasm of low malignant potential at low **(A)** and high **(B)** magnification.

Table 6-7 ■ PAPILLARY UROTHELIAL NEOPLASMS: ARCHITECTURAL FEATURES

	PUNLMP*	Low Grade	High Grade
Papillae	Delicate	Delicate	Delicate
	Rarely fused	Occasionally fused	Fused and branching
Organization	Polarity normal	Predominantly ordered with minimal crowding and loss of polarity	Predominantly disordered with crowding, overlapping cells and loss of polarity
	Any thickness	Any thickness	Any thickness—may be single cells (denuding)
	Most increased	Most increased	
	Cohesive cells	Cohesive cells	Often discohesive

*Papillary urothelial neoplasm of low malignant potential.

These tumors have a significantly higher recurrence rate than for papillary urothelial neoplasm of low malignant potential and similar to high-grade papillary carcinomas.[9] They also have a higher rate of stage progression than papillary urothelial neoplasm of low malignant potential but significantly lower than for high-grade papillary carcinoma.[9,19,34] Low-grade tumors can be invasive though this is distinctly uncommon. A review of the literature revealed a mean recurrence rate of 50% and mean stage progression rate of 10%.[13] In the large series of Pan et al.[213] these accounted for 60% of noninvasive papillary tumors and had recurrence and progression rates of 35% and 6.5%, respectively. At last follow-up, 2% of patients presenting with low-grade papillary carcinoma had died of bladder cancer.[213] Patients with these tumors require close clinical follow-up though recently it has been suggested that this can be less frequent than for patients with high-grade tumors.[21] A single dose of intravesical therapy (most often mitomycin-C) is optional but maintenance intravesical therapy is not recommended.[23]

The papillae are largely delicate and separate, but some fusion may be seen. At low magnification, there is a generally ordered architectural appearance to the cells within the epithelium (Figs. 6-37A and 6-38A). There is, however, an impression of increased cellularity with increased nuclear density. The nuclei tend to be uniformly enlarged and retain the elongated to oval shape of normal urothelial cells. The chromatin remains fine with small and generally inconspicuous nucleoli. There is often some variability with scattered hyperchromatic nuclei (Figs. 6-37B and 6-38B). Mitoses may be present but are few and generally remain basally located (Tables 6-7 and 6-8).

Papillary Urothelial Carcinoma, High Grade

As previously discussed, many WHO grade 2 (1973) tumors (roughly the upper one-half to one-third) have a significant risk of invasion and biologically have more in common with the grade 3 tumors. These tumors not only have a significant risk of recurrence but have a substantial risk of invasion and progression to muscle-invasive disease. For this reason, the consensus was that these were better included in a high-grade category with the WHO grade 3 (1973) neoplasms. The overall progression rate (to invasive carcinoma) ranges from 15% to 40%. Of the patients initially presenting with high-grade papillary carcinoma in the Pan et al.[213] series, 22% died of bladder cancer. For high-grade Ta tumors, intravesical BCG therapy with an induction course and maintenance is recommended.[23]

Heterogeneity of grade is recognized in papillary lesions,[214,215] and the consensus is that tumors should be graded on the basis of the worst grade present (Fig. 6-39). There is no consensus on a minimum quantity that should be present to assign a higher grade in cases such as this. Some authors have used a 5% cutoff for recognition of a higher-grade component.[215,216] After reviewing this topic, the recent International Consultation on Urologic Diseases concluded that there is some evidence to indicate that pure

Table 6-8 ■ PAPILLARY UROTHELIAL NEOPLASMS: NUCLEAR FEATURES

	PUNLMP*	Low Grade	High Grade
Size	Mildly enlarged	Enlarged	Enlarged
	Uniform	Some variation	Marked variability
Shape	Elongated	Elongated, oval, or round	Pleomorphic
	Uniform	Slight variation	
Chromatin	Fine	Fine with some variation	Frequently coarse with marked variation
Nucleoli	Absent to inconspicuous	Usually inconspicuous	Prominent
			Single to multiple
Mitoses	Rare	Infrequent	Frequent
	Basal if present	Most basal if present	Any level

*Papillary urothelial neoplasm of low malignant potential.

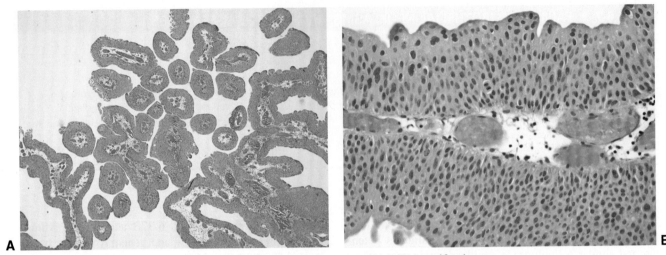

FIGURE 6-37 ■ Low-grade papillary urothelial carcinoma at low **(A)** and high **(B)** magnification.

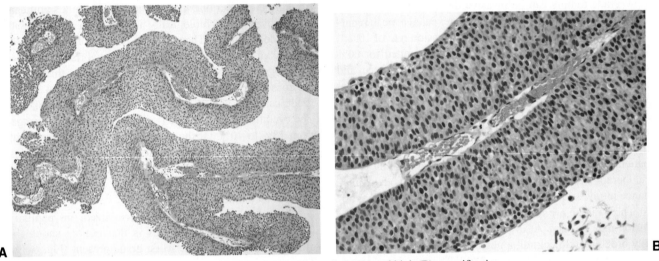

FIGURE 6-38 ■ Low-grade papillary urothelial carcinoma at medium **(A)** and high **(B)** magnification.

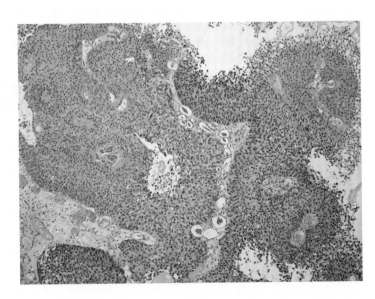

FIGURE 6-39 ■ Papillary urothelial carcinoma with low-grade **(left)** and high-grade **(right)** areas.

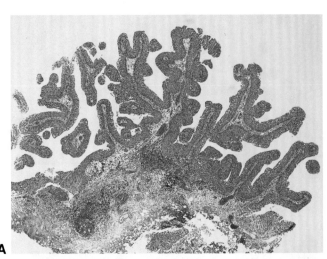
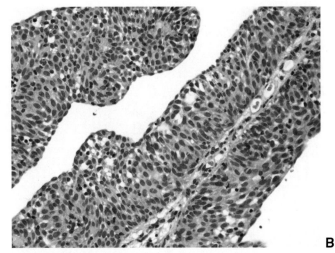

A

B

FIGURE 6-40 ■ High-grade papillary urothelial carcinoma at low **(A)** and high **(B)** magnification.

high-grade tumors are more aggressive than mixed low- and high-grade ones.[27] This is a subject that is in need of further study.[8,14,172] Our current approach is to assign the worst grade present, irrespective of quantity, but to include a note indicating that there is grade heterogeneity and which grade is predominant.

The papillae are frequently fused forming apparently solid masses. The overall impression is one of disordered growth (Figs. 6-40A and 6-41A). The epithelium is of variable thickness and may resemble "denuding carcinoma in situ" in some instances. Individual cells are haphazardly arranged within the epithelium and have a generally discohesive nature. Nuclei are hyperchromatic and pleomorphic. The chromatin is dense, irregularly distributed, and often clumped. Nucleoli may be single or multiple and are often prominent (Figs. 6-40B and 6-41B). Mitoses are generally frequent and may be seen at any level of the epithelium. Abnormal mitoses are often present (Tables 6-7 and 6-8). CIS can be present in the adjacent mucosa.

Cytologic Features

The sensitivity of cytology for detecting papillary tumors is strongly correlated with the tumor grade. There is a low degree of sensitivity for papillary urothelial neoplasms of low malignant potential and low-grade papillary urothelial carcinoma. Particularly in bladder washings, fragments of papillary tumors can be obtained and these are very helpful in making the diagnosis. The presence of papillary fragments in voided urine in the absence of inflammation or lithiasis is suspicious for papillary urothelial neoplasia. In these fragments an increased cellularity and crowding of nuclei may be evident (Fig. 6-42). The umbrella cells are variably preserved. The nuclei are uniformly enlarged with an increased nuclear to cytoplasmic ratio. The chromatin tends to be uniformly distributed with inconspicuous or small nucleoli. The nuclear membranes show variable thickening and there is irregularity of nuclear shape. Nuclear membrane features have been reported to be most helpful in identifying low-grade lesions.[217] The cytoplasm

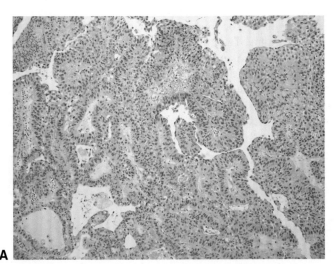
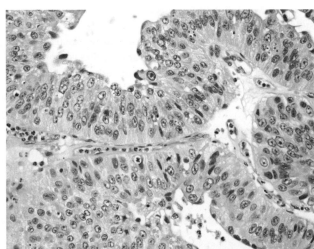

A

B

FIGURE 6-41 ■ High-grade papillary urothelial carcinoma at low **(A)** and high **(B)** magnification.

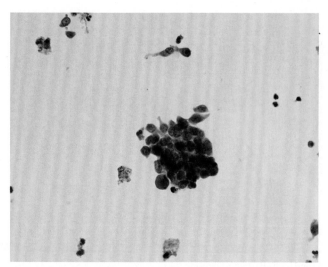

FIGURE 6-42 ■ Bladder washing specimen from a low-grade papillary urothelial carcinoma.

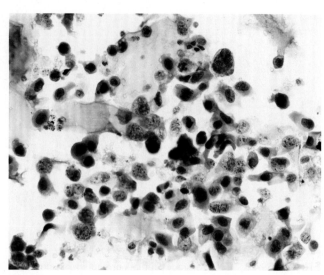

FIGURE 6-43 ■ Bladder washing specimen from a high-grade papillary urothelial carcinoma.

is homogeneous and lacks vacuolization. Mitoses are absent or infrequent.

In high-grade papillary tumors, the most identifying feature to distinguish from low-grade tumors is the presence of nuclear pleomorphism. The cells are markedly enlarged and are present as cohesive groups and as single cells (Fig. 6-43). There is an increased nuclear to cytoplasmic ratio. The nuclei are hyperchromatic with irregular clumped chromatin and prominent nucleoli. The nuclear membranes are thick and irregular. Mitoses are frequent. Umbrella cells are absent. The cytoplasm is not homogeneous, and cytoplasmic features may indicate squamous or glandular differentiation.

Differential Diagnosis

There are several benign processes in the urinary bladder that can mimic papillary urothelial neoplasms (Table 6-9). Papillary hyperplasia is discussed above. Nephrogenic adenoma is covered in the section on clear cell adenocarcinoma. Condyloma acuminatum is discussed in the section on squamous papilloma.

Papillary/polypoid cystitis is a condition characteristically associated with indwelling catheter and is reported to occur in up to 80% of patients with catheters.[37,38,207,218,219] These lesions may also occur in other settings related to

chronic irritation, such as fistula and long-standing urinary tract obstruction. By cystoscopy, polypoid cystitis appears as exophytic lesions that may be large and polypoid, or somewhat narrower mimicking papillary structures. Histologically, the typical finding is that of marked edema of the lamina propria resulting in exophytic polypoid projections. The overlying urothelium ranges from flattened and attenuated to normal to hyperplastic, but shows no significant cytologic or architectural atypia. In some cases, the stroma may be less edematous resulting in a more papillary appearance (so-called papillary cystitis). There always continues to be some stroma present frequently with interspersed inflammatory cells and small capillaries.

Fibroepithelial polyp can occur throughout the urinary tract and over a wide age range from children to adults.[220–222] In the pediatric population, fibroepithelial polyp is the second most common mass in the bladder (after rhabdomyosarcoma).[222] These are considered to be nonneoplastic lesions that can be congenital or acquired and may represent a hamartoma. There is a male predominance. Presentation is variable but includes obstruction (particularly in urethral and ureteral lesions), hematuria, and pain. Grossly these are polypoid structures that can have multiple finger-like projections (Box 6-2). The overall polypoid appearance distinguishes these from papillary urothelial neoplasms.

Table 6-9 ■ MIMICS OF PAPILLARY NEOPLASMS
Papillary urothelial hyperplasia
Nephrogenic adenoma
Polypoid cystitis
Papillary cystitis
Fibroepithelial polyp
Condyloma acuminatum

Box 6-2 ● FIBROEPITHELIAL POLYP—CLUES TO DIAGNOSIS
Finger-like projections
Fibrous stroma
Attenuated to hyperplastic urothelium
Variable inflammation

The finger-like projections have central fibrous cores covered by attenuated to hyperplastic urothelium with a scattered inflammatory infiltrate. These can simulate papillary neoplasia; however, the fibrous cores tend to be wider and are more dense and fibrotic in nature than papillary neoplasms. Atypical stromal cells can be present.[223] In a minority of cases, the urothelium proliferates producing complex anastomosing nests. These can mimic inverted papilloma. In fibroepithelial polyp the anastomosing nests of urothelium are embedded in a fibrous stroma and are more irregular and less "solid" than is seen in inverted papilloma.

Invasive Urothelial Carcinoma

Gross Features

Invasive urothelial carcinoma can be unifocal or multifocal. In most cases the invasive carcinoma forms a single mass. Additional foci, when present, are often noninvasive papillary tumors, papillary tumors with invasion, or areas of CIS. The latter may be appreciated as hemorrhagic or red mucosa. Invasive carcinoma can be polypoid, sessile, or ulceroinfiltrative (Figs. 6-44 to 6-46). Polypoid growth is most often associated with the sarcomatoid variant and these can be attached to the bladder wall by a narrow pedicle. Invasive tumors are solid, gray-white, and poorly circumscribed with infiltrative borders. In cases with extensive squamous differentiation there can be abundant keratinous

debris on the surface. Invasive carcinomas developing from papillary tumors often have a sessile appearance and there may be papillary structures evident on the surface or at the lateral mucosal margins. In some cases there is diffuse thickening of the bladder wall resembling linitis plastica, a pattern most often associated with the plasmacytoid and micropapillary variants. An ulcero-infiltrative pattern of growth may grossly resemble a site of prior TURBT. These areas can be deceiving with the poorly defined lesion representing scarring and secondary changes rather than solid tumor.

Microscopic Features

Invasive urothelial carcinoma is most remarkable for the diversity of histologic patterns that can be found. Many of these are so distinctive that they are now recognized as specific variants, some of which have significant clinical characteristics. These are discussed in detail in a following section. The architectural patterns of invasive carcinoma include solid sheets, large and small nests, trabeculae, cords, and single cells (Box 6-3) (Figs. 6-47 to 6-51). In larger nests, the cells at the periphery may have palisading of the nuclei with a pattern of maturation toward the center reminiscent of normal urothelium. In most cases, however, the urothelial nature of the tumor is assumed based on the absence of another specific histology. The pattern of invasion has been linked to prognosis with tumors having well-defined nests,

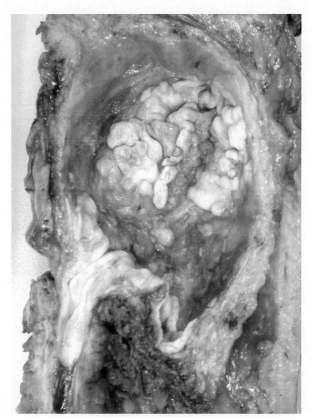

FIGURE 6-44 ■ Invasive (pT2b) high-grade urothelial carcinoma with a somewhat polypoid appearance.

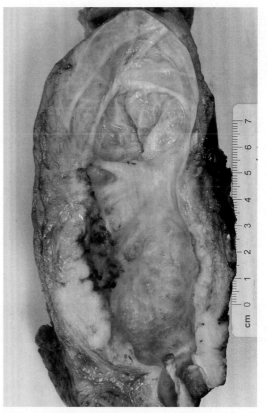

FIGURE 6-45 ■ Invasive (pT3b) high-grade urothelial carcinoma.

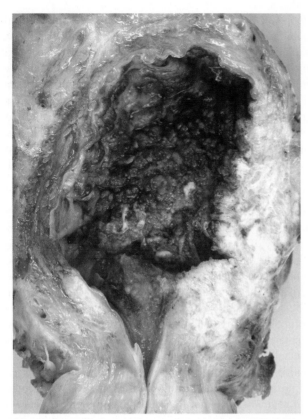

FIGURE 6-46 ■ Invasive (pT3b) high-grade urothelial carcinoma.

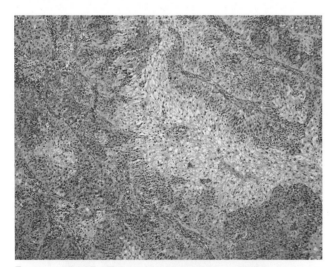

FIGURE 6-47 ■ Invasive high-grade urothelial carcinoma growing in large nests. Note the squamoid appearance.

Box 6-3 ● INVASIVE UROTHELIAL CARCINOMA—GROWTH PATTERNS

Inverted—pushing
Solid
Variably sized nests
Trabecular
Cords
Single cells

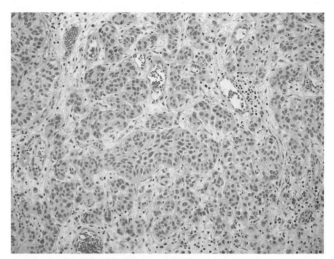

FIGURE 6-48 ■ Invasive high-grade urothelial carcinoma with small variably shaped nests.

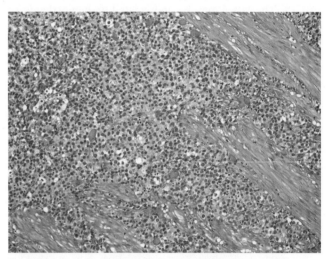

FIGURE 6-49 ■ Invasive high-grade urothelial carcinoma growing as a solid sheet of cells.

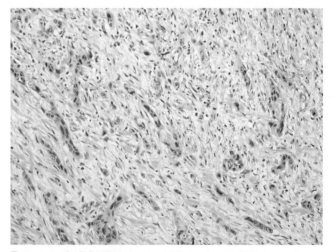

FIGURE 6-50 ■ Invasive high-grade urothelial carcinoma forming small cords in a desmoplastic stromal background.

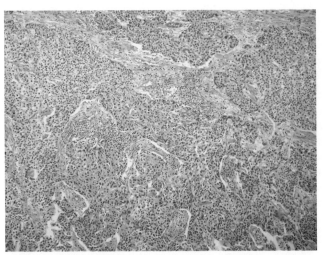

FIGURE 6-51 ■ Invasive high-grade urothelial carcinoma with a trabecular architecture.

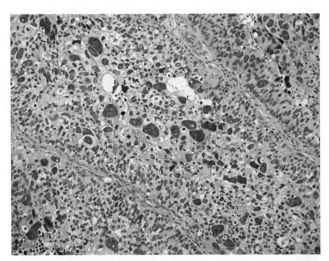

FIGURE 6-53 ■ Invasive high-grade urothelial carcinoma with bizarre pleomorphic nuclei.

trabeculae, and pushing borders behaving better outcome than those with infiltrating nests, cords, and single cells.[224,225]

The majority of invasive carcinomas are high grade and this is reflected in striking nuclear pleomorphism manifest by variability in nuclear size and shape, nuclear chromatin pattern, and presence or absence of single or multiple nucleoli (Fig. 6-52). Nuclear contours are often irregular with sharp angles. Bizarre giant tumor nuclei and multinucleated tumor giant cells can be present (Fig. 6-53). Mitotic activity is variable but in most cases mitoses are frequent and abnormal mitotic figures are identifiable. There is generally moderate to abundant cytoplasm that is eosinophilic. In many cases this results in a squamoid appearance to the tumor. In other tumors the cytoplasm can be basophilic. Cytoplasmic vacuoles can occur and cytoplasmic mucin may be visible. Mucin stains are positive for cytoplasmic mucin in up to 60% of invasive high-grade tumors (Fig. 6-54).[226] The presence of mucin does not indicate glandular differentiation;

the latter diagnosis is reserved for tumors with the presence of well-formed glandular structures. Cytoplasmic clearing due to the accumulation of glycogen is another feature that can be present. This is usually focal but when more extensive has been described as the clear cell variant of urothelial carcinoma.[227]

In most cases of invasive carcinoma, there is a desmoplastic stromal response (Fig. 6-55). This can be quite prominent and in some cases consists of a cellular pseudosarcomatous spindle cell stroma mimicking sarcomatoid carcinoma.[228] The stroma can also be myxoid, and in some tumors, this myxoid background becomes a predominant part of the tumor (Fig. 6-56).[229] Benign osseous metaplasia can develop and should not be confused with a heterologous element of sarcomatoid carcinoma.[230,231] Retraction of the stroma away from invasive tumor nests is also a characteristic feature of urothelial carcinoma. This can be a particularly helpful feature in foci of early invasion. In most tumors this is a focal finding, when prominent a diagnosis of the micropapillary variant of urothelial carcinoma should be considered. It also creates a problem in distinguishing retraction artifact from lymph–vascular invasion.[232] Invasion of the stroma by tumor can be accompanied by an associated inflammatory infiltrate that can be polymorphous or predominantly lympho-plasmacytic (Fig. 6-57). In some cases, this is particularly intense and obscures the tumor resulting in a lymphoepithelioma-like morphology.[233]

Cytologic Features

Cytology is highly sensitive in cases of invasive urothelial carcinoma. These tumors are almost always high grade. Cells are shed singly and in cohesive groups; the latter are most apparent in specimens obtained at cystoscopy (Fig. 6-58). The cells are markedly enlarged and have increased nuclear to cytoplasmic ratios. Nuclei are large, hyperchromatic, and have coarsely clumped chromatin and single to multiple nucleoli. The nuclear membranes are thick and irregular.

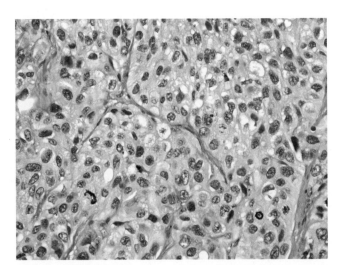

FIGURE 6-52 ■ Invasive high-grade urothelial carcinoma with nuclear pleomorphism.

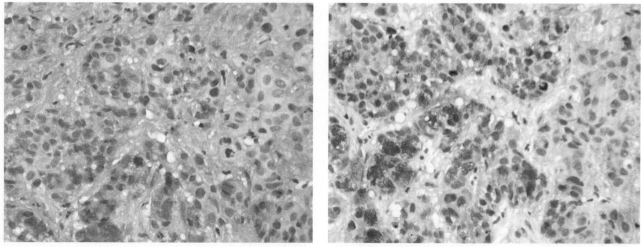

A **B**

FIGURE 6-54 ■ Mucin positivity (**A**, Alcian blue pH 2.4; **B**, mucicarmine) in an otherwise typical high-grade urothelial carcinoma.

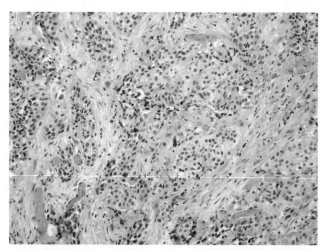

FIGURE 6-55 ■ Invasive high-grade urothelial carcinoma with desmoplastic stroma.

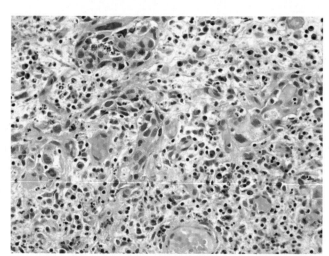

FIGURE 6-57 ■ Invasive high-grade urothelial carcinoma with inflammation including lymphocytes, plasma cells, and eosinophils.

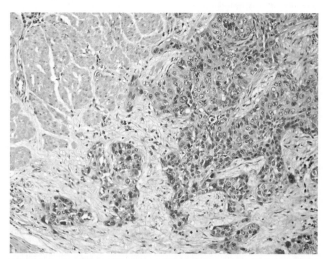

FIGURE 6-56 ■ Invasive high-grade urothelial carcinoma with myxoid stroma.

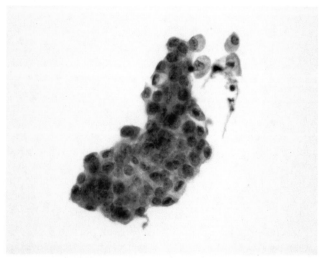

FIGURE 6-58 ■ High-grade urothelial carcinoma in a voided urine specimen.

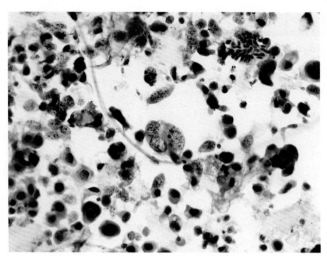

FIGURE 6-59 ■ High-grade urothelial carcinoma in a bladder wash specimen.

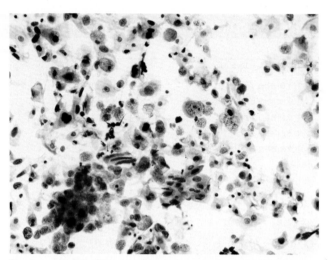

FIGURE 6-60 ■ High-grade urothelial carcinoma in a bladder wash specimen.

There is striking nuclear pleomorphism (Fig. 6-59). Mitotic figures are common. The background is typically bloody with inflammation and necrotic tissue fragments (Fig. 6-60). Cytoplasmic features are variable and can reflect squamous or glandular differentiation. Features of specific histologic variants can be present.

Differential Diagnosis

The differential diagnosis of invasive urothelial carcinoma includes benign conditions that can mimic invasive carcinoma, nonurothelial carcinomas, other primary tumors, and secondary tumors (either direct invasion from another site or metastases). Benign proliferations that can mimic urothelial carcinoma such as von Brunn's nest hyperplasia and proliferative cystitis are discussed in the section on the nested variant of urothelial carcinoma. Inverted papilloma is dealt with in the section on urothelial carcinoma with inverted papilloma-like architecture. Nephrogenic adenoma is reviewed in the section on clear cell adenocarcinoma. Other benign glandular lesions are discussed in the nonurachal adenocarcinoma section. Other tumors such as paraganglioma are covered in the relevant section. Secondary involvement of the bladder is covered in detail in the section on secondary neoplasms.

Pseudocarcinomatous Proliferations. Baker and Young[234] first described the occurrence of benign reactive epithelial proliferations that mimic invasive urothelial carcinoma in the setting of radiation therapy. Subsequently similar lesions have been described following chemotherapy or without any evident pathogenic factor.[235,236]

These lesions are characterized by irregular nests of urothelium extending into the lamina propria simulating invasive carcinoma. This is often accompanied by cytologic atypia and mitotic figures as well as cytoplasmic eosinophilia, all typical of invasive carcinoma. A key clue to recognition is the impression of an inflammatory background with stromal hemorrhage, fibrin, edema, hemosiderin

deposition, and inflammation. There are often prominent ectatic vascular structures. In the setting of radiation the typical vascular changes may be evident as well as stromal cell atypia. There may be overlying mucosal ulceration. If a lesion reminds you of a urethral caruncle, think of this as a possibility.

Immunohistochemistry

Immunohistochemistry can play a vital role in the diagnosis and differential diagnosis of urothelial carcinoma.[237,238] Given the diversity of the morphologic manifestations of urothelial carcinoma, not surprisingly a large number of immunohistochemical markers can be expressed by these tumors (Table 6-10). It is important to recognize that the reported frequency of expression is often dependent on the type of cases studied. For example, in one study thrombomodulin was expressed by 86% of papillary urothelial neoplasms of low malignant potential but only 39% of invasive urothelial carcinomas.[244] The immunohistochemical profiles of urothelial carcinoma variants are discussed in the specific sections below and are not repeated here. Immunohistochemistry is also included in the differential diagnosis sections throughout this chapter and the reader is referred to those discussions for specific questions.

There are markers that are used to assist in identifying a tumor as being of urothelial origin. Uroplakin III has been reported to be 100% specific in some studies but its usefulness is somewhat limited by low sensitivity (57% to 60%).[241,244,255] Expression decreases with increasing grade and so in the types of tumors most often causing difficulty, it is least often expressed.[244] Thrombomodulin has also been used as a specific marker of urothelial carcinomas. It is expressed by 49% to 91% of tumors with expression decreasing in invasive high-grade tumors.[241,244,254] It is not as specific as uroplakin III and is also expressed in some cases of squamous cell carcinoma, mesothelioma, and adenocarcinoma

Table 6-10 ■ IMMUNOHISTOCHEMISTRY OF UROTHELIAL CARCINOMA (USUAL TYPE)

Marker	Positive (%)	Comments
Cytokeratin 5/6[239,240]	6–75	
Cytokeratin 7[241,242]	87–94	
Cytokeratin 8/18[239,243]	83–87	
Cytokeratin 19[239]	92	
Cytokeratin 20[239,241,244]	25–67	
Cytokeratin 34βE12[244,245]	65–97	
EMA[246]	80–94	
Vimentin[239,247]	11–33	
P63[242,247,248]	81–100	
P16[249,250]	30–50	
P53[208,251]	34–68	Higher percent positive with higher-grade and nonpapillary type
CD10[252,253]	54–67	Predominantly cytoplasmic
Thrombomodulin[241,244,254]	49–91	Lower % positive with invasive carcinomas
Uroplakin III[241,244,255]	57–60	Lower % positive with higher grade
GATA3[256]	67	
CD117[246]	30	
AMACR (racemase)[242,257]	31–36	
S100P[256,258]	71–78	
TTF-1[259]	5	
Calretinin[260]	5	
Hepatocyte nuclear factor-1β[261]	3	
PAX-2[247,262]	0–6	
PAX-8[247,263,264]	0–17	Results appear antibody-dependent
PSA[241,242]	0	
PAP[241,242]	0–11	
PSMA[265,266]	0–13	Weak in one case of urothelial carcinoma; may be + with glandular differentiation
Prostein (P501S)[258,267]	0–6	
NKX3.1[258]	0	
CDX-2[268]	0	Positive with enteric-type glandular differentiation
Estrogen receptor-β[269,270]	63–80	
Estrogen receptor-α[270,271]	1.4–4.5	
Progesterone receptor[271]	0	
HMB-45[272]	0	
Melan-A[273]	0	
Synaptophysin[248]	6	Rare cells
CD56[248]	0	
Chromogranin-A[248]	0	

of the bladder, lung, ovary, pancreas, and breast among others.[244,254] More recently, GATA3 has been shown to be expressed in 67% of urothelial carcinomas.[256] In an extensive tissue microarray study, Higgins et al.[256] found only ductal adenocarcinoma of the breast to also express GATA3 indicating a high degree of specificity for this marker. These authors also reported expression of S100P in 78% of bladder urothelial carcinomas but this marker was less specific with gastrointestinal tract adenocarcinoma, hepatocellular carcinoma, ovarian carcinoma, and rarely (2%) prostatic adenocarcinoma also being positive.[256]

The expression of cytokeratins is also of interest in urothelial carcinoma. The urothelium is a stratified epithelium and as such has some similarities with squamous cell carcinoma. One characteristic is the expression of high molecular weight cytokeratins. One of the more frequently studied high molecular weight cytokeratin clones, 34βE12, is expressed in 65% to 97% of cases (Fig. 6-61A and B).[242,244,245,274] Urothelial carcinoma is also one of the tumors that coexpress cytokeratins 7 and 20 (Fig. 6-61C and D). There has, however, been wide variation in the literature with the reported frequency of this ranging from

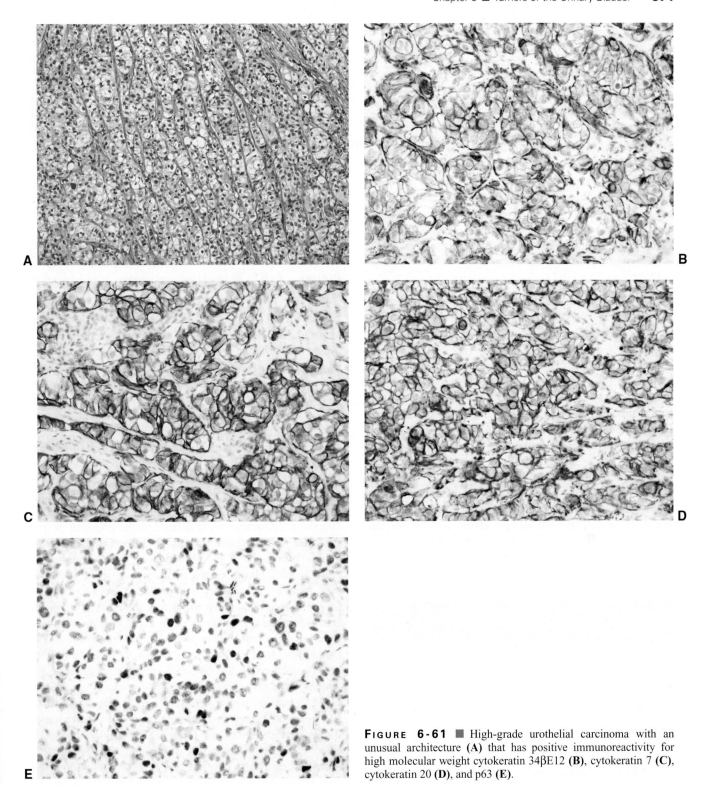

FIGURE 6-61 ■ High-grade urothelial carcinoma with an unusual architecture (**A**) that has positive immunoreactivity for high molecular weight cytokeratin 34βE12 (**B**), cytokeratin 7 (**C**), cytokeratin 20 (**D**), and p63 (**E**).

50% to 62%.[241,242] Up to 14% of high-grade urothelial carcinomas do not express either cytokeratin 7 or 20.[241,275] The results are highly dependent on case selection as cytokeratin 20 expression is much less often present in invasive and metastatic urothelial carcinomas (44%).[244]

Lastly p63 has become a useful marker of urothelial carcinoma. It is expressed in 81% to 92% of high-grade urothelial carcinomas (Fig. 6-61E).[242,248] This marker is also consistently expressed in squamous and basal cell carcinomas. Its value in the urinary bladder has been primarily related to assisting in the differential diagnosis with prostatic adenocarcinoma[242] and its expression in the spindle cell component of sarcomatoid carcinomas.

Histologic Variants of Urothelial Carcinoma

The morphologic diversity of tumors arising from the urothelium is well recognized and is reflected in the current classification system.[14,15,53,276] In this section, the focus will be on those tumors that are considered variants of urothelial carcinoma. Other epithelial tumors such as squamous cell carcinoma, adenocarcinoma, and small cell carcinoma that can develop in the urinary tract are not considered. Table 6-11 provides a modified listing of these variants as described within the WHO classification scheme[14] as well as in more recent publications.[53,276]

Urothelial Carcinoma with Mixed Differentiation

Urothelial tumors have a great capacity for divergent differentiation.[277] Squamous differentiation, defined by the presence of intercellular bridges and/or keratinization, occurs in up to 40% of urothelial carcinomas (Fig. 6-62).[53,276,278–280] For this reason, the diagnosis of squamous cell carcinoma is reserved for pure lesions without any associated urothelial component, including urothelial CIS.[14,15,280] Tumors with any identifiable urothelial element are classified as urothelial carcinoma with squamous differentiation. Some authors will classify urothelial carcinoma with extensive squamous differentiation as squamous cell carcinoma (but we prefer to continue to follow the WHO guidelines).[281] The clinical significance of squamous differentiation remains uncertain; it has been reported to be an unfavorable prognostic feature in patients undergoing radical cystectomy, possibly because of its association with high-grade urothelial carcinoma.[282] Mixed differentiation in transurethral resection specimens

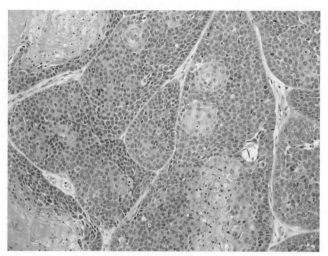

FIGURE 6-62 ■ Urothelial carcinoma with squamous differentiation.

has been associated with a higher frequency of muscle invasion and extravesical extension, but not decreased survival.[279] Squamous differentiation has been reported in a limited number of reports to be predictive of a poor response to radiation therapy and has been associated with a poor response to systemic chemotherapy.[282–284] There is no association with HPV infection.[285] Immunohistochemical markers of squamous differentiation such as caveolin-1 and -2, MAC387, and desmocolin-2 can identify this component in urothelial carcinoma.[278,286,287] We currently report the percentage of the squamous component in cases with mixed differentiation.

Glandular differentiation is less common than squamous differentiation, being present in up to 18% of cases.[14,279] Glandular differentiation is defined as the presence of true glandular spaces within the tumor.[14,280] In most cases, these glands have an enteric morphology (Fig. 6-63). Tumors with a mucinous (colloid) carcinoma or signet ring cell adenocarcinoma component are also included. Pseudoglandular spaces caused by necrosis or artifact should not be considered evidence of glandular differentiation. Mucin-containing cells are common in high-grade urothelial carcinoma. Donhuijsen et al.[226] found mucin-positive cells in 14% of grade 1, 49% of grade 2, and 63% of grade 3 urothelial carcinomas. The presence of cytoplasmic mucin is not considered evidence of glandular differentiation. The diagnosis of adenocarcinoma is reserved for pure tumors[14,288] and a tumor with mixed glandular and urothelial differentiation is classified as urothelial carcinoma with glandular differentiation regardless of the extent of the glandular differentiation. The clinical significance of glandular differentiation and mucin positivity in urothelial carcinoma remain uncertain. In one study, the presence of glandular differentiation was associated with a poorer response to systemic chemotherapy.[283] In another report, mixed differentiation in transurethral resection specimens was associated with a higher frequency of muscle invasion and extravesical extension, but not survival.[279] Immunohistochemistry for MUC5AC-apomucin may be an indicator of glandular differentiation.[41] In cases

Table 6-11 ■ VARIANTS OF UROTHELIAL CARCINOMA
Mixed differentiation
With squamous differentiation
With glandular differentiation
With small cell differentiation
Nested
Microcystic
Micropapillary
Lymphoepithelioma-like
Plasmacytoid
Inverted papilloma-like carcinoma
Giant cell carcinoma
Urothelial carcinoma with trophoblastic differentiation
Clear cell (glycogen-rich) urothelial carcinoma
Lipid-rich (lipoid) urothelial carcinoma
Sarcomatoid carcinoma (carcinosarcoma)
Undifferentiated carcinoma

Adapted from Eble J, Epstein J, Sauter G, et al. *World Health Organization Histologic and Genetic Typing of Tumours of the Kidney, Urinary Bladder, Prostate Gland and Testis.* Lyon, France: IARC Press; 2004.

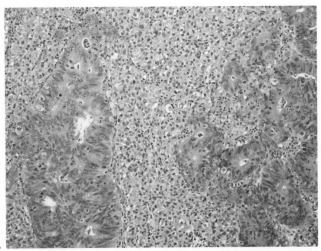
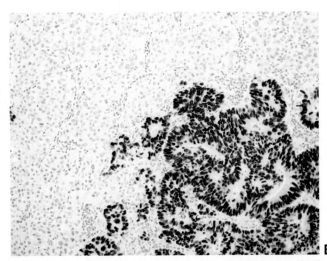

FIGURE 6-63 ■ Urothelial carcinoma with glandular differentiation (**A**). The glandular component has positive immunoreactivity for CDX2 (**B**).

with glandular differentiation, we report the percentage of the glandular component.

Small cell differentiation histologically identical to that occurring in the lung is estimated to account for approximately 0.5% of bladder tumors.[289,290] In about 50% of cases it is pure and in the others mixed with other histologic types.[291] In contrast to the way squamous and glandular differentiation is reported, given the clinical significance of this diagnosis, we report these mixed tumors as small cell carcinoma and then indicate the percentage of the small cell and urothelial components. This topic is covered in detail in the section on small cell carcinoma later in the chapter.

Nested Variant

In 1992, Murphy and Deana[292] described four cases of invasive urothelial carcinoma with a distinctive growth pattern of small nests, a pattern that had also been described by Talbert and Young.[293] There are no specific clinical or epidemiologic characteristics. These are invasive carcinomas. Larger series have confirmed the aggressive nature of this tumor despite its deceptively benign morphology.[294–297] Some studies have suggested these are more aggressive than usual urothelial carcinoma.[295-297] In the largest series to date, Wasco et al.[297] reported lymph node metastases in 67% of the 30 cases undergoing cystectomy.

This variant of urothelial carcinoma is characterized by infiltrating discrete nests made up of uniform

benign-appearing urothelial cells, closely resembling von Brunn nests (Box 6-4) (Fig. 6-64). The nests can be closely packed or more scattered and haphazard and can show considerable size variation (Fig. 6-65). There is often no associated stromal response. Some nests have small tubular lumens. This can result in focal areas resembling cystitis cystica or glandularis. In some areas the nests become more complex or confluent, features that are helpful when present (Fig. 6-66). Nuclei generally show little or no atypia but are often considerably enlarged when compared to normal urothelial cells (Fig. 6-67). Invariably the tumor also contains foci of unequivocal cancer with more variable nuclear size, enlarged nucleoli, and a coarse chromatin pattern. Increasing levels of atypia are often identified in the deeper portions of the tumor. Invasion of the muscular propria is common and when identified is diagnostic of carcinoma. There may be an associated typical urothelial carcinoma component and/or urothelial CIS.

Box 6-4 ● NESTED VARIANT—CLUES TO DIAGNOSIS

Nuclear enlargement with variable atypia
Haphazard arrangement of nests
Infiltrative growth
Confluence of nests
Deep lamina propria involvement
Involvement of muscularis propria

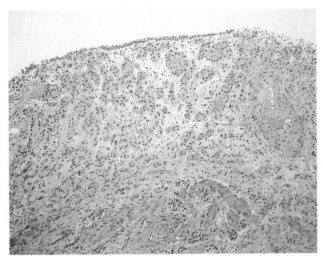

FIGURE 6-64 ■ Nested variant of urothelial carcinoma with infiltrating small nests of cells.

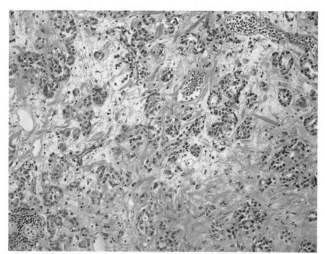

FIGURE 6-65 ■ Nested variant of urothelial carcinoma with a more obvious high-grade component.

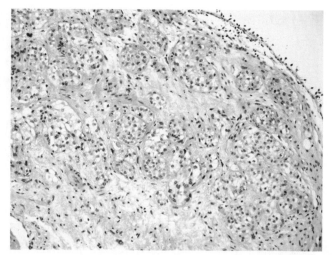

FIGURE 6-67 ■ Nested variant of urothelial carcinoma with uniform nests and uniform round nuclei.

The immunohistochemical profile is typical of urothelial carcinoma with cytokeratin 7 (93%), cytokeratin 20 (68%), high molecular weight cytokeratin (34βE12; 92%), and p63 (92%) positivity.[297] Overexpression of p53 was found in 25% of cases in one series.[298]

The major differential diagnosis is with benign mimics such as prominent von Brunn nest or von Brunn nest hyperplasia (proliferative cystitis).[54] Useful features in recognizing this lesion as malignant are the closely packed and haphazard arrangement of the nests, tendency for increasing cellular anaplasia in the deeper portions of the lesion, the infiltrative nature, and the presence of deep lamina propria and muscle invasion. Von Brunn nests tend to extend downward to a consistent level forming almost a linear edge to the proliferation with the cells maintaining the features of urothelium and with minimal cytologic atypia. In von Brunn nests, the cells mature toward the center, a feature not seen in the nested variant. Although Ki-67 (MIB-1) staining

generally shows a higher rate of positive cells in carcinoma than in proliferative cystitis, there is sufficient overlap such that this is not a reliable criteria to base the diagnosis on.[54,298] Similarly, overexpression of p53 protein does not seem to have value in this distinction.[54]

The nested variant of urothelial carcinoma may mimic paraganglioma or paraganglionic tissue; the prominent vascular network of paraganglioma that surrounds individual nests is different than in carcinoma.[299] Rare carcinoid tumors in the bladder can have a nested architecture and bland cytologic features. Immunohistochemistry can distinguish carcinoma from paraganglionic tissue, paraganglioma, and carcinoid tumor in difficult cases. Another mimic is nephrogenic adenoma that can have solid nests and an apparent infiltrative growth; recognition of other architectural patterns including tubules, microcysts, and surface papillary component lead to the correct diagnosis. Prominent basement membranes around the nests and hobnail-type cells further indicate a diagnosis of nephrogenic adenoma.[300,301]

Microcystic Variant

Young and Zukerberg[302] described four cases of invasive urothelial carcinoma characterized by the formation of microcysts. The pattern was similar to some foci of tubular differentiation included in the "nested variant" of Murphy and Deana and "deceptively benign-appearing" bladder cancer of Talbert and Young.[293] The cases included lesions with intermediate- to high-grade urothelial carcinoma having areas of microcystic and/or macrocystic change or tubular (glandular) differentiation. Microcysts can be identified in up to 1% of urothelial carcinomas, most of which are high grade and high stage.[303,304] The cysts and tubules may be empty, or contain necrotic debris or mucin (Fig. 6-68). In my experience the nested and microcystic patterns often coexist. If the lining cells become flattened with scant cytoplasm, the spaces can mimic lymph–vascular channels (Fig. 6-69).

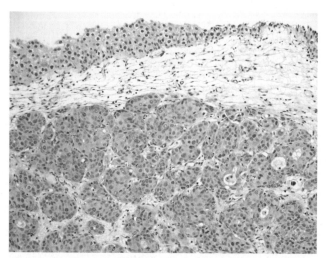

FIGURE 6-66 ■ Nested variant of urothelial carcinoma with the nests focally becoming confluent.

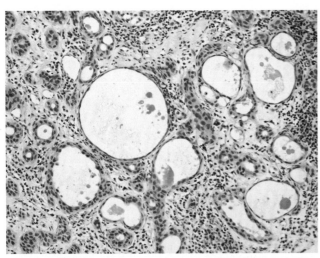

FIGURE 6-68 ■ Microcystic variant of urothelial carcinoma with variably sized cystic spaces and some solid nests.

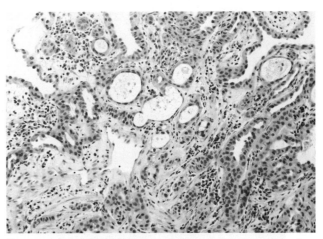

FIGURE 6-70 ■ Urothelial carcinoma with tubule formation. This case mimics nephrogenic adenoma.

It is important to distinguish cystic change in urothelial carcinoma from benign and malignant mimics. It may be confused with benign proliferations such as cystitis cystica and glandularis and nephrogenic adenoma. Clues to nephrogenic adenoma include the presence of a papillary component (papillae covered by a single layer of cells), prominent basement membrane around the tubules, and a heterogeneous lining with attenuated, cuboidal, and hobnail cells.[300,301] There can be a fibromyxoid background that could be confused with a stromal response to tumor invasion.[305] The presence of significant nuclear atypia at least focally and areas of typical invasive urothelial carcinoma allow accurate separation. More problematic is the separation of the microcystic pattern of urothelial carcinoma and adenocarcinoma of the bladder. The diagnosis of adenocarcinoma should be restricted to pure tumors with true gland formation.[14,15] In microcystic urothelial cancer, the lining cells are urothelial

and the spaces formed are pseudoglandular and not true glands.

Urothelial Carcinoma with Small Tubules

In some cases of urothelial carcinoma there are areas of the tumor with the formation of small- to medium-sized tubular structures, some of which can be elongated (Fig. 6-70).[172,306] The tubules are lined by urothelial cells and show some degree of nuclear pleomorphism. This generally occurs in the setting of a usual type of urothelial carcinoma but in limited biopsy material it is possible that this could be diagnostically challenging. There is considerable overlap between this feature and the microcystic pattern described above. The major differential diagnosis is with cystitis glandularis and nephrogenic adenoma. These tumors are distinguished from benign conditions using the same features already described in the preceding sections on the nested and microcystic variants. In one reported example the tubular pattern closely resembled prostatic adenocarcinoma.[307]

Micropapillary Variant

The occurrence of this distinctive morphologic variant of carcinoma in the urinary bladder was first presented in detail by Amin et al.[308] in a description of 18 patients. A recent review article summarized 268 cases of micropapillary urothelial carcinoma (including those originating in the ureter and renal pelvis) culled from the literature.[309] There are no distinctive epidemiologic features. Although one series suggests that the greater the proportion of the micropapillary component the more aggressive the tumor,[310] most recommend diagnosing this variant irrespective of the proportion present.[311] It is estimated to constitute 0.6% to 1.0% of urothelial carcinomas[53] and is clinically significant for its aggressive clinical course and propensity for extensive and deep invasion.[308–314] Cases with as little as 10% micropapillary morphology have been shown to have this aggressive behavior.[315] The tumor has been described elsewhere in the urothelial tract.[309,316,317] When seen in biopsy or transurethral

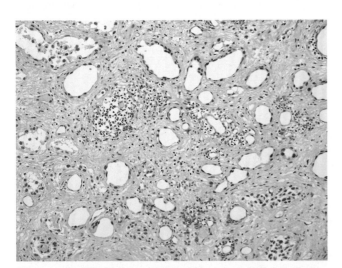

FIGURE 6-69 ■ Microcystic variant of urothelial carcinoma with the tumor cells having scant cytoplasm producing structures that mimic lymph–vascular spaces.

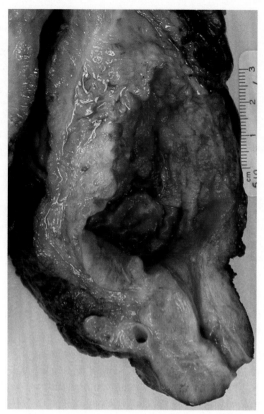

FIGURE 6-71 ■ Micropapillary variant of urothelial carcinoma. The tumor in this case was 90% micropapillary.

resection specimens, a repeat resection of the area is indicated if muscle invasion is not demonstrable in the original material. Occult lymph node metastases were present in 27% of cases at the time of cystectomy in one series.[311] Some authors have advocated immediate cystectomy in T1 cases.[318]

There are no unique gross pathologic features although these can produce a diffuse thickening of the bladder wall similar to linitis plastica (Fig. 6-71). The tumor is composed of cytologically malignant cells arranged in small pseudopapillary clusters. A similar pattern is identifiable in urine cytology specimens.[317] At low magnification, the striking pattern of small tumor cell nests with prominent tissue retraction is immediately evident (Box 6-5) (Figs. 6-72 and 6-73). The cells often have the nuclei toward the outer aspect of the nests with a tapering of cytoplasm centrally (Fig. 6-74). This mimics a papillary structure; however, a true fibrovascular core is absent (Fig. 6-75). It has been hypothesized that this

---

**Box 6-5 ● MICROPAPILLARY VARIANT —
CRITERIA FOR DIAGNOSIS**

Diffuse retraction artifact
Multiple nests in some spaces
Small size of nests
Peripheral location of nuclei
Epithelial ring forms

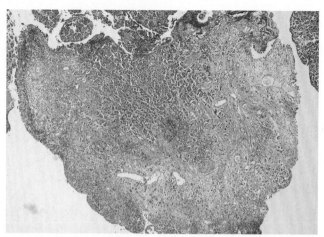

FIGURE 6-72 ■ Micropapillary variant of urothelial carcinoma in a TURBT chip.

architectural growth is related to an inversion (reverse apical) of the location of the MUC1 protein.[319] These clusters are usually floating free in an empty space suggesting lymph–vascular invasion. Although most of these spaces appear related to tissue retraction artifact, extensive lymph–vascular invasion is generally present (Fig. 6-76). The tumor is often associated with overlying CIS. In some cases the pattern mimics adenocarcinoma and combined with the frequent expression of CA125, it has been suggested that this may represent a type of glandular differentiation.[320] A surface micropapillary pattern has been described in some cases with slender delicate filiform projections that lack a central fibrovascular core. These tumors are often quite extensive at the time of resection and can spread widely. Care should be taken when evaluating ureter resection margins at frozen section as the tumor can be found in the periureteral soft tissue (Fig. 6-77). The tumor retains this distinctive morphology in metastases. This is important when a biopsy from a lymph node or other presumed metastasis shows this morphology (Fig. 6-78). In cases of an unknown primary,

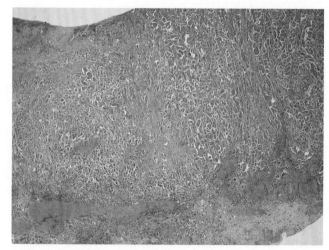

FIGURE 6-73 ■ Micropapillary variant of urothelial carcinoma in a section from a cystectomy specimen.

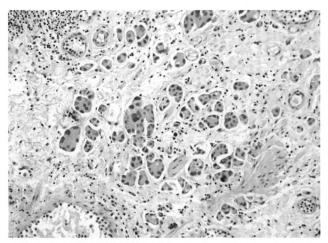

FIGURE 6-74 ■ Micropapillary variant of urothelial carcinoma in the lamina propria.

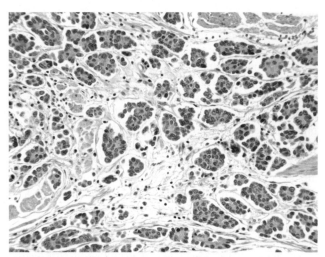

FIGURE 6-75 ■ Micropapillary variant of urothelial carcinoma with prominent peripheral location of nuclei.

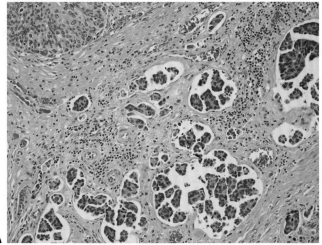

A

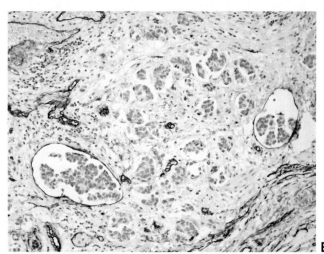

B

FIGURE 6-76 ■ Micropapillary variant of urothelial carcinoma **(A)** with some of the nests in spaces lined by CD34-positive cells **(B)**. Note the usual urothelial carcinoma component in the upper left.

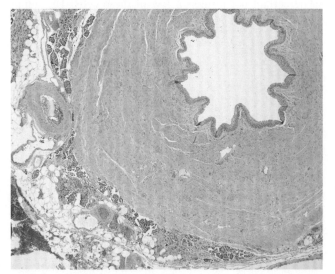

FIGURE 6-77 ■ Micropapillary variant of urothelial carcinoma involving a ureter resection margin (the surgeon could not get a clear margin in this case).

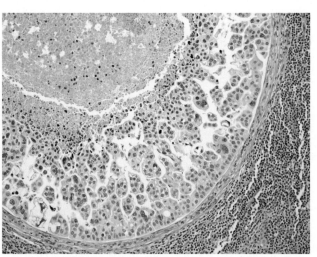

FIGURE 6-78 ■ Micropapillary variant of urothelial carcinoma metastatic to a pelvic lymph node.

bladder origin should be considered and secondly in cases with known bladder cancer this could represent a metastasis from the known primary.

The immunophenotype is similar to usual urothelial carcinoma with most expressing cytokeratin 7 (100%), cytokeratin 20 (54% to 90%), high molecular weight cytokeratin (34βE12, 15% to 54%), p63 (27%), epithelial membrane antigen (EMA) (100%), CEA (65%), thrombomodulin (23%), and uroplakin III (77% to 92%).[53,244,310,312,314,321,322] The vast majority are MUC1 and MUC2 positive[314,319,321] although this does not distinguish the micropapillary variant from usual urothelial carcinoma with retraction artifact. There is no expression of MUC5A, MUC6, or CDX2.[314] P53 overexpression is present in up to 100% of cases.[314]

Morphologically, the tumor bears a striking resemblance to serous papillary carcinoma of the ovary, a differential diagnosis that may require clinical correlation for exclusion in female patients. One feature of note is that psammoma bodies are extremely rare in the bladder tumor. The presence of a typical urothelial carcinoma component in the invasive carcinoma and/or the presence of a surface component would support interpretation as a bladder primary. Immunohistochemistry could also be of assistance with cytokeratin 20 and uroplakin positivity supporting a bladder origin and WT-1 positivity supporting a serous ovarian carcinoma.[322] Metastatic micropapillary carcinoma from other organs where this histology occurs such as lung and breast should also be considered. Clinical correlation may be necessary in some cases; immunohistochemistry for TTF-1 (lung) and mammaglobin (breast) may be of value.[322] A small percentage (5%) of urothelial carcinomas will express TTF-1.[259]

The micropapillary variant must also be distinguished from retraction artifact in usual urothelial carcinoma. In the latter, this is typically focal and scattered, whereas in the micropapillary variant, the clefts surround virtually all of the tumor nests. The features that best distinguish this from usual urothelial carcinoma with retraction artifact are multiple nests in single spaces, peripherally located nuclei, intracytoplasmic vacuolization, back-to-back spaces, epithelial ring forms, small nests (<4 cells across), and extensiveness of the spaces.[323]

Plasmacytoid Variant

Rare carcinomas of the urinary bladder can mimic malignant lymphoma. Small cell carcinoma and lymphoepithelioma-like carcinoma are discussed elsewhere. Zukerberg et al.[324] described two cases of bladder carcinoma that diffusely permeated the bladder wall and were composed of cells with a monotonous appearance mimicking lymphoma. Similar tumors have been referred to as plasmacytoid or lobular carcinoma-like and have been included in some series as signet ring carcinomas.[325–330] In the original description of signet ring cell carcinoma of the bladder, Saphir[331] reported two cases of signet ring cell carcinoma that contained "monocyte-like" cells. The resemblance to lobular carcinoma of the breast has also been noted.[328] These are aggressive tumors with over 95% of cases locally advanced (T3/4) and/or with lymph node metastases at the time of presentation.[325–327,329,332] In the 16 cases with follow-up reported by Nigwekar et al.,[329] 11 patients were dead from disease (1 to 43 months; median, 6 months) and the remaining 5 were alive but with known disease. These also have an unusual predilection for involving peritoneal surfaces.[333]

These tumors may not produce a discrete mass but rather produce thickening of the bladder wall with a linitis plastica-like appearance. Edema of the mucosa can be present. This feature is important; in a bladder biopsy or transurethral resection with a clinical impression of a tumor, the presence of mucosal edema should raise this possibility and a careful examination for rare tumor cells should be undertaken (Fig. 6-79). In some instances, it may be appropriate to use immunohistochemistry with a pancytokeratin antibody to be certain not to miss a few of these cells. The tumor

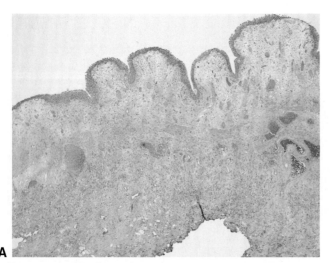
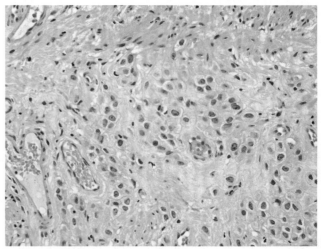

FIGURE 6-79 ■ Plasmacytoid variant of urothelial carcinoma in a TURBT specimen. The mucosa is edematous (**A**) with the tumor cells in the deep lamina propria (**B**).

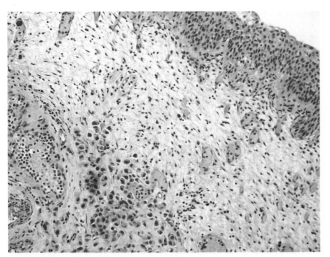

FIGURE 6-80 ■ Plasmacytoid variant of urothelial carcinoma in the lamina propria.

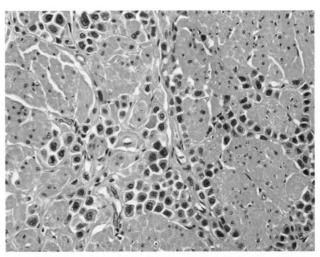

FIGURE 6-82 ■ Plasmacytoid variant of urothelial carcinoma infiltrating between smooth muscle bundles of the muscularis propria.

cells are medium sized with pale eosinophilic cytoplasm and eccentric nuclei producing the plasmacytoid appearance (Fig. 6-80). The appearance can be strikingly plasma cell-like such that plasmacytoma is strongly considered in the differential diagnosis.[334] In some cases, the cytoplasm is more basophilic. Many cells have an area of perinuclear clearing that may be mucin positive. In all cases, a minority of cells have true signet ring morphology. The nuclei tend to be round or indented with prominent nucleoli in a minority. Overall there is a more uniform nuclear appearance than typical of urothelial carcinoma (Fig. 6-81). The cells tend to infiltrate as single cells (Fig. 6-82) or cords of cells but can also form nests and sheets (Fig. 6-83). The diffusely permeative nature results in the tumor being more extensive than appreciated clinically or on gross examination. These can be extremely challenging at frozen section evaluation of ureter margins, and knowledge of the histology is very helpful in avoiding false-negative interpretations. Typical urothelial

carcinoma, often a surface papillary carcinoma, is present in the majority of cases. The diagnosis of carcinoma can be confirmed by positive immunoreactivity for cytokeratin, EMA, and CEA with negative reactivity for lymphoid markers.

The differential diagnostic considerations are plasmacytosis, lymphoma, and multiple myeloma. Identification of an epithelial component confirms the diagnosis. If immunohistochemistry is needed, a pancytokeratin is most useful. These tumors have been reported to be immunoreactive for CD138, a plasma cell marker, in over 90% of cases (Fig. 6-84).[329,335] The possibility of metastasis from another site can also be considered in pure tumors. These tumors have an immunohistochemical profile similar to usual urothelial carcinoma with expression of cytokeratins 7 (70% to 100%) and 20 (31% to 100%), p63, and uroplakin III (11%) (Fig. 6-85).[326–329] In one study, all 5 cases showed loss of E-cadherin expression,[327] and in another, 7 of 10 lacked

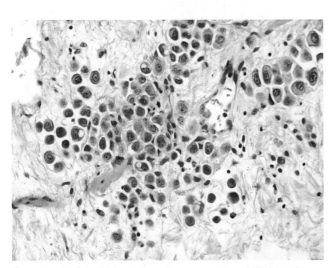

FIGURE 6-81 ■ Plasmacytoid variant of urothelial carcinoma illustrating the morphologic range of the individual cells. A few tumor cells have cytoplasmic vacuoles.

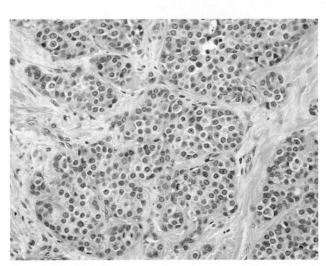

FIGURE 6-83 ■ Plasmacytoid variant of urothelial carcinoma with the cells forming more defined nests.

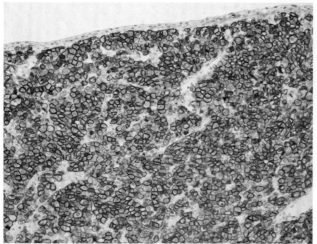

FIGURE 6-84 ■ Plasmacytoid variant of urothelial carcinoma with strong immunoreactivity for CD138.

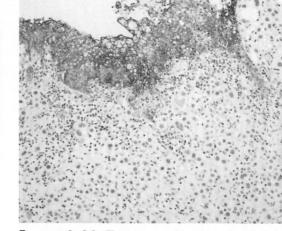

FIGURE 6-86 ■ Plasmacytoid variant of urothelial carcinoma with loss of expression of E-cadherin.

E-cadherin expression (Fig. 6-86).[328] Like urothelial carcinoma, these tumors can express estrogen and progesterone receptors in a minority of cases,[328] an important feature to recognize if the possibility of metastatic carcinoma of the breast is considered.

Lymphoepithelioma-like Variant

Carcinoma that histologically resembles lymphoepithelioma of the nasopharynx has been described in the urinary tract.[233,336–341] It is more common in men than in women, occurs in late adulthood, and is not associated with Epstein-Barr

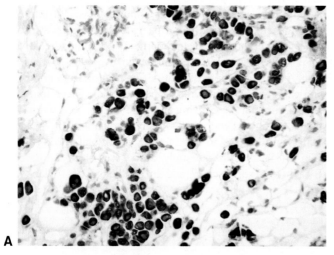

A

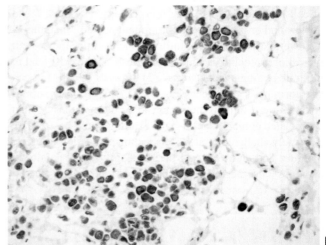

B

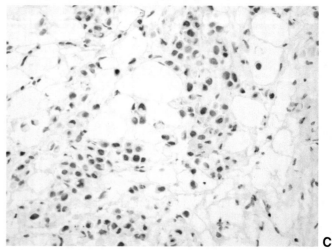

C

FIGURE 6-85 ■ Plasmacytoid variant of urothelial carcinoma with positive immunoreactivity for cytokeratins 7 **(A)** and 20 **(B)** but not for p63 **(C)**.

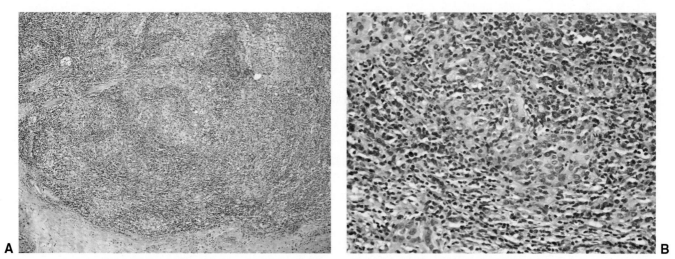

FIGURE 6-87 ■ Lymphoepithelioma-like variant of urothelial carcinoma at low **(A)** and high **(B)** magnification.

virus infection.[338,339,341–343] The clinical significance of lymphoepithelioma-like carcinoma rests with its apparent responsiveness to chemotherapy. In four cases reported from the MD Anderson Cancer Center, there was complete response to transurethral resection combined with chemotherapy, allowing preservation of the bladder.[336] Some subsequent reports have confirmed this apparent distinct responsiveness[339,341] while others have not.[339] This response is related to tumors with pure or predominantly lymphoepithelioma-like histology; tumors with a significant urothelial component behave as usual urothelial carcinoma.[341] It is important to report whether these case are pure or mixed; if mixed it is helpful to indicate the proportion of the typical urothelial component.

The tumor usually presents as a sessile mass. Histologically it may be pure or mixed with typical urothelial carcinoma, the latter being focal and inconspicuous in some instances. It can be limited to urothelial CIS on the surface. Glandular and squamous differentiation can be seen. The tumor is composed of nests, sheets, and cords of undifferentiated cells with large

pleomorphic nuclei and prominent nucleoli. The cytoplasmic borders are poorly defined, giving a syncytial appearance (Fig. 6-87). The background consists of a prominent lymphoid stroma that includes lymphocytes, plasma cells, histiocytes, and occasional neutrophils or eosinophils. The inflammatory cells can spare the syncytial islands or can be admixed with the epithelial element obscuring it (Fig. 6-88).

Immunohistochemical studies show an expression pattern consistent with urothelial origin (Fig. 6-89). The carcinoma cells express pancytokeratin (AE1/AE3; 100%), cytokeratin 7 (majority, 100%), cytokeratin 20 (15% to 100%), and EMA (100%).[233,337,339,340] The lymphoid cells express both B- and T-cell markers.[233]

The major differential diagnostic considerations are poorly differentiated urothelial carcinoma, squamous cell carcinoma, and lymphoma, with the latter being most important. Differentiation from lymphoma may be difficult, but the presence of a syncytial pattern of large malignant cells with a dense polymorphous lymphoid background is an important clue.

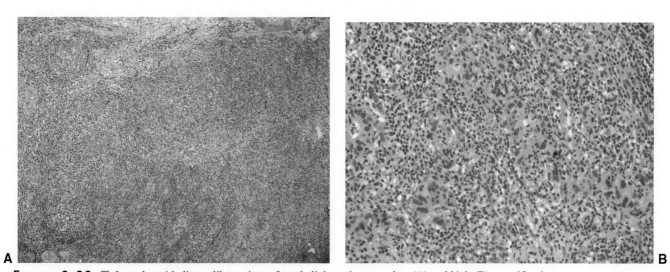

FIGURE 6-88 ■ Lymphoepithelioma-like variant of urothelial carcinoma at low **(A)** and high **(B)** magnification.

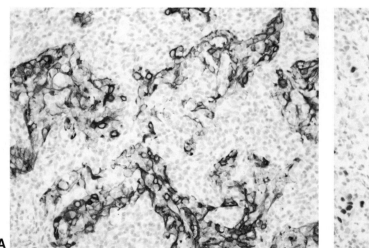

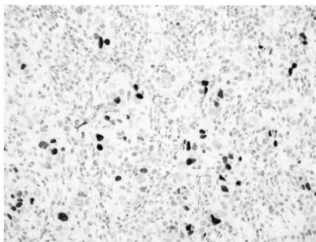

FIGURE 6-89 ■ Lymphoepithelioma-like variant of urothelial carcinoma with positive immunoreactivity for high molecular weight cytokeratin 34βE12 **(A)** and p63 **(B)**.

Immunohistochemistry shows cytokeratin expression in the malignant cells. It is possible to overlook the malignant cells in the background of inflamed bladder mucosa and misdiagnose the condition as florid chronic cystitis. Cases submitted by the urologist as "tumors" or "masses" should be carefully evaluated for the presence of malignant cells; in difficult cases, immunohistochemistry should be employed as an adjunct to define an epithelial component within the inflammation.

Inverted Papilloma-like Urothelial Carcinoma (Urothelial Carcinoma with Inverted Features)

In 1976, Cameron and Lupton[40] described two cases of urothelial carcinoma that mimicked inverted papilloma architecturally, but possessed high-grade cytologic abnormalities. There are no specific epidemiologic features to this variant.[52] The high frequency of *FGFR3* gene mutations in these tumors indicates that the majority of these tumors likely represent a variant of papillary urothelial carcinoma.[48] A proposed classification for inverted papilloma-like carcinoma is presented in Table 6-12. There is insufficient published data to indicate whether these behave in a manner different than what would be expected with usual urothelial carcinoma on a stage for stage basis.[47] There is data in the literature stating that urothelial carcinomas that invade with a pushing front have a better outcome than those with a more infiltrative pattern of growth.[224,225]

The potential for misinterpretation of such cases as inverted papilloma has been confirmed by other authors.[48,52] In a few cases, the tumor architecture is almost identical to inverted papilloma. In most cases, however, these carcinomas grow with more of a broad pushing front (Fig. 6-90) or variably sized nests (Box 6-6; Fig. 6-91). In the latter, the nests are both discrete and confluent. The amount of stroma tends to be variable from area to area in contrast to inverted papilloma where there is minimal stroma. Trabecular architecture when present is much more variable with respect to the size and width of the trabeculae when compared to inverted papilloma (Fig. 6-92). By definition, this variant of urothelial carcinoma has significant nuclear pleomorphism, mitotic figures, and architectural disruption. The well-defined palisading of the basal layer nuclei, maturation

Table 6-12 ■ CLASSIFICATION OF INVERTED UROTHELIAL TUMORS

Inverted urothelial papilloma
Inverted papillary urothelial neoplasm of low malignant potential
Inverted papillary urothelial carcinoma, low grade, noninvasive
Inverted papillary urothelial carcinoma, high grade, noninvasive
Inverted papillary urothelial carcinoma, high grade, invasive

Modified from Epstein J, Amin M, Reuter V. *Bladder Biopsy Interpretation.* Philadelphia, PA: Lippincott Williams & Wilkins; 2010.

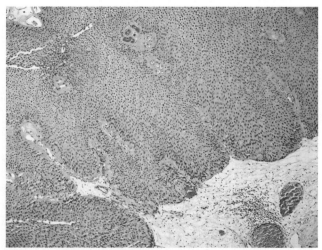

FIGURE 6-90 ■ Inverted papilloma-like variant of urothelial carcinoma with broad pushing borders.

toward the center of the trabeculae, and spindling of the cells typical of inverted papilloma is absent or at most poorly developed. In most, the overlying epithelium has similar abnormalities. The complex anastomosing trabecular architecture typical of inverted papilloma is rarely a feature. An exophytic papillary or typical invasive component is often associated with the inverted element (Fig. 6-93). In contrast, the coexistence of inverted papilloma with papillary carcinoma is exceedingly rare. In contrast to inverted papilloma, these tumors harbor the cytogenetic changes of urothelial carcinoma.[48] In contrast to inverted urothelial carcinoma, immunohistochemical studies have shown inverted papilloma to have a low proliferation rate with Ki-67, a normal expression pattern of cytokeratin 20, and no overexpression of p53.[48]

More problematic than distinguishing these from inverted papilloma is determining if there is invasion present or if the tumor is a noninvasive low-grade papillary urothelial carcinoma with inverted architecture.[52] Features of invasion are discussed in detail later in the chapter in a section devoted to this topic and are not repeated in detail here. Clues to the presence of invasion in this specific setting include more irregular contours to the nests with more variable size and shape including the presence of jagged edges.[47]

Giant Cell Variant

Giant cells have been reported in bladder tumors in a variety of different contexts. Giant cell carcinoma with malignant

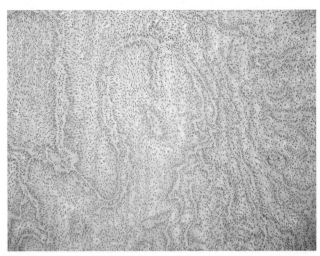

FIGURE 6-92 ■ Inverted papilloma-like variant of urothelial carcinoma with trabecular architecture closely mimicking inverted papilloma. Not the marked variability in the size of the trabeculae.

epithelial giant cells has been described.[344–346] There are insufficient cases in the literature to make any major conclusions regarding epidemiologic aspects of this tumor. Most have occurred in older men and have been associated with a very poor prognosis.

Morphologically, these tumors have similarity to giant cell carcinoma of the lung. There are no characteristic gross features. In most cases there is an associated usual urothelial carcinoma component although one case of pure giant cell carcinoma is described.[346] The giant cells may have single nuclei or be multinucleated with marked nuclear pleomorphism and frequent mitoses including abnormal forms (Fig. 6-94). The tumors can be solid or composed of smaller infiltrating nests. Immunohistochemistry shows expression of cytokeratins and EMA in the giant cells with variable expression of p63, thrombomodulin, and uroplakin.[346]

The major differential diagnosis includes other situations in which giant cells can be present in association with

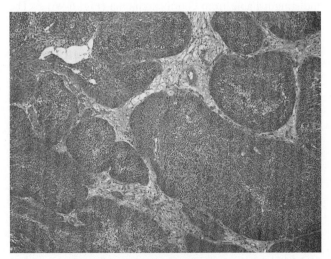

FIGURE 6-91 ■ Inverted papilloma-like variant of urothelial carcinoma with large variably shaped nests.

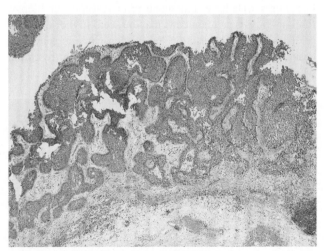

FIGURE 6-93 ■ Inverted papilloma-like variant of urothelial carcinoma with prominent trabecular architecture and a minor exophytic papillary component.

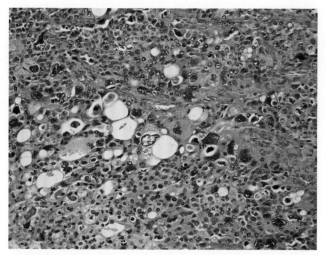

FIGURE 6-94 ■ Giant cell variant of urothelial carcinoma.

urothelial carcinoma (Table 6-13). Most frequently, benign giant cells normally present to varying degrees in the lamina propria could be confused with tumor giant cells.[347] In the past, the term "giant cell cystitis" has been applied when these cells were particularly prominent.[348] These cells tend to be stellate in shape with multiple small nuclei. They may be more prominent in the vicinity of tumors and in patients treated with radiation or chemotherapy.[347]

Rarely osteoclastic giant cells occur in invasive high-grade urothelial carcinoma.[349,350] These giant cells have abundant eosinophilic cytoplasm and numerous small, round, regular nuclei and stain positively for vimentin and tartrate-resistant acid phosphatase but not for epithelial markers.

Giant cells are also seen in association with urothelial carcinoma in three other situations. Urothelial carcinoma can show trophoblastic differentiation with formation of syncytiotrophoblastic giant cells. In patients who have received BCG therapy, a granulomatous response that includes Langhans giant cells can be seen. These are well-formed granulomas that do not show caseous necrosis. Also, in patients who have undergone prior resection or biopsy, foreign body–type giant cells may be seen. In the setting of prior transurethral resection these often contain cauterized tissue fragments allowing the inference of a prior resection when no history has been provided.

Table 6-13 ■ DIFFERENTIAL DIAGNOSIS OF UROTHELIAL CARCINOMA WITH GIANT CELLS

Benign giant cells
    Multinucleated stromal giant cells
    Foreign body giant cells (associated with prior instrumentation)
    Langhans giant cells in granulomas following BCG therapy
    Osteoclastic giant cells
Malignant giant cells
    Pleomorphic carcinoma giant cells (giant cell carcinoma)
    Sarcomatoid carcinoma with pleomorphic spindle cells
Syncytiotrophoblastic giant cells

Urothelial Carcinoma with Trophoblastic Differentiation

Giant cells may also be found in urothelial carcinoma associated with human chorionic gonadotropin (HCG) production, and are indicative of syncytiotrophoblastic differentiation.[351] Some patients with significant β-HCG production have developed gynecomastia. Production of HCG by urothelial carcinoma can be frequently demonstrated by immunohistochemistry (up to 35%) and can be detected in the serum of bladder cancer patients. In one study, 20% of patients with metastatic urothelial carcinoma had an elevated serum β-HCG.[352] In another report, serum β-HCG was elevated in 76% of patients with metastatic disease compared with 3% of those with localized tumors.[353] In patients treated with chemotherapy, the serum β-HCG decreased in parallel with tumor response and subsequently increased when the therapy failed.[352] These and other studies led to the interest in the utility of serum β-HCG in patient management.[354] These observations reflect the immunohistochemical studies showing a strong correlation between histologic grade and stage and expression of HCG.[351,355,356] The clinical significance of this finding is uncertain. There have been reports that tumors expressing HCG are more resistant to external beam radiotherapy.[284] It has also been demonstrated that β-HCG production by epithelial tumors can act as an autocrine growth factor inhibiting apoptosis.[357] The presence of choriocarcinoma in the bladder is associated with a highly aggressive clinical course.

Tumors with choriocarcinomatous differentiation have frequently been described as hemorrhagic. Histologically, many tumors expressing β-HCG have no morphologic features distinct from any other high-grade urothelial carcinoma.[284,351] In other cases, pleomorphic tumor giant cells that are present are positive (Fig. 6-95); in far fewer cases there are β-HCG-positive cells present that morphologically resemble syncytiotrophoblastic giant cells. In the latter instance, the combination of mononuclear and multinucleated trophoblastic cells produces areas that histologically are indistinguishable from choriocarcinoma (Fig. 6-96).[351] The β-HCG-producing variant of urothelial carcinoma can be present with other variant histology including micropapillary and plasmacytoid.[358,359] Identification of β-HCG expression by immunohistochemistry does not currently have any known clinical significance and so routine staining of high-grade tumors is not indicated. The presence of true trophoblastic differentiation does seem to indicate a poor prognosis and if present should be diagnosed.

In cases with pure trophoblastic histology the differential diagnosis of primary or metastatic choriocarcinoma should be considered. A diagnosis of a pure choriocarcinoma requires exclusion of an urothelial component. It does appear that true primary choriocarcinoma of the bladder exists with the demonstration of isochromosome 12 in one such tumor.[360] Careful clinical evaluation is required to exclude the possibility of metastasis from a gonadal or extragonadal germ cell tumor.

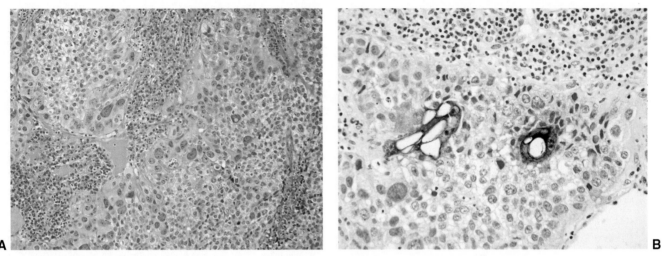

FIGURE 6-95 ■ Urothelial carcinoma with pleomorphic tumor cells **(A)** that react positively for β-HCG **(B)**.

Urothelial Carcinoma with Osteoclastic Giant Cells

Osteoclastic giant cells can be found in some cases of bladder carcinoma. Fewer than 20 such cases have been reported in the literature at the time of this writing.[172] There are no specific epidemiologic features with most being reported in older men.[349,350,361–365] There are a disproportionate number of cases that have arisen in the renal pelvis.[350,366] Based on the limited available data, it is difficult to ascertain with certainty the clinical significance of these tumors.[350,362,364] In one review, the authors conclude that these are aggressive tumors with a

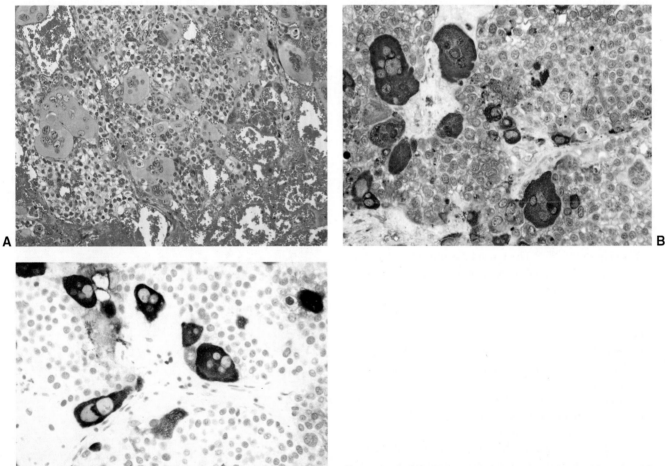

FIGURE 6-96 ■ Urothelial carcinoma with trophoblastic differentiation mimicking choriocarcinoma **(A)**. The giant cells show positive immunoreactivity for β-HCG **(B)** and inhibin **(C)**.

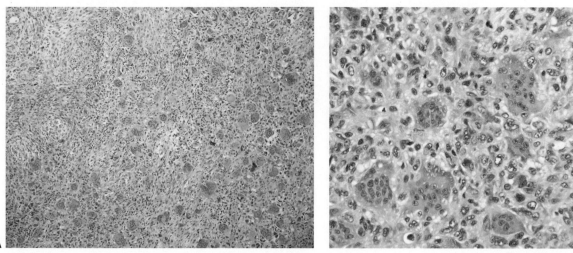

FIGURE 6-97 ■ Sarcomatoid urothelial carcinoma with osteoclastic giant cells at low (**A**) and high (**B**) magnification.

"dismal prognosis"[350] while in a second review, the authors conclude that prognosis is dependent on the features of the associated urothelial tumor and that the giant cell tumor component itself carries a good prognosis.[365] For cases arising in the urinary bladder where follow-up information was available, there were six patients alive with no evidence of disease (follow-up of 2, 8, 12, 18, 35, and 42 months)[344,349,365,367]; one patient developed recurrent urothelial carcinoma following TURBT and was alive without evidence of disease in the second year,[350] one case had local recurrence requiring exenteration with no further recurrence at 6 months[362]; one patient died of an unrelated cause at 33 months with no tumor found at autopsy[368]; and lastly one patient died of disease at 1 year.[350]

Many of these tumors have a polypoid appearance on gross examination. Histologically, a variety of patterns can be seen with all having in common the presence of osteoclastic giant cells. The giant cells are large and multinucleated with numerous small round nuclei that tend to be clustered in one part of the cell (Fig. 6-97). There is no pleomorphism of the nuclei. Histochemistry has demonstrated the presence of tartrate-resistant acid phosphatase.[349,361] By immunohistochemistry they express CD68, CD51, and CD54 (Fig. 6-98).[350,361] These results confirm that these are histiocytic in nature and more specifically have features of normal bone osteoclasts.

Osteoclastic giant cells can be present in association with usual urothelial carcinoma including papillary tumors and CIS. In over 90% of reported cases, there is an associated urothelial carcinoma component.[350] In several examples, the giant cell tumor–like process was identified underlying a noninvasive low-grade papillary urothelial carcinoma. In other cases, they are present with a sarcomatoid carcinoma composed of malignant spindle cells arranged in fascicles or with a myxoid background. Finally, the giant cells may be embedded in a background of mononuclear cells that can have variable degrees of nuclear pleomorphism. Cases with areas closely resembling the histology of giant cell tumors of bone are also described.[361] In all of these situations, the background cells were epithelial in derivation and showed variable immunoreactivity for epithelial markers (cytokeratins including pancytokeratin, cytokeratins 7 and 20, and high molecular weight cytokeratin).[350] Positivity for p63 can be found.

Diagnostic terminology for these tumors has been varied. In the presence of an identifiable urothelial component we refer to these as urothelial carcinoma with osteoclastic giant cells; if a sarcomatoid component is present, then this is also included. The term osteoclast-rich undifferentiated carcinoma has also been advocated.[350] In the six cases reported by Baydar et al.,[350] all had a recognizable urothelial carcinoma component. We would limit the term undifferentiated carcinoma to cases with a background of mononuclear epithelial-derived cells without a recognizable urothelial or sarcomatoid component and lacking a urothelial carcinoma immunohistochemical expression pattern.

The differential diagnosis includes tumors with other types of giant cells including benign giant cells such as the

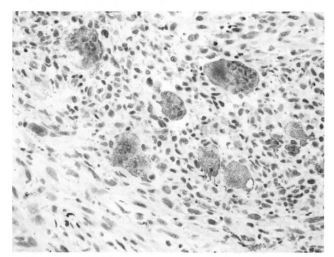

FIGURE 6-98 ■ The osteoclastic giant cells show positive immunoreactivity for CD68.

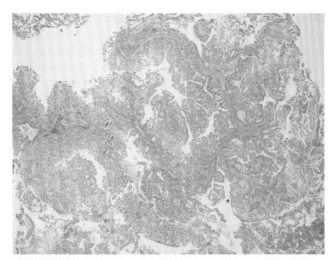

FIGURE 6-99 ■ Urothelial carcinoma with villoglandular differentiation.

normal multinucleated stromal cells, foreign body giant cells, and giant cells of BCG-related granulomas. Malignant tumor giant cells and syncytiotrophoblastic giant cells should also be considered.

Urothelial Carcinoma with Villoglandular Differentiation

Some urothelial carcinomas have a component characterized by fine filiform papillae covered by a glandular epithelium.[65] The epidemiologic features are identical to usual urothelial carcinoma, and there is no specific clinical significance attributed to this histologic variant.

This histology has always accompanied usual urothelial carcinoma including noninvasive papillary carcinoma but is more often associated with invasive carcinomas including tumors with glandular differentiation and other variant histology. The most characteristic feature is the presence of exophytic finger-like or long filiform processes on the tumor surface (Fig. 6-99). The glandular epithelium contains true

glandular spaces and mucin-secreting cells. These glands are often lined by a columnar or cuboidal epithelium. A cribriform architecture is present in many while others have slit-like glandular spaces (Fig. 6-100). In cases with a high-grade papillary component, the glandular epithelium is intermingled with the high-grade urothelial component.

The differential diagnosis includes adenocarcinoma in situ. We reserve this term for pure glandular in situ lesions that in the bladder manifest most often as high-grade dysplastic change in areas of intestinal metaplasia. These can also present as villous adenoma with high-grade dysplasia. Urothelial carcinoma with villoglandular differentiation has a urothelial component and the finger-like processes are not covered by an enteric type of adenomatous epithelium. The presumed in situ pattern of micropapillary carcinoma has small thin delicate filiform processes but these are covered by cells having eosinophilic to clear cytoplasm and glandular features are not present.[53] Urothelial carcinoma with glandular differentiation is most often applied to invasive urothelial carcinoma. In cases of urothelial carcinoma with villoglandular differentiation, and with glandular differentiation in the invasive component, use of both designations would be appropriate. In limited biopsies where there is no urothelial component present, it may not be possible to exclude secondary involvement of the bladder by an adenocarcinoma of colorectal origin without clinical correlation.

Urothelial Carcinoma with Abundant Myxoid Stroma

Invasive urothelial carcinoma typically has a stromal response that can vary from desmoplastic to myxoid. In some cases, the myxoid stroma is pronounced with abundant extracellular mucin.[229] The epidemiologic features are similar to usual urothelial carcinoma and there is no specific clinical significance to this histology.

This term has been applied to cases of invasive urothelial carcinoma where the myxoid stoma consists predominantly of mucinous material (Fig. 6-101). The urothelial

FIGURE 6-100 ■ Urothelial carcinoma with villoglandular differentiation.

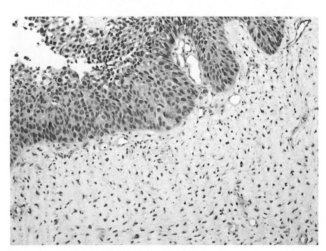

FIGURE 6-101 ■ Noninvasive high-grade papillary urothelial carcinoma with abundant myxoid stroma.

carcinoma can have any morphologic pattern, but cases with glandular differentiation are excluded as these are more correctly classified in the mixed differentiation category. The carcinoma grows in variably sized nests, trabeculae, cords, or as single cells. The cells have moderate to abundant eosinophilic cytoplasm and most do not contain obvious cytoplasmic mucin. When the cells have scant cytoplasm and are ranged in a more filigree or anastomosing cord-like architecture the term "chordoid" is applied. Most have high-grade cytology though cases with histology reminiscent of the nested variant can have this stroma. Mucin stains (Alcian blue, mucicarmine, periodic acid–Schiff [PAS]) will highlight the extracellular mucin and demonstrate cytoplasmic positivity. The immunohistochemical profile reflects the urothelial nature.[229] These tumors also express MUC2 and MUC3 and are CDX2 negative.[229]

The major differential diagnosis is with urothelial carcinoma with glandular differentiation. These tumors can have a mucinous or colloid pattern, but the cells take on a glandular morphology that is most often enteric in type. Secondary involvement of the bladder by a mucinous carcinoma originating elsewhere could be considered. Mucinous carcinoma of the gastrointestinal tract has an enteric-type epithelium in contrast to urothelial carcinoma with myxoid stroma where the carcinoma looks urothelial. In mucinous carcinoma of the prostate the glands typically look like usual prostatic adenocarcinoma glands with uniform nuclei and a single prominent nucleolus. If this is seriously entertained, immunohistochemistry will readily resolve the case.

Urothelial Carcinoma with Chordoid Features

In some cases of urothelial carcinoma with myxoid stroma, the carcinoma grows as cords within the myxoid matrix producing a pattern highly reminiscent of that seen in chordoma.[369] There are no specific epidemiologic features and no known specific prognostic significance to this morphologic variant.

This pattern has always had an associated component of typical invasive high-grade urothelial carcinoma. The cells are small with scant eosinophilic to pale cytoplasm and are arranged in thin cords (Fig. 6-102). There is a mucinous background that has a basophilic hue. The pattern is striking in its

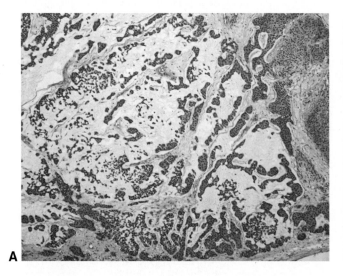

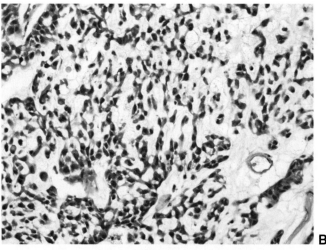

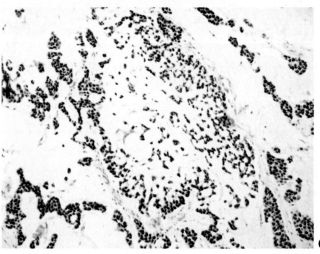

FIGURE 6-102 ■ Urothelial carcinoma with chordoid features at low **(A)** and high **(B)** magnification; the tumor expresses p63 protein **(C)**.

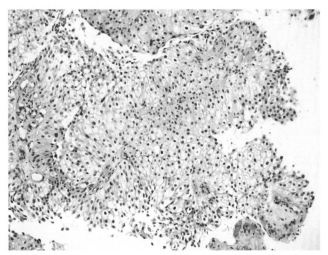

FIGURE 6-103 ■ Clear cell variant of urothelial carcinoma that in this case was a noninvasive papillary tumor.

resemblance to chordoma or yolk sac tumor. The mucinous material in the background is positive with colloidal iron and Alcian blue but not PAS.[369] Cytoplasmic mucin is not present. This morphology may be retained in metastases. These tumors express usual urothelial carcinoma markers including p63 (100%) and high molecular weight cytokeratin (100%).[369]

The differential diagnosis is as discussed in the section on urothelial carcinoma with abundant myxoid stoma above.[229] In addition, sarcomatoid urothelial carcinoma should also be considered in the differential diagnosis since they can have a myxoid pattern to the sarcomatoid component.[370,371] In these cases, the cells have marked nuclear pleomorphism and cellular spindle cell areas are present. Myxoid mesenchymal tumors, particularly myxoid leiomyosarcoma, occur in the bladder.[372] These would lack an epithelial component and would express smooth muscle markers.

Clear Cell (Glycogen-rich) Urothelial Carcinoma

It is important to recognize that urothelial carcinoma can occasionally show prominent cytoplasmic clearing due to the presence of glycogen.[227] This can occur in papillary tumors as well as invasive carcinomas. This is part of the morphologic diversity of urothelial carcinoma and has no specific epidemiologic or clinical features.

The gross features reflect the tumor in which the cytoplasmic clearing is occurring. Generally the tumor retains the architectural characteristics of the urothelial carcinoma. It can be seen in noninvasive papillary carcinoma (Fig. 6-103) and in invasive carcinoma (Fig. 6-104). In most cases, the histology is reminiscent of a glycogenated squamous epithelium of the female genital tract forming large islands or sheets. In rare examples, a nested morphology resembling renal cell carcinoma is present focally (Fig. 6-105). Glycogen can be demonstrated by histochemistry (Fig. 6-106). The immunohistochemical profile is that of urothelial carcinoma.

The differential diagnosis includes clear cell adenocarcinoma of the urethra/bladder[373,374] or metastatic clear cell renal cell carcinoma.[375] Clear cell adenocarcinoma has papillary, solid, and tubular architecture with pleomorphic cells including cells with hobnail morphology. In general the cytoplasm tends to be more eosinophilic than clear. Metastatic clear cell renal cell carcinoma usually shows small nests or alveoli with a prominent sinusoidal vascular pattern. Cautery can also result in cytoplasmic clearing and should not be confused with variant histology.

Lipid-rich (Lipoid) Urothelial Carcinoma

Rare cases of bladder carcinoma having cells containing cytoplasmic lipid have been reported.[376,377] These are too rare for any specific clinical significance to have been attributed to them; however, the prognosis in cases reported to date has been poor.[377]

The individual tumor cells can mimic lipoblasts or signet ring cells with multiple intracytoplasmic vacuoles distorting

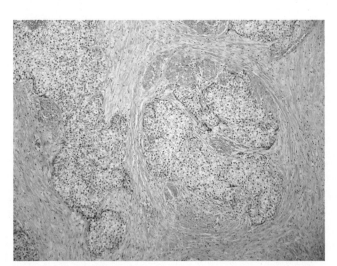

FIGURE 6-104 ■ Clear cell variant of urothelial carcinoma invading as solid nests.

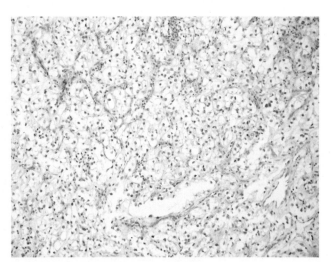

FIGURE 6-105 ■ Clear cell variant of urothelial carcinoma that in some areas had small nests mimicking clear cell renal cell carcinoma.

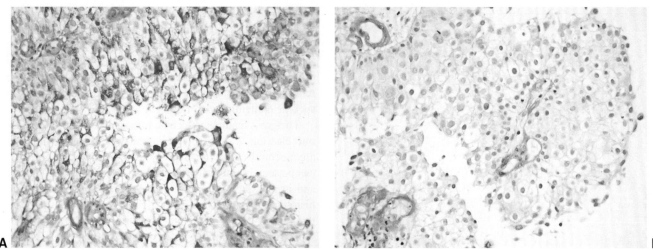

FIGURE 6-106 ■ Clear cell variant of urothelial carcinoma (same case as Fig. 6-103) with demonstrable cytoplasmic glycogen (**A**, PAS; **B**, PAS with diastase digestion).

the nucleus (Fig. 6-107). The tumors are solid or infiltrative. The lipid cell component can make up to 50% of the tumor volume with all cases reported to date having an associated typical urothelial carcinoma component. Stains for mucin and glycogen are negative. By immunohistochemistry the profile is similar to high-grade urothelial carcinoma with variable expression of cytokeratins 7 and 20, high molecular weight cytokeratin, and thrombomodulin (Fig. 6-108). There is no immunoreactivity for S100 protein. Analysis using loss of heterozygosity has demonstrated similar abnormalities in the lipid cell component to the associated urothelial carcinoma.[377]

The differential diagnosis includes other patterns of urothelial carcinoma with signet ring cells. Signet ring cell adenocarcinoma can occur as a pure tumor or mixed with urothelial carcinoma. In both the tumor cells contain mucin and have a single large mucin vacuole in the cytoplasm. In some cases the cytoplasm has a bubbly appearance. Mucin stains will resolve the differential diagnosis with the lipoid

cell variant. Sarcomatoid carcinoma with heterologous elements can include a liposarcomatous component. In these, the sarcomatous element will form a distinct component of the tumor rather than scattered lipoblast-like cells within usual urothelial carcinoma. The plasmacytoid variant of urothelial carcinoma also can have cells with cytoplasmic vacuoles in a minority of cells. The cells are small and discohesive and the vacuoles represent mucin. Finally examples of primary liposarcoma of the bladder are described but this is excluded from consideration because of the epithelial nature of the lipoid variant.

Urothelial Carcinoma with Rhabdoid Features

Urothelial carcinoma with morphologic features reminiscent of rhabdoid tumor of the kidney is well described.[378–382] There are no specific epidemiologic features associated with this variant. One case has been described in a 2-year-old girl.[379] There are too few documented cases to indicate

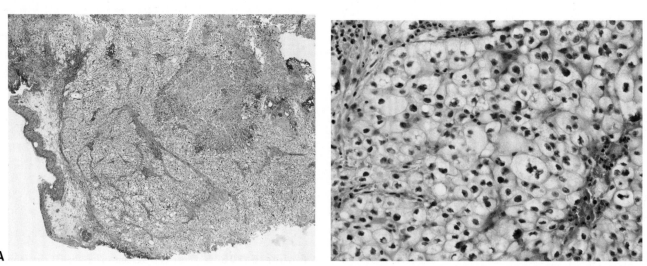

FIGURE 6-107 ■ Lipid-rich variant of urothelial carcinoma at low (**A**) and high (**B**) magnification. Note the microvesicular character of the cytoplasm.

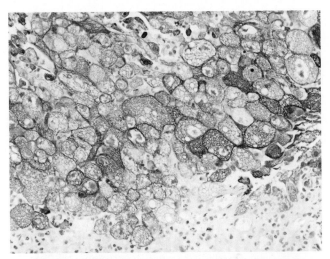

FIGURE 6-108 ■ Lipid-rich variant of urothelial carcinoma with positive immunoreactivity for cytokeratin 7. The reactivity pattern highlights the microvesicular character of the cytoplasm.

clinical behavior, but in several cases patients died shortly after diagnosis.[380,382] It is likely that many of these cases have been classified as sarcomatoid carcinoma without the specific rhabdoid designation.

Grossly, these tumors can produce a polypoid mass. In most cases, they have been associated with invasive high-grade urothelial carcinoma but pure rhabdoid morphology can be seen.[378,381] Other variant histology including sarcomatoid carcinoma[379,380] and small cell carcinoma have been reported associated with this subtype. The rhabdoid component is characterized by large, poorly cohesive cells with abundant eosinophilic cytoplasmic and eccentric nuclei having a single prominent macronucleolus (Fig. 6-109). The cytoplasm contains a large finely fibrillar eosinophilic inclusion. The cells occur singly, in small clusters, or in sheets. In most cases cytokeratin expression can be demonstrated with pancytokeratins or low molecular weight cytokeratin antibodies (cam 5.2).[382] Other epithelial markers such as EMA

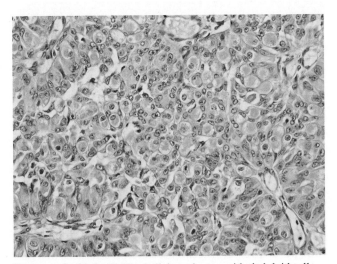

FIGURE 6-109 ■ Urothelial carcinoma with rhabdoid cells.

can be positive. The cells do not express muscle markers or S100 protein.[382]

The differential diagnosis includes rhabdomyosarcoma and sarcomatoid carcinoma with rhabdomyosarcomatous differentiation. In both, the rhabdoid cells would express markers of muscle rather than epithelial differentiation. A case of true extrarenal rhabdoid tumor of the urinary bladder has been reported.[383] True rhabdoid tumors have mutation or loss of the *INI1* gene on chromosome 22q11.[384] This can be demonstrated by loss of nuclear expression of INI1 by immunohistochemistry.[385] We would be reluctant to make a diagnosis of extrarenal rhabdoid tumor in the urinary bladder without loss of INI1 staining by immunohistochemistry.

Sarcomatoid Urothelial Carcinoma (Carcinosarcoma)

Tumors of the urinary tract can contain both malignant epithelial and malignant spindle cell components. In a report from a SEER (Surveillance Epidemiology and End Results Program) database, sarcomatoid carcinoma/carcinosarcoma was reported in 0.6% of patients with urothelial carcinoma.[386] Various terms have been used for these neoplasms, including carcinosarcoma, sarcomatoid carcinoma, pseudosarcomatous transitional cell carcinoma, malignant mesodermal mixed tumor, spindle cell and giant cell carcinoma, and malignant teratoma.[272,370,371,386–389] A common histogenesis for the epithelial and stromal elements of these tumors has been demonstrated.[390,391] It is currently recommended that these be reported under the term sarcomatoid carcinoma with the added descriptor of "with or without heterologous differentiation."[14] When present, the heterologous element(s) should be specified.

Sarcomatoid carcinoma affects males more frequently than females (2-3:1) and tends to occur in older patients (seventh and eighth decades), with only rare cases in patients under the age of 50 years. Sarcomatoid urothelial carcinoma is highly malignant, with crude 1- and 2-year survivals of about 50% and 25%, respectively. A comparison of survival for 32 cases without heterologous elements and 24 cases with heterologous elements culled from the literature showed no significant difference between the two types.[280] This was also the conclusion of Lopez-Beltran et al.[388] in an analysis of 41 cases. Using a SEER database, Wright and Black reported that patients with carcinosarcoma have a significantly worse prognosis than those with sarcomatoid carcinoma (overall 1- and 5-year survivals of 48% and 17% compared with 54% and 37%). These data are limited by the lack of pathology review and the inconsistent use of terminology by pathologists. Presently these tumors are treated the same as high-grade urothelial carcinoma; in the MD Anderson Cancer Center series, many of the patients received adjuvant or neo-adjuvant chemotherapy.[389]

Sarcomatoid carcinoma is usually exophytic, often with a polypoid or pedunculated growth pattern (Figs. 6-110 and 6-111). Histologically, the tumors contain a mixture of carcinoma and malignant spindle cells (Fig. 6-112). The epithelial component is most often urothelial with squamous

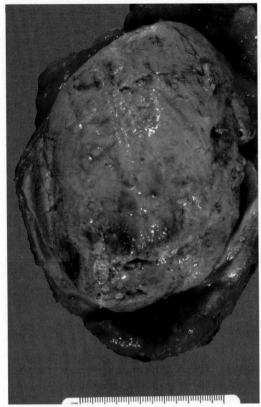

FIGURE 6-110 ■ Sarcomatoid urothelial carcinoma. The tumor forms a large polypoid mass.

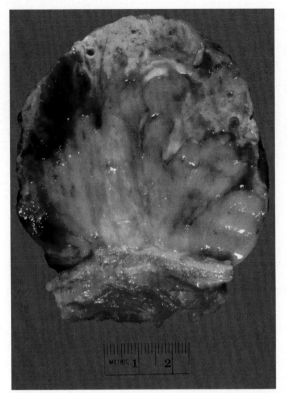

FIGURE 6-111 ■ Sarcomatoid urothelial carcinoma. A cross section from a sarcomatoid carcinoma highlighting the polypoid growth and in this case a narrow pedicle attached to the bladder wall.

being the next most frequent; adenocarcinoma and small cell carcinoma can also occur (Figs. 6-113 and 6-114). In some cases, the epithelial component consists only of CIS, while in others the epithelial component cannot be recognized histologically, and special studies are required to prove the epithelial nature of the spindle cells.

In most cases, the spindle cell component consists of pleomorphic cells in poorly formed fascicles without a specific pattern of differentiation. In some cases the fascicles closely resemble those of leiomyosarcoma. In others, the fascicles are shorter and produce a storiform pattern. The individual cells can be rounded or elongate with abundant eosinophilic cytoplasm resembling rhabdomyosarcoma.[382] In some cases, the architecture can even simulate angiosarcoma.[392] Sclerosing and myxoid patterns can also be seen (Fig. 6-115).[370] Individual cells usually have moderate to

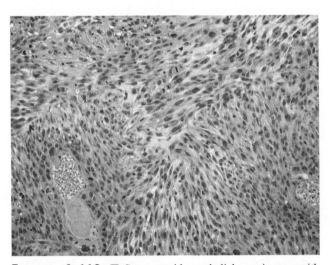

FIGURE 6-112 ■ Sarcomatoid urothelial carcinoma with interweaving fascicles of spindle cells.

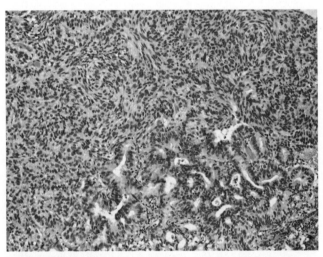

FIGURE 6-113 ■ Sarcomatoid urothelial carcinoma with gandular differentiation.

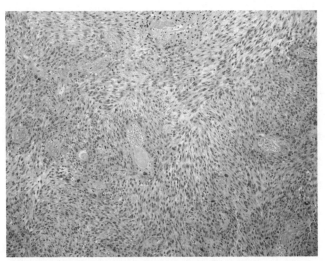

FIGURE 6-114 ■ Sarcomatoid urothelial carcinoma where the tumor also showed squamous differentiation.

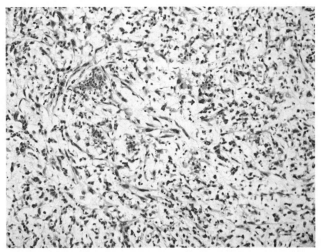

FIGURE 6-115 ■ Sarcomatoid urothelial carcinoma with a myxoid appearance.

severe nuclear atypia with frequent mitoses including abnormal forms. Infrequently the cells can be relatively bland. The merging of the epithelial and spindle cell components is helpful in the diagnosis. In some cases the epithelial element appears as discrete nests in a background of malignant spindle cells. Heterologous differentiation, when present, usually consists of chondrosarcoma (Fig. 6-116) (47%), osteosarcoma (31%), or rhabdomyosarcoma (24%). Other histologic types including leiomyosarcoma, malignant fibrous histiocytoma, fibrosarcoma, and liposarcoma can also occur.[388,393]

Immunohistochemical studies have found the spindle cell element to express cytokeratin at least focally, although in some cases cytokeratin has not been demonstrable (Fig. 6-117A and B).[272,370,371,394,395] Other epithelial markers such as EMA may also be expressed although less consistently. There is expression of p63 in about 50% of cases

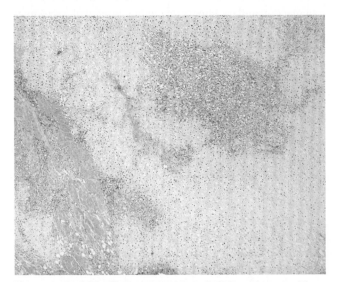

FIGURE 6-116 ■ Sarcomatoid urothelial carcinoma with an extensive chondrosarcomatous component.

(Fig. 6-117C). Coexpression of vimentin in the spindle cell component is usual. Occasionally, the spindle cells express muscle-specific actin, but are negative for desmin. There is no overexpression of ALK-1.[395] Heterologous elements express markers appropriate to the type of differentiation.

In cases with carcinoma and an atypical spindle cell component, the major differential diagnostic consideration is urothelial carcinoma with pseudosarcomatous stroma. In these cases, the reactive stroma can show sufficient cellularity and atypia to raise a serious concern of sarcomatoid carcinoma.[228,389,394,396] The stroma varies from myxoid with stellate or multinucleated cells to cellular and spindled with fascicle formation. By immunohistochemistry, the stromal cells show fibroblastic and myofibroblastic differentiation with vimentin and actin immunoreactivity; desmin is usually negative. The cells also express low molecular weight but not high molecular weight keratins.

Osseous metaplasia is present in some cases of urothelial carcinoma, and this should be differentiated from an osteosarcoma component.[230,397,398] This finding has also been described in metastatic urothelial carcinoma. The metaplastic bone is histologically benign, with a normal lamellar pattern; it is usually found adjacent to areas of hemorrhage. The cells in the adjacent stroma are cytologically benign.

The giant cells of so-called giant cell cystitis should not be confused with sarcomatoid carcinoma. These cells typically have several small, round uniform nuclei and scant cytoplasm.

In cases without obvious carcinoma, the main differential diagnostic considerations are sarcoma or a benign spindle cell proliferation (postoperative spindle cell nodule or inflammatory myofibroblastic pseudotumor). Because of the rarity of primary bladder sarcoma, a malignant spindle cell tumor in the urinary bladder of an adult should be considered sarcomatoid carcinoma until proven otherwise. Extensive sectioning of the tumor and surrounding mucosa may reveal an in situ or invasive epithelial component. The

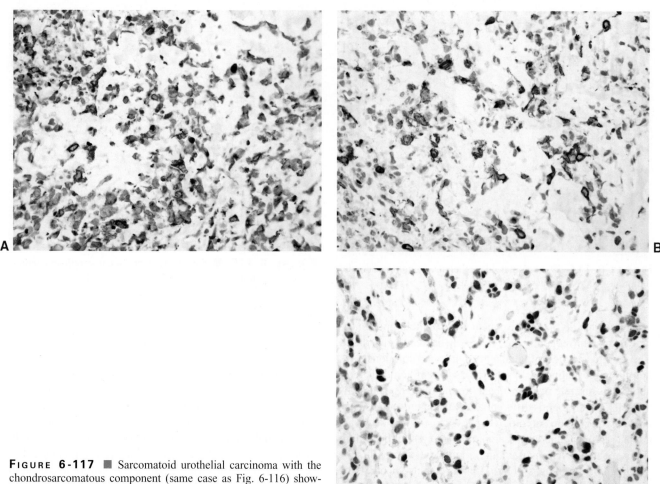

FIGURE 6-117 ■ Sarcomatoid urothelial carcinoma with the chondrosarcomatous component (same case as Fig. 6-116) showing positive immunoreactivity for cytokeratin 7 **(A)**, high molecular weight cytokeratin 34βE12 **(B)**, and p63 **(C)**.

most common primary sarcoma of the bladder in adults is leiomyosarcoma though virtually all sarcoma types are described.[389] Immunohistochemical studies with antibodies to low molecular weight cytokeratin may give evidence of epithelial differentiation; ultrastructural studies can also be helpful.

Both postoperative spindle cell nodule and inflammatory myofibroblastic pseudotumor are characterized by a mixture of compact spindle cells with fascicle formation and more myxoid areas with long, tapered or stellate spindle cells.[389,399] There is often a sprinkling of inflammatory cells in the background. There is minimal cytologic atypia, but mitotic activity can be brisk. By immunohistochemistry, the cells react like myofibroblasts, but cytokeratin expression can be strong and diffuse.[395] In some cases, there is overexpression of ALK-1.[395,400] These entities are dealt with in greater detail in Chapter 5.

Prognosis and Predictive Factors

Grading of Urothelial Carcinoma

Grading of urothelial carcinoma has largely focused on papillary tumors. As discussed in the section on classification,

this has been an area of controversy and change. What is certain for papillary tumors is that histologic grade is a powerful predictor of tumor behavior. The current grading system places papillary tumors (excluding urothelial papilloma) into three categories: papillary urothelial neoplasm of low malignant potential, low-grade papillary urothelial carcinoma, and high-grade papillary urothelial carcinoma. These categories and the significance of each are detailed in the section on papillary tumors.

Grading of invasive urothelial carcinoma has had much less of an impact. In most urologic pathologists' hands, the vast majority of invasive tumors are considered high grade. For example in a series of 201 consecutive invasive urothelial carcinomas, Jordan et al.[4] considered 97% to be grade 3 and 3% grade 2. Jimenez et al. graded 15 of 93 (16%) cases of muscle-invasive urothelial carcinoma as grade 2B and the remaining 78 (84%) as grade 3 using the Malmström system.[9,224] These would all be considered high grade in the current WHO (2004) system. The literature contains numerous publications where the study set includes many grade 1 and grade 2 invasive tumors. The existence of invasive grade 1 tumors has been challenged. In a review of cases of invasive grade 1 tumors reported to a tumor data registry, Mikulowski and Hellsten[401] concluded that these were all either higher grade or noninvasive. The 1973 WHO grade 2 category included tumors ranging from low to high grade and not surprisingly many grade 2 tumors were invasive. One of the major goals of the 1998 WHO/ISUP proposals was to place these tumors into the high-grade category. This aim has largely been achieved but with the result that very few invasive carcinomas are now considered to be low grade. It has been suggested that other features such as growth pattern could be incorporated in a new grading scheme specifically to address this limitation. This topic is discussed in more detail in a following section on pattern of invasion.[224]

Lymph–Vascular Invasion

In 1971 Bell et al.[402] reported that vascular invasion was a significant prognostic factor in bladder cancer. Since that time there have been many reports that have in general confirmed the significance of lymph–vascular invasion in specific subsets of patients[403] and in both TURBT and cystectomy specimens.[404–407] In general, assessment of lymph–vascular invasion has been based on assessment of the hematoxylin and eosin–stained sections.[402,404,406,407] In one study, a subset of cases was evaluated by immunohistochemistry for CD31 and D2-40[405]; in that study, 2 of 25 TURBT cases with lymph–vascular invasion on hematoxylin and eosin had the finding confirmed by immunohistochemistry. An additional case with lymph–vascular invasion was identified by immunohistochemistry that had not been recognized on hematoxylin and eosin.

Identification of lymph–vascular invasion is problematic in urinary bladder specimens (Fig. 6-118). Invasive urothelial carcinoma has a propensity for tissue retraction resulting in nests of cells mimicking involvement of endothelial line spaces. This difficulty was nicely illustrated in a study by Larsen et al.[232] where immunohistochemistry confirmed the presence of lymph–vascular invasion in only 5 of 36 cases reported on hematoxylin and eosin as having this finding. Algaba[408] recommended specific morphologic features of true lymph–vascular invasion including (i) presence in spaces with an unequivocal endothelial cell lining, preferably with adjacent arteriole, (ii) tumor floating freely in the vessel space with fibrin and/or red blood cells around it, and (iii) tumor cells that are tightly cohesive with a smooth border and cells at the periphery that have a shell-like morphology.

The independent value of lymph–vascular invasion as a prognostic feature has not been generally accepted[409] although a majority of reports have indicated its significance in certain populations including T1 tumors and in patients treated by cystectomy when the lymph nodes are negative for metastases.[27] The current CAP guidelines recommend the routine reporting of lymph–vascular invasion but not the routine application of immunohistochemistry.[26] This was also the conclusion of the pathology panel in the International Consultation of Urologic Diseases review.[27] In contrast, in one European proposal this is recommended to be routinely reported, including the application of immunohistochemistry as needed.[410] We currently report lymph–vascular invasion when it is present and considered unequivocal on hematoxylin and eosin–stained sections, but do not routinely utilize immunohistochemistry. It would, however, be reasonable to include the routine use of immunohistochemistry as part of a standard therapeutic algorithm in a clinical trial or at an individual institution level.

Pattern of Invasion

The pattern of invasion in urothelial carcinoma has been evaluated as a potential prognostic indicator. Jimenez et al.[224] assigned three patterns of invasion to 93 patients undergoing cystectomy for muscle-invasive urothelial carcinoma. The patterns were nodular, trabecular, and infiltrative; each represented the predominant pattern in 14%, 42%, and 44% of cases, respectively (Fig. 6-119). The median survival for patients with any amount of the infiltrative pattern was 29 months compared with 85 months for patients without. Subsequent studies using this classification in the urinary bladder[225,411,412] and upper urinary tract[413] have confirmed

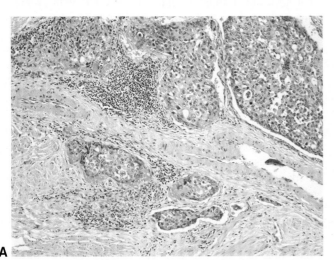
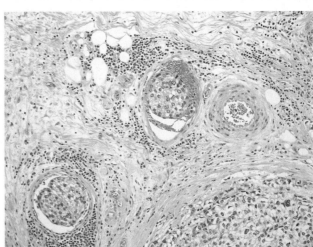

FIGURE 6-118 ■ Invasive high-grade urothelial carcinoma with lymph–vascular invasion **(A,B).**

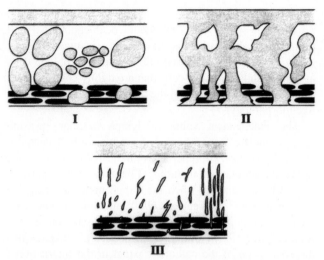

FIGURE 6-119 ■ Architectural patterns of growth: (*I*) nodular; (*II*) trabecular; and (*III*) infiltrative. (From Jimenez RE, Gheiler E, Oskanian P, et al. Grading the invasive component of urothelial carcinoma of the bladder and its relationship with progression-free survival. *Am J Surg Pathol* 2000;24:980–987, with permission.)

these findings. In the study by Bircan et al.,[412] invasive tumors with an infiltrative growth pattern were infrequently T1 at diagnosis (11%) compared to those with trabecular (72%) and nodular (77%) patterns. In a study limited to T1 tumors, Denzinger et al.[225] reported a cancer-specific survival of 60% in cases with an infiltrative architecture versus 86% and 91% for the trabecular and nodular patterns. Finally, in a study of upper tract tumors, Langner et al.[413] reported actuarial 5-year metastasis-free survivals of 94%, 74%, and 12% for cases with nodular, trabecular, and infiltrative growth patterns, respectively. In that report, the presence of an infiltrative growth pattern and pT stage were the two independent predictors of metastasis-free survival.

Molecular and Genetic Markers

There have been innumerable studies evaluating potential molecular and genetic markers for their potential as prognostic markers. More recently studies have begun to focus on markers that could have a role in predicting response to therapy. It is beyond the scope of this chapter to provide a detailed review of these. The reader is referred to many comprehensive review articles available in the literature.[414–416] The recognition of at least two distinct pathways of urothelial tumorigenesis and the prognostic significance of those pathways is discussed in the genetics section of this chapter and is not repeated here. In this section, a few of the most extensively studied and promising individual markers are briefly reviewed. The 2012 International Consultation on Bladder Cancer concluded that as yet there are no molecular or genetic markers with sufficient evidence to support routine use in surgical pathology practice.[27]

TP53 and Cell Cycle Regulators. Perhaps no marker has been as extensively studied in bladder cancer as the *Tp53* gene and its product.[415–417] The *p53* gene plays a central role in

one of the two pathways of bladder tumor development (see Cytogenetics section) and in particular the pathway associated in general with the development of more aggressive urothelial carcinomas. It has been found in many studies to be a significant predictor of recurrence for noninvasive and T1 tumors,[418,419] for progression of noninvasive and T1 tumors to muscle-invasive tumors,[201,420,421] and for survival.[418,422] In one meta-analysis that comprised over 10,000 patients, the authors concluded that "evidence is not sufficient to conclude whether changes in *p53* act as markers of outcome in patients with bladder cancer."[417] The *retinoblastoma* (*Rb*) gene has had tremendous interest as a prognostic marker in bladder cancer for many years. Loss of *Rb* gene expression has also been correlated with recurrence, progression, and survival in bladder cancer.[423,424] In some studies the evaluation of both p53 and Rb in combination with other cell cycle–related proteins yields more powerful prognostic information.[251,425,426] Studies of many other cell cycle–related markers including p21 and p27 have also generated data suggesting their potential values as prognostic markers in bladder cancer.[251,425–427]

Cellular Proliferation. Cellular proliferation has been extensively studied in bladder cancer beginning with mitosis counting[418,428] and now most often with Ki-67 (MIB1) labeling.[418,429,430] These studies have consistently demonstrated a significant association between high proliferation rates and high tumor grade,[429–431] and increased risk of progression[418,429–431] and of bladder cancer death.[418,429,432] Most recently, proliferation has been combined with *FGFR3* status to produce a molecular grade.[429] The significance of cellular proliferation has been demonstrated in noninvasive papillary tumors,[418,430,433] T1 tumors,[418,429,434] and muscle-invasive bladder cancers.[432] The independent prognostic value has been demonstrated in large, multi-institutional studies.[432]

Apoptosis-Related. There has also been considerable interest in apoptosis and genes that have a role in apoptosis as prognostic indicators in bladder cancer. There are studies that have found apoptotic index to correlate with progression and outcome.[431] A number of apoptosis-related genes including *bcl-2*,[435,436] *Fas*,[437] *caspase-3*,[436] *mdm-2*,[438] and *survivin*,[439,440] among others, have also had some reports indicating potential prognostic value. Overexpression of bcl-2 has been shown to be associated with higher stage and increased risk of progression[436] as has loss of Fas[437] and caspase-3 expression.[436] Survivin expression has been shown is several studies to be associated with higher stage and an increased risk of progression in urothelial carcinoma.[439–441] Survivin has been used as a part of a marker panel (with cathepsin E, maspin, and Plk1) to produce "risk signatures" for tumor progression and survival.[441] Survivin can also be detected in the urine and has been studied as a urine-based test for the detection of bladder cancer.[128]

Signaling Proteins and Receptors. There is an extensive literature regarding a variety of signaling proteins and their receptors in urothelial carcinoma. The fibroblast growth factor receptor gene (*FGFR3*) has already been extensively discussed because of its central role in the pathogenesis of papillary neoplasia (see genetics section).[102,103] Similarly, members of the *ras* gene family are also considered to be critical factors in the development of a subset of urothelial tumors.[102,103] Among the many other genes in this category that have been studied, a few comments regarding *EGFR* and epidermal growth factor receptor 2 (*HER-2*) are warranted. Expression of EGFR is found in up to 70% of invasive urothelial carcinomas.[442,443] Studies of the prognostic significance of EGFR expression have indicated an association with recurrence and survival[444] but these not been consistently found[443]; however, EGFR expression may be of greater relevance as it relates to treatment. Studies have demonstrated that in urothelial carcinoma expression of EGFR is not related to mutations of the *EGFR* gene.[445] There have also been several reports of the overexpression of HER2 in urothelial carcinoma.[446-449] This is more frequent in high-grade and high-stage tumors with an overall frequency in the 20% to 40% range. Although some studies have reported HER2 overexpression to indicate a worse prognosis,[446-448] others have not.[449] Targeted therapies aimed at these and the related pathways are under active study.

Angiogenesis-Related. Some early studies of microvessel density in invasive urothelial carcinoma indicated that this had potential as a prognostic parameter[450]; however, the initial results were not consistently found by other investigators.[451] There are several genes, however, including vascular endothelial growth factor (*VEGF*),[451,452] basic fibroblast growth factor,[451] and thrombospondin-1,[451,453,454] that are related to angiogenesis that have been studied with promising results.

Gene Expression and Molecular Profiling. The last several years have seen numerous studies using a variety of techniques to produce genetic profiles of tumors that can be used to diagnose urothelial carcinoma and to predict tumor, recurrence, progression, and survival.[27] Some of these reports have produced a small number of markers that can then be evaluated and used to generate expression patterns. For example, using an analysis of 24 genes, Birkhahn et al.[455] developed a panel of three markers (HRAS, VEGF, and VEGFR2) that produced a model with 81% sensitivity and 94% specificity for predicting recurrence in noninvasive papillary urothelial carcinoma. In contrast, using oligonucleotide arrays, Sanchez-Carbayo et al.[456] developed a molecular profile that incorporated 174 probes to identify patients with lymph node metastases and poor survival. In a different approach, Lindgren et al. used whole genome array–comparative genomic hybridization (CGH) combined with mutation analysis to evaluate a panel of eight genes (*FGFR3, PIK3CA, KRAS, HRAS, NRAS, TP53, CDKN2A,* and *TSC1*). Applying hierarchical clustering they then developed a model with two subtypes (NS1 and MS2) that predicted tumor grade and stage and had a significant correlation with

progression, metastasis, and survival in three different data sets.[457] These and many other studies have highlighted the potential for these approaches in the future.

Treatment

The treatment of bladder cancer continues to evolve. Both the AUA and the European Association of Urology (EAU) publish guidelines that provide insights into the current thinking regarding areas of general agreement and areas of uncertainty in the management of these patients.[23,24,458] In reviewing these, it is immediately apparent that the pathologist plays a critical role in choice of therapy with histologic grade and tumor stage being the primary drivers of treatment choice. The current AJCC/TNM staging system is presented in Tables 6-14 and 6-15. Pathologic staging remains a powerful prognostic parameter in invasive bladder cancer[459]; nonetheless, various details about the T categories continue to be put to critical evaluation.[460,461]

Follow-up is also a major part of the management of patients being treated with transurethral resection with or

Table 6-14 ■ AJCC—TNM PATHOLOGIC STAGING—URINARY BLADDER (2010)

Primary Tumor (T)

TX	Primary tumor cannot be assessed
T0	No evidence of primary tumor
Ta	Noninvasive papillary carcinoma
Tis	Carcinoma *in situ* "flat tumor"
T1	Tumor invades subepithelial connective tissue
T2a	Tumor invades superficial muscularis propria (inner one-half)
T2b	Tumor invades deep muscularis propria (outer one-half)
T3a	Tumor invades perivesical tissue—microscopically
T3b	Tumor invades perivesical tissue—macroscopically (extravesical mass)
T4a	Tumor invades any of the following: prostatic stroma, seminal vesicles, uterus, vagina
T4b	Tumor invades pelvic wall, abdominal wall

Regional Lymph Nodes (N)

NX	Lymph nodes cannot be assessed
N0	No lymph node metastasis
N1	Single regional lymph node metastasis in the true pelvis (hypogastric, obturator, external iliac, or presacral lymph node)
N2	Multiple regional lymph node metastasis in the true pelvis (hypogastric, obturator, external iliac, or presacral lymph node metastases)
N3	Lymph node metastasis to the common iliac lymph nodes

Distant Metastases (M)

M0	No distant metastasis
M1	Distant metastasis

From Edge S, Byrd D, Compton C, et al., eds. *AJCC Cancer Staging Manual.* 7th ed. New York: Springer; 2009:497–505.

Table 6-15 ■ AJCC-TNM STAGING OF BLADDER CARCINOMA (2010)—STAGE GROUPINGS

Stage	T	N	M
Stage 0a	Ta	N0	M0
Stage 0is	Tis	N0	M0
Stage I	T1	N0	M0
Stage II	T2a	N0	M0
	T2b	N0	M0
Stage III	T3a	N0	M0
	T3b	N0	M0
	T4a	N0	M0
Stage IV	T4b	N0	M0
	Any T	N1-3	M0
	Any T	Any N	M1

From Edge S, Byrd D, Compton C, et al., eds. *AJCC Cancer Staging Manual.* 7th ed. New York: Springer; 2009:497–505.

without intravesical therapy. The frequency is dependent on the risk of progression and recurrence as discussed below. For all patients, the first follow-up cystoscopy is at 3 months, and the findings at that time are important in predicting the subsequent course of the disease.[458] Tumor recurrence in low-risk patients is almost always also low-risk, and so recurrences of low-grade papillary tumors present no immediate danger to the patient. For this reason, their early detection is not necessary for successful treatment.[462]

Noninvasive Papillary Tumors (Ta). The choice of therapy in these cases is dependent on assessment of the risk for recurrence and progression. In the EAU guidelines for treatment, the most important factors for determining risk are the number of tumors, tumor diameter, prior tumor recurrence rate, concomitant CIS, and histologic grade.[458] Of these, the number of tumors and prior recurrence rate are given the greatest significance for recurrence while concomitant CIS and histologic grade are the most significant for progression.

For patients with low-risk tumors, complete transurethral resection alone may be sufficient or the addition of a single dose of intravesical chemotherapy can be included. In this setting the agents of choice include mitomycin-C, epirubicin, or doxorubicin. Ideally the instillation is given within 24 hours of resection and this has been shown to reduce recurrences but not risk of progression.[463] These agents have a very low risk of significant complications. Intravesical BCG has been shown to significantly reduce the risk of recurrences[464] and to reduce the risk of progression or at least to delay it.[465,466] Treatment with BCG requires both an induction course and a maintenance therapy to maximize its effect. This treatment does, however, have significant toxicity with serious side effects occurring in <5% of patients.[467] For intermediate-risk patients, either chemotherapy or BCG can be selected. For high-risk patients, the use of BCG is considered standard. For patients with multifocal high-grade tumors, some authors would recommend repeat resection to rule out the presence of invasive disease. Cystectomy is considered an option for patients with multiple recurrent high-grade tumors or with high-grade tumors and concomitant CIS.[458]

Carcinoma In Situ. CIS, whether primary or in association with papillary urothelial carcinoma, is the single most important predictor of progression to invasive disease. For that reason, BCG therapy is the standard approach for these patients.[458] This has been shown to reduce the risk of recurrence and to reduce the risk of progression or delay the time to progression.[465] Treatment is for at least a year with close follow-up by cystoscopy. For patients that fail BCG with persistent CIS or progression to invasive disease, cystectomy is recommended.[458]

Lamina Propria Invasion (T1). Perhaps the stage of greatest interest and controversy is T1. The presence of lamina propria invasion adds significantly to the above features in assigning risk for the progression to muscle-invasive disease. Standard therapy for T1 tumors has been transurethral resection combined with intravesical therapy.[23,458] This requires complete transurethral resection of the tumor. Because of the significant risk for understaging at the time of initial transurethral resection, a repeat resection is recommended if the treatment choice is less than cystectomy.[458,468,469] The intravesical agent of choice is BCG. For patients not tolerant of BCG, other intravesical chemotherapy agents can be used, but these are less effective.[458] Long-term follow-up studies show that approximately 20% to 50% of these patients will die of bladder cancer.[470–472]

The T1 category is one where early cystectomy has been demonstrated to improve survival in some but not all institutional studies and remains controversial. One major problem with clinical T1 disease is that a substantial proportion are upstaged (up to 50%) or are found to have aggressive histologic features when cystectomy is performed.[468,471,472] It should be recognized that the understaging is partly an issue of pathologic interpretation. In centrally reviewed pathology material approximately 10% of muscle invasion had not been recognized by the diagnosing pathologist.[473] In one series of 167 patients undergoing cystectomy for clinical T1 disease, 18% had lymph node metastases.[468] In another large multi-institutional study of 1,136 patients, 50% were upstaged with 29% having pT3/4 tumors and 16% lymph node metastases.[472]

There have been several reports documenting improved survival for patients with high-grade T1 tumors treated by immediate cystectomy,[471] but others have not shown a benefit.[195,474] This has led to great interest in identifying patients with "high-risk" T1 tumors that might benefit most from early cystectomy.[472,475] Factors such as histologic grade, depth of invasion, presence of lymph–vascular invasion, and selected variant histologies have all been proposed as pathologic features that can be used for this purpose. In addition, a large number of other markers such as p53 and retinoblastoma expression, and others have been suggested.

In one thought-provoking analysis, between 32% and 47% of bladder cancer deaths were judged to be potentially avoidable.[476] Not surprisingly, most of these are in patients with lower-stage disease who are hypothesized to have had an improved survival with earlier aggressive intervention.

Muscle Invasion (T2/3). Documentation of muscle-invasive disease remains one of the most important aspects in the evaluation of tumor biopsy or transurethral resection specimens. For most patients it is this finding that leads to the decision to proceed with definitive local therapy (cystectomy).[24,477] Radical cystectomy is considered the standard therapy for localized muscle-invasive bladder cancer.[24] In the male, radical cystectomy includes removal of the urinary bladder, the prostate gland with seminal vesicles, and the distal most portions of both ureters. In female patients, the resection includes the urinary bladder, the uterus and adnexae, portions of the urethra and vaginal mucosa (variable), and the distal most portions of both ureters. Lymphadenectomy is routinely performed, and recent literature advocates a more extended lymph node dissection. The choice of type of urinary diversion or neobladder construction is based on multiple factors beyond the scope of this discussion.[478] The presence of CIS at the urethral resection margin is a relative contraindication to use of a neobladder and for this reason frozen sections may be requested to assess the margin status. Patients with diffuse CIS or involvement of the prostatic urethra are at a particularly high risk for this. For similar reason frozen section evaluation of ureteral margins is routinely performed. The actual value of these frozen sections has been questioned in the literature.[479]

The published results of radical cystectomy are quite variable and are dependent on multiple factors. In general, the 5- and 10-year recurrence-free survival is in the 66% to 68% and 60% to 73% range, respectively. The overall 5- and 10-year survivals are reported to be 58% to 66% and 43% to 49%, respectively.[480]

The role of neoadjuvant chemotherapy prior to radical cystectomy is unresolved at this time.[24,481] Recent reports indicate a 5% to 8% overall survival benefit with neoadjuvant cisplatin-based chemotherapy leading some groups to recommend this routinely for patients with good performance scores who can tolerate the treatment.[24] A role for adjuvant chemotherapy seems less well defined and is currently recommended only in the setting of clinical trials.[24]

An alternate approach that has played a secondary role is the use of combined chemotherapy and radiation therapy with bladder preservation.[482,483] Studies have demonstrated that this approach can be used successfully in selected patients with about one-half of patients keeping their bladder.[483,484] This treatment strategy has not been widely used and is largely restricted to institutions with highly committed multidisciplinary teams.

Metastatic Disease (M1). Urothelial carcinoma has been recognized as being responsive to chemotherapy for over two decades. The greatest success and most experience has been with cisplatin-based protocols.[283,485,486] Response rates are in the 48%

range, and survival has been prolonged by about 14 months. Long-term survivals in the 20% range have been achieved.

SQUAMOUS CELL CARCINOMA

Epidemiology

The prevalence of squamous cell carcinoma varies among different parts of the world. In areas where schistosomiasis is endemic, it had accounted for up to 73% of bladder cancer; however, this proportion is changing.[487–489] In contemporary series, urothelial carcinoma is the most common histologic type accounting for three-quarters of cases.[488,489] In one study, the percentage of squamous cell carcinomas changed from 78% in 1980 to 28% in 2005.[488] This change has been attributed largely to the success of public health efforts in reducing schistosomiasis and to increasing use of tobacco. In series from England and the United States, squamous cell carcinoma comprises only 3% to 6% of bladder malignancies.[281,490–493] In the United States and Europe, the male:female ratio is 1.7:1, with ages ranging from 30 to 90 years (mean, 66 years).[281,491,494] In one registry study, squamous cell carcinoma was more common in women than men.[492] A higher incidence of squamous cell carcinoma has been reported in African Americans compared to Caucasian Americans.[495,496]

Many patients with squamous cell carcinoma have a history of long-standing bladder irritation caused by infection,[497,498] stones,[497,499] indwelling catheters,[500] intermittent self-catheterization,[498,501] or urinary retention (Box 6-7).[499] Smoking is also a risk factor. In patients with neurogenic bladder there is an increased risk of bladder cancer with squamous cell carcinoma being the most common type accounting for over 50% of cases in some series.[502,503] Squamous cell carcinoma has also been described following radiation therapy[504] and treatment with cyclophosphamide.[505] Keratinizing squamous metaplasia is an important risk factor for the development of squamous cell carcinoma.[503,506] In one series, 33 of 78 patients with keratinizing squamous metaplasia had simultaneous or subsequent carcinoma. In those who subsequently developed cancer, the tumor developed an average of 12 years after the diagnosis of metaplasia. Many tumors arising in bladder diverticula are squamous cell carcinoma.[507,508]

Schistosome infection is a worldwide medical problem and its role in the pathogenesis of bladder cancer in endemic areas is of considerable interest.[88,487,509] There are three major species pathogenic to humans: *Schistosoma mansoni*, *Schistosoma japonicum*, and *S. haematobium*. Only

---

Box 6-7 ● MAJOR RISK FACTORS FOR SQUAMOUS CELL CARCINOMA

Schistosomiasis infection
Chronic infection—other causes
Bladder lithiasis
Other chronic irritants
Nonfunctioning bladder

S. haematobium causes bladder cancer.[510] In a series of 1,095 cases of bladder cancer from Egypt, schistosome eggs were identified in the bladder wall in 902 cases (82%).[487] Bladder infection by *S. haematobium* may result in polyposis, ulceration, urothelial hyperplasia and metaplasia, dysplasia, or carcinoma.[511] Although squamous cell carcinoma is the most frequent type of cancer, a relatively high prevalence of adenocarcinoma (6%) is also seen.[487] Studies of HPV in both schistosomiasis- and non–schistosomiasis-related tumors have for the most part been negative.[512,513]

Clinical Features

Most patients present with hematuria (63% to 100%) and/or irritative symptoms (33% to 67%).[509] Other symptoms often associated with advanced disease include weight loss, back and pelvic pain, or symptoms related to obstruction.[509] Cases with associated hypercalcemia have been described.[514,515] A high proportion of patients have advanced cancer at the time of diagnosis.[490,494,516] Rare tumors arising in bladder exstrophy and in the urachus are squamous cell carcinoma.[517–519]

At cystoscopy, the tumors are usually single and located in the trigone or posterior wall region.[509] An exophytic solid or ulceroinfiltrative pattern is most common. Keratin debris can be present on the surface. Leukoplakia can be present in the adjacent mucosa.

Pathology

Most squamous cell carcinomas are bulky, polypoid, solid, necrotic masses, often filling the bladder lumen, although

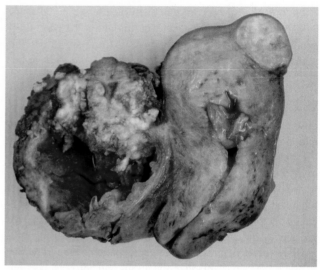

FIGURE 6-121 ■ Squamous cell carcinoma of the bladder.

some are predominantly flat and irregularly bordered or ulcerated and infiltrating (Figs. 6-120 and 6-121).[490,520,521] The presence of necrotic material and keratin debris on the surface is relatively constant.

In the current classification scheme, the diagnosis of squamous cell carcinoma is restricted to pure tumors.[14,15] The surface can have a papillary or verruciform surface and superficial biopsies can have a deceptively benign appearance (Fig. 6-122). The tumors may be well differentiated with well-defined islands of squamous cells with keratinization, prominent intercellular bridges, and minimal nuclear pleomorphism, or poorly differentiated, with marked nuclear pleomorphism and only focal evidence of squamous differentiation (Fig. 6-123). Basaloid squamous cell carcinoma histologically identical to tumors of the upper aerodigestive tract has been described.[522] There can be lymph–vascular invasion and perineural invasion.[523]

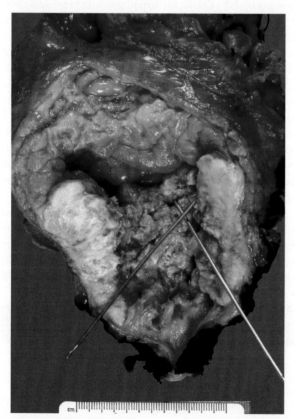

FIGURE 6-120 ■ Squamous cell carcinoma of the bladder.

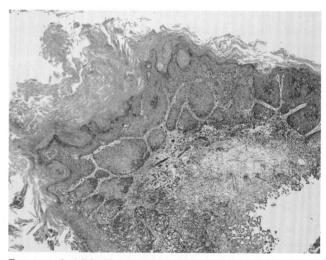

FIGURE 6-122 ■ Invasive squamous cell carcinoma with a well-differentiated verruciform surface.

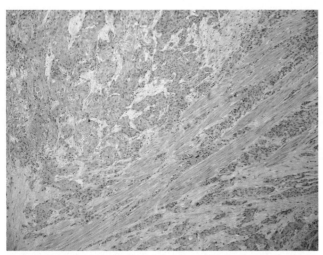

FIGURE 6-123 ■ Invasive squamous cell carcinoma involving the muscularis propria.

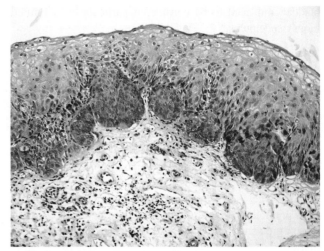

FIGURE 6-125 ■ Squamous metaplasia with high-grade dysplasia.

Necrosis is common. Squamous metaplasia is identifiable in the adjacent epithelium in 17% to 65% of cases.[281,497,520] This can be keratinizing, nonkeratinizing, or verrucous squamous hyperplasia (Fig. 6-124).[281] There can be varying degrees of atypia ranging up to squamous CIS present in some (Fig. 6-125).

Histologic grade may correlate with stage and outcome although this has not been uniform.[497,520,524] In one study, DNA ploidy was a powerful predictor of progression with 35%, 45%, and 92% of patients with diploid, tetraploid, and aneuploid tumors progressing, respectively.[516]

Differential Diagnosis

Lesions with squamous differentiation that occur in the urinary bladder are listed in Table 6-16. The major differential

diagnostic consideration for squamous cell carcinoma is urothelial carcinoma with squamous differentiation, which occurs in up to 40% of high-grade urothelial carcinomas.[278,279,525,526] In North America, Europe, and other regions where squamous cell carcinoma is uncommon, such tumors should be carefully studied for an urothelial component. The presence of keratinizing squamous metaplasia, especially if associated with dysplasia, would support a diagnosis of squamous cell carcinoma. There are no immunohistochemical markers to reliably distinguish these two possibilities. When a biopsy or transurethral resection contains pure squamous cell carcinoma, a comment can be added indicating that the possibility of urothelial carcinoma with squamous differentiation cannot be excluded without examination of the entire tumor. Secondary invasion of the bladder by an adjacent primary such as squamous cell carcinoma of the cervix or vagina should always be considered and excluded clinically. Immunohistochemical staining cannot reliably distinguish primary from secondary squamous cell carcinoma. Demonstration of HPV DNA in a female patient would strongly favor a genital tract origin.[513,527] A variety of benign squamous lesions can be seen in the

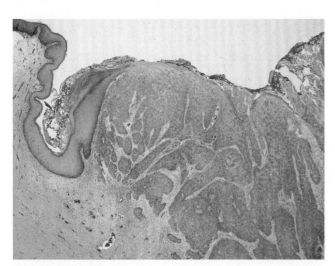

FIGURE 6-124 ■ Invasive squamous cell carcinoma with keratinizing squamous cell metaplasia of the adjacent mucosa.

Table 6-16 ■ SQUAMOUS LESIONS OF THE URINARY BLADDER
Squamous metaplasia
Nonkeratinizing
Keratinizing
Normal adult female
Condyloma acuminatum
Squamous papilloma
Urothelial carcinoma with squamous differentiation
Verrucous carcinoma
Squamous cell carcinoma

bladder and need to be considered particularly in limited biopsy specimens.[67]

Treatment and Natural History

The treatment of choice for pure squamous cell carcinoma of the bladder has been radical cystectomy or cystoprostatectomy.[528] Radiation therapy alone is not effective.[494] Some reports suggest that preoperative radiation therapy, with or without neoadjuvant chemotherapy, may be useful.[529,530] Chemotherapy is ineffective in dealing with metastatic squamous cell carcinoma of the bladder. Tumor stage is the most important prognostic indicator for squamous cell carcinoma.[490,497] As noted above, histologic grade and possibly DNA ploidy are other prognostic markers.

Overall the prognosis for patients with squamous cell carcinoma is poor. In a study of newly diagnosed invasive bladder cancer from the Netherlands Cancer Registry, 88% of squamous cell carcinomas were muscle invasive compared with 52% of urothelial carcinomas.[492] The relative 5-year survival rate was only 23% for cases with T2 or greater stage.[492] In a 1976 series from the MD Anderson Cancer Center, 5- and 10-year survivals were only 14% and 53%, respectively.[521] A more recent series for the same institution reported 2-year overall and recurrence-free survivals of 48% and 33%.[491] Other studies have reported 5-year survivals ranging from 7% to 50%.[281,499,530] The highest survival was in a small series of patients treated with preoperative radiation and radical cystectomy.[530] The biologic behavior of squamous cell carcinoma is different than that of urothelial carcinoma. In most patients, death is due to local recurrence rather than metastatic cancer.[499,530] Metastases show a striking predilection for bone.[490,499]

Verrucous Carcinoma

Rare cases of verrucous carcinoma of the urinary bladder have been described.[531–535] One case in the urinary bladder developed in a patient with long-standing anogenital condyloma acuminatum, suggesting a possible link with the bladder tumor.[533] Analysis for HPV when performed has been negative, however.[535] One case reported as verrucous carcinoma invaded in nests with areas of perineural invasion, and probably represented typical squamous cell carcinoma.[536] Verrucous carcinoma is more common in patients with schistosomiasis, accounting for 3% of bladder cancers.[487,537] This cancer appears as an exophytic, papillary, or "warty" mass with epithelial acanthosis and papillomatosis, minimal nuclear and architectural atypia, and rounded, pushing, deep borders. It can extend through the full thickness of the bladder wall.[534] Treatment is with surgical resection.[534] In other organs, verrucous carcinoma has a good prognosis, but results in the bladder are limited. In a series of 19 cases

from Egypt treated by cystectomy, no lymph node metastases were present.[537] To date, no case with metastases has been reported.

PRIMARY ADENOCARCINOMA

Primary adenocarcinoma accounts for <2% of malignant bladder tumors in Europe and North America[14,15,492,538,539] and up to 5% of cases in the Egyptian literature.[540,541] The largest published series with 185 and 192 cases, respectively, were reported by El-Mekresh et al.[541] and Zaghloul et al.[540] Both series are from Egypt. The largest North American series included 72 cases.[288] Adenocarcinoma of the bladder is divided into two major categories: those arising in the urachus and those developing in the bladder proper (Table 6-17). For clinical and pathologic reasons, these are addressed in separate sections. Specific variants of clinical significance (signet ring cell adenocarcinoma, clear cell adenocarcinoma, and hepatoid adenocarcinoma) are dealt with individually.

Nonurachal Adenocarcinoma

Clinical Features

Nonurachal adenocarcinoma accounts for 61% to 80% of primary bladder adenocarcinomas.[280,542,543] These occur over a wide age range, with a mean of 59 years, and are more common in males than in females (3:1).[280,288,538,540–542,544,545]

Table 6-17 ■ COMPARISON OF URACHAL AND NONURACHAL ADENOCARCINOMA

Feature	Urachal	Nonurachal
Age (mean)	52 y	62 y
Sex (male:female ratio)	1–1.5:1	3:1
Mucusuria	Common	Infrequent
Stage at diagnosis	50% advanced	75% advanced
Histologic type (frequency)		
Enteric	30%	15%
Mucinous	50%	10%
Signet ring	<5%	10%
NOS	<5%	40%
Mixed	10%	25%
Treatment	Partial or radical cystectomy with resection of urachal tract	Radical cystectomy
Survival		
5-y	37%–51%	17%–50%
10-y	17%–42%	11%–28%

Hematuria is the most common presentation, followed by irritative symptoms and rarely mucusuria.[280] The tumors are often advanced, with metastases in up to 40% of patients at the time of presentation.[280,540,546]

Most cases of nonurachal adenocarcinoma arise from intestinal metaplasia of the urothelium. Support for this mechanism comes from cases arising in patients with long-standing diffuse intestinalization of the bladder mucosa associated with a nonfunctioning bladder, chronic irritation, obstruction, and cystocele (Fig. 6-126). Cystitis glandularis is present in 4% to 7% of patients with nonurachal adenocarcinoma.[539,547] Origin from metaplasia is also considered to be the mechanism in patients with exstrophy.[548,549] Most cancers arising in association with exstrophy are adenocarcinoma. The risk of adenocarcinoma in patients with exstrophy is in the range of 4% to 7%.[549,550] There is also an increased risk of adenocarcinoma in patients with pelvic lipomatosis, and this is attributed to its association with cystitis glandularis.[551,552] Adenocarcinoma also arises in patients with *S. hematobium* infection.[487,540,541] Rare cases of adenocarcinoma[553,554] and adenosarcoma[555] have arisen in association with endometriosis involving the bladder.

Pathology

Nonurachal adenocarcinoma can appear as an exophytic, papillary, solid, sessile, ulcerating, or infiltrative mass (Fig. 6-127). The signet ring variant frequently shows diffuse thickening of the bladder wall, producing a linitis plastica–like appearance (see below).

There has been some variability in defining adenocarcinoma in the literature. Most have excluded any case containing a recognizable urothelial carcinoma component, preferring to classify these as urothelial carcinoma with glandular differentiation.[15,288] The current WHO classification follows this approach.[14] Grignon et al.[288] recognized six

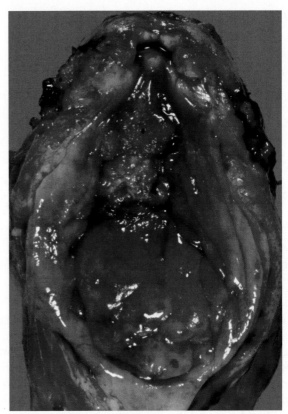

FIGURE 6-127 ■ Primary nonurachal adenocarcinoma with an ulcerated infiltrative appearance.

histologic variants of adenocarcinoma of the urinary bladder; (i) adenocarcinoma of no specific type when the tumor did not resemble another recognized pattern; (ii) enteric, when the cancer was composed of pseudostratified columnar cells forming glands, often with central necrosis, typical of colonic adenocarcinoma (Fig. 6-128); (iii) mucinous (colloid), when the tumor cells were single or in nests floating

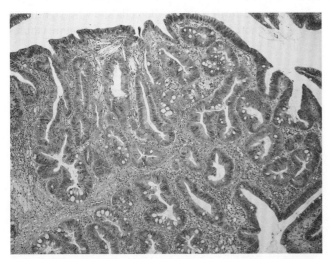

FIGURE 6-126 ■ An area of extensive cystitis glandularis with intestinal metaplasia that shows dysplasia similar to that seen in adenomatous polyps of the gastrointestinal tract.

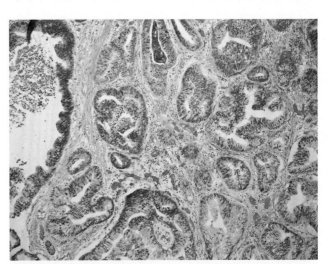

FIGURE 6-128 ■ Nonurachal adenocarcinoma of bladder with enteric-like morphology.

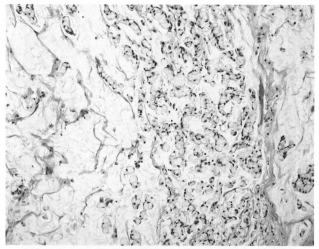

FIGURE 6-129 ■ Nonurachal adenocarcinoma of bladder with mucinous (colloid) morphology.

in extracellular mucin (Fig. 6-129); (iv) signet ring, when the tumor consisted of signet ring cells diffusely infiltrating the bladder wall; (v) clear cell, when the tumor was composed of papillary and tubular structures with cytologic features identical to mesonephric adenocarcinoma; and (vi) mixed, when two or more of the described patterns were found (Fig. 6-130). For nonurachal adenocarcinoma, the enteric type is most common. Immunohistochemical findings are similar to those described below for urachal adenocarcinoma.

A uniform grading system has not been applied to adenocarcinoma of the bladder.[539,556] Anderstrom et al.[556] found grade to be a significant prognostic indicator while others did not.[539,540] In the former system, grade was assessed based on the degree of gland formation with two specific histologic subtypes (pure colloid and signet ring) considered to be poorly differentiated. The histologic pattern did not correlate with outcome in the MD Anderson Cancer Center

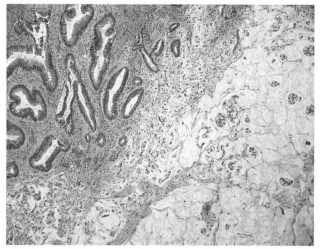

FIGURE 6-130 ■ Nonurachal adenocarcinoma with mixed enteric and mucinous appearance.

series, although the poor prognosis of the signet ring variant was noted.[288] In contrast, Zaghloul et al.[540] applied the classification scheme of Grignon et al.[288] and found it to have prognostic value.

Chan and Epstein[557] reported 19 cases of what they referred to as "adenocarcinoma in situ." In 17 cases, these most likely represented urothelial CIS with glandular or pseudoglandular differentiation, a well-described pattern in urothelial CIS. In these, the term adenocarcinoma in situ is not appropriate and is potentially confusing. This term should be reserved for true cases of adenocarcinoma in situ with colonic-type epithelium having severe dysplastic change.[558]

Differential Diagnosis

The differential diagnosis of adenocarcinoma is extensive due to the range of glandular lesions that can occur in the urinary bladder (Table 6-18). First, benign mimics of adenocarcinoma need to be excluded.[301] Cystitis cystica and cystitis glandularis may be florid, producing pseudopapillary or polypoid lesions that can mimic a tumor. The benign cytology of the lining cells and lack of invasion are important features.[558] In unusual cases of intestinal metaplasia, extracellular mucin is present.[558] In these cases, careful evaluation for malignant cells suspended in the mucin is required. Patients with long-standing intestinal metaplasia are at risk for the development of adenocarcinoma, and such cases should be carefully evaluated for early evidence of neoplastic transformation. Villous adenoma occurs rarely in the urinary bladder and shows the cytologic and architectural abnormalities of adenomatous epithelium without stromal invasion.[58,59] Invasive adenocarcinoma is often associated with villous adenoma and should be looked for carefully. Nephrogenic adenoma must be distinguished from adenocarcinoma, particularly the clear cell variant (see below). Endometriosis, endocervicosis, and müllerianosis can mimic adenocarcinoma.[301,559] These lesions can be quite infiltrative and form masses. The cells show no significant atypia, and more than anything the diagnosis requires thinking about the possibility.

Table 6-18 ■ GLANDULAR LESIONS OF THE URINARY BLADDER
Urachal remnant
Ectopic prostate tissue
Cystitis cystica/glandularis
Intestinal metaplasia
Nephrogenic adenoma
Müllerianosis
Endocervicosis
Endometriosis
Endosolpingosis
Villous adenoma
Adenocarcinoma (urachal and nonurachal)
Urothelial carcinoma with glandular differentiation
Secondary adenocarcinoma

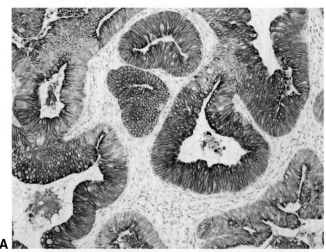
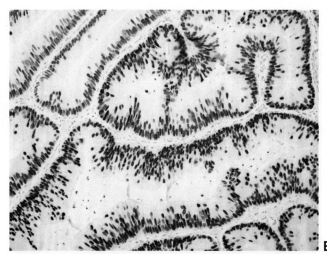

FIGURE 6-131 ■ ■ Nonurachal adenocarcinoma of bladder that shows strong expression of cytokeratin 7 **(A)** and CDX2 **(B)**.

Secondary involvement of the bladder must always be excluded and requires clinicopathologic correlation. The majority of primary bladder adenocarcinomas have an enteric, mucinous, signet ring or a combination of these patterns making secondary involvement by an adenocarcinoma of the gastrointestinal tract a major consideration. Mucin histochemistry does not distinguish urachal adenocarcinoma or nonurachal adenocarcinoma from colorectal adenocarcinoma.[560] Immunohistochemistry has been reported to be of some value in the distinction of primary adenocarcinoma from secondary colonic adenocarcinoma with the latter being CK20 positive and CK7 negative in the majority of cases and with primary adenocarcinoma being variably reactive to both CK7 and CK20 (Fig. 6-131A).[561–564] There is expression of CDX2 in both (Fig. 6-131B)[563] although loss of CDX2 may be more frequent in primary bladder tumors.[564,565] Some reports have suggested that villin-1 may be more useful with absence of villin-1 expression in some primary bladder adenocarcinomas,[565] but this has not been confirmed by others.[563,566] Absence of nuclear β-catenin was also been reported in primary bladder adenocarcinoma,[561] but this also has not been found by others.[563] Thrombomodulin is reported to be positive in primary but not secondary tumors.[561] In individual cases, however, there is sufficient overlap to limit the practical application of immunohistochemistry.

Treatment and Natural History

Nonurachal adenocarcinoma is staged using the standard AJCC–TNM staging system.[567] Stage is considered to be the most significant prognostic indicator in bladder adenocarcinoma. Surgery is the preferred therapy for nonurachal adenocarcinoma with radical cystectomy or cystoprostatectomy with pelvic lymph node dissection.[528] Adjuvant radiotherapy is also used in some series for locally advanced disease.[540] There is very limited information on the role of chemotherapy in these tumors.[568] Prognosis for this tumor is poor.

The overall 5- and 10-year survivals for the 48 cases of nonurachal adenocarcinoma reported by Grignon et al.[288] were 31% and 28%, respectively. These data indicate that most patients dying of this tumor do so in the first 5 years, with uncommon late recurrences and deaths. In more contemporary series survivals in the 40% to 50% range have been reported[540,541] with others having much worse outcomes.[546] In patients treated by cystectomy, the outcome is significantly worse for adenocarcinoma as compared to urothelial carcinoma.[546]

Urachal Adenocarcinoma

Diagnostic Criteria

The separation of urachal from nonurachal adenocarcinoma requires correlation of clinical and pathologic findings.[542,547,569,570] A variety of criteria have been suggested over the years with those proposed by Johnson et al.[571] being perhaps most practical: the tumor should be located anteriorly or in the dome, there should be a sharp demarcation between tumor and normal epithelium, and a primary elsewhere must be excluded. There are no specific pathologic features that distinguish urachal from nonurachal tumors.

The pathogenesis of urachal adenocarcinoma is believed to be similar to primary nonurachal adenocarcinoma of the bladder with intestinal metaplasia being the intermediary step.[572] Cases arising from villous adenoma of the urachus have been described.[573]

Clinical Features

Urachal adenocarcinoma occurs throughout adulthood and the youngest case was that of a 15-year-old girl.[574] The majority occur in the fifth and sixth decades, with a mean age in the mid-50s in most series years, approximately 10 years younger than the mean for nonurachal adenocarcinoma. There is also a predominance of men over women

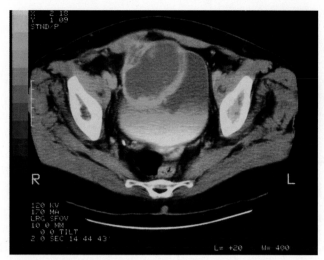

FIGURE 6-132 ■ Computed tomography of a urachal adeno-carcinoma of the bladder.

(1.8 to 1), which is lower than the 3:1 ratio for nonurachal adenocarcinoma.[280,288,538,542,570,575–577] The most frequent presenting symptoms are hematuria, pain, and irritative symptoms. Mucusuria occurs in up to 25% of patients.[280,576]

Cystoscopy most often reveals a polypoid mass in the bladder dome or anterior wall that may be covered by an intact or ulcerated mucosa.[576] Imaging studies localize the tumor to the bladder dome region (Fig. 6-132). A plain film x-ray may show characteristic stippled calcifications.

Pathology

Most urachal adenocarcinomas form discrete masses in the dome of the bladder. The tumors appear to have an epicenter in the wall of the bladder, rather than being mucosal based (Fig. 6-133). The bladder mucosa can be intact or ulcerated. The cut surface usually has a glistening mucoid appearance due to abundant mucus production (Fig. 6-134). The tumor can extend along the urachal tract and the tumor may be found within the abdominal wall (Fig. 6-135). Although some authors have excluded cases where there is associated cystitis glandularis or intestinal metaplasia, this may be too restrictive as these lesions are relatively frequent in the bladder.[570] In the majority of cases, urachal remnants can be identified.

Urachal adenocarcinoma has a variety of histologic appearances. The most frequent is mucinous (colloid) carcinoma with nests and single cells floating in extracellular mucin (Fig. 6-136). The cells may have a signet ring or columnar morphology. The next most frequent pattern is enteric adenocarcinoma with features typical of colorectal adenocarcinoma, and can include Paneth cells and argyrophil neuroendocrine cells.[578,579] An uncommon pattern is linitis plastica–like signet ring cell carcinoma.[330] The presence of signet ring cells has been found to predict a poor prognosis.[580]

Not all carcinomas arising in the urachus are adenocarcinoma. All other histologic types of bladder carcinoma occur in this site with urothelial carcinoma being the second most

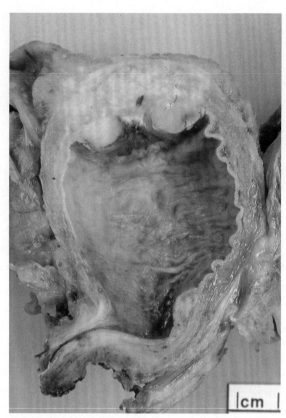

FIGURE 6-133 ■ Urachal adenocarcinoma arising within the wall of the bladder. In this case the tumor is solid. The ulcerated area is the site of the TURBT procedure.

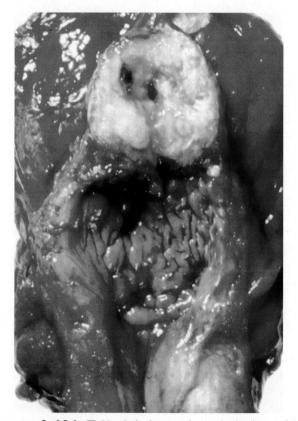

FIGURE 6-134 ■ Urachal adenocarcinoma in the dome of the bladder. The cut surface has a glistening mucoid appearance.

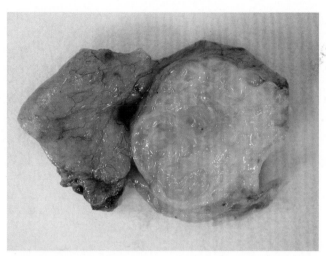

FIGURE 6-135 ■ Urachal adenocarcinoma arising in the extravesical portion of the urachal tract. The mucinous surface reflects the mucinous histology of the tumor.

frequent followed by squamous cell carcinoma and small cell carcinoma.[519,576,581] A variety of sarcomas have also been reported to have arisen in the urachus.[581]

Histochemical stains reveal neutral and acid (sulfated and nonsulfated) mucin.[288,560] Urachal adenocarcinoma expresses cytokeratin, CEA, Leu-M1, and EMA.[202,288,570] The tumors express cytokeratin 20 (100%), cytokeratin 7 (50%), high molecular weight cytokeratin (34βE12, 67%), and CDX2 (100%, variable intensity).[570] The majority of cases (75%) lack nuclear expression of β-catenin.[570]

Differential Diagnosis

The major differential diagnostic consideration is nonurachal adenocarcinoma. This distinction requires clinicopathologic correlation. Urachal adenocarcinoma should be distinguished from urachal villous adenoma; this rare lesion is histologically identical to those found in the gastrointestinal tract.[55,573] The presence of invasion indicates malignancy. Secondary invasion of the bladder by adenocarcinoma arising elsewhere, particularly the gastrointestinal tract, must always be excluded clinically. As presented in detail in the preceding section, immunohistochemistry cannot reliably distinguish primary adenocarcinoma of the bladder (of either urachal or nonurachal type) from secondary involvement from the gastrointestinal tract.

Treatment and Natural History

Most authorities recommend segmental resection of the tumor or radical cystectomy with en bloc resection of the urachus and umbilicus.[528,575,576,582] Adjuvant chemotherapy and radiation therapy have been used in patients with locally advanced or metastatic disease.[575,576] A role for these treatment approaches remains to be clarified. Urachal adenocarcinoma has been staged with the same systems used for urothelial bladder cancer.[288,545] Application of these systems is problematic because, by virtue of their anatomic origin, all urachal adenocarcinomas are muscles invasive. Sheldon et al.[517] proposed a system specific for urachal tumors. Stage I is confined to the urachal mucosa; stage II is invasive but confined to the urachus; stage III includes local extension to bladder (IIIA), abdominal wall (IIIB), peritoneum (IIIC), or viscera other than the bladder (IIID); and stage IV includes metastases to regional lymph nodes (IVA) or distant sites (IVB). This system with some modification has proven to be a significant predictor of outcome in one series.[576,580]

The reported prognosis for these tumors also varies considerably. Survival curves, based on 71 patients reported in the literature, combined with raw data obtained from Grignon et al.[288] revealed 5- and 10-year survivals of 37% and 17%, respectively.[280] Patients with localized disease have a significantly better prognosis; in the Mayo Clinic series the median survival time was 11 years for stage I and II disease.[576] In a population-based study, the 5- and 10-year overall survivals were 51% and 42%, respectively.[577] In a study limited to signet ring cell adenocarcinoma of the bladder, Grignon et al.[330] reported a significantly better survival for those originating in the urachus than elsewhere in the bladder.

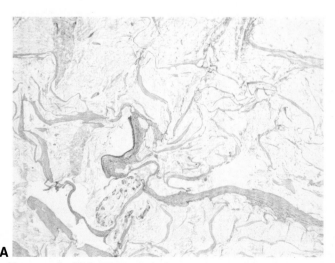

A

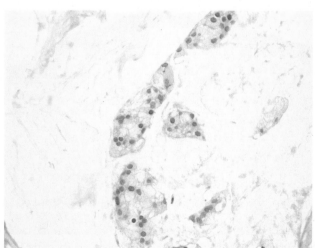

B

FIGURE 6-136 ■ Urachal adenocarcinoma with mucinous appearance **(A,B)**.

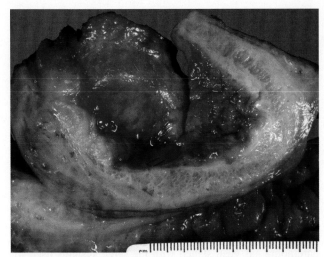

FIGURE 6-137 ■ Signet ring cell adenocarcinoma of the bladder producing a thickened bladder wall with a mucoid cut surface.

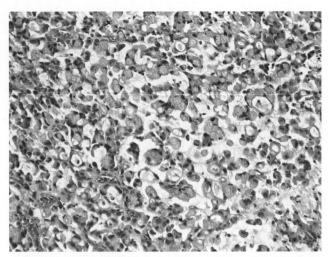

FIGURE 6-138 ■ Signet ring cell carcinoma of the bladder with tumor cells containing bubbly mucin.

Signet Ring Cell Adenocarcinoma

Clinical Features

The first report of the signet ring variant of bladder adenocarcinoma as a distinct clinicopathologic entity is attributed to Saphir in 1955.[331] Grignon et al.[330] reported 12 cases and reviewed 56 cases from the literature. Since that review additional small series have been described.[583–585] Grignon et al.[330] restricted the diagnosis to bladder adenocarcinomas with at least a focal component of diffuse linitis plastica–like signet ring cell adenocarcinoma and excluded cases with a urothelial carcinoma component. Urothelial carcinoma with glandular differentiation includes cases where the glandular component is manifest as a signet ring cell adenocarcinoma.[583]

There are no specific epidemiologic characteristics to these patients. The median age of presentation is in the sixth decade and men are more frequently affected than women (approximately 3:1). Gross hematuria and irritative symptoms are the most common presentation. In up to 50% of cases, cystoscopy does not show a mucosal or mass lesion with the mucosa most often being described as "edematous" or "bullous." The significance of this subtype of adenocarcinoma is the extremely poor prognosis.[330,586] A high proportion of patients present with advanced disease. The 5-year survival for patients with a pure signet ring pattern was only 13% whereas it was 33% in tumors with a mixed pattern in one comprehensive review.[330] Stage is the best predictor of outcome.[583]

Pathology

Grossly, signet ring cell adenocarcinoma causes diffuse thickening of the bladder wall in a linitis plastic–like pattern (Fig. 6-137). The cut surface may have a mucoid consistency. There is often edema of the mucosa. Histologically, there is diffuse permeation of the bladder wall by single signet ring cells. Most of the cells have a single cytoplasmic vacuole and others a bubbly cytoplasm (Fig. 6-138). In some cases, the cytoplasm is pale and eosinophilic with the nucleus pushed to one end, a pattern referred to as monocytoid (Fig. 6-139).[330,331] These tumors have abundant cytoplasmic mucin when evaluated with mucin stains. Many of

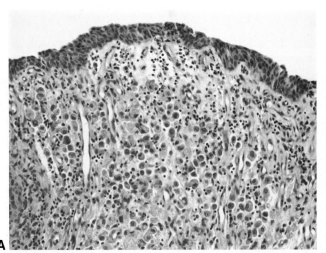

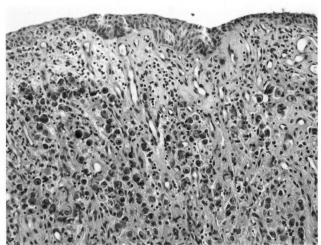

FIGURE 6-139 ■ Signet ring cell adenocarcinoma of the bladder with many but not all cells having bubbly cytoplasm (**A**); there is, however, diffuse positivity for cytoplasmic mucin (**B:** Alcian blue, pH 2.5).

these latter cases are now reported as the plasmacytoid variant of urothelial carcinoma.

Differential Diagnosis

The major differential diagnosis is with urothelial carcinoma with mixed differentiation, the plasmacytoid variant of urothelial carcinoma and secondary involvement of the bladder by a signet ring cell adenocarcinoma from another site. In the current classification the term signet ring cell adenocarcinoma is reserved for pure tumors; cases with a definite urothelial carcinoma component are included in the mixed differentiation category. Tumors where the cells have a predominantly plasmacytoid or monocytoid morphology with only scattered signet ring cells and little cytoplasmic mucin are now placed in the plasmacytoid variant of urothelial carcinoma. Differentiation of metastatic signet ring cell carcinoma of gastrointestinal origin from primary signet ring cell adenocarcinoma requires clinical correlation. Immunohistochemistry cannot reliably distinguish between these two possibilities (see section on immunohistochemistry of adenocarcinoma above).[563] Prostatic adenocarcinoma can also have a signet ring–like morphology. These are extraordinarily rare as pure tumors and are almost always mixed with usual acinar prostatic adenocarcinoma. The signet ring–like cells of prostatic origin are almost always mucin-negative and express prostatic markers by immunohistochemistry.[587]

Clear Cell Adenocarcinoma

Clinical Features

Primary clear cell adenocarcinoma of the urinary bladder is rare, with only a limited number of well-documented cases in the English language literature.[373,553,588–592] In contrast to the bladder, the urethra is a relatively frequent site for clear cell adenocarcinoma, particularly in females.[374] These tumors occur over a wide age range with a mean age of 62 years.[591] They occur more commonly in females than in males (3:2).[591] The bladder neck is reported to be the most common site. The prognosis is uncertain; in one review 50% of patients were alive and disease free with a median follow-up of 31 months.[591]

The pathogenesis of clear cell adenocarcinoma in the bladder remains unresolved. Origin from embryonic rests of mesoderm from the mesonephric ducts had been favored,[593] but this has been challenged and a metaplastic origin from urothelium suggested.[588,590,594] The occurrence of urothelial carcinomas with areas having characteristic morphologic features of clear cell adenocarcinoma supports this hypothesis.[594] Further, molecular studies have also supported an urothelial origin for these tumors.[594] Cases reported in association with endometriosis and müllerian remnants suggest a müllerian origin in at least some instances.[373,553,595,596] The latter hypothesis was supported by Drew et al.,[589] who studied six clear cell adenocarcinomas of the lower urinary tract by histochemistry and immunohistochemistry; all six

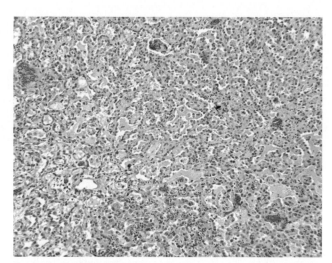

FIGURE 6-140 ■ Clear cell adenocarcinoma of the bladder with tubular architecture.

cases demonstrated positivity for CA-125. Clear cell adenocarcinomas have also been shown to consistently express hepatocyte nuclear factor-1β (100%) compared to expression in <5% of urothelial carcinomas.[261] This marker is also expressed in tumors of müllerian origin adding additional support to a müllerian origin for clear cell adenocarcinoma. A clear cell adenocarcinoma arising in a müllerian duct cyst has also been described.[597]

Pathology

These tumors are solid or papillary, and located in the trigone or posterior wall. The majority form a single mass. Histologically, all have a tubular component, some of which are cystically dilated (Fig. 6-140). Papillary (Fig. 6-141) and diffuse patterns (Fig. 6-142) can also be present. The tubulocystic areas have basophilic or eosinophilic luminal secretions. The lining cells are flattened, cuboidal, or columnar with clear cytoplasm and at least focally have characteristic

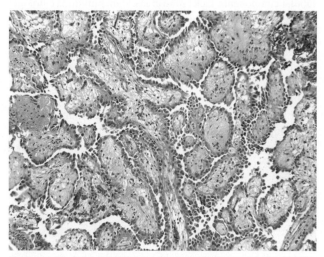

FIGURE 6-141 ■ Clear cell adenocarcinoma of the bladder with papillary architecture.

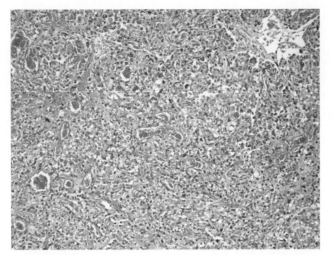

FIGURE 6-142 ■ Clear cell adenocarcinoma of the bladder with solid growth.

"hobnail" cells. The cells have significant nuclear pleomorphism with frequent mitotic figures. There are cases of clear cell adenocarcinoma with less severe cytologic atypia and lacking solid areas.[598] Special stains demonstrate abundant cytoplasmic glycogen in most but not all, and, in most, focal cytoplasmic and luminal mucin.

Immunohistochemical studies show that the tumors are usually cytokeratin 7 positive with variable reactivity for cytokeratin 20.[373] Most are negative or only weakly positive for high molecular weight cytokeratin (34βE12).[599] There is positive immunoreactivity for Ca-125.[589] Expression of PAX8 has been reported.[600] The tumors do not express PSA, prostatic acid phosphatase, estrogen receptor, or progesterone receptor.[599]

Differential Diagnosis

The major differential diagnostic considerations are nephrogenic adenoma and metastatic clear cell carcinoma. Nephrogenic adenoma is typically small, has both papillary and tubular components, lacks solid areas, shows minimal cytologic atypia, and has no or rare mitotic figures.[300,301,601] Infrequently, more severe cytologic atypia can be seen, but this does not approach that of clear cell adeno carcinoma.[602] Nephrogenic adenoma can infiltrate the muscular wall, and the presence of this feature should not be used as a diagnostic criterion for malignancy.[300,601] A clinical history of trauma or instrumentation may be helpful. Most clear cell adeno carcinomas express p53 while nephrogenic adenoma is consistently negative for p53.[599] Proliferation markers show high expression in clear cell adenocarcinoma compared to low expression in nephrogenic adenoma.[599] These lesions also express markers such as PAX2, PAX8, and p504s (racemase), reflecting their origin from renal tubular epithelial cells.[262,600,603] Nephrogenic adenoma can recur and so recurrence does not indicate malignancy.

Direct extension of a urethral adenocarcinoma arising in a urethral diverticulum should be considered in any female patient with a tumor presenting in the bladder neck or trigone region.[374,604] Clear cell adenocarcinoma of the urethra, and specifically a urethral diverticulum, is much more common than primary clear cell adenocarcinoma of the bladder. Metastatic or direct extension of clear cell (mesonephric) carcinoma should also be excluded in all female patients. Renal cell carcinoma can metastasize to the bladder and also needs to be considered.[375] Recognition of the typical sinusoidal vascular pattern, lack of tubular differentiation, absence of mucin, and clinical features should resolve this differential.

Hepatoid Adenocarcinoma

Rare cases of tumors arising in the urinary bladder mimicking hepatocellular carcinoma have been reported.[605–607] Cases have been described in five men and one woman with ages ranging from 61 to 85 years. In three of the five cases with follow-up, the patients died 12, 14, and 19 months after diagnosis; a fourth patient was alive with metastatic disease at 4 months; the final patient was alive at 26 months.

These tumors are composed of cells with abundant eosinophilic cytoplasm arranged in sheets and trabeculae with focal formation of glandular structures. Cytoplasmic hyaline globules were present in all five reported tumors. In three cases bile production was present. Expression of alpha-fetoprotein, alpha-1-antitrypsin, and HepPar-1 was demonstrated by immunohistochemistry. CEA immunohistochemistry demonstrated a canalicular pattern typical of hepatocellular carcinoma in all cases.

SMALL CELL CARCINOMA

Pathogenesis

The currently favored pathogenesis of small cell carcinoma is origin from multipotential undifferentiated or stem cells present in the urothelium.[608–610] The frequent association of this tumor with other histologic variants such as urothelial carcinoma and adenocarcinoma supports this theory.[611] Further, in cases with mixed differentiation, the small cell component harbors the same cytogenetic abnormalities as the urothelial carcinomas indicating a common origin.[291] Other hypotheses are origin from neuroendocrine cells within normal[610] or metaplastic urothelium[612] or from an undefined population of submucosal neuroendocrine cells.[613]

Clinical Features

Small cell carcinoma of the bladder, histologically identical to that occurring in the lung, is being reported with increasing frequency, with over 500 cases now described.[289,290,608,614–618] The tumor has been estimated to represent 0.5% of bladder malignancies but this is probably an underestimate.[608] It develops much more frequently in men than women (ratio, 4:1) and is essentially a tumor of older patients (range, 20 to 85 years; mean, 66 years).[614] Hematuria is the most frequent presentation (90% of cases), with symptoms of bladder irritability or obstruction occurring less commonly. The

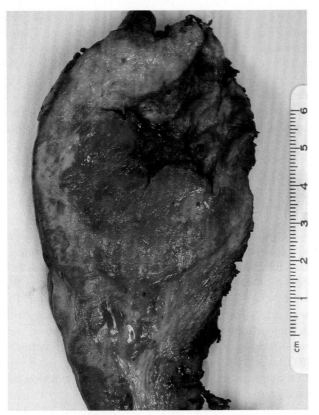

FIGURE 6-143 ■ Small cell carcinoma of the bladder forming a solid invasive tumor.

patients often present with locally advanced or metastatic cancer. Paraneoplastic syndromes rarely occur, including ectopic adrenocorticotropic hormone production,[619] hypercalcemia,[608] and hypophosphatemia.[612]

Pathology

There are no specific gross features separating small cell carcinoma from other carcinomas of the bladder (Fig. 6-143).

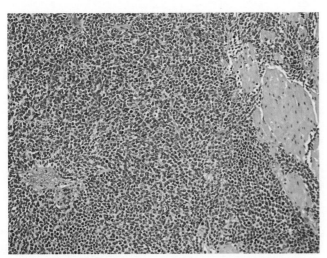

FIGURE 6-144 ■ Small cell carcinoma of the bladder with typical histologic features.

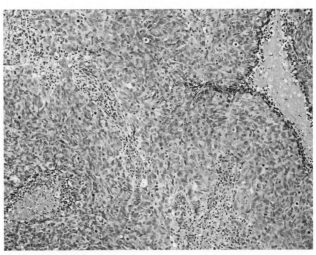

FIGURE 6-145 ■ Small cell carcinoma of the bladder with larger cells, some of which have a more fusiform nuclear shape.

This tumor ranges in size and shape from 2-cm polypoid lesions to solid masses of up to 10 cm. It can develop at any location including the dome and within bladder diverticula.

Approximately 50% of cases have pure small cell histology without an identifiable urothelial component. In mixed tumors a common origin has been demonstrated.[291] The small cell areas fulfill the light microscopic criteria used for small cell carcinoma of the lung. It can show either an oat cell or intermediate cell pattern, and both may be present in the same tumor. The "oat cell" type consists of a relatively uniform population of cells with scant cytoplasm, hyperchromatic nuclei with dispersed chromatin, and absent or inconspicuous nucleoli (Fig. 6-144). The intermediate cell type has more abundant cytoplasm, larger nuclei with less hyperchromasia, and similar chromatin pattern and nucleolar features. In some cases, the intermediate type of small cell carcinoma contains elongate or spindled cells (Fig. 6-145). Both types have extensive necrosis (Fig. 6-146), prominent nuclear molding, frequent mitotic figures, prominent

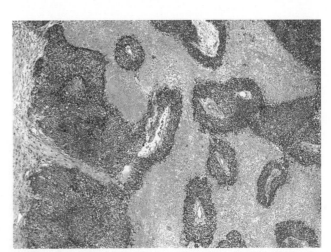

FIGURE 6-146 ■ Small cell carcinoma of the bladder with extensive necrosis resulting in a pattern mimicking a papillary appearance.

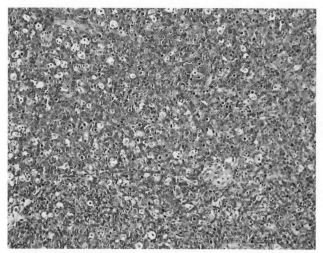

FIGURE 6-147 ■ Small cell carcinoma of the bladder with prominent apoptosis.

apoptosis (Fig. 6-147), and may have DNA encrustation of blood vessel walls (Azzopardi phenomenon). A large cell neuroendocrine carcinoma phenotype has been described, and the presence of scattered cells with "monstrous nuclei" occurs.[620] Skeletal muscle differentiation can occur.[621]

Between 23% and 67% of cases are mixed with other histologic patterns.[611,620] A urothelial carcinoma component (papillary or nonpapillary) is most common, but glandular and squamous differentiation has been observed (Fig. 6-148). One case of small cell carcinoma arose in association with urachal adenocarcinoma.[622]

In cases studied by electron microscopy, dense core neurosecretory granules have been found.[620] In most cases evidence of neuroendocrine differentiation can be found by immunohistochemistry with neuron-specific enolase immunoreactivity being most frequent; other neuroendocrine markers are less often positive, with CD56 being most sensitive (Fig. 6-149A to C).[248,610,615,618,623] Although cytokeratin is present in most tumors, some are nonreactive.[615,620,623] The

presence of a "dot-like" pattern for cytokeratin has been noted (Fig. 6-149D).[620] The tumors are infrequently cytokeratin 20 or p63 positive with most positive for cytokeratin 7.[248,624] Cells of the associated urothelial carcinoma can be both cytokeratin 20 and p63 positive, and these can be admixed with the small cell carcinoma and should not result in altering the diagnosis if morphologically the tumor is consistent with small cell carcinoma. Most cases are p16 positive, but this can also expressed by urothelial carcinoma.[248] Uroplakin has been reported to be negative in the cases evaluated.[624]

Differential Diagnosis

The major differential diagnostic considerations are small cell carcinoma from other sites and malignant lymphoma. In about 50% of prostatic small cell carcinomas, there is a coexistent adenocarcinoma component; positive staining of this element for PSA and PSAP indicates prostatic origin. The small cell component, however, is characteristically negative for these markers, so in pure cases clinical correlation may be essential to separate prostate from bladder primaries.[625] Metastases from other sites also need to be considered; interestingly, symptomatic bladder metastasis from bronchogenic small cell carcinoma is a rare occurrence.[626] Primary small cell carcinoma of the bladder can express TTF-1, so this marker is not helpful in this differential diagnosis.[624] The identification of a urothelial component, including urothelial CIS, would strongly support primary bladder origin.[620] Malignant lymphoma should be distinguishable in most cases on histologic grounds, but immunohistochemical staining for cytokeratin and leukocyte common antigen in difficult cases should readily distinguish the two.[620]

Treatment and Prognosis

The aggressive behavior of this tumor has been noted repeatedly, and overall survival is poor.[289] There are several reports

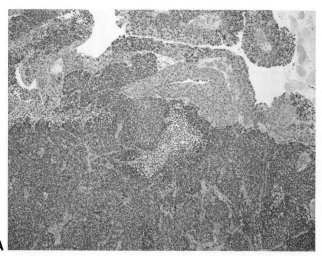

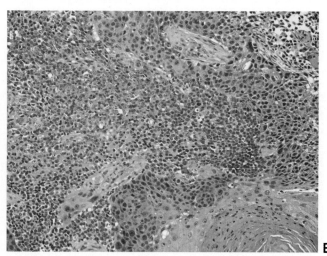

FIGURE 6-148 ■ Small cell carcinoma of the bladder mixed with high-grade papillary urothelial carcinoma **(A)** and squamous cell carcinoma **(B)**.

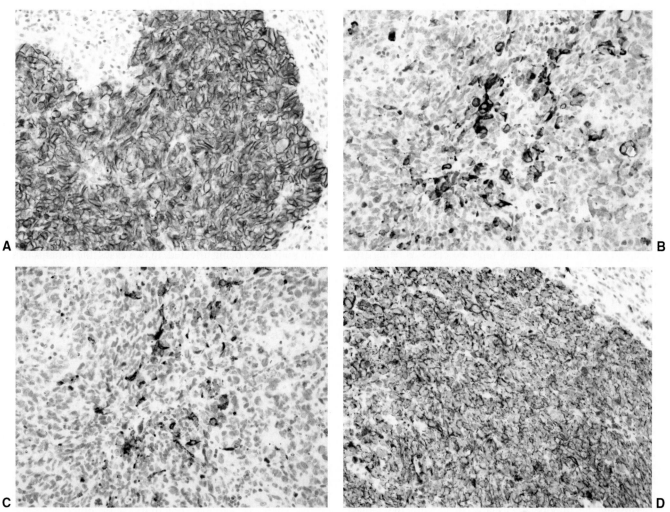

FIGURE 6-149 ■ Small cell carcinoma of the bladder with positive immunoreactivity for CD56 **(A)**, synaptophysin **(B)**, chromogranin A **(C)**, and cytokeratin (AE1/AE3, **D**).

indicating that patients may respond to aggressive combination therapy if given at the time of diagnosis.[289,618,620,627] In a series from the MD Anderson Cancer Center, 26 patients treated with cystectomy or cystoprostatectomy alone had a 36% 5-year disease-free survival compared to 78% for surgery combined with neoadjuvant and adjuvant multiagent chemotherapy.[618] Others have used sequential chemotherapy and radiation therapy for these patients with success.[628] These reports underscore the importance of recognizing this distinct form of bladder cancer, which may respond to aggressive therapy. In contrast to the way squamous and glandular differentiation are reported, given the clinical significance of this diagnosis, we report these mixed tumors as small cell carcinoma and then indicate the percentage of the small cell and urothelial components.

Large Cell Neuroendocrine Carcinoma

A few examples of large cell neuroendocrine carcinoma arising in the urinary bladder have been reported.[622,629–636] The majority have occurred in males with ages ranging from 19 to 82 years. All have presented with hematuria. There is insufficient information to comment specifically on treatment and outcome. To date, most cases have been aggressive with rapid growth and early metastases. Follow-up has been short in those patients reported to be alive and well at last follow-up.

Pathologically, the tumor cells are arranged in sheets, trabeculae, or nests. An organoid pattern can be present. Individual cells are large and polygonal with abundant eosinophilic cytoplasm resulting in a low nuclear to cytoplasmic ratio. Nuclei are large with coarse chromatin and variably prominent nucleoli. Mitotic figures (>10 per 10 high power fields) and apoptotic bodies are frequent. Necrosis can be focal or diffuse. Bizarre tumor giant cells can be seen. In over half of the reported cases the tumor has been mixed with other histologies including urothelial carcinoma, squamous carcinoma,[629] lymphoepithelioma-like carcinoma,[633] sarcomatoid carcinoma,[636] and adenocarcinoma.[622,630] The typical appearance of the cells has been described in a urine cytology specimen.[634]

The tumors demonstrate neuroendocrine differentiation by immunohistochemistry with variable expression of synaptophysin, chromogranin, CD56, and neuron-specific enolase. Cytokeratin positivity with a distinct perinuclear dot-like pattern can be seen.[630] Expression of cytokeratin 20 and TTF-1 has been reported.[631] The cells are nonreactive for prostatic markers. Ultrastructural examination shows the cells have cytoplasmic processes and contain neurosecretory granules.[630]

Carcinoid Tumor

Rare examples of better differentiated neuroendocrine neoplasms showing histologic features of carcinoid tumor, without associated urothelial carcinoma, have been described.[637–644] In a critical review of the literature, Martignoni and Eble[641] accepted only four previously reported cases as being true pure carcinoid tumors.[637–640] Since then, at least three additional convincing cases have been added.[642–644] These have occurred over a wide age range (29 to 75 years) and have been more common in males. Hematuria and irritative symptoms are most common. No cases with the carcinoid syndrome have been reported. Most cases have been cured by transurethral resection, but recurrences have been documented and malignant behavior has been reported.[645,646] One of these cases had a small cell carcinoma component,[646] and in the other cases the pathologic description and images are insufficient to be certain of the accuracy of the classification.[645] The presence of carcinoid-like areas in small cell carcinoma has been recognized, and these cases should be classified as small cell carcinoma rather than carcinoid tumor.[611]

Grossly the tumors are usually small with the largest reported tumor measuring 4 cm. The typical microscopic features of carcinoid tumor are the organoid, glandular, or trabecular growth pattern (Fig. 6-150). Tumor cells are moderate in size with abundant cytoplasm. A case with oncocytic cells has been described.[642] Nuclei are small and uniform with finely stippled chromatin and inconspicuous nucleoli. Necrosis is not a feature. The tumor cells consistently express neuroendocrine markers including synaptophysin, chromogranin, and neuron-specific enolase.[641,643] Positive immunoreactivity for cytokeratin 7, TTF-1, and β-HCG has been reported in some cases.[641] Prostate markers are negative.[641]

Primitive Neuroectodermal Tumor/Ewing Sarcoma

Several examples of these tumors, confirmed by demonstrating expression of CD99 or demonstration of the *EWS/FLI1* fusion transcript, have been described arising in the urinary bladder.[647–654] These have occurred over a wide age range with both sexes being affected. In two cases, the patients had previously received chemotherapy.[647,654] Presentation is usually with hematuria and/or irritative symptoms. Treatment has varied but has included resection and chemotherapy. There are too few cases to determine the prognosis. There have been four cases where the patients were alive and free of disease at the time of last follow-up[648,649,653,654] and two patients who died of disease.[650,652]

The tumors have ranged from 3 cm to very large. Histologically, the typical features of primitive neuroectodermal tumor are present. Cells are arranged in sheets, trabeculae, or lobules. Nuclei are small with fine chromatin and inconspicuous or small nucleoli. There is scant pale to clear cytoplasm. Rosettes are occasionally present. Mitoses are frequent and necrosis is present. The tumor is positive for CD99 with a prominent membranous pattern. There is variable reactivity with other markers; positive reactivity for CD117 and vimentin has also been described. Neuroendocrine markers can also be positive in some cases. A small percentage of cases can be cytokeratin positive. Molecular analysis demonstrates the *EWS-FLI1* fusion transcript.

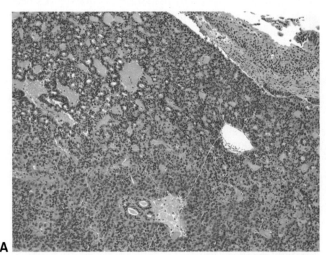 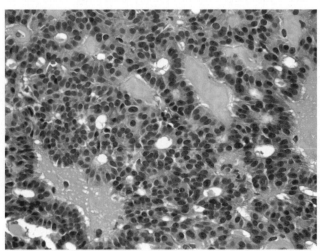

A   B

FIGURE 6-150 ■ Carcinoid tumor arising in the urinary bladder at low **(A)** and high **(B)** magnification.

MESENCHYMAL TUMORS—BENIGN

Benign soft tissue tumors are uncommon in the bladder with leiomyoma, hemangioma, or neurofibroma representing the majority. In a review of all newly diagnosed bladder tumors, Melicow[655] reported that benign soft tissue tumors accounted for only 0.9% of all primary bladder lesions. In addition to those detailed below, rare examples of other benign soft tissue tumors have been reported including lymphangioma,[656] benign fibrous histiocytoma,[657,658] aggressive angiomyxoma,[659] and ganglioneuroma.[660,661]

Leiomyoma

Clinical Features

In a comprehensive literature review, leiomyoma was the most common benign mesenchymal tumor of the urinary bladder accounting for 47% of published cases.[662] In 1986, Knoll et al.[663] reviewed the literature and provided an analysis of 155 cases they identified. Recent series have added significantly to this total.[664,665] Leiomyoma is more common in women (male:female ratio, 1:2) and the majority occur in adults, although rare examples in children have been reported.[666] These have been described in the setting of von Recklinghausen disease.[667] Obstructive symptoms are most common, due to a ball-valve effect of a pedunculated tumor.[668] These can be a cause of acute urinary retention.[669] Less often, it produces pelvic pain or ureteral obstruction with hydronephrosis. Bladder leiomyoma may be associated with paraurethral leiomyoma.

Treatment of leiomyoma is conservative. Depending on the tumor size, transurethral resection or segmental resection is indicated. In cases with atypical features, resection with frozen sections to ensure negative margins may be appropriate.[372] In most cases, treatment is curative, although leiomyoma can recur if incompletely resected. No case of malignant change developing in a leiomyoma has been reported.[665]

Pathology

Leiomyoma is submucosal in two-thirds of cases, producing a polypoid or pedunculated mass (Fig. 6-151). Less commonly, it arises within the wall or in a subserosal location. The overlying epithelium is usually intact. Most are small, measuring 1 to 4 cm in greatest dimension, although cases up to 25 cm have been described; multiple lesions can be present.[665,670] The cut surface is circumscribed and bulging, with a whorled gray-white appearance. Histologically, the characteristic features of leiomyoma are identified, including fascicles of spindle-shaped cells with fusiform, blunt-ended nuclei and eosinophilic cytoplasm (Fig. 6-152). There is minimal atypia and only rare mitotic figures. Morphologic variants such as epithelioid leiomyoma can occur.[671] In a few cases, the degenerative nuclear atypia present as seen in symplastic leiomyoma can be present in leiomyomas of the bladder.[665]

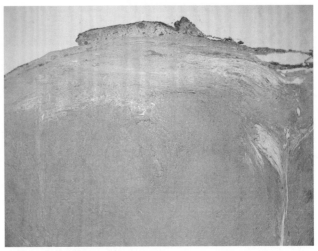

FIGURE 6-151 ■ Leiomyoma of the bladder forming a circumscribed submucosal mass.

Differential Diagnosis

The major differential diagnosis is with leiomyosarcoma but other spindle cell lesions may be considered (Table 6-19). In most cases this distinction is straightforward. Mills et al.[672] considered leiomyoma to be characterized by a sharply circumscribed margin, little or no mitotic activity, and minimal cytologic atypia. Further, they suggest that a smooth muscle tumor with rare or absent mitotic figures and an infiltrative pattern should be considered as a low-grade leiomyosarcoma.[672] These criteria have been supported in subsequent series.[664,665] Although focal myxoid change can occur in a leiomyoma, prominent myxoid stroma is more likely in leiomyosarcoma; although these tumors may be otherwise cytologically quite bland.[372]

Other benign mesenchymal tumors such as schwannoma and neurofibroma can also be considered in the differential diagnosis. Generally the morphologic features will be sufficient for distinguishing between these, but if needed, immunohistochemistry will resolve the differential diagnosis (Table 6-19).

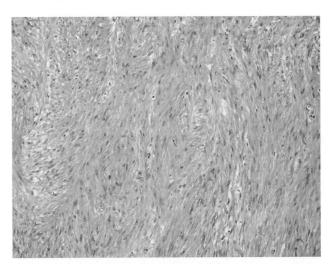

FIGURE 6-152 ■ Leiomyoma of the bladder.

Table 6-19 ■ DIFFERENTIAL DIAGNOSIS OF SPINDLE CELL LESIONS

Benign
    Postoperative spindle cell nodule
    Inflammatory myofibroblastic tumor
    Leiomyoma
    Other benign mesenchymal tumors
Malignant
    Urothelial carcinoma with pseudosarcomatous stroma
    Sarcomatoid carcinoma
    Leiomyosarcoma
    Other sarcoma types

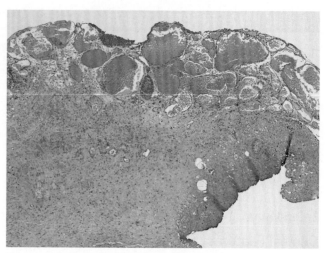

FIGURE 6-153 ■ Hemangioma of the bladder.

Hemangioma

Clinical Features

In 1991, Jahn and Nissen[673] reviewed the literature on hemangioma of the urinary tract and identified 106 cases in the bladder. Since that report, numerous additional examples have been described.[674–678] In the large series reported by Melicow,[655] hemangioma accounted for 40% of benign mesenchymal tumors, and 0.6% of primary bladder tumors. It occurs at any age, with the majority presenting prior to age 30. There is a slight male preponderance. Although they tend to present in adults it is generally believed that these are congenital in nature.[678] Most patients present with hematuria that can occasionally be life threatening, but irritation, pain, and obstructive symptoms may occur. Up to 30% of patients also have cutaneous hemangiomas.[679] Bladder hemangioma occurs in 3% to 6% of patients with Klippel-Trenaunay syndrome; it is also reported in patients with Sturge-Weber syndrome.[680] Cystoscopically, hemangioma appears purple, multilobulated, and sessile and may be mistaken for endometriosis, melanoma, or sarcoma.[673]

Treatment depends on the size and location of the hemangioma. Most authors recommend partial cystectomy or local excision.[673] Biopsy and transurethral resection carry a significant risk for massive hemorrhage[673]; management with the Nd:YAG laser has been successfully applied.[679] There is a risk of local recurrence if the resection is incomplete.[673]

Pathology

Hemangiomas may be single (66%) or multiple, and be superficial or extend through the full thickness of the bladder wall.[676] The majority are small (1 to 2 cm), although cases up to 10 cm have been described. It is soft, spongy, and hemorrhagic. Histologically, they are characterized by vascular spaces containing blood and thrombi. Depending on the pattern, hemangioma is classified as cavernous, capillary, venous, or racemose with cavernous being most common (Fig. 6-153). The lesion is usually restricted to the submucosa without involvement of the muscularis propria.[678] The endothelial cells show no cytologic atypia.

Differential Diagnosis

The major differential diagnostic considerations are arteriovenous malformation and angiosarcoma. Arteriovenous malformation has often been included within the category of hemangioma in the literature.[678] These have variably sized vascular spaces with thin and thick walls having features of venous and arterial channels. Angiosarcoma typically has significant nuclear pleomorphism and numerous mitotic figures.[681] Bladder involvement by Kaposi sarcoma in AIDS patients has also been described.[682] Rare cases of hemangiopericytoma (solitary fibrous tumor) arise in the bladder, although this tumor is more cellular than hemangioma and has a characteristic vascular pattern.[683] Epithelioid hemangioendothelioma has also been described in the bladder.[673,678] These have the typical features seen elsewhere with epithelioid and spindle cells having abundant eosinophilic cytoplasm, vesicular nuclei, and intracytoplasmic lumens containing red blood cells. Discrete vascular channels are present in a myxoid or hyalinized stroma. Finally papillary endothelial hyperplasia has been described in patient previously treated with radiation therapy.[678] These have dilated vascular channels with papillary proliferations of plump endothelial cells. There is minimal cytologic atypia, with no mitoses and no necrosis.

Neurofibroma

Clinical Features

In 1986, Ogawa and Watanabe[684] described a case of neurofibroma in the bladder, and reviewed approximately 50 other reported cases. The contemporary literature contains several additional examples.[685,686] The majority develop in patients with von Recklinghausen disease,[686–688] although many cases occur in the absence of this syndrome.[685,689] Neurofibroma can present at any age, including infancy, and is slightly more common in males. The majority of patients complain of hematuria, dysuria, or irritative symptoms. In some cases, there is concomitant involvement of other genitourinary sites including the ureter, spermatic cord, penis, and scrotum.

The treatment of neurofibroma is controversial. For localized lesions transurethral resection or partial cystectomy is adequate. For diffuse involvement by plexiform neurofibroma most authors recommend radical resection with urinary diversion due to the high rate of recurrence with partial resection. Urinary diversion alone may be useful in cases with extensive involvement, although conservative management has been advocated by some until the tumor becomes too extensive for transurethral resection or until ureteral obstruction develops. Despite the benign histology, neurofibroma can recur and can cause death by urinary obstruction and renal failure.

Pathology

Grossly, neurofibroma may be single or multiple, consisting of discrete variably sized nodules within the wall or submucosa and may be polypoid or pedunculated (Fig. 6-154). Most are small, but some may be up to several centimeters in diameter. It can also appear as diffuse thickening of the bladder wall without discrete margins; this pattern corresponds to the plexiform variant characteristically associated with von Recklinghausen disease. In these patients, the tumor may extensively invade the bladder wall, ureters, and adjacent soft tissues. Histologically, neurofibroma of the bladder is identical to those occurring elsewhere, composed of interweaving fascicles of elongated spindle-shaped cells with thin wavy hyperchromatic nuclei in a collagenized and fibrillar background. Nuclear atypia can be present but mitotic activity is absent or rare at most. Small nerve fibers are usually present within the mass. Myxoid areas may be present. Some tumors are circumscribed but not encapsulated. Malignant

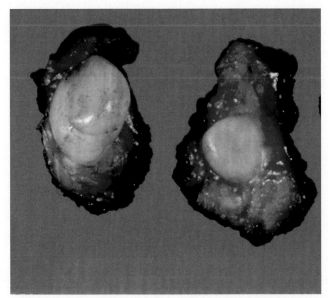

FIGURE 6-154 ■ Gross photo of a 1.2-cm neurofibroma of the bladder that was submucosal in location.

transformation is indicated by more diffuse and marked nuclear atypia, high cellularity, and increased mitoses.[661,690] Immunohistochemical results are similar to neurofibroma elsewhere with essentially all cases having S100 protein positivity. A case of ganglioneuromatosis in association with plexiform neurofibroma has been described in a child with neurofibromatosis.[691]

Differential Diagnosis

The differential diagnostic considerations with neurofibroma include other benign spindle cell lesions such as leiomyoma, schwannoma, and inflammatory myofibroblastic pseudotumor. The majority of leiomyomas in the bladder show typical features, and separation should be straightforward.[665] In problem cases, immunohistochemistry reveals evidence of muscle differentiation. Inflammatory myofibroblastic pseudotumor is characterized by cytologically benign spindle or stellate cells in a loose myxoid background mixed with inflammatory cells.[399,692] The spindle cells contain vimentin and actin, reflecting their fibroblastic and myofibroblastic nature. Since most bladder neurofibromas occur in patients with von Recklinghausen disease, clinical history should be obtained when this diagnosis is entertained. Schwannoma is usually well circumscribed and may be encapsulated. Both Antoni A and Antoni B areas are usually evident.[685]

Schwannoma

Schwannoma is much less common than neurofibroma with only a handful of cases described in the urinary bladder.[685,693–697] These have occurred in adult patients, with both males and females affected. These are benign lesions and are cured by local resection. The tumors are sharply circumscribed and gray-white.[694] The histology is typical of schwannoma. Spindle-shaped cells are present in a loose matrix with a well-defined capsule. Cellularity is variable and nuclear palisading is prominent with both Antoni A and B patterns present. An epithelioid morphology can be present.[685,697] So-called ancient schwannomas have been described here.[693] There is no significant nuclear pleomorphism or necrosis and minimal mitotic activity. The tumors strongly express S100 protein with variable expression of Leu-7 and glial fibrillary acidic protein.[698] There is no reactivity for smooth muscle actin, CD117, or cytokeratin.[694]

Granular Cell Tumor

Several cases of granular cell tumor involving the urinary bladder have been described.[699–704] These occur over a wide range including one case present at the time of birth.[701] Gross hematuria is the most common presentation with females being affected more often than males.[699] It can occur in patients with von Recklinghausen disease.[702] All cases in the contemporary literature have been considered benign except for one. In that case the tumor was considered malignant based on nuclear pleomorphism and a mitotic rate of 2 to 3 per 10 high-power fields. The patient was free of disease 8 years after radical cystectomy.[699] There is one case that recurred following transurethral resection in a patient with multiple lesions.[702] The tumors can be relatively well or poorly circumscribed with infiltration of the bladder wall. It is composed of round to polyhedral cells with abundant granular eosinophilic cytoplasm. Nuclei are small to medium in size and round to oval with vesicular chromatin. There is mild nuclear pleomorphism and mitoses are rare. The cells are arranged in nests or cords. The overlying urothelium can show pseudoepitheliomatous hyperplasia.[700] Immunohistochemistry demonstrates positive reactivity for S100 protein, CD68, laminin, and neuron-specific enolase.[698] The cells contain lysosomes and are strongly positive for CD68.[698] There is no expression of cytokeratins or muscle markers.

Lipoma

A few examples of lipoma involving the bladder wall have been reported.[705–709] These have all occurred in adults and have presented with hematuria or urinary frequency. These have been small lesions (<2 cm), and radiologic evaluation has demonstrated well-circumscribed masses with fat density on computed tomography. Small polypoid protrusions into the bladder are present at cystoscopy. Microscopically the lesions have been well-circumscribed proliferations of mature adipose tissue.

Solitary Fibrous Tumor

Solitary fibrous tumor can arise within the wall of the urinary bladder. These are uncommon with <20 examples described in the English language literature.[710–714] Most patients are older with the majority of tumors involving males. They can present with hematuria or pain; a few cases have been incidental findings. In some cases the actual origin of the tumor is uncertain with some arising in the soft tissue adjacent to the urinary bladder. There are too few cases that have been reported to ascertain whether features of malignancy used at other sites are applicable in the urinary bladder.

The tumors are well circumscribed, and most have been submucosal. Size has ranged up to 20 cm. The tumor is composed of spindle-shaped cells haphazardly arranged (patternless pattern) in a variably collagenized stroma or with fascicle formation. There is variable cellularity. The background includes areas with dense collagen deposition. A hemangiopericytoma-like vascular pattern is characteristic. The possibility of malignancy should be considered when high cellularity and mitotic activity, significant nuclear pleomorphism, or necrosis is present. Immunohistochemistry demonstrates positive reactivity for CD34, bcl-2, and CD99.[698] Other markers expressed to a lesser degree include EMA and actin. Desmin, S100 protein, and cytokeratin are usually negative.

MESENCHYMAL TUMORS—MALIGNANT

Primary sarcoma of the urinary bladder is uncommon and there is a distinctive age distribution according to histologic type. Rhabdomyosarcoma is the most frequent tumor of the bladder in childhood, whereas leiomyosarcoma is the most frequent sarcoma in adults.[662,665,715] In the review by Melicow,[655] sarcoma accounted for 2.7% of all primary bladder neoplasms. In addition to these, virtually all other types of sarcoma including malignant fibrous histiocytoma,[716] osteogenic sarcoma,[717] chondrosarcoma,[718,719] fibrosarcoma,[720] malignant mesenchymoma,[721] angiosarcoma,[678,722] hemangiopericytoma,[683] liposarcoma,[723] perivascular epithelioid cell tumor (PEComa),[724] and rhabdoid tumor[725] have been described.[726] Any diagnosis of a malignant mesenchymal tumor requires exclusion of a sarcomatoid urothelial carcinoma.

Leiomyosarcoma

Clinical Features

Leiomyosarcoma is the most common sarcoma of the bladder in adults.[280,664,665,672,715,727,728] In a recent literature review, leiomyosarcoma accounted for 57% of published primary bladder sarcomas (excluding rhabdomyosarcoma).[662] There is a wide age range (7 to 81 years) with a mean age of 52 years, with some cases occurring in patients under the age of 21 years. Several cases have developed following cyclophosphamide therapy for other conditions.[729] The most common presentation is hematuria and obstructive symptoms.

Leiomyosarcoma is treated by partial cystectomy for localized tumors or radical cystectomy for more extensive ones.[665,698,715,727] The use of combined chemotherapy has been advocated.[727] Many authors have commented on the aggressive nature of these lesions, but a review of 62 cases with outcome data reported between 1960 and 1992 revealed crude 2- and 5-year survivals of 81% and 67%, respectively; none of the eight patients under the age of 21 years with available follow-up died of leiomyosarcoma.[280] More recent reports have shown similar outcomes with high-grade tumors having a worse prognosis.[665,715]

Pathology

Leiomyosarcoma is most often lobulated or polypoid, and may be ulcerated (Fig. 6-155). A "mushroom shape" at cystoscopy is typical. Most tumors are 2 to 5 cm in greatest dimension but may measure up to 13 cm. Histologically, the majority have the typical appearance of leiomyosarcoma, composed of interweaving fascicles of spindle-shaped cells with long blunt-ended nuclei and eosinophilic cytoplasm (Fig. 6-156). Nuclear pleomorphism is variable (Fig. 6-157) as is the mitotic rate (Fig. 6-158). Necrosis may be present (Fig. 6-159). In a few cases, the tumor has been myxoid (Fig. 6-160).[372,665] Epithelioid leiomyosarcoma has also been described in the urinary bladder.[665] Ultrastructural studies

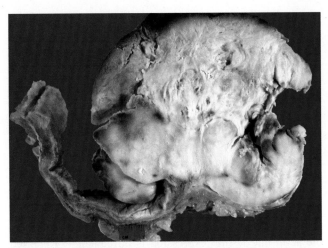

FIGURE 6-155 ■ Leiomyosarcoma of the bladder producing a polypoid mass protruding into the bladder lumen.

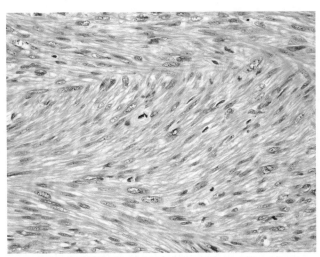

FIGURE 6-158 ■ Leiomyosarcoma of the bladder with minimal nuclear pleomorphism but having mitotic activity.

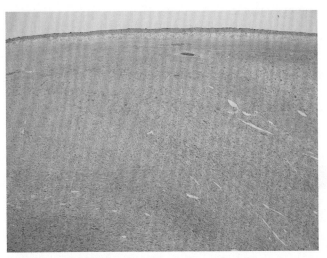

FIGURE 6-156 ■ Leiomyosarcoma of the bladder with the overlying urothelium.

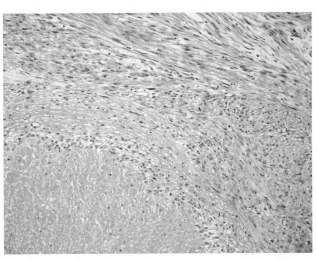

FIGURE 6-159 ■ Leiomyosarcoma of the bladder with areas of necrosis.

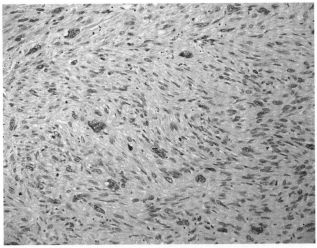

FIGURE 6-157 ■ Leiomyosarcoma of the bladder with the tumor cells showing nuclear pleomorphism.

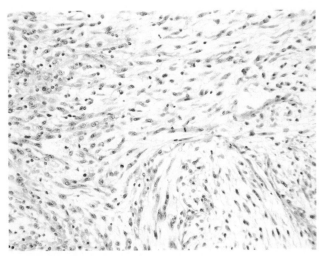

FIGURE 6-160 ■ Leiomyosarcoma of the bladder with a myxoid appearance.

show features typical of smooth muscle cells, including thin filaments with dense bodies and pinocytotic vesicles.

Cases evaluated by immunohistochemistry have shown cytokeratin immunoreactivity for pancytokeratins and for low molecular weight cytokeratin in a minority of cases.[395] The expression is typically weak and focal. There is no expression of high molecular weight cytokeratins (cytokeratin 5/6, 34βE12).[395] Markers of muscle differentiation including muscle-specific actin and desmin are positive in the majority.[395,400,672] Expression of p63 is present in a small percentage; there is no expression of ALK-1.[395,400]

In a series from the Mayo Clinic, tumors were divided into low- and high-grade categories based on nuclear pleomorphism, mitotic activity, and necrosis. A tumor was low grade if it had mild to moderate nuclear pleomorphism and <5 mitoses per 10 high-power fields and necrosis involving <25% of the tumor.[664] A more recent series supports the Mayo Clinic criteria with only one patient with a low-grade tumor recurring but without metastases compared to 50% mortality in the high-grade group.[665] Grade can be heterogeneous, and so low-grade histology on a biopsy or transurethral resection does not exclude a high-grade tumor.[665]

Differential Diagnosis

The differential diagnosis of spindle cell lesions in the bladder is extensive (Table 6-19).[395] If the tumor is clearly malignant, the major considerations are other types of sarcoma and sarcomatoid carcinoma. Other sarcomas are distinguished by histologic features and immunohistochemical findings. Sarcomatoid carcinoma may mimic high-grade leiomyosarcoma. In most cases, extensive sampling reveals a recognizable epithelial component; however, there are cases of sarcomatoid carcinoma without foci of identifiable carcinoma, and immunohistochemistry is invaluable in such cases (Table 6-20).[395] The majority of cases of sarcomatoid carcinoma express cytokeratin at least focally in the spindle cell component including expression of high molecular weight cytokeratins in some (cytokeratin 5/6; 34βE12). They also can express p63 in about 50% of the cases. Sarcomatoid carcinoma frequently expresses smooth muscle actin but desmin expression is infrequent.[395] Reported desmin positivity is related to the presence of heterologous rhabdomyosarcomatous elements in most sarcomatoid carcinomas.[730] This distinction is not merely academic; sarcomatoid carcinoma has a much poorer prognosis than leiomyosarcoma.[388,389]

In any spindle cell lesion in the bladder, the possibility of a benign process should be considered. Several entities produce spindle cell proliferations that can be quite alarming in their histologic appearance. Pseudosarcomatous fibromyxoid tumor or inflammatory myofibroblastic pseudotumor is typically polypoid and can be quite large.[399,692] Postoperative spindle cell nodule can also mimic leiomyosarcoma. It is

Table 6-20 ■ DIFFERENTIAL DIAGNOSIS OF SPINDLE CELL LESIONS

Feature	Post-op Spindle Cell Nodule	Inflammatory Myofibroblastic Pseudotumor	Sarcomatoid Carcinoma	Leiomyosarcoma
Age	Older adults	Children, young adults	Older adults	Adults
Sex	M > F	F > M	M > F	M = F
Gross pathology	Small (most < 1 cm)	Small to large (4 to 5 cm)	Large	Large
	Nodular	Polypoid	Polypoid	Polypoid
Histology				
Cellularity	High	Low	High (low with myxoid)	High
Pleomorphism	Minimal	Minimal	Marked	Variable
Mitotic rate	High	Low	High	Variable
Abnormal MF	No	No	Yes	Yes/No
Vessels	Granulation tissue–like	Slit-like	Not specific	Not specific
Growth pattern	Fascicles	Haphazard—myxoid	Fascicles or haphazard	Fascicles or haphazard myxoid
Heterologous elements	No	No	Yes or No	No
IHC				
Vimentin	+++	+++	+++	+++
Actin	++	++	+/−	++
Desmin	− (few +)	− (few +)	−	++
Keratin (pan)	+ (>50%)	+ (>50%)	+ (>90%)	− (+ <10%)
CK (34βE12)	−	−	+/−	−
P63	−	−	++ (>50%)	− (few +)
ALK-1	− (<10% +)	++ (50%)	−	− (<5% +)

most often incidental and develops following surgery or trauma.[731] Because of the overlapping histologic and immunohistochemical findings, some authors consider inflammatory myofibroblastic pseudotumor and postoperative spindle cell nodule as a single entity while others argue that these should be kept as separate entities. Inflammatory myofibroblastic tumor usually has a loose myxoid appearance with numerous slit-like blood vessels and a background of acute and chronic inflammatory cells. Individual cells are spindle-shaped or stellate with little nuclear pleomorphism, although occasional bizarre nuclei may be seen; mitotic figures are infrequent and abnormal forms are absent. The process is infiltrative and can involve muscle, a feature making distinction from myxoid leiomyosarcoma difficult and, on small samples often impossible.[672,732] Postoperative spindle cell nodule is similar to inflammatory myofibroblastic pseudotumor but the spindle-shaped cells tend to be arranged in short haphazard fascicles reminiscent of granulation tissue. Cellularity is high and mitotic activity can be brisk, but abnormal mitotic figures and nuclear pleomorphism are not found. With adequate sampling, the latter should show features diagnostic of leiomyosarcoma. Immunohistochemistry of both conditions is similar. The majority demonstrate strong expression of cytokeratins.[395,399,692] Expression of high molecular weight cytokeratins (cytokeratin 5/6, 34βE12) is, however, absent.[395] EMA reactivity has been reported in a small percentage of case.[733] Expression of smooth muscle actin is consistently present, and most are also desmin positive.[395,399,692] Calponin and caldesmon can also be positive.[692] There is expression of ALK-1 in about 50% of cases.[395,399,692] In one study there was no reactivity for p63.[395]

Distinction from leiomyoma in most instances is not difficult. The presence of significant nuclear pleomorphism, high mitotic rate, infiltrative growth, and necrosis suggest malignancy. Mills et al.[672] considered any tumor with 5 or more mitotic figures per 10 high-power fields to be leiomyosarcoma, and cautioned that a tumor with even 0 or 1 mitotic figures should be considered malignant if it had an infiltrative growth pattern. Caution is indicated in calling any mitotically active smooth muscle tumor of the bladder benign. The degenerative nuclear atypia of symplastic leiomyoma can be seen in leiomyoma of the urinary bladder.[665] Necrosis is not a feature of leiomyoma.

Rhabdomyosarcoma

Clinical Features

In general, rhabdomyosarcoma accounts for between 4% and 8% of all malignant tumors in children under the age of 15 years.[734] Not all malignant neoplasms of the bladder in children are rhabdomyosarcoma; however, other types of sarcoma and a variety of epithelial tumors have also been described.[735] Rhabdomyosarcoma of the bladder is rare in adult patients.[736–739] In children, it occurs more frequently in boys (ratio of 3:2), and most develop before age 5. It most often presents because of hematuria and bladder neck

Table 6-21 ■ IRS-TNM STAGING SYSTEM FOR URINARY BLADDER RHABDOMYOSARCOMA

Characteristic	Definition
Tumor	
T1	Confined to urinary bladder
T1a	≤5 cm in diameter
T1b	>5 cm in diameter
T2	Extension and/or fixation to surrounding tissue
T2a	≤5 cm in diameter
T2b	>5 cm in diameter
Regional nodes	
N0	Not clinically involved
N1	Clinically involved by tumor
NX	Clinical status of regional nodes unknown
Metastasis	
M0	No distant metastasis
M1	Metastasis present

Reprinted from Lawrence W, Jr., Anderson JR, Gehan EA, et al. Pretreatment TNM staging of childhood rhabdomyosarcoma: a report of the Intergroup Rhabdomyosarcoma Study Group. Children's Cancer Study Group. Pediatric Oncology Group. *Cancer* 1997;80:1165–1170, with permission, Ref.[742]

obstruction. Cystoscopically, the characteristic finding is a polypoid mass filling the bladder lumen.

Historically, rhabdomyosarcoma had a dismal prognosis, but combinations of surgery, radiation therapy, and chemotherapy have markedly improved survival.[740,741] Important features predicting outcome are tumor size, stage, and histologic type (alveolar vs. other types). A staging system specific for rhabdomyosarcoma has been developed (Table 6-21). In a recent review of 4 protocols treating 379 patients with bladder or prostate rhabdomyosarcoma, the overall 5-year survival for patients with localized embryonal rhabdomyosarcoma was 84%.[741]

Pathology

For genitourinary rhabdomyosarcoma as a group, the embryonal type is most common (71%) followed by botryoid (20%), alveolar (2%), and pleomorphic (<1%); the remaining 7% do not fall into the above categories.[743] In the bladder, rhabdomyosarcoma forms polypoid masses that may be single or multiple producing a "sarcoma botryoides" (grape-like) appearance (Fig. 6-161). The trigone is the most common location. Embryonal rhabdomyosarcoma is characterized by a diffuse infiltration of small blue round cells with scant cytoplasm with alternating cellular and myxoid zones. The nuclei are small and hyperchromatic and the cells are oval to spindle shaped. Cytoplasm varies from scant to more abundant and eosinophilic characteristic of rhabdomyoblasts (Fig. 6-162). Cross striations can be identified in 50% to 60% of cases.[698] Rarely these tumors have more of a spindle cell pattern. In the sarcoma botryoides type, the

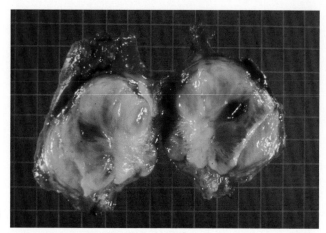

FIGURE 6-161 ■ Rhabdomyosarcoma of the bladder in a child.

cells are scattered in a loose myxoid stroma, with condensation of rhabdomyoblasts beneath the surface epithelium in a cambium layer. Classification as a botryoid rhabdomyosarcoma requires this subepithelial condensation of tumor cells separated from the overlying epithelium by a zone of loose stroma. The cells range from small cells with hyperchromatic nuclei and scant cytoplasm to cells with features of rhabdomyoblasts. The cells scattered in the loose myxoid stroma often have a stellate appearance. In most cases immunohistochemistry is used to confirm the diagnosis. Electron microscopic examination can also identify definitive rhabdomyoblastic differentiation.

In almost all cases muscle differentiation is demonstrable by immunohistochemistry.[698] Desmin and actin expression is present in close to 100% of tumors but is not specific. The myogenic regulatory proteins myogenin and MyoD1 are most specific and are quite sensitive in the embryonal and botryoid types of rhabdomyosarcoma (>95% positive). Myoglobin can be demonstrated in approximately 50% of cases. Rhabdomyosarcoma can infrequently express cytokeratin, S100 protein, and CD99.

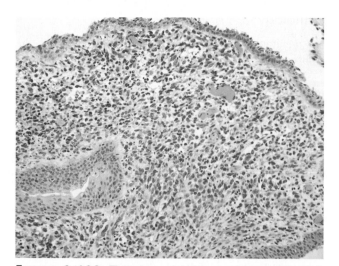

FIGURE 6-162 ■ Embryonal rhabdomyosarcoma of the bladder with concentration of tumor cells in the subepithelial area.

Differential Diagnosis

In the pediatric age group the differential diagnosis includes other small blue round cell tumors. In most cases the presence of rhabdomyoblasts and positive immunoreactivity for desmin, myogenin, and MyoD1 will resolve the case. Particularly in small biopsies the typical morphology may be unapparent and consideration should be given to other possibilities. In the pediatric population, a number of other small blue round cell tumors have been reported with the urinary bladder as the site of origin including primitive neuroendocrine tumor/Ewing sarcoma,[654] neuroblastoma,[744] and malignant lymphoma/leukemia.[745,746] A case with synchronous presentation of nephroblastoma in the kidney and urinary bladder has been described.[747] In any small blue round cell tumor other than rhabdomyosarcoma, the possibility of metastasis from another site must be considered. Myofibroblastic proliferations occur in the pediatric population and also need to be considered.[748] Fibroepithelial polyps also develop in this age group, and a case with atypical stromal cells that raised the differential diagnosis of rhabdomyosarcoma has been reported.[223]

In the adult patient, the majority of tumors with rhabdomyosarcoma differentiation will be sarcomatoid carcinoma with heterologous elements.[730] This should be the working diagnosis until excluded by careful histologic examination for an epithelial component. In the absence of identifiable carcinoma, the epithelial nature of the sarcomatoid component can be demonstrated by immunohistochemistry. Small cell carcinoma should also be considered in cases with pure alveolar histology. In about one-half of these cases there is another type of carcinoma present, a finding that would exclude rhabdomyosarcoma. Small cell carcinoma can have skeletal muscle differentiation, but this has only been reported once in the urinary bladder.[621] The presence of expression of epithelial and neuroendocrine markers and absence of muscle markers would for practical purposes confirm the diagnosis of small cell carcinoma.[739]

Angiosarcoma

Clinical Features

Primary angiosarcoma is a rare tumor in the urinary bladder. In a comprehensive review published in 2006, Seethala et al.[749] identified eight cases they considered acceptable and added one of their own. A few additional cases have appeared subsequently.[678,715,750,751] These have all occurred in adult patients with a male predominance. Hematuria is the most common presentation. In several cases there is a prior history of radiation.[678,749] These have generally been treated with resection with or without adjuvant radiation therapy. Prognosis is poor with most patients dying of their disease and only a few long-term survivors.[751]

Pathology

Grossly the tumors have tended to be large, exophytic, and hemorrhagic. Microscopically most have areas of classic angiosarcoma with solid areas not being uncommon. Spindled and epithelioid histology or a combination is seen. There is significant cytologic atypia with mitotic activity. There is invasion of the bladder wall including extension to the perivesical adipose tissue in most. Most of the cases studied have expressed endothelial cell markers (CD31, CD34, and factor VIII–related antigen).[678,749]

Differential Diagnosis

Hemangioma is much more common and should be considered prior to making a diagnosis of angiosarcoma. Cases of angiosarcoma in the literature have been unequivocally malignant and so this should in the majority of instances not be problematic. The solid areas of angiosarcoma can mimic any malignant spindle cell tumor including sarcomatoid carcinoma. The latter will usually have a recognizable carcinoma component and the spindle cells will express epithelial rather than endothelial cell markers. A case of angiosarcoma with associated urothelial carcinoma has been described.[678] An example of a malignant epithelioid hemangioendothelioma has been described in a child.[752]

Perivascular Epithelioid Cell Tumors

Rare examples of PEComas primary in the urinary bladder have been described in the literature.[724,753–756] In a recent report, Sukov et al.[724] added three cases and summarized four additional published cases. The cases have occurred in young adults (age range 19 to 48 years) with both males and females affected. None of the cases had associated tuberous sclerosis.

The tumors have ranged from 3.0 to 5.0 cm with both circumscribed and infiltrative growth. The histology has included both the epithelioid and spindle cell patterns. Individual cells have pale to clear cytoplasm and mild nuclear atypia. In the epithelioid areas, the cells are arranged in nests and in the spindle cell areas into fascicles. The tumors have been uniformly positive for HMB-45 with variable reactivity for Melan A, MiTF, actin, and desmin. Cytokeratins have been negative. The differential diagnosis includes epithelioid leiomyosarcoma, urothelial carcinoma, paraganglioma, and inflammatory myofibroblastic tumor.

HEMATOPOIETIC AND LYMPHOID TUMORS

Malignant Lymphoma

Clinical Features

Involvement of the bladder by malignant lymphoma is usually secondary to systemic lymphoma. In autopsy series of patients dying with non-Hodgkin lymphoma, bladder involvement has been identified in up to 13% of the cases.[757,758] The majority of patients are asymptomatic. Much less frequent is the development of primary malignant lymphoma in the bladder in the absence of systemic lymphoma.[759–762] Such cases account for only 0.2% of all cases of extranodal malignant lymphoma. Ohsawa et al.[762] reported three cases and

critically reviewed the world literature, identifying 27 additional examples. The majority of patients with primary lymphoma of the bladder are women (male:female ratio, 1:6.5), usually in the seventh and eighth decades (median age, 64 years).[762] Most patients present with gross hematuria but may complain of dysuria or irritative symptoms. Cystoscopically, the tumor is single or multiple, and sessile or polypoid. In a few cases, diffuse involvement without formation of a discrete mass may be seen. The presence of intact mucosa overlying the mass is a useful clue to the diagnosis.

The treatment of choice for these tumors is radiotherapy. In cases with tumor outside the bladder, systemic therapy may be indicated. Although the prognosis for these patients has historically been poor, it is now clear that patients presenting with disease limited to the bladder have a good outcome following radiotherapy. In 27 cases summarized by Ohsawa et al.,[762] only three died of tumor, and the 5-year survival was 82%.

Pathology

Lymphoma appears as a solid mass, forming sessile or polypoid lesions. Treatment is medical, and pathologic material is usually a biopsy or transurethral resection specimen. Histologically, the tumor consists of a diffuse, infiltrative proliferation of lymphoid cells surrounding and permeating normal structures rather than replacing them. The most common type of primary lymphoma is considered to be low-grade mucosa-associated lymphoid tissue (MALT) lymphoma (Fig. 6-163).[760] Other types reported include diffuse large cell and small lymphocytic lymphoma; less frequently, follicular, plasmacytoid, mantle zone, and monocytoid are found. Cases studied with immunohistochemistry have all been of B-cell origin.[762] Very rare T-cell lymphomas have been reported[763,764] including one case with a sarcomatoid morphology.[765] Primary Hodgkin disease involving the bladder is extremely rare.[762]

Differential Diagnosis

The major differential diagnostic considerations of malignant lymphoma are a florid chronic inflammatory process, small cell carcinoma, and lymphoma-like carcinoma. Inflammatory processes should not be a significant problem; these lesions contain a polymorphous infiltrate without formation of a mass lesion, and immunohistochemistry, documenting polyclonality, may be helpful. Small cell carcinoma is increasingly reported in the bladder.[623] It has histologic features identical to small cell carcinoma elsewhere. The presence of a cohesive growth pattern, prominent nuclear molding, and an identifiable urothelial or other epithelial component in up to one-half of cases should allow for its diagnosis. In biopsies, the use of immunohistochemistry can be helpful; lymphoma should be cytokeratin negative and leukocyte common antigen positive. Most cases of small cell carcinoma are cytokeratin positive and all should be leukocyte common antigen negative. Several examples of carcinoma other than the small cell type resembling malignant lymphoma have been described.[324] Examples of lymphoepithelioma-like carcinoma resembling nasopharyngeal carcinoma are well

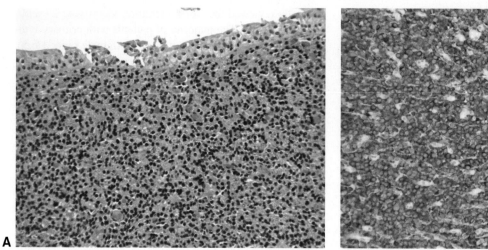

FIGURE 6-163 ■ Malignant lymphoma of the bladder showing the typical histology of a MALT-type lymphoma **(A)** and with strong expression of CD79A **(B)**.

described.[233,339] This tumor has syncytial groups of cytokeratin-positive carcinoma cells in a polymorphous inflammatory background. Awareness of the entity, combined with immunohistochemical results, should prevent misdiagnosis.

Leukemia

Clinical Features

Involvement of the bladder is identified at the time of autopsy in 15% to 26% of patients dying with leukemia.[757,758] It is, however, an infrequent cause of symptomatic involvement during the course of disease.[745] In patients with leukemia involving the bladder, significant symptoms including severe hematuria can occur.[745,766] In patients treated by bone marrow transplantation, hemorrhagic cystitis is a significant complication in up to 8% of patients and is not related to recurrence of the leukemia in the bladder, but is usually drug related or due to viral infection.[767,768] Occasionally urinary bladder involvement may be the initial presentation of leukemia. Almost all of these have been in cases of acute myeloid

leukemia with initial presentation as hematuria and a bladder mass (granulocytic sarcoma).[769–771]

Pathology

The histologic features are dependent on the type of leukemia (Fig. 6-164). In general the bladder wall is diffusely infiltrated by tumor cells. This is the typical pattern present for lymphocytic leukemia. The infiltrating cells are discohesive and uniform with the cytologic features specific for the type of acute lymphocytic leukemia.

In cases of acute myeloid leukemia a mass may develop. Several examples of myeloid (granulocytic) sarcoma have been described[769,770] including in nonleukemic patients.[771] In these cases there is a proliferation of myeloblasts. The cells will appear more monotonous than in a high-grade urothelial carcinoma, with less cytoplasm and evidence of myeloid differentiation with cells having coarse eosinophilic cytoplasmic granules. Immunohistochemical studies will demonstrate expression of myeloid markers such as CD68 and CD117. A myeloperoxidase stain will also be positive.[769]

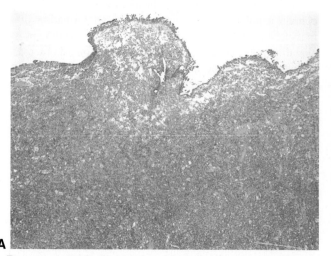
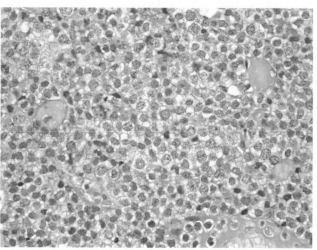

FIGURE 6-164 ■ Acute myeloid leukemia involving the bladder at low **(A)** and high **(B)** magnification.

Differential Diagnosis

For lymphocytic leukemias the differential diagnosis includes malignant lymphoma, small cell carcinoma, or a high-grade urothelial carcinoma. The latter is particularly important for granulocytic sarcoma. The key to avoiding a misdiagnosis of urothelial carcinoma is thinking of the possibility in a tumor with unusual morphology.[770]

Plasmacytoma

Clinical Features

Extramedullary plasmacytoma has been described in the urinary bladder.[772–776] These have occurred in adults, over a wide age range, with a female preponderance. A case has been described post renal transplantation.[777] Hematuria is the most common presentation.[778] Plasmacytomas occur as isolated lesions without associated multiple myeloma or can develop in patients with known systemic disease. A variety of treatments have been applied including radiation and surgery. Prognosis has generally been favorable with a minority of patients presenting as isolated masses subsequently developing systemic disease. Multiple myeloma can also involve the urinary bladder in patients known to have the disease.[779]

Pathology

The tumor can be quite large (up to 4 cm) and well-circumscribed.[776] Microscopically there is a proliferation of plasma cells with varying degrees of differentiation within the bladder wall. The cells are poorly cohesive, a feature that may be best appreciated at the edge of the lesion. These have been recognized in urine cytology specimens.[775,776]

Differential Diagnosis

The major differential diagnoses are malignant lymphoma and plasmacytoid urothelial carcinoma. Plasmacytoma expresses lymphoid and plasma cell markers such as pan-B-cell markers and kappa or lambda light chains. Plasmacytoid urothelial carcinoma can be recognized by obvious epithelial areas in most cases. In difficult cases immunohistochemistry is diagnostic; plasmacytoid carcinoma expresses epithelial markers including pancytokeratin, cytokeratin 7, and cytokeratin 20.[329] Plasmacytoid carcinoma can express CD138, a marker also expressed by plasma cells.[329]

OTHER TUMORS

Malignant Melanoma

Clinical Features

Primary malignant melanoma of the urinary tract is rare with the urethra being the most common site; the urinary bladder is involved less frequently.[780–782] A comprehensive review published in 2006 identified 18 acceptable cases.[783]

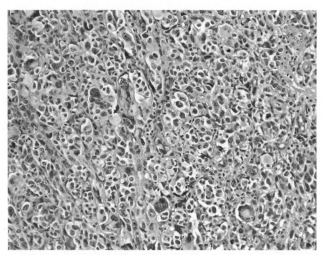

FIGURE 6-165 ■ Malignant melanoma involving the bladder (this case was metastatic).

The pathogenesis is uncertain but these may be related to rare examples of melanosis involving the bladder.[784,785] Melanosis of the bladder is characterized by multifocal and diffuse pigmentation of the bladder mucosa. The tumors occur in approximately equal numbers between men and women over a wide age range. Hematuria is the most common presentation. A case diagnosed by urinary cytology has been described.[782] Treatment has been primarily surgical; the prognosis is poor.

Pathology

There are no specific gross pathologic features. Microscopically the tumors have typical features of melanoma with nests of large pleomorphic cells with macronuclei and prominent nucleoli (Fig. 6-165). Melanin pigment is present in variable quantities. Melanosis has been present in some cases. Immunohistochemical studies show typical features of melanoma with positivity for HMB45, melan-A, and S100 protein with no expression of epithelial markers.

Differential Diagnosis

The major differential diagnosis is with metastatic melanoma, which is much more common than primary tumors.[786] Because of this, strict criteria have been proposed for the diagnosis of primary melanoma in the urinary tract (Box 6-8).[787] These include (i) no history of cutaneous

---

Box 6-8 ● DIAGNOSTIC CRITERIA FOR PRIMARY BLADDER MELANOMA

No history of melanoma
Negative physical exam for other primary
No subsequent primary elsewhere
Spread consistent with bladder origin
Intramucosal component

melanoma, (ii) a negative physical examination of the skin and mucosal surfaces, (iii) no subsequent development of melanoma at a more common primary site, (iv) a pattern of recurrence consistent with origin in the urinary bladder, and (v) the presence of intramucosal atypical melanocytes at the tumor edge.

Other tumors with a nested pattern of growth including urothelial carcinoma and paraganglioma should also be considered. These can be readily distinguished by immunohistochemical studies.

Paraganglioma

Paraganglioma is believed to arise from paraganglionic tissue that can be found in the wall of the urinary bladder.[788] Paraganglionic tissue is most often present in the anterior or posterior walls and can be found anywhere within the wall. The most frequent genetic abnormalities in paraganglioma involve the succinate dehydrogenase family of genes (*SDHA*, *SDHB*, *SDHC*, and *SDHD*). Mutation of the *SDHB* (1p35-p36.1), *SDHC* (1q21), and *SDHD* (11q23) genes have all been identified in paraganglioma, most often in young patients, familial syndromes, malignant tumors and intra-abdominal tumors.[789] These have less often been documented in sporadic pheochromocytoma.[789] The *SDHB* gene has most often been implicated in extra-adrenal paraganglioma.[790]

Clinical Features

The first description of paraganglioma in the urinary bladder is credited to Zimmerman et al.[791] These occur at any age though they are distinctly uncommon in children[792]; there is a slight female predominance.[299,793–796] It accounts for <0.1% of bladder neoplasms.[3] Paraganglioma arises sporadically or develops in certain inherited conditions including von Recklinghausen disease, multiple endocrine neoplasia type 2, and von Hippel-Lindau disease.[789] For paragangliomas of the urinary bladder there are no known predisposing conditions, with only rare cases reported in patients with von Recklinghausen disease[797] and von Hippel-Lindau disease.[798]

Hematuria is the most common presenting feature but a significant number of patients report episodic headache, palpitations, and sweating related to micturition. There may be a history of systemic hypertension. Catecholamine elevation can be demonstrated in most patients. By cystoscopy the mass is intramural; ulceration of the overlying mucosa can be present. Diagnosis is made on biopsy or transurethral resection.

Treatment of urinary bladder paraganglioma is primarily surgical by transurethral resection, partial cystectomy, or radical cystectomy. A review of 246 cases culled from the literature found 14% to be malignant with spread beyond the urinary bladder and/or metastases.[662] Predicting malignant behavior remains uncertain.[794,799–801] In general metastatic paraganglioma has not been very responsive to

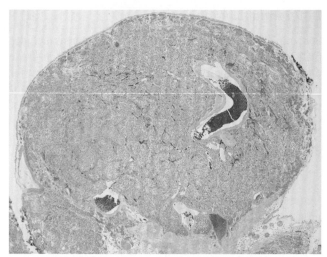

FIGURE 6-166 ■ Paraganglioma of the bladder producing a submucosal mass.

chemotherapy. Recent reports indicate that a higher level of responsiveness may be seen with tyrosine kinase inhibitors such as sunitinib.[802]

Pathology

The tumor is characteristically intramural in location (Fig. 6-166). Paraganglioma is relatively well circumscribed with most ranging from several millimeters to 5 cm in greatest dimension though much large tumors have been described.[803]

The histology is similar to paraganglioma at other locations. The cells are arranged in variably sized nests (zellballen) with a prominent vascular network in the background (Figs. 6-167 and 6-168). There are two cell types present. The cells in the nests have moderate to abundant pale eosinophilic to clear cytoplasm. The cells can have an oncocytic appearance.[804] Nuclei tend to be oval and occasional pleomorphic nuclei are present. At the periphery of the nests a second population of flattened cells (sustentacular cells) can

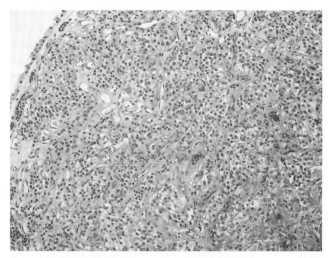

FIGURE 6-167 ■ Paraganglioma of the bladder with overlying urothelium.

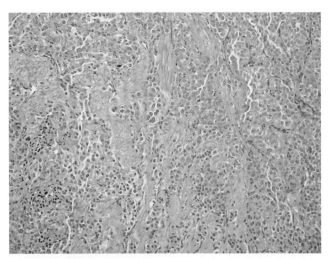

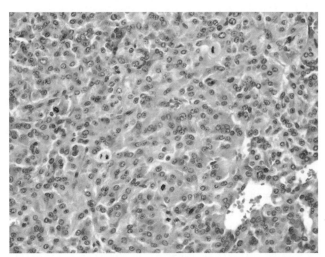

FIGURE 6-168 ■ Paraganglioma of the bladder involving the muscularis propria.

FIGURE 6-169 ■ Paraganglioma of the bladder with frequent mitoses.

often be appreciated. Mitotic activity is variable (Fig. 6-169). Calcification can be prominent.[805] Rare examples of composite paraganglioma–ganglioneuroma and paraganglioma with neuroblastoma-like foci have been described.[806–808]

Immunohistochemical studies demonstrate consistent positivity with neuroendocrine markers (chromogranin, synaptophysin, neuron-specific enolase) (Fig. 6-170A).[299,795,799,809] The sustentacular cells express the S100 protein (Fig. 6-170B).[801] There is no immunoreactivity for cytokeratins or other epithelial markers.[299,801] Ultrastructural examination demonstrates neurosecretory granules.[794,799,809] DNA ploidy analysis has been shown to be of limited value in predicting behavior.[794,795,799,801]

Differential Diagnosis

The major differential diagnoses are nonneoplastic paraganglionic tissue and urothelial carcinoma.[299] In limited biopsies, the possibility of normally present paraganglionic tissue should always be considered prior to rendering a diagnosis of paraganglioma. Invasive urothelial carcinoma can grow as variably sized nests both in the nested variant and in usual carcinoma.[296] The nested variant is characterized by small nests of cells that are infiltrative and lack the prominent vascular network of paraganglioma. In contrast to paraganglioma the nests do not form a circumscribed mass and are usually separated by variable amounts of stromal tissue. The nuclei in the nested variant tend to be relatively uniform and lack the degree of pleomorphism often present in paraganglioma. Cytoplasmic characteristics may be similar between urothelial carcinoma and paraganglioma. Cautery artifact in small samples can result in misdiagnosis.[299] Immunohistochemistry can readily differentiate these two.

Other considerations in the differential diagnosis should include granular cell tumor, alveolar soft part sarcoma, and metastatic renal cell carcinoma. Granular cell tumors are

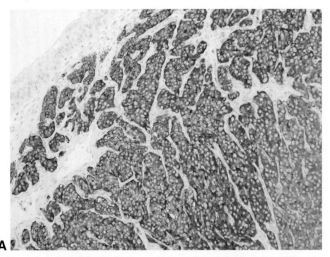

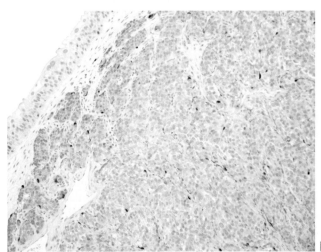

A | **B**

FIGURE 6-170 ■ Paraganglioma of the bladder with diffuse immunoreactivity for synaptophysin **(A)** and a few S100-positive sustentacular cells **(B)**.

typically small and infiltrative and will diffusely express the S100 protein. Alveolar soft part sarcoma does not express neuroendocrine markers.[810] Metastatic renal cell carcinoma will express cytokeratins and not neuroendocrine markers.

GERM CELL TUMORS

Trophoblastic Tumors

The older literature contains several reports of primary choriocarcinoma of the urinary bladder. As noted by Eble and Young,[811] since the recognition that trophoblastic differentiation occurs in urothelial carcinoma, such reports have largely disappeared from the recent literature. The identification of isochromosome 12 in a case of choriocarcinoma in the bladder does support its rare occurrence as a primary in the bladder.[360] Prior to accepting the diagnosis the possibility of urothelial carcinoma with trophoblastic differentiation must be excluded. In most cases the urothelial carcinoma component will be evident. When typical syncytiotrophoblastic giant cells are found, the background cells will most often be pleomorphic and not have features of cytotrophoblasts. Metastatic choriocarcinoma requires clinical correlation for exclusion.

Dermoid Cyst or Teratoma

There have been a handful of reports of dermoid cysts occurring in the bladder of female patients.[812–815] In one case, the lesion presented as an intraluminal mass mimicking a bladder stone.[814] Secondary involvement of the bladder by direct invasion from dermoid cyst of the ovary is well-described[816] and should be excluded before accepting a lesion as being primary. Dermoid cysts in the bladder are similar to those developing elsewhere with keratinizing squamous epithelium and skin adnexal structures. In the bladder most have contained hair and have been calcified.[814]

Cases of teratoma distinct from dermoid cyst have also been described in the urinary bladder.[817,818] One of these occurred in an 8-year-old girl with no evidence of teratoma at another site.[816]

Yolk Sac Tumor

A single example of yolk sac tumor arising in the bladder proper has been described. The tumor presented as a large polypoid mass in a 1-year-old boy.[819]

Three cases of yolk sac tumor developing in the urachus have also been reported.[820–822] Two developed in children (7-month-old male and 2-year-old child) and one in a 44-year-old woman. These cases have demonstrated typical histologic features of yolk sac tumor with elevated serum alpha-fetoprotein levels. No tumor at another site was found with 3 years' and 3 years, 8 months' follow-up, respectively, in the 7-month-old and 2-year-old children, respectively.

SECONDARY TUMORS

Clinical Features

Secondary involvement of the bladder by tumors from other sites can occur by direct extension or by metastatic spread.[655,823,824] These account for approximately 2.3% of surgical bladder tumor specimens.[825] Direct extension is most frequent, accounting for 70% of cases, with carcinomas of the prostate gland, colorectal region, and uterine cervix being most important.[825] Blood-borne metastases to the bladder can originate in many sites with the stomach, malignant melanoma, lung, breast, and kidney being most frequent.[375,825,826] Rare examples from almost any other origin can be found in the literature.

The possibility of a secondary tumor should always be considered when the morphologic features do not fit with those of urothelial carcinoma or one of its variants. Tumors that do not appear to be mucosa based or that have predominant or pure vascular space involvement may indicate origin elsewhere. In one large series the majority (97%) of secondary tumors produced a single mass.[825] For nonurothelial carcinoma the possibility of secondary involvement is always a consideration. Detailed discussion of these is found in the sections on primary adenocarcinoma, squamous cell carcinoma, and small cell carcinoma, respectively. In this section, common sites of origin are discussed individually.

Prostatic Adenocarcinoma

Involvement of the bladder by prostatic adenocarcinoma most often occurs in the setting of known locally advanced disease or recurrence following prior therapy (most often radiation therapy). In these cases the serum PSA may not be elevated. Secondary involvement is almost always by direct invasion, making the bladder neck and trigone the preferred location.

In most cases, the diagnosis of prostatic adenocarcinoma is apparent based on morphologic features alone (Fig. 6-171).

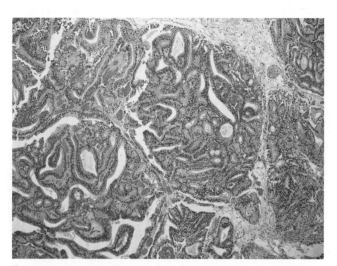

FIGURE 6-171 ■ Prostatic adenocarcinoma involving the bladder; the morphology is readily identifiable as prostatic.

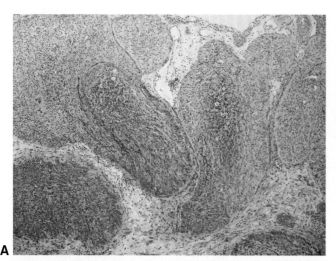 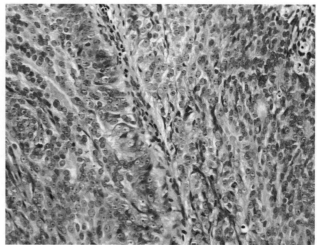

FIGURE 6-172 ■ Prostatic adenocarcinoma in the bladder that was misdiagnosed as urothelial carcinoma **(A)**. The nuclear features are an important clue to the correct diagnosis **(B)**.

The ductal variant of prostatic adenocarcinoma frequently has a complex papillary component that can mimic urothelial carcinoma. Further, these tumors can have a cribriform architecture that mimics enteric adenocarcinoma, a pattern that can be present in urothelial carcinoma with glandular differentiation. Cribriform architecture without an enteric look would be extremely unusual in urothelial carcinoma. In both of these, the nuclear morphology is an important clue with the uniformity of the nuclei and often a single prominent nucleolus in contrast to the greater degree of pleomorphism typical of urothelial carcinoma (Fig. 6-172). In mucinous prostatic adenocarcinoma, the glands suspended in the extravasated mucin look like prostate cancer glands with small fused acini having uniform nuclei with single prominent nucleoli. Urothelial carcinoma with glandular differentiation and mucin production typically has an enteric appearance. Signet ring–like adenocarcinoma of the prostate is rare and almost always mixed with more typical prostatic adenocarcinoma. One characteristic feature is that these are usually mucin negative in contrast with signet ring carcinomas of urothelial origin.[587]

Most problematic is poorly differentiated carcinoma without features typical of either urothelial carcinoma or prostatic adenocarcinoma. In these cases, the presence of nuclear uniformity should raise the suspicion of prostatic origin. The cytoplasm in prostatic carcinoma is often pale or even slightly foamy in contrast with the more dense and eosinophilic cytoplasm of urothelial carcinoma. Squamoid features or squamous differentiation would strongly favor urothelial origin. It should be remembered that both urothelial carcinoma and prostatic adenocarcinoma can coexist and collision tumors in the urinary bladder have been described.[827]

In many difficult cases, immunohistochemistry is necessary to resolve the differential diagnosis. Over 90% of poorly differentiated prostatic adenocarcinoma cases will stain, at least focally for PSA and/or PSAP.[258,828] Some tumors that are nonreactive for PSA and PSAP will demonstrate positive immunoreactivity for p501s or PSMA.[258] These markers are uniformly negative in urothelial carcinoma although a few reports have appeared over the years describing variable expression of these markers in a handful of cases of primary adenocarcinoma of the bladder.[172] Approximately 80% of urothelial carcinomas express p63 while poorly differentiated prostatic adenocarcinoma is negative. GATA3 is expressed by 67% of urothelial carcinomas but not by prostatic adenocarcinoma.[256] Placental S100 (S100P) has been reported to be positive in 78% of urothelial carcinomas compared to 2% in prostatic adenocarcinomas.[256] High molecular weight cytokeratin is expressed by up to 90% of urothelial carcinomas; it has been reported to be focally expressed in <10% of prostatic adenocarcinoma.[258,829] Both cytokeratin 7 and 20 are commonly expressed by urothelial carcinoma (approximately 90% and 60%, respectively) but can also be expressed by prostatic adenocarcinoma (approximately 15% and 20%, respectively) and so are of limited value in individual cases.[258,274,275]

Colorectal Adenocarcinoma

Direct invasion of the urinary bladder by adenocarcinoma of the gastrointestinal tract occurs with sufficient frequency to create diagnostic problems (Fig. 6-173).[566,830] In most cases, the problem is the distinction of these tumors from primary adenocarcinoma of the bladder. This topic has been covered in detail earlier in the section on primary adenocarcinoma and is not repeated here.

Uterine Cervix and Endometrial Carcinoma

Carcinoma of the uterine cervix and endometrium can invade directly into the wall of the urinary bladder (Fig. 6-174). This is frequent enough with cervical carcinoma that cystoscopy may be a regular part of the workup for patients with bulky or locally advanced disease.[831,832] Currently the major use of cystoscopy is to confirm balder invasion suspected

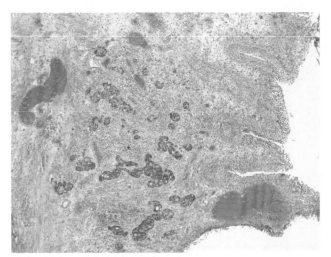

FIGURE 6-173 ■ Colonic adenocarcinoma metastasis to the bladder.

on imaging examinations.[832] For squamous cell carcinoma of the cervix, there are no reliable morphologic criteria to distinguish these from primary squamous cell carcinoma of the urinary bladder. This distinction largely requires correlation with the clinical impression and radiologic findings that in most cases can determine the epicenter and likely origin of the lesion. Although the finding of keratinizing squamous metaplasia with dysplasia of the urothelium may suggest bladder origin, this is not absolute and should not be relied upon. Cervical squamous cell carcinoma and urothelial carcinoma frequently express p16 (60% vs. 30% to 50%), making this marker of no value in the differential diagnosis.[249,250] In situ hybridization for HPV DNA could be helpful as this can be detected in the majority of cervical but not bladder squamous cell carcinomas.[513,527]

Adenocarcinoma of the uterine cervix is most often endocervical in type with complex and branching glandular

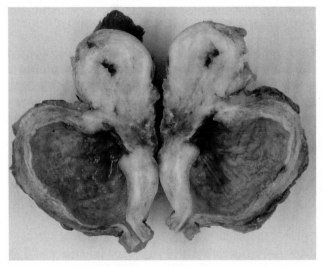

FIGURE 6-174 ■ Endometrial adenocarcinoma invading the bladder wall.

structures lined by columnar mucin-secreting cells with basally located nuclei. This morphology would be highly unusual in either urothelial carcinoma with glandular differentiation or primary adenocarcinoma of the bladder. Less frequent patterns such as papillary serous adenocarcinoma, endometrioid adenocarcinoma, and clear cell adenocarcinoma would have much more potential for morphologic overlap with primary bladder carcinomas. Immunohistochemistry demonstrates expression of p16 and in situ hybridization is positive for HPV DNA in a high percentage of cervical adenocarcinomas.[833] Urothelial carcinoma and bladder adenocarcinoma can also express p16.[834,835] HPV has not been demonstrated to be involved in the development of bladder cancers though there is no data on HPV DNA expression in primary bladder adenocarcinoma or urothelial carcinoma with glandular differentiation. Nonetheless, demonstration of HPV DNA in a problem case would strongly support an endocervical origin. Correlation with the clinical findings would be needed to fully resolve the differential diagnosis.

Malignant Melanoma

Primary malignant melanoma of the urinary bladder is extremely rare, and so, any involvement of the bladder should be considered a metastasis until proven otherwise.[786] The presence of an in situ component with intraepithelial atypical melanocytes would suggest a primary in the bladder while the presence of multiple nodules and a prominent intravascular component would favor metastasis. Irrespective of the pathologic features, careful clinical evaluation is necessary prior to diagnosing the lesion as primary or secondary.

Breast Carcinoma

There have been several examples of metastatic breast carcinoma involving the urinary bladder reported.[826,836–838] The breast is estimated to account for approximately 2.5% of cases of metastatic tumors to the bladder.[825] Most cases occur in the setting of known carcinoma of the breast and typically in patients with advanced disease.[836] Rare examples of breast carcinoma presenting with urinary symptoms have been described.[839] Even with a known history, the morphology may be similar to primary urothelial carcinoma and cause diagnostic difficulty. The plasmacytoid variant of urothelial carcinoma has overlapping morphologic features with lobular carcinoma of the breast and has been reported under the term "lobular carcinoma–like urothelial carcinoma."[328] Most cases of plasmacytoid urothelial carcinoma are mixed with a more typical component and when present would lead to the correct diagnosis. The "targetoid" cytoplasmic inclusions typical of lobular carcinoma are not a feature of plasmacytoid carcinoma and if present would favor a breast primary.

Positive reactivity for p63 and/or high molecular weight cytokeratin would favor urothelial origin. Expression of both estrogen and progesterone receptors would support a breast origin but is not specific; estrogen receptor has been reported to be expressed by up to 80% of invasive urothelial carcinomas.[269–271] It appears that this is due to expression of the β form with expression of estrogen receptor-α being infrequent. In one study estrogen receptor-β was detected in 63% of 140 tumors studied compared to only 1.4% for estrogen receptor-α.[270] In another report, estrogen receptor-α was detected in 4.5% of 198 tumors examined.[271] There is much less information on progesterone receptor expression. Bolenz et al.[271] did not detect any immunoreactivity for progesterone receptor in 198 specimens. In a study of 10 cases of plasmacytoid urothelial carcinoma (lobular carcinoma–like urothelial carcinoma), 20% of cases expressed estrogen and/or progesterone receptors.[328]

Renal Cell Carcinoma

The literature contains numerous reports of metastatic renal cell carcinoma involving the urinary bladder[375,840–842] with a recent review identifying fewer than 40 cases in total.[842] The majority occur in the setting of known metastatic disease. These can appear many years after nephrectomy for the primary tumor.[843] It has been hypothesized that some of these are due to seeding of the bladder by cells transiting within the urinary tract.[844] Most cases are associated with gross hematuria. Cystoscopy shows sessile or spherical protrusions into the bladder lumen. Microscopically the tumor shows the typical features of clear cell renal cell carcinoma.

The major differential diagnosis is with the clear cell variant of urothelial carcinoma. In most cases of urothelial carcinoma, the clear cytoplasm occurs in large tumor nests with a squamoid morphology that does not have the typical sinusoidal vascular pattern of clear cell renal cell carcinoma. Unusual examples of urothelial carcinoma focally can have small nests of cells with clear cytoplasm and a prominent vascular network that does mimic renal cell carcinoma. Immunohistochemistry can readily distinguish the two with urothelial carcinoma expressing cytokeratins 7 and 20, p63, and high molecular weight cytokeratin. Clear cell renal cell carcinoma lacks expression of these markers but does express the renal cell carcinoma antigen and PAX 8.

Other Sites of Origin

Metastasis from serous carcinoma of the female genital tract can closely mimic the micropapillary variant of urothelial carcinoma.[322] Psammomatous microcalcifications are typical of serous carcinoma and are not seen in micropapillary urothelial carcinoma. In difficult cases, immunohistochemistry is helpful with serous carcinoma expressing WT-1 and PAX 8, markers not found in urothelial carcinoma.[322]

Metastatic non–small cell carcinomas of lung origin will reflect the histology of the primary type. In some cases, this could mimic urothelial carcinoma. The majority of carcinomas of lung origin are TTF-1 positive while urothelial carcinoma infrequently expresses TTF-1.[259] Metastatic small cell carcinoma of lung origin is discussed in the section on primary small cell carcinoma.

STAGING

Malignant epithelial tumors of the urinary bladder are staged according to the AJCC/TNM staging system. The most recent version (2010) of the staging system has not changed since the prior (2002) version in terms of the T category definition (Tables 6-14 and 6-15).[567] As discussed earlier, stage is arguably the most powerful prognostic indicator and is critically important in therapeutic decision making. The pathologist plays a central role in the assignment of local clinical (T) and ultimately a final pathologic stage (pT). In the following sections individual issues related to the assessment of bladder cancer specimens as related to accurate assignment of stage are discussed.

Diagnosis of Invasion

Having made a diagnosis of either a papillary neoplasm or CIS, the next decision that must be reached is whether there is or is not invasion of the underlying tissue. In most cases this is straightforward; however, it is not uncommon to face cases where this can be quite problematic. Several reports have documented significant differences in the diagnosis of the presence or absence of invasion and in the presence or absence of muscularis propria invasion.[5,845–847] In two large series, 35% and 53% of cases reported to be T1 were considered to be noninvasive on review.[5,847] The literature contains many series that include grade 1 tumors reported to be invasive (T1); the existence of such cases has been challenged.[4,401] In my experience, all tumors reported as grade 1 T1 have been either noninvasive or higher grade. The diagnosis of invasion should always be made with caution in low-grade papillary tumors. In contrast, any case of high-grade papillary carcinoma or CIS should be studied with the mindset that invasion is common and must be excluded. For papillary lesions invasion can occur at the tumor base or within the fibrovascular cores so both areas must be evaluated.

A variety of histologic features are clues to invasion into the underlying lamina propria/submucosa (Table 6-22).[52,172,848] With even early invasion, individual tumor cells often have different morphologic features than the in situ tumor including more abundant eosinophilic cytoplasm or higher nuclear grade (Fig. 6-175). An associated stromal response including desmoplasia, edema (myxoid), fibrosis, and inflammation is frequently but not always present (Fig. 6-176). Retraction artifact around small clusters of cells suggests that they are invasive (Fig. 6-177). In some cases, the small size of the nests or presence of single cells is not compatible with tangential sectioning of an overlying papillary tumor (Fig. 6-178). The type of stromal reaction has not been found to have prognostic significance in T1 tumors.[849] If there is a marked inflammatory infiltrate,

Table 6-22 ■ CRITERIA FOR THE DIAGNOSIS OF INVASION INTO THE LAMINA PROPRIA BY UROTHELIAL CARCINOMA

Histologic grade
- Invasion much more frequent in high-grade lesions (but not exclusively)

Epithelial features
- Irregularly shaped nests
- Single cell infiltration
- Irregular or absent basement membrane
- Tentacular finger-like projections
- Invading cells with more abundant eosinophilic cytoplasm "paradoxical differentiation"

Stromal features
- Desmoplasia or fibrosis
- Myxoid stroma
- Pseudosarcomatous stroma
- Retraction artifact
- Inflammation
- No stromal change

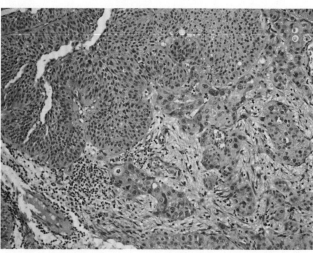

FIGURE 6-176 ■ Invasive urothelial carcinoma. Note the irregular shape of the nests, the change in morphology of the invasive tumor, and the myxoid stromal reaction.

care must be taken to look carefully for obscured tumor cells or nests of cells, and occasionally a cytokeratin stain is needed to clarify the nature of suspicious cells. Certain variants of urothelial carcinoma can mimic lymphoid lesions including so-called lymphoma-like patterns,[324] plasmacytoid urothelial carcinoma,[329] and lymphoepithelioma-like carcinoma.[233]

Muscularis Propria Invasion

Having determined that invasion is present, the next most critical feature is assessing the specimen for muscularis propria invasion. This is often viewed as the most critical parameter in treatment algorithms with T1 tumors managed primarily by transurethral resection and intravesical therapy (most often BCG) and T2 tumors by cystectomy;

as noted in the section on treatment, cystectomy is increasingly being performed for T1 disease.[23,458] Muscularis propria must be distinguished from muscularis mucosae.[850,851] The former is characterized by thick, compact bundles of smooth muscle cells forming a "solid" tissue (Figs. 6-179 and 6-180). In contrast, muscularis mucosae is characterized by wispy collections of smooth muscle cells that only rarely form a "solid" layer (Fig. 6-181). The muscularis mucosae layer is typically associated with large vascular channels (Fig. 6-182). Infrequently the muscularis mucosae can be thickened or form better-developed round bundles of smooth muscle (Fig. 6-183). The trigone region is problematic in that the muscularis propria has a pattern of interweaving smooth muscle bundles with a thin submucosa. In this region, the muscularis mucosae is for practical purposes impossible to define.[851] Overdiagnosis of muscularis propria invasion has been documented to occur in

FIGURE 6-175 ■ Invasive urothelial carcinoma. Note the change in morphology of the invasive tumor from the overlying high-grade papillary tumor and the focal clefting around smaller invasive nests.

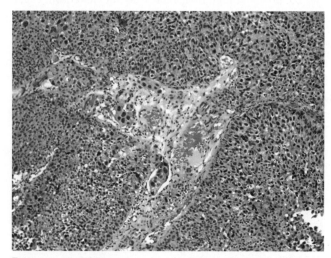

FIGURE 6-177 ■ Invasive urothelial carcinoma. Note the small irregular nests and the clefting around one nest.

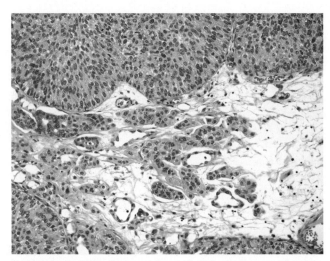

FIGURE 6-178 ■ Invasive urothelial carcinoma. Note the small nests, clusters of three or four cells, and focal clefting around nests.

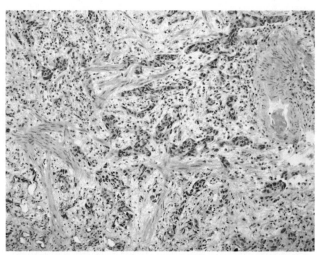

FIGURE 6-181 ■ Urothelial carcinoma invading the muscularis mucosae. The smooth muscle cells form thin tapered bundles.

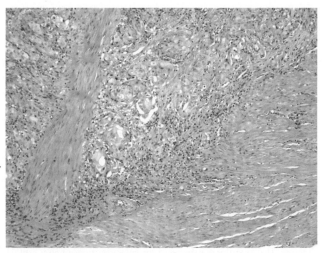

FIGURE 6-179 ■ Urothelial carcinoma invading the muscularis propria. Note the thick, dense smooth muscle.

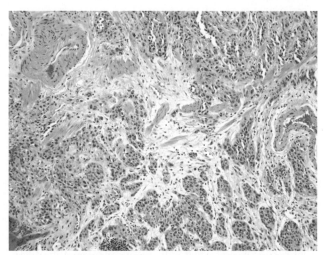

FIGURE 6-182 ■ Urothelial carcinoma invading the muscularis mucosae. There are thick-walled blood vessels in the area of the muscularis mucosae.

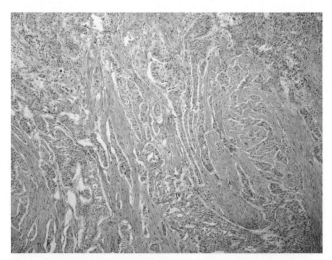

FIGURE 6-180 ■ Urothelial carcinoma invading and disrupting the muscularis propria. Although many of the individual bundles are thin, they retain the characteristic density of the muscularis propria.

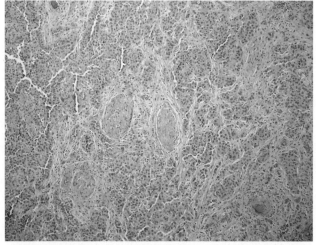

FIGURE 6-183 ■ Urothelial carcinoma invading the muscularis mucosae. Infrequently the muscularis mucosae is composed of better-defined round smooth muscle bundles.

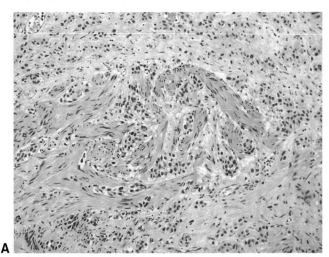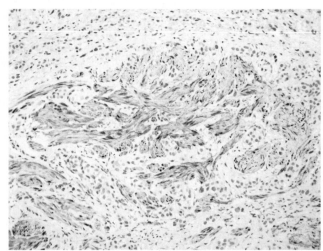

A   **B**

FIGURE 6-184 ■ Invasive urothelial carcinoma splaying apart smooth muscle bundles that could represent muscularis mucosae or muscularis propria **(A)**. Positive immunoreactivity for smoothelin **(B)** suggests that this is muscularis propria.

a significant number of cases.[5,845] The potential for using the smooth muscle marker smoothelin has been reported to preferentially stain the smooth muscle cells of the muscularis propria (Fig. 6-184).[852,853] Evaluation of problem cases has, however, shown limitations of the use of this antibody in daily practice.[854,855] Vimentin has been reported in one study to be expressed much more intensely by the smooth muscle cells of the muscularis mucosae than the muscularis propria.[853]

Thermal artifact related to cautery can also result in the submucosa having a dense eosinophilic appearance mimicking the muscularis propria. In cases where muscularis propria involvement is strongly suspected, a trichrome stain can be helpful. Desmin will also mark smooth muscle fibers but will not distinguish the layer of muscle. Actin should not be used for this purpose as it will strongly stain myofibroblasts and could lead to misinterpretation.

Depth of Invasion

If no muscularis propria invasion is present, the concept of substaging T1 tumors has been advocated. Two approaches have been taken. In 1982, Farrow et al.[856] introduced the term microinvasion based on measuring the depth of invasion, with invasions <5 mm considered microinvasive. Cheng et al.,[857] applying a similar approach to a study of transurethral resection specimens, found invasion deeper than 4 mm to be the best cutoff for predicting the likelihood of extravesical extension in the subsequent cystectomy specimen. In another study, van der Aa et al.[858] found 5 mm to be a significant cut point for predicting an increased risk of progression to muscle-invasive disease. Two other recent reports have found that more than even a single 200× field[859] or two or less high-power fields[860] indicate a higher risk of progression. At present there is no accepted definition of microinvasion though this may eventually be defined with increased experience and study.

Using the muscularis mucosae as a layer to substage T1 tumors was first proposed by Younes et al.,[861] who reported that tumors invading to the level of the muscularis mucosae or deeper behaved more like pT2 tumors than those with invasion superficial to this layer (Fig. 6-185). Many studies have subsequently repeated this analysis with most having similar results.[862] Angulo et al.[863] also found this to be a powerful predictor of progression but noted that in many cases it was not possible to accurately apply this method of substaging. Others have found substaging to be possible in up to 87% of cases.[862]

Given the current interest in identifying patients with T1 disease at high risk for progression in order to consider early cystectomy, it is appropriate to provide at least some descriptive information regarding the depth or volume of invasive disease. If muscularis mucosae invasion is present in a specimen it may be appropriate to specifically report it. Further, if there is minimal invasion, terms such as superficial invasion

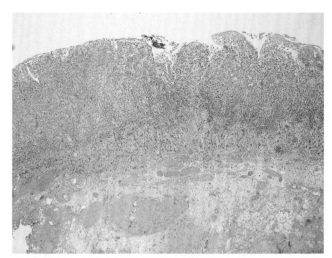

FIGURE 6-185 ■ Invasive urothelial carcinoma extending down just to the level of the muscularis mucosae.

with a clarifier such as <1 mm or invasion superficial to the muscularis mucosae can be applied.

Identification of T3 or T4 Disease

The diagnosis of T3 disease in biopsy or transurethral material is complicated by the fact that fat can be present throughout the bladder wall, including the lamina propria.[864] For this reason, it is not possible to confirm T3 disease without examination of a cystectomy or partial cystectomy specimen.

SPECIMEN HANDLING AND REPORTING

Guidelines for the handling and reporting of tumor-containing specimens obtained from the urinary bladder are available.[26,27,410,865,866] These include contributions from the European Society of Uropathology,[410] the CAP,[26] and the International Consultation on Bladder Cancer.[27] In this section, the guidelines published by the CAP[26] will form the basis for the reporting recommendations (Tables 6-23 and 6-24).

Table 6-23 ■ CAP GUIDELINES FOR REPORTING OF TUMOR CONTAINING BIOPSY AND TRANSURETHRAL RESECTION SPECIMENS

Histologic Type

_____ Urothelial (transitional cell) carcinoma

_____ Urothelial (transitional cell) carcinoma with squamous differentiation

_____ Urothelial (transitional cell) carcinoma with glandular differentiation

_____ Urothelial (transitional cell) carcinoma with variant histology (specify): _____

_____ Squamous cell carcinoma, typical

_____ Squamous cell carcinoma, variant histology (specify): _____

_____ Adenocarcinoma, typical

_____ Adenocarcinoma, variant histology (specify): _____

_____ Small cell carcinoma

_____ Undifferentiated carcinoma (specify): _____

_____ Mixed cell type (specify): _____

_____ Other (specify): _____

_____ Carcinoma, type cannot be determined

*Associated Epithelial Lesions (check all that apply)

*_____ None identified

*_____ Urothelial (transitional cell) papilloma (WHO/ISUP, 1998)

*_____ Urothelial (transitional cell) papilloma, inverted type

*_____ Papillary urothelial (transitional cell) neoplasm, low malignant potential (WHO/ISUP 1998)

*_____ Cannot be determined

Histologic Grade

_____ Not applicable

_____ Cannot be determined

Urothelial Carcinoma (WHO/ISUP, 1998)

_____ Low-grade

_____ High-grade

_____ Other (specify): _____

Adenocarcinoma and Squamous Carcinoma

_____ GX: Cannot be assessed

_____ G1: Well differentiated

_____ G2: Moderately differentiated

_____ G3: Poorly differentiated

_____ Other (specify): _____

*Tumor Configuration (check all that apply)

*_____ Papillary

*_____ Solid/nodule

*_____ Flat

*_____ Ulcerated

*_____ Indeterminate

*_____ Other (specify): _____

Adequacy of Material for Determining T Category

_____ Muscularis propria (detrusor muscle) absent

_____ Muscularis propria (detrusor muscle) present

_____ Indeterminate

Lymph–Vascular Invasion

_____ Not identified

_____ Present

_____ Indeterminate

Microscopic Eextent of Tumor (select all that apply)

_____ Cannot be assessed

_____ Noninvasive papillary carcinoma

_____ Flat CIS

_____ Tumor invades subepithelial connective tissue (lamina propria)

_____ Tumor invades muscularis propria (detrusor muscle)

_____ Urothelial CIS involving prostatic urethra in prostatic chips sampled by TURBT

_____ Urothelial CIS involving prostatic ducts and acini in prostatic chips sampled by TURBT

_____ Urothelial carcinoma invasive into prostatic stroma in prostatic chips sampled by TURBT

*Additional Pathologic Findings (check all that apply)

*_____ Urothelial dysplasia (low-grade intraurothelial neoplasia)

*_____ Inflammation/regenerative changes

*_____ Therapy-related changes

*_____ Cautery artifact

*_____ Cystitis cystica glandularis

*_____ Keratinizing squamous metaplasia

*_____ Intestinal metaplasia

*_____ Other (specify): _____

Comment(s)

Reproduced from Amin M, Delahunt B, Bochner B, et al. Protocol for the examination of specimens from patients with carcinoma of the urinary bladder. In: Washington K, ed. *Reporting on Cancer Specimens. Case Summaries and Background Documentation.* Northfield, IL: College of American Pathologists; 2012, with permission.

Table 6-24 ■ CAP GUIDELINES FOR REPORTING OF TUMOR IN PARTIAL OR RADICAL CYSTECTOMY AND ANTERIOR EXENTERATION SPECIMENS

Specimen

_____ Bladder

_____ Other (specify)

_____ Not specified

Procedure

_____ Partial cystectomy

_____ Total cystectomy

_____ Radical cystectomy

_____ Radical cystoprostatectomy

_____ Anterior exenteration

_____ Other (specify)

_____ Not specified

*Tumor Site (select all that apply)

*_____ Trigone

*_____ Right lateral wall

*_____ Left lateral wall

*_____ Anterior wall

*_____ Posterior wall

*_____ Dome

*_____ Other (specify)

*_____ Not specified

Tumor size

Greatest dimension: _____ cm

* Additional dimensions: _____ × _____ cm

_____ Cannot be determined (see comment)

Histologic type

_____ Urothelial (transitional cell) carcinoma

_____ Urothelial (transitional cell) carcinoma with squamous differentiation

_____ Urothelial (transitional cell) carcinoma with glandular differentiation

_____ Urothelial (transitional cell) carcinoma with variant histology (specify): _____

_____ Squamous cell carcinoma, typical

_____ Squamous cell carcinoma, variant histology (specify): _____

_____ Adenocarcinoma, typical

_____ Adenocarcinoma, variant histology (specify): _____

_____ Small cell carcinoma

_____ Undifferentiated carcinoma (specify): _____

_____ Mixed cell type (specify): _____

_____ Other (specify): _____

_____ Carcinoma, type cannot be determined

Associated Epithelial Lesions (check all that apply)

_____ None identified

_____ Urothelial (transitional cell) papilloma (WHO/ISUP, 1998)

_____ Urothelial (transitional cell) papilloma, inverted type

_____ Papillary urothelial (transitional cell) neoplasm, low malignant potential (WHO/ISUP 1998)

_____ Cannot be determined

Histologic Grade

_____ Not applicable

_____ Cannot be determined

Urothelial Carcinoma (WHO/ISUP, 1998)

_____ Low-grade

_____ High-grade

_____ Other (specify): _____

Adenocarcinoma and Squamous Carcinoma

_____ GX: Cannot be assessed

_____ G1: Well differentiated

_____ G2: Moderately differentiated

_____ G3: Poorly differentiated

_____ Other (specify): _____

*Tumor Configuration (check all that apply)

*_____ Papillary

*_____ Solid/nodule

*_____ Flat

*_____ Ulcerated

*_____ Indeterminate

*_____ Other (specify): _____

Microscopic Tumor Extension (select all that apply)

_____ None identified

_____ Perivesical fat

_____ Rectum

_____ Prostate stroma

_____ Seminal vesicle (specify laterality)

_____ Vagina

_____ Uterus and adnexae

_____ Pelvic side wall (specify laterality)

_____ Ureter (specify laterality)

_____ Other (specify)

Margins (select all that apply)

_____ Cannot be assessed

_____ Margins uninvolved by invasive carcinoma

    * Distance of invasive carcinoma from closest margin _____ mm

    * Specify margins

_____ Margin(s) involved by invasive carcinoma

    Specify _____

_____ Margin(s) uninvolved by CIS

_____ Margin(s) involved by CIS

    Specify _____

Lymph–Vascular Invasion

_____ Not identified

_____ Present

_____ Indeterminate

Pathologic Staging (see Table 6.14)

Additional Pathologic Findings (select all that apply)

_____ Adenocarcinoma of prostate (use protocol for carcinoma of the prostate)

Continued

Table 6-24 ■ CAP GUIDELINES FOR REPORTING OF TUMOR IN PARTIAL OR RADICAL CYSTECTOMY AND ANTERIOR EXENTERATION SPECIMENS (*Continued*)

_____ Urothelial (transitional cell) carcinoma involving urethra, prostatic ducts and acini, with or without stromal invasion (use protocol for carcinoma of the urethra)

* _____ Urothelial dysplasia (low-grade intraurothelial neoplasia)

* _____ Inflammation/regenerative changes

* _____ Therapy-related changes

* _____ Cystitis cystica/glandularis

* _____ Intestinal metaplasia

* _____ Keratinizing squamous metaplasia

*Comments:

Reproduced from Amin M, Delahunt B, Bochner B, et al. Protocol for the examination of specimens from patients with carcinoma of the urinary bladder. In: Washington K, ed. *Reporting on Cancer Specimens. Case Summaries and Background Documentation.* Northfield, IL: College of American Pathologists; 2012, with permission.

Biopsy Specimens

Biopsies are obtained by urologists using cold cup forceps, diathermy forceps, or a small diathermy loop; the former is preferred as the least artifact is introduced. These biopsies may be directed at a visible lesion, randomly obtained in a patient with hematuria or abnormal cytology in the absence of a visible lesion, or be random samples of "normal" mucosa in a patient with known urothelial carcinoma to assess for the presence or absence of associated CIS. These biopsies should be immediately placed in fixative unless there is a specific protocol in place for another method. All submitted tissue should be processed for evaluation. Although some groups have recommended examination to determine the mucosal surface and embedding "on edge,"[27] most randomly embed these specimens. At least two or three levels should be prepared for microscopic examination.[26,865] In cases with tumor present, the CAP synoptic reporting guidelines include all essential information (Table 6-23).

Not infrequently, these specimens have partial or even complete absence of the surface urothelium. In these situations the concern is that CIS is present but the malignant cells have been lost, so-called denuding cystitis.[867] In patients in whom there is a suspicion of malignancy, cutting deeper levels is recommended.[27] Deeper levels can identify tumor in von Brunn nests in some cases even when there is complete denudation of the surface epithelium. In other situations, routinely obtaining additional levels is not necessary. Correlation with urine cytology can be helpful; urine cytology is almost always positive in cases of denuding CIS. Parwani et al.[868] reported positive urinary cytology in 54% of cases with a denuded biopsy specimen. None of the patients in this study with negative urine cytology and a denuded biopsy subsequently developed urothelial carcinoma during the follow-up period. In another study of 44 patients with denuded bladder biopsies, 31% of patents were diagnosed with CIS within 24 months.[869] In that study, the most significant predictors for CIS were a history of CIS and the biopsy having been obtained by the cold cup method. The latter is less likely to result in a denuded surface in the absence of significant pathology.

In biopsies with denuded surface epithelium, a diagnosis of "negative for malignancy" should not be made.[869] Most urologists are aware of this issue, and reporting the biopsy as having denuded surface epithelium will alert them to the fact that the status of the urothelium remains uncertain. The absence of invasive carcinoma can be indicated and this information does have clinical value.

Transurethral Resection Specimens

In most situations where a visible tumor is present at the time of cystoscopy the urologist will elect to resect it using a transurethral resectoscope. This instrument has a diathermy loop and tends to remove tissue in strips with cautery artifact along the cutting edge. The TURBT is for diagnosis and may be therapeutic. The key information to be gleaned from these specimens is reflected in the CAP-recommended synoptic report (Table 6-23). The amount of tissue removed can vary from a few small fragments to literally hundreds of grams. The specimen should be placed in fixative at the time of resection unless a specific protocol for receiving the specimen fresh is in place.

For smaller specimens all of the tissue removed should be submitted for histologic evaluation. For large specimens, an initial partial sampling is recommended. No optimal sampling strategy has been determined. Approaches such as one block for every centimeter of aggregated chips up to a maximum of 10 blocks have been suggested.[27,865] If the initial sample shows an invasive high-grade tumor with invasion of the muscularis propria, no further sampling is required. Any lesser degree of abnormality will require examination of the entire specimen. An initial sample showing a noninvasive low-grade papillary urothelial carcinoma could still harbor a high-grade tumor with or without invasion. In a noninvasive high-grade tumor, invasion can be focal and cannot be excluded until the entire specimen has been examined. Similarly, an invasive high-grade tumor can have demonstrable muscularis propria invasion in only a single tissue fragment.

Partial Cystectomy Specimens

Partial cystectomy has only a very limited role in the treatment of urothelial carcinoma and is an uncommon specimen in this setting.[870] It can be used in selected patients with a tumor localized to a part of the bladder with a "free wall" including the dome or high on the anterior or lateral walls. The presence of CIS is a relative contraindication.[871,872] It is frequently used in patients with tumors arising in diverticula.[873] This approach is most often used in the setting of nonurothelial tumors including urachal adenocarcinoma and mesenchymal neoplasmas.

These specimens are handled much the same way as radical cystectomy specimens with sampling aimed at accurately staging the tumor. The assessment of the mucosal and soft tissue margins is much more relevant in these cases and often the margins will be evaluated by frozen section at the time of surgery. These are reported using the same template as for radical cystectomy specimens (Table 6-24).

Radical Cystectomy Specimens

Radical cystectomy in male patients includes removal of the urinary bladder, segments of both ureters, the prostate gland, both seminal vesicles, and a minimal amount of the urethra. Frozen section examination of the ureter margins is considered standard although the urology literature does include a number of reports questioning the value of this.[874–876] In some cases, particularly when a neobladder is being created, the surgeon may request a frozen section on the urethral margin. Radical cystectomy in females most often involves performance of an anterior exenteration with removal of the urinary bladder, segments of both ureters, the urethra with a portion of the vaginal wall, the uterus, cervix, and both fallopian tubes and ovaries (when present). In selected patients, an orthotopic bladder reconstruction approach is being used in women with preservation of the urethra and without resection of vaginal tissue.[877,878] In these cases, frozen section assessment of the urethra is critical at the time of surgery.

The approach to the examination of the cystectomy specimen is determined by the significant information to be gained regarding the patients' prognosis and indications for further therapy. The gross examination should include documentation of the various components received and the relevant organ measurements. The external surfaces should be evaluated for areas of possible tumor involvement. Soft

tissue resection margins should be inked; in males the external surface of the prostate should also be inked preferably with different colors to allow later orientation if necessary. If the specimen is fixed prior to dissection, inflating the bladder with fixative can produce superior fixation and subsequent sections (Fig. 6-186). Unless the situation indicates an alternate approach, the specimen is usually opened along the anterior surface (Fig. 6-187). Alternately, the specimen can be bisected using a probe in the urethra to guide the blade (Fig. 6-186). The location and size of grossly visible tumors or defects related to prior transurethral resection should be documented. The mucosa should be evaluated for any abnormalities including reddened or indurated areas, granularity, or ulcerations (Fig. 6-188). Sections through the tumor are examined for gross evaluation of the tumor extent; substaging of the pT3 category is based on gross versus microscopic involvement of the perivesical fat (Fig. 6-189). Sections are submitted to confirm the gross impression. If the tumor grossly extends close to or appears to involve a margin this should be stated in the gross description and sections submitted to document the observation. In males, if the tumor is in the trigone or bladder neck, sections should be submitted to show the relationship of the tumor to the prostate gland (Fig. 6-190). In female patients, cystectomy specimens usually include a portion of the vagina, the uterus and cervix, and possibly the fallopian tubes and ovaries. Areas suspicious for involvement of these organs by direct tumor extension should be sampled (Fig. 6-191).

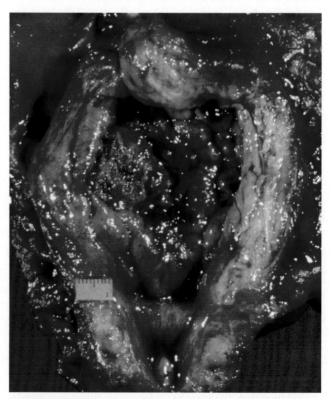

FIGURE 6-187 ■ Cystectomy specimen that was opened along the midline anterior wall with a small "Y" cut producing the tongue of anterior wall at the top of the photo.

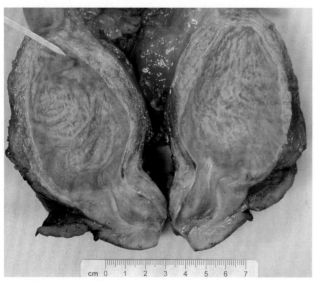

FIGURE 6-186 ■ Cystectomy specimen that was inflated with formalin and allowed to partially fix prior to bivalving it.

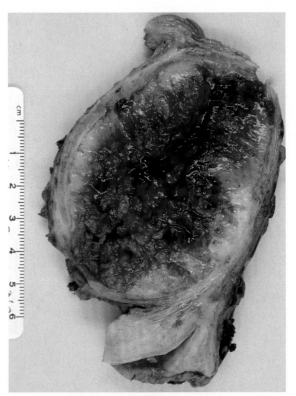

FIGURE 6-188 ■ Cystectomy specimen with extensive mucosal hemorrhage and ulceration. There was only focal invasion into the deep muscularis propria present (pT2b).

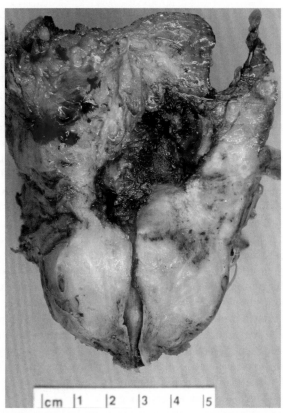

FIGURE 6-190 ■ Cystoprostatectomy specimen with a large tumor that grossly seems to directly invade the prostate gland (pT4a).

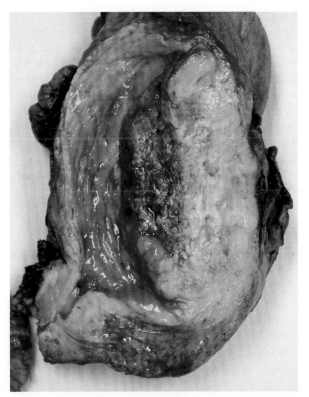

FIGURE 6-189 ■ Cystectomy specimen with a large tumor that grossly involves the perivesical fat (pT3b). The tumor also appears to extend to the inked margin focally.

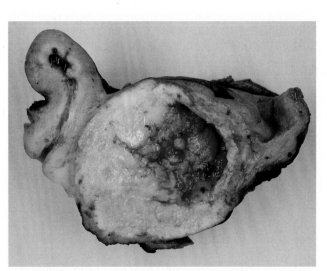

FIGURE 6-191 ■ Cystectomy specimen with a large urothelial carcinoma (predominantly sarcomatoid histology) that is invading to the lower uterine segment. Histologic examination confirmed invasion of the cervix stroma (pT4a).

The examination of the tumor includes a re-evaluation of the histologic type such as identification of a variant histology that was not present or recognized in the biopsy or transurethral resections specimen (e.g., micropapillary variant or presence of a small cell component) or reclassification of the tumor (e.g., initial specimen reported as squamous cell carcinoma but identification of a urothelial component changes classification to urothelial carcinoma with squamous differentiation). Perhaps more important is the determination of the pathologic stage. Other significant pathologic features related to the tumor such as associated CIS and its extent if present are important prognostically and are also indicators of an increased risk of prostatic involvement[193] or upper tract recurrence.[879,880] Documentation of multifocality in the bladder is important as this is also a significant risk factor for subsequent urethral[881] and upper tract recurrence.[880] One of the purposes of submitting sections from uninvolved areas of the bladder is to assess for these features. Finally surgical margins need to be assessed. Identification and sampling of the ureters is not critical if these have been evaluated separately at frozen section or in segments submitted without frozen sections having been performed. The urethral margin needs to be evaluated if not sampled for frozen section. The soft tissue margins are also important, and surgical margins should be inked prior to sectioning.

In male patients, the prostate must be examined for involvement by the bladder carcinoma and for other significant pathology. The prostatic urethra is often involved by urothelial carcinoma at the time of cystectomy for urothelial carcinoma of the bladder. In one study that completely submitted the prostate glands using whole mount sections, prostatic involvement was found in 38%.[882] This was more frequent through spread along the urethra (83%) than by direct extension (17%). Involvement of the prostate gland has possible prognostic significance and is the most important risk factor for subsequent urethral recurrence.[881,883] When the prostate gland is directly invaded by the tumor this is considered pT4 disease; however, if the involvement is through the urethral route the prostate involvement is staged separately using the urethral staging protocol.[26]

It is not uncommon with current urologic practice to have no residual tumor in the bladder at cystectomy. In one contemporary large series there was no residual tumor in 11% of 1,104 cystectomy specimens.[884] These are variably referred to in the literature as "P0" or "pT0." The former is a reasonable way to identify these cases but the latter is not an appropriate application of the TNM system and should not be used.[567] The pathologic stage is correctly determined by using the findings from the transurethral resection combined with the cystectomy pathology.[567] For example, if muscularis propria invasion is documented in the transurethral resection and there is no residual tumor at cystectomy, the pathologic stage is pT2 (the cystectomy findings having excluded a higher stage). The gross appearance of a transurethral resection site is typically that of a depressed ulcer or crater (Fig. 6-192). The surrounding tissue often is interpreted as being

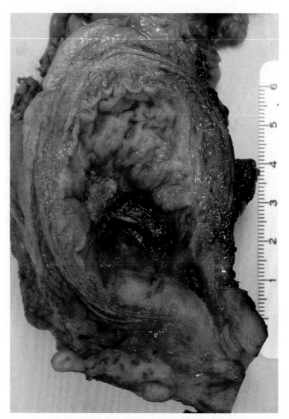

FIGURE 6-192 ■ Cystectomy specimen with area of ulceration and calcific material on the surface typical of a TURBT site. Microscopic examination showed no residual tumor.

tumor due to the firm white appearance. If the area is small and can be completely submitted in four or five sections, that is how we approach these. For larger abnormalities, a similar number of sections are submitted. When no tumor is found, additional sections can be submitted, but it is not necessary to extensively sample normal appearing areas in a search for tumor. There are several reports indicating that patients with no residual tumor at cystectomy have a significantly better survival than those with residual tumor of a presumed similar stage.[480,884]

The CAP recommendations for the reporting of radical cystectomy specimens are presented in Table 6-24.

Lymph Node Specimens

The resection of regional lymph nodes is a standard procedure performed during a radical cystectomy for bladder cancer. The role of lymphadenectomy as a therapeutic procedure and as a critical part of prognostication has received considerable attention in the last decade. Currently most authorities advocate an extended lymphadenectomy procedure that increases the number of lymph nodes removed and extends the dissection beyond the initial landing site of lymph node metastases.[885,886] Contemporary reviews of this literature have concluded that the extended lymph node dissection approach "can be curative in patients with metastasis or micrometastasis to a few nodes."[887–889] There are inconsistent data that for patients with negative lymph nodes, the greater the number of nodes sampled the better the prognosis.[887,890,891] In the study by Koppie et al.,[891] the predicted probability of 5-year survival was 50% for patients with 8 lymph nodes removed versus 68% if 32 nodes were obtained. For patients with lymph node metastases there are data indicating that the larger the number of nodes removed the better the prognosis.[887,892] For example, in one report of patients with lymph node metastases, the median survival was 13 months if 5 or fewer nodes were removed compared to 23 months if more than 16 had been resected ($p < 0.0001$).[892] The percent of lymph nodes positive (often referred to as the lymph node density) has also been reported to be prognostically significant in several but not all studies.[887,892] Lastly there are conflicting data on the significance of extranodal extension in patients with lymph node metastases.[893,894]

This intensive interest in lymph node status has led to questions regarding the adequacy of lymph node dissection. Despite extensive discussion in the clinical literature, no consensus has emerged though numbers in the range of 16 to 24 seem to be most often cited.[891,895] It has also been suggested that the number of lymph nodes removed could be a quality monitor for surgical technique. For the pathologist this has led, as in other organs, to clinician pressure to maximize the identification of lymph nodes. Meticulous dissection combined with use of a clearing agent can significantly improve lymph node yield.

REFERENCES

1. Grignon DJ. The current classification of urothelial neoplasms. *Mod Pathol* 2009;22:S60–S69.
2. Mostofi F, Sobin L. *Histologic Typing of Urinary Bladder Tumors.* Geneva, Switzerland: World Health Organization; 1973.
3. Murphy W, Beckwith J, Farrow G. *Atlas of Tumor Pathology: Tumors of the Kidney, Bladder, and Related Structures.* Washington, DC: American Registry of Pathology; 1994.
4. Jordan AM, Weingarten J, Murphy WM. Transitional cell neoplasms of the urinary bladder. Can biologic potential be predicted from histologic grading? *Cancer* 1987;60:2766–2774.
5. Witjes JA, Moonen PMJ, van der Heijden AG. Review pathology in a diagnostic bladder cancer trial: effect of patient risk category. *Urology* 2006;67:751–755.
6. Kiemeney LA, Witjes JA, Verbeek AL, et al. The clinical epidemiology of superficial bladder cancer. Dutch South-East Cooperative Urological Group. *Br J Cancer* 1993;67:806–812.
7. Bostwick DG, Mikuz G. Urothelial papillary (exophytic) neoplasms. *Virchows Arch* 2002;441:109–116.
8. Epstein JI, Amin MB, Reuter VR, et al. The World Health Organization/International Society of Urological Pathology consensus classification of urothelial (transitional cell) neoplasms of the urinary bladder. Bladder Consensus Conference Committee. *Am J Surg Pathol* 1998;22:1435–1448.
9. Malmström PU, Busch C, Norlen BJ. Recurrence, progression and survival in bladder cancer. A retrospective analysis of 232 patients with greater than or equal to 5-year follow-up. *Scand J Urol Nephrol* 1987;21:185–195.
10. Mostofi F, Davis CJ, Sesterhenn I. *Histologic Typing of Urinary Bladder Tumors: International Histological Classification of Tumors.* Geneva, Switzerland: World Health Organization; 1999.
11. Cheng L, Bostwick DG. World Health Organization and International Society of Urological Pathology classification and two-number grading system of bladder tumors: reply. *Cancer* 2000;88:1513–1516.
12. Oyasu R. World Health Organization and International Society of Urological Pathology classification and two-number grading system of bladder tumors. *Cancer* 2000;88:1509–1512.
13. Lopez-Beltran A, Montironi R. Non-invasive urothelial neoplasms: according to the most recent WHO classification. *Eur Urol* 2004;46:170–176.
14. Eble J, Epstein J, Sauter G, et al. *World Health Organization Histologic and Genetic Typing of Tumours of the Kidney, Urinary Bladder, Prostate Gland and Testis.* Lyon, France: IARC Press; 2004.
15. Murphy W, Grignon D, Perlman E. *Atlas of Tumor Pathology: Tumors of the Kidney, Bladder, and Related Urinary Structures.* Washington, DC: American Registry of Pathology; 2004.
16. Reuter VE. The pathology of bladder cancer. *Urology* 2006;67:11–17.
17. Samaratunga H, Makarov DV, Epstein JI. Comparison of WHO/ISUP and WHO classification of noninvasive papillary urothelial neoplasms for risk of progression. *Urology* 2002;60:315–319.
18. Yin H, Leong ASY. Histologic grading of noninvasive papillary urothelial tumors: validation of the 1998 WHO/ISUP system by immunophenotyping and follow-up. *Am J Clin Pathol* 2004;121:679–687.
19. Herr HW, Donat SM, Reuter VE. Management of low grade papillary bladder tumors. *J Urol* 2007;178:1201–1205.
20. Burger M, van der Aa MNM, van Oers JMM, et al. Prediction of progression of non-muscle-invasive bladder cancer by WHO 1973 and 2004 grading and by FGFR3 mutation status: a prospective study. *Eur Urol* 2008;54:835–843.
21. Herr HW. Low risk bladder tumors—less is more! *J Urol* 2008;179:13–14.
22. Nieder AM, Soloway MS. Eliminate the term "superficial" bladder cancer. *J Urol* 2006;175:417–418.
23. Hall MC, Chang SS, Dalbagni G, et al. Guideline for the management of nonmuscle invasive bladder cancer (stages Ta, T1, and Tis): 2007 update. *J Urol* 2007;178:2314–2330.
24. Stenzl A, Cowan NC, De Santis M, et al. The updated EAU guidelines on muscle-invasive and metastatic bladder cancer. *Eur Urol* 2009;55:815–825.
25. Amin MB, Srigley JR, Grignon DJ, et al. Updated protocol for the examination of specimens from patients with carcinoma of the urinary bladder, ureter, and renal pelvis. *Arch Pathol Lab Med* 2003;127:1263–1279.
26. Amin M, Delahunt B, Bochner B, et al. Protocol for the Examination of Specimens from Patients with Carcinoma of the Urinary Bladder; 2012. Available from College of American Pathologists Web site.
27. Amin M, Reuter V, Epstein J, et al. Consensus of guidelines by the pathology of bladder cancer workgroup. In: Soloway M, Khoury S, eds. *Bladder Cancer: 2nd International Consultation on Bladder Cancer—Vienna.* 2nd ed. Paris, France: ICUD-EAU; 2012.
28. Eble JN, Young RH. Benign and low-grade papillary lesions of the urinary bladder: a review of the papilloma-papillary carcinoma controversy, and a report of five typical papillomas. *Semin Diagn Pathol* 1989;6:351–371.
29. Mostofi FK. Pathological aspects and spread of carcinoma of the bladder. *JAMA* 1968;206:1764–1769.
30. van Rhijn BWG, Montironi R, Zwarthoff EC, et al. Frequent FGFR3 mutations in urothelial papilloma. *J Pathol* 2002;198:245–251.
31. McKenney JK, Amin MB, Young RH. Urothelial (transitional cell) papilloma of the urinary bladder: a clinicopathologic study of 26 cases. *Mod Pathol* 2003;16:623–629.
32. Magi-Galluzzi C, Epstein JI. Urothelial papilloma of the bladder: a review of 34 de novo cases. *Am J Surg Pathol* 2004;28:1615–1620.
33. Cheng L, Darson M, Cheville JC, et al. Urothelial papilloma of the bladder. Clinical and biologic implications. *Cancer* 1999;86:2098–2101.
34. Oosterhuis JWA, Schapers RFM, Janssen-Heijnen MLG, et al. Histological grading of papillary urothelial carcinoma of the bladder: prognostic value of the 1998 WHO/ISUP classification system and comparison with conventional grading systems. *J Clin Pathol* 2002;55:900–905.
35. van Oers JMM, Wild PJ, Burger M, et al. FGFR3 mutations and a normal CK20 staining pattern define low-grade noninvasive urothelial bladder tumours. *Eur Urol* 2007;52:760–768.

36. van Rhijn BWG, Vis AN, van der Kwast TH, et al. Molecular grading of urothelial cell carcinoma with fibroblast growth factor receptor 3 and MIB-1 is superior to pathologic grade for the prediction of clinical outcome. *J Clin Oncol* 2003;21:1912–1921.

37. Young RH. Papillary and polypoid cystitis. A report of eight cases. *Am J Surg Pathol* 1988;12:542–546.

38. Lane Z, Epstein JI. Polypoid/papillary cystitis: a series of 41 cases misdiagnosed as papillary urothelial neoplasia. *Am J Surg Pathol* 2008;32:758–764.

39. Taylor DC, Bhagavan BS, Larsen MP, et al. Papillary urothelial hyperplasia. A precursor to papillary neoplasms. *Am J Surg Pathol* 1996;20:1481–1488.

40. Cameron KM, Lupton CH. Inverted papilloma of the lower urinary tract. *Br J Urol* 1976;48:567–577.

41. Kunze E, Schauer A, Schmitt M. Histology and histogenesis of two different types of inverted urothelial papillomas. *Cancer* 1983;51:348–358.

42. Sung M-T, Eble JN, Wang M, et al. Inverted papilloma of the urinary bladder: a molecular genetic appraisal. *Mod Pathol* 2006;19:1289–1294.

43. Cheng CW, Chan LW, Chan CK, et al. Is surveillance necessary for inverted papilloma in the urinary bladder and urethra? *ANZ J Surg* 2005;75:213–217.

44. Witjes JA, van Balken MR, van de Kaa CA. The prognostic value of a primary inverted papilloma of the urinary tract. *J Urol* 1997;158:1500–1505.

45. Cheville JC, Wu K, Sebo TJ, et al. Inverted urothelial papilloma: is ploidy, MIB-1 proliferative activity, or p53 protein accumulation predictive of urothelial carcinoma? *Cancer* 2000;88:632–636.

46. Asano K, Miki J, Maeda S, et al. Clinical studies on inverted papilloma of the urinary tract: report of 48 cases and review of the literature. *J Urol* 2003;170:1209–1212.

47. Hodges KB, Lopez-Beltran A, Maclennan GT, et al. Urothelial lesions with inverted growth patterns: histogenesis, molecular genetic findings, differential diagnosis and clinical management. *BJU Int* 2011;107:532–537.

48. Jones TD, Zhang S, Lopez-Beltran A, et al. Urothelial carcinoma with an inverted growth pattern can be distinguished from inverted papilloma by fluorescence in situ hybridization, immunohistochemistry, and morphologic analysis. *Am J Surg Pathol* 2007;31:1861–1867.

49. Gould VE, Schmitt M, Vinokurova S, et al. Human papillomavirus and p16 expression in inverted papillomas of the urinary bladder. *Cancer Lett* 2010;292:171–175.

50. Broussard JN, Tan PH, Epstein JI. Atypia in inverted urothelial papillomas: pathology and prognostic significance. *Hum Pathol* 2004;35:1499–1504.

51. Fine SW, Epstein JI. Inverted urothelial papillomas with foamy or vacuolated cytoplasm. *Hum Pathol* 2006;37:1577–1582.

52. Amin MB, Gomez JA, Young RH. Urothelial transitional cell carcinoma with endophytic growth patterns: a discussion of patterns of invasion and problems associated with assessment of invasion in 18 cases. *Am J Surg Pathol* 1997;21:1057–1068.

53. Amin MB. Histological variants of urothelial carcinoma: diagnostic, therapeutic and prognostic implications. *Mod Pathol* 2009;22:S96–S118.

54. Volmar KE, Chan TY, De Marzo AM, et al. Florid von Brunn nests mimicking urothelial carcinoma: a morphologic and immunohistochemical comparison to the nested variant of urothelial carcinoma. *Am J Surg Pathol* 2003;27:1243–1252.

55. Eble JN, Hull MT, Rowland RG, et al. Villous adenoma of the urachus with mucusuria: a light and electron microscopic study. *J Urol* 1986;135:1240–1244.

56. Assor D. A villous tumor of the bladder. *J Urol* 1978;119:287–288.

57. Miller DC, Gang DL, Gavris V, et al. Villous adenoma of the urinary bladder: a morphologic or biologic entity? *Am J Clin Pathol* 1983;79:728–731.

58. Cheng L, Montironi R, Bostwick DG. Villous adenoma of the urinary tract: a report of 23 cases, including 8 with coexistent adenocarcinoma. *Am J Surg Pathol* 1999;23:764–771.

59. Seibel JL, Prasad S, Weiss RE, et al. Villous adenoma of the urinary tract: a lesion frequently associated with malignancy. *Hum Pathol* 2002;33:236–241.

60. Thomas AA, Rackley RR, Lee U, et al. Urethral diverticula in 90 female patients: a study with emphasis on neoplastic alterations. *J Urol* 2008;180:2463–2467.

61. Yip SK, Wong MP, Cheung MC, et al. Mucinous adenocarcinoma of renal pelvis and villous adenoma of bladder after a caecal augmentation of bladder. *Aust N Z J Surg* 1999;69:247–248.

62. Channer JL, Williams JL, Henry L. Villous adenoma of the bladder. *J Clin Pathol* 1993;46:450–452.

63. Lane Z, Hansel DE, Epstein JI. Immunohistochemical expression of prostatic antigens in adenocarcinoma and villous adenoma of the urinary bladder. *Am J Surg Pathol* 2008;32:1322–1326.

64. Tzortzis V, Ioannou M, Melekos MD. Villous adenoma of the urachus: a case with prostate specific antigen immunoreactivity. *J Urol* 2003;170:1302–1303.

65. Lim M, Adsay NV, Grignon D, et al. Urothelial carcinoma with villoglandular differentiation: a study of 14 cases. *Mod Pathol* 2009;22:1280–1286.

66. Cheng L, Leibovich BC, Cheville JC, et al. Squamous papilloma of the urinary tract is unrelated to condyloma acuminata. *Cancer* 2000;88:1679–1686.

67. Guo CC, Fine SW, Epstein JI. Noninvasive squamous lesions in the urinary bladder: a clinicopathologic analysis of 29 cases. *Am J Surg Pathol* 2006;30:883–891.

68. Del Mistro A, Koss LG, Braunstein J, et al. Condylomata acuminata of the urinary bladder. Natural history, viral typing, and DNA content. *Am J Surg Pathol* 1988;12:205–215.

69. Parkin DM, Bray F, Ferlay J, et al. Global cancer statistics, 2002. *CA Cancer J Clin* 2005;55:74–108.

70. Parkin DM. The global burden of urinary bladder cancer. *Scand J Urol Nephrol Suppl* 2008:12–20.

71. Wu X, Ros MM, Gu J, et al. Epidemiology and genetic susceptibility to bladder cancer. *BJU Int* 2008;102:1207–1215.

72. Siegel R, Naishadham D, Jemal A. Cancer statistics, 2013. *CA Cancer J Clin* 2013;63:11–30.

73. Prout GR Jr, Wesley MN, McCarron PG, et al. Survival experience of black patients and white patients with bladder carcinoma. *Cancer* 2004;100:621–630.

74. Paner GP, Zehnder P, Amin AM, et al. Urothelial neoplasms of the urinary bladder occurring in young adult and pediatric patients: a comprehensive review of literature with implications for patient management. *Adv Anat Pathol* 2011;18:79–89.

75. Zeegers MP, Tan FE, Dorant E, et al. The impact of characteristics of cigarette smoking on urinary tract cancer risk: a meta-analysis of epidemiologic studies. *Cancer* 2000;89:630–639.

76. Bjerregaard BK, Raaschou-Nielsen O, Sorensen M, et al. The effect of occasional smoking on smoking-related cancers: in the European Prospective Investigation into Cancer and Nutrition (EPIC). *Cancer Causes Control* 2006;17:1305–1309.

77. Brennan P, Bogillot O, Cordier S, et al. Cigarette smoking and bladder cancer in men: a pooled analysis of 11 case-control studies. *Int J Cancer* 2000;86:289–294.

78. Vineis P, Simonato L. Proportion of lung and bladder cancers in males resulting from occupation: a systematic approach. *Arch Environ Health* 1991;46:6–15.

79. King WD, Marrett LD. Case-control study of bladder cancer and chlorination by-products in treated water (Ontario, Canada). *Cancer Causes Control* 1996;7:596–604.

80. Villanueva CM, Cantor KP, Cordier S, et al. Disinfection byproducts and bladder cancer: a pooled analysis. *Epidemiology* 2004;15:357–367.

81. Chen CJ, Chuang YC, You SL, et al. A retrospective study on malignant neoplasms of bladder, lung and liver in blackfoot disease endemic area in Taiwan. *Br J Cancer* 1986;53:399–405.

82. Riboli E, Norat T. Epidemiologic evidence of the protective effect of fruit and vegetables on cancer risk. *Am J Clin Nutr* 2003;78:559S–569S.

83. Garcia-Closas R, Garcia-Closas M, Kogevinas M, et al. Food, nutrient and heterocyclic amine intake and the risk of bladder cancer. *Eur J Cancer* 2007;43:1731–1740.

84. Steinmaus CM, Nunez S, Smith AH. Diet and bladder cancer: a meta-analysis of six dietary variables. *Am J Epidemiol* 2000;151:693–702.

85. Holick CN, De Vivo I, Feskanich D, et al. Intake of fruits and vegetables, carotenoids, folate, and vitamins A, C, E and risk of bladder cancer among women (United States). *Cancer Causes Control* 2005;16:1135–1145.

86. Ferrucci L, Sinha R, Ward M, et al. Meat and components of meat and the risk of bladder cancer in the NIH-AARP Diet and Health Study. *Cancer* 2010;116:4345–4353.

87. Kang D, Park SK, Beane-Freeman L, et al. Cancer incidence among pesticide applicators exposed to trifluralin in the Agricultural Health Study. *Environ Res* 2008;107:271–276.

88. Bedwani R, Renganathan E, El Kwhsky F, et al. Schistosomiasis and the risk of bladder cancer in Alexandria, Egypt. *Br J Cancer* 1998;77:1186–1189.

89. Gelfand M, Weinberg RW, Castle WM. Relation between carcinoma of the bladder and infestation with *Schistosoma haematobium*. *Lancet* 1967;1:1249–1251.

90. Lucas SB. Squamous cell carcinoma of the bladder and schistosomiasis. *East Afr Med J* 1982;59:345–351.

91. Johansson SL, Cohen SM. Epidemiology and etiology of bladder cancer. *Semin Surg Oncol* 1997;13:291–298.

92. Kiemeney L. Hereditary bladder cancer. *Scand J Urol Nephrol Suppl* 2008:110–115.

93. Aben KKH, Witjes JA, Schoenberg MP, et al. Familial aggregation of urothelial cell carcinoma. *Int J Cancer* 2002;98:274–278.

94. Murta-Nascimento C, Silverman DT, Kogevinas M, et al. Risk of bladder cancer associated with family history of cancer: do low-penetrance polymorphisms account for the increase in risk? *Cancer Epidemiol Biomarkers Prev* 2007;16:1595–1600.

95. Gripp KW. Tumor predisposition in Costello syndrome. *Am J Med Genet C Semin Med Genet* 2005;137C:72–77.

96. van der Post R, Kiemeney L, Ligtenberg M, et al. Risk of urothelial bladder cancer in Lynch syndrome is increased, in particular among MSH2 mutation carriers. *J Med Genet* 2010;47:464–470.

97. Grignon DJ, Shum DT, Bruckschwaiger O. Transitional cell carcinoma in the Muir-Torre syndrome. *J Urol* 1987;138:406–408.

98. Fortuny J, Kogevinas M, Garcia-Closas M, et al. Use of analgesics and nonsteroidal anti-inflammatory drugs, genetic predisposition, and bladder cancer risk in Spain. *Cancer Epidemiol Biomarkers Prev* 2006;15:1696–1702.

99. Travis LB, Curtis RE, Glimelius B, et al. Bladder and kidney cancer following cyclophosphamide therapy for non-Hodgkin's lymphoma. *J Natl Cancer Inst* 1995;87:524–530.

100. Kaldor JM, Day NE, Kittelmann B, et al. Bladder tumours following chemotherapy and radiotherapy for ovarian cancer: a case-control study. *Int J Cancer* 1995;63:1–6.

101. Lin J, Dinney CP, Grossman HB, et al. Personal permanent hair dye use is not associated with bladder cancer risk: evidence from a case-control study. *Cancer Epidemiol Biomarkers Prev* 2006;15:1746–1749.

102. Cordon-Cardo C. Molecular alterations associated with bladder cancer initiation and progression. *Scand J Urol Nephrol Suppl* 2008:154–165.

103. Knowles MA. Bladder cancer subtypes defined by genomic alterations. *Scand J Urol Nephrol Suppl* 2008:116–130.

104. Czerniak B, Cohen GL, Etkind P, et al. Concurrent mutations of coding and regulatory sequences of the Ha-ras gene in urinary bladder carcinomas. *Hum Pathol* 1992;23:1199–1204.

105. Dalbagni G, Presti J, Reuter V, et al. Genetic alterations in bladder cancer. *Lancet* 1993;342:469–471.

106. Billerey C, Chopin D, Aubriot-Lorton MH, et al. Frequent FGFR3 mutations in papillary non-invasive bladder (pTa) tumors. *Am J Pathol* 2001;158:1955–1959.

107. van Rhijn BW, Lurkin I, Radvanyi F, et al. The fibroblast growth factor receptor 3 (FGFR3) mutation is a strong indicator of superficial bladder cancer with low recurrence rate. *Cancer Res* 2001;61:1265–1268.

108. Jebar AH, Hurst CD, Tomlinson DC, et al. FGFR3 and Ras gene mutations are mutually exclusive genetic events in urothelial cell carcinoma. *Oncogene* 2005;24:5218–5225.

109. Aveyard JS, Skilleter A, Habuchi T, et al. Somatic mutation of PTEN in bladder carcinoma. *Br J Cancer* 1999;80:904–908.

110. Williamson MP, Elder PA, Shaw ME, et al. p16 (CDKN2) is a major deletion target at 9p21 in bladder cancer. *Hum Mol Genet* 1995;4:1569–1577.

111. Cairns P, Shaw ME, Knowles MA. Initiation of bladder cancer may involve deletion of a tumour-suppressor gene on chromosome 9. *Oncogene* 1993;8:1083–1085.

112. McGarvey TW, Maruta Y, Tomaszewski JE, et al. PTCH gene mutations in invasive transitional cell carcinoma of the bladder. *Oncogene* 1998;17:1167–1172.

113. Habuchi T, Luscombe M, Elder PA, et al. Structure and methylation-based silencing of a gene (DBCCR1) within a candidate bladder cancer tumor suppressor region at 9q32-q33. *Genomics* 1998;48:277–288.

114. Hornigold N, Devlin J, Davies AM, et al. Mutation of the 9q34 gene TSC1 in sporadic bladder cancer. *Oncogene* 1999;18:2657–2661.

115. Cordon-Cardo C, Zhang ZF, Dalbagni G, et al. Cooperative effects of p53 and pRB alterations in primary superficial bladder tumors. *Cancer Res* 1997;57:1217–1221.

116. Esrig D, Elmajian D, Groshen S, et al. Accumulation of nuclear p53 and tumor progression in bladder cancer. *N Engl J Med* 1994;331:1259–1264.

117. Hopman AHN, Kamps MAF, Speel EJM, et al. Identification of chromosome 9 alterations and p53 accumulation in isolated carcinoma in situ of the urinary bladder versus carcinoma in situ associated with carcinoma. *Am J Pathol* 2002;161:1119–1125.

118. Zieger K, Dyrskjot L, Wiuf C, et al. Role of activating fibroblast growth factor receptor 3 mutations in the development of bladder tumors. *Clin Cancer Res* 2005;11:7709–7719.

119. Mian C, Maier K, Comploj E, et al. uCyt+/ImmunoCyt in the detection of recurrent urothelial carcinoma: an update on 1991 analyses. *Cancer* 2006;108:60–65.

120. Grossman HB, Soloway M, Messing E, et al. Surveillance for recurrent bladder cancer using a point-of-care proteomic assay. *JAMA* 2006;295:299–305.

121. Tritschler S, Scharf S, Karl A, et al. Validation of the diagnostic value of NMP22 BladderChek test as a marker for bladder cancer by photodynamic diagnosis. *Eur Urol* 2007;51:403–407.

122. Van Le T-S, Miller R, Barder T, et al. Highly specific urine-based marker of bladder cancer. *Urology* 2005;66:1256–1260.

123. van Rhijn BWG, van der Poel HG, van der Kwast TH. Urine markers for bladder cancer surveillance: a systematic review. *Eur Urol* 2005;47:736–748.

124. Tetu B. Diagnosis of urothelial carcinoma from urine. *Mod Pathol* 2009;22:S53–S59.

125. Passerotti CC, Bonfim A, Martins JRM, et al. Urinary hyaluronan as a marker for the presence of residual transitional cell carcinoma of the urinary bladder. *Eur Urol* 2006;49:71–75.

126. Fernandez-Gomez J, Rodriguez-Martinez JJ, Barmadah SE, et al. Urinary CYFRA 21.1 is not a useful marker for the detection of recurrences in the follow-up of superficial bladder cancer. *Eur Urol* 2007;51:1267–1274.

127. Bian W, Xu Z. Combined assay of CYFRA21-1, telomerase and vascular endothelial growth factor in the detection of bladder transitional cell carcinoma. *Int J Urol* 2007;14:108–111.

128. Shariat SF, Casella R, Khoddami SM, et al. Urine detection of survivin is a sensitive marker for the noninvasive diagnosis of bladder cancer. *J Urol* 2004;171:626–630.

129. Weikert S, Christoph F, Schrader M, et al. Quantitative analysis of survivin mRNA expression in urine and tumor tissue of bladder cancer patients and its potential relevance for disease detection and prognosis. *Int J Cancer* 2005;116:100–104.

130. Eissa S, Swellam M, Ali-Labib R, et al. Detection of telomerase in urine by 3 methods: evaluation of diagnostic accuracy for bladder cancer. *J Urol* 2007;178:1068–1072.

131. Rieger-Christ KM, Mourtzinos A, Lee PJ, et al. Identification of fibroblast growth factor receptor 3 mutations in urine sediment DNA samples complements cytology in bladder tumor detection. *Cancer* 2003;98:737–744.

132. Eissa S, Salem AM, Zohny SF, et al. The diagnostic efficacy of urinary TGF-beta1 and VEGF in bladder cancer: comparison with voided urine cytology. *Cancer Biomark* 2007;3:275–285.

133. Caraway NP, Khanna A, Payne L, et al. Combination of cytologic evaluation and quantitative digital cytometry is reliable in detecting recurrent disease in patients with urinary diversions. *Cancer* 2007;111:323–329.

134. van der Aa MNM, Zwarthoff EC, Steyerberg EW, et al. Microsatellite analysis of voided-urine samples for surveillance of low-grade non-muscle-invasive urothelial carcinoma: feasibility and clinical utility in a prospective multicenter study (Cost-Effectiveness of Follow-Up of Urinary Bladder Cancer trial [CEFUB]). *Eur Urol* 2009;55:659–667.

135. Moonen PMJ, Merkx GFM, Peelen P, et al. UroVysion compared with cytology and quantitative cytology in the surveillance of non-muscle-invasive bladder cancer. *Eur Urol* 2007;51:1275–1280.

136. Jones JS. DNA-based molecular cytology for bladder cancer surveillance. *Urology* 2006;67:35–45.

137. Vrooman OPJ, Witjes JA. Molecular markers for detection, surveillance and prognostication of bladder cancer. *Int J Urol* 2009;16:234–243.

138. de Bekker-Grob EW, van der Aa MNM, Zwarthoff EC, et al. Non-muscle-invasive bladder cancer surveillance for which cystoscopy is partly replaced by microsatellite analysis of urine: a cost-effective alternative? *BJU Int* 2009;104:41–47.

139. Horstmann M, Patschan O, Hennenlotter J, et al. Combinations of urine-based tumour markers in bladder cancer surveillance. *Scand J Urol Nephrol* 2009;43:461–466.

140. Mowatt G, Zhu S, Kilonzo M, et al. Systematic review of the clinical effectiveness and cost-effectiveness of photodynamic diagnosis and urine biomarkers (FISH, ImmunoCyt, NMP22) and cytology for the detection and follow-up of bladder cancer. *Health Technol Assess* 2010;14:1–331, iii–iv.

141. Nieder AM, Soloway MS, Herr HW. Should we abandon the FISH test? *Eur Urol* 2007;51:1469–1471.

142. Hong YM, Loughlin KR. Economic impact of tumor markers in bladder cancer surveillance. *Urology* 2008;71:131–135.

143. Ku J, Godoy G, Amiel G, et al. Urine survivin as a diagnostic biomarker for bladder cancer: a systematic study. *BJU Int* 2012;110:630–636.

144. Allard P, Bernard P, Fradet Y, et al. The early clinical course of primary Ta and T1 bladder cancer: a proposed prognostic index. *Br J Urol* 1998;81:692–698.

145. Allard P, Fradet Y, Tetu B, et al. Tumor-associated antigens as prognostic factors for recurrence in 382 patients with primary transitional cell carcinoma of the bladder. *Clin Cancer Res* 1995;1:1195–1202.

146. Schwarz S, Rechenmacher M, Filbeck T, et al. Value of multicolour fluorescence in situ hybridisation (UroVysion) in the differential diagnosis of flat urothelial lesions. *J Clin Pathol* 2008;61:272–277.

147. Laudadio J, Keane TE, Reeves HM, et al. Fluorescence in situ hybridization for detecting transitional cell carcinoma: implications for clinical practice. *BJU Int* 2005;96:1280–1285.

148. Sarosdy MF, Kahn PR, Ziffer MD, et al. Use of a multitarget fluorescence in situ hybridization assay to diagnose bladder cancer in patients with hematuria. *J Urol* 2006;176:44–47.

149. Tetu B, Tiguert R, Bernier V, et al. ImmunoCyt(TM) improves the accuracy of urine cytology. *Histopathology* 2002;41:409–414.

150. Skacel M, Fahmy M, Brainard JA, et al. Multitarget fluorescence in situ hybridization assay detects transitional cell carcinoma in the majority of patients with bladder cancer and atypical or negative urine cytology. *J Urol* 2003;169:2101–2105.

151. Schlomer BJ, Ho R, Sagalowsky A, et al. Prospective validation of the clinical usefulness of reflex fluorescence in situ hybridization assay in patients with atypical cytology for the detection of urothelial carcinoma of the bladder. *J Urol* 2010;183:62–67.

152. Nieder A, Soloway M. Cystoscopy. In: Lerner S, Schoenberg M, Sternberg C, eds. *Textbook of Bladder Cancer*. 1st ed. Chicago, IL: Taylor & Francis; 2006:179–185.

153. Cauberg ECC, de Bruin DM, Faber DJ, et al. A new generation of optical diagnostics for bladder cancer: technology, diagnostic accuracy, and future applications. *Eur Urol* 2009;56:287–296.

154. Carter H, Chan D. Basic instrumentation and cystoscopy. In: Wein A, Kavoussi L, Novick A, et al., eds. *Campbell-Walsh Urology*. 9th ed. Philadelphia, PA: Saunders Elsevier; 2007:161–170.

155. Wedderburn AW, Ratan P, Birch BR. A prospective trial of flexible cystodiathermy for recurrent transitional cell carcinoma of the bladder. *J Urol* 1999;161:812–814.

156. May F, Treiber U, Hartung R, et al. Significance of random bladder biopsies in superficial bladder cancer. *Eur Urol* 2003;44:47–50.

157. Kiemeney LA, Witjes JA, Heijbroek RP, et al. Dysplasia in normal-looking urothelium increases the risk of tumour progression in primary superficial bladder cancer. *Eur J Cancer* 1994;30A:1621–1625.

158. Herr H, Al-Ahmadie H, Dalbagni G, et al. Bladder cancer in cystoscopically normal-appearing mucosa: a case of mistaken identity? *BJU Int* 2010;106:1502–1507.

159. Herr HW. Does cystoscopy correlate with the histology of recurrent papillary tumours of the bladder? *BJU Int* 2001;88:683–685.

160. Zaak D, Hungerhuber E, Schneede P, et al. Role of 5-aminolevulinic acid in the detection of urothelial premalignant lesions. *Cancer* 2002;95:1234–1238.

161. Jocham D, Stepp H, Waidelich R. Photodynamic diagnosis in urology: state-of-the-art. *Eur Urol* 2008;53:1138–1148.

162. Riedl CR, Plas E, Pfluger H. Fluorescence detection of bladder tumors with 5-amino-levulinic acid. *J Endourol* 1999;13:755–759.

163. Filbeck T, Roessler W, Knuechel R, et al. 5-aminolevulinic acid-induced fluorescence endoscopy applied at secondary transurethral resection after conventional resection of primary superficial bladder tumors. *Urology* 1999;53:77–81.

164. Herr HW. Narrow-band imaging cystoscopy to evaluate the response to bacille Calmette-Guérin therapy: preliminary results. *BJU Int* 2010;105:314–316.

165. Bryan RT, Billingham LJ, Wallace DMA. Narrow-band imaging flexible cystoscopy in the detection of recurrent urothelial cancer of the bladder. *BJU Int* 2008;101:702–705.

166. Lagerveld BW, Koot RAC, Smits GAHJ. Thermal artifacts in bladder tumors following loop endoresection: electrovaporization v electrocauterization. *J Endourol* 2004;18:583–586.

167. Wang DS, Bird VG, Leonard VY, et al. Use of bipolar energy for transurethral resection of bladder tumors: pathologic considerations. *J Endourol* 2004;18:578–582.

168. Richards B, Parmar MK, Anderson CK, et al. Interpretation of biopsies of "normal" urothelium in patients with superficial bladder cancer. MRC Superficial Bladder Cancer Sub Group. *Br J Urol* 1991;67:369–375.

169. Robertson AJ, Beck JS, Burnett RA, et al. Observer variability in histopathological reporting of transitional cell carcinoma and epithelial dysplasia in bladders. *J Clin Pathol* 1990;43:17–21.

170. Hartmann A, Moser K, Kriegmair M, et al. Frequent genetic alterations in simple urothelial hyperplasias of the bladder in patients with papillary urothelial carcinoma. *Am J Pathol* 1999;154:721–727.

171. van Oers JMM, Adam C, Denzinger S, et al. Chromosome 9 deletions are more frequent than FGFR3 mutations in flat urothelial hyperplasias of the bladder. *Int J Cancer* 2006;119:1212–1215.

172. Epstein J, Amin M, Reuter V. *Bladder Biopsy Interpretation*. Philadelphia, PA: Wolters Kluwer/Lippincott Williams & Wilkins; 2010.

173. Cheng L, Cheville JC, Neumann RM, et al. Flat intraepithelial lesions of the urinary bladder. *Cancer* 2000;88:625–631.

174. Hodges KB, Lopez-Beltran A, Davidson DD, et al. Urothelial dysplasia and other flat lesions of the urinary bladder: clinicopathologic and molecular features. *Hum Pathol* 2010;41:155–162.

175. Obermann EC, Junker K, Stoehr R, et al. Frequent genetic alterations in flat urothelial hyperplasias and concomitant papillary bladder cancer as detected by CGH, LOH, and FISH analyses. *J Pathol* 2003;199:50–57.

176. Murphy WM, Busch C, Algaba F. Intraepithelial lesions of urinary bladder: morphologic considerations. *Scand J Urol Nephrol Suppl* 2000:67–81.

177. Lopez-Beltran A, Cheng L, Andersson L, et al. Preneoplastic non-papillary lesions and conditions of the urinary bladder: an update based on the Ancona International Consultation. *Virchows Arch* 2002;440:3–11.

178. Harewood LM. The significance of urothelial dysplasia as diagnosed by cup biopsies. *Aust N Z J Surg* 1986;56:199–203.

179. Kakizoe T, Matumoto K, Nishio Y, et al. Significance of carcinoma in situ and dysplasia in association with bladder cancer. *J Urol* 1985;133:395–398.

180. Wolf H, Hojgaard K. Urothelial dysplasia in random mucosal biopsies from patients with bladder tumours. *Scand J Urol Nephrol* 1980;14:37–41.

181. Cheng L, Cheville JC, Neumann RM, et al. Natural history of urothelial dysplasia of the bladder. *Am J Surg Pathol* 1999;23:443–447.

182. Harnden P, Eardley I, Joyce AD, et al. Cytokeratin 20 as an objective marker of urothelial dysplasia. *Br J Urol* 1996;78:870–875.

183. Mallofre C, Castillo M, Morente V, et al. Immunohistochemical expression of CK20, p53, and Ki-67 as objective markers of urothelial dysplasia. *Mod Pathol* 2003;16:187–191.

184. McKenney JK, Desai S, Cohen C, et al. Discriminatory immunohistochemical staining of urothelial carcinoma in situ and non-neoplastic urothelium: an analysis of cytokeratin 20, p53, and CD44 antigens. *Am J Surg Pathol* 2001;25:1074–1078.

185. Hartmann A, Schlake G, Zaak D, et al. Occurrence of chromosome 9 and p53 alterations in multifocal dysplasia and carcinoma in situ of human urinary bladder. *Cancer Res* 2002;62:809–818.

186. Farrow GM. Pathology of carcinoma in situ of the urinary bladder and related lesions. *J Cell Biochem Suppl* 1992;16I:39–43.

187. Orozco RE, Martin AA, Murphy WM. Carcinoma in situ of the urinary bladder. Clues to host involvement in human carcinogenesis. *Cancer* 1994;74:115–122.

188. Nese N, Gupta R, Bui MHT, et al. Carcinoma in situ of the urinary bladder: review of clinicopathologic characteristics with an emphasis on aspects related to molecular diagnostic techniques and prognosis. *J Natl Compr Canc Netw* 2009;7:48–57.

189. Cheng L, Cheville JC, Neumann RM, et al. Survival of patients with carcinoma in situ of the urinary bladder. *Cancer* 1999;85:2469–2474.

190. Gofrit ON, Pode D, Pizov G, et al. The natural history of bladder carcinoma in situ after initial response to bacillus Calmette-Guérin immunotherapy. *Urol Oncol* 2009;27:258–262.

191. Sylvester RJ, van der Meijden A, Witjes JA, et al. High-grade Ta urothelial carcinoma and carcinoma in situ of the bladder. *Urology* 2005;66:90–107.

192. Witjes JA. Bladder carcinoma in situ in 2003: state of the art. *Eur Urol* 2004;45:142–146.

193. Nixon RG, Chang SS, Lafleur BJ, et al. Carcinoma in situ and tumor multifocality predict the risk of prostatic urethral involvement at radical cystectomy in men with transitional cell carcinoma of the bladder. *J Urol* 2002;167:502–505.

194. Zincke H, Garbeff PJ, Beahrs JR. Upper urinary tract transitional cell cancer after radical cystectomy for bladder cancer. *J Urol* 1984;131:50–52.

195. Dalbagni G. The management of superficial bladder cancer. *Nat Clin Pract Urol* 2007;4:254–260.

196. Stein JP. Indications for early cystectomy. *Urology* 2003;62:591–595.

197. McKenney JK, Gomez JA, Desai S, et al. Morphologic expressions of urothelial carcinoma in situ: a detailed evaluation of its histologic patterns with emphasis on carcinoma in situ with microinvasion. *Am J Surg Pathol* 2001;25:356–362.

198. Patriarca C, Colombo P, Pio Taronna A, et al. Cell discohesion and multifocality of carcinoma in situ of the bladder: new insight from the adhesion molecule profile (e-cadherin, Ep-CAM, and MUC1). *Int J Surg Pathol* 2009;17:99–106.

199. Lopez-Beltran A, Jimenez RE, Montironi R, et al. Flat urothelial carcinoma in situ of the bladder with glandular differentiation. *Hum Pathol* 2011;42:1653–1659.

200. Yin H, He Q, Li T, et al. Cytokeratin 20 and Ki-67 to distinguish carcinoma in situ from flat non-neoplastic urothelium. *Appl Immunohistochem Mol Morphol* 2006;14:260–265.

201. Sarkis AS, Dalbagni G, Cordon-Cardo C, et al. Association of P53 nuclear overexpression and tumor progression in carcinoma in situ of the bladder. *J Urol* 1994;152:388–392.

202. McKenney JK, Amin MB. The role of immunohistochemistry in the diagnosis of urinary bladder neoplasms. *Semin Diagn Pathol* 2005;22:69–87.

203. Yin M, Bastacky S, Parwani AV, et al. p16ink4 immunoreactivity is a reliable marker for urothelial carcinoma in situ. *Hum Pathol* 2008;39:527–535.

204. Shariat SF, Pahlavan S, Baseman AG, et al. E-cadherin expression predicts clinical outcome in carcinoma in situ of the urinary bladder. *Urology* 2001;57:60–65.

205. Li L, Xu H, Spaulding BO, et al. Expression of RNA-binding protein IMP3 (KOC) in benign urothelium and urothelial tumors. *Hum Pathol* 2008;39:1205–1211.

206. Jones EC. Urinary bladder. Mimics of neoplasia and new pathologic entities. *Urol Clin North Am* 1999;26:509–534.

207. Cheng L, Bostwick DG. Overdiagnosis of bladder carcinoma. *Anal Quant Cytol Histol* 2008;30:261–264.

208. Cina SJ, Lancaster-Weiss KJ, Lecksell K, et al. Correlation of Ki-67 and p53 with the new World Health Organization/International Society of Urological Pathology Classification System for Urothelial Neoplasia. *Arch Pathol Lab Med* 2001;125:646–651.

209. Cheng L, Neumann RM, Bostwick DG. Papillary urothelial neoplasms of low malignant potential. Clinical and biologic implications. *Cancer* 1999;86:2102–2108.

210. Holmang S, Andius P, Hedelin H, et al. Stage progression in Ta papillary urothelial tumors: relationship to grade, immunohistochemical expression of tumor markers, mitotic frequency and DNA ploidy. *J Urol* 2001;165:1124–1128.

211. Campbell PA, Conrad RJ, Campbell CM, et al. Papillary urothelial neoplasm of low malignant potential: reliability of diagnosis and outcome. *BJU Int* 2004;93:1228–1231.

212. Barbisan F, Santinelli A, Mazzucchelli R, et al. Strong immunohistochemical expression of fibroblast growth factor receptor 3, superficial staining pattern of cytokeratin 20, and low proliferative activity define those papillary urothelial neoplasms of low malignant potential that do not recur. *Cancer* 2008;112:636–644.

213. Pan C-C, Chang Y-H, Chen K-K, et al. Prognostic significance of the 2004 WHO/ISUP classification for prediction of recurrence, progression, and cancer-specific mortality of non-muscle-invasive urothelial tumors of the urinary bladder: a clinicopathologic study of 1,515 cases. *Am J Clin Pathol* 2010;133:788–795.

214. Pich A, Chiusa L, Formiconi A, et al. Biologic differences between noninvasive papillary urothelial neoplasms of low malignant potential and low-grade (grade 1) papillary carcinomas of the bladder. *Am J Surg Pathol* 2001;25:1528–1533.

215. Cheng L, Neumann RM, Nehra A, et al. Cancer heterogeneity and its biologic implications in the grading of urothelial carcinoma. *Cancer* 2000;88:1663–1670.

216. May M, Brookman-Amissah S, Roigas J, et al. Prognostic accuracy of individual uropathologists in noninvasive urinary bladder carcinoma: a multicentre study comparing the 1973 and 2004 World Health Organisation classifications. *Eur Urol* 2010;57:850–858.

217. Raab SS, Lenel JC, Cohen MB. Low grade transitional cell carcinoma of the bladder. Cytologic diagnosis by key features as identified by logistic regression analysis. *Cancer* 1994;74:1621–1626.

218. Buck EG. Polypoid cystitis mimicking transitional cell carcinoma. *J Urol* 1984;131:963.

219. Ekelund P, Anderstrom C, Johansson SL, et al. The reversibility of catheter-associated polypoid cystitis. *J Urol* 1983;130:456–459.

220. Chang HH, Ray P, Ockuly E, et al. Benign fibrous ureteral polyps. *Urology* 1987;30:114–118.

221. Tsuzuki T, Epstein JI. Fibroepithelial polyp of the lower urinary tract in adults. *Am J Surg Pathol* 2005;29:460–466.

222. Huppmann AR, Pawel BR. Polyps and masses of the pediatric urinary bladder: a 21-year pathology review. *Pediatr Dev Pathol* 2011;14:438–444.

223. Young RH. Fibroepithelial polyp of the bladder with atypical stromal cells. *Arch Pathol Lab Med* 1986;110:241–242.

224. Jimenez RE, Gheiler E, Oskanian P, et al. Grading the invasive component of urothelial carcinoma of the bladder and its relationship with progression-free survival. *Am J Surg Pathol* 2000;24:980–987.

225. Denzinger S, Burger M, Fritsche H-M, et al. Prognostic value of histopathological tumour growth patterns at the invasion front of T1G3 urothelial carcinoma of the bladder. *Scand J Urol Nephrol* 2009;43:282–287.

226. Donhuijsen K, Schmidt U, Richter HJ, et al. Mucoid cytoplasmic inclusions in urothelial carcinomas. *Hum Pathol* 1992;23:860–864.

227. Kotliar SN, Wood CG, Schaeffer AJ, et al. Transitional cell carcinoma exhibiting clear cell features. A differential diagnosis for clear cell adenocarcinoma of the urinary tract. *Arch Pathol Lab Med* 1995;119:79–81.

228. Young RH, Wick MR. Transitional cell carcinoma of the urinary bladder with pseudosarcomatous stroma. *Am J Clin Pathol* 1988;90:216–219.

229. Tavora F, Epstein JI. Urothelial carcinoma with abundant myxoid stroma. *Hum Pathol* 2009;40:1391–1398.

230. Eble JN, Young RH. Stromal osseous metaplasia in carcinoma of the bladder. *J Urol* 1991;145:823–825.

231. Nese N, Kandiloglu AR, Atesci YZ. Nested variant of transitional cell carcinoma with osseous metaplasia of the urinary bladder: a case report and review of published reports. *Int J Urol* 2007;14:365–367.

232. Larsen MP, Steinberg GD, Brendler CB, et al. Use of Ulex europaeus agglutinin I (UEAI) to distinguish vascular and "pseudovascular" invasion in transitional cell carcinoma of bladder with lamina propria invasion. *Mod Pathol* 1990;3:83–88.

233. Amin MB, Ro JY, Lee KM, et al. Lymphoepithelioma-like carcinoma of the urinary bladder. *Am J Surg Pathol* 1994;18:466–473.

234. Baker PM, Young RH. Radiation-induced pseudocarcinomatous proliferations of the urinary bladder: a report of 4 cases. *Hum Pathol* 2000;31:678–683.

235. Chan TY, Epstein JI. Radiation or chemotherapy cystitis with "pseudocarcinomatous" features. *Am J Surg Pathol* 2004;28:909–913.

236. Lane Z, Epstein JI. Pseudocarcinomatous epithelial hyperplasia in the bladder unassociated with prior irradiation or chemotherapy. *Am J Surg Pathol* 2008;32:92–97.

237. Coleman JF, Hansel DE. Utility of diagnostic and prognostic markers in urothelial carcinoma of the bladder. *Adv Anat Pathol* 2009;16:67–78.

238. Hodges KB, Lopez-Beltran A, Emerson RE, et al. Clinical utility of immunohistochemistry in the diagnoses of urinary bladder neoplasia. *Appl Immunohistochem Mol Morphol* 2010;18:401–410.

239. Skinnider BF, Folpe AL, Hennigar RA, et al. Distribution of cytokeratins and vimentin in adult renal neoplasms and normal renal tissue: potential utility of a cytokeratin antibody panel in the differential diagnosis of renal tumors. *Am J Surg Pathol* 2005;29:747–754.

240. Chu PG, Weiss LM. Expression of cytokeratin 5/6 in epithelial neoplasms: an immunohistochemical study of 509 cases. *Mod Pathol* 2002;15:6–10.

241. Mhawech P, Uchida T, Pelte M-F. Immunohistochemical profile of high-grade urothelial bladder carcinoma and prostate adenocarcinoma. *Hum Pathol* 2002;33:1136–1140.

242. Kunju LP, Mehra R, Snyder M, et al. Prostate-specific antigen, high-molecular-weight cytokeratin (clone 34betaE12), and/or p63: an optimal immunohistochemical panel to distinguish poorly differentiated prostate adenocarcinoma from urothelial carcinoma. *Am J Clin Pathol* 2006;125:675–681.

243. Thomas P, Battifora H. Keratins versus epithelial membrane antigen in tumor diagnosis: an immunohistochemical comparison of five monoclonal antibodies. *Hum Pathol* 1987;18:728–734.

244. Parker DC, Folpe AL, Bell J, et al. Potential utility of uroplakin III, thrombomodulin, high molecular weight cytokeratin, and cytokeratin 20 in noninvasive, invasive, and metastatic urothelial (transitional cell) carcinomas. *Am J Surg Pathol* 2003;27:1–10.

245. Lindeman N, Weidner N. Immunohistochemical profile of prostatic and urothelial carcinoma: impact of heat-induced epitope retrieval and presentation of tumors with intermediate features. *Appl Immunohistochem* 1996;4:264–275.

246. Kobayashi N, Matsuzaki O, Shirai S, et al. Collecting duct carcinoma of the kidney: an immunohistochemical evaluation of the use of antibodies for differential diagnosis. *Hum Pathol* 2008;39:1350–1359.

247. Carvalho JC, Thomas DG, McHugh JB, et al. p63, CK7, PAX8 and INI-1: an optimal immunohistochemical panel to distinguish poorly differentiated urothelial cell carcinoma from high-grade tumours of the renal collecting system. *Histopathology* 2012;60:597–608.

248. Buza N, Cohen PJ, Pei H, et al. Inverse p16 and p63 expression in small cell carcinoma and high-grade urothelial cell carcinoma of the urinary bladder. *Int J Surg Pathol* 2010;18:94–102.

249. Cioffi-Lavina M, Chapman-Fredricks J, Gomez-Fernandez C, et al. P16 expression in squamous cell carcinomas of cervix and bladder. *Appl Immunohistochem Mol Morphol* 2010;18:344–347.

250. Nakazawa K, Murata S-I, Yuminamochi T, et al. p16(INK4a) expression analysis as an ancillary tool for cytologic diagnosis of urothelial carcinoma. *Am J Clin Pathol* 2009;132:776–784.

251. Shariat SF, Ashfaq R, Sagalowsky AI, et al. Predictive value of cell cycle biomarkers in nonmuscle invasive bladder transitional cell carcinoma. *J Urol* 2007;177:481–487.

252. Murali R, Delprado W. CD10 immunohistochemical staining in urothelial neoplasms. *Am J Clin Pathol* 2005;124:371–379.

253. Chu P, Arber DA. Paraffin-section detection of CD10 in 505 nonhematopoietic neoplasms. Frequent expression in renal cell carcinoma and endometrial stromal sarcoma. *Am J Clin Pathol* 2000;113:374–382.

254. Ordonez NG. Thrombomodulin expression in transitional cell carcinoma. *Am J Clin Pathol* 1998;110:385–390.

255. Kaufmann O, Volmerig J, Dietel M. Uroplakin III is a highly specific and moderately sensitive immunohistochemical marker for primary and metastatic urothelial carcinomas. *Am J Clin Pathol* 2000;113:683–687.

256. Higgins JPT, Kaygusuz G, Wang L, et al. Placental S100 (S100P) and GATA3: markers for transitional epithelium and urothelial carcinoma discovered by complementary DNA microarray. *Am J Surg Pathol* 2007;31:673–680.

257. Jiang Z, Fanger GR, Woda BA, et al. Expression of alpha-methylacyl-CoA racemase (P504s) in various malignant neoplasms and normal tissues: a study of 761 cases. *Hum Pathol* 2003;34:792–796.

258. Chuang A-Y, DeMarzo AM, Veltri RW, et al. Immunohistochemical differentiation of high-grade prostate carcinoma from urothelial carcinoma. *Am J Surg Pathol* 2007;31:1246–1255.

259. Matoso A, Singh K, Jacob R, et al. Comparison of thyroid transcription factor-1 expression by 2 monoclonal antibodies in pulmonary and nonpulmonary primary tumors. *Appl Immunohistochem Mol Morphol* 2010;18:142–149.

260. Lugli A, Forster Y, Haas P, et al. Calretinin expression in human normal and neoplastic tissues: a tissue microarray analysis on 5233 tissue samples. *Hum Pathol* 2003;34:994–1000.

261. Brimo F, Herawi M, Sharma R, et al. Hepatocyte nuclear factor-1beta expression in clear cell adenocarcinomas of the bladder and urethra: diagnostic utility and implications for histogenesis. *Hum Pathol* 2011;42:1613–1619.

262. Tong G-X, Melamed J, Mansukhani M, et al. PAX2: a reliable marker for nephrogenic adenoma. *Mod Pathol* 2006;19:356–363.

263. Tong G-X, Yu WM, Beaubier NT, et al. Expression of PAX8 in normal and neoplastic renal tissues: an immunohistochemical study. *Mod Pathol* 2009;22:1218–1227.

264. Tacha D, Zhou D, Cheng L. Expression of PAX8 in normal and neoplastic tissues: a comprehensive immunohistochemical study. *Appl Immunohistochem Mol Morphol* 2011;19:293–299.

265. Silver DA, Pellicer I, Fair WR, et al. Prostate-specific membrane antigen expression in normal and malignant human tissues. *Clin Cancer Res* 1997;3:81–85.

266. Mhawech-Fauceglia P, Zhang S, Terracciano L, et al. Prostate-specific membrane antigen (PSMA) protein expression in normal and neoplastic tissues and its sensitivity and specificity in prostate adenocarcinoma: an immunohistochemical study using multiple tumour tissue microarray technique. *Histopathology* 2007;50:472–483.

267. Kalos M, Askaa J, Hylander BL, et al. Prostein expression is highly restricted to normal and malignant prostate tissues. *Prostate* 2004;60:246–256.

268. Moskaluk CA, Zhang H, Powell SM, et al. Cdx2 protein expression in normal and malignant human tissues: an immunohistochemical survey using tissue microarrays. *Mod Pathol* 2003;16:913–919.

269. Kaufmann O, Baume H, Dietel M. Detection of oestrogen receptors in non-invasive and invasive transitional cell carcinomas of the urinary bladder using both conventional immunohistochemistry and the tyramide staining amplification (TSA) technique. *J Pathol* 1998;186:165–168.

270. Shen SS, Smith CL, Hsieh J-T, et al. Expression of estrogen receptors-alpha and -beta in bladder cancer cell lines and human bladder tumor tissue. *Cancer* 2006;106:2610–2616.

271. Bolenz C, Lotan Y, Ashfaq R, et al. Estrogen and progesterone hormonal receptor expression in urothelial carcinoma of the bladder. *Eur Urol* 2009;56:1093–1095.

272. Ikegami H, Iwasaki H, Ohjimi Y, et al. Sarcomatoid carcinoma of the urinary bladder: a clinicopathologic and immunohistochemical analysis of 14 patients. *Hum Pathol* 2000;31:332–340.

273. Loy TS, Phillips RW, Linder CL. A103 immunostaining in the diagnosis of adrenal cortical tumors: an immunohistochemical study of 316 cases. *Arch Pathol Lab Med* 2002;126:170–172.

274. Genega EM, Hutchinson B, Reuter VE, et al. Immunophenotype of high-grade prostatic adenocarcinoma and urothelial carcinoma. *Mod Pathol* 2000;13:1186–1191.

275. Bassily NH, Vallorosi CJ, Akdas G, et al. Coordinate expression of cytokeratins 7 and 20 in prostate adenocarcinoma and bladder urothelial carcinoma. *Am J Clin Pathol* 2000;113:383–388.

276. Lopez-Beltran A, Cheng L. Histologic variants of urothelial carcinoma: differential diagnosis and clinical implications. *Hum Pathol* 2006;37:1371–1388.

277. Grace DA, Winter CC. Mixed differentiation of primary carcinoma of the urinary bladder. *Cancer* 1968;21:1239–1243.

278. Lopez-Beltran A, Requena MJ, Alvarez-Kindelan J, et al. Squamous differentiation in primary urothelial carcinoma of the urinary tract as seen by MAC387 immunohistochemistry. *J Clin Pathol* 2007;60:332–335.

279. Wasco MJ, Daignault S, Zhang Y, et al. Urothelial carcinoma with divergent histologic differentiation (mixed histologic features) predicts the presence of locally advanced bladder cancer when detected at transurethral resection. *Urology* 2007;70:69–74.

280. Grignon D. Neoplasms of the urinary bladder. In: Bostwick D, Eble J, eds. *Urologic Surgical Pathology*. 1st ed. St. Louis, MO: Mosby Year Book Inc; 1997:214–305.

281. Lagwinski N, Thomas A, Stephenson AJ, et al. Squamous cell carcinoma of the bladder: a clinicopathologic analysis of 45 cases. *Am J Surg Pathol* 2007;31:1777–1787.

282. Akdas A, Turkeri L. The impact of squamous metaplasia in transitional cell carcinoma of the bladder. *Int Urol Nephrol* 1991;23:333–336.

283. Logothetis CJ, Dexeus FH, Chong C, et al. Cisplatin, cyclophosphamide and doxorubicin chemotherapy for unresectable urothelial tumors: the M.D. Anderson experience. *J Urol* 1989;141:33–37.

284. Martin JE, Jenkins BJ, Zuk RJ, et al. Human chorionic gonadotrophin expression and histological findings as predictors of response to radiotherapy in carcinoma of the bladder. *Virchows Arch A Pathol Anat Histopathol* 1989;414:273–277.

285. Alexander R, Hu Y, Kum J, et al. p16 expression is not associated with human papilloma virus (HPV) in urinary bladder squamous cell carcinoma. *Mod Pathol* 2012;25:1526–1533.

286. Fong A, Garcia E, Gwynn L, et al. Expression of caveolin-1 and caveolin-2 in urothelial carcinoma of the urinary bladder correlates with tumor grade and squamous differentiation. *Am J Clin Pathol* 2003;120:93–100.

287. Hayashi T, Sentani K, Oue N, et al. Desmocollin 2 is a new immunohistochemical marker indicative of squamous differentiation in urothelial carcinoma. *Histopathology* 2011;59:710–721.

288. Grignon DJ, Ro JY, Ayala AG, et al. Primary adenocarcinoma of the urinary bladder. A clinicopathologic analysis of 72 cases. *Cancer* 1991;67:2165–2172.

289. Choong NWW, Quevedo JF, Kaur JS. Small cell carcinoma of the urinary bladder. The Mayo Clinic experience. *Cancer* 2005;103:1172–1178.

290. Abrahams NA, Moran C, Reyes AO, et al. Small cell carcinoma of the bladder: a contemporary clinicopathological study of 51 cases. *Histopathology* 2005;46:57–63.

291. Cheng L, Jones TD, McCarthy RP, et al. Molecular genetic evidence for a common clonal origin of urinary bladder small cell carcinoma and coexisting urothelial carcinoma. *Am J Pathol* 2005;166:1533–1539.

292. Murphy WM, Deana DG. The nested variant of transitional cell carcinoma: a neoplasm resembling proliferation of Brunn's nests. *Mod Pathol* 1992;5:240–243.

293. Talbert ML, Young RH. Carcinomas of the urinary bladder with deceptively benign-appearing foci. A report of three cases. *Am J Surg Pathol* 1989;13:374–381.

294. Drew PA, Furman J, Civantos F, et al. The nested variant of transitional cell carcinoma: an aggressive neoplasm with innocuous histology. *Mod Pathol* 1996;9:989–994.

295. Holmang S, Johansson SL. The nested variant of transitional cell carcinoma—a rare neoplasm with poor prognosis. *Scand J Urol Nephrol* 2001;35:102–105.

296. Dhall D, Al-Ahmadie H, Olgac S. Nested variant of urothelial carcinoma. *Arch Pathol Lab Med* 2007;131:1725–1727.

297. Wasco MJ, Daignault S, Bradley D, et al. Nested variant of urothelial carcinoma: a clinicopathologic and immunohistochemical study of 30 pure and mixed cases. *Hum Pathol* 2010;41:163–171.

298. Lin O, Cardillo M, Dalbagni G, et al. Nested variant of urothelial carcinoma: a clinicopathologic and immunohistochemical study of 12 cases. *Mod Pathol* 2003;16:1289–1298.

299. Zhou M, Epstein JI, Young RH. Paraganglioma of the urinary bladder: a lesion that may be misdiagnosed as urothelial carcinoma in transurethral resection specimens. *Am J Surg Pathol* 2004;28:94–100.

300. Oliva E, Young RH. Nephrogenic adenoma of the urinary tract: a review of the microscopic appearance of 80 cases with emphasis on unusual features. *Mod Pathol* 1995;8:722–730.

301. Young RH. Tumor-like lesions of the urinary bladder. *Mod Pathol* 2009;22:S37–S52.

302. Young RH, Zukerberg LR. Microcystic transitional cell carcinomas of the urinary bladder. A report of four cases. *Am J Clin Pathol* 1991;96:635–639.

303. Paz A, Rath-Wolfson L, Lask D, et al. The clinical and histological features of transitional cell carcinoma of the bladder with microcysts: analysis of 12 cases. *Br J Urol* 1997;79:722–725.

304. Sari A, Uyaroglu MA, Ermete M, et al. Microcystic urothelial carcinoma of the urinary bladder metastatic to the penis. *Pathol Oncol Res* 2007;13:170–173.

305. Hansel DE, Nadasdy T, Epstein JI. Fibromyxoid nephrogenic adenoma: a newly recognized variant mimicking mucinous adenocarcinoma. *Am J Surg Pathol* 2007;31:1231–1237.

306. Young RH, Oliva E. Transitional cell carcinomas of the urinary bladder that may be underdiagnosed. A report of four invasive cases exemplifying the homology between neoplastic and non-neoplastic transitional cell lesions. *Am J Surg Pathol* 1996;20:1448–1454.

307. Huang Q, Chu PG, Lau SK, et al. Urothelial carcinoma of the urinary bladder with a component of acinar/tubular type differentiation simulating prostatic adenocarcinoma. *Hum Pathol* 2004;35:769–773.

308. Amin MB, Ro JY, el-Sharkawy T, et al. Micropapillary variant of transitional cell carcinoma of the urinary bladder. Histologic pattern resembling ovarian papillary serous carcinoma. *Am J Surg Pathol* 1994;18:1224–1232.

309. Watts KE, Hansel DE. Emerging concepts in micropapillary urothelial carcinoma. *Adv Anat Pathol* 2010;17:182–186.

310. Samaratunga H, Khoo K. Micropapillary variant of urothelial carcinoma of the urinary bladder; a clinicopathological and immunohistochemical study. *Histopathology* 2004;45:55–64.

311. Kamat AM, Dinney CPN, Gee JR, et al. Micropapillary bladder cancer: a review of the University of Texas M. D. Anderson Cancer Center experience with 100 consecutive patients. *Cancer* 2007;110:62–67.

312. Johansson SL, Borghede G, Holmang S. Micropapillary bladder carcinoma: a clinicopathological study of 20 cases. *J Urol* 1999;161: 1798–1802.

313. Maranchie JK, Bouyounes BT, Zhang PL, et al. Clinical and pathological characteristics of micropapillary transitional cell carcinoma: a highly aggressive variant. *J Urol* 2000;163:748–751.

314. Lopez-Beltran A, Montironi R, Blanca A, et al. Invasive micropapillary urothelial carcinoma of the bladder. *Hum Pathol* 2010;41:1159–1164.

315. Compérat E, Roupret M, Yaxley J, et al. Micropapillary urothelial carcinoma of the urinary bladder: a clinicopathological analysis of 72 cases. *Pathology* 2010;42:650–654.

316. Guo CC, Tamboli P, Czerniak B. Micropapillary variant of urothelial carcinoma in the upper urinary tract: a clinicopathologic study of 11 cases. *Arch Pathol Lab Med* 2009;133:62–66.

317. Ylagan LR, Humphrey PA. Micropapillary variant of transitional cell carcinoma of the urinary bladder: a report of three cases with cytologic diagnosis in urine specimens. *Acta Cytol* 2001;45:599–604.

318. Kamat AM, Gee JR, Dinney CPN, et al. The case for early cystectomy in the treatment of nonmuscle invasive micropapillary bladder carcinoma. *J Urol* 2006;175:881–885.

319. Nassar H, Pansare V, Zhang H, et al. Pathogenesis of invasive micropapillary carcinoma: role of MUC1 glycoprotein. *Mod Pathol* 2004;17:1045–1050.

320. Kuroda N, Tamura M, Ohara M, et al. Invasive micropapillary carcinoma of the urinary bladder: an immunohistochemical study of neoplastic and stromal cells. *Int J Urol* 2006;13:1015–1018.

321. Sangoi AR, Higgins JP, Rouse RV, et al. Immunohistochemical comparison of MUC1, CA125, and Her2Neu in invasive micropapillary carcinoma of the urinary tract and typical invasive urothelial carcinoma with retraction artifact. *Mod Pathol* 2009;22:660–667.

322. Lotan TL, Ye H, Melamed J, et al. Immunohistochemical panel to identify the primary site of invasive micropapillary carcinoma. *Am J Surg Pathol* 2009;33:1037–1041.

323. Sangoi AR, Beck AH, Amin MB, et al. Interobserver reproducibility in the diagnosis of invasive micropapillary carcinoma of the urinary tract among urologic pathologists. *Am J Surg Pathol* 2010;34:1367–1376.

324. Zukerberg LR, Harris NL, Young RH. Carcinomas of the urinary bladder simulating malignant lymphoma. A report of five cases. *Am J Surg Pathol* 1991;15:569–576.

325. Mai KT, Park PC, Yazdi HM, et al. Plasmacytoid urothelial carcinoma of the urinary bladder report of seven new cases. *Eur Urol* 2006;50:1111–1114.

326. Ro JY, Shen SS, Lee HI, et al. Plasmacytoid transitional cell carcinoma of urinary bladder: a clinicopathologic study of 9 cases. *Am J Surg Pathol* 2008;32:752–757.

327. Fritsche HM, Burger M, Denzinger S, et al. Plasmacytoid urothelial carcinoma of the bladder: histological and clinical features of 5 cases. *J Urol* 2008;180:1923–1927.

328. Baldwin L, Lee AHS, Al-Talib RK, et al. Transitional cell carcinoma of the bladder mimicking lobular carcinoma of the breast: a discohesive variant of urothelial carcinoma. *Histopathology* 2005;46:50–56.

329. Nigwekar P, Tamboli P, Amin MB, et al. Plasmacytoid urothelial carcinoma: detailed analysis of morphology with clinicopathologic correlation in 17 cases. *Am J Surg Pathol* 2009;33:417–424.

330. Grignon DJ, Ro JY, Ayala AG, et al. Primary signet-ring cell carcinoma of the urinary bladder. *Am J Clin Pathol* 1991;95:13–20.

331. Saphir O. Signet-ring cell carcinoma of the urinary bladder. *Am J Pathol* 1955;31:223–231.

332. Keck B, Stoehr R, Wach S, et al. The plasmacytoid carcinoma of the bladder—rare variant of aggressive urothelial carcinoma. *Int J Cancer* 2011;129:346–354.

333. Ricardo-Gonzalez RR, Nguyen M, Gokden N, et al. Plasmacytoid carcinoma of the bladder: a urothelial carcinoma variant with a predilection for intraperitoneal spread. *J Urol* 2012;187:852–855.

334. Sahin AA, Myhre M, Ro JY, et al. Plasmacytoid transitional cell carcinoma. Report of a case with initial presentation mimicking multiple myeloma. *Acta Cytol* 1991;35:277–280.

335. Patriarca C, Di Pasquale M, Giunta P, et al. CD138-positive plasmacytoid urothelial carcinoma of the bladder. *Int J Surg Pathol* 2008;16:215–217.

336. Dinney CP, Ro JY, Babaian RJ, et al. Lymphoepithelioma of the bladder: a clinicopathological study of 3 cases. *J Urol* 1993;149:840–841.

337. Holmang S, Borghede G, Johansson SL. Bladder carcinoma with lymphoepithelioma-like differentiation: a report of 9 cases. *J Urol* 1998;159:779–782.

338. Izquierdo-Garcia FM, Garcia-Diez F, Fernandez I, et al. Lymphoepithelioma-like carcinoma of the bladder: three cases with clinicopathological and p53 protein expression study. *Virchows Arch* 2004;444:420–425.

339. Tamas EF, Nielsen ME, Schoenberg MP, et al. Lymphoepithelioma-like carcinoma of the urinary tract: a clinicopathological study of 30 pure and mixed cases. *Mod Pathol* 2007;20:828–834.

340. Lopez-Beltran A, Luque RJ, Vicioso L, et al. Lymphoepithelioma-like carcinoma of the urinary bladder: a clinicopathologic study of 13 cases. *Virchows Arch* 2001;438:552–557.

341. Williamson SR, Zhang S, Lopez-Beltran A, et al. Lymphoepithelioma-like carcinoma of the urinary bladder: clinicopathologic, immunohistochemical, and molecular features. *Am J Surg Pathol* 2011;35:474–483.

342. Gulley ML, Amin MB, Nicholls JM, et al. Epstein-Barr virus is detected in undifferentiated nasopharyngeal carcinoma but not in lymphoepithelioma-like carcinoma of the urinary bladder. *Hum Pathol* 1995;26:1207–1214.

343. Chikwava KR, Gingrich JR, Parwani AV. Lymphoepithelioma-like carcinoma of the urinary bladder. *Pathology* 2008;40:310–311.

344. Kitazawa M, Kobayashi H, Ohnishi Y, et al. Giant cell tumor of the bladder associated with transitional cell carcinoma. *J Urol* 1985;133:472–475.

345. Serio G, Zampatti C, Ceppi M. Spindle and giant cell carcinoma of the urinary bladder: a clinicopathological light microscopic and immunohistochemical study. *Br J Urol* 1995;75:167–172.

346. Lopez-Beltran A, Blanca A, Montironi R, et al. Pleomorphic giant cell carcinoma of the urinary bladder. *Hum Pathol* 2009;40:1461–1466.

347. Ohtsuki Y, Furihata M, Iwata J, et al. Multinucleated giant cells in submucosal layer of human urinary bladder: an immunohistochemical and electron microscopic study. *Pathol Res Pract* 2000;196:293–298.

348. Wells H. Giant cells in cystitis. *Arch Pathol Lab Med* 1938;26:32–43.

349. Zukerberg LR, Armin AR, Pisharodi L, et al. Transitional cell carcinoma of the urinary bladder with osteoclast-type giant cells: a report of two cases and review of the literature. *Histopathology* 1990;17:407–411.

350. Baydar D, Amin MB, Epstein JI. Osteoclast-rich undifferentiated carcinomas of the urinary tract. *Mod Pathol* 2006;19:161–171.

351. Grammatico D, Grignon DJ, Eberwein P, et al. Transitional cell carcinoma of the renal pelvis with choriocarcinomatous differentiation.

Immunohistochemical and immunoelectron microscopic assessment of human chorionic gonadotropin production by transitional cell carcinoma of the urinary bladder. *Cancer* 1993;71:1835–1841.

352. Dexeus F, Logothetis C, Hossan E, et al. Carcinoembryonic antigen and beta-human chorionic gonadotropin as serum markers for advanced urothelial malignancies. *J Urol* 1986;136:403–407.

353. Iles RK, Jenkins BJ, Oliver RT, et al. Beta human chorionic gonadotrophin in serum and urine. A marker for metastatic urothelial cancer. *Br J Urol* 1989;64:241–244.

354. Iles RK, Butler SA. Human urothelial carcinomas—a typical disease of the aged: the clinical utility of human chorionic gonadotrophin in patient management and future therapy. *Exp Gerontol* 1998;33:379–391.

355. Dirnhofer S, Koessler P, Ensinger C, et al. Production of trophoblastic hormones by transitional cell carcinoma of the bladder: association to tumor stage and grade. *Hum Pathol* 1998;29:377–382.

356. Hotakainen K, Lintula S, Jarvinen R, et al. Overexpression of human chorionic gonadotropin beta genes 3, 5 and 8 in tumor tissue and urinary cells of bladder cancer patients. *Tumour Biol* 2007;28:52–56.

357. Iles RK. Ectopic hCGbeta expression by epithelial cancer: malignant behaviour, metastasis and inhibition of tumor cell apoptosis. *Mol Cell Endocrinol* 2007;260–262:264–270.

358. Regalado JJ. Mixed micropapillary and trophoblastic carcinoma of bladder: report of a first case with new immunohistochemical evidence of urothelial origin. *Hum Pathol* 2004;35:382–384.

359. Shimada K, Nakamura M, Ishida E, et al. Urothelial carcinoma with plasmacytoid variants producing both human chorionic gonadotropin and carbohydrate antigen 19-9. *Urology* 2006;68:891.e7–e10.

360. Hanna NH, Ulbright TM, Einhorn LH. Primary choriocarcinoma of the bladder with the detection of isochromosome 12p. *J Urol* 2002;167:1781.

361. Amir G, Rosenmann E. Osteoclast-like giant cell tumour of the urinary bladder. *Histopathology* 1990;17:413–418.

362. O'Connor RC, Hollowell CMP, Laven BA, et al. Recurrent giant cell carcinoma of the bladder. *J Urol* 2002;167:1784.

363. Garcia Garcia F, Garcia Ligero J, Martinez Diaz F, et al. [Bladder carcinoma with osteoclast-type giant cells. A case with a rare presentation. Review of the literature]. *Actas Urol Esp* 2003;27:317–320.

364. Kruger S, Johannisson R, Kausch I, et al. Papillary urothelial bladder carcinoma associated with osteoclast-like giant cells. *Int Urol Nephrol* 2005;37:61–64.

365. Behzatoglu K. Osteoclast-rich undifferentiated carcinoma of the urinary bladder: is it really an entity? *Adv Anat Pathol* 2010;17:288.

366. McCash SI, Unger P, Dillon R, et al. Undifferentiated carcinoma of the renal pelvis with osteoclast-like giant cells: a report of two cases. *APMIS* 2010;118:407–412.

367. Lidgi S, Embon OM, Turani H, et al. Giant cell reparative granuloma of the bladder associated with transitional cell carcinoma. *J Urol* 1989;142:120–122.

368. Holtz F, Fox JE, Abell MR. Carcinosarcoma of the urinary bladder. *Cancer* 1972;29:294–304.

369. Cox RM, Schneider AG, Sangoi AR, et al. Invasive urothelial carcinoma with chordoid features: a report of 12 distinct cases characterized by prominent myxoid stroma and cordlike epithelial architecture. *Am J Surg Pathol* 2009;33:1213–1219.

370. Jones EC, Young RH. Myxoid and sclerosing sarcomatoid transitional cell carcinoma of the urinary bladder: a clinicopathologic and immunohistochemical study of 25 cases. *Mod Pathol* 1997;10:908–916.

371. Torenbeek R, Blomjous CE, de Bruin PC, et al. Sarcomatoid carcinoma of the urinary bladder. Clinicopathologic analysis of 18 cases with immunohistochemical and electron microscopic findings. *Am J Surg Pathol* 1994;18:241–249.

372. Young RH, Proppe KH, Dickersin GR, et al. Myxoid leiomyosarcoma of the urinary bladder. *Arch Pathol Lab Med* 1987;111:359–362.

373. Oliva E, Amin MB, Jimenez R, et al. Clear cell carcinoma of the urinary bladder: a report and comparison of four tumors of mullerian origin and nine of probable urothelial origin with discussion of histogenesis and diagnostic problems. *Am J Surg Pathol* 2002;26:190–197.

374. Oliva E, Young RH. Clear cell adenocarcinoma of the urethra: a clinicopathologic analysis of 19 cases. *Mod Pathol* 1996;9:513–520.

375. Sim SJ, Ro JY, Ordonez NG, et al. Metastatic renal cell carcinoma to the bladder: a clinicopathologic and immunohistochemical study. *Mod Pathol* 1999;12:351–355.

376. Leroy X, Gonzalez S, Zini L, et al. Lipoid-cell variant of urothelial carcinoma: a clinicopathologic and immunohistochemical study of five cases. *Am J Surg Pathol* 2007;31:770–773.

377. Lopez-Beltran A, Amin MB, Oliveira PS, et al. Urothelial carcinoma of the bladder, lipid cell variant: clinicopathologic findings and LOH analysis. *Am J Surg Pathol* 2010;34:371–376.

378. Duvdevani M, Nass D, Neumann Y, et al. Pure rhabdoid tumor of the bladder. *J Urol* 2001;166:2337.

379. Inagaki T, Nagata M, Kaneko M, et al. Carcinosarcoma with rhabdoid features of the urinary bladder in a 2-year-old girl: possible histogenesis of stem cell origin. *Pathol Int* 2000;50:973–978.

380. Harris M, Eyden BP, Joglekar VM. Rhabdoid tumour of the bladder: a histological, ultrastructural and immunohistochemical study. *Histopathology* 1987;11:1083–1092.

381. Kumar S, Kumar D, Cowan DF. Transitional cell carcinoma with rhabdoid features. *Am J Surg Pathol* 1992;16:515–521.

382. Parwani AV, Herawi M, Volmar K, et al. Urothelial carcinoma with rhabdoid features: report of 6 cases. *Hum Pathol* 2006;37:168–172.

383. Chang JH, Dikranian AH, Johnston WH, et al. Malignant extrarenal rhabdoid tumor of the bladder: 9-year survival after chemotherapy and partial cystectomy. *J Urol* 2004;171:820–821.

384. Versteege I, Sevenet N, Lange J, et al. Truncating mutations of hSNF5/INI1 in aggressive paediatric cancer. *Nature* 1998;394:203–206.

385. Hoot AC, Russo P, Judkins AR, et al. Immunohistochemical analysis of hSNF5/INI1 distinguishes renal and extra-renal malignant rhabdoid tumors from other pediatric soft tissue tumors. *Am J Surg Pathol* 2004;28:1485–1491.

386. Wright JL, Black PC, Brown GA, et al. Differences in survival among patients with sarcomatoid carcinoma, carcinosarcoma and urothelial carcinoma of the bladder. *J Urol* 2007;178:2302–2306.

387. Ro J, Ayala A, Wishnow K, et al. Sarcomatoid bladder carcinoma: clinical, pathologic and immunohistochemical study. *Surg Pathol* 1988;1:359–374.

388. Lopez-Beltran A, Pacelli A, Rothenberg HJ, et al. Carcinosarcoma and sarcomatoid carcinoma of the bladder: clinicopathological study of 41 cases. *J Urol* 1998;159:1497–1503.

389. Spiess PE, Tuziak T, Tibbs RF, et al. Pseudosarcomatous and sarcomatous proliferations of the bladder. *Hum Pathol* 2007;38:753–761.

390. Sung MT, Wang M, MacLennan GT, et al. Histogenesis of sarcomatoid urothelial carcinoma of the urinary bladder: evidence for a common clonal origin with divergent differentiation. *J Pathol* 2007;211:420–430.

391. Cheng L, Zhang S, Alexander R, et al. Sarcomatoid carcinoma of the urinary bladder: the final common pathway of urothelial carcinoma dedifferentiation. *Am J Surg Pathol* 2011;35:e34–e46.

392. Pitt MA, Morphopoulos G, Wells S, et al. Pseudoangiosarcomatous carcinoma of the genitourinary tract. *J Clin Pathol* 1995;48:1059–1061.

393. Bloxham CA, Bennett MK, Robinson MC. Bladder carcinosarcomas: three cases with diverse histogenesis. *Histopathology* 1990;16:63–67.

394. Bannach B, Grignon D, Shum D. Sarcomatoid transitional cell carcinoma versus pseudosarcomatous stromal reaction in bladder carcinoma. *J Urol Pathol* 1993;1:105–119.

395. Westfall DE, Folpe AL, Paner GP, et al. Utility of a comprehensive immunohistochemical panel in the differential diagnosis of spindle cell lesions of the urinary bladder. *Am J Surg Pathol* 2009;33:99–105.

396. Jao W, Soto JM, Gould VE. Squamous carcinoma of bladder with pseudosarcomatous stroma. *Arch Pathol Lab Med* 1975;99:461–466.

397. Nakachi K, Miyamoto I, Kuroda J, et al. [A case of transitional cell carcinoma of the bladder with heterotopic bone formation]. *Acta Urol Jpn* 1988;34:1651–1655.

398. Toma H, Yamashita N, Nakazawa H, et al. Transitional cell carcinoma with osteoid metaplasia. *Urology* 1986;27:174–176.

399. Harik LR, Merino C, Coindre J-M, et al. Pseudosarcomatous myofibroblastic proliferations of the bladder: a clinicopathologic study of 42 cases. *Am J Surg Pathol* 2006;30:787–794.

400. Sukov WR, Cheville JC, Carlson AW, et al. Utility of ALK-1 protein expression and ALK rearrangements in distinguishing inflammatory myofibroblastic tumor from malignant spindle cell lesions of the urinary bladder. *Mod Pathol* 2007;20:592–603.

401. Mikulowski P, Hellsten S. T1 G1 urinary bladder carcinoma: fact or fiction? *Scand J Urol Nephrol* 2005;39:135–137.

402. Bell JT, Burney SW, Friedell GH. Blood vessel invasion in human bladder cancer. *J Urol* 1971;105:675–678.

403. Lopez JI, Angulo JC. The prognostic significance of vascular invasion in stage T1 bladder cancer. *Histopathology* 1995;27:27–33.

404. Lotan Y, Gupta A, Shariat SF, et al. Lymphovascular invasion is independently associated with overall survival, cause-specific survival, and local and distant recurrence in patients with negative lymph nodes at radical cystectomy. *J Clin Oncol* 2005;23:6533–6539.

405. Kunju LP, You L, Zhang Y, et al. Lymphovascular invasion of urothelial cancer in matched transurethral bladder tumor resection and radical cystectomy specimens. *J Urol* 2008;180:1928–1932.

406. Canter D, Guzzo T, Resnick M, et al. The presence of lymphovascular invasion in radical cystectomy specimens from patients with urothelial carcinoma portends a poor clinical prognosis. *BJU Int* 2008;102:952–957.

407. Streeper NM, Simons CM, Konety BR, et al. The significance of lymphovascular invasion in transurethral resection of bladder tumour and cystectomy specimens on the survival of patients with urothelial bladder cancer. *BJU Int* 2009;103:475–479.

408. Algaba F. Lymphovascular invasion as a prognostic tool for advanced bladder cancer. *Curr Opin Urol* 2006;16:367–371.

409. Reuter VE. Lymphovascular invasion as an independent predictor of recurrence and survival in node-negative bladder cancer remains to be proven. *J Clin Oncol* 2005;23:6450–6451.

410. Lopez-Beltran A, Bassi PF, Pavone-Macaluso M, et al.; European Society of Uropathology, Uropathology Working Group. Handling and pathology reporting of specimens with carcinoma of the urinary bladder, ureter, and renal pelvis. A joint proposal of the European Society of Uropathology and the Uropathology Working Group. *Virchows Arch* 2004;445:103–110.

411. Kruger S, Noack F, Bohle A, et al. Histologic tumor growth pattern is significantly associated with disease-related survival in muscle-invasive transitional cell carcinoma of the urinary bladder. *Oncol Rep* 2004;12:609–613.

412. Bircan S, Candir O, Kapucuoglu N. The effect of tumor invasion patterns on pathologic stage of bladder urothelial carcinomas. *Pathol Oncol Res* 2005;11:87–91.

413. Langner C, Hutterer G, Chromecki T, et al. Patterns of invasion and histological growth as prognostic indicators in urothelial carcinoma of the upper urinary tract. *Virchows Arch* 2006;448:604–611.

414. Netto GJ, Epstein JI. Theranostic and prognostic biomarkers: genomic applications in urological malignancies. *Pathology* 2010;42:384–394.

415. Netto GJ, Cheng L. Emerging critical role of molecular testing in diagnostic genitourinary pathology. *Arch Pathol Lab Med* 2012;136:372–390.

416. Cheng L, Zhang S, MacLennan GT, et al. Bladder cancer: translating molecular genetic insights into clinical practice. *Hum Pathol* 2011;42:455–481.

417. Malats N, Bustos A, Nascimento CM, et al. P53 as a prognostic marker for bladder cancer: a meta-analysis and review. *Lancet Oncol* 2005;6:678–686.

418. Liukkonen T, Rajala P, Raitanen M, et al. Prognostic value of MIB-1 score, p53, EGFr, mitotic index and papillary status in primary superficial (Stage pTa/T1) bladder cancer: a prospective comparative study. The Finnbladder Group. *Eur Urol* 1999;36:393–400.

419. Pfister C, Moore L, Allard P, et al. Predictive value of cell cycle markers p53, MDM2, p21, and Ki-67 in superficial bladder tumor recurrence. *Clin Cancer Res* 1999;5:4079–4084.

420. Sarkis AS, Dalbagni G, Cordon-Cardo C, et al. Nuclear overexpression of p53 protein in transitional cell bladder carcinoma: a marker for disease progression. *J Natl Cancer Inst* 1993;85:53–59.

421. Pycha A, Mian C, Posch B, et al. Numerical chromosomal aberrations in muscle invasive squamous cell and transitional cell cancer of the urinary bladder: an alternative to classic prognostic indicators? *Urology* 1999;53:1005–1010.

422. Sarkis AS, Bajorin DF, Reuter VE, et al. Prognostic value of p53 nuclear overexpression in patients with invasive bladder cancer treated with neoadjuvant MVAC. *J Clin Oncol* 1995;13:1384–1390.

423. Kubota Y, Miyamoto H, Noguchi S, et al. The loss of retinoblastoma gene in association with c-myc and transforming growth factor-beta 1 gene expression in human bladder cancer. *J Urol* 1995;154:371–374.

424. Cote RJ, Dunn MD, Chatterjee SJ, et al. Elevated and absent pRb expression is associated with bladder cancer progression and has cooperative effects with p53. *Cancer Res* 1998;58:1090–1094.

425. Chatterjee SJ, Datar R, Youssefzadeh D, et al. Combined effects of p53, p21, and pRb expression in the progression of bladder transitional cell carcinoma. *J Clin Oncol* 2004;22:1007–1013.

426. Shariat SF, Bolenz C, Godoy G, et al. Predictive value of combined immunohistochemical markers in patients with pT1 urothelial carcinoma at radical cystectomy. *J Urol* 2009;182:78–84.

427. Rabbani F, Koppie TM, Charytonowicz E, et al. Prognostic significance of p27Kip1 expression in bladder cancer. *BJU Int* 2007;100:259–263.

428. Bol MGW, Baak JPA, Rep S, et al. Prognostic value of proliferative activity and nuclear morphometry for progression in TaT1 urothelial cell carcinomas of the urinary bladder. *Urology* 2002;60:1124–1130.

429. van Rhijn BW, Zuiverloon TC, Vis AN, et al. Molecular grade (FGFR3/MIB-1) and EORTC risk scores are predictive in primary non-muscle-invasive bladder cancer. *Eur Urol* 2010;58:433–441.

430. Quintero A, Alvarez-Kindelan J, Luque RJ, et al. Ki-67 MIB1 labelling index and the prognosis of primary TaT1 urothelial cell carcinoma of the bladder. *J Clin Pathol* 2006;59:83–88.

431. Gonzalez-Campora R, Davalos-Casanova G, Beato-Moreno A, et al. Apoptotic and proliferation indexes in primary superficial bladder tumors. *Cancer Lett* 2006;242:266–272.

432. Margulis V, Lotan Y, Karakiewicz PI, et al. Multi-institutional validation of the predictive value of Ki-67 labeling index in patients with urinary bladder cancer. *J Natl Cancer Inst* 2009;101:114–119.

433. Pich A, Chiusa L, Formiconi A, et al. Proliferative activity is the most significant predictor of recurrence in noninvasive papillary urothelial neoplasms of low malignant potential and grade 1 papillary carcinomas of the bladder. *Cancer* 2002;95:784–790.

434. Lopez-Beltran A, Luque RJ, Alvarez-Kindelan J, et al. Prognostic factors in survival of patients with stage Ta and T1 bladder urothelial tumors: the role of G1-S modulators (p53, p21Waf1, p27Kip1, cyclin D1, and cyclin D3), proliferation index, and clinicopathologic parameters. *Am J Clin Pathol* 2004;122:444–452.

435. Kong G, Shin KY, Oh YH, et al. Bcl-2 and p53 expressions in invasive bladder cancers. *Acta Oncol* 1998;37:715–720.

436. Karam JA, Lotan Y, Karakiewicz PI, et al. Use of combined apoptosis biomarkers for prediction of bladder cancer recurrence and mortality after radical cystectomy. *Lancet Oncol* 2007;8:128–136.

437. Yamana K, Bilim V, Hara N, et al. Prognostic impact of FAS/CD95/APO-1 in urothelial cancers: decreased expression of Fas is associated with disease progression. *Br J Cancer* 2005;93:544–551.

438. Maluf FC, Cordon-Cardo C, Verbel DA, et al. Assessing interactions between mdm-2, p53, and bcl-2 as prognostic variables in muscle-invasive bladder cancer treated with neo-adjuvant chemotherapy followed by locoregional surgical treatment. *Ann Oncol* 2006;17:1677–1686.

439. Shariat SF, Ashfaq R, Karakiewicz PI, et al. Survivin expression is associated with bladder cancer presence, stage, progression, and mortality. *Cancer* 2007;109:1106–1113.

440. Shariat SF, Karakiewicz PI, Godoy G, et al. Survivin as a prognostic marker for urothelial carcinoma of the bladder: a multicenter external validation study. *Clin Cancer Res* 2009;15:7012–7019.

441. Fristrup N, Ulhoi BP, Birkenkamp-Demtroder K, et al. Cathepsin E, maspin, Plk1, and survivin are promising prognostic protein markers for progression in non-muscle invasive bladder cancer. *Am J Pathol* 2012;180:1824–1834.

442. Kiyoshima K, Oda Y, Kinukawa N, et al. Overexpression of laminin-5 gamma2 chain and its prognostic significance in urothelial carcinoma of urinary bladder: association with expression of cyclooxygenase 2, epidermal growth factor receptor and human epidermal growth factor receptor 2. *Hum Pathol* 2005;36:522–530.

443. Colquhoun AJ, Sundar S, Rajjayabun PH, et al. Epidermal growth factor receptor status predicts local response to radical radiotherapy in muscle-invasive bladder cancer. *Clin Oncol (R Coll Radiol)* 2006;18:702–709.

444. Kassouf W, Luongo T, Brown G, et al. Schedule dependent efficacy of Gefitinib and Docetaxel for bladder cancer. *J Urol* 2006;176:787–792.

445. Chaux A, Cohen J, Schultz L, et al. High epidermal growth factor receptor immunohistochemical expression in urothelial carcinoma of the bladder is not associated with *EGFR* mutations in exons 19 and 21: a study using formalin-fixed, paraffin-enbedded archival tissues. *Hum Pathol* 2012;43:1590–1595.

446. Jimenez RE, Hussain M, Bianco FJ Jr, et al. Her-2/neu overexpression in muscle-invasive urothelial carcinoma of the bladder: prognostic significance and comparative analysis in primary and metastatic tumors. *Clin Cancer Res* 2001;7:2440–2447.

447. Kruger S, Weitsch G, Buttner H, et al. HER2 overexpression in muscle-invasive urothelial carcinoma of the bladder: prognostic implications. *Int J Cancer* 2002;102:514–518.

448. Kolla SB, Seth A, Singh MK, et al. Prognostic significance of Her2/neu overexpression in patients with muscle invasive urinary bladder cancer treated with radical cystectomy. *Int Urol Nephrol* 2008;40: 321–327.

449. Memon AA, Sorensen BS, Meldgaard P, et al. The relation between survival and expression of HER1 and HER2 depends on the expression of HER3 and HER4: a study in bladder cancer patients. *Br J Cancer* 2006;94:1703–1709.

450. Bochner BH, Cote RJ, Weidner N, et al. Angiogenesis in bladder cancer: relationship between microvessel density and tumor prognosis. *J Natl Cancer Inst* 1995;87:1603–1612.

451. Shariat SF, Youssef RF, Gupta A, et al. Association of angiogenesis related markers with bladder cancer outcomes and other molecular markers. *J Urol* 2010;183:1744–1750.

452. Miyata Y, Kanda S, Ohba K, et al. Lymphangiogenesis and angiogenesis in bladder cancer: prognostic implications and regulation by vascular endothelial growth factors-A, -C, and -D. *Clin Cancer Res* 2006;12:800–806.

453. Ioachim E, Michael MC, Salmas M, et al. Thrombospondin-1 expression in urothelial carcinoma: prognostic significance and association with p53 alterations, tumour angiogenesis and extracellular matrix components. *BMC Cancer* 2006;6:140.

454. Grossfeld GD, Ginsberg DA, Stein JP, et al. Thrombospondin-1 expression in bladder cancer: association with p53 alterations, tumor angiogenesis, and tumor progression. *J Natl Cancer Inst* 1997;89:219–227.

455. Birkhahn M, Mitra AP, Williams AJ, et al. Predicting recurrence and progression of noninvasive papillary bladder cancer at initial presentation based on quantitative gene expression profiles. *Eur Urol* 2010;57:12–20.

456. Sanchez-Carbayo M, Socci ND, Lozano J, et al. Defining molecular profiles of poor outcome in patients with invasive bladder cancer using oligonucleotide microarrays. *J Clin Oncol* 2006;24:778–789.

457. Lindgren D, Frigyesi A, Gudjonsson S, et al. Combined gene expression and genomic profiling define two intrinsic molecular subtypes of urothelial carcinoma and gene signatures for molecular grading and outcome. *Cancer Res* 2010;70:3463–3472.

458. Babjuk M, Oosterlinck W, Sylvester R, et al. EAU guidelines on non-muscle-invasive urothelial carcinoma of the bladder. *Eur Urol* 2008;54:303–314.

459. Dalbagni G, Genega E, Hashibe M, et al. Cystectomy for bladder cancer: a contemporary series. *J Urol* 2001;165:1111–1116.

460. Boudreaux KJ Jr, Clark PE, Lowrance WT, et al. Comparison of American Joint Committee on Cancer pathological stage T2a versus T2b urothelial carcinoma: analysis of patient outcomes in organ confined bladder cancer. *J Urol* 2009;181:540–545.

461. Boudreaux KJ Jr, Chang SS, Lowrance WT, et al. Comparison of American Joint Committee on Cancer pathologic stage T3a versus T3b urothelial carcinoma: analysis of patient outcomes. *Cancer* 2009;115:770–775.

462. Gofrit ON, Pode D, Lazar A, et al. Watchful waiting policy in recurrent Ta G1 bladder tumors. *Eur Urol* 2006;49:303–306.

463. Sylvester RJ, Oosterlinck W, van der Meijden APM. A single immediate postoperative instillation of chemotherapy decreases the risk of recurrence in patients with stage Ta T1 bladder cancer: a meta-analysis of published results of randomized clinical trials. *J Urol* 2004;171:2186–2190.

464. Han RF, Pan JG. Can intravesical bacillus Calmette-Guérin reduce recurrence in patients with superficial bladder cancer? A meta-analysis of randomized trials. *Urology* 2006;67:1216–1223.

465. Sylvester RJ, van der Meijden APM, Lamm DL. Intravesical bacillus Calmette-Guérin reduces the risk of progression in patients with superficial bladder cancer: a meta-analysis of the published results of randomized clinical trials. *J Urol* 2002;168:1964–1970.

466. Bohle A, Jocham D, Bock PR. Intravesical bacillus Calmette-Guérin versus mitomycin C for superficial bladder cancer: a formal meta-analysis of comparative studies on recurrence and toxicity. *J Urol* 2003;169:90–95.

467. van der Meijden APM, Sylvester RJ, Oosterlinck W, et al.; EORTC Genito-Urinary Track Cancer Group. Maintenance bacillus Calmette-Guérin for Ta T1 bladder tumors is not associated with increased toxicity: results from a European Organisation for Research and Treatment of Cancer Genito-Urinary Group Phase III Trial. *Eur Urol* 2003;44:429–434.

468. Gupta A, Lotan Y, Bastian PJ, et al. Outcomes of patients with clinical T1 grade 3 urothelial cell bladder carcinoma treated with radical cystectomy. *Urology* 2008;71:302–307.

469. Schwaibold HE, Sivalingam S, May F, et al. The value of a second transurethral resection for T1 bladder cancer. *BJU Int* 2006;97: 1199–1201.

470. Herr HW. Tumour progression and survival in patients with T1G3 bladder tumours: 15-year outcome. *Br J Urol* 1997;80:762–765.

471. Raj GV, Herr H, Serio AM, et al. Treatment paradigm shift may improve survival of patients with high risk superficial bladder cancer. *J Urol* 2007;177:1283–1286.

472. Fritsche H-M, Burger M, Svatek RS, et al. Characteristics and outcomes of patients with clinical T1 grade 3 urothelial carcinoma treated with radical cystectomy: results from an international cohort. *Eur Urol* 2010;57:300–309.

473. Donat SM, Shabsigh A, Savage C, et al. Potential impact of postoperative early complications on the timing of adjuvant chemotherapy in patients undergoing radical cystectomy: a high-volume tertiary cancer center experience. *Eur Urol* 2009;55:177–185.

474. Emiliozzi P, Pansadoro A, Pansadoro V. The optimal management of T1G3 bladder cancer. *BJU Int* 2008;102:1265–1273.

475. Kulkarni GS, Hakenberg OW, Gschwend JE, et al. An updated critical analysis of the treatment strategy for newly diagnosed high-grade T1 (previously T1G3) bladder cancer. *Eur Urol* 2010;57:60–70.

476. Morris DS, Weizer AZ, Ye Z, et al. Understanding bladder cancer death: tumor biology versus physician practice. *Cancer* 2009;115: 1011–1020.

477. Thalmann GN, Stein JP. Outcomes of radical cystectomy. *BJU Int* 2008;102:1279–1288.

478. Gschwend JE. Bladder substitution. *Curr Opin Urol* 2003;13: 477–482.

479. Donat SM. Argument against frozen section analysis of distal ureters in transitional cell bladder cancer. *Nat Clin Pract Urol* 2008;5:538–539.

480. Stein JP, Lieskovsky G, Cote R, et al. Radical cystectomy in the treatment of invasive bladder cancer: long-term results in 1,054 patients. *J Clin Oncol* 2001;19:666–675.

481. Milowsky MI, Stadler WM, Bajorin DF. Integration of neoadjuvant and adjuvant chemotherapy and cystectomy in the treatment of muscle-invasive bladder cancer. *BJU Int* 2008;102:1339–1344.

482. Herr HW, Bajorin DF, Scher HI. Neoadjuvant chemotherapy and bladder-sparing surgery for invasive bladder cancer: ten-year outcome. *J Clin Oncol* 1998;16:1298–1301.

483. Shipley WU, Kaufman DS, Zehr E, et al. Selective bladder preservation by combined modality protocol treatment: long-term outcomes of 190 patients with invasive bladder cancer. *Urology* 2002;60:62–67.

484. Herr HW. Transurethral resection of muscle-invasive bladder cancer: 10-year outcome. *J Clin Oncol* 2001;19:89–93.

485. Sternberg CN, de Mulder P, Schornagel JH, et al. Seven year update of an EORTC phase III trial of high-dose intensity M-VAC chemotherapy and G-CSF versus classic M-VAC in advanced urothelial tract tumours. *Eur J Cancer* 2006;42:50–54.

486. von der Maase H, Sengelov L, Roberts JT, et al. Long-term survival results of a randomized trial comparing gemcitabine plus cisplatin, with methotrexate, vinblastine, doxorubicin, plus cisplatin in patients with bladder cancer. *J Clin Oncol* 2005;23:4602–4608.

487. El-Bolkainy MN, Mokhtar NM, Ghoneim MA, et al. The impact of schistosomiasis on the pathology of bladder carcinoma. *Cancer* 1981;48:2643–2648.

488. Felix AS, Soliman AS, Khaled H, et al. The changing patterns of bladder cancer in Egypt over the past 26 years. *Cancer Causes Control* 2008;19:421–429.

489. Fedewa SA, Soliman AS, Ismail K, et al. Incidence analyses of bladder cancer in the Nile delta region of Egypt. *Cancer Epidemiol* 2009;33:176–181.

490. Sarma KP. Squamous cell carcinoma of the bladder. *Int Surg* 1970;53:313–319.

491. Kassouf W, Spiess PE, Siefker-Radtke A, et al. Outcome and patterns of recurrence of nonbilharzial pure squamous cell carcinoma of the bladder: a contemporary review of The University of Texas M D Anderson Cancer Center experience. *Cancer* 2007;110:764–769.

492. Ploeg M, Aben KK, Hulsbergen-van de Kaa CA, et al. Clinical epidemiology of nonurothelial bladder cancer: analysis of the Netherlands Cancer Registry. *J Urol* 2010;183:915–920.

493. Dahm P, Gschwend JE. Malignant non-urothelial neoplasms of the urinary bladder: a review. *Eur Urol* 2003;44:672–681.

494. Rundle JS, Hart AJ, McGeorge A, et al. Squamous cell carcinoma of bladder. A review of 114 patients. *Br J Urol* 1982;54:522–526.

495. Porter MP, Voigt LF, Penson DF, et al. Racial variation in the incidence of squamous cell carcinoma of the bladder in the United States. *J Urol* 2002;168:1960–1963.

496. Schroder LE, Weiss MA, Hughes C. Squamous cell carcinoma of bladder: an increased incidence in blacks. *Urology* 1986;28:288–291.

497. Faysal MH. Squamous cell carcinoma of the bladder. *J Urol* 1981;126:598–599.

498. Pattison S, Choong S, Corbishley CM, et al. Squamous cell carcinoma of the bladder, intermittent self-catheterization and urinary tract infection—is there an association? *BJU Int* 2001;88:441.

499. Bessette PL, Abell MR, Herwig KR. A clinicopathologic study of squamous cell carcinoma of the bladder. *J Urol* 1974;112:66–67.

500. Groah SL, Weitzenkamp DA, Lammertse DP, et al. Excess risk of bladder cancer in spinal cord injury: evidence for an association between indwelling catheter use and bladder cancer. *Arch Phys Med Rehabil* 2002;83:346–351.

501. Kaye MC, Levin HS, Montague DK, et al. Squamous cell carcinoma of the bladder in a patient on intermittent self-catheterization. *Cleve Clin J Med* 1992;59:645–646.

502. Kalisvaart JF, Katsumi HK, Ronningen LD, et al. Bladder cancer in spinal cord injury patients. *Spinal Cord* 2010;48:257–261.

503. Delnay KM, Stonehill WH, Goldman H, et al. Bladder histological changes associated with chronic indwelling urinary catheter. *J Urol* 1999;161:1106–1108.

504. Sheaff M, Jenkins BJ. Squamous cell carcinoma of the bladder following radiotherapy for transitional cell carcinoma. *Br J Urol* 1994;74:131–132.

505. Stein JP, Skinner EC, Boyd SD, et al. Squamous cell carcinoma of the bladder associated with cyclophosphamide therapy for Wegener's granulomatosis: a report of 2 cases. *J Urol* 1993;149:588–589.

506. Roehrborn CG, Teigland CM, Spence HM. Progression of leukoplakia of the bladder to squamous cell carcinoma 19 years after complete urinary diversion. *J Urol* 1988;140:603–604.

507. Shirai T, Arai M, Sakata T, et al. Primary carcinomas of urinary bladder diverticula. *Acta Pathol Jpn* 1984;34:417–424.

508. Tamas EF, Stephenson AJ, Campbell SC, et al. Histopathologic features and clinical outcomes in 71 cases of bladder diverticula. *Arch Pathol Lab Med* 2009;133:791–796.

509. Shokeir AA. Squamous cell carcinoma of the bladder: pathology, diagnosis and treatment. *BJU Int* 2004;93:216–220.

510. Nash TE, Cheever AW, Ottesen EA, et al. Schistosome infections in humans: perspectives and recent findings. NIH conference. *Ann Intern Med* 1982;97:740–754.

511. Smith JH, Christie JD. The pathobiology of *Schistosoma haematobium* infection in humans. *Hum Pathol* 1986;17:333–345.

512. Cooper K, Haffajee Z, Taylor L. Human papillomavirus and schistosomiasis associated bladder cancer. *Mol Pathol* 1997;50:145–148.

513. Westenend PJ, Stoop JA, Hendriks JG. Human papillomaviruses 6/11, 16/18 and 31/33/51 are not associated with squamous cell carcinoma of the urinary bladder. *BJU Int* 2001;88:198–201.

514. Wolchok JD, Herr HW, Kelly WK. Localized squamous cell carcinoma of the bladder causing hypercalcemia and inhibition of PTH secretion. *Urology* 1998;51:489–491.

515. Desai PG, Khan SA, Jayachandran S, et al. Paraneoplastic syndrome in squamous cell carcinoma of urinary bladder. *Urology* 1987;30:262–264.

516. Winkler HZ, Nativ O, Hosaka Y, et al. Nuclear deoxyribonucleic acid ploidy in squamous cell bladder cancer. *J Urol* 1989;141:297–302.

517. Sheldon CA, Clayman RV, Gonzalez R, et al. Malignant urachal lesions. *J Urol* 1984;131:1–8.

518. Chow YC, Lin WC, Tzen CY, et al. Squamous cell carcinoma of the urachus. *J Urol* 2000;163:903–904.

519. Fujiyama C, Nakashima N, Tokuda Y, et al. Squamous cell carcinoma of the urachus. *Int J Urol* 2007;14:966–968.

520. Newman DM, Brown JR, Jay AC, et al. Squamous cell carcinoma of the bladder. *J Urol* 1968;100:470–473.

521. Johnson DE, Schoenwald MB, Ayala AG, et al. Squamous cell carcinoma of the bladder. *J Urol* 1976;115:542–544.

522. Vakar-Lopez F, Abrams J. Basaloid squamous cell carcinoma occurring in the urinary bladder. *Arch Pathol Lab Med* 2000;124:455–459.

523. Guo CC, Gomez E, Tamboli P, et al. Squamous cell carcinoma of the urinary bladder: a clinicopathologic and immunohistochemical study of 16 cases. *Hum Pathol* 2009;40:1448–1452.

524. Richie JP, Waisman J, Skinner DG, et al. Squamous carcinoma of the bladder: treatment by radical cystectomy. *J Urol* 1976;115:670–672.

525. Martin JE, Jenkins BJ, Zuk RJ, et al. Clinical importance of squamous metaplasia in invasive transitional cell carcinoma of the bladder. *J Clin Pathol* 1989;42:250–253.

526. Sakamoto N, Tsuneyoshi M, Enjoji M. Urinary bladder carcinoma with a neoplastic squamous component: a mapping study of 31 cases. *Histopathology* 1992;21:135–141.

527. Kraus I, Molden T, Holm R, et al. Presence of E6 and E7 mRNA from human papillomavirus types 16, 18, 31, 33, and 45 in the majority of cervical carcinomas. *J Clin Microbiol* 2006;44:1310–1317.

528. Abol-Enein H, Kava BR, Carmack AJK. Nonurothelial cancer of the bladder. *Urology* 2007;69:93–104.

529. Patterson JM, Ray EH Jr, Mendiondo OA, et al. A new treatment for invasive squamous cell bladder cancer: the Nigro regimen: preoperative chemotherapy and radiation therapy. *J Urol* 1988;140:379–380.

530. Swanson DA, Liles A, Zagars GK. Preoperative irradiation and radical cystectomy for stages T2 and T3 squamous cell carcinoma of the bladder. *J Urol* 1990;143:37–40.

531. Wyatt JK, Craig I. Verrucous carcinoma of urinary bladder. *Urology* 1980;16:97–99.

532. Holck S, Jorgensen L. Verrucous carcinoma of urinary bladder. *Urology* 1983;22:435–437.

533. Walther M, O'Brien DP III, Birch HW. Condylomata acuminata and verrucous carcinoma of the bladder: case report and literature review. *J Urol* 1986;135:362–365.

534. Ellsworth PI, Schned AR, Heaney JA, et al. Surgical treatment of verrucous carcinoma of the bladder unassociated with bilharzial cystitis: case report and literature review. *J Urol* 1995;153:411–414.

535. Lewin F, Cardoso APG, Simardi LH, et al. Verrucous carcinoma of the bladder with koilocytosis unassociated with vesical schistosomiasis. *Sao Paulo Med J* 2004;122:64–66.

536. Boileau M, Hui KK, Cowan DF. Invasive verrucous carcinoma of urinary bladder treated by irradiation. *Urology* 1986;27:56–59.

537. El-Sebai I, Sherif M, El-Bolkainy MN, et al. Verrucose squamous carcinoma of bladder. *Urology* 1974;4:407–410.

538. Jacobo E, Loening S, Schmidt JD, et al. Primary adenocarcinoma of the bladder: a retrospective study of 20 patients. *J Urol* 1977;117:54–56.

539. Thomas DG, Ward AM, Williams JL. A study of 52 cases of adenocarcinoma of the bladder. *Br J Urol* 1971;43:4–15.

540. Zaghloul MS, Nouh A, Nazmy M, et al. Long-term results of primary adenocarcinoma of the urinary bladder: a report on 192 patients. *Urol Oncol* 2006;24:13–20.

541. El-Mekresh MM, El-Baz MA, Abol-Enein H, et al. Primary adenocarcinoma of the urinary bladder: a report of 185 cases. *Br J Urol* 1998;82:206–212.

542. Mostofi FK, Thomson RV, Dean AL Jr. Mucous adenocarcinoma of the urinary bladder. *Cancer* 1955;8:741–758.

543. von Garrelts B, Moberg A, Ohman U. Carcinoma of the urachus. Review of the literature and report of two cases. *Scand J Urol Nephrol* 1971;5:91–95.

544. Kamat MR, Kulkarni JN, Tongaonkar HB. Adenocarcinoma of the bladder: study of 14 cases and review of the literature. *Br J Urol* 1991;68:254–257.

545. Wilson TG, Pritchett TR, Lieskovsky G, et al. Primary adenocarcinoma of bladder. *Urology* 1991;38:223–226.

546. Rogers CG, Palapattu GS, Shariat SF, et al. Clinical outcomes following radical cystectomy for primary nontransitional cell carcinoma of the bladder compared to transitional cell carcinoma of the bladder. *J Urol* 2006;175:2048–2053.

547. Abenoza P, Manivel C, Fraley EE. Primary adenocarcinoma of urinary bladder. Clinicopathologic study of 16 cases. *Urology* 1987;29:9–14.

548. O'Kane HO, Megaw JM. Carcinoma in the exstrophic bladder. *Br J Surg* 1968;55:631–635.

549. Engel RM, Wilkinson HA. Bladder exstrophy. *J Urol* 1970;104:699–704.

550. Goyanna R, Emmett JL, McDonald JR. Exstrophy of the bladder complicated by adenocarcinoma. *J Urol* 1951;65:391–400.

551. Heyns CF, De Kock ML, Kirsten PH, et al. Pelvic lipomatosis associated with cystitis glandularis and adenocarcinoma of the bladder. *J Urol* 1991;145:364–366.

552. Gordon NS, Sinclair RA, Snow RM. Pelvic lipomatosis with cystitis cystica, cystitis glandularis and adenocarcinoma of the bladder: first reported case. *Aust N Z J Surg* 1990;60:229–232.

553. Chor PJ, Gaum LD, Young RH. Clear cell adenocarcinoma of the urinary bladder: report of a case of probable mullerian origin. *Mod Pathol* 1993;6:225–228.

554. Yoshimura S, Ito Y. Malignant transformation of endometriosis of the urinary bladder; case report [Japanese text]. *Gann* 1951;42:334–335.

555. Vara AR, Ruzics EP, Moussabeck O, et al. Endometrioid adenosarcoma of the bladder arising from endometriosis. *J Urol* 1990;143:813–815.

556. Anderstrom C, Johansson SL, von Schultz L. Primary adenocarcinoma of the urinary bladder. A clinicopathologic and prognostic study. *Cancer* 1983;52:1273–1280.

557. Chan TY, Epstein JI. In situ adenocarcinoma of the bladder. *Am J Surg Pathol* 2001;25:892–899.

558. Jacobs LB, Brooks JD, Epstein JI. Differentiation of colonic metaplasia from adenocarcinoma of urinary bladder. *Hum Pathol* 1997;28:1152–1157.

559. Hao H, Tsujimoto M, Tsubamoto H, et al. Immunohistochemical phenotype of the urinary bladder endocervicosis: comparison with normal endocervix and well-differentiated mucinous adenocarcinoma of uterine cervix. *Pathol Int* 2010;60:528–532.

560. Nakanishi K, Tominaga S, Kawai T, et al. Mucin histochemistry in primary adenocarcinoma of the urinary bladder (of urachal or vesicular origin) and metastatic adenocarcinoma originating in the colorectum. *Pathol Int* 2000;50:297–303.

561. Wang HL, Lu DW, Yerian LM, et al. Immunohistochemical distinction between primary adenocarcinoma of the bladder and secondary colorectal adenocarcinoma. *Am J Surg Pathol* 2001;25:1380–1387.

562. Torenbeek R, Lagendijk JH, Van Diest PJ, et al. Value of a panel of antibodies to identify the primary origin of adenocarcinomas presenting as bladder carcinoma. *Histopathology* 1998;32:20–27.

563. Thomas AA, Stephenson AJ, Campbell SC, et al. Clinicopathologic features and utility of immunohistochemical markers in signet-ring cell adenocarcinoma of the bladder. *Hum Pathol* 2009;40:108–116.

564. Raspollini MR, Nesi G, Baroni G, et al. Immunohistochemistry in the differential diagnosis between primary and secondary intestinal adenocarcinoma of the urinary bladder. *Appl Immunohistochem Mol Morphol* 2005;13:358–362.

565. Suh N, Yang XJ, Tretiakova MS, et al. Value of CDX2, villin, and alpha-methylacyl coenzyme A racemase immunostains in the distinction between primary adenocarcinoma of the bladder and secondary colorectal adenocarcinoma. *Mod Pathol* 2005;18:1217–1222.

566. Tamboli P, Mohsin SK, Hailemariam S, et al. Colonic adenocarcinoma metastatic to the urinary tract versus primary tumors of the urinary tract with glandular differentiation: a report of 7 cases and investigation using a limited immunohistochemical panel. *Arch Pathol Lab Med* 2002;126:1057–1063.

567. Edge S, Byrd D, Compton C, et al., eds. *AJCC Cancer Staging Manual.* 7th ed. New York: Springer; 2010.

568. De Santis M, Bachner M. New developments in first- and second-line chemotherapy for transitional cell, squamous cell and adenocarcinoma of the bladder. *Curr Opin Urol* 2007;17:363–368.

569. Jones WA, Gibbons RP, Correa RJ Jr, et al. Primary adenocarcinoma of bladder. *Urology* 1980;15:119–122.

570. Gopalan A, Sharp DS, Fine SW, et al. Urachal carcinoma: a clinicopathologic analysis of 24 cases with outcome correlation. *Am J Surg Pathol* 2009;33:659–668.

571. Johnson DE, Hogan JM, Ayala AG. Primary adenocarcinoma of the urinary bladder. *South Med J* 1972;65:527–530.

572. Begg R. The colloid adenocarcinomata of the bladder vault arising from the epithelium of the urachal canal: with a critical survey of the tumours of the urachus. *Br J Surg* 1931;18:422–464.

573. Lucas D, Lawrence W, McDevitt W, et al. Mucinous papillary adenocarcinoma of the bladder arising within a villous adenoma of urachal remnants: an immunohistochemical and ultrastructural study. *J Urol Pathol* 1994;2:173.

574. Cornil C, Reynolds CT, Kickham CJ. Carcinoma of the urachus. *J Urol* 1967;98:93–95.

575. Siefker-Radtke A. Urachal carcinoma: surgical and chemotherapeutic options. *Expert Rev Anticancer Ther* 2006;6:1715–1721.

576. Molina JR, Quevedo JF, Furth AF, et al. Predictors of survival from urachal cancer: a Mayo Clinic study of 49 cases. *Cancer* 2007;110:2434–2440.

577. Pinthus JH, Haddad R, Trachtenberg J, et al. Population based survival data on urachal tumors. *J Urol* 2006;175:2042–2047.

578. Pallesen G. Neoplastic Paneth cells in adenocarcinoma of the urinary bladder: a first case report. *Cancer* 1981;47:1834–1837.

579. Satake T, Matsuyama M. Neoplastic nature of argyrophil cells in urachal adenocarcinoma. *Acta Pathol Jpn* 1986;36:1587–1592.

580. Nakanishi K, Kawai T, Suzuki M, et al. Prognostic factors in urachal adenocarcinoma. A study in 41 specimens of DNA status, proliferating cell-nuclear antigen immunostaining, and argyrophilic nucleolar-organizer region counts. *Hum Pathol* 1996;27:240–247.

581. Ghazizadeh M, Yamamoto S, Kurokawa K. Clinical features of urachal carcinoma in Japan: review of 157 patients. *Urol Res* 1983;11:235–238.

582. Santucci RA, True LD, Lange PH. Is partial cystectomy the treatment of choice for mucinous adenocarcinoma of the urachus? *Urology* 1997;49:536–540.

583. Akamatsu S, Takahashi A, Ito M, et al. Primary signet-ring cell carcinoma of the urinary bladder. *Urology* 2010;75:615–618.

584. Daljeet S, Amreek S, Satish J, et al. Signet ring cell adenocarcinoma of the urachus. *Int J Urol* 2004;11:785–788.

585. Holmang S, Borghede G, Johansson SL. Primary signet ring cell carcinoma of the bladder: a report on 10 cases. *Scand J Urol Nephrol* 1997;31:145–148.

586. Yamamoto S, Ito T, Akiyama A, et al. Primary signet-ring cell carcinoma of the urinary bladder inducing renal failure. *Int J Urol* 2001;8:190–193.

587. Ro JY, El-Naggar A, Ayala AG, et al. Signet-ring-cell carcinoma of the prostate: electron-microscopic and immunohistochemical studies of eight cases. *Am J Surg Pathol* 1988;12:453–460.

588. Young RH, Scully RE. Clear cell adenocarcinoma of the bladder and urethra. A report of three cases and review of the literature. *Am J Surg Pathol* 1985;9:816–826.

589. Drew PA, Murphy WM, Civantos F, et al. The histogenesis of clear cell adenocarcinoma of the lower urinary tract. Case series and review of the literature. *Hum Pathol* 1996;27:248–252.

590. Suttmann H, Holl-Ulrich K, Peter M, et al. Mesonephroid adenocarcinoma arising from mesonephroid metaplasia of the urinary bladder. *Urology* 2006;67:846.e7–e8.

591. Kosem M, Sengul E. Clear cell adenocarcinoma of the urinary bladder. *Scand J Urol Nephrol* 2005;39:89–92.

592. Adeniran AJ, Tamboli P. Clear cell adenocarcinoma of the urinary bladder: a short review. *Arch Pathol Lab Med* 2009;133:987–991.

593. Kanokogi M, Uematsu K, Kakudo K, et al. Mesonephric adenocarcinoma of the urinary bladder: an autopsy case. *J Surg Oncol* 1983;22:118–120.

594. Sung M-T, Zhang S, MacLennan GT, et al. Histogenesis of clear cell adenocarcinoma in the urinary tract: evidence of urothelial origin. *Clin Cancer Res* 2008;14:1947–1955.

595. Mai KT, Yazdi HM, Perkins DG, et al. Multicentric clear cell adenocarcinoma in the urinary bladder and the urethral diverticulum: evidence of origin of clear cell adenocarcinoma of the female lower urinary tract from Mullerian duct remnants. *Histopathology* 2000;36:380–382.

596. Balat O, Kudelka AP, Edwards CL, et al. Malignant transformation in endometriosis of the urinary bladder: case report of clear cell adenocarcinoma. *Eur J Gynecol Oncol* 1996;17:13–16.

597. Novak RW, Raines RB, Sollee AN. Clear cell carcinoma in a Mullerian duct cyst. *Am J Clin Pathol* 1981;76:339–341.

598. Herawi M, Drew PA, Pan C-C, et al. Clear cell adenocarcinoma of the bladder and urethra: cases diffusely mimicking nephrogenic adenoma. *Hum Pathol* 2010;41:594–601.

599. Gilcrease MZ, Delgado R, Vuitch F, et al. Clear cell adenocarcinoma and nephrogenic adenoma of the urethra and urinary bladder: a histopathologic and immunohistochemical comparison. *Hum Pathol* 1998;29:1451–1456.

600. Tong G-X, Weeden EM, Hamele-Bena D, et al. Expression of PAX8 in nephrogenic adenoma and clear cell adenocarcinoma of the lower urinary tract: evidence of related histogenesis? *Am J Surg Pathol* 2008;32:1380–1387.

601. Ford TF, Watson GM, Cameron KM. Adenomatous metaplasia (nephrogenic adenoma) of urothelium. An analysis of 70 cases. *Br J Urol* 1985;57:427–433.

602. Cheng L, Cheville JC, Sebo TJ, et al. Atypical nephrogenic metaplasia of the urinary tract: a precursor lesion? *Cancer* 2000;88:853–861.

603. Amin W, Parwani AV. Nephrogenic adenoma. *Pathol Res Pract* 2010;206:659–662.

604. Meis JM, Ayala AG, Johnson DE. Adenocarcinoma of the urethra in women. A clinicopathologic study. *Cancer* 1987;60:1038–1052.

605. Lopez-Beltran A, Luque RJ, Quintero A, et al. Hepatoid adenocarcinoma of the urinary bladder. *Virchows Arch* 2003;442:381–387.

606. Sinard J, Macleay L Jr, Melamed J. Hepatoid adenocarcinoma in the urinary bladder. Unusual localization of a newly recognized tumor type. *Cancer* 1994;73:1919–1925.

607. Burgues O, Ferrer J, Navarro S, et al. Hepatoid adenocarcinoma of the urinary bladder. An unusual neoplasm. *Virchows Arch* 1999;435:71–75.

608. Blomjous CE, Vos W, De Voogt HJ, et al. Small cell carcinoma of the urinary bladder. A clinicopathologic, morphometric, immunohistochemical, and ultrastructural study of 18 cases. *Cancer* 1989;64:1347–1357.

609. Podesta AH, True LD. Small cell carcinoma of the bladder. Report of five cases with immunohistochemistry and review of the literature with evaluation of prognosis according to stage. *Cancer* 1989;64:710–714.

610. Wang X, MacLennan GT, Lopez-Beltran A, et al. Small cell carcinoma of the urinary bladder—histogenesis, genetics, diagnosis, biomarkers, treatment, and prognosis. *Appl Immunohistochem Mol Morphol* 2007;15:8–18.

611. Mills SE, Wolfe JT III, Weiss MA, et al. Small cell undifferentiated carcinoma of the urinary bladder. A light-microscopic, immunocytochemical, and ultrastructural study of 12 cases. *Am J Surg Pathol* 1987;11:606–617.

612. Cramer SF, Aikawa M, Cebelin M. Neurosecretory granules in small cell invasive carcinoma of the urinary bladder. *Cancer* 1981;47:724–730.

613. Oesterling JE, Brendler CB, Burgers JK, et al. Advanced small cell carcinoma of the bladder. Successful treatment with combined radical cystoprostatectomy and adjuvant methotrexate, vinblastine, doxorubicin, and cisplatin chemotherapy. *Cancer* 1990;65:1928–1936.

614. Angulo J, Lopez J, Sanches-Chapado M, et al. Small cell carcinoma of the urinary bladder: a report of two cases with complete remission and a comprehensive literature review with emphasis on therapeutic decisions. *J Urol Pathol* 1996;5:1–19.

615. Trias I, Algaba F, Condom E, et al. Small cell carcinoma of the urinary bladder. Presentation of 23 cases and review of 134 published cases. *Eur Urol* 2001;39:85–90.

616. Cheng L, Pan C-X, Yang XJ, et al. Small cell carcinoma of the urinary bladder: a clinicopathologic analysis of 64 patients. *Cancer* 2004;101:957–962.

617. Sved P, Gomez P, Manoharan M, et al. Small cell carcinoma of the bladder. *BJU Int* 2004;94:12–17.

618. Siefker-Radtke AO, Dinney CP, Abrahams NA, et al. Evidence supporting preoperative chemotherapy for small cell carcinoma of the bladder: a retrospective review of the M. D. Anderson cancer experience. *J Urol* 2004;172:481–484.

619. Partanen S, Asikainen U. Oat cell carcinoma of the urinary bladder with ectopic adrenocorticotrophic hormone production. *Hum Pathol* 1985;16:313–315.

620. Grignon DJ, Ro JY, Ayala AG, et al. Small cell carcinoma of the urinary bladder. A clinicopathologic analysis of 22 cases. *Cancer* 1992;69:527–536.

621. Yajima N, Mizukami H, Wada R, et al. Small cell carcinoma with skeletal muscle differentiation of urinary bladder. *Pathol Int* 2009;59:748–751.

622. Abenoza P, Manivel C, Sibley RK. Adenocarcinoma with neuroendocrine differentiation of the urinary bladder. Clinicopathologic, immunohistochemical, and ultrastructural study. *Arch Pathol Lab Med* 1986;110:1062–1066.

623. Alijo Serrano F, Sanchez-Mora N, Angel Arranz J, et al. Large cell and small cell neuroendocrine bladder carcinoma: immunohistochemical and outcome study in a single institution. *Am J Clin Pathol* 2007;128:733–739.

624. Jones TD, Kernek KM, Yang XJ, et al. Thyroid transcription factor 1 expression in small cell carcinoma of the urinary bladder: an immunohistochemical profile of 44 cases. *Hum Pathol* 2005;36:718–723.

625. Tetu B, Ro JY, Ayala AG, et al. Small cell carcinoma of the prostate. Part I. A clinicopathologic study of 20 cases. *Cancer* 1987;59: 1803–1809.

626. Coltart RS, Stewart S, Brown CH. Small cell carcinoma of the bronchus: a rare cause of haematuria from a metastasis in the urinary bladder. *J R Soc Med* 1985;78:1053–1054.

627. Matsui Y, Fujikawa K, Iwamura H, et al. Durable control of small cell carcinoma of the urinary bladder by gemcitabine and paclitaxel. *Int J Urol* 2002;9:122–124.

628. Bex A, de Vries R, Pos F, et al. Long-term survival after sequential chemoradiation for limited disease small cell carcinoma of the bladder. *World J Urol* 2009;27:101–106.

629. Akamatsu S, Kanamaru S, Ishihara M, et al. Primary large cell neuroendocrine carcinoma of the urinary bladder. *Int J Urol* 2008;15:1080–1083.

630. Evans AJ, Al-Maghrabi J, Tsihlias J, et al. Primary large cell neuroendocrine carcinoma of the urinary bladder. *Arch Pathol Lab Med* 2002;126:1229–1232.

631. Lee KH, Ryu SB, Lee MC, et al. Primary large cell neuroendocrine carcinoma of the urinary bladder. *Pathol Int* 2006;56:688–693.

632. Lee WJ, Kim CH, Chang SE, et al. Cutaneous metastasis from large-cell neuroendocrine carcinoma of the urinary bladder expressing CK20 and TTF-1. *Am J Dermatopathol* 2009;31:166–169.

633. Dundr P, Pesl M, Povysil C, et al. Large cell neuroendocrine carcinoma of the urinary bladder with lymphoepithelioma-like features. *Pathol Res Pract* 2003;199:559–563.

634. Oshiro H, Gomi K, Nagahama K, et al. Urinary cytologic features of primary large cell neuroendocrine carcinoma of the urinary bladder: a case report. *Acta Cytol* 2010;54:303–310.

635. Hailemariam S, Gaspert A, Komminoth P, et al. Primary, pure, large-cell neuroendocrine carcinoma of the urinary bladder. *Mod Pathol* 1998;11:1016–1020.

636. Li Y, Outman JE, Mathur SC. Carcinosarcoma with a large cell neuroendocrine epithelial component: first report of an unusual biphasic tumour of the urinary bladder. *J Clin Pathol* 2004;57:318–320.

637. Colby TV. Carcinoid tumor of the bladder. A case report. *Arch Pathol Lab Med* 1980;104:199–200.

638. Burgess NA, Lewis DC, Matthews PN. Primary carcinoid of the bladder. *Br J Urol* 1992;69:213–214.

639. Walker BF, Someren A, Kennedy JC, et al. Primary carcinoid tumor of the urinary bladder. *Arch Pathol Lab Med* 1992;116:1217–1220.

640. Stanfield BL, Grimes MM, Kay S. Primary carcinoid tumor of the bladder arising beneath an inverted papilloma. *Arch Pathol Lab Med* 1994;118:666–667.

641. Martignoni G, Eble JN. Carcinoid tumors of the urinary bladder. Immunohistochemical study of 2 cases and review of the literature. *Arch Pathol Lab Med* 2003;127:e22–e24.

642. McCabe JE, Das S, Dowling P, et al. Oncocytic carcinoid tumour of the bladder. *J Clin Pathol* 2005;58:446–447.

643. Mascolo M, Altieri V, Mignogna C, et al. Calcitonin-producing well-differentiated neuroendocrine carcinoma (carcinoid tumor) of the urinary bladder: case report. *BMC Cancer* 2005;5:88.

644. Sugihara A, Kajio K, Yoshimoto T, et al. Primary carcinoid tumor of the urinary bladder. *Int Urol Nephrol* 2002;33:53–57.

645. Hemal AK, Singh I, Pawar R, et al. Primary malignant bladder carcinoid—a diagnostic and management dilemma. *Urology* 2000;55:949.

646. Anichkov N, Nikonov A, Veresh I. Malignant carcinoid tumor of the bladder. *Arkh Patol* 1979;41:46–49.

647. Desai S. Primary primitive neuroectodermal tumour of the urinary bladder. *Histopathology* 1998;32:477–478.

648. Banerjee SS, Eyden BP, McVey RJ, et al. Primary peripheral primitive neuroectodermal tumour of urinary bladder. *Histopathology* 1997;30:486–490.

649. Gousse AE, Roth DR, Popek EJ, et al. Primary Ewing's sarcoma of the bladder associated with an elevated antinuclear antibody titer. *J Urol* 1997;158:2265–2266.

650. Mentzel T, Flaschka J, Mentzel HJ, et al. [Primary primitive neuroectodermal tumor of the urinary bladder. Clinicopathologic case report and differential small cell tumor diagnosis of this site]. *Pathologe* 1998;19:154–158.

651. Colecchia M, Dagrada GP, Poliani PL, et al. Immunophenotypic and genotypic analysis of a case of primary peripheral primitive neuroectodermal tumour (pPNET) of the urinary bladder. *Histopathology* 2002;40:108–109.

652. Kruger S, Schmidt H, Kausch I, et al. Primitive neuroectodermal tumor (PNET) of the urinary bladder. *Pathol Res Pract* 2003;199: 751–754.

653. Lopez-Beltran A, Perez-Seoane C, Montironi R, et al. Primary primitive neuroectodermal tumour of the urinary bladder: a clinicopathological study emphasising immunohistochemical, ultrastructural and molecular analyses. *J Clin Pathol* 2006;59:775–778.

654. Osone S, Hosoi H, Tanaka K, et al. A case of a Ewing sarcoma family tumor in the urinary bladder after treatment for acute lymphoblastic leukemia. *J Pediatr Hematol Oncol* 2007;29:841–844.

655. Melicow MM. Tumors of the urinary bladder: a clinico-pathological analysis of over 2500 specimens and biopsies. *J Urol* 1955;74: 498–521.

656. Bolkier M, Ginesin Y, Lichtig C, et al. Lymphangioma of bladder. *J Urol* 1983;129:1049–1050.

657. Karol JB, Eason AA, Tanagho EA. Fibrous histiocytoma of bladder. *Urology* 1977;10:593–595.

658. Kunze E, Theuring F, Kruger G. Primary mesenchymal tumors of the urinary bladder. A histological and immunohistochemical study of 30 cases. *Pathol Res Pract* 1994;190:311–332.

659. May F, Luther A, Mohr W, et al. Recurrent aggressive angiomyxoma of the urinary bladder. Case report and review of the literature. *Urol Int* 2000;65:57–59.

660. Wyman H, Chappell B, Jones WJ. Ganglioneuroma of bladder: report of a case. *J Urol* 1950;63:526–532.

661. Kalafatis P, Kavantzas N, Pavlopoulos PM, et al. Malignant peripheral nerve sheath tumor of the urinary bladder in von Recklinghausen disease. *Urol Int* 2002;69:156–159.

662. Petersen R, Sesterhenn I, Davis C. *Urologic Pathology.* 3rd ed. Philadelphia, PA: Wolters Kluwer, Lippincott Williams & Wilkins; 2009.

663. Knoll LD, Segura JW, Scheithauer BW. Leiomyoma of the bladder. *J Urol* 1986;136:906–908.

664. Martin SA, Sears DL, Sebo TJ, et al. Smooth muscle neoplasms of the urinary bladder: a clinicopathologic comparison of leiomyoma and leiomyosarcoma. *Am J Surg Pathol* 2002;26:292–300.

665. Lee TK, Miyamoto H, Osunkoya AO, et al. Smooth muscle neoplasms of the urinary bladder: a clinicopathologic study of 51 cases. *Am J Surg Pathol* 2010;34:502–509.

666. Mutchler RW Jr, Gorder JL. Leiomyoma of the bladder in a child. *Br J Radiol* 1972;45:538–540.

667. Dauth TL, Conradie M, Chetty R. Leiomyoma of the bladder in a patient with von Recklinghausen's neurofibromatosis. *J Clin Pathol* 2003;56:711–712.

668. Kabalin JN, Freiha FS, Niebel JD. Leiomyoma of bladder. Report of 2 cases and demonstration of ultrasonic appearance. *Urology* 1990;35:210–212.

669. Saunders SE, Conjeski JM, Zaslau S, et al. Leiomyoma of the urinary bladder presenting as urinary retention in the female. *Can J Urol* 2009;16:4762–4764.

670. Chavez CA, Neto M. Multiple leiomyomata of the urinary bladder. *J Kans Med Soc* 1984;85:298–299.

671. Soloway D, Simon MA, Milikowski C, et al. Epithelioid leiomyoma of the bladder: an unusual cause of voiding symptoms. *Urology* 1998;51:1037–1039.

672. Mills SE, Bova GS, Wick MR, et al. Leiomyosarcoma of the urinary bladder. A clinicopathologic and immunohistochemical study of 15 cases. *Am J Surg Pathol* 1989;13:480–489.

673. Jahn H, Nissen HM. Haemangioma of the urinary tract: review of the literature. *Br J Urol* 1991;68:113–117.

674. Fernandes ET, Manivel JC, Reinberg Y. Hematuria in a newborn infant caused by bladder hemangioma. *Urology* 1996;47:412–415.

675. Mor Y, Hitchcock RJ, Zaidi SZ, et al. Bladder hemangioma as a cause of massive hematuria in a child. A case report and literature review. *Scand J Urol Nephrol* 1997;31:305–307.

676. Suzuki Y, Kaneko H, Kubota Y, et al. Hemangioma of the bladder with extravesical extension. *Urol Int* 1997;59:125–128.

677. Cheng L, Nascimento AG, Neumann RM, et al. Hemangioma of the urinary bladder. *Cancer* 1999;86:498–504.

678. Tavora F, Montgomery E, Epstein JI. A series of vascular tumors and tumorlike lesions of the bladder. *Am J Surg Pathol* 2008;32:1213–1219.

679. Hockley NM, Bihrle R, Bennett RM III, et al. Congenital genitourinary hemangiomas in a patient with the Klippel-Trenaunay syndrome: management with the neodymium:YAG laser. *J Urol* 1989;141:940–941.

680. Hall BD. Bladder hemangiomas in Klippel-Trenaunay-Weber syndrome. *N Engl J Med* 1971;285:1032–1033.

681. Stroup RM, Chang YC. Angiosarcoma of the bladder: a case report. *J Urol* 1987;137:984–985.

682. Schwartz RA, Kardashian JF, McNutt NS, et al. Cutaneous angiosarcoma resembling anaplastic Kaposi's sarcoma in a homosexual man. *Cancer* 1983;51:721–726.

683. Sutton R, Hopper IP, Munson KW. Haemangiopericytoma of the bladder. *Br J Urol* 1989;63:548–549.

684. Ogawa A, Watanabe K. Genitourinary neurofibromatosis in a child presenting with an enlarged penis and scrotum. *J Urol* 1986;135:755–757.

685. Wang W, Montgomery E, Epstein JI. Benign nerve sheath tumors on urinary bladder biopsy. *Am J Surg Pathol* 2008;32:907–912.

686. Cheng L, Scheithauer BW, Leibovich BC, et al. Neurofibroma of the urinary bladder. *Cancer* 1999;86:505–513.

687. Aygun C, Tekin MI, Tarhan C, et al. Neurofibroma of the bladder wall in von Recklinghausen's disease. *Int J Urol* 2001;8:249–253.

688. Chakravarti A, Jones MA, Simon J. Neurofibromatosis involving the urinary bladder. *Int J Urol* 2001;8:645–647.

689. Kramer SA, Barrett DM, Utz DC. Neurofibromatosis of the bladder in children. *J Urol* 1981;126:693–694.

690. Hulse CA. Neurofibromatosis: bladder involvement with malignant degeneration. *J Urol* 1990;144:742–743.

691. Scheithauer BW, Santi M, Richter ER, et al. Diffuse ganglioneuromatosis and plexiform neurofibroma of the urinary bladder: report of a pediatric example and literature review. *Hum Pathol* 2008;39:1708–1712.

692. Montgomery EA, Shuster DD, Burkart AL, et al. Inflammatory myofibroblastic tumors of the urinary tract: a clinicopathologic study of 46 cases, including a malignant example inflammatory fibrosarcoma and a subset associated with high-grade urothelial carcinoma. *Am J Surg Pathol* 2006;30:1502–1512.

693. Ng KJ, Sherif A, McClinton S, et al. Giant ancient schwannoma of the urinary bladder presenting as a pelvic mass. *Br J Urol* 1993;72:513–514.

694. Gafson I, Rosenbaum T, Kubba F, et al. Schwannoma of the bladder: a rare pelvic tumour. *J Obstet Gynecol* 2008;28:241–243.

695. Cummings JM, Wehry MA, Parra RO, et al. Schwannoma of the urinary bladder: a case report. *Int J Urol* 1998;5:496–497.

696. Geol H, Kim DW, Kim TH, et al. Laparoscopic partial cystectomy for schwannoma of urinary bladder: case report. *J Endourol* 2005;19:303–306.

697. Kindblom LG, Meis-Kindblom JM, Havel G, et al. Benign epithelioid schwannoma. *Am J Surg Pathol* 1998;22:762–770.

698. Weiss S, Goldblum J. *Enzinger and Weiss's Soft Tissue Tumors.* 5th ed. Philadelphia, PA: Mosby Elsevier; 2008.

699. Abbas F, Memon A, Siddiqui T, et al. Granular cell tumors of the urinary bladder. *World J Surg Oncol* 2007;5:33.

700. Eandi JA, Asuncion A, Vandewalker KN, et al. Granular cell tumor of the urinary bladder with pseudoepitheliomatous hyperplasia and colocalization with adenocarcinoma. *Int J Urol* 2007;14:862–864.

701. Park SH, Kim TJ, Chi JG. Congenital granular cell tumor with systemic involvement. Immunohistochemical and ultrastructural study. *Arch Pathol Lab Med* 1991;115:934–938.

702. Kontani K, Okaneya T, Takezaki T. Recurrent granular cell tumour of the bladder in a patient with von Recklinghausen's disease. *BJU Int* 1999;84:871–872.

703. Yoshida T, Hirai S, Horii Y, et al. Granular cell tumor of the urinary bladder. *Int J Urol* 2001;8:29–31.

704. Kang H-W, Kim Y-W, Ha Y-S, et al. Granular cell tumor of the urinary bladder. *Korean J Urol* 2010;51:291–293.

705. Eggener SE, Hairston J, Rubenstein JN, et al. Bladder lipoma. *J Urol* 2001;166:1395.

706. Meraj S, Narasimhan G, Gerber E, et al. Bladder wall lipoma. *Urology* 2002;60:164.

707. Kunkle DA, Mydlo JH. Bladder wall lipoma in patient with irritative voiding symptoms. *Urology* 2005;66:653–654.

708. Lang EK. Symptomatic bladder lipomas. *J Urol* 2005;174:313.

709. Brown C, Jones A. Bladder lipoma associated with urinary tract infection. *Scientific World Journal* 2008;8:573–574.

710. Bainbridge TC, Singh RR, Mentzel T, et al. Solitary fibrous tumor of urinary bladder: report of two cases. *Hum Pathol* 1997;28:1204–1206.

711. Westra WH, Grenko RT, Epstein J. Solitary fibrous tumor of the lower urogenital tract: a report of five cases involving the seminal vesicles, urinary bladder, and prostate. *Hum Pathol* 2000;31:63–68.

712. Corti B, Carella R, Gabusi E, et al. Solitary fibrous tumour of the urinary bladder with expression of bcl-2, CD34, and insulin-like growth factor type II. *Eur Urol* 2001;39:484–488.

713. Heinzelbecker J, Becker F, Pflugmann T, et al. Solitary fibrous tumour of the urinary bladder in a young woman presenting with haemodynamic-relevant gross haematuria. *Eur Urol* 2008;54:1188–1191.

714. Tzelepi V, Zolota V, Batistatou A, et al. Solitary fibrous tumor of the urinary bladder: report of a case with long-term follow-up and review of the literature. *Eur Rev Med Pharmacol Sci* 2007;11:101–106.

715. Spiess PE, Kassouf W, Steinberg JR, et al. Review of the M.D. Anderson experience in the treatment of bladder sarcoma. *Urol Oncol* 2007;25:38–45.

716. Egawa S, Uchida T, Koshiba K, et al. Malignant fibrous histiocytoma of the bladder with focal rhabdoid tumor differentiation. *J Urol* 1994;151:154–156.

717. Young RH, Rosenberg AE. Osteosarcoma of the urinary bladder. Report of a case and review of the literature. *Cancer* 1987;59:174–178.

718. Ikemoto S, Sugimura K, Yoshida N, et al. Chondrosarcoma of the urinary bladder and establishment of a human chondrosarcoma cell line (OCUU-6). *Hum Cell* 2004;17:93–96.

719. Torenbeek R, Blomjous CE, Meijer CJ. Chondrosarcoma of the urinary bladder: report of a case with immunohistochemical and ultrastructural findings and review of the literature. *Eur Urol* 1993;23:502–505.

720. Suster S, Huszar M, Bubis JJ, et al. Fibrosarcoma of the urinary bladder. Study of a case showing extensive chondroid differentiation. *Arch Pathol Lab Med* 1987;111:767–770.

721. Terada Y, Saito I, Morohoshi T, et al. Malignant mesenchymoma of the bladder. *Cancer* 1987;60:858–863.

722. Williams S, Romaguera R, Kava B. Angiosarcoma of the bladder: case report and review of the literature. *Scientific World Journal* 2008;8:508–511.

723. Rosi P, Selli C, Carini M, et al. Myxoid liposarcoma of the bladder. *J Urol* 1983;130:560–561.

724. Sukov WR, Cheville JC, Amin MB, et al. Perivascular epithelioid cell tumor (PEComa) of the urinary bladder: report of 3 cases and review of the literature. *Am J Surg Pathol* 2009;33:304–308.

725. McBride J, Ro J, Hicks J, et al. Malignant rhabdoid tumor of the bladder in an adolescent: case report and discussion of extrarenal rhabdoid tumor. *J Urol Pathol* 1994;2:255–263.

726. Lott S, Lopez-Beltran A, Montironi R, et al. Soft tissue tumors of the urinary bladder Part II: malignant neoplasms. *Hum Pathol* 2007;38:963–77.

727. Ahlering TE, Weintraub P, Skinner DG. Management of adult sarcomas of the bladder and prostate. *J Urol* 1988;140:1397–1399.

728. Ozteke O, Demirel A, Aydin NE, et al. Bladder leiomyosarcoma: report of three cases. *Int Urol Nephrol* 1992;24:393–396.

729. Kawamura J, Sakurai M, Tsukamoto K, et al. Leiomyosarcoma of the bladder eighteen years after cyclophosphamide therapy for retinoblastoma. *Urol Int* 1993;51:49–53.

730. Perret L, Chaubert P, Hessler D, et al. Primary heterologous carcinosarcoma (metaplastic carcinoma) of the urinary bladder: a clinicopathologic, immunohistochemical, and ultrastructural analysis of eight cases and a review of the literature. *Cancer* 1998;82:1535–1549.

731. Huang WL, Ro JY, Grignon DJ, et al. Postoperative spindle cell nodule of the prostate and bladder. *J Urol* 1990;143:824–826.

732. Jones E, Young R. Nonneoplastic and neoplastic spindle cell proliferations and mixed tumors of the urinary bladder. *J Urol Pathol* 1994;2:105–134.

733. Jones EC, Clement PB, Young RH. Inflammatory pseudotumor of the urinary bladder. A clinicopathological, immunohistochemical, ultrastructural, and flow cytometric study of 13 cases. *Am J Surg Pathol* 1993;17:264–274.

734. Kaplan WE, Firlit CF, Berger RM. Genitourinary rhabdomyosarcoma. *J Urol* 1983;130:116–119.

735. Dehner L. Pathology of the urinary bladder in children. In: Young R, ed. *Pathology of the Urinary Bladder*. New York: Churchill Livingstone; 1989:179–211.

736. Ziari M, Sonpavde G, Shen S, et al. Patients with unusual bladder malignancies and a rare cause of splenomegaly. Case 2. Rhabdomyosarcoma of the urinary bladder in an adult. *J Clin Oncol* 2005;23:4459–4460.

737. Aydoganli L, Tarhan F, Atan A, et al. Rhabdomyosarcoma of the urinary bladder in an adult. *Int Urol Nephrol* 1993;25:159–161.

738. Henriksson C, Zetterlund CG, Boiesen P, et al. Large rhabdomyosarcoma of the urinary bladder in an adult. Case report. *Scand J Urol Nephrol* 1985;19:237–239.

739. Paner GP, McKenney JK, Epstein JI, et al. Rhabdomyosarcoma of the urinary bladder in adults: predilection for alveolar morphology with anaplasia and significant morphologic overlap with small cell carcinoma. *Am J Surg Pathol* 2008;32:1022–1028.

740. Meza JL, Anderson J, Pappo AS, et al.; Children's Oncology Group. Analysis of prognostic factors in patients with nonmetastatic rhabdomyosarcoma treated on intergroup rhabdomyosarcoma studies III and IV: the Children's Oncology Group. *J Clin Oncol* 2006;24:3844–3851.

741. Rodeberg D, Anderson JR, Arndt C, et al. Comparison of outcomes based on treatment algorithms for rhabdomyosarcoma (RMS) of the bladder/prostate (BP): combined results from the Children's Oncology Group (COG), German Cooperative Soft Tissue Sarcoma Society (CWS), Italian Cooperative Group (ICG), and International Society of Pediatric Oncology (SAIOP) Malignant Mesenchymal Tumors (MMT) Committee. *Int J Cancer* 2010;128:1232–1239.

742. Lawrence W Jr, Anderson JR, Gehan EA, et al. Pretreatment TNM staging of childhood rhabdomyosarcoma: a report of the Intergroup Rhabdomyosarcoma Study Group. Children's Cancer Study Group. Pediatric Oncology Group. *Cancer* 1997;80:1165–1170.

743. Newton WA Jr, Soule EH, Hamoudi AB, et al. Histopathology of childhood sarcomas, Intergroup Rhabdomyosarcoma Studies I and II: clinicopathologic correlation. *J Clin Oncol* 1988;6:67–75.

744. Entz-Werle N, Marcellin L, Becmeur F, et al. The urinary bladder: an extremely rare location of pediatric neuroblastoma. *J Pediatr Surg* 2003;38:E10–E12.

745. Chang C-Y, Chiou T-J, Hsieh Y-L, et al. Leukemic infiltration of the urinary bladder presenting as uncontrollable gross hematuria in a child with acute lymphoblastic leukemia. *J Pediatr Hematol Oncol* 2003;25:735–739.

746. Schniederjan SD, Osunkoya AO. Lymphoid neoplasms of the urinary tract and male genital organs: a clinicopathological study of 40 cases. *Mod Pathol* 2009;22:1057–1065.

747. Zhang D-Y, Lin T, Wei G-H, et al. A rare case of simultaneous occurrence of Wilms' tumor in the left kidney and the bladder. *Pediatr Surg Int* 2010;26:319–322.

748. Hojo H, Newton WA Jr, Hamoudi AB, et al. Pseudosarcomatous myofibroblastic tumor of the urinary bladder in children: a study of 11 cases with review of the literature. An Intergroup Rhabdomyosarcoma Study. *Am J Surg Pathol* 1995;19:1224–1236.

749. Seethala RR, Gomez JA, Vakar-Lopez F. Primary angiosarcoma of the bladder. *Arch Pathol Lab Med* 2006;130:1543–1547.

750. Kulaga A, Yilmaz A, Wilkin RP, et al. Epithelioid angiosarcoma of the bladder after irradiation for endometrioid adenocarcinoma. *Virchows Arch* 2007;450:245–246.

751. Pazona JF, Gupta R, Wysock J, et al. Angiosarcoma of bladder: long-term survival after multimodal therapy. *Urology* 2007;69:575.e9–e10.

752. Geramizadeh B, Banani A, Foroutan H, et al. Malignant epithelioid hemangioendothelioma of the bladder: the first case report in a child. *J Pediatr Surg* 2009;44:1443–1445.

753. Pan C-C, Yu IT, Yang A-H, et al. Clear cell myomelanocytic tumor of the urinary bladder. *Am J Surg Pathol* 2003;27:689–692.

754. Kalyanasundaram K, Parameswaran A, Mani R. Perivascular epithelioid tumor of urinary bladder and vagina. *Ann Diagn Pathol* 2005;9:275–278.

755. Parfitt JR, Bella AJ, Wehrli BM, et al. Primary PEComa of the bladder treated with primary excision and adjuvant interferon-alpha immunotherapy: a case report. *BMC Urol* 2006;6:20.

756. Weinreb I, Howarth D, Latta E, et al. Perivascular epithelioid cell neoplasms (PEComas): four malignant cases expanding the histopathological spectrum and a description of a unique finding. *Virchows Arch* 2007;450:463–470.

757. Givler RL. Involvement of the bladder in leukemia and lymphoma. *J Urol* 1971;105:667–670.

758. Sufrin G, Keogh B, Moore RH, et al. Secondary involvement of the bladder in malignant lymphoma. *J Urol* 1977;118:251–253.

759. Abraham NZ Jr, Maher TJ, Hutchison RE. Extra-nodal monocytoid B-cell lymphoma of the urinary bladder. *Mod Pathol* 1993;6:145–149.

760. Kempton CL, Kurtin PJ, Inwards DJ, et al. Malignant lymphoma of the bladder: evidence from 36 cases that low-grade lymphoma of the MALT-type is the most common primary bladder lymphoma. *Am J Surg Pathol* 1997;21:1324–1333.

761. Bates AW, Norton AJ, Baithun SI. Malignant lymphoma of the urinary bladder: a clinicopathological study of 11 cases. *J Clin Pathol* 2000;53:458–461.

762. Ohsawa M, Aozasa K, Horiuchi K, et al. Malignant lymphoma of bladder. Report of three cases and review of the literature. *Cancer* 1993;72:1969–1974.

763. Mourad WA, Khalil SM, Radwi A, et al. Primary T-cell lymphoma of the urinary bladder. *Am J Surg Pathol* 1998;22:373–377.

764. Wang L, Cao ZZ, Qi L. Primary T-cell lymphoma of the urinary bladder presenting with haematuria and hydroureteronephrosis. *J Int Med Res* 2011;39:2027–2032.

765. Allory Y, Merabet Z, Copie-Bergman C, et al. Sarcomatoid variant of anaplastic large cell lymphoma mimics ALK-1-positive inflammatory myofibroblastic tumor in bladder [comment]. *Am J Surg Pathol* 2005;29:838–839.

766. Grooms AM, Morgan SK, Turner WR Jr. Hematuria and leukemic bladder infiltration. *JAMA* 1973;223:193–194.

767. Cesaro S, Brugiolo A, Faraci M, et al. Incidence and treatment of hemorrhagic cystitis in children given hematopoietic stem cell transplantation: a survey from the Italian association of pediatric hematology oncology-bone marrow transplantation group. *Bone Marrow Transplant* 2003;32:925–931.

768. Cheuk DKL, Lee TL, Chiang AKS, et al. Risk factors and treatment of hemorrhagic cystitis in children who underwent hematopoietic stem cell transplantation. *Transpl Int* 2007;20:73–81.

769. Al-Quran SZ, Olivares A, Lin P, et al. Myeloid sarcoma of the urinary bladder and epididymis as a primary manifestation of acute myeloid leukemia with inv(16). *Arch Pathol Lab Med* 2006;130:862–866.

770. Aki H, Baslar Z, Uygun N, et al. Primary granulocytic sarcoma of the urinary bladder: case report and review of the literature. *Urology* 2002;60:345.

771. Meis JM, Butler JJ, Osborne BM, et al. Granulocytic sarcoma in non-leukemic patients. *Cancer* 1986;58:2697–2709.

772. Matsumiya K, Kanayama Y, Yamaguchi S, et al. Extramedullary plasmacytoma (EMP) of urinary bladder. *Urology* 1992;40:67–70.

773. Ho DS, Patterson AL, Orozco RE, et al. Extramedullary plasmacytoma of the bladder: case report and review of the literature. *J Urol* 1993;150:473–474.

774. Lopez A, Mendez F, Puras-Baez A. Extramedullary plasmacytoma invading the bladder: case report and review of the literature. *Urol Oncol* 2003;21:419–423.

775. Mokhtar GA, Yazdi H, Mai KT. Cytopathology of extramedullary plasmacytoma of the bladder: a case report. *Acta Cytol* 2006;50:339–343.

776. Farinola MA, Lawler LP, Rosenthal D. Plasmacytoma with involvement of the urinary bladder. Report of a case diagnosed by urine cytology. *Acta Cytol* 2003;47:787–791.

777. Takahashi R, Nakano S, Namura K, et al. Plasmacytoma of the urinary bladder in a renal transplant recipient. *Int J Hematol* 2005;81:255–257.

778. Shpilberg O, Raviv G, Ramon J, et al. Massive hematuria due to extramedullary plasmacytoma invading the bladder. *Med Pediatr Oncol* 1993;21:67–69.

779. Neal MH, Swearingen ML, Gawronski L, et al. Myeloma cells in the urine. *Arch Pathol Lab Med* 1985;109:870–872.

780. De Torres I, Fortuno MA, Raventos A, et al. Primary malignant melanoma of the bladder: immunohistochemical study of a new case and review of the literature. *J Urol* 1995;154:525–527.

781. Tainio HM, Kylmala TM, Haapasalo HK. Primary malignant melanoma of the urinary bladder associated with widespread metastases. *Scand J Urol Nephrol* 1999;33:406–407.

782. Khalbuss WE, Hossain M, Elhosseiny A. Primary malignant melanoma of the urinary bladder diagnosed by urine cytology: a case report. *Acta Cytol* 2001;45:631–635.

783. Pacella M, Gallo F, Gastaldi C, et al. Primary malignant melanoma of the bladder. *Int J Urol* 2006;13:635–637.

784. Rossen K, Petersen MM. Simple melanosis of the bladder. *J Urol* 1999;161:1564.

785. Talmon G, Khan A, Koerber R, et al. Simple melanosis of the bladder: a rare entity. *Int J Surg Pathol* 2010;18:547–549.

786. Morichetti D, Mazzucchelli R, Lopez-Beltran A, et al. Secondary neoplasms of the urinary system and male genital organs. *BJU Int* 2009;104:770–776.

787. Ainsworth AM, Clark WH, Mastrangelo M, et al. Primary malignant melanoma of the urinary bladder. *Cancer* 1976;37:1928–1936.

788. Honma K. Paraganglia of the urinary bladder. An autopsy study. *Zentralbl Pathol* 1994;139:465–469.

789. Pasini B, Stratakis CA. SDH mutations in tumorigenesis and inherited endocrine tumours: lesson from the phaeochromocytoma-paraganglioma syndromes. *J Intern Med* 2009;266:19–42.

790. Timmers HJLM, Gimenez-Roqueplo A-P, Mannelli M, et al. Clinical aspects of SDHx-related pheochromocytoma and paraganglioma. *Endocr Relat Cancer* 2009;16:391–400.

791. Zimmerman I, Biron R, MacMahon H. Pheochromocytoma of the urinary bladder. *N Engl J Med* 1953;249:26.

792. Mou JWC, Lee KH, Tam YH, et al. Urinary bladder pheochromocytoma, an extremely rare tumor in children: case report and review of the literature. *Pediatr Surg Int* 2008;24:479–480.

793. Shono T, Sakai H, Minami Y, et al. Paraganglioma of the urinary bladder: a case report and review of the Japanese literature. *Urol Int* 1999;62:102–105.

794. Grignon DJ, Ro JY, Mackay B, et al. Paraganglioma of the urinary bladder: immunohistochemical, ultrastructural, and DNA flow cytometric studies. *Hum Pathol* 1991;22:1162–1169.

795. Kato H, Suzuki M, Mukai M, et al. Clinicopathological study of pheochromocytoma of the urinary bladder: immunohistochemical, flow cytometric and ultrastructural findings with review of the literature. *Pathol Int* 1999;49:1093–1099.

796. Kovacs K, Bell D, Gardiner GW, et al. Malignant paraganglioma of the urinary bladder: immunohistochemical study of prognostic indicators. *Endocr Pathol* 2005;16:363–369.

797. Khan O, Williams G, Chisholm GD, et al. Phaeochromocytomas of the bladder. *J R Soc Med* 1982;75:17–20.

798. Athyal RP, Al-Khawari H, Arun N, et al. Urinary bladder paraganglioma in a case of von Hippel-Lindau disease. *Australas Radiol* 2007;51 Spec No.:B67–B70.

799. Brown HM, Komorowski RA, Wilson SD, et al. Predicting metastasis of pheochromocytomas using DNA flow cytometry and immunohistochemical markers of cell proliferation: a positive correlation between MIB-1 staining and malignant tumor behavior. *Cancer* 1999;86:1583–1589.

800. John H, Ziegler WH, Hauri D, et al. Pheochromocytomas: can malignant potential be predicted? *Urology* 1999;53:679–683.

801. Cheng L, Leibovich BC, Cheville JC, et al. Paraganglioma of the urinary bladder: can biologic potential be predicted? *Cancer* 2000;88:844–852.

802. Joshua AM, Ezzat S, Asa SL, et al. Rationale and evidence for sunitinib in the treatment of malignant paraganglioma/pheochromocytoma. *J Clin Endocrinol Metab* 2009;94:5–9.

803. Lam KY, Chan AC. Paraganglioma of the urinary bladder: an immunohistochemical study and report of an unusual association with intestinal carcinoid. *Aust N Z J Surg* 1993;63:740–745.

804. Cammassei F, Bosman C, Corsi A, et al. Oncocytic paraganglioma of the urinary bladder. *J Urol Pathol* 1998;8:8.

805. Singh DV, Seth A, Gupta NP, et al. Calcified nonfunctional paraganglioma of the urinary bladder mistaken as bladder calculus: a diagnostic pitfall. *BJU Int* 2000;85:1152–1153.

806. Usuda H, Emura I. Composite paraganglioma-ganglioneuroma of the urinary bladder. *Pathol Int* 2005;55:596–601.

807. Dundr P, Dudorkinova D, Povysil C, et al. Pigmented composite paraganglioma-ganglioneuroma of the urinary bladder. *Pathol Res Pract* 2003;199:765–769.

808. Chen CH, Boag AH, Beiko DT, et al. Composite paraganglioma-ganglioneuroma of the urinary bladder: a rare neoplasm causing hemodynamic crisis at tumour resection. *Can Urol Assoc J* 2009;3:E45–E48.

809. Salo JO, Miettinen M, Makinen J, et al. Pheochromocytoma of the urinary bladder. Report of 2 cases with ultrastructural and immunohistochemical analyses. *Eur Urol* 1989;16:237–239.

810. Amin MB, Patel RM, Oliveira P, et al. Alveolar soft-part sarcoma of the urinary bladder with urethral recurrence: a unique case with emphasis on differential diagnoses and diagnostic utility of an immunohistochemical panel including TFE3. *Am J Surg Pathol* 2006;30:1322–1325.

811. Eble JN, Young RH. Carcinoma of the urinary bladder: a review of its diverse morphology. *Semin Diagn Pathol* 1997;14:98–108.

812. Cauffield EW. Dermoid cysts of the bladder. *J Urol* 1956;75:801–804.

813. Kuyumcuoglu U, Kale A. Unusual presentation of a dermoid cyst that derived from the bladder dome presenting as subserosal leiomyoma uteri. *Clin Exp Obstet Gynecol* 2008;35:309–310.

814. Okeke L, Ogun G, Etikakpan B, et al. Dermoid cyst of the urinary bladder as a differential diagnosis of bladder calculus: a case report. *J Med Case Reports* 2007;1:32.

815. Agrawal S, Khurana N, Mandhani A, et al. Primary bladder dermoid: a case report and review of the literature. *Urol Int* 2006;77:279–280.

816. Tandon A, Gulleria K, Gupta S, et al. Mature ovarian dermoid cyst invading the urinary bladder. *Ultrasound Obstet Gynecol* 2010;35:751–753.

817. Misra S, Agarwal PK, Tandon RK, et al. Bladder teratoma: a case report and review of literature. *Indian J Cancer* 1997;34:20–21.

818. Bhalla S, Masih K, Rana RS. Teratomas of rare sites: a review of ten cases. *J Indian Med Assoc* 1991;89:291–294.

819. Taylor G, Jordan M, Churchill B, et al. Yolk sac tumor of the bladder. *J Urol* 1983;129:591–594.

820. D'Alessio A, Verdelli G, Bernardi M, et al. Endodermal sinus (yolk sac) tumor of the urachus. *Eur J Pediatr Surg* 1994;4:180–181.

821. Romero-Rojas A, Messa-Botero O, Melo-Uribe M, et al. Primary yolk sac tumor of the urachus. *Int J Surg Pathol* 2010;19:658–661.

822. Huang H-Y, Ko S-F, Chuang J-H, et al. Primary yolk sac tumor of the urachus. *Arch Pathol Lab Med* 2002;126:1106–1109.

823. Velcheti V, Govindan R. Metastatic cancer involving bladder: a review. *Can J Urol* 2007;14:3443–3448.

824. Klinger M. Secondary tumors of the genito-urinary tract. *J Urol* 1951;65:144–153.

825. Bates AW, Baithun SI. Secondary neoplasms of the bladder are histological mimics of nontransitional cell primary tumours: clinicopathological and histological features of 282 cases. *Histopathology* 2000;36:32–40.

826. Silverstein LI, Plaine L, Davis JE, et al. Breast carcinoma metastatic to bladder. *Urology* 1987;29:544–547.

827. Mai KT, Nguyen B. Urothelial carcinoma and prostatic adenocarcinoma presenting as collision tumors. *Can J Urol* 2009;16:4850–4853.

828. Keillor JS, Aterman K. The response of poorly differentiated prostatic tumors to staining for prostate specific antigen and prostatic acid phosphatase: a comparative study. *J Urol* 1987;137:894–896.

829. Varma M, Jasani B. Diagnostic utility of immunohistochemistry in morphologically difficult prostate cancer: review of current literature. *Histopathology* 2005;47:1–16.

830. Silver SA, Epstein JI. Adenocarcinoma of the colon simulating primary urinary bladder neoplasia: a report of nine cases. *Am J Surg Pathol* 1993;17:171–178.

831. Liang CC, Tseng CJ, Soong YK. The usefulness of cystoscopy in the staging of cervical cancer. *Gynecol Oncol* 2000;76:200–203.

832. Sharma DN, Thulkar S, Goyal S, et al. Revisiting the role of computerized tomographic scan and cystoscopy for detecting bladder invasion in the revised FIGO staging system for carcinoma of the uterine cervix. *Int J Gynecol Cancer* 2010;20:368–372.

833. Kong CS, Beck AH, Longacre TA. A panel of 3 markers including p16, ProExC, or HPV ISH is optimal for distinguishing between primary endometrial and endocervical adenocarcinomas. *Am J Surg Pathol* 2010;34:915–926.

834. Abdulamir AS, Hafidh RR, Kadhim HS, et al. Tumor markers of bladder cancer: the schistosomal bladder tumors versus non-schistosomal bladder tumors. *J Exp Clin Cancer Res* 2009;28:27.

835. Yang C-C, Chu K-C, Chen H-Y, et al. Expression of p16 and cyclin D1 in bladder cancer and correlation in cancer progression. *Urol Int* 2002;69:190–194.

836. Gatti G, Zurrida S, Gilardi D, et al. Urinary bladder metastases from breast carcinoma: review of the literature starting from a clinical case. *Tumori* 2005;91:283–286.

837. Lin W-C, Chen J-H. Urinary bladder metastasis from breast cancer with heterogeneic expression of estrogen and progesterone receptors. *J Clin Oncol* 2007;25:4308–4310.

838. Fisher MB, Weise AJ, Powell IJ. Breast carcinoma metastatic to the bladder and renal pelvis requiring fulguration. *Clin Breast Cancer* 2005;6:173–174.

839. Soon PSH, Lynch W, Schwartz P. Breast cancer presenting initially with urinary incontinence: a case of bladder metastasis from breast cancer. *Breast* 2004;13:69–71.

840. Matsuo M, Koga S, Nishikido M, et al. Renal cell carcinoma with solitary metachronous metastasis to the urinary bladder. *Urology* 2002;60:911–912.

841. Dogra P, Kumar A, Singh A. An unusual case of von Hippel Lindau (VHL) syndrome with bilateral multicentric renal cell carcinoma with synchronous solitary urinary bladder metastasis. *Int Urol Nephrol* 2007;39:11–14.

842. McAchran SE, Williams DH, MacLennan GT. Renal cell carcinoma metastasis to the bladder. *J Urol* 2010;184:726–727.

843. Shiraishi K, Mohri J, Inoue R, et al. Metastatic renal cell carcinoma to the bladder 12 years after radical nephrectomy. *Int J Urol* 2003;10:453–455.

844. Raviv S, Eggener SE, Williams DH, et al. Long-term survival after "drop metastases" of renal cell carcinoma to the bladder. *Urology* 2002;60:697.

845. Abel PD, Henderson D, Bennett MK, et al. Differing interpretations by pathologists of the pT category and grade of transitional cell cancer of the bladder. *Br J Urol* 1988;62:339–342.

846. Tosoni I, Wagner U, Sauter G, et al. Clinical significance of interobserver differences in the staging and grading of superficial bladder cancer. *BJU Int* 2000;85:48–53.

847. van der Meijden A, Sylvester R, Collette L, et al. The role and impact of pathology review on stage and grade assessment of stages Ta and T1 bladder tumors: a combined analysis of 5 European Organization for Research and Treatment of Cancer Trials. *J Urol* 2000;164:1533–1537.

848. Grignon D, Sakr W. Pathologic stage T1 carcinoma of the bladder: clinical implications and prognostic significance. *Pathol Case Rev* 1997;2:107–114.

849. Samaratunga H, Fairweather P, Purdie D. Significance of stromal reaction patterns in invasive urothelial carcinoma. *Am J Clin Pathol* 2005;123:851–857.

850. Ro JY, Ayala AG, El-Naggar A. Muscularis mucosa of urinary bladder. Importance for staging and treatment. *Am J Surg Pathol* 1987;11:668–673.

851. Paner GP, Ro JY, Wojcik EM, et al. Further characterization of the muscle layers and lamina propria of the urinary bladder by systematic histologic mapping: implications for pathologic staging of invasive urothelial carcinoma. *Am J Surg Pathol* 2007;31:1420–1429.

852. Paner GP, Shen SS, Lapetino S, et al. Diagnostic utility of antibody to smoothelin in the distinction of muscularis propria from muscularis mucosae of the urinary bladder: a potential ancillary tool in the pathologic staging of invasive urothelial carcinoma. *Am J Surg Pathol* 2009;33:91–98.

853. Council L, Hameed O. Differential expression of immunohistochemical markers in bladder smooth muscle and myofibroblasts, and the potential utility of desmin, smoothelin, and vimentin in staging of bladder carcinoma. *Mod Pathol* 2009;22:639–650.

854. Paner GP, Brown JG, Lapetino S, et al. Diagnostic use of antibody to smoothelin in the recognition of muscularis propria in transurethral resection of urinary bladder tumor (TURBT) specimens. *Am J Surg Pathol* 2010;34:792–799.

855. Miyamoto H, Sharma RB, Illei PB, et al. Pitfalls in the use of smoothelin to identify muscularis propria invasion by urothelial carcinoma. *Am J Surg Pathol* 2010;34:418–422.

856. Farrow GM, Utz DC, Rife CC. Morphological and clinical observations of patients with early bladder cancer treated with total cystectomy. *Cancer Res* 1976;36:2495–2501.

857. Cheng L, Weaver AL, Bostwick DG. Predicting extravesical extension of bladder carcinoma: a novel method based on micrometer measurement of the depth of invasion in transurethral resection specimens. *Urology* 2000;55:668–672.

858. van der Aa MNM, van Leenders GJLH, Steyerberg EW, et al. A new system for substaging pT1 papillary bladder cancer: a prognostic evaluation. *Hum Pathol* 2005;36:981–986.

859. Chang W-C, Chang Y-H, Pan C-C. Prognostic significance in substaging of T1 urinary bladder urothelial carcinoma on transurethral resection. *Am J Surg Pathol* 2012;36:454–461.

860. Bertz S, Denzinger S, Otto W, et al. Substaging by estimating the size of invasive tumour can improve risk stratification in pT1 urothelial bladder cancer-evaluation of a large hospital-based single-centre series. *Histopathology* 2011;59:722–732.

861. Younes M, Sussman J, True LD. The usefulness of the level of the muscularis mucosae in the staging of invasive transitional cell carcinoma of the urinary bladder. *Cancer* 1990;66:543–548.

862. Orsola A, Trias I, Raventos CX, et al. Initial high-grade T1 urothelial cell carcinoma: feasibility and prognostic significance of lamina propria invasion microstaging (T1a/b/c) in BCG-treated and BCG-non-treated patients. *Eur Urol* 2005;48:231–238.

863. Angulo JC, Lopez JI, Grignon DJ, et al. Muscularis mucosa differentiates two populations with different prognosis in stage T1 bladder cancer. *Urology* 1995;45:47–53.

864. Philip AT, Amin MB, Tamboli P, et al. Intravesical adipose tissue: a quantitative study of its presence and location with implications for therapy and prognosis. *Am J Surg Pathol* 2000;24:1286–1290.

865. Cheng L, Montironi R, Davidson DD, et al. Staging and reporting of urothelial carcinoma of the urinary bladder. *Mod Pathol* 2009;22:S70–S95.

866. Lopez-Beltran A, Bassi P, Pavone-Macaluso M, et al. Handling and pathology reporting of specimens with carcinoma of the urinary bladder, ureter, and renal pelvis. *Eur Urol* 2004;45:257–266.

867. Elliott GB, Moloney PJ, Anderson GH. "Denuding cystitis" and in situ urothelial carcinoma. *Arch Pathol Lab Med* 1973;96:91–94.

868. Parwani AV, Levi AW, Epstein JI, et al. Urinary bladder biopsy with denuded mucosa: denuding cystitis-cytopathologic correlates. *Diagn Cytopathol* 2004;30:297–300.

869. Levi AW, Potter SR, Schoenberg MP, et al. Clinical significance of denuded urothelium in bladder biopsy. *J Urol* 2001;166:457–460.

870. Efstathiou J, Quinn D, Stenzl A, et al. Muscle-invasive, presumably regional, tumor. In: Soloway M, Khoury S, eds. *Bladder Cancer: 2nd International Consultation on Bladder Cancer—Vienna.* Paris, France: ICUD-EAU; 2012:269–341.

871. Kassouf W, Swanson D, Kamat AM, et al. Partial cystectomy for muscle invasive urothelial carcinoma of the bladder: a contemporary review of the M. D. Anderson Cancer Center experience. *J Urol* 2006;175:2058–2062.

872. Smaldone MC, Jacobs BL, Smaldone AM, et al. Long-term results of selective partial cystectomy for invasive urothelial bladder carcinoma. *Urology* 2008;72:613–616.

873. Golijanin D, Yossepowitch O, Beck SD, et al. Carcinoma in a bladder diverticulum: presentation and treatment outcome. *J Urol* 2003;170:1761–1764.

874. Schumacher MC, Scholz M, Weise ES, et al. Is there an indication for frozen section examination of the ureteral margins during cystectomy for transitional cell carcinoma of the bladder? *J Urol* 2006;176:2409–2413.

875. Tollefson MK, Blute ML, Farmer SA, et al. Significance of distal ureteral margin at radical cystectomy for urothelial carcinoma. *J Urol* 2010;183:81–86.

876. Touma N, Izawa JI, Abdelhady M, et al. Ureteral frozen sections at the time of radical cystectomy: reliability and clinical implications. *Can Urol Assoc J* 2010;4:28–32.

877. Stein JP, Penson DF, Wu SD, et al. Pathological guidelines for orthotopic urinary diversion in women with bladder cancer: a review of the literature. *J Urol* 2007;178:756–760.

878. Bhatta Dhar N, Kessler TM, Mills RD, et al. Nerve-sparing radical cystectomy and orthotopic bladder replacement in female patients. *Eur Urol* 2007;52:1006–1014.

879. Huguet-Perez J, Palou J, Millan-Rodriguez F, et al. Upper tract transitional cell carcinoma following cystectomy for bladder cancer. *Eur Urol* 2001;40:318–323.

880. Volkmer BG, Schnoeller T, Kuefer R, et al. Upper urinary tract recurrence after radical cystectomy for bladder cancer—who is at risk? *J Urol* 2009;182:2632–2637.

881. Boorjian SA, Kim SP, Weight CJ, et al. Risk factors and outcomes of urethral recurrence following radical cystectomy. *Eur Urol* 2011;60:1266–1272.

882. Mazzucchelli R, Barbisan F, Santinelli A, et al. Prediction of prostatic involvement by urothelial carcinoma in radical cystoprostatectomy for bladder cancer. *Urology* 2009;74:385–390.

883. Huguet J, Monllau V, Sabate S, et al. Diagnosis, risk factors, and outcome of urethral recurrences following radical cystectomy for bladder cancer in 729 male patients. *Eur Urol* 2008;53:785–792.

884. Kassouf W, Spiess PE, Brown GA, et al. P0 stage at radical cystectomy for bladder cancer is associated with improved outcome independent of traditional clinical risk factors. *Eur Urol* 2007;52:769–774.

885. Herr HW. Extent of pelvic lymph node dissection during radical cystectomy: where and why! *Eur Urol* 2010;57:212–213.

886. Dalbagni G. Editorial comment on: the extent of lymphadenectomy seems to be associated with better survival in patients with non-metastatic upper-tract urothelial carcinoma: how many lymph nodes should be removed? *Eur Urol* 2009;56:519.

887. Karl A, Carroll PR, Gschwend JE, et al. The impact of lymphadenectomy and lymph node metastasis on the outcomes of radical cystectomy for bladder cancer. *Eur Urol* 2009;55:826–835.

888. Dhar NB, Klein EA, Reuther AM, et al. Outcome after radical cystectomy with limited or extended pelvic lymph node dissection. *J Urol* 2008;179:873–878.

889. Abol-Enein H, Tilki D, Mosbah A, et al. Does the extent of lymphadenectomy in radical cystectomy for bladder cancer influence disease-free survival? A prospective single-center study. *Eur Urol* 2011;60:572–577.

890. Leissner J, Hohenfellner R, Thuroff JW, et al. Prognostic significance of histopathological grading and immunoreactivity for p53 and p21/WAF1 in grade 2 pTa transitional cell carcinoma of the urinary bladder. *Eur Urol* 2001;39:438–445.

891. Koppie TM, Vickers AJ, Vora K, et al. Standardization of pelvic lymphadenectomy performed at radical cystectomy: can we establish a minimum number of lymph nodes that should be removed? *Cancer* 2006;107:2368–2374.

892. Wright JL, Lin DW, Porter MP. The association between extent of lymphadenectomy and survival among patients with lymph node metastases undergoing radical cystectomy. *Cancer* 2008;112:2401–2408.

893. Kassouf W, Leibovici D, Luongo T, et al. Relevance of extracapsular extension of pelvic lymph node metastasis in patients with bladder cancer treated in the contemporary era. *Cancer* 2006;107:1491–1495.

894. Fleischmann A, Thalmann GN, Markwalder R, et al. Extracapsular extension of pelvic lymph node metastases from urothelial carcinoma of the bladder is an independent prognostic factor. *J Clin Oncol* 2005;23:2358–2365.

895. Fang AC, Ahmad AE, Whitson JM, et al. Effect of a minimum lymph node policy in radical cystectomy and pelvic lymphadenectomy on lymph node yields, lymph node positivity rates, lymph node density, and survivorship in patients with bladder cancer. *Cancer* 2010;116:1901–1908.

Pathology of the Male and Female Urethra

JESSE K. McKENNEY and ESTHER OLIVA

ANATOMY AND HISTOLOGY

The urethra is a long muscular tube that carries urine from the urinary bladder to the external urethral orifice for excretion. In males, it also provides the conduit for semen, which enters the urethra through the ejaculatory ducts within the prostate. The urethra consists of an epithelial-lined mucosal surface enveloped by a supporting connective tissue/smooth muscle coat.

The male urethra is 15 to 20 cm in length and is divided descriptively into four regions/segments: preprostatic (intramural or within the bladder neck), prostatic, membranous (intermediate), and penile (spongy or cavernous).[1–3] The prostatic urethra is located in the pelvis, while the membranous and penile regions are in the perineum. The shortest segment (1.0 to 1.5 cm), is the preprostatic or intramural urethra, which runs from the bladder neck to the superior aspect of the prostate. The second segment, the prostatic urethra, is approximately 3 cm in length and begins at the internal urethral orifice at the apex of the bladder trigone. It courses through the prostate, making an anteriorly concave bend, ending where the urethra penetrates the fascia of the urogenital diaphragm, and enters the perineum. The posterior wall of the prostatic urethra has several unique features related to prostatic secretory function. It contains a longitudinal ridge, the urethral crest, lined by two adjacent grooves, the prostatic sinuses.[4]

The prostatic ducts enter the urethra predominantly in the sinuses with fewer entering along the lateral aspects of the crest. The urethral crest also has a midline protuberance, the seminal colliculus or verumontanum, which contains a 5 mm vestigial opening called the prostatic utricle. The ejaculatory ducts open on each side of the utricle. The prostatic urethra receives blood supply from a branch of the inferior vesical artery, the urethral artery. Venous drainage occurs via the periprostatic plexus, while lymphatic drainage is primarily through the obturator and internal iliac nodes. Sympathetic and parasympathetic innervation of the prostate is derived from the pelvic plexus through the cavernous nerves. The third portion, the membranous urethra,

is approximately 2.0 cm in length and extends from the apex of the prostate to the perineal membrane at the bulb of the penis within the deep perineal space. It is surrounded by the striated external urethral sphincter. The small bulbourethral glands, the Cowper glands, are located on each side of the membranous urethra. In the membranous (intermediate) urethra, the striated sphincter corresponds to the location of peak urethral closing pressure. Innervation to this muscle is supplied by the pudendal nerve,[5] but a branch of the sacral plexus has also been identified as a second source of innervation.[6,7] Blood is supplied via the artery to the bulb and the urethral artery, and lymphatic drainage is also to the obturator and internal iliac nodes. The distal segment, the penile or spongy urethra, is the longest, approximately 15 to 16 cm. It courses through the bulb of the penis and corpus spongiosum to its end at the external urethral orifice (meatus). The ducts of the bulbourethral glands open into the proximal (bulbar) portion of the penile urethra, approximately 2.5 to 3 cm distal to the perineal membrane. The ducts of the urethral (Littre) glands also open into the penile urethra and are concentrated on the dorsal surface of the penile urethra. There are also multiple mucosal recesses, or lacunae, within the penile urethra. The distal region of the penile urethra within the glans penis is a saccular expansion referred to as the fossa navicularis; it contains the largest lacuna, the lacuna magnum. The blood supply to the penile urethra is delivered by the internal pudendal artery and veins, while innervation is provided by branches of the pudendal nerve. The lymphatics of the distal penile urethra drain to the superficial inguinal lymph nodes.

The *female urethra* is shorter, measuring on average 4 cm in length, and extends from the bladder neck to the external urethral orifice in the vaginal vestibule. It is divided into two regions. The proximal portion corresponds to the prostatic urethra and the distal portion to the membranous urethra. The bulbar and pendulous regions of the penile urethra are androgen dependent and, therefore, are not present in the female. Urethral glands are located along the wall of the urethra, particularly in the superior portion. One group of glands, the paraurethral (Skene) glands, represent the homolog of the prostate and are located on each side of the urethra. The paraurethral glands share a common duct on each side, the paraurethral ducts, which enter the urethra near the external urethral orifice. The female urethra receives blood circulation from the vaginal and internal pudendal arteries and veins, while it is innervated by the pudendal nerve. Lymphatic drainage courses to the internal iliac and sacral lymph nodes, with some drainage to the inguinal lymph nodes.

In the male, the preprostatic, prostatic, and membranous urethra regions have an epithelial lining identical to that of the urinary bladder with a stratified layer of urothelium and a superficial umbrella cell layer (Fig. 7-1A). The prostatic urethral lining may also contain admixed prostatic secretory cells. The lamina propria within these regions consists of loose collagenous tissue and small thin-walled blood vessels. The deeper structures of the penile urethra (corpus

spongiosum, tunica albuginea, and Buck fascia) are described in the penile chapter. The pendulous and bulbar regions of the penile urethra are lined by a stratified layer of small columnar epithelial cells that are distinct from bladder urothelium. This distinctive epithelium is 4 to 15 cells in thickness and lacks an umbrella layer. The fossa navicularis is lined by a stratified nonkeratinizing squamous epithelium that is continuous with the squamous epithelium of the glans penis (Fig. 7-1B). In the female, the urethral lining is urothelial proximally with a transition to squamous distally; however, nonkeratinizing squamous metaplasia of the urothelial regions is common. The posterolateral bulbourethral (Cowper) glands have a lobular arrangement with central ducts lined by a cuboidal layer of epithelial cells and surrounding clusters of tubuloalveolar glands lined by mucin distended columnar cells (Fig. 7-1C). The urethral (Littre and Skene) glands consist of small aggregates of mucous glands (Fig. 7-1D).

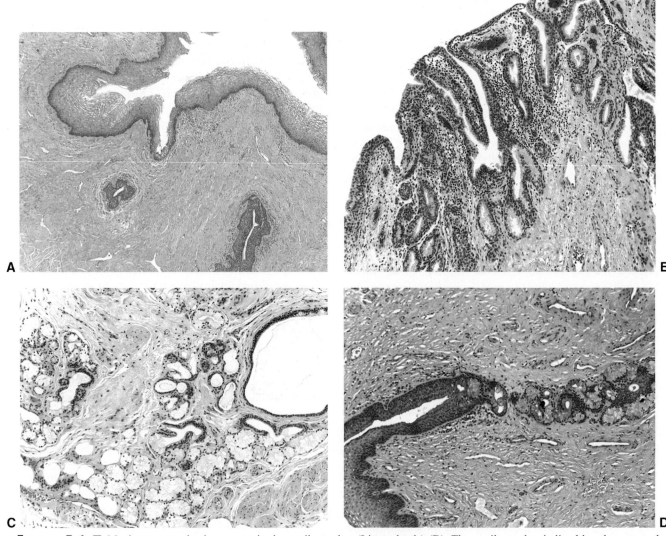

FIGURE 7-1 ■ Mucinous-type glands are seen in the penile urethra (Littre glands) **(D)**. The penile urethra is lined by glycogenated squamous epithelium **(A)** while the prostatic urethra shows alternating patches of urothelial and prostatic epithelium **(B)**. Cowper glands show a lobular arrangement with central ducts (lined by urothelium) and glands lined by mucinous cells **(C)**.

EMBRYOLOGY

The epithelium of the female urethra develops from the endodermal urogenital sinus, which is the anterior portion of the cloaca after it becomes separated from the posterior anorectal canal at 4 to 7 weeks' gestation. The connective tissue and smooth muscle derive from the splanchnic mesoderm. Similarly in the male urethra, the epithelium of the prostatic and membranous portions of the urethra originates from the urogenital sinus and the connective tissue and smooth muscle are also derived from the splanchnic mesoderm.[8–10] In the male, the bulbar and pendulous regions of the penile urethra are derived from the urethral plate on the ventral aspect of the genital tubercle. The epithelium of the fossa navicularis has historically been described as originating distally from ectodermal ingrowth of the glans penis[9]; however, more recent studies have suggested differentiation from the proximal endoderm.[11]

CONGENITAL ABNORMALITIES

Posterior Urethral Valves

This is the most common congenital cause of urethral obstruction leading to bilateral renal failure. It typically occurs in boys with an approximate incidence between 1:3,000 and 1:8,000 male births.[2] Posterior urethral valves may be associated with hypospadias, ureteropelvic junction stenosis, imperforate anus, dysgenetic kidney, or congenital heart disease and very rarely with the prune belly syndrome.[12]

The clinical presentation is variable. Newborns with severe obstruction may present with urinary retention, enlarged bladder, hydronephrosis, uni- or bilateral reflux, and a history of prenatal in utero oligohydramnios associated with pulmonary hypoplasia. Older patients usually have a history of urinary tract infections, urinary retention, pyelonephritis, hematuria, and/or urinary incontinence.[13] Cystography frequently shows dilatation of the urethra above the valves, bladder hypertrophy and dilation, bladder diverticula, tortuous dilated ureters, and varying degrees of hydronephrosis (Fig. 7-2).[12,14,15] Three types of valves have been described. Type I, which is the most common, consists of two posterior folds extending from the verumontanum downward to fuse anteriorly, which has been also described as a complete diaphragm with a central pinhole (depending if a catheter has been put in previously).[16] The folds are usually lined by urothelium, and variable degrees of inflammation may be seen associated with it or present in the lamina propria. Type II is the least common and consists of vertical folds between the verumontanum and proximal urethra and bladder neck. Typre III shows concentrick disk within the prostatic urerthra, either below or verumontanum and it is frequently associated with renal impression.

The treatment of posterior urethral valves is surgical. Mortality associated with this congenital abnormality is currently <5%.[16] As the prenatal diagnosis of posterior urethral valves may be difficult, most deaths occur in newborns

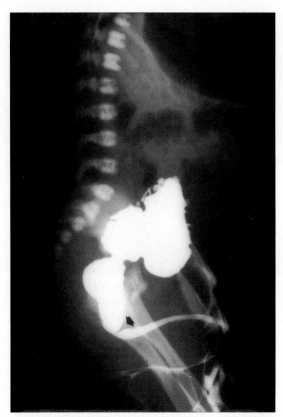

FIGURE 7-2 ■ Type I posterior urethral valves in a newborn. There is marked dilation of the posterior urethra and severe bladder trabeculation. (Courtesy Dr. R Pieretti.)

with severe bilateral renal dysplasia, pulmonary hypoplasia, electrolyte imbalances, or sepsis but may also occur in older children secondary to renal insufficiency.[14,17]

Anterior Urethral Diverticulum and Valve

These congenital abnormalities frequently occur together as it has been hypothesized that commonly one of the walls of the diverticulum acts as an obstructive valve.[18,19] They are rarer than posterior urethral valves with an approximate incidence of 1 in 5,000 to 8,000 male births,[20] are not associated with other defects, and typically occur secondary to a defect of the corpus spongiosum. They occur more frequently in the bulbous region of the penile urethra.[21] Clinical manifestations vary with age; neonates (secondary to severe obstruction) may present with hydronephrosis; however, older boys typically present with repetitive infections or voiding symptoms including incontinence, retention, or thin urine stream.[22] Surgery is the mainstay of treatment. Complications secondary to obstruction may occur as described in posterior urethral valves including end stage renal disease, but they are much less common.[23]

Urethral Duplication

This is a rare congenital malformation that typically occurs in males and occasionally may be associated with bladder duplication.[24] If both urethra and bladder are affected, patients also have other congenital anomalies, more

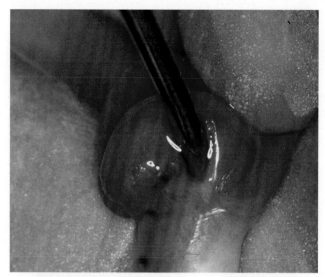

FIGURE 7-3 ■ Urethral duplication is identified by a catheter and urethral sound. (Courtesy Dr. R Pieretti.)

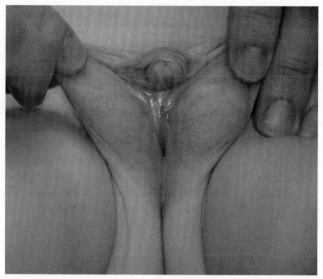

FIGURE 7-4 ■ Penoscrotal hypospadias. Extreme ectopic urethral opening is present close to the perianal orifice. (Courtesy Dr. R Pieretti.)

frequently involving external genitalia and gastrointestinal tract.[25] Most urethral duplications occur in the same sagittal plane (dorsal or ventral to the urethra), and they are classified as complete (with one or two orifices) or incomplete (with a distal or proximal blind end) or may be part of an incomplete or complete caudal duplication (Fig. 7-3).[26] This anomaly may be asymptomatic or be associated with infections, incontinence, or even double stream of urine if the duplication is complete.[26] Histologically, the anomalous urethra is lined by urothelium that may be associated to variable degrees of inflammation in the lamina propria. In symptomatic cases, surgery is the treatment of choice.

Megalourethra

This entity is characterized by absence of the corpus spongiosum or absence of both the corpus spongiosum and corpora cavernosa depending on the degree of severity.[18,27] It may be seen in association with the VATER syndrome, prune belly syndrome (characterized by congenital absence or hypoplasia of the abdominal wall musculature, bilateral cryptorchidism, and anomalies of the urinary tract), or other isolated genitourinary anomalies.[28] An enlarged and deformed penis can be noted in neonates. It is always important to perform a thorough evaluation of the urinary tract due to the high percentage of associated urinary anomalies. Surgical reconstruction depends on the degree of absence of penile tissue.

Hypospadias

This congenital abnormality is one of the most common in the United States with an approximate frequency of 1 in 125 male births.[29] It occurs secondarily to arrest of the urethral development with incomplete fusion of the urethral folds resulting in an ectopic urethral opening on the ventral

surface of the penis, scrotum, or perineum (Fig. 7-4). It is typically associated with an abnormal ventral curvature of the penis and an abnormal distribution of the foreskin around the area.[30] Although the etiology of this condition is unknown, multiple factors have been related to it including maternal (advanced age and primiparity), endocrine (defects in testosterone metabolism or receptors), environmental, and inherited factors.[29,31,32] Hypospadias may be an isolated defect or part of an intersex status. The diagnosis is established in most cases on physical examination, except the very minor forms that may require ultrasound. The defect is treated successfully with surgery.[30,31]

Prostatic Utricle Cyst

These are cysts centered in the prostatic midline, around the area of the verumontanum, and arise from the prostatic utricle. They are typically seen in adult males, and in most instances, they represent an incidental finding during screening for other reasons.[33] As occurs with the prostatic utricle, these cysts are typically connected to the urethra but not to the prostatic ducts.[34] Prostatic utricle cysts are lined by cuboidal to columnar cells histologically similar to those lining the prostatic ducts and acini,[35] and they frequently stain for prostatic-specific antigen (PSA).[35,36] There seems to be some controversy regarding the embryogenesis of these cysts. In the past, they were thought to derive from müllerian remnants, but recent studies have shown that they may have an origin from both müllerian remnants and the urogenital sinus, hence their histologic and immunohistochemical characteristics.[36] Prostatic utricle cyst should be distinguished from the so-called enlarged prostatic utricle, an anomaly frequently seen in the pediatric age group, typically associated with other genitourinary abnormalities, most commonly hypospadias or intersex.[37]

Other Congenital Abnormalities

Other rare urethral congenital anomalies include narrowing of the bulbar portion of the urethra (Cobb collar),[38] Cowper syringocele, and lacuna magna.[23,39]

INFLAMMATION AND INFECTION

Urethritis

Nonspecific Urethritis

Nonspecific urethritis is defined as the finding of irritative urethral symptoms such as burning micturition without evidence of an infectious etiology. With new molecular assays, many cases that might have been previously diagnosed as nonspecific urethritis are now found to have infectious etiology. Nonspecific urethritis has been reported in association with drug exposure including isotretinoin and alcohol and with contact to chemical irritants such as spermicides.[40,42] Nonspecific urethritis may also be part of the spectrum of Reiter syndrome (triad of urethritis, conjunctivitis, and arthritis), typically following dysenteric infections such as *Shigella* or *Salmonella*.[43]

Papillary and Polypoid Urethritis

Papillary and polypoid urethritis is a nonneoplastic lesion that is usually secondary to an inflammatory process; however, unlike the bladder, it is not commonly associated with a catheter.[44,45] Irritative urinary symptoms and hematuria are common presenting signs. Characteristically, the exophytic appearance results from edema in the lamina propria (Fig. 7-5A), but variable fibrosis, chronic inflammation, and associated dilated blood vessels are also present.[46] Older lesions tend to have less edema with more stromal fibrosis. The papillary component is usually broader at the base, but

may also have a bulbous tip. Reactive urothelial changes are frequent and include urothelial hyperplasia, prominent nucleoli, and mitotic activity. The main differential consideration is a papillary urothelial neoplasm, but the inflammatory background and the simple papillary architecture usually aid in this distinction (Fig. 7-5B). These lesions usually regress with resolution of the inciting inflammatory condition.

Infections

Human Papillomavirus Associated Lesions

Human papillomavirus (HPV) is a common source of urethritis.[47] HPV-related squamous dysplasia in the urethra is usually present in continuity with lesions of the external genitalia, anus, or perineum. Flat lesions range from low-grade squamous dysplasia with koilocytotic atypia to high-grade squamous dysplasia identical to that seen in the cervix. Flat intraepithelial squamous dysplasia is rarely biopsied de novo because most urethral lesions are subclinical[48,49]; however, it is common to find squamous dysplasia adjacent to invasive squamous cell carcinoma. Condyloma acuminatum is the most common HPV-related lesion, especially in the male urethra, and it commonly comes to clinical attention because of its intraluminal location with a resultant mass lesion, voiding symptoms, or bleeding.[50] These lesions are morphologically identical to the more common perineal counterparts and are characterized by an exophytic squamous proliferation with hyperkeratosis, prominent granular layer, and typical cytologic features of HPV infection (perinuclear halos, binucleation, nuclear hyperchromasia, and irregular nuclear membranes) (Fig. 7-6A and B). HPV types 6 and 11 are most commonly found in association with condyloma, but other types have been also reported.[51,52] For condyloma acuminatum, the main differential diagnosis is the rare squamous papilloma of the urothelial tract. The latter occur predominantly in elderly women and are characterized by fibrovascular cores

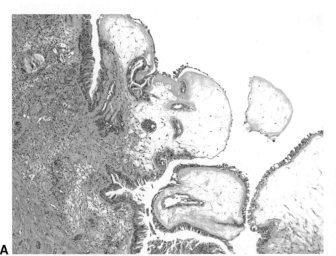

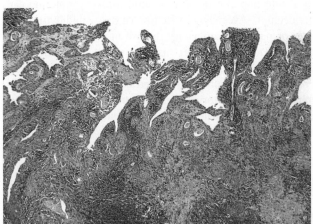

A   B

FIGURE 7-5 ■ Polypoid cystitis. Bulbous and edematous papillae are lined by reactive-appearing urothelium **(A)**. Papillary cystitis. Irregular thin papillae lined by two to three layers of urothelium are associated with prominent inflammatory background in the lamina propria **(B)**.

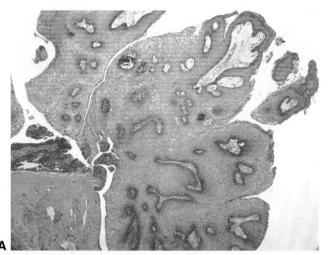
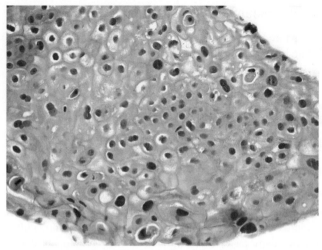

FIGURE 7-6 ■ Condyloma acuminatum. A striking papillary architecture is seen **(A)** with the squamous cells showing striking koilocytic changes **(B)**.

lined by benign-appearing squamous epithelium without viral cytopathic effect; they are also HPV negative by in situ hybridization studies.[53] As in other sites, HPV-associated squamous dysplasia may progress to invasive squamous cell carcinoma, often associated with high-risk HPV types 16, 18, 31, 33, or 35. Therapy for squamous intraepithelial lesions is typically ablative, by surgery, laser, or topical agents.[54]

Gonococcus

Gonorrhea is a sexually transmitted infection caused by *Neisseria gonorrhoeae*, which is a Gram-negative diplococcus. Gonococcal urethritis typically affects teenagers or young adults. Patients typically present 2 to 5 days following infection with burning urination or a purulent urethral discharge.[55] Gonorrhea may be diagnosed by culture, but ELISA and molecular diagnostic testing are also available.[56,57] Tissue biopsy evaluation is not performed routinely. Urethral fluid sampling typically yields neutrophils, and Gram stain may reveal intracellular diplococci. The most significant complication is urethral stricture. Patients with chronic gonorrheal infection also develop urethral fistulae ("watering can perineum"). Ascending infection causing epididymitis in men or pelvic inflammatory disease in women may occur. *Chlamydia* coinfection is also common. Antibiotic therapy is curative, but drug-resistant strains are emerging.[58] Postgonococcal urethritis is defined as persistent signs, symptoms, and/or laboratory evidence of urethritis 4 to 7 days following antibiotic treatment for documented gonorrhea. Most cases result from coinfection with *Chlamydia* or *Ureaplasma* infections; thus, the use of prophylactic multidrug treatment is advocated to cover possible coinfections.[59]

Chlamydia

Urethritis secondary to *Chlamydia trachomatis*, an obligate intracellular bacteria, is a sexually transmitted disease common in teenagers and young adults. *Chlamydia* is the most common sexually transmitted disease in the United States

with over 1,000,000 infections reported to the Center for Disease Control in 2006.[60] *Chlamydia* is asymptomatic in many patients but may present with painful/burning urination or urethral discharge 1 to 3 weeks after exposure.[61] The diagnosis of *Chlamydia* may be based on culture, antigen detection by ELISA or direct fluorescent antibody (DFA), and/or molecular identification with methods such as nucleic acid amplification. The long-term complications of untreated cases are similar to gonorrhea, including epididymitis and pelvic inflammatory disease. In addition, genital chlamydial infection may be associated with urethritis, conjunctivitis, and arthritis (i.e., Reiter syndrome)[62] or with reactive arthritis alone. *Chlamydia* is curable with antibiotic therapy.

Other

Other bacteria responsible for infectious urethritis include *Ureaplasma urealyticum* and *Mycoplasma genitalium*. Evidence suggests that *Ureaplasma parvum* commonly colonizes the urethra without resultant clinical symptoms.[63] Viral etiologies of urethritis include HSV-1 and adenovirus, and being both associated with oral sexual habits.[64] Urethral tuberculosis is exceedingly rare (male > female) and occurs secondarily to infection of the upper urinary (most commonly prostate) or female genital tracts. Predisposing factors include previous infection, immunosuppression, or prior BCG treatment for bladder carcinoma. In the urethra, the most common presentation is acute urethritis with or without discharge, or if untreated, stricture and/or fistulae. The microscopic appearance is characteristic and shows caseating granulomas. If chronic, extensive fibrosis may be seen. The standard treatment requires the use of antituberculous drugs for up to 9 months. However, as often patients present with complications, surgery is still a mainstay of treatment.[65] Wegener granulomatosis can also rarely affect the urethra. Patients may have a known history but occasionally, this location may be the first manifestation of the disease. In males, the gross appearance can be quite worrisome,

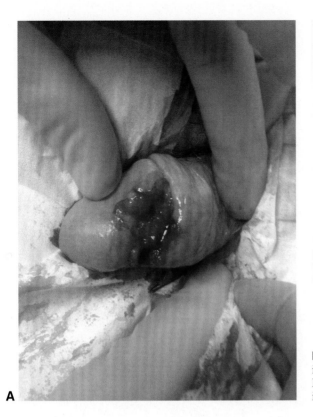

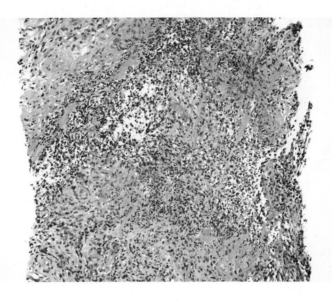

FIGURE 7-7 ■ Wegener granulomatosis. A deep ulcer is present involving the penile urethra and surrounding tissues **(A)**. (Courtesy Dr. F McGovern.) On microscopic examination, the lesion granulomatous inflammation with microabscesses and eosinophils **(B)**.

and clinically misdiagnosed as carcinoma, especially in the penile urethra where Wegener granulomatosis may present as painful fungating mass or extensive ulceration (Fig. 7-7A). Histologic examination may not be diagnostic, only showing extensive necrosis as oftentimes the first diagnostic procedure is a biopsy (Fig. 7-7B). However, the classical morphology includes geographic areas of eosinophilic necrosis associated with palisading histiocytes. Vascular involvement typically shows granulomatous vasculitis with giant cells, but it is not always seen. Methotrexate is the treatment of choice, but patients still often require surgery due to local complications.[66–68] The urethra is the least common site of involvement by sarcoidosis in the genitourinary tract. On gross examination, it may grossly simulate cancer.[69] The morphology is that of noncaseating loose granulomas, but this histologic appearance is nondiagnostic and can be seen in infections and other processes including malignancy (typically at its periphery). However, these patients often have a well-established history of sarcoidosis.[70]

METAPLASIA AND HYPERPLASIA

Squamous Metaplasia

Nonkeratinizing squamous metaplasia is a physiologic phenomenon in women. It is common in the trigone of the bladder, but may also involve the proximal urethra. Nonkeratinizing metaplasia is also reported in men following estrogen therapy.[71] Urethral keratinizing squamous

metaplasia may be seen in association with chronic trauma or chronic inflammatory conditions such as recurring infection, calculi, diverticula, or repeated instrumentation.[72] Extensive and multifocal keratinizing squamous metaplasia may be associated with dysplasia and development of penile carcinoma (more frequently verrucous); thus, patients need to be closely followed.[73]

Glandular Metaplasia

This type of metaplasia is similarly related to a chronic irritative process. It most commonly involves the bladder but may extend into the urethra. Morphologically, glandular metaplasia is typically characterized by columnar epithelium with goblet cells (intestinal metaplasia).

Flat Urothelial Hyperplasia

As in the bladder, the urothelium of the proximal urethra may become markedly thickened. In the absence of cytologic atypia, this is termed flat urothelial hyperplasia.[74] In isolation, urothelial hyperplasia is not regarded as a neoplastic precursor lesion, but it may be seen adjacent to low-grade papillary urothelial neoplasms.[75]

von Brunn Nests, Urethritis Cystica, Urethritis Glandularis

von Brunn nests represent a normal variation of urothelial histology that may result from a prior inflammatory insult. They are characterized by well-circumscribed, evenly spaced

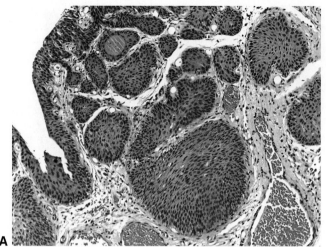

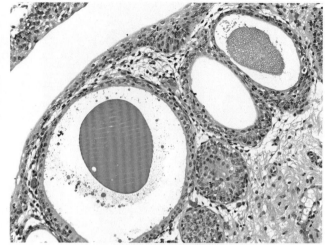

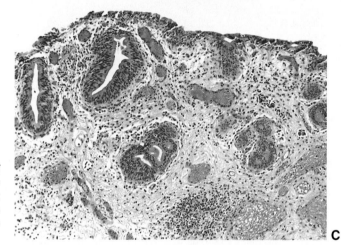

FIGURE 7-8 ■ von Brunn nests are composed of solid nests of benign-appearing urothelium (**A**), Urtheritis cystica, shows cystic dilatation of the glands with abundant eosinophilic contents present in the lumens (**B**). Urtheritis glandularis, conventional type displays glandular metaplasia with a columnar or cuboidal appearance of the luminal cells (**C**).

nests of invaginated urothelium in the lamina propria. The nests typically have smooth, rounded contours and are often clustered in groups, but the connection with the overlying urothelium may not be identifiable (Fig. 7-8A). They are usually located in the superficial lamina propria, but they may deeper however, they are never present in the muscularis propria.

The term "urethritis cystica" is used when the von Brunn nests become cystically dilated with an inner luminal cell layer (Fig. 7-8B). When the inner adluminal cells show glandular metaplasia with a columnar or cuboidal appearance and prominent apical cytoplasm, the term urethritis cystica glandularis is used (Fig. 7-8C). Finally, the presence of admixed intestinal-type goblet cells within the von Brunn nests warrants the designation cystitis cystica glandularis with intestinal metaplasia. These lesions are not regarded as obligate precursors of adenocarcinoma.[76,77]

The main differential diagnosis of von Brunn nests, urethritis cystica, urethritis glandularis are "deceptively benign" urothelial carcinomas that includes nested, microcystic, or tubular variants.[78] In general, these carcinomas have architecturally complex, branching and crowded epithelial proliferations, at least focally, but individual cases may be morphologically indistinguishable from florid von Brunn or urtheritis glanduloris on a superficial biopsy. The identification of stromal reaction, cleft-like spaces surrounding the nests, an irregular infiltrative border, or invasion into the muscularis propria are the most helpful findings for recognizing subtle urothelial carcinomas. In contrast, the nests and glands of urethritis cystica, glandularis are superficial and have a sharp border with the lamina propria. Occasionally, the distinction from inverted papilloma (with a cystitis cystica–like pattern) may be somewhat arbitrary.[79] Inverted papillomas typically show an anastomosing pattern of the epithelial nests and retain the peripheral palisading of cells even when central lumina are present. Occasionally, urothelial carcinoma in situ may extend into von Brunn nests and mimic invasion. The smooth round contour of the nests, the absence of surrounding retraction spaces, the lobular or linear arrangement of the nests with a noninfiltrative base, and the absence of a stromal reaction should aid in that distinction. Rarely, urothelial (transitional cell) carcinomas may grow as large regular nests with minimal cytologic atypia also mimicking von Brunn nests. However, they often also display irregularly infiltrating nests, some associated with desmoplastic reaction and others with muscularis propria invasion.[80]

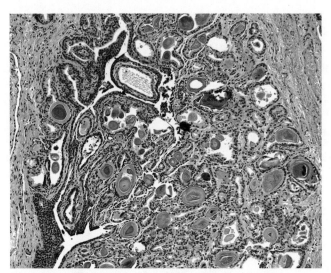

FIGURE 7-9 ■ Verumontanum hyperplasia. Closely packed and small prostatic acini can cause concern for prostatic carcinoma in a small sample.

Cowper Gland Hyperplasia

One case of extensive Cowper gland hyperplasia presenting as a 6-cm urethral mass has been reported.[81] Morphologically, it was characterized by greatly increased number of acini with banal cytologic features maintaining a lobular configuration. In a small biopsy specimen, Cowper glands may raise the differential diagnosis with prostatic carcinoma; however, negative immunohistochemical stains for PSA and prostatic acid phosphatase are helpful to rule out the diagnosis of carcinoma.[82]

Verumontanum Gland Hyperplasia

The verumontanum is an elevation present in the wall of the distal third of the prostatic urethra containing the prostatic utricle flanked by the ejaculatory ducts. This region of the prostate is infrequently biopsied. Verumontanum hyperplasia can be confused with prostatic adenocarcinoma on a biopsy as it shows an increased number of prostatic acini, which are crowded and small (Fig. 7-9). However, the epithelial cells have frequently cuboidal eosinophilic or, more frequently, pale cytoplasm with small nuclei and tiny to absent nucleoli, and the basal cell layer is preserved. Corpora amylacea with concentric laminations that can be fragmented are commonly seen.[83]

POLYPS, CYSTS, AND PSEUDOTUMOROUS LESIONS

Polyps

Caruncle

This benign lesion occurs mainly in women between 20 and 60 years of age (Table 7-1). It appears to be reactive and frequently related to trauma.[84] Patients may present with dysuria or spotting or be asymptomatic. Caruncles are typically seen at the posterior wall of the urethra near the meatus. Grossly, they are pedunculated or broad-based with a dusky red or gray appearance. From the histologic point of view, three patterns have been recognized in the older literature: (a) granulomatous where the granulation tissue is the most striking component, (b) papillomatous with a prominent lobulated growth of the epithelium, and (c) angiomatous or telangiectatic rich in blood vessels.[84] However, this classification is not used in routine practice as it lacks clinical or pathologic significance. Caruncles are typically lined by urothelium or less commonly squamous epithelium that may be hyperplastic (Fig. 7-10A). Metaplastic epithelial changes (intestinal glands) have been reported. The lamina propria is typically rich in acute and chronic inflammatory cells that are associated with abundant small blood vessels and edema (Fig. 7-10A). In some instances, atypical spindled to round mononucleated or rarely binucleated stromal cells arranged either in clusters or diffusely and showing large nuclei and prominent nucleoli may be seen (Fig. 7-10B).[85,86] Myeloid metaplasia has been reported.[87] The urothelial hyperplasia and striking invaginations of the surface epithelium frequently associated with caruncles may raise the possibility of a low-grade urothelial carcinoma. However, there is a bulbous rather than delicate papillary architecture, the nests of epithelium seen in the superficial stroma are rounded and do not elicit stromal response, and the cells lack any degree of cytologic atypia. When atypical cells are present in the stroma, the differential diagnosis include lymphoma,[88,89] malignant melanoma,[90] and even more rarely, spindle cell sarcoma.[85] The small size of the lesion, scarcity of mitotic activity, as well as immunostaining limited to vimentin, smooth muscle actin, and rarely desmin exclude these possibilities.[85] Surgical excision is the treatment of choice.

Prostatic-type Polyp

This benign papillary lesion occurs in adult males. It is typically found in the posterior urethra (more frequently in the verumontanum and prostatic urethra) and less commonly in the bladder or ureteral orifice.[91–95] It often presents with painless gross or microscopic hematuria, voiding symptoms, or hematospermia[91,96–98] although it may be an incidental finding.[94] Grossly, it appears as an exophytic papillary to filiform or infrequently sessile lesion <1 cm in size.[94] Histologically, prostatic-type polyps are composed of irregular polypoid growths or papillary fronds lined by a double layer of cells identical to that seen in prostatic acini with cuboidal to columnar cells displaying basally located nuclei and abundant clear to slightly eosinophilic cytoplasm overlying flattened basal cells (Fig. 7-11A). Urothelium may be interspersed with the prostatic epithelium on the surface. The underlying stroma may contain prostatic acini that may show luminal corpora amylacea. The prostatic epithelium is positive for PSA and prostatic acid phosphatase (Fig. 7-11B).[94,99–102]

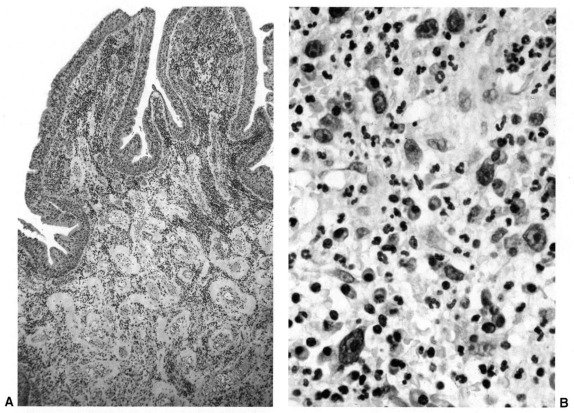

FIGURE 7-10 ■ Caruncle. A striking papillary growth is seen associated with prominent vessels in the lamina propria **(A)**. Atypical stromal cells with enlarged nuclei and prominent nucleoli are admixed with a prominent inflammatory infiltrate **(B)**.

Table 7-1 ■ URETHRAL POLYPS AND CYSTS

Urethral polyps:
  Caruncle
    Frequently related to trauma
    Posterior wall
    May have atypical stromal cells
    Often associated urothelial hyperplasia
  Prostatic-type polyp
    Verumontanum and prostatic urethra in males
    <1 cm
    Lined by prostatic epithelium that may alternate with transitional epithelium
    Differential diagnosis: prostatic ductal carcinoma
  Fibroepithelial polyp
    Mostly males, first decade
    <4 cm
    Club-like projections most common pattern
    Lined by unremarkable urothelium
Urethral cysts:
  Cowper gland duct cyst
    Congenital (children) or acquired (adults)
    May be associated with other abnormalities (more frequently urinary tract)
    Typically confirmed by urethrography
  Skene duct cyst
    Most often secondary to infection and obstruction
    Lined by stratified squamous epithelium
    Differential diagnosis: Urethral diverticulum

This benign lesion should be distinguished from prostatic adenocarcinoma, especially in older that secondary involve the urethra[101]; however, in the latter, prostatic acini are lined by a single layer of malignant epithelial cells with prominent nucleoli. Ductal carcinoma, the most common variant of prostate carcinoma, if low grade, may enter in the differential diagnosis of a prostatic-type polyp. Grossly, the tumor may be seen as an exophytic mass protruding into the prostatic urethra, although it is typically larger than prostatic-type polyps.[103] Cytologically, even though the tumor forms glands that may superficially mimic the low-power appearance seen in a prostatic-type polyp, in contrast to the latter, there is often some degree of cytologic atypia and absence of basal cells. Furthermore, in most cases, a component of acinar carcinoma may be seen. From the immunohistochemical point of view, 34bE12 is helpful to separate ductal carcinoma (except when intraductal) from a prostatic-type polyp, as the former lacks basal cells.[103] Rarely, a primary papillary adenocarcinoma of the urethra or the bladder may enter in the differential diagnosis, but these lesions typically display higher degree of cytologic atypia. The histogenesis of this benign polyp is a matter of debate. It has been postulated that it may represent either a metaplastic process (supported by the fact that the prostate normally develops from an anlage of the urothelium of the urethra) or a defect of embryogenesis.[94] Surgical excision is the treatment of choice with only rare recurrences being reported.

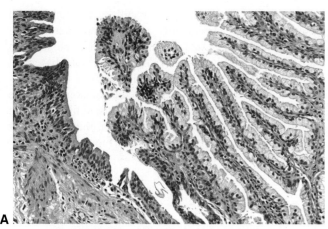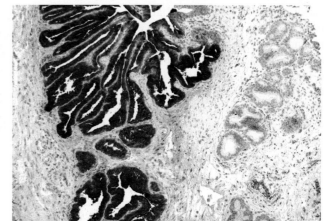

FIGURE 7-11 ■ Prostatic-type polyp. Irregular fronds of prostatic-type epithelium are intermixed with transitional epithelium **(A)**. The prostatic cells are PSA positive **(B)**.

Fibroepithelial Polyp

This is a nonneoplastic lesion with a marked male predominance occurring typically in the first decade of life[92,104]; however, it can also be seen in adult and female patients.[105–107] It is more often located in the urethra (verumontanum) and urinary bladder.[106,107] The most common clinical manifestations include hematuria and obstructive symptoms, but it may be an incidental finding.[104,107,108] On gross examination, fibroepithelial polyps are typically polypoid, soft, and <4 cm in dimension.[92,105,107,109] Histologically, at low power magnification, they may display (a) club-like projections (most common pattern) associated with florid cystitis cystica and glandularis in the stalk; (b) abundant small, plump and rounded fibrovascular cores associated with abundant connective tissue; and (c) simple finger-like projections. They are lined by unremarkable urothelium, but rarely columnar epithelium may be seen.[107] Surface squamous metaplasia and ulceration may occur. Infrequently, the nonsurface epithelial component may show anastomosing nests of urothelium or back to back glands. The stroma may be edematous and may contain atypical stromal cells and calcifications. Entities that more commonly may cause problems in differential diagnosis include florid cystitis glandularis cystica, polypoid or papillary cystitis, and urothelial papilloma. Distinguishing features include absent polypoid or papillary architecture (florid cystitis glandularis); prominent edema and inflammation; and history of instrumentation/trauma (polypoid or papillary cystitis), more delicate stalks or/and associated connective tissue (urothelial papilloma). As this lesion occurs more frequently in early childhood, the differential diagnosis should include botryoid embryonal rhabdomyosarcoma. However, the latter is characterized by a dense "blue" cambium layer under the surface epithelium composed of small immature cells with high nuclear to cytoplasmic ratio and frequent mitotic activity that may alternate with fully developed rhabdomyoblasts showing prominent eosinophilic cytoplasm and cross-striations.[110] After surgical excision, these lesions generally do not recur.

Cowper Gland Duct Cyst

Cowper glands, or bulbourethral glands, are present as paired glands in the bulbomembranous urethra, to which they are connected through small ducts. Their acini form small lobules and are composed of cells with abundant mucin.[111] Cowper gland cyst, also known as syringocele, is a cystic dilatation of the main ducts. It is typically detected in children (congenital) or young adult males (acquired) who present with lower urinary tract symptoms including frequency, urgency, dysuria, postvoid incontinence, recurrent infections and/or hematuria, but it may be asymptomatic.[112–116] In children, it may be associated with other congenital abnormalities, most often of the urinary tract.[113] The diagnosis is easily confirmed by urethrography,[112] and rarely, these specimens undergo pathologic examination. Histologically, the wall of the syringocele may be denuded and associated with prominent inflammation as well as fibrosis of the wall. Treatment consists of marsupialization, and follow-up is uneventful.[39,112]

Skene Duct Cyst

Skene glands and ducts, the homologue of the male prostate gland, are located in the floor of the distal urethra.[117] Skene cysts are rare and frequently occur due to obstruction of the ducts most often secondary to infection. They are seen in female patients who may present with dysuria or obstructive voiding symptoms or be asymptomatic.[118] Grossly, the cysts vary in size, and on microscopic examination they are lined by stratified squamous epithelium.[119] The most common differential diagnosis is with a urethral diverticulum, a distinction that should be made on cystourethroscopy and pelvic MRI findings. Other entities to consider include cystocele and Gartner duct cyst.[118] Surgical excision is the treatment of choice.

Nephrogenic Adenoma

This is a rare pseudoneoplastic lesion that occurs most commonly in adult males, although it can be seen in children and females, in the latter frequently in association with a urethral diverticulum.[120–122] The urethra is the second most frequent location (15%) following the bladder.[123] In most instances, nephrogenic adenoma is an incidental finding at cystoscopy performed for other reasons, but if large it may cause symptoms related to obstruction. In these cases, it may be potentially confused with a malignant tumor, most commonly a low-grade papillary urothelial carcinoma. On microscopic examination, nephrogenic

adenoma shows tubular, cystic, papillary, and rarely solid growths, but not infrequently an admixture thereof.[122,123] The tubules vary in size and shape and may be solid on rare occasions (Fig. 7-12A). An appreciable basement membrane may be seen surrounding some of the tubules. Of note, the tubules of nephrogenic adenoma may be intermixed with muscle fibers of the muscle fibers present in the wall of the prostatic urethra when the specimen is obtained from transurethral resection (Fig. 7-12B).[120,124,125]

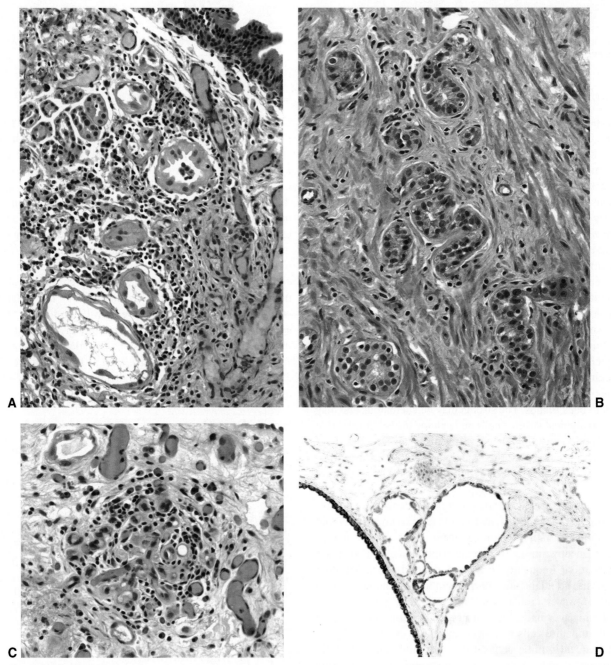

FIGURE 7-12 ■ Nephrogenic adenoma. Tubules and cysts are lined by one layer of cells **(A)**. Tubules are present between muscle fibers mimicking invasive prostatic carcinoma **(B)**. Signet ring–like cells with basophilic intracellular material are set in an edematous and inflammatory stroma **(C)**. The cells are P504s positive **(D)**.

Recently, a fibromyxoid variant of nephrogenic adenoma has been reported characterized by very small tubules associated with prominent fibromyxoid background that may closely mimic the appearance of an infiltrating carcinoma (Chapter 5).[126] Cysts are frequently admixed with tubules, but they are not striking in most cases (Fig. 7-12A). The papillae are simple without branching, and they are rarely seen in the absence of tubules. The solid pattern is very rare and, when present, typically represents a minor component. The cells of nephrogenic adenoma are cuboidal to columnar to flattened with variable eosinophilic to slightly clear and granular cytoplasm, and exceptionally they may be spindled.[126] Hobnail cells are typically present, most often lining the cysts, but are rarely conspicuous.[123,127] The cells lining tiny tubules have a compressed nucleus with a single vacuole containing basophilic material resembling signet ring cells (Fig. 7-12C). The nuclei are round to oval with minimal cytologic atypia. Nucleoli are inconspicuous, and mitotic figures are rare (<1/10 HPFs) and seen in 5% of the lesions.[123] The term "atypical nephrogenic adenoma," has been used for lesions characterized by nuclear enlargement, nuclear hyperchromasia, and enlarged nucleoli.[127] There is no known clinical or biologic significance to this designation. The stroma associated with nephrogenic adenoma is focally edematous and contains variable amounts of inflammatory cells. Stromal calcification may be seen.

The immunohistochemical profile of nephrogenic adenoma includes positivity for CK7, epithelial membrane antigen (EMA), vimentin, and PAX2 and PAX8 (the latter two, antigens expressed during embryogenesis),[128–130] common positivity for racemase (p504s) (Fig. 7-12D)[131,132] and CA-125, but less frequently for CK20, CD10, CEA, and renal cell carcinoma antigen (RCC).[133] Nephrogenic adenoma is positive for aquaporin 1 (marker of proximal and descending thin limb of Henle loop renal tubular cells)[134] and may express different lectins,[135] but it is negative for uroplakin[133], p63,[131,132] Ki67 and p53.[127,136]

When involving the urethra, the main differential diagnosis includes prostatic adenocarcinoma as nephrogenic adenoma may show a pseudoinfiltrative growth with the tubules being intercalated between the muscle fibers.[120,124–125,137] The lumens of the tubules may contain mucinous secretions, and the cells may show prominent nucleoli.[120,138] It is important to keep in mind the possibility of nephrogenic adenoma before establishing the diagnosis of prostatic adenocarcinoma in the setting of a transurethral resection. Immunohistochemical stains for p63, 23βE12, and racemase (p504s) are not helpful in this differential diagnosis in many instances.[131,132] It appears that urethral nephrogenic adenomas more often express p504s when compared to bladder nephrogenic adenomas. The most helpful immunostains are PSA and prostate-specific acid phosphatase (PSAP) (36% and 55%, respectively—typically focal) as most prostatic adenocarcinomas show diffuse and strong positivity for these markers in sharp contrast with nephrogenic adenoma, which may only show focal and weak staining 36 and 55% respectively.[120] A new antibody, S100A1, a calcium-binding protein, has been shown to be positive in most nephrogenic adenomas but negative in prostatic carcinoma.[139] Furthermore, to other typical architectural patterns of nephrogenic adenoma are commonly observed, the cytologic atypia is frequently of the degenerative type, and the stroma frequently shows some degree of inflammation.[123] Another entity in the differential diagnosis is clear cell carcinoma.[138,140,141] This malignant tumor is more frequently seen in older women; it forms large masses and may show areas of hemorrhage and necrosis. On microscopic examination, the histologic patterns of clear cell carcinoma overlap with those seen in nephrogenic adenoma, although a solid growth is more common, papillae tend to branch and may contain hyalinized fibrovascular cores, and the degree of cytologic atypia and mitotic activity are clearly evident[138,140,141] However, some of these tumors may have bland cytologic features throughout and even more closely mimic the morphologic appearance of nephrogenic adenoma.[142] PAX2 and PAX8, two recent antibodies reported to be expressed in nephrogenic adenoma, are also expressed in clear cell carcinoma; thus, they are not helpful in this differential diagnosis.[130] CD10, estrogen receptor, p63, high-molecular weight keratin, and P504s are not helpful either to separate clear cell carcinoma from nephrogenic adenoma. Only ki67 may be helpful as clear cell carcinomas typically show >25% positivity rate compared to <5% in nephrogenic adenoma.[142]

Even though nephrogenic adenoma may recur (rates ranging from 28% to almost 90%),[143–145] there is no proof that nephrogenic adenoma may undergo malignant transformation or is in fact related to clear cell carcinoma.

Malakoplakia

This is a common tumor-like condition of the urinary tract that only rarely involves the urethra.[146–152] Not infrequently, urethral malakoplakia is associated with bladder involvement.[146,150,152] The urethral meatus is the most common location, and exceptionally malakoplakia has been described within a urethral diverticulum.[153] It occurs more frequently in females than males (female/male ratio 6 to 4:1), being more common during adult life.[146–149] It is more often seen in patients with diabetes mellitus or immunocompromised patients. Malakoplakia may be asymptomatic or present with voiding symptoms, hematuria, or dysuria.[147,150–152] An associated urinary infection is detected in a number of patients, more commonly by *Escherichia coli*.[149] Grossly, malakoplakia may be seen as single or multiple white to yellow plaques or polypoid lesions. On microscopic examination, sheets of histiocytes (Von Hansemann cells) admixed with chronic inflammatory cells (lymphocytes and plasma cells) expand the lamina propria. The histiocytes have abundant eosinophilic and granular cytoplasm and contain Michaelis-Gutmann bodies which can also be seen outside the cells. Michaelis-Gutmann bodies have a targetoid and basophilic appearance due to concentric lamination and they can be visualized by von Kossa (calcium) or Prussian blue (iron) stain. Although Michaelis-Gutmann bodies are characteristic of malakoplakia they are not required for its diagnosis. The overlying epithelium may be hyperplastic, ulcerated or atrophic if it is associated with prominent scarring. Several hypotheses have been postulated to elucidate the pathogenesis of this condition including infections (more commonly by *E. coli*, *Mycobacterium tuberculosis*, *Proteus*, and *Staphylococcus aureus*), an altered immune response, and finally, an abnormal macrophage response. Macrophages are able to phagocytose but not digest bacteria due to low levels of intracellular cyclic guanosine monophosphate and diminished release of β-glucuronidase.[154] Patients are best treated with antibiotics and surgery, but recurrences may occur.[149]

Amyloidosis

Primary localized amyloidosis of the urethra is very rare. It occurs more commonly in adult men.[155–156] Patients may present with obstructive and irritative voiding symptoms as well as hematuria. In a number of patients, a prior gonococcal infection has been documented.[101] On cystoscopic or gross examination, primary localized amyloidosis may be seen as a poorly defined firm white nodule or plaque or be may associated with a stricture and confused with malignancy.[155,157] On microscopic examination, extracellular dense amorphous deposits of eosinophilic material frequently associated with variable number of chronic inflammatory cells and foreign-body giant cells are present beneath the urothelium. A Congo red stain shows the characteristic apple green birefringence of this material using a polarized microscope. In most cases, amyloid deposits show a polyclonal protein composition (non-AA, non-AL) indicating that the process is not related to either primary or secondary systemic disease.[155] Electron microscopy displays amyloid fibers. Treatment of isolated urethral amyloidosis is either conservative or surgical if obstructive symptoms are present.[155,158]

Endometriosis

Involvement of the urinary tract by endometriosis is uncommon, occurring in 1% to 3%, of patients but urethral endometriosis is extremely rare.[159] Women between menarche and menopause are most often affected. They may present with dyspareunia, dysmenorrhea, urinary frequency, or lower pelvic pain.[160] The lesions may or not be seen grossly depending on size and location within the urethra. If superficial, endometriosis may be seen as black to red to white areas. On microscopic examination, two of the three following components should be seen to establish the diagnosis of endometriosis: (a) endometrial-type glands, (b) endometrial-type stroma, (c) recent or old hemorrhage (Fig. 7-13). Cyclic changes as seen in normal endometrium may not be as notable, and old endometriosis may lead to prominent scarring and/or elastosis as the sole microscopic finding. Endometriosis may undergo malignant transformation, more commonly clear cell carcinoma.[142,161] Conservative treatment is often effective, but if symptoms are important, surgical treatment may be necessary.

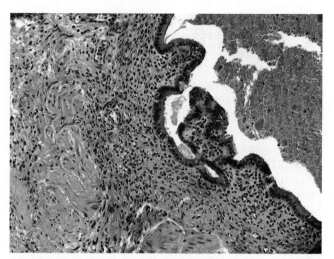

FIGURE 7-13 ■ Endometriosis. Endometrial-type glands and stroma associated with hemosiderin-laden macrophages are present in the urethral wall.

Radiation-Induced Changes

The range of changes seen with radiation therapy is time dependent and very similar to those observed in the bladder mainly secondary to treatment of urothelial carcinoma.[162] In the acute phase, there may be ulceration of the urothelium accompanied by fibrin deposition, acute and chronic inflammation, and/or hemorrhage. Urothelial cells are typically enlarged, displaying abundant cytoplasm and nucleomegaly with prominent nucleoli associated with degenerative chromatin; however, the nucleus to cytoplasmic ratio is preserved. The urothelium may be replaced by metaplastic squamous epithelium, and over time, any epithelium may be associated with pseudocarcinomatous hyperplasia.[163,164] In the stroma, fibroblasts appear plump, some showing multinucleation, associated with edema, vascular changes (congestion, fibrinoid necrosis, wall thickening, and lumen obliteration and/or recanalization), chronic inflammation, and late fibrosis with secondary stricture.[165]

Urethral Diverticulum

This abnormality may be congenital or acquired. Even though preponderant in female patients, presenting more commonly between the third and fifth decades, it may also be seen in neonates and men.[166,167] In most cases, urethral diverticula result as a complication from infections of the paraurethral glands and less frequently from trauma.[168] The pathognomonic presentation of postvoid dribbling, urethral pain, tender periurethral mass, or expression of pus from the urethra is uncommon. Most frequently, patients complain of a variety of chronic or recurrent lower urinary tract symptoms. The diagnosis is made with voiding cystourethrography.[169] In most instances, gross examination is not helpful as the specimen is received fragmented; however, the presence of any exophytic, nodular, or indurated area should raise suspicion for an associated malignancy, and these areas should be carefully sampled. On microscopic examination, a variably thickened wall is lined by either urothelium or squamous epithelium that may show hyperplastic and/or reactive changes. Ulceration and underlying acute, chronic inflammation and fibrosis are often present. Urethral diverticulum can be associated with nephrogenic adenoma and carcinoma, including urothelial, squamous and clear cell types.[161] Surgery is the treatment of choice.

NEOPLASMS

Epithelial

Benign

Squamous Papilloma

This is a rare benign proliferative squamous lesion occurring more commonly in females who may be asymptomatic or present with irritative urinary symptoms or hematuria. Patients typically do not have history of genital, perineal, or perianal condylomas.[53] The lesions are small and polypoid, and, on microscopic examination, fibrovascular fronds are lined by mature squamous epithelium lacking morphologic features of HPV infection.[170] Even though in the past these lesions have been thought to represent part of the spectrum that also includes condyloma acuminatum and low-grade squamous cell carcinoma, recent data do not support this hypothesis as squamous papillomas have been shown to be negative for HPV 6/11, 16/18, and 31/33; show absent to very low p53 expression; are diploid; and do not recur.[53]

Urothelial (Transitional Cell) Papilloma

Conventional urothelial (transitional cell) papillomas of the urethra are very rare. In contrast, inverted papillomas have been more often reported, typically occurring in the prostatic urethra of men.[171–174] Patients may present with gross or microscopic hematuria and/or irritative urinary symptoms, but the lesion may be an incidental finding. Urethral or urothelial papilloma has an appearance identical to that described in the urinary bladder. It shows a simple to complex (branching) papillary architecture with fibrovascular cores that range from delicate to stubby secondary to edema or marked dilated lymphatics. The fibrovascular cores are covered by normal-appearing urothelium. The umbrella cells appear to show the most distinctive features including increased cytoplasm, vacuolization, and striking nuclear atypia of the degenerative type.[175,176] In contrast, inverted papillomas appear as polypoid to pedunculated lesions growing beneath unremarkable surface urothelium. There is a characteristic endophytic growth with anastomosing cords and trabeculae of variable thickness. Frequent features include palisading of the urothelial cells at the periphery and streaming of the cells towards the center of the nests and trabeculae. Squamous metaplasia may be seen. The cells are cytologically banal, although has degenerative-type atypia including multinucleated cells have been reported.[171,177] Some tumors may have a more prominent

glandular architecture in the center of the nests as reported in the urinary bladder.[178] An exophytic component may be focally seen.[171] CK20 pattern of positivity is similar to that of normal urothelium with expression limited to umbrella cells. Typical urothelial (transitional cell) papilloma should be differentiated from a low-grade papillary urothelial carcinoma; however, the latter usually is composed of longer and slender papillae, it shows variable degree of hyperplasia of the lining urothelium, and it may have some degree of cytologic atypia. Inverted urothelial (transitional cell) papilloma should be distinguished from von Brunn nests, which usually do not show trabecular arrangement, and most importantly from inverted urothelial (transitional cell) carcinoma. The latter is typically associated with a more complex architecture displaying broad rounded nests and trabeculae, may be associated with focal desmoplastic reaction, lacks palisading and streaming of the cells, and shows cytologic atypia albeit focal. Furthermore, urothelial (transitional cell) carcinoma with an inverted growth pattern but not inverted papilloma demonstrates gains of chromosomes 3, 7, and 17 and loss of chromosome 9p21 abnormalities.[27] Rarely, carcinoma has been described to arise or follow an inverted papilloma.[179] MIB-1, p53 expression and ploidy have been unable to predict any association between inverted papilloma and the development of urothelial (transitional cell) carcinoma.[180] These lesions rarely recur and the treatment of choice is transurethral resection.[171,174,181]

Villous Adenoma

The urethra is an infrequent location for villous adenoma.[182–185] At this site, it occurs more commonly in the bulbous or prostatic urethra of males. Patients may be asymptomatic or present with hematuria or irritative urinary symptoms. Grossly, a delicate papillary lesion without associated hemorrhage or necrosis may be seen.[183] On microscopic examination, villous adenoma is composed of villiform papillae lined by columnar cells including goblet cells containing abundant mucin. The nuclei are oval and pseudostratified with mild to moderate degree of cytologic atypia and scattered mitoses. Invaginations of the epithelium into the underlying stroma may be present, which may be associated with pools of extravasated mucin imparting a pseudoinfiltrative appearance. Other benign processes, including urethritis glandularis, may be seen in its vicinity.[183,185] Villous adenoma is positive for CK20 and CEA, frequently positive for CK7, and CDX2 negative and much less commonly for EMA CDX2 is negative.[183] Malignant transformation, including in situ and invasive carcinoma (either transitional or glandular), has been reported.[183,185,186] In these cases, direct extension from a colonic carcinoma always has to be excluded. Villous adenoma has to be distinguished from prostatic ductal carcinoma, although the latter lacks intracytoplasmic mucin and is positive for PSA and PSAP.[187] High-grade prostatic ductal carcinoma can be CDX2 positive.[188] In general, when dealing with a small transurethral biopsy showing a villous adenoma-like morphology, the pathologist should be aware of any relevant clinical history of the patient and gross findings and use a descriptive nomenclature especially if the lesion has not been completely excised. A comment should be added to the fact that invasive adenocarcinoma either primary or rarely metastatic from the colon may present showing a villous histology only replacing the urethral lining. When in its pure form, villous adenoma has an excellent prognosis.

Malignant

Urothelial (Transitional Cell) Carcinoma

Primary isolated urothelial (transitional cell) carcinoma of the urethra is rare occurring more commonly in association with a synchronous or metachronous urothelial carcinoma of the urinary bladder.[189] It more commonly affects patients in their sixth and seventh decades. In men, the prostatic urethra is more commonly involved as this is the anatomic region typically lined by urothelium.[190,191] In women, urothelial carcinoma typically involves the proximal third of the urethra.[192] In both, it is the second most common carcinoma following squamous cell carcinoma. Patients present with a palpable mass, irritative or obstructive urinary complaints, and less commonly hematuria. On gross examination, the tumors may have an exophytic (Fig. 7-14A) or endophytic growth, or both. On microscopic examination, in situ, papillary (Fig. 7-14B), or nonpapillary invasive urothelial carcinoma may be seen. Glandular, squamous, and sarcomatoid differentiation, especially in high-grade tumors, has been reported.[190] The tumors may secondarily populate the periurethral glands (Fig. 7-14C) and also prostatic ducts and acini; however, this finding should not be confused with urethral or prostatic stromal invasion as it does not affect prognosis. A pagetoid growth of malignant cells intermingled with preexistent urothelial can also be present. This phenomenon may be seen in sections of margins of a cystoprostatectomy specimen, and especially it may be a subtle finding at frozen section, thus becoming a pitfall in evaluation of such margins. Prior to establishing a diagnosis of primary urothelial carcinoma of the urethra, it is important to rule out a primary bladder tumor especially when an in situ or pagetoid component is identified.[189] Primary urothelial carcinoma of the prostate ducts is rare, and it is frequently associated with urinary bladder or urethral urothelial carcinoma; thus, before establishing this

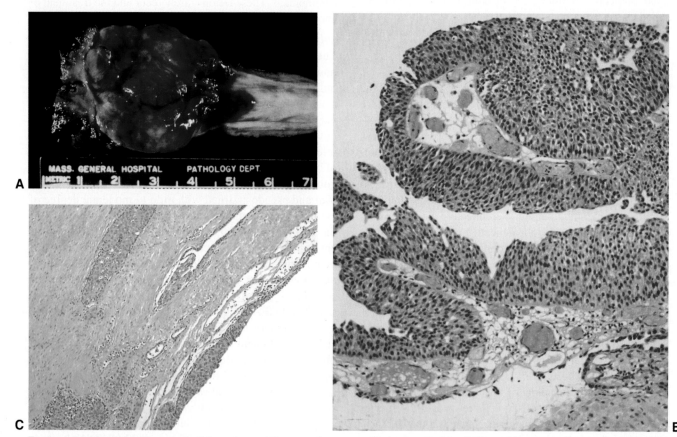

FIGURE 7-14 ■ Papillary urothelial carcinoma. The tumor has an exophytic growth and a fleshy and hemorrhagic cut surface **(A)**. The papillae are lined by multiple layers of atypical urothelium **(B)**. Urothelial carcinoma cells extend to and replace periurethral glands, but no stromal invasion is seen **(C)**.

Box 7-1 ● URETHRAL CARCINOMA

Female

Squamous cell carcinoma	70% (distal and meatus)
Urothelial carcinoma	20% (proximal)
Adenocarcinoma	10% (proximal)
Conventional	60%
Clear cell type	40%

Male

Squamous cell carcinoma	75% (penile and membranous)
Urothelial carcinoma	17% (prostatic)
Adenocarcinoma, conventional	8% (bulbomembranous)

diagnosis, origin in these other sites should be excluded.[193] Urothelial carcinomas of the prostate are classified following the TNM classification of urethral carcinoma. For treatment purposes, as multifocal urothelial carcinoma of the bladder in males and females, either invasive or in situ, predisposes to concomitant urethral involvement or subsequent recurrence, urethrectomy at the time of cystectomy or close surveillance of the urethra is recommended.[194,195] The prognosis of patients with isolated urothelial carcinoma of the urethra is, in general, better than for patients with squamous cell carcinoma, and it is mostly stage related (Box 7-1).[191]

Squamous Cell Carcinoma

This is a very rare malignant epithelial tumor; however, it accounts for approximately 75% of all carcinomas of the male urethra, more frequently involving the bulbomembranous or penile regions,[196–198] and also 70% of all urethral carcinomas in women, typically located in the distal two thirds of the urethra. Patients are frequently diagnosed with urethral stenosis. On gross examination, squamous cell carcinomas are frequently exophytic but may be ulcerative and may show a white scaly surface. On microscopic examination, they may be keratinizing or nonkeratinizing, while the majority are moderately differentiated and deeply invasive into adjacent structures. Secondary extension from a primary penile or vulvar squamous cell carcinoma should be excluded although direct urethral invasion is present in only 25% of primary penile squamous cell carcinomas.[73,199] The differential diagnosis also includes a primary urothelial carcinoma with extensive squamous differentiation, especially in biopsy or transurethral specimens. In these cases, as the material is limited, the diagnosis should be that of high-grade malignant urothelial neoplasm with extensive squamous differentiation and in a note comment about the two existent possibilities, namely a urothelial carcinoma with massive squamous differentiation or a pure squamous cell carcinoma. HPV 6 and 16 have been detected in these tumors.[200–202] Squamous cell carcinoma is associated with a very poor outcome.[203]

Adenocarcinoma, Not Otherwise Specified

Although rare, primary urethral adenocarcinoma, not otherwise specified (NOS), occurs much more frequently in females, accounting for approximately 10% of all malignant urethral tumors. In females, they are seen more commonly in the proximal urethra,[204,205] while in males, these tumors are more frequently located in the bulbomembranous urethra. It appears to be the most common histologic subtype in patients with an urethral diverticulum.[206] Urethral adenocarcinoma can arise from patches of pseudostratified epithelium on the surface or from paraurethral glands (Skene [in females] or Littre [in males]).[207] Women most commonly present with irritative symptoms, repetitive infections, hematuria, or a prolapsing mass,[208] while in men the symptoms are nonspecific.[209] In females, these tumors are not infrequently misdiagnosed as a urethral caruncle. On gross examination, they can form a mass or be ulcerated. On microscopic examination, adenocarcinomas may be subclassified as mucinous (colloid), signet ring, and not otherwise specified.[204,210–212] They display glandular (Fig. 7-15), papillary, or cribriform/solid architecture or admixture thereof. The lining cells frequently have eosinophilic or amphophilic columnar cytoplasm that may contain abundant mucin and nuclei with varying degrees of cytologic atypia and mitotic activity, although most tumors are moderately differentiated.[190,204] The overall morphologic appearance overlaps with that seen in endocervical or colonic carcinomas.[213] Rare tumors have a resemblance to prostate carcinoma.[206,213] From the immunohistochemical point of view, they are positive for CEA and negative for PSA (except tumors arising from Skene glands with a prostatic-like morphology).[206] As primary urethral adenocarcinoma is rare, the possibility of a urothelial carcinoma with extensive glandular differentiation, extension from a primary bladder adenocarcinoma, or metastases (more commonly from the colon) should be ruled out, especially in biopsy specimens.[214,215] Tumors

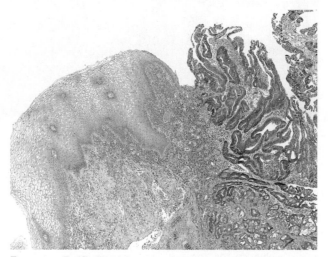

FIGURE 7-15 ■ Littre adenocarcinoma. The tumor forms glands and it is ulcerating the overlaying squamous epithelium.

with an intestinal appearance have displayed a CK7/CK20 positive immunoprofile; however, they have been negative for CDX2 and b-catenin.[210] In men, secondary extension to the urethra by acinar- or ductal-type prostate carcinoma should also be ruled out.[216,217] There is controversy regarding the origin of urethral adenocarcinomas. Although in the past, these tumors were thought to arise from the periurethral glands (Skene glands), it is now accepted that urethral adenocarcinomas may have more than one origin[213] including origin from preexisting villous adenoma that undergo secondary malignant transformation[186] or urethritis glandularis.[164,210] Prognosis is related to stage and location of the tumor. Patients with urethral adenocarcinoma frequently present at advanced stage.[204] When centered in the distal urethra (anterior), patients have a better prognosis compared to tumors located in the proximal urethra (posterior) with the overall survival being low (<30% at 5 years).[218,219]

Clear Cell Carcinoma

This tumor resembles its müllerian counterpart and accounts approximately for 15% of all urethral adenocarcinomas.[204,220] It occurs more frequently in older women

with a female-to-male ratio of 3:1.[221] Patients frequently present with gross or microscopic hematuria or lower urinary tract symptoms. Tumors often form a visible mass (Fig. 7-16A).[138,140,161] On microscopic examination, clear cell carcinoma frequently has a prominent polypoid growth, and it shows tubulocystic (Fig. 7-16B), papillary (Fig. 7-16C) or solid patterns or admixture thereof. The papillae may have hyalinized fibrovascular cores. Tubules, cysts, and papillae are lined by columnar to cuboidal to flat (more commonly in cysts) cells with moderate amount of eosinophilic to clear cytoplasm. Hobnail cells are a frequent finding but may not be conspicuous in a given neoplasm (Fig. 7-16B). The tumor cells show prominent nuclear pleomorphism and brisk mitotic activity. Areas of hemorrhage and necrosis are common. Tumors express low molecular weight keratins, CK7 and CK20, but are negative for estrogen and progesterone receptors, PSA, PSAP, and racemase (p504S).[127,140,161,222,223] There is a striking association of clear cell carcinoma with urethral diverticulum.[161] The most common problem in differential diagnosis is nephrogenic adenoma, as both have a common association with a diverticulum, similar growth patterns, and the finding of hobnail and

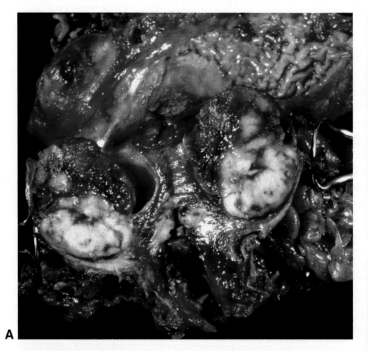
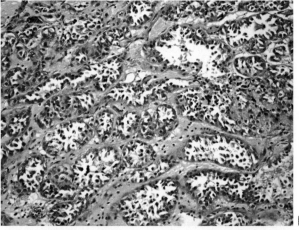
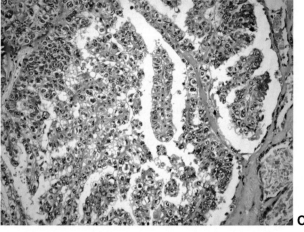

FIGURE 7-16 ■ Clear cell carcinoma. The tumor forms a large exophytic mass, and it is present within a diverticulum. The tumor is composed of tubules and cysts display hobnail cells (**B**). The tumor cells also form papillae lined by clear cells (**C**). (**A**, From Oliva E, Amin MB, Jimenez R, et al. Clear cell carcinoma of the urinary bladder: a report and comparison of four tumors of müllerian origin and nine of probable urothelial origin with discussion of histogenesis and diagnostic problems. *Am J Surg Pathol* 2002;26(2):190–197, with permission.)

clear cells.[121,122,141,161,224] Furthermore, a subset of clear cell carcinomas may diffusely mimic nephrogenic adenoma.[142] Even though clear cell carcinoma may focally have a subtle appearance, the presence of any degree of cytologic atypia or mitotic activity should raise suspicion for malignancy.[138,140,161] It has been postulated by some investigators that nephrogenic adenoma may be the precursor lesion of clear cell carcinoma[225]; however, this hypothesis has never been proven. Immunohistochemical stains are not helpful in this differential diagnosis as both lesions show an overlapping immunohistochemical profile including expression of PAX2 and PAX8.[123,127,130,140,141] Other entities in the differential diagnosis include metastatic clear cell carcinoma of the gynecologic tract (PAX8 positive),[226] metastatic renal cell clear cell carcinoma (PAX2 and PAX8 positive)[226–228] (clinical history being very important in both), urothelial carcinoma with cysts or clear cells[229,230] (typically negative for hepatocyte nuclear factor-1β in contrast to clear cell carcinoma),[231] and the rare tubulocystic clear cell carcinoma arising in the prostate.[232] Even though an origin of these tumors from Skene glands has been proposed, it has not been supported to date. Clear cell carcinoma has a relatively good prognosis that correlates with stage at the time of diagnosis linked to the fact that many of the tumors have an exophytic growth and do not penetrate deep into the urethral wall and that many of them originate within a diverticulum.[123,204]

Adenocarcinoma of Accessory Glands

Adenocarcinoma arising from Skene glands of the female urethra or Littre or Cowper glands in the male urethra has also been reported, but they are exceedingly rare.[233–237] In females they can arise anywhere in the urethra, but they are more commonly seen in its distal segment. In contrast, adenocarcinoma arising from Littre glands is typically centered in the penile urethra, while Cowper gland adenocarcinoma grows in the bulbomembranous urethra. Presenting symptoms are nonspecific. The gross and histologic appearance of the tumors is similar to that described for urethral adenocarcinoma, NOS (Fig. 7-15); however, in female patients, the tumors may have a morphology that is similar to prostatic adenocarcinoma including staining for prostatic markers.[206,238] Furthermore, adenoid cystic carcinoma arising from Skene glands has been reported. The tumors typically form a well-circumscribed mass (Fig. 7-17A) with a suburethral location and no direct continuity with the urethra.[239] On sectioning, they have a homogeneous gray to white, firm cut surface (Fig. 7-17A). On microscopic examination, the tumors display variably sized nests with prominent cribriforming (Fig. 7-17B), tubules, and cords and infrequently may have a solid pattern as seen in their salivary gland counterpart. The cribriform spaces are filled with eosinophilic or basophilic acellular basement-like material which is highlighted with PAS-D (Fig. 7-17B). The cells are uniform and small displaying eosinophilic cytoplasm and round nuclei. The intervening stroma may be hyalinized. Perineural invasion is a frequent finding. As these tumors tend to occur in the distal portion of the female urethra, a Bartholin gland origin should be excluded. The tumor reported in the literature was positive for keratins, CEA, and S100.[239] In most instances, it is impossible to determine with certainty the origin of these carcinomas as at the time of surgery the tumor has destroyed any preexistent histologic evidence. Only when the tumor is seen in close association with periurethral glands, an origin from these glands can be considered (Box 7-2).

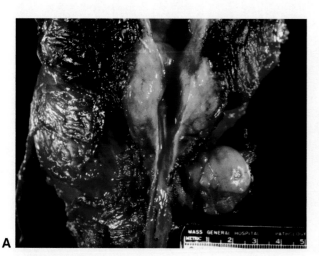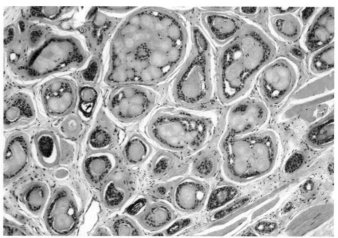

FIGURE 7-17 ■ Adenoid cystic carcinoma. The tumor has a paraurethral location **(A)**. It is composed of nests with cribriform spaces that are filled with eosinophilic or basophilic acellular basement-like material **(B)**.

Box 7-2 ● URETHRAL ADENOCARCINOMA

1. Primary
   Conventional:
   In females: proximal urethra most common
   In males: bulbomembranous urethra most common
   Most frequent carcinoma within diverticulum
   Subtypes:
   NOS
   Mucinous (colloid)
   Signet ring
   Typically CEA positive and PSA negative
   If intestinal differentiation CDX2 positive
   Differential diagnosis:
   Urothelial carcinoma with extensive glandular
   differentiation
   Urinary bladder adenocarcinoma with secondary urethral
   extension
   Prostate carcinoma
   Overall poor survival (<30% at 5 years)
   Clear cell
   Female 3:1 Male
   Polypoid growth
   Frequent association with diverticulum
   Tubulocystic, papillary, solid growths frequently admixed
   CK7, CK20, HNF-β1, PAX2, PAX8 positive
   ER, PR, PSA, PSAP, racemase negative
   Differential diagnosis:
   Nephrogenic adenoma
   Metastatic clear cell carcinoma gynecologic tract
   Metastatic renal cell clear cell carcinoma
   Prognosis related to stage
   Adenocarcinoma of accessory glands
   In females: more common in distal urethra
   In males: more common in penile and bulbomembra-
   nous urethra
   Histologically similar to conventional urethral
   adenocarcinoma
   Uncommon variant: Adenoid cystic carcinoma

2. Secondary
   Prostatic
   Colorectal
   Other

Other Malignant Epithelial Tumors

Other malignant epithelial tumors, either primary or metastatic to the urethra, have been reported including small cell carcinoma,[240–243] metastatic colon (Fig. 7-18), prostate, and renal carcinoma[214,244,245] as well as carcinoid tumors.[246]

Mesenchymal

Benign

Leiomyoma

Although mesenchymal neoplasms of the urethra are exceedingly rare, leiomyomas are by far the most common subtype in adults, being more often encountered in females than males.[247–249] They may be asymptomatic or present with urinary symptoms such as hematuria, obstruction, or dysuria. The gross and microscopic features are identical to their uterine counterparts. They are typically well circumscribed with a bulging white, whorled cut surface. They are composed of compact intersecting fascicles of spindled cells with cytoplasmic eosinophilia, oval-shaped nuclei with blunted ends, and fine nuclear chromatin (Fig. 7-19). Mitotic activity is typically low to absent, and tumor cell necrosis and nuclear pleomorphism are lacking; however, symplastic nuclei can be seen on occasion as it has been reported in the urinary bladder.[250]

The differential diagnosis of urethral leiomyoma includes postoperative spindle cell nodule or pseudosarcomatous myofibroblastic proliferation and genital stromal tumors such as angiomyofibroblastoma, cellular angiofibroma, and aggressive angiomyxoma, given their possible anatomic proximity to the urethra. Most problematic may be the differential diagnosis with leiomyosarcoma, especially in small biopsies as infiltrative growth, necrosis, or cytologic atypia may not be uniformly present. Primary urethral leiomyosarcoma is exceedingly rare. It is typically associated with poor circumscription, ulceration, necrosis, and hemorrhage. On microscopic examination, the presence of any degree of cytologic atypia and mitotic activity should raise concern for malignancy. Leiomyomas show immunoreactivity for smooth muscle actin and desmin, and estrogen receptor expression has also been reported.[251] Urethral leiomyomas are typically cured by conservative excision with only rare local recurrences reported.

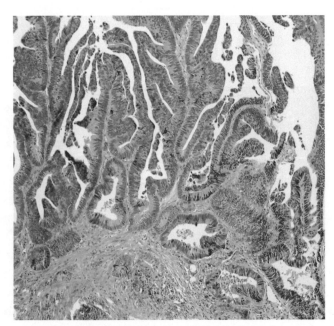

FIGURE 7-18 ■ Metastatic colonic carcinoma. The tumor shows papillary and glandular arrangements, and the cells have pseudostratified nuclei.

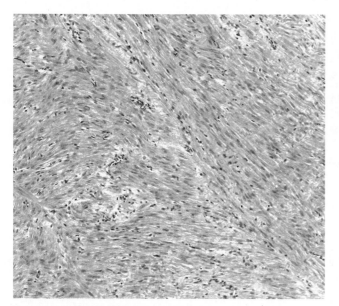

FIGURE 7-19 ■ Leiomyoma. The bland spindled tumor cells with pink cytoplasm and "cigar-shaped" nuclei form long fascicles.

Neurofibroma

Neurofibromas of the urethra are rare, and most reported cases have occurred in the setting of neurofibromatosis.[252–254] Their presentation is nonspecific and includes obstruction or other urinary symptoms. Urethral neurofibromas have an appearance identical to those in other anatomic sites, characterized by a hypocellular proliferation of spindle cells arranged in loose and disorganized fascicles with scattered, variably shaped bundles of collagen (Fig. 7-20). They may be extensively myxoid or collagenized. The cells have scant cytoplasm and small bland nuclei with curved or wavy contours containing a tiny nucleolus.

The most important differential diagnosis is botryoid rhabdomyosarcoma as hypocellular areas in this tumor may

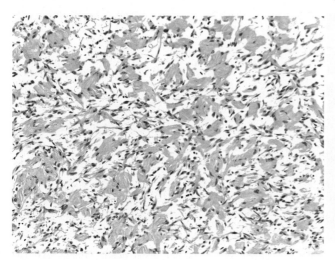

FIGURE 7-20 ■ Neurofibroma. Spindle cells are arranged in loose and disorganized short fascicles set in an edematous background.

closely mimic a neurofibroma. Both cytoplasmic and nuclear immunoreactivity for S100 protein help to confirm the diagnosis of neurofibroma. These tumors are benign and can be treated with surgical excision.

Hemangioma and Vascular Malformation. Although urethral hemangiomas have been frequently reported in the literature,[255–257] most of these lesions are currently considered vascular or lymphatic malformations following most recent classifications.[258] They may affect patients of any age who frequently present with bleeding. Grossly, a multilobated submucosal hemorrhagic mass is seen, and large-caliber vessels may be identifiable. These lesions are morphologically heterogeneous but typically have variably sized, irregularly formed blood or lymphatic vessels which may be thrombosed. Generally, conservative local excision is performed to alleviate symptoms and preserve function.

Other Tumors

Granular cell tumors may occur throughout the genitourinary tract but are extremely rare in the urethra.[259] They are similar to those seen in other sites with eosinophilic granules filling the cytoplasm, round nuclei, and an association with pseudo-epitheliomatous hyperplasia in some cases. Other reported but uncommon urethral mesenchymal tumors include Masson tumor (papillary endothelial hyperplasia)[260,261] and paraganglioma.[262]

Malignant

Rhabdomyosarcoma

Rhabdomyosarcoma is the most common soft tissue sarcoma in children, and the genitourinary tract is a frequent location.[110,263,264] Grossly, these tumors present as polypoid, predominantly intraluminal masses. Morphologically, the main diagnostic feature is the finding of a "cambium layer" where spindle cells condense underneath the surface urothelial or squamous lining epithelium. The spindle cells show varying degrees of differentiation ranging from small undifferentiated mesenchymal cells (Fig. 7-21A) to fully developed rhabdomyoblasts with prominent eosinophilic cytoplasm and cross-striations. At low-power magnification, these hypercellular areas alternate with hypocellular areas composed of loose myxoid/edematous stroma with relatively bland spindle cells (Fig. 7-21B). This morphologic appearance is characteristic of the botryoid subtype rhabdomyosarcoma. Desmin and nuclear myogenin or MyoD1 expression confirms the diagnosis. The clinical differential diagnosis is usually straightforward in children. Embryonal rhabdomyosarcoma may closely mimic a benign process such as neurofibroma or postoperative spindle cell nodule/pseudosarcomatous myofibroblastic proliferation especially when only small biopsies showing the hypocellular areas are provided. It should also be distinguished from alveolar rhabdomyosarcoma, which is relatively infrequent in the genitourinary tract, especially in children.[110,264]

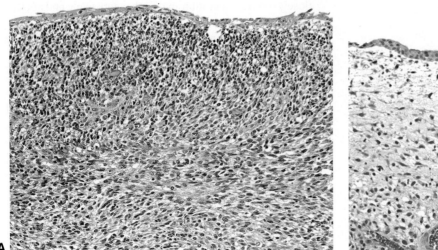
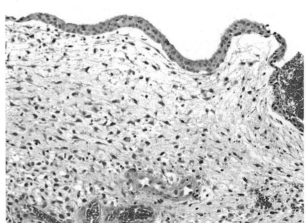

FIGURE 7-21 ■ Botryoid Rhabdomyosarcoma. The tumor has highly cellular areas with primitive-appearing cells **(A)** alternating with hypocellular and myxoid areas **(B)**.

Treatment consists of multimodality therapy including chemotherapy, surgery, and radiation, with cure rates over 80% in the botryoid embryonal rhabdomyosarcoma.[265]

Other Malignant Mesenchymal Tumors

Other malignant mesenchymal tumors of the urethra and periurethral region are extremely rare and include Kaposi sarcoma of the urethral meatus.[266]

Melanoma

The urethra is the preferred site for primary malignant melanoma in the urinary tract accounting for 4% of urethral cancers and 0.2% of all melanomas.[267] It is more common in females than males (3:1), more frequent in the white population, and most often diagnosed after the fifth decade.[268–270] The distal urethra is affected most often in both genders. In men >50% melanomas occur in the fossa navicularis, 5% in

the urethral meatus, and 15% in the pendulous and prostatic urethra respectively.[271,272] If the glans penis is involved, it may be difficult to determine if the tumor is primary in the glans or urethra, but primary tumors of the glans are approximately twice as common as those of the urethra.[273] If multifocal, suspicion for spread from an occult primary elsewhere should be high. Presenting symptoms are nonspecific, but occasionally patients may present with melanuria.[274] Urethral malignant melanomas rarely arise in association with nevi. On cystoscopic examination, the tumors are commonly confused with urothelial carcinomas. On gross examination, the tumors are often polypoid, and a dark or black color may be appreciable (Fig. 7-22A). Although less frequently, they can present as macules along the urethral mucosa or as ulcerated lesions.[275] Urethral malignant melanoma shows a wide histologic spectrum including diffuse, nested, fascicular, or storiform

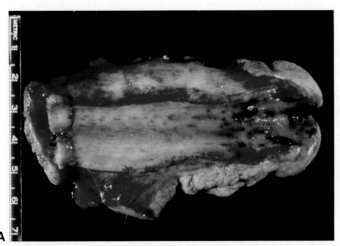
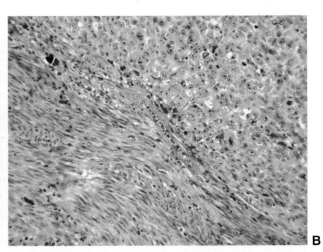

FIGURE 7-22 ■ Malignant melanoma. Multiple dark brown irregular lesions are present in the distal penile urethra **(A)**. The tumor shows a biphasic epithelioid and spindled growth. Notice the presence of melanin pigment **(B)**. (**A**, From Oliva E, Quinn TR, Amin MB, et al. Primary malignant melanoma of the urethra: a clinicopathologic analysis of 15 cases. *Am J Surg Pathol* 2000;24: 785–796, with permission.)

growths of usually pleomorphic tumor cells (Fig. 7-22B). Pseudoglandular or follicle-like spaces can be seen. The tumor cells usually have abundant eosinophilic cytoplasm (epithelioid appearance) with or without melanin pigment (Fig. 7-22B), but they can also have a rhabdoid, clear, or even vacuolated appearance. No histologic differences between primary or metastatic melanomas exist; thus, careful clinical information is crucial in determining the origin of the neoplasm.[275,276]

The differential diagnosis includes most commonly urothelial carcinoma, either poorly differentiated (if solid growth) or papillary (if pseudopapillary pattern and cells devoid of melanin). Careful search for melanoma in situ, melanin pigment, or findings that rule out melanoma such as focal squamous or glandular differentiation are helpful. Furthermore, urothelial carcinoma is positive for CK7 and CK20 and uroplakin.[275,277,278] Extramammary Paget disease extending from the vulva in females or the scrotum or penis in males may be confused with the radial growth phase of malignant melanoma. Cells in Paget disease have abundant vacuolated cytoplasm and large vesicular nuclei, and the atypical cells tend to cluster at the tips of the rete ridges whereas melanoma cells are situated at the squamous–mucosal junction. Paget cells are found above a preserved basal cell layer. These atypical cells contain mucin in their cytoplasm, which is PAS-D resistant; they are also CEA and EMA positive. This immunohistochemical profile coupled with negativity for S100 and HMB-45 staining points toward a diagnosis of Paget disease.[279] Other entities in the differential diagnosis include genital lentiginosis, atypical lentiginous hyperplasia, and melanocytic nevi of the genital area.[280,281] Electron microscopy may aid by demonstrating melanosomes in different stages of maturation, especially when dealing with amelanotic neoplasms.[282]

Urethral malignant melanoma has a worse prognosis than does its cutaneous counterpart, in part as a result of delay in diagnosis that is associated with extension outside the urethra. Most patients do not survive more than 3 years. There appears to be no correlation between tumor stage and survival even though most tumors are not deeply invasive into the urethral wall because of their polypoid growth (low stage).[275,283]

Hematopoietic and Lymphoid Neoplasms

The urethra is the least common organ of the urinary tract to be involved by lymphoma. Non-Hodgkin lymphomas are more frequent, diffuse large B-cell lymphoma (Fig. 7-23) representing 50% of all of them, followed by extranodal marginal zone lymphoma,[284–289] and plasmacytomas.[290] Patients most often present with nonspecific symptoms/ signs including hematuria, dysuria, obstruction, or a mass. When lymphomas have a polypoid growth, they may mimic the appearance of a urethral caruncle. Furthermore, the atypical stromal cells in this pseudoneoplastic lesion may be confused with lymphoma cells.[85] Although these tumors have been reported to have an overall good prognosis, especially for plasmacytoma, experience is very limited, and some patients have died.

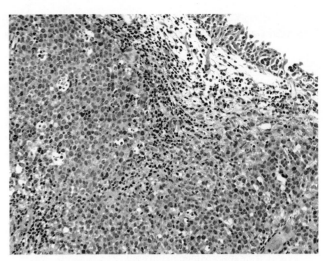

FIGURE 7-23 ■ Diffuse large B-cell Lymphoma. Sheets of large lymphoid cells with irregular nuclei are admixed with tingible body macrophages.

Secondary Neoplasms

Because of the anatomic proximity of the urethra to other organs, extension of an adjacent neoplasm to involve the urethra is not infrequent. In females, primary neoplasms of the gynecologic tract, such as cervicovaginal squamous cell carcinoma, are most common. In males, high-stage penile squamous cell carcinoma and prostatic ductal carcinoma may involve the urethra.

STAGING OF PRIMARY MALIGNANT EPITHELIAL AND MESENCHYMAL TUMORS OF THE URETHRA

Specimen Handling

In females, the surgical treatment for urethral malignant tumors often includes urethrectomy as well as cystectomy as the urethra is very short, and in cases of advanced disease an exenteration may be performed. In contrast, as the urethra in men is much longer, depending on the location of the tumor, different types of specimens may be obtained. However, in all cases, as assignment of stage is based on depth of invasion, it is extremely important to properly orient these specimens. After inking the surgical margins and opening the urethra longitudinally, pinning of the specimen to a firm surface may be helpful to ensure appropriate orientation. Consecutive sections perpendicular to the pong axis of the urethra should be performed in order to preserve orientation and relationship of tumor to adjacent structures and for estimation of size and depth of invasion. After proper fixation, sections should be taken indicating orientation from proximal to distal or vice versa in a section code. If the tumor is very close to the distal or proximal urethral margin, radial rather than en face sections of that margin ensure proper visualization of the surgical margin. It is important to take

Box 7-3 ● TNM STAGING SYSTEM FOR URETHRAL TUMORS MALIGNANT

TX	Primary tumor cannot be assessed
T0	No evidence of primary tumor
Ta	Noninvasive papillary, polypoid, or verrucous carcinoma
Tis	Carcinoma in situ
T1	Tissue invades subepithelial connective tissue
T2	Tumor invades any of the following: corpus spongiosum, prostate, periurethral muscle
T3	Tumor invades any of the following: corpus cavernosum, beyond prostatic capsule, anterior vagina, bladder neck
T4	Tumor invades other adjacent organs

Urothelial Carcinoma of the Prostate

Tis pu	Carcinoma in situ, involvement of the prostatic urethra
Tis pd	Carcinoma in situ, involvement of the prostatic ducts
T1	Tumor invades subepithelial connective tissue
T2	Tumor invades any of the following: prostatic stroma, corpus spongiosum, periurethral muscle
T3	Tumor invades any of the following: corpus cavernosum, beyond prostatic capsule, bladder neck (extraprostatic extension)
T4	Tumor invades other adjacent organs (invasion of the bladder)

Regional Lymph Nodes (N)

NX	Regional lymph nodes cannot be assessed
N0	No regional lymph node metastasis
N1	Metastasis in a single lymph node 2 cm or less in greatest dimension
N2	Metastasis in a single node more than 2 cm in greatest dimension, or in multiple nodes

sections that include tumor and nontumor mucosa in order to identify potential precursor lesions (Box 7-3).

Specimen Reporting

A complete report should include tumor type, including secondary types of differentiation if present; grade of differentiation; depth of invasion including secondary organs affected; presence of lymphovascular invasion and/or perineural invasion; and status of the surgical margins. In some cases, an underlying precursor lesion may be identified, and it is of interest to include it in the report as it may be helpful for ulterior clinical management of the patient. It is important that if the specific T stage is not provided, all elements that are necessary for proper staging are listed in the report in a clear manner. If ancillary techniques are performed in

order to properly classify the tumor, this information may be reported in a note (Box 7-3 and 7-4).

Box 7-4 ●

PATHOLOGY REPORTING FOR URETHRAL CARCINOMA
(*):
Tumor size
Tumor type, including secondary types of differentiation if present (not required)
Grade of differentiation (not required)
Depth of invasion
Tumor extension to adjacent organs
Presence of lymphovascular invasion (not required)
Status of surgical margins
Presence of underlying precursor lesion (not required)
Pathologic staging (pTNM)
Protocol for the Examination of Specimens from Patients with Carcinoma of the Urethra. http://www.cap.org/apps/docs/committees/cancer/cancer_protocols/2011/urethra_11protocol.pdf

REFERENCES

1. Brooks JD. Anatomy of the lower urinary tract and male genitalia. In: Weiner E, ed. *Campbell-Walsh Urology*. 9th ed. Philadelphia, PA: Saunders Elsevier; 2007.
2. Krishnan A, de Souza A, Konijeti R, et al. The anatomy and embryology of posterior urethral valves. *J Urol* 2006;175:1214–1220.
3. Moore KL, Dalley AF. *Clinically Oriented Anatomy*. 5th ed. Philadelphia, PA: Lippincott; 2006.
4. McNeal JE. The prostate and prostatic urethra: a morphologic synthesis. *J Urol* 1972;107:1008–1016.
5. Tanagho EA, Schmidt RA, de Araujo CG. Urinary striated sphincter: what is its nerve supply? *Urology* 1982;20:415–417.
6. Lawson JO. Pelvic anatomy. I. Pelvic floor muscles. *Ann R Coll Surg Engl* 1974;54:244–252.
7. Zvara P, Carrier S, Kour NW, et al. The detailed neuroanatomy of the human striated urethral sphincter. *Br J Urol* 1994;74:182–187.
8. Glenister TW. The origin and fate of the urethral plate in man. *J Anat* 1954;88:413–425.
9. Moore KL, Persaus TVN. *The Developing Human. Clinically Oriented Embryology*. 8th ed. Philadelphia, PA: Saunders; 2008.
10. Park JM. Normal development of the urogenital system. In: Wein AJ, Kavoussi LR, Novick AC, et al, eds. *Campbell-Walsh Urology*. Philadelphia: Elsevier, 2007:3121–3148.
11. Kurzrock EA, Baskin LS, Cunha GR. Ontogeny of the male urethra: theory of endodermal differentiation. *Differentiation* 1999;64:115–122.
12. Montagnino B. Posterior urethral valves: pathophysiology and clinical implications. *ANNA J* 1994;21:26–30, 8; quiz 1–2.
13. Eckoldt F, Heling KS, Woderich R, et al. Posterior urethral valves: prenatal diagnostic signs and outcome. *Urol Int* 2004;73:296–301.
14. Dinneen MD, Duffy PG. Posterior urethral valves. *Br J Urol* 1996;78:275–281.
15. Imaji R, Moon DA, Dewan PA. Congenital posterior urethral membrane: variable morphological expression. *J Urol* 2001;165:1240–1242; discussion 2–3.

16. Yohannes P, Hanna M. Current trends in the management of posterior urethral valves in the pediatric population. *Urology* 2002;60:947–953.

17. Walker RD, Padron M. The management of posterior urethral valves by initial vesicostomy and delayed valve ablation. *J Urol* 1990;144:1212–1214.

18. Karnak I, Senocak ME, Buyukpamukcu N, et al. Rare congenital abnormalities of the anterior urethra. *Pediatr Surg Int* 1997;12:407–409.

19. Tank ES. Anterior urethral valves resulting from congenital urethral diverticula. *Urology* 1987;30:467–469.

20. Jehannin B. [Congenital obstructive valves and diverticula of the anterior urethra]. *Chir Pediatr* 1990;31:173–180.

21. Scherz HC, Kaplan GW, Packer MG. Anterior urethral valves in the fossa navicularis in children. *J Urol* 1987;138:1211–1213.

22. Paulhac P, Fourcade L, Lesaux N, et al. Anterior urethral valves and diverticula. *BJU Int* 2003;92:506–509.

23. Kajbafzadeh A. Congenital urethral anomalies in boys. Part II. *Urol J* 2005;2:125–131.

24. Prasad N, Vivekanandhan KG, Ilangovan G, et al. Duplication of the urethra. *Pediatr Surg Int* 1999;15:419–421.

25. Berrocal T, Novak S, Arjonilla A, et al. Complete duplication of bladder and urethra in the coronal plane in a girl: case report and review of the literature. *Pediatr Radiol* 1999;29:171–173.

26. Singh G, Murray K. Distal urethral duplication—a case report and literature review. *Scand J Urol Nephrol* 1996;30:149–151.

27. Jones EA, Freedman AL, Ehrlich RM. Megalourethra and urethral diverticula. *Urol Clin North Am* 2002;29:341–348, vi.

28. Vaux KK, Jones MC, Benirschke K, et al. Megalourethra: a report of three cases associated with maternal diabetes and a review of the literature—is sonic hedgehog the common pathway? *Am J Med Genet A* 2005;132A:314–317.

29. Paulozzi LJ, Erickson JD, Jackson RJ. Hypospadias trends in two US surveillance systems. *Pediatrics* 1997;100:831–834.

30. Mouriquand PD, Persad R, Sharma S. Hypospadias repair: current principles and procedures. *Br J Urol* 1995;76(suppl 3):9–22.

31. Baskin LS. Hypospadias and urethral development. *J Urol* 2000;163:951–956.

32. Wang MH, Baskin LS. Endocrine disruptors, genital development, and hypospadias. *J Androl* 2008;29:499–505.

33. Coppens L, Bonnet P, Andrianne R, et al. Adult mullerian duct or utricle cyst: clinical significance and therapeutic management of 65 cases. *J Urol* 2002;167:1740–1744.

34. Kato H, Hayama M, Furuya S, et al. Anatomical and histological studies of so-called mullerian duct cyst. *Int J Urol* 2005;12:465–468.

35. Kato H, Komiyama I, Maejima T, et al. Histopathological study of the mullerian duct remnant: clarification of disease categories and terminology. *J Urol* 2002;167:133–136.

36. Wernert N, Kern L, Heitz P, et al. Morphological and immunohistochemical investigations of the utriculus prostaticus from the fetal period up to adulthood. *Prostate* 1990;17:19–30.

37. Devine CJ Jr, Gonzalez-Serva L, Stecker JF Jr, et al. Utricular configuration in hypospadias and intersex. *J Urol* 1980;123:407–411.

38. Dewan PA. A study of the relationship between syringoceles and Cobb's collar. *Eur Urol* 1996;30:119–124.

39. Maizels M, Stephens FD, King LR, et al. Cowper's syringocele: a classification of dilatations of Cowper's gland duct based upon clinical characteristics of 8 boys. *J Urol* 1983;129:111–114.

40. Edwards S, Sonnex C. Urethritis associated with isotretinoin therapy. *Acta Derm Venereol* 1997;77:330.

41. Kellock DJ, Parslew R, Mendelsohn SS, et al. Non-specific urethritis—possible association with isotretinoin therapy. *Int J STD AIDS* 1996;7:135–136.

42. Saborio DV, Kennedy WA II, Hoke GP. Acute urinary retention secondary to urethral inflammation from a vaginal contraceptive suppository in a 17-year-old boy. *Urol Int* 1997;58:128–130.

43. Amor B. Reiter's syndrome. Diagnosis and clinical features. *Rheum Dis Clin North Am* 1998;24:677–695, vii.

44. Lane Z, Epstein JI. Polypoid/papillary cystitis: a series of 41 cases misdiagnosed as papillary urothelial neoplasia. *Am J Surg Pathol* 2008;32:758–764.

45. Schinella R, Thurm J, Feiner H. Papillary pseudotumor of the prostatic urethra: proliferative papillary urethritis. *J Urol* 1974;111:38–40.

46. Young RH. Papillary and polypoid cystitis. A report of eight cases. *Am J Surg Pathol* 1988;12:542–546.

47. Shigehara K, Sasagawa T, Kawaguchi S, et al. Prevalence of human papillomavirus infection in the urinary tract of men with urethritis. *Int J Urol* 2010;17:563–568.

48. Kotoulas IG, Cardamakis E, Relakis K, et al. Peoscopic diagnosis of flat condyloma and penile intraepithelial neoplasia. IV. Urethral reservoir. *Gynecol Obstet Invest* 1996;41:55–60.

49. Schneede P, Munch P, Wagner S, et al. Fluorescence urethroscopy following instillation of 5-aminolevulinic acid: a new procedure for detecting clinical and subclinical HPV lesions of the urethra. *J Eur Acad Dermatol Venereol* 2001;15:121–125.

50. Kilciler M, Bedir S, Erdemir F, et al. Condylomata acuminata of external urethral meatus causing infravesical obstruction. *Int Urol Nephrol* 2007;39:107–109.

51. Del Mistro A, Braunstein JD, Halwer M, et al. Identification of human papillomavirus types in male urethral condylomata acuminata by in situ hybridization. *Hum Pathol* 1987;18:936–940.

52. Melchers WJ, Schift R, Stolz E, et al. Human papillomavirus detection in urine samples from male patients by the polymerase chain reaction. *J Clin Microbiol* 1989;27:1711–1714.

53. Cheng L, Leibovich BC, Cheville JC, et al. Squamous papilloma of the urinary tract is unrelated to condyloma acuminata. *Cancer* 2000;88:1679–1686.

54. Zaak D, Hofstetter A, Frimberger D, et al. Recurrence of condylomata acuminata of the urethra after conventional and fluorescence-controlled Nd:YAG laser treatment. *Urology* 2003;61:1011–1015.

55. Pelouze PS. *Gonorrhea in the Male and Female*. Philadelphia, PA: Saunders; 1941.

56. Fredlund H, Falk L, Jurstrand M, et al. Molecular genetic methods for diagnosis and characterisation of *Chlamydia trachomatis* and *Neisseria gonorrhoeae*: impact on epidemiological surveillance and interventions. *APMIS* 2004;112:771–784.

57. O'Mahony C, Reeve-Fowkes A, Worthen E, et al. Three years of using Aptima Combo 2 (AC2) transcription-mediated amplification for gonorrhoea in a district hospital genitourinary medicine clinic shows it to be superior to culture and has a specificity of almost 100%. *Int J STD AIDS* 2008;19:67–69.

58. De Jongh M, Dangor Y, Adam A, et al. Gonococcal resistance: evolving from penicillin, tetracycline to the quinolones in South Africa—implications for treatment guidelines. *Int J STD AIDS* 2007;18:697–699.

59. Yokoi S, Maeda S, Kubota Y, et al. The role of *Mycoplasma genitalium* and *Ureaplasma urealyticum* biovar 2 in postgonococcal urethritis. *Clin Infect Dis* 2007;45:866–871.

60. Prevention CfDCa. *Sexually Transmitted Disease Survelliance, 2006*. Atlanta, GA: U.S. Department of Health and Human Services; 2007.

61. Swartz SL, Kraus SJ. Persistent urethral leukocytosis and asymptomatic Chlamydial urethritis. *J Infect Dis* 1979;140:614–617.

62. Martin DH, Pollock S, Kuo CC, et al. *Chlamydia trachomatis* infections in men with Reiter's syndrome. *Ann Intern Med* 1984;100:207–213.

63. Yoshida T, Deguchi T, Meda S, et al. Quantitative detection of *Ureaplasma parvum* (biovar 1) and *Ureaplasma urealyticum* (biovar 2) in urine specimens from men with and without urethritis by real-time polymerase chain reaction. *Sex Transm Dis* 2007;34:416–419.

64. Bradshaw CS, Tabrizi SN, Read TR, et al. Etiologies of nongonococcal urethritis: bacteria, viruses, and the association with orogenital exposure. *J Infect Dis* 2006;193:336–345.

65. Gupta N, Mandal AK, Singh SK. Tuberculosis of the prostate and urethra: a review. *Indian J Urol* 2008;24:388–391.

66. Adam R, Katz S, Lee K, et al. Wegener's granulomatosis of the penis: diagnosis and management. *Can J Urol* 2004;11:2341–2343.

67. Davenport A, Downey SE, Goel S, et al. Wegener's granulomatosis involving the urogenital tract. *Br J Urol* 1996;78:354–357.

68. Stone JH, Millward CL, Criswell LA. Two genitourinary manifestations of Wegener's granulomatosis. *J Rheumatol* 1997;24:1846–1848.

69. Ho KL, Hayden MT. Sarcoidosis of urethra simulating carcinoma. *Urology* 1979;13:197–199.

70. Carr LK, Honey RJ, Sugar L. Diagnosis and management of urethral sarcoidosis. *J Urol* 1995;153:1612–1613.

71. Russell GA, Crowley T, Dalrymple JO. Squamous metaplasia in the penile urethra due to oestrogen therapy. *Br J Urol* 1992;69:282–285.

72. Bailey DM, Foley SJ, McFarlane JP, et al. Histological changes associated with long-term urethral stents. *Br J Urol* 1998;81:745–749.

73. Velazquez EF, Soskin A, Bock A, et al. Epithelial abnormalities and precancerous lesions of anterior urethra in patients with penile carcinoma: a report of 89 cases. *Mod Pathol* 2005;18:917–923.

74. Epstein JI. Urothelial hyperplasia. In: Eble JN, Sauter G, Epstein JI, et al., eds. *Pathology & Genetics Tumours of the Urinary System and Male Genital Organs*. Lyon, France: IARC Press; 2004:111.

75. Obermann EC, Junker K, Stoehr R, et al. Frequent genetic alterations in flat urothelial hyperplasias and concomitant papillary bladder cancer as detected by CGH, LOH, and FISH analyses. *J Pathol* 2003;199:50–57.

76. Corica FA, Husmann DA, Churchill BM, et al. Intestinal metaplasia is not a strong risk factor for bladder cancer: study of 53 cases with long-term follow-up. *Urology* 1997;50:427–431.

77. Smith AK, Hansel DE, Jones JS. Role of cystitis cystica et glandularis and intestinal metaplasia in development of bladder carcinoma. *Urology* 2008;71:915–918.

78. Volmar KE, Chan TY, De Marzo AM, et al. Florid von Brunn nests mimicking urothelial carcinoma: a morphologic and immunohistochemical comparison to the nested variant of urothelial carcinoma. *Am J Surg Pathol* 2003;27:1243–1252.

79. Kunze E, Schauer A, Schmitt M. Histology and histogenesis of two different types of inverted urothelial papillomas. *Cancer* 1983;51:348–358.

80. Cox R, Epstein JI. Large nested variant of urothelial carcinoma: 23 cases mimicking von Brunn nests and inverted growth pattern of noninvasive papillary urothelial carcinoma. *Am J Surg Pathol* 2011;35:1337–1342.

81. Young RH, Srigley JR, Amin MB, et al. Tumor-like lesions of the prostate. In: Rosai J, Sobin LH, eds. *Tumors of the Prostate Gland, Seminal Vesicles, Male Urethra and Penis*. Washington, DC: Armed Forces Institute of Pathology; 2000.

82. Paner GP, Luthringer DJ, Amin MB. Best practice in diagnostic immunohistochemistry: prostate carcinoma and its mimics in needle core biopsies. *Arch Pathol Lab Med* 2008;132:1388–1396.

83. Gagucas RJ, Brown RW, Wheeler TM. Verumontanum mucosal gland hyperplasia. *Am J Surg Pathol* 1995;19:30–36.

84. Palmer JK, Emmett JL, Mc DJ. Urethral caruncle. *Surg Gynecol Obstet* 1948;87:611–620.

85. Young RH, Oliva E, Garcia JA, et al. Urethral caruncle with atypical stromal cells simulating lymphoma or sarcoma—a distinctive pseudoneoplastic lesion of females. A report of six cases. *Am J Surg Pathol* 1996;20:1190–1195.

86. Young RH, Scully RE. Pseudosarcomatous lesions of the urinary bladder, prostate gland, and urethra. A report of three cases and review of the literature. *Arch Pathol Lab Med* 1987;111:354–358.

87. Balogh K, O'Hara CJ. Myeloid metaplasia masquerading as a urethral caruncle. *J Urol* 1986;135:789–790.

88. Atalay AC, Karaman MI, Basak T, et al. Non-Hodgkin's lymphoma of the female urethra presenting as a caruncle. *Int Urol Nephrol* 1998;30:609–610.

89. Khatib RA, Khalil AM, Tawil AN, et al. Non-Hodgkin's lymphoma presenting as a urethral caruncle. *Gynecol Oncol* 1993;50:389–393.

90. Lopez JI, Angulo JC, Ibanez T. Primary malignant melanoma mimicking urethral caruncle. Case report. *Scand J Urol Nephrol* 1993;27:125–126.

91. Chan JK, Chow TC, Tsui MS. Prostatic-type polyps of the lower urinary tract: three histogenetic types? *Histopathology* 1987;11:789–801.

92. Isaac J, Snow B, Lowichik A. Fibroepithelial polyp of the prostatic urethra in an adolescent. *J Pediatr Surg* 2006;41:e29–e31.

93. Ishikawa J, Yasuno H, Higuchi A, et al. Benign polyp with prostatic-type epithelium of the urinary bladder: a case report. *Hinyokika Kiyo* 1990;36:1463–1465.

94. Remick DG Jr, Kumar NB. Benign polyps with prostatic-type epithelium of the urethra and the urinary bladder. A suggestion of histogenesis based on histologic and immunohistochemical studies. *Am J Surg Pathol* 1984;8:833–839.

95. Sekine H, Mine M, Kaneoya F, et al. Benign polyp with prostatic-type epithelium in the anterior urethra accompanied with urethral stricture. *Urol Int* 1993;50:114–116.

96. Craig JR, Hart WR. Benign polyps with prostatic-type epithelium of the urethra. *Am J Clin Pathol* 1975;63:343–347.

97. Furuya S, Ogura H, Shimamura S, et al. [Clinical manifestations of 25 patients with prostatic-type polyps in the prostatic urethra]. *Hinyokika Kiyo* 2002;48:337–342.

98. Herman TE, Siegel MJ. Special imaging casebook. Congenital polyp of prostatic urethra. *J Perinatol* 1997;17:500–502.

99. Anjum MI, Ahmed M, Shrotri N, et al. Benign polyps with prostatic-type epithelium of the urethra and the urinary bladder. *Int Urol Nephrol* 1997;29:313–317.

100. Fan K, Schaefer RF, Venable M. Urethral verumontanal polyp: evidence of prostatic origin. *Urology* 1984;24:499–501.

101. Walker AN, Mills SE, Fechner RE, et al. Epithelial polyps of the prostatic urethra. A light-microscopic and immunohistochemical study. *Am J Surg Pathol* 1983;7:351–356.

102. Yuhara K, Ishida K, Kanimoto Y. [A case of benign polyp with prostatic-type epithelium in the bulbar urethra]. *Hinyokika Kiyo* 2004;50:873–875.

103. Humphrey PA. Histological variants of prostatic carcinoma and their significance. *Histopathology* 2012;60:59–74.

104. Downs RA. Congenital polyps of the prostatic urethra. A review of the literature and report of two cases. *Br J Urol* 1970;42:76–85.

105. Aita GA, Begliomini H, Mattos D Jr. Fibroepithelial polyp of the urethra. *Int Braz J Urol* 2005;31:155–156.

106. Demircan M, Ceran C, Karaman A, et al. Urethral polyps in children: a review of the literature and report of two cases. *Int J Urol* 2006;13:841–843.

107. Tsuzuki T, Epstein JI. Fibroepithelial polyp of the lower urinary tract in adults. *Am J Surg Pathol* 2005;29:460–466.

108. De Castro R, Campobasso P, Belloli G, et al. Solitary polyp of posterior urethra in children: report on seventeen cases. *Eur J Pediatr Surg* 1993;3:92–96.

109. Lanzas Prieto JM, Menendez Fernandez CL, Perez Garcia FJ, et al. [Fibroepithelial polyp of the urethra in an adult]. *Actas Urol Esp* 2003;27:654–656.

110. Leuschner I, Harms D, Mattke A, et al. Rhabdomyosarcoma of the urinary bladder and vagina: a clinicopathologic study with emphasis on recurrent disease: a report from the Kiel Pediatric Tumor Registry and the German CWS Study. *Am J Surg Pathol* 2001;25:856–864.

111. Bourne CW, Kilcoyne RF, Kraenzler EJ. Prominent lateral mucosal folds in the bulbous urethra. *J Urol* 1981;126:326–330.

112. Bevers RF, Abbekerk EM, Boon TA. Cowper's syringocele: symptoms, classification and treatment of an unappreciated problem. *J Urol* 2000;163:782–784.

113. Campobasso P, Schieven E, Fernandes EC. Cowper's syringocele: an analysis of 15 consecutive cases. *Arch Dis Child* 1996;75:71–73.

114. Kajiwara M, Inoue K, Kato M, et al. Anterior urethral valves in children: a possible association between anterior urethral valves and Cowper's duct cyst. *Int J Urol* 2007;14:156–160.

115. Richter S, Shalev M, Nissenkorn I. Late appearance of Cowper's syringocele. *J Urol* 1998;160:128–129.

116. Watson RA, Lassoff MA, Sawczuk IS, et al. Syringocele of Cowper's gland duct: an increasingly common rarity. *J Urol* 2007;178:285.

117. Eilber KS, Raz S. Benign cystic lesions of the vagina: a literature review. *J Urol* 2003;170:717–722.

118. Miller EV. Skene's duct cyst. *J Urol* 1984;131:966–967.

119. Satani H, Yoshimura N, Hayashi N, et al. [A case of female paraurethral cyst diagnosed as epithelial inclusion cyst]. *Hinyokika Kiyo* 2000;46:205–207.

120. Allan CH, Epstein JI. Nephrogenic adenoma of the prostatic urethra: a mimicker of prostate adenocarcinoma. *Am J Surg Pathol* 2001;25:802–808.

121. Ford TF, Watson GM, Cameron KM. Adenomatous metaplasia (nephrogenic adenoma) of urothelium. An analysis of 70 cases. *Br J Urol* 1985;57:427–433.

122. Medeiros LJ, Young RH. Nephrogenic adenoma arising in urethral diverticula. A report of five cases. *Arch Pathol Lab Med* 1989;113:125–128.

123. Oliva E, Young RH. Nephrogenic adenoma of the urinary tract: a review of the microscopic appearance of 80 cases with emphasis on unusual features. *Mod Pathol* 1995;8:722–730.

124. Malpica A, Ro JY, Troncoso P, et al. Nephrogenic adenoma of the prostatic urethra involving the prostate gland: a clinicopathologic and immunohistochemical study of eight cases. *Hum Pathol* 1994;25:390–395.

125. Young RH. Nephrogenic adenomas of the urethra involving the prostate gland: a report of two cases of a lesion that may be confused with prostatic adenocarcinoma. *Mod Pathol* 1992;5:617–620.

126. Hansel DE, Nadasdy T, Epstein JI. Fibromyxoid nephrogenic adenoma: a newly recognized variant mimicking mucinous adenocarcinoma. *Am J Surg Pathol* 2007;31:1231–1237.

127. Cheng L, Cheville JC, Sebo TJ, et al. Atypical nephrogenic metaplasia of the urinary tract: a precursor lesion? *Cancer* 2000;88:853–861.

128. Ozcan A, Shen SS, Hamilton C, et al. PAX 8 expression in non-neoplastic tissues, primary tumors, and metastatic tumors: a comprehensive immunohistochemical study. *Mod Pathol* 2011;24:751–764.

129. Tong GX, Melamed J, Mansukhani M, et al. PAX2: a reliable marker for nephrogenic adenoma. *Mod Pathol* 2006;19:356–363.

130. Tong GX, Weeden EM, Hamele-Bena D, et al. Expression of PAX8 in nephrogenic adenoma and clear cell adenocarcinoma of the lower urinary tract: evidence of related histogenesis? *Am J Surg Pathol* 2008;32:1380–1387.

131. Gupta A, Wang HL, Policarpio-Nicolas ML, et al. Expression of alpha-methylacyl-coenzyme A racemase in nephrogenic adenoma. *Am J Surg Pathol* 2004;28:1224–1229.

132. Skinnider BF, Oliva E, Young RH, et al. Expression of alpha-methylacyl-CoA racemase (P504S) in nephrogenic adenoma: a significant immunohistochemical pitfall compounding the differential diagnosis with prostatic adenocarcinoma. *Am J Surg Pathol* 2004;28:701–705.

133. Oliva E, Moch H, Cabrera R, et al. Nephrogenic adenoma (NA): an immunohistochemical (ICH) study of 40 cases. *Mod Pathol* 2003;16.

134. Mazal PR, Schaufler R, Altenhuber-Muller R, et al. Derivation of nephrogenic adenomas from renal tubular cells in kidney-transplant recipients. *N Engl J Med* 2002;347:653–659.

135. Devine P, Ucci AA, Krain H, et al. Nephrogenic adenoma and embryonic kidney tubules share PNA receptor sites. *Am J Clin Pathol* 1984;81:728–732.

136. Pycha A, Mian C, Reiter WJ, et al. Nephrogenic adenoma in renal transplant recipients: a truly benign lesion? *Urology* 1998;52:756–761.

137. Daroca PJ, Martin AW, Reed RJ, et al. Urethral nephrogenic adenoma; a report of three cases, including a case with infiltration of the prostatic stroma. *J Urol Pathol* 1993;1:157.

138. Young RH, Scully RE. Clear cell adenocarcinoma of the bladder and urethra. A report of three cases and review of the literature. *Am J Surg Pathol* 1985;9:816–826.

139. Cossu-Rocca P, Contini M, Brunelli M, et al. S-100A1 is a reliable marker in distinguishing nephrogenic adenoma from prostatic adenocarcinoma. *Am J Surg Pathol* 2009;33:1031–1036.

140. Gilcrease MZ, Delgado R, Vuitch F, et al. Clear cell adenocarcinoma and nephrogenic adenoma of the urethra and urinary bladder: a histopathologic and immunohistochemical comparison. *Hum Pathol* 1998;29:1451–1456.

141. Oliva E, Amin MB, Jimenez R, et al. Clear cell carcinoma of the urinary bladder: a report and comparison of four tumors of mullerian origin and nine of probable urothelial origin with discussion of histogenesis and diagnostic problems. *Am J Surg Pathol* 2002;26:190–197.

142. Herawi M, Drew PA, Pan CC, et al. Clear cell adenocarcinoma of the bladder and urethra: cases diffusely mimicking nephrogenic adenoma. *Hum Pathol* 2010;41:594–601.

143. Ducrocq S, Bruniau A, Cordonnier C, et al. [Bladder nephrogenic metaplasia: circumstances of discovery, predisposing factors, and clinical course in 7 cases diagnosed between 1988 and 2000]. *Prog Urol* 2003;13:613–617.

144. Fournier G, Menut P, Moal MC, et al. Nephrogenic adenoma of the bladder in renal transplant recipients: a report of 9 cases with assessment of deoxyribonucleic acid ploidy and long-term followup. *J Urol* 1996;156:41–44.

145. Tse V, Khadra M, Eisinger D, et al. Nephrogenic adenoma of the bladder in renal transplant and non-renal transplant patients: a review of 22 cases. *Urology* 1997;50:690–696.

146. Bessim S, Heller DS, Dottino P, et al. Malakoplakia of the female genital tract causing urethral and ureteral obstruction. A case report. *J Reprod Med* 1991;36:691–694.

147. Karaiossifidi H, Kouri E. Malacoplakia of the urethra: a case of unique localization with followup. *J Urol* 1992;148:1903–1904.

148. Long JP Jr, Althausen AF. Malacoplakia: a 25-year experience with a review of the literature. *J Urol* 1989;141:1328–1331.

149. Love KD, Chitale SV, Vohra AK, et al. Urethral stricture associated with malacoplakia: a case report and review of the literature. *Urology* 2001;57:169.

150. McClure J. A case of urethral malacoplakia associated with vesical disease. *J Urol* 1979;122:705–706.

151. Sharma TC, Kagan HN, Sheils JP. Malacoplakia of the male urethra. *J Urol* 1981;125:885–886.

152. Sloane BB, Figueroa TE, Ferguson D, et al. Malacoplakia of the urethra. *J Urol* 1988;139:1300–1301.

153. Rosales Leal JL, Cozar Olmo JM, Vicente Prados FJ, et al. [Malacoplakia within a female urethral diverticulum]. *Arch Esp Urol* 2004;57:162–165.

154. Yousef GM, Naghibi B, Hamodat MM. Malakoplakia outside the urinary tract. *Arch Pathol Lab Med* 2007;131:297–300.

155. Crook TJ, Koslowski M, Dyer JP, et al. A case of amyloid of the urethra and review of this rare diagnosis, its natural history and management, with reference to the literature. *Scand J Urol Nephrol* 2002;36:481–486.

156. Provet JA, Mennen J, Sabatini M, et al. Primary amyloidosis of urethra. *Urology* 1989;34:106–108.

157. Ichioka K, Utsunomiya N, Ueda N, et al. Primary localized amyloidosis of urethra: magnetic resonance imaging findings. *Urology* 2004;64:376–378.

158. Miyamoto S, Tamiya T, Takatsuka K, et al. Primary localized amyloidosis of urethra. *Urology* 1991;37:576–578.

159. Comiter CV. Endometriosis of the urinary tract. *Urol Clin North Am* 2002;29:625–635.

160. Chowdhry AA, Miller FH, Hammer RA. Endometriosis presenting as a urethral diverticulum: a case report. *J Reprod Med* 2004;49:321–323.

161. Oliva E, Young RH. Clear cell adenocarcinoma of the urethra: a clinicopathologic analysis of 19 cases. *Mod Pathol* 1996;9:513–520.

162. Marks LB, Carroll PR, Dugan TC, et al. The response of the urinary bladder, urethra, and ureter to radiation and chemotherapy. *Int J Radiat Oncol Biol Phys* 1995;31:1257–1280.

163. Baker PM, Young RH. Radiation-induced pseudocarcinomatous proliferations of the urinary bladder: a report of 4 cases. *Hum Pathol* 2000;31:678–683.

164. Chan YM, Ka-Leung Cheng D, Nga-Yin Cheung A, et al. Female urethral adenocarcinoma arising from urethritis glandularis. *Gynecol Oncol* 2000;79:511–514.

165. Lopez-Beltran A, Luque RJ, Mazzucchelli R, et al. Changes produced in the urothelium by traditional and newer therapeutic procedures for bladder cancer. *J Clin Pathol* 2002;55:641–647.

166. Ballesteros Sampol JJ, Cortadellas Angel R, Juanpere Rodero N. [Acquired male urethra diverticula. Report of seven cases. Bibliographic review]. *Arch Esp Urol* 2008;61:1–6.

167. Davis BL, Robinson DG. Diverticula of the female urethra: assay of 120 cases. *J Urol* 1970;104:850–853.

168. Khati NJ, Javitt MC, Schwartz AM, et al. MR imaging diagnosis of a urethral diverticulum. *Radiographics* 1998;18:517–522.

169. Romanzi LJ, Groutz A, Blaivas JG. Urethral diverticulum in women: diverse presentations resulting in diagnostic delay and mismanagement. *J Urol* 2000;164:428–433.

170. Helpap B. Squamous cell papilloma. In: Eble JN, Sauter G, Epstein JI, Sesterhenn IA, eds. *Pathology & Genetics: Tumours of the Urinary System and Male Genital Organs.* Lyon, France: IARC Press; 2004.

171. Fine SW, Chan TY, Epstein JI. Inverted papillomas of the prostatic urethra. *Am J Surg Pathol* 2006;30:975–979.

172. Occhipinti K, Kutcher R, Gentile RL. Prolapsing inverted papilloma of the prostatic urethra: diagnosis by transrectal sonography. *AJR Am J Roentgenol* 1992;159:93–94.

173. Ojea Calvo A, Alonso Rodrigo A, Rodriguez Iglesias B, et al. [Inverted papilloma of the urethra]. *Actas Urol Esp* 1993;17:193–195.

174. Sung MT, Maclennan GT, Lopez-Beltran A, et al. Natural history of urothelial inverted papilloma. *Cancer* 2006;107:2622–2627.

175. Magi-Galluzzi C, Epstein JI. Urothelial papilloma of the bladder: a review of 34 de novo cases. *Am J Surg Pathol* 2004;28:1615–1620.

176. McKenney JK, Amin MB, Young RH. Urothelial (transitional cell) papilloma of the urinary bladder: a clinicopathologic study of 26 cases. *Mod Pathol* 2003;16:623–629.

177. Broussard JN, Tan PH, Epstein JI. Atypia in inverted urothelial papillomas: pathology and prognostic significance. *Hum Pathol* 2004;35:1499–1504.

178. Lopez JI, Ereno C. Glandular-type inverted papilloma of the prostatic urethra. *Arch Anat Cytol Pathol* 1997;45:227–229.

179. Cheng CW, Chan LW, Chan CK, et al. Is surveillance necessary for inverted papilloma in the urinary bladder and urethra? *ANZ J Surg* 2005;75:213–217.

180. Cheville JC, Wu K, Sebo TJ, et al. Inverted urothelial papilloma: is ploidy, MIB-1 proliferative activity, or p53 protein accumulation predictive of urothelial carcinoma? *Cancer* 2000;88:632–636.

181. Renfer LG, Kelley J, Belville WD. Inverted papilloma of the urinary tract: histogenesis, recurrence and associated malignancy. *J Urol* 1988;140:832–834.

182. Algaba F, Matias-Guiu X, Badia F, Sole-Balcells F. Villous adenoma of the prostatic urethra. *Eur Urol* 1988;14:255–257.

183. Cheng L, Montironi R, Bostwick DG. Villous adenoma of the urinary tract: a report of 23 cases, including 8 with coexistent adenocarcinoma. *Am J Surg Pathol* 1999;23:764–771.

184. Morgan DR, Dixon MF, Harnden P. Villous adenoma of urethra associated with tubulovillous adenoma and adenocarcinoma of rectum. *Histopathology* 1998;32:87–89.

185. Seibel JL, Prasad S, Weiss RE, et al. Villous adenoma of the urinary tract: a lesion frequently associated with malignancy. *Hum Pathol* 2002;33:236–241.

186. Tran KP, Epstein JI. Mucinous adenocarcinoma of urinary bladder type arising from the prostatic urethra. Distinction from mucinous adenocarcinoma of the prostate. *Am J Surg Pathol* 1996;20:1346–1350.

187. Sato K, Tachibana H, Tsuzuki T, et al. Prostatic ductal adenocarcinoma mimicking villous adenoma of the urethra. *Virchows Arch* 2006;449:597–599.

188. Herawi M, De Marzo AM, Kristiansen G, et al. Expression of CDX2 in benign tissue and adenocarcinoma of the prostate. *Hum Pathol* 2007;38:72–78.

189. Kakizoe T, Tobisu K. Transitional cell carcinoma of the urethra in men and women associated with bladder cancer. *Jpn J Clin Oncol* 1998;28:357–359.

190. Amin MB, Young RH. Primary carcinomas of the urethra. *Semin Diagn Pathol* 1997;14:147–160.

191. Dalbagni G, Zhang ZF, Lacombe L, et al. Male urethral carcinoma: analysis of treatment outcome. *Urology* 1999;53:1126–1132.

192. Johnson DE, O'Connell JR. Primary carcinoma of female urethra. *Urology* 1983;21:42–45.

193. Cheville JC, Dundore PA, Bostwick DG, et al. Transitional cell carcinoma of the prostate: clinicopathologic study of 50 cases. *Cancer* 1998;82:703–707.

194. De Paepe ME, Andre R, Mahadevia P. Urethral involvement in female patients with bladder cancer. A study of 22 cystectomy specimens. *Cancer* 1990;65:1237–1241.

195. Hardeman SW, Soloway MS. Urethral recurrence following radical cystectomy. *J Urol* 1990;144:666–669.

196. Dinney CP, Johnson DE, Swanson DA, et al. Therapy and prognosis for male anterior urethral carcinoma: an update. *Urology* 1994;43:506–514.

197. Kim SJ, MacLennan GT. Tumors of the male urethra. *J Urol* 2005;174:312.

198. Urrutia Alonso J, Machuca Santacruz J, Tallada Bunuel M, et al. [Epidermoid carcinoma of the male urethra. Our experience in 5 cases]. *Arch Esp Urol* 1995;48:355–363.

199. Chaux A, Reuter V, Lezcano C, et al. Autopsy findings in 14 patients with penile squamous cell carcinoma. *Int J Surg Pathol* 2011;19:164–169.

200. Cupp MR, Malek RS, Goellner JR, et al. Detection of human papillomavirus DNA in primary squamous cell carcinoma of the male urethra. *Urology* 1996;48:551–555.

201. Grussendorf-Conen EI, Deutz FJ, de Villiers EM. Detection of human papillomavirus-6 in primary carcinoma of the urethra in men. *Cancer* 1987;60:1832–1835.

202. Wiener JS, Liu ET, Walther PJ. Oncogenic human papillomavirus type 16 is associated with squamous cell cancer of the male urethra. *Cancer Res* 1992;52:5018–5023.

203. Tazi K, Moudouni S, Karmouni T, et al. [Epidermoid carcinoma of the male urethra]. *Prog Urol* 2000;10:600–602.

204. Meis JM, Ayala AG, Johnson DE. Adenocarcinoma of the urethra in women. A clinicopathologic study. *Cancer* 1987;60:1038–1052.

205. Roberts TW, Melicow MM. Pathology and natural history of urethral tumors in females: review of 65 cases. *Urology* 1977;10:583–589.

206. Murphy DP, Pantuck AJ, Amenta PS, et al. Female urethral adenocarcinoma: immunohistochemical evidence of more than 1 tissue of origin. *J Urol* 1999;161:1881–1884.

207. Mostofi FK, Davis CJ Jr, Sesterhenn IA. Carcinoma of the male and female urethra. *Urol Clin North Am* 1992;19:347–358.

208. Abascal Junquera JM, Cecchini Rosell L, Martos Calvo R, et al. [Presentation of a new case of primary clear cell adenocarcinoma of the urethra and its surgical management]. *Actas Urol Esp* 2007;31:411–416.

209. Hopkins SC, Nag SK, Soloway MS. Primary carcinoma of male urethra. *Urology* 1984;23:128–133.

210. Osunkoya AO, Epstein JI. Primary mucin-producing urothelial-type adenocarcinoma of prostate: report of 15 cases. *Am J Surg Pathol* 2007;31:1323–1329.

211. Suzuki K, Morita T, Tokue A. Primary signet ring cell carcinoma of female urethra. *Int J Urol* 2001;8:509–512.

212. Yvgenia R, Ben Meir D, Sibi J, et al. Mucinous adenocarcinoma of posterior urethra. Report of a case. *Pathol Res Pract* 2005;201:137–140.

213. Dodson MK, Cliby WA, Pettavel PP, et al. Female urethral adenocarcinoma: evidence for more than one tissue of origin? *Gynecol Oncol* 1995;59:352–357.

214. Chang YH, Chuang CK, Ng KF, et al. Urethral metastasis from a colon carcinoma. *Urology* 2007;69:575.e1–575.e3.

215. Dougherty KR, Khettry U, Stoffel JT, et al. Rectal adenocarcinoma with metachronous metastases to the urethra. *Am Surg* 2009;75:265–266.

216. Bostwick DG, Kindrachuk RW, Rouse RV. Prostatic adenocarcinoma with endometrioid features. Clinical, pathologic, and ultrastructural findings. *Am J Surg Pathol* 1985;9:595–609.

217. Zaloudek C, Williams JW, Kempson RL. "Endometrial" adenocarcinoma of the prostate: a distinctive tumor of probable prostatic duct origin. *Cancer* 1976;37:2255–2262.

218. Ray B, Canto AR, Whitmore WF Jr. Experience with primary carcinoma of the male urethra. *J Urol* 1977;117:591–594.

219. Zaino RJ. Carcinoma of the vulva, urethra, and Bartholin's gland. In: WIlkerson EJ, ed. *Contemporary Issues in Surgical Pathology: Vulva, Vagina.* New York: Churchill Livingstone; 1987:119–153.

220. Grabstald H. Proceedings: tumors of the urethra in men and women. *Cancer* 1973;32:1236–1255.

221. Miller J, Karnes RJ. Primary clear-cell adenocarcinoma of the proximal female urethra: case report and review of the literature. *Clin Genitourin Cancer* 2008;6:131–133.

222. Kawano K, Yano M, Kitahara S, et al. Clear cell adenocarcinoma of the female urethra showing strong immunostaining for prostate-specific antigen. *BJU Int* 2001;87:412–413.

223. Sun K, Huan Y, Unger PD. Clear cell adenocarcinoma of urinary bladder and urethra: another urinary tract lesion immunoreactive for P504S. *Arch Pathol Lab Med* 2008;132:1417–1422.

224. Young RH, Scully RE. Nephrogenic adenoma. A report of 15 cases, review of the literature, and comparison with clear cell adenocarcinoma of the urinary tract. *Am J Surg Pathol* 1986;10:268–275.

225. Alsanjari N, Lynch MJ, Fisher C, et al. Vesical clear cell adenocarcinoma. V. Nephrogenic adenoma: a diagnostic problem. *Histopathology* 1995;27:43–49.

226. Laury AR, Perets R, Piao H, et al. A comprehensive analysis of PAX8 expression in human epithelial tumors. *Am J Surg Pathol* 2011;35:816–826.

227. Gokden N, Gokden M, Phan DC, et al. The utility of PAX-2 in distinguishing metastatic clear cell renal cell carcinoma from its morphologic mimics: an immunohistochemical study with comparison to renal cell carcinoma marker. *Am J Surg Pathol* 2008;32:1462–1467.

228. Ozcan A, Zhai Q, Javed R, et al. PAX-2 is a helpful marker for diagnosing metastatic renal cell carcinoma: comparison with the renal cell carcinoma marker antigen and kidney-specific cadherin. *Arch Pathol Lab Med* 2010;134:1121–1129.

229. Kotliar SN, Wood CG, Schaeffer AJ, et al. Transitional cell carcinoma exhibiting clear cell features. A differential diagnosis for clear cell adenocarcinoma of the urinary tract. *Arch Pathol Lab Med* 1995;119:79–81.

230. Young RH, Zukerberg LR. Microcystic transitional cell carcinomas of the urinary bladder. A report of four cases. *Am J Clin Pathol* 1991;96:635–639.

231. Brimo F, Herawi M, Sharma R, et al. Hepatocyte nuclear factor-1beta expression in clear cell adenocarcinomas of the bladder and urethra: diagnostic utility and implications for histogenesis. *Hum Pathol* 2011;42:1613–1619.

232. Pan CC, Chiang H, Chang YH, et al. Tubulocystic clear cell adenocarcinoma arising within the prostate. *Am J Surg Pathol* 2000;24:1433–1436.

233. Bourque JL, Charghi A, Gauthier GE, et al. Primary carcinoma of Cowper's gland. *J Urol* 1970;103:758–7561.

234. Sacks SA, Waisman J, Apfelbaum HB, et al. Urethral adenocarcinoma (possibly originating in the glands of Littre). *J Urol* 1975;113:50–55.

235. Svanholm H, Andersen OP, Rohl H. Tumour of female paraurethral duct. Immunohistochemical similarity with prostatic carcinoma. *Virchows Arch A Pathol Anat Histopathol* 1987;411:395–398.

236. Taylor RN, Lacey CG, Shuman MA. Adenocarcinoma of Skene's duct associated with a systemic coagulopathy. *Gynecol Oncol* 1985;22:250–256.

237. Zaviacic M, Sidlo J, Borovsky M. Prostate specific antigen and prostate specific acid phosphatase in adenocarcinoma of Skene's paraurethral glands and ducts. *Virchows Arch A Pathol Anat Histopathol* 1993;423:503–505.

238. Dodson MK, Cliby WA, Keeney GL, et al. Skene's gland adenocarcinoma with increased serum level of prostate-specific antigen. *Gynecol Oncol* 1994;55:304–307.

239. Ali SZ, Smilari TF, Gal D, et al. Primary adenoid cystic carcinoma of Skene's glands. *Gynecol Oncol* 1995;57:257–261.

240. Altintas S, Blockx N, Huizing MT, et al. Small-cell carcinoma of the penile urethra: a case report and a short review of the literature. *Ann Oncol* 2007;18:801–804.

241. Rudloff U, Amukele SA, Moldwin R, et al. Small cell carcinoma arising from the proximal urethra. *Int J Urol* 2004;11:674–677.

242. Yoo KH, Kim GY, Kim TG, et al. Primary small cell neuroendocrine carcinoma of the female urethra. *Pathol Int* 2009;59:601–603.

243. Chen YB, Epstein JI. Primary carcinoid tumors of the urinary bladder and prostatic urethra: a clinicopathologic study of 6 cases. *Am J Surg Pathol* 2011;35:442–446.

244. Llarena Ibarguren R, Vesga Molina F, Acha Perez M, et al. [Urethral metastases of prostatic adenocarcinoma]. *Arch Esp Urol* 1993;46:779–782.

245. Senzaki H, Okamura T, Tatsura H, et al. Urethral metastasis from renal cell carcinoma. *Int J Urol* 2003;10:661–663.

246. Murali R, Kneale K, Lalak N, et al. Carcinoid tumors of the urinary tract and prostate. *Arch Pathol Lab Med* 2006;130:1693–1706.

247. Cornella JL, Larson TR, Lee RA, et al. Leiomyoma of the female urethra and bladder: report of twenty-three patients and review of the literature. *Am J Obstet Gynecol* 1997;176:1278–1285.

248. Leidinger RJ, Das S. Leiomyoma of the female urethra. A report of two cases. *J Reprod Med* 1995;40:229–231.

249. Leung YL, Lee F, Tam PC. Leiomyoma of female urethra causing acute urinary retention and acute renal failure. *J Urol* 1997;158:1911–1192.

250. Lee TK, Miyamoto H, Osunkoya AO, et al. Smooth muscle neoplasms of the urinary bladder: a clinicopathologic study of 51 cases. *Am J Surg Pathol* 2010;34:502–509.

251. Alvarado-Cabrero I, Candanedo-Gonzalez F, Sosa-Romero A. Leiomyoma of the urethra in a Mexican woman: a rare neoplasm associated with the expression of estrogen receptors by immunohistochemistry. *Arch Med Res* 2001;32:88–90.

252. Brown JA, Levy JB, Kramer SA. Genitourinary neurofibromatosis mimicking posterior urethral valves. *Urology* 1997;49:960–962.

253. Gersell DJ, Fulling KH. Localized neurofibromatosis of the female genitourinary tract. *Am J Surg Pathol* 1989;13:873–878.

254. Shah S, Murthy PV, Gopalkrishnan G, et al. Neurofibromatosis of the bladder and urethra presenting as obstructive uropathy. *Br J Urol* 1988;61:364–365.

255. Saito S. Posterior urethral hemangioma: one of the unknown causes of hematuria and/or hematospermia. *Urology* 2008;71:168.e11–168.e14.

256. Steinhardt G, Perlmutter A. Urethral hemangioma. *J Urol* 1987;137:116–117.

257. Tabibian L, Ginsberg DA. Thrombosed urethral hemangioma. *J Urol* 2003;170:1942.

258. North PE, Mihm MC Jr. Histopathological diagnosis of infantile hemangiomas and vascular malformations. *Facial Plast Surg Clin North Am* 2001;9:505–524.

259. Yokoyama H, Kontani K, Komiyama I, et al. Granular cell tumor of the urethra. *Int J Urol* 2007;14:461–462.

260. Barua R, Munday RN. Intravascular angiomatosis in female urethral mass. Masson intravascular hemangioendothelioma. *Urology* 1983;21:191–193.

261. Nevin DT, Palazzo J, Petersen R. A urethral mass in a 67-year-old woman. Papillary endothelial hyperplasia (Masson tumor). *Arch Pathol Lab Med* 2006;130:561–562.

262. Badalament RA, Kenworthy P, Pellegrini A, et al. Paraganglioma of urethra. *Urology* 1991;38:76–78.

263. Arndt CA, Crist WM. Common musculoskeletal tumors of childhood and adolescence. *N Engl J Med* 1999;341:342–352.

264. Newton WA Jr, Gehan EA, Webber BL, et al. Classification of rhabdomyosarcomas and related sarcomas. Pathologic aspects and proposal for a new classification—an Intergroup Rhabdomyosarcoma Study. *Cancer* 1995;76:1073–1085.

265. Crist WM, Anderson JR, Meza JL, et al. Intergroup rhabdomyosarcoma study-IV: results for patients with nonmetastatic disease. *J Clin Oncol* 2001;19:3091–3102.

266. Millan-Rodriguez F, Montlleo-Gonzalez M, Rosales-Bordes A, et al. Kaposi's sarcoma of the urethral meatus: management by urethral dilatation. *Br J Urol* 1995;75:558.

267. Nakamoto T, Inoue Y, Ueki T, et al. Primary amelanotic malignant melanoma of the female urethra. *Int J Urol* 2007;14:153–155.

268. Dasgupta T, Grabstald H. Melanoma of the genitourinary tract. *J Urol* 1965;93:607–614.

269. Fernandez Madrigal F, Junquera Villa JM. [Primary melanoma of the male urethra. A review of the literature]. *Actas Urol Esp* 1984;8:221–224.

270. Garcia Riestra V, Fernandez Garcia ML, Varela Salgado M. [Primary malignant melanoma of the female urethra]. *Arch Esp Urol* 1995;48:403–405.

271. Gupta R, Bhatti SS, Dinda AK, et al. Primary melanoma of the urethra: a rare neoplasm of the urinary tract. *Int Urol Nephrol* 2007;39: 833–836.

272. Morita T, Suzuki H, Goto K, et al. Primary malignant melanoma of male urethra with fistula formation. *Urol Int* 1991;46:114–115.

273. Manivel JC, Fraley EE. Malignant melanoma of the penis and male urethra: 4 case reports and literature review. *J Urol* 1988;139: 813–816.

274. Calcagno L, Casarico A, Bandelloni R, et al. Primary malignant melanoma of male urethra. *Urology* 1991;37:366–368.

275. Oliva E, Quinn TR, Amin MB, et al. Primary malignant melanoma of the urethra: a clinicopathologic analysis of 15 cases. *Am J Surg Pathol* 2000;24:785–796.

276. Nakhleh RE, Wick MR, Rocamora A, et al. Morphologic diversity in malignant melanomas. *Am J Clin Pathol* 1990;93:731–740.

277. Radhi JM. Urethral malignant melanoma closely mimicking urothelial carcinoma. *J Clin Pathol* 1997;50:250–252.

278. Rashid AM, Williams RM, Horton LW. Malignant melanoma of penis and male urethra. Is it a difficult tumor to diagnose? *Urology* 1993;41:470–471.

279. Ro JY, Amin MB. Penis and scrotum. In: Bostwick DG, Eble JN, eds. *Urologic Surgical Pathology*. St. Louis, MO: Mosby; 1997:713.

280. Barnhill RL, Albert LS, Shama SK, et al. Genital lentiginosis: a clinical and histopathologic study. *J Am Acad Dermatol* 1990;22:453–460.

281. Clark WH Jr, Hood AF, Tucker MA, et al. Atypical melanocytic nevi of the genital type with a discussion of reciprocal parenchymal-stromal interactions in the biology of neoplasia. *Hum Pathol* 1998;29: S1–S24.

282. Begun FP, Grossman HB, Diokno AC, et al. Malignant melanoma of the penis and male urethra. *J Urol* 1984;132:123–125.

283. Sanchez-Ortiz R, Huang SF, Tamboli P, et al. Melanoma of the penis, scrotum and male urethra: a 40-year single institution experience. *J Urol* 2005;173:1958–1965.

284. Hatcher PA, Wilson DD. Primary lymphoma of the male urethra. *Urology* 1997;49:142–144.

285. Hofmockel G, Dammrich J, Manzanilla Garcia H, et al. Primary non-Hodgkin's lymphoma of the male urethra. A case report and review of the literature. *Urol Int* 1995;55:177–180.

286. Masuda A, Tsujii T, Kojima M, et al. Primary mucosa-associated lymphoid tissue (MALT) lymphoma arising from the male urethra. A case report and review of the literature. *Pathol Res Pract* 2002;198: 571–575.

287. Ohsawa M, Mishima K, Suzuki A, et al. Malignant lymphoma of the urethra: report of a case with detection of Epstein-Barr virus genome in the tumour cells. *Histopathology* 1994;24:525–529.

288. Richter LA, Hegde P, Taylor JA III. Primary non-Hodgkin's B-cell lymphoma of the male urethra presenting as stricture disease. *Urology* 2007;70:1008.e11–1008.e12.

289. Vapnek JM, Turzan CW. Primary malignant lymphoma of the female urethra: report of a case and review of the literature. *J Urol* 1992;147:701–703.

290. Witjes JA, De Vries JD, Schaafsma HE, et al. Extramedullary plasmacytoma of the urethra: a case report. *J Urol* 1991;145:826–828.

Nonneoplastic Diseases of the Prostate and Seminal Vesicles

PETER A. HUMPHREY

PROSTATE

Introduction

Nonneoplastic diseases of the prostate are common afflictions of men. Prostatitis and benign prostatic hyperplasia (BPH) in particular are highly prevalent clinical disorders. About one in nine men aged 25 to 80 have clinical prostatitis-like symptoms.[1,2] Moderate to severe lower urinary tract symptoms, which are clinical hallmarks of BPH, are found in one-quarter of men in their 50s, one-third of men in their 60s, and about one-half of men 80 years or older.[3] Histologic detection of inflammation and BPH (nodular glandular and/or stromal hyperplasia) in prostatic tissues is even more common. In contrast, nonneoplastic diseases of the seminal vesicles are distinctly uncommon to rare. In this chapter, benign nonneoplastic conditions of the prostate and seminal vesicles are surveyed, with a focus on pathologic diagnosis and differential diagnosis, with clinicopathologic correlations.

Nonneoplastic diseases of the prostate are also important since several nonneoplastic lesions can be misdiagnosed as prostate cancer, and are therefore pseudoneoplasms or benign mimickers of prostate cancer (Table 8-1). Foremost amongst these histologic benign mimickers are prostatic atrophy, atypical adenomatous hyperplasia (AAH) (adenosis), basal cell hyperplasia, and inflammatory atypia.[4–7] In the seminal vesicle a classical pitfall is the misinterpretation of normal nuclear atypia as malignancy, and in particular, prostatic carcinoma.

Function

The prostate is one of the male sex accessory tissues, which include the prostate, seminal vesicles, and bulbourethral glands. The main function of the prostate is to form secretions that constitute one-half to two-thirds of the 3 mL volume of the ejaculate.[8] The biologic role of many biochemical substances found in the semen is unknown. A well-defined function has been established for several enzymes that participate in the clotting and lysis of the seminal vesicle clot. One of these enzymes is prostate specific antigen (PSA), which is a serine protease and esterase that cleaves semenogelin, a protein involved in clotting. Additional substances found in high concentration include potassium, zinc, citric acid, spermine, amino acids, prostaglandins, and a number of enzymes. These secretory products enhance fertility by promoting sperm viability and motility. An antimicrobial role has been suggested for zinc, spermine, and proteases. Physically, by mass effect, musculature, and location, the prostate may contribute to urine flow from the bladder. The prostate is not essential for life. Removal of the entire gland by surgery (radical prostatectomy) can be accomplished without consequences. In some men, there may be complications of incontinence and impotence, the latter being due to damage to periprostatic neurovascular bundles. Failure of the gland to form, as seen in 5α-reductase deficiency[9] and testicular feminization,[10] is not lethal.

Normal Embryology, Anatomy, and Histology

Embryology

The prostate is derived from the urogenital sinus and is first recognizable at 9 to 10 weeks of development.[11] Testosterone from the embryonic testis stimulates ingrowth of endodermal buds into urogenital sinus mesenchyme. It is thought that there is a reciprocal interaction of epithelium and mesenchyme during development by which, under the influence of androgens, urogenital sinus mesenchyme induces urogenital sinus epithelium to undergo prostatic ductal morphogenesis and differentiation.[12] The differentiating prostatic epithelium in turn signals the urogenital mesenchyme to differentiate

Table 8-1 ■ PSEUDONEOPLASMS OF THE PROSTATE

Atrophy*
Atypical adenomatous hyperplasia (adenosis)*
Basal cell hyperplasia*
Cribriform hyperplasia
Nephrogenic metaplasia (adenoma)
Verumontanum mucosal gland hyperplasia
Squamous metaplasia
Urothelial metaplasia
Radiation atypia
Prostatitis (especially xanthogranulomatous)
Malacoplakia
Endometriosis
Postoperative spindle cell nodule
Atypical stromal cells
Extramedullary hematopoiesis
Cowper glands
Paraganglia in prostate
Benign glands adjacent to nerves and skeletal muscle
Signet ring change in stromal nodule
Crowded benign glands
Seminal vesicle/ejaculatory duct epithelium

*Most likely to be misdiagnosed as carcinoma.

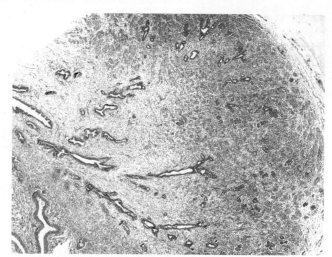

FIGURE 8-1 ■ Fetal prostate at 33 weeks with dominance of stroma and immature epithelium.

into smooth muscle cells that closely surround the epithelial ducts. This dynamic dance of tissue remodeling entails coordinated temporal and spatial processes of ductal budding, branching morphogenesis, cellular proliferation, and secretory function.[13] By 13 weeks some 70 primary ducts are present. Three stages of development from 20 weeks' gestation to 1 month of age have been delineated.[14] The bud stage at 20 to 30 weeks' gestation exhibits solid cellular buds at the end of ducts, with spindled cells in the center and columnar cells at the periphery. The bud–tubule stage at 31 to 36 weeks shows small collections of cellular buds and acinar structures (Figs. 8-1 and 8-2). The third stage is characterized by more distinct lobular organization of acinotubular clusters. Squamous metaplasia of prostatic ducts and urethra is a common finding in the fetal prostate. This metaplasia is gradually lost after birth.

The immunophenotype of fetal prostatic epithelial cells is similar to the rare adult transiently amplifying epithelial cells, which show coexpression of basal and luminal cytokeratins, high proliferation, and lack of p27 expression.[15]

Molecular pathways thought to be important in prostate organogenesis and morphogenesis include those regulated by androgens, hedgehog, p63, Nkx3.1, Sox9, Noggin, fibroblast growth factor receptor, forkhead transcription factor, Notch, and BMP7. Most of this work, with a few exceptions,[16] has been done in rodent model systems. Interestingly, some of these molecules have been implicated in human prostate cancer biologic behaviors.[17] The definitive identification of prostatic epithelial stem cells involved in prostate gland

development has not yet been realized, but cell populations enriched for cells exhibiting stem cell characteristics express the stem cell markers CD133(+), alpha2beta1(hi), CD44, and Sca-1 along with embryonic stem cell factors including Oct-1, Nanog, Sox2, and nestin.[18]

The seminal vesicles, epididymis, vas deferens, and ejaculatory ducts are formed from Wolffian (mesonephric) ducts under the influence of testosterone. It has been proposed that the central zone of the prostate is also of mesodermal Wolffian duct origin.[11] In this model the prostate gland is of dual embryonic derivation.

Anatomy

From birth to age 10 to 12 years there is an infantile resting phase where prostate size remains stable at about 1 to 1.4 g. During this time there is continual duct formation, solid budding at the periphery, and branching morphogenesis.[13] From

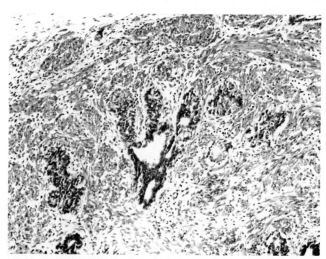

FIGURE 8-2 ■ Fetal prostate at 33 weeks with small glands and solid cellular buds.

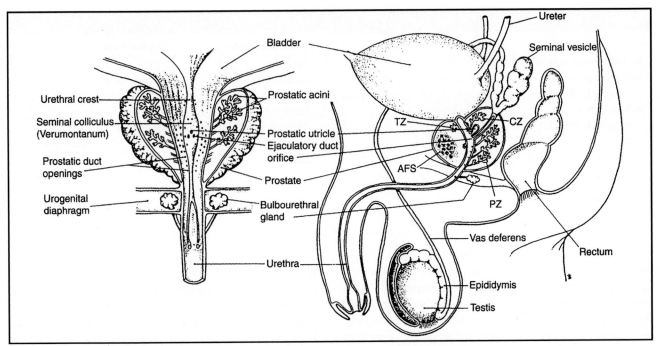

FIGURE 8-3 ■ Anatomical relationships of prostate from the frontal **(left)** and coronal **(right)** perspectives. TZ, transition zone; CZ, central zone; PZ, peripheral zone; AFS, anterior fibromuscular stroma. (From Timms BG. Anatomical perspectives of prostate development. In: Naz RK, ed. *Prostate: basic and clinical aspects.* New York: CRC Press; 1997:36, figure 4-A).

12 to 18 years of age there is a pubertal maturation period with a significant increase in gland size, to 11 to 18 g by age 18. This period is characterized by androgen-driven gland branching, and differentiation of immature prostatic epithelium into adult-type basal and secretory cells.

The adult prostate gland surrounds the urethra immediately below the base of the urinary bladder and is located posterior to the inferior symphysis pubis, superior to the urogenital diaphragm, and anterior to the rectum (Figs. 8-3 and 8-4). It has a shape like a truncated cone or a top lying on its side. It measures 5 cm × 4 cm × 3 cm and weighs 20 g from ages 20 to 50, with an increase to 30 g from ages 60 to 80.

Historically, the prostate was thought to have anywhere from two to five lobes.[19,20] The five-lobe model was utilized in the first half of the 20th century, until 1954, when Franks[21] forwarded the concept of an outer gland, where carcinomas arose, and a periurethral inner gland. Further modeling evolution occurred when McNeal developed the three-zone model, which defines the central zone, the transition zone, and the peripheral zone (Fig. 8-4). It may be difficult in some cases to grossly and microscopically recognize a sharp demarcation between these zones, but these zones do have structural differences, and disease differentially affects these zones (Table 8-2). Carcinoma tends to arise in the peripheral zone (although about 20% of carcinomas do arise in the transition zone) and BPH is typically a transition zone process, while the central zone is remarkably resistant to disease. The prostatic urethra is formed at the bladder neck, turns anteriorly 35 degrees at its midpoint (the urethral angle), and exits the prostate at the apex, where it is

continuous with the membranous urethra. The urethral angle can vary between 0 degree and 90 degrees and divides the urethra into proximal (so-called preprostatic) and distal (so-called prostatic) segments. The transition zone, which normally makes up 5% of prostate gland volume, wraps around

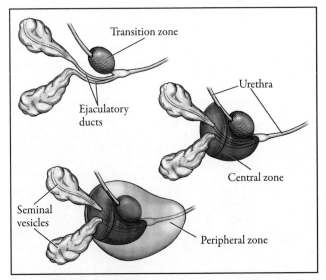

FIGURE 8-4 ■ Anatomical relationships of the adult prostate. The prostate has three zones: central zone (CZ, through which the ejaculatory ducts course), transition zone (TZ, site of benign prostatic hyperplasia nodules), and the peripheral zone (PZ), where most carcinomas arise. (Modified from Cancer: Principles and Practice of Oncology, 4th edition, Lippincott Williams and Wilkins).

Table 8-2 ■ COMPARISON OF THE THREE ZONES OF THE PROSTATE

	Peripheral Zone	Transition Zone	Central Zone
Percentage of normal prostate	70%	5%	25%
Embryologic origin	Urogenital sinus	Urogenital sinus	Wolffian duct
Anatomic location	Posterior, lateral, and apical	Around proximal urethra	Posterior cone-like structure
Inflammation	Common	Common	Rare
Hyperplasia (BPH)	Uncommon	Common	Rare
PIN	Common	Uncommon	Rare
Percentage of cases of adenocarcinoma	70%	20%	5%
Gland:stroma ratio	1:1	1:1	2:1
Epithelium	Irregular small acini	Irregular small acini	Larger, darker, complex glands
Stroma	Loose fibromuscular	Compact fibromuscular	Compact fibromuscular

the proximal urethra (Fig. 8-4). The main ducts of this zone drain into posterolateral recesses of the urethra at a point just proximal to the urethral angle. Some of the more medial ducts penetrate through the thick smooth muscle bundles of preprostatic sphincter. Also found in the smooth muscle of the preprostatic sphincter are minute ducts and abortive acinar arrangements of periurethral glands, which constitute only about 1% of the total glandular volume of the prostate. The central zone makes up about 25% of the entire prostate gland and is a posteriorly situated cone-like structure with the base of the cone projecting toward the base of the bladder. The paired ejaculatory ducts (Fig. 8-5) run through the central zone from the seminal vesicles to their exit at the posterior urethral protuberance, known as the verumontanum (or colliculus seminalis) (Fig. 8-6). Within the verumontanum is a cul-de-sac, the prostatic utricle, located between the ejaculatory ducts (Fig. 8-7). It may also lie deep to the ejaculatory ducts or may be embedded as a tiny cavity in the prostatic parenchyma.[22] The ducts from the central zone drain into the urethra via orifices positioned just next to the ejaculatory duct orifices on the verumontanum. The peripheral zone of

the prostate gland is the bulk of the posterior, lateral, and apical portion of the prostate gland and accounts for 70% of the total gland volume. The ducts of this zone empty into the posterior urethral recesses or grooves in a double row from the verumontanum to the prostatic apex. Finally, a patch of nonglandular tissue called the anterior fibromuscular stroma is present anteriorly over the prostate and extends from the bladder neck to the apex of the prostate.

Histology/Immunohistology

Epithelium

Microscopically, the normal adult prostate is a branching duct–acinar glandular system embedded in a dense fibromuscular stroma (Fig. 8-8). Zonal architectural differences can be appreciated. Normally, the peripheral zone ducts and acini are evenly distributed but are irregular in size and shape. Normal transition zone glands are similar to those of the peripheral zone. Central zone glands are more densely arranged than peripheral and transition zone glands. The epithelial–stromal ratio in the central zone is 2:1, compared

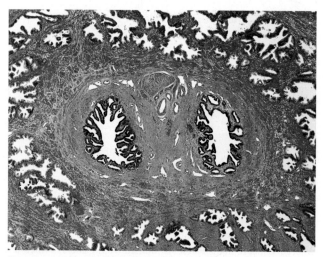

FIGURE 8-5 ■ Paired ejaculatory ducts that run through the central zone of the prostate.

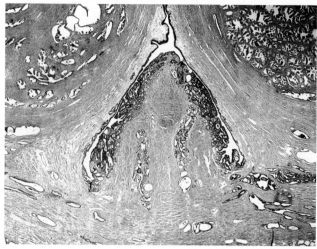

FIGURE 8-6 ■ Verumontanum of prostate—a mound of tissue protruding into the urethral lumen.

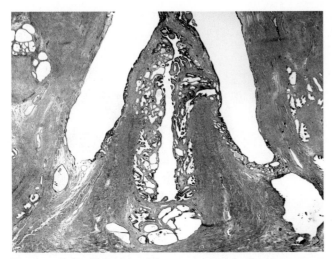

FIGURE 8-7 ■ Utricle of the prostate in the verumontanum.

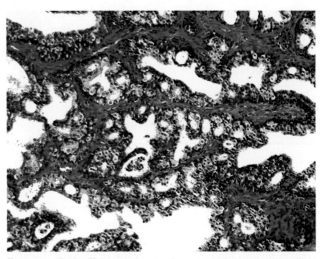

FIGURE 8-9 ■ Normal central zone epithelium with cribriform growth and Roman bridge formation.

with 1:1 for the peripheral and transition zones. Also, central zone glands are larger and display intraluminal projections with fibrovascular cores. Central zone epithelium displays tall columnar cells with eosinophilic cytoplasm, a prominent basal cell layer, and on occasion complex intraluminal architecture such as Roman bridge and cribriform formations (Fig. 8-9). These findings can be misdiagnosed as atypia or prostatic intraepithelial neoplasia (PIN).[23] Central zone epithelium is distinctive in its selective expression of pepsinogen II, lactoferrin, and lectin-binding sites.[7] Central zone epithelium also differs from epithelium in other zones in proteomic profile.[24]

The normal epithelium of the prostate is classically defined as having two cell layers: a luminal or secretory cell layer and a basal cell layer (Fig. 8-10). A third cell type in normal prostatic epithelium is the neuroendocrine cell, which is rare

(Box 8-1). The secretory or luminal cells of the normal prostate glandular epithelium make up the bulk (73%) of the epithelial volume. The secretory cells are cuboidal to columnar with nuclei positioned in the basal to midportion of the cell. Cleared cytoplasm is a hallmark of normal prostatic secretory cells because of the presence of a large number of small clear secretory vacuoles. The central zone secretory cell cytoplasm is somewhat denser because it contains a smaller number of theses vacuoles.[7] Mucin is not usually seen in H&E-stained sections of normal glands, but histochemical stains for mucins reveal neutral mucins (with periodic acid–Schiff [PAS] with diastase positivity), whereas neoplastic glands demonstrate neutral and acidic mucin staining. Pigment is common in the cytoplasm of normal prostatic secretory epithelial cells. These granules are 1 to 3 μm in diameter, are apical or subnuclear, and are yellow-brown to gray-brown to blue by

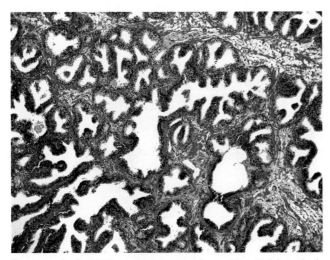

FIGURE 8-8 ■ Normal prostate with complex glands embedded in a fibromuscular stroma.

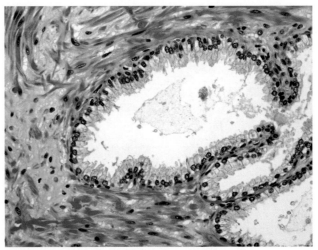

FIGURE 8-10 ■ Normal prostatic epithelium with a secretory luminal cell layer and basal cell layer.

hematoxylin and eosin (H&E) staining (Fig. 8-11).[25] The histochemical staining characteristics, including positivity for Fontana-Masson, PAS with diastase, Congo red, Luxol fast blue, and Oil-Red-O, and autofluorescence of the pigment are consistent with lipofuscin. This lipofuscin pigment can also be found in the cytoplasm of seminal vesicle and ejaculatory duct epithelium, where it is more abundant, coarser, and more refractile. The nuclei of normal prostatic secretory epithelial cells are small and round with fine, evenly dispersed chromatin. Nucleoli usually are not evident or are pinpoint in size. Nuclei in the central zone usually are larger than those in the peripheral zone and also appear crowded. This results in a pseudostratified nuclear appearance in the central zone and along with the aforementioned denser cytoplasm may yield a false impression of PIN.[23] Normal secretory cells are immunoreactive for pan-cytokeratins, cytokeratins 8 and 18, PSA (Fig. 8-12), prostate-specific acid phosphatase (PSAP) (Fig. 8-13), and the androgen receptor. Of diagnostic significance, immunostains for α-methylacyl–coenzyme A racemase (alpha methylacyl CoA racemase [AMACR]; also known as P504S), a marker for prostatic neoplasia, can be focally positive in secretory cells in normal glands, but this staining should be focal and noncircumferential within normal and benign glands (Fig. 8-14).[26] Additional prostate markers that have been utilized in diagnostic immunohistochemistry to assess for prostate versus nonprostate carcinoma

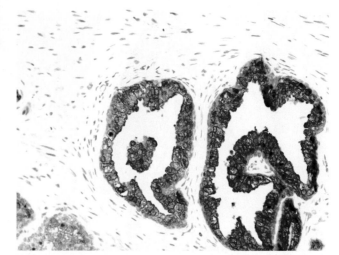

FIGURE 8-12 ■ Prostate-specific antigen immunoreactivity in normal prostatic epithelium.

include prostate-specific membrane antigen (PSMA), prostein (P501S) (Fig. 8-15), proPSA, and NKX3.1. In normal prostatic tissues PSMA is weakly expressed in benign luminal cells.[27,28] P501S is strongly expressed in benign luminal cells, with prominent dot-like Golgi complex staining[29,30] (Fig. 8-15). Two different proPSA molecular forms differ in expression in benign glands, with strong or moderate/diffuse [−5/−7]proPSA expression and negative or weak [−2] proPSA expression.[31] NKX3.1 immunostains show intense labeling of most secretory luminal cell nuclei, with weak staining of basal cell nuclei.[32]

The basal cell layer separates the secretory cells from the basement membrane and is nearly continuous (Figs. 8-10, 8-16, and 8-17). Basal cells in the prostatic epithelium often appear as rounded or oblong cells, but can also be flattened, spindled, cuboidal, and triangular.[33] Basal cells have a scant amount of dense cytoplasm and small, hyperchromatic nuclei. The immunophenotype of basal cells is distinctive, is different

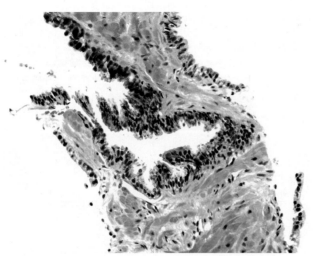

FIGURE 8-11 ■ Lipofuscin pigment in benign prostatic epithelium.

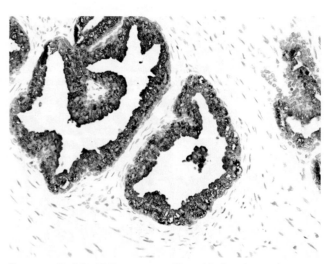

FIGURE 8-13 ■ Prostate-specific acid phosphatase immunoreactivity in normal prostatic epithelium.

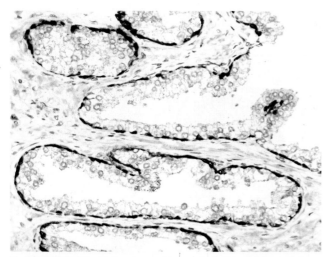

FIGURE 8-14 ■ Focal, noncircumferential AMACR immunoreactivity in benign prostatic epithelium. *Red*, AMACR signal; *brown*, 34βE12/p63 cocktail antibody binding to basal cells.

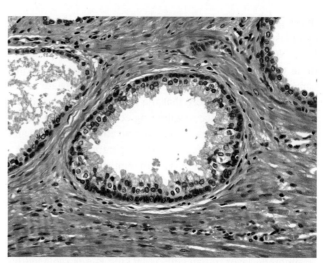

FIGURE 8-16 ■ Continuous prominent basal cell layer in a benign prostatic gland.

from luminal secretory cells, and can be of diagnostic utility. The most commonly employed basal cell–specific antibodies are those that react with p63 and high-molecular-weight cytokeratins, especially 1, 5, 10, and 14 that are detected by mouse monoclonal antibody 34βE12 (also known as CK903).[26] A cocktail consisting of 34βE12 and p63 antibodies slightly improves the detection of basal cells (Fig. 8-12).[34] Immunostaining of basal cells can also be achieved using antibodies directed against cytokeratins 5/6.[26] It should be noted that discontinuity or even focal lack of basal cell staining may be seen in a minority of entirely normal glands.[35] The precise function of basal cells is unsettled, but they represent the proliferative component of prostatic epithelium. Stem cells may reside within the basal cell population.

Neuroendocrine (endocrine-paracrine) cells constitute a third population of cells in normal prostatic epithelium.[36] These cells are a small minority at about 0.4% of the total

adult prostatic epithelial cell population. This is a terminally differentiated, postmitotic cell population that variably expresses androgen receptor and the secretory products PSA and PSAP. The keratin expression pattern is more like luminal than basal cells. These neuroendocrine cells are usually recognizable only by histochemical (Fontana-Masson argentaffin and Churukian-Schenk argyrophil) or immunohistochemical staining. By immunohistochemical detection of chromogranin and neuron-specific enolase, these cells may be found throughout the prostate but are at highest concentrations in the periurethral region and prostatic ducts.[37] A variety of neuroendocrine markers, including chromogranin, neuron-specific enolase, serotonin, thyroid-stimulating hormone–like peptide, calcitonin, bombesin, gastrin-releasing peptide, somatostatin, parathormone-related protein, and neurotensin, have been identified in these cells by immunohistochemistry.[36] These immunostains highlight the highly

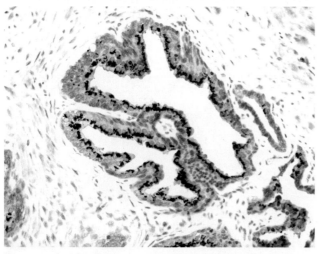

FIGURE 8-15 ■ Prostein (P501S) immunoreactivity in normal prostatic epithelium. Note granular perinuclear cytoplasmic pattern.

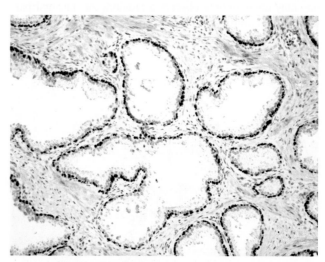

FIGURE 8-17 ■ Continuous basal cell layer in normal prostatic epithelium, as highlighted by a p63 immunohistochemical stain.

interdigitating nature of these cells, which exhibit slender, cytoplasmic dendritic process that may be up to 200 μm long. Neurosecretory granules of varying sizes are found in these cells by electron microscopy. The functional significance of neuroendocrine cells in the normal prostate is not clear, but it seems likely that the neuroendocrine products of these cells influence neighboring cells through the elaborate dendritic processes via a paracrine effect. Autocrine and endocrine influences may also be in operation.

Urothelium is another type of epithelial cell normally found in the prostate. In addition to lining the prostatic urethra, urothelium also normally lines major prostatic ducts (Fig. 8-18). This ductal lining is variable in extent from one man to the next. The urothelium in the prostatic ducts differs from such lining elsewhere in the urinary tract in that an umbrella layer of cap cells is lacking and is replaced by secretory cells that are PSA-positive. The urothelial cells are PSA-negative. Recognition of urothelium usually is straightforward: this is a multilayered epithelium with rounded to elongated nuclei, some of which possess nuclear grooves. A degree of cytoplasmic clearing usually is evident. When urothelium involves acini in the peripheral aspects of the prostate gland, the designation urothelial metaplasia is applied.[38] Here, unlike the normal ductal urothelial epithelial lining, there is often an associated acute or chronic inflammatory cell infiltrate.[38]

Intraluminal contents of normal prostatic glands include shed and degenerating epithelial cells, corpora amylacea, and calculi. Corpora amylacea are extremely common in the normal prostate and are found in up to 78% of benign prostates.[39] They are inspissated secretions that often assume a concentrically lamellar appearance[40] like rings in a tree (Fig. 8-19). They are mainly rounded and may vary widely in size and shape (Fig. 8-20). Corpora amylacea usually are pink to purple but may be yellow-gold to orange, particularly in verumontanum glands. Although corpora amylacea usually have a concentrically lamellar structure, one may uncommonly observe a radiating or starburst pattern within corpora amylacea. Sometimes corpora amylacea

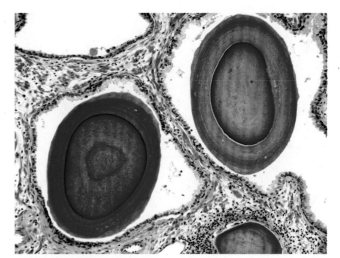

FIGURE 8-19 ■ Corpora amylacea.

can be seen in atrophic glands, with only a thin atrophic epithelial lining surrounding them, and in spaces without an obvious epithelial lining, or they can be seen in stroma, with or without associated giant cells. They often calcify and probably contribute to the formation of prostatic calculi. Prostatic corpora amylacea possess many cellular constituents, including RNA, DNA, lipid, mucopolysaccharide, and protein[41,42]; by electron microscopy they show interwoven fibrils arranged in rings.[43] Prostatic calculi are also extremely common, being detectable in 75% to 100% of men by ultrasonography.[44] They are typically found in central, large prostatic ducts. These stones vary in size from microscopic to 4 cm in size and grossly are usually multiple, round or ovoid, and brown, with variable white or gray areas.[39] Prostatic stones mainly contain calcium phosphate, but calcium oxalate, carbonate–apatite, and hydroxyapatite may also be present. Prostatic calculi are most often seen as incidental findings in the setting of inflammation and BPH. The diagnostic impact of corpora amylacea, microcalcifications, and calculi is that they are all more common in benign glands, but their presence does not rule

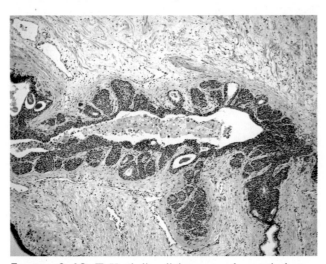

FIGURE 8-18 ■ Urothelium lining a normal prostatic duct.

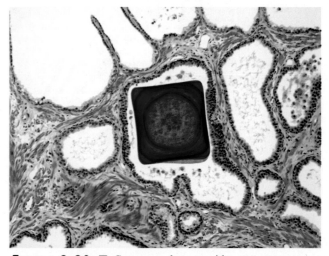

FIGURE 8-20 ■ Corpus amylaceum with square appearance.

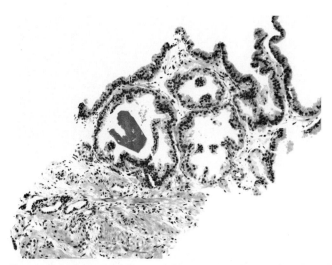

FIGURE 8-21 ■ Crystalloid in lumen of benign gland.

out malignancy. Corpora amylacea have been reported in 13% of carcinomas,[45] and calculi are found associated with 6% of prostate cancers.[46]

Other intraluminal materials are, conversely, rare in normal gland lumina but are more common in neoplastic processes. These intraluminal materials include pink amorphous acellular secretions, intraluminal wispy blue mucin (also known as blue-tinged mucinous secretions), and crystalloids. Identification of these secretions, mucin, or crystalloids[47] in benign prostatic tissue from needle biopsy (Fig. 8-21) is not an indication for rebiopsy.

Nonprostatic epithelium that can be seen associated with all prostatic tissue samples includes ejaculatory duct and seminal vesicle epithelium and colorectal epithelium. This last epithelium is frequently seen in needle biopsies of the prostate and is often of colonic glandular type, but squamous epithelium can also be observed. Distorted rectal tissue can potentially be confused with prostatic adenocarcinoma due to intraluminal blue mucin, prominent nucleoli, mitotic activity, and the immunoprofile of negative 34βE12 and p63

immunoreactivity, with positive staining for alpha-methylacyl CoA racemase.[48]

Stroma

Other structures of the prostate include the capsule, preprostatic sphincter, striated sphincter, anterior fibromuscular stroma, and intraglandular stroma, including smooth muscle cells, fibroblasts, vasculature, and nerves.[11] There are zonal differences in stromal density. The normal peripheral zone stroma is fibromuscular and loosely woven (Fig. 8-22A), whereas normal transition zone stroma is more compact, with interlacing smooth muscle bundles (Fig. 8-22B). Rarely, adipocytes can be seen in the prostate,[49,50] including in needle biopsy.[51] For practical purposes, carcinoma in fat should be viewed as extraprostatic extension.[50]

"Capsule"

The outer prostatic "capsule" is actually a band of concentrically placed fibrovascular tissue that is inseparable from prostatic stroma[11,52] and surrounding fasciae. Outside the prostate, this band is also continuous with pelvic fascia and rectovesical fascia (of Denonvilliers). Denonvilliers fascia is a sheath between the rectum and prostate that covers the posterior aspect of the prostate and seminal vesicles.

The fibromuscular band ("capsule") of the prostate is 0.5 to 3 mm thick and is incomplete, being absent at the apex.[52–54] It is composed mainly of transversely disposed bundles of smooth muscle and collagen. Smooth muscle bundles course between the gland and periepithelial stroma inside the prostate gland, without obeying any sort of boundary (Fig. 8-23). Also, the concentration of smooth muscle fibers in the band and prostatic stroma is identical. Glands from the prostate approach this band, but the border between the outer limit of epithelium and the band is not often clearly definable under the light microscope. Posteriorly, the band fuses with Denonvilliers fascia and does not clearly separate prostate from seminal vesicle.

Posterolaterally, peripheral gaping blood vessels have been used as a demarcation landmark between intraprostatic

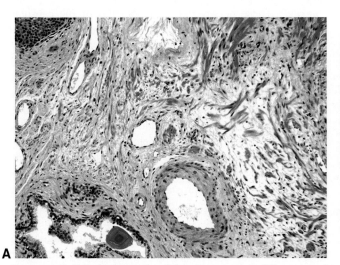
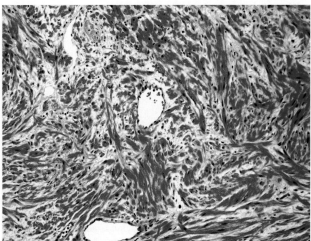

A **B**

FIGURE 8-22 ■ Normal peripheral zone stroma (**A**) compared to denser normal transition zone stroma (**B**).

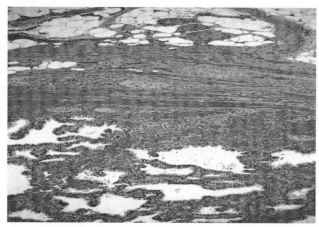

FIGURE 8-23 ■ Fibromuscular sling or "capsule" surrounding the prostate is ill defined.

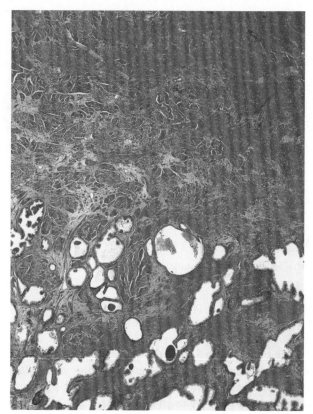

FIGURE 8-25 ■ Boundary between prostate (**below**) and urinary bladder neck (**top**): absence of a capsule.

and extraprostatic tissue, but such vessels clearly can extend into the substance of the prostate and therefore are unreliable as a capsular marker. Anteriorly and anterolaterally, the band blends with the pelvic fascia. Apically, the band is no longer present, and instead there is a jumble of smooth muscle, skeletal muscle, and fibroelastic fibers. Here, it is important to know that the urethral striated sphincter (rhabdosphincter) is in direct continuity with the prostate, and indeed skeletal muscle fibers can normally be found, at an anterior and apical location, within the substance of the gland itself (Fig. 8-24).[55] At the bladder neck, a capsular separation of bladder and prostate also does not exist; rather, there is a fusion of smooth muscle bundles (Fig. 8-25).

Smooth Muscle, Fibroblasts, Extracellular Matrix, and Basement Membrane

The stroma in the prostate gland consists chiefly of smooth muscle cells and fibroblasts, with ramifications of blood and lymph vessels as well as nerve bundles and axons.[11] The extracellular stromal matrix of the prostate is primarily collagen of types I and III, complex polysaccharides, and glycosaminoglycans such as dermatan sulfate, heparin, chondroitin, and hyaluronic acid.[8] Fibronectin and tenascin polypeptides are also found in prostatic stroma.[56,57] Abutting prostatic glands is a think, delicate basement membrane, that, at 100-nm thickness, is too small to be seen in H&E-stained sections.

Nerves

The prostate gland has a rich nerve supply, with sympathetic and parasympathetic innervation arising from the pelvic plexus.[58] These nerves run with branches of the capsular artery and penetrate the prostate, where parasympathetic fibers course to acini and stimulate secretion and where sympathetic fibers cause contraction of outer band "capsular" and intraprostatic smooth muscle. Innervation of the peripheral zone and posterior "capsule" is significantly higher than that of the transition zone and anterior "capsule."[59] Histologically, nerves are seen in the periprostatic neurovascular bundle, in the outer fibromuscular band, and in the prostate itself. Ganglia and paraganglia (Fig. 8-26) are usually found outside the gland but may also be found in the outer fibromuscular band and within the prostate itself. Paraganglia are most often located in or adjacent to the lateral neurovascular bundles.[60] They should not be confused with "hypernephroid" prostatic carcinoma. Because ganglia and paraganglia can be found inside the prostate and in the outer fibromuscular

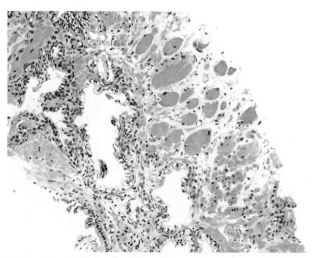

FIGURE 8-24 ■ Benign prostatic glands admixed with skeletal muscle in needle biopsy tissue.

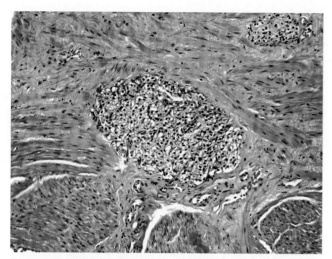

FIGURE 8-26 ■ Paraganglion in smooth muscle tissue.

band, carcinoma invading around these structures should not necessarily be equated with extraprostatic extension of malignancy. Another diagnostic pitfall is the relationship of normal and benign prostatic glands to intraprostatic nerves. Benign prostatic glands can abut nerves[61–63] (Fig. 8-27) and can even be found within nerves.[63,64] Such glands should not be considered automatically malignant, and a constellation of histomorphologic traits should be used in diagnosis, not solely the physical proximity of prostatic glands and nerves.

Lymphatics and Blood Vessels

The blood supply to the prostate is from the inferior vesical artery. By light microscopy, intraglandular blood vessels are easily seen in prostatic stroma, but capillaries adjacent to normal glands are not so readily appreciated on H&E sections, probably because a large number have closed lumina.[65] There is a network of intraprostatic lymphatics that drain principally into obturator and then internal iliac

lymph nodes. A minor amount of drainage occurs through the presacral group and external iliac nodes. An uncommon site of flow is through periprostatic or periseminal vesicle lymph nodes, which are found in about 4% of radical prostatectomy specimens.[66]

Periprostatic Adipose Tissue

Outside the prostate in posterolateral sites one can find neurovascular bundles and abundant adipose tissue, although the amount and distribution of periprostatic adipose tissue in radical prostatectomy specimens is quite variable. Assessment of this periprostatic adipose tissue for invasion by carcinoma is essential for pathologic staging. One can also find periprostatic adipose tissue in some needle biopsy cases.

Cowper Glands

Cowper bulbourethral glands are extrinsic to the prostate gland but are discussed here because these normal anatomic structures can be misdiagnosed as prostatic adenocarcinoma[67,68] (Table 8-1). They are located in the urogenital diaphragm, just inferior to the prostate gland and lateral to the membranous urethra. These small structures measure on average 10 mm × 6 mm × 5 mm in adult men. Cowper glands can be incidentally and inadvertently sampled by needle biopsy directed at the prostate gland,[67] by transurethral resection of the prostate,[69] and by cystoprostatectomy.[70] The incidental sampling in needle biopsy is a rare event, with an incidence of 0.006%.[67] Microscopically, Cowper glands are compound tubuloalveolar glands composed of lobules of acini, admixed with excretory ducts and ductules (Fig. 8-28). Skeletal muscle fibers are seen associated with Cowper gland in all needle biopsy cases.[67] The acinar lumens are small to occluded. Cuboidal to columnar pale-staining mucinous cells form the acini, whereas more flattened hybrid mucinous-ductal cells line the ducts and ductules. The mucinous cells are distended, with bluish,

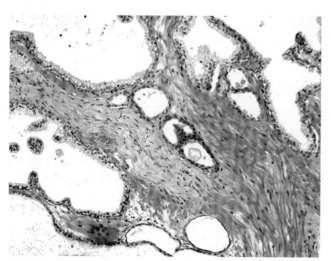

FIGURE 8-27 ■ Benign perineural glands.

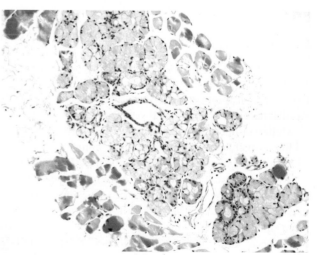

FIGURE 8-28 ■ Cowper glands with mucinous acini, central duct, and surrounding skeletal muscle tissue.

foamy cytoplasm, and possess small, bland, basally situated nuclei. An acinar basal cell layer often is not apparent on H&E-stained sections. Immunohistochemical studies have produced mixed findings. In particular, studies have found luminal cells in the acini to be PSA positive[67,70] or PSA negative[68] and PSAP positive[70] or PSAP negative.[68] Also unsettled is whether the basal epithelial cells express high-molecular-weight cytokeratins recognized by antibody 34βE12. The acini can be negative with 34βE12 immunolabeling.[68] In most cases the basal cells are highlighted by antibodies to smooth muscle actin (SMA), which can be useful in the differential diagnosis with prostatic adenocarcinoma, although Cowper glands can usually be recognized by examination of H&E-stained slides without use of immunostains.

Malformations

Clinically manifest developmental abnormalities of the prostate itself are rare and include agenesis, hypoplasia, cystic change, and abnormal persistence and hyperplasia of mesonephric remnants. Ectopic prostatic tissue is another form of maldevelopment.

Agenesis and Hypoplasis

Agenesis and hypoplasia of the prostate occur in several conditions including 5α-reductase deficiency,[10] testicular feminization,[71] and prune belly syndrome.[72] Congenital 5α-reductase deficiency results in a rare form of pseudohermaphroditism in which patients have ambiguous external genitalia and small or undetectable prostates. In males with testicular feminization, the androgen receptor is defective, and the prostate is entirely absent. In the prune belly syndrome the prostate is hypoplastic and may not be grossly evident.[72] Histologically, there is a pronounced reduction in epithelial elements, a reduction in smooth muscle fibers, and increased fibrous tissue. Concomitantly, the seminal vesicles can be rudimentary or absent and the vas deferens segmentally atretic. The prostatic urethra is markedly dilated in these cases.

Congenital Cysts

Congenital cysts in the prostate region may be classified as utricular (of endodermal origin),[73] müllerian duct cysts (which are of mesodermal origin), ejaculatory duct cysts, vas deferens cysts, and seminal vesicle cysts.

Müllerian duct cysts and utricular cysts are uncommon midline structures that rarely produce clinical symptoms. The embryologic origin of the prostatic utricle is controversial, with suggested contributions from müllerian duct and urogenital sinus, with recent evidence suggesting a urogenital sinus origin.[74] The incidence of utricular cystic dilatation (congenital or postinflammatory) is estimated at 7% (5/70) in newborns and young infants and 1% (7/678) in adults.[75] Utricular dilatation and cyst formation are associated with intersex abnormalities and hypospadias, whereas true

müllerian duct cysts are not.[76] Considering the two together, the median age at presentation is 26 to 39 years, and symptomatic patients present most often with hematospermia, recurrent testicular or pelviperineal pain, and irritative lower urinary tract symptoms such as frequency, dysuria, and urgency.[73,77] These cysts may also be associated with infertility due to ejaculatory duct obstruction.[73] Aspiration fluid or portions of the cyst obtained by transurethral resection "unroofing," or a complete cyst, removed by open surgery, may be received in the anatomic pathology laboratory.[78] Grossly, incidentally detected utricular cysts are 2 to 3 cm in greatest dimension, with a smooth inner wall.[75] The ejaculatory ducts are displaced laterally, with compression of their lumens. Microscopically, the epithelium lining the cystic cavity has been described as columnar or cuboidal (32% of cases), although it may be stratified squamous (19%), urothelial (10%), or devoid of epithelium (19%).[73,75] The cyst walls are composed of smooth muscle or fibrous tissue. In 25% of cases, acini with columnar epithelium have been noted in the cyst wall near the connection with the urethra. Aspiration fluid should not reveal any sperm (unlike the ejaculatory duct cyst). The fluid has been characterized as clear[75] or whitish to brown,[73] with old blood and cellular debris.[79] Stones have been found in these cysts. Treatment depends on symptoms, cyst size, and location. Options range from observation for asymptomatic patients to aspiration to surgery.[73,77] A rare complication in these cysts is the occurrence of malignancy. A few cases of ductal adenocarcinoma,[80–82] squamous cell carcinoma,[83] and clear cell adenocarcinoma[84] arising in müllerian duct or utricular cysts have been reported.

Congenital seminal vesicle cysts and ejaculatory duct cysts are also in the differential diagnosis of cystic change in the prostatic region. Congenital ejaculatory duct cysts are rare; in one series where vesiculography was performed in infertile men, the incidence was 0.6% (1/158).[85] Minor congenital anatomic variations of the ejaculatory duct include caudal formation of ejaculatory ducts within the central zone (18% of cases), abnormal posterior penetration of the ejaculatory ducts at the rectal surface (12%), abnormally large muscle bundles in the duct sheath (6%), and ductal dilatation (7%).[86]

Mesonephric Remnants

As a developmental anomaly, rare examples of mesonephric remnants have been recognized in the prostate, where they may assume pseudoneoplastic status due to florid hyperplasia[87–90] (see Hyperplasia section below). The incidence of nonhyperplastic mesonephric remnants in the prostate is unknown.

Prostatic Tissue Ectopia

Ectopic benign prostatic tissue in males has been found in a number of extraprostatic locations including testis, epididymis, processus vaginalis, urinary bladder, penile urethra, seminal vesicle, root of the penis, subvesical space, retrovesical space, pericolic fat, anal submucosa, perirectal fat, urachal remnant, and spleen.[91–103] The most frequently cited type of prostatic ectopia is in the prostatic urethra in the form of prostatic urethral polyps. However, because prostatic epithelium normally can line the urethra in the verumontanum region, one could argue that these polyps do not represent ectopia.

Prostatic tissue has been reported in females in the posterior wall of the distal urethra, in paraurethral Skene glands,[104] in ovarian hilar mesonephric rests,[105] in ovarian teratomas,[106] and in the vagina, vulva, and cervix.[104,107] In the vagina, tubulosquamous polyps may display prostatic differentiation, as substantiated by PSA and PSAP immunostains.[104,107] A single case of ovarian teratoma with prostatic tissue with morphologic features of prostatic carcinoma has been published.[106]

Mature-appearing prostatic tissue has also been rarely reported in neoplasms, including a retroperitoneal lipoma[108] and a testicular teratoma.[109]

Ectopic prostatic tissue usually presents as an incidental finding but can manifest clinically as a mass[110] or as urinary frequency, voiding difficulty, dysuria, or hematuria. Although these patients could conceivably present with serum PSA elevation due to ectopic prostate, this has not been reported. By cystoscopy, ectopic prostatic tissue in the bladder may be confused with cystitis cystica.[92] Benign adenomatous[110] and malignant[111] changes have been described in ectopic prostatic tissue. The precise mechanisms for the formation of ectopic prostatic tissue are not definitely established. An embryologic remnant of the ventral portion of the cloaca is favored, and urothelial metaplasia has also been forwarded. For the lower female genital tract, a developmental anomaly, metaplasia of preexisting endocervical glands, and derivation from mesonephric remnants have been raised as possibilities.[94] The presence of prostatic tissue in ovarian teratomas could be caused by induction by locally-produced androgen or tissue-specific genomic imprinting, but this is speculative.

Inflammation and Infection

Inflammation of the prostate (prostatitis) and infection of the prostate are common clinical problems. It is important for histopathologists to appreciate the National Institutes of Health's (NIH's) definition of prostatitis,[112] and to not necessarily equate histologic evidence of prostatic inflammation ("histologic prostatitis") with clinical prostatitis. Infections of the prostate are most often bacterial and are diagnosed clinically. Histopathologic detection of inflammatory cells in the prostate is common, but histologic identification of specific infectious agents in prostatic tissues is rare.

Prostatitis: Introduction

Clinical prostatitis is a major health problem and has been considered to be the third most important disease of the

---

Box 8-2 ● PROSTATITIS: SUMMARY

Diagnosis of chronic prostatitis is typically based on quantitative bacterial cultures and microscopic examination of fractionated urine specimens (first 10 mL of urine is urethral, midstream urine is from bladder) and expressed prostatic secretions

Definition of bacterial prostatitis: >10 WBC/HPF in prostatic secretions without pyuria; prostatic secretion cultures should have bacterial counts 10x urethral/bladder cultures

Clinical: inflammation can produce elevated PSA

Treatment of chronic bacterial prostatitis: difficult because antibiotics penetrate poorly into prostate

Micro: macrophages in stroma, neutrophils in ducts/acini and usually localized; lymphoid aggregates are common with aging and nodular hyperplasia and not specific for prostatitis

---

prostate gland after BPH and cancer.[113] In the United States it accounts for 2 million annual doctor visits and 25% of all office visits for genitourinary-related complaints.[114] The estimated community-based prevalence of clinical prostatitis is 10% to 16%,[113,115] which is of a magnitude similar to that of diabetes and ischemic heart disease.[116] Compared with BPH and prostate cancer, prostatitis is far more likely to affect younger men (18 to 50 years of age).

From a strict definitional standpoint, prostatitis is inflammation of the prostate. However, clinical use of the term prostatitis is not confined to cases with inflammation. Conversely, when histopathologists see inflammation in, for example, a prostate needle biopsy, a diagnosis of prostatitis, although histologically correct, does not usually correlate with the clinical concept of prostatitis (Box 8-2).

In the 1999 NIH consensus statement, prostatitis and prostatitis-like symptoms were classified into four broad categories (Table 8-3).[112] This is now the most widely accepted classification system. Note that only category IV has a tissue-based component in the clinical diagnosis. Category III prostatitis, known as chronic prostatitis/chronic pelvic pain syndrome, is by far the most common form of prostatitis, comprising 90% of all prostatitis cases.[117] These patients

---

Table 8-3 ■ NIH CLASSIFICATION OF PROSTATITIS SYNDROMES

Category I	Acute bacterial prostatitis
Category II	Chronic bacterial prostatitis
Category III	Chronic abacterial prostatitis/chronic pelvic pain syndrome
Category IIIa	Inflammatory chronic pelvic pain syndrome
Category IIIb	Non-inflammatory chronic pelvic pain syndrome
Category IV	Asymptomatic inflammatory prostatitis

present with pelvic pain localized to the prostate, perineum, or urethra, and a variable degree of voiding abnormalities such as urinary frequency, and sexual dysfunction.[118] The etiology is unknown and optimal treatment has not been established.[118] Acute bacterial prostatitis (category I) (usually due to *Escherichia coli*), is rare, being diagnosed in 0.02% of all prostatitis patients and chronic bacterial prostatitis affects 5% to 10% of patients with chronic prostatitits.[119] Acute bacterial prostatitis is usually readily diagnosed clinically by the sudden onset of urogenital and often systemic symptoms, such as fever, chills, irritative voiding symptoms, and pain in the lower back, rectum, and perineum, along with bacteriuria.[120] Treatment is with systemic antibiotic therapy.[120] Patients with chronic bacterial prostatitis (category II), in contrast, experience prolonged or recurrent symptoms and relapsing bacteriuria. Treatment is more difficult and requires selection of an antibiotic with properties that allow for penetration into the prostate.[120] Prostate biopsy is contraindicated in patients with acute bacterial prostatitis due to the risk of septicemia and prostate biopsy for patients with chronic prostatitis/chronic pelvic pain syndrome is currently a research tool only.[121] Asymptomatic inflammatory prostatitis (category IV) is an incidental finding of unknown clinical significance, except that such inflammation can be associated with an elevated serum PSA.[121]

Histologic Acute Inflammation

An acute inflammatory cell infiltrate made up of neutrophils is common in prostatic tissue samples acquired for reasons not related to clinical prostatitis. In needle biopsy tissue taken to rule out prostate cancer, up to 50% of cases harbor acute inflammation,[122] while 20% to 98% of transurethral and open prostatectomy cases have acute inflammatory infiltrates.[123–125] Microscopically, the acute inflammation is often intraluminal (Fig. 8-29) and varies in extent from a few scattered neutrophils to microabscesses. Neutrophilic infiltrates

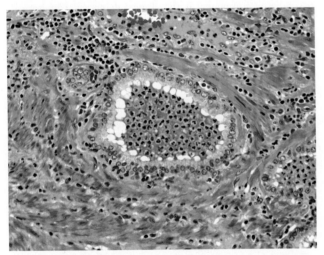

FIGURE 8-29 ■ Intraluminal acute inflammation in a benign gland with reactive nuclear atypia, including visible nucleoli.

in the prostate can be associated with intraluminal necrotic debris, duct rupture, and epithelial alterations, especially atrophy and hyperplasia. Squamous metaplasia in the prostate can also be acutely inflamed, but neoplastic proliferations—PIN and carcinoma—rarely exhibit neutrophilic infiltrates. The main differential diagnostic difficulty with neutrophilic infiltrates is the distinction of reactive, inflammatory nuclear atypia from prostatic adenocarcinoma. The diagnostician should be aware that prominent nucleoli (of >1 μm) are detectable in almost one-half of cases of acutely inflamed atrophy.[126] Special studies generally are of limited value in assessing histologic acute inflammation of the prostate. The one special study that can be diagnostically beneficial is immunohistochemical staining to confirm basal cell presence (using p63 and/or 34βE12 immunostains) in acutely inflamed, reactive, benign glands, but this is not usually necessary. One need not apply histochemical stains for organisms to sections of prostate with acute inflammation.

Histologic Chronic Inflammation

Chronic inflammatory cell infiltrates, consisting of lymphocytes, histiocytes, and plasma cells, are extremely common in all types of prostatic tissue samples, being found in the majority of needle biopsy and prostatectomy cases.[121,123,124]

Microscopically, several patterns of chronic inflammatory cell involvement of benign prostatic tissue have been described.[124,127,128] Lymphocytic and plasmacytic chronic inflammatory cell infiltrates, in contrast to acute inflammation, tend to be stromal-based and periglandular. Admixture with other inflammatory cell types is common. In tissue from the peripheral zone chronic inflammation is often associated with atrophy (Fig. 8-30A and B).

In hyperplastic TURP tissue, a very common pattern seen in 85% of TURP chips is dilated glands containing cell debris, foamy macrophages, neutrophils, and pink proteinaceous material, associated with surrounding periglandular lymphocytes and plasma cells (Fig. 8-31).[124] A second highly common arrangement is a periglandular, lymphoplasmacytic infiltrate in the absence of intraluminal inflammatory cells. Another morphologic presentation is a more diffuse stromal extension by the lymphocytes and plasma cells. Lymphoid aggregates and even lymphoid follicles (Fig. 8-32) may be seen. In the glandulocentric infiltrates of lymphocytes or plasma cells, direct extension of lymphocytes into benign prostatic epithelium commonly occurs, sometimes with perilymphocytic clearing that allows for recognition of intraepithelial lymphocytes. Scattered single lymphocytes can also be noted, especially in nodules of stromal hyperplasia (stromal nodules). Additionally, perivenular lymphocytic cuffs can be observed; it is thought that these venules are an avenue of entry for the lymphocytes into the prostate gland.[129]

Mast cells, eosinophils, and macrophages are cell types that can also be identified in histologic prostatitis. Mast cells are difficult to discover in prostatic tissues without

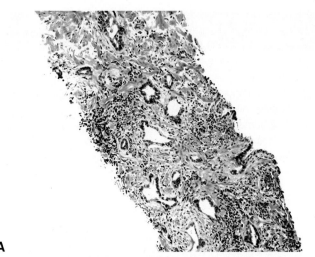
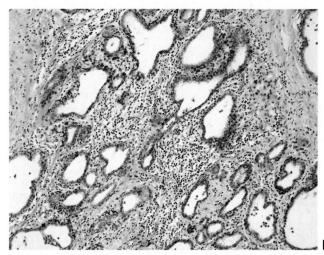

A   B

FIGURE 8-30 ■ Chronic inflammation associated with atrophy in needle biopsy tissue **(A)** and in the whole gland **(B)**.

histochemical stains. They increase in number with age[130] but are not associated with any specific disease process.[130,131] Eosinophils can nonspecifically accompany other inflammatory cells in histologic prostatitis (Fig. 8-33). The designation of eosinophilic (allergic) prostatitis should be reserved for those rare patients with a hypersensitivity disorder (such as asthma), peripheral eosinophilia, and large numbers of eosinophils admixed with granulomas.[132–136] Macrophages can be found in dilated glands surrounding ruptured ducts and acini and in granulomatous prostatitis.

Benign prostatic epithelium in the setting of chronic histologic inflammation may display a range of reactive alterations. Secretory epithelial cells can lose cytoplasmic volume, some of the cells become cuboidal instead of columnar, and the cytoplasm becomes more dense and eosinophilic rather than clear to granular.[124,129] This lends an atrophic appearance to these glands. Basal cell hyperplasia is often involved by lymphocytes.[137,138] Urothelial metaplasia, nephrogenic

adenoma, and squamous cell metaplasia in the prostate are also often associated with inflammation. Reactive nuclear atypia in the chronically inflamed epithelium generally is mild[128] and is regularly manifested as crowded, enlarged nuclei with small nucleoli. These nucleoli are usually small, but in inflamed basal cell hyperplasia and in some inflamed atrophic or squamous metaplastic cells larger nucleoli may be seen.

Stromal alterations are less well described in chronic prostatic inflammation, but stromal sclerosis can definitely occur,[128] particularly in response to gland rupture.

Inflammation in the prostate involves neoplastic epithelium less often than benign epithelium.[129] Rarely is high-grade PIN involved by abundant inflammation,[139] whereas a minor lymphocytic infiltrate is common in prostatic carcinoma.[140] Of note, when urothelial carcinoma of the urethra or urinary bladder extends into the prostate, it can exhibit an exuberant peritumoral inflammatory and sclerotic response.

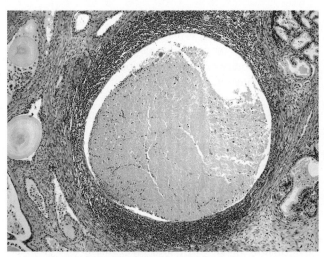

FIGURE 8-31 ■ Dilated benign prostatic gland with surrounding band of chronic inflammatory cells.

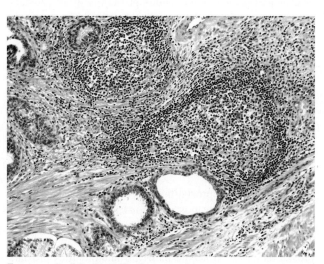

FIGURE 8-32 ■ Follicular prostatitis.

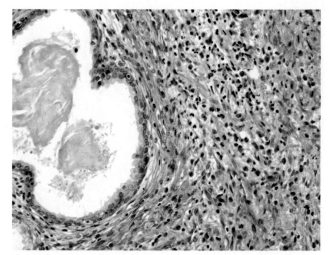

FIGURE 8-33 ■ Eosinophils in nonspecific inflammation in the prostate.

Benign lymphocytes in the prostate may be mistaken for malignant cells of epithelial or hematopoietic types. Arrangement of lymphocytes in cords, linear arrays, or sheets may cause confusion with high-grade Gleason pattern 4 or 5 adenocarcinoma, prostatic small cell carcinoma, or lymphoma at low magnification. Higher-power examination will allow for identification of small bland lymphocytic nuclei. Lymphocytes with crush/distortion artifact or thermal damage may on occasion be difficult to distinguish from carcinoma, especially when such distorted lymphocytes are present around nerves or at the margin of radical prostatectomy tissue sections. Thermal damage at TURP can induce signet ring change in benign lymphocytes,[141] mimicking signet ring carcinoma.

Granulomatous Prostatitis

Granulomatous prostatitis is a distinctive form of prostatitis that can be mistaken for carcinoma clinically,[142–144] radiologically (by ultrasound),[145,146] and histopathologically.[147] The incidence of granulomatous prostatitis in all prostatic samples ranges from 0.4% to 4%.[124,128,148,149] The incidence in needle biopsy is <1%.[148] Most patients are 50 to 70 years of age (mean = 62 years; range = 18 to 86 years) and present with irritative or obstructive voiding symptoms, fever, and chills. Consistent with this presentation, most patients had a urinary tract infection 1 to 8 weeks before diagnosis. Clinical concerns for malignancy are raised in granulomatous prostatitis because of an elevated total serum PSA, a low percentage free PSA, hypoechoic lesions on ultrasound, and a hard, fixed, indurated prostate gland on digital rectal examination.[144,146,148]

Granulomatous prostatitis can be classified based on cause (Table 8-4). The most common cause of granulomatous prostatitis is so-called nonspecific granulomatous prostatitis, which accounts for about three quarters of granulomatous prostatitis cases. In needle biopsy, granulomatous prostatitis is categorized as nonspecific in 77% of cases, infectious

Table 8-4 ■ GRANULOMATOUS PROSTATITIS: CLASSIFICATION

I. Nonspecific (due to duct/acinar rupture)
  Usual type
  Xanthogranulomatous
  Nodular histiocytic prostatitis
  Xanthoma
II. Infectious
  A. Bacterial
    Tuberculosis
    Brucellous
  B. Spirochetal
    Syphilis
  C. Fungal
    Coccidioidomycosis
    Cryptococcosis
    Blastomycosis
    Histoplasmosis
    Paracoccidioidomycosis
    Candidiasis
    Aspergillosis
  D. Parasitic
    Schistosomiasis
  E. Viral
    Herpes zoster
III. Postbiopsy/resection
IV. Malakoplakia
V. Systemic granulomatous disease
  Allergic (eosinophilic)
  Sarcoidosis
  Wegener granulomatosis
VI. Foreign body
  Teflon
  Hair

Modified from reference Roberts RO, Lieber MM, Bostwick DG, et al. A review of clinical and pathological prostatitis syndromes. *Urology* 1997;49:809.

in 18% of cases, and indeterminate in 4% of cases.[148] The infectious agent here is bacille Calmette-Guerin (BCG), used in therapy for urothelial carcinoma. In larger tissue samples, postbiopsy and postresection granulomas are more common, being diagnosed in 25% of all granulomatous prostatitis cases.[149] The other listed causes of granulomatous prostatitis in Table 8-4 are uncommon to rare.

Nonspecific Granulomatous Prostatitis

Nonspecific granulomatous prostatitis is termed nonspecific because it is not considered secondary to a specific agent but rather it is viewed as representing a foreign body-type response to prostatic secretions, with associated duct or acinar rupture.[150,151] Yet some patients have positive urine cultures (mainly for *E. coli*), such that some of this response may also be caused by bacterial products. Impairment of drainage, perhaps secondary to BPH, and infection seem to

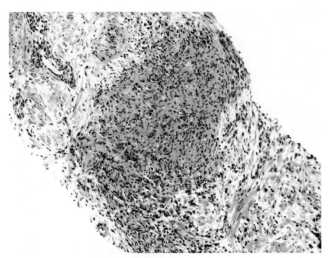

FIGURE 8-34 ■ Nonspecific granulomatous prostatitis that is noncaseating with lobular pattern.

FIGURE 8-35 ■ Nonspecific granulomatous prostatitis with a mixed inflammatory cell infiltrate comprising lymphocytes, plasma cells, histiocytes, and multinucleated giant cells.

be pathogenetic components.[144,151] The serum PSA is often significantly elevated, with a mean of around 13 ng/mL (range 0.4 to 114 ng/mL).[148,152]

Grossly, nonspecific granulomatous prostatitis appears as small, firm, yellow granular nodules.[144] Microscopically, the usual type of nonspecific granulomatous prostatitis is a lobulocentric noncaseating granulomatous inflammatory cell infiltrate (Fig. 8-34). The inflammation is centered on ducts and glands, which exhibit a variable degree of destruction. Liquefactive necrosis has been reported in the center of the inflammatory infiltrate,[132] although other series do not allow necrosis.[149] Necrosis raises the possibility of specific infectious granulomatous prostatitis and is not usually seen in nonspecific granulomatous prostatitis. The granulomas can be focal or diffuse. In needle biopsy, more than one core is involved in most cases.[148] The lobulocentricity of the granulomas can be appreciated in some needle biopsy cases, where smaller granulomas are present, but in other cases the granulomatous inflammation can appear more sheet-like because of partial sampling of larger granulomas. In TURP and simple prostatectomy tissues, the granulomas can be extremely focal, can form a discrete mass, or can be a diffuse spread of fused nodules. The cellular infiltrate in usual nonspecific granulomatous prostatitis is mixed, with epithelioid histiocytes, lymphocytes, neutrophils, eosinophils, plasma cells, and multinucleated giant cells (Fig. 8-35). The giant cells can be of foreign body, Langhans, and Touton types.[153] They can be difficult to detect in needle biopsies. Lymphocytic infiltrates, sometimes with lymphoid follicle formation, surround the granulomatous nodules. Perinodular stromal fibrosis and scarring can ensue in some cases.[144]

The spectrum of morphologic abnormalities in nonspecific granulomatous prostatitis also includes "xanthogranulomatous prostatitis," "nodular histiocytic prostatitis," and "prostatic xanthoma." The first two designations are applied when the epithelioid histiocytes possess a cleared to vacuolated cytoplasm (due to lipid accumulation).[153–156] In prostatic xanthoma there is a solitary, microscopic aggregate of foamy histiocytes (Fig. 8-36).[157,158] This is a rare entity that is usually an incidental finding in peripheral zone tissues removed to evaluate for BPH or carcinoma. Only one patient had hyperlipidemia.

Sheets or cords of epithelioid histiocytes in nonspecific granulomatous prostatitis or xanthoma can masquerade as poorly differentiated carcinoma or carcinoma with hormonal treatment effect.[148,149,158] This is particularly problematic when histiocytes predominate in nonspecific granulomatous prostatitis, without significant numbers of giant cells, plasma cells, lymphocytes, eosinophils, or neutrophils. Also, the epithelioid histiocytes can display prominent nucleoli, which can cause concern for malignancy. An immunohistochemical marker panel can be helpful in defining the differentiation status of the atypical epithelioid cells. Negative

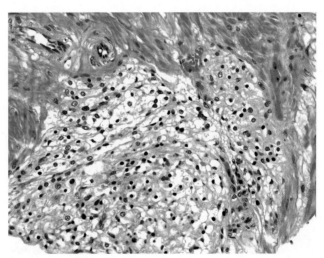

FIGURE 8-36 ■ Xanthoma of prostate consisting of a small aggregate of foamy histiocytes.

immunoreactions for pan-cytokeratin, PSA, and PSAP, with immunopositivity for CD68 and lysozyme in the epithelioid cells are useful in establishing a diagnosis of granulomatous prostatitis in this context.[147,148,158]

Infectious Granulomatous Prostatitis

Specific infectious types of granulomatous prostatitis include bacterial, fungal, parasitic, and viral prostatitis (Table 8-4).

BCG Granulomatous Prostatitis

The most common type of infectious granulomatous inflammation is that due to BCG therapy for urothelial carcinoma (usually of the bladder). In fact, every case of infectious granulomatous prostatitis in one needle biopsy series was caused by BCG treatment.[148] Whereas only 10% of men treated with intravesical BCG for superficial urinary bladder carcinoma develop clinically symptomatic BCG prostatitis,[159] a substantial percentage (80% to 100%) of patients have histologic evidence of BCG granulomatous prostatitis.[159–161] Grossly, the cut surfaces of prostate glands in radical cystoprostatectomies from patients treated with BCG show multiple, firm, white nodules or soft, yellowish-gray nodules with granular centers, central caseation, and focal cavitation.[160] In exceedingly rare cases abscess formation can occur.[162] The large, confluent granulomas can measure up to 1.6 cm in greatest dimension.[160] Microscopically the granulomas, particularly the larger ones, are of the typical caseating, tuberculoid type (Fig. 8-37). Smaller (<1 mm) granulomas composed predominantly of histiocytes can lack giant cells and caseous necrosis. Indeed, in needle biopsy up to one-quarter of BCG granulomatous prostatitis cases lack caseous necrosis.[148] The smaller granulomas are periglandular (Fig. 8-38), often with intraluminal protrusion. With a history of previous BCG treatment, it is not necessary to stain sections with Ziehl-Neelsen for acid-fast organisms. If the stain is performed, 40% to 77% of cases demonstrate mycobacteria in the granulomas.[160,163]

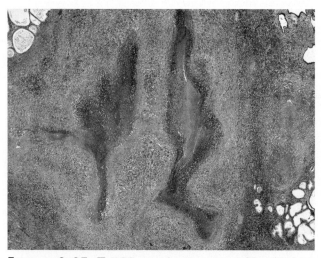

FIGURE 8-37 ■ BCG granulomatous prostatitis with large geographic areas of caseating granulomas.

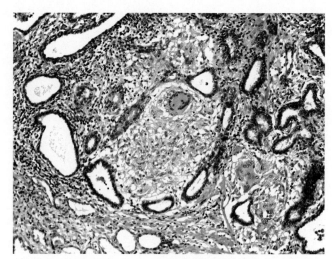

FIGURE 8-38 ■ BCG granulomatous prostatitis with small periglandular epithelioid granuloma without caseation.

Infectious Granulomatous Prostatitis: Non-BCG Types

Mycobacterial prostatitis due to *Mycobacterium tuberculosis* or atypical species is rare,[164–168] with an incidence of 3% of all examples of granulomatous prostatitis.[165] The spread to the prostate is hematogenous, usually from active pulmonary disease. The prostate is nodular to palpation. Grossly, yellow to grayish-yellow nodules are located in the peripheral zone.[167] Larger lesions exhibit caseation, but caseation is minimal in the "small yellow tubercle" granulomas.[167] The granulomas are similar to those in BCG granulomatous prostatitis, including lack of caseous necrosis in some examples in needle biopsy. Presentation as an incidental finding in TURP chips has also been a mode of diagnosis.[164] For patients without a history of BCG treatment and those in whom tuberculosis is clinically suspected, special stains for acid-fast bacilli and fungi should be performed.

Isolated case reports of prostatic brucellosis[144] and prostatic syphillis[169] indicate that these organisms can also elicit a granulomatous prostatitis.

Fungal, parasitic, and viral granulomatous prostatitis due to specific organisms is also rare.[170–179] Predisposing conditions for prostatic fungal infection include immunosuppression, prolonged antibiotic use, diabetes mellitus, malignancy, and an indwelling bladder catheter.[177,180,181] Even in disseminated fungal infections, the prostate is uncommonly invaded. Fungi detected in the prostate include *Cryptoccocus,*[178,182,183] *Paracoccidioides,*[184] *Coccidioides* (Fig. 8-39A and B),[172,173] *Histoplasma,*[185] *Blastomyces,*[186] *Candida,*[170,176,177] and *Aspergillus.*[149] Among cases of granulomatous prostatitis, fungal granulomatous prostatitis accounted for 1 in 200 (0.5%) of cases.[133] In patients with the aforementioned predisposing conditions, and granulomatous prostatitis or necrotizing granulomas in the absence of BCG therapy, special histochemical stains for fungal organisms and acid-fast bacilli should be

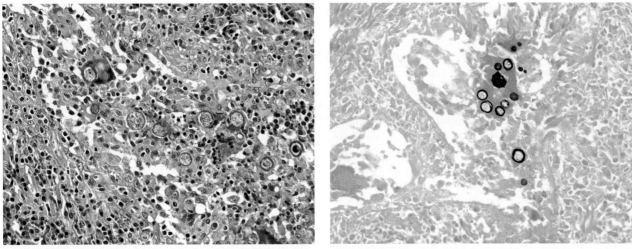

FIGURE 8-39 ■ *Coccidioides immitis* granulomatous prostatitis (**A**) with spherules highlighted by Gomori methenamine-silver histochemical stain (**B**).

performed. PCR specific for cryptococcal 18S rDNA from fixed prostate tissue was performed in one case.[183]

Granulomatous prostatitis due to parasitic infection can occur in schistosomiasis. Eggs of *Schistosoma* (usually *haematobium*) are deposited in the prostate of about 20% of African men with schistosomiasis, but this rarely gives rise to prostate-related symptoms.[175]

Necrotizing, focally granulomatous prostatitis has been reported in two patients in association with herpes zoster infection.[174]

Postbiopsy and Postresection Granulomatous Prostatitis

The incidence of this kind of granulomatous prostatitis is highly variable, depending on the type of tissue sample. Amongst cases of granulomatous prostatitis, the incidence in needle biopsy was 0%,[148] whereas in another series that included TURP chips, the incidence was 25%.[149] This is so because this granulomatous process tends to be central, involving periurethral transition zone tissue, which is readily sampled by TURP, as opposed to involvement of the peripheral zone, which is most often the target of needle biopsies. Amongst all cases of prostatitis, it made up 7.1%.[128] Patients were 51 to 87 years of age and had undergone TURP 7 days to 3 years previously.[132,187–190] Two patients had a history of needle biopsy of only the prostate.[190] Patients present for repeat TURP (or initial TURP in the needle biopsy patients) because of persistent prostatism, urinary obstruction or retention, and hematuria. It is noteworthy that TURP does not always seem to elicit such a granulomatous response, as 12 of 23 patients in one repeat TURP series[191] did not have detectable granulomas, but the possibility remains that with additional chip sampling more granulomas might have been detected. The basis for the development of post-TURP granulomas appears to be a response to altered and cauterized prostatic epithelium and stroma, secretions, urine, or even metal from the diathermy instruments used for resection.[192]

Grossly, no difference is recognized in chips with or without postbiopsy or postresection granulomas.[188] Microscopically, the granulomas assume a variety of shapes, including round, ovoid, elongated, stellate, serpiginous, triangular, slit-like, and rectangular forms (Fig. 8-40). Almost all of the granulomas demonstrate a connection with a cauterized TURP chip surface. A common finding is the base of a wedge-shaped granuloma at the edge of a TURP chip.[132] The granulomas measure 0.5 mm to 2 mm[190] and are usually multiple, with an average of 4 to 5 per case, but can be single.[132,191] The granulomas are characterized by a fibrinoid central zone and surrounding, palisaded epithelioid histiocytes and fibroblasts. A rim of lymphocytes (which mark as T cells) is present outside the palisaded cell layer. Admixed with the lymphocytes are occasional plasma cells and eosinophils. The eosinophils may be numerous if the previous TURP was performed earlier than 2 months.[132,187] Multinucleated giant cells are observed in some but not all cases and are usually of foreign body type but can also be of Touton or Langhans types.[191] Occasional giant cells

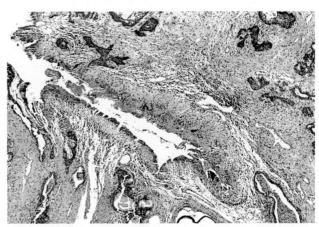

FIGURE 8-40 ■ Post-TURP granuloma with central fibrinoid necrosis.

contain brown pigment related to cautery-induced tissue carbonization.[191] Older granulomas exhibit both central and peripheral hyalinization.

Reactive changes often are visualized in epithelium and stroma adjacent to postbiopsy TURP granulomas. Prostatic glands adjacent to the granulomas may appear compressed and reactive with slight to moderate nuclear atypia and small nucleoli, but macronucleoli are generally absent. Squamous metaplasia can be seen in about one-half of cases.[191] Postbiopsy and post-TURP granulomas have been found in chips with both BPH and carcinoma. Localized vasculitis confined to the prostate has been reported in association with a few cases of post-TURP granulomas.[153,189]

Postbiopsy and post-TURP granulomas have been misdiagnosed as rheumatoid nodules and as tuberculous granulomatous prostatitis. A history of a previous procedure, in conjunction with the appearance of a palisading, fibrinoid granuloma, is most helpful in establishing the diagnosis of postbiopsy or post-TURP granulomatous prostatitis. In this setting it is not necessary to stain for organisms. Histochemical stains for organisms in these cases have been uniformly negative. Also, invariably negative are examinations for birefringent material with polarized light. Other types of granulomas are also in the differential diagnosis, such as allergic (eosinophilic) granulomatous prostatis and nonspecific granulomatous prostatitis.[132] The former entity may overlap morphologically with early post-TURP granulomas in having numerous eosinophils, but allergic granulomatous prostatitis is seen in a different clinical context, with a clinical history of a hypersensitivity disorder (such as asthma) and a peripheral eosinophilia. Unlike nonspecific granulomatous prostatitis, postbiopsy and post-TURP granulomas are not centered on ducts and acini and also possess a striking fibrinoid central zone.

Malakoplakia

Malakoplakia uncommonly involves the prostate, with only about 30 cases reported to date.[193–202] In one review of malakoplakia occurring at all sites, the prostate was primarily involved in 10% of all cases.[197] Although uncommon, malakoplakia, like other forms of granulomatous prostatitis, can be misdiagnosed as carcinoma by DRE, transrectal ultrasound (TRUS), and histopathologic examination.[198–200] Patients with prostatic malakoplakia usually are in their 60s (range 49 to 85) and present with voiding symptoms (dysuria, frequency, urinary retention) and an enlarged, firm to hard prostate by DRE. There is almost always an associated urinary tract infection with *E. coli*. Immunosuppression has been associated with malakoplakia in general,[197] but only two patients with prostatic malakoplakia were known to be immunosuppressed.[201,202]

Grossly, malakoplakia appears as soft, yellowish nodules in the prostate.[195] Resected prostatic chips involved by malakoplakia are soft and yellow-brown to gray.[200] Microscopically, there are sheets of macrophages, effacing normal prostatic architecture, with smaller numbers of lymphocytes, plasma cells, eosinophils, and neutrophils. The macrophages (also known as von Hansemann cells) contain round, often concentrically lamellated, basophilic intracytoplasmic inclusions that are 2 to 10 μm in diameter. They look targetoid, with a central basophilic body surrounded by a clear zone. These are the characteristic Michaelis-Gutmann bodies that represent calcified bacterial debris within phagolysosomes. These structures can also be extracellular.

The essential differential diagnostic distinction is the separation of malakoplakia from poorly differentiated carcinoma. There are three published cases in which an initial diagnosis of carcinoma was rendered.[198–200] As in other types of granulomatous prostatitis, the diffuse growth of epithelioid histiocytes creates diagnostic difficulty. In one case misdiagnosed as clear cell carcinoma, the malakoplakia was diffuse and extensive, involving 60% of the TURP chips.[200] The aforementioned immunohistochemical marker panel of pan-cytokeratin, PSA, PSAP, CD68, and lysozyme can also be diagnostically beneficial in selected cases. The presence of Michaelis-Gutmann bodies distinguishes malakoplakia from other types of granulomatous prostatitis.

Treatment is directed toward control of urinary tract infection.[197] In one patient, failure of control resulted in a fatal prostate–rectal fistula.[195] Overall, prognosis is related to extent of malakoplakia in the urinary tract and especially extent of renal involvement.[197]

Systemic Granulomatous Disease Affecting the Prostate

Several systemic granulomatous diseases can involve the prostate and even present primarily as a prostatic disorder (Table 8-4). All of these are uncommon to rare.

Allergic (eosinophilic) granulomatous prostatitis must be clearly defined and distinguished from other types of prostatitis that have eosinophils.[132,148,149] The mere finding of eosinophils, even numerous eosinophils, does not equate with a diagnosis of allergic prostatitis. Rather, a histopathologic diagnosis of allergic (eosinophilic) granulomatous prostatitis should incorporate clinical findings of a hypersensitivity disorder (usually asthma or drug allergy), with or without a peripheral eosinophilia. Peripheral eosinophila without documented clinical hypersensitivity is not sufficient. Allergic (eosinophilic) granulomatous prostatitis is a rare condition, with an incidence of 0.06% in 3,600 TURP chip cases. Not a single case was diagnosed in 25,852 needle biopsies.[148] It accounts for 1% of all cases of granulomatous prostatitis.[149] Only a handful of cases have been well documented.[132] Microscopically, the prototypical case has central fibrinoid necrosis with surrounding, palisaded epithelioid histiocytes and numerous eosinophils. No Charcot-Leyden crystals are seen. The differential diagnosis of allergic (eosinophilic) granulomatous prostatitis mainly includes other types of granulomatous prostatitis. Significant numbers of eosinophils can be seen in nonspecific granulomatous prostatitis (68% of cases), postbiopsy TURP cases, and less frequently in infectious granulomatous prostatitis (12% of cases).[148]

Sarcoidosis rarely involves the prostate, with only a few case reports.[203–205] The noncaseating granulomas have been detected in needle biopsy,[203,205] at radical prostatectomy,[204] and at autopsy.

Wegener granulomatosis usually involves the upper respiratory tract, lungs, and kidneys, but in 2.7% to 7.4% of patients, prostatic involvement can occur.[206–209] Prostatic involvement at autopsy was seen in 7.4% of all Wegener cases,[206] but only about 20 patients with Wegener granulomatosis have had symptoms referable to the prostate gland in the form of symptomatic prostatitis with urinary frequency, dysuria, hematuria, lower back pain, or acute urinary retention. Only a few patients ($n = 10$) had these prostatitis symptoms at initial clinical presentation.[208,209] In a few patients localized induration on the DRE has caused clinical concern for carcinoma.[209] Acute necrotizing granulomas have been detected in patients with prostatic Wegener granulomatosis in needle biopsy, in TURP chips, and at autopsy. An important microscopic finding is that of vasculitis, and this discovery, in conjunction with the necrotizing granulomas, should prompt a workup for Wegener granulomatosis in these rare patients who present with Wegener granulmatosis in the prostate. As in other anatomic sites, it is important to exclude infectious granulomatous disease before diagnosing Wegener granulomatosis, and so performance of histochemical stains for organisms is obligatory.

Foreign Body Granulomatous Prostatitis

A few examples of specific foreign body granulomatous reaction to Teflon (polytetrafluorethylene)[210] and hair[211–213] have been described. Teflon injection has been used to treat urinary incontinence, and this can cause prostatic nodularity by DRE and elevated serum PSA.[210] Prostate needle biopsy demonstrates an exuberant foreign body giant cell reaction to the refractile, irregular fragments of Teflon. With polarization, the Teflon is highly birefringent. Detection of a Teflon granuloma does not rule out the coexistence of epithelial proliferative abnormalities. In one reported case, high-grade PIN was found, and in a second there was an associated Gleason score 7 adenocarcinoma.[210] Hair granulomas with prostatic hair implantation due to long-term catheterization[211] or perineal prostatic biopsy[213] have also been seen.

Vasculitis

Inflammation of vessels in the prostate can represent a vasculitis confined to or isolated in the prostate or can represent a manifestation of systemic or nonprostatic confined vasculitis. Examples of localized vasculitis include vasculitis in post-TURP granulomatous prostatitis, giant cell arteritis (one case),[214] and isolated nonfibrinoid arteritis in BPH (significance unknown). Systemic diseases that can produce vasculitis in the prostate include polyarteritis nodosa,[215–217] Wegener granulomatosis, and hypersensitivity disorders causing allergic (eosinophilic) granulomatous prostatitis. Radiation therapy directed toward the prostate can also result in vasculitis in the prostate.

Infectious Prostatitis: Additional Types

Additional specific infections of the prostate have been reported for both immunocompetent and immunosuppressed patients. These include rare cases of prostatic actinomycosis,[218] amebic prostatitis,[219] *Pseudomonas pseudomallei* prostatitis,[220] and prostatic *Echinococcus*[221,222] in immunocompetent men. Microscopically, the prostatic response to these organisms is variable. For example, prostatic acute and chronic inflammation with fibrosis, granulation tissue, and abscess formation (with sulfur granules present) are evident in prostatic actinomycosis. A chronic, fibrosing prostatitis with eosinophils has been reported for echinococcal prostatic infection.[221] It is uncertain how often sexually transmitted infections of the prostate by *Neisseria gonorrhoeae* and human papillomavirus occur and whether this is a clinical problem.[223]

In immunosuppressed patients, viral, bacterial, fungal, and parasitic prostatitis can occur. Most of these reports are of patients with acquired immunodeficiency syndrome (AIDS), although most cases of cytomegalovirus (CMV) prostatitis have been observed in patients undergoing immunosuppressive therapy following organ transplantation.[224] In AIDS, patients can experience bacterial prostatitis, with progression toward abscess formation.[225] Opportunistic infectious agents that have been reported in the prostates of patients with AIDS include CMV, *Mycobacterium, Histoplasma, Candida, Pneumocystis,* adenovirus, and *Cryptococcus.* Cryptococcal organisms may be sequestered in the prostate of patients with AIDS and thereby act as a reservoir for persistent infection.[226] Microscopically, organisms can be identified in expressed prostatic secretions, prostate needle biopsy, or prostate glands from postmortem examination. The prostatic response to infection in patients with AIDS is variable and can be lacking,[227] or there can be necrosis or abscess formation.[228]

Atrophy and Its Variants

Atrophy in the prostate is a common, age-related process that represents one of the benign lesions most often misdiagnosed as carcinoma.[4–6] Prostatic atrophy begins at an early age and there is an increase in incidence and extent with age[229,230]; 67% of men aged 19 to 29 have atrophy and this increases to nearly 100% for men over 70.[230,231] In needle biopsy, atrophy is an extremely common finding, detectable in 90% of peripheral zone biopsies.[138] Atrophy in TURP chips usually represents cystic atrophy in nodular hyperplasia. In whole prostate glands, atrophy is principally localized to the peripheral zone.[229]

The cause of age-related atrophy is unknown. Factors that have been invoked include compression by hyperplastic nodules, inflammation, hormones, obstruction, nutritional deficiency, and systemic or local ischemia, such as that induced by arteriosclerosis.[230–234] Atrophy in the prostate can also be caused by treatment, including radiation therapy and androgen deprivation therapy.

There are no clinical or radiologic features specific for atrophy although ultrasound examination may demonstrate cystic change that can be cystic atrophy.

Grossly, atrophy is visible only when there is cyst formation. Such cystic atrophy can occur in both the transition zone in BPH and the peripheral zone. However, atrophy is only definable at the light microscopic level, and it is not possible to tell macroscopically whether prostatic cysts are atrophic or not. These cysts have been termed retention cysts[235] and impart a sponge-like appearance. Their size can range up to 2 cm in greatest diameter.[235]

Histologic classification of atrophy is useful for reasons of diagnostic awareness and differential diagnosis, but it is not absolutely necessary to subtype atrophy because there is currently no known clinical significance in doing so. For diagnostic recognition and research purposes atrophy may be classified as simple atrophy, simple atrophy with cyst formation, postatrophic hyperplasia (PAH), and partial atrophy.[236] These patterns are often admixed. Sclerotic atrophy and proliferative atrophy (PA)/proliferative inflammatory atrophy (PIA) are also discussed here. The essential, unifying feature of all forms of atrophy is reduction of cytoplasmic volume of luminal epithelial cells (Box 8-3).

Simple Atrophy

Simple atrophy can be found in the peripheral zone with or without cyst formation. This is the most common type of atrophy, occurring in 89% of prostates with atrophy, sometimes alone and sometimes in combination with other types of atrophy.[229] Simple atrophy is most often seen in combination with PAH (hyperplastic atrophy) and sclerotic atrophy.[230] Microscopically, atrophy can be focal, involving just a few lobules, or it can involve virtually the entire peripheral zone. Simple acinar atrophy usually involves an entire lobule, with retention of a lobular architecture (Fig. 8-41). In noncystic atrophy there are aggregates of small dark acini with open lumens. The acini are rounded to angular in shape and are not crowded. Atrophic ducts ramifying into atrophic acini can be noted. Corpora amylacea are common in atrophic glands but crystalloids and intraluminal wispy blue mucin are decidedly uncommon. The stroma in the lobule is often altered with pale fibrosis and sometimes with a thickening of periacinar collagen (Fig. 8-42).[232] Sclerosis around ducts can be marked (Fig. 8-43). Acute inflammation (of a moderate to severe grade) is observed in 15% of simple atrophy cases, whereas moderate to severe

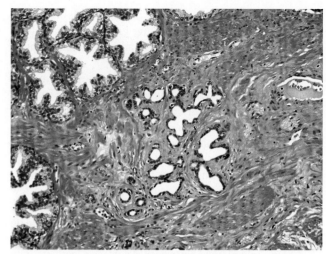

FIGURE 8-41 ■ Simple atrophy, with a lobular configuration. Compare scant cytoplasm in atrophy versus adjacent benign nonatrophic glands where the luminal cells have a moderate amount of cytoplasm.

chronic inflammation is seen in 30% of cases (Fig. 8-44).[126] The luminal epithelial cells in the atrophic foci are cuboidal (Fig. 8-45) to flattened (Fig. 8-46) and have a high nuclear/cytoplasmic ratio. The nuclei are typically not enlarged but are often deeply staining, with condensed chromatin. However, nuclear atypia can be seen (Fig. 8-47), with prominent (>1 μm) nucleoli detectable in a minority of cases.[126]

In needle biopsy, simple atrophy is eye-catching because it is often characterized by a haphazard distribution of small glands (Fig. 8-48). At higher magnifications, the small acini are seen to have distorted and angulated outer contours. This appearance, along with the stromal fibrosis of the atrophic lobule, and even chain-like (Fig. 8-47) and cord-like structures (Fig. 8-49) simulate an infiltrative process.

Simple Atrophy with Cystic Change

Cystic change in simple atrophy is a fairly common alteration, with gland size varying from mild dilatation to medium sized

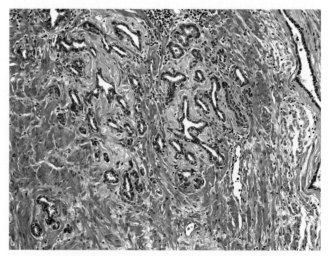

FIGURE 8-42 ■ Atrophy with adjacent sclerotic stroma.

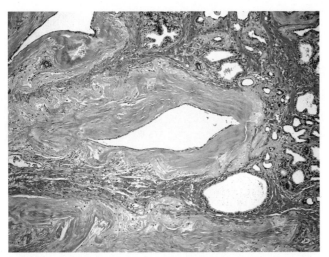

FIGURE 8-43 ■ Atrophic prostatic duct with surrounding sclerosis.

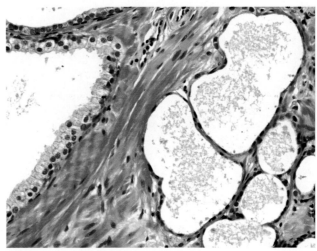

FIGURE 8-46 ■ Atrophy with marked cytoplasmic volume loss and nuclear flattening.

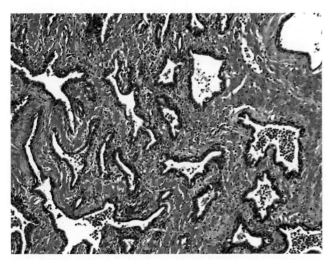

FIGURE 8-44 ■ Atrophy with associated acute and chronic inflammation.

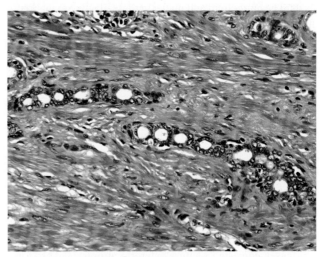

FIGURE 8-47 ■ Atrophy with chain-like appearance and nuclear atypia with nuclear enlargement and nucleoli.

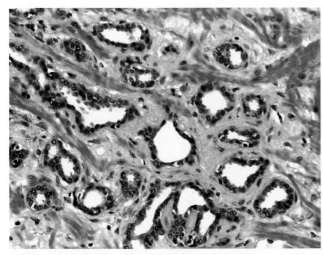

FIGURE 8-45 ■ Atrophy with cytoplasmic volume loss.

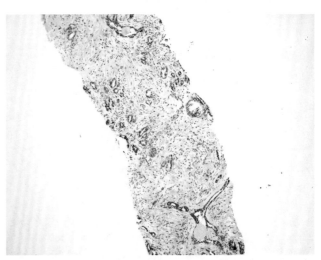

FIGURE 8-48 ■ Atrophy with irregular distribution of small acini.

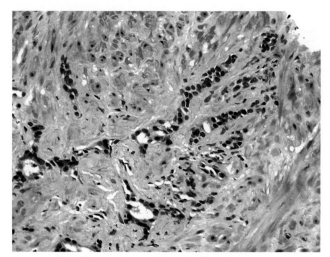

FIGURE 8-49 ■ Atrophy with cord-like structures.

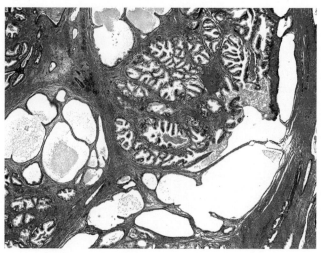

FIGURE 8-51 ■ Cystic atrophy in BPH.

to larger cysts (Fig. 8-50), including the aforementioned 2-cm cysts. The epithelium and nuclei in these glands are markedly flattened. In the peripheral zone, a lobular arrangement of the cystically dilated, atrophic glands is sometimes evident, but with distortion the cystic, atrophic glands appear haphazardly arranged. Glands with cystic atrophy can masquerade as vessels. Simple cystic atrophy can also occur in areas of nodular hyperplasia in the transition zone (Fig. 8-51), where a flattened, atrophic-appearing epithelium can be found in nodules of usual epithelial and stromal hyperplasia.

Sclerotic Atrophy

Sclerotic atrophy is a frequently detected type of peripheral zone atrophy, having been found in 74% of cases of atrophy in the whole gland.[229] Like simple atrophy, it is usually admixed with other types of atrophy, and only 11% of atrophy cases consisted of pure sclerotic atrophy.[230] This form of atrophy is remarkable for the lobular acinar disarray due to exuberant fibrosis. Accompanying chronic inflammation with often large collections of lymphocytes and histiocytes

can be present. The acinar distortion and angulation in a background of stromal sclerosis can produce an infiltrative appearance (Fig. 8-52), especially in needle biopsy. Such an image may be highly alarming in needle biopsy, where lobular arrangements may be difficult or impossible to visualize. Yet, cytologically, the lining cells are small and bland; basal cells can be identified in some glands but not in all, owing to nuclear compression and crowding.

Partial Atrophy

Partial atrophy is a variant of atrophy in which the atrophic glands have relatively scant cytoplasm, but the glands appear as a crowded collection of pale glands rather than dark glands (Fig. 8-53).[237,238] In many needle biopsies with partial atrophy, fully developed atrophy is also present.[237,238] In about one-third of cases there is a disorganized rather than circumscribed growth pattern.[238] Unlike other types of atrophy, stromal sclerosis is generally lacking and inflammation is rarely detected.[238] The glandular outlines in partial atrophy vary from straight luminal borders to more undulating

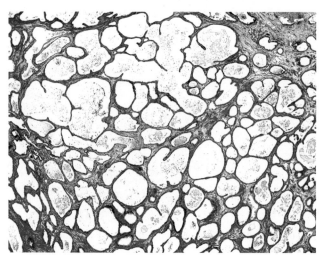

FIGURE 8-50 ■ Cystic change in atrophy.

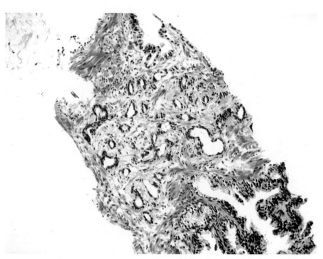

FIGURE 8-52 ■ Sclerotic atrophy simulating an infiltrative process.

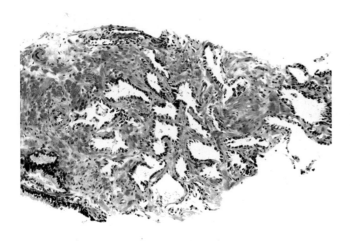

FIGURE 8-53 ■ Partial atrophy in needle biopsy tissue.

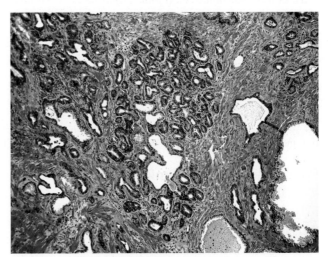

FIGURE 8-55 ■ Partial atrophy with nuclear elongation in some of the cells.

luminal surfaces and papillary projections. A stellate shape is assumed by some glands (Fig. 8-54). Intraluminal pale amorphous debris was observed in 33% of cases but intraluminal wispy blue mucin (blue-tinged mucinous secretions) and crystalloids, which are more often present in malignant than in benign glands, are not seen.[237,238] Nuclear/cytoplasmic ratios are 1:2 for most constituent epithelial cells, compared with 1:1 for fully developed atrophy. The nuclei of these cells are often abnormal, with an elongated, cylindrical shape (Fig. 8-55) and with nuclear and nucleolar enlargement in 15% to 25% of cases.[237,238] The enlarged nucleoli did not, however, assume the size seen in some prostatic adenocarcinomas[238] and specifically, none were macronucleoli, defined as nucleoli easily seen at 10× magnification.[239]

Postatrophic Hyperplasia

PAH was originally felt to represent atrophic prostatic epithelium that underwent hyperplasia.[232] Accordingly, another term that has been used for PAH is hyperplastic atrophy.[230] (Of course, it is impossible to prove that this process is atrophy in hyperplastic acini or hyperplasia in atrophy.) Subtyping into categories of lobular hyperplasia and sclerotic atrophy with hyperplasia (postsclerotic hyperplasia) was proposed[232] but has not been routinely applied. PAH has an incidence of 2% to 4% in needle biopsy cases[240] and 13% to 78% in whole prostate glands.[230,240–242] Most (about 90% of) foci are identified in the peripheral zone,[241,243] and this type of atrophy is always found admixed with another type of atrophy (usually simple).[230] In addition, PAH is multicentric in 16% of needle biopsy cases[240] and in 44% of whole glands.[242]

Microscopically, PAH has a lobular outline, with a central duct surrounded by small, fairly regular, and closely packed acini (Fig. 8-56).[232] The central "feeder" duct can show some slight cystic change and has a low, atrophic epithelium. The surrounding, clustered acini number from about 10 to 20 (with a range of 5 to 88) and appear to bud from the central duct.[240,242] The acini are mainly small and oval to round,

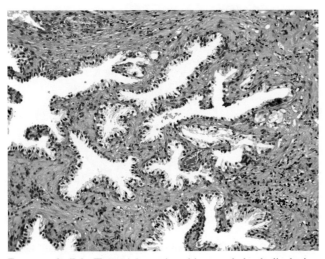

FIGURE 8-54 ■ Partial atrophy with several glands displaying a stellate shape.

FIGURE 8-56 ■ Post-atrophic hyperplasia with lobular arrangement of crowded small acini.

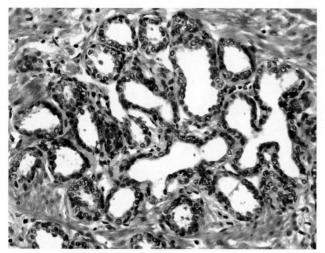

FIGURE 8-57 ■ Post-atrophic hyperplasia with nuclear enlargement and several visible nucleoli.

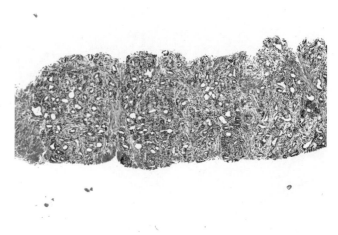

FIGURE 8-58 ■ Post-atrophic hyperplasia in needle biopsy tissue, with crowded small acini in partially sampled lobules.

but there is variability in size and shape; a minority of acini show cystic change and round, oval, elongated, slit-like, and stellate glands may be observed.[240] The acinar epithelium is low cuboidal, and the luminal epithelial cell nuclei are mildly enlarged with fine, granular chromatin and small nucleoli (Fig. 8-57).[232,242] Prominent (>1 μm) nucleoli can be noted in up to 26% of PAH cases, particularly when acute inflammation is present.[126] The tinctorial character of the luminal cell cytoplasm is often condensed and basophilic but can be eosinophilic, finely granular, and clear. Basal cells can usually be seen in PAH using H&E-stained sections, although, as for other forms of atrophy, their detection becomes difficult (or impossible) when epithelial cell flattening occurs. Basal cells are highlighted in all foci with use of 34βE12 high-molecular-weight cytokeratin or p63 immunostains, although it is important to note that in about one-quarter of cases, occasional glands will lack any staining at all.[240] Intracytoplasmic blue mucin representing mucinous metaplasia can be found in PAH foci. Basal cell hyperplasia has also been seen in PAH, as has transitional cell (urothelial) metaplasia. Stromal alterations occur commonly in PAH and vary from smooth muscle atrophy to dense sclerosis[242] and elastosis.[244] In needle biopsy, lobules of PAH may be sampled nearly in toto or partially (Fig. 8-58). Without such lobularity, these crowded glands can be mistaken for adenocarcinoma (Fig. 8-59). PAH contains moderate to severe acute and chronic inflammatory cell infiltrates in about one-third of needle biopsy cases.[126] In the whole gland, PAH displays associated chronic inflammation in 43% to 88% of foci.[241,243]

Proliferative Atrophy/Proliferative Inflammatory Atrophy

PA and PIA refer to forms of atrophy with an increased proliferation index relative to normal epithelium. The use of these terms is currently considered optional.[236] Several of the above-discussed histologic types of atrophy, including

simple atrophy and PAH, can represent PA or PIA,[236] but this is difficult to ascertain in each individual case based on examination of H&E-stained sections alone, without performance of MIB-1 immunostaining.

PIA was originally forwarded as a regenerative lesion that was a potential precursor to PIN and carcinoma.[245] The hypothesis that carcinogenesis (and possibly atrophy) in the prostate might be related to oxidative damage secondary to inflammation[245,246] is intriguing and warrants further investigation. Diagnosis of isolated PA or PIA in prostate tissue from needle biopsy or transurethral resection has not been shown to be a risk factor for the subsequent detection of carcinoma of the prostate.

Ancillary and Special Studies in Atrophy

Immunohistochemical stains for basal cells and AMACR can be misleading when applied to foci of atrophy since the

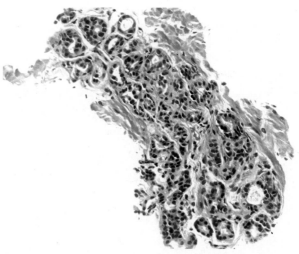

FIGURE 8-59 ■ Post-atrophic hyperplasia in small tissue fragment. This case had been misdiagnosed as adenocarcinoma.

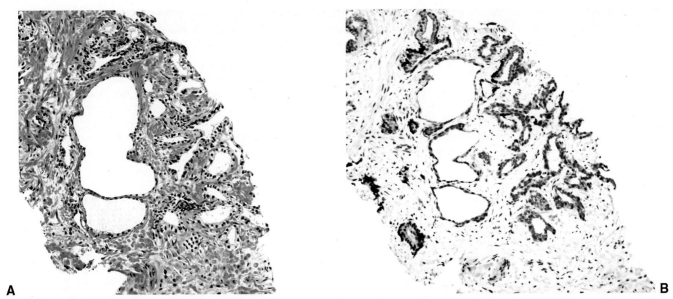

FIGURE 8-60 ■ Partial atrophy **(A)** with a fragmented to absent basal cell layer, as demonstrated by 34βE12/p63 cocktail immunohistochemical staining (*brown* chromogen) and AMACR overexpression (*red* chromogen) **(B)**.

immunoprofile can overlap with that of carcinoma. Specifically, atrophy often displays a patchy or fragmented basal cell layer and scattered atrophic glands can be completely negative for 34βE12 and p63 basal cell immunostains in 6% to 23% of cases[238–240,247,248] (Fig. 8-60). Also, AMACR can be positive in 4% of all atrophy cases[249] and 10% to 79% of partial atrophy cases.[26,238,239,248] In one study, a cocktail immunostain consisting of 34βE12, p63, and AMACR antibodies demonstrated a cancer-like immunoreactivity pattern (p63⁻, 34βE12⁻, AMACR⁺) in 24% of cases of partial atrophy (Fig. 8-60).[238]

Molecular and genetic abnormalities have been demonstrated in some cases of atrophy compared to nonatrophic benign prostatic epithelium, but none are used diagnostically. These abnormalities include reduced Nkx3.1[32] and p27Kip1[245] expression; overexpression of cyclooxygenase-2,[250] bcl-2,[245] GSTP1,[245] p53,[251] and p16[252]; gains of 8q24[253] and chromosome X[254]; and an increased proliferation index that is 2 to 11 times that of nonatrophic benign glands.[126,243,245,255] Gene expression profiling of atrophy has identified differentially expressed genes in atrophy compared to normal prostatic epithelium, PIN, and carcinoma,[256] including cytoglobin, which is a stress response hemoprotein, related to oxidative damage. Many of the above-cited molecular abnormalities have been found specifically in PA. TMPRSS2-ERG gene fusion, a common molecular abnormality in prostatic carcinoma, has not been identified in atrophy (PIA).[257]

Differential Diagnosis of Atrophy

The differential diagnosis of benign prostatic atrophy versus prostatic adenocarcinoma is one of the most important in diagnostic surgical pathology of the prostate. The differential distinction of prostatic atrophy and carcinoma should rely on a constellation of light microscopic findings

(Table 8-5). One should be cognizant, as noted above, of the diagnostic traps that exist with basal cell and AMACR immunostains. Finally, prostatic adenocarcinoma with atrophic features,[258] including atrophic and microcystic features,[259] is in the differential diagnosis with benign atrophy. Atrophic change can occur in both treated and untreated prostatic adenocarcinoma. The absence of infiltrative growth, macronucleoli, and nucleomegaly and the presence of basal cells are factors with the greatest power in diagnosing benign atrophy.[258] Cystic change can be seen in both benign atrophy and the uncommon microcystic adenocarcinoma of the prostate.[259]

Clinical Significance and Reporting of Atrophy

The histopathologic identification of atrophy in prostate needle core tissue is not associated with an increased risk of subsequent detection of prostate cancer,[260] so currently, reporting of atrophy in any prostatic tissue sample is not necessary.

Metaplasia

Metaplasia, or change in cell type, can affect benign prostatic epithelium or prostatic urethral urothelium. Metaplastic change is usually secondary to inflammation, alteration in the hormonal milieu, or injury. Metaplasia can also occur as a result of therapy, such as hormonal therapy, radiation therapy, TURP, and cryosurgery. Four major categories of prostatic glandular cell metaplasia are presented here: squamous cell metaplasia, urothelial metaplasia, mucinous metaplasia, and Paneth cell–like and eosinophilic metaplasia. The diagnostic significance of metaplasia resides in its pseudoneoplastic status. That is, it is possible to mistake some forms of metaplasia

Table 8-5 ■ DIFFERENTIAL DIAGNOSIS OF ATROPHY VERSUS ADENOCARCINOMA

Histologic Feature	Atrophy	Adenocarcinoma
Architecture	Lobular or disordered	Infiltrative (except for circumscribed, well-differentiated, Gleason score 2–4 carcinomas)
Low-power image	Clusters of dark, small, acini	Low grade[*]: aggregate of pale, small acini Intermediate grade[†]: haphazardly arranged single, separate small glands
Luminal cell nuclei	Typically slightly enlarged with small nucleoli	Nucleomegaly and nucleolomegaly
Luminal cell cytoplasm	Scanty to minimal, basophilic to cleared[‡]	Moderate amount, cleared to amphophilic
Apoptotic bodies	Rare	Present in one-third of cases
Basal cells		
H&E	Present, but may be inconspicuous	Absent
34βE12 and/or p63 IHC[§]	Usually continuous, occasionally fragmented, absent in scattered glands	Absent
Luminal contents		
Corpora amylacea	Common	Uncommon
Crystalloids	Rare	May be present
Wispy blue mucin	Rare	May be present
Stromal response		
Sclerosis	Present	Variable, usually absent
Inflammation	Common	Uncommon
AMACR[¶] IHC	Positive in a minority, especially partial atrophy	Positive in 90% of cases

[*]Low-grade carcinoma, well differentiated; Gleason score, 2–4.
[†]Intermediate-grade carcinoma, moderately differentiated; Gleason score, 5–6.
[‡]Cytoplasm is cleared in partial atrophy.
[§]IHC, immunohistochemistry.
[¶]AMACR, alpha methylacyl CoA racemase (P5045).

for neoplastic growth. These metaplastic proliferations are not precursors for prostatic carcinoma and do not constitute a risk factor for detection of carcinoma.

Squamous Cell Metaplasia

The most common clinical settings for the occurrence of squamous cell metaplasia in the nontreated prostate are prostatitis and BPH. Histologically, squamous cell metaplasia is most often an incidental finding associated with inflammation and infarction in BPH nodules. Inflammation and BPH, with or without infarction, can elevate serum PSA levels and prompt needle biopsy, leading to detection of squamous cell metaplasia. The incidence of squamous cell metaplasia varies from 5% to 94%, depending on the type of tissue sample and the clinical and histologic context.[261–269] The incidence in core needle biopsies is 5%,[249] and the highest incidence is in the setting of BPH with infarction, where the incidence varies from 37% to 94%.

Treatment generally produces a higher incidence of squamous cell metaplasia than in nontreated glands, with the exception of infarcts. Surgical, medical (androgen deprivation), and radiation treatments can all induce squamous cell metaplasia.[270–278] For patients who underwent repeat TURP for BPH, 52% had a squamous cell metaplastic epithelium in the second set of TURP chips,[278] and squamous cell metaplasia was noted in 21% to 23% of needle biopsies after cryosurgery.[271,275]

Squamous cell metaplastic epithelium in the prostate is not grossly evident.[278] Microscopically, the presence of small, solid nests with admixed inflammation is one low-magnification clue to the presence of squamous cell metaplasia. This is usually a focal finding unless the patient has been treated. Glands may be partially or completely involved by squamous cell metaplasia (Fig. 8-61). Sometimes only a small glandular lumen persists. The involved glands can be atrophic. At higher-power scrutiny, intercellular bridges

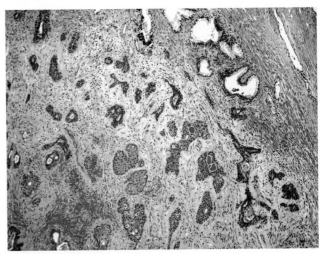

FIGURE 8-61 ■ Squamous metaplasia of the prostate with complete and partial gland involvement.

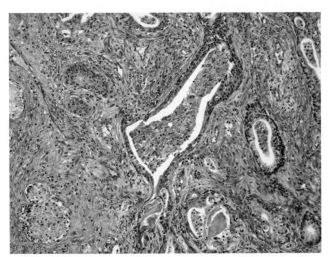

FIGURE 8-62 ■ Squamous metaplasia adjacent to prostatic infarct.

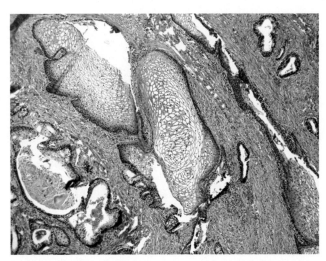

FIGURE 8-64 ■ Squamous metaplasia with glycogenated cytoplasm, postestrogen therapy.

and an eosinophilic, squamoid cytoplasm are indicators of squamous cell metaplasia. So-called immature squamous cell metaplasia has much less squamoid cytoplasm. Keratin pearls can be found but are unusual.[278] Squamous cell metaplasia can also be found lining large, central prostatic ducts containing stones and cellular debris.

Squamous cell metaplasia associated with infarcts is first seen at about 4 days as a reactive rim immediately adjacent to infarcted hyperplasic tissue. Here the metaplastic epithelium is arranged as irregularly shaped, solid islands, partially involved glands, nests with central degenerated cells, and distorted groups (Fig. 8-62). The cells are polygonal and often pavemented, with distinct intercellular borders. The cytoplasm is acidophilic or vacuolated, with large nuclei. True macronucleoli can be seen (Fig. 8-63), along with squamous cell cytologic atypia and mitotic figures. With healing, the necrotic tissue is replaced by fibrous tissue, which can contain persistent solid or acinar nests of metaplastic cells.[265]

Squamous cell metaplasia induced by radiation and hormonal therapy is often of the immature type,[277,279] with less abundant, nonglycogenated cytoplasm, larger nuclei, and absence of keratinization. An exception to this is use of estrogen as hormonal therapy (a common form of prostate cancer therapy in the past), which can cause diffuse squamous cell metaplasia with glycogenated cytoplasm and small, shrunken nuclei (Fig. 8-64).[266,270] Prostatic urethral urothelium and prostatic ducts and acini can all be involved by such glycogenated mature squamous cell metaplasia. Previous needle biopsy can induce a squamous cell metaplastic response in glands entrapped or immediately adjacent to the fibrous needle track (Box 8-4).

The differential diagnosis of squamous cell metaplasia centers on carcinoma, and mainly squamous cell carcinoma. Squamous cell carcinoma does occur in the prostate, but it is rare and should be diagnosed with caution. Diagnostic difficulties arise if reactive, metaplastic squamous epithelium is viewed out of context. Therefore, if inflammation or an adjacent infarct is ignored and reactive, metaplastic squamous epithelium is studied at high-power magnification, the reactive, nuclear atypia could be misinterpreted as evidence of malignancy. Architecturally, the nests of metaplastic squamous epithelium adjacent to infarcts or TURP sites may appear to be arranged in a disordered way (Fig. 8-65), but infiltration into tissue surrounding the reactive rim does not

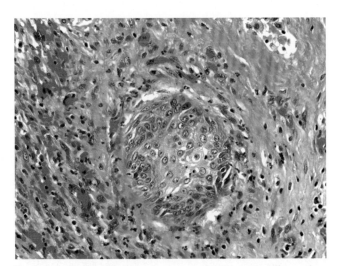

FIGURE 8-63 ■ Squamous metaplasia nest with nuclear atypia, next to infarct.

Box 8-4 ● CAUSES OF SQUAMOUS METAPLASIA IN THE PROSTATE
Inflammation
Infarction
Post-biopsy/transurethral resection
Radiation therapy
Cryosurgery
Androgen deprivation therapy

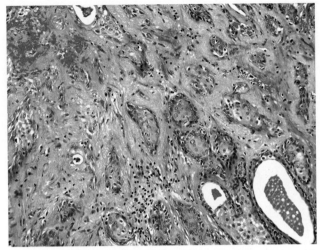

FIGURE 8-65 ■ Squamous metaplasia in fibrotic stroma, with pseudoinfiltrative appearance, adjacent to a previous TURP site.

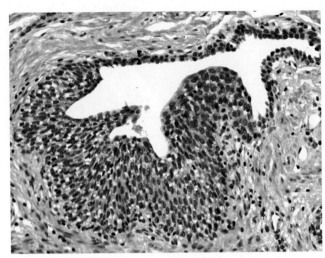

FIGURE 8-66 ■ Urothelial metaplasia with partial gland involvement.

occur.[265] Also, the individual metaplastic cells do not show anaplasia, hyperchromatism, or abnormal mitotic figures.[265] Prominent nucleoli in this situation should not be misconstrued as evidence of malignancy. In the framework of treatment effect, there is even a greater diagnostic conundrum because glandular disarray, squamous epithelial cell cytologic atypia, and fibrosis can be found. For example, interpretation of prostate needle biopsies after radiation therapy can be difficult because almost every case with squamous cell metaplasia had cytologic atypia.[272] Immunohistohemical evaluation using 34βE12 and AMACR immunostains[276,280,281] can be invaluable in difficult cases to confirm the presence of immature squamous cell metaplasia in these patients after radiation treatment. Other special studies are not of diagnostic relevance.

Urothelial Metaplasia

Urothelial cells normally line the prostatic urethra and extend for a variable distance into the main prostatic ducts.[233] Because of this variability, there can be difficulty in determining whether a urothelial proliferation represents a variation of normal anatomy or a metaplastic process. There is a wide variation in the reported incidence of transitional cell metaplasia, from 3% to 34%.[273,282,283] The development of urothelial metaplasia may be related to epithelial damage or androgen deprivation because about one-third of cases are associated with inflammation,[283] and urothelial metaplasia has been detected adjacent to infarcts,[265] after cryosurgery,[271] and after androgen deprivation hormonal therapy.[273] No clinical or radiologic findings are specific for urothelial metaplasia. It is usually a focal, incidental histologic finding. It has a low proliferation index of 0.3%[282] and no premalignant potential.

Histologically, usually only a few glands are involved in a single focus, but extent ranges from partial gland involvement (Fig. 8-66) to more florid gland involvement (Fig. 8-67). At low magnification the glands stand out because they

are hypercellular and appear dark. Small, solid nests are commonly noted, but often there is preservation of a small central lumen (Fig. 8-68). The glands exhibit proliferation of elongated cells beneath a bland-appearing luminal secretory cell layer. The nuclei are elongated and are arranged perpendicular to the basal membrane. Because of the elongation and stratification, the cells can appear to stream toward the luminal surface. At high power, the elongated nuclei have frequent nuclear grooves, and the faint eosinophilic cytoplasm exhibits frequent perinuclear clearing.[283] The nuclei are cytologically small and bland, with inconspicuous nucleoli and little to no mitotic activity.

The most important entity in the differential diagnosis is PIN. High-grade PIN does not, in contrast, exhibit solid cell nests, and does show appreciable nuclear atypia. The other neoplastic proliferation in the differential diagnosis is urothelial carcinoma, but most urothelial carcinomas that involve the prostate are cytologically high-grade and are unlikely to

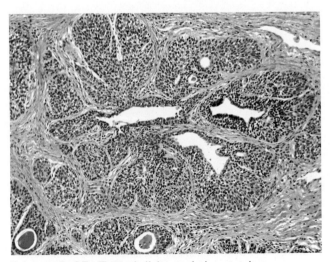

FIGURE 8-67 ■ Urothelial metaplasia, extensive.

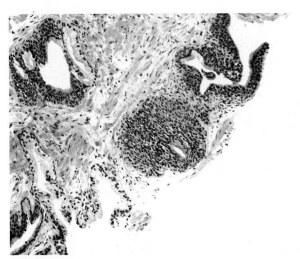

FIGURE 8-68 ■ Urothelial metaplasia, with partial gland involvement. One gland shows preservation of a small central lumen lined by secretory cells.

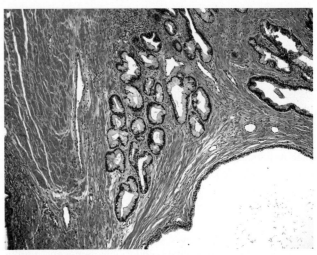

FIGURE 8-69 ■ Mucinous metaplasia in a small cluster of glands.

be mistaken for urothelial metaplasia. Basal cell hyperplasia and squamous cell metaplasia could also be confused with transitional cell metaplasia, but basal cell hyperplasia nuclei are typified by a rounded profile and lack nuclear grooves. The cells of squamous cell metaplasia can have distinct intercellular borders, as do the cells in urothelial metaplasia, but in squamous cell metaplasia there are intercellular bridges, and the cells have a more densely eosinophilic cytoplasm without perinuclear clearing. On occasion, urothelial metaplasia can merge with squamous cell metaplasia or basal cell hyperplasia. Special studies are not indicated in the evaluation of transitional cell metaplasia.

Mucinous Metaplasia

Mucinous metaplasia, which has also been called mucous gland metaplasia, may be defined as the replacement of usual benign luminal epithelium by benign mucin-secreting cells.[284–287] This alteration most often refers to cellular changes detected with H&E-stained sections, but some have used histochemical staining for intracytoplasmic mucin to define mucinous metaplasia.[284] Mucin production by benign prostatic luminal epithelial cells is common when histochemical methods are used to detect it.[288,289] This mucin is predominantly neutral and can be highlighted with a PAS stain, with prior diastase digestion. Mucinous metaplasia is uncommon in benign glands by H&E staining, with an incidence of 1% to 8%.[285–287] No specific clinical or radiologic features are associated with mucinous metaplasia. Mucinous metaplasia has no known premalignant potential. Mucinous PIN and mucinous carcinoma of the prostate do not have a reported association with mucinous metaplasia.[290,291] Finally, mucinous metaplasia occurred with equal frequency in needle biopsies with and without carcinoma,[286] and this also points to a lack of association with malignancy.

Mucinous metaplasia is a focal, incidental histologic finding. It can be located centrally or peripherally.[287]

Microscopically, the metaplastic cells are grouped in clusters of 5 to 10 (Fig. 8-69), although occasionally individual, isolated glands or cells can be found.[266] Rare foci are extensive, with only a few examples >1 mm². The constituent cells are cuboidal to tall and columnar, with a cytoplasm filled with bluish mucin (Fig. 8-70). A suggestion of goblet cell–like vacuolization may be seen in a few cells, but mostly the cytoplasm has a diffuse granular blue character. Rarely, this mucin is released into the glandular lumen. The nuclei of the metaplastic cells are small, dark, and basally situated. Mucinous metaplasia is most often found in a background of atrophy, including both sclerotic and PAH types, urothelial metaplasia, usual epithelial hyperplasia, and basal cell hyperplasia. Basal cells usually are seen easily, although difficulty may arise because of the basal distribution of the nuclei of the metaplastic cells.

Special stains are not usually needed to diagnose mucinous metaplasia. The mucin is of mixed neutral and acidic types,

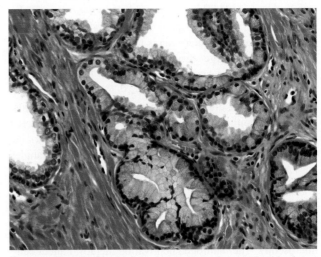

FIGURE 8-70 ■ Mucinous metaplasia characterized by intracytoplasmic mucin granules.

as indicated by positive PAS and Alcian blue (pH 2.5) stains, respectively. These mucinous cells are nonreactive, using antibodies directed against PSA and PSAP.[284,285,287] An intact basal cell layer can be confirmed by 34βE12 or p63 immunostains.

The entity of greatest import in the differential diagnosis is adenocarcinoma, although intracytoplasmic mucin, as identified on H&E staining, is rare in prostatic adenocarcinoma. Mucinous adenocarcinoma is not in the differential diagnosis because a substantial volume (at least 25%) of such tumors is made up of extracellular lakes of mucin with embedded tumor cells. Extracellular, stromal-based lakes of mucin are not seen in mucinous metaplasia. Mucinous high-grade PIN is not a prominent consideration because the mucin in these glands is intraluminal rather than intracytoplasmic,[271] and because the high-grade PIN nuclei are atypical, with nucleomegaly and nucleolomegaly, unlike mucinous metaplasia. Finally, the epithelium that mucinous metaplasia most resembles is that of Cowper glands, which differ in being mucinous glands in a complete lobule, often with a central feeder duct and surrounding skeletal muscle. Cowper glands are not seen against a background of hyperplasia, atrophy, or urothelial metaplasia, as mucinous metaplasia can be. The lectin-binding profile of mucinous metaplasia differs from that of Cowper glands,[287] but such lectin histochemical stains are not needed because this differential is best addressed with H&E-stained sections.

Eosinophilic Metaplasia and Paneth Cell–Like Change

This cellular alteration is characterized by the presence of large, cytoplasmic, eosinophilic granules. This cytoplasmic granularity seems to result from several different processes. It has been proposed that the basis for this morphologic appearance may depend on the nature of epithelial proliferation.[292–300] Thus, in benign epithelium it may be caused by exocrine differentiation with lysosome-like granules,[24,297,299] whereas in PIN and carcinoma the granules appear to reflect neuroendocrine differentiation.[292,293,300] Accordingly, for Paneth cell–like change in prostatic adenocarcinoma, the name "neuroendocrine cells with large eosinophilic granules" has been proposed. Eosinophilic metaplasia is the designation for benign epithelium with large eosinophilic granules (Fig. 8-71).[299] The incidence of eosinophilic granules in benign prostatic epithelium ranges from 0% to 23%.[24,255,301] These supranuclear eosinophilic granules are more commonly seen in prostatic ductal epithelium than in acinar epithelium. Epithelial involvement is usually focal and is associated with variable degrees of chronic inflammation and atrophy.[301] The granules are PAS positive, diastase-resistant, and immunopositive for PSA, PSAP, lysozyme, and α-1 antichymotrypsin while failing to stain for chromogranin, serotonin, and neuron-specific enolase by immunohistochemistry. Exocrine-like granules 400 to 690 nm in diameter have been observed by electron microscopy. After androgen deprivation therapy, Paneth cell–like change is uncommon,[273] whereas these cells were found

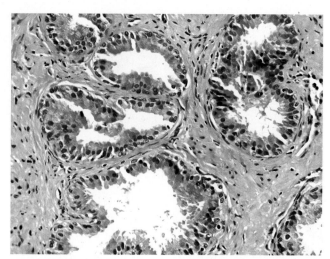

FIGURE 8-71 ■ Eosinophilic metaplasia in benign glands with intracytoplasmic brightly eosinophilic granules.

in 32% of postradiation biopsies and were always found in benign epithelium.[295,302] In the latter posttherapy setting, this cellular change indicates neuroendocrine differentiation rather than exocrine secretory granules because almost all cells are chromogranin positive and lysozyme negative in immunohistochemistry.

The differential diagnosis of eosinophilic granules in benign prostatic epithelium centers on the distinction from high-grade PIN and adenocarcinoma with neuroendocrine cells with large eosinophilic granules. The granules are seen in 15% of prostatic adenocarcinomas.[292] This intracytoplasmic pigment should also be distinguished from other prostatic cytoplasmic inclusions, such as lipofuscin pigment and viral inclusions.

Nephrogenic Adenoma

Nephrogenic adenoma is a benign lesion of the urinary tract that occurs in a setting of damage to the urothelium such as that secondary to surgery, trauma, mechanical irritation, inflammation, and calculi.[303] For a long time it was considered a metaplasia of urothelium, although more recently it has been shown that, at least for transplant patients, the constituent cells originated from detached renal tubular epithelial cells that implanted at sites of urinary tract injury.[304] Nephrogenic metaplasia/adenoma is most common in the urinary bladder, with 4% of all cases found in the prostatic urethra.[305] About 70 cases of nephrogenic metaplasia/adenoma in the prostatic urethra have been reported.[306–309] It is discussed in this chapter since nephrogenic adenoma arising in the prostatic urethra extends into smooth muscle and the prostate in 60% of cases.[306]

Typically, men in their 60s or 70s (range 44 to 79) present 1.5 to 10 years after TURP with hematuria and urinary obstruction.[306] At cystoscopy/urethroscopy papillary urethral lesions can be visualized. In other cases nephrogenic adenoma is an incidental finding. The lesions tend to be

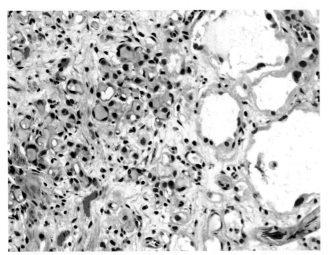

Figure 8-72 ■ Nephrogenic adenoma of prostatic urethra with small tubules containing intraluminal blue mucin.

small with a mean size of 3 mm (range 1 to 9 mm)[310]; rarely they are quite large, with one lesion measuring 7.8 cm.[311] Microscopically, the classical patterns of growth are tubular (Fig. 8-72), tubulocystic, and papillary/polypoid.[303] In the prostatic urethra the most common pattern is tubular, followed by a vascular-like pattern.[310] The tubules are usually small, solid to hollow and are lined by cuboidal epithelium with eosinophilic to cleared cytoplasm. There may be intraluminal eosinophilic secretions imparting a thyroid-like look ("thyroidization") and intraluminal blue mucin (Fig. 8-72). Thick hyalinized peritubular sheaths may be noted. Cells lining the vessel-like spaces may be flattened or assume a hobnail appearance. Additional arrangements include cords, papillary/polypoid configurations, and single cells, with rare signet ring–like cells seen.[310] Nuclear atypia may be evident and is usually of the degenerative type, with smudged chromatin, although prominent nucleoli may be focally present in a subset of cases. Mitotic activity is absent.

Immunohistochemical stains may be diagnostically misleading due to a degree of immunophenotypic overlap with adenocarcinoma of the prostate.[26] Specifically, basal cell markers may be absent in nephrogenic metaplasia/adenoma, especially with p63 immunostains. 34βE12 immunoreactivity is variable and is absent in about one-half of cases. Another pitfall is that nephrogenic adenoma expresses AMACR in a majority of cases.[309,312,313] So, nephrogenic metaplasia/adenoma presenting as small tubules in the prostate, with negative basal cell/positive AMACR immunostains, may be misdiagnosed as acinar adenocarcinoma of the prostate. The most useful immunostains are those with antibodies directed against PSA, PSAP, PAX2, PAX8, and S-1001A. Expression of PSA and PSAP is lacking or is weak in nephrogenic adenoma, while gland-forming adenocarcinomas are characteristically positive. S-100A1 immunoreactivity is found in 78% of nephrogenic adenoma cases, and

is absent in prostatic adenocarcinoma.[314] PAX2 and PAX8 proteins are sensitive and specific markers for nephrogenic adenoma in the differential diagnosis with adenocarcinoma of the prostate: a nuclear signal is seen in all cases of nephrogenic adenoma and is negative in adenocarcinoma of the prostate.[307,315,316] Additional markers positive in nephrogenic adenoma include pan-cytokeratin, cytokeratin 7, epithelial membrane antigen, and CA-125. Uroplakin immunostains are negative.

The most important differential diagnostic consideration for nephrogenic adenoma in the prostatic parenchyma is prostatic adenocarcinoma, as just discussed. Intraprostatic extension of urethral clear cell carcinoma and the nested variant of urothelial carcinoma, with or without tubule formation, should also be entertained.[303]

Stromal Metaplasia

There is a single case report of cartilaginous stromal metaplasia.[317] This 69-year-old man had hematuria, was clinically diagnosed with BPH, and underwent TURP. Microscopically, glandular and stromal hyperplasia and "a few foci of well-differentiated adenocarcinoma" were identified. Benign cartilaginous stroma in transition with benign fibrous tissue was noted. Other forms of mesenchymal metaplasia are not known to occur. It is not known if adipocytes in the prostate parenchyma, a rare finding (see above section on normal microanatomy of prostatic stroma), represent metaplasia, a malformation, or a variation of normal anatomy.

Hyperplasia

Benign Prostatic Hyperplasia

Definition and Incidence

Nodular hyperplasia (BPH) is one of the most common diseases to affect men. Precisely how common depends on the definition used for BPH. One way to classify BPH is a microscopic BPH, macroscopic BPH, and clinical BPH.[318–320] In this conceptual framework, microscopic BPH is the histologic diagnosis of usual glandular and/or stromal hyperplasia. Macroscopic BPH describes an enlarged prostate, which can be detected by DRE or by radiologic means, usually transrectal ultrasonography (TRUS) or, less commonly, magnetic resonance imaging. Clinical BPH is a diagnosis based on urinary tract symptoms and bladder dysfunction.[318,319] It is important to note that BPH contributes to, but is not the sole cause of, lower urinary tract symptoms.[319] In fact, the clinical diagnosis of BPH is often made by a combination of assessments for macroscopic and clinical BPH, which includes evaluation of prostate size, urinary symptoms, and reduced urinary flow rate.[319] The diagnosis of BPH is a clinical one. A histologic diagnosis of BPH is not needed for treatment.

Histologic evidence of BPH at autopsy is found in a majority of men over 60 years of age.[264] This proliferative process is strongly related to age, with only a few percent of men under 40 having histologic BPH, whereas almost all men (88%) over 80 have histologic BPH.[264,321] The prevalence of histologic BPH at autopsy is the same in different countries around the world.[318]

BPH is a common clinical diagnosis,[319] with the prevalence dependent on the clinical criteria used. Some studies have used only symptoms in its definition, whereas other studies have included prostate size or urinary flow rates. To assess symptom severity and frequency the American Urological Association International Prostate Symptom Score, which is based on a self-administered questionnaire, is frequently used.[319,322] Bother and interference with daily quality of life are also important clinical considerations.[319]

Etiology and Epidemiology

Established etiologic risk factors for BPH are aging and an intact androgen axis.[319,320,323] Patients castrated before puberty do not develop BPH. The role of androgens in the development of BPH is felt to be permissive rather than directly causative. Another risk factor for BPH is a positive family history, indicative of an inheritable genetic basis, with an autosomal dominant mode of inheritance.[324–326] As is common with inherited disease, hereditary BPH tends to strike younger patients: It is estimated that about 50% of men under 60 years of age who undergo surgery (prostatectomy) for BPH could have hereditary BPH, whereas only about 9% of men over 60 with BPH have the inherited form of the disease.[326] Men with hereditary BPH have larger prostate glands, with a mean volume of 83 cm^3, compared with a mean volume of 56 cm^3 for men with sporadic BPH.[326] The gene (or, more likely, genes) responsible for hereditary BPH have not been identified. Smoking, alcohol intake, vasectomy, and sexual activity have little or no association with BPH.[319,320] Histologically, hereditary BPH exhibits a higher stromal–epithelial ratio than sporadic BPH nodules.[325]

The molecular pathogenesis of BPH has not been fully elucidated, but epithelial–stromal cellular interactions and various growth-promoting molecules, including androgens, estrogens, and polypeptide growth factors, are probably involved.[319] Because BPH is a benign increase in cell number, it fundamentally must represent an imbalance between cell proliferation and cell death. Therefore, it is probably a combination of growth promotion and impaired programmed cell death (apoptosis) that leads to BPH. Gene expression profiling has identified hundreds of genes up-regulated or down-regulated in BPH compared to normal prostatic tissue.[327] Despite these perturbations of normal growth pathways, BPH is not a risk factor for development of carcinoma.

Clinical Presentation

Patients with BPH present with symptoms often called prostatism, which can be separated into obstructive and irritative symptoms. Obstructive symptoms include hesitancy, postvoid dribbling, sensation of incomplete bladder emptying, and urinary retention. Irritative symptoms include frequency, urgency, nocturia, urge incontinence, and dysuria.[328,329] Symptoms of prostatism are not specific for BPH, and other diseases must be ruled out in the workup for BPH. For example, urinary tract infections and bladder cancer may produce symptoms such as frequency and urgency that mimic BPH. Other diseases that can clinically simulate BPH include urethral stricture, bladder neck contracture, bladder calculus, and neurogenic bladder.[328] Prostate size and histologic BPH presence correlate poorly with the degree of obstruction and these clinical symptoms.[319,328]

Treatment

Treatment options for patients with BPH include watchful waiting, medical therapy (including but not limited to α-adrenergic receptor blockers and 5α-reductase inhibitors),[330] and minimally invasive therapies such as high-intensity focused ultrasound, laser therapy, transurethral balloon dilatation thermotherapy, transurethral electrovaporization, intraurethral stents, and transurethral needle ablation of the prostate.[319] Surgical therapy includes TURP and open (simple) prostatectomy.[319]

Usual Nodular Epithelial and Stromal Hyperplasia

This type of prostatic hyperplasia typically forms BPH nodules. Usual prostatic hyperplasia can be diagnosed in all types of prostatic tissue samples, but its recognition is most straightforward in tissue samples larger than the needle core biopsy. Hyperplasia is actually uncommon in prostatic needle biopsy because the zone of origin of BPH—the transition zone—is usually not biopsied and because hyperplasia is uncommon in the peripheral zone, which is targeted. Histopathologists should not diagnose hyperplasia when benign, complex glands are appreciated in a needle biopsy since normal glands also have this appearance. Also, it is not possible to recognize the nodularity of BPH glands in needle biopsy. Finally, it is not necessary to diagnose usual prostatic hyperplasia in needle biopsy because treatment of BPH is driven by the clinical diagnosis.

Grossly, nodule formation is the hallmark of usual prostatic hyperplasia. Such nodularity can be seen in TURP chips, simple prostatectomy specimens, and whole glands (from radical prostatectomy, cystoprostatectomy, and autopsy specimens) but not needle biopsies. In TURP chips, most nodules (more than 80%) are <4 mm in diameter, whereas in simple prostatectomies (enucleations), most nodules are >4 mm (Fig. 8-73).[331] In the whole gland, most nodules are found in the transition zone or periurethral areas, with peripheral zone hyperplastic nodules detected in 0.1% to 19% of prostate.[264,332–335] Periurethral and peripheral zone hyperplastic nodules tend to be smaller than the transition zone nodules.[264,332,333] Transition zone and periurethral area nodules are typically multiple, whereas peripheral zone nodules are usually solitary.[332,336] The number and size of

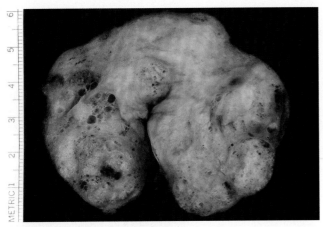

FIGURE 8-73 ■ BPH nodules in a simple prostatectomy specimen. Solid and cystic features are evident.

Box 8-5 ● HISTOLOGIC VARIANTS OF PROSTATIC HYPERPLASIA

Usual patterns
  Glandular
  Stromal
    Leiomyomatous
    Leiomyomatous with symplastic atypia
    Myxoid
  Mixed glandular and stromal
    Fibroadenomatous nodule
Special patterns
  Basal cell hyperplasia
  Cribriform clear cell hyperplasia

hyperplastic nodules increases with age,[21,336] with the greatest number of large nodules found in men over 60 years of age. Transition zone nodules exhibit expansile growth, and larger ones in the transition zone can compress the urethra and peripheral zone. In the periurethral zone, the nodules are randomly scattered along the length of the proximal segment of the urethra, with extension to the bladder neck. When these proximal periurethral nodules become significantly enlarged, the mass can project into the bladder as an enlarged median or middle lobe (Fig. 8-74), which can obstruct the urethra in a ball-and-valve–like fashion. Peripheral zone nodules can produce a subcapsular bulge that can simulate carcinoma by DRE and TRUS. The gross appearance and texture of the nodules depend on the histologic cellular composition. Periurethral nodules made up of pure stromal cells are round, elliptical, dense, white nodules with a suggestion of a fibrillary or whorled cut surface.[264] The whorled look is reminiscent of a leiomyoma. Mixed glandular and stromal nodules may be hard or soft; the more epithelial ones can seem spongy with cystic change (Fig. 8-73).

Microscopically, usual prostatic hyperplasia is a proliferation of either pure stromal cells or epithelial and stromal cells (Box 8-5). Pure stromal cell hyperplasias may be either nodular or diffuse.[21,331] Stromal cell nodules, which are thought to represent the first signs of BPH, are found predominantly in suburothelial tissues above the distal region of the verumontanum but have also been reported in the central zone, and a few examples have been found in the peripheral zone.[337] They are characterized by a well-circumscribed mass of spindled to star-shaped cells embedded in a myxoid (Fig. 8-75) or, more commonly, hyalinized matrix (Fig. 8-76). The spindled cells in the more hyalinized nodules can be arranged in bundles or whorls. Some cells have a denser, more eosinophilic cytoplasm. There is a prominent vasculature that is made up of capillaries in the myxoid nodules and thick-walled vessels in the more hyalinized form. Singly dispersed mature, small lymphocytes (which are mainly T lymphocytes) are common in stromal nodules. Cytologic atypia and mitoses are lacking.[337] Rare cases may show focal symplastic, degenerative-type nuclear atypia with enlarged nuclei displaying smudged

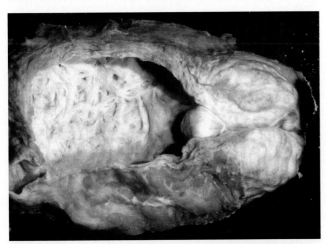

FIGURE 8-74 ■ BPH with prominent median lobe protruding into urinary bladder. (Reprinted from Royal College of Surgeons of England Slide Atlas of Pathology, 1985, slide 100.)

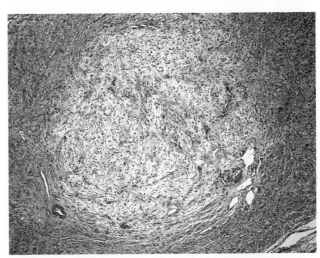

FIGURE 8-75 ■ Stromal hyperplasia in periurethral zone, with myxoid matrix.

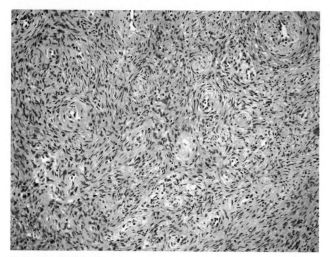

FIGURE 8-76 ■ Stromal hyperplasia in periurethral zone, with sclerotic stroma and prominent blood vessels.

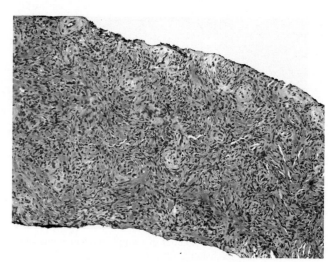

FIGURE 8-78 ■ Stromal hyperplasia in needle core tissue.

chromatin. Another rare finding in stromal nodules is the presence of signet ring cell change in stromal cells.[338] These signet ring stromal cells are likely myofibroblasts, based on the immunohistochemical profile of vimentin positive and weak desmin positivity, with negative immunostains for PSA and PSAP. Stromal nodules have been classified as fibrous or fibrovascular, fibromuscular, and muscular[21] or as fibroblastic, fibromuscular, smooth muscular, and immature mesenchymal.[337] Another classification is leiomyomatous (Fig. 8-77), leiomyomatous with symplastic change, and myxoid pattern (Fig. 8-75). This ordering is not diagnostically necessary but rather speaks to mesenchymal cell types that are part of these nodules. Diffuse stromal hyperplasia is less common than the nodular form and is distinguished from stromal nodules only by being larger and having a border that merges gradually with surrounding normal smooth muscle stroma. Stromal hyperplasia can be seen in needle biopsies (Fig. 8-78).

Glandular nodules, which are a variable mixture of epithelial and stromal hyperplastic cells, are usually found in the transition zone but can also be seen in the periurethral area, central zone, and peripheral zone (Fig. 8-79). The smallest or earliest growths can be difficult to identify because there is only an increased density of small glands with little in the way of an expansile border.

Larger and better-developed glandular nodules are readily appreciated at scanning magnification (Fig. 8-80). The variable amount of hyperplastic epithelium and stroma can also be noted at this level of examination. Epithelial-predominant nodules (Fig. 8-80) have an epithelial–stromal ratio of about 2:1, whereas for stromal predominant nodules the ratio is reversed at 1:2 (Fig. 8-81).[331] The epithelial hyperplasia in glandular nodules is typified by a complex, branching arrangement of glands.[339] Variable size and shape of glands, with complexity, true papillary projections, luminal undulations, and branching are all emblems of epithelial hyperplasia in the prostate (Figs. 8-82 and 8-83). Smaller glands may be seen (Fig. 8-84) but when they are abundant one should consider a diagnosis of AAH (see below section on Atypical

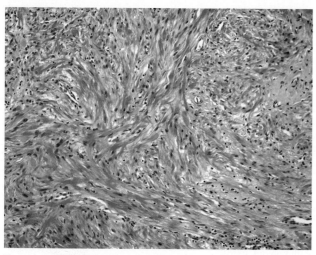

FIGURE 8-77 ■ Stromal hyperplasia of leiomyomatous type.

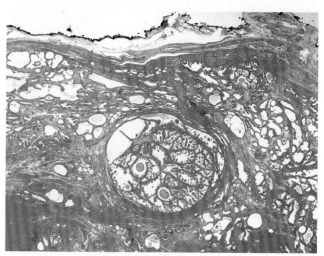

FIGURE 8-79 ■ Small BPH nodule in peripheral zone.

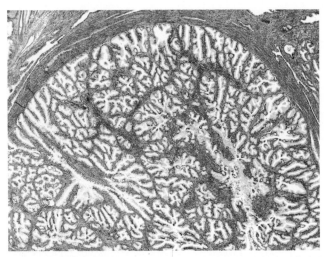

FIGURE 8-80 ■ Nodular glandular and stromal hyperplasia, with predominance of epithelium.

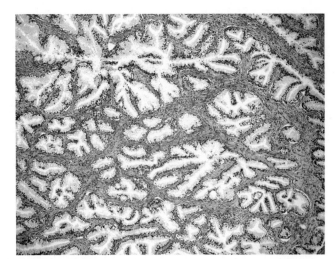

FIGURE 8-82 ■ Hyperplastic nodule with typical glandular complexity.

Adenomatous Hyperplasia), especially if the small acini are rounded without luminal complexity. The constituent epithelial cells of the glandular hyperplastic nodule include high columnar luminal cells and basal cells. In cystically dilated glands, the lining can be flattened and atrophic (Fig. 8-85). Basal cells are readily detected in hyperplastic nodules, and not uncommonly this epithelial population also shows hyperplasia (see below section on Basal Cell Hyperplasia). Mitotic figures and apoptotic bodies in the hyperplastic luminal and basal cells are exceedingly rare. The luminal contents of hyperplastic glands include shed epithelial cells and corpora amylacea, while intraluminal findings such as crystalloids and wisp blue mucin are rare. The appearance of stroma in glandular hyperplastic nodules varies from narrow smooth muscle bands between glands to broad bands to most of the nodules being composed of bland spindled cells similar to those in stromal nodules.

It is not necessary for diagnostic purposes to subtype the glandular hyperplastic nodules. One scheme[21] uses the terms

fibromyoepithelial nodule and fibroadenomatous nodule. Foci resembling the mammary fibroadenoma do occur within the spectrum of nodular prostatic hyperplasia (Fig. 8-86), but this is uncommon, with an incidence of 1%.[340]

Secondary histologic alterations in hyperplastic nodules include cystic change, inflammation, duct or acinar rupture, squamous cell metaplasia, and infarction. Cystic glandular dilatation is common in BPH (Fig. 8-73). As noted, the epithelial lining of the cysts is often flattened, with an atrophic appearance (Fig. 8-85). Inflammation is also common in BPH. The mixed inflammatory cell infiltrate includes T lymphocytes (in 81% of cases), B lymphocytes (in 52% of cases), and macrophages (in 82% of cases).[341] Duct or acinar expansion by inflammatory exudate can be associated with this inflammatory infiltrate (Fig. 8-87). Squamous cell metaplasia can be found in inflamed or infarcted BPH areas.

Infarction is a reasonably common histologic finding in large BPH tissue samples (TURP chips, simple prostatectomy specimens, and whole glands from autopsy), with an

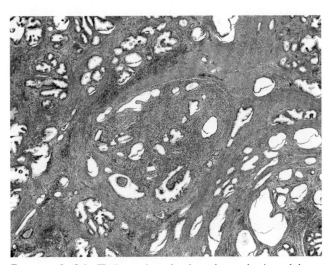

FIGURE 8-81 ■ Stromal-predominant hyperplastic nodule.

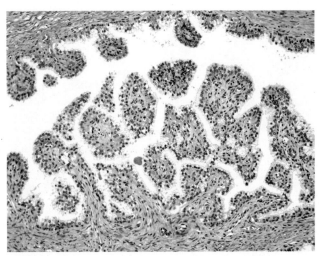

FIGURE 8-83 ■ Papillary structures in hyperplasia.

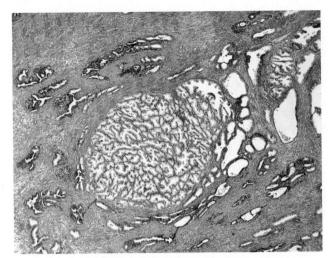

FIGURE 8-84 ■ Epithelial-predominant hyperplastic nodule comprising smaller glands.

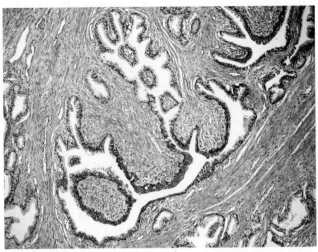

FIGURE 8-86 ■ Fibroadenomatous features in a hyperplastic nodule.

overall incidence of 18% (451 of 2,563 cases), with a range of 3% to 85%.[261,264,267,268] However, infarcts are rarely identified in needle biopsy tissue,[301] mainly because the transition zone, where BPH arises, typically is not targeted by needle biopsy. Infarction is clinically associated with acute urinary retention, gross hematuria, advanced patient age, and large volume BPH.[261,342] Clinically, infarcts can mimic prostate cancer because they can present (rarely) as a palpable nodule or be associated with an elevated serum PSA,[343,344] which can range from 6.9 ng/mL to 287 ng/mL, the latter level often being associated with metastatic prostate carcinoma. Grossly, prostatic infarcts in BPH appear bright and red to mottled, dull, reddish-brown or gray, and round to oval (Fig. 8-88). They can be single or multiple and measure up to several centimeters in diameter.[261] Microscopically, the appearance depends on the age of the infarct.[268] Coagulative necrosis, with a ghost-like outline of hyperplastic glands, is typical (Fig. 8-89). During the first 1 to 2 days, neutrophilic

infiltrates are minimal. By day 4 neutrophilic infiltrates, stromal edema, and parenchymal necrosis are maximal.[268] Hemorrhage and squamous cell metaplasia are common in the border zone between necrotic and viable tissue. Hemorrhagic infarcts can also be seen. Repair takes place during the third to 6th week, with the only residue being squamous cell metaplasia, lymphocytes, and fibrosis.[264,268]

The differential diagnosis of usual prostatic hyperplasia can be divided into stromal-based and epithelial-based lists. For stromal hyperplasia of the prostate, the main differential diagnostic considerations are bland spindle cells in normal, reactive, and reparative prostatic stroma, benign mesenchymal neoplasms such as leiomyoma and neurofibroma (both rare), postoperative spindle cell nodule/ inflammatory myofibroblastic tumor (IMT), stromal tumors of uncertain malignant potential (STUMP), prostatic sarcomas, and the spindle cell component of homologous sarcomatoid carcinomas. Reactive or reparative spindled granulation tissue, fibrosis,

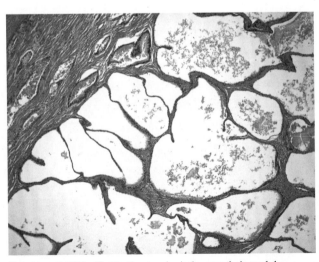

FIGURE 8-85 ■ Cystic atrophy in hyperpalstic nodule.

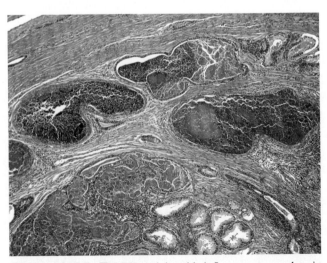

FIGURE 8-87 ■ BPH nodule with inflammatory exudate in dilated glands.

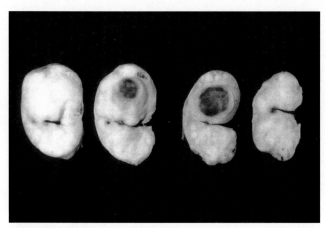

FIGURE 8-88 ■ Infarct in hyperplasia. (Reprinted from Royal College of Surgeons of England Slide Atlas of Pathology, 1985, slide 99.)

and postoperative spindle cell nodules could mimic prostatic stromal hyperplasia, but the former two entities are not usually nodular. Cases diagnosed as leiomyoma of the prostate probably represent the leiomyomatous variant of nodular stromal hyperplasia. Myxoid neurofibroma could be simulate myxoid stromal nodules but these are exceedingly rare in the prostate. Postoperative spindle cell nodules and IMT of the prostate, also known as pseudosarcomatous fibromyxoid tumor, are probably the same entity and may be neoplastic.[345] This pseudosarcomatous myofibroblastic proliferation can involve the prostate but differs from stromal hyperplasia in having a background of granulation tissue-like vascularity, with inflammation.[346] Some cases of pseudosarcomatous myofibroblastic proliferation can show hypercellular areas with fascicular growth, infiltration, and necrosis, unlike prostatic stromal hyperplasia. STUMPs with scattered degenerative-appearing nuclei with smudged chromatin and mutlinucleation that are found between benign glands[347] have also been termed stromal hyperplasia with atypia.[348] STUMPS are considered neoplasms,[347] although it has also been suggested

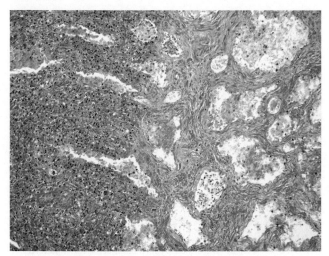

FIGURE 8-89 ■ Infarcted hyperplastic nodule.

that those cases with the dispersed degenerative nuclei are a variant of usual hyperplasia[349] or a reactive or degenerative process occurring in association with usual stromal hyperplasia.[348] In needle biopsy of myxoid stromal proliferations, prominent round vessels and chronic inflammation argue for myxoid pattern of usual stromal hyperplasia rather than myxoid STUMP.[350] Prostatic sarcomas and spindle cell elements of sarcomatoid carcinoma, in contrast to prostatic stromal hyperplasia, show nuclear atypia, invasiveness or stromal overgrowth, necrosis, and mitotic activity.

The main differential diagnostic concerns for usual epithelial hyperplasia in the prostate are normal prostatic epithelium, PIN, AAH (adenosis), and pseudohyperplastic and microcystic adenocarcinoma. Normal prostatic epithelium and hyperplastic epithelium can both have complex configurations, with papillary infoldings, branching, and luminal undulations, but normal epithelium does not form nodules and does not have admixed stromal hyperplasia. Usual epithelial hyperplasia may be difficult to distinguish from low-grade PIN but low-grade PIN glands will show luminal cell nuclear enlargement and size variability. This distinction is not necessary since low-grade PIN need not be reported since it is not a risk factor for detection of malignancy. High-grade PIN is readily distinguished from epithelial hyperplasia based on its malignant-appearing luminal cell nuclei in glands with a tufted, micropapillary, cribriform, and/or flat architecture. A few small acinar buds in usual glandular hyperplasia can raise the possibility of AAH (adenosis) but AAH has a greater number and density of small, closely packed glands. Also, intraluminal crystalloids are more common in AAH glands and AAH glands have a fragmented basal cell layer. The variants of prostatic adenocarcinoma most likely to be confused with epithelial hyperplasia are pseudohyperplastic[258,351] and microcystic[259] adenocarcinoma of the prostate. At low magnifications usual epithelial hyperplasia and pseudohyperplastic adenocarcinoma can appear nearly identical. When cystic change is present in the transition zone, consideration should be given to cystic epithelial hyperplasia versus microcystic adenocarcinoma. Gland crowding, continuity with usual small acinar adenocarcinoma, nuclear atypia, complete absence of basal cells, and AMACR positivity will indicate a diagnosis of pseudohyperplastic or microcystic adenocarcinoma in this setting.

Diagnostic difficulties can arise in the diagnosis of usual epithelial hyperplasia secondary to thermal damage in prostate chips from TURP. Architectural and nuclear distortion as a consequence of thermal injury can render interpretation difficult to impossible, especially at the edge of the prostatic chips. Levels and/or basal cell and AMACR immunostains can on occasion help resolve concern for high-grade PIN or carcinoma, when such concern exists. Another diagnostic problem due to heat effect on tissue is the generation of signet ring change in lymphocytes.[141] If cell type is in doubt, immunostains for lymphocyte markers such as CD45, with negative PSA and PSAP immunostains, can confirm the nature of the signet ring cells.

Special studies are rarely required to diagnose usual prostatic hyperplasia. If adenosis (see below) or pseudo-hyperplastic/microcystic adenocarcinoma are possibilities, immunostains for basal cells (34βE12 and/or p63) and AMACR may be helpful. Usual epithelial hyperplasia may demonstrate focal basal cell loss, but the basal cell layer is not fragmented, as in adenosis, or completely absent, as in pseudohyperplastic and microcystic adenocarcinoma. AMACR immunostains can be focally positive in usual hyperplasia, can be strongly positive in 8% of cases of adenosis, and are positive in most cases of pseudohyperplastic and microcystic adenocarcinoma.

Basal Cell Hyperplasia

Basal cell hyperplasia is an increase in the number of benign basal cells.[137,138,352–363] Basal cell hyperplasia is uncommon, with an incidence of 3% to 15%.[138,141,355,357] Though often viewed as a transition zone proliferation found in the setting of usual epithelial hyperplasia, it can also be found in the peripheral zone, associated with inflammation.[138] Finally, basal cell hyperplasia is a common reactive response to therapy of the prostate.

Basal cell hyperplasia is an incidental histologic finding in TURP chips[354,356,358] or needle biopsies of the peripheral zone performed to rule out carcinoma.[138] Patients typically are 60 to 80 years of age and present with prostatism symptoms that result in transurethral resection or open prostatectomy, or with an abnormal DRE or serum PSA that results in needle biopsy.

Histologically, basal cell hyperplasia is often multifocal and is characterized by two or more layers of basal cells with a range of growth features. These glands or nests are often focal but can form nodules.[334] In some cases the glands can appear to infiltrate between normal or hyperplastic glands (Fig. 8-90). The glandular forms vary from tubular to cribriform to solid configurations (Figs. 8-91 to 8-93). The patterns vary from focal, eccentric, partial gland involvement

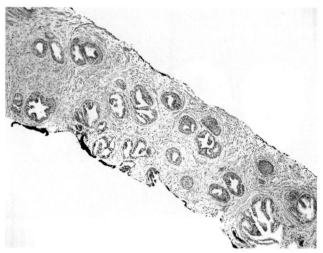

FIGURE 8-91 ■ Basal cell hyperplasia, with some of the glands having a tubular appearance.

to a symmetric, circumferential proliferation with central retention of secretory cell layer, to nearly complete, luminal obliteration. Solid, small nests are also common and these can occasionally demonstrate peripheral palisading. The cribriform (adenoid basal cell) pattern has been reported to be rare.[356,361] Cribriform structures can resemble adenoid cystic carcinoma, hence the term adenoid cystic-like hyperplasia.[363] These cases demonstrate transition zone location, mutifocality, and lobulation, with squamous metaplasia and a myxoid stroma occasionally seen.[363] Additional unusual morphologic patterns include basal hyperplasia within intracytoplasmic globules and squamous features.[361] The surrounding stroma may be similar to adjacent uninvolved prostate,[352] may reveal a few concentric layers of cellular or myxoid compressed stroma, or may show a hypercellular, hyperplastic stroma, which has been called sclerosing basal cell hyperplasia.[356] Microcalcifications are seen in nests in about one-half of cases (Fig. 8-94).[357] Cytologically, the

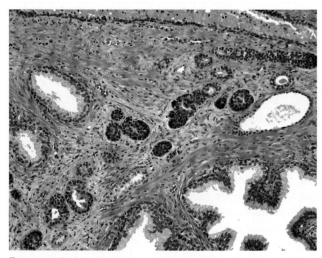

FIGURE 8-90 ■ Basal cell hyperplasia, with pseudoinfiltrative pattern.

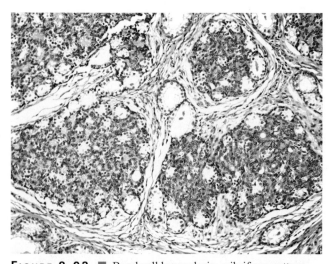

FIGURE 8-92 ■ Basal cell hyperplasia, cribriform pattern.

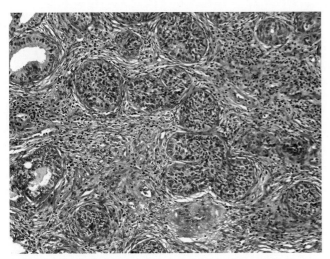

FIGURE 8-93 ■ Basal cell hyperplasia, solid nested pattern.

basal cells are ovoid to occasionally elongated. Cytoplasmic volume is scanty and usually dense, but some cells can have cytoplasmic clearing. The nuclei are uniform, with finely dispersed chromatin and usually without prominent (>1 μm) nucleoli or pleomorphism. In a small minority of basal cell hyperplasia foci there are prominent nucleoli.[137,138,356,361,364] The designation of "atypical basal cell hyperplasia" should not be applied in these cases since there is no evidence that this finding constitutes a risk factor for subsequent detection of carcinoma. Mitoses are rare. Lymphocytes are commonly found in foci of basal cell hyperplasia, suggesting that some foci may be a reactive proliferation. No physical transition between basal cell hyperplasia and neoplasia, including PIN and carcinoma, has been noted.[138]

Special histochemical stains have shown acid and neutral mucin in basal cell hyperplasia,[357] whereas immunohistochemical stains demonstrate an immunophenotype similar to normal basal cells. Of diagnostic importance, immunolabeling using p63 and 34βE12 antibodies is found.[26,356,357] Immunostains for AMACR are negative.[362] Weak to absent PSA and PSAP immunoreactivity in basal cells has been reported,[356,357] and preserved secretory cells are strongly positive for these two markers. Rare basal cells have stained for chromogranin, neuron-specific enolase, and SMA.[356,357,360] BCL2 immunostains are negative to weakly positive, and weakly positive p53 immunoreactivity has been detected.[364] The mean proliferation index for usual basal cell hyperplasia (based on Ki-67 immunopositive cells) has been quantitated at 1.3%.[138,364] Compared with normal basal cells, basal cell hyperplasia exhibits a coordinate increase in proliferation index and a decrease in apoptotic index, which may account for the increased cell number in basal cell hyperplasia.[138,365]

The differential diagnosis for basal cell hyperplasia centers mainly on high-grade PIN, particularly when nucleoli are present, but basal cell hyperplasia is a uniform cell population and does not exhibit the tufted and micropapillary patterns commonly present in PIN. Urothelial metaplasia, when florid, can on occasion exhibit overlapping features with basal cell hyperplasia but urothelial cells have more elongated nuclei, sometimes with nuclear grooves and cytoplasmic clearing. As far as malignancy, basal cell hyperplasia should not be misdiagnosed as adenocarcinoma or the rare basal cell carcinoma in the prostate. Tubular and cribriform basal cell hyperplasia can be mistaken for adenocarcinoma but again the multilayered uniform basaloid cell population is the key finding that aids in diagnostic recognition. Basal cell hyperplasia lacks the infiltrative growth, extraprostatic extension, perineural invasion, and stromal desmoplasia seen in basal cell carcinoma. The adenoid cystic-like hyperplasia pattern of basal cell hyperplasia additionally differs from the adenoid cystic pattern of basaloid carcinoma in being associated with usual basal cell hyperplasia, and lacking mitoses, apoptosis, and sebaceous differentiation.[363,366] Immunostains for BCL2 and Ki-67 can help in the distinction of basal cell hyperplasia and basaloid carcinoma in difficult cases, where BCL2 negativity and a Ki-67 index <20% favors basal cell hyperplasia over basal cell carcinoma.[364]

Cribriform Hyperplasia

Cribriform hyperplasia is a variant of usual epithelial hyperplasia that is found in about 8% of untreated prostate glands.[273] Although they are called clear cell cribriform hyperplasia,[367,368] not all such proliferations have cleared cells, so the term cribriform hyperplasia is preferable. These proliferations appear to be completely benign and do not constitute a risk factor for subsequent development of neoplasia.

Patients with cribriform hyperplasia are of a mean age of 64 to 72 years and usually present with a clinical diagnosis of BPH. Almost all of the initially reported cases of cribriform hyperplasia were TURP chip cases[367,368]; cribriform hyperplasia can also be detected in needle biopsy,[368] radical prostatectomy,[273] and cystoprostatectomy tissues.[368]

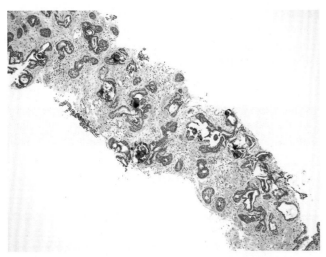

FIGURE 8-94 ■ Basal cell hyperplasia, with calcifications.

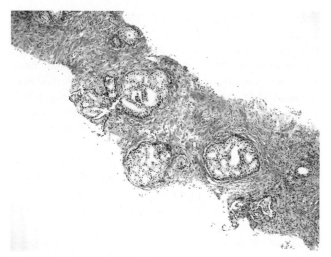

FIGURE 8-95 ■ Cribriform hyperplasia in prostate needle biopsy tissue.

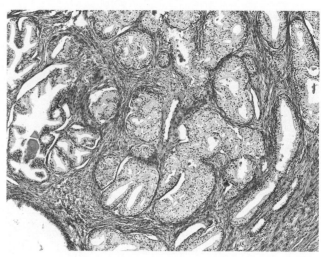

FIGURE 8-97 ■ Cribriform hyperplasia in a hyperplastic nodule.

Histologically, cribriform hyperplasia is usually seen in nodules of hyperplasia in the transition zone and is characterized by a sieve-like glandular profile (Figs. 8-95 to 8-97), with or without admixed papillary proliferations. This can be a single focus or multiple foci. Partial gland involvement is possible. The constituent cells have bland nuclei with only rare, small, inconspicuous nucleoli and cleared cytoplasm (Fig. 8-96). A peripheral basal cell layer is readily detected on H&E sections (Fig. 8-96) and by 34βE12 and/ or p63 immunostains. On occasion this basal cell layer can be hyperplastic. No necrosis or mitotic figures should be evident. The DNA content of cribriform hyperplastic nuclei is diploid, whereas that of cribriform carcinoma is often aneuploid.[368]

The differential diagnosis of cribriform hyperplasia centers on other cribriform proliferations in the prostate. One must be aware that central zone epithelium can normally form cribriform glands. Basal cell hyperplasia can be found admixed with cribriform hyperplasia, and pure cribriform basal cell hyperplasia does exist but is unusual. These basaloid cells have a much smaller volume of cytoplasm than clear cell cribriform hyperplasia. Unlike cribriform high-grade PIN, the cells forming the round, regular glands in cribriform hyperplasia do not exhibit nuclear atypia. Also, although clear cell change can occur in PIN, the cytoplasm of PIN cells is usually amphophilic. Intraductal carcinoma also has neoplastic nuclear atypia in luminal cells,[369,370] unlike cribriform hyperplasia. Ductal adenocarcinomas with characteristic cribriform, papillary, comedo, and/or solid cylinder growth patterns have a particular propensity for intraductal spread. Finally, in contrast to cribriform hyperplasia, invasive cribriform carcinoma, which can be acinar or ductal in type, displays nuclear atypia and is often admixed with an adjacent small acinar or papillary ductal adenocarcinomatous component, and lacks a basal cell layer.[371] Cribriform carcinoma can also be found surrounding the central necrosis of comedocarcinoma (Box 8-6).

Mesonephric Remnant Hyperplasia

Mesonephric remnant hyperplasia is well known in the female genital tract but is an uncommon proliferation in the prostate and periprostatic tissues, with 27 cases reported.[87–90,372] The incidence in TURP cases is estimated to be 0.6% (4/698).[90]

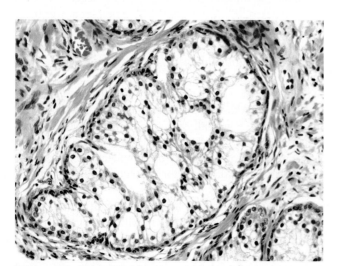

FIGURE 8-96 ■ Cribriform hyperplasia with circumferential basal cell layer and bland luminal cell nuclei.

Box 8-6 ● DIFFERENTIAL DIAGNOSIS OF CRIBRIFORM GLANDS IN THE PROSTATE

Normal central zone glands
Cribriform clear cell hyperplasia
Basal cell hyperplasia
PIN
Intraductal carcinoma
Acinar adenocarcinoma
Ductal adenocarcinoma

It is always an incidental histologic finding. The mean patient age is 70 (range 50 to 85), and most patients present with prostatism with subsequent TURP. A few patients had the proliferation detected in radical prostatectomy tissues, and one patient had these glands in needle biopsy performed to rule out prostate cancer. The clinical and pathologic significance of this proliferation is that it can be confused microscopically with adenocarcinoma. Indeed, this happened in one case, and the patient underwent an unnecessary radical prostatectomy.[87]

Histologically, mesonephric remnant hyperplasia is most often characterized by a vaguely lobular or infiltrative growth of small tubules with cuboidal epithelium (Fig. 8-98) and intraluminal, eosinophilic colloid-like secretions. These tubules can infiltrate prostatic tissue, in and around smooth muscle bundles of the bladder neck, and in periprostatic soft tissue. In three cases,[75,76] there was an association with nerve tissue. Sometimes the tubules form aggregates or can stream in columns. The tubules have a single-cell-lining layer and are usually simple acini, but intraluminal micropapillary projections can be seen in some instances. The lining epithelium is most often cuboidal but can be flattened and atrophic, especially in medium-sized tubules, with cystic dilatation. Cytologically, the cells are bland, usually with no evidence of nuclear enlargement or prominent nucleoli. Occasionally, "punctate" or "conspicuous" nucleoli are visualized. There is generally not a stromal proliferation or response to the acini. Immunohistochemically, the critical finding is lack of staining for PSA and PSAP. Variable results have been obtained with the 34βE12 immunostain, which can be negative in mesonephric hyperplasia.

Verumontanum Mucosal Gland Hyperplasia

This is a benign microacinar proliferation of the verumontanum and adjacent posterior urethra where the ejaculatory ducts and utricle empty into the urethra.[373] Its incidence in whole glands (from radical prostatectomies

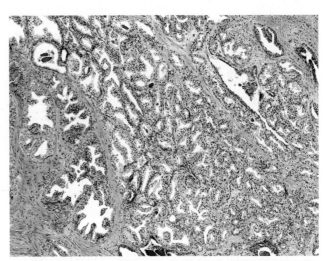

FIGURE 8-99 ■ Verumontanum mucosal gland hyperplasia.

and cystoprostatectomies) is 14%.[373] Although it has been reported in needle biopsies,[374] the incidence in this type of tissue specimen and in TURP chips has not been defined. Verumontanum mucosal gland hyperplasia is an incidental histologic finding in men 47 to 87 years of age.[373] Its clinical and pathologic significance is that it can potentially mimic small acinar prostatic adenocarcinoma.

Histologically, verumontanum mucosal gland hyperplasia (Fig. 8-99) is more often multifocal than solitary. In needle biopsy the mean focus size is 2.9 mm. Most foci in the whole gland are <1 mm and contain 6 to 25 glands.[373] The glands exhibit a nodular growth, regularly centered around ejaculatory or prostatic ducts. Urothelium is identified immediately adjacent to hyperplastic verumontanum mucosal gland nodules in both needle biopsy and the whole gland. The small acini are positioned back to back with scanty, interspersed stroma. These acini are lined by cuboidal to columnar cells with small bland nuclei and rare, small nucleoli. Basal cells are readily recognized. Numerous intraluminal, small, fragmented orange-red concretions and corpora amylacea are present, but crystalloids and wispy blue mucin are absent to rare, respectively. Immunohistochemically, the luminal cells are strongly positive for PSA, and the basal cells mark with 34βE12. Verumontanum mucosal gland hyperplasia has been associated with the presence of AAH (adenosis),[375] but it is not a risk factor for malignancy.

Atypical Adenomatous Hyperplasia (Adenosis)

AAH, also known as adenosis, is a small glandular proliferation that has been defined as "a localized proliferation of small glands within the prostate that may be mistaken for carcinoma"[376] or "a relatively well-circumscribed nodule of closely packed glands with a lobular growth pattern."[377–381] A variant, known as diffuse adenosis of the peripheral zone, is not circumscribed.[382]

AAH is invariably an incidental histologic finding. There are no clinical findings that are specific for AAH. The mean

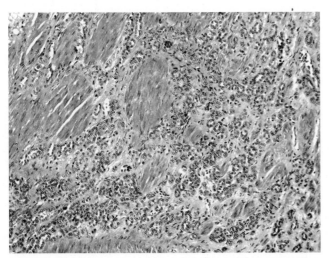

FIGURE 8-98 ■ Mesonephric remnant hyperplasia: infiltrative-appearing small tubules.

age of patients diagnosed with AAH is 64 to 70 years, with a range of 45 to 83 years.[377,383,384] The volume of AAH and the number of AAH foci increase with age.[384] It is not known whether AAH can elevate the serum PSA or produce a mass palpable by DRE. Except for a few examples of larger-volume AAH cases, production of a mass seems unlikely because most AAH foci are microscopic in size.

The incidence of AAH depends on the type of tissue sample,[375,377,383–390] with a wide range from <1% on needle biopsies[383,387] to 22% to 60% in whole glands.[375,384,389,390] In transurethral and simple prostatectomy specimens, there is an intermediate incidence of 2% to 16%.[377,385,386,388]

Grossly, AAH is not recognizable because it is usually a minute proliferation. The largest reported AAH nodule (at 21 cm^3) was not macroscopically distinguishable from other large hyperplastic nodules in the same 124-cm^3 prostate.[391] Microscopically, most foci of AAH are extremely small, as the mean diameter in needle biopsy is 1.4 mm and in TURP chips, 2.5 mm.[377,383] In radical prostatectomy tissues the average volume is 0.029 cm^3.[384] Multifocality is found in a majority of TURP chips but only in a minority of needle biopsy and radical prostatectomy tissues. Most AAH foci (86% to 100%) are discovered in the periurethral or transition zone region, with a minority in the peripheral and central zones.[384,390]

Histologically, usual AAH typically is a well-circumscribed collection of densely packed small, pale, acini, which merge with larger, more complex glands (Figs. 8-100 to 8-107). Diffuse adenosis of the peripheral zone, as the name indicates, is not circumscribed.[382] The periphery of aggregates of usual AAH is characteristically rounded (Figs. 8-100 to 8-102 and 8-104) but in a minority of cases, the small acini can extend into surrounding stroma in a pseudoinfiltrative pattern (Figs. 8-103 and 8-105). The small acini in AAH can be localized to the periphery of the nodule in ring-like or crescentic fashion, or can be intermixed with the larger, complex glands. The number of small acini is variable, and they can make up a minority or majority of the glandular

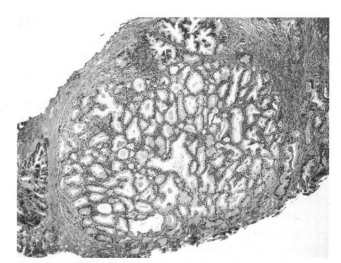

FIGURE 8-101 ■ AAH in TURP chip. In this case the smaller glands predominate.

proliferation. Many of these small glands are round and regular (Fig. 8-104), or elongated, with open lumens. There is usually little intervening stroma, but this is not an absolute diagnostic requirement. A transition is present between the small AAH glands and larger, usual hyperplastic glands with luminal undulations, branching, and papillary infoldings. These larger glands clearly possess basal cells and on occasion basal cell prominence, or cystic change can be noted. Of critical diagnostic importance, the small, tubular acini have a fragmented basal layer. Basal cells can be found in the majority of foci of adenosis (78% in one needle biopsy study)[383] by careful scrutiny of H&E-stained sections, but they can be difficult to discern in some foci. Confirmation of a discontinuous basal cell layer can be accomplished by use of immunohistochemical staining with antibody 34βE12 or a p63 immunostain. On average, more than one-half of the glands in a particular focus are positive with this immunostain, but the range is 10% to 90%.[376,383] Also of substantial

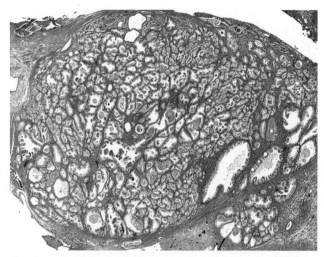

FIGURE 8-100 ■ AAH: a nodule with admixed small acini and larger, more complex glands.

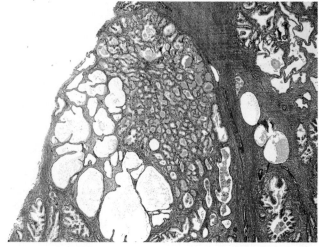

FIGURE 8-102 ■ AAH with closely packed small acini adjacent to cystically dilated glands.

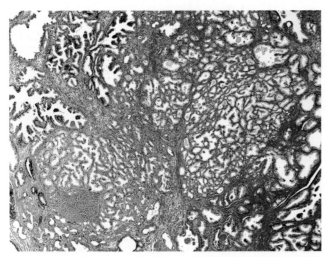

FIGURE 8-103 ■ AAH with a degree of nodularity but also with small acini extending beyond the nodules.

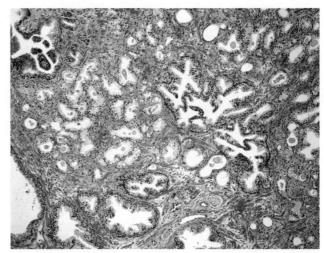

FIGURE 8-105 ■ AAH with pseudoinfiltrative growth.

importance, the nuclei of AAH and diffuse adenosis of the peripheral zone should be bland. That is, the nuclei should be small with little variation in size and shape, and most detectable nucleoli should be small. The nuclei in the small acini should appear similar to those of complex, benign-appearing glands both within the AAH focus and distant from the AAH focus. However, a degree of nuclear atypia is allowable in AAH, and very focal nuclear atypia can also be seen in diffuse adenosis of the peripheral zone. The nucleoli in AAH are usually inconspicuous, but in 13% to 28% of cases, prominent nucleoli (>1 μm in diameter) are present. Additional atypical features that can be found in a minority of AAH cases include intraluminal crystalloids, mitotic figures, and intraluminal wispy blue mucin. Attempts have been made to grade AAH based on the degree of the atypical findings,[392,393] but grading of AAH is not necessary.

The differential diagnostic list for usual AAH is dominated by well-differentiated, Gleason score 2 to 4 adenocarcinoma. Both are circumscribed proliferations of small, pale glands, but AAH merges with hyperplastic-appearing glands, whereas most well-differentiated carcinomas consist of tubular glands with straight luminal borders. Also, the high-power identification of basal cells and bland luminal cell nuclei in AAH allows separation of these entities in most cases, based on examination of H&E-stained slides alone. Difficulty arises when atypical features such as pseudoinfiltrative growth, prominent nucleoli, intraluminal crystalloids, and intraluminal wispy blue mucin are detected. Diffuse adenosis of the peripheral zone can be a diagnostic challenge since the small glands can appear infiltrative like Gleason pattern 3 adenocarcinoma and also since it can be extensive in needle core tissue. Here, the absence or only very focal presence of nuclear atypia is helpful in diagnostic recognition.[382] In needle biopsy, the typical lobular character of AAH can be difficult to appreciate because in only 7% of foci is the entire lobular lesion sampled (Fig. 8-106).

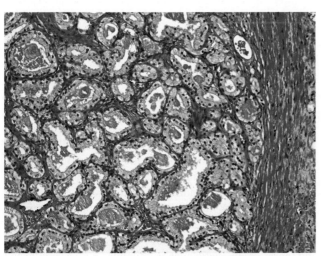

FIGURE 8-104 ■ AAH with a crowded small acinar component.

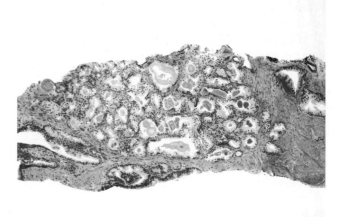

FIGURE 8-106 ■ AAH in needle prostate biopsy. The nodule has been transected.

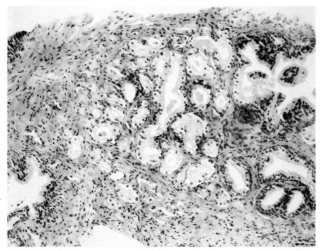

FIGURE 8-107 ■ AAH in needle biopsy tissue: a crowded small pale acinar proliferation.

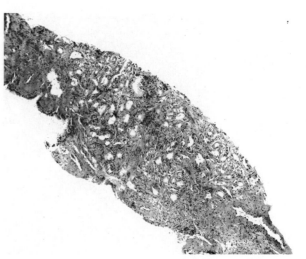

FIGURE 8-108 ■ Sclerosing adenosis in prostate needle biopsy tissue.

In about one-half of needle cases, AAH extends to both sides of the needle core,[383] and this can cause concern for invasion. Furthermore, in some cases, basal cells can be a challenge to definitively identify on H&E-stained sections. In such cases, immunohistochemical staining for basal cells using 34βE12 and/or p63 antibodies can help confirm basal cell presence. Overall, however, only a minority (15% to 20%) of adenosis cases warrants a basal cell immunostain,[394] and the diagnosis can usually be established with H&E-stained slides. Also in the differential diagnosis is pseudohyperplastic prostatic carcinoma.[258,351] Here, there can be an admixture of small, pale glands and complex hyperplastic-appearing glands. Yet these glands completely lack basal cells, and the nuclei exhibit substantial nucleomegaly with macronucleoli.

The most important special study, as noted above, is immunohistochemistry (p63 and/or 34βE12) for basal cells. AMACR immunostains are generally not helpful in the differential diagnosis of AAH versus adenocarcinoma since AAH can be positive for AMACR in a minority (8% to 18%) of cases.[395] Morphometric analysis, histochemistry, immunophenotype, and genetic abnormalities such as DNA ploidy[396] and allelic loss[385,397] do not discriminate between AAH and adenocarcinoma.

Morphologic linkage of usual AAH to PIN and carcinoma is weak to absent. Follow-up of a limited number of patients suggests a benign outcome.[398] If detected in TURP or needle biopsy tissue, clinical follow-up, but not necessarily rebiopsy, might be prudent. An exception to this approach might be when diffuse adenosis of the peripheral zone is diagnosed. In an initial study,[382] there does appear to be an increased risk for subsequent detection of carcinoma, so that after diffuse adenosis is diagnosed in needle biopsy, rebiopsy should be considered.

Sclerosing Adenosis

Sclerosing adenosis is also adenotic in being a compact small gland proliferation.[399–403] This benign, nodular, small acinar proliferation is embedded in a spindle cell background

(Fig. 8-108). Most cases have been diagnosed incidentally in TURP chips from men in their 60s or 70s with clinical symptoms related to BPH. Serum PSA elevations have been reported,[399] probably due to coexisting BPH. The incidence of sclerosing adenosis in TURP chips, simple prostatectomy, and radical cystoprostatectomy is 2%.[399,403] Rare cases have been reported in needle biopsy.[401] Microscopically, most nodules are only a few millimeters in greatest dimension (range 2 to 11 mm). They can be solitary or multifocal. The small glands are crowded and irregular with rounded, oval, and compressed profiles that are often encircled by a thick eosinophilic membrane. Compression of acini can produce the appearance of epithelial cords, small clusters, and single cells. In a minority of cases cystic glandular dilatation is found. The cytoplasm of the luminal cells is cuboidal to scanty and amphophilic to vacuolated. The vacuolated cytoplasm can occasionally impart a signet ring–like image.[401] Cytoplasmic volume loss can generate an atrophic appearance in some glands. The luminal cell nuclei are round to oval and in usual sclerosing adenosis cases there may be a slight degree of atypia. Significant nuclear atypia with enlarged, hyperchromatic nuclei with prominent nucleoli has been seen in a few cases and designated as atypical sclerosing adenosis.[404] Mitotic figures are rare to absent. Glandular luminal secretions are typically not present but can be eosinophilic or basophilic; intraluminal wispy blue mucin can be present. The spindled stroma is highly cellular and is composed of cytologically bland spindle cells set within a collagenous or myxoid, lightly basophilic matrix.[401] Occasional stromal lymphocytes or plasma cells may be noted. The constituent cells mark as myoepithelial cells, with positive immunoreactions for muscle-specific actin, S100 protein, and high-molecular-weight cytokeratin. Some intra-acinar myoepithelial cells, along with standard basal cells, are detectable by immunohistochemical stains. This immunophenotype excludes adenocarcinoma, including those rare prostatic adenocarcinomas with a spindle cell stroma simulating sclerosing adenosis at the H&E level.[405]

Similarly, atypical sclerosing adenosis glands have a basal cell layer and are also negative for AMACR in immunohistochemistry.[404] Sclerosing adenosis of the prostate is benign, with no known malignant potential. Follow-up of atypical sclerosing adenosis has also demonstrated a benign course for these patients.

Miscellaneous Unusual Conditions

Postoperative Spindle Cell Nodule

Postoperative spindle cell nodule is now thought to represent a subset of IMT, which is also known as pseudosarcomatous fibromyxoid tumor, myofibroblastoma, pseudosarcomatous myofibroblastic proliferation, and inflammatory pseudotumor. These prostatic postoperative spindle cell nodules, which follow transurethral resection for BPH, do not differ from IMTs without prior surgery in morphologic, immunohistochemical, and molecular features, or clinical outcome.[406] It is not established as to whether these proliferations are true neoplasms or exuberant reactions[345]; some consider IMTs to be neoplasms of uncertain malignant potential.[407]

About 11 cases of IMT involving the prostate have been reported,[408–411] with 7 of these cases designated as postoperative spindle cell nodule.[408,410] These seven men were of an average age of 65 (range 45 to 79) and presented with obstruction and hematuria at a mean of 2 months (range 1 to 3 months) after TURP or transurethral resection of the urinary bladder. The gross appearance by cystoscopic examination was that of an "unusual-appearing mass or heaped-up tumor."[408] The tumors measure from 0.5 to 4 cm in greatest dimension. Microscopically, there is an infiltrative, uniform, spindle cell proliferation that can infiltrate and efface stroma. Interlacing fascicles can be formed by the plump spindle cells, which have cytologically bland nuclei, and abundant eosinophilic to amphophilic cytoplasm. There is a background of delicate blood vessels, with edema, focal hemorrhage, and scattered chronic inflammatory cells typically present. The mitotic rate is variable but can be extremely high, ranging up to 25 mitotic figures per 10 high-power fields. Abnormal mitoses should not be seen. Vimentin, SMA, and desmin immunostains are positive. The most important differential diagnostic consideration is a prostatic sarcoma, and indeed, five of the seven cases were initially diagnosed as leiomyosarcoma. Sarcomatoid carcinoma is also in the differential diagnosis but both prostatic sarcomas and sarcomatoid carcinomas should display a greater degree of nuclear atypia than prostatic IMT and additionally may exhibit necrosis and atypical mitotic figures. Furthermore, sarcomatoid carcinoma may possess an epithelioid component. The immunophenotype of IMT can overlap with leiomyosarcoma and sarcomatoid carcinoma, with desmin, vimentin, SMA, and cytokeratin expression potentially found in all three entities. ALK immunostaining and FISH for ALK gene breakapart rearrangements can be helpful in diagnosis of IMT[407]; sarcomas and sarcomatoid carcinomas will lack these ALK abnormalities. IMTs of the prostate usually follow a benign course, although incomplete surgical excision can lead to recurrence in about one-quarter of cases.

Pigment Disorders

Melanosis, blue nevus, and ochronosis are benign pigmentary conditions found in the prostate.

Melanosis is defined as the appearance of melanin in glandular epithelium, with or without stromal melanocytes. In the past, cases of lipofuscin pigment in prostatic epithelium have been mistaken for melanosis, due to interpretation of a positive Lillie's ferrous iron stain and positive Fontana-Masson stains as being indicative of melanin, but these stains are not specific for melanin. (A Luxol fast blue histochemical stain will distinguish lipofuscin from melanin, with lipofuscin staining blue and melanin being negative.) True melanosis with an ultrastructural finding of melanosomes in prostatic epithelium is extremely rare, with two reported cases.[412,413] These two men, aged 64 and 75 years, underwent TURP for BPH symptoms. Grossly, the prostatic chips were black. Microscopically, finely granular brown to black pigment was present in the cytoplasm of stromal cells and in the cytoplasm of benign and malignant epithelial cells. The stromal cells were rounded, polygonal, or spindled, with dendritic cytoplasmic processes.[412] The pigmented stromal cells were S100 positive in immunohistochemistry and by electron microscopy contained melanosomes of differing maturation states, while the epithelial cells harbored mature stage IV melanosomes.[412,413] It was suggested that melanin in the prostatic epithelium was a result of transfer from the stromal melanocytes.

Blue nevus in the prostate is similar to its counterpart in the dermis of the skin, with the presence of stromal melanin-laden spindle cells. About 24 cases of prostatic blue nevus have been reported in detail.[412,414–416] It is an incidental histologic finding, usually seen in patients who underwent transurethral or simple prostatectomy for BPH symptoms. The average age at detection is 66 (range 50 to 80 years). Grossly, brown to black areas measuring 0.1 to 2 cm in greatest dimension can be visualized. Microscopically, finely granular brown to black pigment is identified in stromal cells and sometimes in extracellular matrix (Fig. 8-109). The pigmented stromal cells are often haphazardly dispersed with single cells and clumps of cells. A pattern of concentric arrangement around glands and vessels has also been described. These pigment-laden cells are spindled, with bipolar, long, dendritic, cytoplasmic processes but the cell shape can also be round, ovoid, or polygonal. Useful histochemical reactions include Fontana-Masson positivity with loss of staining after potassium permanganate bleaching, coupled with a negative Luxol fast blue stain. The pigmented cells are positive by S100 immunohistochemistry. Ultrastructural examination shows melanosomes of variable maturation in the cytoplasm. Blue nevus is not a risk factor for subsequent development of malignancy, such as melanoma.

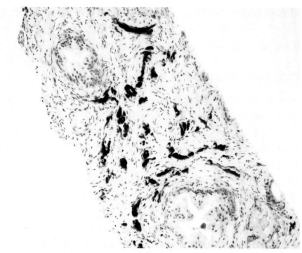

FIGURE 8-109 ■ Blue nevus in the prostate: marked melanin pigmentation in single spindle cells and clumps of stromal cells.

The major entities in differential diagnosis of melanosis and blue nevus are stromal hemosiderin-laden macrophages, epithelial lipofuscin, and malignant melanoma. Hemosiderin forms larger aggregates of golden yellow pigment and an iron histochemical stain is positive. The histochemical distinction of lipofuscin and melanin can be accomplished, as noted above, with a Luxol fast blue stain. Malignant melanoma can rarely be seen in the prostate, but the clinical context is usually a patient with known widespread metastases.

Ochronosis of the prostate has been reported in a single patient.[417] Ochronosis is the clinical sequela of alkaptonuria, a rare hereditary metabolic disorder. The patient had a rock-hard prostate by DRE and sections of needle biopsy tissues showed dark brown melanin-like pigment, representing homogentisic acid, in corpora amylacea and prostatic epithelium.

Amyloid

Amyloid can be found in the prostate as an incidental finding in corpora amylacea, stroma, and blood vessels.[418–423] Amyloid in corpora amylacea is detected by Congo red staining, with apple-green birefringence obtained by crossed polarizing filters. The amyloid proteins in prostatic corpora amylacea are β2 microglobulin and S100A8/A9 proteins.[419,420] The reported incidence of prostatic amyloid is 0.6%[421] to 10%[418]; the reason for this wide range is not clear. The average age of patients with prostatic amyloidosis ranges from 66[418] to 86.[422] Secondary, incidental amyloidosis has been reported in patients with multiple myeloma, with an incidence of 38%.[418] No gross abnormalities attributable to prostatic amyloid deposition have been described. Microscopically, amyloid in prostatic stroma presents as irregular nodules of amorphous, highly eosinophilic material.[421] The amount and location of the stromal amyloid are variable. Congo red and crystal violet histochemical stains have been used in the identification of prostatic amyloid. The pathogenetic basis for primary accumulation of amyloid in the prostate is not known.

Endometriosis

A single case of endometriosis in the prostate has been reported.[424] This 78-year-old man was diagnosed with prostatic adenocarcinoma and then took the estrogen chlorotrianisene for almost 6 years before developing hematuria. A transurethral resection of a small, raised prostatic urethral nodule was performed and microscopic examination of the prostatic chip sections revealed endometriotic stroma and hemosiderin.

Extramedullary Hematopoiesis

Extramedullary hematopoiesis in the prostate was reported in a 75-year-old man with an 8-year history of myelofibrosis, with massive splenomegaly and a 5-year history of bladder outlet obstruction symptoms.[425] TURP produced chips that showed, on microscopic examination, increased stromal cellularity due to immature granulocytes, erythroid precursors, and atypical megakaryocytes. These immature hematopoietic elements were observed in perivascular and intravascular locations. A chloroacetate esterase (Leder) stain was positive in the immature granulocytes. The atypical megakaryocytes initially were concerning for a stromal neoplasm; identification of associated erythroid and myeloid precursors was crucial in ruling out a stromal neoplasm.

Diagnostic and Treatment-Related Alterations in Benign Prostate

Biopsy and Surgery

Diagnostic needle biopsy can rarely induce granulomatous inflammation as noted above. More commonly there is a fibroinflammtory response to the needle biopsy procedure, with granulation tissue formation, and generation of a fibrous needle track scar (Fig. 8-110), sometimes with

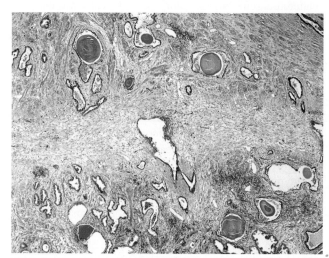

FIGURE 8-110 ■ Needle track scar in radical prostatectomy tissue.

creation of a cavity.[426] Reparative epithelial atypia, including squamous metaplasia with atypia, may be seen at the edges of the fibrous scar. It is uncommon to visualize a long segment of the scar; usually only focal scarring is seen, representing oblique sectioning of a small portion of the linear fibrous track. It is likely that adjacent hemorrhage and acute inflammation are also induced by needle biopsy. Needle track seeding of benign tissue by carcinoma can occur but is rare with use of 18-gauge needles.[426,427]

TURP can also induce distinctive granulomatous inflammation (see above section of postresection granulomatous inflammation for details). Post-TUR there can also be formation of central cavity, with squamous metaplasia of the prostatic urethra and surrounding periurethral fibrosis. In the TURP chips benign tissue at the edge of the chips can exhibit distortion and thermal injury (cautery)—induced changes. At times, this damage can cause difficulty in ascertainment of the nature of the cauterized/distorted epithelium. On occasion, when there is suspicion of malignancy, examination of additional H&E-stained levels and/or immunohistochemical stains for basal cells[34] and AMACR can be diagnostically helpful in arguing for or against a diagnosis of carcinoma in the setting of cautery/distortion damage.

Similarly, crushed, distorted cells/glands at the edge of radical prostatectomy margin sections secondary to the surgical procedure can be difficult to interpret as benign or malignant. Again, study of H&E-stained levels and/or employment of an AMACR/p63/34βE12 cocktail immunostain can be diagnostically advantageous.[428]

Hormonal Therapy

Endocrine or androgen deprivation therapy is a common treatment modality for patients with locally advanced or metastatic prostate cancer. The major methods of androgen deprivation include orchiectomy, estrogen therapy, luteinizing-releasing hormone agonists, steroidal antiandrogens (such as cyproterone and megestrol), nonsteroidal antiandrogens (such as flutamide, nilutamide, and bicalutamide), and nonclassical antiandrogens (such as ketoconazole, aminoglutethimide, and the 5α-reductase inhibitors finasteride and dutasteride).

The pathologic effects of different androgen deprivation therapies on benign prostatic tissue are similar, with the exceptions of estrogen therapy and 5α-reductase inhibitor use.[429,430] Grossly, prostates treated with neoadjuvant hormonal therapy are small and nodules of hyperplasia are more difficult to identify compared with untreated glands.[431] Microscopically, the general impression at scanning magnification is stromal dominance (Fig. 8-111). This is due to a global decrease in size and number of benign prostatic glands.[432] Normal[433] and hyperplastic glands are simplified in that they lose their branching complexity and intraluminal undulations and appear small, ovoid, round, or comma-shaped (Fig. 8-112). The secretory luminal epithelium is often atrophic, with loss of cytoplasmic volume, and displays nuclear pyknosis and cytoplasmic clearing. Basal cell prominence and hyperplasia are

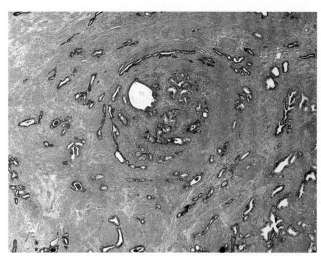

FIGURE 8-111 ■ Androgen deprivation therapy effect on benign prostate: stromal dominance with diffuse glandular atrophy. The whorled structure in the center of the field is a BPH nodule with hormonal therapy effect.

also characteristic responses of benign glands to withdrawal of androgens (Fig. 8-112). The frequency of squamous metaplasia is variable, depending on the study, ranging from 0%[434] to 53%.[273] Urothelial metaplasia is not usually associated with androgen deprivation therapy but was common in one series.[273] Stromal changes other than the relative increase in area are not prominent. Focal stromal hyperplasia and scattered lymphocytes have been reported.[431] Androgen deprivation causes epithelial involution in BPH nodules by a combined reduction in proliferative activity and enhancement of apoptosis. The histomorphologic effects of androgen deprivation therapy can persist for years. Estrogen therapy, in addition to these changes, can result in glycogenated squamous metaplasia (Fig. 8-64). Atrophy and basal cell hyperplasia caused by androgen deprivation should not be confused with adenocarcinoma. The same principles in differential diagnosis as for atrophy and basal

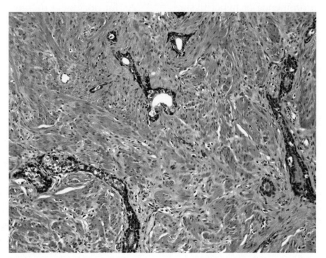

FIGURE 8-112 ■ Androgen deprivation therapy effect on benign prostate: atrophy and basal cell prominence.

cell hyperplasia seen in the absence of androgen deprivation therapy (see above sections) should be employed. p63 and high-molecular-weight cytokeratin expression is not altered by hormonal therapy and are valuable basal cell markers in this setting.

The 5α-reductase inhibitors finasteride (which inhibits the type 2 isoenzyme) and dutasteride (which inhibits both the type 1 and type 2 isozymes) have been used to treat BPH and in prostate cancer chemoprevention clinical trials. Their histologic effects are more pronounced on benign prostatic tissue compared to PIN and carcinoma. These drugs decrease gland size, with an estimated 20% to 30% reduction in volume.[431] Microscopically, atrophy and smaller nuclei and nucleoli have been described in benign prostatic glands.[435–441] Secretory cells with treatment effect exhibit shrunken nuclei, condensed chromatin, inconspicuous nucleoli, and cytoplasmic clearing. Basal cell prominence may be seen. Finasteride induces prostatic involution in benign tissues via atrophy and cell death.[435] Apoptotic cell death is seen at 16 to 18 days[435] and long-term treatment of 24 to 40 months leads to progressive contraction of both transition zone and peripheral zone epithelium.[438] There is a corresponding increase in stromal–epithelial ratio. Dutasteride-treated benign prostatic tissue shows similar features, with a significant decrease in epithelial cell height and width.[442,443]

Radiation Therapy

Radiation therapy changes are seen most commonly in prostate needle cores procured in rebiopsy procedures after radiation therapy for established prostate cancer. Whole prostate glands are available for examination when radical salvage radical prostatectomy is performed for radioresistant locally recurrent prostate cancer. This salvage procedure is uncommonly done, and these patients have often been treated with both radiation and hormonal therapy prior to surgery. Microscopically, radiation-treated benign prostatic tissue shows extensive atrophy, cytologic atypia, and basal cell prominence or hyperplasia.[433,444–447] As for hormonal therapy effect, the glandular atrophy generates an appearance of stromal dominance (Fig. 8-113). Both the size and number of benign glands are reduced. Atrophy is evident in the form of glandular luminal cytoplasmic volume loss. Basal cells are often prominent or hyperplastic and can display pronounced nuclear atypia, with nucleomegaly and nucleolomegaly (Fig. 8-114). Nuclear pleomorphism can also be striking with variations in nuclear size and shape. In addition to enlargement, some nuclei may be shrunken and pyknotic.[444,445] The atypical nuclei may have a vacuolated or smudged hyperchromatic appearance.[295] Cytoplasmic changes include vacuolization, mucinous metaplasia, and squamous metaplasia. The stroma is fibrotic and may show chronic inflammation, foreign body giant cell reaction to extruded corpora amylacea, and, in a minority of cases, edema, calcification, and atypical radiation fibroblasts. Severe vascular damage with intimal and media thickening, medial hyalinization, and luminal narrowing is often noted. The degree of radiation-related change

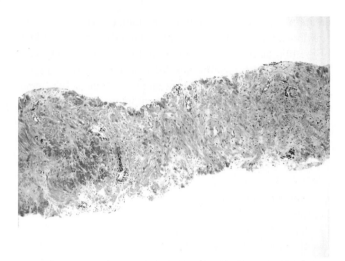

FIGURE 8-113 ■ Radiation treatment effect on benign prostate: stromal dominance with glandular atrophy.

is related to the dose and duration of radiation, method of radiation therapy delivery (brachytherapy and/or external beam radiotherapy), and time from radiotherapy.[449] There is a greater degree of stromal fibrosis and glandular epithelial atypia in patients treated with brachytherapy or combined brachytherapy/external beam radiotherapy compared to external beam therapy alone.[449] For external beam radiation therapy, there is less atypia after 4 years.

The differential diagnosis of irradiated, atypical benign glands centers on adenocarcinoma. Irradiated benign glands can appear infiltrative, especially when they are atrophic and distorted by stromal sclerosis. The nuclear atypia in irradiated benign glands can be significant and indeed in one morphometric study the nuclear size of irradiated benign glandular nuclei was actually greater than that of irradiated prostatic adenocarcinoma nuclei. The nuclear atypia in basal cells, which can be mistaken for neoplastic-type nuclear atypia, can persist for years.[449] Immunohistochemical stains can be extremely valuable in the diagnostic distinction of

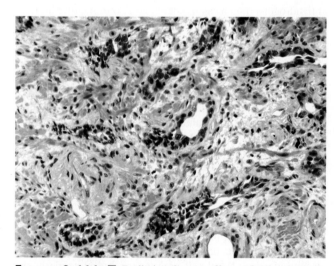

FIGURE 8-114 ■ Radiation therapy effect on benign prostatic epithelium: nuclear atypia.

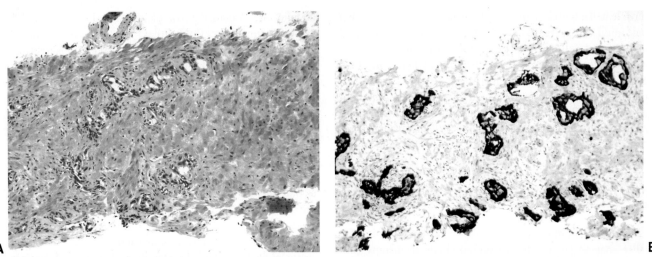

FIGURE 8-115 ■ Radiation therapy effect on benign prostate **(A)** with confirmation of basal cell presence using "triple stain" immunohistochemistry with AMACR, 34βE12, and p63 antibodies **(B)**. Brown—basal cell staining. Red stain indicating AMACR expression is absent **(B)**.

radiation atypia in benign glands versus adenocarcinoma. Many of the atypical epithelial cells are basal cells and so will be highlighted by p63 and 34βE12 immunostains (Fig. 8-115).[281,295,444,446-448] A negative AMACR immunostain can also be contributory; expression of this enzyme is maintained in most irradiated prostatic carcinomas and is negative in benign irradiated glands.[450] PSA and PSAP immunostains will tend to mark adenocarcinoma rather than irradiated benign glands[446,451–454] but these immunostains are not usually necessary when p63/34βE12 and AMACR immunostaining is done. Immunostains are not needed in every case with radiation atypia but one should have a low threshold for performance of such ancillary staining.

Cryotherapy

Cryotherapy to treat prostate cancer involves freezing the prostate gland, creating an intraprostatic ice ball by use of cryoprobes placed under ultrasound guidance.[455] Ultrasound is used to monitor the size of the ice ball. Histologic changes in benign prostatic tissue depend on the time of tissue sampling after treatment. Edema and hemorrhage are seen immediately after freezing and in the first posttreatment week.[456] Necrosis is found 10 days to 30 weeks after freezing.[275,456] Reparative alterations with stromal fibrosis, hyalinization, and inflammation predominate after 10 weeks.[456] At 5 to 48 weeks after cryotherapy the most common microscopic findings in prostate needle biopsy tissue sections are stromal fibrosis and hyalinization (Fig. 8-116), basal cell hyperplasia, coagulative necrosis, and inflammation.[271,275,457] This tissue damage can persist beyond 1 year.[457] Immunostains for basal cells and AMACR can be useful tools in confirming a benign diagnosis in cases with reactive epithelial atypia.[431]

Chemotherapy

Chemotherapy and in particular docetaxel is usually reserved for patients with castration-resistant (hormone-refractory)

metastatic prostate cancer although it has also been used in neoadjuvant protocols prior to radical prostatectomy. In these trials docetaxel has been used as a single agent, or in combination with hormones or etoposide. Only one report on use of docetaxel as a single agent prior to radical prostatectomy describes the effect on benign prostatic tissue.[458] Most benign prostatic glands showed prominent basal cells and urothelial metaplasia after docetaxel treatment.

Medical Therapy for BPH

Medical therapies for BPH include α-adrenergic blockers, aromatase inhibitors, and various plant extracts, and 5α-reductase inhibitors (discussed above).[459] Little is known of the histologic changes, if any, induced by the first three of these therapies. Alpha-adrenoreceptor antagonists cause relaxation of prostate and bladder neck smooth muscle. There is a suggestion that doxazosin and terazosin can induce apoptosis in prostatic epithelial and smooth

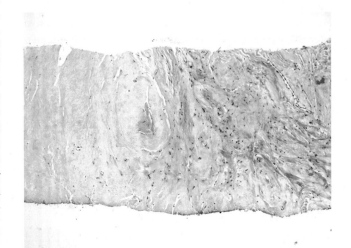

FIGURE 8-116 ■ Cryotherapy effect on benign prostate: hyalinization and fibrosis.

muscle cells, with loss of smooth muscle cells,[460,461] and that naftopidil can decrease cell proliferation index in epithelial and stromal cells.[462] A large number of plant extracts are available to treat symptoms of BPH.[459] In two studies on *Sabal serrulata* (saw palmetto) there a reduction in stromal edema and inflammation, and an increase in epithelial atrophy.[463,464] However, a recent clinical trial of saw palmetto showed no improvement of symptoms or objective measures of BPH,[465] so the clinical significance of the histologic alterations is unclear.

Minimally Invasive Therapy for BPH and Prostate Cancer

There are a number of minimally invasive therapies for BPH that serve as alternatives to medical therapy and TURP. These include laser therapy, transurethral microwave therapy, transurethral balloon dilation of the prostate, transurethral electrovaporization, transurethral needle ablation, water-induced thermotherapy, transurethral ethanol ablation of the prostate, and intraurethral stents.[466] The first two of these have also been used on an experimental basis to treat prostate cancer, as have radiofrequency interstitial tumor ablation and high-intensity focused ultrasound. In many of these procedures, tissue is not submitted for examination, although needle biopsy could be performed in follow-up of treatment for prostate cancer so it is important to be aware of treatment effects on benign tissue. Heat-induced damage from laser therapy, microwave therapy, ultrasound hyperthermia, balloon thermotherapy, and radiofrequency is manifest as sharply circumscribed hemorrhagic coagulative necrosis, with subsequent formation of granulation tissue[431] and fibrosis. As a specific example, consider the hyperthermia damage caused by laser treatment. Lasers introduced into the prostatic urethra can induce prostate ablation via coagulative necrosis, incision, or contact vaporization of tissues. The histomorphologic effects are variable and dependent on the amount of energy delivered, tissue contact, and time after treatment.[467,468] Immediately after therapy a black eschar can be seen.[467] At 24 hours, acute inflammation and edema are noted.[468] By 1 week there are wide zones of coagulative necrosis, with a rim of inflammation and hemorrhage; dilated vessels, vascular thrombosis, and squamous metaplasia are seen adjacent to the necrotic tissue. Sloughing of the coagulated tissue occurs by 7 weeks. At 10 to 12 weeks a periurethral cavity can be found[467] with a reepithelialized surface and a rim of inflammation and squamous metaplasia. At 1 year, ischemic damage and squamous metaplasia persist.[468]

THE SEMINAL VESICLES

Function

The physiologic function of the seminal vesicle is to secrete fluid that is important for sperm function.[469,470] These secretions, which constitute the majority of the ejaculate volume, contain ions, fructose, prostaglandins, and proteins such as semenogelin, the scaffold protein for the semen coagulate and substrate for PSA. Seminal vesicle secretions appear to function specifically in nutrition and modification of sperm motility, in formation of the seminal coagulum, and possibly in immunosuppression and antibacterial actions.

Normal Embryology, Anatomy, and Histology

Embryology

The seminal vesicles begin initial development at 12 weeks as outpouchings or bulbous swellings of the lower portion of the Wolffian ducts near the urogenital sinus.[471] The tubular vesicle then elongates and numerous diverticula form. This branching morphogenesis requires androgens as well as bidirectional paracrine signaling involving members of the fibroblast growth factor, Hedgehog, and transforming growth factor-beta families.[472] Mucosal folding and complexity increase in the reproductive years until around age 45.[471] The central zone of the prostate, ejaculatory duct, and the seminal vesicles share a common origin from the Wolffian ducts.

Anatomy

The seminal vesicles are paired, coiled, and tubular male sex accessory glands.[469,470,473,474] They lie posterolateral to the base of the urinary bladder and anterior to Denonvilliers fascia (Figs. 8-2 and 8-3). A short excretory duct from the seminal vesicle joins the ampulla of the vasa differentia to form the paired ejaculatory ducts, which course through the base and central zone of the prostate to the prostatic urethra. The normal adult seminal vesicle is 3.5 to 7.5 cm in length and 1.2 to 2.4 cm in width. The mean weight is 7.5 g (range 5.8 to 8.8 g).[470] Cut surfaces show luminal convolutions and a thick muscular wall (Fig. 8-117). The blood supply to the seminal vesicle is from the vesiculodeferential artery, a branch of the umbilical artery, with an occasional contribution from the inferior vesicle artery.[470] Venous drainage is via the vesiculodeferential veins and inferior vesical veins. Lymphatic

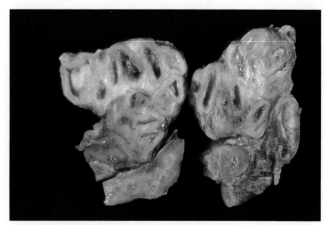

FIGURE 8-117 ■ Seminal vesicle: cut surfaces show convolutions and smooth muscle wall surrounding luminal spaces.

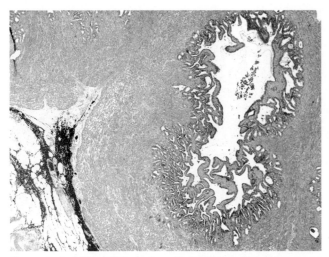

FIGURE 8-118 ■ Normal seminal vesicle with luminal space and mucosa, with surrounding smooth muscle wall and periseminal vesicle adipose tissue.

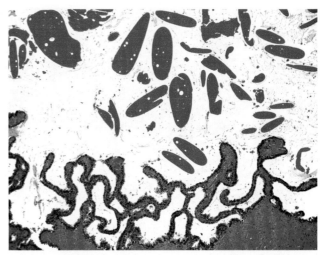

FIGURE 8-120 ■ Intraluminal seminal vesicle crystalloids.

drainage is to the internal iliac lymph nodes.[470] Innervation is by the pelvic nerve and hypogastric nerve. Microscopically, nerves can be seen in soft tissue surrounding the seminal vesicle and in the smooth muscle wall of the seminal vesicle.

Histology

Microscopically, there are four major anatomic compartments—the lumen, the mucosa, the smooth muscle wall, and surrounding fibroadipose tissue (Figs. 8-118 and 8-119). The seminal vesicle displays a large central lumen with six to eight primary branches and several secondary branches.[474] The luminal space may contain proteinaceous fluid, sloughed epithelial cells and cellular debris, refluxed spermatozoa, and crystalloids.[471,474,475] These seminal vesicle crystalloids are larger with curved or blunt angles and plate-like secretions (Fig. 8-120) compared to prostatic intraluminal crystalloids.[475]

The seminal vesicle epithelium is composed of ducts and acini with a two-cell-lining layer of secretory cells and basal cells (Fig. 8-121). Many of the secretory cells harbor a large amount of intracytoplasmic pigment that varies in coloration from golden yellow (Fig. 8-122) to pale brown to gray-brown, blue, or pink. This pigment is not specific for seminal vesicle epithelium and may also be seen in epithelium of the ejaculatory ducts and the ampulla of the vas deferens and also in prostatic epithelium.[25,476] The seminal vesicle golden-yellow lipofuscin pigment is more abundant, coarser, larger, and more refractile than the prostatic epithelial pigment.[25,476] Luminal cell nuclei are variable in appearance, with scattered nuclei exhibiting enlargement and marked degenerative-type hyperchromasia[477,478] (Figs. 8-121 to 8-123). This variability in nuclear features can help distinguish seminal vesicle epithelium from prostatic epithelium,

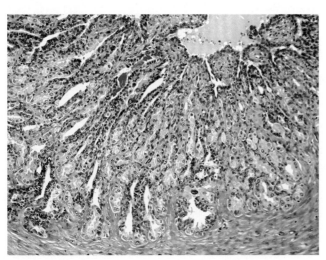

FIGURE 8-119 ■ Normal seminal vesicle mucosa with crowded acini.

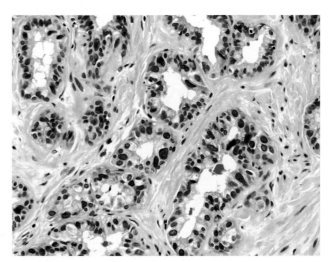

FIGURE 8-121 ■ Benign seminal vesicle epithelium with nuclear atypia. Basal cells may be difficult to identify on H&E-stained sections.

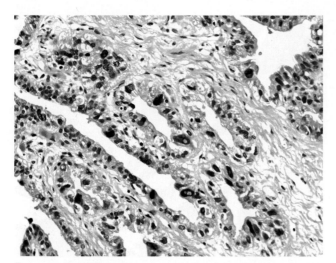

FIGURE 8-122 ■ Benign seminal vesicle with intracytoplasmic pigment and nuclear atypia.

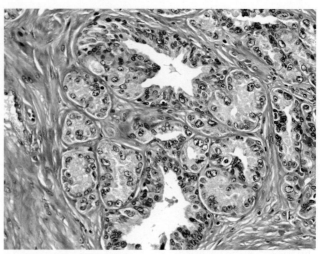

FIGURE 8-124 ■ Prominent nucleoli in benign seminal vesicle epithelium.

both neoplastic and nonneoplastic, which displays more uniform nuclei. Giant cell carcinomas of the prostate do exist but are exceedingly rare and the giant cells do not have the smudged chromatin of the large normal seminal vesicle epithelial cells. Seminal vesicle nuclei may harbor prominent nucleoli (Fig. 8-124), which can be confused with prostatic neoplastic nuclei. Another characteristic of secretory cell nuclei is the presence of intranuclear cytoplasmic protrusions, which are seen in a few cells in most seminal vesicles. The seminal vesicle nuclear atypia does not indicate dysplasia or malignancy.

The smooth muscle wall of the seminal vesicle has a thin external longitudinal layer and a thicker internal circular layer (Fig. 8-125). Uncommonly, small hyaline globules are seen in the wall. These structures probably represent degenerated smooth muscle cells. Two cases of intracellular stromal lipofuscinosis have been reported.[479] This finding should not be mistaken for a melanocytic process.

Fibroadipose tissue with blood vessels and nerves is identified at the base of the seminal vesicles excised in radical prostatectomy specimens (Fig. 8-126).

Immunohistology

The seminal vesicle epithelial basal cells are positive for high-molecular-weight cytokeratins[480] and p63 (Fig. 8-127). The luminal cells in the epithelium react with AE1/AE3 and CAM5.2 cytokeratin antibodies and with antibodies to MUC6 and PAX-2. These latter two markers are present in seminal vesicle and ejaculatory duct epithelium but not in prostatic adenocarcinoma.[481,482] AMACR, also known as P504S, is negative in seminal vesicle epithelium and positive in most prostatic adenocarcinomas.[483] An AMACR/p63 or AMACR/p63/34betaE12 cocktail immunostain is useful in distinguishing seminal vesicle epithelium from prostatic carcinoma[484] (Fig. 8-128). PSA and PSAP immunostains are also negative

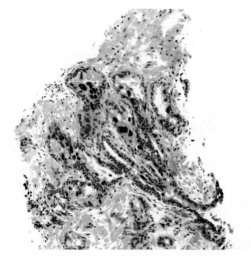

FIGURE 8-123 ■ Benign seminal vesicle epithelium, with nuclear atypia, inadvertently sampled in biopsy of prostate gland.

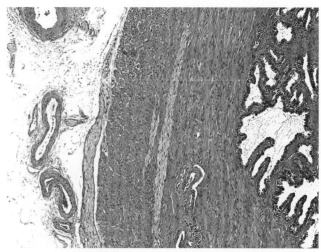

FIGURE 8-125 ■ Normal seminal vesicle smooth muscle wall with inner circular and outer longitudinal layers. Note peripheral nerve inside wall and also in periseminal vesicle soft tissue.

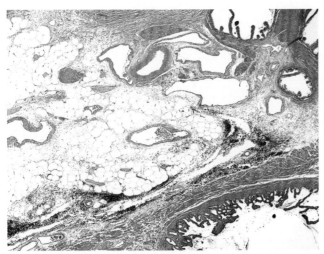

FIGURE 8-126 ■ Triangular-shaped soft tissue between prostate **(upper right)** and seminal vesicle **(lower right)**. A common mode of spread of prostatic carcinoma into the seminal vesicle is via extraprostatic extension into this soft tissue, with growth into the outer aspect of the seminal vesicle wall.

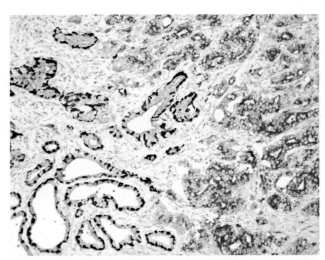

FIGURE 8-128 ■ Seminal vesicle wall invasion by prostatic adenocarcinoma, as demonstrated by "triple stain." Benign seminal vesicle epithelium, with basal cells marked by *brown* chromogen, is on left. AMACR-positive (*red* chromogen), basal cell–negative prostatic adenocarcinoma is invading the seminal vesicle wall on the right.

in seminal vesicle epithelium, as long as monoclonal rather than polyclonal antibodies are used.[476,481,485,486]

Ultrastructural Features

The columnar secretory cells have microvilli, numerous mitochondria, and a well-developed rough endoplasmic reticulum.

Malformations

Developmental abnormalities of the seminal vesicle are rare. In one large postmortem examination series, the incidence was 0.05%.[487] The incidence is higher in infertile patients,

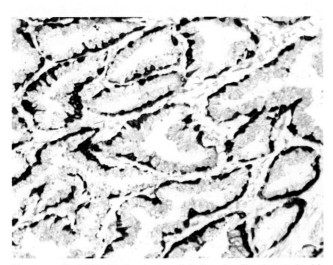

FIGURE 8-127 ■ Seminal vesicle basal cells, detected with "triple stain" comprising 34βE12 and p63 antibodies (*brown* chromogen). The AMACR antibody is nonreactive with normal seminal vesicle epithelium; a positive reaction is *red*.

at about 6%.[85,488] Radiologic imaging, especially magnetic resonance imaging, is useful in clinical diagnosis of congenital anomalies of the seminal vesicle.[489]

Agenesis, or absence of seminal vesicle due to failure to form, may be unilateral or bilateral. Unilateral agenesis of the seminal vesicle is frequently associated with an ipsilateral absence of the vas deferens and kidney, and may be associated with ipsilateral central zone agenesis.[490] These anomalies occur when an embryologic insult affects the ureteric bud and mesonephric duct prior to their separation at 7 weeks of gestation.[491] Bilateral absence of the seminal vesicles is often present in conjunction with a bilateral absence of the vas deferens in men who are carriers for the cystic fibrosis transmembrane conductance regulator (CTFR) gene mutation in cystic fibrosis.[492,493] Anywhere from 60% to 100% of men with bilateral seminal vesicle agenesis are carriers of a CTFR mutation. A high percentage of men with overt cystic fibrosis have congenital bilateral absence of vas deferens and lack a seminal vesicle.[492] A few cases of seminal vesicle hypoplasia,[85] fusion,[85] and duplications[85,494] have been reported.

Ureterovesicular fistulas can occur as malformations and represent implantation and drainage of an ectopic ureter into the seminal vesicles.[495,496] This anomaly is caused by an abnormally high cranial origin of the ureteric bud on the mesonephric duct, with resultant delayed absorption and ectopic insertion of the ureter into the posterior urethra, vas deferens, ejaculatory ducts, or seminal vesicle.[496] The ectopic ureter often drains into a cystic seminal vesicle.

Other forms of ectopia in the seminal vesicle include rare examples of vasa deferentia opening into a seminal vesicle cyst[497] and benign prostatic tissue in a seminal vesicle wall (Fig. 8-129). There are two reported cases of benign ectopic prostatic tissue in the seminal vesicle.[99,498]

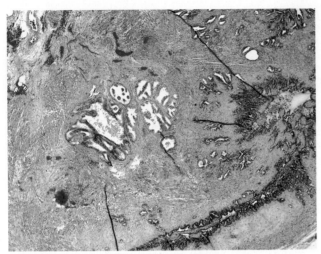

FIGURE 8-129 ■ Ectopic benign prostatic tissue in seminal vesicle wall: a rare finding.

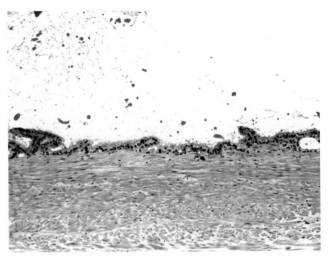

FIGURE 8-130 ■ Seminal vesicle cyst with flattened seminal vesicle mucosa.

Benignancy in one case was substantiated by the histomorphologic appearance in conjunction with basal cell presence as verified by 34βE12 immunohistochemistry.[99] The glands formed a 5-mm nodule in the seminal vesicle wall, had a cribriform pattern, resembled benign central zone glands, and were PSA and PSAP positive. In contrast, prostatic adenocarcinoma would exhibit nuclear atypia and basal cell absence.

Cysts

Seminal vesicle cysts are rare, with an incidence of 0.001%.[499] About 135 cases have been reported. Seminal vesicle cysts may be congenital or acquired.[500] Acquired cysts are often bilateral and typically develop due to ejaculatory duct obstruction secondary to chronic prostatitis or prostate surgery. Congenital cysts are associated with anomalies of the ipsilateral mesonephric duct, such as ipsilateral renal agenesis and ureteral ectopia in the cyst.[501,502] Seminal vesicle cysts are also linked with autosomal dominant polycystic kidney disease.[503,504] From 20% to 60% of patients with autosomal dominant polycystic kidney disease have seminal vesicle cysts. Other associations include hemivertebra, infertility, absence or atresia of the vas deferens, and ipsilateral absence of the testis.[500]

Most seminal vesicle cysts are <5 cm, unilateral, and asymptomatic. These cysts are usually detected incidentally as a palpable abdominal mass or as a fluctuant mass on DRE. Symptomatic men present in the second to fourth decades of life (range 3 to 63 years). Symptoms include dysuria, frequency, hematuria, perineal pain, postejaculatory pain, and scrotal pain.[502] Cysts >12 cm have been designated giant cysts and these patients often present with symptoms related to urinary bladder and/or colonic obstruction secondary to mass effect.[501] Ultrasound and MRI examinations are diagnostic.[489] Surgical excision is usually reserved for symptomatic cysts.

Histologic sections of seminal vesicle cysts show a unilocular cyst with a flattened mucosa (Fig. 8-130) and epithelium, with or without ulceration.[505] Acute and chronic inflammatory cell infiltrates may be seen in a fibrotic wall. The cyst lumen may contain red blood cells, inflammatory cells, and/or spermatozoa.[505] In five cases a neoplasm has been discovered in a benign seminal vesicle cyst.[506–510] Four cases were carcinoma and one was classified as a "mesonephroid tumor."[510] The carcinomas were squamous cell carcinoma,[509] papillary/mucinous adenocarcinoma,[506] papillary adenocarcinoma,[508] and tubulopapillary adenocarcinoma.[507] Of note, the last two cases were of young patients aged 17 and 19 years.

The differential diagnosis for benign seminal vesicle cysts should focus on prostatic cysts and müllerian duct cysts. Seminal vesicle cysts are lateral, like prostatic cysts, but unlike prostatic cysts, sperm is present in the cyst contents of seminal vesicle cysts. Also, symptomatic seminal vesicle cysts tend to occur in younger patients (second to fourth decades) compared to prostatic cysts, which are usually found in patients over 50 years of age. Finally, the lining layer in seminal vesicle cysts is PSA and PSAP negative while prostatic cyst epithelial linings are PSA and PSAP positive in immunohistochemistry. In contrast to seminal vesicle cysts, müllerian duct cysts are midline and lack sperm in the cystic cavity.

Inflammation and Infection

Clinical seminal vesiculitis is rare in the United States. Incidental histologically detected inflammatory cell infiltrates (Fig. 8-131) are also uncommon, in stark contrast to the common finding of incidental histologic inflammation in the prostate. Clinical prostatitis and epididymitis are associated with seminal vesiculitis.[511] In patients with prostatitis, the seminal vesiculitis is frequently due to enteric bacteria. Seminal vesicle abscess formation is rare.[500,512] Patients with

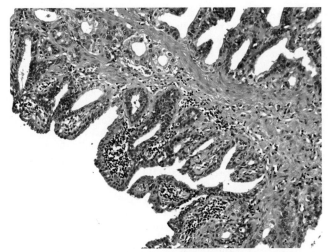

FIGURE 8-131 ■ Chronic seminal vesiculitis.

diabetes, urinary tract infection, prolonged catheterization, and anatomical anomalies are also predisposed to abscess development.[500] MRI is the modality of choice for visualization of seminal vesicle abscess. Abscess aspiration or puncture followed by culture has demonstrated that *Staphylococcus aureus* and *E. coli* are the most common organisms in the abscesses. Other organisms that have been identified in a few cases of seminal vesicle abscess include *Mycobacteria*,[513] CMV,[514] *Schistosoma*,[515] and *Echinococcus*.[516] One case was polymicrobial in a renal transplant patient.[517] Single cases of infectious agent–associated histologic entities include seminal vesicle malakoplakia[518] and seminal vesicle BCG granulomas.[519]

Inflammation of the seminal vesicle blood vessels has been reported as an incidental finding in two radical prostatectomy cases.[520] This necrotizing vasculitis was not associated with a systemic vasculitis.

Calcification and Calculi

Dystrophic calcification in the wall of the seminal vesicle is clinically rare,[521] but is common as an incidental histologic finding.[522] Clinically, it is often associated with calcification of the vas deferens, particularly in diabetic patients. The histologic incidence is 58% in radical prostatectomy and cystoprostatectomy specimens.[522] Microscopically, calcifications can be found in glands and/or stroma, and are usually mild in degree of calcium deposition.[522] Bony metaplasia has also been found in a few patients.[523] Calcification in the seminal vesicle has no known functional or clinical significance.

Stones are also rare in the seminal vesicle.[524–526] Seminal vesicle lithiasis is usually due to obstruction and/or infection.[524,525] The stones are smooth, hard, and are composed of a nucleus of epithelial cells, mucoid material, and a covering of lime salts. Size ranges from 1 mm to 3 cm.[526] Symptomatic stones are treated by open vesiculectomy.

Amyloid

Amyloid deposition in the wall of the seminal vesicle may be seen as an incidental, localized finding in 5% to 10% of prostates from radical prostatectomy and autopsy.[527–530] The incidence range at autopsy is 1% to 19%. Incidence is related to age, with the highest incidence reported for men over 75.[529] Amyloid in the seminal vesicle is almost always asymptomatic although there are rare exceptions.[531] Radiologically, by MR imaging, seminal vesicles involved by amyloid demonstrate diffuse wall thickening that can often mimic tumor invasion by prostate cancer.[532] Grossly, seminal vesicles with amyloid typically appear normal, although in a few cases the wall is thickened and firm.[530] Microscopically, both seminal vesicles are involved by a subepithelial, nodular to strand-like deposition of pink, homogeneous extracellular material[529,530,533] (Figs. 8-132 and 8-133). The luminal space of the seminal vesicle may be narrowed as a consequence of the amyloid accumulation (Fig. 8-132). In the vast majority of cases seminal vesicle amyloid is localized without evidence of systemic amyloidosis. One should specifically assess perivesicular vessels for amyloid. Detection of amyloid in vessel walls suggests systemic amyloidosis.[529,533] The presence of amyloid in the seminal vesicle is indicative of ejaculatory system amyloid, with amyloid also being found in the vasa deferentia and ejaculatory ducts. Congo red and crystal violet histochemical stains are positive, with Congo red staining displaying a typical green birefringence. Immunohistochemical stains of sections of localized seminal vesicle amyloid are positive for the P component and lactoferrin, with negative staining for AA amyloid, β2 microglobulin, prealbumin, and kappa and lambda light chains.[533,534] In contrast, in the few reported cases of systemic amyloidosis involving the seminal vesicle, the immunophenotype is different, with stains for prealbumin transthyretin type of amyloid[535] and AA amyloid[533] being

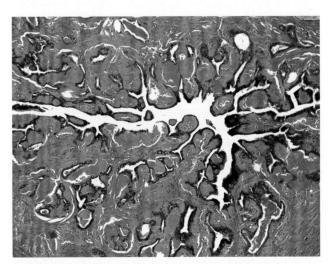

FIGURE 8-132 ■ Amyloid deposition in seminal vesicle, with luminal narrowing.

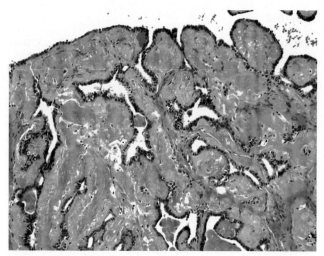

FIGURE 8-133 ■ Amyloid deposition in seminal vesicle.

positive. Ultrastructural examination of seminal vesicle amyloid shows characteristic 7.5- to 10-nm rigid, linear, and nonbranching fibrils.[534]

Muscular/Fibromuscular Hyperplasia

There are three reported cases of hyperplasia of mesenchymal cells in the seminal vesicle wall.[536–538] Two cases represent fibromuscular hyperplasia and one is likely smooth muscle hyperplasia of the seminal vesicle wall. The first case of fibromuscular hyperplasia was seen in a 27-year-old man. CT scan showed unilateral seminal vesicle enlargement and histologically the basis for the enlargement was fibromuscular hyperplasia of the seminal vesicle wall.[536] The second case of fibromuscular hyperplasia was seen in the setting of a large congenital seminal vesicle cyst. The last case, which was considered to be adenomyosis, was diagnosed in a 62-year-old man who presented with hematospermia. An ultrasound showed an enlarged right seminal vesicle.[537] Sections of the excised seminal vesicle showed adenomyosis, which may represent smooth muscle hyperplasia with entrapped seminal vesicle glands. These glands in the wall of the seminal vesicle should not be misdiagnosed as adenocarcinoma.

REFERENCES

1. Krieger JN, Lee SW, Jeon J, et al. Epidemiology of prostatitis. *Int J Antimicrob Agents* 2008;31(suppl 1):S85.
2. Clemens JQ, Meenan RT, O'Keeffe-Rosetti MC, et al. Prevalence of prostatitis-like symptoms in a managed care population. *J Urol* 2006;176:593.
3. McVary KT. BPH: epidemiology and comorbidities. *Am J Manag Care* 2006;12(5 suppl):S122.
4. Srigley JR. Benign mimickers of prostatic adenocarcinoma. *Mod Pathol* 2004;17:328.
5. Herawi M, Parwani AV, Irie J, et al. Small glandular proliferations on needle biopsies: most common benign mimickers of prostatic adenocarcinoma sent in for expert second opinion. *Am J Surg Pathol* 2005;29:874.
6. Bostwick DG, Cheng L. Overdiagnosis of prostatic adenocarcinoma. *Semin Urol Oncol* 1999;17:199.
7. Hameed O, Humphrey PA. Pseudoneoplastic mimics of prostate and bladder carcinomas. *Arch Pathol Lab Med* 2010;134:427.
8. Partin AW, Coffey DS. The molecular biology, endocrinology, and physiology of the prostate and seminal vesicles. In: Walsh PC, Retik AB, Vaughan ED Jr, et al., eds. *Campbell's Urology*. 8th ed. Philadelphia, PA: Saunders; 2002.
9. Wilson JD, Griffin JE, Leshin M, et al. Role of gondal hormones in development of the sexual phenotypes. *Hum Genet* 1981;58:78.
10. Imperato-McGinely J, Guerrero L, Gautier T, et al. Steroid 5alpha-reductase deficiency in man: an inherited form of male pseudohermaphroditism. *Science* 1974;186:1213.
11. McNeal JE. Prostate. In: Mills SE, ed. *Histology for Pathologists*. 3rd ed. Philadelphia, PA: Lippincott Williams & Wilkins; 2007.
12. Cunha GR, Ricke W, Thomson A, et al. Hormonal, cellular, and molecular regulation of normal and neoplastic prostatic development. *J Steroid Biochem Mol Biol* 2004;92:221.
13. Timms BG, Lee CW, Aumüller G, et al. Instructive induction of prostate growth and differentiation by a defined urogenital sinus mesenchyme. *Microsc Res Tech* 1995;30:319.
14. Xia T, Blackburn WR, Gardner WA Jr. Fetal prostate growth and development. *Pediatr Pathol* 1990;10:527.
15. Letellier G, Perez MJ, Yacoub M, et al. Epithelial phenotypes in the developing human prostate. *J Histochem Cytochem* 2007;55:885.
16. Zhu G, Zhau HE, He H, et al. Sonic and desert hedgehog signaling in human fetal prostate development. *Prostate* 2007;67:674.
17. Shen MM, Abate-Shen C. Roles of the Nkx.3 homeobox gene in prostate organogenesis and carcinogenesis. *Dev Dyn* 2003;228:767.
18. Kasper S. Exploring the origins of the normal prostate and prostate cancer stem cell. *Stem Cell Rev* 2008;4:193.
19. LeDuc IE. The anatomy of the prostate and the pathology of early benign hypertrophy. *J Urol* 1939;42:1217.
20. Lowsley OS. The development of the human prostate gland with reference to the development of the other structures at the neck of the urinary bladder. *Am J Anat* 1912;13:299.
21. Franks LM. Benign nodular hyperplasia of the prostate: a review. *Ann R Coll Surg Engl* 1954;14:92.
22. Oh C-S, Chung I-H, Won H-S, et al. Morphologic variants of the prostatic utricle. *Clin Anat* 2009;22:358.
23. Srodon M, Epstein JI. Central zone histology of the prostate: a mimicker of high-grade prostatic intraepithelial neoplasia. *Hum Pathol* 2002;33:518.
24. Lexander H, Franzén B, Hirschberg D, et al. Differential protein expression in anatomical zones of the prostate. *Proteomics* 2005;5:2570.
25. Amin MB, Bostwick DG. Pigment in prostatic epithelium and adenocarcinoma: a potential source of diagnostic confusion with seminal vesicular epithelium. *Mod Pathol* 1996;9:791.
26. Hameed O, Humphrey PA. Immunohistochemistry in diagnostic surgical pathology of the prostate. *Semin Diagn Pathol* 2005;22:88.
27. Sweat SD, Pacelli A, Murphy GP, et al. Prostate-specific membrane antigen expression is greatest in prostate adenocarcinoma and lymph node metastases. *Urology* 1998;52:637.
28. Marchal C, Redondo M, Padilla M, et al. Expression of prostate specific membrane antigen (PSMA) in prostatic adenocarcinoma and prostatic intraepithelial neoplasia. *Histol Histopathol* 2004;19:715.
29. Xu J, Kalos M, Stolk JA, et al. Identification and characterization of prostein, a novel prostate-specific protein. *Cancer Res* 2001;61:1563.
30. Kalos M, Askaa J, Hylander BL, et al. Prostein expression is highly restricted to normal and malignant prostate tissues. *Prostate* 2004;60:246.
31. Chan TY, Mikolajczyk SD, Lecksell K, et al. Immunohistochemical staining of prostate cancer with monoclonal antibodies to the precursor of prostate-specific antigen. *Urology* 2003;62:177.
32. Bethel CR, Faith D, Li X, et al. Decreased NKX3.1 protein expression in focal prostatic atrophy, prostatic intraepithelial neoplasia, and adenocarcinoma: association with Gleason score and chromosome 8p deletion. *Cancer Res* 2006;66:10683.

33. Srigley JR, Dardick I, Hartwick RWJ, et al. Basal epithelial cells of human prostate gland are not myoepithelial cells. *Am J Pathol* 1990;136:957.

34. Zhou M, Shah R, Shen R, et al. Basal cell cocktail (34betaE12 and p63) improves the detection of prostate basal cells. *Am J Surg Pathol* 2003;27:365.

35. Goldstein NS, Underhill J, Roszka J, et al. Cytokeratin 34 beta E-12 immunoreactivity in benign prostatic acini. Quantitation, pattern assessment, and electron microscopic study. *Am J Clin Pathol* 1999;112:69.

36. di Sant'Agnese PA. Neuroendocrine differentiation in prostatic carcinoma. Recent findings and new concepts. *Cancer* 1995;75:1850.

37. Cohen RJ, Glezerson G, Taylor LF, et al. The neuroendocrine cell population of the human prostate gland. *J Urol* 1993;150:365.

38. Yantiss RK, Young RH. Transitional cell "metaplasia" in the prostate gland. A survey of its frequency and features based on 103 consecutive prostatic biopsy specimens. *J Urol Pathol* 1997;7:71.

39. Humphrey PA, Vollmer RT. Corpora amylacea in adenocarcinoma of the prostate: prevalence in 100 prostatectomies and clinicopathologic correlations. *Surg Pathol* 1990;3:133.

40. Moore RA. Morphology of prostatic corpora amylacea and calculi. *Arch Pathol* 1936;22:24.

41. Seaman AR. Cytochemical observations on corpora amylacea of human prostate gland. *J Urol* 1956;76:99.

42. Moore RA, Hanzel BF. Chemical composition of prostatic corpora amylacea and calculi. *Arch Pathol* 1936;22:41.

43. Marx AJ, Moskal JF, Gueft B. Prostatic corpora amylacea. A study with the electron microscope and electron probe. *Arch Pathol* 1965;80:487.

44. Peeling WB, Griffiths GJ. Imaging of the prostate by ultrasound. *J Urol* 1984;132:217.

45. Woods JE, Soh S, Wheeler TM. Distribution and significance of microcalcifications in the neoplastic and nonneoplastic prostate. *Arch Pathol Lab Med* 1998;122:152.

46. Cristol DS, Emmett JL. The incidence of coincident calculi, prostatic hyperplasia and carcinoma of the prostate gland. *JAMA* 1944;124:646.

47. Henneberry JM, Kahane H, Humphrey PA, et al. The significance of intraluminal crystalloids in benign prostatic glands on needle biopsy. *Am J Surg Pathol* 1997;21:725.

48. Schowinsky JT, Epstein JI. Distorted rectal tissue on prostate needle biopsy: a mimicker of prostate cancer. *Am J Surg Pathol* 2006; 30:866.

49. Cohen RJ, Stables S. Intraprostatic fat. *Hum Pathol* 1998;29:424.

50. Sung MT, Eble JN, Cheng L. Invasion of fat justifies assignment of stage pT3a in prostatic adenocarcinoma. *Pathology* 2006;38:309.

51. Joshi A, Shah V, Varma M. Intraprostatic fat in a needle biopsy: a case report and review of the literature. *Histopathology* 2009;54:912.

52. Ayala AG, Ro JY, Babaian R, et al. The prostatic capsule: does it exist? Its importance in the staging and treatment of prostatic carcinoma. *Am J Surg Pathol* 1989;13:21.

53. DiLollo S, Menchi I, Brizzi E, et al. The morphology of the prostatic capsule with particular regard to the posterosuperior region: an anatomical and clinical problem. *Surg Radiol Anat* 1997;19:143.

54. Sattar AA, Noel JC, Vanderhaegen JJ, et al. Prostate capsule: computerized morphometric analysis of its components. *Urology* 1995;46:178.

55. Manley CB Jr. The striated muscle of the prostate. *J Urol* 1966;45:234.

56. Ibrahim SN, Lightner VA, Ventimiglia JB, et al. Tenascin expression in prostatic hyperplasia, intraepithelial neoplasia, and carcinoma. *Hum Pathol* 1993;24:982.

57. Xue Y, Li J, Latijnhouwers MA, et al. Expression of periglandular tenascin-C and basement membrane laminin in normal prostate, benign prostatic hyperplasia and prostate carcinoma. *Br J Urol* 1998;81:844.

58. McVary KT, McKenna KE, Lee C. Prostate innervation. *Prostate Suppl* 1998;8:2.

59. Powell MS, Li R, Dai H, et al. Neuroanatomy of the normal prostate. *Prostate* 2005;65:52.

60. Ostrowski ML, Wheeler TM. Paraganglia of the prostate. Location, frequency and differentiation from prostatic adenocarcinoma. *Am J Surg Pathol* 1994;18:412.

61. Carstens PH. Perineural glands in normal and hyperplastic prostate. *J Urol* 1980;123:686.

62. McIntire TL, Franzini DA. The presence of benign prostatic glands in perineural spaces. *J Urol* 1986;135:507.

63. Ali TZ, Epstein JI. Perineural involvement by benign prostatic glands on needle biopsy. *Am J Surg Pathol* 2005;29:1159.

64. Cramer SF. Benign glandular inclusion in prostatic nerve. *Am J Clin Pathol* 1981;75:854.

65. Montironi R, Galluzzi CM, Diamanti L, et al. Prostatic intra-epithelial neoplasia. Qualitative and quantitative analyses of the blood capillary architecture on thin tissue sections. *Pathol Res Pract* 1993;189:542.

66. Kothari PS, Scardino PT, Ohori M, et al. Incidence, location, and significance of periprostatic and periseminal vesicle lymph nodes in prostate cancer. *Am J Surg Pathol* 2001;25:1429.

67. Cina SJ, Silberman MA, Kahane H, et al. Diagnosis of Cowper's glands on prostate needle biopsy. *Am J Surg Pathol* 1997;21:550.

68. Saboorian MH, Huffman H, Ashfaq R, et al. Distinguishing Cowper's glands from neoplastic and pseudoneoplastic lesions of prostate: immunohistochemical and ultrastructural studies. *Am J Surg Pathol* 1997;21:1069.

69. Melcher MP. Bulbourethral glands of Cowper [letter]. *Arch Pathol Lab Med* 1986;110:991.

70. Elgamal AA, Van de Voorde W, Van Poppel H, et al. Immunohistochemical localization of prostate-specific markers within the accessory male sex glands of Cowper, Littre, and Morgagni. *Urology* 1994;44:84.

71. Griffin JE, Wilson JD. Disorders of androgen receptor function. *Ann N Y Acad Sci* 1984;438:61.

72. Popek EJ, Tyson RW, Miller GJ, et al. Prostate development in prune belly syndrome (PBS) and posterior urethral valves (PUV): etiology of PBS-lower urinary tract obstruction or primary mesenchymal defect? *Pediatr Pathol* 1991;11:1.

73. Schuhrke TD, Kaplan GW. Prostatic utricle cysts (Müllerian duct cysts). *J Urol* 1978;119:765.

74. Shapiro E, Huang H, McFadden DE, et al. The prostate utricle is not a Mullerian duct remnant: immunohisotchmeical evidence for a distinct urothenital sinus origin. *J Urol* 2004;172:1753.

75. Moore RA. Pathology of the prostatic utricle. *Arch Pathol* 1937;23:517.

76. Devine CJ Jr, Gonzalez-Serva L, Stecker JF Jr, et al. Utricular configuration in hypospadias and intersex. *J Urol* 1980;123:407.

77. Coppens L, Bonnet P, Andrianne R, et al. Adult müllerian duct or utricle cyst: clinical significance and therapeutic management of 65 cases. *J Urol* 2002;167:1740.

78. Shabsigh R, Lerner S, Fishman IJ, et al. The role of transrectal ultrasonography in the diagnosis and management of prostatic and seminal vesicle cysts. *J Urol* 1989;141:1206.

79. Sanchez-Chapado M, Angulo JC. Giant Müllerian duct cyst mimicking prostatic malignancy. *Scand J Urol Nephrol* 1995;29:229.

80. Barringer BS. Papillary intracystic adenocarcinoma of prostate and massive benign prostatic cyst. *Am J Surg* 1933;20:51.

81. Nogueira March JL, Figueiredo L, Mata J, et al. Coexisting cyst of the utricle and carcinoma of the endometrial type in the prostate. *Eur Urol* 1982;8:42.

82. Xing JP, Dang JG, Wu PP, et al. Papillary cystadenocarcinoma in a Müllerian duct cyst: report of a case with literature review [Chinese]. *Zhonghua Nan Ke Xue* 2006;12:218.

83. Szemes GC, Rubin DJ. Squamous cell carcinoma in a Mullerian duct cyst. *J Urol* 1968;100:40.

84. Gualco G, Ortega V, Ardao G, et al. Clear cell adenocarcinoma of the prostate utricle in an adolescent. *Ann Diagn Pathol* 2005;9:153.

85. Malatinsky E, Labady F, Lepies P, et al. Congenital anomalies of the seminal ducts. *Int Urol Nephrol* 1987;19:189.

86. Villers A, Terris MK, McNeal JE, et al. Ultrasound anatomy of the prostate: the normal gland and anatomical variations. *J Urol* 1990; 143:732.

87. Gikas PW, Del Buono EA, Epstein JI. Florid hyperplasia of mesonephric remnants involving prostate and periprostatic tissue. Possible confusion with adenocarcinoma. *Am J Surg Pathol* 1993;17:454.

88. Jimenez RE, Raval MFT, Spanta R, et al. Mesonephric remnants hyperplasia: a pitfall in the diagnosis of prostatic adenocarcinoma. *J Urol Pathol* 1998;9:83.

89. Val-Bernal JF, Gomez-Ortega JM. Hyperplasia of prostatic mesonephric remnants: a potentitial pitfall in the evaluation of prostate gland biopsy. *J Urol* 1995;154:1138.

90. Bostwick DG, Qian J, Ma J, et al. Mesonephric remnants of the prostate: incidence and histologic spectrum. *Mod Pathol* 2003;16:630.

91. Bromberg WD, Kozlowski JM, Oyasu R. Prostate-type gland in the epididymis. *J Urol* 1991;145:1273.

92. Ewing R, Harnden-Mayor P, Mason MK, et al. Extra-urethral ectopic prostate. *Br J Urol* 1987;60:433.

93. Fulton RS, Rouse RV, Ranheim EA. Ectopic prostate: case report of a presacral mass presenting with obstructive symptoms. *Arch Pathol Lab Med* 2001;125:286.

94. Kanomata N, Eble JN, Ohbayashi C, et al. Ectopic prostate in the retrovesical space. *J Urol Pathol* 1997;7:121.

95. Klein HZ, Rosenberg ML. Ectopic prostatic tissue in bladder trigone. Distinctive cause of hematuria. *Urology* 1984;23:81.

96. Milburn JM, Bluth EI, Mitchell WT Jr. Ectopic prostate in the testicle: an unusual cause of a solid testicular mass on ultrasonography. *J Ultrasound Med* 1994;13:578.

97. Morey AF, Kreder KJ, Wikert GA, et al. Ectopic prostate tissue at the bladder dome. *J Urol* 1989;141:942.

98. Morgan MB. Ectopic prostatic tissue of the anal canal. *J Urol* 1992;147:165.

99. Salem CE, Gibbs PM, Highshaw RA, et al. Benign ectopic prostatic tissue involving the seminal vesicle in a patient with prostate cancer: recognition and implications for staging. *Urology* 1996;48:490.

100. Spiro LH, Levine B. Ectopic subvesical prostatic tissue. *J Urol* 1994;112:631.

101. Vogel U, Negri G, Bültmann B. Ectopic prostatic tissue in the spleen. *Virchows Arch* 1996;427:543.

102. Bellezza G, Sidoni A, Cavaliere H. Ectopic prostatic tissue in the bladder. *Int J Urol* 2005;12:1066.

103. Van Beek CA, Peters CA, Vargas SO. Ectopic prostate tissue within the processus vaginalis: insights into prostate embryogenesis. *Pediatr Dev Pathol* 2005;8:379.

104. Kazakov DV, Stewart CJR, Kacerovska D, et al. Prostatic-type tissue in the lower female genital tract: a morphologic spectrum, including vaginal tubulosquamous polyp, adenomyomatous hyperplasia of paraurethral Skene glands (female prostate), and ectopic lesion in the vulva. *Am J Surg Pathol* 2010;34:950.

105. Smith CET, Toplis PJ, Nogales FF. Ovarian prostatic tissue originating from hilar mesonephric nests. *Am J Surg Pathol* 1999;23:232.

106. Halabi M, Oliva E, Mazal PR, et al. Prostatic tissue in mature cystic teratomas. A report of 4 cases, including 1 with features of prostatic adenocarcinoma, and cytogenetic studies. *Int J Gynecol Pathol* 2002;21:267.

107. McCluggage WG, Ganesan R, Hirschowitz L, et al. Ectopic prostatic tissue in the uterine cervix and vagina: report of a series with a detailed immunohistochemical analysis. *Am J Surg Pathol* 2006;30:209.

108. Tokumitsu S, Tokumitsu K, Takeya M, et al. Developmentally heterotopic urogenital tissues in a retroperitoneal lipoma with hematopoiesis. *Acta Pathol Jpn* 1981;31:289.

109. Roma AA, Humphrey PA. Prostatic tissue in testicular teratoma. A clinicopathologic and immunohistochemical study. *Ann Diagn Pathol* 2013;17:10.

110. Yasukawa S, Aoshi H, Takamatsu M. Ectopic prostatic adenoma in retrovesical space. *J Urol* 1987;137:998.

111. Adams JR Jr. Adenocarcinoma in ectopic prostatic tissue. *J Urol* 1993;150:1253.

112. Krieger JN, Nyberg L, Nickel JC. NIH consensus definition and classification of prostatitis. *JAMA* 1999;281:236.

113. Roberts RO, Lieber MM, Bostwick DG, et al. A review of clinical and pathological prostatitis syndromes. *Urology* 1997;49:809.

114. NCHS (National Center for Health Statistics). Advance data from vital and health statistics. Nos. 61-70 *Vital Health Stat* 1993;16.

115. Collins MM, Meigs JB, Barry MJ, et al. Prevalence and correlates of prostatitis in the health professionals follow-up study cohort. *J Urol* 2002;167:1362.

116. Roberts RO, Lieber MM, Rhodes T, et al. Prevalence of a physician-assisted diagnosis of prostatitis: the Olmsted County study of urinary symptoms and health status among men. *Urology* 1998;51:578.

117. Pontari MA. Chronic prostatitis/chronic pelvic pain syndrome. *Urol Clin North Am* 2008;35:81.

118. Strauss AC, Dimitrakov JD. New treatments for chronic prostatitis/chronic pelvic pain syndrome. *Nat Rev Urol* 2010;7:127.

119. Benway BM, Moon TD. Bacterial prostatitis. *Urol Clin Am* 2008;35:23.

120. Lipsky BA, Byren I, Hoey CT. Treatment of bacterial prostatitis. *Clin Infect Dis* 2010;50:1641.

121. True LD, Berger RE, Rothman I, et al. Prostate histopathology and the chronic prostatitis/chronic pelvic pain syndrome: a prospective biopsy study. *J Urol* 1999;162:2014.

122. Nadler RB, Humphrey PA, Smith DS, et al. Effect of inflammation and benign prostatic hyperplasia on elevated serum prostate specific antigen levels. *J Urol* 1995;154:407.

123. Brawer MK, Rennels MS, Nagle RB, et al. Serum prostate-specific antigen and prostate pathology in men having simple prostatectomy. *Am J Clin Pathol* 1989;92:760.

124. Hasui Y, Marutsuka K, Asada Y, et al. Relationship between serum prostate specific antigen and histological prostatitis in patients with benign prostatic hyperplasia. *Prostate* 1994;25:91.

125. Kohnen PE, Drach GW. Patterns of inflammation in prostatic hyperplasia: a histologic and bacteriologic study. *J Urol* 1979;121:755.

126. Ruska KM, Sauvageot J, Epstein JI. Histology and cellular kinetics of prostate atrophy. *Am J Surg Pathol* 1998;22:1073.

127. Nickel JC, True LD, Krieger JN, et al. Consensus development of a histopathological classification system for chronic prostatic inflammation. *BJU Int* 2001;87:797.

128. Helpap B. Histological and immunohistochemical study of chronic prostatic inflammation with and without benign prostatic hyperplasia. *J Urol Pathol* 1994;2:49.

129. Blumenfeld W, Tucci S, Narayan P. Incidental lymphocytic prostatitis. Selective involvement with nonmalignant glands. *Am J Surg Pathol* 1992;16:975.

130. Gupta RK. Mast cell variations in prostate and urinary bladder. *Arch Pathol* 1970;89:302.

131. de Rosario AD, Ross JS. Stromal mast cell density (MCD) in benign and malignant prostatic lesions (abstract). *Mod Pathol* 1998;11:80A.

132. Epstein JI, Hutchins GM. Granulomatous prostatitis: posttransurethral resection lesions. *Hum Pathol* 1984;15:818.

133. Towfighi J, Sadeghee S, Wheeler JE, et al. Granulomatous prostatitis with emphasis on the eosinophilic variety. *Am J Clin Pathol* 1972;58:630.

134. Melicow MM. Allergic granulomas of the prostate. *J Urol* 1951;65:288.

135. Stewart MJ, Wray S, Hull M. Allergic prostatitis in asthmatics. *J Pathol Bacteriol* 1954;67:423.

136. Kelalis PP, Harrison EG Jr, Greene LF. Allergic granulomas of the prostate in asthmatics. *JAMA* 1964;188:963.

137. Epstein JI, Armas OA. Atypical basal cell hyperplasia of the prostate. *Am J Surg Pathol* 1992;16:1205.

138. Thorson P, Swanson PE, Vollmer RT, et al. Basal cell hyperplasia in the peripheral zone of the prostate. *Mod Pathol* 2003;16:598.

139. Bostwick DG, Amin MB, Dundore P, et al. Architectural patterns of high-grade prostatic intraepithelial neoplasia. *Hum Pathol* 1993;24:298.

140. Vesalainen S, Lipponen P, Talja M, et al. Histological grade, perineural infiltration, tumor-infiltrating lymphocytes and apoptosis as determinants of long term prognosis in prostatic adenocarcinoma. *Eur J Cancer* 1994;30A:1797.

141. Alguacil-Garcia A. Artifactual changes mimicking signet ring cell carcinoma in transurethral prostatectomy specimens. *Am J Surg Pathol* 1986;10:795.

142. Taylor EW, Whelis RF, Correa RJ Jr, et al. Granulomatous prostatitis: confusion clinically with carcinoma of the prostate. *J Urol* 1977;117:316.

143. Thompson GJ, Albers DO. Granulomatous prostatitis: condition which clinically may be confused with carcinoma of prostate. *J Urol* 1953;69:530.

144. Kelalis PP, Greene LF, Harrison EG Jr. Granulomatous prostatitis. A mimic of carcinoma of the prostate. *JAMA* 1965;191:287.

145. Bude R, Bree RL, Adler RS, et al. Transrectal ultrasound appearance of granulomatous prostatititis. *J Ultrasound Med* 1990;9:677.

146. Rubenstein JB, Swayne LC, Magidson JG, et al. Granulomatous prostatitis: a hypoechoic lesion of the protate. *Urol Radiol* 1991;13:119.

147. Presti B, Weidner N. Granulomatous prostatitis and poorly differentiated prostate carcinoma. Their distinction with the use of immunohistochemical methods. *Am J Clin Pathol* 1991;95:330.

148. Oppenheimer JR, Kahane H, Epstein JL. Granulomatous prostatitis on needle biopsy. *Arch Pathol Lab Med* 1997;121:724.

149. Stillwell TJ, Engen DE, Farrow GM. The clinical spectrum of granulomatous prostatitis: a report of 200 cases. *J Urol* 1987;138:320.

150. Schmidt JD. Non-specific granulomatous prostatitis: classification, review and report of cases. *J Urol* 1965;94:607.

151. O'Dea MJ, Hunting DB, Green LF. Non-specific granulomatous prostatits. *J Urol* 1977;118:58.

152. Pavlica P, Barozzi L, Bartolone A, et al. Nonspecific granulomatous prostatitis. *Ultraschall Med* 2005;26:203.

153. Bryan RL, Newman J, Campbell A, et al. Granulomatous prostatitis: a clinicopathologic study. *Histopathology* 1991;19:453.

154. Fox H. Nodular histocytic prostatitis. *J Urol* 1966;96:372.

155. Matsumoto T, Sakamoto N, Kimiya K, et al. Nonspecific granulomatous prostatitis. *Urology* 1992;39:420.

156. Miekos E, Wlodarczyk W, Szram S. Xanthogranulomatous prostatitis. *Int Urol Nephrol* 1986;18:433.

157. Sebo TJ, Bostwick DG, Farrow GM, et al. Prostatic xanthoma: a mimic of prostatic adenocarcinoma. *Hum Pathol* 1994;25:386.

158. Chuang AY, Epstein JI. Xanthoma of the prostate: a mimicker of high-grade prostate adenocarcinoma. *Am J Surg Pathol* 2007;31:1225.

159. Lamm DL, Stogdill VD, Stogdill BJ, et al. Complications of bacillus Calmette-Guerin immunotherapy in 1,278 patients with bladder cancer. *J Urol* 1986;135:272.

160. LaFontaine P, Middleman BR, Graham SD Jr, et al. Incidence of granulomatous prostatitis and acid-fast bacilli after intravesical BCG therapy. *Urology* 1997;49:363.

161. Mukamel E, Konichezky M, Engelstein D, et al. Clinical and pathological findings in prostate following intravesical bacillus Calmette-Guerin instillations. *J Urol* 1990;144:1399.

162. Matlaga BR, Veys JA, Thacker CC, et al. Prostate abscess following intravesical bacillus Calmette-Guerin treatment. *J Urol* 2002;167:251.

163. Miyashita H, Tronsco P, Babaian RJ. BCG-induced granulomatous prostatitis: a comparative ultrasound and pathologic study. *Urology* 1992;39:364.

164. Kostakopoulos A, Economou G, Pieramenos D, et al. Tuberculosis of the prostate. *Int Urol Nephrol* 1998;30:153.

165. Lee LW, Burgher LW, Price EB Jr, et al. Granulomatous prostatitis: association with isolation of *Mycobacterium kamasii* and *Mycobacterium fortuitum*. *JAMA* 1987;237:2408.

166. Mikolich DJ, Mates SM. Granulomatous prostatitis due to *Mycobacterium avium* complex. *Clin Infect Dis* 1992;14:589.

167. Moore RA. Tuberculosis of the prostate gland. *J Urol* 1937;37:372.

168. Tamsel S, Killi R, Ertan Y, et al. A rare case of granulomatous prostatitis caused by *Mycobacterium tuberculosis*. *J Clin Ultrasound* 2007;35:58.

169. Thompson L. Syphillis of the prostate. *Am J Syph* 1920;4:323.

170. Bartkowski DP, Lanesky JR. Emphysematous prostatitis and cystitis secondary to *Candida albicans*. *J Urol* 1988;139:1063.

171. Bissada NK, Finkbeiner AE, Redman JF. Prostate mycosis. Nonsurgical diagnosis and management. *Urology* 1977;9:327.

172. Sohail MR, Andrews PE, Blair JE. Coccidioidomycosis of the male genital tract. *J Urol* 2005;173:1978.

173. Yurkanin JP, Ahmann F, Dalkin BL. Coccidioimycosis of the prostate: a determination of incidence, report of 4 cases, and treatment recommendations. *J Infect* 2006;52:e19.

174. Clason AE, McGeorge A, Garland C, et al. Urinary retention and granulomatous prostatitis following sacral herpes zoster infection. A report of 2 cases with a review of the literature. *Br J Urol* 1982;54:166.

175. Gelfand M, Ross CMD, Blair DM, et al. Schistosomiasis of the male pelvic organs. Severity of infection as determined by digestion of tissue and histologic methods in 300 cadavers. *Am J Trop Med Hyg* 1970;19:799.

176. Golz R, Mendling W. Candidosis of the prostate: a rare form of endomycosis. *Mycoses* 1991;34:381.

177. Haas CA, Bodner DR, Hampel N, et al. Systemic candidiasis presenting with prostatic abscess. *Br J Urol* 1998;82:450.

178. Salyer WR, Salyer DC. Involvement of the kidney and prostate in cryptococcosis. *J Urol* 1973;109:695.

179. Symmers WSTC. Two cases of eosinophilic prostatitis due to metazoan infestation with *Oxyuris vermicularis*, and with a larva of *Linguatula serata*. *J Pathol Bacteriol* 1957;73:549.

180. Abbas F, Kamal MK, Talati J. Prostatic aspergillosis. *J Urol* 1995;153:748.

181. Campbell TB, Kaufman L, Cook JL. Aspergillosis of the prostate associated with an indwelling bladder catheter: case report and review. *Clin Infect Dis* 1992;14:942.

182. Caballes RL, Cabelles RA Jr. Primary cryptococcal prostatitis in an apparently uncompromised host. *Prostate* 1999;39:119.

183. Wada R, Nakano N, Yajima N, et al. Granulomatous prostatitis due to *Cryptococcus neoformans*: diagnostic usefulness of special stains and molecular analysis of 18S rDNA. *Prostate Cancer Prostatic Dis* 2008;11:203.

184. Melo CR, Melo JS, Cerski CT. Leukemic infiltration, paracoccidiodomycosis and nodular hyperplasia of the prostate. *Br J Urol* 1992;70:329.

185. Rubin H, Furcolow ML, Yates JL, et al. The course and prognosis of histoplasmosis. *Am J Med* 1959;27:278.

186. Eickenberg HU, Amin H, Lich R Jr. Blastomycosis of the genitourinary tract. *J Urol* 1975;113:650.

187. Hedelin H, Johansson S, Nilsson S. Focal prostatic granulomas. A sequel to transurethral resection. *Scand J Urol Nephrol* 1981;15:193.

188. Helpap B, Vogel J. TUR-prostatitis. Histological and immunohistochemical observations in a special type of granulomatous prostatitis. *Pathol Res Pract* 1986;181:301.

189. Kopolovic J, Rivkind A, Sherman Y. Granulomaous prostatitis with vasculitis. A sequel to transurethral prostatic resection. *Arch Pathol Lab Med* 1984;108:732.

190. Mies C, Balogh K, Stadeker M. Palisading prostate granulomas following surgery. *Am J Surg Pathol* 1984;8:217.

191. Pieterse AS, Aarons I, Jose JS. Focal prostatic granulomas. Rheumatoid-like-probably iatrogenic in origin. *Pathology* 1984;16:174.

192. Henry L, Wagner B, Faulkner MK, et al. Metal deposition in postsurgical granulomas of the urinary tract. *Histopathology* 1993;22:457.

193. Wagner D, Joseph J, Huang J, et al. Malakoplakia of the prostate on needle core biopsy: a case report and review of the literature. *Int J Surg Pathol* 2007;15:86.

194. Thrasher JB, Sutherland RS, Limoge JP, et al. Transrectal ultrasound in diagnosis of malakoplakia of prostate. *Urology* 1992;39:262.

195. Andersen T, Kristiansen W, Ruge S, et al. Malakoplakia of the prostate causing fatal fistula to rectum. *Scand J Urol Nephrol* 1986;20:153.

196. Arena F, Fortunati C, di Stefano C, et al. Prostatic malacoplakia associated with prostatic abscess: diagnosis and treatment. *Urol Int* 2001;66:212.

197. Stanton MJ, Maxted W. Malakoplakia: a study of the literature and current concepts of pathogenesis. *J Urol* 1981;125:139.

198. Rubenstein M, Bucy JG. Malakoplakia of the prostate. *South Med J* 1977;70:351.

199. Coup AJ. Malakoplakia of the prostate. *J Pathol* 1976;119:119.

200. Ferreira AA, Alvarenga M. Malacoplakia of the prostate confused with clear cell carcinoma. *J Urol* 1976;116:828.

201. Konnak JW, Hart WR. Malacoplakia of the prostate in an immunosuppressed patient. *J Urol* 1976;116:830.

202. Sujka SK, Malin BT, Asirwatham JE. Prostatic malakoplakia associated with prostatic adenocarcinoma and multiple prostatic abscesses. *Urology* 1989;34:159.

203. Morris SB, Gordon EM, Corbishley CM. Prostatic sarcoidosis. Review of genitourinary sarcoidosis. *Br J Urol* 1993;72:462.

204. Furusato B, Koff S, McLeod DG, et al. Sarcoidosis of the prostate. *J Clin Pathol* 2007;60:325.

205. Mulpuru SK, Gujja K, Pai VM, et al. A rare and unusual cause of PSA elevation: sarcoidosis of the prostate. *Am J Med Sci* 2008;335:246.

206. Yalowitz PA, Greene L, Sheps SG, et al. Wegener's granulomatosis involving the prostate gland: report of a case. *J Urol* 1966;96:801.

207. Stillwell TJ, DeRemee RA, McDonald TJ, et al. Prostatic involvement in Wegener's granulomatosis. *J Urol* 1987;138:1251.

208. Branner A, Tzankov A, Akkad T, et al. Wegener's granulomatosis presenting with gross hematuria due to prostatitis. *Virchows Arch* 2004;444:92.

209. Huong DLT, Papo T, Piette JC, et al. Urogenital manifestations of Wegener granulomatosis. *Medicine* 1995;74:152.

210. Orozco RE, Peters RL. Teflon granuloma of the prostate mimicking adenocarcinoma. *J Urol Pathol* 1995;3:365.

211. White J, Chan YF. Hair granuloma in the prostate. *Br J Urol* 1994;74:260.

212. Day DS, Carpenter HD, Allsbrook WC Jr. Hair granuloma of the prostate. *Hum Pathol* 1998;27:196.

213. Ventura L, Martini E, Di Nicola G, et al. Hair granuloma of the prostate. A clinically silent, under-recognized complication of needle core biopsy. *Histopathology* 2006;49:654.

214. Bretal-Laranga M, Insua-Vilarino S, Blanco-Rodriquez J, et al. Giant cell arteritis limited to the prostate. *J Rheumatol* 1995;22:566.

215. Balague F, Humair L, de Torrente A. Periarteritis nodosa in a patient carrying simultaneously HBs, HBc, and HBe antigens and anti-HBs antibodies [in French]. *Schweiz Med Wochenschr* 1983;113:1201.

216. Genesca J, Esteban R, Cervantes M, et al. Prostatic vasculitis, an unusual beginning for panarteritis nodosa [in Spanish]. *Med Clin (Barc)* 1984;83:545.

217. Cheatum De, Sowell DS, Dulany RB. Hepatitis B antigen associated periarteritis nodosa with prostatic vasculitis. *Arch Intern Med* 1981;141:107.

218. de Souza E, Katz DA, Dworzack DL, et al. Actinomycosis of the prostate. *J Urol* 1985;133:290.

219. Goff DA, Davisdon RA. Amebic prostatitis. *South Med J* 1984;77:1053.

220. Kan SK, Kay RW. Melioidosis presenting as prostatitis: a case report from Subah. *Trans R Soc Trop Med Hyg* 1978;72:522.

221. Deklotz RJ. Echinococcal cyst involving the prostate and seminal vesicles: a case report. *J Urol* 1976;115:116.

222. Houston W. Primary hydatid cyst of the prostate gland. *J Urol* 1975;113:732.

223. Zambrano A, Kalantari M, Simoneau A, et al. Detection of human polyomaviruses and papillomaviruses in prostatic tissue reveals the prostate as a habitat for multiple viral infections. *Prostate* 2002;53:263.

224. Yoon GS, Nagar MS, Tavora F, et al. Cytomegalovirus prostatitis: a series of 4 cases. *Int J Surg Pathol* 2010;18:55.

225. Kwan DJ, Lowe FC. Genitourinary manifestations of the acquired immunodeficiency syndrome. *Urology* 1995;45:13.

226. Ndimbie OK, Dekker A, Martinez AJ, et al. Prostatic sequestration of *Cryptococcus neoformans* in immunocompromised persons treated for cryptococcal meningoencephalitis. *Histol Histopathol* 1994;9:643.

227. Benson BJ, Smith CS. Cytomegalovirus prostatitits. *Urology* 1992;40:165.

228. Marans HY, Mandell W, Kislak JW, et al. Prostatic abscess due to *Histoplasma capsulatum* in acquired immunodeficiency syndrome. *J Urol* 1991;145:1275.

229. Billis A. Prostatic atrophy: an autopsy study of a histologic mimic of adenocarcinoma. *Mod Pathol* 1998:114:47.

230. Liavåg I. Atrophy and regeneration in the pathogenesis of prostate carcinoma. *Acta Pathol Microbiol Scand* 1968;73:338.

231. Gardner WA Jr, Culberson DE. Atrophy and proliferation in the young adult prostate. *J Urol* 1987;137:53.

232. Franks LM. Atrophy and hyperplasia in the prostate proper. *J Pathol Bacteriol* 1954;68:617.

233. McNeal JE. Normal histology of the prostate. *Am J Surg Pathol* 1988;12:619.

234. Moore RA. The evolution and involution of the prostate gland. *Am J Pathol* 1936;12:599.

235. Emmett JL, Braasch WF. Cysts of the prostate gland. *J Urol* 1936;36:236.

236. De Marzo AM, Platz EA, Epstein JI, et al. A working group classification of focal prostate atrophy lesions. *Am J Surg Pathol* 2006;30:1281.

237. Oppenheimer JR, Wills ML, Epstein JI. Partial atrophy in prostate needle cores: another diagnostic pitfall for the surgical pathologist. *Am J Surg Pathol* 1998;22:440.

238. Wang W, Sun X, Epstein JI. Partial atrophy on prostate needle biopsy cases: a morphologic and immunohistochemical study. *Am J Surg Pathol* 2008;32:851.

239. Przybycin CG, Kunju LP, Wu AJ, et al. Partial atrophy in prostate needle biopsies: a detailed analysis of its morphology, immunophenotype, and cellular kinetics. *Am J Surg Pathol* 2008;32:58.

240. Amin MB, Tamboli P, Varma M, et al. Post-atrophic hyperplasia of the prostate gland: a detailed analysis of its morphology in needle biopsy specimens. *Am J Surg Pathol* 1999;23:925.

241. Anton RC, Kattan MW, Chakraborty S, et al. Postatrophic hyperplasia of the prostate. *Am J Surg Pathol* 1999;23:932.

242. Cheville JC, Bostwick DG. Postatrophic hyperplasia of the prostate: a histologic mimic of prostatic adenocarcinoma. *Am J Surg Pathol* 1995;19:1068.

243. Shah R, Mucci NR, Amin A, et al. Postatrophic hyperplasia of the prostate gland: neoplastic precursor or innocent bystander? *Am J Pathol* 2001;158:1767.

244. Billis A, Magna LA. Prostate elastosis: a microscopic feature useful for the diagnosis of posatrophic hyperplasia. *Arch Pathol Lab Med* 2000;124:1308.

245. De Marzo AM, Marchi VL, Epstein JI, et al. Proliferative inflammatory atrophy of the prostate: implications for prostatic carcinogenesis. *Am J Pathol* 1999;155:1985.

246. De Marzo AM, Nakai Y, Nelson WG. Inflammation, atrophy, and prostate carcinogenesis. *Urol Oncol* 2007;25:398.

247. Hedrick L, Epstein JI. Use of keratin 903 as an adjunct in the diagnosis of prostate carcinoma. *Am J Surg Pathol* 1989;13:369.

248. Adley BP, Yang XJ. α-methylacyl coenzyme A racemase immunoreactivity in partial atrophy of the prostate. *Am J Clin Pathol* 2006;126:849.

249. Hameed O, Sublett J, Humphrey PA. Immunohistochemical stains for p63 and alpha-methylacyl-CoA racemase, versus a cocktail comprising both, in the diagnosis of prostatic carcinoma: a comparison of the immunohistochemical staining of 430 foci in radical prostatectomy and needle biopsy tissues. *Am J Surg Pathol* 2005;29:579.

250. Zha S, Gage WR, Sauvageot J, et al. Cyclooxygenase-2 is upregulated in proliferative inflammatory atrophy of the prostate, but not in prostate carcinoma. *Cancer Res* 2001;61:8617.

251. Wang W, Bergh A, Damber J-A. Increased p53 immunoreactivity in proliferative inflammatory atrophy of prostate is related to focal acute inflammation. *APMIS* 2009;117:185.

252. Faith D, Han S, Lee DK, et al. p16 is upregulated in proliferative inflammatory atrophy of the prostate. *Prostate* 2005;65:73.

253. Yildiz-Sezer S, Verdorfer I, Schäfer G, et al. Assessment of aberrations of chromosome 8 in prostatic atrophy. *BJU Int* 2006;98:184.

254. Yildiz-Sezer S, Verdorfer I, Schäfer G, et al. Gain of chromosome X in prostatic atrophy detected by CGH and FISH analyses. *Prostate* 2007;67:433.

255. Feneley MR, Young MPA, Chinyama C, et al. Ki-67 expression in early prostate cancer and associated pathological lesions. *J Clin Pathol* 1996;49:741.

256. Mogal AP, Watson MA, Ozsolak F, Salavaggione L, Humphrey PA. Gene expression profiles and differential cytoglobin expression in atrophy and adenocarcinoma of the prostate. *Prostate* 2012;72:931.

257. Perner S, Mosquera JM, Demichelis F, et al. TMPRSS2-ERG fusion prostate cancer: an early molecular event associated with invasion. *Am J Surg Pathol* 2007;31:882.

258. Kaleem Z, Swanson PE, Vollmer RT, et al. Prostatic adenocarcinoma with atrophic features: a study of 202 consecutive, completely-embedded radical prostatectomy specimens. *Am J Clin Pathol* 1998;109:695.

259. Yaskiv O, Cao D, Humphrey PA. Microcystic adenocarcinoma of the prostate. A variant of pseudohyperplastic and atrophic patterns. *Am J Surg Pathol* 2010;34:556.

260. Postma R, Schröder FH, van der Kwast TH. Atrophy in prostate needle biopsy cores and its relationship to prostate cancer incidence in screened men. *Urology* 2005;65:745.

261. Golden MR, Abeshouse BS. A further clinical and pathological study of prostatic infarction. *J Urol* 1953;70:930.

262. Culp OS. Squamous metaplasia, simulating carcinoma, associated with prostatic infarction. *Bull Johns Hopkins Hosp* 1939;65:1239.

263. Kasman LP, Gold J. Metaplastic changes in the prostate gland. *J Lab Clin Med* 1933;19:301.

264. Moore RA. Benign hypertrophy of the prostate. A morphological study. *J Urol* 1943;50:680.

265. Mostofi FK, Morse WH. Epithelial metaplasia in "prostatic infarction." *Arch Pathol* 1951;51:340.

266. Nanson EM. Squamous metaplasia of the prostate gland. *J Urol* 1950;22:394.

267. Roth RB. Prostatic infarction. *J Urol* 1949;62:474.

268. Spiro LH, Labay G, Orkin LA. Prostatic infarction: role in acute urinary retention. *Urology* 1974;3:345.

269. Helpap B. Treated prostatic carcinoma. Histological, immunohistochemical and cell kinetic studies. *Appl Pathol* 1985;3:230.

270. Bainborough AR. Squamous metaplasia of prostate following estrogen therapy. *J Urol* 1952;66:329.

271. Borkowski P, Robinson MI, Poppiti RJ, et al. Histologic findings in postcryosurgical prostatic biopsies. *Mod Pathol* 1996;9:807.

272. Bostwick DG, Egbert BM, Fajardo LF. Radiation injury of the normal and neoplastic prostate. *Am J Surg Pathol* 1982;6:541.

273. Civantos F, Marcial MA, Banks ER, et al. Pathology of androgen deprivation therapy in prostate carcinoma. *Cancer* 1995;75:1634.

274. Montironi R, Diamanti L. Morphologic changes in benign prostatic hyperplasia following chronic treatment with the 5-alpha-reductase inhibitor finasteride. Comparison with the effect of combination endocrine therapy. *J Urol Pathol* 1996;4:123.

275. Shabaik A, Wilson S, Bidair M, et al. Pathologic changes in prostate biopsies following cryoablation therapy of prostate carcinoma. *J Urol Pathol* 1995;3:183.

276. Sheaff MT, Baithun SI. Effects of radiation on the normal prostate gland. *Histopathology* 1997;30:341.

277. Vaillancourt L, Têtu B, Fradet Y, et al. Effect of neoadjuvant endocrine therapy (combined androgen blockade) on normal prostate and prostatic carcinoma. A randomized study. *Am J Surg Pathol* 1996;20:86.

278. Sutton EB, McDonald JR. Metaplasia of the prostatic epithelium: a lesion sometimes mistaken for carcinoma. *Am J Clin Pathol* 1943;13:607.

279. Têtu B, Srigley JR, Boivin JC, et al. Effect of combination endocrine therapy (LHRH agonist and flutamide) on normal prostate and prostatic adenocarcinoma. A histopathologic and immunohistochemical study. *Am J Surg Pathol* 1991;15:111.

280. Yang X, Laven B, Tretiakova M, et al. Detection of alpha-methylacyl-coenzyme A racemase in postradiation prostatic adenocarcinoma. *Urology* 2003;62:282.

281. Brawer MK, Nagle RB, Pitts W, et al. Keratin immunoreactivity as an aid to the diagnosis of persistent adenocarcinoma in irradiated human prostate. *Cancer* 1989;63:454.

282. Helpap B, Stiens R. The cell proliferation of epithelial metaplasia in the prostate gland. An autoradiographic in vitro study. *Virchows Arch B Cell Pathol* 1975;19:69.

283. Yantiss RK, Young RH. Transitional cell "metaplasia" in the prostate gland. A survey of its frequency and features based on 104 consecutive prostatic biopsy specimens. *J Urol Pathol* 1997;7:71.

284. Gal R, Koren R, Nofech-Mozes S, et al. Evaluation of mucinous metaplasia of the prostate gland by mucin histochemistry. *Br J Urol* 1996;77:113.

285. Grignon DJ, O'Malley FP. Mucinous metaplasia in the prostate gland. *Am J Surg Pathol* 1993;17:287.

286. Hu JC, Palpattu GS, Kattan MW, et al. The association of selected pathological features with prostate cancer in a single-needle biopsy accession. *Hum Pathol* 1998;29:1536.

287. Shiraishi T, Kusano I, Watanabe M, et al. Mucous gland metaplasia of the prostate. *Am J Surg Pathol* 1993;17:618.

288. Franks LM, O'Shea JD, Thomson AER. Mucin in the prostate: a histochemical study in normal glands, latent, clinical, and colloid cancers. *Cancer* 1964;17:983.

289. Hukill PB, Vidone RA. Histochemistry of mucus and other polysaccharides in tumors. II carcinoma of the prostate. *Lab Invest* 1967;16:395.

290. Reyes AO, Swanson PE, Carbone JM, et al. Unusual histologic types of high-grade prostatic intraepithelial neoplasia. *Am J Surg Pathol* 1997;21:1215.

291. Grignon DJ. Unusual subtypes of prostate cancer. *Mod Pathol* 2004;17:316.

292. Adlakha H, Bostwick DG. Paneth cell-like change in prostatic adenocarcinoma represents neuroendocrine differentiation. Report of 30 cases. *Hum Pathol* 1994;25:135.

293. di Sant'Agnese PA. Neuroendocrine differentiation in prostatic adenocarcinoma does not represent true Paneth cell differentiation [editorial]. *Hum Pathol* 1994;25:115.

294. Frydman CP, Bleiweiss IJ, Unger PD, et al. Paneth cell-like metaplasia of the prostate gland. *Arch Pathol Lab Med* 1992;116:274.

295. Gaudin PB, Zelefsky MJ, Leibel SA, et al. Histopathologic effects of three-dimensional conformal external beam radiation therapy on benign and malignant prostate tissue. *Am J Surg Pathol* 1999;23:1021.

296. van de Voorde W, van Poppel H, Haustermans K, et al. Mucin-secreting adenocarcinoma of the prostate with neuroendocrine differentiation and Paneth-like cells. *Am J Surg Pathol* 1994;18:200.

297. Weaver MG, Abdul-Karim FW, Srigley JR. Paneth cell-like change and small cell carcinoma of the prostate. Two divergent forms of prostatic neuroendocrine differentiation. *Am J Surg Pathol* 1992;16:1013.

298. Dikov D, Vassilev I, Dimitrakov J. Nonspecific granulomatous prostatitis with calculous ductal ectasia and extensive Paneth cell-like epithelial metaplasia. Case report. *APMIS* 2005;113:564.

299. Cheng L, MacLennan GT, Abdul-Karim FW, et al. Eosinophilic metaplasia of the prostate: a newly described lesion distinct from other eosinophilic changes in prostatic epithelium. *Anal Quant Cytol Histol* 2008;30:226.

300. Tamas EF, Epstein JI. Prognostic significance of Paneth cell-like neuroendocrine differentiation in adenocarcinoma of the prostate. *Am J Surg Pathol* 2006;30:980.

301. Milford RA, Kahane H, Epstein JI. Infarct of the prostate gland: experience on needle biopsy specimens. *Am J Surg Pathol* 2000; 24:1378.

302. Gaudin PB, Zelefsky MJ, Hutchinson B, et al. Paneth cell-like change in benign prostatic ducts and acini post-radiation therapy represents neuroendocrine differentiation [abstract]. *Mod Pathol* 1998;11:83A.

303. Rahmetullah A, Oliva E. Nephrogenic adenoma: an update on an innocuous but troublesome entity. *Adv Anat Pathol* 2006;13:247.

304. Mazal PR, Schaufler R, Altenhuber-Muller R, et al. Derivation of nephrogenic adenomas from renal tubular cells in kidney transplant recipients. *N Engl J Med* 2002;347:653.

305. McIntire TL, Soloway MS, Murphy WM. Nephrogenic adenoma. *Urology* 1987;29:237.

306. Humphrey PA. Prostatic urethra. In: *Prostate Pathology.* Chicago, IL: ASCP Press; 2004, Table 23.5:527.

307. Tong GX, Melamed J, Mansukhani M, et al. PAX2: a reliable marker for nephrogenic adenoma. *Mod Pathol* 2006;19:356.

308. Hansel DE, Nadasdy T, Epstein JI. Fibromyxoid nephrogenic adenoma: a newly recognized variant mimicking mucinous adenocarcinoma. *Am J Surg Pathol* 2007;31:1231.

309. Xiao GQ, Burstein DE, Miller LK, et al. Nephrogenic adenoma: immunohistochemical evaluation for its etiology and differentiation from prostatic adenocarcinoma. *Arch Pathol Lab Med* 2006;130:805.

310. Allan CH, Epstein JI. Nephrogenic adenoma of the prostatic urethra: a mimicker of prostate adenocarcinoma. *Am J Surg Pathol* 2001;25:802.

311. Piper NY, Thompson IM. Large nephrogenic adenoma following transurethral resection of the prostate. *J Urol* 1999;161:605.

312. Gupta A, Wanh HL, Policarpio-Nicolas ML, et al. Expression of alpha-methylacyl-coenzyme A racemase in nephrogenic adenoma. *Am J Surg Pathol* 2004;28:1224.

313. Skinnider BF, Oliva E, Young RH, et al. Expression of alpha-methylacyl-CoA racemase (P504S) in nephrogenic adenoma: a significant immunohistochemical pitfall compounding the differential diagnosis with prostatic adenocarcinoma. *Am J Surg Pathol* 2004;28:701.

314. Cossu-Rocca P, Contini M, Brunelli M, et al. S100A1 is a reliable marker in distinguishing nephrogenic adenoma from prostatic adenocarcinoma. *Am J Surg Pathol* 2009;33:1031.

315. Zhai QJ, Ozcan A, Hamilton C, et al. PAX-2 expression in non-neoplastic, primary neoplastic, and metastatic neoplastic tissue: a comprehensive immunohistochemical study. *Appl Immunohistochem Mol Morphol* 2010;18:323.

316. Tong GX, Weeden EM, Hamele-Bena D, et al. Expression of PAX8 in nephrogenic adenoma and clear cell adenocarcinoma of the lower urinary tract: evidence of related histogenesis? *Am J Surg Pathol* 2008;32:1380.

317. Bedrosian SA, Goldman RL, Sung MA. Heterotopic cartilage in prostate. *Urology* 1983;21:536.

318. Isaacs JT, Coffey DS. Etiology and disease process of benign prostatic hyperplasia. *Prostate Suppl* 1989;2:33.

319. Roehrborn CG, McConnell JD. Benign prostatic hyperplasia: etiology, pathophysiology, epidemiology, and natural history. In: Wein AJ, ed-in-chief. *Campbell-Walsh Urology.* 9th ed. Philadelphia, PA: Saunders Elsevier; 2007.

320. Bushman W. Etiology, epidemiology, and natural history of benign prostatic hyperplasia. *Urol Clin North Am* 2009;36:403.

321. Berry SJ, Coffy DS, Walsh PC, et al. The development of human benign prostatic hyperplasia with age. *J Urol* 1984;132:474.

322. Kok ET, Bohnen AM, Jonkheijm R, et al. Simple case definition of clinical benign prostatic hyperplasia, based on International Prostate Symptom Score, predicts general practioner consultaiton rates. *Urology* 2006;68:784.

323. Foster CS. Pathology of benign prostatic hyperplasia. *Prostate Suppl* 2000;9:4.

324. Partin AW, Page WF, Lee BR, et al. Concordance rates for benign prostatic disease among twins suggest hereditary influence. *Urology* 1994;44:646.

325. Sanda MG, Doehring CB, Binkowitz B, et al. Clinical and biological characterization of familial benign prostatic hyperplasia. *J Urol* 1997;157:876.

326. Sanda MG, Beaty TH, Stutzman RE, et al. Genetic susceptibility of benign prostatic hyperplasia. *J Urol* 1994;152:115.

327. Endo T, Uzawa K, Suzuki H, et al. Characteristic gene expression profiles of benign hypertrophy and prostate cancer. *Int J Oncol* 2009;35:499.

328. Madsen FA, Bruskewitz RC. Clinical manifestations of benign prostatic hyperplasia. *Urol Clin North Am* 1995;22:291.

329. Thorner DA, Weiss JP. Benign prostatic hyperplasia: symptoms, symptom scores, and outcome measures. *Urol Clin North Am* 2009;36:417.

330. Auffenberg GB, Hefland BT, McVary KT. Established medical therapy for benign prostatic hyperplasia. *Urol Clin North Am* 2009;36:443.

331. Price H, McNeal JE, Stamey TA. Evolving patterns of tissue composition in benign prostatic hyperplasia as a function of specimen size. *Hum Pathol* 1990;21:578.

332. Kerley SW, Corica FA, Qian J, et al. Peripheral zone involvement by prostatic hyperplasia. *J Urol Pathol* 1997;6:87.

333. Ohori M, Egawa S, Wheeler TM. Nodules resembling nodular hyperplasia in the peripheral zone of the prostate gland. *J Urol Pathol* 1994;2:223.

334. Oyen R, Van de Voorde W, Van Poppel H, et al. Benign hyperplastic nodules that originate in the peripheral zone of the prostate gland. *Radiology* 1993;189:707.

335. Van de Voorde W, Oyen R, Van Poppel H, et al. Peripherally localized benign prostatic nodules of the prostate. *Mod Pathol* 1995;8:46.

336. McNeal JE. Origin and evolution of benign prostatic enlargement. *Invest Urol* 1978;15:340.

337. Bierhoff E, Vogel J, Benz M, et al. Stromal nodules in benign prostatic hyperplasia. *Eur Urol* 1996;24:345.

338. Wang HL, Humphrey PA. Exaggerated signet-ring cell change in stromal nodule of prostate: a pseudoneoplastic proliferation. *Am J Surg Pathol* 2002;26:1066.

339. McNeal JE. The prostate gland: morphology and pathobiology. *Monogr Urol* 1983;4:3.

340. Katandaris PM, Polyzonis MB. Fibroadenoma-like foci in human prostatic nodular hyperplasia. *Prostate* 1983;4:33.

341. Robert G, Descazeaud A, Nicolaiew N, et al. Inflammation in benign prostatic hyperplasia: a 282 patients' immunohistochemical analysis. *Prostate* 2009;69:1774.

342. Baird HH, McKay HW, Kimmelstiel P. Ischemic infarction of the prostate gland. *South Med J* 1950;43:234.

343. Brawn PN, Foster DM, Kuhl D, et al. Characteristics of prostatic infarcts and their effect on serum prostate-specific antigen and prostatic acid phosphatase *Urology* 1994;44:71.

344. Garvin TJ. Prostatic infarction associated with aortic and iliac aneurysm repair (letter). *J Urol* 1990;144:1485.

345. Harik LR, Merino C, Coindre JM, et al. Pseudosarcomatous myofibroblastic proliferations of the bladder: a clinicopathologic study of 42 cases. *Am J Surg Pathol* 2006;30:787.

346. Ro JY, el-Naggar AK, Amin MB, et al. Pseudosarcomatous fibromyxoid tumor of the urinary bladder and prostate: immunohistochemical, ultrastructural, and DNA flow cytometric analyses of nine cases. *Hum Pathol* 1993;24:1203.

347. Herawi M, Epstein JI. Specialized stromal tumors of the prostate: a clinicopathologic study of 50 cases. *Am J Surg Pathol* 2006;30:694.

348. Hossain D, Meiers I, Qian J, et al. Prostatic stromal hyperplasia with atypia. Follow-up study of 18 cases. *Arch Pathol Lab Med* 2008;132:1729.

349. Young RH, Srigley JR, Amin MB, et al. Miscellaneous tumors of the prostate. In: *Tumors of the Prostate Gland, Seminal Vesicles, Male Urethra, and Penis.* Washington, DC: Armed Forces Institute of Pathology; 2000:257.

350. Hansel DE, Herawi M, Montgomery E, et al. Spindle cell lesions of adult prostate. *Mod Pathol* 2007;20:148.

351. Levi AW, Epstein JI. Pseudohyperplastic prostatic adenocarcinoma on needle biopsy and simple prostatectomy. *Am J Surg Pathol* 2000;24:1039.

352. Bennett BD, Gardner WA Jr. Embryonal hyperplasia of the prostate. *Prostate* 1985;7:411.

353. Bonkhoff H, Stein U, Remberger K. The proliferative function of basal cells in the normal and hyperplastic human prostate. *Prostate* 1994;24:114.

354. Cleary KR, Choi HY, Ayala AG. Basal cell hyperplasia of the prostate. *Am J Clin Pathol* 1983;80:850.

355. Derner GB. Basal cell proliferation in benign prostatic hyperplasia. *Cancer* 1978;41:1857.

356. Devaraj LT, Bostwick DG. Atypical basal cell hyperplasia of the prostate. Immunophenotypic profile and proposed classification of basal cell proliferations. *Am J Surg Pathol* 1993;17:645.

357. Grignon DJ, Ro JY, Ordonez NG, et al. Basal cell hyperplasia, adenoid basal cell tumor, and adenoid cystic carcinoma of the prostate gland: an immunohistochemical study. *Hum Pathol* 1988;19:1425.

358. Mittal BV, Amin MB, Kinare SG. Spectrum of histological lesions in 185 consecutive prostatic specimens. *J Postgrad Med* 1989;35:157.

359. Sarma DP, Guileyardo JM. Basal cell hyperplasia of the prostate. *J La State Med Soc* 1982;134:23.

360. van de Voorde W, Baldewijns M, Lauweryns J. Florid basal cell hyperplasia of the prostate. *Histopathology* 1994;24:341.

361. Rioux-Leclercq N, Epstein JI. Unusual morphologic patterns of basal cell hyperplasia of the prostate. *Am J Surg Pathol* 2002;26:237.

362. Hosler GA, Epstein JI. Basal cell hyperplasia: an unusual diagnostic dilemma on prostate needle biopsies. *Hum Pathol* 2005;36:480.

363. McKenney JK, Amin MB, Srigley JR, et al. Basal cell proliferations of the prostate other than usual basal cell hyperplasia: a clinicopathologic study of 23 cases, including four carcinomas, with a proposed classification. *Am J Surg Pathol* 2004;28:1289.

364. Yang XJ, McEntee M, Epstein JI. Distinction of basaloid carcinoma of the prostate from benign basal cell lesions using immunohistochemistry for bcl-2 and Ki-67. *Hum Pathol* 1998;29:1447.

365. Kyprianou N, Tu H, Jacobs SC. Apoptotic versus proliferative activities in human benign prostatic hyperplasia. *Hum Pathol* 1996; 27:668.

366. Young RH, Srigley JR, Amin MB, et al. Tumor-like lesions of the prostate. In: *Tumors of the Prostate Gland, Seminal Vesicles, Male Urethra, and Penis*. Washington, DC: Armed Forces Institute of Pathology; 2000:308, Table 7-2.

367. Ayala AG, Srigley JR, Ro JY, et al. Clear cell cribriform hyperplasia of prostate. Report of 10 cases. *Am J Surg Pathol* 1986;10:665.

368. Frauenhoffer EE, Ro JY, El-Naggar AK, et al. Clear cell cribriform hyperplasia of the prostate. Immunohistochemical and DNA flow cytometric study. *Am J Clin Pathol* 1991;95:446.

369. Shah RB, Magi-Galluzzi C, Han B, et al. Atypical cribriform lesions of the prostate: relationship to prostatic carcinoma and implication for diagnosis in prostate biopsies. *Am J Surg Pathol* 2010;34:470.

370. Guo CC, Epstein JI. Intraductal carcinoma of the prostate on needle biopsy: histologic features and clinical significance. *Mod Pathol* 2006;19:1528.

371. Amin MB, Schultz DS, Zarbo RJ. Analysis of cribriform morphology in prostatic neoplasia using antibody to high-molecular-weight cytokeratins. *Arch Pathol Lab Med* 1994;110:260.

372. Chen YB, Fine SW, Epstein JI. Mesonephric remnant hyperplasia involving prostate and periprostatic tissue: findings at radical prostatectomy. *Am J Surg Pathol* 2011;35:1054.

373. Gagucas RJ, Brown RW, Wheeler TM. Verumontanum mucosal gland hyperplasia. *Am J Surg Pathol* 1995;19:30.

374. Gaudin PB, Wheeler TM, Epstein JI. Verumontanum mucosal gland hyperplasia in prostatic needle biopsy specimens. A mimic of low grade prostatic adenocarcinoma. *Am J Clin Pathol* 1995;104:620.

375. Muezzinoglu B, Erdamar S, Chakraborty S. Verumontanum mucosal gland hyperplasia is associated with atypical adenomatous hyperplasia of the prostate. *Arch Pathol Lab Med* 2001;125:358.

376. Bostwick DG, Srigley J, Grignon D, et al. Atypical adenomatous hyperplasia of the prostate: morphologic criteria for its distinction from well-differentiated carcinoma. *Hum Pathol* 1993;24:819.

377. Gaudin PB, Epstein JI. Adenosis of the prostate. Histologic features in transurethral resection specimens. *Am J Surg Pathol* 1994;18:863.

378. Amin MB, Ro JY, Ayala AG. Putative precursor lesions of prostatic adenocarcinoma: fact or fiction? *Mod Pathol* 1993;6:476.

379. Bostwick DG. Prospective origins of prostate carcinoma. Prostatic intraepithelial neoplasia and atypical adenomatous hyperplasia. *Cancer* 1996;78:330.

380. Epstein JI. Adenosis (atypical adenomatous hyperplasia): histopathology and relationship to carcinoma. *Pathol Res Pract* 1995; 191:888.

381. Grignon DJ, Sakr WA. Atypical adenomatous hyperplasia of the prostate: a critical review. *Eur Urol* 1996;30:206.

382. Lotan TL, Epstein JI. Diffuse adenosis of the peripheral zone in prostate needle biopsy and prostatectomy specimens. *Am J Surg Pathol* 2008;32:1360.

383. Gaudin PB, Epstein JI. Adenosis of the prostate. Histologic features in needle biopsy specimens. *Am J Surg Pathol* 1995;19:737.

384. Bostwick DG, Qian J. Atypical adenomatous hyperplasia of the prostate. Relationship with carcinoma in 217 whole-mount radical prostatectomies. *Am J Surg Pathol* 1995;19:506.

385. Doll JA, Zhu X, Furman J, et al. Genetic analysis of protatic atypical adenomatous hyperplasia (adenosis). *Am J Pathol* 1999;155:967.

386. Mai KT, Isotalo PA, Green J, et al. Incidental prostatic adenocarcinomas and putative premalignant lesions in TURP specimens collected before and after introduction of prostate specific antigen screening. *Arch Pathol Lab Med* 2000;124:1454.

387. Reyes AO, Humphrey PA. Diagnostic effect of complete histologic sampling of prostate needle biopsy specimens. *Am J Clin Pathol* 1998:109:416.

388. Skjorten F, Berner A, Harvei S, et al. Prostatic intraepithelial neoplasia in surgical resections: relationship to coexistent adenocarcinoma and atypical adenomatous hyperplasia of the prostate. *Cancer* 1997;79:1172.

389. Srigley J, Toth P, Hartwick RWJ. Atypical histological patterns in cases of benign prostatic hyperplasia [abstract]. *Lab Invest* 1984;60:90A.

390. Troncoso P, Ordonez NG, Ayala AG. Atypical adenomatous hyperplasia in radical prostatectomy and cystoprostatectomy specimens [abstract]. *Mod Pathol* 1995;8:44A.

391. Humphrey PA, Zhu X, Crouch EC, et al. Mass-formative atypical adenomatous hyperplasia of prostate. *J Urol Pathol* 1998;9:73.

392. Helpap B, Riede C. Nucleolar and AgNOR-analysis of prostatic intraepithelial neoplasia (PIN) atypical adenomatous hyperplasia (AAH) and prostatic carcinoma. *Pathol Res Pract* 1995;191:381.

393. Brawn PN. Adenosis of the prostate: a dysplastic-lesion that can be confused with prostate adenocarcinoma. *Cancer* 1982;49:826.

394. Wojno KJ, Epstein JI. The utility of basal cell-specific anti-cytokeratin antibody (34βE12) in the diagnosis of prostate cancer. A review of 228 cases. *Am J Surg Pathol* 1995;19:251.

395. Yang XJ, Wu CL, Woda BA, et al. Expression of α-methylacyl-CoA racemase (P504S) in atypical adenomatous hyperplasia of the prostate. *Am J Surg Pathol* 2002;26:921.

396. Lopez-Beltran A, Qian J, Montironi R, et al. Atypical adenomatous hyperplasia (adenosis) of the prostate: DNA ploidy analysis and immunophenotype. *Int J Surg Pathol* 2005;13:167.

397. Cheng L, Shan A, Cheville JC, et al. Atypical adenomatous hyperplasia of the prostate: a premalignant lesion? *Cancer Res* 1998;58:389.

398. Meyer F, Têtu B, Bairati I, et al. Prostatic intraepithelial neoplasia in TURP specimens and subsequent prostate cancer. *Can J Urol* 2006;13:3255.

399. Sakamoto N, Tsuneyoshi M, Enjoji M. Sclerosing adenosis of the prostate. Histopathologic and imunohistochemical analysis. *Am J Surg Pathol* 1991;15:660.

400. Collina G, Botticelli AR, Martinelli AM, et al. Sclerosing adenosis of the prostate. Report of three cases with electron microscopy and immunohistochemical study. *Histopathology* 1991;20:505.

401. Jones EC, Clement PB, Young RH. Sclerosing adenosis of the prostate gland. A clinicopathlogic and immunohistochemical study of 11 cases. *Am J Surg Pathol* 1991;151:1171.

402. Young RH, Clement PB. Sclerosing adenosis of the prostate. *Arch Pathol Lab Med* 1987;111:363.

403. Grignon DJ, Ro JY, Srigley JR, et al. Sclerosing adenosis of the prostate. A lesion showing myoepithelial differentiation. *Am J Surg Pathol* 1992;16:383.

404. Cheng L, Bostwick DG. Atypical sclerosing adenosis of the prostate: a mimic of adenocarcinoma. *Histopathology* 2010;56:627.

405. Young RH, Srigley JR, Amin MB, et al. Carcinoma of the prostate. In: *Tumors of the Prostate Gland, Seminal Vesicles, Male Urethra, and Penis*. Washington, DC: Armed Forces Institute of Pathology; 2000:153,155.

406. Epstein JI, Netto GJ. Mesenchymal tumors and tumor-like conditions. In: *Biopsy Interpretation of the Prostate*. Philadelphia, PA: Wolters Kluwer/Lippincott Williams & Wilkins; 2008:284–287.

407. Cheng L, Foster SR, MacLennan GT, et al. Inflammatory myofibroblastic tumors of the genitourinary tract—single entity or continuum? *J Urol* 2008;180:1235.

408. Proppe KH, Scully RE, Rosai J. Postoperative spindle cell nodules of genitourinary tract resembling sarcomas. *Am J Surg Pathol* 1984;2:101.

409. Ro JY, el-Naggar AK, Amin MB, et al. Pseudosarcomatous fibromyxoid tumor of the urinary bladder and prostate: immunohistochemical, ultrastructural, and DNA flow cytometric analyses of nine cases. *Hum Pathol* 1993;24:1203.

410. Huang WL, Ro JY, Grignon DJ, et al. Postoperative spindle cell nodule of the prostate and bladder. *J Urol* 1990;143:824.

411. Montgomery EA, Shuster DD, Burkart AL, et al. Inflammatory myofibroblastic tumors of the urinary tract: a clinicopathologic study of 46 cases, including a malignant example inflammatory fibrosarcoma and a subset associated with high-grade urothelial carcinoma. *Am J Surg Pathol* 2006;30:1502.

412. Ro JY, Grignon DJ, Ayala AG, et al. Blue nevus and melanosis of the prostate. Electron-microscopic and immunohistochemical studies. *Am J Clin Pathol* 1988;90:530.

413. Aguilar M, Gaffney EF, Finnerty DP. Prostatic melanosis with involvement of benign and malignant epithelium. *J Urol* 1982;128:825.

414. Langley JW, Weitzner S. Blue nevus and melanosis of the prostate. *J Urol* 1974;112:359.

415. Humphrey PA. Unusual benign conditions. In: *Prostate Pathology*. Chicago, IL: ASCP Press; 2004:167, Table 9.2.

416. Kudva R, Hegde P. Blue nevus of the prostate. *Indian J Urol* 2010;26:301.

417. Suarez GM, Roberts JA. Ochronosis of prostate presenting as advanced carcinoma. *Urology* 1983;32:168.

418. Wilson SK, Buchanan RD, Stone SK, et al. Amyloid deposition in the prostate. *J Urol* 1973;110:322.

419. Cross PA, Bartley CJ, McClure J. Amyloid in prostatic corpora amylacea. *J Clin Pathol* 1992;45:894.

420. Yanamandra K, Alexeyev O, Zamotin V, et al. Amyloid formation by the pro-inflammatory S100A8/A9 proteins in the ageing prostate. *PLoS One* 2009;4:e5562.

421. McDonald JH, Heckel NJ. Primary amyloidosis of lower genitourinary tract. *J Urol* 1956;75:122.

422. Lupovitch A. The prostate and amyloidosis. *J Urol* 1972;108:301.

423. Tripathi VNP, Desautels RE. Primary amyloidosis of the urogenital system: a study of 16 cases and brief review. *J Urol* 1969;102:96.

424. Beckman EN, Pintado SO, Lenard GL, et al. Endometriosis of the prostate. *Am J Surg Pathol* 1985;9:374.

425. Humphrey PA, Vollmer RT. Extramedullary hematopoiesis in the prostate. *Am J Surg Pathol* 1991;15:486.

426. Bostwick DG, Vonk JB, Picado A. Pathologic changes in the prostate following contemporary 18-gauge needle biopsy. No apparent risk of local cancer seeding. *J Urol Pathol* 1994;2:203.

427. Bastacky SS, Walsh PC, Epstein JI. Needle biopsy associated tumor tracking of adenocarcinoma of the prostate. *J Urol* 1991;145; 1003.

428. Daoud NA, Li G, Evans AJ, van der Kwast TH. The value of triple antibody (34βE12 + p63 + AMACR) cocktail in radical prostatectomy specimens with crushed surgical margins. *J Clin Pathol* 2012;65:437.

429. Shelley MD, Kumar S, Wilt T, et al. A systematic review and meta-analysis of randomized trials of neo-adjuvant hormone therapy for localized and locally advanced prostate carcinoma. *Cancer Treat Res* 2009;35:9.

430. Petraki CD, Sifkas CP. Histopathological changes induced by therapies in the benign prostate and prostate adenocarcinoma. *Histol Histopathol* 2007;22:107.

431. Bostwick DG, Meiers I. Diagnosis of prostatic carcinoma after therapy. *Arch Pathol Lab Med* 2007;131:360–371.

432. Armas OA, Aprikian AG, Melamed J, et al. Clinical and pathological effects of neoadjuvant total ablation therapy on clinically localized prostatic adenocarcinoma. *Am J Surg Pathol* 1994;18:879.

433. Gaudin PB. Histopathologic effects of radiation and hormonal therapies on benign and malignant prostate tissues. *J Urol Pathol* 1998;8:55.

434. De Voot HJ, Rao BR, Geldof AA, et al. Androgen action blockade does not result in reduction in size but changes histology of the normal human prostate. *Prostate* 1987;11:305.

435. Rittmaster RS, Norman RW, Thomas LN, et al. Evidence for atrophy and apoptosis in the prostates of men given finasteride. *J Clin Endocrinol Metab* 1996;81:814.

436. Montironi R, Valli M, Fabris G. Treatment of benign prostatic hyperplasia with 5-alpha-reductase inhibitor: morphological changes in patients who fail to respond. *J Clin Pathol* 1996;49:324.

437. Civantos F, Watson RB, Pinto JE, et al. Finasteride effect on benign prostatic hyperplasia and prostate cancer. A comparative clinic-pathologic study of radical prostatectomies. *J Urol Pathol* 1997;6:1–8.

438. Marks LS, Partin AW, Dorey FJ, et al. Long-term effects of finasteride on prostate tissue composition. *Urology* 1999;53:574.

439. Sacz C, Gonzalez-Baena AC, Japon MA, et al. Regressive changes in finasteride-treated human hyperplastic prostates correlate with an upregulation of TGF-beta receptor expression. *Prostate* 1998;37:84.

440. Pomante R, Santinelli A, Muzzonigro G, et al. Nodular hyperplasia of the prostate. Quantitative evaluation of secretory cell changes after treatment with finasteride. *Anal Quant Cytol Histol* 1999;21:63.

441. Thomas LN, Wright AS, Lazier CB, et al. Prostatic involution in men taking finasteride is associated with elevated levels of insulin-like growth factor-binding proteins (IGFBPs)-2, -4, and -5. *Prostate* 2000;42:203.

442. Iczkowski KA, Qiu J, Qian J, et al. The dual 5-alpha-reductase inhibitor dutasteride induces atrophic changes and decreases relative cancer volume in human prostate cancer. *Urology* 2005;65:76.

443. Andriole GL, Humphrey P, Ray P, et al. Effect of the dual 5alpha-reductase inhibitor dutasteride on markers of tumor regression in prostate cancer. *J Urol* 2004;172:915.

444. Cheng L, Cheville JC, Bostwick DG. Diagnosis of prostate cancer in needle biopsies after radiation therapy. *Am J Surg Pathol* 1999;23:1173.

445. Dhom G, Degro S. Therapy of prostatic carcinoma and histopathologic follow-up. *Prostate* 1982;3:531.

446. Crook JM, Bahadur YA, Robertson SJ, et al. Evaluation of radiation effect, tumor differentiation, and prostate specific antigen staining in sequential prostate biopsies after external beam radiotherapy for patients with prostate carcinoma. *Cancer* 1997;79:81.

447. Goldstein NS, Martinez A, Vicini FA, et al. The histology of radiation therapy effect on prostate adenocarcinoma as assessed by needle biopsy after brachytherapy boost. Correlation with biochemical failure. *Am J Clin Pathol* 1998;110:765.

448. Grignon DJ, Sakr WA. Histologic effects of radiation therapy and total androgen blockade on prostate cancer. *Cancer* 1995;75:1837.

449. Magi-Galluzzi C, Sanderson H, Epstein JI. Atypia in nonneoplastic prostate glands after radiotherapy for prostate cancer. *Am J Surg Pathol* 2003;27:206.

450. Yang XY, Laven B, Tretiakova M, et al. Detection of alpha-methyl-acyl-conezyme A racemase in postradiation prostatic adenocarcinoma. *Urology* 2003;62:282.

451. Grob BM, Schellhammer PF, Brassil DN, et al. Changes in immunohistochemical staining of PSA, PSAP, and TURP-27 following irradiation therapy for clinically localized prostate cancer. *Urology* 1994;44:525.

452. Helpap B, Koch V. Histological and immunohistochemical findings of prostatic carcinoma after external or interstitial radiotherapy. *J Cancer Res Clin Oncol* 1991;117:608.

453. Ljung G, Norberg M, Holmberg L, et al. Characterization of residual tumor cells following radiation therapy for prostatic adenocarcinoma, immunohistochemical expression of prostate-specific antigen, prostatic acid phosphatase, and cytokeratin 8. *Prostate* 1997;31:91.

454. Mahan DE, Bruce AW, Manley PN, et al. Immunohistochemical evaluation of prostatic carcinoma before and after radiotherapy. *J Urol* 1980;124:488.

455. Lam JS, Psiters LL, Belldegrun AS. Cryotherapy for prostate cancer. In: Wein AJ, Kavoussi LR, Novick AC, et al., eds. *Campbell's Urology.* 9th ed. Philadelphia, PA: Saunders; 2007:3032–3052.

456. Petersen DS, Milleman LA, Rose EF, et al. Biopsy and clinical course after cryosurgery for prostatic cancer. *J Urol* 1978;120:308.

457. Izawa JI, Busby JE, Morganstern N, et al. Histological changes in prostate biopsies after salvage cryotherapy: effect of chronology and the method of biopsy. *BJU Int* 2006;98:554.

458. Magi-Galluzzi C, Zhou M, Reuther AM, et al. Neoadjuvant docetaxel treatment for locally advanced prostate cancer. A clinicopathologic study. *Cancer* 2007;110:1248.

459. Kirby R, Lepor H. Evaluation and nonsurgical management of benign prostatic hyperplasia. In: Wein AJ, Kavoussi LR, Novick AC, et al., eds. *Campbell's Urology.* 9th ed. Philadelphia, PA: Saunders; 2007:2776–2802.

460. Chon JK, Borkowski A, Partin AW, et al. Alpha 1-adrenorecptor antagonists terazosin and doxazosin induce prostate apoptosis without affecting cell proliferation in patients with benign prostatic hyperplasia. *J Urol* 1999;161:2002.

461. Kyprianou N, Benning CM. Induction of prostate apoptosis by doxazosin in benign prostatic hyperplasia. *J Urol* 1998;159:1810.

462. Kojima Y, Sasaki S, Oda N, et al. Prostate growth inhibition by subtype-selective alpha(1)-adrenoceptor antagonist naftopidil in benign prostatic hyperplasia. *Prostate* 2009;69:1521.

463. Helpap B, Oehler U, Weisser H, et al. Morphology of benign prostatic hyperplasia after treatment with Sabal Extract IDS 89 or placebo. *J Urol Pathol* 1995;3:175.

464. Marks LS, Partin AW, Epstein JI, et al. Effects of saw palmetto herbal blend in men with sympromatic benign prostatic hyperplasia. *J Urol* 2000;163:1451.

465. Bent S, Kane C, Shinohara K, et al. Saw palmetto for benign prostatic hyperplasia. *N Engl J Med* 2006;354:557.

466. Fitzpatrick JM. Minimally invasive and endoscopic management of benign prostatic hyperplasia. In: Wein AJ, Kavoussi LR, Novick AC, et al., eds. *Campbell's Urology.* 9th ed. Philadelphia, PA: Saunders; 2007:2803–2844.

467. Cowan DF, Orihuela E, Montamedi M, et al. Histoapthologic effects of laser radiation on the human prostate. *Mod Pathol* 1995;8:716.

468. Costello AJ, Bolton DM, Ellis D, et al. Histopathological changes in human prostate adenoma following neodymium: YAG laser ablation therapy. *J Urol* 1994;152:1526.

469. Aumuller G, Riva A. Morphology and functions of the human seminal vesicle. *Andrologia* 1992;24:183–196.

470. Sandlow JI, Winfield HN, Goldstein M. Surgery of the scrotum and seminal vesicles. In: Wein AJ, Kavoussi LR, Novick AC, et al., eds. *Campbell's Urology.* 9th ed. Philadelphia, PA: Saunders; 2007: 1109–1125.

471. Brewster SF. The development and differentiation of human seminal vesicles. *J Anat* 1985;143:43.

472. Thomson AA, Marker PC. Branching morphogenesis in the prostate gland and seminal vesicle. *Differentiation* 2006;74:382.

473. Aboul-Azm TE. Anatomy of the human seminal vesicles and ejaculatory ducts. *Arch Androl* 1979;3:287–292.

474. Trainer TD. Testis and excretory duct system. In: Mills SE, ed. *Histology for Pathologists.* 3rd ed. Philadelphia, PA: Lippincott Williams & Wilkins; 2007:957–958.

475. Shah RB, Lee MW, Giraldo AA, et al. Histologic and histochemical characterization of seminal intraluminal secretions. Particlular emphasis on their crystalloid morphology. *Arch Pathol Lab Med* 2001;125:141.

476. Shidham VB, Lindholm PF, Kajdacsy-Balla A, et al. Prostate-specific antigen expression and lipochrome pigment granules in the differential diagnosis of prostatic adenocarcinoma versus seminal vesicle-ejaculatory duct epithelium. *Arch Pathol Lab Med* 1999;123:1093.

477. Arias-Stella J, Takano-Moron J. Atypical epithelial changes in seminal vesicles. *Arch Pathol* 1958;66:761.

478. Kuo TT, Gomez LB. Monstrous epithelial cells in human epididymis and seminal vesicles. A pseudomalignant change. *Am J Surg Pathol* 1981;5:483–490.

479. Schned AR, Brennick JB, Gonzalez JL. Stromal lipofuscinosis of the seminal vesicle [letter]. *Pathology* 2010;42:177.

480. Laczko I, Hudson DL, Freeman A, et al. Comparison of the zones of the human prostate with the seminal vesicle: morphology, immuno-histochemistry, and cell kinetics. *Prostate* 2005;62:260.

481. Leroy X, Ballereau C, Villers A, et al. MUC6 is a marker of seminal vesicle-ejaculatory duct epithelium and is useful for the differential diagnosis with prostate adenocarcinoma. *Am J Surg Pathol* 2003;27:519.

482. Quick CM, Gokden N, Sangoi AR, et al. The distribution of PAX-2 immunoreactivity in the prostate gland, seminal vesicle, and ejaculatory duct: comparison with prostatic adenocarcinoma and discussion of prostatic zonal embryogenesis. *Hum Pathol* 2010;41:1145.

483. Beach R, Gown AM, De Peralta-Venturina MN, et al. P504S immunohistochemical detection in 405 prostatic specimens including 376 18-gauge needle biopsies. *Am J Surg Pathol* 2002;26:1588.

484. Harvey AM, Grice B, Hamilton C, et al. Diagnostic utility of P504S/ p63 cocktail, prostate-specific antigen, and prostatic acid phosphatase in verifying prostatic carcinoma involvement in seminal vesicles. A study of 57 cases of radical prostatectomy specimens of pathologic stage pT3b. *Arch Pathol Lab Med* 2010;134:983.

485. Grob BM, Haley C, Schellhammer PE, et al. The detection of prostate specific antigen, MHS-5, and other markers in invasive prostate cancer and seminal vesicle. *J Urol* 1992;147:1435.

486. Varma M, Morgan M, Jasani B, et al. Polyclonal anti-PSA is more sensitive but less specific than monoclonal anti-PSA. *Am J Clin Pathol* 2002;118:202.

487. Meiraz D, Fischelovitch J, Lazebnik J. Agenesis of the kidney associated with congenital malformation of the seminal vesicle. *Br J Urol* 1973;45:451.

488. Dominguez C, Boronat F, Cunat E, et al. Agenesis of seminal vesicles in infertile males: ultrasonic diagnosis. *Eur Urol* 1991;20:129.

489. Kim B, Kawashima A, Ryu JA, et al. Imaging of the seminal vesicle and vas deferens. *Radiographics* 2009;29:1105.

490. Argani P, Walsh PC, Epstein JI. Analysis of the prostatic central zone in patients with unilateral absence of wolffian duct structures: further evidence of the mesodermal origin of the prostatic central zone. *J Urol* 1998;160:2126.

491. Hall S, Oates RD. Unilateral absence of the scrotal vas deferens associated with contralateral mesonephric duct anomalies resulting in infertility: laboratory, physical and radiographic findings, and therapeutic alternatives. *J Urol* 1993;150:1161.

492. Holsclaw DS, Perlmutter AD, Jockin H, et al. Genital abnormalities in male patients with cystic fibrosis. *J Urol* 1971;106:568.

493. De la Taille A, Rigot JM, et al. Correlation between genito-urinary anomalies, semen analysis and CTFR genotype in patients with congenital bilateral absence of the vas deferens. *Br J Urol* 1998;81:614.

494. Christiano AP, Palmer JS, Chekmareva MA, et al. Duplicated seminal vesicle. *Urology* 1999;54:162.

495. Kaneti J, Lissmer L, Smailowitz Z, et al. Agenesis of kidney associated with malformations of the seminal vesicle. Various clinical presentations. *Int Urol Nephrol* 1988;20:29.

496. MacDonald GR. The ectopic ureter in men. *J Urol* 1986;135:1269.

497. Negi SC, Dhiman ML, Gupta R. Larger seminal vesicle cyst obstructing the ureter of a solitary kidney. *Br J Urol* 1998;82:446.

498. Lau SK, Chu PG. Prostatic tissue ectopia within the seminal vesicle: a potential source of confusion with seminal vesicle involvement by prostatic adenocarcinoma. *Virchows Arch* 2006;449:600.

499. Ogreid P, Hatteland K. Cyst of seminal vesicle associated with ipsilateral renal agenesis. *Scand J Urol Nephrol* 1979;13:113.

500. Patel B, Gujral S, Jefferson K, et al. Seminal vesicle cysts and associated anomalies. *BJU Int* 2002;90:265.

501. Heaney JA, Pfister RC, Meares EM. Giant cyst of the seminal vesicle with renal agenesis. *AJR Am J Roentgenol* 1987;149:139.

502. Van den Ouden D, Blom JHM, Bangma C, et al. Diagnosis and management of seminal vesicle cysts associated with ipsilateral renal agenesis: a pooled analysis of 52 cases. *Eur Urol* 1998;33:433.

503. Belet U, Danaci M, Sarikaya S, et al. Prevalence of epididymal, seminal vesicle, prostate, and testicular cysts in autosomal dominant polycystic kidney disease. *Urology* 2002;60:138.

504. Torra R, Sarquella J, Calabia J, et al. Prevalence of cysts in seminal tract and abnormal semen parameters in patients with autosomal dominant polycystic kidney disease. *Clin J Am Soc Nephrol* 2008;3:790.

505. Hart JB. A case of cyst or hydrops of the seminal vesicle. *J Urol* 1961;86:137.

506. Lee BH, Seo JW, Han YH, et al. Primary mucinous adenocarcinoma of a seminal vesicle cyst associated with ectopic ureter and ipsilateral renal agenesis: a case report. *Korean J Radiol* 2007;8:258.

507. Atobe T, Naoe S, Taguchi K, et al. Primary seminal vesicle carcinoma in a 19-year-old male [in Japanese]. *Gan No Rinsho* 1984;30:205.

508. Okada Y, Tanaka H, Takeuchi H, et al. Papillary adenocarcinoma in a seminal vesicle cyst associated with ipsilateral renal agenesis. *J Urol* 1992;148:1543.

509. Yanagisawa N, Saegusa M, Yoshida T, et al. Squamous cell carcinoma arising from a seminal vesicle cyst: possible relationship between chronic inflammation and tumor development. *Pathol Int* 2002;52:244.

510. Bagley DH, Javadpour N, Witebsky FG, et al. Seminal vesicle cyst containing mesonephroid tumor. *Urology* 1975;5:147.

511. Furuya R, Takahashi S, Furuya S, et al. Is seminal vesiculitis a discrete disease entity? Clinical and microbiological study of seminal vesiculitis in patients with acute epididymitis. *J Urol* 2004;171:1550.

512. Pandy P, Peters J, Shingleton WB. Seminal vesicle abscess: a case report and review of the literature. *Scand J Urol Nephrol* 1995;29:521.

513. Eastham JA, Spires KS, Abreo F, et al. Seminal vesicle abscess due to tuberculosis: role of tissue culture in making the diagnosis. *South Med J* 1999;92:328.

514. Kimura M, Maekura S, Satou T, et al. Cytomegaloviral inclusions detected in the seminal vesicle, ductus deferens and lungs in an autopsy case of lung cancer [in Japanese]. *Rinsho Byori* 1993;41:1059.

515. Al Adnani MS. Schistosomiasis, metaplasia and squamous cell carcinoma of the prostate: histogenesis of the squamous cancer cells determined by localization of specific markers. *Neoplasma* 1985;326:613.

516. Sagglam M, Tasar M, Bulakbasi N, et al. TRUS, CT, and MRI findings of hydatid disease of the seminal vesicles. *Eur Radiol* 1998;8:933.

517. Wadei HM, Brumble L, Broderick GA, et al. Polymicrobial seminal vesicle abscess in a kidney transplant recipient. *Urology* 2008;72:296.

518. Sanchez Chapado M, Angulo Cuesta J, Guil Cid M, et al. Malacoplakia of the prostate and seminal vesicle. Ultrastructural study and review of the literature [in Spanish]. *Arch Esp Urol* 1995;48:775.

519. Kim K, Cho YM, Hong YO, et al. Bacillus calmette-guerin granuloma in seminal vesicle: report of the first case in the English literature. *Int J Clin Exp Pathol* 2009;2:599.

520. Argani P, Carter HB, Epstein JI. Isolated vasculitis of the seminal vesicle. *Urology* 1998;52:131.

521. Schned AR, Cozzolino DJ. Idiopathic dense calcification of the seminal vesicles. *J Urol* 1997;157:2263.

522. Suh JH, Gardner JM, Kee KH, et al. Calcifications in prostate and ejaculatory system: a study on 298 consecutive whole mount sections of prostate from radical prostatectomy or cystoprostatectomy specimens. *Ann Diag Pathol* 2008;12:165.

523. George S. Calcification of the vas deferens and seminal vesicles. *JAMA* 1906;47:103.

524. Li YK. Diagnosis and management of large seminal vesicle stones. *Br J Urol* 1991;68:322.

525. Wilkinson AG. Case report: calculus in the seminal vesicle. *Pediatr Radiol* 1993;23;327.

526. Corriere JN Jr. Painful ejaculation due to seminal vesicle calculi. *J Urol* 1997;157:626.

527. Kee KH, Lee MJ, Shen SS, et al. Amyloidosis of seminal vesicles and ejaculatory ducts: a histologic analysis of 21 cases among 447 prostatectomy specimens. *Ann Diagn Pathol* 2008;12:235.

528. Tsutsumi Y, Serizawa A, Hori S. Localized amyloidosis of the seminal vesicle: identification of lactoferrin immunoreactivity in the amyloid material. *Pathol Int* 1996;46:491.

529. Pitkanen P, Westermark P, Cornwell GG III, et al. Amyloid of the seminal vesicles. A distinctive and common localized form of senile amyloidosis. *Am J Pathol* 1989;110:64.

530. Goldman H. Amyloidosis of seminal vesicles and vas deferens. *Arch Pathol* 1963;75:94.

531. Carris CK, McLaughlin AP, Gittes RF. Amyloidosis of the lower genitourinary tract. *J Urol* 1976;115:423.

532. Ramchandani P, Schnall MD, LiVolsi VA, et al. Senile amyloidosis of the seminal vesicles mimicking metastatic spread of prostatic carcinoma on MR images. *AJR Am J Roentgenol* 1993;161:99.

533. Coyne JD, Kealy WF. Seminal vesicle amyloidosis: morphological, histochemical and immunohistochemical observations. *Histopathology* 1993;22:173.

534. Unger PD, Wang Q, Gordon RE, et al. Localized amyloidosis of the seminal vesicle. Possible association with hormonally treated prostatic adenocarcinoma. *Arch Pathol Lab Med* 1997;121:1265.

535. Suess K, Moch H, Eppert R, et al. Heterogeneity of seminal vesicle amyloid. Immunohistochemical detection of lactoferrin and amyloid of the prealbumin-transthyretin type [in German]. *Pathologe* 1998;19:115.

536. Hatcher PA, Tucker JA, Carson CC. Fibromuscular hyperplasia of the seminal vesicle. *J Urol* 1989;141:957.

537. Fujisawa M, Ishigami J, Kamidono S, et al. Adenomyosis of the seminal vesicle with hematospermia. *Hinyokika Kiyo* 1993;39:73.

538. Lissidini G, Greco L, Gurrado A, et al. Bowel obstruction caused by primitive fibromuscular hyperplasia of the seminal vesicle in the elderly. *Int Surg* 2008;93:192.

Adenocarcinoma of the Prostate

GLADELL P. PANER, CRISTINA MAGI-GALLUZZI, MAHUL B. AMIN, and JOHN R. SRIGLEY

INTRODUCTION

Prostatic adenocarcinoma, the commonest noncutaneous malignancy in humans, is a significant cause of morbidity and mortality in men. Adenocarcinomas account for >99.5% of carcinomas of the prostate gland, and as such, population statistics on prostate cancer essentially reflect adenocarcinoma. The diagnosis and treatment of prostatic adenocarcinoma generates significant workload for the surgical pathologist. Prostatic needle biopsies and radical prostatectomy (RP) specimens are very common specimens in most pathology laboratories. It has been estimated that upwards of a million prostate biopsies are done annually in the United States.[1] Adenocarcinoma of the prostate has a wide spectrum of clinical presentations ranging from the identification of a small focus of low-grade carcinoma in the asymptomatic patient with a prostate-specific antigen (PSA) elevation to widely metastatic carcinoma in a patient with bone pain. The architectural patterns of adenocarcinoma are diverse, and certain morphologies are predictive of clinical outcome and help explain, at least in part, the heterogeneous behavior of this tumor. The complexity of reporting both biopsy and radical resection specimens has increased in recent years, and there is an expectation on the part of urologists and oncologists that the surgical pathology report will include not just the diagnostic information but also all relevant prognostic data related to grade, extent, stage, margin status, and other information in selected cases.

In view of the sheer volume of prostatic cancer cases handled by pathologists, the morphologic heterogeneity of adenocarcinoma and the clinical impact of this diagnosis and associated prognostic factors, it was decided to devote an entire chapter to this tumor. Acinar adenocarcinoma and its variations (e.g., atrophic, pseudohyperplastic) and special variants of adenocarcinoma including ductal, mucinous, and signet-ring carcinoma are discussed here. Other rare carcinomas including basaloid, squamous (adenosquamous), sarcomatoid, small cell, large cell neuroendocrine, and urothelial carcinoma are presented in Chapter 10.

EPIDEMIOLOGY

Incidence and Prevalence

Prostate cancer is the second most common and sixth leading cause of cancer death in men with an estimated 899,000 new cases and 258,000 deaths in the world in 2008.[2] In the United States, in 2013, it is estimated that there will be 238,590 new cases and 29,720 deaths from prostate cancer with age-adjusted incidence rate of 154.8 cases per 100,000 men.[3,4] Due to the high incidence and absolute mortality rates, considerable resources have been allocated to prostate cancer, with approximately $9.9 billion spent each year on treatment in the United States alone.[5] In 2009, the National Cancer Institute invested $293.9 million on prostate cancer research.[6]

Unlike other common visceral organ malignancies, prostate cancer diagnoses far outweigh the number of cancer-related deaths. This is due to its long latency period and the fact that most tumors are low-grade organ-confined tumors. In the United States, the ratio of new prostate cancer diagnosed to total number of deaths in a year is 8:1 in contrast to much higher ratios for other common tumors such as lung cancer (1.4:1) and colon cancer (2:1).[4] The high incidence of prostate cancer has been attributed to widespread serum PSA screening introduced in the early 1990s. This had led to increased detection of indolent tumors resulting in long lead-time bias (of at least about 10 years) in survival proportions and no significant effect on the time of death.[7,8] Some authors consider this phenomenon as "overdiagnosis," and it is estimated that 23% to 42% of prostate cancer in the United States and Europe is overdiagnosed because of PSA screening.[8,9] Currently, controversy surrounds the use of population-based PSA screening, discussed later in details.[10–12]

Most patients with prostate cancer, due to its long latency, survive the disease, and many eventually die of other nonrelated causes, mostly from cardiovascular disease. As a result, prostate cancer is the most prevalent cancer in men (43%), a figure that is striking in comparison with

Table 9-1 ■ AGE OF DIAGNOSIS OF PROSTATE CANCER

Age in Years	Diagnosis Rates (%)
<20	0
20–34	0
35–44	0.6
45–54	9.5
55–64	31.6
65–74	35.5
75–84	18.6
85+	4.1

Reprinted from *SEER Stat Fact Sheets: Prostate.* 2012, with permission.

the percentage prevalence of colorectal cancer (9%) and melanoma of the skin (7%).[13] United States statistics for 2009 indicate that there were approximately 2,496,784 men alive who had a history of prostate cancer.[3]

Age

Prostate cancer is considered a disease of older men, and notably among all cancers, the incidence increases dramatically with age (Table 9-1).[3] The median age of diagnosis is 67 years. Incidence is remarkably low in men <50 years old, and about 60% of cases occur in men ≥65 years old. Diagnosis rates peak in men 65 to 74 years old, whereas in men ≤54 years old, the rate is about 10%.

Lifetime Risk

It is estimated that one in six men born today will be diagnosed with prostate cancer at some time during his lifetime.[3] The lifetime risk also markedly increases with age, from 1:1,000 in men <40 years old to 1:8 in men 60 to 79 years old. It is estimated that 8.5% of men will develop prostate cancer between their 50th and 70th birthdays.

Ethnic Relationship

In the United States, African-Americans have the highest incidence rates, which are about 60% higher than in Caucasians, and rates are much lower in Asian Americans and Native Americans and Alaskans (Table 9-2).[4] Interestingly,

differences among ethnic groups are also documented in other parts of the world, such as in Brazil and Europe. It is not fully understood why the incidence rate is very high in black men in the United States and some Caribbean countries, and perhaps it could be due to inherent genetic factors.[14–16]

Mortality

In the United States, the age-adjusted death rate for prostate cancer is 23.6 per 100,000 men per year.[3] From 2005 to 2009, the median age at death for prostate cancer is 80 years. Mortality rate is highest in African Americans (54.9 per 100,000 men) and lowest in Asian Americans and Pacific Islanders (Table 9-3). Mortality also increases with age; prostate cancer is the third and second most common cause of cancer death in men 60 to 79 years old and ≥80 years old, respectively, but is not even in the top five causes of cancer death in men 40 to 59 years old.

Worldwide Geographical Distribution

Incidence Rate

The incidence of prostate cancer differs worldwide, and these variations can be attributed to several factors including detection rates of clinically latent tumors, ethnicity, and environmental factors.[2] Prostate cancer incidence rates have been increasing in many countries with no notable decrease reported in any nation.[17] Incidence rates are highest in more developed or higher-resourced countries such as the United States, Canada, Australia and New Zealand, western Europe and Scandinavia, and the Caribbean and are lowest in south central and eastern Asia and northern Africa (Fig. 9-1).[17] Prostate cancer in South Korea, Thailand, and Chennai, India, is as low as <10 per 100,000 men.[17] These worldwide disparities can be attributed, at least in part, to variations in practice of PSA screening. Differences may also be related to diet, as incidence is usually low in regions with mainly low fat and plant-based diet and higher with westernized diet.

Mortality Rate

Mortality rates also tend to be higher in less-developed parts of the world including the Caribbean, some countries in southern and western Africa, and in South America, and the lowest

Table 9-2 ■ PROSTATE CANCER INCIDENCE BY RACE

Ethnicity	Incidence
African American	228.7 per 100,000
White	141.0 per 100,000
Hispanic/Latino	124.9 per 100,000
American Indian or Alaskan Native	98.8 per 100,000
Asian American or Pacific Islander	77.2 per 100,000

Reprinted from Siegel R, Naishadham D, Jemal A. Cancer statistics, 2013. *CA Cancer J Clin* 2013;63(1):11–30, with permission.

Table 9-3 ■ PROSTATE CANCER MORTALITY BY RACE

Ethnicity	Mortality
African American	53.1 per 100,000
White	21.7 per 100,000
American Indian or Alaskan Native	19.7 per 100,000
Hispanic/Latino	17.8 per 100,000
Asian American or Pacific Islander	10.0 per 100,000

Reprinted from Siegel R, Naishadham D, Jemal A. Cancer statistics, 2013. *CA Cancer J Clin* 2013;63(1):11–30, with permission.

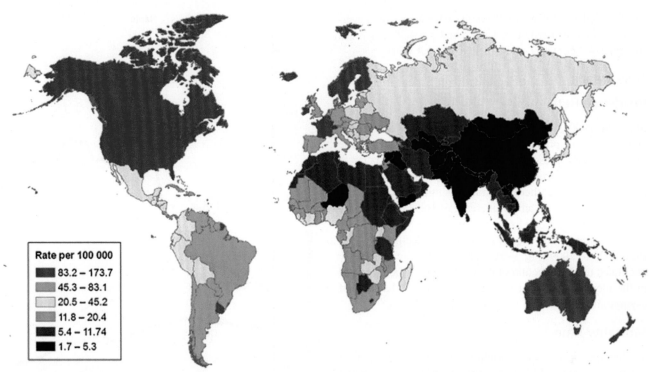

FIGURE 9-1 ■ Worldwide variation in age-standardized prostate cancer incidence rates 2008. (Reprinted from Center MM, et al. International variation in prostate cancer incidence and mortality rates. *Eur Urol* 2012;61(6):1079–1092, with permission.)

mortality rates are observed in most parts of Asia, northern Africa, and North America (Fig. 9-2).[17] Differences overall are less marked for mortality compared to incidence, but are high in Trinidad and Tobago (53.6 per 100,000 men), which are twice the rate of second place Cuba (22.6 per 100,000 men) and

25 times that of lowest place Uzbekistan (1.6 per 100,00 men). During the past several years, prostate cancer mortality rates have been decreasing in many countries, but also increasing in some nations.[17] High average increases in mortality rates occurred in Korea (7.8% per year), Moldova (6.5% per year),

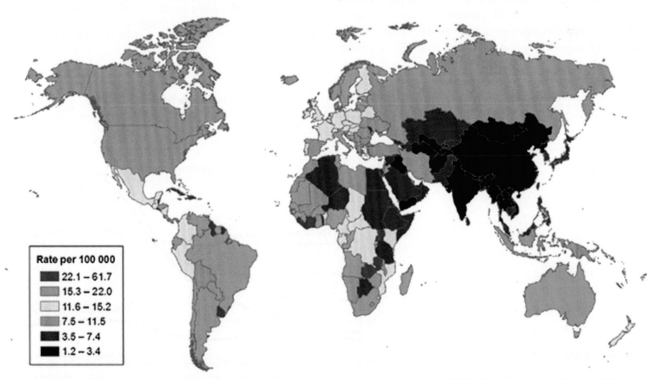

FIGURE 9-2 ■ Worldwide variation in age-standardized prostate cancer mortality rates 2008. (Reprinted from Center MM, et al. International variation in prostate cancer incidence and mortality rates. *Eur Urol* 2012;61(6):1079–1092, with permission.)

and Trinidad and Tobago (4.5% per year), whereas high average decreases occurred in the United States (−4.3% per year), Austria (−4% per year), and Israel (−3.7% per year).

Time Trends

Incidence Rate

Since the 1990s, in the United States, there was a dramatic 40% decline in prostate cancer deaths and 75% decrease in symptomatic presentation attributed by most experts to earlier tumor detection from widespread PSA screening.[18] From 1988 to 1992, there was a large surge in prostate cancer diagnosis with an annual increase of 16.5% followed by an annual increase of 11.6% in 1992 to 1995, followed by relative stability, and then a small annual decline of 1.9% from 2000 to 2009 (Fig. 9-3).[3,4] The initial surge essentially paralleled the introduction of PSA screening, which resulted in the identification of a substantial prevalence backlog of asymptomatic cases that later evened out with time.

Mortality Rate

Worldwide, decreasing mortality rates are also seen in many developed and high-resource countries. In the United States, mortality rates from prostate cancer increased from 1975 to 1991 and declined since the mid-1990s that was greatest and most sustained in men >75 years old.[19] In both the United States and the United Kingdom, prostate cancer mortality peaked in the early 1990s at almost identical rates, but age-adjusted mortality in the United States subsequently declined by 4.2% per year, four times the rate of decline in the United Kingdom (1.1%).[19] Decline in prostate cancer mortality can be attributed to several factors including improved treatments such as RP, radiation, and hormonal therapies (Fig. 9-4).[746] Widespread PSA screening

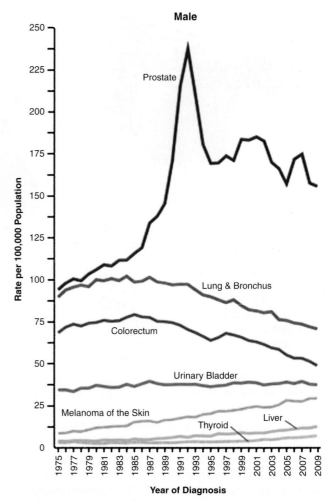

FIGURE 9-3 ■ Cancer trends for men in the United States from 1975 to 2008. (Reprinted from Siegel R, Naishadham D, Jemal A. Cancer statistics, 2013. *CA Cancer J Clin* 2013;63(1):11–30, with permission.)

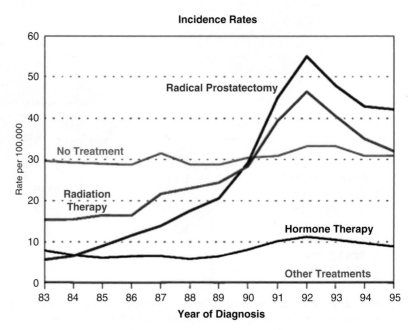

FIGURE 9-4 ■ Incidence over time of prostate cancer treatment. (Reprinted from Stanford JL, Stephenson RA, Coyle LM, et al. *Prostate Cancer Trends 1973–1995*, SEER Program, National Cancer Institute, NIH Pub. No. 99-4543, Bethesda, MD, 1999, with permission.)

is indirectly linked as a reason for decrease prostate cancer mortality. However, this is currently controversial, as recent large randomized PSA screening studies for prostate cancer in the United States did not show benefit and, in Europe, only 20% reduction in mortality.[10,11] Further, decline in prostate cancer mortality was observed even in countries with low PSA screening such as United Kingdom.[20]

ETIOPATHOGENESIS

Introduction

The exact cause of prostate cancer remains elusive despite extensive research carried out in this field. Currently, older age, ethnicity (black race), and family history, which are all nonmodifiable factors, are well-established risks for prostate cancer.[21] Epidemiologic studies show that immigrants from low-incidence regions acquire intermediate-risk level after migrating to high-risk areas suggesting also a role for environmental factors.

There is no single identified genetic event that can cause prostate cancer, and perhaps, neoplastic growth arises from multiple genetic alterations and/or epigenetic factors. It remains poorly understood why most of the prostate cancer diagnosed exhibits long latency and only a subset unpredictably transforms into clinically aggressive disease. Similar to nodular hyperplasia, growth and development of prostate cancer is dependent on androgen signaling. However, a subset of prostate cancer may progress even with an absent or suppressed level of androgen hormone (castration-resistant state), and these are generally incurable. The mechanism of evolution to androgen independence by prostate cancer is currently an intense area of research.

Risk Factors

Age

As discussed above, the incidence of prostate cancer sharply increases with age with about 60% of cases diagnosed in men >65 years old. Interestingly based on these statistics, if men live up to 100 years old, almost all will have prostate cancer.

Ethnicity

As discussed above, the incidence of prostate cancer is much greater in African-American men, which is 1.6 and 2.8 times higher than in whites and Asian Americans, respectively. Likewise, death from prostate cancer in African-American men is less than two times and about five times higher than in whites and Asian Americans, respectively. There is also an increased likelihood of a high Gleason score and more rapid tumor growth with earlier transformation from latent to aggressive disease in black than in white men.[22,23]

Several studies suggest that the higher incidence and mortality from prostate cancer in black men are partly due to genetic susceptibility.[21,24] Genetic differences such as variants in alleles on chromosomes including 8q24 and 17q21–22, which are associated with increased risk for prostate cancer, are suggested to be higher in men of African descent.[25–28] Microsatellite marker DG8S737 on chromosome 8q24 has a population attributable risk of 16% in African Americans, which is higher than in European men (5% to 11%).[28] The frequency of risk allele in 17q21 is about 5% in men of African descent, whereas it is rare in other races (<1%).[25] Variant G allele of *CYP3A4* associated with aggressive prostate cancer progression is much more frequent in African-American men (81%) than in white men (8%).[29,30] Polymorphism of CYP17 may have a role in the susceptibility to prostate cancer in men of African but not of European descent.[31] Mutation in ephB2 gene is associated with prostate cancer risk in African-American men with a family history of prostate cancer but is not found in white men.[32]

Family History

Familial association in prostate cancer is well documented.[33,34] There is a twofold increased risk if 1 first-degree relative and a 9 times increased risk if 3 first-degree relatives are diagnosed with prostate cancer. Risk also increases inversely with age of diagnosis in relatives. If the age of onset is 50 years old, the relative risk is increased 7 times.

There are compelling evidence to suggest a genetic basis for familial predisposition in prostate cancer. High-risk alleles are identified with either autosomal dominant or X-linked mode of inheritance. Implicated genetic factors for hereditary prostate cancer include *BRCA2* on chromosome 13q12, *ELAC2* on chromosome 17p, *RNASEL* on chromosome 1q25, *MSR1* on chromosome 8p22–23, *NBS1* on chromosome 5, and *CHEK2* on chromosome 22q.[35,36]

Diet

There is a positive association of prostate cancer with consumption of animal products, particularly red meat cooked at high temperatures.[37–39] This association is suggested to be due to heterocyclic amine content in meat.[38] A recent large prospective study suggested little or no association between fruit and vegetable intake and prostate cancer risk.[40] In the large Selenium and Vitamin E Cancer Prevention Trial (SELECT) of 35,533 men, neither vitamin E nor selenium supplementation was shown to be significantly associated with prostate cancer risk.[41]

Obesity and Metabolic Syndrome

Several studies suggest obesity as a risk factor for prostate cancer.[42,43] Elevated body mass index (BMI) increases the risk of prostate cancer mortality in prospective cohort studies and biochemical recurrence in prostate cancer patients.[43] Adipose tissue may influence circulating levels of several bioactive substances that may affect the risk of developing prostate cancer.[42] It is also suggested that obesity may modify genes of periprostatic adipose tissue to promote a favorable environment for prostate cancer progression.[44] Overall, the highly prevalent metabolic syndrome including central obesity, insulin resistance, dyslipidemia, and hypertension is suggested to have an association with prostate cancer.[45]

Environmental Factors

Increased risk for prostate cancer has been proposed with exposures to cadmium, pesticides, rubber, textile, and chemicals.[46–49] Vitamin D deficiency has been implicated as a risk for prostate cancer and may explain geographic differences in incidence due to light exposure, as ecologic studies have shown that mortality rates from prostate cancer are inversely correlated with levels of ultraviolet radiation.[50] Earlier mortality analysis suggested a higher risk for prostate cancer in atomic energy workers, but this was seen to be declining.[51] Farming is suggested as a risk factor for prostate cancer, but this increased risk may not be due to pesticide exposure.[52]

Vasectomy

There is conflicting evidence suggesting vasectomy as a risk factor for prostate cancer, although more recent data support a lack of association.[53–58]

Others

There is a controversial association of xenotropic murine leukemia-related virus (XMRV) to prostate cancer after XMRV DNA was isolated in 6% of prostate cancer.[59–63] Other later studies however did not show XMRV infection in prostate, and it is being suggested that the identification may be due to sample contamination.

Cell of Origin

The luminal acinar secretory cells were thought to be the cell of origin of prostate cancer since this tumor is characterized by phenotypic similarity to acinar cells (PSA positive, p63/ HMWK negative) and absence of basal cells. Recent in vitro studies in animal models however suggest that basal cells are more likely the precursor cells of prostate adenocarcinoma.[64] The cooperative effects of AKT via loss of *PTEN*, *ERG*, and androgen receptor (AR) in basal cells were able to reproduce the histologic and molecular features of prostate cancer including absence of basal cells and overexpression of alpha-methyl-CoA racemase (AMACR).[64]

Molecular and Genomic Basis

Prostate cancer, like most other cancers, exhibits multiple genomic alterations such as point mutations, microsatellite sequence changes, and chromosomal rearrangements (e.g., translocations, insertions, duplications, and deletions).[36,65–69] The most common chromosomal alterations in prostate cancer are losses at 1p, 6q, 8p, 10q, 13q, 16q, and 18q and gains at 1q, 2p, 7, 8q, and Xq.[66,70] Rearrangement in chromosome 22 between *TMPRSS2* and *ERG* is seen in about half of prostate cancers and is discussed below in detail.[71,72]

Multiple putative prostate cancer susceptibility loci have been identified by linkage analysis including the HPC1 locus on 1q23–25 (*RNASEL*), HPC2 locus on 17p (*ELAC2*), PCAP locus on 1q42–43, CAPB locus on 1p36, HPC20 locus on 20q13, and HPCX locus on Xq27–28.[30,73–79] Analysis among 426 families with hereditary prostate cancer identified a susceptibility region at 17q22 (*BRCA1*).[80] Genome-wide association study identified a variant on 8q24 containing *MYC* oncogene that confers risk for prostate cancer.[28] Nine SNP loci identified at this chromosome region were independently associated with prostate cancer risk.[65] Another genome-wide association study identified 7 new prostate cancer susceptibility loci at 2p11, 3q23, 3q26, 5p12, 6p21, 12q13, and Xq12.59.[81] About 50 prostate cancer susceptibility loci have now been identified.[65]

Multiple somatic genetic alterations in prostate cancer may result in inactivation of tumor suppressor gene or activation of oncogenes (Table 9-4).[30,36,65] Among implicated in prostate carcinogenesis includes tumor suppressor genes *GSTP1*, *PTEN*, *CDKN1B*, *NKX3.1*, *KLF6*, *Rb*, and *p53* and oncogenes *c-myc*, *bcl-2*, *c-kit*, and *STAT5*.[36]

PTEN is mutated in about 20% to 40% of prostate cancers (often 10q23 deletion), more identified in advanced prostate cancer suggesting a role in cancer progression.[66,69,82] *PTEN* is present in normal prostatic epithelial cells and high-grade prostatic intraepithelial neoplasia (HGPIN) and is reduced in prostate cancers with high grade and stage.[83,84] There is a significant co-occurrence of *TMPRSS2:ERG* and *PTEN* loss in prostate cancer, suggesting the possibility of *PTEN* loss as a late genetic event or "second hit" after *ERG* rearrangement.[85] *SPOP* is the most frequent nonsynonymous mutated gene in prostate cancer, detected in 6% to 13% of prostate cancers.[69] Interestingly, unlike *PTEN* loss, *SPOP* alterations are present in *TMPRSS2:ETS*-negative prostate cancer and may represent a different class of prostate cancers.[65] The mutually exclusive occurrence of *TMPRSS2:ERG* and *SPOP* forms the basis for a possible molecular classification of prostate cancer (Fig. 9-5).

Alterations in AR may lead to AR activation in prostate cancer that may allow them to survive in an environment deprived of androgen hormone (castration resistant).[86] AR is mutated or amplified in 20% to 30% of castration-resistant prostate cancers.[87,88] Polymorphisms are also observed in genes associated with androgen biosynthesis.[65]

Hedgehog signaling pathway has been shown to play a role in growth and metastasis of prostate cancer.[89,90]

Gene Fusion

The first chromosome translocation identified in prostate cancer was t(6;16), which results in the *TPC:HPR* fusion.[91]

Fusion of *TMPRSS2* and *ETS* gene family is specific for prostate cancer detected in about 50% of cases.[71,72,92–94] *TMPRSS2* encodes for serine protease secreted by prostatic cells in response to androgen exposure, and this explains why the gene fusion leads to androgen-responsive expression of

Table 9-4 ■ MUTATED GENES IN PROSTATE CANCER

Gene	Chromosome
CHD5	1p36.31
SDF4	1p36.33
EPHB2	1p36.12
SPTA1	1q23.1
SRD5A2	2p23.1
THSD7B	2q22.1
SCN11A	3p22.2
PLXNB1	3p21.31
PRKCI	3q26.2
PIK3CA	3q26.32
ZNF595	4p16.3
CHD1	5q15–q21.1
APC	5q22.2
HSP90AB1	6p21.1
DLK2	6p21.1
HDAC9	7p21.1
EGFR	7p11.2
BRAF	7q34
HSPA5	9q33.3
KLF6	10p15.1
PTEN	10q23.31
CDKN1B	12p13.1
KRAS	12p12.1
MLL2	12q13.12
RB1	13q14.2
GPC6	13q31.3–32.1
FOXA1	14q21.1
HSPA2	14q23.3
DICER	14q31.13
MYH11	16p13.11
ZFHX3	16q22.2–q22.3
TP53	17p13.1
CDK12	17q12
SPOP	17q21.33
ASXL1	20q11.21
CHEK2	22q12.1
KDM6A	Xp11.3
AR	Xq12
MED12	Xq13.1
HPRT1	Xq26.2–q26.3

Reprinted from Boyd LK, Mao X, Lu YJ. The complexity of prostate cancer: genomic alterations and heterogeneity. *Nat Rev Urol* 2012; 9(11):652–664, with permission.

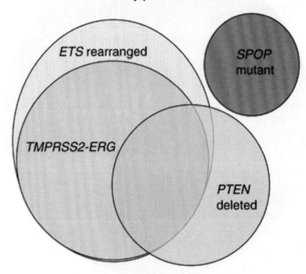

FIGURE 9-5 ■ Molecular classification of prostate cancer. About 50% of prostate cancers harbor *ETS* rearrangement, and majority of these are *TMPRSS2:ERG*. *PTEN* is deleted in 20% to 40% prostate cancers, with significant overlap to *ETS* rearrangements. *SPOP* mutation is mutually exclusive with *ETS* rearrangement. (Reprinted from Barbieri CE, Demichelis F, Rubin MA. Molecular genetics of prostate cancer: emerging appreciation of genetic complexity. *Histopathology* 2012;60(1):187–198, with permission.)

Fusion of the two genes occurs by intra- and interchromosomal genetic rearrangements. In about two-thirds of cases, fusion results from deletion of the intervening 3 Mb between *TMPRSS2* and *ERG* (Fig. 9-6).[94] Fusion may also occur by more complex rearrangements such as translocation. The most commonly reported fusion transcript is between exon 1 of *TMPRSS2* and exon 4 of *ERG*. About 20 *TMPRSS2:ERG* transcripts have now been identified. Morphologic features of prostate cancer associated with *TMPRSS2:ERG* include blue-tinged mucin, cribriform pattern, intraductal spread, macronucleoli, and signet ring cells.[97] Only 24% of tumors without any of these features displayed *TMPRSS2:ERG*, whereas 93% of cases with three or more features harbor the fusion.[97] The clinical significance of this gene fusion on prostate cancer behavior is not yet fully understood, and studies correlating it with outcome and pathologic variables have conflicting results.[98–107]

CLINICAL FEATURES

Symptoms and Signs

In the United States, the vast majority of prostate cancers are diagnosed in asymptomatic patients through early detection programs. The main reasons for performing prostate

ETS transcription factors.[95,96] *ETS* family of transcription factors includes *ERG*, *ETV1*, *ETV4*, and *ETV5* as 3′ end fusion partners, and *ERG* is the most commonly fused gene at 5′ end with *TMPRSS2* comprising about 90% of cases. Several other 5′ end fusion partners of *ETS* gene have been identified (Table 9-5). With fusion, *ERG* is brought under the control of an androgen-regulated promoter causing overexpression.

Table 9-5 ■ DETECTED ETS GENE FUSIONS IN PROSTATE CANCER

5′ Partner	3′ Partner
TMPRSS2	ERG
HERPUD1	ERG
SLC45A3	ERG
NDRG1	ERG
FKBP5	ERG
TMPRSS2	ETV4
DDX5	ETV4
CANT1	ETV4
KLK2	ETV4
TMPRSS2	ETV5
SLC45A3	ETV4
SLC45A3	ETV1
SLC45A3	ETV1
TMPRSS2	ETV1
SLC45A3	ETV1
C15orf21	ETV1
HNRPA2B1	ETV1
FLJ35294	ETV1
ACSL3	ETV1
EST14	ETV1
HERVK17	ETV1
HERVK22Q11.23	ETV1
FOXP1	ETV1
KLK2	ETV1
FUBP1	ETV1
SNURF	ETV1

Reprinted from Spans L, et al. The genomic landscape of prostate cancer. *Int J Mol Sci* 2013;14(6):10822–10851, with permission.

biopsies leading to cancer diagnoses are elevated PSA and/or abnormal digital rectal examination. Prostate cancer is also a common incidental finding in 28.5% cystoprostatectomy specimens, of which only 25.3% are considered clinically significant, defined by most experts as tumors with a volume of 0.5 mL or more and Gleason score of 7 or higher.[106,107]

In symptomatic patients, prostate cancer usually manifests with symptoms indicative of advanced disease. Presentations may include irritative (e.g., frequency, urgency) or obstructive (e.g., hesitancy, dribbling) voiding symptoms. Cancers located in transition zone may manifest earlier because of its proximity to the urethra. These lower urinary tract symptoms, however, are not specific for prostate cancer and, when encountered, are more often attributed to hyperplasia. About 10% to 15% of transurethral resection specimens performed for hyperplasia however may contain incidental prostate cancer. Local extension of tumor to structures adjacent to prostate may produce pelvic pain. Skeletal metastasis may result to bone pain and tenderness, spinal cord compression, weakness of lower extremities, and urinary or fecal incontinence. Metastasis to lymph nodes may produce adenopathy, and lower extremity lymphedema in there is inguinal

lymph node involvement. Rarely, advanced prostate cancer may present as disseminated intravascular coagulation, nonbacterial thrombotic endocarditis, malignant ascites, or pleural effusion from tumor dissemination. Paraneoplastic syndrome (e.g., syndrome of inappropriate ADH secretion, hypercalcemia, DIC, thrombotic thrombocytopenic purpura, neurologic syndromes) may occur with prostate cancer and is seen more often, but not always, when the histology contains small cell carcinoma component.

The hallmark physical finding for prostate cancer is the presence of palpable prostatic nodule or firmness on rectal examination. It should be noted that most patients with prostate cancer have normal rectal exams. In about 25% of cases, serum PSA is not elevated, and abnormal rectal exams is the reason for prostate biopsy. Other signs of prostate cancer are related to advanced stage such as hyperreflexia and increased bulbocavernosus reflex from cord compression of bone metastasis.

Aside from serum PSA elevation detailed below, abnormal laboratory findings in prostate cancer may reflect presence of advanced disease. These include azotemia (increase BUN and creatinine) from bilateral urinary obstruction, increased alkaline phosphatase from bone metastasis, and anemia and rarely low platelets from DIC or TTP.

Prostate-Specific Antigen

Prostate-specific antigen (PSA) is currently the most widely used tumor biomarker in medicine. PSA is an androgen-regulated serine protease of the human kallikrein (hK) family located on chromosome 19q13.4.[108] PSA is synthesized by secretory cells of normal, hyperplastic, or malignant prostatic acinar cells. Thus, while detectable levels are considered specific for prostatic origin, it is not a specific marker for cancer of the prostate. Nonneoplastic causes of PSA elevation include BPH, inflammation or prostatitis, ejaculation, and injury or manipulation (e.g., recent needle biopsy, bicycle ride).

When prostate cancer disrupts the basement membrane, there is leakage of PSA into the peripheral blood. Most of the circulating PSA (about 70% to 90%) is bound to α1-antichymotrypin and a subset with other protease inhibitors such as α2-macroglobulin and α1-antityrpsin. Most antibodies currently used in PSA assays detect free and most of the bound form, except for that, which is complexed with α2-macroglobulin. Detection by PSA elevation is more sensitive than rectal examination in detecting prostate cancer. The introduction of PSA as an oncologic marker and its integration into practice with rectal examination and transrectal ultrasound allow for the detection of early-stage curable prostate cancer. Serum PSA level is also a good measure in monitoring response after treatment and to diagnose disease recurrence.

Certain factors may influence PSA level. 5α-reductase inhibitors (finasteride) may cause artificial lowering of PSA level by about 50%. Patients with a high BMI may have lower PSA values because of hemodilution.[109] Some modifications of measurement and interpretation in PSA are being

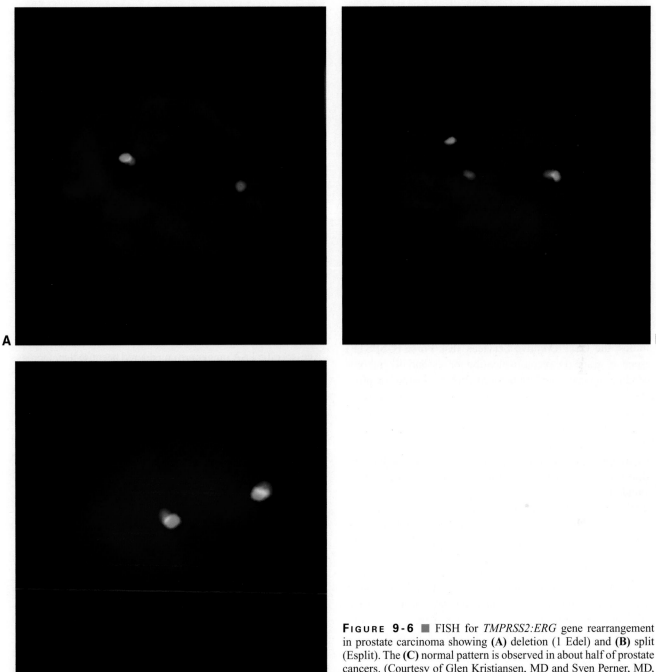

FIGURE 9-6 ■ FISH for *TMPRSS2:ERG* gene rearrangement in prostate carcinoma showing **(A)** deletion (1 Edel) and **(B)** split (Esplit). The **(C)** normal pattern is observed in about half of prostate cancers. (Courtesy of Glen Kristiansen, MD and Sven Perner, MD, PhD.)

used to enhance sensitivity and specificity in diagnosis of prostate cancer discussed below.

PSA Screening

The aim of screening programs for a particular cancer is to ultimately reduce cancer-related deaths. PSA screening in asymptomatic men is currently controversial because of the lack of definitive evidence in reducing prostate cancer mortality.[10–12,110–112] Amidst the ongoing controversy, most urology experts advocate PSA screening mainly because (a) there was a 40% decline in prostate cancer mortality since the widespread application of PSA screening from the early 1990s, (b) most tumors detected by PSA screening are low-grade low-volume tumors that can be cured, and (c) treatment options are available for these tumors.

In 2009, the two largest randomized studies on population-based PSA screening in the United States and Europe showed no or only limited benefit in reducing prostate cancer mortality.[10,11] The Prostate, Lung, Colorectal, and Ovarian Cancer Screening Trial (PLCO) in the United States included 76,693 men randomized for PSA screening (38,343 men) and usual care as control (38,350 men).[10] After 7- to 10-year follow-up, the death rate from prostate cancer in the PCLO study was very low and did not differ significantly between the study and control groups. In a larger European Randomized Study of Screening for Prostate Cancer (ERSPC) study that involved 7 countries, 162,243 men were randomized to care with and without PSA testing.[11] Results of the ERSPC study with median follow-up of 9 years showed that PSA-based screening reduced prostate cancer death rates by 20% but was associated with high detection and treatment of indolent tumors. In practical terms, 1,410 men must be screened, and additional 48 men must be treated to prevent one death from prostate cancer.[11]

Another study from Sweden of 9,026 men with longer follow-up of 20 years also did not show a significant difference in deaths between men with and without PSA screening.[12] In ERSPC, a subset study in Rotterdam showed that disease-specific survival of men with interval cancer screened every 4 years was similar with and without PSA screening.[111] Few other, but lesser quality, studies showed benefits of PSA screening such as in Quebec City involving 46,486 men showed significant reduction in prostate cancer mortality in the PSA-screened group versus the nonscreened group.[113]

In great part due to the concurrent PCLO and ERSPC studies, the US Preventive Services Task Force (USPSTF) issued a grade D recommendation or essentially recommending against population-based PSA screening for prostate cancer.[114] The USPSTF recommendation is to avoid unnecessary over treatment of prostate cancer leading to complications; the latter should be weighed against the benefit of PSA screening. This recommendation received strong opposition from urology advocate groups such as the American Urological Association (AUA), Prostate Cancer Foundation, Large Urology Group Practice Association, Men's Health Network, and others.[115,116] Arguments against the studies included high (50%) contamination rate by PSA measurement in the PCLO control group (essentially making the study one of regular versus inconsistent PSA screening), whereas the ERSCP did not specify contamination, many subjects with abnormal PSA tests did not have prompt biopsy, the follow-up was relatively short considering the long latency of prostate cancer, and that there was no consideration of high-risk groups particularly black men.[116]

PSA Cutoff

Currently, most guidelines recommend PSA screening in men between 40 and 50 years old, and the younger age will have less confounding effect of hyperplasia.[117–120] Some recommend PSA screening only in men with longer life expectancy (>10 years expectancy or <75 years old), since these patients will likely die of other reasons and not from prostate cancer.[117,120] Yearly PSA testing is recommended, although may opt for follow-up testing at longer intervals if PSA level is low (<1 ng/mL).

The traditional cutoff for PSA elevation to do prostate biopsy is 4 ng/mL. This cutoff has a sensitivity of about 20% and specificity of 60% to 70% for prostate cancer. Lower PSA cutoffs are considered in higher-risk individuals such

as African-American men or those with family histories of prostate cancer. Higher cutoff increases the predictive value; a cutoff of 10 ng/mL has a positive predictive value of 42% to 71%. Of note, no level of PSA is risk free and that the PSA value represents a risk continuum. The AUA in particular does not recommend any PSA cutoff value to prompt a biopsy and recommends that other factors such as family history, ethnicity, and rectal examination findings be taken into account.

Posttherapy PSA Monitoring

After therapy of localized prostate cancer, PSA is expected to decline to a nadir of <0.2 ng/mL, which is used to determine cure. PSA nadir is usually achieved 6 weeks after RP since all benign glands and cancer are removed, but is much longer with radiotherapy (about 27 weeks) as it takes time for cancer to degenerate. PSA elevation afterward (≥0.2 ng/mL on two occasions) is considered biochemical recurrence.[121]

Other PSA Measurements

Age-Specific PSA Ranges

Age-specific PSA ranges are considered because they increase the sensitivity in detection in younger men and increase the specificity for prostate cancer in older men. The prostate is usually larger in older male because of hyperplasia; thus, higher PSA value is permissible (e.g., 6.5 ng/mL for men 70 to 79 years old versus 2.5 ng/mL for men 40 to 49 years old) to perform biopsy. However, use of age-specific PSA ranges is controversial particularly in older men because increasing the cutoff value may lead to missing significant numbers of clinically important cancer.

PSA Dynamics (Velocity, Doubling Time)

Changes in PSA level over time may be used to stratify risk for prostate cancer including in predicting response to therapy. PSA velocity refers to the relative change in time of PSA value.[122–124] An increase of >0.75 ng/mL/y is considered a significant risk factor for prostate cancer that would prompt a prostate biopsy. It is important that the same laboratory is used to measure PSA levels over a period of at least 18 months. A very rapid rise in PSA value can be seen in prostatitis.[125] PSA doubling time refers to the amount of time required for PSA to double.[126,127] Use of pretreatment PSA velocity and doubling time is currently controversial. While both are associated with outcome, there is no clear evidence that they improve outcome prediction beyond pretreatment PSA alone.[125,128]

PSA Density

PSA density takes into account the variation in size of the prostate that may influence the PSA level. PSA density is serum PSA divided by the prostate gland volume, and a higher value suggests increase risk for prostate cancer. A PSA density of >0.15 ng/mL/cm^3 would be the recommended cutoff to perform a biopsy. Others however have found this test to be inaccurate. The problems are that the prostate may have a larger size also because of increase in stromal volume and TRUS is not accurate in measuring prostate volume. The positive predictive value of PSA density is only slightly higher than the 4 ng/mL cutoff for serum PSA. Further, performing TRUS is still an uncomfortable procedure for the patient even without biopsy. A modification of PSA density adjusts for the transition zone volume.

Free PSA (fPSA)

About 90% of PSA in circulation is bound to α1-antichymotrypsin, and a smaller amount is bound to other serum protease inhibitors. Unbound PSA is known as fPSA. Low level (<10%) of fPSA is associated with a higher risk of prostate cancer and can be useful in monitoring patients after therapy. A large multicenter study in men with normal rectal examinations and PSA of 4 to 10 ng/mL showed that fPSA with cutoff of 25% was able to detect 95% of cancers while avoiding 20% of unnecessary biopsies.[129] Another approach is to determine the ratio of fPSA to total PSA, and lower value increases the specificity in diagnosing cancer.

PUTATIVE PRECURSOR LESIONS

High-Grade Prostatic Intraepithelial Neoplasia

Introduction

Since 1926, the model for the transition of benign acinar epithelium to malignant cellular change via intermediate "atypical glands" in the prostate has been proposed by several authors. In 1949, Andrews illustrated precancerous conditions, which he identified in 70% of the glands in the prostate containing carcinoma compared to only 26% of glands without carcinoma.[130] The atypical glandular foci were characterized by cellular stratification, papillary formation, nuclear enlargement, and mitotic activity—many features that in contemporary practice would be identified in prostatic intraepithelial neoplasia (PIN). McNeal's landmark work in 1965 described the morphogenetic origin of prostate carcinoma that became the foundation for our current understanding of PIN.[131,132] In 1986, McNeal and Bostwick[133] characterized this premalignant lesion as "intraductal dysplasia" describing it to be present in more than half of carcinomatous prostates. One year later, Bostwick and Brawer[134] introduced the now preferred term "prostatic intraepithelial neoplasia," in part, to recognize that this lesion may arise from either the prostatic acini or ducts, which are often indistinguishable from each other. In 1989, the term PIN was endorsed in a consensus conference and since then became the terminology uniformly used in the literature.[135]

PIN is defined as a noninvasive neoplastic transformation of the epithelium of preexisting prostatic ducts and acini.[136–141] Originally, PIN was divided in three grades (PIN I, II, and III) based on a spectrum of architectural and cytologic abnormalities,[133] with the suggestion that PIN III was equivalent to carcinoma in situ. At the 1989 consensus meeting, PIN was condensed into low grade (I) and high grade (II and III) because of poor diagnostic reproducibility.[135] The separation of low- and high-grade PIN was based on a number of criteria but especially the presence of nucleolar prominence in the latter. The reporting of low-grade PIN eventually fell into disfavor due to its poor diagnostic reproducibility and the lack of clinical relevance including its questionable association with prostate cancer.[142,143] Nowadays, the word PIN is used almost synonymously to refer to HGPIN.

Epidemiology

HGPIN is a common finding in routine prostate pathology specimens, identified as an isolated diagnosis in up to 16% of needle core biopsies (NCBs) (usually 5% to 10%) and 1% to 5% of TUR specimens.[144,145] Approximately, 115,000 new cases of isolated HGPIN are diagnosed each year in the United States.[137,146] There is a significant variation in the reporting of HGPIN of 0.7% to 20% in needle biopsies and 3% to 33% in TURs that can be attributed to interpretation discrepancies and varied application of morphologic criteria.[139] The incidence is much higher at 80% to 100% in prostatectomies harboring adenocarcinoma compared to 43% of age-matched nontumorous controls. The incidence of HGPIN, like that of adenocarcinoma, increases with age although with somewhat earlier onset, beginning in the third decade of life reaching about 67% in white men by the eighth decade of life.[147,148] Like prostate adenocarcinoma, the incidence is higher in African Americans compared to other races.[149–152] The lesion is usually more diffuse and presents earlier in African Americans compared to Caucasian Americans. HGPIN is detected with increasing incidence in African Americans with rates of 7%, 26%, 46%, 72%, 75%, and 91% from the third through the eight decade.[148] This strong association with race is not limited to the United States, as similar higher incidence is reported among black Brazilian men compared to white Brazilian men.[153]

PIN as a Precursor for Cancer

There is much evidence supporting PIN as a precursor lesion for prostate cancer,[145] including (a) the spatial relationship of HGPIN to foci of carcinoma, including the budding off of early invasive glands; (b) HGPIN is more common and multifocal in prostates containing carcinoma[154–157]; (c) a significant subset of HGPIN and carcinoma harbor similar molecular alterations (e.g., TMPRSS2:ERG fusion,[72,158] AMACR overexpression[159,160]); (d) both HGPIN and carcinoma incidence increase with age and are more common in black men; and (e) appearance of HGPIN in the prostate precedes carcinoma by about 10 years.

Historically, the diagnosis of isolated HGPIN in a prostate biopsy would prompt repeat biopsy, with carcinoma being detected in 40% to 60% of cases.[161–168] However, contemporary data in the era of extended prostate biopsy sampling have shown that the risk of cancer following diagnosis of HGPIN is between 21% and 27.5%.[144,169] This risk of finding cancer after unifocal HGPIN is not significantly different from the risk following a benign diagnosis.[144,155,156] Extended biopsy sampling has resulted in higher sensitivity for cancer detection, and therefore, less carcinoma is detected on subsequent samples.[155]

However, patients with multifocal HGPIN (i.e., present in more than 2 cores), bilateral HGPIN, and those associated with an atypical small acinar proliferation (ASAP) diagnosis on biopsy have a higher risk of harboring concomitant prostate carcinoma and should be more aggressively followed.[154–157,170–173] Multifocal and bilateral HGPIN are considered adverse features significantly increasing the risk of prostate cancer detection; other clinical variables such as serum PSA and abnormal rectal examination are taken into account.[174] The estimated probabilities in detecting cancer 1 and 5 years after a benign diagnosis are 3.7% and 22.5% and are much higher with multifocal HGPIN at 9.1% and 47.8% and bilateral multifocal HGPIN at 12.5% and 57.8%, respectively.[174]

Molecular Biology

There is genetic evidence associating HGPIN and prostate carcinoma. HGPIN and cancer share similar chromosomal anomalies, telomere shortening, alterations in members of the *bcl-2* gene family, decreased expression of NKX3.1 and p27, and overexpression of p16, p53, *MYC*, and AMACR.[160,175–186] *TMPRSS2:ERG* fusion, which is seen in about half of clinically localized prostate cancers, can also be detected in 16% to 21% of HGPIN that is usually intermingling with cancer foci.[72,158,187] When *TMPRSS2:ERG* is detected in cancer and in HGPIN in the same prostate, the matching lesions usually share the same fusion pattern.[158] Sixty percent of *TMPRSS2:ERG* fusion-negative prostate cancer has also concomitant fusion-negative HGPIN.[158]

DNA aneuploidy is common in both HGPIN (65%) and cancer (62%).[185] There is high correlation (75% of cases) in ploidy and pattern of cytogenetic alterations between HGPIN and paired prostate cancer foci in the same specimen.[185] Numeric alterations of chromosomes 7, 8, 10, 12, and Y are common in both HGPIN and carcinoma, although the mean overall number of alterations is higher in carcinoma.[175] Chromosome 8p deletion is the most commonly detected allelic loss, present in both HGPIN and carcinoma.[146] A genetic pathway for prostate carcinogenesis has been proposed with two distinct initiating events, namely, 8p and 13q losses.[188] Loss of 8p leads to development of HGPIN and carcinoma, whereas loss of 13q leads to carcinoma without the presence of HGPIN. These primary chromosomal imbalances are then preferentially followed by 8q gain; 6q, 16q, and 18q losses; and a set of late events that make recurrent and metastatic prostate cancers genetically more complex.[188] Nuclear morphometric studies also show no significant difference in nuclear volume between HGPIN and cancer, but both show significant increments from benign prostatic glands.[189,190] p53 mutation is suggested to be an early change in prostate carcinogenesis, and p53 overexpression associated with chromosomal instability is greater in HGPIN foci intermingled with cancer compared to HGPIN away from cancer.[186] Hypermethylation of glutathione *S*-transferase, considered to be a major event in prostate carcinogenesis, can be detected in HGPIN.[191,192]

Clinical Features

Isolated HGPIN does not cause any specific symptoms. The lesion is encountered as an incidental finding in prostate specimens, often in biopsies performed for an abnormal serum PSA level. It is however debatable whether or not HGPIN is the actual cause of the elevated PSA since it is difficult to exclude an undetected coexistent carcinoma, and in some cases, the PSA elevation may relate to BPH or inflammation. By ultrasound, it has been suggested that HGPIN may be associated with a hypoechoic pattern in the peripheral zone similar to carcinoma.[193,194]

No treatment (e.g., surgery, radiotherapy, hormonal therapy) is warranted for HGPIN, unless a concomitant carcinoma is identified. Several clinical trials are being undertaken targeting HGPIN using different agents, including antiandrogens, 5α-reductase inhibitors, and even dietary nutrients and supplements, as chemopreventive measures for the development of prostate carcinoma.[137]

As discussed above, the current clinical practice is to perform a repeat biopsy after a diagnosis of HGPIN when it is multifocal, bilateral, or associated with ASAP.[155,157] If carcinoma is detected on repeat biopsy, it may or it may not be present in or adjacent to quadrant where HGPIN was detected.[165,167,195] In 40% to 74% of cases, the carcinoma will be detected at the area of HGPIN.[165,167,196] On average, 30% of carcinomas are found on the contralateral side.[144] The incidence of detection of subsequent carcinoma in patients with isolated HGPIN increases when rebiopsy is performed at 1 and 3 years. At mean biopsy intervals of 34 months (first rebiopsy) and 66 months (second rebiopsy), cancer was detected at 22% and 23%, respectively, with a high likelihood for organ-confined and clinically significant disease.[197] Thus, while rebiopsy within 1 year may not be that crucial, biopsy at longer intervals can be beneficial and should be considered as a valid follow-up option.

Pathology

HGPIN is not associated with any recognizable gross findings. Histologically, PIN consists of preexisting ducts and acini, usually of medium to large size, lined by crowded secretory cells with abnormal cytologic features. PIN is divided into low and high grade. Low-grade PIN exhibits tufted or micropapillary patterns with nuclear crowding, stratification, and irregular spacing. Nuclei are mildly enlarged, and, in particular, nucleoli are inconspicuous to only rarely prominent.

HGPIN shows proliferation of medium- to large-sized glands. The cells have increased basophilia or amphophilia that can readily be detected at low-power magnification. The nuclei are larger, are round, show overlapping, are hyperchromatic, have nuclear membrane irregularity, and, most importantly, show prominent nucleoli easily appreciable at 20× magnification (Fig. 9-7). Multiple nucleoli may be present and, similar to carcinoma, are occasionally peripherally situated close to the nuclear membrane. The diagnostic threshold for HGPIN varies, as some individuals require all cells to be atypical and others require at least 10% of the cells to have prominent nucleoli. If the cytologic threshold for diagnosis is doubtful or borderline, our practice bias is not to consider the lesion as HGPIN. A preserved or discontinuous basal cell layer may be readily identified on routine slides or with use of basal cell–specific immunostains.

PIN may exhibit several architectural and cytologic features (Table 9-6). There are four major architectural patterns described for HGPIN, namely, tufted, micropapillary, cribriform, and flat HGPIN (Fig. 9-8).[198] Multiple patterns of HGPIN may be seen concurrently within a specimen. Tufted PIN is the most common pattern seen in 87% of PIN and is characterized by stratification of acinar cells imparting luminal undulations or folds (Fig. 9-8A). Micropapillary PIN is also common (85%), which shows nuclear stratification forming intraluminal slender filiform projections and cellular budding (Fig. 9-8B). Cribriform PIN (32%) shows complex intraluminal proliferation resulting in multiple irregular or round punched-out lumina (Fig. 9-8C). Cribriform PIN in particular may show "cellular maturation" wherein peripheral cells show greater nuclear atypia (i.e., nucleomegaly, prominent nucleoli) than do cells at the luminal or central

Table 9-6 ■ COMMON AND UNUSUAL PATTERNS OF HGPIN
Basic Architecture
Tufted
Micropapillary
Cribriform
Flat
Other Patterns
Foamy
Inverted or "hobnail"
Small cell
Signet ring
Mucinous
PIN with squamous differentiation
Miscellaneous Features
Apocrine snouts
Cytoplasmic lipochrome
Paneth cell–like change

aspect. Flat PIN (25%) lacks significant cellular stratification and is composed of only 1 or 2 cell layers (Fig. 9-8D). Other uncommon types have been described such as foamy (Fig. 9-9), inverted or "hobnail" (Fig. 9-10), small cell (Fig. 9-11), signet ring, mucinous, and PIN with squamous differentiation.[199–202] Rarely, PIN may involve large cystic glands and glands in nodular hyperplasia and exhibit mucinous metaplasia.[198] Central necrosis is not a feature of HGPIN, and its presence should raise concern for an invasive or intraductal carcinoma (IDC).

Several other features may be present in HGPIN including luminal cytoplasmic blebs, epithelial arches, cellular trabecular epithelial bars, "Roman" bridges, partial gland involvement, and basal cell layer disruption with glandular budding. Additionally, luminal cytoplasmic blebs, cytoplasmic lipochrome deposits (Fig. 9-12), and scattered Paneth-like cells (Fig. 9-13) may be present in HGPIN. Small round blue-tinged vacuoles (so-called blue blobs) are present in increased frequency in HGPIN compared to nonneoplastic glands. Rarely, HGPIN may also exhibit apical snouts (Fig. 9-14). A variety of luminal features may also be observed in HGPIN such as amorphous proteinaceous secretions, corpora amylacea, exfoliated cells, and rarely crystalloids. The basic approach for diagnosis is to screen for HGPIN at low-power magnification and to confirm the cytologic features at high-power, similar to cancer. Interobserver reproducibility for the diagnosis of HGPIN is fairly high among urologic pathologists and is moderate among general surgical pathologists.[144] HGPIN is noninvasive and must be associated with of basal cells (Fig. 9-15). The basal cells can be continuous and readily apparent on hematoxylin and eosin (H&E) sections or discontinuous. A discontinuous basal cell layer may not be appreciable in a particular plane of section, compounding the differential diagnosis with carcinoma. Use of basal cell markers (p63, CK5/6, HMWK [keratin 34βE12]) may highlight the

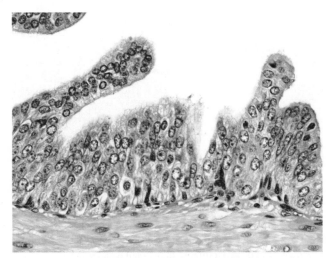

FIGURE 9-7 ■ HGPIN is characterized by presence of high-grade nuclei.

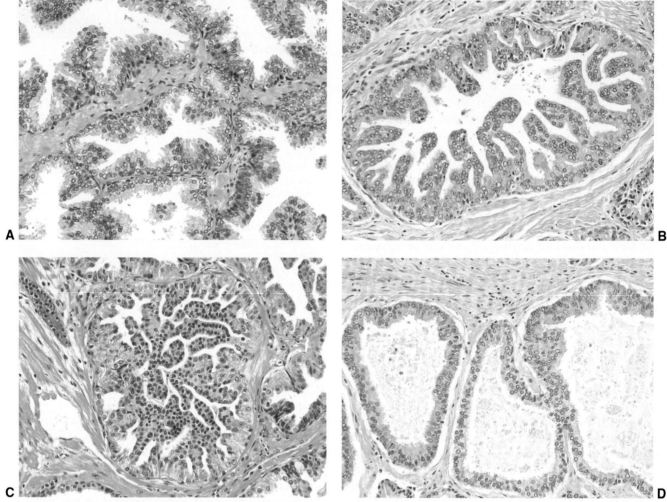

FIGURE 9-8 ■ Basic patterns of HGPIN include **(A)** tufted, **(B)** micropapillary, **(C)** cribriform, and **(D)** flat architectures. Note the presence of cell maturation in cribriform HGPIN.

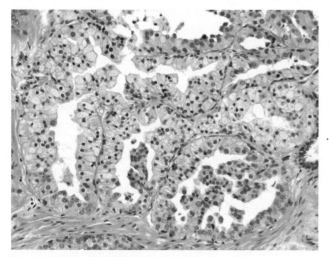

FIGURE 9-9 ■ HGPIN with foamy cells.

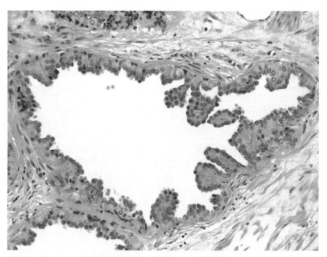

FIGURE 9-10 ■ HGPIN with inverted pattern.

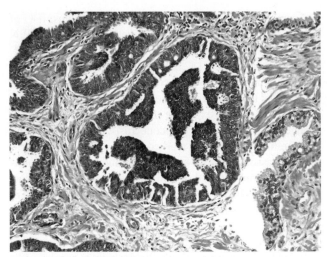

FIGURE 9-11 ■ Small cell HGPIN. The small cells do not express neuroendocrine markers.

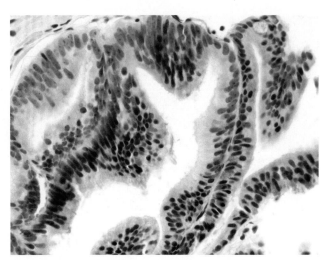

FIGURE 9-13 ■ HGPIN with scattered Paneth-like cells.

discontinuous basal cell layer around the involved acini or ducts.[203] AMACR stains the dysplastic or neoplastic cells, but immunostaining can be variable at 44% to 90%.[159,204–207] HGPIN cells stain positively for PSA, prostate-specific acid phosphatase (PSAP), prostate-specific membrane antigen (PSMA), and pro-PSA.[204,208,209] Small cell HGPIN does not show reactivity for synaptophysin and chromogranin, suggesting that it is not a manifestation of neuroendocrine differentiation.[210]

If HGPIN (without invasive foci) is found in prostate needle biopsy specimens, it is prudent to consider performing deeper sections particularly if HGPIN is extensive or associated with ASAP (glandular atypia). If isolated HGPIN is detected in a TUR, further sampling of the specimen may be considered depending on factors such as the patient's age and PSA value. The presence of HGPIN in biopsies without concomitant invasive foci should be reported. The site and number of biopsy cores involved by HGPIN should also be

documented. Further, the number of foci of HGPIN (e.g., isolated, focal, multifocal, extensive) should be reflected in the report. In the presence of carcinoma in or a needle biopsy (resection), reporting of HGPIN becomes optional. However, in the setting of a small focus of carcinoma, the presence of extensive HGPIN may be taken into account in determining treatment.

Differential Diagnosis

A variety of carcinomas especially adenocarcinoma variants enter the differential diagnosis of HGPIN, and distinction among these can be difficult, particularly in limited samples. Of note, acinar adenocarcinoma with a cribriform pattern, ductal adenocarcinoma, and IDC (intraductal spread of cancer) may cause diagnostic difficulties. High-grade acinar carcinoma with a cribriform pattern (Gleason grade 4 or 5) shows architectural overlap with cribriform HGPIN. Unlike HGPIN,

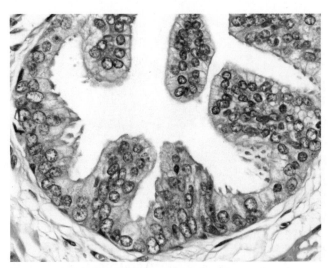

FIGURE 9-12 ■ Lipochrome pigments may sometimes be seen in HGPIN.

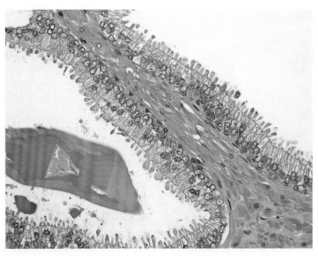

FIGURE 9-14 ■ HGPIN with cells with apical snouts.

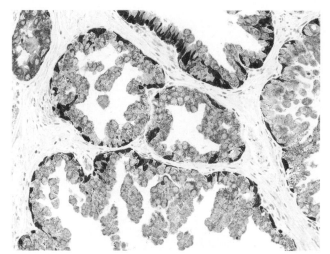

FIGURE 9-15 ■ Cocktail of AMACR, HMWK, and p63 on HGPIN shows the presence of basal cells (*brown*) and increased AMACR expression (*red*).

cribriform adenocarcinoma exhibits more complexity including the presence of large expansile glands (bigger than preexisting glands), confluence or back-to-back glands, consistent cribriform architecture, and associated solid nests or may have intraluminal necrosis (Gleason pattern 5). Basal cells are absent in invasive cribriform carcinoma, but this may need to be confirmed with basal cell immunostains. Ductal adenocarcinoma may resemble the different architectures of HGPIN. Ductal adenocarcinoma is characteristically composed of tall columnar cells that are frequently pseudostratified and can be mitotically active. Unlike HGPIN, ductal adenocarcinoma may have large expansile glands and papillae with true fibrovascular stalks, and the cells do not exhibit luminal "maturation." Invasive features such as crowded back-to-back glands, stromal fibrosis, perineural invasion (PNI), and extraprostatic extension (EPE) are present in ductal adenocarcinoma. Basal cells are absent in the majority of ductal adenocarcinomas

that can be confirmed with basal cell immunostains. IDC of the prostate can be very difficult to distinguish from HGPIN due to the lack of a consistent morphologic cutoff separating these two entities. IDC like HGPIN involves large glands containing markedly atypical cells and notably has preserved basal cells (see subsequent section). Unlike HGPIN, the glands of IDC can be expansile and show extensive cribriform change, sometimes with comedonecrosis. A lumen-spanning proliferation of cells with marked atypia and mitoses is usually seen associated with high-volume and high-grade carcinoma (Gleason pattern 4 or 5). However, without an invasive focus, IDC can be very difficult to distinguish from HGPIN in limited biopsy material. Sometimes, a descriptive term such as "markedly atypical cribriform proliferation" or "atypical cribriform lesion" can be used and the differential diagnosis explained in a comment. Generally such cases require additional biopsies.

In needle biopsy, when an atypical small glandular focus is identified next to HGPIN (so-called PIN-ATYP or PIN-ASAP), distinction should be made between a tangentially sectioned outpouching of HGPIN (so-called transitive glands) and a small focus of low-grade acinar adenocarcinoma (Gleason pattern 3) (Fig. 9-16). Immunostains are useful only if basal cells are demonstrated in the small glands, confirming outpouching of HGPIN. Even if no basal cells are present, they still could represent HGPIN, as the basal cell layer can be discontinuous or markedly attenuated. If a definitive diagnosis cannot be reached, our approach is to label the entire focus as "HGPIN with an atypical small acini suspicious but not diagnostic for carcinoma" or similar terminology.

Other malignant differential diagnoses for PIN include stratified or "PIN-like" adenocarcinoma, basal cell/adenoid cystic carcinoma, and urothelial carcinoma spreading through prostatic ducts and acini. "PIN-like" adenocarcinoma has stratified epithelium and may form medium-sized glands and, as the name implies, resemble HGPIN particularly flat or tufted patterns. Unlike HGPIN, "PIN-like"

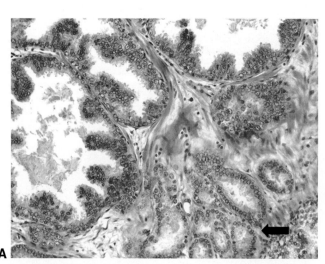

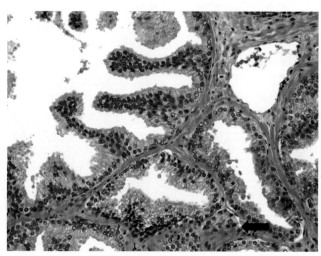

FIGURE 9-16 ■ Examples of **(A)** HGPIN with adjacent Gleason pattern 3 carcinoma (*arrow*) and **(B)** HGPIN with adjacent atypical glands that may represent outpouching (HGPIN-ATYP).

adenocarcinoma has no basal cells and may be associated or mingled with typical acinar carcinoma. Basal cell/adenoid cystic carcinoma contains basaloid-appearing cells with smaller nuclei and exhibits solid or adenoid cystic patterns and basement membrane material. Unlike HGPIN, basal cell/adenoid cystic carcinoma expresses p63 and keratin 34βE12 and is usually negative for PSA and PSAP. Urothelial carcinoma originating in the urethra or prostate may spread within the prostatic ducts and acini without invading stroma and thus mimic HGPIN. Urothelial carcinoma, however, tends to fill and expand the ductal or acinar lumen exhibiting solid growth and has significant cell pleomorphism and increased mitotic activity. The cells of urothelial carcinoma may have dense eosinophilic cytoplasm and may show squamoid features. Randomly distributed atypical cells with a pagetoid pattern may be present in glands involved by urothelial carcinoma. Urothelial carcinoma, unlike HGPIN, expresses GATA3 positivity and p63, HMCK (34βE12) staining in the nonbasally situated cells. PSA and PSAP stains are negative.

Several benign structures and processes in the prostate may also mimic HGPIN. Prostate central zone glands show architectural complexity including cribriform and Roman bridges, but lack the typical nuclear changes of HGPIN. Seminal vesicle/ejaculatory duct epithelium shows more pleomorphism than HGPIN with spotty cellular atypia, nuclear pseudoinclusions, degenerative nuclear changes, and coarse cytoplasmic lipofuscin pigment. The distinction between HGPIN and reactive atypia requires stringent criteria especially when infarction, inflammation, or a history of radiation is present. The architectural features of HGPIN tend to be absent in reactive glandular mimics. Urothelial metaplasia has multilayered cells or solid nests lacking the typical patterns of HGPIN. Cells are uniform and smaller with nuclear grooves, and a native secretory cell layer may be focally present. Nodular hyperplasia with prominent papillary infolding is often located in the transition zone, has background hyperplastic stroma, and lacks the nuclear changes of HGPIN. Cribriform hyperplasia is also in the transition zone, frequently shows clear cytoplasm without amphophilia, and lacks the nuclear changes of HGPIN. Atypical basal cell hyperplasia shows atypical nuclei in basal cells and not the secretory cells, and lumina are frequently obliterated not demonstrating the usual architecture of HGPIN.

Atypical Adenomatous Hyperplasia

Introduction

Atypical adenomatous hyperplasia (AAH), also known as adenosis, has been described under different terms such as atypical adenosis, small acinar atypical hyperplasia, and atypical hyperplasia. A consensus statement in 1994 recommended the use of the term AAH, although both AAH and adenosis are still used interchangeably.[211] AAH is characterized by small to medium size acini usually forming a well-circumscribed nodule in the transition zone associated with hyperplasia, but does not fulfill the cytologic criteria of carcinoma.[212–217] Unlike PIN, the evidence linking AAH to prostate carcinoma is weak at best and is still debated. It has been suggested that some well-differentiated adenocarcinomas (Gleason patterns 1 and probably some 2) originally described before the era of immunohistochemistry were perhaps examples of AAH.[218] The greater significance of AAH in current practice is as a differential diagnosis or potential pitfall for cancer in the setting of small atypical glandular lesions in needle biopsy.[203,219]

Epidemiology

AAH is detected more commonly in older men (mean 64 to 70 years old), similar to carcinoma and BPH.[214–216] AAH is relatively common in resection specimens and can be present in up to 19.6% of TUR and 23% of RP specimens.[215,219] The lesion is usually found in the transition zone and less commonly in peripheral zone and can be multifocal. Only about 3% of AAH foci are exclusively seen in nontransition zones.[215] AAH is seen in only 2% of biopsies mainly because the transition zone is often less sampled.[216]

Molecular Biology

One study on chromosomes 7q, 8p, 8q, and 18q demonstrated allelic imbalance in 47% of AAH, which are also genetic changes present in early prostate carcinogenesis that suggested a link.[220] One study showed a lower rate of allelic imbalance at 12%, with loss only within chromosomes 8p11–12.[221] By fluorescence in situ hybridization (FISH), chromosomal anomalies were seen in 9% of AAH cases compared to 55% in prostatic carcinoma.[222]

AAH as Risk for Carcinoma

There is minimal evidence to suggest that AAH is a precursor of adenocarcinoma, including low-grade transition zone carcinoma.[145] Thus far, evidence is circumstantial, mostly based on morphologic findings, with little supportive molecular or clinical data. It was reported in an earlier study that 6.4% of patients with AAH developed carcinoma compared to only 3.7% for patients with nodular hyperplasia; however, the diagnosis of AAH in some cases was thought by experts to represent carcinoma.[223] The estimation of nuclear volume is able to discriminate AAH and nodular hyperplasia from well-differentiated prostate adenocarcinoma suggesting that AAH is probably a variant of BPH.[224] AAH, nodular hyperplasia, and carcinoma show similar DNA ploidy status (diploid), and these three lesions are not discriminated by a panel of Ki-67, mib1, bcl-2, and c-erbB-2.[225] Nuclear Ki-67 labeling discriminates AAH from nodular hyperplasia but not from carcinoma, and microvessel density is different for AAH and carcinoma but not for AAH and nodular hyperplasia.[225] Interestingly, about half of AAH foci exhibit stronger and more extensive AMACR expression when associated with prostatic adenocarcinoma.[226]

Clinical Features

AAH is an incidental histologic finding that usually comes to attention in routine practice as mimicker of prostate cancer in needle biopsy. There is no specific gross abnormality for AAH other than the presence of associated nodular hyperplasia in the transition zone. Reporting of AAH is optional, and no treatment or follow-up is warranted.

Pathology

At low-power, AAH exhibits a relatively well-circumscribed nodular proliferation of tightly packed small- to medium-sized glands sometimes associated with a parent duct (Fig. 9-17). The lesion is in the transition zone and is admixed with typical hyperplastic nodules. Nuclear and nucleolar enlargement if present are only mild. Some glands at the periphery of the nodule infiltrate the surrounding stroma, tending to merge with adjacent benign glands. Usually the glands at the centers of the nodules are larger or dilated. Secretory cells with pale or clear cytoplasm, round uniform nuclei, and inconspicuous nucleoli line the glands (Fig. 9-18). The basal cells are discontinuous and may not be easily discernible, often requiring immunostains to be detected (Fig. 9-19). The lumina of glands occasionally contain eosinophilic secretions, crystalloids, and, uncommonly, basophilic mucin, features that are often seen in cancer. In addition, corpora amylacea may also be present in 43% of cases.[216]

By immunostaining, basal cell markers (p63, HMWK) frequently show a discontinuous layer of basal cells, which may also be absent in occasional to many acini within the focus.[226,227] AMACR is focally positive in 10% of cases and can be diffusely positive in up to 7.5% of AAH.[227] There is generally less luminal accentuation of AMACR staining in AAH compared to adenocarcinoma.

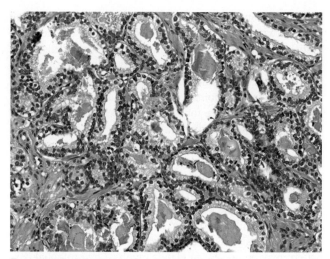

FIGURE 9-18 ■ Glands of AAH are often crowded and may contain luminal eosinophilic materials and crystalloids, mimicking carcinoma.

Differential Diagnosis

The diagnosis of AAH in prostate resection specimens is usually straightforward since the entire nodule can be appreciated as well as background hyperplasia and the transition zone location. However, the diagnosis may be difficult when only part of the nodule is sampled in needle biopsy. The periphery of an AAH focus may show glands with limited infiltration, and further individual glands may contain intraluminal mucin, crystalloids, or eosinophilic secretions, mimicking microacinar (Gleason pattern 3) adenocarcinoma. In contrast, carcinoma exhibits nucleomegaly, prominent nucleoli, and often amphophilic cytoplasm. Basal cell immunomarkers should be carefully interpreted in AAH since some of the acini may have patchy or absent staining. All atypical glands within a focus of concern on H&E

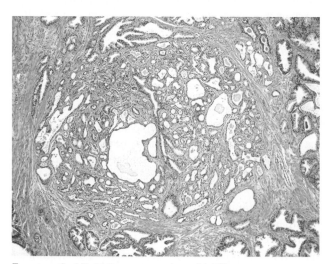

FIGURE 9-17 ■ Low-power view of AAH.

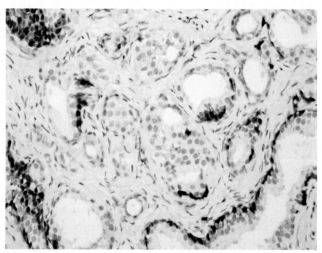

FIGURE 9-19 ■ Cocktail of AMACR, HMWK, and p63 on AAH shows patchy basal cell immunostaining (*brown*). AMACR can be positive in a small subset of AAH like in this case.

should have complete abscence of basal cell immunostaining in order to support a diagnosis of adenocarcinoma.

Other benign processes in the prostate may mimic AAH (see Chapter 8). Usual nodular hyperplasia has better circumscribed nodules with no stromal infiltration of the glands at the periphery. Ordinary hyperplastic glands are larger in caliber, more uniform in size and shape and usually have luminal papillary infoldings. Stromal proliferation is usually present. Sclerosing adenosis is associated with dense fibroblastic spindle cell stroma. The glands are more irregular, angulated, or pointed and may have budding, and the basal cells are usually easy to recognize. The glands exhibit thickened basement membranes and may have surrounding rims of hyalinized stroma. Mesonephric remnants are lined by cuboidal to flattened cells and contain dense eosinophilic colloid-like material in the lumina. Mesonephric glands are less circumscribed and are more haphazardly arranged. Verumontanum mucosal gland hyperplasia is often subjacent to urothelium, and the glands often contain dark orange or brown concretions.

Atrophy and Proliferative Inflammatory Atrophy

Some authors have previously considered focal glandular atrophy as a possible precursor of prostate cancer. Focal atrophy similarly occurs commonly in the peripheral zone where most cancer arises. But so far, there is no strong evidence linking pure glandular atrophy to carcinoma. However, atrophy associated with inflammation has been raised as a risk for prostate carcinoma development.[228] Simple atrophy or postatrophic hyperplasia occurring in association with inflammation that appears to be regenerating or proliferating is referred to as "proliferative inflammatory atrophy" (PIA) (Fig. 9-20). A topographic study showed that PIA appears to merge with HGPIN in 42.5% of HGPIN lesions and is seen adjacent to carcinoma in 30%.[229] Areas of presumed low-grade PIN are also found in association with HGPIN

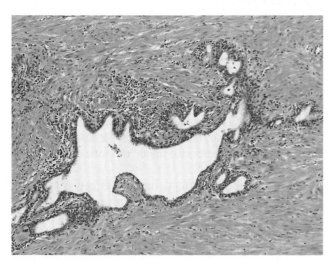

FIGURE 9-20 ■ PIA lesion shows glandular atrophy with associated chronic inflammation. Ki-67 shows increase nuclear labeling (not shown).

and PIA suggesting progression from PIA to PIN and/or carcinoma.[229] Clusters of atypical epithelial cells with nuclear enlargement, hyperchromasia, and enlarged nucleoli can also be associated with PIA.[230] Cells that are phenotypically intermediate between basal and secretory cells (CK5, GSTP1, c-MET, and C/EBPbeta expression) are enriched in PIA lesions.[230,231] Somatic inactivation of glutathione S-transferase-pi gene (GSTP1) via CpG island hypermethylation occurs early during prostate carcinogenesis, which is present in about 70% of HGPIN and more than 90% of carcinomas. GSTP1 CpG island hypermethylation can also be detected in some PIA lesions but not in normal or hyperplastic epithelium.[232] Half of p53-positive PIA epithelial cells express diffuse GSTP1 immunostaining and may play a role in induction of p53 overexpression.[233] NKX3.1 and p27, which are lost or down-regulated in cancer and HGPIN, are also down-regulated in atrophy.[182,228] Currently, more evidence is required to definitively establish or disprove a relationship between PIA and cancer.

PATHOLOGY OF ACINAR ADENOCARCINOMA

Macroscopic Features

Prostatic adenocarcinomas are often not recognized at the macroscopic level especially when they are small. In TUR samples, gross examination of chips is of little value.[234,235] In rare cases, usually with extensive tumor, the carcinomatous chips may be harder and have a yellow or orange color compared to the spongy tan-brown chips of nodular hyperplasia.[236] The color and texture of chips, however, are nonspecific, and conditions such as granulomatous prostatitis can be associated with firm yellow fragments.

In RP specimens, carcinomas are sometimes visualized but usually only when the tumor is large. In general, lesions, <5mm in diameter are not detectable.[237] Carcinomas were commonly visualized in the pre-PSA screening era when many patients presented with large-volume stage cT2 disease. In one study from 1998, 63% of carcinomas were identified in a consecutive series of RPs.[238] Importantly, there was a false-positivity rate of 19%. The detected tumors were larger and of higher stage and grade than the more subtle ones. In recent years, with the higher proportion of cT1c disease, carcinoma is grossly recognized in a minority of cases, perhaps 30% of cases in our experience. Palpation of the gland is generally not helpful unless there is a significant peripheral nodule.

When grossly recognized on transverse sections, carcinoma usually involves the posterior or posterolateral peripheral zone just beneath the capsule (Fig. 9-21). Anterior involvement may be seen, but this is often difficult to recognize because of admixed stromal tissue. It is useful to compare the right and left sides of the gland in transverse sections looking for asymmetry and subtle color differences.

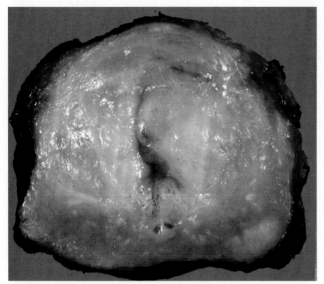

FIGURE 9-21 ■ Transverse section of RP specimen showing peripheral nodule, right. Periurethral nodularity corresponding to a nodular hyperplasia is also noted.

The tumor tissue has a smoother and more solid appearance and firmer texture than the spongy or sometimes cystic benign tissue. Carcinoma often has a yellow, yellow-orange, white, or gray color compared to the tan or beige appearance of benign prostate. The edges of the lesion are often indistinct, and microscopy usually reveals more tumor than was appreciated grossly. Extensive tumor can be overlooked since the whole gland may have a uniform appearance (Fig. 9-22). Many benign lesions such as stromal nodules, infarcts, and areas of prostatitis and atrophy may be grossly mistaken for carcinoma attesting to the nonspecificity of the macroscopic findings.[236] Sometimes, extension of tumor beyond the confines of the gland may be seen macroscopically, but the observation may not be accurate, and it always requires histologic

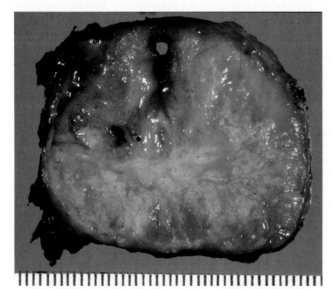

FIGURE 9-22 ■ Transverse section of RP. Note widespread irregular yellow areas corresponding to extensive adenocarcinoma.

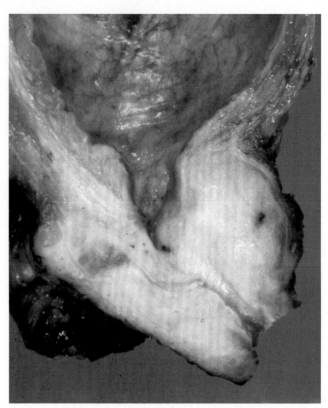

FIGURE 9-23 ■ Parasagittal section of radical cystoprostatectomy showing adenocarcinoma extending around the seminal vesicle.

confirmation (Fig. 9-23). In one study,[238] only one-half of carcinomas thought to show gross extension demonstrated EPE or margin positivity microscopically. In another study, 80% of cases with extraprostatic or margin involvement were correctly identified on gross assessment.[239] Necrosis and hemorrhage are rarely seen in prostate carcinoma.

Tumor Location

About 70% of prostatic adenocarcinomas are located in the peripheral zone, mostly in posterior and posterolateral locations.[240,241] (A small number are located in the anterior horns of the peripheral zone.)[242] Ten percent to twenty-five percent of adenocarcinomas have an epicenter in the transition zone, and some of these also have peripheral zone involvement.[240,241] Tumors uncommonly arise in the central zone, about 5% in two studies.[240,241] In some cases, especially where there is more extensive tumor, the zone of origin cannot be determined.

There are clinicopathologic differences between tumors arising in the peripheral and transition zones.[241,243] Peripheral zone carcinomas are more commonly detected by needle biopsy, show higher Gleason scores, and are more likely to be extraprostatic than transition zone carcinomas.[244,245] The latter are more likely to be detected in TUR specimens, have lower Gleason scores and be organ confined. Nevertheless, some high-grade transition zone tumors may be encountered, and some may be difficult to detect because of biopsy

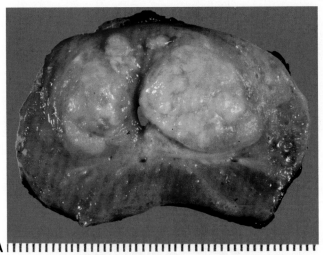
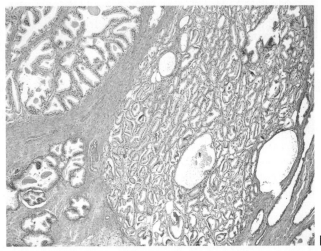

FIGURE 9-24 ■ Transverse section of RP showing prominent periurethral nodular lesions, which corresponded to extensive transition zone adenocarcinoma. **A:** Transverse section of RP specimen. Note yellow-tan nodular lesions in transition zone corresponding to extensive adenocarcinoma. **B:** Low-grade adenocarcinoma (Gleason score 6) involving transition zone.

sampling protocols.[246] Additionally, low-grade, high-volume transition zone tumors may be found, and these cases may be present with a high serum PSA (Fig. 9-24).[247] Some have suggested that transition zone tumors have a distinct appearance with acini lined by columnar cells with basally located nuclei, but this latter can be seen in peripheral zone carcinomas as well.[248] Interestingly, there have been some papers discussing differences in biomarker and molecular genetic findings between zones, but all of these changes may be related to the underlying Gleason score.[249] The outcome data on differences between peripheral and transition zone tumors are mixed, some studies showing better outcomes and others showing no difference at all.[249,250] Central zone carcinomas are uncommon and, in at least one study, have been associated with high Gleason score and high rates of extraprostatic involvement.[251] The specific location of a tumor does not appear to have any independent prognostic significance.

Tumor Focality

Adenocarcinomas are commonly multifocal in 50% to >90% of cases.[252–255] The additional tumors are often small and are often located at the apex. Commonly, the multifocal tumors involve both peripheral and transition zones (Fig. 9-25). Analysis of histologic and molecular features in multifocal tumors shows significant heterogeneity.[256,257] There is a suggestion based on comparative genomic hybridization and gene rearrangement studies (*TMPRSS2*) that multifocal prostatic adenocarcinomas arise from independent clones.[258]

General Approach to Microscopic Diagnosis

Major Diagnostic Criteria

The diagnosis of adenocarcinoma of the prostate is based on the careful analysis of H&E-stained slides using a systematic approach. The slides are derived from a variety of specimen types including thin-core needle biopsies, prostatic chips, suprapubic and RPs, and, at times, metastatic sites. Time-tested morphologic criteria are analyzed in an algorithmic fashion starting from scanning power to high magnification. The histologic diagnosis of adenocarcinoma involves the assessment of overall glandular architecture, the cellular composition of individual architectural structures, and the cytologic features of constituent cells. The criteria advanced by Arthur Purdy Stout et al.[259] are as applicable today as they were in the 1950s. They include (a) glandular pattern usually manifest by small irregular glands without any particular relation to adjacent glands or stroma, (b) arrangement of glandular epithelium with a lack of basal cells, and (c) cellular details including large deeply staining nucleoli. This morphologic triad constituted the major diagnostic criteria proposed by Algaba.[260] In

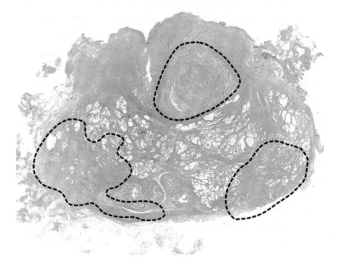

FIGURE 9-25 ■ Diagram of RP showing multifocal adenocarcinoma with involvement of transition and peripheral zones. (Reprinted from Eggener S, et al. Focal therapy for prostate cancer: possibilities and limitations. *Eur Urol* 2010;58(1):57–64, with permission.)

Table 9-7 ■ MICROSCOPIC DIAGNOSIS OF ADENOCARCINOMA

Major Diagnostic Criteria

1. Disordered glandular architecture
2. Tinctorial alteration
3. Absence of basal cells
4. Nuclear atypia including nucleolar enlargement

Minor Diagnostic Criteria

1. Eosinophilic luminal secretion
2. Basophilic luminal mucus
3. Luminal crystalloids
4. Mitotic figures
5. Apoptotic bodies
6. Smooth rigid luminal borders
7. Associated high-grade PIN

that study, minor criteria included basophilic luminal secretions, pink amorphous secretions, intraluminal crystalloids, amphophilic cytoplasm, mitotic figures, and adjacent high-grade PIN. Our approach to diagnosing prostatic adenocarcinoma also utilizes major and minor criteria (Table 9-7). In addition to architectural pattern, absence of basal cells, and nuclear abnormalities including nucleolar enlargement, we include tinctorial alteration as a major criterion for diagnosis. Tinctorial changes are usually appreciated on scanning magnification, and like architectural disarray, they often draw one's attention to sometimes subtle glandular abnormalities.

The usual architectural patterns of prostatic adenocarcinoma are best described by referring to the classical Gleason drawing (Fig. 9-26).[261] This diagram not only has formed the historical basis for grading prostate cancer (see page 64) but also is important in discussing the fundamentals of diagnosis and differential diagnosis. In this context, the architectural features are presented focusing on the original nine patterns (1; 2; 3A,B,C; 4A,B; 5A,B) described by Gleason. The subsequent section on Gleason grading deals with the substantial modifications of the original system for the purposes of contemporary grading.

Most prostatic adenocarcinomas are composed of separate small- to medium-sized atypical acini permeating between nonneoplastic glands (Gleason pattern 3A, 3B). Less commonly, separate acini are arranged in tight or loose clusters or more randomly in stroma without admixed nonneoplastic glands. When individual acini are uniform in size and shape and show little intervening stroma and the edge of the proliferation is rounded and "pushing" without admixed nonneoplastic glands, the pattern conforms to Gleason pattern 1. This diagnosis of adenocarcinoma, of course, would require other criteria including an absence of basal cells and other cytologic criteria (see later section). Gleason pattern 1 is nonexistent in needle biopsies and vanishingly rare in other specimen types, and many experts deny its existence arguing that the application of Gleason criteria as strictly written essentially eliminates the possibility of making this diagnosis since there is almost always some degree of nonuniformity

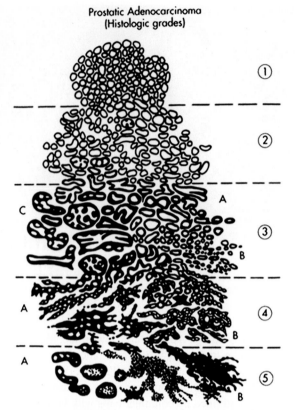

Prostatic Adenocarcinoma
(Histologic grades)

FIGURE 9-26 ■ Gleason diagram showing 9 distinct patterns arranged in 5 grades. (Reprinted from Gleason DF. Histologic grading of prostate cancer: a perspective. *Hum Pathol* 1992;23:273–279, with permission.)

in the small gland proliferation. Nevertheless, one occasionally encounters a tightly packed proliferation of uniform small neoplastic acini in the transition zone in TURs or RP specimen (Fig. 9-27).[236]

Gleason pattern 2 also involves small- to medium-sized acini without admixed nonneoplastic ones. There is more variation in acinar size and shape than grade 1, and the edge

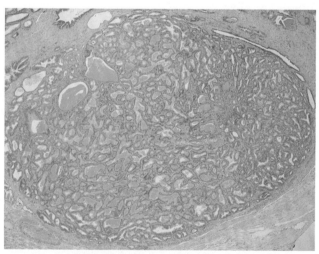

FIGURE 9-27 ■ Gleason pattern 1. Closely packed small- to medium-sized acini show only slight size and shape variation. The edge of the lesion is visualized as a smooth pushing interface with stroma.

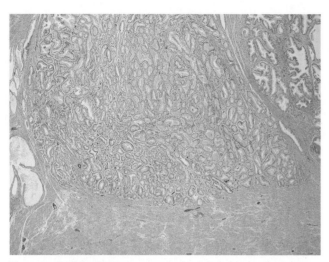

FIGURE 9-28 ■ Gleason pattern 2 adenocarcinoma in the lesion is well circumscribed but contains acini showing some size and shape variation with more interweaving stroma than in Gleason pattern 1.

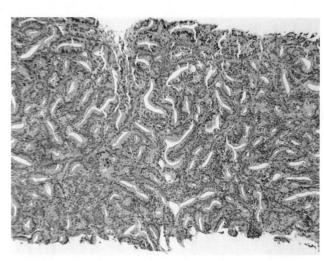

FIGURE 9-30 ■ Pattern 3A adenocarcinoma showing focal glandular angulation.

of the lesion is more irregular. Furthermore, there is more intervening stroma between proliferating glands in Gleason pattern 2 compared to pattern 1 (Fig. 9-28). Gleason pattern 2 is an uncommon pattern of carcinoma that may be seen in the transition zone and is therefore identified in prostatic chips, enucleations, and RP specimens. In modern practice, Gleason grade 2 is virtually never diagnosed in prostate needle biopsy specimens.[262]

The adenocarcinomas that constitute Gleason patterns 3A and 3B show a greater degree of infiltrative growth than pattern 2 tumors, and in fact, they are the commonest patterns of prostate carcinoma. There is a greater degree of size and shape variation compared to Gleason pattern 2 tumors especially in the 3A tumors, and there is greater separation of acini (Fig. 9-29). The 3A tumors include small to mostly medium and sometimes large acini that are irregular and commonly show angulation and branching (Fig. 9-30).

The 3B tumors are composed of small to tiny acini, some with lumina and others without, displaying an infiltrative growth pattern (Fig. 9-31). The most frequent pattern of invasion for these 3A/3B tumors is irregular infiltration between nonneoplastic glands (Fig. 9-32). This is the typical pattern recognized as a cardinal diagnostic criterion by Stout and others in the early days. Generally, the pattern is easily appreciated on low power especially if there is a reasonable amount of tumor. Another pattern seen with these tumors is a haphazard infiltration of stroma without any nearby nonneoplastic glands (Fig. 9-33). There is an irregular distribution of glands and splitting of stroma that is readily appreciated on low power (Fig. 9-34). The neoplastic acini of Gleason grade 3 tumors can be associated with periacinar clefts leaving a peculiar halo-like effect (Fig. 9-35).[236,263–265] This observation while uncommon is more likely associated with carcinoma than benign glandular processes.

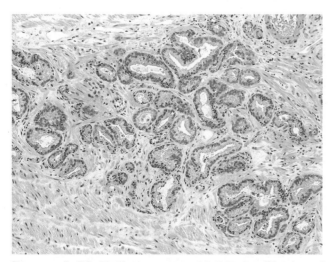

FIGURE 9-29 ■ Gleason pattern 3A. Note proliferation of single separate acini showing size and shape variation. This lesion is more irregular and infiltrative than Gleason pattern 2.

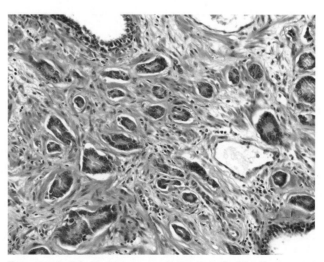

FIGURE 9-31 ■ Gleason pattern 3B. Note small irregular acini infiltrating between nonneoplastic ones. All acini have at least partially discernable lumina.

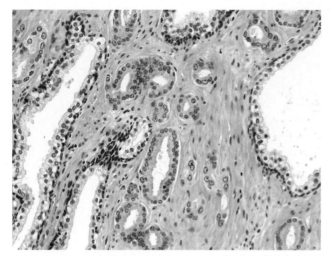

FIGURE 9-32 ■ Gleason pattern 3 adenocarcinoma showing infiltrations between nonneoplastic glands.

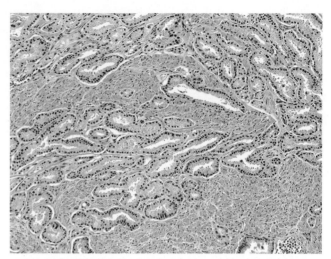

FIGURE 9-34 ■ Gleason pattern 3 adenocarcinoma showing splitting and permeation between stromal muscle elements.

While separate acini constitute the commonest morphology of adenocarcinoma, there are additional architectural patterns including cribriform, papillary, fused acinar, cord-like, solid, and single cell that must be recognized. These account for the intermediate- and high-grade patterns in the Gleason system. Gleason pattern 3C in the original description consists of smoothly contoured glandular aggregates with punched-out relatively uniform lumina creating a sieve-like pattern (Fig. 9-36). Similarly rounded glands with a papillary architecture were also included in this category. Confluence of aggregates, solid cylinders, and necrosis was not allowable in the 3C category. Sometimes, there is difficulty in separating Gleason pattern 3C from other patterns including cribriform high-grade PIN and cribriform hyperplasia (Fig. 9-37). Immunohistochemistry stains looking for the presence of basal cells may be required in some cases.[203,266,267] While it is important to appreciate the diagnostic significance of the cribriform pattern of adenocarcinoma, recent studies suggest that pathologists, for the most part, include any significant amount of cribriform tumor in a higher-grade (Gleason 4) category for the purpose of prognostication[268] (see grading section).

The original Gleason grade 4 comprised two patterns, 4A and 4B. Pattern 4A consists of fused glandular aggregates or chains and cords of neoplastic cells with little or no intervening stroma (Figs. 9-38 to 9-40). The fused glands can have a rounded edge or one that is more ragged. Stromal invasion is usually readily seen in Gleason pattern 4. Large and irregular cribriform masses are also part of the original Gleason pattern 4 (Fig. 9-41). The cells comprising most Gleason 4A tumors have relatively scant cytoplasm, which is usually amphophilic or sometimes eosinophilic. Rarely, Gleason 4 tumors consist of masses and sheets of fused or poorly formed glands with abundant clear cytoplasm. These so-called hypernephroid carcinomas (Gleason pattern 4B)

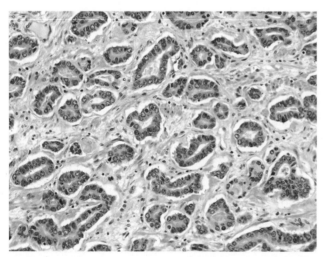

FIGURE 9-33 ■ Adenocarcinoma characterized by irregular permeation of stroma without any nearby nonneoplastic glands.

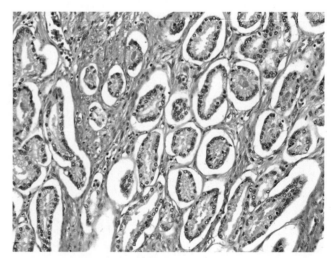

FIGURE 9-35 ■ Gleason pattern 3 adenocarcinoma showing prominent periglandular spaces.

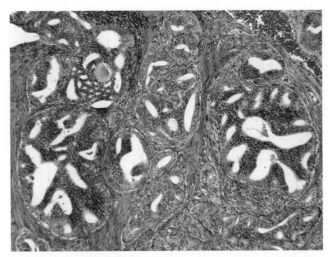

FIGURE 9-36 ■ Classic Gleason pattern 3C rounded cribriform glands with punched-out lumina. In contemporary useage, this pattern is considered grade 4.

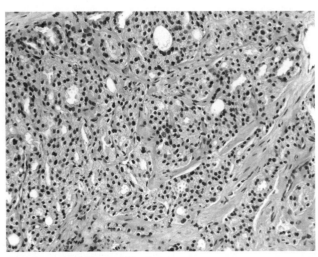

FIGURE 9-39 ■ Gleason pattern 4A. Note striking fusion of acini and formation of occasional elongated acinar chains (**lower right**).

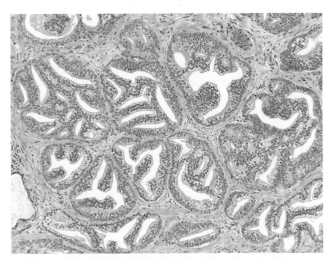

FIGURE 9-37 ■ Rounded cribriform structures showing stromal infiltration. No basal cells identified. These cribriform structures are considered Gleason pattern 4.

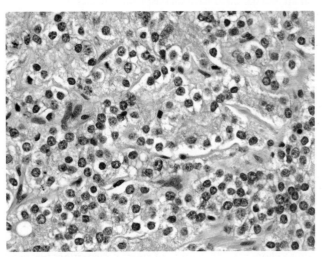

FIGURE 9-40 ■ Gleason pattern 4A. Note prominent fusion with virtually no lumen formation.

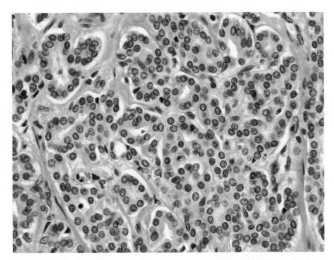

FIGURE 9-38 ■ Gleason pattern 4A. Note prominent acinar fusion.

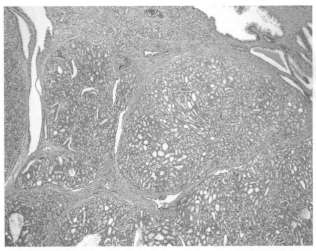

FIGURE 9-41 ■ Gleason pattern 4A. Note large irregular and consulate cribriform structures with extensive infiltration of stroma.

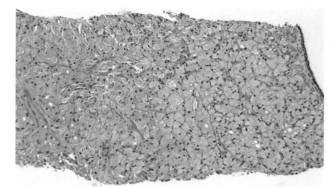

Figure 9-42 ■ Gleason pattern 4B in needle biopsy. Note a fused acinar morphology with little or no gland formation. Individual cells have abundant clear to foamy cytoplasm and small dark nucleoli.

bear a passing resemblance to renal clear cell carcinoma (Fig. 9-42). Interestingly, the nuclei in such cases may be small and dark and have inconspicuous nucleoli.

The highest grade in the Gleason system includes a variety of patterns including tumors composed of rounded solid cylinders and cribriform structures with central comedo-like necrosis (Fig. 9-43). The comedocarcinoma may look similar to ductal carcinoma of the breast (Fig. 9-44). Often, there is a spectrum of cribriform tumor ranging from cribriform pattern 4 blending imperceptively into more solid cribriform areas (Gleason 5A). The most poorly differentiated tumors are composed of solid sheets, aggregates, cords, and single cells sometimes with vacuolated cytoplasm (signet ring cells) but without well-defined lumens (Figs. 9-45 to 9-47). Solid masses, trabeculae, and sheets of tumor with rosette-like structures may also be seen. Grade 5 tumors often show extensive stromal invasion.

The architectural patterns of adenocarcinoma as described above show varying degrees of stromal disruption; however, stromal reaction is unusual especially in the lower grades of carcinoma. A desmoplastic reaction may rarely be seen in

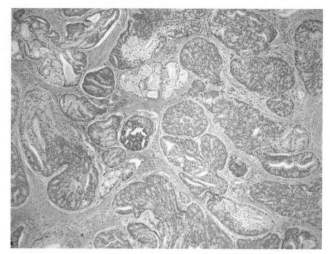

Figure 9-44 ■ Cribriform carcinoma. Note extensive infiltration of stroma by cylindrical and sheet-like cribriform structures.

Gleason grade 3 carcinomas but is more commonly noted in higher-grade patterns (Fig. 9-48). Stromal reaction may be difficult to appreciate on routine slides.[269] Lymphocytic reactions are rarely seen in prostate carcinoma. A neutrophilic response is highly unusual except if there is superimposed acute bacterial prostatitis. A granulomatous stromal reaction is rarely seen. Sometimes, one can see a layered fibrous reaction at the advancing edge of the carcinoma especially in RP specimens when the tumor is beyond the prostatic capsule (Fig. 9-49).

In addition to the above patterns that conform to the original Gleason diagram, there are other uncommon patterns of prostate adenocarcinoma that may be underrecognized because of their resemblance to common nonneoplastic conditions including atrophy and hyperplasia. These variations, which include atrophic, pseudohyperplastic, cystic, foamy gland, and stratified (PIN-like) adenocarcinoma, are detailed in the next section of the chapter.

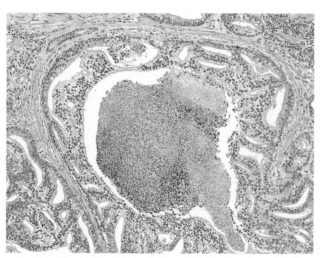

Figure 9-43 ■ Gleason pattern 5A. Note rounded cribriform structures with prominent central comedonecrosis.

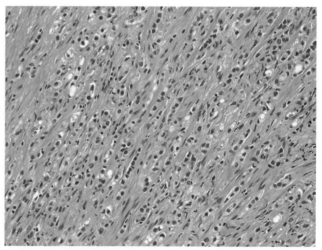

Figure 9-45 ■ Gleason pattern 5B. Note extensive tissue involvement by Indian file–like cords and spindle cells.

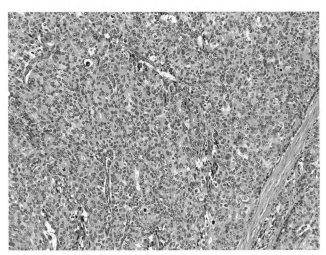

FIGURE 9-46 ■ Gleason 5B. Note solid sheet of tumor with only focal lumens.

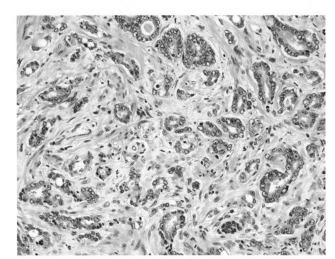

FIGURE 9-48 ■ Adenocarcinoma showing a desmoplastic stromal reaction.

While the architectural pattern is the most common and most important low-power manifestation of prostatic carcinoma, tinctorial alteration is another frequent phenomenon that can be appreciated at scanning magnification. Sometimes, the tinctorial change is more obvious than any architectural disturbance, and we consider the glandular color change to be a major diagnostic criterion of adenocarcinoma. The tinctorial quality of glands is somewhat dependent on fixation and staining. In applying this criterion, it is important to have a histology laboratory that produces consistent H&E staining. Tinctorial alteration is always judged in relation to nearby nonneoplastic glands, and while the change is usually manifested by increasing degrees of amphophilia (Fig. 9-50), this is not always the case. Sometimes, the neoplastic glands are clearer than the nearby nonneoplastic ones (Fig. 9-51). Rarely, the neoplastic glands have an eosinophilic hue. In addition to the general

difference in "color temperature," the neoplastic cells may show more specific cytoplasmic changes including Paneth cell–like alteration, which usually indicates neuroendocrine differentiation (Fig. 9-52). Paneth cell–like change when present is usually focal, but in rare cases, it may be extensive. Neoplastic glandular cells may have a microvacuolated appearance (so-called foamy gland or xanthomatous change) or a macrovacuolated (signet ring–like cell) morphology (see later section). In very rare instances, the cells may display an oncocytic look with abundant granular eosinophilic cytoplasm (Fig. 9-53).

A third major criterion for the diagnosis of adenocarcinoma is an absence of basal cells, often but not always resulting in single cell–layered glands. Most normal and hyperplastic glands show a double layer with luminal secretory cells enveloped by basal cells.[270] The basal cell layer may be complete or discontinuous, a feature that is often

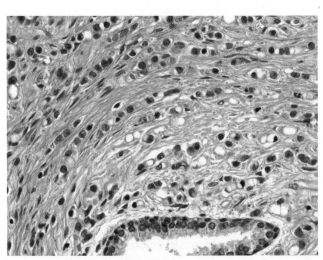

FIGURE 9-47 ■ Gleason pattern 5. Note poorly differentiated cells arranged in cords, and individually. Many cells show prominent signet ring cell change.

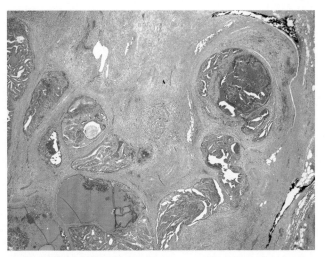

FIGURE 9-49 ■ Fibrous reaction at advancing edge of carcinoma in extra-prostatic extension.

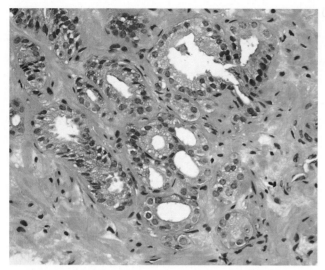

FIGURE 9-50 ■ Gleason pattern 3 adenocarcinoma showing cytoplasmic amphophilia.

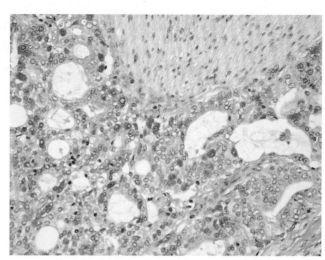

FIGURE 9-52 ■ Adenocarcinoma with prominent Paneth-like cells.

difficult to discern with an H&E-stained slide. Most benign mimickers of adenocarcinoma have complete or incomplete layers of basal cell.[203,266,271] The usual patterns of complete atrophy show complete basal cell layers, while partial atrophy, postatrophic hyperplasia, and AAH typically have a discontinuous layer.[214,216,272–277] Some benign glands especially in areas of partial atrophy totally lack a basal cell layer, and therefore, an absence of basal cells is not a specific criterion of malignancy.[274–276,278] Nevertheless, in adenocarcinoma, basal cells are absent, and this feature is an important aid in establishing a malignant diagnosis (Fig. 9-54).

Careful microscopy at medium to high power is often required to appreciate the basal cell layer. Basal cells are darker than secretory cells, have relatively high nuclear to cytoplasmic ratios and may have a variety of shapes including cuboidal, triangular, and elongated forms (Fig. 9-55). The last may be difficult to separate from periglandular stromal

cells, which may be closely apposed to glands. Additionally, distorted or poorly preserved neoplastic glands may simulate basal cells. Most small acinar carcinomas display a single layer of abnormal cells; however, some carcinomas show cellular overlapping creating a double layer with an apparent basal cell component (Fig. 9-56). Careful inspection in these cases shows nuclear atypia in all cells including the basally located ones, thus helping to confirm a malignant diagnosis. While it is clear that the absence of basal cells is important in acinar carcinoma, it is also critical in the analysis of atypical cribriform and papillary proliferations. Invasive cribriform carcinoma may be difficult to separate from high-grade intraepithelial neoplasia and intraductal spread of adenocarcinoma (see later section). The complete lack of basal cells is important in arriving at a correct diagnosis.

The observation of basal cell absence can be judged on routine slides in most cases; however, one may need to

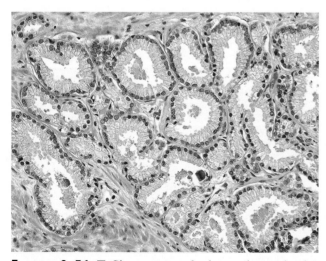

FIGURE 9-51 ■ Gleason pattern 3 adenocarcinoma showing abundant pale cytoplasm.

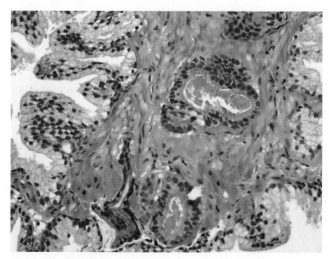

FIGURE 9-53 ■ Adenocarcinoma composed of cells with abundant eosinophilic cytoplasm.

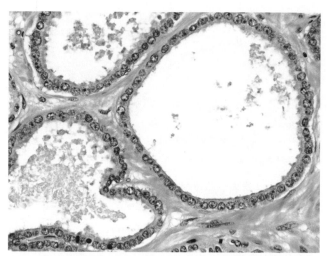

FIGURE 9-54 ■ Adenocarcinoma composed of single-layered glands with no basal cells identified.

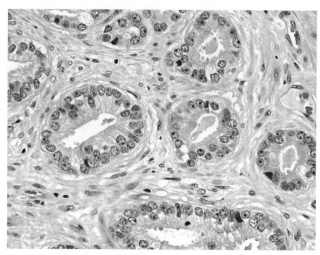

FIGURE 9-56 ■ Adenocarcinoma showing cellular overlapping with no basal cells.

employ basal cell markers (see later section) in some cases especially when the issue of periglandular stromal cells is a problem or when there is more than one layer with cellular overlapping or in situations where there are only very few glands on which to base a judgment (Fig. 9-57). A basal cell marker should not be considered a "malignant stain" since one is looking for a negative observation, a finding that may also be rarely seen in benign glands.[203,266]

Nuclear atypia is the fourth major criterion for diagnosing malignancy. It is usually manifested by nuclear and nucleolar enlargement. Historically, the latter has been emphasized as a key feature of adenocarcinoma; however, the finding while helpful may not always be present.[279–283] Prominent nucleoli are generally defined as ones measuring 1 to 3 μm in diameter, and they have an amphophilic or eosinophilic coloration (Fig. 9-58). The absence of prominent nucleoli may result from a number of factors including

poor fixation or processing, type of fixative, thick sectioning, and overstaining. Some fixatives such as Bouin or B5 can lead to nucleolar prominence even in normal and hyperplastic glands. The use of such fixatives is discouraged in prostate biopsy pathology. While enlarged nucleoli are typical of carcinoma, they may be seen in other conditions such as high-grade PIN, radiation effects, inflamed glands, and basal cell hyperplasia.[284,285] Multiple nucleoli are seen in malignancy more often than in benign lesions; however, they are not considered a specific malignant feature (Fig. 9-59).[279,286] In addition to the technical factors that may obscure nucleoli in malignant glands, there are some carcinomas that are considered nucleolus poor (Fig. 9-60).[280] In one study of limited carcinoma, one-quarter of cases lacked prominent nucleoli.[282] In another analysis of low-grade adenocarcinoma, 8% of cases lacked nucleoli, and a further 20% only showed rare prominent nucleoli.[280] Furthermore, certain

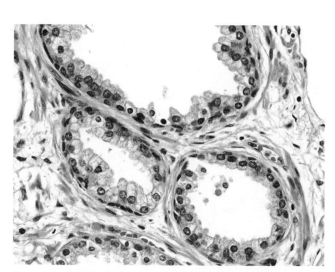

FIGURE 9-55 ■ Nonneoplastic prostatic glands showing prominent basal cells with elongate and triangular forms.

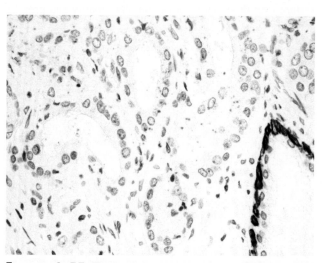

FIGURE 9-57 ■ Gleason pattern 3 adenocarcinoma showing absence of basal cells with basal cell marker. Note the useful internal positive control of positive staining in basal cells of a nonneoplastic gland (**lower right**).

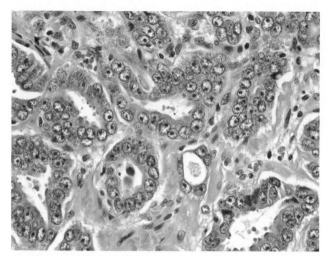

FIGURE 9-58 ■ Adenocarcinoma showing prominent cytoplasmic amphophilia and enlarged nuclei with large inclusion-like nucleoli.

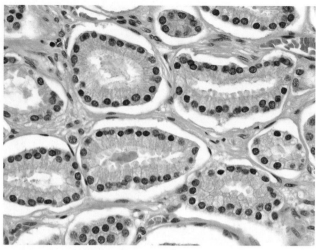

FIGURE 9-60 ■ Gleason pattern 3 adenocarcinoma showing mildly enlarged nuclei without prominent nucleoli.

patterns of adenocarcinoma, especially hypernephroid carcinoma (Gleason pattern 4B), and the nuclei are often dark and have a pyknotic appearance with inconspicuous nucleoli (Fig. 9-61). The key point here is that the nuclear atypia does not always equate to nucleolar prominence.[282] In the absence of the latter, there are other important attributes of nuclear atypia to look for including nuclear enlargement, nuclear shape and membrane irregularities, hyperchromasia, and parachromatin clearing (Fig. 9-62). These features need to be assessed using high-power microscopy.

Minor Diagnostic Criteria

The minor diagnostic features generally occur more frequently in adenocarcinoma than in benign lesions and are useful as sentinels for a malignant diagnosis especially when other criteria may not, at least initially, be obvious. A minor feature may draw one's eyes to an abnormality and prompt

a closer look at a given group of glands. The minor criteria are listed in Table 9-8.

Amorphous eosinophilic secretions are more commonly seen in carcinomatous glands than in benign ones.[281] The flocculent secretions are pink to red and often have a granular appearance (Fig. 9-63). In occasional cases, nuclear debris may be seen but not to the extent seen in comedocarcinoma (Fig. 9-64). The secretions do not have the well-defined structure of corpora amylacea, and the exact nature of the secretory material or its relationship with neoplasia is unclear. Eosinophilic secretions may be found in up to 84% of adenocarcinomas in prostatectomy specimens and 53% to 73% of minimal carcinomas in needle biopsies.[282,287] Eosinophilic secretions are commonly seen in high-grade PIN and occasionally in benign glands including atrophic ones.

Basophilic luminal mucin (blue mucin) is more frequent in malignant glands than in benign ones.[288] The mucin is often focal and present as wispy small strands, or it may fill lumina

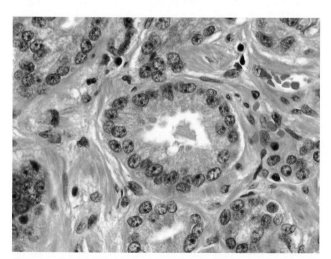

FIGURE 9-59 ■ Adenocarcinoma showing prominent nucleoli including spindle cells with multiple nucleoli.

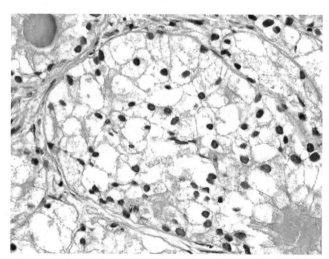

FIGURE 9-61 ■ Gleason pattern 4B adenocarcinoma composed of cells with small dark nuclei with no nucleoli.

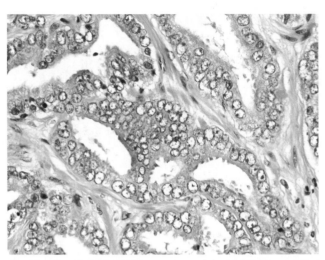

FIGURE 9-62 ■ High-power photomicrograph showing marked nuclear atypia. Note nuclear membrane irregularities, prominent parachromatic clearing, and focally prominent nucleoli.

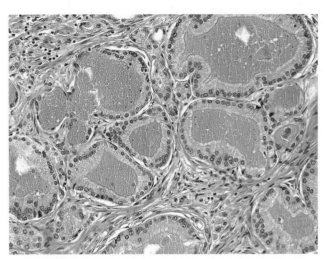

FIGURE 9-63 ■ Gleason pattern 3 adenocarcinoma with prominent granular eosinophilic secretions. A crystalloid is seen on the right.

and distend glands (Fig. 9-65). On occasion, there is extensive involvement of acini (Fig. 9-66). The mucin stains with Alcian blue at pH 2.5 indicating its acidic nature. The blue mucin can be present on its own, or it may be accompanied by granular eosinophilic secretions or crystalloids. Blue mucin is present in up to 72% of completely embedded RP specimens and in 18% to 32% of limited adenocarcinomas in needle biopsies.[282,287] Blue mucin is not specific for carcinoma and may be seen in a variety of other processes including mucinous metaplasia, basal cell hyperplasia, sclerosing adenosis, and high-grade PIN.[288] Importantly, basophilic mucin may also be seen occasionally in atrophy and AAH (adenosis), both of which are common mimickers of small acinar carcinoma[289] (Fig. 9-67).

Intraluminal eosinophilic crystalloids occur more often in malignant than in benign glands.[282,287,290,291] They are nonbirefringent brightly eosinophilic structures, which have a variety of shapes including needle-like, rectangular, and triangular ones (Fig. 9-68). Rarely, a crystalloid is seen in the prostatic stroma. They differ from corpora amylacea, which are laminated structures usually but not always with rounded contours. Corpora amylacea may have odd triangular or rectangular shapes, but they tend to conform to the shapes of glandular lumina and they are less brightly eosinophilic than crystalloids. Corpora amylacea are uncommon in acinar carcinomas but are regularly seen in benign glands (Fig. 9-69). Crystalloids are commonly associated with flocculent eosinophilic secretions

and may be associated with basophilic mucin as well. When all three luminal products are present, there is a very high likelihood that the glands are neoplastic (Fig. 9-70). Crystalloids are more commonly present in low-grade acinar carcinomas and are rarely seen in Gleason grade 4 and 5 tumors. The composition and mechanism of formation of crystalloids are poorly understood although they are known to contain a high content of sulfur.[292,293] Like other minor diagnostic criteria, crystalloids often draw the pathologist's attention to an area of abnormality.

Mitotic figures are rarely detectable in benign glands but may occur more often in reactive epithelium and high-grade PIN. In needle biopsies, they are present in about 10% of Gleason 6 adenocarcinomas and more commonly in high-grade tumors.[282,287] Mitotic figures are uncommon in the low- to intermediate-grade (Fig. 9-71) (Gleason scores 2 to 7)

Table 9-8 ■ SPECIFIC DIAGNOSTIC CRITERIA OF CARCINOMA

1. Atypical glands in extraprostatic location
2. Lymphovascular space invasion
3. Circumferential perineural invasion
4. Collagenous micronodules (Mucinous fibroplasia)
5. Intraglandular glomerulations

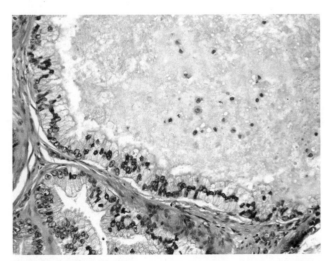

FIGURE 9-64 ■ High-powered photomicrograph of carcinomatous glands showing eosinophilic luminal secretions and scattered nuclear debris.

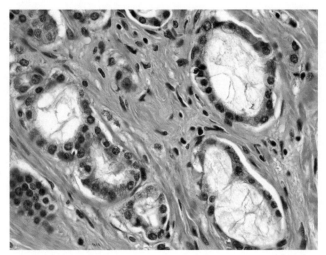

FIGURE 9-65 ■ Adenocarcinoma Gleason pattern 3 showing luminal basophilic mucin.

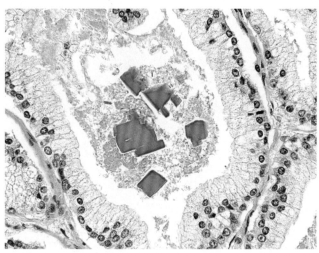

FIGURE 9-68 ■ High-power photomicrograph showing prominent crystalloids of varying shapes.

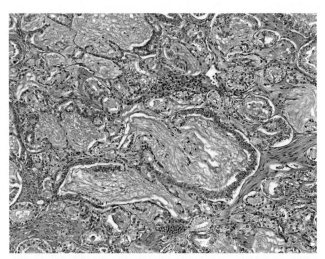

FIGURE 9-66 ■ Adenocarcinoma showing extensive luminal mucin.

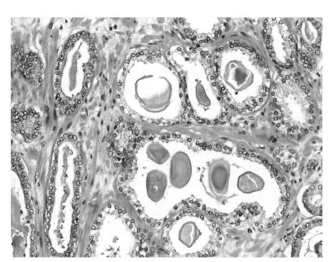

FIGURE 9-69 ■ Adenocarcinoma, Gleason pattern 3 with numerous corpora amylacea.

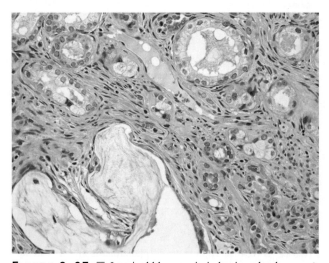

FIGURE 9-67 ■ Luminal blue mucin in benign glands.

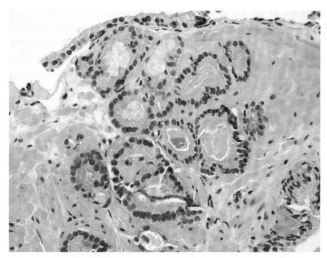

FIGURE 9-70 ■ Admixed luminal products—eosinophilic material, basophilic mucin, crystalloids.

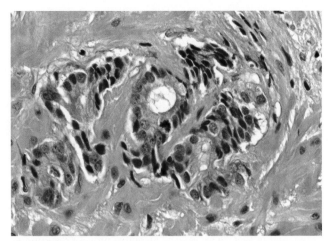

FIGURE 9-71 ■ High-powered photomicrograph of adenocarcinoma showing a mitotic figure.

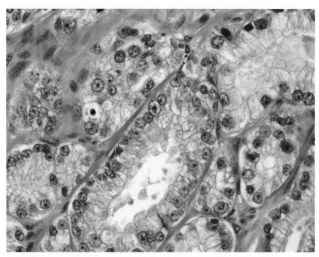

FIGURE 9-73 ■ Adenocarcinoma showing a few apoptotic bodies.

carcinomas and more likely to be seen in Gleason grade 8 to 10 tumors.[294] Atypical mitotic figures are almost never identified except in high grade tumors (Fig. 9-72). Overall, the finding of a mitotic figure is neither sensitive nor specific for a diagnosis of adenocarcinoma, but it should prompt the pathologist to take a closer look at the involved gland and nearby ones.

Some authors have found the presence of apoptotic bodies useful (Fig. 9-73).[286] Apoptotic bodies are found in decreasing frequency in carcinoma, high-grade PIN, and benign glands, respectively.[295–297]

With respect to cytoplasmic membrane features, it has been suggested that neoplastic acini have a more "rigid" appearance with smooth sharp cytoplasmic borders (Fig. 9-74). While this feature is common, it is not specific for carcinoma and indeed some benign glands, especially in atrophy will also demonstrate smooth luminal borders. Furthermore, some carcinomas have irregular and undulating luminal edges.

The presence of high-grade PIN should heighten the pathologist's suspicion that carcinoma may be present in the immediately adjacent tissue or in a separate fragment. In one

study, 47% of patients with high-grade PIN in one core had carcinoma in a separate core compared to 31% of cases without high-grade PIN.

Putatively-Specific Diagnostic Criteria

The presence of abnormal prostatic acini outside the prostate gland is a definitive indicator of malignancy with a few caveats. Ectopic prostate tissue may be found in a variety of sites including bladder, seminal vesicle, retrovesical space, and pericolonic fat, to name a few. The prostate epithelium in these cases can appear normal, atrophic, or hyperplastic. Therefore, it is important to recognize that the glands in question have some degree of abnormality, as defined above, in order to use this criterion. When neoplastic acini are outside the prostate gland, they usually involve periprostatic connective tissue, which generally contains fat. On rare occasions, one may see atypical acini in fibroadipose tissue at the tip of a core biopsy that is otherwise free of carcinoma (Fig. 9-75). While no tumor is present in the prostate

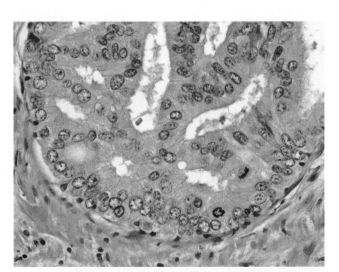

FIGURE 9-72 ■ Atypical mitotic figures in high-grade carcinoma.

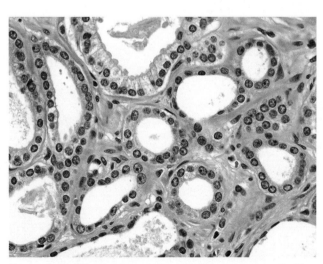

FIGURE 9-74 ■ Adenocarcinoma, Gleason pattern 3. Note smooth "rigid" luminal cytoplasmic borders.

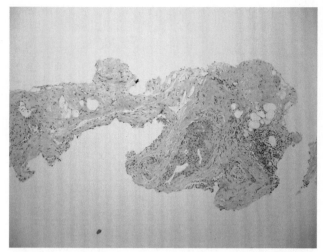

FIGURE 9-75 ■ Low-power photomicrograph showing adenocarcinoma in periprostatic fibroadipose connective tissue. No actual involvement of prostate parenchyma was present.

proper, this finding is generally diagnostic of prostatic carcinoma and suggests that the intraprostatic tumor has not been sampled. One must be cautious in such situations since metastatic carcinoma (e.g., gastrointestinal signet-ring carcinoma) may also present in this fashion, so prostatic marker studies may be useful. It is important to be aware that intraprostatic fat can rarely be seen. Involvement of seminal vesicle or bladder tissue by atypical prostatic glands is a good indicator of malignancy.

Lymphovascular space invasion is considered a specific criterion for malignancy; however, it is rarely seen and, when present, is usually associated with high-grade carcinoma that is diagnostically obvious (Fig. 9-76). We are not personally aware of a case in which lymphovascular involvement by tumor was the only criterion of malignancy, but it remains a theoretical possibility.

With the exception of seeing abnormal acini clearly beyond the confines of the prostate or as an isolated finding in lymphovascular spaces, there are three reasonably specific criteria diagnostic of carcinoma. They are circumferential PNI, collagenous micronodules, and intraglandular glomerulations.

PNI has historically been recognized as a common feature of adenocarcinoma and one that is important for diagnosis. In RP specimens, PNI is present in up to 94% of cases. A recent pooled analysis of biopsy studies shows that 22% of adenocarcinomas exhibit PNI.[298] The likelihood of seeing perineural invasion is related to the grade and amount of tumor. In minimal carcinomas, the frequency of PNI has been reported to be as low as 2%. In rare cases, a small focus of perineural carcinoma is the only feature identified (Fig. 9-77). Originally, it was thought that PNI represented perineural lymphatic space invasion, but this hypothesis has been disproven. The nerves represent a pathway of least resistance for spread of carcinoma, and in fact, there may be an active process resulting in a tropism of carcinoma cells for nerves.[299] Perineural "invasion" can have a number of patterns ranging from tumor cells abutting or indenting nerves to true circumferential involvement (Figs. 9-78 and 9-79). It is only the latter that should be considered a specific diagnostic criterion of malignancy.[300,301] Normal, hyperplastic, and occasionally atrophic glands may abut or indent intraprostatic nerves. Likewise, while intraneural involvement suggests malignancy, however, there are rare examples of intraneural benign glands, so one should exercise caution in using this situation.[300]

PNI can have many forms. Circumferential involvement can be seen in transverse or longitudinal sections (Fig. 9-80). Partial circumferential involvement is sometimes manifested as crescentic extension of neoplastic glands around nerves. Peninsular or knob-like patterns of PNI may also be noted (Fig. 9-81). Neoplastic glands can directly invade nerves and can be completely surrounded by nerve tissue. Involvement of ganglia may also accompany neural invasion (Fig. 9-82). The perineural involvement may involve separate acini or fused glands and cribriform structures. In some cases, the involvement is subtle and may resemble hyperplasia or PIN (Fig. 9-83). The latter may have a micropapillary appearance with a nerve being in a papillary core. On occasion,

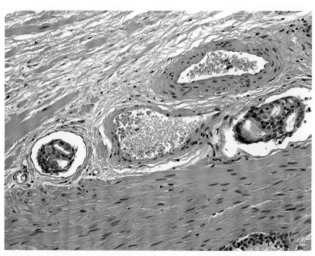

FIGURE 9-76 ■ Intralymphatic adenocarcinoma.

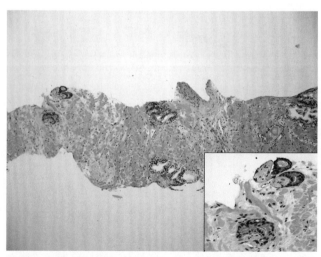

FIGURE 9-77 ■ Low-power photomicrograph of prostatic core. Note perineural carcinoma near tip on left (**inset**).

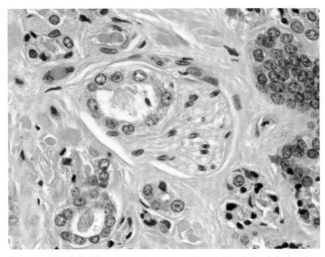

FIGURE 9-78 ■ Adenocarcinoma, Gleason pattern 3 indenting a small nerve.

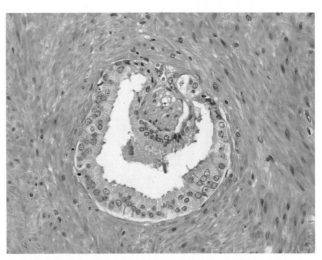

FIGURE 9-81 ■ Partial encasement of a small nerve by adenocarcinoma creating a peninsular pattern.

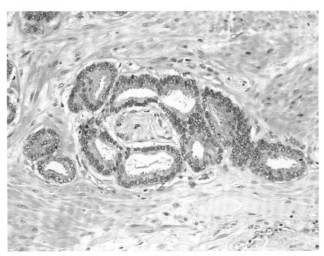

FIGURE 9-79 ■ Circumferential perineural involvement by atypical glands is diagnostic of adenocarcinoma.

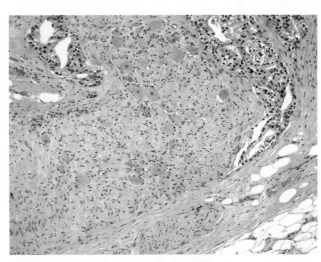

FIGURE 9-82 ■ Adenocarcinoma infiltrating around a large ganglion.

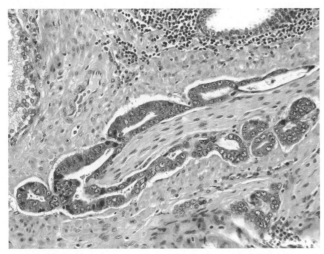

FIGURE 9-80 ■ Circumferential perineural invasion in longitudinal section.

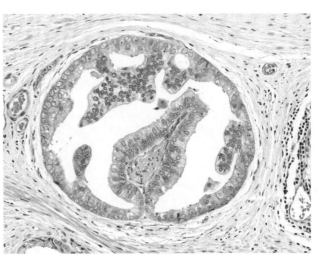

FIGURE 9-83 ■ Perineural adenocarcinoma with PIN-like pattern.

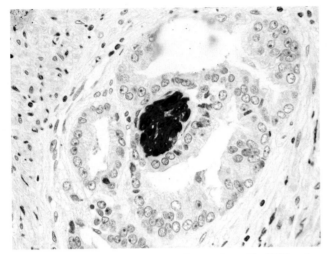

FIGURE 9-84 ■ Perineural invasion confirmed by S100 stain.

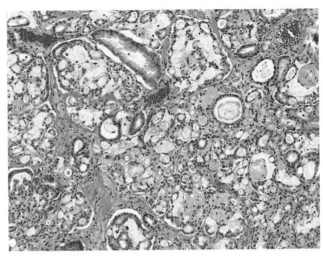

FIGURE 9-86 ■ Adenocarcinoma with extensive collagenous micronodules (mucinous fibroplasia).

the glands around an involved nerve may show cystic dilatation. Crushed cells can be seen around nerves, and this can lead to problems in differential diagnosis. Lymphocytes can be distributed in a perineural location, and when crushed, they can mimic the appearance of distorted tumor cells. Immunohistochemistry may be required to make a correct diagnosis. Sometimes stromal cells or aggregates of extracellular material such as one sees in collagenous micronodules may simulate PNI and, in selected cases immunostains for S-100, may be useful to confirm the presence of neural tissue (Fig. 9-84).

Collagenous micronodules also referred to as musinous micronodules consist of rounded collections of hyalinized stroma admixed with or surrounded by abnormal acini.[302,303] Sometimes, the micronodules are actually within the lumina of neoplastic glands. They are composed of collagen and often show a few admixed fibroblast nuclei (Fig. 9-85). Collagenous micronodules are commonly associated with mucin-producing areas and likely represent a peculiar fibrous

organization of mucus. While usually rounded, the collagenous formations may be present as strands or larger lobulated masses (Fig. 9-86). Collagenous micronodules have not been identified in benign glandular lesions and are considered pathognomonic of adenocarcinoma. Unfortunately, this feature only presents in 1% to 5 % of needle biopsies with carcinoma and is rarely present in cases of limited carcinoma.[271] Collagenous micronodules are more commonly found in totally embedded prostatectomy specimens.

Intraglandular glomerulations are considered a relatively specific feature of adenocarcinoma. The ball-like tufts of fused cribriform glands project into lumina surrounded by crescentic spaces bearing superficial resemblance to Bowen spaces (Fig. 9-87). One or sometimes multiple points of attachment to the surrounding gland may be seen. Glomerulations are present in 3% to 15% of carcinomas in needle biopsies although our personal experience would be the lower end of that range.[304] They are extremely rare in limited carcinoma.[287]

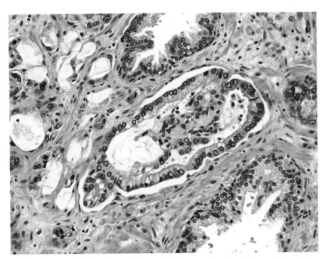

FIGURE 9-85 ■ Adenocarcinoma with fused small collagenous micronodules.

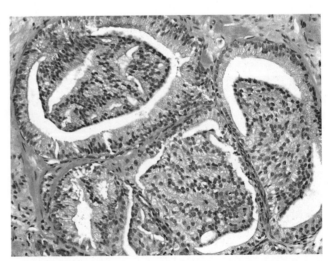

FIGURE 9-87 ■ Adenocarcinoma with prominent intraluminal glomerulations. This is a specific diagnostic feature of carcinoma.

Ancillary Studies

Immunohistochemistry is a valuable adjunct to routine microscopy in prostatic pathology. In particular, basal cell markers and racemase (AMACR) are useful to confirm the presence of adenocarcinoma, especially in small foci of atypical glands.[203,266] It has been recognized for over 25 years that high molecular weight cytokeratin (HMWCK) decorated by antibody 34βE12 [CK903], is preferentially expressed in prostatic basal cells rather than luminal secretory cells.[305] In more recent years, other basal cell–specific markers such as cytokeratin 5/6 and p63 have also been successfully used in clinical practice (Fig. 9-88).[306–308] Cocktails including antibodies to p63 and 34BE12 or CK5/6 are sometimes used. The staining is more intense because both nuclear and cytoplasmic domains are being decorated. However, at a practical level, the cocktails have no major advantage over single stains.[309] The sensitivity and specificity of p63 and 34BE12 are similar in needle biopsies but, for TURs p63, may have better sensitivity.[310] There are numerous factors that may interfere with successful immunohistochemical staining, and it is important to carefully assess internal and external controls when looking at basal cell markers. Factors such as time to fixation, time in fixative, and type of fixation can have an effect on immunostaining. The antibody should be optimized for the conditions within the individual laboratory, and there should be a good system of quality control. Antibodies such as 34BE12 work well in formalin-fixed paraffin-embedded tissues. Antigen retrieval using protease digestion or heat-induced or microwave techniques is generally employed. The stains can be done on stored intervening unstained sections or fresh sections cut from the block. Stains can also be carried out on destained H&E slides although the technique can be tricky and the staining reactions are usually not as strong as one sees with fresh sections.[311] Ideally there should be internal nonneoplastic (normal or hyperplastic)

glands for comparison. The benign glands should show strong basal cell staining, and it is very helpful when the nonneoplastic glands are close by the abnormal glands in question.

Basal cells markers should be incorporated into an algorithmic approach to the diagnosis of adenocarcinoma. They always need to be assessed in conjunction with the H&E sections and should not be ordered indiscriminately. Minimal adenocarcinoma can be diagnosed in needle biopsies without the use of immunostains[278]; however, in many practices, basal cell markers are used routinely in putative limited carcinomas as a confirmatory measure.

The absence of basal cells is a major criterion used to diagnose adenocarcinoma. Usually, this observation can be made using routine slides, but sometimes, the absence of basal cells must be confirmed. This is especially the case with tiny foci of putative carcinoma in needle biopsies specimens or when the abnormal glands are distorted. Periacinar stromal cells may simulate basal cells as can carcinoma cells when they are distorted, overlapping, or tangentially cut (Fig. 9-89). Basal cell markers will be negative in those situations. A negative basal cell stain on its own is not diagnostic of carcinoma. This observation has to be linked with the other morphologic features as noted earlier. One should exert caution since there may be other technical factors that result in a negative stain. To quote Peter Humphrey, "absence of proof is not proof of absence" (personal communication). While most benign glandular patterns have a continuous or discontinuous pattern of basal cell staining, some small acinar lesions such as partial atrophy show a complete absence of basal cells despite having completely banal cytoarchitectural features. Additionally, lesions such as AAH, partial atrophy, and postatrophic hyperplasia may show mixtures of small acini with basal cells and others without them. Scattered negative acini have been found in 11% to 23% of

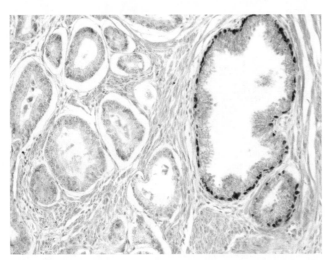

FIGURE 9-88 ■ p63 staining in adenocarcinoma case. Note absence of p63-positive basal cells in adenocarcinoma (**upside**) and internal control positivity in nonneoplastic glands on right.

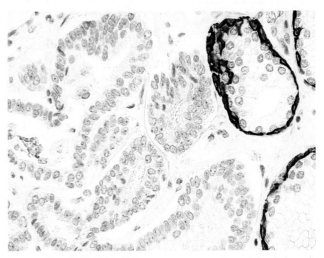

FIGURE 9-89 ■ 34βE12 stain showing strong control positivity in basal cells in nonneoplastic glands (**right**) and negative staining in the glands on left, which display nuclear overlapping, a feature that can simulate basal cells on H&E.

atrophic foci.[312,313] In an early study, looking at the utility of 34βE12 staining in small foci of atypical glands, the stain established a diagnosis of carcinoma in 14% of cases and was confirmatory for carcinoma in 58% of cases, equivocal in 18%, and of no value in 8%.[305]

Basal cell staining is also useful in the differential diagnosis of carcinoma and can be used to support a diagnosis of atrophy, postatrophic hyperplasia, AAH (adenosis), basal cell hyperplasia, and PIN.[203,266,314] Radiation effects can be problematic, and basal cell stains can help to identify residual or recurrent carcinoma. Small atypical pseudoinfiltrative glands can be seen with radiation effects. Nuclear atypia and nucleolar prominence may be present. The presence of basal cell staining in these glands helps to confirm them as altered nonneoplastic acini. Furthermore, basal cell stains can be used in cribriform intraglandular lesions to separate cribriform PIN from invasive cribriform carcinoma (see earlier discussion).

There are rare reports of focal 34BE12 positive cells in prostatic adenocarcinoma.[315] Additionally, p63-positive adenocarcinomas have also been identified (Fig. 9-90).[316] In the latter cases, the neoplastic cells displaying varying degree of nuclear positivity. Despite these rare exceptions, basal cell

markers are important adjunctive stains that are regularly useful to establish or confirm a malignant diagnosis.

Over the last decade, AMACR (P504S), an enzyme involved in the B-oxidation of fatty acids, has emerged as an important immunomarker in prostate pathology. In contrast to the basal cell markers where one is looking for a negative result, racemase is a "positive cancer stain." Using high-throughput gene expression studies, the P504S gene was found to be overexpressed in prostatic adenocarcinomas but not in benign prostate glands.[317] The protein, identified by immunohistochemistry, is overexpressed in 75% to 95% of adenocarcinomas.[318–321] Racemase can be used as an individual stain or in cocktails. Cocktails of two antibodies (racemase and p63) using single- or dual-color detection systems or three antibodies (racemase, p63, 34βE12) with a dual-color detection kit may be employed.[266,322–325] These cocktails allow the detection of cytoplasmic racemase positivity and an absence of basal cells in the same glands (Fig. 9-91). Racemase staining is cytoplasmic, often with luminal membranous and submembranous enhancement (Fig. 9-92). In carcinomas, the staining is usually extensive with circumferential luminal border enhancement, and the intensity, while varying somewhat from case to case,

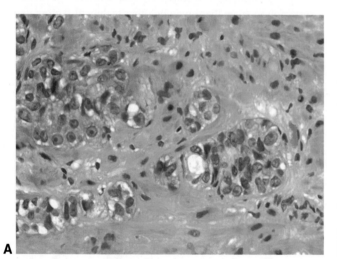

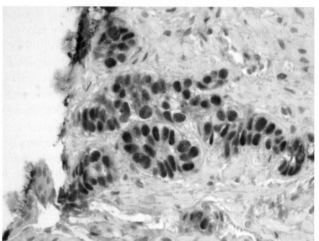

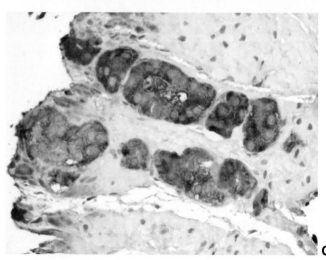

FIGURE 9-90 ■ p63-positive prostatic adenocarcinoma. **A.** Note nests and poorly formed glands. **B.** Diffusely positive p63 nuclear staining. **C.** Strong racemase staining in atypical cells.

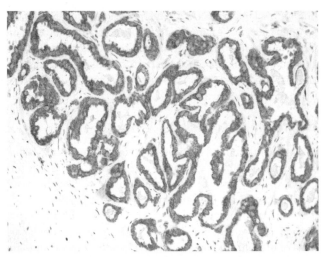

FIGURE 9-91 ■ p63/racemase cocktail stains showing absence of basal cells and strong cytoplasmic racemase positivity (*red marker*).

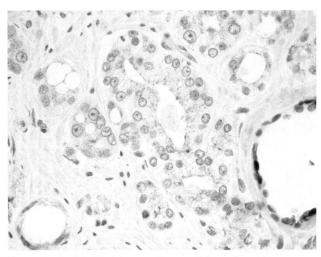

FIGURE 9-93 ■ Adenocarcinoma with weak to absent racemase staining.

is usually relatively strong. Technical issues can result in variations in staining intensity, and it is important to optimize the stain and use the appropriate controls. Racemase is a reasonably sensitive marker (80% to 95%) for usual adenocarcinoma, but the sensitivity is lower in variant histology including pseudohyperplastic, atrophic, and foamy gland patterns (Fig. 9-93).[326,327] Racemase is not specific for adenocarcinoma and is often present in high-grade PIN.[207] Racemase positivity may be seen in a wide variety of benign processes and mimickers of carcinoma including nonneoplastic benign glands, atrophy especially partial atrophy, and AAH.[203,227,266,276,320,328–330] The staining is usually more focal, weaker, and less circumferential in these conditions than in carcinoma. Nephrogenica adenoma, which may affect the prostatic urethra and prostate proper, shows strong and diffuse racemase positivity (Fig. 9-94).[331,332] This could result in the overdiagnosis of nephrogenic adenoma (metaplasia) as small acinar carcinoma. Just like the

basal cell markers, racemase must be utilized in the appropriate histologic context. It is usually used to help establish a malignant diagnosis when one encounters a small focus of atypical glands. The presence of cytoplasmic racemase positivity and negative basal cell markers can support a malignant interpretation especially in the setting of limited adenocarcinoma.[203,266,333]

There are other diagnostically useful immunohistochemical stains. Keratin stains such as cytokeratin AE1/AE3 and Cam5.2 can be useful in the diagnosis of high-grade carcinoma versus conditions such as inflammation with crush artifact, and nonspecific granulomatous and xanthomatous inflammation. Hematolymphoid markers such as CD45 and CD68 may also help in these situations. Keratin stains may also be useful to highlight clandestine tumor cells in patients treated with radiation and hormones (Fig. 9-95).[203,334]

Prostate lineage-specific markers are useful in the diagnosis and differential diagnosis of prostatic adenocarcinoma.

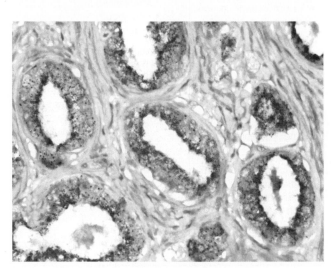

FIGURE 9-92 ■ Racemase stains showing luminal membranous and submembranous enhancement.

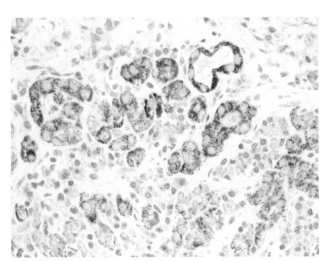

FIGURE 9-94 ■ Nephrogenic adenoma showing strong cytoplasmic racemase positivity.

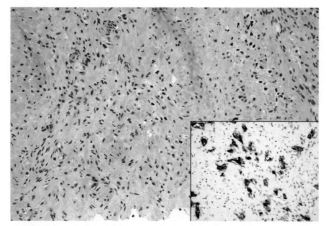

FIGURE 9-95 ■ Discreet individual neoplastic cells in a setting of hormonal therapy, highlighted by cytokeratin AE1/AE3 (**inset**).

The older markers, PSA and PSAP, can be used to confirm the prostatic origin of an acinar lesion and rule out mimickers such as seminal vesicle/ejaculatory duct (Fig. 9-96), Cowper glands, nephrogenic adenoma, mesonephric gland hyperplasia, and paraganglion.

The lineage markers are also useful in confirming the prostatic origin of a tumor when the differential diagnosis includes secondary involvement of the prostate by carcinoma or other tumors such as metastatic melanoma.

PSMA initially showed promise as a diagnostic marker but now has been shown not to be prostate-specific.[335–337] Two more recent promising lineage markers are prostein and NKX3.1, both of which have been shown to discriminate between prostatic and urothelial carcinomas.[338–342]

In regard to DNA flow cytometric, cytogenetic, or molecular genetic testing, there are currently no tests that are useful to establish a diagnosis of a prostatic adenocarcinoma or to discriminate between a possible focus of adenocarcinoma and the protean benign mimickers. There is an older

literature related to DNA cytometry as a prognostic factor in prostate cancer.[343] There is an evolving literature however on the potential importance of molecular testing for prognosis and prediction of response to certain therapies. Markers such as TMPRRS2 gene fusion products are showing some promise in the prognostic arena.

Differential Diagnosis

The broad differential diagnosis of prostatic adenocarcinoma can be distilled into three major categories: (a) benign mimickers, (b) PIN, and (c) other malignancies, especially other carcinomas. There are few other (if any) epithelial tumors that have as many benign mimickers as prostatic adenocarcinoma. This relates in part to the wide range of growth patterns of prostatic carcinoma and the fact that other histologic processes including atrophy, inflammation, and hyperplasia commonly affect the prostate gland. Furthermore, anatomic structures like the seminal vesicles, ejaculatory ducts, prostatic urethra, and periurethral (including Cowper) glands are adjacent to or integrated within the prostate and may be sampled during the course of prostatic biopsy or resection. The benign mimickers are shown in Table 9-9. Much has been written pertaining to mimickers and the differential diagnosis of prostatic carcinoma.[203,219,344–347]

The benign mimickers of adenocarcinoma can logically be discussed in relation to the diverse architectural patterns as outlined in the classical Gleason diagram. The drawing can be further simplified into four basic architectural patterns, namely, small gland, large gland, fused gland, and solid

Table 9-9 ■ CLASSIFICATION OF BENIGN MIMICKERS OF ADENOCARCINOMA	
Histoanatomic structures • Seminal vesicle/ejaculatory duct • Cowper gland • Paraganglion • Verumontanum mucosal glands (hyperplasia) • Mesonephric remnant gland (hyperplasia) *Atrophy* • Simple • Partial • Postatrophic • Sclerotic • Linear (streaming) *Inflammation* • Usual prostatitis with preservation artifacts • Granulomatous prostatitis, nonspecific • Xanthogranulomatous prostatitis (xanthoma) • Malakoplakia	*Reactive atypia* • Inflammatory • Ischemic • Radiation *Metaplasia* • Mucinous • Nephrogenic adenoma *Prostatic hyperplasia* • Basal cell hyperplasia • Benign nodular hyperplasia, small gland pattern • Clear cell cribriform hyperplasia • Sclerosing adenosis *AAH (adenosis)*

Reprinted from Srigley JR. Benign mimickers of prostatic adenocarcinoma. *Mod Pathol*, 2004;17:328–348, with permission.

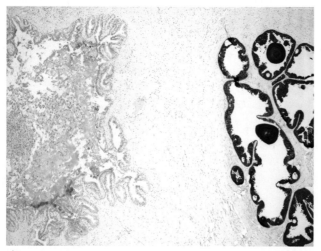

FIGURE 9-96 ■ PSA stain showing negativity in glandular the seminal vesicle (**left**) and strong positivity in prostatic glands (**right**).

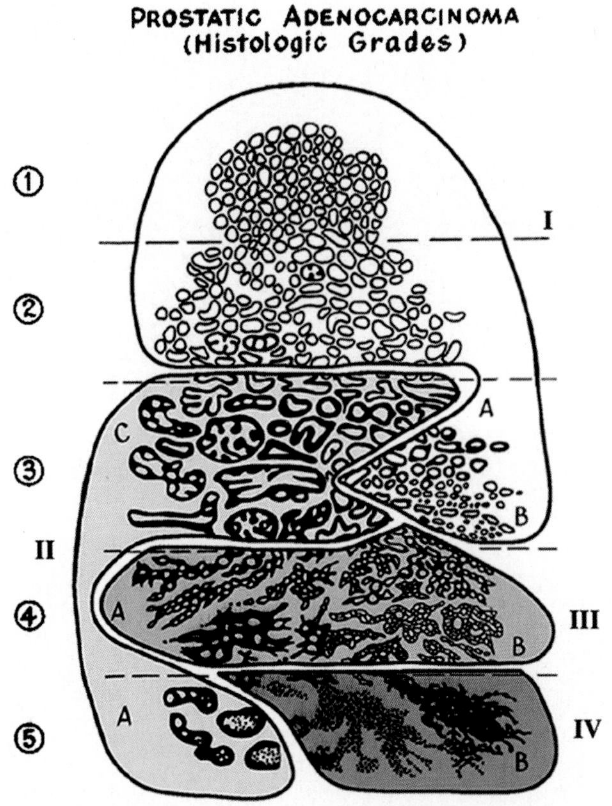

PROSTATIC ADENOCARCINOMA
(Histologic Grades)

FIGURE 9-97 ■ Gleason diagram divided into four major architectural patterns. (Reprinted from Srigley JR. Benign mimickers of prostatic adenocarcinoma. *Mod Pathol* 2004;17:328–348, with permission.)

(Fig. 9-97 and Table 9-10). This approach provides a conceptual framework to discuss differential diagnosis. There are numerous benign processes and histologic patterns that may be confused with each of the major architectures of carcinoma (Table 9-11). The benign mimickers are individually discussed in detail in Chapter 12. In this section, general comments on differential diagnosis in relation to some common mimickers will be made.

The small acinar pattern of carcinoma has the greatest number of mimickers, the most common ones being atrophy

Table 9-10 ■ MAJOR GROWTH PATTERNS OF ADENOCARCINOMA

	Growth Pattern	Gleason Patterns	Descriptors
I	Small gland	1, 2, 3A, 3B	Tiny, small, medium, separate acini
II	Large gland	3A, 3C, 5A	Simple, papillary, cribriform, comedo
III	Fused gland	4A, 4B	Coalescing acini, amphophilic or clear (hypernephroid)
IV	Solid	5B	Sheets, cords, single cells

Reprinted from Srigley JR. Benign mimickers of prostatic adenocarcinoma. *Mod Pathol* 2004;17:328–348, with permission.

Table 9-11 ■ BENIGN MIMICKERS IN RELATION TO MAJOR GROWTH PATTERNS OF PROSTATE ADENOCARCINOMA

Small gland pattern
- Seminal vesicle
- Cowper gland
- Atrophy
- Postatrophic hyperplasia
- Nephrogenic adenoma
- Basal cell hyperplasia
- Benign nodular hyperplasia
- Sclerosing adenosis
- Verumontanum mucosal gland hyperplasia
- Mesonephric gland hyperplasia
- AAH

Large gland pattern
- Clear cell cribriform hyperplasia
- Adenoid cystic-like basal cell hyperplasia
- Reactive atypia

Fused gland pattern
- Paraganglion
- Xanthogranulomatous inflammation (xanthoma)
- Malakoplakia

Solid gland pattern
- Idiopathic prostatitis with crush artifacts
- Idiopathic granulomatous prostatitis
- Signet ring–like change in lymphocytes and stromal cells

Reprinted from Srigley JR. Benign mimickers of prostatic adenocarcinoma. *Mod Pathol* 2004;17:328–348, with permission.

(complete and partial), postatrophic hyperplasia and adenosis (AAH), and seminal vesicle (Fig. 9-98).[219,273-278,344-347] The most common small acinar pattern (Gleason 3B) consists of infiltrating small glands invading between nonneoplastic glands or stroma indiscriminately. Complete and partial atrophy and postatrophic hyperplasia can have a pseudoinvasive architecture, especially in needle biopsies where the organized, lobular appearance of the atrophy may not always be appreciated. The atrophic glands are small, dark, and shrunken, and the basal cell layer may not be identified. The atrophic glands can have irregular luminal contours especially in cases of partial atrophy and postatrophic hyperplasia. There may be admixed small dark acini and ones with more abundant clear cytoplasm, especially in partial atrophy. Mild nuclear atypia may be seen. Additionally, luminal features such as eosinophilic secretions, basophilic mucins, and crystalloids may occasionally be seen in atrophy, although if all three of these features are present in the same focus, adenocarcinoma is the more likely diagnosis. Some small acinar carcinomas are composed of small shrunken cells simulating atrophy.[425-427] The atrophic pattern may be focal or rarely extensive. These "atrophic carcinomas" can be a particular challenge in differential diagnosis (see later section). The key features to support a diagnosis of carcinoma include the degree of infiltration beyond what could be acceptable for atrophy and the presence of nuclear atypia. Basal cell markers will be completely negative in atrophic carcinoma, and often, racemase overexpression is noted, although some studies have suggested that atrophic carcinomas are less likely to express racemase than nonatrophic ones. It should be noted that in partial atrophy,

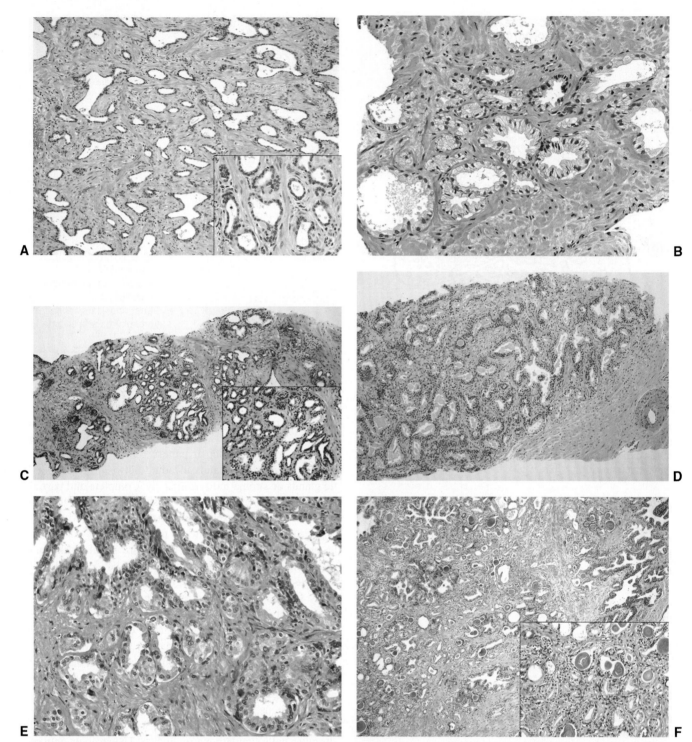

Figure 9-98 ■ Benign mimickers of prostate cancer with small gland pattern. Atrophy with pseudoinfiltrative growth (**A and inset**), partial atrophy (**B**), postatrophic hyperplasia (**C and inset**), atypical adenomatous hyperplasia (**D**), seminal vesicle epithelium (**E**), and verumontanum mucosal gland hyperplasia (**F and inset**).

one may see an absence of basal cells and some racemase overexpression, although the staining pattern of the latter is usually more patchy and weaker and displays less luminal/subluminal accentuation than carcinoma.

Adenosis (AAH) consists of a completely or partially circumscribed proliferation of small glands lined by cuboidal clear cells with bland nuclear features.[212-217,277] Basal cells are

present, but they may be difficult to appreciate on routine stains. This lesion can mimic small acinar carcinoma. Key points separating adenosis from carcinoma are the relative circumscription of the proliferating small glands and their relationship to larger parent glands along with the bland appearance of the acinar lining cells. Some examples of adenosis may show abnormal luminal contents (eosinophilic secretions, mucin, crystalloids), but these are more commonly present in carcinoma. Basal cell markers are useful in establishing a correct diagnosis. The acini in adenosis usually have a discontinuous pattern of basal cells. Sometimes, individual acini may lack basal cells, but these are admixed with other acini displaying a complete or incomplete basal cell layer. It is important not to overinterpret a few small glands without basal cells as malignant ones. Racemase staining may be seen in 18% of examples of AAH although the staining pattern is usually weak and focal.

Seminal vesicle, especially in needle biopsies, can be confused with small glandular carcinoma especially when this tissue is crushed or tangentially cut.[219] The seminal vesicle is composed of ducts with surrounding acinar tissue. The central often dilated glands of seminal vesicle may not be appreciated in small biopsy cores, and only the peripheral acini are seen. Atypical epithelial lining cells are often noted. This pattern can be overdiagnosed as carcinoma. The low-power architecture, the spotty distribution of atypical epithelial cells, and the presence of prominent cytoplasmic lipochrome pigment point to a diagnosis of seminal vesicle. Immunohistochemistry can be helpful as well. Seminal vesicle epithelium stains positively for PSA, and basal cells are identified with the appropriate markers.

Carcinomas can be composed of medium to large simple glands with an amphophilic or clear appearance. The tumor may exhibit a vaguely or on rare occasion, a distinct nodular appearance and may show cystic dilatation of glands. These patterns of carcinoma may simulate nodular hyperplasia, and hence, terms such as pseudohyperplastic and cystic carcinoma have been used (see later section).[420-422] Pseudohyperplastic carcinoma is often difficult to diagnose in needle biopsies. The acini show less circumscription than typical nodular hyperplasia, and sometimes, a subtle pattern of infiltration between nonneoplastic glands is present. Both hyperplasia and pseudohyperplastic carcinomas contain tall cuboidal to columnar cells often with abundant clear cytoplasm, but nodular hyperplasia displays a basal cell layer. The nuclei of hyperplasia are bland, while those of carcinoma show nuclear atypia with prominent nucleoli. Abnormal luminal products are often present in the pseudohyperplastic carcinoma, and it may be the secretion that draws one's eyes to the glands in question. Basal cell markers and racemase may assist in arriving at the correct diagnosis.

Large glands with a cribriform morphology are typical of clear cell cribriform hyperplasia and in some forms of basal cell hyperplasia, especially those with an adenoid cystic-like morphology (Fig. 9-99). Both of these patterns of hyperplasia have a nodular low-power morphology, and they are

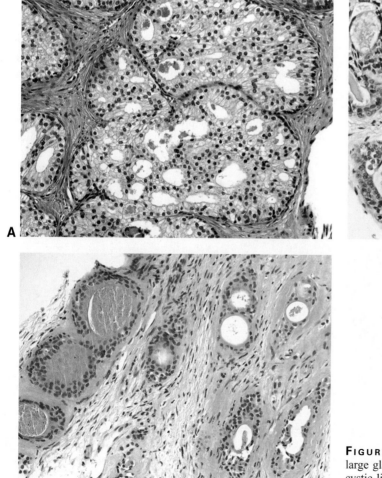

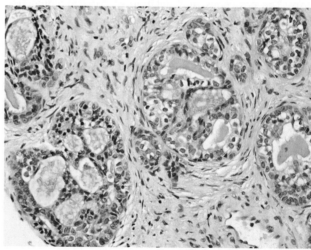

FIGURE 9-99 ■ Benign mimickers of prostate cancer with large gland pattern. Clear cell cribriform hyperplasia (**A**), adenoid cystic-like basal cell hyperplasia (**B**), and reactive atypia in the setting of ischemia (**C**).

usually associated with some degree of stromal hyperplasia as well. In clear cell cribriform hyperplasia, the architecture and cytology are very uniform. Basal cell hyperplasia with cribriform morphology may show some degree of nuclear atypia, but the usual high-grade nuclear changes seen in cribriform carcinoma are not present. The latter tumors usually have medium to large amphophilic glands and show significant architectural and cytologic irregularity. Large glands with reactive features associated with inflammation or ischemia may also simulate malignancy. The glands may be somewhat distorted and cytologically atypical, but they do not show true infiltration, and the associated benign process (if recognized) points to a correct diagnosis.

Some benign mimickers may be mistaken for the fused glandular pattern of carcinoma (Fig. 9-100).[219] For instance, a paraganglion is composed of very tightly packed cell clusters, often with an amphophilic color. On cursory inspection, this structure may be interpreted as a focus of fused carcinoma. Careful inspection of paraganglia, however, shows that the cell clusters are separated by a very delicate network of capillaries. The cells of paraganglia are bland and show no nuclear atypia. On occasion, there may be some admixed ganglion cells, and these can have a large central nucleolus and may be mistaken for carcinoma cells. Often, there are associated nerves, which help to establish the correct diagnosis. The erroneous interpretation of paraganglionic tissue not only can lead to a false-positive diagnosis but can also result in grading and staging errors. For instance, when there is a carcinoma composed of separate acini (Gleason 3) and a paraganglion is interpreted as Gleason 4, the tumor would be erroneously graded as Gleason score 7 (primary 3, secondary 4). Furthermore, if a tumor was otherwise organ confined except for a periprostatic paraganglion incorrectly interpreted as carcinoma, then the tumor would be incorrectly staged as pT3a rather than pT2.

Xanthogranulomatous inflammation (prostatic xanthoma) and malakoplakia rarely affect the prostate gland, and both of these lesions may, at least on low power, resemble Gleason pattern 4B (hypernephroid) carcinoma. This pattern may, on occasion, display rather bland nuclear features, which adds to the challenge. Both forms of granulomatous inflammation and 4B carcinoma can have an irregular growth pattern, but the carcinoma shows more destructive features and generally shows at least focal atypia. The xanthoma cells have very tiny dark nuclei with no appreciable atypia. The von Hansemann histiocytes of malakoplakia will often be mixed with other inflammatory cells including neutrophils, lymphocytes, and plasma. Furthermore, the telltale Michaelis-Gutmann bodies are generally found on closer inspection. In some difficult cases, immunohistochemistry for epithelial and macrophage markers will resolve the differential diagnosis.

Other inflammatory processes such as usual idiopathic granulomatous prostatitis or nonspecific prostatitis with crush artifacts may resemble solid high-grade (Gleason 5) adenocarcinoma (Fig. 9-101). Likewise, stromal cells and lymphocytes may undergo degenerative changes and have signet ring–like appearance, thus simulating a Gleason 5 carcinoma composed of dissociated single cells with an infiltrative appearance. Usually, the above changes are recognized as benign and inflammatory, but in some cases, immunohistochemistry for keratins, prostatic epithelial markers, and lymphohistiocytic markers is necessary to make a correct diagnosis.

The distinction between adenocarcinoma and HGPIN including topics such as atypical acini immediately adjacent to HGPIN (PIN-ATYP or PIN-ASAP) and PIN-like patterns of adenocarcinoma has been discussed in the earlier section on precursor lesions.[144,171]

There are other malignancies that occasionally enter the differential diagnosis of prostatic carcinoma. The prostate gland may be invaded by urothelial carcinoma of the bladder

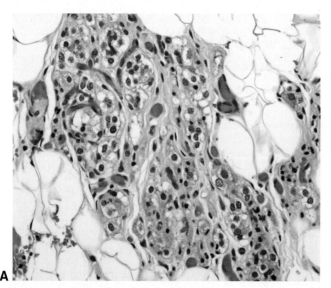

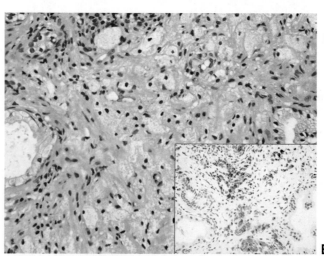

FIGURE 9-100 ■ Benign mimickers of prostate cancer with fused gland patterns. Paraganglion and **(A)** xanthoma confirmed by CD68 immunostaining **(inset) (B)**.

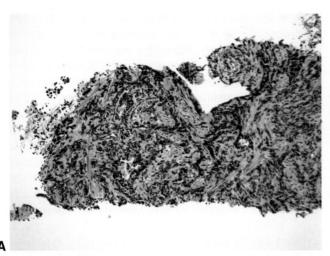
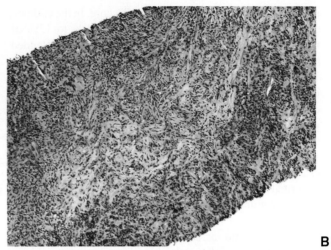

FIGURE 9-101 ■ Benign mimickers of prostate cancer with solid patterns. Usual prostatitis with crush artifacts and **(A)** idiopathic granulomatous prostatitis **(B)**.

or urethra or, on rare occasion, may be primarily involved by urothelial carcinoma (see Chapter 10). Such tumors may be mistaken for high-grade prostatic adenocarcinoma. Glandular differentiation in the urothelial carcinoma can add further confusion to this picture. While both high-grade urothelial carcinoma and solid prostate carcinoma can have sheet-like diffuse growth patterns, the urothelial carcinomas tend to be composed of cells with more polygonal shapes compared to the rounded shapes of prostatic carcinoma. Urothelial carcinomas also show a greater degree of nuclear pleomorphism and less regularly prominent nucleoli than high-grade prostate carcinoma. Sometimes, urothelial carcinoma in situ is present in prostatic ducts and acini, and this is a helpful feature supporting a diagnosis of urothelial carcinoma. In some cases, the two tumors can have an identical appearance on routine staining, and in those situations, marker studies are required to arrive at a correct diagnosis. Prostatic epithelial markers (PSA, PAP, prostein, NKX3.1) and urothelial markers (34BE12, CK7, uroplakin, GATA3) are included in a panel to resolve this differential diagnosis. It is important to get the correct diagnosis since urothelial carcinoma and prostatic carcinoma have completely different therapeutic approaches.

Colorectal adenocarcinoma can involve the prostate gland directly or by metastasis. The resultant pattern can resemble the large glandular (ductal) pattern of prostatic carcinoma. The elongated cigar-shaped nuclei and "dirty" necrosis favor a diagnosis of colonic carcinoma. A marker panel including prostatic epithelial markers and lower gastrointestinal tract markers (CK20, CDX2) may be used on difficult cases. On very rare occasions, one can have a primary urothelial-type adenocarcinoma involving the prostate gland.[348,349] These tumors can resemble secondary colonic carcinoma, and it is important to rule out the latter by radiologic and endoscopic means.

Metastatic involvement of the prostate by signet-ring carcinoma can simulate primary signet-ring carcinoma of the prostate. Clinical information can support the former. Metastatic signet-ring carcinoma of the prostate may originate in the stomach, elsewhere in the gastrointestinal tract, or in the bladder. When seen in the prostate, it does not usually have accompanying typical patterns of prostatic carcinoma that may be found in association with the primary signet-ring carcinomas of the prostate.[415,416] Furthermore, the vacuoles in metastatic signet-ring carcinoma are mucin positive, while those in signet-ring prostate carcinoma are usually mucin negative. Immunohistochemistry can be used to resolve difficult cases. Secondary renal carcinoma, especially clear cell carcinoma, can be confused with the hypernephroid pattern of prostatic carcinoma (Gleason 4B). Both can have sheet-like growth patterns, and both may show relatively bland nuclear features. In metastases, one can often identify lymphovascular space involvement, a finding that is uncommon in primary prostate carcinoma. Clinical history and immunohistochemical markers will generally resolve the differential diagnosis.

In addition to carcinomas, other tumors such as metastatic melanoma and large cell lymphoma may rarely affect the prostate gland and enter the differential diagnosis of a high-grade solid carcinoma. Usually, these tumors bear only a superficial resemblance to carcinoma, and one should have a high index of suspicion in such cases. Careful routine microscopy coupled with knowledge of the clinical history and an appropriate panel of immunohistochemical markers will lead to the right diagnosis.

Diagnosis of Minimal Adenocarcinoma and Atypical Small Acinar Proliferation (Glandular Atypia)

The diagnosis of a minute focus of adenocarcinoma is often a challenge, especially when it represents the only evidence of malignancy.[271,272,282] Minimal or limited adenocarcinoma can be defined as a solitary tumor focus measuring <1 mm in length and/or <5% of the length of the core. In the authors' experience, minimal cancers account for 10% to 15% of newly diagnosed adenocarcinomas in the era of extended biopsy samples (10 to 14 cores).[154]

Small atypical glandular foci should be approached in a logical, algorithmic fashion. The importance of technically excellent histology cannot be overemphasized, especially when dealing with thin-core needle biopsies. Careful and consistent fixation, embedding, microtomy, and staining are required to produce the high-quality slides necessary to establish a definitive diagnosis when there is only a small abnormal focus. It is especially important to be conservative in microtomy and not to cut excessively deep sections, thereby trimming through a small area of concern. Many histology laboratories save intervening unstained sections between the usual H&E-stained levels so that immunohistochemistry can be performed if required.

Careful, systematic screening of the sections using low-power microscopy will generally identify the focus of concern. The major and minor diagnostic criteria, as described above, are used to establish a diagnosis of minimal carcinoma, and in many cases, immunohistochemistry is also carried out. In most instances, this approach will allow one to make a confident diagnosis of adenocarcinoma. In the great majority of cases, the abnormal lesion consists of single separate acini (Gleason pattern 3); however, in about 10% of cases, the atypical focus consists of higher-grade patterns including poorly formed, fused, and cribriform glands or solid, cord-like, and single cell morphologies. Before making a definitive diagnosis of adenocarcinoma, it is important to remember the diverse benign mimickers and other neoplastic conditions that may simulate adenocarcinoma (see above section) and to make sure that the lesion of concern does not represent one of those conditions.

The issue of quantity of abnormality often arises, especially when assessing a tiny focus of atypical single separate glands. Most minimal carcinomas consist of 10 to 20 abnormal glands. Is there a minimum number of atypical acini required to make a diagnosis of adenocarcinoma? This question is difficult to address and should dealt with on a case-by-case basis. In some instances, especially if there is obvious cancer in other cores, a diagnosis of microfocal carcinoma can be made on the basis of a single atypical acinus. However, if an initial diagnosis of carcinoma is being made, one may want to be more conservative. Notwithstanding a few very rare situations, most urologic pathologists like to see two or more atypical acini preferably with supportive marker studies, to establish a diagnosis of carcinoma.

In situations where one cannot confidently diagnose an atypical focus as carcinoma, the term ASAP or glandular atypia may be used.[144,154,161,163,165,168,169,621,622] In primary biopsy practices, ASAP accounts for 1% to 5% of cases.[144,161] Rates higher than 5% suggest that minimal carcinomas are likely being underdiagnosed. In the authors' experience, the ASAP rate is about 2% or one in fifty cases.[154]

It is important to understand that ASAP is not a specific diagnosis; it is a term indicating to the urologist or oncologist uncertainty regarding a diagnosis of carcinoma. The term is used because an abnormality is very limited in amount and/or a confounding factor such as crush artifact or obscuring inflammation is present. In most instances, ASAP represents undersampled carcinoma, but in some cases, it represents a benign mimicker that is not clearly diagnostic (Figs. 9-102 to 9-104). ASAP is not a term that should be used loosely for any "atypical" lesion. It should be reserved for reasonably worked-up cases where there are insufficient criteria to confidently diagnose either carcinoma or a specific mimicker such as partial atrophy. Undoubtedly, one pathologist's ASAP is another pathologist's minimal carcinoma, as evidenced by the range of prevalence rates. In the experience of the authors, many consultation cases with diagnoses of ASAP are converted to limited carcinomas or benign mimickers, especially partial atrophy or adenosis.

What is a reasonable workup in a case of putative ASAP? Additional "gentle" block levels are sometimes useful in clarifying the morphology. Marker studies carried out on additional sections or saved intervening sections often help one make a definitive diagnosis. Basal cell markers and racemase stains are very useful in establishing a definitive diagnosis. Consultation with a colleague, especially one with expertise in urologic pathology, or obtaining a formal external consultation can be useful.

Patients with a diagnosis of ASAP are often rebiopsied in 3 to 12 months. Follow-up biopsies show adenocarcinoma in 35% to 60% of cases. When ASAP is accompanied by multifocal high-grade PIN, the likelihood of detecting carcinoma is even higher.[154,169,171,622,623] Some authors have subdivided ASAP into cases that are suspicious for malignancy and those of uncertain significance, but this subclassification does not appear to have any prognostic significance. If the specific location of the ASAP is known, it is useful to suggest that the subsequent biopsies be directed at the site of abnormality and that additional cores be taken from the involved site and the immediately adjacent ones. Patients who have negative second biopsies can generally be followed with clinical exam and serum PSA, and a decision regarding further biopsies can be based on changes in those parameters. Some patients with ASAP and high PSA may be pursued more aggressively with techniques such as saturation biopsies. Radical treatment procedures should not be performed on the basis of an ASAP diagnosis. Such therapies should only be entertained when there is an established malignant diagnosis.

Intraductal Carcinoma of the Prostate

Background

Intraepithelial spread of prostatic carcinoma within preexisting nonneoplastic ducts or acini is known as IDC.[350-353] This phenomenon is characterized by preservation of basal cells and is now widely regarded as tumor progression succedent to prostate cancer invasion. The alternate hypothesis

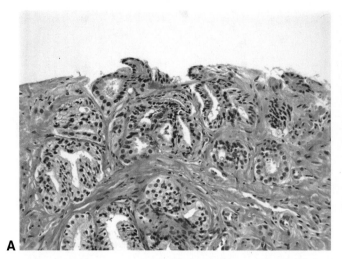

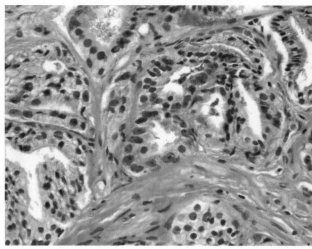

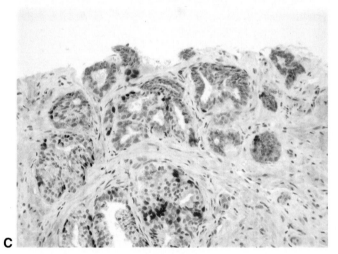

FIGURE 9-102 ■ **A–C:** Atypical small acinar proliferation. **A,B:** Some small atypical glands show nucleomegaly and prominent nucleoli. **C:** Despite AMACR overexpression, some glands exhibit basal cell marker staining.

of IDC as carcinomatous evolution from HGPIN preceding invasion is less accepted, since IDC is more often seen in higher-grade and higher-stage cancers.[354] Diagnosis of IDC in routine practice has so far been limited by its problematic distinction from HGPIN and its almost invariable coexistence with high-grade invasive cancers where IDC is likely to be discounted. IDC as an isolated finding is rare, and its clinical implication is still currently under discussion.

The first description of IDC is credited to Kovi et al.[355] in 1985, wherein they reported 48% of 123 prostate glands with cancer to contain IDC. IDC patterns were likely to have been accounted previously as Gleason pattern 4 or 5 invasive cancers. Identification and subsequent characterization of IDC have been greatly facilitated with the advent of immunostaining for basal cells.[354] And for a while, IDC was mired with controversy because of its overlap with the putative cancer precursor lesion HGPIN (or intraductal dysplasia), both distinguished from invasive cancer by retention of basal cells. In fact, initial studies have lumped HGPIN and IDC together, particularly in those that exhibit cribriform architectures.[355–357] As detailed below, IDC and HGPIN have differing molecular biology and associated pathologic variables. IDC was initially distinguished from HGPIN by the

presence of intraluminal encroachment of tumor mass.[354,358] More contemporary criteria for morphologic diagnosis of IDC,[359,360] mainly to differentiate from HGPIN, and understanding its adverse pathologic variables and poorer behavior[355,356,358,359,361–363] have led to better recognition of this entity.

Incidence

IDC is often encountered admixed with invasive cancer and is reported in 18% of RP with cancers.[361] The incidence of IDC is higher in RP with higher-stage (pT3) cancers at 43%.[362] Only three cases of IDC without concurrent invasive cancer on RP have been described, including one that spread outside of the prostate via the ejaculatory ducts.[363,364]

Early studies preceding the PSA era identified IDC in 20% of needle biopsies with cancers.[355] More contemporary studies reported an overall incidence of 2.8% for IDC in needle biopsies.[365] IDC as an isolated finding is even rarer, reported in only 0.26% of needle biopsies.[365]

Clinical Significance

Distinction of IDC from HGPIN is critical because of the adverse pathologic variables associated with IDC. Studies

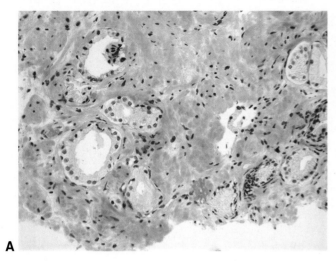

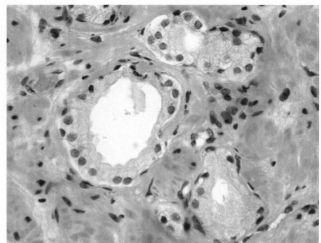

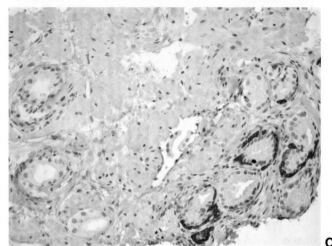

FIGURE 9-103 ■ **A-C:** ASAP, favor benign. **A,B:** Small crowded glands, luminal undulations, and pale cytoplasm (resembling partial atrophy). **C:** The atypical glands lack basal cell marker staining.

had shown a strong association between IDC and high Gleason score, large tumor volume, advanced tumor stage, positive surgical margin, extensive PNI, and treatment failure.[355,356,358,361,362] Multivariate analysis confirms IDC as an independent prognostic indicator in prostate cancer over preoperative serum PSA, Gleason score, tumor volume and stage.[356,361,362] These findings warrant that IDC should be lumped clinically with invasive cancers.

Interestingly, in neoplasia with cribriform patterns, IDC was shown to have higher risk for PSA failure than cribriform cancer.[356] This suggests that IDC may represent a more advanced tumor progression than cribriform cancer without ductal/acinar spread. Further, although IDC is associated with larger tumor volume, serum PSA is lower compared to cancers without ductal/acinar spread.[361]

Only a few studies have examined IDC as an isolated finding in needle biopsy.[359,363] Isolated IDC in needle biopsy treated with definitive therapy after diagnosis resulted in 12% disease progression, 6% metastasis, and additional 6% with PSA failure after follow-up.[363] Corresponding RP of needle biopsies with isolated IDC showed higher-stage cancers including 38% with EPE and 14% with seminal vesicle extension.[363]

There is controversy regarding the management of IDC encountered in NCB without invasive cancer. Some advocate definitive management including resection, hormonal therapy, or radiation therapy (RT) immediately following diagnosis of IDC even without invasive cancer,[359,360,363] while some suggest immediate repeat biopsy be performed,[366] which very likely will result to detection and definitive diagnosis of invasive cancer. This latter approach may prevent the serious consequence of overtreating a misdiagnosed HGPIN as IDC.

Morphology

The criteria for histologic diagnosis of IDC proposed by Cohen et al.[360] are presented in Table 9-12. The first four major criteria are always present, and the minor criteria are helpful in making the diagnosis.[360] A more simplified diagnostic approach to IDC proposed by Guo and Epstein[359] is by identifying large acini and ducts containing basal cells filled with malignant epithelial cells that show solid or dense cribriform patterns. If the luminal pattern is loose cribriform or micropapillary, marked nuclear atypia (≥6×) or nonfocal comedonecrosis is required.[359] These criteria are essentially

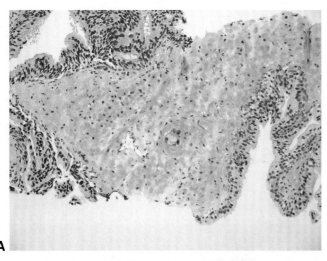

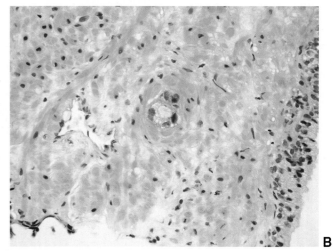

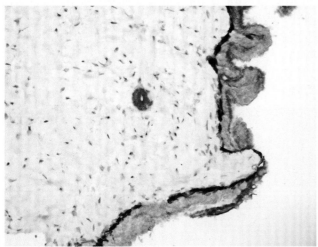

FIGURE 9-104 ■ ASAP, highly suspicious for carcinoma. A single small gland with nucleomegaly, prominent nucleoli, luminal mucin **(A,B)**, AMACR overexpression, and absent basal cell marker staining is likely undersampled carcinoma **(C)**.

for distinction of IDC from HGPIN, and the high threshold is meant to avoid overdiagnosis of HGPIN as IDC.

IDC is often encountered associated with invasive prostate cancer (Fig. 9-105). Glands of IDC are larger, are expansile, may be irregularly shaped, and may exhibit extension or gland branching (Fig. 9-106). The architecture of IDC is most commonly cribriform, that is, either dense (small holes, 70%) or loose (large holes, 63%), and can be solid (44%) or micropapillary (19%) (Fig. 9-107).[359] There can be overlap in patterns of HGPIN and IDC, but when

the nuclear atypia far exceeds HGPIN, the lesion is considered IDC (Fig. 9-108). Luminal necrosis may occur in IDC (Fig. 9-109). The presence of basal cells is *sine qua non* to the diagnosis of IDC. Using the proposed criteria, diagnoses of IDC can be made readily when surrounding basal cells

Table 9-12 ■ CRITERIA FOR DIAGNOSIS OF IDC
Major Criteria
Large glands (>2× normal), presence of basal cells (confirmed by immunohistochemistry), cytologically malignant cells with frequent mitosis, cells spanning gland lumen, comedonecrosis
Minor Criteria
Right-angle gland branching, round smooth gland contour, frequently two population of cells

Reprinted from Cohen RJ, et al. A proposal on the identification, histologic reporting, and implications of intraductal prostatic carcinoma. *Arch Pathol Lab Med* 2007;131:1103–1109, with permission.

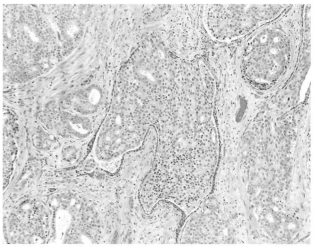

FIGURE 9-105 ■ IDC with associated invasive adenocarcinoma.

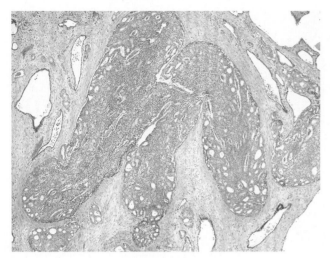

FIGURE 9-106 ■ IDC filling large ducts.

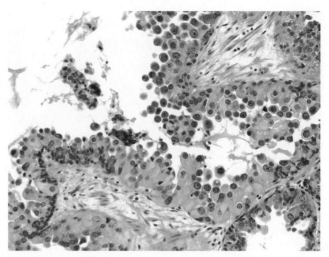

FIGURE 9-108 ■ IDC with nonpapillary growth and marked nuclear atypia.

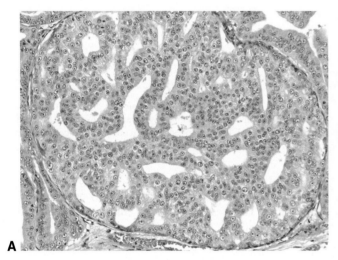

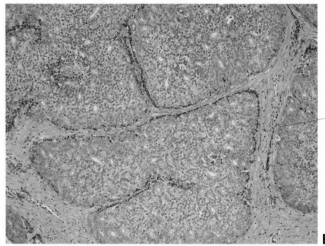

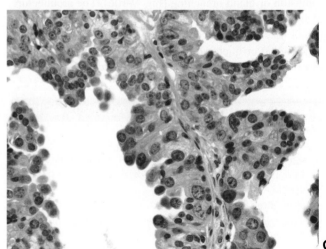

FIGURE 9-107 ■ Different patterns of IDC. Cribriform **(A)**, solid **(B)**, and micropapillary **(C)**.

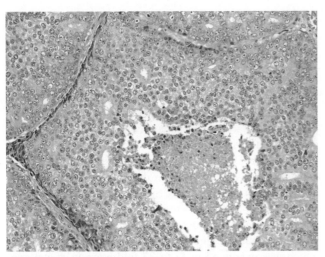

FIGURE 9-109 ■ IDC with central tumor cell necrosis.

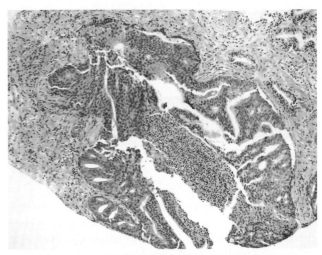

FIGURE 9-111 ■ IDC with central necrosis in needle biopsy.

are obvious on H&E, but this is not always the case. Prior to the advent of immunostaining, IDC with less discernible basal cells may easily be called as Gleason pattern 3 or 4 (i.e., cribriform) or 5 (i.e., solid or comedonecrosis) cancers. Basal cell marker immunostains (e.g., p63, HMWK) in IDC may show complete or partial basal cells, both acceptable in the diagnosis. Similar to cancer and HGPIN, racemase is overexpressed in IDC (Fig. 9-110).

IDC is a rare finding in needle biopsy (Fig. 9-111). Isolated large glands with cribriform architecture in needle biopsy may have problematic features borderline between IDC and HGPIN. An alternative diagnostic term of *atypical cribriform lesion* has been proposed for this lesion and should warrant a repeat biopsy.[350,367] Ductal adenocarcinoma occasionally contains basal cells and is distinguished from cribriform or micropapillary IDC by its tall columnar and pseudostratified cells. Intraductal spread of poorly differentiated urothelial carcinoma may mimic solid IDC. Urothelial carcinoma expresses p63 and HMWK, which are expressed in basal cells of IDC. Benign differential diagnoses of IDC such as cribriform hyperplasia and central zone glands do not exhibit the high-grade cytology of IDC.

At this juncture, the concept of intraductal or acinar spread of cancer is still evolving, and several issues in IDC remain unresolved. It is unclear if IDC should be diagnosed separately in RP with Gleason 4 or 5 cancers that would warrant basal cell immunostaining. Whether to retain Gleason grading of IDC based on its intraluminal patterns similar to invasive cancers is not settled. Further, it is unclear if unusual forms such as partial ducts/acini involvement, simpler spread (e.g., flat or tufted), or low-grade cytology occur in IDC. Although these are theoretically possible, the answers may remain elusive until separation between spread and de novo evolution of cancer within ducts/acini can be made with certainty.

Molecular Features

Certain molecular features distinguish IDC from HGPIN and invasive cancers.[368–371] LOH studies showed 60% allelic loss in IDC compared to only 9% in HGPIN.[368] Multiple allelic losses are usual in IDC than in HGPIN.[368] By CGH, most IDC has chromosomal imbalance, mainly losses, which in one study was absent in HGPIN.[369] LOH of *TP53* is present in 60% of IDC and in only 30% of HGPIN, and LOH of *RB1* is present in 81% of IDC and 53% of HGPIN.[369] *PTEN* is down-regulated in IDC, and 84% shows loss of cytoplasmic PTEN expression, which is not observed in HGPIN.[369,370] Immunohistochemical detection of PTEN can be useful to distinguishing IDC from HGPIN,[370] although this needs to be validated.

The main genomic difference between IDC and HGPIN is in the occurrence of TMPRSS2:ERG fusion. Most IDC (75%) shows ERG rearrangement which is detected in only approximately 20% of HGPIN and shown to be absent in isolated HGPIN.[371]

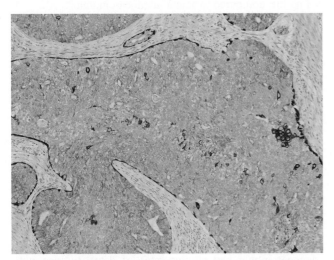

FIGURE 9-110 ■ Immunostain cocktail for HMWK, p63, and AMACR in IDC shows an intact basal cell layer (*brown*) and increased expression of AMACR (*red*).

Interestingly, LOH studies showed higher allelic loss and LOH of TP53 and RB1 in IDC than invasive cancers.[368,369] This further supports the idea that IDC represents a more advanced form of tumor progression than invasive cancer.

SPECIAL VARIANTS AND VARIATIONS OF ADENOCARCINOMA

Ductal Adenocarcinoma

Introduction

Ductal adenocarcinoma is a carcinoma of prostatic epithelial cell origin characterized by large glandular and papillary growths that (by definition) are lined by tall columnar cells that often exhibit nuclear pseudostratification or palisading.[372–381] This tumor was previously referred to as endometrioid adenocarcinoma of the prostate because of its morphologic resemblance to female endometrioid carcinoma.[374–376,378,382] Initially, ductal adenocarcinoma was thought to arise from the müllerian-derived prostatic utricle, and some tumors do occur at the central aspect of the prostate encompassing the area of utricle.[372,373,382] It is now widely accepted that ductal adenocarcinoma is of prostatic acinar cell origin supported by its overlap in zonal derivation (some arises also in the peripheral zone), spatial relationship (commonly mixed), similar immunohistochemical profile, and molecular concordance with acinar adenocarcinoma.[374,375,378–380,383–385] Ductal adenocarcinoma may occur either as a pure ductal tumor or more commonly in combination with acinar adenocarcinoma, reported in 47% to 80% of cases.[372,374,375,378,381] Diagnosis as ductal adenocarcinoma requires a predominant (>80%) or pure histology of the entire tumor when appreciated in TUR or RP specimens. Thus, definitive diagnosis in needle biopsy is not tenable and diagnosis of "adenocarcinoma with ductal features" is recommended.

Epidemiology

Ductal adenocarcinoma is rare, yet it is considered to be the most common histologic variant of prostatic adenocarcinoma. "Pure" ductal adenocarcinoma accounts for 0.2% to 1.3% of all prostate cancers.[372,374,377] Mixed ductal and acinar adenocarcinoma is more common and is reported in 1.7% to 5% of prostate cancers.[377,380] More contemporary studies show presence of ductal component in 0.5% to 12.7% of prostate cancers.[386,387] The patients' mean age is 60 to 72 years with range of 41 to 89 years or of similar age group to acinar adenocarcinoma.[372,374,375,377–381,387] Interestingly, SEER data show that ductal adenocarcinoma is more common than acinar adenocarcinoma in patients above 70 years old in the United States.[388]

Molecular Biology

It is unclear if there are significant differences in TMPRSS2:ERG gene rearrangement between ductal and acinar adenocarcinoma. One study identified TMPRSS2:ERG fusion less frequently in pure ductal adenocarcinoma (11%) and mixed ductal and acinar adenocarcinoma (5%) compared to pure acinar adenocarcinoma (45%).[383] When present in ductal adenocarcinoma, 75% of TMPRSS2:ERG fusions occur through deletion.[383] Another concurrent study however identified TMPRSS2:ERG fusion in ductal adenocarcinoma at about the same frequency (50%) as acinar adenocarcinoma.[385] Ductal and acinar adenocarcinomas have similer DNA ploidy abnormalities.[377] Interestingly, analysis from whole sections of ductal and acinar adenocarcinomas identified only 25 gene transcripts whose expression was significantly different, showing striking similarities between these two tumors at the level of gene expression.[389] One differentially expressed transcript is prolactin receptor, which was expressed in 5- to 27-fold more in ductal adenocarcinoma.[389] SPINK1, which is overexpressed in about 11% of ETS fusion-negative prostate carcinomas and suggested to be an unfavorable clinical parameter, was shown to be overexpressed in 22% of ETS fusion-negative ductal adenocarcinomas.[385]

Clinical Features

Ductal adenocarcinoma arises in the central and peripheral aspects of the prostate and may manifest accordingly in two clinical forms. Centrally located tumors involve the periurethral area and transition zone and can be encountered in TUR specimens. The tumor may also occasionally protrude into the urethra as a cystoscopically visible polypoid mass. Peripheral tumors primarily involve the peripheral zone but may also extend into the transition zone. Central or periurethral tumors may present with obstructive symptoms and hematuria, whereas peripherally located tumors may be detected on abnormal DRE and elevated serum PSA levels. A majority of patients with ductal adenocarcinoma have elevated serum PSA but are 2.4 times more likely to have PSA < 4 ng/mL compared to acinar adenocarcinoma.[388]

Ductal adenocarcinoma is suggested to have a more aggressive clinical behavior than acinar adenocarcinoma.[376,377,381,386–388,390] More patients with ductal adenocarcinoma present with higher-stage disease. A ductal adenocarcinoma component on biopsy, particularly if comprising >10% of the tumor, is significantly associated with EPE and seminal vesicle invasion (SVI) on subsequent prostatectomy.[386,387] EPE and seminal vesicle involvement are encountered in 64% and 12% of prostatectomy specimens, respectively.[386] Also, the presence of ductal morphology in biopsies indicates a shortened progression time compared to Gleason 7 or less acinar adenocarcinoma.[386] In a report of 371 ductal adenocarcinomas, a higher rate of distant metastasis was encountered in ductal (12%) than acinar (4%) adenocarcinoma.[388] Data from SEER show that men with ductal adenocarcinoma had similar rates of death to men with Gleason 4 + 4 acinar adenocarcinoma.[390] The overall 5-year survival rate of ductal adenocarcinoma in older series was only 15% to 24%.[372,374] Metastasis is encountered in 12% to 50% of ductal adenocarcinoma, mostly to the lymph nodes, bone, and lungs.[377–379,381] Control of localized ductal adenocarcinoma with prostatectomy with radiotherapy and endocrine therapy yields disease-free survival, similar to acinar adenocarcinoma.[391,392] Ductal adenocarcinoma appears to be sensitive to hormonal manipulation.[378,392]

Pathology

Macroscopically, centrally located tumors can have exophytic friable fronds protruding into the urethral lumen around the prostatic utricle or verumontanum. Peripherally located tumors are most often situated posteriorly and can be appreciated as firm gray white parenchymal masses similar to acinar adenocarcinoma. These tumors are often grossly visible because of the higher stage of presentation.

Histologically, the main architectures of ductal adenocarcinomas are papillary, cribriform, individual glands, or solid growth patterns (Fig. 9-112). Combination of different patterns is common, often with papillary and cribriform patterns. Papillary and cribriform patterns are seen in 65% and 59% of peripherally situated ductal adenocarcinoma, respectively.[380] The neoplastic cells are distinctively tall columnar that can be in a single or pseudostratified cell layer (Fig. 9-113). The cytoplasm is usually amphophilic but can be pale or clear. The nucleus of ductal adenocarcinoma cells appears "higher-grade" compared to acinar adenocarcinoma (Fig. 9-114). The nucleus is typically elongated and usually has a prominent nucleolus. There is a greater degree of chromatin irregularities in ductal adenocarcinoma. Mitotic figures can be occasional or frequent. The tumor may also grow intraluminally into preexisting ducts retaining a "native" basal cell layer. An invasive component must be present to make the diagnosis of ductal adenocarcinoma. Negative staining for basal cell markers (e.g., HMWK, p63) immunohistochemistry is a must in the invasive component. The glands can also be very large, expansile, and crowded back-to-back. Evidence of invasiveness can be obvious such as background stromal fibrosis or PNI. About half of ductal adenocarcinomas are admixed with acinar adenocarcinoma (Fig. 9-115). Concomitant acinar adenocarcinomas are

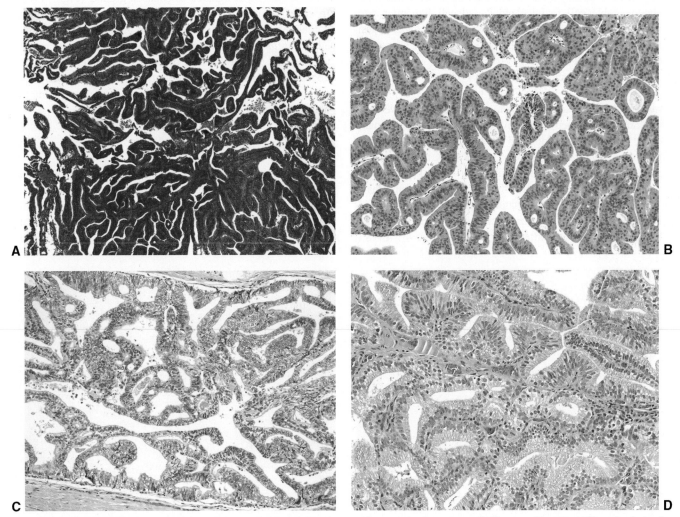

FIGURE 9-112 ■ Ductal adenocarcinoma exhibits papillae **(A)** with central cores **(B)**, cribriform architecture **(C)** and admixed individual glands **(D)**.

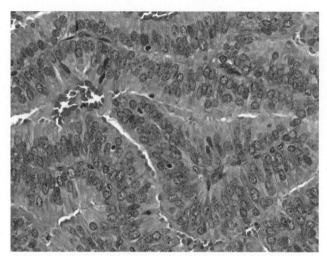

FIGURE 9-113 ■ Ductal adenocarcinoma is characterized by tall columnar cells with elongated nuclei that often exhibit pseudostratification.

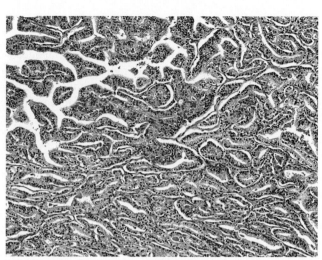

FIGURE 9-115 ■ Mixture of ductal adenocarcinoma (**top left**) and acinar adenocarcinoma (**bottom and right**). Ductal adenocarcinoma is distinguished by the tall columnar cells and papillae.

usually Gleason pattern 3.[381] Other rarer patterns have been described such as ductal adenocarcinoma with mucinous change, goblet cell, foamy gland, Paneth cell–like, micropapillary, and cystic change.[393,394] A subset of ductal adenocarcinomas may present as urethral polyps that can be adequately treated with TUR alone (Fig. 9-116).[395,396]

Ductal adenocarcinoma expresses PSA and PSAP.[374,378,379] AMACR is overexpressed in 77% of tumors (Fig. 9-117).[384] The majority of ductal adenocarcinomas lack basal cell layers and this can be confirmed by negative staining for basal cell markers.[384,397] By immunostaining, 31% of ductal adenocarcinomas have detectable basal cells by p63 or HMWK that are usually patchy or discontinuous in distribution.[386] This component is regarded as an intraductal growth of ductal adenocarcinoma.

According to the International Society of Urological Pathology (ISUP) consensus, ductal adenocarcinoma should be graded as Gleason pattern 4 or Gleason score $4 + 4 = 8$ if

the tumor is pure.[218] If luminal necrosis is present, then the focus should be designated as Gleason grade 5 (Fig. 9-118). In cases of mixed histology, the ductal adenocarcinoma component is to be assigned Gleason grade 4 and the acinar adenocarcinoma component graded according to its architecture, and the proportion of each component should be documented. Because of the common admixture with acinar adenocarcinoma, the diagnosis of ductal adenocarcinoma in needle biopsy is not possible (Fig. 9-119).

Differential Diagnosis

Distinction between ductal adenocarcinoma and HGPIN can be very difficult in limited samples. The micropapillary, cribriform, and flat patterns of HGPIN can mimic ductal adenocarcinoma due to overlap in architecture. Unlike ductal adenocarcinoma, HGPIN typically lacks the predominance

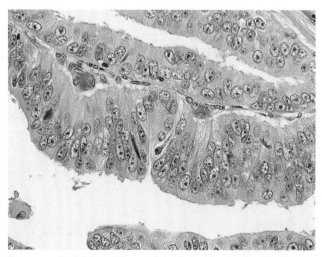

FIGURE 9-114 ■ The nuclei of ductal adenocarcinoma are typically "higher grade" compared to acinar adenocarcinoma.

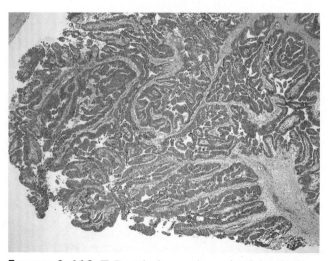

FIGURE 9-116 ■ Ductal adenocarcinoma involving the prostatic urethra.

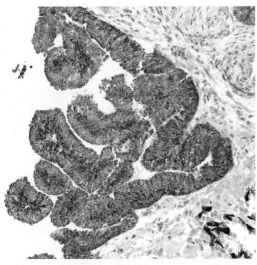

FIGURE 9-117 ■ Cocktail of HMWK, p63 (*brown*), and AMACR (*red*) shows overexpression of AMACR and complete absence of basal cells in this adenocarcinoma with ductal features in biopsy.

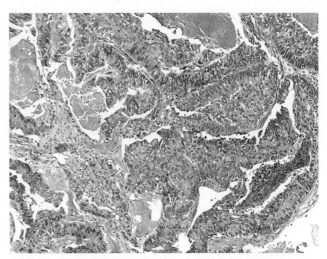

FIGURE 9-118 ■ Gleason pattern 5 ductal adenocarcinoma with abundant comedo necrosis.

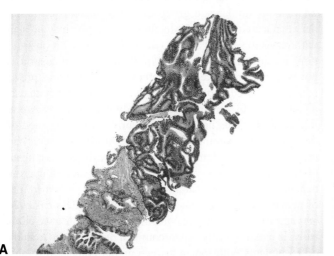

A

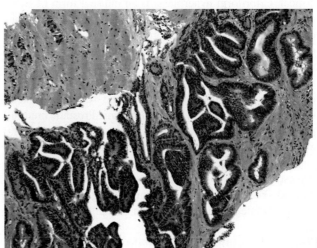

B

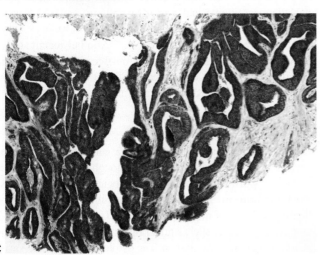

C

FIGURE 9-119 ■ Needle biopsies of adenocarcinoma with ductal features show cribriform patterns and papillae **(A,B)** with individual glands lined by tall columnar cells **(B)**. Diagnosis is confirmed by overexpression of AMACR and absence of basal cell immunostaining **(C)**.

of tall columnar cells and expansile large glandular growth pattern (not larger than native glands). Invasive features such as crowded back-to-back glands, stromal fibrosis, or PNI are absent in HGPIN. Among the patterns, micropapillary HGPIN cellular fronds lack a true fibrovascular core. Occasionally, the cells at the center of cribriform HGPIN glands tend to have lower nuclear grade. HGPIN consistently contains a basal cell layer highlighted by basal cell markers such as p63 or HMWK, in contrast to ductal adenocarcinoma where it is absent in a significant proportion of the glands.

Distinction from cribriform pattern (Gleason grade 4 or 5 if with necrosis), acinar adenocarcinoma can be problematic. There may be a significant overlap or perhaps a continuum between ductal adenocarcinoma and cribriform acinar adenocarcinoma within a tumor focus. Similar to ductal adenocarcinoma, cribriform acinar adenocarcinoma shows invasive features including large expansile growth and crowding. The morphologic definition of cribriform acinar adenocarcinoma is limited to invasive large cribriform glands lacking a "true" papillary component and tall columnar cells.

Some benign lesions in the prostate may also mimic ductal adenocarcinoma, and their distinction is much more critical. Cribriform hyperplasia is an unusual form of BPH composed of crowded cribriform glands. This lesion typically has a nodular pattern of growth. Unlike ductal adenocarcinoma, cribriform hyperplasia is composed of cells with uniformly bland cytology and often with clear cytoplasm and absent nucleoli. The basal cell layer is present and often discernible in cribriform hyperplasia, and basal cell markers are frequently not needed for confirmation. Prostatic urethral polyp is a reactive papillary lesion that grows into the urethra and is lined by cuboidal to columnar prostatic acinar cells and may mimic a centrally located ductal adenocarcinoma. Prostatic urethral polyp is more commonly seen in younger patients. These lesions have benign cytologic features (e.g., lack nucleomegaly, hyperchromasia, and high mitotic rate).

Mucinous (Colloid) Carcinoma

Introduction

Intraluminal mucin is a common finding and a helpful feature for detection and diagnosis of acinar adenocarcinoma. Mucin is detected in 38% to 93% of all prostatic carcinomas depending on which special staining technique is used.[398–401] Prostatic adenocarcinoma glands that secrete mucin may also develop a stromal reaction of fibrillary and nodular collagen deposits called collagenous micronodules which are considered one of the pathognomonic features of carcinoma and appreciated in 12.7% of cases.[302,303,402,403] Diagnosis of mucinous carcinoma however requires more copious extracellular mucin and follows strict criteria.[404–409] The diagnosis of mucinous carcinoma is made if (a) at least 25% of tumor cells are seen floating in lakes of extracellular mucin, (b) dilated or nondilated glands containing intraluminal mucinous materials are not accounted, (c) and extraprostatic origin of the tumor is ruled out. By these criteria, mucinous carcinoma is

rare comprising only 0.38% to 0.43% of all prostate carcinomas.[406–408] It is apparent with these criteria that the diagnosis of mucinous carcinoma is possible only in RP specimens, where examination of entire tumor can be made. In biopsies, the diagnosis of "adenocarcinoma with mucinous features" should be rendered. Interestingly, there seems to be a spatial association between collagenous micronodules and mucinous carcinoma seen in 64% of cases.[405]

Molecular Biology

TMPRSS2–ERG fusion is detected in mucinous carcinoma with a higher incidence of 83% compared to approximately 50% in acinar adenocarcinoma.[385] Interestingly, mucin production is one of the morphologic features shown to be associated with the presence of TMPRSS2–ERG fusion in prostate carcinoma.[97] As a consequence of the gene fusion, overexpression of ERG protein is confirmed to be present in 75% of mucinous carcinomas.[410]

Clinical Features

The patients' mean age is 56 years with a range of 44 to 70 years, a similar age group to that of patients with acinar adenocarcinoma.[405,406] Mucinous carcinoma may present with elevated serum PSA or symptomatically with obstruction, hematuria, or irritative symptoms.[407,408] Mucosuria is not typically encountered. Mucinous carcinoma was previously considered to be an aggressive variant of prostate carcinoma.[407,408] In an earlier small study before the PSA era, five of six patients had recurrence or metastasis or died of the disease.[408] In another study from 1990, all 12 patients had metastasis at presentation and 7 died of the disease at a mean of 56 months.[407] However, more recent data suggest that the behavior of mucinous carcinoma is probably similar to that of acinar adenocarcinoma when treated with RP or is even less aggressive.[405,406] More contemporary patients have clinically or pathologically organ-confined disease.[405,406] A study of 14 patients with mucinous carcinoma compared to acinar adenocarcinoma had 5-year overall survival and 5-year biochemical recurrence-free survival of 100% versus 93.8% and 100% versus 68%, respectively.[406] Another recent study showed a 5-year actuarial progression-free risk of 97.2% for mucinous carcinoma compared to 85.4% for nonmucinous prostate cancers (by Kattan nomogram).[405]

Pathology

Grossly, the tumor may have mucoid or gelatinous appearance particularly if mucin is abundant, although many tumors are without any distinctive features. Histologically, the tumor cells exhibit cribriform, anastomosing nests, tubules, or cords seen floating in pools of mucin (Fig. 9-120). Unlike mucinous carcinomas from other sites, signet ring cells are rarely present in prostatic mucinous carcinoma. The cytologic features are variable, and nuclei may have prominent nucleoli. Mitotic figures are not frequently seen. PAS, mucicarmine, and Alcian blue pH

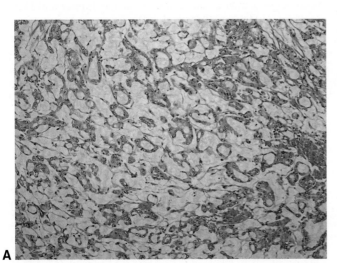
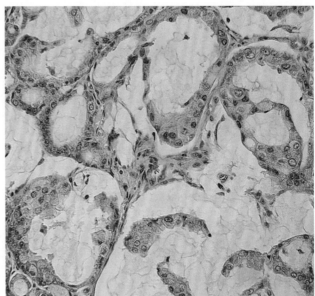

FIGURE 9-120 ■ Mucinous carcinoma of the prostate shows **(A)** copious amount of extracellular mucin and **(B)** fused or cribriform glands floating in mucin pools.

2.5 highlight the mucin in the tumor, which is often not necessary. Alcian blue reaction is decreased at pH 0.9 indicating presence of nonsulfated mucin. The vast majority of tumors are Gleason score 7 or higher, with 3 + 4 = 7 in 78.7% of cases.[405,406] ISUP consensus recommends grading pure irregular cribriform glands floating in mucin as 4 + 4 = 8.[218] However, there is no consensus on grading individual discrete glands present in mucin,[218] perhaps influenced by the contrasting tumor behavior shown in earlier and more recent studies. Mucinous carcinoma is invariably associated with acinar adenocarcinoma. The amount of the mucinous component varies and ranges from 25% to 90% (mean 52%). EPE is common with mucinous carcinoma and is nonfocal or established in 25.5% of cases.[405]

Mucinous carcinoma expresses PSA and PSAP and can be helpful in diagnosis of tumors at metastatic sites.[407,408] MUC2 is also expressed in mucinous carcinoma in contrast to nonmucinous prostatic carcinomas.[405,411]

Differential Diagnosis

Mucinous carcinoma may arise from other visceral organ sites such as urinary bladder, urachus, urethra, and large bowel, and secondary involvement of the prostate must be ruled out.[404] Mucinous carcinomas of colorectal and bladder origin usually exhibit intestinal-type appearances (i.e., tall columnar palisading or stratified cells) and express CDX2 and not PSA and PSAP, in contrast to prostatic mucinous carcinoma. Finding dysplastic glands or urothelial carcinoma (in cases of mixed tumor) at the urethra or urinary bladder surface mucosa is helpful in establishing such sites as the origin of a secondary prostatic tumor. Urinary bladder primary adenocarcinoma usually expresses CK7 and not CK20, whereas colorectal adenocarcinoma expresses CK20 and not CK7. Nuclear β-catenin is expressed in a subset of

colorectal adenocarcinomas, although its ubiquitous cytoplasmic staining makes interpretation difficult.

Mucinous metaplasia may occur in benign prostatic glands, but the mucin is intracellular and focal, and the cells contain unenlarged round regular nuclei and have discernible basal cells. Cowper gland has a lobular arrangement of glands composed of benign cells with intracellular mucin encountered at the apex often seen intermingled with sphincteric skeletal muscle cells.

Signet-Ring Cell Carcinoma

Introduction

Signet-ring cell carcinoma of the prostate is an aggressive and rare variant with only <60 cases reported in the literature.[412–416] The estimated incidence is 30 per 100,000 cases of prostate cancer.[416] This tumor is considered a variant of high-grade prostatic adenocarcinoma. There is no uniformity in the literature in terms of the amount of signet ring cells required to make the diagnosis. A cutoff of more than 25% of resected tumor showing signet ring cell morphology is being used as an arbitrary definition, since most of the published cases (85%) fulfill this definition.

Clinical Features

The patient ages are similar to those with acinar adenocarcinoma (range 50 to 85 years), and serum PSA is often elevated (mean 95.3 ng/mL).[416] The clinical presentation is also similar to acinar adenocarcinoma, but with a tendency to present at higher stage, including some presenting with metastasis. One meta-analysis and review of cases showed that 34% of patients had stage IV disease at presentation.[416] Prognosis is reported to be poor with a mean survival of only 29 months.

Pathology

The cells contain optically clear vacuoles that displace the nuclei and are widely infiltrative (Fig. 9-121). The intracytoplasmic vacuoles enlarge the cells, often with a single hole that displaces the nucleus. Most signet-ring cell carcinomas lack intracytoplasmic mucinous content, but some may have mucin either obvious or discernible with mucin stains. It is not clear if mucinous and nonmucinous signet-ring cell carcinomas are clinically distinct.[417] Typically, the tumors may have concurrent high-grade acinar adenocarcinoma (usually Gleason grade 4 or 5). The amount of signet ring cell component varies and may compose up to 80% of the tumor. The Gleason score ranges from 6 to 10 and is most commonly 8 (33%). HGPIN with optically clear vacuoles may also be seen associated with invasive tumor.

Differential Diagnosis

Morphologically, signet-ring cell carcinoma of the prostate if seen purely is indistinguishable from signet-ring cell carcinoma from the bladder or stomach. In the prostate, primary signet-ring cell carcinoma usually is admixed with acinar adenocarcinoma and expresses PSA and PSAP. Signet ring cell change may occur in lymphocytic infiltrates in chronic prostatitis or lymphoma involving the prostate, which is considered an artifactual change.[418,419] Lymphocytes expresses leukocyte common antigen (CD45) and is negative for epithelial marker, PSA or PSAP.

Pseudohyperplastic Carcinoma

Introduction

Pseudohyperplastic prostate carcinoma is a variant composed of enlarged and sometimes complex malignant glands that architecturally, and to a certain extent cytologically, resembles hyperplasia.[420–422] Pseudohyperplastic carcinoma is uncommon, encountered in 2% of cancers in needle biopsy and 11% of cancers in RP.[420–422] Because of its deceptive low-power magnification appearance, the diagnosis may become problematic, particularly in needle biopsy and TUR specimens. About half (45% to 57%) of pseudohyperplastic carcinomas may arise from the transition zone, which is the usual site for hyperplasia.[421,422] This variant invariably coexists with acinar adenocarcinoma often seen as contiguous foci or can be situated elsewhere in the prostate. When present, the amount of pseudohyperplastic features ranges from 2% to 80% (mean 22%) of the carcinoma.[422]

Clinical Features

The patient age ranges from 52 to 80 years (mean 64 years), which is a similar age group to that of patients with acinar adenocarcinoma.[422] Clinical follow-up studies are limited, and presentation may not be different from acinar adenocarcinoma. Since about half of the tumors are situated in the transition zone, it may present as an incidental finding in TUR specimens performed for BPH. One review of TUR specimens identified 1.3% with pseudohyperplastic carcinoma initially misdiagnosed as hyperplasia.[420] The clinical behavior is still unclear and perhaps is equivalent to that of Gleason score 6 carcinomas and also is influenced by the amount and grade of coexistent nonpseudohyperplastic carcinoma. One series identified EPE in 43% of cases.[422] In a few cases with follow-up, metastases were documented 3 to 4 years after diagnosis in needle biopsy.[420]

Pathology

The tumor is often nodular, particularly in the transition zone or clustered when in the peripheral zone, consisting of large-sized or dilated glands that may be branching or with papillary infoldings (Fig. 9-122). Tall columnar cells with abundant pale to slightly granular cytoplasm with basally situated nuclei along the basement membrane line the glands. Corpora amylacea may be seen in the lumens of 20% of cases further confounding its overlap with epithelial hyperplasia.[421]

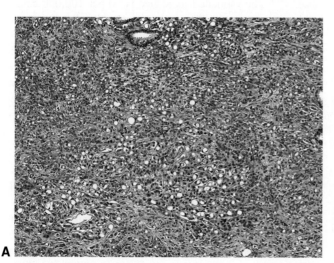
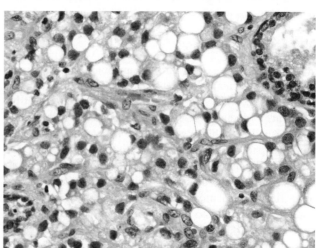

A   **B**

FIGURE 9-121 ■ Signet-ring cell carcinoma with **(A)** diffuse infiltrative growth characterized by the presence of **(B)** tumor cells with intracytoplasmic vacuolations.

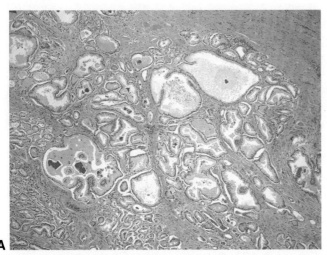
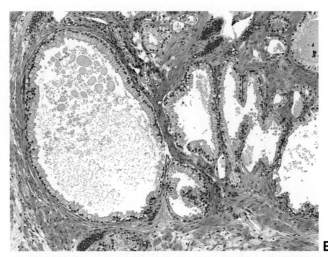

FIGURE 9-122 ■ Pseudohyperplastic variant of prostate carcinoma shows **(A)** large-sized glands with occasional luminal infoldings mimicking hyperplasia. Note the presence of luminal amorphous material and crystalloids. The nuclei are typically basally oriented **(B)**.

Malignant nuclear features are present such as nucleomegaly and nucleolomegaly, which are key in its diagnosis (Fig. 9-123). Similar to nonpseudohyperplastic carcinomas, gland lumina may also contain luminal eosinophilic amorphous secretions, crystalloids, and uncommonly mucin. Infiltrative growth is not a common feature and is seen in only 27% of cases.[422] Likewise, PNI is seen in only 5% to 9% of cases.[421,422] Pseudohyperplastic carcinoma is often admixed and shows transition or continuity with acinar adenocarcinoma (Fig. 9-124). Most carcinomas are Gleason grade 3 + 3 = 6, and if part of a well-circumscribed nodule, the grade may include a component of pattern 2 (i.e., 3 + 2 = 5 or 2 + 3 = 5).

Recently, a subset of these tumors was described to exhibit microcystic dilatations that are sometimes lined by atrophic-appearing cells, in addition to other features of pseudohyperplastic carcinoma, and mimic cystic atrophy and hyperplasia.[423]

AMACR is expressed in 70% to 83% of pseudohyperplastic carcinomas usually exhibiting homogenous staining, and basal cell marker HMWK is not expressed, which may help in confirmation of the diagnosis (Fig. 9-125).[422,424]

Differential Diagnosis

The nodular growth, gland architecture, pale columnar cells with basally oriented nuclei, occasional corpora amylacea, and infrequency of other usual features of cancer such as small glandular infiltration, mucin, and PNI in pseudohyperplastic carcinoma give the deceptive appearance of hyperplasia (including AAH) on low-power view. Detection of other luminal features of cancer such as crystalloids and amorphous materials is often helpful, and recognition of malignant nuclear features helps make the diagnosis. In addition, acinar adenocarcinoma is often seen adjacent to

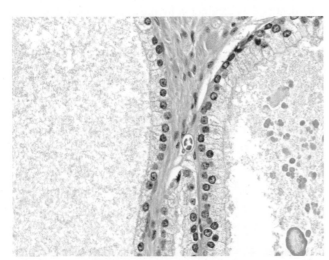

FIGURE 9-123 ■ Key in making the diagnosis of the pseudo-hyperplastic variant of prostate carcinoma is the presence of malignant nuclear features.

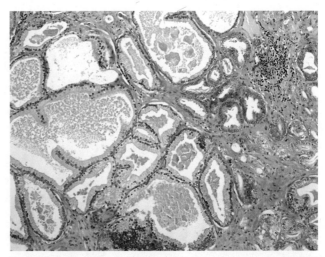

FIGURE 9-124 ■ Mixed pseudohyperplastic variant (**left**) and acinar adenocarcinoma (**right**).

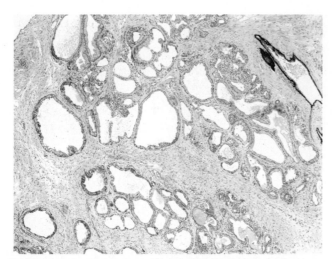

FIGURE 9-125 ■ Cocktail of HMWK, p63, and AMACR in the pseudohyperplastic variant shows expression of AMACR (*red*) and absence of basal cell immunostaining (*brown*) including in large glands.

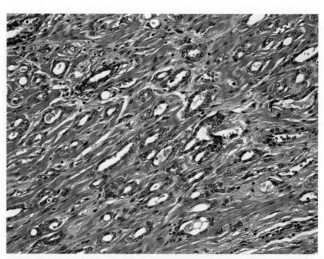

FIGURE 9-126 ■ Atrophic variant of prostate carcinoma showing infiltrative growth. Note the presence of intraluminal mucin.

these tumors. If necessary, AMACR expression and lack of basal cell marker staining confirm the diagnosis of the pseudohyperplastic variant.

Atrophic Carcinoma

Introduction

Prostatic carcinoma glands may have a lining composed of flattened cells with scanty cytoplasm resembling atrophic benign glands.[425–427] An atrophic-appearing pattern in adenocarcinoma may also be seen in posttreatment setting, particularly with antiandrogen therapy. Those that occur without prior therapy are referred to as the atrophic variant. This deceptive pattern often occurs admixed with acinar adenocarcinoma, with the atrophic pattern comprising 10% to 60% (mean 27%) of the tumor.[427] Some authors require at least 50% of the tumor to have the atrophic pattern for diagnosis as the atrophic variant.[426]

Clinical Features

Atrophic carcinoma is reported in 2% of carcinomas in prostatic needle biopsies and 3% to 16% of carcinomas in RP specimens.[425,427] Patients with atrophic carcinoma range in age from 48 to 73 years (mean of 60 to 65 years), a similar age group to those with acinar adenocarcinoma.[426,427] Patients may also present with elevated serum PSA.[427] The histologic grade, tumor volume, and pathologic stage are similar to acinar carcinomas, suggesting that the behavior is not different from acinar adenocarcinoma.[425]

Pathology

Atrophic carcinoma is characterized by malignant glands composed of cells with scanty cytoplasm and high nuclear to cytoplasmic ratio, giving the appearance of atrophy on low-power magnification (Figs. 9-126 and 9-127). These glands are identified as carcinoma by presence of other malignant

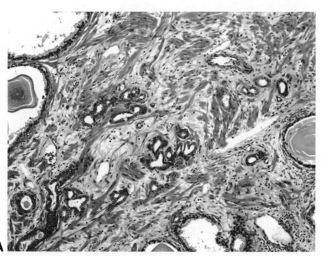

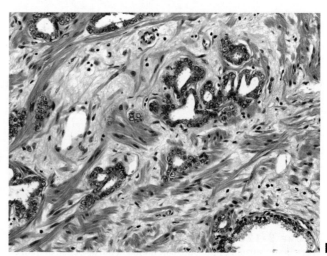

FIGURE 9-127 ■ Atrophic variant of prostate carcinoma **(A)** present between benign glands mimicking focal atrophy. A key feature to diagnosis is the presence of malignant nuclear features **(B)**.

features, mainly by nucleomegaly and prominent nucleoli and by the presence of infiltrative growth. In addition, luminal features of cancer such as eosinophilic proteinaceous materials, blue mucin, and crystalloids may also be present. Most glands are well formed with lumina (Gleason grade 3) and less often exhibit fusion (Gleason grade 4). AMACR is overexpressed in 69.6% of atrophic carcinomas, which is lower compared to acinar adenocarcinoma.[327]

Differential Diagnosis

Retention of nuclear and luminal features of cancer allows distinction of atrophic carcinoma from benign atrophic glands. Simple atrophy shows a lobular growth and does not exhibit gland infiltration. Atrophic carcinoma is often seen admixed with acinar adenocarcinoma which may also aid in its diagnosis. Beware that 30% of atrophic carcinomas may not express AMACR, further confounding its morphologic overlap with the AMACR-negative benign atrophy.[327] It is also important to note that benign atrophy may have discontinuous or patchy staining for basal cell markers. Atrophic carcinoma should completely lack basal cell marker staining. The mean Ki-67 proliferation index of atrophic carcinoma is 4% compared to 1.2% for benign atrophic glands and 5.3% for nonatrophic carcinoma.[425]

Foamy Gland (Xanthomatous) Carcinoma

Introduction

Foamy gland carcinoma is characterized by cells with abundant foamy cytoplasm and small pyknotic-appearing nuclei.[428–432] Foamy gland carcinoma can be seen admixed with acinar adenocarcinoma in 14% to 23% of RPs.[428] The foamy gland component varies and ranges from 1% to 90% of carcinoma in RP and 5% to 100% of carcinoma in biopsies.[201,429,431] The lack of typical malignant nuclear features (i.e., nucleomegaly and prominent nucleoli) makes the diagnosis as carcinoma difficult in limited samples. By electron

microscopy, the foamy cytoplasm is seen to be due to abundant microvesicles and polyribosomes, and the cytoplasm lacks lipid, glycogen, or neutral mucin content; thus strictly speaking these are not "xanthomatous" cells.[431,432] *TMPRSS2:ERG* fusion was identified in 29% (5/17) of foamy gland carcinomas, which is lower than acinar adenocarcinoma.[97]

Clinical Features

The patient ages range from 42 to 78 years (mean 62 years), similar to the age group of patients with acinar adenocarcinoma.[428] Some patients may present with elevated serum PSA and average from 8.4 to 15.2 ng/mL.[201,429,430,432] It is unclear if tumor behavior is different from acinar adenocarcinoma. Initial series had shown non–organ-confined disease in 67% to 83% which suggested a more aggressive behavior,[201,431] but later studies suggest that its behavior is not different from acinar adenocarcinoma.[428] Foamy gland and non–foamy gland carcinomas appear to have about similar recurrence rates (23% versus 22%) and average time to PSA recurrence.[428]

Pathology

This carcinoma variant is distinguished by having cells with abundant voluminous pale foamy cytoplasm (Fig. 9-128). Malignant nuclear features (i.e., nucleomegaly and prominent nucleoli) are not always present, as nuclei may be small or pyknotic (Fig. 9-129). Architectures include discrete well-formed glands, fused or ill-defined glands, cribriform structures, and nests or single cells with confluence. The glands are usually crowded and infiltrative. In cases of higher-grade architectural patterns, the nuclei occasionally show nucleolar prominence. The glandular lumina may contain pink amorphous secretions, which are common in discrete gland patterns. Other features of carcinoma such as mitosis, blue mucin, crystalloids, PNI, and associated HGPIN are not commonly present. The ISUP consensus on Gleason grading recommends discounting

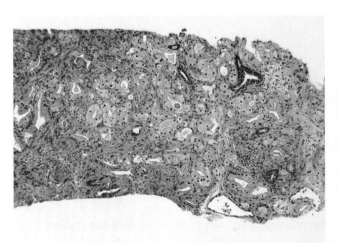
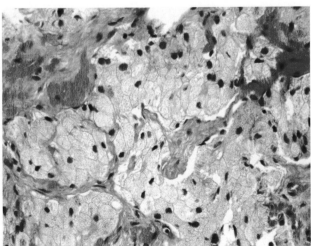

A   **B**

FIGURE 9-128 ■ Foamy gland carcinoma with **(A)** individual gland and **(B)** fused gland patterns.

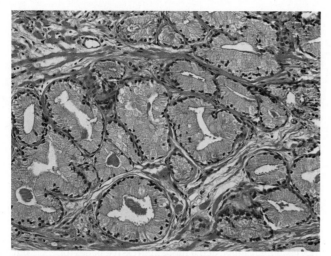

FIGURE 9-129 ■ Nuclei of foamy gland carcinoma are typically small dark and without nucleolar prominence.

foamy cytoplasm and assigning a grade based on the tumor architecture.[218] Gleason score varies from 6 to 10, and most are Gleason score 7 (64%).[428,429] Metastatic carcinoma cells from the same tumor also exhibit similar foamy cytoplasm. AMACR is expressed in 68% of foamy gland carcinomas, which can be heterogeneous, and basal cell marker staining is absent.[424]

Differential Diagnosis

Distinction of foamy gland carcinoma should be made from its benign mimickers including prostatic xanthoma, Cowper gland, mucinous metaplasia, and clear cell cribriform hyperplasia and can be difficult in biopsy samples. Prostate xanthoma shares a similar cytoplasmic appearance with foamy gland carcinoma.[433,434] However, xanthoma occurs purely as a single cell or cluster of cells that does not form any glands. It should be noted that a small subset of foamy gland carcinoma might also have infiltrative (non–gland-forming)

pattern. Use of epithelial markers and CD68, which are not expressed and which are expressed in xanthoma cells, respectively, may aid in their distinction. Beware that about 10% or less of xanthoma may show nonspecific staining to PSA, PSAP, or AMACR.[433] Cowper gland has lobular appearance and lacks the infiltrative pattern of foamy gland carcinoma. In addition, luminal features of cancer, particularly amorphous eosinophilic secretion, are not seen in Cowper gland. Cowper gland is usually encountered in apical biopsies, often intermingling with sphincteric skeletal muscles, and does not express PSA. Cribriform clear cell hyperplasia lacks the infiltrative growth and contains basal cells that are often discernible on H&E stain. Interestingly, an uncommon foamy HGPIN was also described, and it is unclear if this pattern has direct relationship to the development of foamy gland carcinoma.

Carcinoma with Stratified Epithelium ("PIN-like")

This is a recently described variant of prostate carcinoma in which the malignant glands exhibit cellular stratification (two or more cell layers thick) and thus morphologically resembles HGPIN.[435,436] Thus, knowledge of the existence of this variant is important to avoid underdiagnoses as HGPIN. Patients range in age from 50 to 91 years (mean 68 years), a similar age group to those with acinar adenocarcinoma.[435] The malignant glands have lumina that may be flat, tufted, micropapillary, or a mixture of these architectures. The neoplastic cells are cuboidal to mostly tall columnar cells with amphophilic cytoplasm and rounded to elongated nuclei (Fig. 9-130). Predominance of stratified tall columnar cells is similar to ductal adenocarcinoma and, thus, is also referred to as "HGPIN-like ductal adenocarcinoma."[435] The tumor lacks solid growth, necrosis, true papillae, and marked cellular pleomorphism. Concurrent acinar adenocarcinoma can be seen in the same prostate gland, but both are often seen as separate nodules. The acinar adenocarcinoma is frequently Gleason score 6. Unlike ductal adenocarcinoma

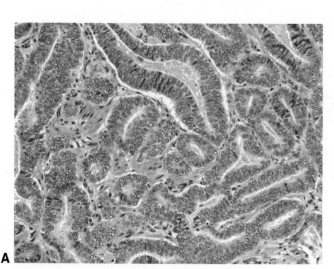

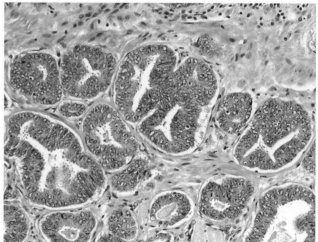

FIGURE 9-130 ■ PIN-like carcinoma with **(A,B)** multilayered growth of tall columnar cells and elongated high-grade nuclei.

that behaves like Gleason score 8 cancers, it is suggested (based on limited follow-up) that carcinoma with stratified epithelium may behave similar to Gleason sore 6 cancers.[435]

This unusual carcinoma variant must be distinguished from flat, tufted, or micropapillary HGPIN. AMACR staining, which is often strong and diffuse, is reported in 93% of cases, similar to HGPIN.[435] Lack of staining for basal cell markers distinguishes carcinoma with stratified epithelium. Ductal adenocarcinoma exhibits true papillary or cribriform patterns, which are not features of PIN-like carcinoma.

Lymphoepithelioma-like Carcinoma

This is an exceedingly rare poorly differentiated carcinoma of the prostate that morphologically resembles lymphoepithelioma of the nasopharyngeal region.[437,438] The tumors were reported in older individuals (66 to 82 years) presenting with obstructive urinary symptoms, elevated PSA, or locally advanced disease. Histologically, the tumor consists of a syncytium of carcinoma cells with indistinct cell borders. Tumor cells exhibit vesicular nuclei and enlarged nucleoli and have abundant mitosis. The carcinoma cells are admixed with abundant lymphocytes and often plasma cells. Neutrophils and eosinophils may also be present. These lymphocytes are polyclonal and are mostly T cells. The poorly differentiated carcinoma component expresses PSA, PSAP, and AMACR. Unlike its nasopharyngeal counterpart, no Epstein-Barr virus is detected in this tumor. Admixed acinar adenocarcinoma is often present and may include discrete Gleason pattern 3 the lymphoepithelioma component varies

from 10% to 90% of the tumor. Additional tumor morphology such as adenosquamous carcinoma was also reported. Lymphoepithelioma-like carcinoma is suggested to have an aggressive behavior.

Oncocytic Carcinoma

This is an exceptionally rare variant of prostate carcinoma characterized by cells that exhibit abundant eosinophilic granular cytoplasm.[439-441] Like oncocytic tumors from other organs, the cells are ultrastructurally rich in mitochondria.[440] The reported cases show infiltrating glands or solid nests or cords (Fig. 9-131). The nuclei are round and small to medium sized. PSA and PSAP are expressed by the tumor. The clinical significance of this variant is still unclear. High-stage disease, metastasis, and death occurred in some of the reported cases.[439,440]

Pleomorphic Giant Cell Adenocarcinoma

An extremely rare type of prostate carcinoma characterized by the presence of large bizarre anaplastic giant cells was described.[442,443] Cases were reported in patients 59 to 76 years old (mean 66 years).[442] This morphology may occur admixed with high-grade prostate carcinoma (mostly Gleason score 9) or other histologies such as ductal adenocarcinoma component, squamous carcinoma, and small cell carcinoma. The pleomorphic cells are positive for epithelial markers, but staining with PSA or PSAP is inconsistent. The tumor is suggested to have an aggressive behavior.

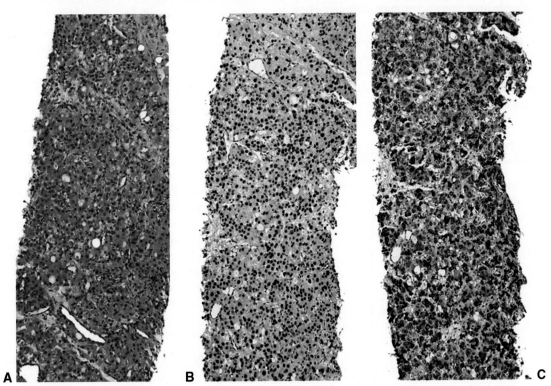

FIGURE 9-131 ■ Prostate carcinoma with oncocytic features. This is a needle core biopsy from a neck mass in a patient with known prostate and renal cancer **(A)**. Immunostains for **(B)** P501S (Prostein) and **(C)** NKX3.1 are positive.

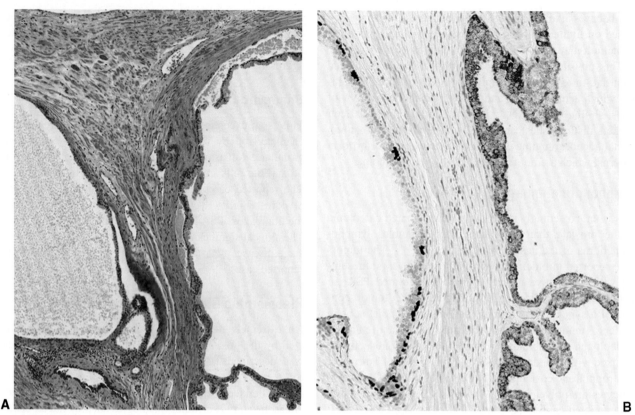

FIGURE 9-132 ■ Prostate carcinoma with cystic change **(A)**, confirmed by absence of p63 immunostaining and AMACR overexpression **(B)**.

Other Unusual Patterns

Microcystic change may rarely occur in prostate carcinoma, and is considered by some as a variant of pseudohyperplastic and atrophic carcinoma (Fig. 9-132).[423] Another pattern is the carcinoid-like prostate carcinoma (Fig. 9-133A and B). Its very unusual neuroendocrine-like features may cause diagnostic problems, particularly at metastatic sites where carcinoid tumor is common (Fig. 9-133C).

GLEASON GRADING

Although in the last three-quarters of the 20th century, numerous histologic grading systems for prostatic adenocarcinoma have been proposed[444]; currently, the most commonly used grading scheme in the Unites States and worldwide is the Gleason system[261,445–448] (Table 9-13).

Gleason Grading System

The Gleason grading system was first developed in 1966 by Donald. F. Gleason, a pathologist at the Minneapolis Veterans Administration Medical Center.[445]

Initially derived from a cohort of only 270 patients, the Gleason system is unique among pathologic grading systems in that it is based solely on the architectural pattern of the tumor evaluated on H&E-stained prostatic tissue sections, at relatively low magnification (4× or 10× lens),

without taking into account cytologic features. In addition, rather than assigning the highest pattern as the grade of the tumor, the grade is defined as the sum of the two most common architectural patterns and reported as Gleason score.

The Gleason grading method is a five-step histologic grading system, which considers only the degree of glandular differentiation of the tumor and its relation to the surrounding prostatic stroma.[261,449] Nine growth patterns are consolidated into five basic grade patterns, in which patterns 1, 2, and 3 represent prostate tumors closely resembling normal prostatic glands and grade 4 and 5 tumors show increasingly abnormal glandular architecture. The five grades are used to generate a histologic score, which can range from 2 to 10, by adding the primary (or predominant) grade and the secondary (second most common) grade. If only one grade is present in the tissue sample, that pattern is multiplied by to give the Gleason score.

Over the years, Gleason's original description of each grade has undergone significant modification (Fig. 9-134), first by Gleason and Mellinger[447] and most recently at the 2005 ISUP Consensus Conference.[218]

Modified Gleason Grading System

More than 40 years have gone by since the introduction of the Gleason grading system. During this time, the clinical and diagnostic steps to detect prostate cancer have changed dramatically. In Gleason's era, there was no screening for prostate cancer other than by DRE, since serum PSA had

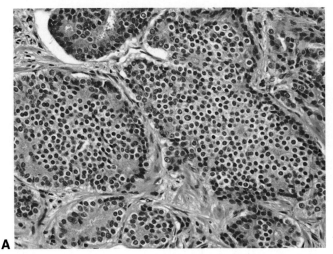

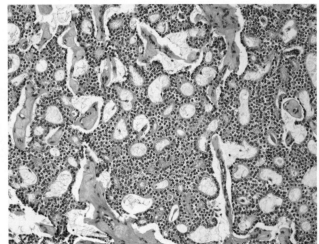

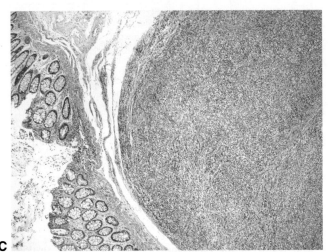

FIGURE 9-133 ■ Carcinoid-like prostate carcinoma **(A,B)** with metastasis to the large bowel **(C)**.

Table 9-13 ■ GLEASON GRADING SYSTEM FOR PROSTATIC ADENOCARCINOMA

Pattern	Tumor Shape	Tumor Borders	Stromal Invasion	Architecture	Gland Size
1	Nodular, well-circumscribed mass	Definite, round, smooth edges	Pushing	Single, round to oval, separated, closely packed glands	Medium
2	Nodular, less well-defined mass	Less sharp but definable edges	Loosely grouped arrangement	Single, round to oval, separated, loosely packed glands with variability in size and shape	Medium
3A	Ill-defined tumor nodule	Infiltrating edges	Irregular extension into stroma	Single glands of irregular shape and spacing, with elongated and angular forms	Medium
3B	Ill-defined tumor nodule	Infiltrating edges	Irregular extension into stroma	Same as 3A, but smaller glands; cords with glandular lumina	Small to very small
3C	Rounded masses	Sharp, smooth rounded edges	Expansile	Cribriform and papillary tumor, without necrosis	Medium to large
4A	Raggedly infiltrative mass	Infiltrative, ragged edges	Diffusely infiltrative	Fused, microacinar, cribriform, or papillary	Small, medium, or large
4B	Raggedly infiltrative mass	Infiltrative, ragged edges	Diffusely infiltrative	Similar to 4A, but cells have clear, pale cytoplasm (hypernephroid).	Small, medium, or large
5A	Rounded masses	Smooth rounded edges	Expansile	Cribriform, papillary, or solid with central necrosis (comedonecrosis)	Variable
5B	Raggedly infiltrative mass	Infiltrative, ragged edges	Diffusely infiltrative	Masses and sheets of anaplastic carcinoma with small glandular lumina or signet ring cells	Small

Original Gleason

ISUP 2005 Gleason

Proposed modification of ISUP
2005 Gleason

**Prostatic adenocarcinoma
(Histologic Patterns)**

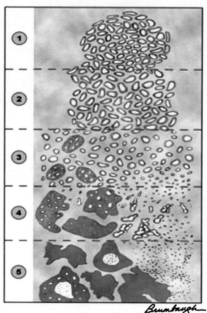

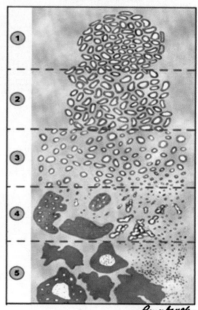

Hum Pathol 1992;23:273–279. *Am J Surg Pathol* 2005;29:1228–1242. *J Urol* 2010;183:433–440.

FIGURE 9-134 ■ Original Gleason system and recent modifications. (Reprinted from Brimo F, et al. Contemporary grading for prostate cancer: implications for patient care. *Eur Urol* 2013;63:892–901, with permission.)

not yet been discovered, and the cases detected tended to be bulky tumors. In 1974, Gleason and Mellinger reported that 86% of men with prostate cancer had advanced disease with extension out of the gland on clinical examination or distant metastases.[447]

The method of obtaining prostate tissue was also different, typically with only a couple of large-gauge needle biopsies taken from an area of palpable abnormality. The use of 18-gauge thin biopsy needle and the practice of sextant needle biopsies to sample the prostate more thoroughly did not develop until the 1980s.[450]

RP was a relatively uncommon procedure in the 1960s, and the prostate was not often removed intact. In addition, the surgical specimens were not processed in their entirety or as extensively, and systematically, as they are currently, hence, grading multiple tumor nodules within the same gland and dealing with the presence of tertiary grade were not addressed in the original Gleason system.

The Gleason system also predated the use of immunohistochemistry: It is likely that with the use of immunoperoxidase staining for basal cell markers, many of the original Gleason score 1 + 1 = 2 carcinomas would currently be regarded as adenosis (AAH). Similarly, many of the cases diagnosed as cribriform Gleason pattern 3 tumors in 1967 would today be diagnosed as either cribriform high-grade PIN or IDC if labeled with basal cell markers.[451]

In addition, new variants and patterns of prostate adenocarcinoma have also been described since the original system.

The 2005 ISUP Consensus Conference

As a result of the changing practice of clinical urology, experts in urologic pathology gradually have adapted the Gleason system to contemporary surgical pathology practice, but without a formal consensus until the 2005 ISUP Consensus Conference, during which the system underwent a major revision.

An international group of more than 70 urologic pathologists convened at the 2005 United States and Canadian Academy Pathology meeting in San Antonio in an attempt to achieve consensus in controversial areas related to the Gleason grading.[218]

The changes proposed at the meeting and implemented in the modified Gleason grade system pertain to both pattern interpretation and reporting.

Change in Pattern Diagnostic Criteria

Gleason Patterns 1 to 2

It was a consensus that a diagnosis of Gleason score 2 to 4 on needle biopsy should be made rarely if ever. For practical purposes, this change has translated into the virtual disappearance of Gleason score 2 to 4 on needle biopsy in contemporary practice. In transurethral resection of prostate (TURP) specimens sampling the transition zone, Gleason score 2 to 4 cancer may still be diagnosed, although it is rare (Fig. 9-135). The virtual absence of Gleason score 2 to 4 has raised the issue as to whether it is more appropriate from the purpose of prognosis and

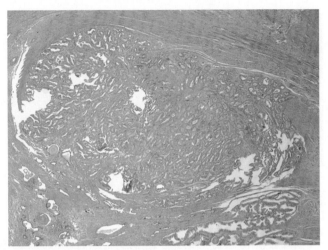

FIGURE 9-135 ■ Adenocarcinoma of the prostate Gleason score 4. The tumor nodule with definable edges consists of round to oval, separated, loosely packed glands with variability in size and shape.

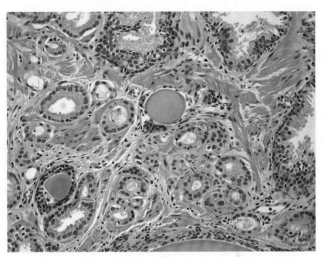

FIGURE 9-137 ■ Gleason grade 3 prostate cancer infiltrating among nonneoplastic prostatic acini.

treatment to state that the Gleason score ranges from 6 to 10 as opposed to 2 to 10.[452,453]

Gleason Grade 3 to 4

Gleason grade 3 prostate cancer is composed of single, well-formed glands (Fig. 9-136) that infiltrate among nonneoplastic prostate acini (Fig. 9-137). A departure from the original Gleason classification system is that "individual cells" would not be allowed within Gleason grade 3.

In addition, the criteria for cribriform pattern three glands were tightened to include only rounded, well-circumscribed cribriform glands of the same size of normal glands. It was the consensus that most (subsequently all) of cribriform patterns be diagnosed as Gleason grade 4.[268] Recently, the validity of including cribriform glands as a component of Gleason grade 3 has been questioned, and it has been recommended that all tumors showing cribriform architecture should be classified as Gleason grade 4[454] (Fig. 9-138A–C).

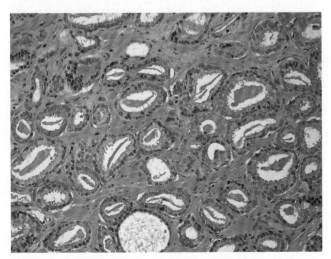

FIGURE 9-136 ■ Adenocarcinoma of the prostate Gleason grade 3 composed of single, well-formed glands.

Ill-defined glands with poorly formed glandular lumina (Fig. 9-139), fused microacinar glands (Fig. 9-140), and hypernephroid tumors with clear, pale cytoplasm (Fig. 9-141) also warrant the diagnosis of Gleason grade 4.

Gleason Pattern 5

For the most part, Gleason original grade 5 has remained unchanged in modern practice. The presence of true comedonecrosis within solid nests (Fig. 9-142) and cribriform masses (Fig. 9-143) should be regarded as Gleason grade 5. However, one must be stringent as to the definition of comedonecrosis, requiring intraluminal necrotic cells and/or karyorrhexis. Masses (Fig. 9-144) and sheets (Fig. 9-145) of anaplastic carcinoma with small glandular lumina or signet ring cells are Gleason grade 5.

Grading Variants of Prostate Cancer

Vacuoles

Adenocarcinomas of the prostate may contain clear cytoplasmic vacuoles, and these should be distinguished from true signet-ring carcinomas, which contain mucin. The consensus was that these tumors should be graded as if the vacuoles were not present, by only evaluating the underlying architectural pattern.

Foamy Gland Carcinoma

Whereas most cases of foamy gland carcinoma would be graded as Gleason score 3 + 3 = 6, higher-grade foamy gland carcinoma exists and should be graded accordingly based on the pattern.

Ductal Adenocarcinoma

Ductal adenocarcinomas are aggressive tumors and should be graded as Gleason score 4 + 4 = 8 (or 9 if comedonecrosis is present), retaining the diagnostic term ductal adenocarcinoma to denote the unique clinical and pathologic findings.[381] However, the recently described PIN-like ductal

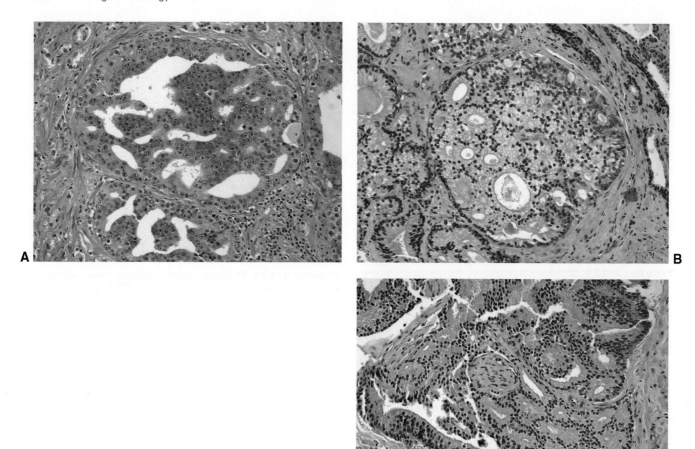

FIGURE 9-138 ■ Adenocarcinoma of the prostate Gleason grade 4 with cribriform architecture (A–C).

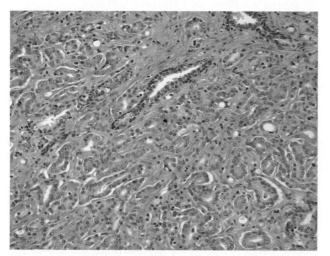

FIGURE 9-139 ■ Adenocarcinoma of the prostate Gleason grade 4 with poorly formed glandular lumina.

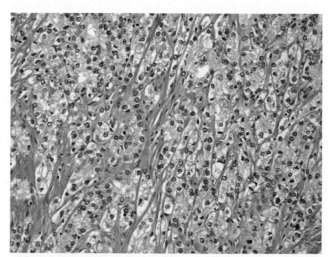

FIGURE 9-140 ■ Adenocarcinoma of the prostate Gleason grade 4 with fused microacinar formation.

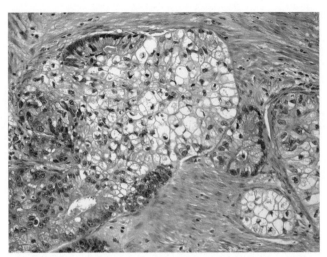

Figure 9-141 ■ Adenocarcinoma of the prostate Gleason grade 4 with clear, pale cytoplasm (hypernephroid).

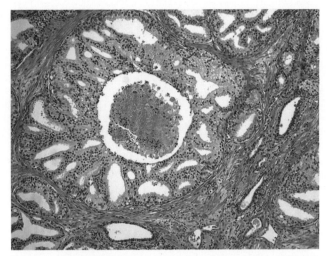

Figure 9-143 ■ Adenocarcinoma of the prostate Gleason grade 5, cribriform gland with central necrosis (comedonecrosis).

adenocarcinoma should be graded as Gleason grade 3 if the glands are discrete as in usual acinar adenocarcinoma.[435]

Colloid (Mucinous) Carcinoma

The majority of cases of colloid carcinoma consists of irregular cribriform or fused glands floating within a mucinous matrix. These cases should be scored as Gleason score 4 + 4 = 8. However, there was no consensus for cases where individual round discrete glands were seen floating within mucinous pools.

Small Cell Carcinoma

Small cell carcinoma of the prostate has unique histologic, immunohistochemical, and clinical features such that it should not be assigned a Gleason grade.

Reporting Limited Secondary Pattern of Lower Grade

In the setting of high-grade cancer, one should ignore lower-grade patterns if they occupy <5% of the tumor area.

For example, a needle biopsy core entirely involved by cancer, with 98% Gleason pattern 4 and 2% Gleason pattern 3, would be diagnosed as Gleason score 4 + 4 = 8. This scoring is a departure from the original Gleason system, which would have resulted in a diagnosis of Gleason score 4 + 3 = 7.

The same 5% cutoff rule for excluding lower-grade tumor also applies for TURP and RP specimens.

Reporting Limited Secondary Pattern of Higher Grade

High-grade tumor of any quantity on needle biopsy, identified at low to medium magnification, should be included within the Gleason score. Consequently, a needle biopsy entirely involved by cancer with 98% Gleason pattern 3 and 2% Gleason pattern 4 would be diagnosed as Gleason score 3 + 4 = 7. This method is unchanged from the original Gleason system.

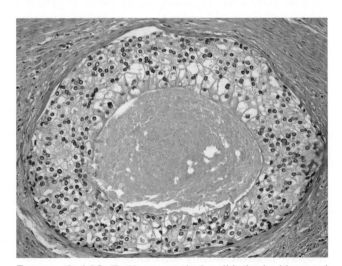

Figure 9-142 ■ Gleason grade 5, solid gland with central necrosis (comedonecrosis).

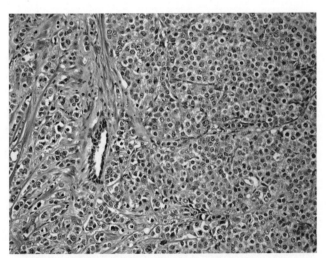

Figure 9-144 ■ Gleason grade 5 adenocarcinoma of the prostate composed of expansile mass of anaplastic tumor cells.

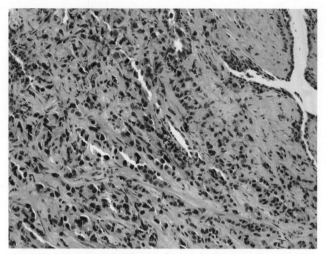

FIGURE 9-145 ■ Gleason grade 5 adenocarcinoma of the prostate composed of sheets of anaplastic tumor cells.

Tertiary Gleason Grade

Needle Biopsy

In the uncommon case in which there are three different grades on needle biopsy, but the third pattern is lower grade, the lower grade should be ignored.

Tumors with grades 3, 4, and 5 should be classified overall as high grade (Gleason score 8 to 10), given the presence of high-grade tumor (patterns 4 and 5) on needle biopsy. For these tumors, both the primary pattern and the highest grade should be recorded. For example, tumors on needle biopsy with Gleason score 3 + 4 with tertiary pattern 5 would be recorded as Gleason score 3 + 5 = 8 (Fig. 9-146). This method is a major departure from the original definition of the Gleason grading system.

Radical Prostatectomy

The definition of tertiary grade is controversial for RP specimens. Prostate cancer is commonly multifocal and the recommendation of the consensus conference was to assign a separate Gleason score to each dominant tumor nodule.

According to some authors, the definition of tertiary grade for RP is the presence of a third pattern higher than the primary and secondary patterns, where the tertiary component is visually estimated to be <5% of the whole tumor.[454] When the third most common component is the highest pattern and occupies >5% of the tumor, some authors would record it as the secondary grade. This definition is not universally accepted, with some pathologists diagnosing the tertiary grade regardless of the proportion.[455,456]

Needle Biopsy with Different Cores Showing Different Grades

When one or more needle biopsy cores show pure high-grade cancer (Gleason score 4 + 4 = 8) and the others show pattern 3 (Gleason score 3 + 3 = 6; 3 + 4 = 7; 4 + 3 = 7), the consensus of the group is to assign individual Gleason scores to separate cores as long as the cores were submitted separately.

When different cores with different grades are submitted in the same container without a site designation, either grading each core separately or giving an overall grade for the involved cores is acceptable.

Impact of the Modified System

Gleason grading remains the single most powerful prognostic parameter in prostate cancer and is used in nomograms, such as the Kattan nomograms[457,458] and the Partin tables,[459] which guide patient treatment decisions. Therefore, preserving the integrity and the prognostic utility of the Gleason system is crucial. Since the publication of the ISUP consensus modification of Gleason scoring, some supporting evidence for these recommendations has been reported.

Upgrading

An important consequence of narrowing the definition of Gleason grade 3 and expanding the definition of pattern 4 has been Gleason grade migration or upgrading. As a consequence, Gleason score 6 prostate cancer, once the most common pattern on needle biopsy, has become less common than Gleason score 7.

In two recent studies comparing the original and modified Gleason systems in needle biopsy specimens, Gleason score 6 tumors decreased from 48% to 22% and from 68% to 55% of the total, whereas Gleason score 7 cases rose from 25% to 68% and from 30% to 43% with the implementation of the modified system.[460,461] In RP specimens, Gleason 7 cases rose from 48% to 60%.[461] In the cohort of patients evaluated by Dong et al.,[462] 34% of patients with original Gleason score 6 prostate cancer were upgraded to modified Gleason score 7 or 8 by the ISUP criteria.

Biopsy–Prostatectomy Agreement

Data are mixed as to whether modified Gleason grading improves biopsy–prostatectomy concordance. One study

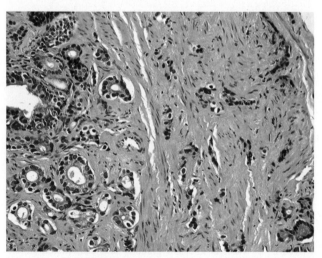

FIGURE 9-146 ■ Adenocarcinoma of the prostate with Gleason grade 3 (**left**) and Gleason grade 5 (**right**).

found a higher percentage agreement by chi-square test ($P <$ 0.001), although κ statistics were not done.[460] The agreement of Gleason score between NCB and RP specimens after modified Gleason grading was more than 85% for Gleason score 7, which is significantly higher than the 45% reported with the old conventional Gleason grading system.[460,463] Another study, using κ statistics and three pathologist evaluators, found no improvement in concordance or in interobserver reproducibility.[464]

Correlation with Outcome and Stage

The important test of the validity of the new Gleason system is its correlation with patient outcomes. In a study of 806 prostatectomy specimens with prostate cancer of original Gleason score 6 or 3 + 4 = 7 and modified Gleason score 6 to 8 with a median follow-up of 12.6 years, patients with classical Gleason score 6 upgraded to modified Gleason score 7 or 8 had intermediate pathologic stage, biochemical progression-free survival, and metastasis-free survival compared with patients with classical and modified Gleason score 6 and patients with classical Gleason score 3 + 4 = 7 and modified Gleason score 7 or 8.[462]

In another study of 204 prostatectomy specimens, the Kaplan-Meier curves showed original Gleason grading to associate with biochemical progression ($P = 0.002$), while the modified Gleason grade did not ($P = 0.393$). However, when scores were grouped (≤6, 7, 8-10), the modified Gleason score improved outcome association from nonsignificant to significant for the distinction between Gleason 6 or lower and Gleason 7 groups, but not between Gleason 7 and Gleason 8 to 10 groups.[465]

It has been shown that for Gleason score 7 tumors, those with tertiary patterns on needle biopsy had a higher risk of PSA recurrence when compared to tumors without tertiary pattern.[466] Similarly, it has been shown that score 7 tumors with tertiary pattern 5 had a time to PSA failure intermediate between Gleason score 8 and Gleason score 9 to 10 tumors.[467]

The limited studies published to date suggest that the presence of a higher-grade tertiary pattern is a marker of more aggressive disease. Additional studies with long-term follow-up are necessary to fully estimate the effect of modified grading on outcome.

Interobserver Reproducibility

The interobserver reproducibility among pathologists using the modified Gleason system, with values around 80%, has improved compared to the old conventional Gleason grading, which has interobserver agreement rates of about 60%.[460,468,469]

While this improvement might in part be due to the decreased diagnosis of low-grade carcinoma on needle biopsy using the modified system, improvement has also been seen in the reproducibility of recognition of Gleason grade 4.[468]

Clinical Implications

One consequence of the modifications of the Gleason system is the increasing difficulty to compare prostate cancer patient outcomes over time. The contemporary cases of Gleason score 6 are a homogeneous group of tumors without cribriform or poorly formed glands and therefore associated with a better prognosis than Gleason score 6 tumors graded under the original Gleason system. The resulting false impression that the survival rate has improved, when in fact much of the change is due to modifications in classification, is referred to as the Will Rogers phenomenon.[470–473]

Whether the Gleason upgrading on prostate cancer needle biopsy is going to affect clinical decision making remains to be seen.

STAGING

Introduction

RP is considered to be the most reliable method of eradication of localized prostate cancer, and the pathologic classification of the specimen following surgery provides important prognostic information. An accurate pathology report is the cornerstone of cancer treatment and follow-up.

The objectives of staging are to group malignancies with similar prognosis and therapeutic approach, to be able to compare clinicopathologic data from different institutions, and to perform clinical trials or research studies on a homogeneous population of patients.

In addition to the preoperative serum PSA, Gleason score on pathology specimen, SVI and lymph node status, EPE, and positive surgical margins are significant predictors of clinical and biochemical recurrence.[474,475]

The reporting of pathologic staging parameters in RP specimens is essential for predicting local and distant disease recurrence and for planning adjuvant treatment.

Clinical and Pathologic Staging

Staging involves determination of the anatomic extent or spread of prostate cancer at the time of diagnosis based on clinical and pathologic criteria. The TNM staging is the most widely used system for prostate cancer staging and assesses the extent of primary tumor (T stage), the absence or presence of regional lymph node involvement (N stage), and the absence or presence of distant metastases (M stage) (Tables 9-14 and 9-15). Once the T, N, and M are determined, a stage of I, II, III, or IV is assigned, with stage I referring to early disease and stage IV referring to advanced disease.

Several modifications have been made over time to the TNM staging system in an attempt to improve the uniformity of patient evaluation and to maintain a clinically relevant classification system. In the most recent American Joint Committee on Cancer (AJCC) classification Gleason score

Table 9-14 ■ DEFINITIONS OF CLINICAL TNM ACCORDING TO AJCC (2010)

Clinical

Primary Tumor (T)

TX	Primary tumor cannot be assessed
T0	No evidence of primary tumor
T1	Clinically inapparent tumor neither palpable nor visible by imaging
T1a	Tumor incidental histologic finding in ≤5% of tissue resected
T1b	Tumor incidental histologic finding in >5% of tissue resected
T1c	Tumor identified by needle biopsy (e.g., because of elevated PSA)
T2	Tumor confined within prostate
T2a	Tumor involves one-half of one lobe or less
T2b	Tumor involves more than one-half of one lobe but not both lobes
T2c	Tumor involves both lobes
T3	Tumor extends through the prostate capsule
T3a	Extracapsular extension (unilateral or bilateral)
T3b	Tumor invades seminal vesicle(s)
T4	Tumor is fixed or invades adjacent structures other than seminal vesicles such as external sphincter, rectum, bladder, levator muscles, and/or pelvic wall

Regional Lymph Nodes (N)

NX	Regional lymph nodes were not assessed
N0	No regional lymph node metastasis
N1	Metastasis in regional lymph node(s)

Distant Metastasis (M)

M0	No distant metastasis
M1	Distant metastasis
M1a	Nonregional lymph node(s)
M1b	Bone(s)
M1c	Other site(s) with or without bone disease

Prostate. In: Edge SB, Byrd DR, Compton CC, eds. *AJCC Cancer Staging Manual.* 7th ed. New York: Springer; 2010:457–468, with permission.

Table 9-15 ■ DEFINITIONS OF PATHOLOGIC TNM ACCORDING TO AJCC (2010)

Pathologic

Primary Tumor (pT)

pT2	Organ confined
pT2a	Unilateral, one-half of one side or less
pT2b	Unilateral, involving more than one-half of one side, but not both sides
pT2c	Bilateral disease
pT3	Extraprostatic extension
pT3a	Extraprostatic extension or microscopic invasion of bladder neck
pT3b	Seminal vesicle invasion
pT4	Invasion of rectum, levator muscles, and/or pelvic wall

Regional Lymph Nodes (pN)

pNX	Regional lymph nodes not sampled
pN0	No positive regional lymph nodes
pN1	Metastases in regional lymph node(s)

Distant Metastasis (pM)

pM0	No distant metastasis
pM1	Distant metastasis
pM1a	Nonregional lymph node(s)
pM1b	Bone(s)
pM1c	Other site(s) with or without bone disease

Prostate. In: Edge SB, Byrd DR, Compton CC, eds. *AJCC Cancer Staging Manual.* 7th ed. New York: Springer; 2010:457–468, with permission.

Substaging of clinical stage T2 prostate cancers is largely based on the extent of the abnormality palpated during a DRE or shown during TRUS in each half of the gland. Prostate cancer extending beyond the boundary of the gland is classified as stage T3; tumors fixed or invading adjacent structures other than seminal vesicles, such as the external sphincter, rectum, bladder, levator muscles, and/or pelvic wall, are considered equivalent to clinical stage T4.[476]

and PSA have been incorporated in the anatomic stage/prognostic groups (Table 9-16).[476]

Clinical T Staging

Clinical staging (cTNM) is performed by the urologist or referring physician during the initial evaluation of the patient or when pathologic classification is not possible. All parameters available before the first definitive treatment may be used for clinical staging and remain unchanged even if pathologic findings differ. Primary tumor assessment includes DRE of the prostate and histologic confirmation of prostate cancer by TRUS-guided biopsy.

Clinical staging stratifies patients based on the tumor detection method, separating nonpalpable "incidental" prostate tumors detected during TUR of the prostate for BPH (classified as stage T1a or T1b) and palpable cancers detected by DRE (stage T2) (Table 9-14). Nonpalpable cancer detected by an elevated serum PSA level or an abnormal TRUS image is classified as stage T1c.

Table 9-16 ■ ANATOMIC STAGE/PROGNOSTIC GROUPS (FROM AJCC 2010)

Group	T	N	M	PSA	Gleason
I	T1a-c	N0	M0	PSA < 10	Gleason ≤ 6
	T2a	N0	M0	PSA < 10	Gleason ≤ 6
	T1-2a	N0	M0	PSA x	Gleason X
IIA	T1a-c	N0	M0	PSA < 20	Gleason 7
	T1a-c	N0	M0	PSA ≥ 10 < 20	Gleason ≤ 6
	T2a	N0	M0	PSA < 20	Gleason ≤ 7
	T2b	N0	M0	PSA < 20	Gleason ≤ 7
	T2b	N0	M0	PSA x	Gleason X
IIB	T2c	N0	M0	Any PSA	Any Gleason
	T1-2	N0	M0	PSA ≥ 20	Any Gleason
	T1-2	N0	M0	Any PSA	Gleason ≥ 8
III	T3a-b	N0	M0	Any PSA	Any Gleason
IV	T4	N0	M0	Any PSA	Any Gleason
	Any T	N1	M0	Any PSA	Any Gleason
	Any T	Any N	M1	Any PSA	Any Gleason

Prostate. In: Edge SB, Byrd DR, Compton CC, eds. *AJCC Cancer Staging Manual.* 7th ed. New York: Springer; 2010:457–468, with permission.

Pathologic T Staging

Pathologic staging (pTNM) is based on the gross and microscopic examination of the prostate gland and is performed after surgical resection of the primary tumor. In general, RP including regional lymph node dissection with comprehensive histologic examination is required for complete pathologic classification.

However, a rectal biopsy positive for prostate cancer allows a pT4 classification without prostatectomy; similarly, a prostate biopsy revealing the presence of cancer glands in extraprostatic tissue or infiltrating seminal vesicles permits a pT3 classification.

Pathologic Stage T2

Within category pT2 prostate cancers, a wide variation in tumor extent may be seen, which varies from single microscopic lesions to large-volume multifocal tumors, often involving both sides of the prostate. In the TNM 2002 staging system, pT2 disease was subdivided into three categories, pT2a, pT2b, and pT2c, as determined by involvement of less than one-half of one side (unilateral disease), more than one-half of one side (unilateral disease), and both sides of the prostate gland (bilateral disease), respectively (Table 9-15).[477] In the TNM 2010 staging system,[478] the clinical and pathologic substaging of pT2 prostate cancers has been retained, although the prognostic value of this has been questioned.[479,480]

In contrast to clinical substaging, pathologic T2 substaging has failed to demonstrate a significant prognostic difference for intermediate-term outcomes between pathologic stage T2a versus T2b versus T2c disease[480–483] and seems to confer no prognostic value for predicting biochemical recurrence after RP. The seventh edition of the AJCC TNM staging system retains the same three pT2 categories as the sixth edition to allow for the accumulation of more data to address this issue, although future staging systems may collapse the substages into a single group.[476]

The 2009 ISUP Consensus Conference on handling and staging of RP specimens, concluded that consensus was reached to discontinue the use of the current pT2 substaging system. In view of the lack of clinical significance of the current (TNM 2002/2010) pT2 subcategories, there was general agreement for the recommendation that the reporting of pT2 substaging of prostate cancers should be optional.[484]

Pathologic Stage T3

Pathologic stage T3 disease is subdivided into two categories as determined by the presence of EPE in any location (pT3a) and the presence of SVI with or without EPE (pT3b).

Extraprostatic Extension (pT3a)

Extraprostatic extension is the preferred terminology and should be used rather than terms such as capsular invasion, capsular penetration, or capsular perforation. EPE is a

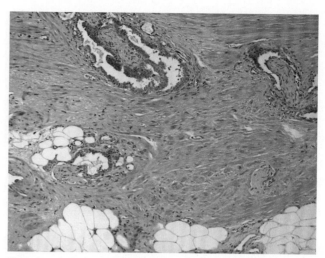

FIGURE 9-147 ■ At low-power magnification, a few cancer glands are noted outside of the confines of the prostate, admixed with periprostatic fat.

well-known adverse prognostic factor in prostate cancer, and accurate identification is required for optimal patient management after RP.[485,486]

EPE is simply defined as the presence of prostate cancer beyond the confines of the prostate, and criteria exist to guide pathologists in its recognition. In the posterior, posterolateral, and lateral aspects of the gland, tumor admixed with periprostatic fat is the most easily recognized manifestation of EPE (Fig. 9-147). However, the prostate gland does not possess a true histologic capsule,[487] and at times, it can be challenging to identify the boundary of the gland, particularly when prostate cancer is associated with a desmoplastic reaction at the periphery.[488,489] The presence of a distinct tumor nodule within desmoplastic stroma that bulges beyond the normal rounded contour of the gland may also be recognized as EPE[489] (Fig. 9-148). EPE in the posterolateral area can be diagnosed when tumor is identified within loose connective tissue or perineural spaces of the neurovascular bundles even in the absence of direct contact between tumor cells and adipocytes (Fig. 9-149).

In the apex, anterior, and bladder neck regions, there is a paucity of fat, and the histologic boundary of the prostate is poorly defined, complicating the assessment of EPE at these sites. At the apex, some authors consider EPE exists when malignant glands touch an inked surgical margin where benign glands have not been similarly cut across or when tumor extends beyond the contour of the normal gland (Fig. 9-150), while others strictly require fat involvement, which is uncommon.[489,490] At the 2009 ISUP Consensus Conference, it was agreed that prostate cancer can be categorized as pT3a in the absence of adipose tissue involvement when cancer bulges beyond the contour of the gland or beyond the condensed smooth muscle of the prostate at posterior and posterolateral sites.[502] At the anterior most part, there is paucity of glandular elements in the anterior fibromuscular stroma creating a gap in the gland contour,

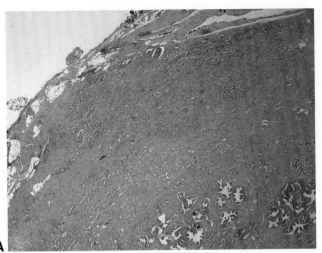
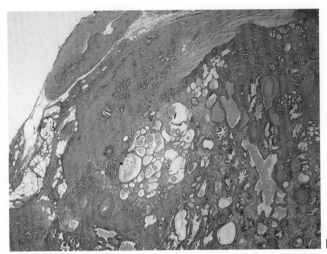

FIGURE 9-148 ■ **A,B:** A tumor nodule within desmoplastic stroma that bulges beyond the normal rounded contour of the gland may also be recognized as EPE.

making assessment of EPE in the absence of fat involvement difficult. Because of the intermingling of benign glands with skeletal muscles at the apex and anteriorly, involvement of skeletal muscle alone at these sites should not be considered as EPE.[489,490]

Substantial variability between experienced and inexperienced pathologists has been reported regarding the diagnosis of EPE.[479,491] It is also important to realize that not all patients with EPE can be accurately identified, particularly when prostate cancer is present at the surgical margin of resection.

Recognizing that more than 50% of patients with EPE at RP do not show tumor progression over a 10-year follow-up period,[492] different methods have been suggested to quantify EPE that will provide more accurate prognostic information in terms of PSA failure and cancer progression. However, no single method has emerged that is objective, practical, and accurate in terms of its ability to predict biochemical failure and disease progression.

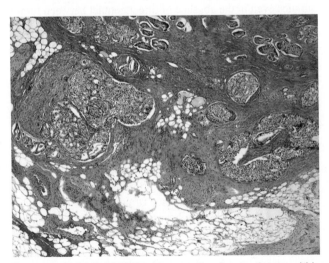

FIGURE 9-149 ■ EPE with prostatic adenocarcinoma within the perineural space of the neurovascular bundle at multiple sites.

In 1993, Epstein et al.[493] suggested to categorize the extent of EPE as focal (Fig. 9-151) or established (Fig. 9-152) (where focal refers to finding a few neoplastic glands outside the prostate and established to anything more than a few glands). Later on, Wheeler et al. subdivided prostate tumors with EPE into two subgroups: focal and established (where focal was defined as extraprostatic tumor occupying less than one high-power field on less than or equal to two separate sections and established as any EPE that was more extensive than focal).[494]

Most recently, Sung et al.[495] have measured the maximum distance of tumor protruding beyond the outer margin of the prostatic stroma (radial extent) in RP specimens. When they systematically compared their approach with other methods of EPE quantification, they found that the radial distance of EPE was the only independent predictor of PSA recurrence in multivariate analysis.[495] However, the accuracy of any method used to quantify EPE is limited by the difficulty pathologists can encounter in identifying the boundary of the prostate gland in some cases.[490]

An overwhelming majority of the 2009 ISUP Consensus Conference delegates supported the suggestion that EPE should be quantitated. However, the delegates could not agree on what specific method should be used to classify EPE as focal.[502]

Microscopic Bladder Neck Invasion (pT3a)

In the sixth edition of AJCC staging, bladder neck involvement was considered as advanced disease and categorized as pT4, based on the belief that tumors that invade surrounding structures are more aggressive and warrant higher staging.[496] This outdated staging system was based upon finding macroscopic invasion of the bladder neck or external sphincter by the urologist.

Today, most prostate cancer patients with bladder neck invasion are detected incidentally after RP. Microscopic bladder neck involvement is defined as the presence of tumor

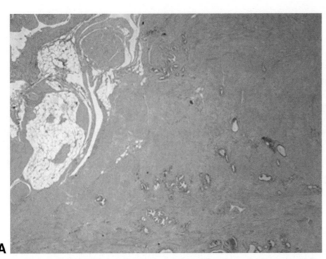
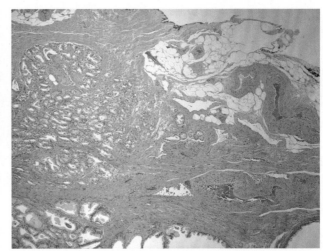

FIGURE 9-150 ■ **A,B:** EPE can be diagnosed at the apex when adenocarcinoma glands extend beyond the contour of the normal gland.

cells within smooth muscle bundles of the bladder neck in absence of benign prostatic glandular tissue on the corresponding slide (Fig. 9-153).[497]

The College of American Pathologists (CAP) practice protocol on prostate and the 7th edition of the AJCC staging system (AJCC 2010)[476] state that microscopic involvement of bladder neck muscle fibers indicates pT3a disease and that gross involvement of the bladder neck is required for pT4 stage.[498] Several recent studies questioning the independent prognostic significance of microscopic bladder neck involvement by PCA have reported a risk of progression similar to EPE and lower than SVI, supporting the notion that bladder neck invasion should be considered as pT3a disease.[497,499–501]

During the 2009 ISUP Consensus Conference, there was consensus that tumor involving the bladder neck, specifically defined as neoplastic cells within thick smooth muscle bundles, should be reported as pT3a. The presence of prostate cancer glands intermixed with benign prostatic glands at the

bladder neck was considered equivalent to capsular incision. It was recommended that if tumor is present at the inked resection margin at the bladder neck, this should be stated in the report.[502]

Seminal Vesicle Invasion (pT3b)

The identification of SVI has an important role in determining a patient's prognosis after RP and may guide appropriate subsequent therapy by use of a number of predictive models.[503]

SVI is defined as invasion of the muscular wall of seminal vesicle by prostate cancer (Fig. 9-154).[504] The variation in the pathologic handling and sampling of seminal vesicles in RP specimens is responsible for the wide range in the percentage of cases with seminal vesicle involvement (5% to 10%) and in the 5-year biochemical recurrence-free survival (5% to 60%) reported in major series.[505–508] SVI is commonly associated with EPE and has been shown to be an adverse prognostic factor.

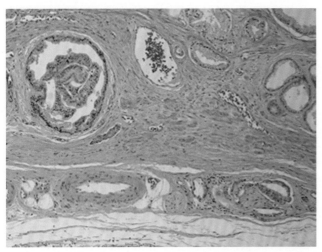

FIGURE 9-151 ■ Focal EPE with few neoplastic glands wrapping around a nerve outside the prostate, at the same level as periprostatic fat.

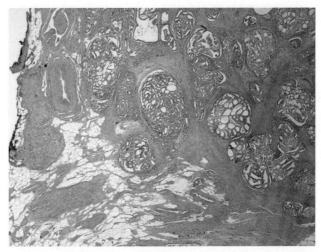

FIGURE 9-152 ■ Established EPE with numerous neoplastic glands extending beyond the contour of the normal prostate and a few glands admixed with periprostatic fat.

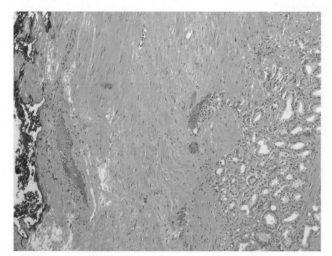

FIGURE 9-153 ■ Prostatic adenocarcinoma microscopically infiltrating among thick muscle bundles of the bladder neck in the absence of benign prostatic glandular tissue.

The junction of the seminal vesicle with the prostate gland should always be assessed for contiguous spread and should be considered the minimum necessary to adequately sample seminal vesicles.[509] At the 2009 ISUP Consensus Conference, it was agreed that only muscular wall invasion of the extraprostatic seminal vesicle should be regarded as SVI.[509]

Stage T4

Pathologic stage T4 prostate cancer is defined by direct rectal involvement, gross invasion of the urinary bladder, external sphincter, levator muscles, and/or pelvic wall, with or without fixation. Since the widespread of PSA screening, clinical stage T4 prostate cancer has become rare, and patients with large bulky masses involving the above-mentioned structures are not typically candidates for surgical treatment.

However, it is reasonable to assign a pT4 stage to a RP specimen with an associated biopsy of rectum, urinary bladder (that is not microscopic invasion of bladder neck), or pelvic side wall positive for prostate cancer, directly invading these structures, as assessed by clinical and/or radiologic means.[502]

Today, prostate cancer with rectal involvement is a clinically late event usually associated with wide EPE and frequently distant metastases and carries a dismal prognosis despite multimodality treatment.[510,511] Urinary bladder and rectum involvement by prostatic carcinoma can also occur via lymphovascular invasion (LVI), without contiguous spread; for these cases, an M1 designation may be more appropriate than pT4.

Surgical Margin Status

Surgical margin status in RP specimens is a prognostic parameter for postoperative biochemical recurrence and disease progression.[489,512]

On pathologic evaluation, a positive surgical margin is defined as the presence of tumor cells reaching the inked surgical margin of resection of the RP specimen (Fig. 9-155).[513] Despite general consensus on the importance and clinical relevance of RP surgical margin status, marked variability still exists in the interpretation of surgical margins by pathologists practicing in different institutions.

The acceptance of considering a surgical margin as negative (Fig. 9-156) as long as cancer cells do not reach the inked surface of the specimen, despite microscopically close distances (<0.1 mm), is supported by the absence of residual tumor and lack of postoperative disease progression in such patients.[489,514]

Interinstitutional variation in the specific classification of margins makes it difficult to compare the location of positive margins in RP specimens in various reported series.[489]

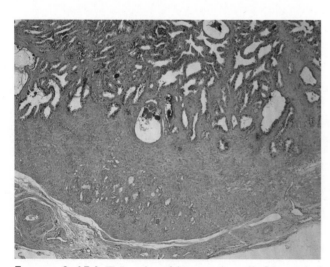

FIGURE 9-154 ■ Invasion of the muscular wall of the seminal vesicle by prostate cancer is stage pT3b.

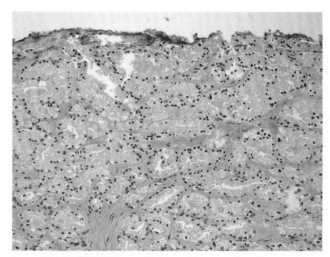

FIGURE 9-155 ■ Positive resection margin. Prostate cancer cells are touching the inked surgical margin of the RP specimen.

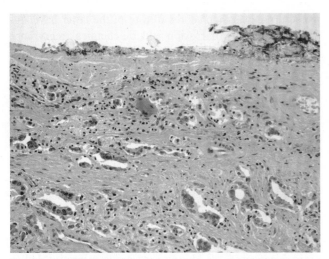

FIGURE 9-156 ■ Negative resection margin. Despite microscopic closeness to the inked surface of the specimen, the cancer glands do not reach the ink.

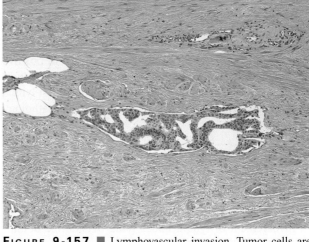

FIGURE 9-157 ■ Lymphovascular invasion. Tumor cells are present within an intraprostatic endothelial-lined space with no underlying muscular wall.

Consensus agreement was reached for the uniform reporting of the location of positive margins as posterior, posterolateral, lateral, and anterior at the the prostatic apex, midprostate, or base.[513]

Several studies have shown that the extent of tumor at the surgical margin correlates with postoperative disease recurrence.[514,515] On the basis of the balance of data available in the literature, there was a consensus that the extent of a positive margin should be recorded as mm of involvement.[513]

Lymphovascular Invasion

LVI is a well-established prognostic factor in a number of human malignancies and is among the histologic variables that the Association of Directors of Anatomic and Surgical Pathology (ADASP) and the CAP recommend to report in RP specimens.[516,517]

LVI is defined as the unequivocal presence of tumor cells within endothelial-lined spaces with no muscular walls (Fig. 9-157) or as the presence of tumor emboli in small intraprostatic vessels.[518,519]

Recently, the incidence of LVI in prostate cancer patients with pT3aN0 disease was found to range between 28% and 35%.[520,521] The prognostic significance of LVI in prostate cancer has been investigated by different groups with conflicting findings. LVI has been significantly associated with regional lymph node metastases[522] and with adverse pathologic features in RP specimens,[490] such as higher Gleason score, positive surgical margins, EPE, and SVI.[519] Multivariate analyses have confirmed that LVI is an independent predictor of disease recurrence.[515,518,523]

At the 2009 ISUP Consensus Conference, there was consensus that LVI should be reported in the routine examination of RP specimens.[502]

Regional Lymph Nodes

The N staging assesses the absence (N0) or presence (N1) of regional lymph node involvement. The spread of any tumor to lymph nodes (Fig. 9-158) indicates tumor dissemination and has an important impact on management and prognosis. Despite recent advances in imaging techniques, pelvic lymph node dissection remains the most accurate staging procedure for the detection of lymph node involvement by prostate cancer.

For prostate cancer, the regional lymph nodes are the nodes of the true pelvis, located below the bifurcation of the common iliac arteries. Laterality does not affect staging. The current AJCC staging manual does not include any stratification of prostate cancer patients according to the number of positive lymph nodes.

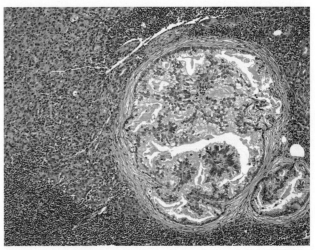

FIGURE 9-158 ■ Metastatic prostate cancer involving a regional lymph node.

The number of lymph nodes obtained in a lymphadenectomy varies widely among centers, which is a function of surgical technique as well as pathologic practice. The diameter of the largest metastasis appears to be more predictive of cancer-specific survival than the number of positive nodes alone.[524,525] At the 2009 ISUP Consensus Conference, there was a consensus that the diameter of the largest lymph node metastasis should be included in the final pathology report.[509]

Metastases

Prostate cancer tends to spread to the regional lymph nodes and bone and, to a lesser degree, to the lung, liver, and brain. Metastases in other locations are exceptional.

Involvement of lymph nodes lying outside the boundaries of the true pelvis is classified as M1a disease. Osteoblastic bone metastases (M1b) are the most common nonnodal site of metastasis with more than 50% of patients with advanced prostate cancer having identifiable lesions (Fig. 9-159).[526] Lung and liver metastases are usually identified late in the course of the disease and classified as M1c.

The presence of bone metastases indicates to a poor prognosis and is one of the major causes of morbidity and mortality in PCA patients.

PROGNOSTIC AND PREDICTIVE FACTORS

Clinicopathologic Factors

Gleason Grade

Gleason grade is one of the most important prognostic factors for prostate cancer. In needle biopsies with cancer, Gleason grade is widely used to choose the mode of therapy. Higher Gleason score (7 to 10) is associated with worse prognosis than scores of 5 to 6; the latter have significantly lower progression and biochemical recurrence rates. Gleason score in NCBs correlates with findings at RP (e.g., stage, Gleason score, tumor volume, and margin status) and outcome after RP, radiotherapy, hormonal therapy, and other treatments, such as cryotherapy and neoadjuvant therapy, or no treatment. In needle biopsies, the predictive value of Gleason score is enhanced when combined with PSA level and DRE findings. In 2005, Gleason grading was updated to its current modified scheme by ISUP via a consensus conference,[218] which further improved its correlation with pathologic stage, margin status, biochemical recurrence, and survival.[453,465,468,471,527–529] The new ISUP modified Gleason grading system caused upgrading across the different grade spectrums, most notably of Gleason score 6 cancers.[453,472] The upward grade migration led to purer Gleason score 6 cancers and enhanced the separation of Gleason grade 3 + 4 = 7 and 4 + 3 = 7 cancers as distinct prognostic groups.[530] Among Gleason score 7 cancers, up to 95% of 3 + 4 = 7 carcinomas are organ-confined tumors, whereas 79% of 4 + 3 = 7 carcinomas are of higher stage.[528] It is unclear, however, if the prognostic difference in Gleason score 7 cancers is also present in needle biopsies that can be used reliably to aid in choosing the type of therapy. Interestingly, a recent study suggested that Gleason 3 + 3 = 6 cancer according to the ISUP modified grading does not show metastasis,[531] precipitating a provocative discussion of whether tumors with this grade should be labeled as cancer.[532] Gleason grade is an integral component of predictive nomograms and TNM stage groupings for prostate cancer, which are important tools in helping clinicians decide on management and follow-up.[458,459,533,534] Gleason grade on biopsy is also incorporated in preoperative nomograms to predict recurrence in patients with localized disease after prostatectomy.[457,534] Gleason grading is covered in detail in the preceding part of this chapter.

Tumor Quantification

Several studies have shown a strong correlation of tumor volume in needle biopsy with RP stage, final tumor volume, Gleason score, margin status, neurovascular bundle involvement, and posttreatment progression.[298,535–537] Higher tumor volume in biopsies is associated with EPE and SVI on RP[298,537] and, more importantly, is predictive of biochemical recurrence. Tumor volume in biopsies is also being incorporated as one of the elements in nomograms to predict biochemical recurrence after RP. Although good correlation is shown with high tumor volume, the presence of a small amount of tumor in biopsies is not always indicative of small tumor volume in RP specimens. This is not unusual particularly in predominantly anterior-based tumors that are not accessed adequately by TRUS-guided biopsy.

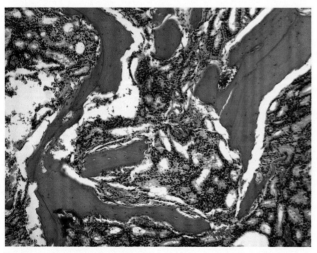

FIGURE 9-159 ■ Metastatic prostate cancer involving femoral head bone.

The different methods of measuring tumor volume in biopsies such as by total percentage of cancer, greatest percentage of cancer per core, total cancer length in millimeters, and fraction of positive cores of needle biopsy are shown to be highly correlated. The fraction of positive cores, total percentage of cancer, and both total and greatest millimeter cancer lengths are most closely associated with pathologic stage and biochemical failure status.[535] In a survey among urologic pathologists, the most common approach of measuring tumor extent in biopsies is to provide the number of cores involved and measurement of tumor in millimeters and/or percentage.[538] Tumor in biopsies can be present as multiple discontinuous foci, thus introducing two possible ways of measuring tumor extent—whether or not to include the intervening stroma. It was shown that measuring the multiple foci as a single connected focus rather than "collapsing" or adding the individual lengths correlates with stage and margin status.[539] However, if the discontinuous tumors are separated by ≤5 mm distance, it does not matter which type of measurement is performed.[535] Quantification of tumor volume in needle biopsies is generally straightforward, but it can be challenging in fragmented cores.[540] Fragmentation is more common in tissue cores containing cancer, and the number of cores submitted and Gleason score contribute to the likelihood of fragmentation.[540]

The percentage of tumor should always be reported in TURP, as tumor volume is a determinant of substaging of cT1 tumors.[541] However, the significance of dividing tumor volume in TURP using the current 5% cutoff in terms of predicting residual tumor and biochemical recurrence is still being debated.[542,543] While waiting for more evidence and optimal tumor volume cutoffs, it is recommended that the number of involved chips and the percentage of involved to total chips should be reported.

Earlier studies have shown correlation of tumor volume in RP with local extension, disease progression, metastasis, and patient survival.[544–548] It was also shown that the tumor percentage is perhaps better than the tumor volume in RP to correlate with pathologic stage and as predictor of tumor progression.[546,547] However, with subsequent studies, the value of tumor volume in RP as a prognostic variable is still being debated, as more contemporary studies are showing contrasting results. While some studies have shown tumor volume to be an independent prognostic factor in RP,[549–552] more studies have shown that it does not provide independent prognostic information beyond Gleason score and pathologic stage.[553–558]

There are different approaches to measuring tumor volume in RP. The most practical and rapid way is by estimation of the percentage of tumor involvement by visual inspection.[484] Other methods have better precision but are more tedious such as by measuring the diameter of the largest focus,[552,553] three-dimensional measurement,[559] computer-assisted image analysis of the maximum tumor area,[560] block counting,[561,562] grid method,[544] point count method,[563,564] and by naked eye visualization after marking the slides.[551] Most urologic pathologists provide the diameter of the largest tumor for size assessment and visual inspection for tumor volume.[484] Tumor dimensions can be directly measured on coronal sections but there may be problems on estimating the third dimension, which relies on the thickness of the sections.

In cases of prostate glands with multifocal cancers, the index tumor was suggested to be the focus or nodule containing the highest grade and/or stage and is considered to be the main determinant of tumor behavior among the several foci.[484] The size of the dominant tumor nodule may be provided in two measured dimensions and/or by number of blocks involved over total number of blocks. However, the concept of index tumor is also being challenged because the largest tumor dimension, as mentioned above, is not independently associated with outcome in more contemporary studies and that the largest size nodule does not always correlate with highest grade on RP. The issues of multifocal cancers and dominant nodules may become more relevant with the emerging treatment strategy of focal therapy for localized prostate cancers.[565]

Measuring the largest tumor dimension is also being considered as a determinant in substaging localized prostate cancer (pT2) in RP.[552,561,566,567] The following cutoffs were proposed: 5 mm or less, 5 to 16 mm, and >16 mm for pT2a, pT2b, and pT2c, respectively.[566] These cutoffs were based on the rationale that tumor dimension of <0.5 mm has tumor volume of <0.5 cm^3, an increase of 10 mm in size increases the recurrence risk by 70%, and that 16 mm was shown to be the median maximum tumor diameter.[541,552,567] However, this substaging proposal has yet to be validated by an independent study.

Extraprostatic Extension

The prostate does not have a true capsule, but instead has an outer rim of condensed fibrous tissue that is contiguous with the stroma. EPE is the preferred term over other ambiguous terms such as "capsular penetration" or "capsular extension."[568,569] Histologically, EPE is defined as tumor involvement of the fat, since fat inside the prostate is vanishingly rare.[489] EPE is reported in about 36% of prostatectomy specimens and is most easily recognizable in the posterior and posterolateral parts where there is abundance of fat. In cases wherein there is no direct contact of tumor to fat, any tumor seen on the outer rim of loose connective tissues at plane of fat is labeled as EPE. However, the amount of extraprostatic fat may vary and may be scant or not present at the apex, anterior, or base that limits the assessment of EPE. Alternatively, it is suggested that for these three regions, that tumor outside the benign glandular confines should be regarded as EPE, although this is controversial. Rarely, fat may be seen around apex making assessment of EPE possible, particularly with robotic-assisted resections. Prostate cancer may extend to extraprostatic tissue by traveling via a nerve, and peri-/intraneural invasion within or in the plane of fat is also considered as EPE. Transition zone cancer when it extends to outside of prostate usually does not travel via the nerve.[489]

It is important to comment on the extent of EPE and if the resection margin is positive for tumor at the site of EPE (noniatrogenic, discussed below). Dividing EPE as focal or nonfocal was shown to have prognostic value.[493,494] EPE is considered focal when tumor extension is less than one high-power field from the prostate outer boundary and is not present in more than two sections.[494] EPE is nonfocal or established with more extensive local tumor spread outside of prostate. The 5-year progression-free survival for focal EPE is 73%, whereas it is 42% for established EPE.[494]

Size estimate of EPE is optional and can be performed by taking the greatest linear dimension with or without the total number of blocks involved. The radial distance of EPE was shown to be an independent predictor of PSA recurrence, compared with the focal and established EPE assessment.[495] Reporting of location of EPE is considered optional. In a 2010 ISUP survey, most expert GU pathologists report the location and number of EPE despite of no proven clinical relevance yet.[484]

Interobserver agreement in calling EPE among expert GU pathologists is good to excellent (κ 0.63).[490] The main reasons for the appreciable interobserver variability among experts include the lack of consistent prostate "capsule" boundary and presence of obscuring desmoplasia.[490]

Comments of EPE may be made in needle biopsy or TURP when the specimen shows fat with involvement by tumor. In needle biopsy, involvement of fat does correlate with findings of EPE in prostatectomy specimens. In biopsy and prostatectomy, involvement of striated muscles (anterior or apex) and/or ganglion cells alone should not be interpreted as EPE. Presence of EPE at needle biopsy is associated with extensive high-grade carcinoma and EPE at prostatectomy, but with relatively limited value when present as an isolated prognostic factor.[570]

Margin Status

A resection margin is considered positive if tumor cells are seen touching the ink or more assertively if the cancer gland is transected at the inked margin.[489,571,572] Positive surgical margin is reported in 11% to 34% of RP specimens.[486,515,571,573–577] Positive surgical margin has been shown to independently predict biochemical recurrence.[512,578] However, this finding is contradicted by other studies.[579] If the tumor is organ confined, the positive surgical margin (i.e., iatrogenic margin) may have no effect on tumor progression.[492] There is higher nonprogression rate or

increase in PSA with negative (83%) than positive (64%) RP margin.[492] Tumor that is only close to the margin (e.g., <0.1 to 5 mm) does not predict PSA recurrence and tumor progression.[514,580,581]

The extent of positive margin should be measured and reported. It was shown in several studies that extent of positive margin may have some predictive value.[514,515,582,583] Using a 3-mm cutoff, recurrence rate was reported as 53% in >3-mm positive margin, whereas it was only <14% in 3-mm or less positive margin.[515] Further, positive surgical margin when stratified into categorical variable (<1, 1 to 3, >3 mm) was shown to be an independent predictor of biochemical recurrence. Interestingly, patients with negative margins and those with a positive margin <1 mm have similar rates of biochemical recurrence (log rank test $P = 0.18$).[578] Most expert GU pathologists prefer to report positive surgical margin in mm.[509]

There are two types of positive margins, iatrogenic or noniatrogenic types, distinguished by presence or absence of complete outer prostate rim and EPE at the tumor transection site. Iatrogenic or capsular incision (pT2, R1) is when tumor is transected at a margin within the prostate. Noniatrogenic is when tumor at EPE is transected at the margin (pT3 R1). Isolated iatrogenic positive margin may have higher recurrence rate than organ-confined or focal EPE margin negative tumors and lower recurrence rate than extensive noniatrogenic positive margin tumor.[584] However, the clinical relevance of these types of positive margin is still being debated.[584,585]

The location of positive margin should also be reported. Common sites of positive margin are the apex, posterior, and posterolateral aspects of prostate.[489,512,573,575,586] The distribution of positive margins for retropubic, perineal, and laparoscopic RPs was apex in 50%, 33.3%, and 44.4%; bladder neck in 29.1%, 41.7%, and 13.9%; and posterolaterally in 20.8%, 25%, and 41.6%, respectively.[575] With robotic prostatectomy, the apex has the highest incidence, which constitutes about half of the positive margins, and the rates are lower than the open prostatectomy approach.[586] The iatrogenic-type positive margin is more common at the posterolateral than apex.[584] Positive margin at the posterolateral may carry a higher risk of progression.[574] Location of positive surgical margin was not proven to be an independent predictor of biochemical recurrence.[578]

The Gleason score of the tumor at the margin is recently considered as another important variable in assessment of positive margin. The Gleason score at the transected site may be similar or lower to that in the main tumor. Gleason score at the margin strongly correlates with preoperative PSA, pathologic stage, and Gleason score of the main tumor, lymph node status, and the linear length of tumor at the positive margin.[587] More importantly, Gleason score at the margin independently predicts biochemical recurrence ($P < 0.05$).[548]

The *multifocality* or number of positive surgical margins may have clinical relevance. Multiple versus solitary positive surgical margins is independently associated with increased risk of biochemical recurrence.[583]

More recent approach in management of positive surgical margin prefers to wait for biochemical recurrence before proceeding with intervention. Some may opt for local RT. Reporting of presence of transected benign glands at the margin including its size and focality (unifocal or multifocal) is optional, as this was not shown to strongly correlate with biochemical recurrence.

Perineural Invasion

PNI is defined as presence of prostate cancer juxtaposed intimately along, around, or within a nerve. PNI is a ubiquitous finding reported in up to 38% of needle biopsy[301] and is one major route for EPE. There appears to be some pathobiologic affinity and enhanced proliferation of prostate carcinoma to nerve, which may explain this phenomenon.[301,588] PNI when present within fat is considered as EPE in prostatectomy or biopsy.

Studies over the last two decades showed varied results regarding the prognostic significance of PNI on needle biopsy, and thus, its value as a prognostic factor still remains controversial.[589–598] More recent studies, however, have shown that patients with PNI were more likely to have adverse pathologic features, including EPE, SVI, and positive surgical margins.[592,594,599] One large study of 3,226 patients identified PNI in 20% of biopsies and was shown to be independently associated with adverse pathologic features and worse survival outcomes after RP.[599] PNI in a needle biopsy has been correlated with recurrence and prostate cancer–specific mortality after RT.[600,601] But given the variable findings from different studies, reporting status of PNI in a biopsy is currently considered optional.

Lymphovascular Invasion

LVI is characterized by presence of tumor cells within an endothelial-lined space in the prostate that is usually devoid of a muscular wall.[518–521,602–608] LVI is reported in the range of 5% to 38% in prostatectomy[518,519,521,602–605,607,609,610]; the wide range reflects the variability and difficulty in interpretation. Distinction between a vessel and a lymphatic channel is often difficult, although distinction between these two structures is of no clinical relevance. Several tissue changes may uncommonly mimic LVI such as retraction artifact, PNI, cancer impinging upon vascular space, tangential sections of endothelium, displacement of benign and collapsed malignant glands, retraction with erythrocytes, intravascular degenerating tumor cells, malignant glands in atrophic ducts, and myofibroblastic proliferation in thrombosed vessels.[608] LVI can be confirmed by the use of endothelial-associated markers such as CD31, CD34, and D2-40, although this is often not necessary.

About half of LVI occurs in the tumor, and about half can be outside at the prostatic stroma.[520,602] Incidence of LVI is higher in higher-volume tumors (7% in <4 mL and 24% higher-volume cancers).[605] LVI was shown to be associated with adverse pathologic variables such as higher PSA, higher Gleason grade, higher percentage of positive biopsy cores, EPE, PNI, seminal vesicle extension, and positive surgical margins.[515,519,523,603,605,610] LVI is also associated with distant metastasis and overall survival after RP.[519,607,609] Several studies have shown LVI as an independent predictor of biochemical failure and disease progression[515,518,523,603,605,610]; thus, reporting of LVI in RP is required.

Seminal Vesicle Invasion

Invasion into seminal vesicle is considered only when prostate carcinoma involves the seminal muscular wall.[504,509] Portion of seminal vesicle may be intraprostatic, and only extraprostatic SVI should be considered. Prognostic distinction however is only scantily addressed in the literature. In needle biopsy specimens, SVI can be diagnosed particularly in biopsies that are directed at the seminal vesicles. However, it is important to remember that there is significant overlap in the histologic features of the seminal vesicles and the ejaculatory ducts including the characteristic features of the epithelium. The muscular wall of the seminal vesicles is thick with dense smooth muscle and a well-defined outer surface. The muscular wall of the ejaculatory ducts is usually thinner, less dense, and less well defined. If benign prostatic glands are in immediate contact with the muscular wall of the structure in question, this would favor ejaculatory duct. In some cases, it is not possible to be certain whether the structure involved is SV or ejaculatory duct, and in this situation, the report should reflect this uncertainty.

There are three mechanisms of SVI by prostate cancer: type 1, direct spread along ejaculatory duct tissue into seminal vesicle; type 2, direct extra- or intraprostatic spread into seminal vesicle; and type 3, noncontiguous metastasis to seminal vesicle. Types 1, 2, and 3 SVI are reported in 26%, 33%, and 13% cases with SVI, respectively.[504] It is unclear, however, if these different types of tumor spread to seminal vesicles have prognostic importance.

SVI overall predicts poor prognosis in terms of biochemical failure[507,508] and is considered as an important variable in staging locally aggressive prostate cancer (pT3b). Differences in how seminal vesicles are sampled and 5-year recurrence-free survival vary from 5% to 60%.[611]

Bladder Neck Invasion

In the recent 2010 AJCC staging, bladder neck invasion by prostate cancer is categorized as pT3.[541] Bladder neck invasion is considered when there is invasion of prostate cancer on bundles of smooth muscles from a section site identified as bladder neck.[501,516,612] Some experts require microscopic invasion in smooth muscle tissue in the absence of benign prostatic glands.[497,613–615] The CAP protocol specifies microscopic invasion of bladder neck muscle as pT3a.[498] Bladder neck invasion is reported in 1.2% to 9% of prostatectomies.[497,501,574,612–617] Most studies show similar prognosis of bladder neck invasion to EPE.[501,574,612–614] Bladder neck invasion is associated with adverse prognostic variable such as higher Gleason grade, larger tumor size, positive margins, higher stage including EPE, and lymph node metastasis.[497,614–616] However, bladder neck invasion is not an independent prognostic predictor when the other adverse prognostic variables are controlled. From a study with a large cohort of 17,000 men, isolated positive bladder neck margin after RP had a 12-year biochemical recurrence-free survival of 37% and cancer-specific survival of 92%, which were similar to patients with SVI (pT3b) and EPE (pT3a), respectively.[617] According to the ISUP consensus, bladder neck involvement is considered as pT3a and that presence of prostate cancer intermixed with benign glands at bladder neck is considered equivalent to capsular incision.[503]

Biomarkers

Prostate cancer is known for its heterogeneous behaviour. Many tumors are detected at an early stages and have ions latency periods. There has been much research attention on identifying biomarkers that can predict progression. Despite extensive research efforts, no biomarker is currently used in routine practice as a prognostic or predictive marker for prostate cancer.

Several review articles dealing with prognostic and predictive markers for prostate cancer including immunohistochemical markers and serum and/or plasma assays are available in the literature.[493,624–630] Table 9-17 summarizes potential prognostic and predictive biomarkers for prostate cancer.

SPECIMEN HANDLING AND REPORTING

Specimen Handling

The routine surgical pathology specimens in prostate cancer practice are usually NCBs and RPs. TURP is mainly used for BPH, and sometimes, specimens harbor incidental prostate cancer. Occasionally, a TURP is performed to relieve obstruction in advanced prostate cancer. Fine needle aspiration of the prostate, while popular in Europe in days past, is rarely done today and is not recommended because the lack of tumor architecture precludes assessment of Gleason grade and there are problems with specificity.

The CAP and ADASP have produced regularly updated guidelines, protocols, checklists, and recommendations for handling and reporting specimens containing prostate cancer.[498,568,569,647,648] More recently, the CAP has become the principal American organization responsible for maintaining these guidelines. This concerted effort has been strengthened by the requirement of the American College of Surgeons Commission on Cancer that the mandatory elements of the CAP cancer checklists be present in at least 90% of pathology reports in cancer facilities seeking CoC accreditation. The Royal Colleges of Pathology in the United Kingdom and Australasia have also been active in the development of data sets and structured reporting guidelines for cancer specimens.[649,650] More recently, the Colleges of Pathology in the United States, United Kingdom, and Australasia together with the Canadian Association of Pathologist have formed the International Collaboration on Cancer Reporting (ICCR).[651] This group is involved in the development of harmonized international cancer reporting data sets based on existing jurisdictional data sets using an evidence-based framework. The data sets contain required and recommended elements and have extensive explanatory notes. Recently, a data set for RPs has been published.[651] These guidelines will be incorporated into the WHO publications in the near future.

In 2011, the ISUP provided comprehensive consensus statements to address the different issues in the handling and reporting of RP specimens.[484,503,509,513,652] A survey was also conducted among European pathologists but mainly on handling and sampling of prostatectomy specimens.[653] Several comprehensive reviews on reporting and handling of prostate specimens are also available in the literature.[487,569,629,654,655]

Needle Core Biopsy

Historically, thick core (14-gauge) digital-guided biopsies were performed to investigate DRE abnormalities. However, these were supplanted in the late 1980s by TRUS-guided thin-core (18-gauge) biopsies, and this technique has stood the test of time.[656] For more than a decade, systematic sextant sampling of the bilateral base, middle, and apical regions was a standard practice. More recently, extended sampling protocols have been used often yielding 10 to 14 cores including ones from wide lateral locations.[629,657] Sometimes, selected samples from the transition zones and/or from nodules detected by DRE or TRUS are also taken. There is little gain in cancer detection when more than 14 cores are obtained.[658] There are many advantages of site-specific labeling, which are shown in Table 9-18. The location and distribution of tumor is used by some urologists and radiation oncologists to plan therapy. This information is of particular importance with emerging focal therapies.[565] When the specific site of an ASAP is known, the follow-up

Table 9-17 ■ SELECTED CANDIDATE BIOMARKERS IN PROSTATE CANCER

Biomarkers	Applications	Assays	Comment
TMPRSS2:ERG[630]	Prognostic	ERG immunohistochemistry, FISH	Reports on prognostic value conflicting
Ki67[630]	Prognostic and predictive	Immunohistochemistry (needle biopsy and RP)	Prognostic for death in patients of watchful waiting cohorts and for biochemical recurrence in patients treated with RP, predictive for disease progression in patients undergoing radiation
AMACR[631]	Prognostic	Immunohistochemistry (needle biopsy and RP)	Lower AMACR expression is associated with increased rate of biochemical recurrence and cancer-specific death in localized prostate cancer.
Annexin A3[632]	Prognostic	Immunohistochemistry (needle biopsy)	Reduced expression in prostate cancer correlated with increasing Gleason score and stage, independent adverse prognostic factor and enabled substratification of group of intermediate-risk patients into high- and low-risk subgroups
Cysteine-rich secretory protein 3 (CRISP-3)[633,634]	Prognostic	Immunohistochemistry (RP)	Independently predicts recurrence after RP for localized prostate cancer
E-cadherin[635, 636, 637, 638]	Prognostic	Immunohistochemistry (RP)	Inverse correlation of E-cadherin expression with Gleason grade and aberrant staining correlated with tumor stage and overall survival
Prostate stem cell antigen (PSCA)[639, 640, 641, 642]	Prognostic	Immunohistochemistry	Expression correlates with tumor stage, grade, and androgen independence.
	Predictive	In situ hybridization (needle biopsy)	Levels suppressed after external beam radiotherapy, and elevated levels after therapy may be a clinically adverse predictor for tumor progression.
Transforming growth factor-β1 (TGF-β1)[643,644]	Prognostic	Immunohistochemistry (RP)	Increased TGF-β1 in prostate tissue correlated with tumor grade and stage and biochemical progression
		Blood assay	Preoperative serum level of TGF-β1 correlated with EPE, seminal vesicle extension, metastasis, and biochemical recurrence
Enhancer of zeste homolog 2 (EZH2)[645,646]	Prognostic	Immunohistochemistry (RP)	Predicts prostate cancer recurrence after RP
		Blood assay	Outperform PSA and Gleason score in determining prostate cancer progression
hK-related peptidase 2	Prognostic	Blood assay	Predictor of stage and biochemical recurrence
Urokinase-type plasminogen activator receptor	Prognostic	Blood assay	High concentration correlates with prostate cancer progression.
Insulin-like growth factors (IGF) and binding proteins (IGFBP)	Prognostic	Blood assay	Increased IGF-1 and decreased IGFBP-3 concentrations have been correlated with increased risk for prostate cancer.
Prostate secretory protein (PSP94)	Prognostic	Blood assay	Ratio of PSP94 to free PSP94 and serum level of PSP94-binding protein associated with Gleason score, biochemical recurrence, and margin status
Chromogranin A	Prognostic	Blood assay	Monitoring of castration-resistant advanced prostate cancer

Table 9-18 ■ ADVANTAGES OF SITE-SPECIFIC LABELING OF BIOPSIES

- Location and distribution of tumor used in treatment decisions
  - Plan radiation fields (e.g., brachytherapy)
  - Laterality useful in planning nerve-sparing RP
  - Basal positivity may influence bladder neck–sparing RP.
  - Critical for emerging focal therapies
- Knowledge of ASAP site allows focused rebiopsy.
- Knowledge of CA site useful in follow-up biopsies for patients on active surveillance
- Knowledge of site of CA allows targeted additional sampling of RP with no apparent cancer.
- Allows detailed correlation with DRE and TRUS
- Knowledge of biopsy sites helps to identify diagnostic pitfalls (e.g., seminal vesicle or central zone in basal sites).
- Less cores per container provides technical advantages for histology.

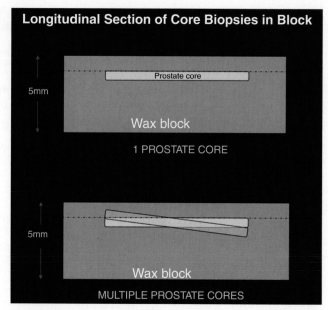

Longitudinal Section of Core Biopsies in Block

5mm — Prostate core — Wax block — 1 PROSTATE CORE

5mm — Wax block — MULTIPLE PROSTATE CORES

FIGURE 9-160 ■ Embedding multiple cores in a paraffin block may create uneven levels among cores, resulting in loss of tissue when cutting.

biopsies can be focused on that site and immediately adjacent ones. Likewise, for minimal cancers on active surveillance protocols, knowledge of the site of initial positivity can allow a more directed approach in the follow-up biopsies. Knowledge of the location of abnormality helps to fine-tune differential diagnosis. For instance, biopsies from the basal region often show prostatic central zone glands, which are architecturally complex and may simulate HGPIN.[659] Importantly, site-specific labeled cases generally have either one or two cores per container, and these are easier for the technologists to handle than cases where there are three or more cores in the container. This increased number of sites per case and the directed sampling has impacted the handling and reporting of biopsy specimens and of course the pathologist's workload.

It is imperative that needle biopsies of the prostate be handled with extreme care by competent technical staff who understand the implications of their work. Misidentification errors are a nightmare for laboratories, pathologists, and clinicians alike. A molecular study of prostate biopsies in a large clinical trial has shown misidentification errors in 0.2% to 0.4% of cases.[660] Wherever possible, a bar-coding system should be used. When accessioning cases, many laboratories avoid sequential numbering of prostate biopsies and separate each prostate biopsy with other biopsy types.

In handling NCBs, one should document the number and lengths of tissue cores and/or core fragments per submitted container. Ideally, there should be one core submitted per container (site). Submitting three or more cores per container can cause problems for the histology laboratory. Only one to two tissue cores per paraffin block are desirable to maximize tissue surface area for analysis. More cores per block may not fully expose all cores on one plane of section and may lead to undesired tissue loss especially when chasing the cores deeper into the block (Fig. 9-160).[661,747] For

the pathologist, reading a few cores at a time also facilitates identification of small atypical glandular foci.[540]

For specimen fixation, neutral buffered formalin is preferred. Bouin solution is not recommended as it alters the nuclear appearance and may enhance the nucleoli even in benign glands. Hematoxylin or other indelible dyes make tissue cores more visible and facilitate cutting of paraffin blocks. Following tissue processing, the embedding, microtomy, and staining should be carried out in a standardized, high-quality fashion. Tissue cores should be embedded flat and straight, if possible, for ease of screening. Microtomy should be done fastidiously with care taken not to exhaust the blocks. Many laboratories save intervening unstained sections for use in immunostaining, if required. This is not necessary in all situations, especially in high-volume prostate laboratories where technologists are highly skilled in tissue core conservation. Generally, two or three slides per block each with two or three sections per slide are presented to the pathologist for reading.

One cannot overemphasize the importance of both thin sections (4 to 5 μm) and standardized consistent H&E staining. Day-to-day variations in staining are to be avoided since the nuclear and cytoplasmic criteria used to make a diagnosis, especially in the case of minimal adenocarcinoma, are dependent on tinctorial consistency and reproducibility.

Transurethral Resection

Prostate cancer is detected in 4% to 16% of TURP, the vast majority incidentally identified.[543,661] TURP is performed mostly to treat BPH although its use is declining because of growing popularity of nonsurgical and ablative therapies. In TURP, cancer detection is also decreasing because of widespread PSA screening and usage of TRUS-guided needle biopsies.[662] TURP specimens mostly contain prostatic transition zone, periurethral glands, and urethral tissues; however, variable amounts of peripheral zone may also be present.

Incidental prostate cancer in TURP specimens is categorized as cT1a when ≤5% and cT1b when >5% of the tissue is involved. Gleason score does not affect the T-category but does affect the stage grouping. Categorical division has been questioned because it is greatly dependent on the amount of tissue recovered at surgery and sampled for histology. Further, this division does not accurately predict the final pathologic stage or correlate with biochemical recurrence after RP, when preoperative variables such as PSA and Gleason grade are taken into account.[542,543,663–665] The cT1b tumors vary considerably in the amount of cancer present, and it has been suggested that stratification of tumor volume is predictive of prostate cancer death.[666] Most incidental cancer detected in TURP samples is organ confined, and in up to 16% of RP cases, no residual cancer (pT0) is detected.[543] The use of serum PSA <1.0 ng/mL is a better predictor for pT0 than cT1a or cT1b categorization.[665]

The CAP has provided some guidance for submitting TURP specimens.[498] If the specimen weighs ≤12 g, the tissue should be submitted entirely. If the specimen is >12 g, 6 to 8 cassettes (roughly equivalent to 12 g) should be submitted, and one may submit 1 cassette for every additional 5 g of tissue. Sensitivity for cancer detection may be increased by selectively submitting tissue fragments that are firm, yellow, or grossly suspicious for cancer; however, the data supporting this statement are scant. If incidental prostate cancer comprises ≤5% of tissue examined, the entire remaining specimen may be submitted, but this decision should be made on a case-by-case basis depending on clinical circumstances. Likewise, if HGPIN is detected without cancer, additional sampling may be undertaken although there is a paucity of data to support this decision, one way or the other.

Radical Prostatectomy

The ISUP made recommendations through consensus conference statements aimed at standardizing the handling, staging, and reporting of RP specimens.[484,503,509,513,652] There is also guidance in various college protocols and guidelines cited earlier.

The RP specimen should be weighed and measured in three dimensions (vertical from base to apex, transverse from right to left, and sagittal from anterior to posterior). Separate dimensions for the seminal vesicles and ejaculatory ducts (if present) should be given. Unless the RP is being sampled in the fresh state for research, it should be fixed in 10%

neutral buffered formalin for 18 to 24 hours prior to sectioning. Sectioning the prostate gland without fixation often results in tissue bulging and retraction of the "capsule" upon immersion in fixative. The number of specimens received fresh without fixative is increasing because of the need for harvesting fresh tissues for molecular studies.[652] It is imperative that sampling for research should not compromise the important variables particularly grading, staging, and margin status. Some authors have suggested that sampling of fresh RPs can be done by ex vivo shaving or punch biopsies.[652,667] Tissue sampling should be performed immediately to assure better quality of DNA, RNA, and proteins.[667–670] Formalin fixation often causes nucleic acid fragmentation and protein cross-linking,[670] but has been shown to have no effect on RNA quality for genomic expression analysis.[671] Alternative ways of fixing RP specimens include microwave-assisted technique or directly injecting fixative to facilitate diffusion.[654,672,673]

The entire outer surface of the prostate should be inked using at least two different colors to identify laterality (right or left) and outer extent or margin of the specimen.[652] Orientation is occasionally challenging, and helpful landmarks include the attached seminal vesicles at the posterosuperior aspect and the smooth fascial plane along the posterior aspect. Furthermore, the verumontanum of the urethra points anteriorly, the ejaculatory ducts are directed posterosuperiorly toward the seminal vesicles, and skeletal muscle can be identified in the anterior fibromuscular region.

When sectioning, the apex, base, and seminal vesicles should be handled in a standardized fashion. It is recommended that every institution and multi-institutional clinical studies should use the same sampling protocol for consistency. Ideally, the apex should be amputated and sectioned perpendicular to the inked surface (Fig. 9-161). Perpendicular

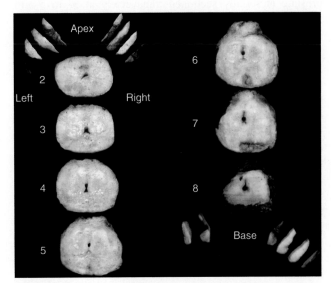

FIGURE 9-161 ■ Gross dissection of the prostate with sectioning of both apex and base in perpendicular fashion (Courtesy of Mark Wahrenbrock, MD).

apical sections may be taken either in a radial manner (similar to cervical cone) or as series of parallel (parasagittal) sections. Most urologic pathologists prefer parasagittal sectioning, which allows more uniform thickness of sections.[652] Shave (en face) sections of the apical margin are not recommended as they may lead to a false-positive margin, since the mere presence of tumor cells on the section is considered transection. Furthermore, assessment of EPE is not possible since only prostatic tissue without the adventitial tissue may be present on superficial cuts. The prostatic urethra often retracts, and urothelium may not be present in the apical sections. This is pertinent only when the prostate or urethra also contains urothelial carcinoma.

The base (bladder neck) can be submitted en face or in a perpendicular fashion with the latter being favored. The base is often irregular, and a shaved (en face) submission may result in a false-positive margin.

The remainder of the prostate gland can be submitted entirely or partially. There are several approaches to partial embedding, and these depend on the clinical stage (cT1c or cT2) or if the cancer is grossly apparent. In one study, complete embedding was not superior to partial embedding for detecting adverse pathologic variables.[674] Partial embedding that includes submission of the grossly visible lesion results in detection of 96% of positive margins and 91% of EPE compared with complete embedding (13 versus 42 blocks).[239] Another study submitting alternate slices showed detection rates for EPE of 15%.[675] Among the partial embedding techniques, submitting the entire posterior and one anterior section from each side or the entire anterior tissue if there is sizeable tumor detected 100% of positive margins and 96% of EPE.[676] While both partial and complete embedding are acceptable, if partial embedding is used, it should be done in a consistent fashion. The middle portion of the prostate is serially sectioned transversely at 3- to 5-mm intervals, and the sections submitted entirely, preferably in quadrants. Partial sampling should be systematic to allow for assessment of volume, multifocality, and orientation. Random sampling precludes tumor measurements, focality determination, and location of positive margin and EPE. Grossly evident tumor should be sampled to include adjacent extraprostatic tissues and inked margins.

Sections of basal prostatic tissue, including the adjacent attached proximal portion of seminal vesicles, are required to demonstrate direct tumor extension. Ideally, the sections should show continuity of the prostate base and seminal vesicle tissue. Of note, SVI is only considered present for staging purposes when the extraprostatic portion of the wall is involved. It is not necessary to submit the entire seminal vesicles. Submission of vas deferens including its margin is optional since cancer spread through this route is highly unusual.

The macroscopic sectioning described above is complex and must be documented in a block legend. This can be done in words or diagrams that may be hand drawn or done with photography. The prostate tissue can also be laid out in an organized fashion on a plexiglass plate containing orientation markers and photocopied for the record.

Few institutions perform whole-mount processing of the prostate.[677] Other than for aesthetics, proponents of this approach report ease in assessing tumor volume, focality, Gleason score in multifocal tumors, and identification of the index tumor. Further, locations of EPE and positive margins are easier to determine. However, whole-mount prostate sectioning is not cost-effective, is technically cumbersome, and requires special histology, and storage equipment.

Specimen Reporting

Detailed recommendations for reporting of prostate cancer specimens have been produced by CAP, RCPath, and RCPA, and more recently, the ICCR has developed a harmonized data set for the RP including both required and recommended elements. These guidelines, protocols, and data sets are updated on a regular basis, and the reader, depending on geographic location, should refer to the appropriate organizational website for the most current version. The specific pathologic elements such as tumor subtype, Gleason grading, tumor staging, and other morphologic prognostics factors are all covered in other sections of this chapter and Chapter 10. For convenience, the current checklist elements from CAP (web posting June 2012) for reporting NCB, TURP, and RP specimens are displayed in Tables 9-19 to 9-21.

TREATMENT EFFECTS

Diverse therapies are used to treat both BPH and adenocarcinoma. Classic treatment options for prostate cancer consist of RP, antiandrogen (or hormonal) therapy, and RT. Hormonal and RT have well-known, often profound effects on the histologic appearance of benign prostate tissue and prostatic carcinoma.[678–680]

The multimodality approach to treat prostate cancer patients at high risk for progression is gaining popularity. The strategies used can include the use of neoadjuvant

---

Table 9-19 ■ IMPORTANT VARIABLES FOR REPORTING OF PROSTATE CANCER IN NEEDLE BIOPSIES

1. Histologic type
2. Histologic grade—primary (predominant), secondary (worst remaining), score
3. Tumor quantitation—number of positive cores and total cores + % prostate tissue involved by tumor and/or total linear mm of carcinoma and total linear mm of core tissue
4. Periprostatic fat invasion*
5. SVI*
6. Lymphovascular invasion†
7. PNI†
8. Additional pathologic findings†

*Documentation required if present.
†Optional.

Table 9-20 ■ IMPORTANT VARIABLES FOR REPORTING OF PROSTATE CANCER IN TUR OR ENUCLEATION SPECIMENS (SUBTOTAL PROSTATECTOMY)

1. Procedure TURP, enucleation
2. Specimen weight and size (enucleation)
3. Histologic type
4. Histologic grade—primary (predominant), secondary (worst remaining), score
5. Tumor quantitation—% tissue involved by tumor (required); number of positive chips and total chips (TURP) and dimensions of tumor nodule (enucleation) are optional.
6. Periprostatic fat invasion*
7. Seminal vesicle invasion*
8. Lymphovascular invasion†
9. Perineural invasion†
10. Additional findings†

*Documentation required if present.
†Optional.

(preoperative) hormonal and/or chemotherapy and a variety of adjuvant approaches including hormonal and external beam radiation.[681–684]

Interest in focal therapy for prostate cancer has recently been renewed owing to downward stage migration, improved biopsy and imaging techniques, and the prevalence of either unifocal cancer or a dominant cancer with secondary tumors of minimal malignant potential.[685] Focal therapy aims to control long-term cancer without the associated morbidity that plagues all radical therapies and is emerging as an alternative to active surveillance for the management of low-risk prostate cancer in carefully selected patients.[686] Different energy modalities have been used to focally ablate cancer tissue, and available techniques include cryotherapy, interstitial laser thermotherapy, high-intensity focused ultrasound (HIFU), vascular-targeted photodynamic therapy (PDT), and microwave thermotherapy.

Table 9-21 ■ IMPORTANT VARIABLES FOR REPORTING OF PROSTATE CANCER IN RADICAL PROSTATECTOMY SPECIMENS

1. Procedure
2. Prostate size—weight, dimensions
3. Lymph node sampling
4. Histologic type—WHO
5. Histologic grade—primary, secondary, tertiary, score
6. Tumor quantification—% prostate involved by tumor and/or greatest dimension of tumor nodule
7. EPE—focal, nonfocal (required); site(optional)
8. SVI
9. Margin including site of positivity; extent margin positivity (optional)
10. Treatment effect on carcinoma
11. Lymphovascular invasion
12. PNI*
13. Pathologic staging—TNM
14. Additional pathologic findings*

*Optional.

The pathologic examination of prostatectomy specimens after treatment shows a recognizable impact on morphology and immunohistochemistry of prostatic adenocarcinoma, and the characteristic morphologic signs of tumor regression may complicate the recognition and grading of treated tumors. The treatment effects may obscure residual carcinoma and make measurements of tumor extent and stage difficult. Pathologists play a central role in documenting the effects of these treatments on normal and malignant prostate tissue.

Radiation Treatment

RT for prostate cancer may be applied in the form of external beam, interstitial implantation (or brachytherapy), or a combination, as a mainstay or adjuvant (external beam) treatment in localized prostate cancer with curative intent. RP and RT have been proven to be effective for long-term survival and probable cure in the management of localized prostate cancer.

Brachytherapy involves the implantation of radioactive seeds in the prostate and is used to treat clinically localized disease. External beam radiotherapy, including conformal and intensity modulated modalities, is more commonly used against locally advanced prostate cancer, and it is often combined with various forms of antiandrogen therapy. Radiosurgery using gamma knife and CyberKnife technology to deliver highly focused beams to selected targets while minimizing the damage to surrounding tissue is currently under development.

Currently, our understanding of the mechanism of radiation-induced death of prostate cancer is limited. The primary effect is the damage of endothelial cells, which causes ischemia that leads to atrophy. However, an increasingly recognized form of radiation-induced death is postmitotic apoptosis.[687] In this process, radiation damages the tumor cell's DNA; the cell then divides prior to completing DNA repair, an event that is lethal.

Although the significance of prostate biopsy status after the completion of radiotherapy as a predictor of outcome has been controversial,[688,689] prostate needle biopsies performed in response to rising posttreatment PSA values are the most commonly encountered post-RT specimen and the only way to directly assess the effectiveness of radiation in eradicating local disease.

Postradiation biopsy has been used as an independent predictor of outcome[690] and of subsequent biochemical disease-free survival.[691] Patients with persistent tumor post-RT are more likely to demonstrate local disease progression and distant metastases and die of disease than those with a negative biopsy.[692–694]

Postradiation biopsies will most commonly be performed 18 to 24 months after the final RT treatment, because of the length of time required for the histologic clearance of tumor. After the confirmation of residual neoplasm, additional treatment may be considered such as androgen ablation or less frequently salvage prostatectomy.

The increased clinical interest in adjunctive therapy for persistent or locally recurrent prostatic cancer mandates accurate postirradiation biopsy specimen diagnosis. However, the interpretation of prostate needle biopsies after treatment such as RT may represent a diagnostic challenge with significant pitfalls, since the morphologic changes in prostate tissue obtained after RT, with or without additional changes induced by combined antiandrogen therapy, can be pronounced. In addition, postradiotherapy prostate biopsies to detect persistent local disease are subject to sampling error. Proper clinical information regarding the patient's treatment history is important for the pathologist to accurately interpret post-RT biopsies.

The effects of radiation on the prostatic tissue are variable and more severe and durable when delivered as seed implants (brachytherapy, either iodine or palladium) than by external beam and also vary with the dose and duration of the irradiation. The changes associated with RT may persist for years after the final radiation treatment.[684]

The interpretation of postirradiation prostate needle biopsy specimens is a diagnostic challenge for pathologists. The difficulty is multifactorial and includes separation of tumor from its mimics, identification of small foci of carcinoma, and separation of treatment effect in benign prostatic glands from recurrent or persistent carcinoma of the prostate.

Effect on Benign Prostate

Morphologic changes caused by radiation can vary markedly within each individual specimen and are often more marked in benign glands than in cancer.[695] The basic histologic changes in normal prostate tissue include variable degrees of glandular atrophy with flattening of the secretory epithelium and prominence of basal cells, distortion of glandular contours, and decreased ratio of acini to stroma (Fig. 9-162). In some cases, the atrophic ducts and acini show a pseudoinfiltrative

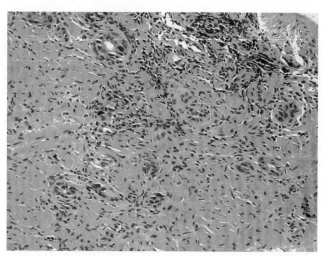

FIGURE 9-163 ■ Prostatic stroma surrounding atrophic glands frequently contains a sparse chronic inflammatory infiltrate.

appearance similar to sclerotic atrophy. The stroma contains a sparse chronic inflammatory infiltrate (Fig. 9-163). These changes can be appreciated at scanning magnification. At intermediate magnification, the basal cells may display vacuolated cytoplasm (Fig. 9-164), marked degenerative atypia with nuclear pleomorphism, hyperchromatic, smudged nuclei (Fig. 9-165), and prominent nucleoli (Fig. 9-166).[696] Basal cell proliferation with prominent nucleoli is a common mimicker of irradiated carcinoma.[697]

Other radiation associated changes include urothelial and squamous cell metaplasia and eosinophilic metaplasia. Squamous metaplasia may be commonly seen in cases where antiandrogen therapy has been combined with radiation.

The stroma may be fibrotic (Fig. 9-167) or edematous with paucicellular scarring and occasional atypical fibroblasts; stromal calcification has been reported, but hemosiderin deposition has not.[697] Vascular changes include intimal thickening and medial fibrosis with luminal narrowing and fibrous obliteration (Fig. 9-168).

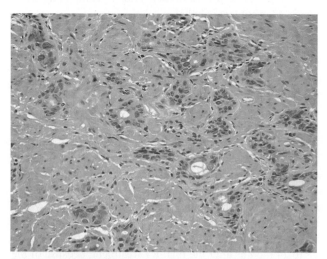

FIGURE 9-162 ■ Benign prostatic glands retain their lobular architecture, although individual glands show variable degrees of glandular atrophy with flattening of the secretory epithelium and prominence of basal cells, distortion of glandular contours, and a decreased ratio of acini to stroma.

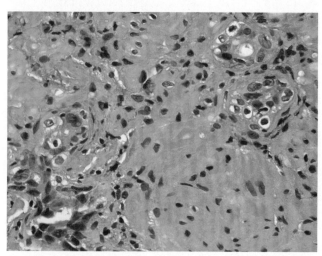

FIGURE 9-164 ■ Basal cells may display vacuolated cytoplasm.

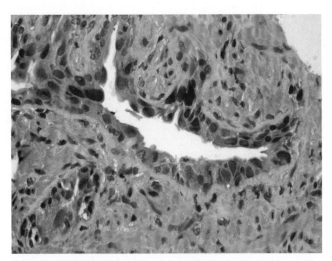

FIGURE 9-165 ■ Basal cells may display marked degenerative atypia with nuclear pleomorphism, and hyperchromatic, smudged nuclei.

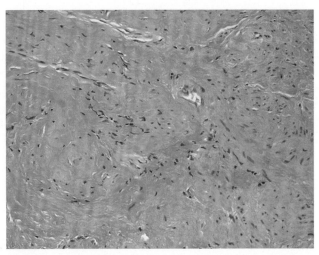

FIGURE 9-167 ■ Prostatic stroma may become fibrotic in response to radiation.

Effect on Prostatic Intraepithelial Neoplasia and Prostate Cancer

Prostate cancer is usually slow to regress, with histologic changes evolving for about 12 months after the completion of external beam RT; therefore, needle biopsy is of limited value prior to about 12 months. The appearance of adenocarcinoma following RT can be highly variable, ranging from no obvious effects to alterations so profound that the affected glands and cells may be difficult to recognize as carcinoma.

The prevalence and extent of HGPIN are diminished in biopsies performed after radiotherapy. However, HGPIN retains characteristic features of untreated PIN, including nuclear crowding, nuclear overlapping and stratification, hyperchromasia, and prominent nucleoli. Occasional cytoplasmic vacuolization or sloughing of epithelium into the lumen has been reported.[696,698]

The histologic appearance of prostate cancer without radiation effect is similar to that of prostate cancer before therapy, and the diagnosis relies on both architectural and cytologic atypia. Radiation causes diminution in the number of neoplastic glands (Fig. 9-169), shrinkage of cancer glands, and loss of cytoplasm: Glands appear as "collapsed" nests of cells or as single cells with small, often punctuate nuclei and inconspicuous nucleoli (Fig. 9-170).

Marked treatment effects typically manifest as haphazardly scattered glands or single cells with pale, voluminous foamy, or vacuolated cytoplasm; nuclei with smudged and distorted chromatin; minimal degrees of pleomorphism; and often inconspicuous nucleoli (Fig. 9-171). Nuclear pyknosis and desmoplasia are often present.[698] The infiltrative growth appearance with haphazard arrangement of glands appreciated at low to intermediate magnification is the key to distinguishing residual adenocarcinoma with treatment effect from benign prostatic glands with radiation-induced atypia (Fig. 9-172). In contrast to irradiated benign glands, nuclear pleomorphism is not common in prostate cancer with therapy effect (Fig. 9-173).

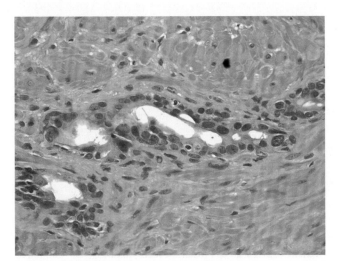

FIGURE 9-166 ■ Prominent nucleoli may be seen in basal cells.

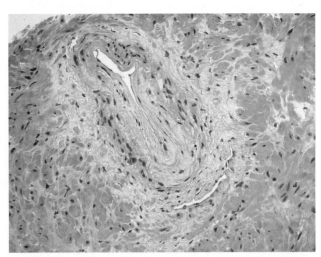

FIGURE 9-168 ■ Intimal thickening with luminal narrowing is a common vascular change associated with RT.

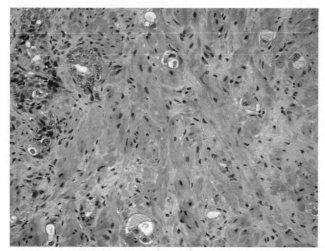

FIGURE 9-169 ■ Prostate cancer with radiation-induced changes is characterized by reduction in number and shrinkage of neoplastic glands.

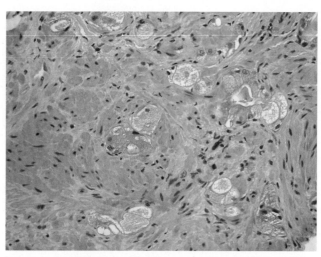

FIGURE 9-171 ■ Prostate cancer glands and single cells with pale, voluminous foamy cytoplasm; minimal degrees of pleomorphism; and inconspicuous nucleoli.

PNI, intraluminal crystalloids, and blue mucin can be helpful in identifying residual malignancy. The cytologic changes of nuclear enlargement and prominent nucleoli are frequently seen in postradiation nonneoplastic prostatic acini, and therefore, these changes alone are not helpful in separating cancer from benign.

Effect on Tumor Grade

Recent studies have shown that the degree of postradiation effect may provide important prognostic information in patients with a positive biopsy.[693,699] Since the histologic effects of systemic therapy on prostate cancer can be remarkable, the general opinion has been that treated prostate cancer should not be graded. However, Gleason score and degree of treatment effect in positive prostate biopsies 2 year post-RT have been shown to be strongly predictive of long-term disease-free survival.[691,700]

Some investigators have recommended grading of treatment effects in prostate specimens after radiotherapy, recognizing that the biologic significance of grade may be different from that in untreated cancer. A 3-point scoring system for nuclear and cytoplasmic postradiation changes has been proposed but has not been universally applied. Briefly, nuclear and cytoplasmic changes are measured separately on a scale of 0 (no effect) to 3 (maximum effect) and then added together to obtain a combined score (range, 0 to 6). The combined scores of 0 to 2, 3 to 4, and 5 to 6 correspond to minimal, moderate, and marked radiation effect, respectively.[693]

Biopsies showing minimal degrees of treatment effect are the only category for which Gleason scores should be applied; such cases are associated with local failure rates in the range of 55%. Biopsies showing tumors with moderate treatment effects have local failure rates in the range of 30%. Prostate tumors showing marked treatment effect

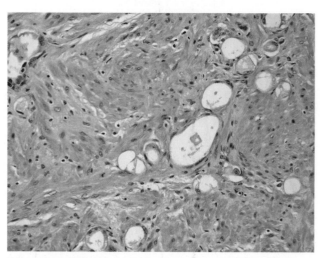

FIGURE 9-170 ■ Prostate cancer glands with marked cytoplasm loss, punctuate nuclei, and inconspicuous nucleoli.

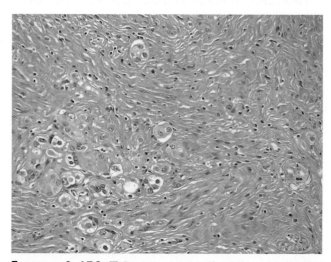

FIGURE 9-172 ■ Prostate cancer showing an infiltrative growth appearance with haphazard arrangement of neoplastic glands.

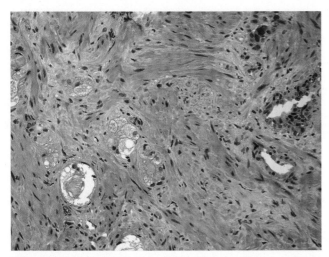

FIGURE 9-173 ■ Nuclear pleomorphism is less common in prostate cancer with therapy effect (**left**) than in irradiated benign glands (**right**).

in 24-month postradiation biopsies have 5-year disease-free survival rates similar to negative biopsies.[691]

Gleason grading is inappropriate for tumors showing RT-related changes, since the therapy-related artifacts simulate high-grade carcinoma. However, in situations where prostate cancer exhibits no, or little, treatment effect, a Gleason grade can be rendered, with a disclaimer that the tumor shows no evidence of or minimum treatment effect.

Ancillary Studies (Immunohistochemistry, Others)

Distinguishing single cancer cells with marked postradiation treatment effect from normal stromal cells with a clear cytoplasm or from histiocytes can be very difficult on H&E stains. In difficult cases, immunohistochemical staining with HMWCK or 34BE12 and/or p63 and racemase (AMACR) can be invaluable in confirming the presence of malignancy, since radiation effects do not change the staining pattern of these markers. PSA stain may be helpful in differentiating tumor cells from histiocytes.

The immunohistochemical profile of irradiated benign glands is similar to that of nonirradiated benign glands but demonstrates a relative preponderance of HMWCK-positive basal cells and a paucity of PSA and PSAP-secretory acinar cells.

Prostate cancer with or without RT effect is immunoreactive for PSA, PSAP, and CAM 5.2 and not for HMWCK.[696,701]

Hormones

Androgen deprivation therapy (ADT) is one of the most popular forms of treatment for prostate cancer, and it may be achieved with castration (orchidectomy), exogenous estrogen administration, drugs with the capacity to deplete the hypothalamus of luteinizing hormone-releasing hormone (LHRH agonists), and antiandrogens.[678] Antiandrogens can be subdivided in two main categories: drugs that block the conversion

of testosterone to its active form of 5α-dihydrotestosterone (i.e., finasteride, dutasteride) and drugs that block the AR on individual cells (i.e., flutamide). To achieve total androgen deprivation, the therapy should be effective in eliminating both testicular and adrenal hormones. These agents are used for treatment of BPH, for neoadjuvant or adjuvant treatment in clinically localized prostate cancer, and as a palliative measure in metastatic prostate cancer.

Therapies targeting the androgen-dependent nature of prostate cancer are widely used and can have profound effects on the histologic appearance of both benign and malignant prostate tissues. The spectrum of characteristic changes associated with androgen ablation varies in relation to the agent(s), dose used, as well as duration of the therapy. Maximal androgen blockade (MAB), combining an LHRH agonist and a pure or nonsteroidal antiandrogen, induces significant morphologic changes in the prostate. Tumor volume, density, EPE, and surgical margin involvement are significantly reduced following such treatment.[702] Nonneoplastic and neoplastic prostatic tissue undergoes marked atrophy and shrinkage of the epithelium, as a result of apoptosis. Monotherapy using a variety of agents causes comparable but often less extensive changes.

Effect on Benign Prostate

Characteristic morphologic changes are present in normal tissue of more than 70% of prostate specimens following MAB. Following MAB, benign and hyperplastic prostatic acini are atrophic and collapsed, typically with prominent basal cell hyperplasia and epithelial cell vacuolization[703] (Fig. 9-174). The altered epithelium displays involution, lobular and acinar atrophy, cytoplasmic clearing and vacuolization, nuclear and nucleolar shrinkage, and chromatin condensation (Fig. 9-175). Decreased glandular elements are accompanied by increased, sometimes hypercellular, stromal tissue with scattered lymphocytic infiltrates (Fig. 9-176).

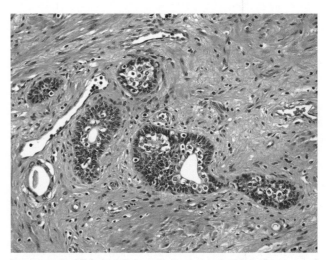

FIGURE 9-174 ■ After ADT, benign prostatic acini are atrophic and collapsed, typically with prominent basal cell hyperplasia and epithelial cell vacuolization.

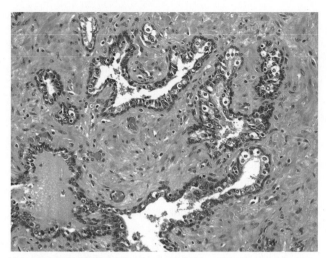

FIGURE 9-175 ■ Benign prostatic epithelium displaying involution, lobular and acinar atrophy, cytoplasmic clearing, and vacuolization.

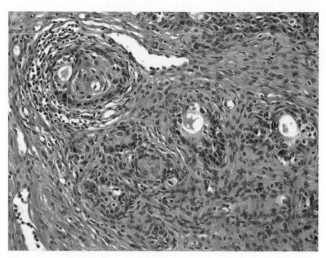

FIGURE 9-177 ■ Atrophic prostatic acini may show squamous metaplasia.

Flattening and rupture of the epithelium of a variable number of benign prostatic glands with possible extravasation of prostatic secretion into the stroma has also been reported.[704] Squamous metaplasia (Fig. 9-177) is not significantly increased with concurrent forms of ADT, but may be remarkable with estrogenic compounds and orchiectomy.

Shrinkage of benign prostate by 5α-reductase inhibitors (finasteride) has been documented in multiple clinical studies.[705,706] The treated secretory cells display shrunken nuclei, condensed chromatin, inconspicuous nucleoli, cytoplasm clearing, and prominent basal cells.

Effect on Prostatic Intraepithelial Neoplasia and Prostate Cancer

Following hormone therapy, HGPIN may be significantly less extensive.[707] However, the criteria used to identify HGPIN should be adapted because of the marked changes

of cell morphology. Undoubtedly, nucleolar prominence, which is the hallmark of HGPIN, is much less evident after hormone therapy. However, HGPIN still presents increased nuclear size, nuclear crowding, anisonucleosis, and disordered nuclear arrangements[708] (Fig. 9-178). The results of 5α-reductase inhibitor treatment on HGPIN are controversial.

ADT substantially reduces the size of the nuclei and nucleoli (Fig. 9-179) and clears the cytoplasm of prostatic adenocarcinoma cells (Fig. 9-180).[709] The most common architectural pattern change induced by androgen deprivation is a decrease in the size and density of the neoplastic glands (the so-called luteinizing hormone-releasing hormone [LHRH] effect). These changes are commonly associated with increased stroma between the dispersed small glands, small cell clusters, and single-file cells[710] (Fig. 9-181).

Another less common pattern consists of branching clefts lined by few scattered tumor cells with pyknotic nuclei and

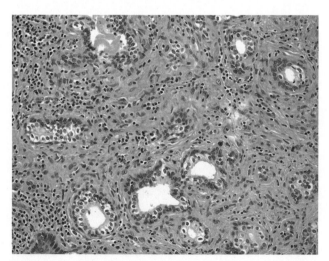

FIGURE 9-176 ■ Prostatic tissue with decreased glandular elements accompanied by increased stromal tissue with scattered lymphocytic infiltrate.

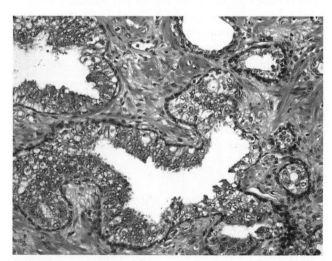

FIGURE 9-178 ■ Following hormone therapy, although less extensive HGPIN still presents increased nuclear size, nuclear crowding, anisonucleosis, and disordered nuclear arrangements.

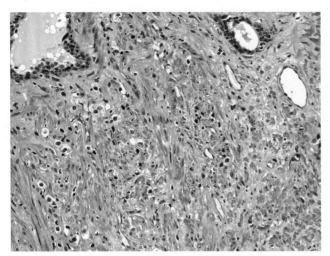

FIGURE 9-179 ■ After ADT, the sizes of the nuclei and nucleoli of prostatic adenocarcinoma are reduced.

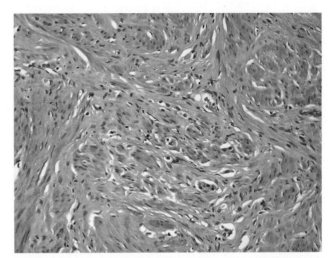

FIGURE 9-181 ■ Prostatic adenocarcinoma with dispersed small cell clusters and single cells associated with increased stroma between them.

degenerated tumor cells with foamy vacuolated cytoplasm (Fig. 9-182). Nuclei are small, round, hyperchromatic, and centrally located. The nucleoli may be large, but are usually inconspicuous and the term "nucleolus-poor" clear cell adenocarcinoma has been applied. Large tumor cells with clear or vacuolated cytoplasm in a dense inflammatory lymphohistiocytic background have been reported in cases with tumor necrosis and scanty residual tumor.[711]

Ruptured malignant glands with mucin extravasation have been seen in up to 77% of cases, with mucin lakes occupying from <5% (Fig. 9-183) to as much as 100% of the tumor.[712] In such cases, the cells of neoplastic glands may be almost completely degenerate, leaving irregular acid mucinous pools with rare cancerous cells (Fig. 9-184).

Some patterns present difficulties in differentiating tumor from treatment-altered benign glands and lymphocytes, or cancer cells can become so inconspicuous as to pose a risk

of underdiagnosis (Fig. 9-185). Occasional cases after ADT display the "vanishing cancer phenomenon," in which no residual cancer is found in the RP specimen.

The changes induced by androgen deprivation with finasteride are less prominent than those seen with other forms of hormonal therapy and, in many instances, are not evident, but, when present, include tumor cells, vacuolization, small tumor glands separated by stroma, empty spaces, and an inflammatory response.[710]

Effect on Tumor Grade

The histologic effects of hormone therapy on prostate cancer can be remarkable. Neoplastic glands are often shrunken and altered and there is increased stroma. There is general agreement that conventional Gleason grading should not be performed.[713]

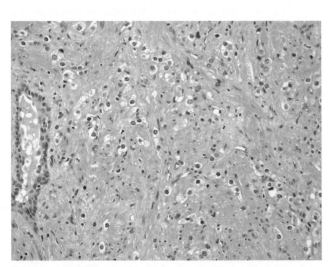

FIGURE 9-180 ■ Prostatic adenocarcinoma showing abundant clear vacuolated cytoplasm and absence of glandular lumina.

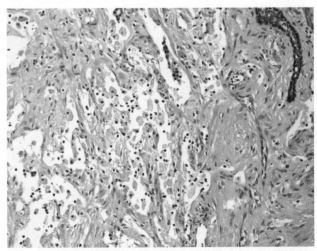

FIGURE 9-182 ■ Prostatic adenocarcinoma with prominent dissolution of neoplastic cells giving rise to branching clefts lined by scattered tumor cells with pyknotic nuclei.

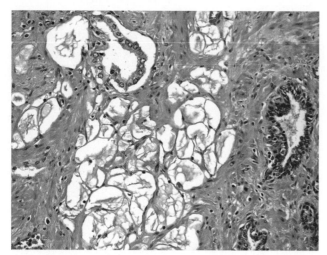

FIGURE 9-183 ■ Rupture of prostatic adenocarcinoma glands with mucin extravasation.

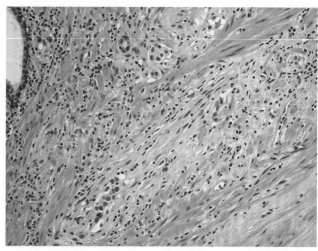

FIGURE 9-185 ■ Sometimes, single cancer cells are widely scattered within lymphocyte-rich stroma resembling histiocytes.

In cases showing marked treatment effect, Gleason score may be falsely increased (artifactual upgrading) and potentially misleading and is not recommended. In situations where prostate cancer exhibits none or little treatment effect, a grade can be rendered. In such cases, the Gleason grade can be reported with a disclaimer that the tumor shows no evidence of treatment effect.

Effect on Tumor Stage and Surgical Margins

Neoadjuvant hormonal therapy has been used to downstage tumors and decrease positive margin rates. Furthermore, shrinkage of the prostate gland could result in better definition of the surgical planes, allowing more complete removal of the tumor. The degree of downstaging varies among different studies.[709] The effects of neoadjuvant hormonal

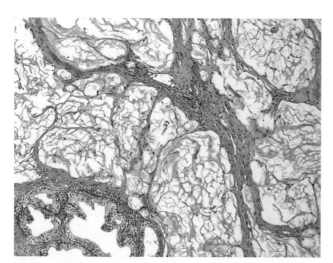

FIGURE 9-184 ■ The neoplastic cells may be almost completely degenerate, leaving irregular mucinous pools with rare cancerous cells.

therapy have been more pronounced after 6 than after 3 months of therapy.

Particularly striking is the significant downstaging of prostate cancer following MAB, due to marked reduction of tumor size. By image analysis on histologic sections, tumor volume is decreased by approximately 44% after 3 months of MAB compared to that of prostate glands not exposed to treatment.[707] In addition, tumor size and density are significantly decreased, and stroma is increased in most patients after treatment.[711] No residual tumor has been found in totally embedded prostates in a percentage of cases (2% to 8%).[714,715]

Most studies have reported an overall 22% decrease of EPE and a statistically significant difference between surgically and hormonally treated patients.[702,716] A 21% net improvement of margin involvement following MAB has been found in different studies.[702] Although these findings are important, the influence of tumor downsizing after several months of neoadjuvant therapy on the prognosis of prostate cancer is still controversial,[717] but most urologists are not currently using neoadjuvant hormonal therapy.

Ancillary Studies (Immunohistochemistry, Others)

The differential diagnosis of isolated cells or groups of tumor cells that have a benign appearances after therapy, from lymphocytes, histiocytes, and stromal fibroblasts, may be extremely challenging. PSA, PSAP, and pankeratin immunoreactivity, as well as the lack of basal cell–specific markers (34βE12 and p63) expression by prostatic cancer cell after therapy, may help in distinguishing cancer from its mimics. However, it is important to keep in mind that PSA, PSAP, and racemase expression decline following long androgen blockade therapy.[718] Most patients experience a drastic reduction of serum PSA as well as a marked decrease in PSA staining by immunohistochemistry.[704,719]

Similarly, a marked decrease in AR expression has been seen after treatment in both normal glands and cancer cells. Keratin 34βE12 and p63 remain negative, regardless of the duration of treatment, confirming an absent basal cell layer.

Cryotherapy

Percutaneous perineal cryoablation of the prostate is a promising technique in the treatment armamentarium for clinically localized prostate cancer and for localized recurrent prostate cancer after RT. Although preliminary results are encouraging, the effectiveness of cryoablation in the treatment of prostate cancer is still unknown, and the method is used only in selected patients.

Cryosurgical ablation refers to rapid deep freezing of the prostate. Multiple cryoprobe needles filled with circulating liquid nitrogen transform the prostate gland into an ice ball, resulting in tissue destruction and death of benign and malignant cells.[686] The liquid nitrogen does not come in contact with the tissue. The flow of liquid nitrogen through the probes can be adjusted to obtain a desired freezing pattern.

Given the focal nature of these treatments, the histologic changes are most likely to be confined to the areas targeted for treatment.

Effect on Benign Prostate

Postcryosurgery prostate tissue shows typical features of repair, including marked stromal fibrosis (Fig. 9-186) and hyalinization (Fig. 9-187), hemosiderin deposition (Fig. 9-188) and/or stromal hemorrhage (Fig. 9-189) inflammation, and squamous metaplasia.[720] Coagulative necrosis (Fig. 9-190) is present between 6 and 30 weeks from therapy, followed by patchy chronic inflammation. Dystrophic calcification is infrequent and usually appears in areas with the

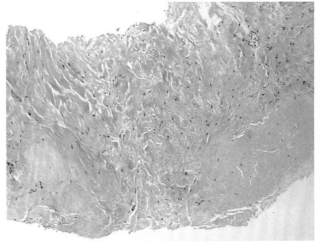

FIGURE 9-187 ■ Postcryosurgery prostate tissue shows marked hyalinization.

greatest reparative response. As the postoperative interval increases, biopsy specimens are more likely to contain unaltered benign prostatic tissue.

The correlation between the histopathologic effects of the above therapies and their clinical significance is not absolutely clear.

Effect on Prostatic Intraepithelial Neoplasia and Prostate Cancer

Atypia and HGPIN are not seen in areas that otherwise show changes of postcryoablation therapy. Biopsies after treatment may reveal no evidence of residual tumor, even in some patients with elevated PSA. Ghosts of malignant cells may be appreciated in areas showing coagulative necrosis.

In some cases, the benign prostate and the prostate cancer after cryoablation show no change in grade or definite evidence of specific tissue response (Fig. 9-191), raising the

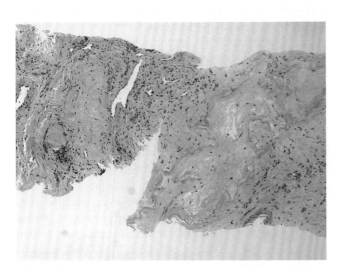

FIGURE 9-186 ■ Prostate biopsy after cryotherapy showing marked stromal fibrosis.

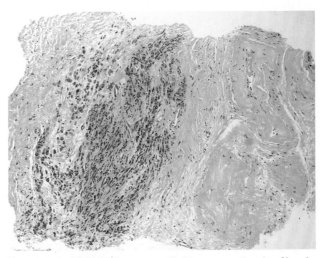

FIGURE 9-188 ■ Prostate needle biopsy core showing fibrosis, and hyalinization, as well as hemosiderin deposition.

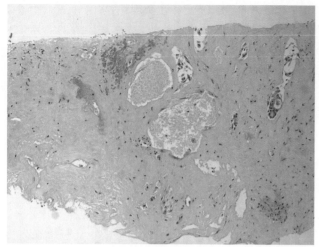

FIGURE 9-189 ■ Stromal hemorrhage can occasionally be present.

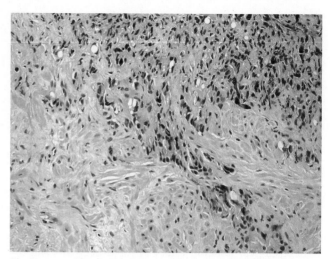

FIGURE 9-191 ■ Residual/recurrent prostatic adenocarcinoma with no definite evidence of specific tissue response.

possibility either that these areas were inadequately frozen or that the treatment was ineffective.

In prostate specimens removed after cryotherapy, pathologists should comment on the presence of residual tumor and whether it appears viable, although, there is no definitive method to assess viability post-cryoablation.

Effect on Tumor Grade

There is no consensus regarding grading prostate cancer after cryoablation therapy, and most pathologists report Gleason grade.

Ancillary Studies (Immunohistochemistry, Others)

PSA and PSAP expression persist in benign and malignant epithelium. Cytokeratin 34βE12, p63, and racemase expression are unaffected in areas with preserved cellularity and are of diagnostic value in separating treated prostate cancer and its mimics.

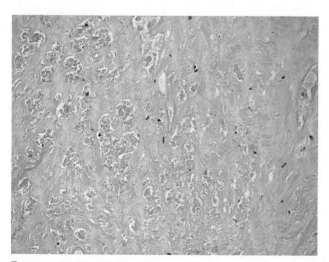

FIGURE 9-190 ■ Coagulative necrosis showing ghost tumor cells.

High-Intensity Focused Ultrasound

HIFU was introduced 15 years ago for the treatment of nodular hyperplasia.[721] This technique is minimally invasive, requires less anesthesia, involves a shorter recovery period than surgery, and can be performed in a day surgery setting, making it an attractive potential option for the treatment of localized prostate cancer.[722] Many studies have been performed to evaluate the use of HIFU for low-grade, localized prostate cancer; HIFU has also been used as salvage therapy after failed radiation. While HIFU appears to provide acceptable short-term local control, it has not been approved as a primary therapy for prostate cancer in the Unites States.

HIFU is a noninvasive method of delivering ultrasonic energy with resultant heat and tissue destruction to a discrete point without damaging intervening tissue or cells in the immediate vicinity of the focal area.[723,724] When applied for the treatment of localized prostate cancer, it uses an ultrasound transducer placed in the rectum to generate acoustic energy that is focused on the tissue target, creating high temperatures and coagulative necrosis.[686,725]

HIFU uses a trackless approach, whereby tissue outside the focal plane is not damaged; the transrectal probe sits on the rectal mucosa and sends acoustic energy through the intervening tissues, only heating the tissue volume targeted by the probe.[726] The probe is repositioned mechanically as needed to target the entire prostate. An automatic cooling device is used during treatment to maintain a constant baseline temperature of <18°C in the transrectal probe, which helps to prevent thermal injury of the rectal mucosa.[727]

HIFU destroys target tissue through the thermal and mechanical effects of nonionizing, acoustic radiation (i.e., sound waves). The thermal effects are achieved by an intense heat impulse (80°C to 200°C) leading to immediate protein denaturation and subsequent cell death. Significant mechanical effects include cavitation, microstreaming, and radiation forces.[728] Cavitation is the creation of movement of gas in an acoustic field: As the tissue compresses and expands with exposure to the acoustic waves, gas is extracted creating bubbles.

The bubbles begin to oscillate violently, collapse, and disrupt cell membranes. Microstreaming refers to the rapid movement of liquid outside an oscillating bubble generated through cavitation forces. Radiation forces are the pressures tissues endure when either absorbing or reflecting sound waves.

The high temperature also induces the creation and release of chemically reactive free radicals, responsible for the induction of apoptosis and activity on nuclear DNA.

Effect on Benign Prostate

The precise histologic changes seen on post-HIFU biopsies, TURP, or RP specimens have not been systematically evaluated. The earliest studies focused on HIFU-induced acute tissue damage, manifested as areas of sharply delineated intraprostatic coagulative necrosis, reliably demonstrable as early as 1 to 2 hours after the procedure.[729,730] Vacuolized cytoplasm, ruptured cell membranes, and destroyed cellular organelles as signs of definitive cell death have been routinely observed in treated tissues regardless of their structure.[729] Careful histologic examination within the area of coagulative necrosis has revealed no remnant viable cells that could potentially escape the therapeutic effect of HIFU.[731]

Recent studies have reported acute and chronic inflammation, glandular atrophy, hemosiderin deposition, focal coagulative necrosis, dense stromal fibrosis, and edema in benign tissue after HIFU treatment.[679,732]

Effect on Prostate Cancer

In areas of viable tumor, there appear to be no post-HIFU histologic changes that would preclude the use of Gleason scoring.[679,732]

The pathologist must be aware of any history of pre-HIFU antiandrogen therapy that may have been used to shrink the gland prior to treatment, in which case Gleason scoring may not be applicable.

Ancillary Studies (Immunohistochemistry, Others)

Immunoperoxidase staining for cytokeratin 34βE12, p63, and racemase (AMACR) is unaffected in areas with preserved cellularity.[679,732]

Photodynamic Therapy, Interstitial Laser Thermotherapy, and Microwave Thermotherapy

The high prevalence of low-risk disease together with an inability to accurately identify men harboring more aggressive prostate cancers has led to tremendous research in low-morbidity focal therapies for prostate cancer.

A promising technique, currently in clinical trials, is vascular-targeted PDT, which has been used for whole gland ablation of locally recurrent cancer after radiotherapy and, more recently, for focal ablation of previously untreated cancer.[685] PDT uses a light-sensitive agent (photosensitizer) that is activated in the prostate by low-power laser light, delivered using optical fibers. The fibers are placed within needles in the prostate, guided by TRUS and a perineal template. Following the activation of the photosensitizer by light and the formation of reactive oxygen species, necrosis occurs at the site of interaction between the photosensitizer, light, and oxygen.[733] This technique does not heat the prostate but destroys the endothelial cells and cancer by activating the photodynamic agent. Damage to surrounding structures appears to be limited and can be controlled by the duration and intensity of the light. Vascular-targeted PDT involves the intravenous administration of a bacteriochlorophyll-derived pharmacologically inactive photosensitizer (WST-09 Tookad, STEBA Biotech, the Netherlands, and WST-11 Stakel, STEBA Biotech) that absorbs light in the visible near-infrared wavelength with maximum light energy absorption at 763 nm.[679] This long light absorption wavelength allows for better light penetration into tissues, resulting in thrombosis and vascular coagulation around the tip of the optic fiber with subsequent localized tissue necrosis within the prostate.[734] The areas of damage are characterized by well-demarcated areas of fibrosis; less frequently organizing granulation tissue or coagulative necrosis is noted. Areas of viable adenocarcinoma located immediately adjacent to the foci of damage show no obvious morphologic changes that would preclude the use of Gleason scoring.[679]

Thermal therapy is used to kill tumors by heating them to temperatures in the range of 50°C to 55°C for an extended period of time (5 to 15 minutes). Cell death results from thermal coagulation. Tissue necrosis and destruction of the prostatic urethra have been identified in RP specimens obtained 1 week after microwave therapy.[735] The energy sources available for this approach include radiofrequency electrodes, microwave antennas, laser fiberoptics, and ultrasound transducers. Each of these modalities has the potential to be delivered in a minimally invasive manner.[736] Thermal and thermal-ablative procedures for treating prostate cancer have been investigated systematically since approximately 1980. Various technologies have been used, including transurethral ablation of prostatic tissue using laser or microwave energy, interstitial application of laser or microwave energy, and inductive heating of previously implanted thermoseeds or injected magnetic nanoparticles in a magnetic field.

Interstitial laser thermotherapy has been performed using laser fibers for photothermal energy. Laser fibers are inserted into the prostate by the perineum and placed at the periphery of the tumor zone to ensure its complete destruction. Magnetic resonance imaging guidance is used to confirm proper placement of the fibers and to obtain real-time temperature monitoring during treatment.[737] The procedure time requires 20 to 30 minutes, heating the tissue to 90°C.[734] The areas targeted for therapy showed well-demarcated foci of necrosis, surrounded by a small rim of hemorrhage. Viable carcinoma in untreated areas of the gland shows no obvious morphology changes that would preclude assigning Gleason scores.[679]

Chemotherapy

Chemotherapy has traditionally been reserved for hormone-refractory metastatic disease and is often used as a palliative measure in combination with corticosteroids or hormonal agents. During the past decade, the role of chemotherapy in the management of advanced prostate cancer has evolved. An increasing numbers of patients with prostate cancer are being treated with chemotherapy, in either a neoadjuvant manner or as second- or third-line therapy for metastatic cancer. The agents used include, but are not limited to, mitoxantrone, etoposide, cisplatin, vinblastine, estramustine, paclitaxel, docetaxel, and everolimus.

A palliative benefit has been reported using the combination of mitoxantrone and prednisone in symptomatic patients with advanced disease.[738] Other antineoplastic agents have also been evaluated, with emphasis on agents that target the nuclear matrix and microtubular function.[739,740] Of these, the taxanes (paclitaxel, docetaxel) have emerged as a highly active class of antineoplastic agents in advanced prostate cancer.[741]

Although the use of neoadjuvant hormonal therapy has been reported to improve the negative surgical margin rate, randomized clinical trials have failed to demonstrate a relapse-free survival or overall survival benefit with this regimen.[742,743]

There is little information on the effect of these agents on the morphology of nonneoplastic and neoplastic prostatic tissue.[744,745] No histologic patterns as distinct as those described for radiation or ADT have been consistently associated with specific chemotherapy regimens.

Effect on Benign Prostate

Some of these agents have essentially no effect on normal prostate tissue when given in a neoadjuvant setting prior to RP. In patients treated with neoadjuvant docetaxel, most benign prostatic glands show prominent basal cells and urothelial metaplasia.[744]

Effect on Prostate Cancer

Histologic changes in prostate tumor cells treated with neoadjuvant docetaxel include cytoplasmic vacuolization (Fig. 9-192) and/or clear cell change, luminal needle-like

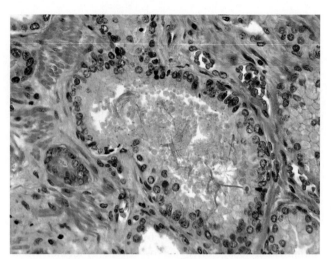

FIGURE 9-193 ■ Luminal needle-like crystalloid structures after neoadjuvant docetaxel treatment.

crystalloid structures (Fig. 9-193), dense intraluminal secretions, and cribriform glands with central necrosis.[744]

In a recent systematic review of 50 high-risk prostate cancers treated with neoadjuvant docetaxel and mitoxantrone, O'Brien et al.[745] evaluated RP specimens and observed at least one of the following distinctive histologic patterns: intraductal growth pattern, prominent cytoplasmic vacuolization (Fig. 9-194), cribriform architecture (Fig. 9-195), inconspicuous collapsed glands, and small inconspicuous tumor cells. Although a few specimens exhibited changes in the preneoadjuvant therapy biopsy that were similar to the histologic changes seen in the corresponding RP, IDC was detected in 20% of prostatectomy specimens but in none of the pretreatment biopsy specimens.

Cribriform pattern and intraductal growth were also detected in half of the RP specimens obtained from patients with high-risk prostate cancer treated with preoperative androgen ablation, alone or in combination with chemotherapy.[713]

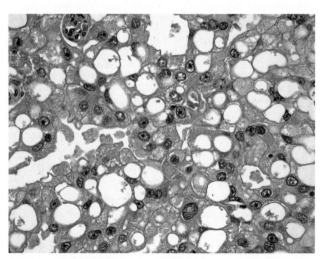

FIGURE 9-192 ■ Prostate tumor cells treated with neoadjuvant docetaxel showing prominent cytoplasmic vacuolization.

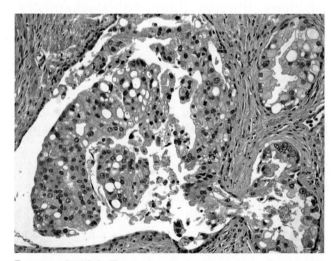

FIGURE 9-194 ■ Intraductal growth pattern and prominent cytoplasmic vacuolization in high-risk prostate cancer treated with neoadjuvant docetaxel.

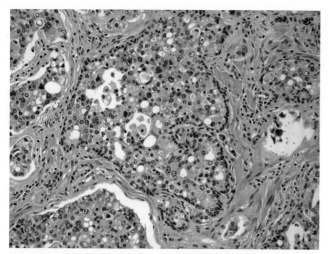

FIGURE 9-195 ■ Intraductal growth pattern and cribriform architecture in high-risk prostate cancer treated with neoadjuvant docetaxel.

Effect on Tumor Grade

Preoperative androgen ablation and chemotherapy affect tumor architecture to render the Gleason score of post therapy specimens nonrepresentative of the disease and therefore not useful for assessing prognosis.

A recent histologic classification has been proposed categorizing pretreated prostate cancer in three morphologically distinct groups: group A, tumor characterized by a predominance of cell clusters, cell cords, and isolated cells; group B, tumors characterized by intact and fused small glands; and group C, tumors with any degree of cribriform growth pattern or intraductal tumor spread.[713] If validated, this classification may introduce uniformity in the assessment of treatment effect and may provide a new prognostic tool for prostate tumors treated with neoadjuvant therapy.

REFERENCES

1. Loeb S, et al. Complications after prostate biopsy: data from SEER-Medicare. *J Urol* 2011;186:1830–1834.
2. Ferlay J, Shin HR, Bray F, et al. *Globocan 2008: Cancer Incidence and Mortality Worldwide*. IARC CancerBase No. 10. Lyon, France: International Agency for Research on Cancer; 2010.
3. *SEER Stat Fact Sheets: Prostate*. 2012 [cited 2012] Available from: http://seer.cancer.gov/statfacts/html/prost.html
4. Siegel R, Naishadham D, Jemal A. Cancer statistics, 2013. *CA Cancer J Clin* 2013;63:11–30.
5. Cancer Trends Progress Report. 2006. Available from: http://progress-report.cancer.gov
6. National Cancer Institute. *A Snapshot of Prostate Cancer*. 2010 [cited 2012] Available from: http://www.cancer.gov/aboutnci/servingpeople/cancer-statistics/snapshots.
7. Draisma G, et al. Lead times and overdetection due to prostate-specific antigen screening: estimates from the European Randomized Study of Screening for Prostate Cancer. *J Natl Cancer Inst* 2003;95:868–878.
8. Draisma G, et al. Lead time and overdiagnosis in prostate-specific antigen screening: importance of methods and context. *J Natl Cancer Inst* 2009;101:374–383.
9. Etzioni R, et al. Overdiagnosis due to prostate-specific antigen screening: lessons from U.S. prostate cancer incidence trends. *J Natl Cancer Inst* 2002;94:981–990.
10. Andriole GL, et al. Mortality results from a randomized prostate-cancer screening trial. *N Engl J Med* 2009;360:1310–1319.
11. Schroder FH, et al. Screening and prostate-cancer mortality in a randomized European study. *N Engl J Med* 2009;360:1320–1328.
12. Sandblom G, et al. Randomised prostate cancer screening trial: 20 year follow-up. *BMJ* 2011;342:d1539.
13. Siegel R, et al. Cancer treatment and survivorship statistics, 2012. *CA Cancer J Clin* 2012;62:220–241.
14. Siegel R, et al. Cancer statistics, 2011: the impact of eliminating socioeconomic and racial disparities on premature cancer deaths. *CA Cancer J Clin* 2011;61:212–236.
15. Bunker CH, et al. High prevalence of screening-detected prostate cancer among Afro-Caribbeans: the Tobago Prostate Cancer Survey. *Cancer Epidemiol Biomarkers Prev* 2002;11:726–729.
16. Glover FE Jr, et al. The epidemiology of prostate cancer in Jamaica. *J Urol* 1998;159:1984–1986; discussion 1986–1987.
17. Center MM, et al. International variation in prostate cancer incidence and mortality rates. *Eur Urol* 2012;61:1079–1092.
18. Etzioni R, et al. Quantifying the role of PSA screening in the US prostate cancer mortality decline. *Cancer Causes Control* 2008;19:175–181.
19. Collin SM, et al. Prostate-cancer mortality in the USA and UK in 1975–2004: an ecological study. *Lancet Oncol* 2008;9:445–452.
20. Gavin A, et al. Evidence of prostate cancer screening in a UK region. *BJU Int* 2004;93:730–734.
21. Leitzmann MF, Rohrmann S. Risk factors for the onset of prostatic cancer: age, location, and behavioral correlates. *Clin Epidemiol* 2012;4:1–11.
22. Fedewa SA, et al. Association of insurance and race/ethnicity with disease severity among men diagnosed with prostate cancer, National Cancer Database 2004–2006. *Cancer Epidemiol Biomarkers Prev* 2010;19:2437–2444.
23. Powell IJ, et al. Evidence supports a faster growth rate and/or earlier transformation to clinically significant prostate cancer in black than in white American men, and influences racial progression and mortality disparity. *J Urol* 2010;183:1792–1796.
24. Powell IJ. Epidemiology and pathophysiology of prostate cancer in African-American men. *J Urol* 2007;177:444–449.
25. Haiman CA, et al. Genome-wide association study of prostate cancer in men of African ancestry identifies a susceptibility locus at 17q21. *Nat Genet* 2011;43:570–573.
26. Haiman CA, et al. Multiple regions within 8q24 independently affect risk for prostate cancer. *Nat Genet* 2007;39:638–644.
27. Okobia MN, et al. Chromosome 8q24 variants are associated with prostate cancer risk in a high risk population of African ancestry. *Prostate* 2011;71:1054–1063.
28. Amundadottir LT, et al. A common variant associated with prostate cancer in European and African populations. *Nat Genet* 2006;38:652–658.
29. Powell IJ, et al. CYP3A4 genetic variant and disease-free survival among white and black men after radical prostatectomy. *J Urol* 2004;172:1848–1852.
30. Bangsi D, et al. Impact of a genetic variant in CYP3A4 on risk and clinical presentation of prostate cancer among white and African-American men. *Urol Oncol* 2006;24:21–27.
31. Ntais C, Polycarpou A, Ioannidis JP. Association of the CYP17 gene polymorphism with the risk of prostate cancer: a meta-analysis. *Cancer Epidemiol Biomarkers Prev* 2003;12:120–126.
32. Kittles RA, et al. A common nonsense mutation in EphB2 is associated with prostate cancer risk in African American men with a positive family history. *J Med Genet* 2006;43:507–511.
33. Lesko SM, Rosenberg L, Shapiro S. Family history and prostate cancer risk. *Am J Epidemiol* 1996;144:1041–1047.
34. Steinberg GD, et al. Family history and the risk of prostate cancer. *Prostate* 1990;17:337–347.

35. Alvarez-Cubero MJ, et al. Genetic analysis of the principal genes related to prostate cancer: a review. *Urol Oncol* 2012. [Epub ahead of print]

36. Hughes C, et al. Molecular pathology of prostate cancer. *J Clin Pathol* 2005;58:673–684.

37. American Institute for Cancer Research (AICR)/World Cancer Research Fund. *Food, Nutrition, Physical Activity, and the Prevention of Cancer: A Global Perspective*. Washington, DC: AICR; 2007.

38. Joshi AD, et al. Red meat and poultry, cooking practices, genetic susceptibility and risk of prostate cancer: results from a multiethnic case–control study. *Carcinogenesis* 2012;33:2108–2118.

39. Major JM, et al. Patterns of meat intake and risk of prostate cancer among African-Americans in a large prospective study. *Cancer Causes Control* 2011;22:1691–1698.

40. Kirsh VA, et al. Prospective study of fruit and vegetable intake and risk of prostate cancer. *J Natl Cancer Inst* 2007;99:1200–1209.

41. Lippman SM, et al. Effect of selenium and vitamin E on risk of prostate cancer and other cancers: the Selenium and Vitamin E Cancer Prevention Trial (SELECT). *JAMA* 2009;301:39–51.

42. Tewari R, et al. Diet, obesity, and prostate health: are we missing the link? *J Androl* 2012;33:763–776.

43. Cao Y, Ma J. Body mass index, prostate cancer-specific mortality, and biochemical recurrence: a systematic review and meta-analysis. *Cancer Prev Res (Phila)* 2011;4:486–501.

44. Ribeiro R, et al. Obesity and prostate cancer: gene expression signature of human periprostatic adipose tissue. *BMC Med* 2012;10:108.

45. De Nunzio C, et al. Metabolic syndrome is associated with high grade Gleason score when prostate cancer is diagnosed on biopsy. *Prostate* 2011;4:486–501.

46. Lin YS, et al. Increased risk of cancer mortality associated with cadmium exposures in older Americans with low zinc intake. *J Toxicol Environ Health A* 2013;76:1–15.

47. Van Maele-Fabry G, et al. Review and meta-analysis of risk estimates for prostate cancer in pesticide manufacturing workers. *Cancer Causes Control* 2006;17:353–373.

48. Delzell E, et al. An updated study of mortality among North American synthetic rubber industry workers. *Res Rep Health Eff Inst* 2006:1–63; discussion 65–74.

49. Gibbs GW, Amsel J, Soden K. A cohort mortality study of cellulose triacetate-fiber workers exposed to methylene chloride. *J Occup Environ Med* 1996;38:693–697.

50. Schwartz GG. Vitamin D, sunlight, and the epidemiology of prostate cancer. *Anticancer Agents Med Chem* 2012;13:45–57.

51. Atkinson WD, Law DV, Bromley KJ. A decline in mortality from prostate cancer in the UK Atomic Energy Authority workforce. *J Radiol Prot* 2007;27:437–445.

52. Ragin C, et al. Farming, reported pesticide use, and prostate cancer. *Am J Mens Health* 2013;7:102–109.

53. Rosenberg L, et al. Vasectomy and the risk of prostate cancer. *Am J Epidemiol* 1990;132:1051–1505; discussion 1062–1065.

54. Giovannucci E, et al. A retrospective cohort study of vasectomy and prostate cancer in US men. *JAMA* 1993;269:878–882.

55. John EM, et al. Vasectomy and prostate cancer: results from a multiethnic case–control study. *J Natl Cancer Inst* 1995;87:662–669.

56. Zhu K, et al. Vasectomy and prostate cancer: a case–control study in a health maintenance organization. *Am J Epidemiol* 1996;144:717–722.

57. Khan MA, Partin AW. Vasectomy and prostate cancer. *Rev Urol* 2004;6:46–47.

58. Holt SK, Salinas CA, Stanford JL. Vasectomy and the risk of prostate cancer. *J Urol* 2008;180:2565–2567; discussion 2567–2568.

59. Kenyon JC, Lever AM. XMRV, prostate cancer and chronic fatigue syndrome. *Br Med Bull* 2011;98:61–74.

60. Lee D, et al. In-depth investigation of archival and prospectively collected samples reveals no evidence for XMRV infection in prostate cancer. *PLoS One* 2012;7:e44954.

61. Schlaberg R, et al. XMRV is present in malignant prostatic epithelium and is associated with prostate cancer, especially high-grade tumors. *Proc Natl Acad Sci U S A* 2009;106:16351–16356.

62. Groom HC, et al. No evidence for infection of UK prostate cancer patients with XMRV, BK virus, *Trichomonas vaginalis* or human papilloma viruses. *PLoS One* 2012;7:e34221.

63. Hong P, Li J. Lack of evidence for a role of xenotropic murine leukemia virus-related virus in the pathogenesis of prostate cancer and/or chronic fatigue syndrome. *Virus Res* 2012;167:1–7.

64. Goldstein AS, et al. Identification of a cell of origin for human prostate cancer. *Science* 2010;329:568–571.

65. Boyd LK, Mao X, Lu YJ. The complexity of prostate cancer: genomic alterations and heterogeneity. *Nat Rev Urol* 2012;9:652–664.

66. Gurel B, et al. Molecular alterations in prostate cancer as diagnostic, prognostic, and therapeutic targets. *Adv Anat Pathol* 2008;15:319–331.

67. Spans L, et al. The genomic landscape of prostate cancer. *Int J Mol Sci* 2013;14:10822–10851.

68. Mackinnon AC, et al. Molecular biology underlying the clinical heterogeneity of prostate cancer: an update. *Arch Pathol Lab Med* 2009;133:1033–1040.

69. Barbieri CE, Demichelis F, Rubin MA. Molecular genetics of prostate cancer: emerging appreciation of genetic complexity. *Histopathology* 2012;60:187–198.

70. Nupponen NN, Visakorpi T. Molecular cytogenetics of prostate cancer. *Microsc Res Tech* 2000;51:456–463.

71. Tomlins SA, et al. Recurrent fusion of TMPRSS2 and ETS transcription factor genes in prostate cancer. *Science* 2005;310:644–648.

72. Perner S, et al. TMPRSS2-ERG fusion prostate cancer: an early molecular event associated with invasion. *Am J Surg Pathol* 2007;31:882–888.

73. Tavtigian SV, et al. A candidate prostate cancer susceptibility gene at chromosome 17p. *Nat Genet* 2001;27:172–180.

74. Smith JR, et al. Major susceptibility locus for prostate cancer on chromosome 1 suggested by a genome-wide search. *Science* 1996;274:1371–1374.

75. Carpten J, et al. Germline mutations in the ribonuclease L gene in families showing linkage with HPC1. *Nat Genet* 2002;30:181–184.

76. Berthon P, et al. Predisposing gene for early-onset prostate cancer, localized on chromosome 1q42.2–43. *Am J Hum Genet* 1998;62:1416–1424.

77. Gibbs M, et al. Evidence for a rare prostate cancer-susceptibility locus at chromosome 1p36. *Am J Hum Genet* 1999;64:776–787.

78. Berry R, et al. Evidence for a prostate cancer-susceptibility locus on chromosome 20. *Am J Hum Genet* 2000;67:82–91.

79. Xu J, et al. Evidence for a prostate cancer susceptibility locus on the X chromosome. *Nat Genet* 1998;20:175–179.

80. Gillanders EM, et al. Combined genome-wide scan for prostate cancer susceptibility genes. *J Natl Cancer Inst* 2004;96:1240–1247.

81. Kote-Jarai Z, et al. Seven prostate cancer susceptibility loci identified by a multi-stage genome-wide association study. *Nat Genet* 2011;43:785–791.

82. Dong JT. Prevalent mutations in prostate cancer. *J Cell Biochem* 2006;97:433–447.

83. McMenamin ME, et al. Loss of PTEN expression in paraffin-embedded primary prostate cancer correlates with high Gleason score and advanced stage. *Cancer Res* 1999;59:4291–4296.

84. Suzuki H, et al. Interfocal heterogeneity of PTEN/MMAC1 gene alterations in multiple metastatic prostate cancer tissues. *Cancer Res* 1998;58:204–209.

85. Han B, et al. Fluorescence in situ hybridization study shows association of PTEN deletion with ERG rearrangement during prostate cancer progression. *Mod Pathol* 2009;22:1083–1093.

86. Vis AN, Schroder FH. Key targets of hormonal treatment of prostate cancer. Part 1: the androgen receptor and steroidogenic pathways. *BJU Int* 2009;104:438–448.

87. Feldman BJ, Feldman D. The development of androgen-independent prostate cancer. *Nat Rev Cancer* 2001;1:34–45.

88. Koivisto P, et al. Androgen receptor gene amplification: a possible molecular mechanism for androgen deprivation therapy failure in prostate cancer. *Cancer Res* 1997;57:314–319.

89. Shaw A, Bushman W. Hedgehog signaling in the prostate. *J Urol* 2007;177:832–838.
90. Karhadkar SS, et al. Hedgehog signalling in prostate regeneration, neoplasia and metastasis. *Nature* 2004;431:707–712.
91. Veronese ML, et al. The t(6;16)(p21;q22) chromosome translocation in the LNCaP prostate carcinoma cell line results in a tpc/hpr fusion gene. *Cancer Res* 1996;56:728–732.
92. Kumar-Sinha C, Tomlins SA, Chinnaiyan AM. Recurrent gene fusions in prostate cancer. *Nat Rev Cancer* 2008;8:497–511.
93. Narod SA, Seth A, Nam R. Fusion in the ETS gene family and prostate cancer. *Br J Cancer* 2008;99:847–851.
94. Tomlins SA, et al. Distinct classes of chromosomal rearrangements create oncogenic ETS gene fusions in prostate cancer. *Nature* 2007;448:595–599.
95. Vaarala MH, et al. The TMPRSS2 gene encoding transmembrane serine protease is overexpressed in a majority of prostate cancer patients: detection of mutated TMPRSS2 form in a case of aggressive disease. *Int J Cancer* 2001;94:705–710.
96. Vaarala MH, et al. Expression of transmembrane serine protease TMPRSS2 in mouse and human tissues. *J Pathol* 2001;193:134–140.
97. Mosquera JM, et al. Morphological features of TMPRSS2-ERG gene fusion prostate cancer. *J Pathol* 2007;212:91–101.
98. Gopalan A, et al. TMPRSS2-ERG gene fusion is not associated with outcome in patients treated by prostatectomy. *Cancer Res* 2009;69:1400–1406.
99. Demichelis F, et al. TMPRSS2:ERG gene fusion associated with lethal prostate cancer in a watchful waiting cohort. *Oncogene* 2007;26:4596–4599.
100. Nam RK, et al. Expression of the TMPRSS2:ERG fusion gene predicts cancer recurrence after surgery for localised prostate cancer. *Br J Cancer* 2007;97:1690–1695.
101. Nam RK, et al. Expression of TMPRSS2:ERG gene fusion in prostate cancer cells is an important prognostic factor for cancer progression. *Cancer Biol Ther* 2007;6:40–45.
102. Attard G, et al. Duplication of the fusion of TMPRSS2 to ERG sequences identifies fatal human prostate cancer. *Oncogene* 2008;27:253–263.
103. Petrovics G, et al. Frequent overexpression of ETS-related gene-1 (ERG1) in prostate cancer transcriptome. *Oncogene* 2005;24:3847–3852.
104. Winnes M, et al. Molecular genetic analyses of the TMPRSS2-ERG and TMPRSS2-ETV1 gene fusions in 50 cases of prostate cancer. *Oncol Rep* 2007;17:1033–1036.
105. Perner S, et al. TMPRSS2:ERG fusion-associated deletions provide insight into the heterogeneity of prostate cancer. *Cancer Res* 2006;66:8337–8341.
106. Lapointe J, et al. A variant TMPRSS2 isoform and ERG fusion product in prostate cancer with implications for molecular diagnosis. *Mod Pathol* 2007;20:467–473.
107. Yoshimoto M, et al. Three-color FISH analysis of TMPRSS2/ERG fusions in prostate cancer indicates that genomic microdeletion of chromosome 21 is associated with rearrangement. *Neoplasia* 2006;8:465–469.
108. Yousef GM, Diamandis EP. The new human tissue kallikrein gene family: structure, function, and association to disease. *Endocr Rev* 2001;22:184–204.
109. Banez LL, et al. Obesity-related plasma hemodilution and PSA concentration among men with prostate cancer. *JAMA* 2007;298:2275–2280.
110. Roobol MJ, et al. Prostate cancer mortality reduction by prostate-specific antigen-based screening adjusted for nonattendance and contamination in the European Randomised Study of Screening for Prostate Cancer (ERSPC). *Eur Urol* 2009;56:584–591.
111. Zhu X, et al. Disease-specific survival of men with prostate cancer detected during the screening interval: results of the European randomized study of screening for prostate cancer-Rotterdam after 11 years of follow-up. *Eur Urol* 2011;60:330–336.
112. Kjellman A, et al. 15-year follow-up of a population based prostate cancer screening study. *J Urol* 2009;181:1615–1621; discussion 1621.
113. Labrie F, et al. Screening decreases prostate cancer mortality: 11-year follow-up of the 1988 Quebec prospective randomized controlled trial. *Prostate* 2004;59:311–318.
114. Moyer VA; U.S. Preventive Services Task Force. Screening for prostate cancer: U.S. Preventive Services Task Force recommendation statement. *Ann Intern Med* 2012;157:120–134.
115. Payton S. Prostate cancer: new PSA screening guideline faces widespread opposition. *Nat Rev Urol* 2012;9:351.
116. Catalona WJ, et al. What the U.S. Preventive Services Task Force missed in its prostate cancer screening recommendation. *Ann Intern Med* 2012;157:137–138.
117. Heidenreich A, et al. EAU guidelines on prostate cancer. Part 1: screening, diagnosis, and treatment of clinically localised disease. *Eur Urol* 2011;59:61–71.
118. Greene KL, et al. Prostate specific antigen best practice statement: 2009 update. *J Urol* 2009;182:2232–2241.
119. NCCN Clinical Practice Guidelines in Oncology (NCCN Guidelines). *Prostate Cancer Early Detection*. 2012 November 23, 2012; Available from: http://www.NCCN.org
120. Basch E, et al. Screening for prostate cancer with prostate-specific antigen testing: American Society of Clinical Oncology Provisional Clinical Opinion. *J Clin Oncol* 2012;30:3020–3025.
121. Cookson MS, et al. Variation in the definition of biochemical recurrence in patients treated for localized prostate cancer: the American Urological Association Prostate Guidelines for Localized Prostate Cancer Update Panel report and recommendations for a standard in the reporting of surgical outcomes. *J Urol* 2007;177:540–545.
122. D'Amico AV, et al. Preoperative PSA velocity and the risk of death from prostate cancer after radical prostatectomy. *N Engl J Med* 2004;351:125–135.
123. D'Amico AV, et al. Pretreatment PSA velocity and risk of death from prostate cancer following external beam radiation therapy. *JAMA* 2005;294:440–447.
124. Yu X, et al. Comparison of methods for calculating prostate specific antigen velocity. *J Urol* 2006;176(6 Pt 1):2427–2431; discussion 2431.
125. Vickers AJ, et al. Prostate-specific antigen velocity for early detection of prostate cancer: result from a large, representative, population-based cohort. *Eur Urol* 2009;56:753–760.
126. Daskivich TJ, Regan MM, Oh WK. Prostate specific antigen doubling time calculation: not as easy as 1, 2, 4. *J Urol* 2006;176:1927–1937.
127. Svatek RS, et al. Critical analysis of prostate-specific antigen doubling time calculation methodology. *Cancer* 2006;106:1047–1053.
128. O'Brien MF, et al. Pretreatment prostate-specific antigen (PSA) velocity and doubling time are associated with outcome but neither improves prediction of outcome beyond pretreatment PSA alone in patients treated with radical prostatectomy. *J Clin Oncol* 2009;27:3591–3597.
129. Catalona WJ, et al. Use of the percentage of free prostate-specific antigen to enhance differentiation of prostate cancer from benign prostatic disease: a prospective multicenter clinical trial. *JAMA* 1998;279:1542–1547.
130. Andrews CS. Latent carcinoma of the prostate. *J Clin Pathol* 1949;2:197–208.
131. McNeal JE. Morphogenesis of prostatic carcinoma. *Cancer* 1965;18:1659–1666.
132. McNeal JE. Origin and development of carcinoma in the prostate. *Cancer* 1969;23:24–34.
133. McNeal JE, Bostwick DG. Intraductal dysplasia: a premalignant lesion of the prostate. *Hum Pathol* 1986;17:64–71.
134. Bostwick DG, Brawer MK. Prostatic intra-epithelial neoplasia and early invasion in prostate cancer. *Cancer* 1987;59:788–794.
135. Drago JR, Mostofi FK, Lee F. Introductory remarks and workshop summary. *Urology* 1989;34(suppl):2–3.

136. Montironi R, et al. Mechanisms of disease: high-grade prostatic intraepithelial neoplasia and other proposed preneoplastic lesions in the prostate. *Nat Clin Pract Urol* 2007;4:321–332.

137. Bostwick DG, Cheng L. Precursors of prostate cancer. *Histopathology* 2012;60:4–27.

138. Clouston D, Bolton D. In situ and intraductal epithelial proliferations of prostate: definitions and treatment implications. Part 1: prostatic intraepithelial neoplasia. *BJU Int* 2012;109(suppl 3):22–26.

139. Zynger DL, Yang X. High-grade prostatic intraepithelial neoplasia of the prostate: the precursor lesion of prostate cancer. *Int J Clin Exp Pathol* 2009;2:327–338.

140. Montironi R, et al. Prostatic intraepithelial neoplasia: its morphological and molecular diagnosis and clinical significance. *BJU Int* 2011;108:1394–1401.

141. Ayala AG, Ro JY. Prostatic intraepithelial neoplasia: recent advances. *Arch Pathol Lab Med* 2007;131:1257–1266.

142. Keetch DW, et al. Morphometric analysis and clinical follow-up of isolated prostatic intraepithelial neoplasia in needle biopsy of the prostate. *J Urol* 1995;154(2 Pt 1):347–351.

143. Epstein JI, et al. Interobserver reproducibility in the diagnosis of prostatic intraepithelial neoplasia. *Am J Surg Pathol* 1995;19:873–886.

144. Epstein JI, Herawi M. Prostate needle biopsies containing prostatic intraepithelial neoplasia or atypical foci suspicious for carcinoma: implications for patient care. *J Urol* 2006;175(3 Pt 1):820–834.

145. Merrimen JL, Evans AJ, Srigley JR. Preneoplasia in the prostate gland with emphasis on high grade prostatic intraepithelial neoplasia. *Pathology* 2013;45:251–263.

146. Bostwick DG, et al. High-grade prostatic intraepithelial neoplasia. *Rev Urol* 2004;6:171–179.

147. Sanchez-Chapado M, et al. Prevalence of prostate cancer and prostatic intraepithelial neoplasia in Caucasian Mediterranean males: an autopsy study. *Prostate* 2003;54:238–247.

148. Sakr WA. Prostatic intraepithelial neoplasia: a marker for high-risk groups and a potential target for chemoprevention. *Eur Urol* 1999;35:474–478.

149. Sakr WA, Grignon DJ, Haas GP. Pathology of premalignant lesions and carcinoma of the prostate in African-American men. *Semin Urol Oncol* 1998;16:214–220.

150. Fowler JE Jr, et al. Prospective study of correlations between biopsy-detected high grade prostatic intraepithelial neoplasia, serum prostate specific antigen concentration, and race. *Cancer* 2001;91:1291–1296.

151. Sakr WA, et al. Age and racial distribution of prostatic intraepithelial neoplasia. *Eur Urol* 1996;30:138–144.

152. Tan PH, et al. Is high-grade prostatic intraepithelial neoplasia on needle biopsy different in an Asian population: a clinicopathologic study performed in Singapore. *Urology* 2006;68:800–803.

153. Billis A. Age and race distribution of high grade prostatic intraepithelial neoplasia: an autopsy study in Brazil (South America). *J Urol Pathol* 1996;5:175–181.

154. Merrimen JL, et al. A model to predict prostate cancer after atypical findings in initial prostate needle biopsy. *J Urol* 2011;185:1240–1245.

155. Merrimen JL, Jones G, Srigley JR. Is high grade prostatic intraepithelial neoplasia still a risk factor for adenocarcinoma in the era of extended biopsy sampling? *Pathology* 2010;42:325–329.

156. Merrimen JL, et al. Multifocal high grade prostatic intraepithelial neoplasia is a significant risk factor for prostatic adenocarcinoma. *J Urol* 2009;182:485–490; discussion 490.

157. Srigley JR, et al. Multifocal high-grade prostatic intraepithelial neoplasia is still a significant risk factor for adenocarcinoma. *Can Urol Assoc J* 2010;4:434.

158. Mosquera JM, et al. Characterization of TMPRSS2-ERG fusion high-grade prostatic intraepithelial neoplasia and potential clinical implications. *Clin Cancer Res* 2008;14:3380–3385.

159. Stewart J, et al. Prognostic significance of alpha-methylacyl-coA racemase among men with high grade prostatic intraepithelial neoplasia in prostate biopsies. *J Urol* 2008;179:1751–1755; discussion 1755.

160. Helpap B. The significance of the P504S expression pattern of high-grade prostatic intraepithelial neoplasia (HGPIN) with and without adenocarcinoma of the prostate in biopsy and radical prostatectomy specimens. *Virchows Arch* 2006;448:480–484.

161. Cheville JC, Reznicek MJ, Bostwick DG. The focus of "atypical glands, suspicious for malignancy" in prostatic needle biopsy specimens: incidence, histologic features, and clinical follow-up of cases diagnosed in a community practice. *Am J Clin Pathol* 1997;108:633–640.

162. Allen EA, Kahane H, Epstein JI. Repeat biopsy strategies for men with atypical diagnoses on initial prostate needle biopsy. *Urology* 1998;52:803–807.

163. Chan TY, Epstein JI. Follow-up of atypical prostate needle biopsies suspicious for cancer. *Urology* 1999;53:351–355.

164. O'Dowd GJ, et al. Analysis of repeated biopsy results within 1 year after a noncancer diagnosis. *Urology* 2000;55:553–559.

165. Borboroglu PG, et al. Repeat biopsy strategy in patients with atypical small acinar proliferation or high grade prostatic intraepithelial neoplasia on initial prostate needle biopsy. *J Urol* 2001;166:866–870.

166. Ouyang RC, et al. The presence of atypical small acinar proliferation in prostate needle biopsy is predictive of carcinoma on subsequent biopsy. *BJU Int* 2001;87:70–74.

167. Park S, et al. Prostate cancer detection in men with prior high grade prostatic intraepithelial neoplasia or atypical prostate biopsy. *J Urol* 2001;165:1409–1414.

168. Iczkowski KA, MacLennan GT, Bostwick DG. Atypical small acinar proliferation suspicious for malignancy in prostate needle biopsies: clinical significance in 33 cases. *Am J Surg Pathol* 1997;21:1489–1495.

169. Schlesinger C, Bostwick DG, Iczkowski KA. High-grade prostatic intraepithelial neoplasia and atypical small acinar proliferation: predictive value for cancer in current practice. *Am J Surg Pathol* 2005;29:1201–1207.

170. Kronz JD, et al. Predicting cancer following a diagnosis of high-grade prostatic intraepithelial neoplasia on needle biopsy: data on men with more than one follow-up biopsy. *Am J Surg Pathol* 2001;25:1079–1085.

171. Kronz JD, Shaikh AA, Epstein JI. High-grade prostatic intraepithelial neoplasia with adjacent small atypical glands on prostate biopsy. *Hum Pathol* 2001;32:389–395.

172. Netto GJ, Epstein JI. Widespread high-grade prostatic intraepithelial neoplasia on prostatic needle biopsy: a significant likelihood of subsequently diagnosed adenocarcinoma. *Am J Surg Pathol* 2006;30:1184–1188.

173. Bishara T, Ramnani DM, Epstein JI. High-grade prostatic intraepithelial neoplasia on needle biopsy: risk of cancer on repeat biopsy related to number of involved cores and morphologic pattern. *Am J Surg Pathol* 2004;28:629–633.

174. Lee MC, et al. Multifocal high grade prostatic intraepithelial neoplasia is a risk factor for subsequent prostate cancer. *J Urol* 2010;184:1958–1962.

175. Qian J, et al. Chromosomal anomalies in prostatic intraepithelial neoplasia and carcinoma detected by fluorescence in situ hybridization. *Cancer Res* 1995;55:5408–5414.

176. Jenkins RB, et al. Detection of c-myc oncogene amplification and chromosomal anomalies in metastatic prostatic carcinoma by fluorescence in situ hybridization. *Cancer Res* 1997;57:524–531.

177. Qian J, Jenkins RB, Bostwick DG. Detection of chromosomal anomalies and c-myc gene amplification in the cribriform pattern of prostatic intraepithelial neoplasia and carcinoma by fluorescence in situ hybridization. *Mod Pathol* 1997;10:1113–1119.

178. Meeker AK, et al. Telomere shortening is an early somatic DNA alteration in human prostate tumorigenesis. *Cancer Res* 2002;62:6405–6409.

179. Koeneman KS, et al. Telomerase activity, telomere length, and DNA ploidy in prostatic intraepithelial neoplasia (PIN). *J Urol* 1998;160:1533–1539.

180. Bostwick DG, Qian J. High-grade prostatic intraepithelial neoplasia. *Mod Pathol* 2004;17:360–379.

181. Krajewska M, et al. Immunohistochemical analysis of bcl-2, bax, bcl-X, and mcl-1 expression in prostate cancers. *Am J Pathol* 1996;148:1567–1576.

182. Bethel CR, et al. Decreased NKX3.1 protein expression in focal prostatic atrophy, prostatic intraepithelial neoplasia, and adenocarcinoma: association with Gleason score and chromosome 8p deletion. *Cancer Res* 2006;66:10683–10690.

183. Henshall SM, et al. Overexpression of the cell cycle inhibitor p16INK4A in high-grade prostatic intraepithelial neoplasia predicts early relapse in prostate cancer patients. *Clin Cancer Res* 2001;7:544–550.

184. Fernandez PL, et al. Expression of p27/Kip1 is down-regulated in human prostate carcinoma progression. *J Pathol* 1999;187:563–566.

185. Alcaraz A, et al. High-grade prostate intraepithelial neoplasia shares cytogenetic alterations with invasive prostate cancer. *Prostate* 2001;47:29–35.

186. Al-Maghrabi J, et al. p53 Alteration and chromosomal instability in prostatic high-grade intraepithelial neoplasia and concurrent carcinoma: analysis by immunohistochemistry, interphase in situ hybridization, and sequencing of laser-captured microdissected specimens. *Mod Pathol* 2001;14:1252–1262.

187. Cerveira N, et al. TMPRSS2-ERG gene fusion causing ERG over-expression precedes chromosome copy number changes in prostate carcinomas and paired HGPIN lesions. *Neoplasia* 2006;8:826–832.

188. Ribeiro FR, et al. Statistical dissection of genetic pathways involved in prostate carcinogenesis. *Genes Chromosomes Cancer* 2006;45:154–163.

189. Montironi R, et al. Nuclear changes in the normal-looking columnar epithelium adjacent to and distant from prostatic intraepithelial neoplasia and prostate cancer. Morphometric analysis in whole-mount sections. *Virchows Arch* 2000;437:625–634.

190. Lopez-Beltran A, et al. Nuclear volume estimates in prostatic intraepithelial neoplasia. *Anal Quant Cytol Histol* 2000;22:37–44.

191. Brooks JD, et al. CG island methylation changes near the GSTP1 gene in prostatic intraepithelial neoplasia. *Cancer Epidemiol Biomarkers Prev* 1998;7:531–536.

192. Bostwick DG, Meiers I, Shanks JH. Glutathione S-transferase: differential expression of alpha, mu, and pi isoenzymes in benign prostate, prostatic intraepithelial neoplasia, and prostatic adenocarcinoma. *Hum Pathol* 2007;38:1394–1401.

193. Ozden E, et al. Transrectal sonographic features of prostatic intraepithelial neoplasia: correlation with pathologic findings. *J Clin Ultrasound* 2005;33:5–9.

194. Lee F, et al. Use of transrectal ultrasound and prostate-specific antigen in diagnosis of prostatic intraepithelial neoplasia. *Urology* 1989;34 (6 suppl):4–8.

195. Kamoi K, Troncoso P, Babaian RJ. Strategy for repeat biopsy in patients with high grade prostatic intraepithelial neoplasia. *J Urol* 2000;163:819–823.

196. Naya Y, et al. Can the number of cores with high-grade prostate intraepithelial neoplasia predict cancer in men who undergo repeat biopsy? *Urology* 2004;63:503–508.

197. Godoy G, et al. Long-term follow-up of men with isolated high-grade prostatic intra-epithelial neoplasia followed by serial delayed interval biopsy. *Urology* 2011;77:669–674.

198. Bostwick DG, et al. Architectural patterns of high-grade prostatic intraepithelial neoplasia. *Hum Pathol* 1993;24:298–310.

199. Reyes AO, et al. Unusual histologic types of high-grade prostatic intraepithelial neoplasia. *Am J Surg Pathol* 1997;21:1215–1222.

200. Argani P, Epstein JI. Inverted (Hobnail) high-grade prostatic intraepithelial neoplasia (PIN): report of 15 cases of a previously undescribed pattern of high-grade PIN. *Am J Surg Pathol* 2001;25:1534–1539.

201. Berman DM, Yang J, Epstein JI. Foamy gland high-grade prostatic intraepithelial neoplasia. *Am J Surg Pathol* 2000;24:140–144.

202. Melissari M, et al. High grade prostatic intraepithelial neoplasia with squamous differentiation. *J Clin Pathol* 2006;59:437–439.

203. Paner GP, Luthringer DJ, Amin MB. Best practice in diagnostic immunohistochemistry: prostate carcinoma and its mimics in needle core biopsies. *Arch Pathol Lab Med* 2008;132:1388–1396.

204. Hull D, et al. Precursor of prostate-specific antigen expression in prostatic intraepithelial neoplasia and adenocarcinoma: a study of 90 cases. *BJU Int* 2009;104:915–918.

205. Murphy AJ, et al. Heterogeneous expression of alpha-methylacyl-CoA racemase in prostatic cancer correlates with Gleason score. *Histopathology* 2007;50:243–251.

206. Ananthanarayanan V, et al. Alpha-methylacyl-CoA racemase (AMACR) expression in normal prostatic glands and high-grade prostatic intraepithelial neoplasia (HGPIN): association with diagnosis of prostate cancer. *Prostate* 2005;63:341–346.

207. Wu CL, et al. Analysis of alpha-methylacyl-CoA racemase (P504S) expression in high-grade prostatic intraepithelial neoplasia. *Hum Pathol* 2004;35:1008–1013.

208. Bostwick DG, et al. Prostate specific membrane antigen expression in prostatic intraepithelial neoplasia and adenocarcinoma: a study of 184 cases. *Cancer* 1998;82:2256–2261.

209. Darson MF, et al. Human glandular kallikrein 2 (hK2) expression in prostatic intraepithelial neoplasia and adenocarcinoma: a novel prostate cancer marker. *Urology* 1997;49:857–862.

210. Lee S, et al. Small cell-like change in prostatic intraepithelial neoplasia, intraductal carcinoma, and invasive prostatic carcinoma: a study of 7 cases. *Hum Pathol* 2013;44:427–431.

211. Bostwick DG, et al. Consensus statement on terminology: recommendation to use atypical adenomatous hyperplasia in place of adenosis of the prostate. *Am J Surg Pathol* 1994;18:1069–1070.

212. Srigley JR. Small-acinar patterns in the prostate gland with emphasis on atypical adenomatous hyperplasia and small-acinar carcinoma. *Semin Diagn Pathol* 1988;5:254–272.

213. Bostwick DG, et al. Atypical adenomatous hyperplasia of the prostate: morphologic criteria for its distinction from well-differentiated carcinoma. *Hum Pathol* 1993;24:819–832.

214. Gaudin PB, Epstein JI. Adenosis of the prostate. Histologic features in transurethral resection specimens. *Am J Surg Pathol* 1994;18:863–870.

215. Bostwick DG, Qian J. Atypical adenomatous hyperplasia of the prostate. Relationship with carcinoma in 217 whole-mount radical prostatectomies. *Am J Surg Pathol* 1995;19:506–518.

216. Gaudin PB, Epstein JI. Adenosis of the prostate. Histologic features in needle biopsy specimens. *Am J Surg Pathol* 1995;19:737–747.

217. Humphrey PA. Atypical adenomatous hyperplasia (adenosis) of the prostate. *J Urol* 2012;188:2371–2372.

218. Epstein JI, et al. The 2005 International Society of Urological Pathology (ISUP) Consensus Conference on Gleason Grading of Prostatic Carcinoma. *Am J Surg Pathol* 2005;29:1228–1242.

219. Srigley JR. Benign mimickers of prostatic adenocarcinoma. *Mod Pathol* 2004;17:328–348.

220. Cheng L, et al. Atypical adenomatous hyperplasia of the prostate: a premalignant lesion? *Cancer Res* 1998;58:389–391.

221. Doll JA, et al. Genetic analysis of prostatic atypical adenomatous hyperplasia (adenosis). *Am J Pathol* 1999;155:967–971.

222. Qian J, Jenkins RB, Bostwick DG. Chromosomal anomalies in atypical adenomatous hyperplasia and carcinoma of the prostate using fluorescence in situ hybridization. *Urology* 1995;46:837–842.

223. Brawn PN. Adenosis of the prostate: a dysplastic lesion that can be confused with prostate adenocarcinoma. *Cancer* 1982;49:826–833.

224. Lopez-Beltran A, et al. Nuclear volume estimates in prostatic atypical adenomatous hyperplasia. *Anal Quant Cytol Histol* 2000;22:438–444.

225. Lopez-Beltran A, et al. Atypical adenomatous hyperplasia (adenosis) of the prostate: DNA ploidy analysis and immunophenotype. *Int J Surg Pathol* 2005;13:167–173.

226. Zhang C, et al. Is atypical adenomatous hyperplasia of the prostate a precursor lesion? *Prostate* 2011;71:1746–1751.

227. Yang XJ, et al. Expression of alpha-methylacyl-CoA racemase (P504S) in atypical adenomatous hyperplasia of the prostate. *Am J Surg Pathol* 2002;26:921–925.

228. De Marzo AM, et al. Proliferative inflammatory atrophy of the prostate: implications for prostatic carcinogenesis. *Am J Pathol* 1999;155:1985–1992.

229. Putzi MJ, De Marzo AM. Morphologic transitions between proliferative inflammatory atrophy and high-grade prostatic intraepithelial neoplasia. *Urology* 2000;56:828–832.

230. Wang W, Bergh A, Damber JE. Morphological transition of proliferative inflammatory atrophy to high-grade intraepithelial neoplasia and cancer in human prostate. *Prostate* 2009;69:1378–1386.

231. van Leenders GJ, et al. Intermediate cells in human prostate epithelium are enriched in proliferative inflammatory atrophy. *Am J Pathol* 2003;162:1529–1537.

232. Nakayama M, et al. Hypermethylation of the human glutathione S-transferase-pi gene (GSTP1) CpG island is present in a subset of proliferative inflammatory atrophy lesions but not in normal or hyperplastic epithelium of the prostate: a detailed study using laser-capture microdissection. *Am J Pathol* 2003;163:923–933.

233. Wang W, Bergh A, Damber JE. Increased p53 immunoreactivity in proliferative inflammatory atrophy of prostate is related to focal acute inflammation. *APMIS* 2009;117:185–195.

234. Mills SE, et al. A symposium on the surgical pathology of the prostate. *Pathol Annu* 1990;25(Pt 2):109–158.

235. Humphrey PA, Walther PJ. Adenocarcinoma of the prostate. I. Tissue sampling considerations. *Am J Clin Pathol* 1993;99:746–759.

236. Young RH, Srigley JR, Amin MB, et al. *Atlas of Tumor Pathology. Tumors of the Prostate Gland, Seminal Vesicles, Male Urethra, and Penis*. Washington, DC: American Registry of Pathology Armed Forces Institute of Pathology; 2000.

237. Furman J, et al. Prostatectomy tissue for research: balancing patient care and discovery. *Am J Clin Pathol* 1998;110:4–9.

238. Renshaw AA, et al. The greatest dimension of prostate carcinoma is a simple, inexpensive predictor of prostate specific antigen failure in radical prostatectomy specimens. *Cancer* 1998;83:748–752.

239. Hall GS, Kramer CE, Epstein JI. Evaluation of radical prostatectomy specimens. A comparative analysis of sampling methods. *Am J Surg Pathol* 1992;16:315–324.

240. McNeal JE, et al. Zonal distribution of prostatic adenocarcinoma. Correlation with histologic pattern and direction of spread. *Am J Surg Pathol* 1988;12:897–906.

241. Erbersdobler A, et al. Prostate cancers in the transition zone: Part 1; pathological aspects. *BJU Int* 2004;94:1221–1225.

242. Al-Ahmadie HA, et al. Anterior-predominant prostatic tumors: zone of origin and pathologic outcomes at radical prostatectomy. *Am J Surg Pathol* 2008;32:229–235.

243. Augustin H, et al. Prostate cancers in the transition zone: Part 2; clinical aspects. *BJU Int* 2004;94:1226–1229.

244. Noguchi M, et al. An analysis of 148 consecutive transition zone cancers: clinical and histological characteristics. *J Urol* 2000;163:1751–1755.

245. McNeal JE, et al. Capsular penetration in prostate cancer. Significance for natural history and treatment. *Am J Surg Pathol* 1990;14:240–247.

246. Shannon BA, McNeal JE, Cohen RJ. Transition zone carcinoma of the prostate gland: a common indolent tumour type that occasionally manifests aggressive behaviour. *Pathology* 2003;35:467–471.

247. Erbersdobler A, et al. Pathological and clinical characteristics of large prostate cancers predominantly located in the transition zone. *Prostate Cancer Prostatic Dis* 2002;5:279–284.

248. Garcia JJ, et al. Do prostatic transition zone tumors have a distinct morphology? *Am J Surg Pathol* 2008;32:1709–1714.

249. Iremashvili V, et al. Prostate cancers of different zonal origin: clinicopathological characteristics and biochemical outcome after radical prostatectomy. *Urology* 2012;80:1063–1069.

250. King CR, Ferrari M, Brooks JD. Prognostic significance of prostate cancer originating from the transition zone. *Urol Oncol* 2009;27:592–597.

251. Villers A, et al. Multiple cancers in the prostate. Morphologic features of clinically recognized versus incidental tumors. *Cancer* 1992;70:2313–2318.

252. Masterson TA, et al. Tumor focality does not predict biochemical recurrence after radical prostatectomy in men with clinically localized prostate cancer. *J Urol* 2011;186:506–510.

253. Wise AM, et al. Morphologic and clinical significance of multifocal prostate cancers in radical prostatectomy specimens. *Urology* 2002;60:264–269.

254. Noguchi M, et al. Prognostic factors for multifocal prostate cancer in radical prostatectomy specimens: lack of significance of secondary cancers. *J Urol* 2003;170(2 Pt 1):459–463.

255. Shekarriz B, et al. Impact of location and multifocality of positive surgical margins on disease-free survival following radical prostatectomy: a comparison between African-American and white men. *Urology* 2000;55:899–903.

256. Arora R, et al. Heterogeneity of Gleason grade in multifocal adenocarcinoma of the prostate. *Cancer* 2004;100:2362–2366.

257. Kobayashi M, et al. Molecular analysis of multifocal prostate cancer by comparative genomic hybridization. *Prostate* 2008;68:1715–1724.

258. Mehra R, et al. Heterogeneity of TMPRSS2 gene rearrangements in multifocal prostate adenocarcinoma: molecular evidence for an independent group of diseases. *Cancer Res* 2007;67:7991–7995.

259. Totten RS, et al. Microscopic differential diagnosis of latent carcinoma of prostate. *AMA Arch Pathol* 1953;55:131–141.

260. Algaba F, et al. Assessment of prostate carcinoma in core needle biopsy—definition of minimal criteria for the diagnosis of cancer in biopsy material. *Cancer* 1996;78:376–381.

261. Gleason D; TVACUR Group. Histologic grading and clinical staging of prostatic carcinoma. In: Tannenbaum M, ed. *Urologic Pathology: The prostate*. Philadelphia PA: Lea & Febiger, 1977:171–198.

262. Epstein JI. Gleason score 2–4 adenocarcinoma of the prostate on needle biopsy: a diagnosis that should not be made. *Am J Surg Pathol* 2000;24:477–478.

263. Kruslin B, et al. Periacinar clefting and p63 immunostaining in prostatic intraepithelial neoplasia and prostatic carcinoma. *Pathol Oncol Res* 2006;12:205–209.

264. Kruslin B, et al. Correlation of periacinar retraction clefting in needle core biopsies and corresponding prostatectomy specimens of patients with prostatic adenocarcinoma. *Int J Surg Pathol* 2005;13:67–72.

265. Kruslin B, et al. Periacinar retraction clefting in the prostatic needle core biopsies: an important diagnostic criterion or a simple artifact? *Virchows Arch* 2003;443:524–527.

266. Hameed O, Humphrey PA. Immunohistochemistry in diagnostic surgical pathology of the prostate. *Semin Diagn Pathol* 2005;22:88–104.

267. Brimo F, Epstein JI. Immunohistochemical pitfalls in prostate pathology. *Hum Pathol* 2012;43:313–324.

268. Latour M, et al. Grading of invasive cribriform carcinoma on prostate needle biopsy: an interobserver study among experts in genitourinary pathology. *Am J Surg Pathol* 2008;32:1532–1539.

269. Yanagisawa N, et al. Stromogenic prostatic carcinoma pattern (carcinomas with reactive stromal grade 3) in needle biopsies predicts biochemical recurrence-free survival in patients after radical prostatectomy. *Hum Pathol* 2007;38:1611–1620.

270. McNeal JE. Normal histology of the prostate. *Am J Surg Pathol* 1988;12:619–633.

271. Humphrey PA. Diagnosis of adenocarcinoma in prostate needle biopsy tissue. *J Clin Pathol* 2007;60:35–42.

272. Epstein JI. Diagnosis of limited adenocarcinoma of the prostate. *Histopathology* 2012;60:28–40.

273. Cheville JC, Bostwick DG. Postatrophic hyperplasia of the prostate. A histologic mimic of prostatic adenocarcinoma. *Am J Surg Pathol* 1995;19:1068–1076.

274. Oppenheimer JR, Wills ML, Epstein JI. Partial atrophy in prostate needle cores: another diagnostic pitfall for the surgical pathologist. *Am J Surg Pathol* 1998;22:440–445.

275. Przybycin CG, et al. Partial atrophy in prostate needle biopsies: a detailed analysis of its morphology, immunophenotype, and cellular kinetics. *Am J Surg Pathol* 2008;32:58–64.

276. Wang W, Sun X, Epstein JI. Partial atrophy on prostate needle biopsy cores: a morphologic and immunohistochemical study. *Am J Surg Pathol* 2008;32:851–857.

277. Epstein JI. Adenosis (atypical adenomatous hyperplasia): histopathology and relationship to carcinoma. *Pathol Res Pract* 1995;191:888–898.

278. Billis A, Meirelles L, Freitas LL. Mergence of partial and complete atrophy in prostate needle biopsies: a morphologic and immunohistochemical study. *Virchows Arch* 2010;456:689–694.

279. Helpap B. Observations on the number, size and localization of nucleoli in hyperplastic and neoplastic prostatic disease. *Histopathology* 1988;13:203–211.

280. Kramer CE, Epstein JI. Nucleoli in low-grade prostate adenocarcinoma and adenosis. *Hum Pathol* 1993;24:618–623.

281. Varma M, et al. Morphologic criteria for the diagnosis of prostatic adenocarcinoma in needle biopsy specimens. A study of 250 consecutive cases in a routine surgical pathology practice. *Arch Pathol Lab Med* 2002;126:554–561.

282. Epstein JI. Diagnostic criteria of limited adenocarcinoma of the prostate on needle biopsy. *Hum Pathol* 1995;26:223–229.

283. Kelemen PR, Buschmann RJ, Weisz-Carrington P. Nucleolar prominence as a diagnostic variable in prostatic carcinoma. *Cancer* 1990;65:1017–1020.

284. Epstein JI, et al. Correlation of prostate cancer nuclear deoxyribonucleic acid, size, shape and Gleason grade with pathological stage at radical prostatectomy. *J Urol* 1992;148:87–91.

285. Armas OA, et al. Nuclear morphology of prostatic carcinoma: comparison of computerized image analysis (CAS 200) versus video planimetry (DynaCELL). *Mod Pathol* 1991;4:763–767.

286. Aydin H, et al. Number and location of nucleoli and presence of apoptotic bodies in diagnostically challenging cases of prostate adenocarcinoma on needle biopsy. *Hum Pathol* 2005;36:1172–1177.

287. Thorson P, et al. Minimal carcinoma in prostate needle biopsy specimens: diagnostic features and radical prostatectomy follow-up. *Mod Pathol* 1998;11:543–551.

288. Ro JY, et al. Mucin in prostatic adenocarcinoma. *Semin Diagn Pathol* 1988;5:273–283.

289. Epstein JI, Fynheer J. Acidic mucin in the prostate: can it differentiate adenosis from adenocarcinoma? *Hum Pathol* 1992;23:1321–1325.

290. Ro JY, et al. Intraluminal crystalloids in whole-organ sections of prostate. *Prostate* 1988;13:233–239.

291. Ro JY, et al. Intraluminal crystalloids in breast carcinoma. Immunohistochemical, ultrastructural, and energy-dispersive x-ray element analysis in four cases. *Arch Pathol Lab Med* 1997;121:593–598.

292. Holmes EJ. Crystalloids of prostatic carcinoma: relationship to Bence-Jones crystals. *Cancer* 1977;39:2073–2080.

293. Ro JY, et al. Intraluminal crystalloids in prostatic adenocarcinoma. Immunohistochemical, electron microscopic, and x-ray microanalytic studies. *Cancer* 1986;57:2397–2407.

294. Vesalainen S, et al. Mitotic activity and prognosis in prostatic adenocarcinoma. *Prostate* 1995;26:80–86.

295. Giannulis I, et al. Frequency and location of mitoses in prostatic intraepithelial neoplasia (PIN). *Anticancer Res* 1993;13:2447–2451.

296. Wheeler TM, et al. Apoptotic index as a biomarker in prostatic intraepithelial neoplasia (PIN) and prostate cancer. *J Cell Biochem Suppl* 1994;19:202–207.

297. Xie W, Wong YC, Tsao SW. Correlation of increased apoptosis and proliferation with development of prostatic intraepithelial neoplasia (PIN) in ventral prostate of the Noble rat. *Prostate* 2000;44:31–39.

298. Bismar TA, et al. Multiple measures of carcinoma extent versus perineural invasion in prostate needle biopsy tissue in prediction of pathologic stage in a screening population. *Am J Surg Pathol* 2003;27:432–440.

299. Ayala GE, et al. In vitro dorsal root ganglia and human prostate cell line interaction: redefining perineural invasion in prostate cancer. *Prostate* 2001;49:213–223.

300. Ali TZ, Epstein JI. Perineural involvement by benign prostatic glands on needle biopsy. *Am J Surg Pathol* 2005;29:1159–1163.

301. Harnden P, et al. The prognostic significance of perineural invasion in prostatic cancer biopsies: a systematic review. *Cancer* 2007;109:13–24.

302. McNeal JE, et al. Mucinous differentiation in prostatic adenocarcinoma. *Hum Pathol* 1991;22:979–988.

303. Baisden BL, Kahane H, Epstein JI. Perineural invasion, mucinous fibroplasia, and glomerulations: diagnostic features of limited cancer on prostate needle biopsy. *Am J Surg Pathol* 1999;23:918–924.

304. Pacelli A, et al. Prostatic adenocarcinoma with glomeruloid features. *Hum Pathol* 1998;29:543–546.

305. Wojno KJ, Epstein JI. The utility of basal cell-specific anti-cytokeratin antibody (34 beta E12) in the diagnosis of prostate cancer. A review of 228 cases. *Am J Surg Pathol* 1995;19:251–260.

306. Abrahams NA, Ormsby AH, Brainard J. Validation of cytokeratin 5/6 as an effective substitute for keratin 903 in the differentiation of benign from malignant glands in prostate needle biopsies. *Histopathology* 2002;41:35–41.

307. Reis-Filho JS, Simpson PT, Martins A, et al. Distribution of p63, cytokeratins 5/6 and cytokeratin 14 in 51 normal and 400 neoplastic human tissue samples using TARP-4 multi-tumor tissue microarray. *Virchows Arch* 2003:443:122–132.

308. Weinstein MH, Signoretti S, Loda M. Diagnostic utility of immunohistochemical staining for p63. *Mod Pathol* 15:1302–1308.

309. Shah RB, Kunju LP, Shen R, et al. Usefulness of basal cell cocktail (34betaE12 + p63) in the diagnosis of atypical prostate glandular proliferations. *Am J Clin Pathol* 2004;122:517–523.

310. Shah RB, Zhou M, LeBlanc M, et al. Comparison of the basal cell-specific markers, 34betaE12 and p63, in the diagnosis of prostate cancer. *Am J Surg Pathol* 2002;26:1161–1168.

311. Dardik M, Epstein JI. Efficacy of restaining prostate needle biopsies with high-molecular weight cytokeratin. *Hum Pathol* 2000;31:1155–1161.

312. Amin MB, et al. Postatrophic hyperplasia of the prostate gland: a detailed analysis of its morphology in needle biopsy specimens. *Am J Surg Pathol* 1999;23:925–931.

313. Hedrick L, Epstein JI. Use of keratin 903 as an adjunct in the diagnosis of prostate carcinoma. *Am J Surg Pathol* 1989;13:389–396.

314. Varma M, Jasani B. Diagnostic utility of immunohistochemistry in morphologically difficult prostate cancer: review of current literature. *Histopathology* 2005;2005:1–16.

315. Ali TZ, Epstein JI. False positive labeling of prostate cancer with high molecular weight cytokeratin: p63 a more specific immunomarker for basal cells. *Am J Surg Pathol* 2008;32:1890–1895.

316. Osunkoya AO, Hansel DE, Sun X, et al. Aberrant diffuse expression of p63 in adenocarcinoma of the prostate on needle biopsy and radical prostatectomy: report of 21 cases. *Am J Surg Pathol* 2008;32:461–467.

317. Xu J, Stolk JA, Zhang X, et al. Identification of differentially expressed genes in human prostate cancer using subtraction and microarray. *Cancer Res* 2000;60:1677–1682.

318. Jiang Z, Woda BA, Rock KL. P504S: a new molecular marker for the detection of prostate carcinoma. *Am J Surg Pathol* 2001;25:1397–1404.

319. Jiang Z, Woda BA, Wu CL, et al. Discovery and clinical application of a novel prostate cancer marker: alpha-methylacyl CoA racemase (P504S). *Am J Clin Pathol* 2004;122:275–289.

320. Beach R, Gown AM, De Peralta-Venturina MN, et al. P504S immunohistochemical detection in 405 prostatic specimens including 376 18-gauge needle biopsies. *Am J Surg Pathol* 2002;26:1588–1596.

321. Jiang Z, Wu CL, Woda BA, et al. P504S/alpha-methylacyl-CoA racemase: a useful marker for diagnosis of small foci of prostatic carcinoma on needle biopsy. *Am J Surg Pathol* 2002;26:1169–1174.

322. Sanderson SO, Sebo TJ, Murphy LM, et al. An analysis of the p63/alpha-methylacyl coenzyme A racemase immunohistochemical cocktail stain in prostate needle biopsy specimens and tissue microarrays. *Am J Clin Pathol* 2004;121:220–225.

323. Molinie V, Fromont G, Sibony M. Diagnostic utility of a p63/alpha-methyl-CoA-racemase (p504s) cocktail in atypical foci in the prostate. *Mod Pathol* 2004;10:1180–1190.

324. Jiang X, Li C, Fischer A, et al. Using an AMACR (P504S)/34betaE12/p63 cocktail for the detection of small focal prostate carcinoma in needle biopsy specimens. *Am J Clin Pathol* 2005;123:231–236.

325. Ng VW, Koh M, Tan SY, et al. Is triple immunostaining with 34betaE12, p63, and racemase in prostate cancer advantageous? A tissue microarray study. *Am J Clin Pathol* 2007;127:248–253.

326. Zhou M, Jiang Z, Esptein JI. Expression and diagnostic utility of alpha-methylacyl-CoA-racemase (P504S) in foamy gland and pseudohyperplastic prostate cancer. *Am J Surg Pathol* 2003;27:772–778.

327. Farinola MA, Epstein JI. Utility of immunohistochemistry for alpha-methylacyl-CoA racemase in distinguishing atrophic prostate cancer from benign atrophy. *Hum Pathol* 2004;35:1272–1278.

328. Hameed O, Sublett J, Humphrey PA. Immunohistochemical stains for p63 and alpha-methylacyl-CoA racemase, versus a cocktail comprising both, in the diagnosis of prostatic carcinoma: a comparison of the immunohistochemical staining of 430 foci in radical prostatectomy and needle biopsy tissues. *Am J Surg Pathol* 2005;29:579–587.

329. Adley BP, Yang XJ. Application of alpha-methylacyl coenzyme A racemase immunohistochemistry in the diagnosis of prostate cancer: a review. *Anal Quant Cytol Histol* 2006;28:1–13.

330. Przybycin CG, Kunju LP, Wu AJ, et al. Partial atrophy in prostate needle biopsies: a detailed analysis of its morphology, immunophenotype, and cellular kinetics. *Am J Surg Pathol* 2008;32:58–64.

331. Skinnider BF, Oliva E, Young RH, et al. Expression of alpha-methylacyl-CoA racemase (P504S) in nephrogenic adenoma: a significant immunohistochemical pitfall compounding the differential diagnosis with prostatic adenocarcinoma. *Am J Surg Pathol* 2004;28:701–705.

332. Gupta A, Wang HL, Policarpio-Nicolas ML, et al. Expression of alpha-methylacyl-coenzyme A racemase in nephrogenic adenoma. *Am J Surg Pathol* 2004;28:1224–1229.

333. Magi-Galluzzi C, Luo J, Isaacs WB, et al. Alpha-methylacyl-CoA racemase: a variably sensitive immunohistochemical marker for the diagnosis of small prostate cancer foci on needle biopsy. *Am J Surg Pathol* 2003;2003:1128–1133.

334. Bazinet M, Zheng W, Began LR, et al. Morphologic changes induced by neoadjuvant androgen ablation may result in underdetection of positive surgical margins and capsular involvement by prostatic adenocarcinoma. *Urology* 1997;49:721–725.

335. Sweat SD, Pacelli A, Murphy GP, et al. Prostate-specific membrane antigen expression is greatest in prostate adenocarcinoma and lymph node metastases. *Urology* 1998;52:637–640.

336. Troyer JK, Beckett ML, Wright GL Jr. Detection and characterization of the prostate-specific membrane antigen (PSMA) in tissue extracts and body fluids. *Int J Cancer* 1995;52:552–558.

337. Wright GL Jr, Haley C, Beckett ML, et al. Expression of prostate-specific membrane antigen in normal, benign, and malignant prostate tissues. *Urol Oncol* 1995;1:18–28.

338. Chuang A, DeMarzo AM, Veltri RW, et al. Immunohistochemical differentiation of high-grade prostate carcinoma from urothelial carcinoma. *Am J Surg Pathol* 2007;31:1246–1255.

339. Srinivasan M, Parwani AV. Diagnostic utility of p63/P501S double sequential immunohistochemical staining in differentiating urothelial carcinoma from prostate carcinoma. *Diagn Cytopathol* 2011;6:67.

340. Gurel B, Ali T, Montgomery EA, et al. NKX3.1 as a marker of prostatic origin in metastatic tumors. *Am J Surg Pathol* 2010;34:1097–1105.

341. Voeller HJ, Augustus M, Madike V, et al. Coding region of NKX3.1, a prostate-specific homeobox gene on 8p21, is not mutated in human prostate cancers. *Cancer Res* 1997;57:4455–4459.

342. Xu J, Kalos M, Stolk JA, et al. Identification and characterization of prostein, a novel prostate-specific protein. *Cancer Res* 2001;61:1563–1568.

343. Bostwick DG, et al. Prognostic factors in prostate cancer. College of American Pathologists Consensus Statement 1999. *Arch Pathol Lab Med* 2000;124:995–1000.

344. Zhou M, Srigley JR. Benign mimickers and potential precursors of prostatic adenocarcinoma. *Diagn Histopathol* 2011;17:434–446.

345. Montironi R, et al. The spectrum of morphology in nonneoplastic prostate including cancer mimics. *Histopathology* 2012;60:41–58.

346. Hameed O, Humphrey PA. Pseudoneoplastic mimics of prostate and bladder carcinomas. *Arch Pathol Lab Med* 2010;134:427–443.

347. Harik LR, O'Toole KM. Nonneoplastic lesions of the prostate and bladder. *Arch Pathol Lab Med* 2012;136:721–734.

348. Curtis MW, Evans AJ, Srigley JR. Mucin-producing urothelial-type adenocarcinoma of prostate: report of two cases of a rare and diagnostically challenging entity. *Mod Pathol* 2005;18:585–590.

349. Osunkoya AO, Epstein JI. Primary mucin-producing urothelial-type adenocarcinoma of prostate: report of 15 cases. *Am J Surg Pathol* 2007;31:1323–1329.

350. Shah RB, Zhou M. Atypical cribriform lesions of the prostate: clinical significance, differential diagnosis and current concept of intraductal carcinoma of the prostate. *Adv Anat Pathol* 2012;19:270–278.

351. Robinson B, Magi-Galluzzi C, Zhou M. Intraductal carcinoma of the prostate. *Arch Pathol Lab Med* 2012;136:418–425.

352. Montironi R, et al. Do not misinterpret intraductal carcinoma of the prostate as high-grade prostatic intraepithelial neoplasia! *Eur Urol* 2012;62:518–522.

353. Henry PC, Evans AJ. Intraductal carcinoma of the prostate: a distinct histopathological entity with important prognostic implications. *J Clin Pathol* 2009;62:579–583.

354. McNeal JE, et al. Cribriform adenocarcinoma of the prostate. *Cancer* 1986;58:1714–1719.

355. Kovi J, Jackson MA, Heshmat MY. Ductal spread in prostatic carcinoma. *Cancer* 1985;56:1566–1573.

356. Rubin MA, et al. Cribriform carcinoma of the prostate and cribriform prostatic intraepithelial neoplasia: incidence and clinical implications. *Am J Surg Pathol* 1998;22:840–848.

357. Kronz JD, Shaikh AA, Epstein JI. Atypical cribriform lesions on prostate biopsy. *Am J Surg Pathol* 2001;25:147–155.

358. McNeal JE, Yemoto CE. Spread of adenocarcinoma within prostatic ducts and acini. Morphologic and clinical correlations. *Am J Surg Pathol* 1996;20:802–814.

359. Guo CC, Epstein JI. Intraductal carcinoma of the prostate on needle biopsy: histologic features and clinical significance. *Mod Pathol* 2006;19:1528–1535.

360. Cohen RJ, et al. A proposal on the identification, histologic reporting, and implications of intraductal prostatic carcinoma. *Arch Pathol Lab Med* 2007;131:1103–1109.

361. Cohen RJ, et al. Prediction of pathological stage and clinical outcome in prostate cancer: an improved pre-operative model incorporating biopsy-determined intraductal carcinoma. *Br J Urol* 1998;81:413–418.

362. Wilcox G, et al. Patterns of high-grade prostatic intraepithelial neoplasia associated with clinically aggressive prostate cancer. *Hum Pathol* 1998;29:1119–1123.

363. Robinson BD, Epstein JI. Intraductal carcinoma of the prostate without invasive carcinoma on needle biopsy: emphasis on radical prostatectomy findings. *J Urol* 2010;184:1328–1333.

364. Cohen RJ, Shannon BA, Weinstein SL. Intraductal carcinoma of the prostate gland with transmucosal spread to the seminal vesicle: a lesion distinct from high-grade prostatic intraepithelial neoplasia. *Arch Pathol Lab Med* 2007;131:1122–1125.

365. Watts KE, Li J, Magi-Galluzzi C. et al., Incidence and clinicopathological characteristics of intraductal carcinoma of the prostate detected in prostate biopsies: a Prospective Cohort study. *Mod Pathol* 2012;25:250A.

366. Pickup M, Van der Kwast TH. My approach to intraductal lesions of the prostate gland. *J Clin Pathol* 2007;60:856–865.

367. Shah RB, et al. Atypical cribriform lesions of the prostate: relationship to prostatic carcinoma and implication for diagnosis in prostate biopsies. *Am J Surg Pathol* 2010;34:470–477.

368. Dawkins HJ, et al. Distinction between intraductal carcinoma of the prostate (IDC-P), high-grade dysplasia (PIN), and invasive prostatic adenocarcinoma, using molecular markers of cancer progression. *Prostate* 2000;44:265–270.

369. Bettendorf O, et al. Chromosomal imbalances, loss of heterozygosity, and immunohistochemical expression of TP53, RB1, and PTEN in intraductal cancer, intraepithelial neoplasia, and invasive adenocarcinoma of the prostate. *Genes Chromosomes Cancer* 2008;47: 565–572.

370. Lotan TL, et al. Cytoplasmic PTEN protein loss distinguishes intraductal carcinoma of the prostate from high-grade prostatic intraepithelial neoplasia. *Mod Pathol* 2013;26:587–603.

371. Han B, et al. ETS gene aberrations in atypical cribriform lesions of the prostate: Implications for the distinction between intraductal carcinoma of the prostate and cribriform high-grade prostatic intraepithelial neoplasia. *Am J Surg Pathol* 2010;34:478–485.

372. Dube VE, Farrow GM, Greene LF. Prostatic adenocarcinoma of ductal origin. *Cancer* 1973;32:402–409.

373. Lemberger RJ, et al. Carcinoma of the prostate of ductal origin. *Br J Urol* 1984;56:706–709.

374. Bostwick DG, Kindrachuk RW, Rouse RV. Prostatic adenocarcinoma with endometrioid features. Clinical, pathologic, and ultrastructural findings. *Am J Surg Pathol* 1985;9:595–609.

375. Epstein JI, Woodruff JM. Adenocarcinoma of the prostate with endometrioid features. A light microscopic and immunohistochemical study of ten cases. *Cancer* 1986;57:111–119.

376. Ro JY, et al. Prostatic duct adenocarcinoma with endometrioid features: immunohistochemical and electron microscopic study. *Semin Diagn Pathol* 1988;5:301–311.

377. Christensen WN, et al. Prostatic duct adenocarcinoma. Findings at radical prostatectomy. *Cancer* 1991;67:2118–2124.

378. Millar EK, Sharma NK, Lessells AM. Ductal (endometrioid) adenocarcinoma of the prostate: a clinicopathological study of 16 cases. *Histopathology* 1996;29:11–19.

379. Oxley JD, et al. Ductal carcinomas of the prostate: a clinicopathological and immunohistochemical study. *Br J Urol* 1998;81:109–115.

380. Bock BJ, Bostwick DG. Does prostatic ductal adenocarcinoma exist? *Am J Surg Pathol* 1999;23:781–785.

381. Brinker DA, Potter SR, Epstein JI. Ductal adenocarcinoma of the prostate diagnosed on needle biopsy: correlation with clinical and radical prostatectomy findings and progression. *Am J Surg Pathol* 1999;23:1471–1479.

382. Zaloudek C, Williams JW, Kempson RL. "Endometrial" adenocarcinoma of the prostate: a distinctive tumor of probable prostatic duct origin. *Cancer* 1976;37:2255–2262.

383. Lotan TL, et al. TMPRSS2-ERG gene fusions are infrequent in prostatic ductal adenocarcinomas. *Mod Pathol* 2009;22:359–365.

384. Herawi M, Epstein JI. Immunohistochemical antibody cocktail staining (p63/HMWCK/AMACR) of ductal adenocarcinoma and Gleason pattern 4 cribriform and noncribriform acinar adenocarcinomas of the prostate. *Am J Surg Pathol* 2007;31:889–894.

385. Han B, et al. Characterization of ETS gene aberrations in select histologic variants of prostate carcinoma. *Mod Pathol* 2009;22: 1176–1185.

386. Amin A, Epstein JI. Pathologic stage of prostatic ductal adenocarcinoma at radical prostatectomy: effect of percentage of the ductal component and associated grade of acinar adenocarcinoma. *Am J Surg Pathol* 2011;35:615–619.

387. Samaratunga H, et al. Any proportion of ductal adenocarcinoma in radical prostatectomy specimens predicts extraprostatic extension. *Hum Pathol* 2010;41:281–285.

388. Morgan TM, et al. Ductal adenocarcinoma of the prostate: increased mortality risk and decreased serum prostate specific antigen. *J Urol* 2010;184:2303–2307.

389. Sanati S, et al. Gene expression profiles of ductal versus acinar adenocarcinoma of the prostate. *Mod Pathol* 2009;22:1273–1279.

390. Meeks JJ, et al. Incidence and outcomes of ductal carcinoma of the prostate in the USA: analysis of data from the Surveillance, Epidemiology, and End Results program. *BJU Int* 2012;109:831–834.

391. Eade TN, et al. Role of radiotherapy in ductal (endometrioid) carcinoma of the prostate. *Cancer* 2007;109:2011–2015.

392. Orihuela E, Green JM. Ductal prostate cancer: contemporary management and outcomes. *Urol Oncol* 2008;26:368–371.

393. Lee TK, Miller JS, Epstein JI. Rare histological patterns of prostatic ductal adenocarcinoma. *Pathology* 2010;42:319–324.

394. Henderson-Jackson E, et al. Cystic prostatic ductal adenocarcinoma: an unusual presentation and cytological diagnosis. *Ann Clin Lab Sci* 2012;42:81–88.

395. Samaratunga H, Letizia B. Prostatic ductal adenocarcinoma presenting as a urethral polyp: a clinicopathological study of eight cases of a lesion with the potential to be misdiagnosed as a benign prostatic urethral polyp. *Pathology* 2007;39:476–481.

396. Aydin H, et al. Ductal adenocarcinoma of the prostate diagnosed on transurethral biopsy or resection is not always indicative of aggressive disease: implications for clinical management. *BJU Int* 2010;105:476–480.

397. Samaratunga H, Singh M. Distribution pattern of basal cells detected by cytokeratin 34 beta E12 in primary prostatic duct adenocarcinoma. *Am J Surg Pathol* 1997;21:435–440.

398. Franks LM, O'Shea JD, Thomson AE. Mucin in the prostate: a histochemical study in normal glands, latent, clinical, and colloid cancers. *Cancer* 1964;17:983–991.

399. Pinder SE, McMahon RF. Mucins in prostatic carcinoma. *Histopathology* 1990;16:43–46.

400. Noiwan S, Rattanarapee S. Mucin production in prostatic adenocarcinoma: a retrospective study of 190 radical prostatectomy and/or core biopsy specimens in department of pathology, Siriraj Hospital, Mahidol University, Thailand. *J Med Assoc Thai* 2011;94: 224–230.

401. Taylor NS. Histochemistry in the diagnosis of early prostatic carcinoma. *Hum Pathol* 1979;10:513–520.

402. Arangelovich V, et al. Pathogenesis and significance of collagenous micronodules of the prostate. *Appl Immunohistochem Mol Morphol* 2003;11:15–19.

403. Bostwick DG, Wollan P, Adlakha K. Collagenous micronodules in prostate cancer. A specific but infrequent diagnostic finding. *Arch Pathol Lab Med* 1995;119:444–447.

404. Bohman KD, Osunkoya AO. Mucin-producing tumors and tumor-like lesions involving the prostate: a comprehensive review. *Adv Anat Pathol* 2012;19:374–387.

405. Osunkoya AO, Nielsen ME, Epstein JI. Prognosis of mucinous adenocarcinoma of the prostate treated by radical prostatectomy: a study of 47 cases. *Am J Surg Pathol* 2008;32:468–472.

406. Lane BR, et al. Mucinous adenocarcinoma of the prostate does not confer poor prognosis. *Urology* 2006;68:825–830.

407. Ro JY, et al. Mucinous adenocarcinoma of the prostate: histochemical and immunohistochemical studies. *Hum Pathol* 1990;21:593–600.

408. Epstein JI, Lieberman PH. Mucinous adenocarcinoma of the prostate gland. *Am J Surg Pathol* 1985;9:299–308.

409. Elbadawi A, et al. Prostatic mucinous carcinoma. *Urology* 1979; 13:658–666.

410. Furusato B, et al. ERG oncoprotein expression in prostate cancer: clonal progression of ERG-positive tumor cells and potential for ERG-based stratification. *Prostate Cancer Prostatic Dis* 2010;13: 228–237.

411. Osunkoya AO, et al. MUC2 expression in primary mucinous and nonmucinous adenocarcinoma of the prostate: an analysis of 50 cases on radical prostatectomy. *Mod Pathol* 2008;21:789–794.

412. Ro JY, et al. Signet-ring-cell carcinoma of the prostate. Electron-microscopic and immunohistochemical studies of eight cases. *Am J Surg Pathol* 1988;12:453–460.

413. Hejka AG, England DM. Signet ring cell carcinoma of prostate. Immunohistochemical and ultrastructural study of a case. *Urology* 1989;34:155–158.

414. Guerin D, Hasan N, Keen CE. Signet ring cell differentiation in adenocarcinoma of the prostate: a study of five cases. *Histopathology* 1993;22:367–371.

415. Torbenson M, et al. Prostatic carcinoma with signet ring cells: a clinicopathologic and immunohistochemical analysis of 12 cases, with review of the literature. *Mod Pathol* 1998;11:552–559.

416. Warner JN, et al. Primary signet ring cell carcinoma of the prostate. *Mayo Clin Proc* 2010;85:1130–1136.

417. Saito S, Iwaki H. Mucin-producing carcinoma of the prostate: review of 88 cases. *Urology* 1999;54:141–144.

418. Schned AR. Artifactual signet ring cells. *Am J Surg Pathol* 1987;11:736–737.

419. Alguacil-Garcia A. Artifactual changes mimicking signet ring cell carcinoma in transurethral prostatectomy specimens. *Am J Surg Pathol* 1986;10:795–800.

420. Arista-Nasr J, et al. Pseudohyperplastic prostatic adenocarcinoma in transurethral resections of the prostate. *Pathol Oncol Res* 2003;9:232–235.

421. Humphrey PA, et al. Pseudohyperplastic prostatic adenocarcinoma. *Am J Surg Pathol* 1998;22:1239–1246.

422. Levi AW, Epstein JI. Pseudohyperplastic prostatic adenocarcinoma on needle biopsy and simple prostatectomy. *Am J Surg Pathol* 2000;24:1039–1046.

423. Yaskiv O, Cao D, Humphrey PA. Microcystic adenocarcinoma of the prostate: a variant of pseudohyperplastic and atrophic patterns. *Am J Surg Pathol* 2010;34:556–561.

424. Zhou M, Jiang Z, Epstein JI. Expression and diagnostic utility of alpha-methylacyl-CoA-racemase (P504S) in foamy gland and pseudohyperplastic prostate cancer. *Am J Surg Pathol* 2003;27:772–778.

425. Kaleem Z, et al. Prostatic adenocarcinoma with atrophic features: a study of 202 consecutive completely embedded radical prostatectomy specimens. *Am J Clin Pathol* 1998;109:695–703.

426. Cina SJ, Epstein JI. Adenocarcinoma of the prostate with atrophic features. *Am J Surg Pathol* 1997;21:289–295.

427. Egan AJ, Lopez-Beltran A, Bostwick DG. Prostatic adenocarcinoma with atrophic features: malignancy mimicking a benign process. *Am J Surg Pathol* 1997;21:931–935.

428. Hudson J, et al. Foamy gland adenocarcinoma of the prostate: incidence, Gleason grade, and early clinical outcome. *Hum Pathol* 2012;43:974–979.

429. Zhao J, Epstein JI. High-grade foamy gland prostatic adenocarcinoma on biopsy or transurethral resection: a morphologic study of 55 cases. *Am J Surg Pathol* 2009;33:583–590.

430. Arista-Nasr J, et al. Foamy gland microcarcinoma in needle prostatic biopsy. *Ann Diagn Pathol* 2008;12:349–355.

431. Nelson RS, Epstein JI. Prostatic carcinoma with abundant xanthomatous cytoplasm. Foamy gland carcinoma. *Am J Surg Pathol* 1996;20:419–426.

432. Tran TT, Sengupta E, Yang XJ. Prostatic foamy gland carcinoma with aggressive behavior: clinicopathologic, immunohistochemical, and ultrastructural analysis. *Am J Surg Pathol* 2001;25:618–623.

433. Chuang AY, Epstein JI. Xanthoma of the prostate: a mimicker of high-grade prostate adenocarcinoma. *Am J Surg Pathol* 2007;31:1225–1230.

434. Sebo TJ, et al. prostatic xanthoma: a mimic of prostatic adenocarcinoma. *Hum Pathol* 1994;25:386–389.

435. Tavora F, Epstein JI. High-grade prostatic intraepithelial neoplasia like ductal adenocarcinoma of the prostate: a clinicopathologic study of 28 cases. *Am J Surg Pathol* 2008;32:1060–1067.

436. Hameed O, Humphrey PA. Stratified epithelium in prostatic adenocarcinoma: a mimic of high-grade prostatic intraepithelial neoplasia. *Mod Pathol* 2006;19:899–906.

437. Lopez-Beltran A, et al. Lymphoepithelioma-like carcinoma of the prostate. *Hum Pathol* 2009;40:982–987.

438. Adlakha K, Bostwick DG. Lymphoepithelioma-like carcinoma of the prostate. *J Urol Pathol* 1994;2:319–325.

439. Ordonez NG, Ro JY, Ayala AG. Metastatic prostatic carcinoma presenting as an oncocytic tumor. *Am J Surg Pathol* 1992;16:1007–1012.

440. Pinto JA, Gonzalez JE, Granadillo MA. Primary carcinoma of the prostate with diffuse oncocytic changes. *Histopathology* 1994;25:286–288.

441. Fiandrino G, et al. Prostatic adenocarcinoma with oncocytic features. *J Clin Pathol* 2011;64:177–178.

442. Parwani AV, Herawi M, Epstein JI. Pleomorphic giant cell adenocarcinoma of the prostate: report of 6 cases. *Am J Surg Pathol* 2006;30:1254–1259.

443. Lopez-Beltran A, Eble JN, Bostwick DG. Pleomorphic giant cell carcinoma of the prostate. *Arch Pathol Lab Med* 2005;129:683–685.

444. Humphrey P. *Grading of Prostatic Carcinoma. Prostate Pathology.* Chicago, IL: ASCP Press; 2003.

445. Gleason DF. Classification of prostatic carcinomas. *Cancer Chemother Rep* 1966;50:125–128.

446. Mellinger GT, Gleason D, Bailar J III. The histology and prognosis of prostatic cancer. *J Urol* 1967;97:331–337.

447. Gleason DF, Mellinger GT. Prediction of prognosis for prostatic adenocarcinoma by combined histological grading and clinical staging. *J Urol* 1974;111:58–64.

448. Gleason DF. Histologic grading of prostate cancer: a perspective. *Hum Pathol* 1992;23:273–279.

449. Gleason DF. Histologic grading of prostate carcinoma. In: Bostwick DG, ed. *Pathology of the Prostate.* Newyork: Churchill Livingstone; 1990:83–93.

450. Hodge KK, et al. Random systematic versus directed ultrasound guided transrectal core biopsies of the prostate. *J Urol* 1989;142:71–74; discussion 74–75.

451. Amin MB, Schultz DS, Zarbo RJ. Analysis of cribriform morphology in prostatic neoplasia using antibody to high-molecular-weight cytokeratins. *Arch Pathol Lab Med* 1994;118:260–264.

452. Berney DM. The case for modifying the Gleason grading system. *BJU Int* 2007;100:725–726.

453. Berney DM, et al. Major shifts in the treatment and prognosis of prostate cancer due to changes in pathological diagnosis and grading. *BJU Int* 2007;100:1240–1244.

454. Epstein JI. An update of the Gleason grading system. *J Urol* 2010;183:433–440.

455. Sim HG, et al. Tertiary Gleason pattern 5 in Gleason 7 prostate cancer predicts pathological stage and biochemical recurrence. *J Urol* 2008;179:1775–1779.

456. Whittemore DE, et al. Significance of tertiary Gleason pattern 5 in Gleason score 7 radical prostatectomy specimens. *J Urol* 2008;179:516–522; discussion 522.

457. Stephenson AJ, et al. Preoperative nomogram predicting the 10-year probability of prostate cancer recurrence after radical prostatectomy. *J Natl Cancer Inst* 2006;98:715–717.

458. Stephenson AJ, et al. Postoperative nomogram predicting the 10-year probability of prostate cancer recurrence after radical prostatectomy. *J Clin Oncol* 2005;23:7005–7012.

459. Makarov DV, et al. Updated nomogram to predict pathologic stage of prostate cancer given prostate-specific antigen level, clinical stage, and biopsy Gleason score (Partin tables) based on cases from 2000 to 2005. *Urology* 2007;69:1095–1101.

460. Helpap B, Egevad L. The significance of modified Gleason grading of prostatic carcinoma in biopsy and radical prostatectomy specimens. *Virchows Arch* 2006;449:622–627.

461. Zareba P, et al. The impact of the 2005 International Society of Urological Pathology (ISUP) consensus on Gleason grading in contemporary practice. *Histopathology* 2009;55:384–391.

462. Dong F, et al. Impact on the clinical outcome of prostate cancer by the 2005 international society of urological pathology modified Gleason grading system. *Am J Surg Pathol* 2012;36:838–843.

463. Lopez-Beltran A, et al. Current practice of Gleason grading of prostate carcinoma. *Virchows Arch* 2006;448:111–118.

464. Veloso SG, et al. Interobserver agreement of Gleason score and modified Gleason score in needle biopsy and in surgical specimen of prostate cancer. *Int Braz J Urol* 2007;33:639–646; discussion 647–651.

465. Tsivian M, et al. Changes in Gleason score grading and their effect in predicting outcome after radical prostatectomy. *Urology* 2009;74:1090–1093.

466. Patel AA, et al. PSA failure following definitive treatment of prostate cancer having biopsy Gleason score 7 with tertiary grade 5. *JAMA* 2007;298:1533–1538.

467. Nanda A, et al. Gleason Pattern 5 prostate cancer: further stratification of patients with high-risk disease and implications for future randomized trials. *Int J Radiat Oncol Biol Phys* 2009;74:1419–1423.

468. Fine SW, Epstein JI. A contemporary study correlating prostate needle biopsy and radical prostatectomy Gleason score. *J Urol* 2008;179:1335–1338; discussion 1338–1339.

469. Melia J, et al. A UK-based investigation of inter- and intra-observer reproducibility of Gleason grading of prostatic biopsies. *Histopathology* 2006;48:644–654.

470. Gofrit ON, et al. The Will Rogers phenomenon in urological oncology. *J Urol* 2008;179:28–33.

471. Billis A, et al. The impact of the 2005 international society of urological pathology consensus conference on standard Gleason grading of prostatic carcinoma in needle biopsies. *J Urol* 2008;180:548–552; discussion 552–553.

472. Egevad L, Mazzucchelli R, Montironi R. Implications of the International Society of Urological Pathology modified Gleason grading system. *Arch Pathol Lab Med* 2012;136:426–434.

473. Delahunt B, et al. Gleason grading: past, present and future. *Histopathology* 2012;60:75–86.

474. McAleer SJ, et al. PSA outcome following radical prostatectomy for patients with localized prostate cancer stratified by prostatectomy findings and the preoperative PSA level. *Urol Oncol* 2005;23:311–317.

475. Isbarn H, et al. Long-term data on the survival of patients with prostate cancer treated with radical prostatectomy in the prostate-specific antigen era. *BJU Int* 2010;106:37–43.

476. Edge SB, et al. AJCC Cancer staging. *From the AJCC Cancer Staging Manual*. 7th ed. New York: Springer-Verlag; 2010:457–468.

477. Sobin LH, Wittekind C, eds.; International Union Against Cancer (UICC). *TNM Classification of Malignant Tumours*. 6th ed. New York: Wiley-Liss; 2002:184–187.

478. Sobin L, Gospodariwicz M, Wittekind C, eds.; International Union Against Cancer (UICC). *TNM Classification of Malignant Tumors*. 7th ed. Oxford, UK: Wiley-Blackwell; 2009.

479. van der Kwast TH. Substaging pathologically organ confined (pT2) prostate cancer: an exercise in futility? *Eur Urol* 2006;49:209–211.

480. van Oort IM, et al. The prognostic role of the pathological T2 subclassification for prostate cancer in the 2002 Tumour-Nodes-Metastasis staging system. *BJU Int* 2008;102:438–441.

481. Freedland SJ, et al. Biochemical failure after radical prostatectomy in men with pathologic organ-confined disease: pT2a versus pT2b. *Cancer* 2004;100:1646–1649.

482. Hong SK, et al. Evaluation of pT2 subdivisions in the TNM staging system for prostate cancer. *BJU Int* 2008;102:1092–1096.

483. Kordan Y, et al. Pathological stage T2 subgroups to predict biochemical recurrence after prostatectomy. *J Urol* 2009;182:2291–2295.

484. van der Kwast TH, et al. International Society of Urological Pathology (ISUP) Consensus Conference on Handling and Staging of Radical Prostatectomy Specimens. Working group 2: T2 substaging and prostate cancer volume. *Mod Pathol* 2011;24:16–25.

485. Kausik SJ, et al. Prognostic significance of positive surgical margins in patients with extraprostatic carcinoma after radical prostatectomy. *Cancer* 2002;95:1215–1219.

486. Swindle P, et al. Do margins matter? The prognostic significance of positive surgical margins in radical prostatectomy specimens. *J Urol* 2005;174:903–907.

487. Ayala AG, et al. The prostatic capsule: does it exist? Its importance in the staging and treatment of prostatic carcinoma. *Am J Surg Pathol* 1989;13:21–27.

488. Chuang AY, Epstein JI. Positive surgical margins in areas of capsular incision in otherwise organ-confined disease at radical prostatectomy: histologic features and pitfalls. *Am J Surg Pathol* 2008;32:1201–1206.

489. Epstein JI, et al. Prognostic factors and reporting of prostate carcinoma in radical prostatectomy and pelvic lymphadenectomy specimens. *Scand J Urol Nephrol Suppl* 2005;34–63.

490. Evans AJ, et al. Interobserver variability between expert urologic pathologists for extraprostatic extension and surgical margin status in radical prostatectomy specimens. *Am J Surg Pathol* 2008;32:1503–1512.

491. Ekici S, et al. The role of the pathologist in the evaluation of radical prostatectomy specimens. *Scand J Urol Nephrol* 2003;37:387–391.

492. Ohori M, et al. Prognostic significance of positive surgical margins in radical prostatectomy specimens. *J Urol* 1995;154:1818–1824.

493. Epstein JI, et al. Influence of capsular penetration on progression following radical prostatectomy: a study of 196 cases with long-term follow-up. *J Urol* 1993;150:135–141.

494. Wheeler TM, et al. Clinical and pathological significance of the level and extent of capsular invasion in clinical stage T1–2 prostate cancer. *Hum Pathol* 1998;29:856–862.

495. Sung MT, et al. Radial distance of extraprostatic extension measured by ocular micrometer is an independent predictor of prostate-specific antigen recurrence: a new proposal for the substaging of pT3a prostate cancer. *Am J Surg Pathol* 2007;31:311–318.

496. Greene FL. The American Joint Committee on Cancer: updating the strategies in cancer staging. *Bull Am Coll Surg* 2002;87:13–15.

497. Rodriguez-Covarrubias F, et al. Invasion of bladder neck after radical prostatectomy: one definition for different outcomes. *Prostate Cancer Prostatic Dis* 2008;11:294–297.

498. Srigley JR, et al. Protocol for the examination of specimens from patients with carcinomas of the prostate gland. *Arch Pathol Lab Med* 2009;133:1568–1576.

499. Ruano T, et al. The significance of microscopic bladder neck invasion in radical prostatectomies: pT4 disease? *Int Urol Nephrol* 2009;41:71–76.

500. Rodriguez-Covarrubias F, et al. Prognostic significance of microscopic bladder neck invasion in prostate cancer. *BJU Int* 2009;103:758–761.

501. Zhou M, et al. Microscopic bladder neck involvement by prostate carcinoma in radical prostatectomy specimens is not a significant independent prognostic factor. *Mod Pathol* 2008;2009;22:385–392.

502. Magi-Galluzzi C, et al. International Society of Urological Pathology (ISUP) Consensus Conference on Handling and Staging of Radical Prostatectomy Specimens. Working group 3: extraprostatic extension, lymphovascular invasion and locally advanced disease. *Mod Pathol* 2011;24:26–38.

503. Walz J, et al. Nomogram predicting the probability of early recurrence after radical prostatectomy for prostate cancer. *J Urol* 2009;181:601–607; discussion 607–608.

504. Ohori M, et al. The mechanisms and prognostic significance of seminal vesicle involvement by prostate cancer. *Am J Surg Pathol* 1993;17:1252–1261.

505. Paul A, et al. Oncologic outcome after extraperitoneal laparoscopic radical prostatectomy: midterm follow-up of 1115 procedures. *Eur Urol* 2010;57:267–272.

506. Touijer K, et al. Oncologic outcome after laparoscopic radical prostatectomy: 10 years of experience. *Eur Urol* 2009;55:1014–1019.

507. Debras B, et al. Prognostic significance of seminal vesicle invasion on the radical prostatectomy specimen. Rationale for seminal vesicle biopsies. *Eur Urol* 1998;33:271–277.

508. Tefilli MV, et al. Prognostic indicators in patients with seminal vesicle involvement following radical prostatectomy for clinically localized prostate cancer. *J Urol* 1998;160(3 Pt 1):802–806.

509. Berney DM, et al. International Society of Urological Pathology (ISUP) Consensus Conference on Handling and Staging of Radical Prostatectomy Specimens. Working group 4: seminal vesicles and lymph nodes. *Mod Pathol* 2011;24:39–47.

510. Guo CC, Pisters LL, Troncoso P. Prostate cancer invading the rectum: a clinicopathological study of 18 cases. *Pathology* 2009;41:539–543.

511. Bowrey DJ, Otter MI, Billings PJ. Rectal infiltration by prostatic adenocarcinoma: report on six patients and review of the literature. *Ann R Coll Surg Engl* 2003;85:382–385.

512. Pettus JA, et al. Biochemical failure in men following radical retropubic prostatectomy: impact of surgical margin status and location. *J Urol* 2004;172:129–132.

513. Tan PH, et al. International Society of Urological Pathology (ISUP) Consensus Conference on Handling and Staging of Radical Prostatectomy Specimens. Working group 5: surgical margins. *Mod Pathol* 2011;24:48–57.

514. Emerson RE, et al. Closest distance between tumor and resection margin in radical prostatectomy specimens: lack of prognostic significance. *Am J Surg Pathol* 2005;29:225–229.

515. Babaian RJ, et al. Analysis of clinicopathologic factors predicting outcome after radical prostatectomy. *Cancer* 2001;91:1414–1422.

516. Epstein JI, et al. Recommendations for the reporting of prostate carcinoma: Association of Directors of Anatomic and Surgical Pathology. *Am J Clin Pathol* 2008;129:24–30.

517. Srigley JR, et al. Updated protocol for the examination of specimens from patients with carcinomas of the prostate gland: a basis for checklists. Cancer Committee. *Arch Pathol Lab Med* 2000;124:1034–1039.

518. May M, et al. Prognostic impact of lymphovascular invasion in radical prostatectomy specimens. *BJU Int* 2007;99:539–544.

519. Shariat SF, et al. Lymphovascular invasion is a pathological feature of biologically aggressive disease in patients treated with radical prostatectomy. *J Urol* 2004;171:1122–1127.

520. Herman CM, et al. Lymphovascular invasion as a predictor of disease progression in prostate cancer. *Am J Surg Pathol* 2000;24:859–863.

521. Yamamoto S, et al. Lymphovascular invasion is an independent predictor of prostate-specific antigen failure after radical prostatectomy in patients with pT3aN0 prostate cancer. *Int J Urol* 2008;15:895–899.

522. Roma AA, et al. Peritumoral lymphatic invasion is associated with regional lymph node metastases in prostate adenocarcinoma. *Mod Pathol* 2006;19:392–398.

523. Ito K, et al. Prognostic implication of microvascular invasion in biochemical failure in patients treated with radical prostatectomy. *Urol Int* 2003;70:297–302.

524. Boormans JL, et al. Histopathological characteristics of lymph node metastases predict cancer-specific survival in node-positive prostate cancer. *BJU Int* 2008;102:1589–1593.

525. Cheng L, et al. Extranodal extension in lymph node-positive prostate cancer. *Mod Pathol* 2000;13:113–118.

526. Rove KO, Crawford ED. Metastatic cancer in solid tumors and clinical outcome: skeletal-related events. *Oncology (Williston Park)* 2009;23(14 suppl 5):21–27.

527. Uemura H, et al. Usefulness of the 2005 International Society of Urologic Pathology Gleason grading system in prostate biopsy and radical prostatectomy specimens. *BJU Int* 2009;103:1190–1194.

528. Helpap B, Egevad L. Correlation of modified Gleason grading with pT stage of prostatic carcinoma after radical prostatectomy. *Anal Quant Cytol Histol* 2008;30:1–7.

529. Eggener SE, et al. Predicting 15-year prostate cancer specific mortality after radical prostatectomy. *J Urol* 2011;185:869–875.

530. Brimo F, et al. Contemporary grading for prostate cancer: implications for patient care. *Eur Urol* 2013;63:892–901.

531. Carter HB, et al. Gleason score 6 adenocarcinoma: should it be labeled as cancer? *J Clin Oncol* 2012;30:4294–4296.

532. Ross HM, et al. Do adenocarcinomas of the prostate with Gleason score (GS) ≤6 have the potential to metastasize to lymph nodes? *Am J Surg Pathol* 2012;36:1346–1352.

533. Partin AW, et al. Combination of prostate-specific antigen, clinical stage, and Gleason score to predict pathological stage of localized prostate cancer. A multi-institutional update. *JAMA* 1997;277:1445–1451.

534. Kattan MW, et al. Development and validation of preoperative nomogram for disease recurrence within 5 years after laparoscopic radical prostatectomy for prostate cancer. *Urology* 2011;77:396–401.

535. Brimo F, et al. Prognostic value of various morphometric measurements of tumour extent in prostate needle core tissue. *Histopathology* 2008;53:177–183.

536. Poulos CK, Daggy JK, Cheng L. Prostate needle biopsies: multiple variables are predictive of final tumor volume in radical prostatectomy specimens. *Cancer* 2004;101:527–532.

537. Quintal MM, et al. Various morphometric measurements of cancer extent on needle prostatic biopsies: which is predictive of pathologic stage and biochemical recurrence following radical prostatectomy? *Int Urol Nephrol* 2011;43:697–705.

538. Egevad L, Allsbrook WC Jr, Epstein JI. Current practice of diagnosis and reporting of prostate cancer on needle biopsy among genitourinary pathologists. *Hum Pathol* 2006;37:292–297.

539. Karram S, et al. Should intervening benign tissue be included in the measurement of discontinuous foci of cancer on prostate needle biopsy? Correlation with radical prostatectomy findings. *Am J Surg Pathol* 2011;35:1351–1355.

540. Fajardo DA, Epstein JI. Fragmentation of prostatic needle biopsy cores containing adenocarcinoma: the role of specimen submission. *BJU Int* 2010;105:172–175.

541. AJCC. *AJCC cancer staging manual.* 7th ed. Springer; 2010.

542. Magheli A, et al. Subclassification of clinical stage T1 prostate cancer: impact on biochemical recurrence following radical prostatectomy. *J Urol* 2007;178(4 Pt 1):1277–1280; discussion 1280–1281.

543. Capitanio U, et al. Radical prostatectomy for incidental (stage T1a-T1b) prostate cancer: analysis of predictors for residual disease and biochemical recurrence. *Eur Urol* 2008;54:118–125.

544. Humphrey PA, Vollmer RT. Intraglandular tumor extent and prognosis in prostatic carcinoma: application of a grid method to prostatectomy specimens. *Hum Pathol* 1990;21:799–804.

545. McNeal JE, et al. Patterns of progression in prostate cancer. *Lancet* 1986;1:60–63.

546. Epstein JI, Oesterling JE, Walsh PC. Tumor volume versus percentage of specimen involved by tumor correlated with progression in stage A prostatic cancer. *J Urol* 1988;139:980–984.

547. Partin AW, et al. Morphometric measurement of tumor volume and per cent of gland involvement as predictors of pathological stage in clinical stage B prostate cancer. *J Urol* 1989;141:341–345.

548. McNeal JE, et al. Stage A versus stage B adenocarcinoma of the prostate: morphological comparison and biological significance. *J Urol* 1988;139:61–65.

549. Stamey TA, et al. Biological determinants of cancer progression in men with prostate cancer. *JAMA* 1999;281:1395–1400.

550. Renshaw AA, et al. Maximum diameter of prostatic carcinoma is a simple, inexpensive, and independent predictor of prostate-specific antigen failure in radical prostatectomy specimens. Validation in a cohort of 434 patients. *Am J Clin Pathol* 1999;111:641–644.

551. Carvalhal GF, et al. Visual estimate of the percentage of carcinoma is an independent predictor of prostate carcinoma recurrence after radical prostatectomy. *Cancer* 2000;89:1308–1314.

552. Eichelberger LE, et al. Maximum tumor diameter is an independent predictor of prostate-specific antigen recurrence in prostate cancer. *Mod Pathol* 2005;18:886–890.

553. Dvorak T, et al. Maximal tumor diameter and the risk of PSA failure in men with specimen-confined prostate cancer. *Urology* 2005;66:1024–1028.

554. Epstein JI, et al. Is tumor volume an independent predictor of progression following radical prostatectomy? A multivariate analysis of 185 clinical stage B adenocarcinomas of the prostate with 5 years of follow-up. *J Urol* 1993;149:1478–1481.

555. Salomon L, et al. Prognostic significance of tumor volume after radical prostatectomy: a multivariate analysis of pathological prognostic factors. *Eur Urol* 2003;43:39–44.

556. Lerner SE, Blute ML, Zincke H. Risk factors for progression in patients with prostate cancer treated with radical prostatectomy. *Semin Urol Oncol* 1996;14(2 suppl 2):12–20; discussion 21.

557. van Oort IM, et al. Maximum tumor diameter is not an independent prognostic factor in high-risk localized prostate cancer. *World J Urol* 2008;26:237–241.

558. Kikuchi E, et al. Is tumor volume an independent prognostic factor in clinically localized prostate cancer? *J Urol* 2004;172:508–511.

559. Chen ME, et al. A streamlined three-dimensional volume estimation method accurately classifies prostate tumors by volume. *Am J Surg Pathol* 2003;27:1291–1301.

560. Renshaw AA, Chang H, D'Amico AV. Estimation of tumor volume in radical prostatectomy specimens in routine clinical practice. *Am J Clin Pathol* 1997;107:704–708.

561. Marks RA, et al. Positive-block ratio in radical prostatectomy specimens is an independent predictor of prostate-specific antigen recurrence. *Am J Surg Pathol* 2007;31:877–881.

562. Jones EC. Resection margin status in radical retropubic prostatectomy specimens: relationship to type of operation, tumor size, tumor grade and local tumor extension. *J Urol* 1990;144:89–93.

563. Billis A, et al. Prostate cancer with bladder neck involvement: pathologic findings with application of a new practical method for tumor extent evaluation and recurrence-free survival after radical prostatectomy. *Int Urol Nephrol* 2004;36:363–368.

564. Billis A, Magna LA, Ferreira U. Correlation between tumor extent in radical prostatectomies and preoperative PSA, histological grade, surgical margins, and extraprostatic extension: application of a new practical method for tumor extent evaluation. *Int Braz J Urol* 2003;29:113–119; discussion 120.

565. Eggener S, et al. Focal therapy for prostate cancer: possibilities and limitations. *Eur Urol* 2010;58:57–64.

566. Cheng L, et al. Staging of prostate cancer. *Histopathology* 2012;60:87–117.

567. Eichelberger LE, et al. Predicting tumor volume in radical prostatectomy specimens from patients with prostate cancer. *Am J Clin Pathol* 2003;120:386–391.

568. Srigley JR, et al. Updated protocol for the examination of specimens from patients with carcinomas of the prostate gland. *Arch Pathol Lab Med* 2006;130:936–946.

569. Srigley JR. Key issues in handling and reporting radical prostatectomy specimens. *Arch Pathol Lab Med* 2006;130:303–317.

570. Miller JS, et al. Extraprostatic extension of prostatic adenocarcinoma on needle core biopsy: report of 72 cases with clinical follow-up. *BJU Int* 2010;106:330–333.

571. Cheng L, et al. Correlation of margin status and extraprostatic extension with progression of prostate carcinoma. *Cancer* 1999;86:1775–1782.

572. Montironi R, et al. Pathological definition and difficulties in assessing positive margins in radical prostatectomy specimens. *BJU Int* 2009;103:286–288.

573. Eastham JA, et al. Prognostic significance of location of positive margins in radical prostatectomy specimens. *Urology* 2007;70:965–969.

574. Obek C, et al. Positive surgical margins with radical retropubic prostatectomy: anatomic site-specific pathologic analysis and impact on prognosis. *Urology* 1999;54:682–688.

575. Salomon L, et al. Location of positive surgical margins after retropubic, perineal, and laparoscopic radical prostatectomy for organ-confined prostate cancer. *Urology* 2003;61:386–390.

576. Sofer M, et al. Positive surgical margins after radical retropubic prostatectomy: the influence of site and number on progression. *J Urol* 2002;167:2453–2456.

577. Watson RB, Civantos F, Soloway MS. Positive surgical margins with radical prostatectomy: detailed pathological analysis and prognosis. *Urology* 1996;48:80–90.

578. Shikanov S, et al. Length of positive surgical margin after radical prostatectomy as a predictor of biochemical recurrence. *J Urol* 2009;182:139–144.

579. Saether T, et al. Are positive surgical margins in radical prostatectomy specimens an independent prognostic marker? *Scand J Urol Nephrol* 2008;42:514–521.

580. Epstein JI, Sauvageot J. Do close but negative margins in radical prostatectomy specimens increase the risk of postoperative progression? *J Urol* 1997;157:241–243.

581. Epstein JI. Evaluation of radical prostatectomy capsular margins of resection. The significance of margins designated as negative, closely approaching, and positive. *Am J Surg Pathol* 1990;14:626–632.

582. Weldon VE, et al. Patterns of positive specimen margins and detectable prostate specific antigen after radical perineal prostatectomy. *J Urol* 1995;153:1565–1569.

583. Stephenson AJ, et al. Location, extent and number of positive surgical margins do not improve accuracy of predicting prostate cancer recurrence after radical prostatectomy. *J Urol* 2009;182:1357–1363.

584. Chuang AY, et al. The significance of positive surgical margin in areas of capsular incision in otherwise organ confined disease at radical prostatectomy. *J Urol* 2007;178(4 Pt 1):1306–1310.

585. Shuford MD, et al. Adverse prognostic significance of capsular incision with radical retropubic prostatectomy. *J Urol* 2004;172:119–123.

586. Smith JA Jr, et al. A comparison of the incidence and location of positive surgical margins in robotic assisted laparoscopic radical prostatectomy and open retropubic radical prostatectomy. *J Urol* 2007;178:2385–2389; discussion 2389–2390.

587. Cao D, et al. The Gleason score of tumor at the margin in radical prostatectomy is predictive of biochemical recurrence. *Am J Surg Pathol* 2010;34:994–1001.

588. Fromont G, et al. Biological significance of perineural invasion (PNI) in prostate cancer. *Prostate* 2012;72:542–548.

589. Villers A, et al. The role of perineural space invasion in the local spread of prostatic adenocarcinoma. *J Urol* 1989;142:763–768.

590. Cannon GM Jr, et al. Perineural invasion in prostate cancer biopsies is not associated with higher rates of positive surgical margins. *Prostate* 2005;63:336–340.

591. O'Malley KJ, et al. Influence of biopsy perineural invasion on long-term biochemical disease-free survival after radical prostatectomy. *Urology* 2002;59:85–90.

592. Loeb S, et al. Does perineural invasion on prostate biopsy predict adverse prostatectomy outcomes? *BJU Int* 2010;105:1510–1513.

593. Egan AJ, Bostwick DG. Prediction of extraprostatic extension of prostate cancer based on needle biopsy findings: perineural invasion lacks significance on multivariate analysis. *Am J Surg Pathol* 1997;21:1496–1500.

594. Katz B, et al. Perineural invasion detection in prostate biopsy is related to recurrence-free survival in patients submitted to radical prostatectomy. *Urol Oncol* 2013;31:175–179.

595. de la Taille A, et al. Perineural invasion on prostate needle biopsy: an independent predictor of final pathologic stage. *Urology* 1999;54:1039–1043.

596. de la Taille A, et al. Can perineural invasion on prostate needle biopsy predict prostate specific antigen recurrence after radical prostatectomy? *J Urol* 1999;162:103–106.

597. Bastacky SI, Walsh PC, Epstein JI. Relationship between perineural tumor invasion on needle biopsy and radical prostatectomy capsular penetration in clinical stage B adenocarcinoma of the prostate. *Am J Surg Pathol* 1993;17:336–341.

598. Elharram M, et al. Perineural invasion on prostate biopsy does not predict adverse pathological outcome. *Can J Urol* 2012;19:6567–6572.

599. Delancey JO, et al. Evidence of perineural invasion on prostate biopsy specimen and survival after radical prostatectomy. *Urology* 2013;81:354–357.

600. Beard C, et al. Perineural invasion associated with increased cancer-specific mortality after external beam radiation therapy for men with low- and intermediate-risk prostate cancer. *Int J Radiat Oncol Biol Phys* 2006;66:403–407.

601. Beard CJ, et al. Perineural invasion is associated with increased relapse after external beam radiotherapy for men with low-risk prostate cancer and may be a marker for occult, high-grade cancer. *Int J Radiat Oncol Biol Phys* 2004;58:19–24.

602. Baydar DE, et al. Prognostic significance of lymphovascular invasion in clinically localized prostate cancer after radical prostatectomy. *ScientificWorldJournal* 2008;8:303–312.

603. Cheng L, et al. Lymphovascular invasion is an independent prognostic factor in prostatic adenocarcinoma. *J Urol* 2005;174:2181–2185.

604. Loeb S, et al. Lymphovascular invasion in radical prostatectomy specimens: prediction of adverse pathologic features and biochemical progression. *Urology* 2006;68:99–103.

605. McNeal JE, Yemoto CE. Significance of demonstrable vascular space invasion for the progression of prostatic adenocarcinoma. *Am J Surg Pathol* 1996;20:1351–1360.

606. Salomao DR, Graham SD, Bostwick DG. Microvascular invasion in prostate cancer correlates with pathologic stage. *Arch Pathol Lab Med* 1995;119:1050–1054.

607. van den Ouden D, et al. Microvascular invasion in prostate cancer: prognostic significance in patients treated by radical prostatectomy for clinically localized carcinoma. *Urol Int* 1998;60:17–24.

608. Kryvenko ON, Epstein JI. Histologic criteria and pitfalls in the diagnosis of lymphovascular invasion in radical prostatectomy specimens. *Am J Surg Pathol* 2012;36:1865–1873.

609. Bahnson RR, et al. Incidence and prognostic significance of lymphatic and vascular invasion in radical prostatectomy specimens. *Prostate* 1989;15:149–155.

610. de la Taille A, et al. Is microvascular invasion on radical prostatectomy specimens a useful predictor of PSA recurrence for prostate cancer patients? *Eur Urol* 2000;38:79–84.

611. Potter SR, Epstein JI, Partin AW. Seminal vesicle invasion by prostate cancer: prognostic significance and therapeutic implications. *Rev Urol* 2000;2:190–195.

612. Poulos CK, et al. Bladder neck invasion is an independent predictor of prostate-specific antigen recurrence. *Cancer* 2004;101:1563–1568.

613. Yossepowitch O, et al. Bladder neck involvement at radical prostatectomy: positive margins or advanced T4 disease? *Urology* 2000;56:448–452.

614. Yossepowitch O, et al. Bladder neck involvement in pathological stage pT4 radical prostatectomy specimens is not an independent prognostic factor. *J Urol* 2002;168:2011–2015.

615. Buschemeyer WC III, et al. Is a positive bladder neck margin truly a T4 lesion in the prostate specific antigen era? Results from the SEARCH Database. *J Urol* 2008;179:124–129; discussion 129.

616. Dash A, et al. Prostate cancer involving the bladder neck: recurrence-free survival and implications for AJCC staging modification. American Joint Committee on Cancer. *Urology* 2002;60:276–280.

617. Pierorazio PM, et al. The significance of a positive bladder neck margin after radical prostatectomy: the American Joint Committee on Cancer Pathological Stage T4 designation is not warranted. *J Urol* 2010;183:151–157.

618. Laurila M, et al. Detection rates of cancer, high grade PIN and atypical lesions suspicious for cancer in the European Randomized Study of Screening for Prostate Cancer. *Eur J Cancer* 2010;46:3068–3072.

619. Herawi M, et al. Risk of prostate cancer on first rebiopsy within 1 year following a diagnosis of high grade prostatic intraepithelial neoplasia is related to the number of cores sampled. *J Urol* 2006;175:121–124.

620. Egevad L, Allsbrook WC, Epstein JI. Current practice of diagnosis and reporting of prostatic intraepithelial neoplasia and glandular atypia among genitourinary pathologists. *Mod Pathol* 2006;19:180–185.

621. Moore CK, et al. Prognostic significance of high grade prostatic intraepithelial neoplasia and atypical small acinar proliferation in the contemporary era. *J Urol* 2005;173:70–72.

622. Scattoni V, et al. Predictors of prostate cancer after initial diagnosis of atypical small acinar proliferation at 10 to 12 core biopsies. *Urology* 2005;66:1043–1047.

623. Alsikafi NF, et al. High-grade prostatic intraepithelial neoplasia with adjacent atypia is associated with a higher incidence of cancer on subsequent needle biopsy than high-grade prostatic intraepithelial neoplasia alone. *Urology* 2001;57:296–300.

624. Sardana G, Dowell B, Diamandis EP. Emerging biomarkers for the diagnosis and prognosis of prostate cancer. *Clin Chem* 2008;54:1951–1960.

625. Nogueira L, Corradi R, Eastham JA. Other biomarkers for detecting prostate cancer. *BJU Int* 2010;105:166–169.

626. Shappell SB. Clinical utility of prostate carcinoma molecular diagnostic tests. *Rev Urol* 2008;10:44–69.

627. Parekh DJ, et al. Biomarkers for prostate cancer detection. *J Urol* 2007;178:2252–2259.

628. Srigley JR, et al. Prognostic and predictive factors in prostate cancer: historical perspectives and recent international consensus initiatives. *Scand J Urol Nephrol Suppl* 2005;8–19.

629. Amin M, et al. Prognostic and predictive factors and reporting of prostate carcinoma in prostate needle biopsy specimens. *Scand J Urol Nephrol Suppl* 2005;20–33.

630. Kristiansen G. Diagnostic and prognostic molecular biomarkers for prostate cancer. *Histopathology* 2012;60:125–141.

631. Rubin MA, et al. Decreased alpha-methylacyl CoA racemase expression in localized prostate cancer is associated with an increased rate of biochemical recurrence and cancer-specific death. *Cancer Epidemiol Biomarkers Prev* 2005;14:1424–1432.

632. Kollermann J, et al. Expression and prognostic relevance of annexin A3 in prostate cancer. *Eur Urol* 2008;54:1314–1323.

633. Bjartell AS, et al. Association of cysteine-rich secretory protein 3 and beta-microseminoprotein with outcome after radical prostatectomy. *Clin Cancer Res* 2007;13:4130–4138.

634. Bjartell A, et al. Immunohistochemical detection of cysteine-rich secretory protein 3 in tissue and in serum from men with cancer or benign enlargement of the prostate gland. *Prostate* 2006;66:591–603.

635. Umbas R, et al. Decreased E-cadherin expression is associated with poor prognosis in patients with prostate cancer. *Cancer Res* 1994;54:3929–3933.

636. Umbas R, et al. Expression of the cellular adhesion molecule E-cadherin is reduced or absent in high-grade prostate cancer. *Cancer Res* 1992;52:5104–5109.

637. De Marzo AM, et al. E-cadherin expression as a marker of tumor aggressiveness in routinely processed radical prostatectomy specimens. *Urology* 1999;53:707–713.

638. Rubin MA, et al. E-cadherin expression in prostate cancer: a broad survey using high-density tissue microarray technology. *Hum Pathol* 2001;32:690–697.

639. Zhigang Z, Wenlu S. External beam radiotherapy (EBRT) suppressed prostate stem cell antigen (PSCA) mRNA expression in clinically localized prostate cancer. *Prostate* 2007;67:653–660.

640. Zhigang Z, Wenlu S. Complete androgen ablation suppresses prostate stem cell antigen (PSCA) mRNA expression in human prostate carcinoma. *Prostate* 2005;65:299–305.

641. Gu Z, et al. Anti-prostate stem cell antigen monoclonal antibody 1G8 induces cell death in vitro and inhibits tumor growth in vivo via a Fc-independent mechanism. *Cancer Res* 2005;65:9495–9500.

642. Gu Z, et al. Prostate stem cell antigen (PSCA) expression increases with high Gleason score, advanced stage and bone metastasis in prostate cancer. *Oncogene* 2000;19:1288–1296.

643. Shariat SF, et al. Tissue expression of transforming growth factor-beta1 and its receptors: correlation with pathologic features and biochemical progression in patients undergoing radical prostatectomy. *Urology* 2004;63:1191–1197.

644. Shariat SF, et al. Early postoperative plasma transforming factor-beta1 is a strong predictor of biochemical progression after radical prostatectomy. *J Urol* 2008;179:1593–1597.

645. Varambally S, et al. The polycomb group protein EZH2 is involved in progression of prostate cancer. *Nature* 2002;419:624–629.

646. Rhodes DR, et al. Multiplex biomarker approach for determining risk of prostate-specific antigen-defined recurrence of prostate cancer. *J Natl Cancer Inst* 2003;95:661–668.

647. Epstein JI, et al. Recommendations for the reporting of prostate carcinoma. *Hum Pathol* 2007;38:1305–1309.

648. Amin MB, et al. Recommendations for the reporting of resected prostate carcinomas. Association of Directors of Anatomic and Surgical Pathology. *Am J Clin Pathol* 1996;105:667–670.

649. Pathologists, R.C.o. Datasets and tissue pathways. 2009; Available from: http://www.rcpath.org/publications-media/publications/datasets

650. Australasia, R.C.o.P.o. Structured pathology reporting of cancer protocols. 2010; Available from: http://www.rcpa.edu.au/Publications/StructuredReporting/cancerprotocols.htm

651. Kench JG, et al. Dataset for reporting of prostate carcinoma in radical prostatectomy specimens: recommendations from the International Collaboration on Cancer Reporting. *Histopathology* 2013;62:203–218.

652. Samaratunga H, et al. International Society of Urological Pathology (ISUP) Consensus Conference on Handling and Staging of Radical Prostatectomy Specimens. Working group 1: specimen handling. *Mod Pathol* 2011;24:6–15.

653. Egevad L, et al. Handling and reporting of radical prostatectomy specimens in Europe: a web-based survey by the European Network of Uropathology (ENUP). *Histopathology* 2008;53:333–339.

654. Egevad L. Handling of radical prostatectomy specimens. *Histopathology* 2012;60:118–124.

655. Fine SW, et al. A contemporary update on pathology reporting for prostate cancer: biopsy and radical prostatectomy specimens. *Eur Urol* 2012;62:20–39.

656. Shariat SF, Roehrborn CG. Using biopsy to detect prostate cancer. *Rev Urol* 2008;10:262–280.

657. Scattoni V, et al. Extended and saturation prostatic biopsy in the diagnosis and characterisation of prostate cancer: a critical analysis of the literature. *Eur Urol* 2007;52:1309–1322.

658. Eichler K, et al. Diagnostic value of systematic biopsy methods in the investigation of prostate cancer: a systematic review. *J Urol* 2006;175:1605–1612.

659. Srodon M, Epstein JI. Central zone histology of the prostate: a mimicker of high-grade prostatic intraepithelial neoplasia. *Hum Pathol* 2002;33:518–523.

660. Marberger M, et al. Biopsy misidentification identified by DNA profiling in a large multicenter trial. *J Clin Oncol* 2011;29:1744–1749.

661. Zigeuner RE, et al. Did the rate of incidental prostate cancer change in the era of PSA testing? A retrospective study of 1127 patients. *Urology* 2003;62:451–455.

662. McVary KT, et al. Update on AUA guideline on the management of benign prostatic hyperplasia. *J Urol* 2011;185:1793–1803.

663. Montironi R, et al. Editorial comment to when should we expect no residual tumor (pT0) once we submit incidental T1a-b prostate cancers to radical prostatectomy? *Int J Urol* 2011;18:153–154.

664. Melchior S, et al. Outcome of radical prostatectomy for incidental carcinoma of the prostate. *BJU Int* 2009;103:1478–1481.

665. Capitanio U, et al. When should we expect no residual tumor (pT0) once we submit incidental T1a-b prostate cancers to radical prostatectomy? *Int J Urol* 2011;18:148–153.

666. Rajab R, et al. An improved prognostic model for stage T1a and T1b prostate cancer by assessments of cancer extent. *Mod Pathol* 2011;24:58–63.

667. Walton TJ, et al. Obtaining fresh prostate cancer tissue for research: a novel biopsy needle and sampling technique for radical prostatectomy specimens. *Prostate* 2005;64:382–386.

668. Huang CY, et al. Molecular alterations in prostate carcinomas that associate with in vivo exposure to chemotherapy: identification of a cytoprotective mechanism involving growth differentiation factor 15. *Clin Cancer Res* 2007;13:5825–5833.

669. True L, et al. A molecular correlate to the Gleason grading system for prostate adenocarcinoma. *Proc Natl Acad Sci U S A* 2006;103:10991–10996.

670. Srinivasan M, Sedmak D, Jewell S. Effect of fixatives and tissue processing on the content and integrity of nucleic acids. *Am J Pathol* 2002;161:1961–1971.

671. Dunn TA, et al. Genome-wide expression analysis of recently processed formalin-fixed paraffin embedded human prostate tissues. *Prostate* 2009;69:214–218.

672. Ruijter ET, et al. Rapid microwave-stimulated fixation of entire prostatectomy specimens. Biomed-II MPC Study Group. *J Pathol* 1997;183:369–375.

673. Jonmarker S, et al. Tissue shrinkage after fixation with formalin injection of prostatectomy specimens. *Virchows Arch* 2006;449:297–301.

674. Hollenbeck BK, et al. Whole mounted radical prostatectomy specimens do not increase detection of adverse pathological features. *J Urol* 2000;164:1583–1586.

675. Cohen MB, Soloway MS, Murphy WM. Sampling of radical prostatectomy specimens. How much is adequate? *Am J Clin Pathol* 1994;101:250–252.

676. Sehdev AE, Pan CC, Epstein JI. Comparative analysis of sampling methods for grossing radical prostatectomy specimens performed for nonpalpable (stage T1c) prostatic adenocarcinoma. *Hum Pathol* 2001;32:494–499.

677. Montironi R, et al. Handling of radical prostatectomy specimens: total embedding with large-format histology. *Int J Breast Cancer* 2012;2012:932784.

678. Petraki CD, Sfikas CP. Histopathological changes induced by therapies in the benign prostate and prostate adenocarcinoma. *Histol Histopathol* 2007;22:107–118.

679. Evans AJ, Ryan P, Van derKwast T. Treatment effects in the prostate including those associated with traditional and emerging therapies. *Adv Anat Pathol* 2011;18:281–293.

680. Srigley JR, Delahunt B, Evans AJ. Therapy-associated effects in the prostate gland. *Histopathology* 2012;60:153–165.

681. Gomella LG, Zeltser I, Valicenti RK. Use of neoadjuvant and adjuvant therapy to prevent or delay recurrence of prostate cancer in patients undergoing surgical treatment for prostate cancer. *Urology* 2003;62(suppl 1):46–54.

682. Kitagawa Y, et al. Pathological effects of neoadjuvant hormonal therapy help predict progression of prostate cancer after radical prostatectomy. *Int J Urol* 2003;10:377–382.

683. Montironi R, Schulman CC. Pathological changes in prostate lesions after androgen manipulation. *J Clin Pathol* 1998;51:5–12.

684. Magi-Galluzzi C, Sanderson H, Epstein JI. Atypia in nonneoplastic prostate glands after radiotherapy for prostate cancer: duration of atypia and relation to type of radiotherapy. *Am J Surg Pathol* 2003;27:206–212.

685. Marberger M, et al. New treatments for localized prostate cancer. *Urology* 2008;72(6 suppl):S36–S43.

686. Lindner U, Trachtenberg J, Lawrentschuk N. Focal therapy in prostate cancer: modalities, findings and future considerations. *Nat Rev Urol* 2010;7:562–571.

687. Garzotto M. Combined androgen deprivation with radiotherapy for prostate cancer: does it make sense? *Mol Urol* 2000;4:209–213; discussion 215.

688. Pollack A, et al. Prostate biopsy status and PSA nadir level as early surrogates for treatment failure: analysis of a prostate cancer randomized radiation dose escalation trial. *Int J Radiat Oncol Biol Phys* 2002;54:677–685.

689. Vance W, et al. The predictive value of 2-year posttreatment biopsy after prostate cancer radiotherapy for eventual biochemical outcome. *Int J Radiat Oncol Biol Phys* 2007;67:828–833.

690. Crook J, et al. Postradiotherapy prostate biopsies: what do they really mean? Results for 498 patients. *Int J Radiat Oncol Biol Phys* 2000;48:355–367.

691. Crook JM, et al. Twenty-four-month postradiation prostate biopsies are strongly predictive of 7-year disease-free survival: results from a Canadian randomized trial. *Cancer* 2009;115:673–679.

692. Scardino PT, et al. The prognostic significance of post-irradiation biopsy results in patients with prostatic cancer. *J Urol* 1986;135:510–516.

693. Crook J. Radiotherapy for prostate cancer: how do we define success? *Can J Urol* 1997;4(2 suppl 1):48–53.

694. Miller EB, et al. Reevaluation of prostate biopsy after definitive radiation therapy. *Urology* 1993;41:311–316.

695. Magi-Galluzzi C. Radiation-induced changes. In: Zhou M, Netto GJ, Epstein JI, eds. *Uropathology: High-Yield Pathology.* Philadelphia, PA: Elsevier Saunders; 2012:104–106.

696. Gaudin PB, et al. Histopathologic effects of three-dimensional conformal external beam radiation therapy on benign and malignant prostate tissues. *Am J Surg Pathol* 1999;23:1021–1031.

697. Cheng L, Cheville JC, Bostwick DG. Diagnosis of prostate cancer in needle biopsies after radiation therapy. *Am J Surg Pathol* 1999;23:1173–1183.

698. Cheng L, et al. Prevalence and distribution of prostatic intraepithelial neoplasia in salvage radical prostatectomy specimens after radiation therapy. *Am J Surg Pathol* 1999;23:803–808.

699. Zelefsky MJ, et al. Dose escalation with three-dimensional conformal radiation therapy affects the outcome in prostate cancer. *Int J Radiat Oncol Biol Phys* 1998;41:491–500.

700. Cheng L, et al. Predictors of survival for prostate carcinoma patients treated with salvage radical prostatectomy after radiation therapy. *Cancer* 1998;83:2164–2171.

701. Ljung G, et al. Characterization of residual tumor cells following radical radiation therapy for prostatic adenocarcinoma; immunohistochemical expression of prostate-specific antigen, prostatic acid phosphatase, and cytokeratin 8. *Prostate* 1997;31:91–97.

702. Têtu B. Morphological changes induced by androgen blockade in normal prostate and prostatic carcinoma. *Best Pract Res Clin Endocrinol Metab* 2008;22:271–283.

703. Magi-Galluzzi C. Hormonal ablation-induced changes. In: Zhou M, Netto GJ, Epstein JI, eds. *Uropathology: High-Yield Pathology.* Philadelphia, PA: Elsevier Saunders; 2012:107–109.

704. Têtu B, et al. Effect of combination endocrine therapy (LHRH agonist and flutamide) on normal prostate and prostatic adenocarcinoma. A histopathologic and immunohistochemical study. *Am J Surg Pathol* 1991;15:111–120.

705. Montironi R, et al. Androgen-deprived prostate adenocarcinoma: evaluation of treatment-related changes versus no distinctive treatment effect with a Bayesian belief network. A methodological approach. *Eur Urol* 1996;30:307–315.

706. Marks LS, et al. Long-term effects of finasteride on prostate tissue composition. *Urology* 1999;53:574–580.

707. Vailancourt L, et al. Effect of neoadjuvant endocrine therapy (combined androgen blockade) on normal prostate and prostatic carcinoma. A randomized study. *Am J Surg Pathol* 1996;20:86–93.

708. van der Kwast TH, Labrie F, Tetu B. Persistence of high-grade prostatic intra-epithelial neoplasia under combined androgen blockade therapy. *Hum Pathol* 1999;30:1503–1507.

709. Bullock MJ, et al. Pathologic effects of neoadjuvant cyproterone acetate on nonneoplastic prostate, prostatic intraepithelial neoplasia, and adenocarcinoma: a detailed analysis of radical prostatectomy specimens from a randomized trial. *Am J Surg Pathol* 2002;26:1400–1413.

710. Civantos F, Soloway MS, Pinto JE. Histopathological effects of androgen deprivation in prostatic cancer. *Semin Urol Oncol* 1996;14(2 suppl 2):22–31.

711. Civantos F, et al. Pathology of androgen deprivation therapy in prostate carcinoma. A comparative study of 173 patients. *Cancer* 1995;75:1634–1641.

712. Tran TA, et al. Pseudomyxoma ovariilike posttherapeutic alteration in prostatic adenocarcinoma: a distinctive pattern in patients receiving neoadjuvant androgen ablation therapy. *Am J Surg Pathol* 1998;22:347–354.

713. Efstathiou E, et al. Morphologic characterization of preoperatively treated prostate cancer: toward a post-therapy histologic classification. *Eur Urol* 2010;57:1030–1038.

714. Witjes WP, Schulman CC, Debruyne FM. Preliminary results of a prospective randomized study comparing radical prostatectomy versus radical prostatectomy associated with neoadjuvant hormonal combination therapy in T2–3 N0 M0 prostatic carcinoma. The European Study Group on Neoadjuvant Treatment of Prostate Cancer. *Urology* 1997;49(3A suppl):65–69.

715. Gleave ME, et al. Biochemical and pathological effects of 8 months of neoadjuvant androgen withdrawal therapy before radical prostatectomy in patients with clinically confined prostate cancer. *J Urol* 1996;155:213–219.

716. Maldonado-Valadez R, et al. The impact of neoadjuvant hormonal therapy on the outcome of laparoscopic radical prostatectomy: a matched pair analysis. *J Urol* 2006;175:2092–2096.

717. Lukka H, et al. Maximal androgen blockade for the treatment of metastatic prostate cancer–a systematic review. *Curr Oncol* 2006;13:81–93.

718. Paterson RF, et al. Immunohistochemical analysis of radical prostatectomy specimens after 8 months of neoadjuvant hormonal therapy. *Mol Urol* 1999;3:277–286.

719. Van de Voorde WM, et al. Morphologic and immunohistochemical changes in prostate cancer after preoperative hormonal therapy. A comparative study of radical prostatectomies. *Cancer* 1994;74:3164–3175.

720. Magi-Galluzzi C. Cryoablation therapy-induced changes. In: Zhou M, Netto GJ, Epstein JI, eds. *Uropathology: High-yield pathology*. Philadelphia, PA: Elsevier Saunders; 2012:110–112.

721. Hou AH, Sullivan KF, Crawford ED. Targeted focal therapy for prostate cancer: a review. *Curr Opin Urol* 2009;19:283–289.

722. Uchida T, et al. Transrectal high-intensity focused ultrasound for treatment of patients with stage T1b-2n0m0 localized prostate cancer: a preliminary report. *Urology* 2002;59:394–398; discussion 398–399.

723. ter Haar G. [Biological effects of hyperthermia and their significance for Doppler ultrasound]. *Ultraschall Med* 1994;15:48–49.

724. Fry FJ. Intense focused ultrasound in medicine. Some practical guiding physical principles from sound source to focal site in tissue. *Eur Urol* 1993;23 (suppl 1):2–7.

725. Rove KO, Flaig TW. A renaissance in the medical treatment of advanced prostate cancer. *Oncology (Williston Park)* 2010;24:1308–1313, 1318.

726. Warwick R, Pond J. Trackless lesions in nervous tissues produced by high intensity focused ultrasound (high-frequency mechanical waves). *J Anat* 1968;102(Pt 3):387–405.

727. Uchida T, et al. Treatment of localized prostate cancer using high-intensity focused ultrasound. *BJU Int* 2006;97:56–61.

728. Rove KO, Sullivan KF, Crawford ED. High-intensity focused ultrasound: ready for primetime. *Urol Clin North Am* 2010;37:27–35, Table of Contents.

729. Susani M, et al. Morphology of tissue destruction induced by focused ultrasound. *Eur Urol* 1993;23(suppl 1):34–38.

730. Madersbacher S, et al. Tissue ablation in benign prostatic hyperplasia with high intensity focused ultrasound. *J Urol* 1994;152(6 Pt 1):1956–1960; discussion 1960–1961.

731. Madersbacher S, et al. Effect of high-intensity focused ultrasound on human prostate cancer in vivo. *Cancer Res* 1995;55:3346–3351.

732. Biermann K, et al. Histopathological findings after treatment of prostate cancer using high-intensity focused ultrasound (HIFU). *Prostate* 2010;70:1196–1200.

733. Moore CM, Pendse D, Emberton M. Photodynamic therapy for prostate cancer–a review of current status and future promise. *Nat Clin Pract Urol* 2009;6:18–30.

734. Polascik TJ, Mouraviev V. Focal therapy for prostate cancer. *Curr Opin Urol* 2008;18:269–274.

735. Huidobro C, et al. Evaluation of microwave thermotherapy with histopathology, magnetic resonance imaging and temperature mapping. *J Urol* 2004;171(2 Pt 1):672–678.

736. Sherar MD, et al. Interstitial microwave thermal therapy for prostate cancer. *J Endourol* 2003;17:617–625.

737. Trachtenberg J, et al. Vascular-targeted photodynamic therapy (padoporfin, WST09) for recurrent prostate cancer after failure of external beam radiotherapy: a study of escalating light doses. *BJU Int* 2008;102:556–562.

738. Tannock IF, et al. Chemotherapy with mitoxantrone plus prednisone or prednisone alone for symptomatic hormone-resistant prostate cancer: a Canadian randomized trial with palliative end points. *J Clin Oncol* 1996;14:1756–1764.

739. Ranganathan S, et al. Altered beta-tubulin isotype expression in paclitaxel-resistant human prostate carcinoma cells. *Br J Cancer* 1998;77:562–566.

740. Laing N, et al. Interaction of estramustine with tubulin isotypes. *Biochemistry* 1997;36:871–878.

741. Obasaju C, Hudes GR. Paclitaxel and docetaxel in prostate cancer. *Hematol Oncol Clin North Am* 2001;15:525–545.

742. Schulman CC, et al. 4-Year follow-up results of a European prospective randomized study on neoadjuvant hormonal therapy prior to radical prostatectomy in T2-3N0M0 prostate cancer. European Study Group on Neoadjuvant Treatment of Prostate Cancer. *Eur Urol* 2000;38:706–713.

743. Aus G, et al. Three-month neoadjuvant hormonal therapy before radical prostatectomy: a 7-year follow-up of a randomized controlled trial. *BJU Int* 2002;90:561–566.

744. Magi-Galluzzi C, et al. Neoadjuvant docetaxel treatment for locally advanced prostate cancer: a clinicopathologic study. *Cancer* 2007;110:1248–1254.

745. O'Brien C, et al. Histologic changes associated with neoadjuvant chemotherapy are predictive of nodal metastases in patients with high-risk prostate cancer. *Am J Clin Pathol* 2010;133:654–661.

746. Stanford JL, Stephenson RA, Coyle LM, et al. *Prostate Cancer Trends 1973–1995*, SEER Program, National Cancer Institute NIH Pub. No. 99-4543, Bethesda, MD, 1999.

747. Kao J, et al. Individual prostate biopsy core embedding facilitates maximal tissue representation. *J Urol* 2002;168:496–499.

Other Tumors of the Prostate Gland and Tumors of the Seminal Vesicle

JONATHAN I. EPSTEIN and FADI BRIMO

OTHER TUMORS OF THE PROSTATE GLAND

Adenosquamous and Squamous Cell Carcinoma

Clinical Features

These are very rare tumors with approximately 55 cases of pure squamous cell and 30 cases of adenosquamous cell carcinoma reported. Risk factors include prior radiation or hormonal therapy, previous history of prostate cancer, and rarely genitourinary schistosomiasis. However, de novo cases without prior history of cancer have been reported. The mean age of diagnosis is 64 years. Patients usually present with obstructive symptoms and sometimes hematuria. While increased prostate-specific antigen (PSA) and acid phosphatase levels is seen more commonly with adenosquamous in comparison to pure squamous cell carcinomas, normal levels are not uncommonly present even with advanced disease.[1]

Pathology

Pure squamous cell carcinoma of the prostate is indistinguishable from squamous carcinoma at other sites. Adenosquamous carcinoma may show an intimate mixture of prostatic acinar adenocarcinoma and squamous cell carcinoma (Fig. 10-1). Alternatively, the two components may be more anatomically distinct with squamous cell carcinoma seen in one area of the specimen and acinar adenocarcinoma in another. The extent of adenocarcinoma varies from 5% to 95% and tends usually to be higher grade tumors with a Gleason score of 7 or higher. The degree of differentiation within the squamous component can also range from well to more poorly differentiated.[1]

Differential Diagnosis

Primary prostatic squamous cell carcinomas must be distinguished on clinical grounds from secondary involvement of the gland by bladder, urethral, or anal pure squamous cell carcinomas. Histologic distinction between those entities is extremely difficult and generally requires clinicopathologic correlation. A more common scenario is secondary invasion by a urothelial carcinoma with squamous differentiation, and in that regard, features that are most consistent with secondary urothelial carcinoma with squamous differentiation rather than a prostatic primary tumor include (1) the presence of a component of usual-type invasive urothelial carcinoma, (2) associated glandular (nonprostatic-type) differentiation, (3) associated urothelial carcinoma in situ or urothelial papillary tumor in the bladder lining. Also, squamous cell carcinoma of the prostate must be differentiated from squamous metaplasia adjacent to a prostatic infarct. In transurethral resections and enucleations, the localized lobular nature of infarcts with the organization from central necrosis and reactive urothelial/squamous islands at the periphery is diagnostic. On needle biopsy, the overall architecture cannot be as easily appreciated. Although the squamous/urothelial nests in an infarct usually lack cytologic atypia, prominent atypia and increased mitotic activity may occasionally be seen. The recognition of adjacent infarcted tissue or the presence of stromal hemorrhage and hemosiderin deposition in the areas adjacent to the infarct is helpful in arriving at the correct diagnosis.

Lastly, squamous changes in benign prostatic tissue following hormonal therapy can be distinguished from carcinoma due to the bland cytological characteristics and the absence of invasive features.

At the immunohistochemical level, while cells in the squamous cell carcinoma component are usually totally negative for prostatic markers (prostate-specific acid phosphatase [PSAP], PSA, prostate-specific membrane antigen [PSMA], prostein) and positive for p63, HMWK, CK5/6, CK14, the glandular component of the adenosquamous cell carcinoma show the opposite pattern of staining.[1]

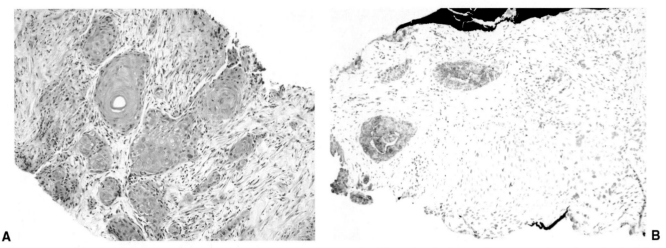

FIGURE 10-1 ■ **A:** Adenosquamous carcinoma of the prostate. Poorly differentiated adenocarcinoma component is at the far left. **B:** Adenosquamous carcinoma of the prostate with PSA staining of adenocarcinoma yet negative immunoreactivity in squamous carcinoma component (*center bottom*).

Prognosis and Treatment

Primary prostatic squamous cell carcinomas have a poor prognosis, with poor response to hormonal therapy, radiation therapy, and chemotherapy. Radical prostatectomy constitutes the only chance of cure, although the majority of cases present with advanced disease.[2] Metastases occur in a third of cases, most commonly to bone and lung. Squamous cell carcinomas develop osteolytic rather than osteoblastic metastases and do not respond to antiandrogen therapy.

Sarcomatoid Carcinoma

Introduction

Some authors restrict the term "carcinosarcoma" for tumors with carcinoma and specific mesenchymal differentiation (i.e., cartilage or osteoid), and designate tumors with only an associated nonspecific malignant spindle cell pattern as "sarcomatoid carcinoma." Given the similar prognosis between these two morphologies and the finding of epithelial differentiation by immunohistochemistry or electron microscopy in the spindle component of some "carcinosarcomas," it is preferable to consider these lesions as one entity.[3]

Clinical Features

Sarcomatoid carcinomas of the prostate are rare with only approximately 100 cases and few reported series.[4–7] Prior history of prostatic adenocarcinoma is present in about half of cases in whom the sarcomatous component develops at a mean of 7 years later (range = 6 months to 16 years). Radiotherapy and/or hormonal therapy are thought to play a role in the development of sarcomatoid carcinoma as some patients have received these treatment modalities prior to the growth of the sarcomatoid component. This being said, sarcomatoid carcinoma may also arise de novo without prior history of adenocarcinoma or previous treatment. Mean age

at diagnosis is 70 years, and the majority of patients present with obstructive urinary symptoms or metastatic disease rather than by being detected by needle biopsy following an increase in serum PSA levels or abnormal digital rectal examination. PSA serum levels may be normal or elevated.

Pathology

Gross findings are often not appreciable as the specimens are typically needle biopsies or transurethral resections. However, tumors removed by radical prostatectomy may resemble sarcomas and present as large white to yellow-tan tumors with necrosis and hemorrhage and fish flesh appearance.

The overall histology shows one of the following three patterns: (1) intimate admixture of carcinoma and sarcomatoid carcinoma with nonspecific spindle cell morphology, this being the most common type, (2) carcinoma admixed with sarcomatous component showing heterologous differentiation, and (3) pure spindle cell tumor. The epithelial component of carcinosarcoma is either moderately or poorly differentiated adenocarcinoma, usually acinar but occasionally ductal, small cell, adenosquamous, or basal cell carcinoma. The acinar adenocarcinoma component is often high-grade (Gleason score 8 to 10). The spindle cell component commonly is undifferentiated, or shows chondroid or osteoid differentiation (Figs. 10-2 to 10-4). Less commonly, the spindle component differentiates toward rhabdomyosarcoma, leiomyosarcoma, or angiosarcoma (Fig. 10-5) and shows variable immunoreactivity for vimentin, desmin, actin, smooth muscle actin (SMA), and S100 protein. Typically, the spindle component is negative for prostatic markers (PSA, PSAP, PSMA, p501s) but may be focally positive. Low molecular weight cytokeratin is virtually always positive although its reaction with other keratin antibodies (PAN-CK, HMWK, CK5/6) is seen in only half of the cases. Vimentin is positive.[7] Electron microscopy of the sarcomatoid areas may reveal desmosomes.

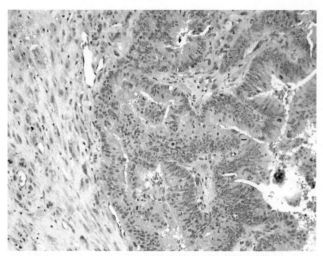

FIGURE 10-2 ■ Sarcomatoid carcinoma with ductal adenocarcinoma (*right*) and undifferentiated malignant spindle cell component (*left*).

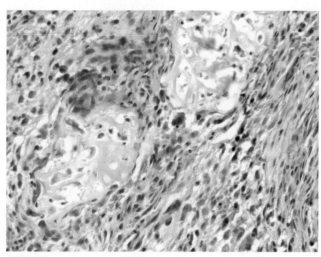

FIGURE 10-4 ■ Sarcomatoid carcinoma with chondrosarcoma component.

Differential Diagnosis

The main differential diagnoses are the following:

(1) Primary sarcoma of the prostate: This occurs in sarcomatoid carcinomas in which the epithelial component is focal or absent. The most common prostatic sarcomas are stromal sarcomas and leiomyosarcomas. In general, extensive sampling and demonstration of an associated epithelial component is consistent with sarcomatoid carcinoma rather than sarcoma. It should be mentioned, however, that stromal sarcoma can have an associated epithelial component in the subtype called "phyllodes-like"; however, the epithelial component is benign in these tumors. Also, stromal sarcomas are keratin-negative and express CD34 and progesterone receptor (PR). Leiomyosarcomas may, however, occasionally show focal keratin positivity, although

diffuse staining is not seen. As a general rule, keratin positivity within the spindle cell component of a lesion, which lacks the typical morphology of one of the sarcomas that can express keratin, is diagnostic of sarcomatoid carcinoma. For example, the sarcomatous component in sarcomatoid carcinoma typically consists of a haphazard array of malignant spindle cells, as opposed to the intersecting parallel bundles of malignant smooth muscle cells seen in leiomyosarcoma. High molecular weight cytokeratin and CK5/6 are two of the better keratins to utilize in this regard.

(2) Inflammatory myofibroblastic tumor (IMT): Features that are distinctive from sarcomatoid carcinoma include the tissue culture–like appearance, the typical granulation tissue–type vascularity and associated inflammatory cells, the lack of nuclear pleomorphism, and hyperchromasia. A further pitfall is that IMTs are positive

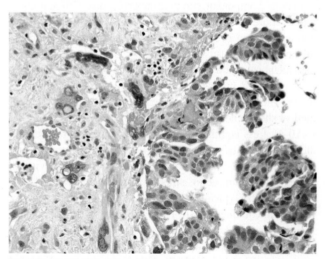

FIGURE 10-3 ■ Sarcomatoid carcinoma with acinar adenocarcinoma (*right*) and undifferentiated sarcomatoid component consisting of malignant giant cells (*left*).

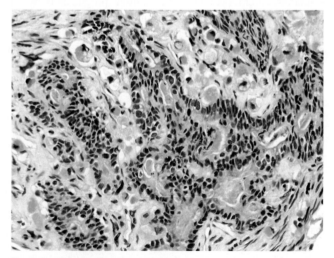

FIGURE 10-5 ■ Sarcomatoid carcinoma with adenocarcinoma and rhabdomyosarcoma components.

for keratin and may express SMA. Approximately two-thirds of IMTs are positive for ALK1, which is diagnostic of IMT. One should, however, be aware of several atypical morphologic features that can be seen in IMT in order not to overdiagnose them as sarcoma or sarcomatoid carcinoma. Those include hypercellularity, infiltrative pattern of growth, necrosis, and increased mitotic activity, although atypical mitotic figures are not seen.

(3) Gastrointestinal stromal tumor (GIST): Rarely those tumors secondarily involve the prostate and are composed of uniform spindle cells with palisading and perinuclear halos, without the pleomorphism of sarcomatoid carcinoma. GISTs are keratin negative and positive for CD117, DOG-1, and CD34.

Prognosis and Treatment

Sarcomatoid carcinomas have an aggressive clinical course and a dismal prognosis with an actuarial risk of death at 1 year up to 20% and 14% survival rates at 7 years postdiagnosis. Metastatic lesions may be purely glandular, mixed carcinosarcomatous, or purely sarcomatous. The treatment is the same as for usual acinar adenocarcinoma of the prostate. However, current therapies, including multimodal approaches, remain ineffective and not standard.

Neuroendocrine Differentiation in Acinar Prostatic Adenocarcinoma

Even in ordinary adenocarcinomas of the prostate without light microscopic evidence of neuroendocrine differentiation, between 30% and 100% show neuroendocrine differentiation when evaluated with immunohistochemistry for multiple neuroendocrine markers. These cells may react with antibodies to chromogranin, serotonin, adrenocorticotropic hormone (ACTH), calcitonin, human chorionic gonadotropin, neuron-specific enolase, somatostatin, leuenkephalin, or beta-endorphin.[8] The vast majority of these cases have no clinical evidence of ectopic hormonal secretion.

Androgen-deprivation therapy is associated with an increased number of neuroendocrine cells.[9] It is suggested that growth-promoting neuropeptides elaborated by the neuroendocrine cells sustain the growth of the nonneuroendocrine carcinoma cells in an androgen-deprived environment.[10–12] Furthermore, androgen depletion may lead to transdifferentiation of carcinoma cells into androgen receptor negative, apoptosis-resistant (bcl-2 positive) neuroendocrine cells.[13,14]

It is controversial whether neuroendocrine differentiation in typical adenocarcinomas worsens prognosis, with some studies suggesting a correlation[8,15,16] yet most others showing no effect of neuroendocrine differentiation on outcome.[17,18] Currently, in accordance with the College of American Pathologists Consensus Statement 1999, neuroendocrine differentiation remains a category III prognostic factor together with other factors not sufficiently studied to demonstrate their prognostic value.[19]

Adenocarcinoma with Paneth Cell–Like Neuroendocrine Differentiation

In histologically typical adenocarcinomas of the prostate and occasionally in high-grade prostatic intraepithelial neoplasia (HGPIN), basally located deeply eosinophilic fine cytoplasmic granules can be identified that are chromogranin positive and contain neurosecretory granules by electron microscopy (Figs. 10-6 and 10-7). The term Paneth cell–like has been used to describe these eosinophilic neuroendocrine cells.[20] Paneth cell–like neuroendocrine differentiation in prostatic adenocarcinoma can be seen as either patchy isolated cells or diffusely involving glands or nests.[21,22] Despite the cells' bland histologic appearance, strictly applying the Gleason grading system one would assign a Gleason pattern 5 to Paneth cell–like foci with no glandular formation (Fig. 10-8). It has been shown that such grade assignment does not reflect the clinical behavior in these cases. It is therefore recommended that Gleason grading in such tumors be assigned only to the areas of conventional adenocarcinoma. If the entire tumor consists of sheets, cords, or nests with Paneth cell–like neuroendocrine differentiation, then a Gleason score should not be assigned and a comment to the generally favorable prognosis of these lesions could be provided.[21]

Carcinoid Tumor

The majority of lesions reported as "carcinoid tumors" of the prostate are merely prostatic adenocarcinomas with neuroendocrine differentiation. Almost all such cases have been positive with antibodies for PSA and PSAP and have clinically behaved like ordinary prostate carcinomas. True carcinoid tumors of the prostate with negative immunoreactivity for PSA and PSAP and otherwise typical carcinoid tumor morphology and immunoprofile are extremely rare (Fig. 10-9).[23–27]

Small Cell Carcinoma

Clinical Features

Although the prostate is one of the most common sites of extrapulmonary small cell carcinoma, prostatic small cell carcinoma is rare, comprising 0.5% to 2% of all prostatic carcinomas. In the largest series of prostatic small cell carcinoma, there was a prior diagnosis of usual adenocarcinoma of the prostate in 42% of cases.[28] The median time interval between the diagnosis of prostate cancer and small cell carcinoma in this study was 25 months with some patients having had a prior history of hormonal therapy. The mean age at presentation is 69 years, and typically patients present with a rapid onset of urinary tract obstruction. Although most cases lack clinically significant hormonal production, some patients present with paraneoplastic symptoms such as ACTH or ADH overproduction or Eaton-Lambert syndrome. Serum PSA levels are variable, and typically are normal. A classic scenario is that patients have very elevated serum PSA levels with metastatic disease and then the PSA levels fall indicating the onset of a small cell component.

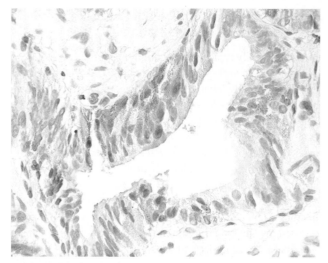

FIGURE 10-6 ■ High-grade prostatic intraepithelial neoplasia with Paneth cell–like neuroendocrine change.

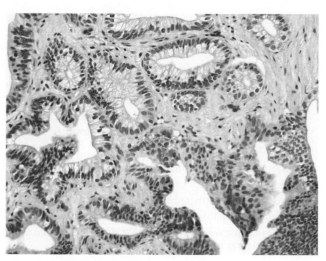

FIGURE 10-7 ■ Prostatic adenocarcinoma with Paneth cell–like neuroendocrine change.

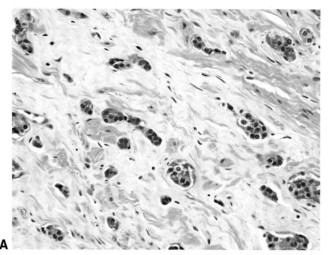

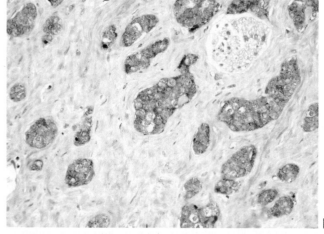

FIGURE 10-8 ■ **A:** Prostatic adenocarcinoma with lack of glandular differentiation showing Paneth cell–like neuroendocrine change. **B:** Strong immunostaining for chromogranin in prostatic adenocarcinoma with Paneth cell–like neuroendocrine change.

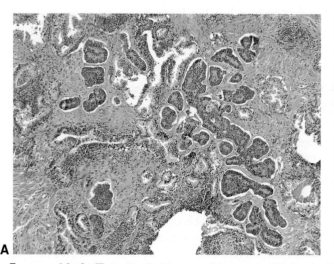

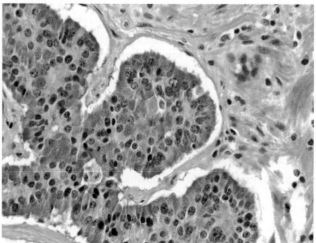

FIGURE 10-9 ■ **A:** Carcinoid tumor of the prostate. **B:** Carcinoid tumor of the prostate with cytoplasmic eosinophilic granules.

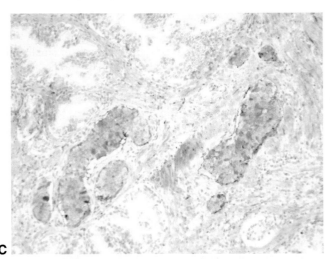

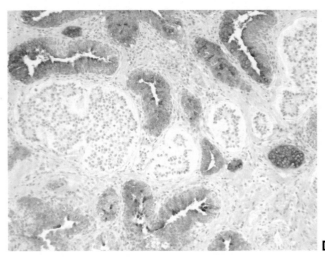

C   **D**

FIGURE 10-9 ■ (*Continued*) **C:** Carcinoid tumor of the prostate positive for chromogranin. **D:** Carcinoid tumor of the prostate negative for PSA.

Pathology

Prostatic and pulmonary small cell carcinomas share the same morphologic features.[29] Classic "oat cell" morphology consists of tumor cells with scant cytoplasm and round, oval, or spindled nuclei usually smaller than three times the size of lymphocytes with fine granular chromatin, and absent or inconspicuous nucleoli, which is the histology seen in two-thirds of prostatic small cell carcinomas (Figs. 10-10 and 10-11). The remaining cases are of the "intermediate cell" variant with slightly more cytoplasm and more visible nucleoli (Fig. 10-12).[30–33] When diagnosing small cell carcinoma in the prostate, morphologic subtyping is not recommended and both subtypes are reported as "small cell carcinoma" as it has been demonstrated that in the lung these two types are clinically indistinguishable.[34] Other features not typically associated with small cell carcinoma, including Indian file formation, giant cells with degenerative atypia, vacuolated cells, and desmoplasia, are seen in a minority of prostatic cases.[28,35]

Pure small cell carcinoma is seen in about one-half of cases with the remaining cases being admixed with prostate adenocarcinoma. In cases with adenocarcinoma, there is a sharp demarcation between small cell carcinoma and adenocarcinoma in about 20% of cases with the remaining cases showing a gradual merging of the two components (Fig. 10-13).[28] Typically the associated acinar adenocarcinoma component is high-grade (Gleason score 8 to 10).

The vast majority (88%) of small cell carcinomas are positive for at least one neuroendocrine marker. In the small cell carcinoma component, 19% are positive for PSA, 28% for prostein (P501s), and 25% for PSMA, although often very focally. Although P501s and PSMA are better than PSA in identifying the prostatic origin of small cell carcinoma, the majority (60%) of prostatic small cell carcinomas are negative for all three markers. Stains for TTF are positive in about one-half of cases. Basal cell (p63, HMWK) and androgen

FIGURE 10-10 ■ Small cell carcinoma of the prostate.

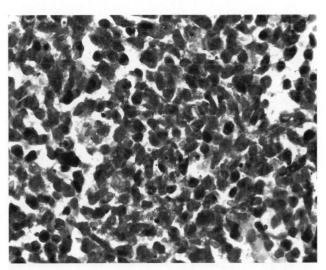

FIGURE 10-11 ■ High magnification of small cell carcinoma of the prostate indistinguishable from small cell carcinomas in other sites.

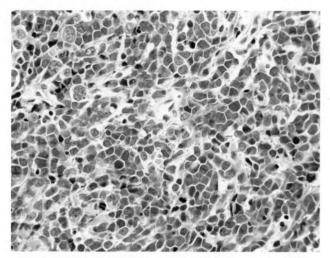

FIGURE 10-12 ■ Small cell carcinoma with more visible nucleoli and slightly more abundant cytoplasm.

receptor markers are typically negative. About 50% of cases are AMACR positive. Small cell carcinoma is typically negative for both CK7 and CK20. Immunoreactivity with PAN-CK shows typical paranuclear dot-like pattern. Ki-67 staining shows >70% of positive cells. CD44 is reported to be positive in small cell prostatic carcinoma, but negative in small cell carcinoma of nonprostatic origin, and is expressed in only rare scattered cells in conventional adenocarcinoma.

Differential Diagnosis

Small cell carcinoma must be differentiated from Gleason score 5 + 5 = 10 usual adenocarcinoma of the prostate. Cases where the small cell carcinoma component merges with non–small cell areas may be more likely to be underdiagnosed as opposed to cases whether there is a sharp demarcation between the two patterns.[36] Also, the intermediate cell variant with more visible cytoplasm and nucleoli is at increased

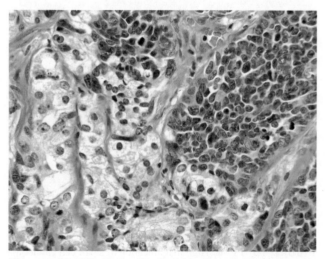

FIGURE 10-13 ■ Small cell carcinoma with sharp demarcation between it and acinar adenocarcinoma of the prostate.

risk of a misdiagnosis of poorly differentiated usual prostate cancer.[28] In part, the likelihood of underdiagnosing small cell carcinoma is due to the rarity of the diagnosis of small cell carcinoma relative to the diagnosis of usual prostate adenocarcinoma. Documentation of neuroendocrine differentiation using immunohistochemistry can help in cases that are ambiguous based on routine hematoxylin and eosin (H&E)-stained sections. It should be noted, however, that synaptophysin can show focal staining in high-grade acinar adenocarcinoma, and therefore the diagnosis should not be entirely based on the expression of neuroendocrine markers. Features that favor high-grade adenocarcinoma over small cell carcinoma are single cell pattern of growth, abundant cytoplasm, prominent nucleoli, absence of nuclear spindling and molding, strong positivity for prostatic markers, negative or focal staining for CD44, <50% of positive cells with Ki-67, and diffuse positivity for PAN-CK markers in contrast to small cell carcinoma in which the staining is dot-like paranuclear.

In general, most cases of small cell carcinoma can be diagnosed on morphologic grounds alone, and immunohistochemistry is reserved for equivocal cases.

Prognosis and Treatment

Over 90% of small cell carcinomas are of advanced stage at time of diagnosis. In most cases with mixed usual adenocarcinoma of the prostate and small cell carcinoma, the metastases are of the small cell component. Treatment consists of combination chemotherapy of the type used in pulmonary small cell carcinoma. The prognosis is dismal with most surviving <2 years.[37] There is no difference in prognosis whether tumors are mixed small cell and usual adenocarcinoma or pure small cell carcinoma. The proportion of small cell carcinoma and whether there is a history of prior usual adenocarcinoma of the prostate also does not affect prognosis. A review of the literature by Mackey et al.[38] of genitourinary small cell carcinoma found cisplatin chemotherapy to be beneficial for bladder tumors but only surgery was prognostic for prostate small cell carcinomas. While this study concluded that hormonal manipulation and systemic chemotherapy had little effect on the natural history of disease in the prostate, the number of patients was small and some suggest that small cell carcinoma of the prostate should be treated with the same combination chemotherapy used to treat small cell carcinomas in other sites.[39–41]

Large Cell Neuroendocrine Carcinoma

Large cell neuroendocrine carcinoma (LCNEC) of prostate is an extremely rare occurrence.[42] Most cases represent progression from prior typical prostate adenocarcinoma following long-standing hormonal therapy, with a median time interval of 4.7 years (range from 2 to 12 years) between the two. The tumors are composed of sheets and ribbons of amphophilic cells with large nuclei, coarse chromatin, and prominent nucleoli with a high mitotic activity and foci of necrosis (Fig. 10-14). The LCNEC component is strongly

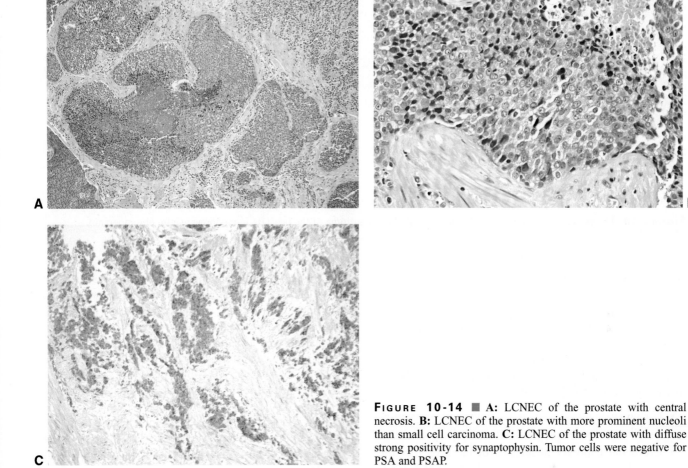

FIGURE 10-14 ■ **A:** LCNEC of the prostate with central necrosis. **B:** LCNEC of the prostate with more prominent nucleoli than small cell carcinoma. **C:** LCNEC of the prostate with diffuse strong positivity for synaptophysin. Tumor cells were negative for PSA and PSAP.

positive various neuroendocrine markers with focal or absent PSA and PSAP immunoreactivity. AMACR may be positive. LCNEC are aggressive tumors that usually present at advanced stage and metastatic disease with patients dying within a year of diagnosis. The importance of distinguishing LCNEC from small cell carcinoma at the therapeutic and prognostic levels is not established. The diagnosis of LCNEC is problematic as usual prostate adenocarcinoma can express neuroendocrine markers. Only when a poorly differentiated carcinoma has a nested or ribbon-like appearance without glands, where the tumor is strongly positive for neuroendocrine markers and negative for prostate markers, can the diagnosis be established.

Lymphoepithelioma-like Carcinoma

Lymphoepithelioma-like carcinomas are very rare tumors with <10 cases reported to date. The mean age at presentation is 76 and patients usually present with urinary obstructive symptoms and elevated serum PSA levels.[43] Histologically the lymphoepithelioma-like component is composed of sheets of undifferentiated cells with indistinct cytoplasmic

borders and a syncytial pattern of growth. The nuclei are high-grade with vesicular chromatin, prominent nucleoli, and numerous mitoses. Typically there is an admixed heavy lymphocytic infiltrate with occasional plasma cells, neutrophils, and eosinophils. The lymphoepithelioma-like component ranges from 10% to 100% of the entire tumor and most cases have an associated acinar adenocarcinoma (most reported with Gleason score 4 + 3) and sometimes ductal adenocarcinoma components. Cells are positive for prostatic markers and AMACR and, when tested, in situ hybridization showed absence of Epstein-Barr virus genome confirming that this is a simply a rare morphologic variant of prostatic carcinoma. All reported cases were associated with an adverse clinical course with death from the disease occurring at a mean follow-up time of 20 months in the largest reported series.[43]

Paraganglioma

A few case reports of paragangliomas originating in the prostate have also been reported, including one in a child (Fig. 10-15).[44-46]

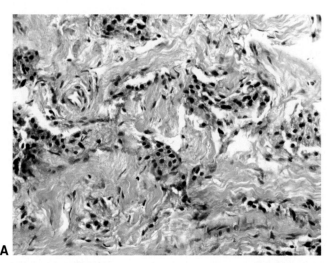
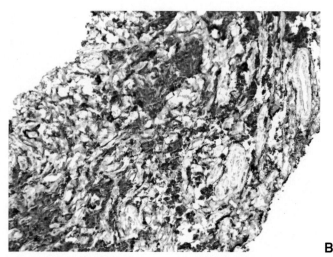

FIGURE 10-15 ■ **A:** Paraganglioma of the prostate. **B:** Paraganglioma of the prostate immunoreactive for chromogranin.

Urothelial Carcinoma

Introduction

Urothelial carcinoma can involve the prostate in the following different manners:

Urothelial neoplasia involving urethra, which may be seen in transurethral resection of the prostate (TURP) specimens. Those can be divided into

- Urethral carcinoma in situ (CIS) in the absence of prostatic duct or stromal involvement.
- Urothelial papillary neoplasms of the prostatic urethra: those lesions range from papilloma to high-grade noninvasive urothelial carcinoma to invasive papillary urothelial carcinoma involving the prostate.

Urothelial neoplasia involving prostatic ducts, acini, or stroma, which may be seen in TURP or needle biopsy specimens. Those can be divided into

- CIS involving ducts and acini without stromal invasion (intraductal urothelial carcinoma).
- CIS involving ducts and acini with stromal invasion.
- Invasive urothelial carcinoma of the bladder with direct invasion of the prostatic stroma.

Clinical Features

The most common scenario for the detection of urothelial carcinoma of the prostate is prostatic involvement in cystoprostatectomies performed for bladder urothelial carcinomas. In that context the most common pattern of involvement is by extension of CIS to the prostatic urethra with secondary prostatic ducts/acinar involvement, which can progress to stromal invasion. A less common pattern of involvement is in advanced invasive bladder urothelial carcinomas that extend directly into the prostate. This latter scenario represents the pathologic stage T4 of the latest bladder

TNM staging system. Random sections of the prostate at the time of cystectomy for urothelial carcinoma show prostatic involvement by urothelial carcinoma in between 12% to 20% of cases. If serial sections of the prostate in cystoprostatectomy specimens with bladder urothelial carcinoma are performed, involvement of the prostate by urothelial carcinoma may be found in 37% to 45% of the cases.[47–49]

Primary prostatic urothelial carcinoma is uncommon and comprises about 2% of prostate cancers in adults. The vast majority of those patients have concomitant bladder urothelial CIS, and prostatic involvement appears to be by direct extension from the overlying urethra, since in the majority of cases the more centrally located prostatic ducts are involved by urothelial neoplasia to a greater extent than the peripheral ducts and acini. However, rarely, primary urothelial carcinomas arise in the prostate without bladder involvement.[47]

Since topical chemotherapy and immunotherapy for superficial bladder carcinomas appear to act by direct contact with neoplastic epithelium, it has become critical to identify those cases of bladder urothelial carcinomas with prostatic involvement, since conservative management will not treat these cases effectively. Currently, biopsies of the prostatic urethra and suburethral prostate tissue may be performed as a staging procedure or in the setting of positive cytology in patients undergoing intravesical treatment for superficial bladder tumors. It is also important to evaluate the urothelium in routine TURP specimens done for benign prostatic hyperplasia (BPH) symptoms, as we have seen several cases of CIS where no history of bladder cancer was present.

Pathology

- **Urethral CIS in the absence of prostatic duct or stromal involvement:** In those lesions, prostatic urethra is replaced by CIS cells. CIS can exhibit different patterns including large cell pleomorphic, large cell nonpleomorphic, small cell, clinging, and pagetoid. Criteria to

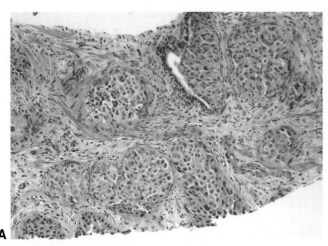
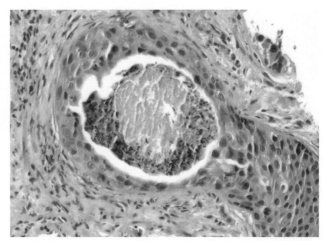

FIGURE 10-16 ■ **A:** Intraductal spread of urothelial carcinoma. **B:** Urothelial carcinoma involving prostatic acini with central comedonecrosis.

distinguish CIS from reactive urothelium are the same as those applied in the bladder.

- **Urothelial papillary carcinoma of the prostatic urethra:** with low- or high-grade histology. Those lesions are usually noninvasive but can show submucosal invasion and even prostatic stromal invasion. For those invasive tumors, the TNM staging system of the urethra rather than the bladder applies and the pathologic stage is T1 for submucosal invasion and T2 for prostatic stromal invasion. T2 tumors are easily diagnosed when invasive tumor is seen infiltrating between prostatic glands; however, the distinction between T1 and T2 lesions when the involved tissue does not contain prostatic glands is not always straightforward due to the lack of clear-cut criteria to distinguish between the two different stages.

- **CIS involving ducts and acini without stromal invasion (intraductal urothelial carcinoma):** Intraductal urothelial carcinoma of the prostatic ducts initially consists of malignant urothelial cells insinuating themselves between the basal cell layer and the columnar to cuboidal luminal epithelium of the prostatic ducts. More peripherally, urothelial carcinoma spreads in a pagetoid fashion within the ducts. Similar to that seen in the breast, large tumor cells with clear cytoplasm are seen in the midst of otherwise normal urothelium. With more extensive involvement, urothelial carcinoma fills and expands ducts and often develops central comedonecrosis (Fig. 10-16). Immunohistochemical stains for basal cells (HMWK, p63) may in some cases outline only the prostatic basal cells and in other cases also label the intraductal urothelial carcinoma. Sometimes the surrounding basal cells may show more intense staining for HMWK than the intraductal carcinoma component (Figs. 10-17 and 10-18).

- **CIS involving ducts and acini with stromal invasion:** Stromal invasion is characterized by the presence of infiltrative small nests and single cells that usually elicit stromal inflammation and desmoplasia and may be accompanied by stromal retraction artifact. Those features along with

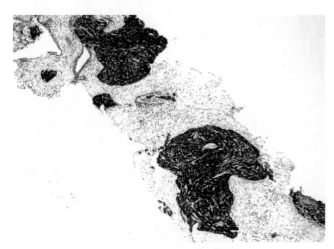

FIGURE 10-17 ■ Intraductal urothelial carcinoma diffusely positive for high molecular weight cytokeratin.

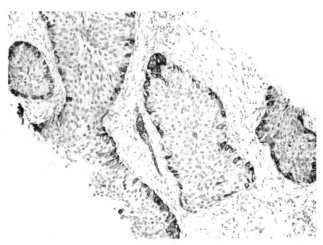

FIGURE 10-18 ■ Intraductal urothelial carcinoma negative for high molecular weight cytokeratin with positivity restricted to residual benign prostatic basal cells.

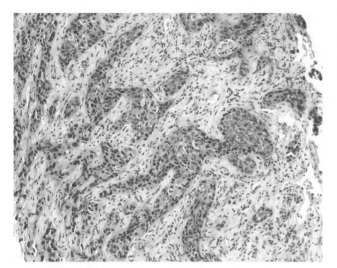

FIGURE 10-19 ■ Nests of infiltrating urothelial carcinoma invading the prostate.

the irregular nests' borders are helpful in the distinction between the invasive and the intraductal components. When urothelial carcinoma invades the prostatic stroma through this route, the urethral tumors staging system applies and the pathologic stage is considered to be T2.

- **Invasive urothelial carcinoma of the bladder with direct invasion of the prostatic stroma:** These cases usually present with invasive urothelial carcinoma invading the prostatic stroma in the absence of an intraductal component or urethral involvement. Infiltrating urothelial carcinoma typically has a different morphology than poorly differentiated adenocarcinoma of the prostate, although there are some cases that show overlap and are impossible to distinguish without ancillary studies. Urothelial cancer tends to grow in nests, even when poorly differentiated (Fig. 10-19). High-grade urothelial carcinomas often reveal marked pleomorphism with tumor giant cells (Fig. 10-20). Urothelial carcinomas may demonstrate hard glassy eosinophilic

Table 10-1 ■ MORPHOLOGIC DISTINCTION OF POORLY DIFFERENTIATED PROSTATIC ADENOCARCINOMA FROM UROTHELIAL CARCINOMA

Prostate Cancer	Urothelial Cancer
Sheets, cords, individual cells	Nests of cells
Microacinar or cribriform pattern	Solid sheets of cells, cribriform pattern rare
Pale delicate cytoplasm	Occasional hard eosinophilic cytoplasm
Typically uniform nuclei	Marked pleomorphism
Central prominent nucleolus	Often marked hyperchromasia
Lacks inflammation	Associated inflammation
Uncommon necrosis	Necrosis more common

cytoplasm or more prominent squamous differentiation. Urothelial carcinoma involving the prostate may contain areas of necrosis or stromal inflammation, which are unusual findings in even high-grade adenocarcinoma of the prostate. The pathologic stage of those tumors is T4 using the bladder TNM staging system.

Differential Diagnosis

The major differential diagnosis for infiltrating urothelial carcinoma involving the prostate is poorly differentiated prostatic adenocarcinoma (Table 10-1). Poorly differentiated prostate cancers may have enlarged nuclei and prominent nucleoli, yet in contrast to urothelial carcinoma there is little variability in nuclear shape or size from one nucleus to another. A subtler finding is that the cytoplasm of prostatic adenocarcinoma is often very foamy and pale imparting a "soft" appearance. Infiltrating cords of cells or focal cribriform or pseudorosette glandular differentiation are other features more typical of prostatic adenocarcinoma than urothelial carcinoma (Fig. 10-21).

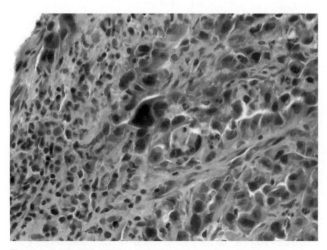

FIGURE 10-20 ■ Urothelial carcinoma with marked pleomorphism and associated inflammation invading the prostate.

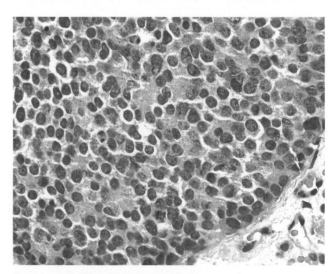

FIGURE 10-21 ■ High-grade acinar adenocarcinoma of the prostate with uniform cytology and subtle microacinar formation.

Although the above distinction between urothelial carcinoma and prostatic adenocarcinoma on H&E-stained sections is valid for almost all cases, we have seen rare cases where prostate adenocarcinoma has marked pleomorphism identical to urothelial carcinoma. Consequently, in a poorly differentiated tumor involving the bladder and prostate without any glandular differentiation typical of prostate adenocarcinoma, the case should be worked up immunohistochemically. Approximately 95% of poorly differentiated prostatic adenocarcinomas show PSA and PSAP staining although it may be focal.[50–52] While some studies claim superiority of PSA over PSAP in staining prostatic carcinoma, other articles have demonstrated poorly differentiated prostatic carcinomas that lacked PSA staining but still maintained their immunoreactivity with antibodies to PSAP.[51–54] In our own hands, PSA has in general been more sensitive. Monoclonal antibodies to PSAP have lower sensitivities than their polyclonal counterparts.[55] In some cases of poorly differentiated prostatic adenocarcinomas, there may be weak or negative PSA staining where the tumor reacts to a greater degree with newer prostate-specific markers including PSMA, p501S (prostein), and NKX 3.1[56] (Table 10-2). However, the lack of immunoreactivity to prostate-specific markers in a poorly differentiated tumor within the prostate, especially if present in limited amount, does not exclude the diagnosis of a poorly differentiated prostatic adenocarcinoma. In a poorly differentiated tumor occurring in the bladder and the prostate where the differential diagnosis is between high-grade prostatic adenocarcinoma and urothelial carcinoma, focal strong staining for prostatic markers can be used reliably to make the diagnosis of prostatic adenocarcinoma, as they have not been convincingly described in urothelial carcinomas.[55,57,58] Almost 50% of cystoprostatectomy specimens performed for urothelial carcinoma also contain adenocarcinoma of the prostate.[47,48,59] Therefore, the finding of a small focus of well-differentiated adenocarcinoma of the prostate in a TURP should not necessarily influence whether a separate focus of poorly differentiated tumor is urothelial carcinoma or adenocarcinoma of the prostate. In general, various cytokeratins (CK7, CK20, high molecular weight cytokeratin) show strong positivity in cases of urothelial carcinoma involving the prostate. Although CK7 and CK20 are more frequently seen in urothelial carcinoma as compared to adenocarcinoma of the prostate, they may also be positive in adenocarcinoma of the prostate.[60,61] The only helpful finding is negative CK7 immunoreactivity, which favors prostatic adenocarcinoma, as it would be unusual for urothelial carcinoma. High molecular weight cytokeratin is positive in more than 90% of urothelial carcinomas.[56,62] In contrast, high molecular weight cytokeratin is only rarely (8%) expressed, and

usually in a very small percentage of cells, in adenocarcinoma of the prostate.[56,63] p63 has a greater specificity albeit lower sensitivity for urothelial carcinoma compared to high molecular weight cytokeratin (100% specificity and 83% sensitivity).[56] Other markers that also appear highly specific but only of modest sensitivity for urothelial carcinoma include uroplakin and thrombomodulin (49% to 69% sensitivity).

Extensive intraductal urothelial carcinoma must be differentiated from invasive urothelial carcinoma. With intraductal urothelial carcinoma of the prostate, nests of urothelial carcinoma have the contours and distribution of prostatic ducts and acini. The nests are circumscribed with a smooth discrete edge between the epithelium and the adjacent stroma, and the stroma lacks a desmoplastic response. Infiltrating urothelial carcinoma is characterized by small cords, nests, or individual cells often with retraction artifact, eliciting a desmoplastic stromal response.

Intraductal urothelial carcinoma must also be differentiated from high-grade prostatic intraepithelial neoplasia. The presence of an intraductal growth where preexisting benign prostate glands are filled with solid nests of tumor differs from HGPIN, which is composed of flat, tufting, papillary, or cribriform patterns. Although the cells of HGPIN are atypical, the presence of pleomorphism and mitoses are uncommon.

Prognosis and Treatment

Patients with prostatic stromal involvement by direct invasion of the bladder urothelial carcinoma (T4) have a worse prognosis than those in whom the invasive prostatic urothelial carcinoma originates from an intraductal component.[64] In the latter scenario, there are typically associated bladder tumors, which may determine the prognosis. Intraductal prostatic urothelial carcinoma with prostatic stromal invasion may also be associated with low-stage (T1, T2) bladder tumors. Prostatic stromal invasion in this setting has a negative effect on prognosis, although the prognosis is less ominous than direct invasion into the prostate from an infiltrating bladder urothelial carcinoma.[64–66]

Most but not all studies have demonstrated that intraductal spread of the prostate by urothelial carcinoma does not adversely affect survival following cystoprostatectomy, which is rather determined by the stage of the bladder tumor.[49,64–67] If intraductal urothelial carcinoma is identified on TURP or transurethral biopsy, patients usually will be recommended for radical cystoprostatectomy. The finding of intraductal urothelial carcinoma has also been demonstrated to increase the risk of urethral recurrence following cystoprostatectomy, such that its identification may also result in prophylactic total urethrectomy.

Table 10-2 ■ IMMUNOHISTOCHEMICAL DISTINCTION OF PROSTATE ADENOCARCINOMA AND UROTHELIAL CARCINOMA						
	PSA	**P501S**	**PSMA**	**HMWCK**	**p63**	**Thrombomodulin**
Prostate carcinoma	37/38 (97%)	38/38 (100%)	35/38 (92%)	3/38 (8%)	0/38 (0%)	2/38 (5%)
Urothelial carcinoma	0/35 (0%)	2/35 (6%)	0/35 (0%)	32/35 (91%)	29/35 (83%)	24/35 (69%)

The overall prognosis of urothelial cell carcinoma diagnosed on prostatic needle biopsy is poor, even in cases without histologic evidence of stromal invasion on biopsy.[63] In these cases with intraductal cancer on biopsy, most likely invasive cancer is present elsewhere in the prostate that was not sampled. Although the prognosis is poor, even with only apparent intraductal involvement, histologic recognition is essential, as the only opportunity for improved outcome is early and aggressive therapy.

Primary urothelial carcinoma of the prostate without bladder involvement is rare.[68–72] A continuum from urothelial hyperplasia without atypia to atypical urothelial hyperplasia to CIS can also be identified.[73] Rarely, urothelial carcinoma may be papillary within enlarged dilated prostatic ducts.[68] Though an older study claimed that one-third of the cases of primary urothelial carcinoma of the prostate have areas of prostatic adenocarcinoma, this number is overstated and this is only uncommonly seen.[68] This study predated the use of immunohistochemistry for PSA and PSAP, and these cases may have been adenocarcinomas of the prostate with areas of poor differentiation, resembling urothelial carcinoma. From a prognostic standpoint, primary prostatic urothelial carcinoma is a heterogeneous disease with higher disease-specific survival rates in cases showing noninvasive carcinoma (CIS of prostatic urethra and/or intraductal carcinoma) in comparison to those showing cancer invading prostatic stroma.[65] Invasive primary urothelial carcinomas of the prostate tend to infiltrate the bladder neck and surrounding soft tissue such that over 50% of the patients present with tumors extending out of the prostate. Twenty percent of the patients present with distant metastases, bone and liver being the most common sites. In contrast to adenocarcinoma of the prostate, bone metastases are usually osteolytic. Rubenstein and Rubnitz described 10 cases of urothelial cell carcinoma arising within the large periurethral prostatic ducts. These patients all died within 2 years of diagnosis, with eight (80%) dying within 1 year.[71] Greene et al. reported a series of 39 patients with primary urothelial cell carcinoma of the prostate. Again, the prognosis was poor with 34 (87%) patients dying within 5 years. Average survival was only 17 months.[68] In their review of three additional cases, Nicolaisen and Williams[70] emphasized clinical presentation (obstructive symptoms in younger patients), an aggressive course with a propensity for local invasion, and stressed radical surgery as the only hope for survival.

Basal Cell Carcinoma

Introduction

Basal cell carcinomas do not appear to arise from basal cell hyperplasia. These lesions express the same immunoprofile as normal basal cells.

Clinical Features

Those are rare tumors with <75 cases reported and a wide age range at presentation (28 to 89 years). Most cases are seen in TURP specimens as these tumors originate in the transition

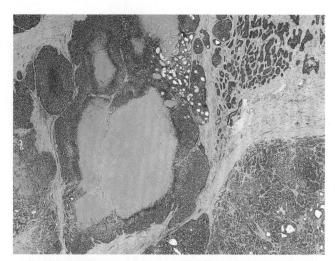

FIGURE 10-22 ■ Basal cell carcinoma with large basaloid nests with central necrosis.

zone and therefore present with urinary obstructive symptoms. Rarely, tumors may be detected on needle biopsies performed during workup of elevated serum PSA levels, although basal cell carcinoma itself does not raise serum PSA levels.

Pathology

Grossly, basal cell carcinomas present with white and fleshy nodules with microcysts, unlike acinar carcinoma, which is usually yellow. It invariably involves the transition zone with or without peripheral zone involvement. Microscopically, it displays different morphologic patterns. It can resemble basal cell carcinoma of the skin with large basaloid nests, cords, or trabeculae showing peripheral palisading and necrosis (Fig. 10-22). Other basal cell carcinomas show an adenoid cystic carcinoma pattern in which the tumor grows in nests with prominent cribriform architecture, the lumina of which may be filled with eosinophilic, hyaline basement membrane–like material or basophilic mucinous secretions (Fig. 10-23).[74–76]

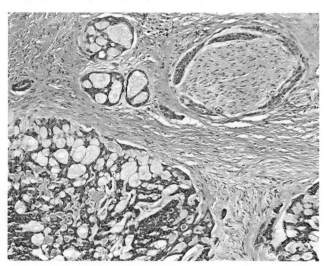

FIGURE 10-23 ■ Adenoid cystic carcinoma pattern of basal cell carcinoma with perineural invasion.

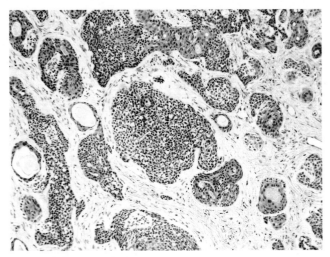

FIGURE 10-24 ■ Basal cell carcinoma with irregular variable-sized basaloid nests with central eosinophilic gland formation.

Table 10-3 ■ FEATURES OF BASAL CELL CARCINOMA
Large basaloid nests often with necrosis
Adenoid cystic-like pattern
Anastomosing nests
Variably sized nests with irregular shapes
Nests or tubules centrally lined by eosinophilic cells
Perineural or vascular invasion
Extraprostatic extension into adipose tissue or seminal vesicles
Invasion of thick muscle bundles of the bladder neck
Widespread infiltration between benign prostatic glands
Prominent desmoplastic or myxoid stromal reaction
Ki67 staining was >20%
Strong diffuse bcl-2 staining

Another pattern unique to basal cell carcinoma are anastomosing basaloid nests and tubules centrally lined by eosinophilic cells, and variably small or medium-sized nests with irregular shapes (Fig. 10-24). Lastly, basal cell carcinoma may also resemble basal cell hyperplasia (Fig. 10-25). Basal cell carcinomas are infiltrative tumors associated with a desmoplastic stromal response, and not uncommonly show extraprostatic or seminal vesicle invasion, along with perineural or lymphovascular invasion. Of note is that Gleason grading does not apply to these tumors.

At the immunohistochemical level, the cells are commonly negative for prostatic markers and positive for basal cells markers (p63, HMWK), which either stain all tumor cell layers or can be restricted to the peripheral aspects of tumor clusters. AMACR is positive in a minority of cases and BCL2 is typically strongly and diffusely positive.

Differential Diagnosis

Basal Cell Hyperplasia

In cases of basal cell carcinoma with overt malignant features, such as necrosis or extension of basal cell carcinoma into periprostatic adipose tissue or seminal vesicles, or perineural invasion, there is no difficulty in differentiating these lesions from basal cell hyperplasia. In other cases, it may be more difficult to diagnose malignancy in a basaloid proliferation (Table 10-3). Extension into the thick muscle bundles of the bladder neck and widespread infiltration of the malignant basal elements between benign prostatic glands is not seen in basal cell hyperplasia (Fig. 10-26). Although florid basal cell hyperplasia may appear infiltrative between benign glands, the nests or tubules of basal cell hyperplasia are more evenly and orderly arranged between benign

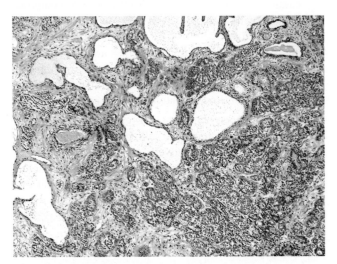

FIGURE 10-25 ■ Basal cell carcinoma resembling basal cell hyperplasia irregularly infiltrating between benign prostate glands.

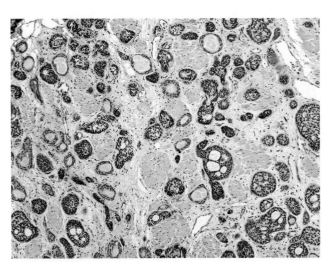

FIGURE 10-26 ■ Basal cell carcinoma infiltrating thick muscle bundles of the bladder neck.

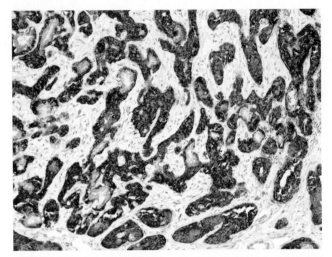

FIGURE 10-27 ■ Diffuse expression of BCL2 in basal cell carcinoma.

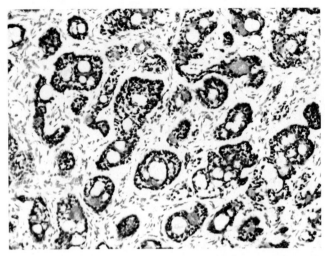

FIGURE 10-29 ■ Basal cell carcinoma diffusely expressing p63.

prostate glands and tend not to infiltrate as isolated units but rather as clusters of nests or tubules. Florid basal cell hyperplasia may have a subtle myxoid stromal reaction but lacks the extensive myxoid or desmoplastic reaction that characterizes some basal cell carcinomas.[77] Other findings that may be seen in association with basal cell carcinoma as well as basal cell hyperplasia include collagenous globules, squamous differentiation, focal microcalcifications and vacuoles. BCL2 labels basal cell carcinoma more strongly and diffusely than basal cell hyperplasia (Fig. 10-27).[78] Ki-67 staining is >20% in approximately one-half of basal cell carcinomas (Fig. 10-28).[76] Immunohistochemistry for Ki-67 can be helpful in differentiating basal cell carcinoma from florid basal cell hyperplasia, as basal cell hyperplasia typically shows <5% positivity.[78] Both high molecular weight cytokeratin and p63 label basal cell carcinoma, although not all the tumor cells are positive (Fig. 10-29).

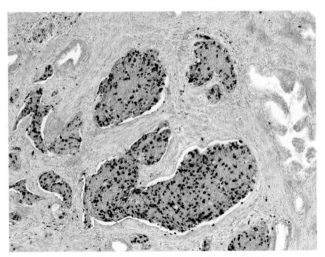

FIGURE 10-28 ■ Basal cell carcinoma with high expression of Ki-67.

Lastly, one should, however, be aware that the presence of cribriform architecture in a proliferative basal cell lesion is not necessarily equivalent to a diagnosis of basal cell carcinoma (adenoid cystic carcinoma pattern) as some cases of florid basal cell hyperplasia show similar structures. In that context, the cribriform nests are small and associated with a background typical of basal cell hyperplasia with lobulocentric growth in the transition zone in which the basaloid structures lack the aforementioned malignant features of carcinoma. Of note is that many cases of basal cell hyperplasia with adenoid cystic pattern were previously reported as basal cell carcinomas in the literature.

1) Cribriform basal cell hyperplasia: The nests are composed of cells with abundant and usually clear cytoplasm and lack the cytologic and invasive features of basal cell carcinomas.

2) Small cell carcinoma: Although small cell carcinoma and basal cell carcinoma share the fact that both are composed of small cells with scant cytoplasm and hyperchromatic nuclei, the latter does not show the typical nuclear molding, salt and pepper chromatin, crush artifact, and single cell necrosis typically present in small cell carcinoma. In addition, small cell carcinomas are positive for neuroendocrine markers and negative for basal cell markers.

3) Acinar adenocarcinoma, Gleason pattern 4 or 5: The cribriform architecture and solid growth seen in Gleason patterns 4 and 5, respectively, may mimic adenoid cystic carcinoma at low magnification. However, acinar adenocarcinoma cells have more cytoplasm and display enlarged nuclei and prominent nucleoli. Basement membrane–like material is absent and cells are positive for prostatic markers and negative for basal cell markers.

4) Poorly differentiated urothelial carcinoma: The context in which invasive urothelial carcinoma is seen invading the prostate is usually in the event of a known concomitant

advanced bladder urothelial carcinoma directly invading the prostate or extensive CIS of the prostatic urethra secondarily involving the prostatic ducts (intraductal urothelial carcinoma), in a way in which basal cell carcinoma is usually not a differential diagnostic possibility. Histologically, however, and similar to basal cell carcinomas, urothelial carcinomas are associated with a desmoplastic stromal reaction, positive staining for basal cell markers, and negative staining for prostatic markers. However, the cells display abundant cytoplasm and pleomorphic features typically not seen in basal cell carcinomas.

Prognosis and Treatment

Most reported cases have been treated with TURP with a subset undergoing radical prostatectomy. Cases with advanced stage are treated with adjuvant radiotherapy and chemotherapy. Overall, a subset of basal cell carcinomas behaves aggressively with local recurrences and distant metastases reported in 30% of cases. In previously reported cases, these have been of the adenoid cystic variant.[75,79,80] Metastases typically involve the lung and liver with rare bone metastasis in comparison to acinar adenocarcinomas. In a recent series, among those with an aggressive behavior the predominant pattern was cases with large solid nests more often with central necrosis, high proliferative index, and less staining with basal cell markers.[76]

Lymphoma

Clinical Features

Lymphomas of the prostate are rare tumors that account for only 0.1% of all newly diagnosed lymphomas.[64,81] They typically present in older men (mean age is 65 years) with urinary obstructive symptoms. Urinary tract infections, or hematuria or may be detected incidentally in biopsies performed during workup of elevated serum PSA levels or even in radical prostatectomies. Systemic symptoms are unusual. Primary prostatic lymphoma with or without pelvic lymph nodal involvement is rarer than secondary involvement of the prostate by systemic lymphoma and accounts for <200 cases reported in the literature.[82] In one of the largest recent series by Chu et al.,[83] only 29 cases were found among over 4,800 cases reviewed (0.6%), including 18 that were primary to the prostate or pelvic lymph nodes. Clinical criteria that have been proposed for a diagnosis of primary prostatic lymphoma include the presence of a histologically proven lymphoma primarily affecting the prostate in the absence of liver, spleen, lymph nodes, and peripheral blood involvement within 1 month of diagnosis.

Pathology

Most reported primary lymphomas have been B-cell lymphomas of the small lymphocytic (small lymphocytic lymphoma [SLL]/chronic lymphocytic leukemia [CLL]), marginal zone, large cell (diffuse large B-cell lymphoma [DLBCL]) and follicular lymphoma, with DLBCL and SLL/CLL being the two most commonly reported subtypes (Fig. 10-30).[84,85] Secondary involvement of the prostate also occurs rarely as part of systemic disease dissemination and in that context, SLL/CLL is the most common subtype. Microscopically, the lymphoid infiltrate typically shows patchy or diffuse interstitial involvement of the prostatic stroma with characteristic preservation of prostatic acini. The infiltrate might also extend to the extraprostatic tissue. Lymphomas with a nodular pattern involving the prostate are seen infrequently. The entire spectrum of malignant lymphomas seen in other sites may become manifest in the prostate. These include undifferentiated (Burkitt-like) lymphomas, mantle cell lymphoma, angiotropic lymphoma, Hodgkin disease and T-cell lymphomas, as well as rare cases of myeloma and pseudolymphoma (Fig. 10-31).[86–92]

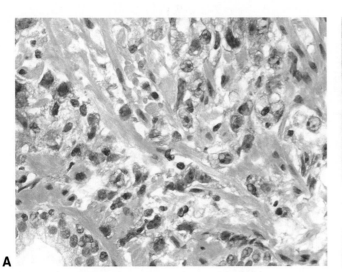
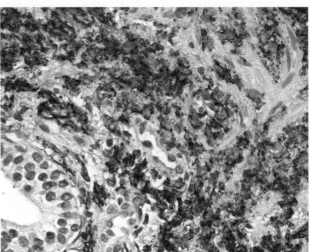

A   B

FIGURE 10-30 ■ **A:** Large cell lymphoma involving the prostate. **B:** CD20 immunoreactivity indicating B-cell differentiation in large cell lymphoma.

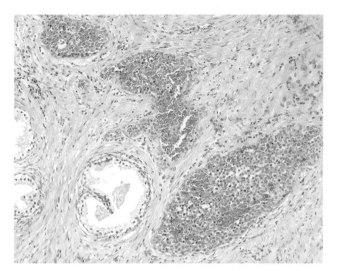

FIGURE 10-31 ■ Intravascular lymphoma involving the prostate.

Differential Diagnosis

The distinction between large cell lymphoma and poorly differentiated prostatic adenocarcinoma can readily be accomplished immunohistochemically with antibodies to keratin, prostatic markers, and lymphoid markers.

Florid chronic inflammation should be differentiated from low-grade lymphoma. In chronic inflammation, the inflammatory infiltrate is typically periglandular and is admixed with plasma cells, whereas low-grade lymphoma shows a more diffuse infiltrate that is not restricted to periglandular location. In addition, the lymphomatous infiltrate is not associated with plasma cells. In problematic cases, immunohistochemistry should be used. Another differential diagnostic possibility is with florid nonspecific granulomatous prostatitis, which in contrast to low-grade lymphomas typically involves the acini and

destroys them and might also be associated with an acute inflammatory infiltrate, both of which are features not seen in lymphoma.

Small cell carcinoma, high-grade stromal sarcoma, and rhabdomyosarcoma are also rarely considered on histologic grounds and their distinction from lymphoma is straightforward using immunohistochemical studies.

Prognosis

Malignant lymphoma involving the prostate is associated with a poor prognosis regardless of patient age, stage of presentation, or treatment regimen, with a disease-specific survival of 64% at 1 year, 33% at 5 years, and 16% at 15 years. There is also no difference in median survival after a diagnosis of prostatic involvement between primary and secondary lymphoma (23 months vs. 28 months, respectively).[84] The poor prognosis of prostatic lymphoma is related to the generalized disease that eventually results rather than to the prostatic involvement. The one exception to the poor prognosis associated with prostatic lymphoma appears to be SLL/CLL, where the prognosis is not affected by the prostatic involvement.

Leukemia

Clinical Features

The most common form of leukemic involvement of the prostate is that of CLL/SLL (Fig. 10-32).[83,93] Most patients, however, with leukemic involvement of the prostate are known leukemics or have their diagnosis established at the time of workup for urinary symptoms. It is often unclear whether the prostatic leukemic infiltrate in CLL is an incidental finding in patients with BPH or the cause of their obstructive symptoms. In other cases the diagnosis of leukemia is established on the prostate specimen usually removed for presumed BPH.

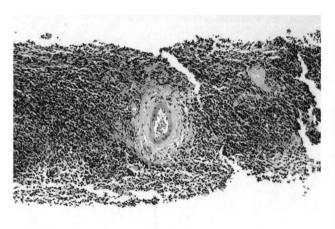

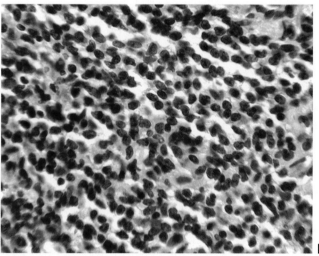

A   B

FIGURE 10-32 ■ **A:** Small lymphocytic lymphoma/chronic lymphocytic leukemia in the prostate. **B:** Monotonous population of small round lymphocytes in SLL/CLL.

Pathology

In CLL, there is a dense infiltrate of small mature round lymphocytes extensively infiltrating the prostatic stroma with preservation of prostatic glands. These lesions differ from nonspecific chronic inflammation in the prostate, where the inflammation tends to remain periglandular, is less dense, and often contains an admixture of plasma cells. Other forms of leukemia that have been described in the prostate include monocytic, granulocytic, and lymphoblastic leukemias.[82,94]

Plasmacytoma/Multiple Myeloma

Multiple myeloma involving the prostate is an extraordinarily rare neoplasm with most cases diagnosed incidentally at autopsy in patients with a known history of multiple myeloma. IgD and IgA myelomas have been described and rarely may cause urinary symptoms.[88,95]

Miscellaneous Primary Tumors

Other malignant tumors of the prostate include reports of a malignant mixed tumor resembling that seen in the salivary gland,[79] endodermal sinus tumor (yolk sac tumor),[96] seminoma[97] (Fig. 10-33), malignant mixed germ cell tumor,[98–100] rhabdoid tumor,[101] papillary cystadenocarcinoma,[102] tubulocystic clear cell adenocarcinoma as seen in the female genital tract (Fig. 10-34),[103] renal-type clear cell carcinoma,[104] ectomesenchymoma with rhabdomyosarcoma and ganglioneuroma,[105] peripheral neuroectodermal tumor primitive neuroectodermal tumor (Fig. 10-35),[106] and malignant perivascular epithelioid cell tumor (PECOMA).[107]

Hemangioma

Albeit rare, involvement of the prostatic urethra by hemangioma has more commonly been reported than primary prostatic hemangioma. Presenting symptoms include obstructive

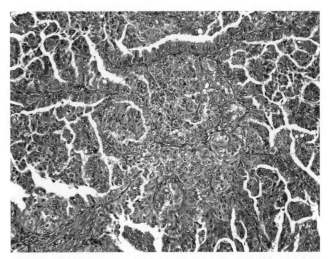

FIGURE 10-34 ■ Tubulopapillary clear cell adenocarcinoma of the prostate.

symptoms, hematuria, hematospermia, or postejaculation urethral bleeding.[108] Histologically, the diagnosis is straightforward and most have been reported as capillary or cavernous hemangiomas. Symptomatic lesions if diagnosed preoperatively should be treated with TURP. Some have recommended laser or bipolar evaporation.

Metastatic Tumors

In addition to urothelial carcinoma, colorectal adenocarcinomas may directly invade the prostate.[109] Usually colorectal adenocarcinomas that invade the prostate are not occult. Adenocarcinoma of the rectum infiltrating the prostate may resemble one of the patterns of prostatic duct adenocarcinomas (Figs. 10-36 and 10-37). Excluding hematopoietic neoplasms, the prostate is rarely involved by metastatic tumor. Metastases from malignant melanoma and carcinoma of the lung predominate (Fig. 10-38).[11]

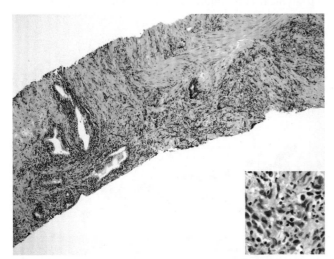

FIGURE 10-33 ■ Seminoma involving the prostate. Tumor cells were negative for epithelial and lymphoid markers and positive for placental alkaline phosphatase.

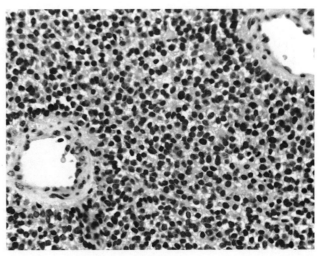

FIGURE 10-35 ■ Primitive neuroectodermal tumor of the prostate. Tumor diffusely expressed CD99.

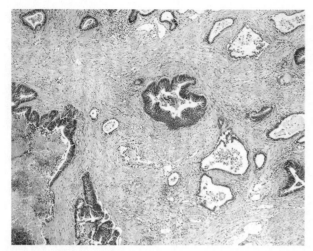

FIGURE 10-36 ■ Colonic adenocarcinoma invading the prostate.

Stromal Tumors of Uncertain Malignant Potential and Stromal Sarcomas

Introduction

Prostatic stromal tumors arising from the specialized prostatic stroma are rare and distinct tumors with diverse histologic patterns. In the past, these tumors have been reported under a variety of terms including atypical stromal (smooth muscle) hyperplasia, phyllodes type of atypical stromal hyperplasia, phyllodes tumor, and cystic epithelial–stromal tumors. As the phyllodes "leaf-like" pattern is only seen in a subset of both benign and malignant stromal tumors, it is preferable to designate stromal tumors of the prostate in more general descriptive terms as STUMPs and stromal sarcomas, as has also been recommended by the 2004 World Health Organization Classification of Tumours of the Urinary System and Male Genital Organs.[3]

Clinical Features

STUMPs have been reported to occur between the ages of 27 and 83 years, with a median age of 58 years and a peak incidence in the sixth and seventh decades.[110–112] Patients present most commonly with lower urinary tract obstruction, followed by an abnormal digital rectal examination, hematuria, hematospermia, rectal fullness, a palpable rectal mass, or less commonly elevated serum PSA levels.

In contrast to STUMPs, stromal sarcomas tend to affect a slightly younger population, with a reported age range of 25 to 86 years. Approximately half of all reported cases of stromal sarcoma occur before the age of 50 years. Stromal sarcomas may arise de novo or may exist in association with either a preexistent or a concurrent STUMP.

Pathology

On gross examination, STUMPs appear white-tan and may demonstrate a solid or solid-cystic pattern with smooth-walled cysts filled with bloody, mucinous, or clear fluid. These tumors may involve either the transition zone or the peripheral zone and may range in size from microscopic lesions (which are typically incidentally found) to large, cystic lesions up to 15 cm in size. Stromal sarcomas manifest as predominantly tan-white, solid, fleshy lesions ranging in size from 2 to 18 cm. Occasionally, areas of edema, hemorrhage, or small cysts may be identified.

Microscopically, four patterns of STUMP have been described and include (1) hypercellular stroma with scattered atypical, but degenerative-appearing cells admixed with benign prostatic glands (Fig. 10-39); (2) hypercellular stroma consisting of bland fusiform stromal cells with eosinophilic cytoplasm admixed with benign glands (Fig. 10-40); (3) leaf-like hypocellular fibrous stroma covered by benign-appearing prostatic epithelium similar in morphology to a benign phyllodes tumor of the breast (Fig. 10-41); and (4) myxoid stroma containing bland stromal cells and often lacking admixed glands (Fig. 10-42). Cases can exhibit a mixture of the above patterns.[112] Approximately half of all reported cases of STUMP demonstrate the first pattern of hypercellular stroma containing atypical cells intermixed with, but not compressing,

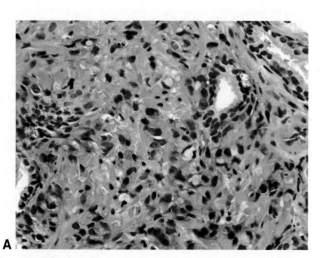

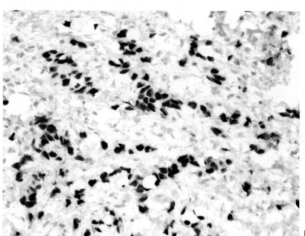

FIGURE 10-37 ■ **A:** Signet ring cell adenocarcinoma of the rectum invading the prostate. **B:** Signet ring cell adenocarcinoma of the rectum positive for CDX2.

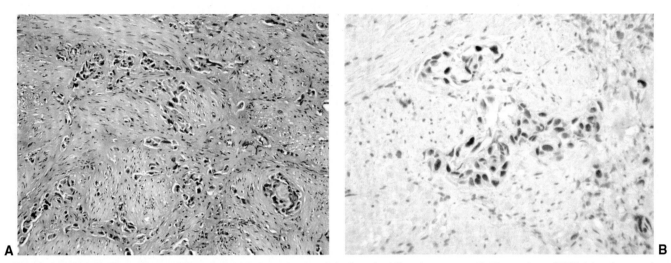

FIGURE 10-38 ■ **A:** Poorly differentiated adenocarcinoma of the lung invading the prostate. **B:** Expression of TTF-1 in adenocarcinoma of the lung invading the prostate.

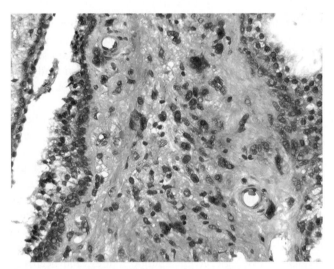

FIGURE 10-39 ■ Stromal tumor of the prostate (STUMP) with stromal cells showing degenerative atypia.

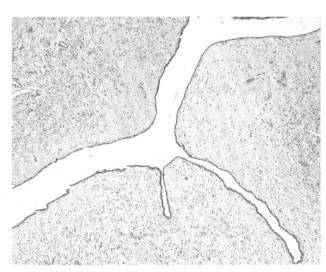

FIGURE 10-41 ■ Phyllodes pattern of STUMP.

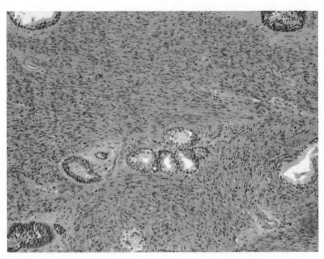

FIGURE 10-40 ■ STUMP composed of hypercellular stroma with prominent eosinophilic cytoplasm.

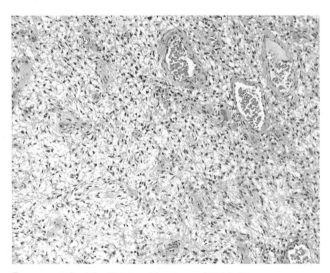

FIGURE 10-42 ■ Myxoid pattern of STUMP.

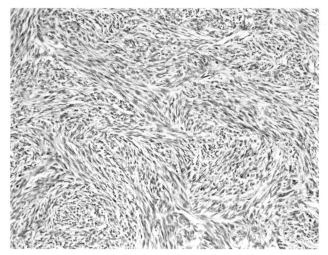

FIGURE 10-43 ■ Stromal sarcoma with storiform pattern.

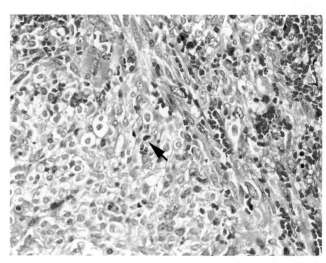

FIGURE 10-44 ■ Stromal sarcoma with epithelioid cells and numerous mitotic figures (*arrow*).

benign glands. The atypical stromal cells in these cases are pleomorphic and hyperchromatic, with a marked degenerative appearance. Mitotic figures are typically absent and atypical mitoses should not be seen. Although the admixed glands resemble normal benign prostatic glands, the glands within a STUMP may appear more crowded than acini in the surrounding uninvolved prostate. Cases of STUMP demonstrating hypercellular, elongated bland stromal cells with admixed glands may be readily misdiagnosed as cellular stroma associated with BPH, although the extent of hypercellularity and often more eosinophilic nature of the cytoplasm is unique. The benign, phyllodes pattern of STUMP may also contain atypical, degenerative-appearing stromal cells and may be associated with a variety of benign epithelial proliferations, including basal cell hyperplasia, adenosis, and sclerosing adenosis.[113]

Finally, the myxoid pattern of STUMP may be confused with stromal nodules of BPH, although the myxoid pattern of STUMP consists of extensive sheets of myxoid stroma without the nodularity identified in BPH. Occasionally the extensive myxoid stroma is admixed with benign prostate glands.

Microscopically, stromal sarcomas demonstrate either a solid growth of neoplastic stromal cells, which may have storiform, epithelioid, fibrosarcomatous, or patternless patterns, or may infiltrate between benign prostatic glands (Figs. 10-43 and 10-44). Less commonly stromal sarcomas may demonstrate leaf-like glands with underlying hypercellular stroma, which is also termed malignant phyllodes tumor (Fig. 10-45). Stromal sarcomas have one or more of the following features within the spindle cell component: hypercellularity, cytologic atypia, mitotic figures, and necrosis.

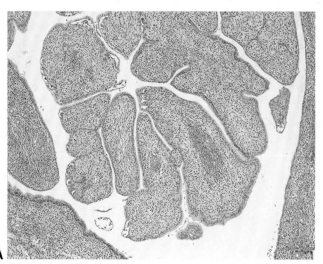

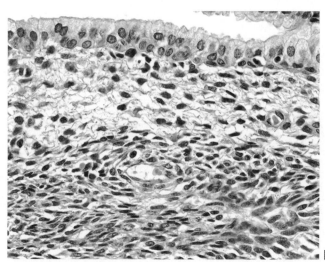

FIGURE 10-45 ■ **A:** Malignant phyllodes pattern of stromal sarcoma. **B:** Higher magnification of malignant phyllodes tumor with increased stromal cellularity beneath benign prostatic glands.

Stromal sarcomas may additionally be subclassified into low and high grades with high-grade tumors defined by moderate-marked pleomorphism and hypercellularity often with increased mitotic activity and occasional necrosis. Rarely, adenocarcinomas of the prostate can involve a stromal sarcoma.

Ancillary Studies

Immunohistochemical studies can be useful in differentiating stromal tumors from other prostatic spindle cell lesions but are not useful in distinguishing STUMP from stromal sarcoma, which relies on morphologic grounds alone. Most cases of STUMP and stromal sarcomas are positive for CD34 and vimentin and variably positive for SMA and desmin (Table 10-4). Progesterone receptor is frequently present on immunostaining, although estrogen receptor is less commonly positive. CKIT and S100 have been negative in all cases examined. In a subset of cases studied, pancytokeratin and CAM5.2 stains were negative.

Differential Diagnosis

Sarcomatoid carcinoma: Can overlap with stromal sarcoma as both show a proliferation of malignant spindle cells. In sarcomatoid carcinoma, however, there is either an associated acinar adenocarcinoma component or a known history of prostatic adenocarcinoma with radiation or hormonal therapy. In addition, the spindle cells are usually positive for cytokeratins HMWK, CK5/6, p63.

Prostatic hyperplasia: Can overlap with STUMP with hypercellular stroma. However, in contrast to BPH, this pattern of STUMP is not associated with the typical small hyalinized blood vessels seen with BPH. In addition, stromal cells of STUMP in this pattern have a distinctive eosinophilic cytoplasm. STUMPs with degenerative atypia may also have florid glandular proliferations mimicking BPH. The key is to recognize scattered stromal cells with atypical but degenerative nuclei. The myxoid pattern of STUMP can also be misdiagnosed as BPH. In contrast to BPH, this pattern of STUMP is not associated with the typical

small hyalinized blood vessels seen with BPH and consists of sheets and sheets of myxoid stromal cells without nodularity.

Smooth muscle tumors: Leiomyosarcoma is the most common sarcoma involving the prostate. It usually shows a distinctive fascicular pattern of growth and typical cigar-shaped nuclei and deeply eosinophilic cytoplasm, which are not typically seen in stromal sarcomas. In contrast to stromal sarcomas, CD34 is negative while desmin and caldesmon are strongly positive. However, PR can be positive and is therefore not very useful in that context, except if totally negative, which goes against a tumor of prostatic stromal origin.

GISTs: Are very rare and characteristically show a relatively bland fascicular spindle cell tumor with nuclear palisading and perinuclear vacuoles, and diffuse and strong staining for CD117 and DOG1. Of note is that CD34 can be positive, and is thus not helpful in differentiation from stromal tumors.

Prognosis and Treatment

Although STUMPs are generally considered to represent a benign neoplastic stromal process, a subset of STUMPs has been associated with stromal sarcoma on concurrent biopsy material or has demonstrated stromal sarcoma on repeat biopsy, suggesting a malignant progression in at least some cases (Fig. 10-46).[112] There appears to be no correlation between the pattern of STUMP and association with stromal sarcoma. As most STUMPs are confined to the prostate and rarely progress to sarcoma, STUMPs are in general associated with a good prognosis. The variability in behavior of STUMPs and stromal sarcomas, and their occasional coexistence, leads to challenges in patient management. Although many STUMPs may behave in an indolent fashion, their unpredictability in a minority of cases and the lack of correlation between different histologic patterns of STUMPs and sarcomatous dedifferentiation

Antibody	GIST	SFT	STUMP	Schwannoma	Smooth Muscle Tumor
C-KIT	+	–	–	–	–
CD34	+	+	+	+/–	–
S100	–	–	–	+	–
Actin	+/–	–	+/–	–	+
Desmin	–	–	+/–	–	+

Table 10-4 ■ IMMUNOHISTOCHEMISTRY IN DIFFERENTIAL DIAGNOSIS OF GIST ON PROSTATE BIOPSY

–, <10% of tumors positive; +/–, 10% to 50% of tumors positive; +, >50% of tumors positive.

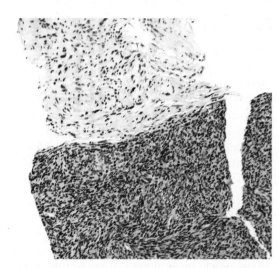

FIGURE 10-46 ■ Needle biopsy of the prostate with high-grade stromal sarcoma (*below*) and STUMP with degenerative atypia (*above*).

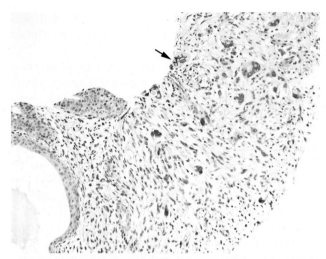

FIGURE 10-47 ■ Stroma sarcoma on prostate needle biopsy. Note atypical mitotic figure (*arrow*).

warrant close follow-up and consideration of definitive resection in younger individuals. Factors to consider in deciding whether to proceed with definitive resection for STUMPs diagnosed on biopsy include patient age and treatment preference, presence and size of the lesion on rectal exam or imaging studies, and extent of the lesion on tissue sampling. Careful review for atypical mitotic figures in what otherwise might appear to be a STUMP with degenerative atypia is essential so as not to underdiagnose a stromal sarcoma on needle biopsy (Fig. 10-47). Expectant management with close clinical follow-up could be considered in an older individual with a limited lesion on biopsy where there is no lesion identified on digital rectal exam or on imaging studies.

Stromal sarcomas can extend out of the prostate and metastasize to distant sites, such as bone, lung, abdomen, and retroperitoneum.

Inflammatory Myofibroblastic Tumor

Introduction

This spindle cell lesion has been described using a variety of terms in the literature, including pseudosarcomatous fibromyxoid tumor, inflammatory pseudotumor, and IMT. In the past, similar lesions that appeared following TURP for nodular hyperplasia were called postoperative spindle cell nodule. Due to significant overlapping morphologic, immunohistochemical, and molecular features, all similar lesions are currently considered to be the same and are called IMTs, whether a previous history of instrumentation is present or not.

Clinical Features

Most cases have been reported in men ranging from 42 to 67 years of age. The lesions range in size from small measuring <1 cm, which can be discovered incidentally on TURP specimens, to large lesions, which can cause obstructive symptoms.

Pathology

Similar to IMTs in other sites, prostatic IMT are composed of intersecting fascicles of spindle cells with haphazard arrangement and tissue culture–like background. Associated granulation tissue–type vascularity, extravasated red blood cells, and inflammatory cells are typical features. Prominent myxoid changes can also be seen. The spindle cells have abundant long tapering cytoplasm and elongated uniform nuclei that display fine chromatin and one or two distinct nucleoli. Mitoses may be seen but atypical mitotic figures are not. These lesions may be infiltrative into and even through the muscularis propria.

Ancillary Studies

IMTs commonly coexpress cytokeratins (low molecular weight form, pancytokeratin) and SMA. They are typically negative for HMWK and CK5/6, and two-thirds express ALK. Desmin reactivity is variable but caldesmon is usually negative.

Differential Diagnosis

The typical cytomorphologic and immunohistochemical features of IMT are usually very helpful in distinguishing them from malignant spindle cell tumors, namely, sarcomatoid carcinoma, leiomyosarcoma, and stromal sarcoma. One should, however, be familiar with the several atypical morphologic features that can be seen in IMTs in order not to overdiagnose them as malignant tumors. Those include hypercellularity, infiltrative pattern of growth, necrosis, and increased mitotic activity, although atypical mitotic figures are not seen. In addition, tumor cells may occasionally show strong keratin expression. In sarcomatoid carcinoma, there is usually an associated acinar adenocarcinoma component or a known history of prostatic adenocarcinoma with radiation or hormonal therapy. IMT features that are distinctive from sarcomatoid carcinoma include the tissue culture appearance, the typical granulation tissue–type vascularity and associated inflammatory cells, and the lack of marked nuclear pleomorphism and hyperchromasia. IMTs express ALK1 in two-thirds of cases in contrast to sarcomatoid carcinoma cells, which are negative. In comparison to IMTs, leiomyosarcomas show a more organized pattern of growth with the interlacing fascicular pattern typical of smooth muscle tumors. Cells of leiomyosarcoma have deeply eosinophilic cytoplasm and show usually high-grade cytologic features with hyperchromatic nuclei and numerous mitotic figures. In contrast to IMTs, they are strongly positive for caldesmon and negative for ALK. Stromal sarcomas are also overtly malignant tumors and display positive CD34 and PR staining and negative staining for ALK and SMA. Table 10-5 includes a detailed morphologic and immunohistochemical comparison of entities with myxoid stroma that overlap with IMT.

Table 10-5 ■ MYXOID LESIONS

	Inflammatory Myofibroblastic Tumor	Sarcomatoid Carcinoma	Myxoid Leiomyosarcoma	Myxoid Rhabdomyosarcoma	Myxoid Undifferentiated Sarcoma	Myxoid Changes of Nodular Hyperplasia	Myxoid STUMP
Associated acinar adenocarcinoma	−	+/−	−	−	−	−	−
Cellularity	Variable, usually low	High	Variable	Variable	Variable	Variable	Variable
Growth pattern	Tissue culture-like	Haphazard arrangement of spindle cells	Intersecting fascicles of spindle cells	Haphazard arrangement of spindle cells with subepithelial condensation	Storiform growth of spindle cells	Nodular growth	Diffuse haphazard growth of spindle cells
Pleomorphism	Usually −, can be + (focal)	++	+	+	+++	−	−
Hyperchromasia	−	+	+	+	+	−	−
Vessels	Slit-like (granulation-tissue like)	Unremarkable	Unremarkable	Unremarkable	Unremarkable	Prominent small round hyalinized vessels	Can have admixed unremarkable vessels
Necrosis	Usually −, can be +	Usually +, can be −	Usually +	Usually +	Usually +	−	−
Mitotic figures	+	+	+	+	++	−	−/+
Atypical mitosis	−	+	+	+	+	−	−
Cytokeratin	+ For low molecular form	+ (Low and high molecular forms)	−/+ (Usually focal)	−	−	+	−
Vimentin	+	+	+	+	+	+	+
Prostatic markers (PSA, PSMA, PSAP, prostein)	−	+/−	−	−	−	−	−
SMA	+	+/−	+	+	−	+/−	+/−
Desmin	+/−	+/−	+	+	−	+/−	+/−
Caldesmon	−	+/−	+	−	−	−	−
Myogenin	−	+/−	−	+	−	−	−
ALK-1	+/−	−	−	−	−	−	−
PR	−	−	−/+	−	−	−	+
CD34	−	−	−	−	−	+	+

Prognosis and Treatment

Most IMTs follow a benign course, although incomplete excision may lead to recurrence. Lesions may extend outside of the prostate and may require definitive cure with radical prostatectomy.

Blue Nevus

Blue nevus may rarely involve the prostate with 28 reported cases to date.[114] They are usually an incidental finding detected either in prostatectomy specimens or in autopsy material. The gross appearance generally consists of multiple brown to black streaks or nodules that can range in size from 0.1 to 2.0 cm. Microscopically, they are composed of stromal cells that contain finely granular brown or black pigment, which may also be seen in the extracellular matrix. The cells can extensively infiltrate the surrounding fibromuscular stroma individually or as irregularly clustered collections. The pigment-laden cells are usually spindle in shape with bipolar, elongated dendritic cytoplasmic processes; they can also be round, ovoid, or polygonal. The nuclei have been described as centrally located and often obscured by the abundant melanin present in the cytoplasm. Cells are positive for S100 and usually lack HMB-45 expression. Another potentially useful immunostain is CD68, which in contrast to the staining in hemosiderin-laden macrophages is negative. Distinction of melanin from lipofuscin or hemosiderin is usually done on morphologic grounds alone. Blue nevus should also be distinguished from malignant melanoma that has overt malignant features and in which cells express HMB-45. Blue nevi are benign lesions that do not progress to melanoma.[114]

Leiomyoma

It is difficult to diagnose a leiomyoma of the prostate, mainly because it is difficult to distinguish from a stromal nodule of hyperplasia (Fig. 10-48).[115] Both entities may contain

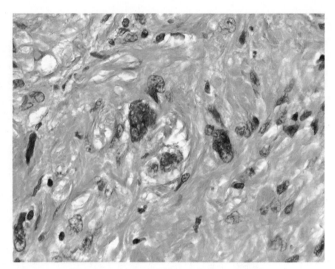

FIGURE 10-49 ■ Leiomyoma of the prostate with low cellularity and degenerative atypia.

abundant smooth muscle, although leiomyomas typically demonstrate well-organized fascicles and may have other degenerative features such as hyalinization and calcification that are not commonly seen in stromal nodules. Large single leiomyomas that are symptomatic are rare.[116,117] Leiomyomas demonstrate virtually no mitotic activity and minimal to no nuclear atypia, with the exception of occasional scattered degenerative nuclei in a normocellular background (Fig. 10-49). The vast majority of leiomyosarcomas of the prostate are high-grade tumors with necrosis, pleomorphism, and mitosis, which makes the distinction from leiomyomas straightforward. However, low-grade leiomyosarcomas exist, and those are distinguished from leiomyomas by a moderate amount of atypia, focal areas of increased cellularity, scattered mitotic figures, and/or a focally infiltrative growth pattern around benign prostatic glands at the periphery.

Solitary Fibrous Tumor

Introduction

There are fewer than 20 cases of solitary fibrous tumor (SFT) involving the prostate reported as single cases and one series of 12 cases.[118] Some older reported cases of hemangiopericytoma of the prostate may also be classified as SFT.

Clinical Features

Prostatic SFTs have been reported in patients ranging in age from 21 to 75 years and the most common clinical findings include lower urinary retention, urinary frequency, dysuria, constipation, incontinence, and groin pain.

Pathology

These tumors have a broad size distribution, ranging from 2 to 14 cm, with many reported to be >5 cm. Microscopically, prostatic SFTs appear similar to those identified in extraprostatic

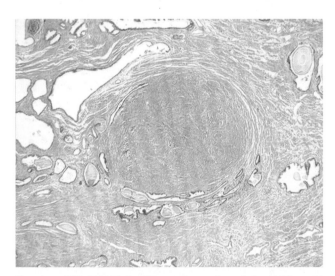

FIGURE 10-48 ■ Small smooth muscle nodule, which could be considered small leiomyoma or smooth muscle nodule of nodular hyperplasia.

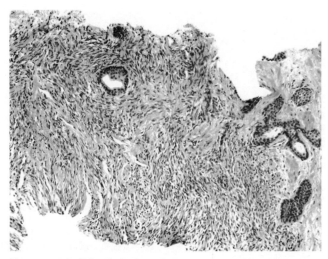

FIGURE 10-50 ■ Solitary fibrous tumor invading the prostate.

sites. Uniform spindle cells with bland nuclei are arranged in a "patternless" pattern in a background of variable ropy collagen (Figs. 10-50 and 10-51). Many cases demonstrate a hemangiopericytomatous appearance. Admixed prostatic tissue is not commonly associated with these lesions.

Ancillary Studies

Immunohistochemistry generally reveals diffuse reactivity for CD34, vimentin, and BCL2, although rare SFTs may lack some of these markers. Staining for CD99, beta-catenin, p53, SMA, and muscle-specific actin have also been reported. These tumors are typically negative for pancytokeratin, S100, and CD117 CKIT (Table 10-4).

Prognosis

None of the prostatic SFTs have behaved in an aggressive fashion. However, based on the behavior of SFTs in other sites and the finding of hypercellularity, pleomorphism, necrosis,

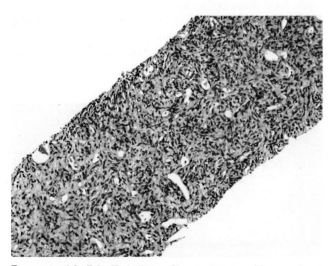

FIGURE 10-51 ■ Solitary fibrous tumor with prominent hemangiopericytomatous pattern invading the prostate.

and infiltrative margins in some prostatic SFTs, careful long-term clinical follow-up is warranted regardless of their histology (Fig. 10-52). It is preferable not to designate them as "benign" or "malignant," but rather note whether there are any features particularly worrisome for aggressive behavior.

Leiomyosarcoma

Introduction

Sarcomas of the prostate account for 0.1% to 0.2% of all malignant prostatic tumors.[119] Leiomyosarcoma is the most common sarcoma involving the prostate in adults, yet is still rare.

Clinical Features

Leiomyosarcoma affects men between the ages of 40 and 78 years. It most frequently presents with urinary obstruction, as well as perineal/pelvic pain, urinary frequency, hematuria, constipation, rectal pain, and pain or burning on ejaculation.[119,120]

Pathology

Lesions range in size from 3 to 21 cm. Microscopically, these hypercellular lesions are composed of intersecting bundles of spindle cells with moderate to severe atypia (Fig. 10-53). The vast majority of leiomyosarcomas in the literature have been high-grade with frequent mitoses and necrosis, although we have also seen rare cases of low-grade prostatic leiomyosarcoma.[121] As opposed to some stromal sarcomas, leiomyosarcomas lack admixed normal glands, except entrapped glands at the periphery.

Ancillary Studies

Leiomyosarcomas commonly express vimentin, actin, and desmin. Cytokeratin expression is observed in about one-quarter of cases.[120] In addition, some leiomyosarcomas have been reported to express the progesterone receptor, similar to STUMPs and stromal sarcomas[122] (Table 10-4).

Prognosis and Treatment

Patients with leiomyosarcoma commonly have a poor outcome, with the clinical course characterized by multiple recurrences. The majority (50% to 75%) of patients die from disease within 2 to 5 years with metastatic spread most commonly to the lungs, often several years following initial diagnosis. In the study by Sexton et al.,[119] the prognosis for leiomyosarcoma of the prostate, as for sarcomas of the prostate in general, was not dependent on stage, with the exception of a better prognosis for those men who presented without distant metastases. The only other variable that these authors found to be predictive of a favorable prognosis was complete surgical resection with microscopically negative margins. Optimal treatment requires a multimodal approach rather than surgery alone. The survival of patients with isolated local recurrences may be prolonged with salvage surgery.

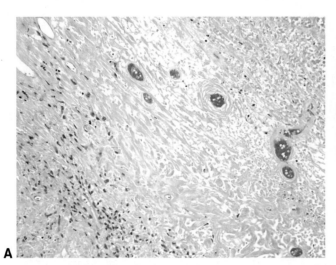

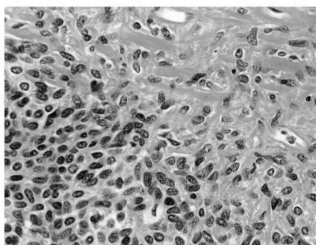

FIGURE 10-52 ■ **A:** Malignant SFT of the prostate with necrosis. **B:** Malignant SFT of the prostate with increased cellularity (*bottom*).

Gastrointestinal Stromal Tumor

Clinical Features

Patients range in age from 42 to 65 years and present with urinary obstructive symptoms, rectal fullness, and abnormal digital rectal examination.[123] Although GIST lesions may clinically present as primary prostatic processes on imaging studies and clinical exam, such cases are typically large masses arising from the rectum or perirectal space that compress but do not invade the prostate (Fig. 10-54). Exceptionally, they may also invade the prostate. Most cases of "prostatic" GISTs are sampled on prostatic needle biopsy, although we have seen one case sampled on a transurethral resection. There is only one prior case reported in the English literature of a GIST that appeared to be localized to the prostate based on computed tomography and magnetic resonance imaging.[124] This patient presented simultaneously with multiple liver metastases and the prostatic mass was not resected. It is doubtful whether this neoplasm was truly a prostatic primary, as studies have demonstrated that imaging studies cannot reliably determine the origin of large GISTs. Consequently, to date there is no fully documented example of a GIST arising within the prostate. Typically, GIST is not considered in the differential diagnosis of spindle cell lesions of the prostate, although the unique management of these tumors underscores the importance of recognizing these tumors. Misdiagnosis of GISTs involving the prostate is not uncommon, and several patients have undergone pelvic exenteration, irradiation, and chemotherapy for a misdiagnosis of pelvic sarcoma.[125]

Pathology

Tumor size ranges from 1 to 14 cm. Microscopically, "prostatic" GISTs are morphologically identical to those found within the gastrointestinal tract. GIST is composed of spindled cells with a fascicular growth pattern (Fig. 10-55). Additional histologic findings include focal epithelioid features, focal dense collagenous stroma, areas with a patternless pattern, and perinuclear halos. When present, a fascicular or palisading growth pattern and perinuclear vacuoles along with a lack of collagen deposition aids in the discrimination of GIST from SFT and STUMP.

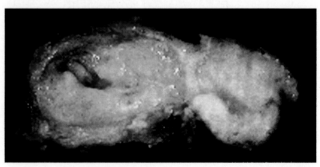

FIGURE 10-53 ■ Leiomyosarcoma of the prostate.

FIGURE 10-54 ■ Gastrointestinal stromal tumor (*right*) adherent to the prostate (*left*).

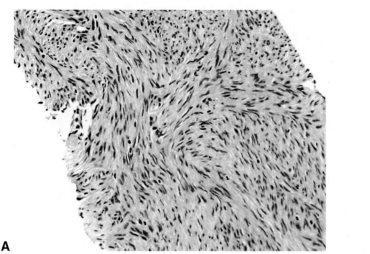

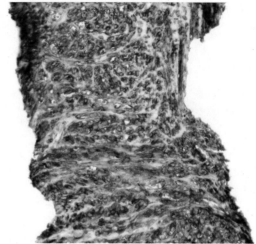

A

B

FIGURE 10-55 ■ **A:** GIST on prostate needle biopsy. **B:** Positivity for CD117 (c-kit) in GIST on prostate biopsy.

Ancillary Studies

CD117/CKIT is uniformly expressed in all cases and CD34 is positive in almost all cases studied (Fig. 10-55) (Table 10-4). S100, desmin, and SMA are negative. On prostate biopsy, it may be difficult to distinguish a GIST from other spindle cell tumors due to limited material. Consequently, prior to rendering a diagnosis of SFT, schwannoma, leiomyosarcoma, or stromal sarcoma, GIST should be considered in the differential diagnosis. Furthermore, immunostains for CD117 should be performed to verify the diagnosis. CD34 is not discriminatory as it is positive in GISTs, SFTs, and specialized prostatic stromal tumors, and variably positive in schwannomas. Strong positive staining for desmin can help discriminate smooth muscle tumors from the other lesions. Similarly, positive immunoreactivity to S100 may aid in diagnosing neural tumors. SMA is typically expressed in smooth muscle tumors, and is variably positive in STUMPs and GISTs and typically negative in SFT and schwannoma.

Prognosis and Treatment

Tumors with malignant potential show elevated mitotic rates of >5 per 50 HPF, cytologically malignant features (high cellularity and overlapping nuclei), or necrosis. A subset of patients treated with the CKIT tyrosine kinase inhibitor imatinib (Gleevec) following the diagnosis of "prostatic" GIST demonstrated a subsequent reduction in tumor size.[123] No long-term follow-up is currently available on these patients to determine if the biologic behavior of GISTs secondarily involving the prostate is different than that described in other sites.

Rhabdomyosarcoma

Clinical Features

The vast majority of rhabdomyosarcomas of the prostate occur in the pediatric population with an average age at diagnosis of 5 years.[126,127] There are <20 prostatic rhabdomyosarcomas

that have been reported in adults ranging in age from 17 to 68 years.[128,129]

Pathology

Because of their large size at the time of diagnosis, distinction between rhabdomyosarcoma originating in the bladder and that originating in the prostate may be difficult. Histologically, most prostate rhabdomyosarcomas are of the embryonal subtype and are considered to be of favorable histology (Figs. 10-56 and 10-57). A single case of the botryoid subtype of embryonal rhabdomyosarcoma has also been reported.[130] Embryonal rhabdomyosarcomas of the prostate are similar to those seen in other organs and may assume a wide variety of histologic patterns. Embryonal rhabdomyosarcoma cells may vary from primitive cells with scant cytoplasm to more well-differentiated tumors with abundant eosinophilic cytoplasm in which cross striations may be seen by light microscopy. Embryonal rhabdomyosarcomas may also assume a cellular spindle cell

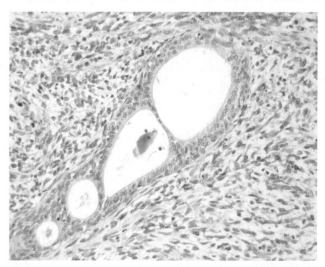

FIGURE 10-56 ■ Embryonal rhabdomyosarcoma infiltrating the prostate.

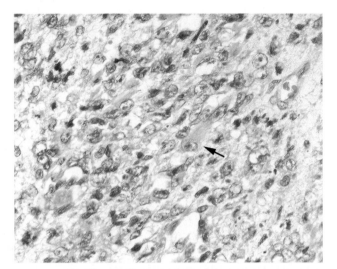

FIGURE 10-57 ■ Embryonal rhabdomyosarcoma with occasional strap cells (*arrow*) infiltrating the prostate.

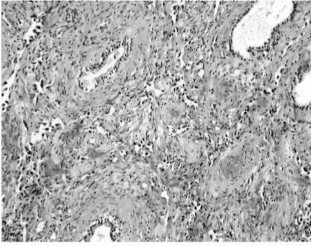

FIGURE 10-59 ■ Vasoformative angiosarcoma infiltrating the prostate.

appearance with a tendency to encircle preserved prostatic glands or a myxoid growth pattern. The use of immunohistochemical, ultrastructural, and molecular techniques may be useful in the diagnosis of embryonal rhabdomyosarcoma involving the prostate. It is important to identify those rare cases of alveolar rhabdomyosarcoma involving the prostate, since this histologic subtype is unfavorable and necessitates more aggressive chemotherapy.

Prognosis

With chemotherapy, the few patients with localized disease (stage 1) or microscopic regional disease (stage 2) stand an excellent chance of being cured. The usual therapy for localized disease is to biopsy or partially excise the tumor, followed by intensive chemotherapy and radiotherapy. If tumor persists despite several courses of this therapy, then radical surgery is performed. Most patients present with stage 3 disease, in which there is gross residual disease following

incomplete resection or biopsy. While the majority of patients with gross residual disease (stage 3) have remained without evidence of disease for a long period of time, approximately 15% to 20% die of their tumor. A smaller but significant proportion of patients present with distant metastases. The prognosis for patients with metastatic tumor (stage 4) is more dismal, with most patients dying of their tumor.

Miscellaneous Mesenchymal Tumors

Other rare mesenchymal lesions of the prostate are hemangioma,[131] chondroma,[132] cartilaginous metaplasia,[133] malignant peripheral nerve sheath tumor,[134] schwannoma,[135] chondrosarcoma,[136] synovial sarcoma (Fig. 10-58),[137–139] granular cell tumor,[140] angiosarcoma (Figs. 10-59 and 10-60),[141] neurofibroma,[142] malignant fibrous histiocytoma,[119,143–145] and hemangiopericytoma.[146] The one case reported of an osteosarcoma was in a patient with a prior history of adenocarcinoma of the prostate treated with radiotherapy and

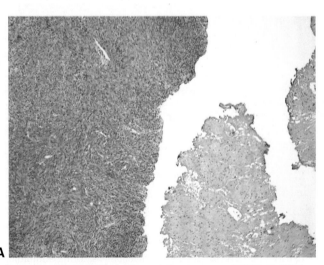

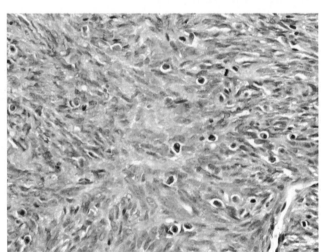

FIGURE 10-58 ■ **A:** Synovial sarcoma on TURP. **B:** Higher magnification of prostatic monophasic synovial sarcoma.

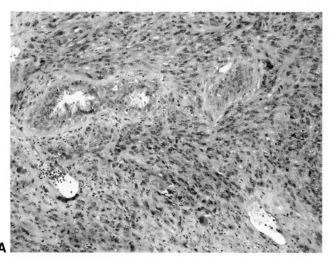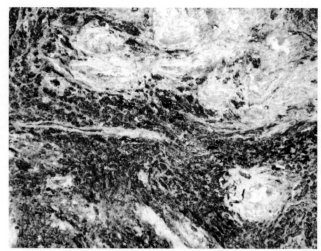

FIGURE 10-60 ■ **A:** Poorly differentiated angiosarcoma involving the prostate. **B:** Strong CD31 immunostaining of prostatic angiosarcoma.

most likely represents a sarcomatoid carcinoma with an osteogenic sarcoma component.[147]

Cystadenoma (Multilocular Cyst)

Introduction

There have been rare reports of multilocular cystic lesions between the bladder and the rectum, which may be separate from the prostate or attached to it by a pedicle. These masses can grow up to 20 cm in diameter.[148]

Clinical Features

Patients present usually present in the late 50s with obstructive urinary symptoms with or without a palpable abdominal mass. The mass is usually palpable by digital rectal examination. Serum PSA levels may be elevated.

Pathology

Microscopically, the cysts are lined by atrophic prostatic epithelium, which reacts with prostatic markers and show the lack of basal cells' immunostaining, leading to a potential erroneous diagnosis of carcinoma on needle biopsies. Focal papillae and even cribriform architecture have been reported within the cysts, and in one case multifocal HGPIN was found in the cysts.[149]

Differential Diagnosis

Nodular hyperplasia, stromal tumor of uncertain malignant potential (STUMP), cystadenocarcinoma, and retrovesical and retroperitoneal multilocular tumors such as multilocular peritoneal inclusion cysts, lymphangiomas, müllerian duct cysts, and seminal vesicle cysts should be considered in the differential diagnosis. Cystadenomas lack the leaf-like projections of STUMP, and the other multilocular tumors can be excluded based on the prostatic epithelial lining in the cystadenoma. The distinction of intraprostatic multilocular cyst from cystic nodular hyperplasia may be difficult, and the

diagnosis of intraprostatic cystadenoma should be restricted to cases where one-half of the prostate resembles normal prostatic tissue and the remaining prostate is enlarged by a solitary encapsulated nodule composed of epithelium and/or cysts.[150] Before diagnosing an intraprostatic cystadenoma one must first exclude a STUMP with prominent epithelial proliferation.[113] Cystadenocarcinoma can be separated from cystadenoma based on malignant-appearing lining epithelium, which is often a papillary adenocarcinoma.

Prognosis and Treatment

Those lesions may recur if incompletely excised and may require extensive surgery because of their large size and impingement on surrounding structures.

TUMORS OF THE SEMINAL VESICLE

Cystadenoma

Clinical Features

Cystadenoma is a rare benign tumor of the seminal vesicles.[151] Patients range in age from 37 to 66 years and may be asymptomatic or symptomatic with bladder outlet obstruction. Ultrasound may reveal a complex, solid-cystic pelvic mass.

Pathology

Microscopically, cystadenomas are well circumscribed and contain variably sized glandular spaces with branching contours and cysts surrounded by a spindle cell stroma. The glands contain pale intraluminal secretions, and are lined by one or two layers of cuboidal to columnar cells. No significant cytologic atypia, mitotic activity, or necrosis is seen.

Prognosis

The tumor has a benign outcome but may recur after incomplete resection.

Adenocarcinoma

Clinical Features

Primary adenocarcinomas of the seminal vesicle are rare with an approximate number of 55 published cases.[152,153] The mean age is 62 years (range 24 to 90 years). Patients usually present with obstructive uropathy due to a nontender perirectal mass and less commonly hematuria or hematospermia. Serum carcinoembryonic antigen may be elevated.

Pathology

Grossly, the tumors are usually large (3 to 5.0 cm) and often invade the bladder, ureter, or rectum. Microscopically, the tumors have nonspecific histologic features with papillary, trabecular, and glandular patterns and varying degrees of differentiation (Figs. 10-61 and 10-62). Rarely, tumors may be undifferentiated, or may produce abundant extracelluar

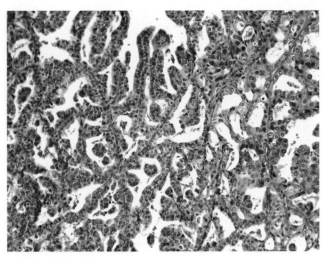

FIGURE 10-61 ■ Seminal vesicle adenocarcinoma with papillary formation.

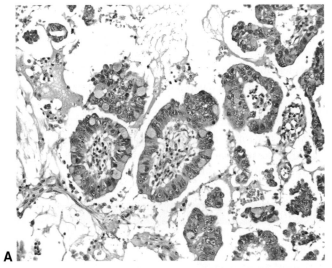

A

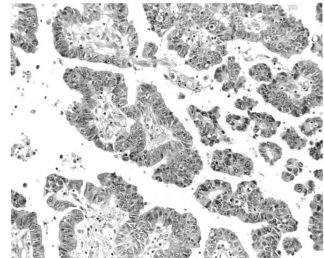

B

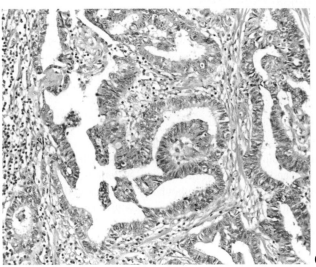

C

FIGURE 10-62 ■ **A:** Seminal vesicle adenocarcinoma. **B:** Papillary seminal vesicle adenocarcinoma without mucin formation. **C:** Seminal vesicle adenocarcinoma with gland formation.

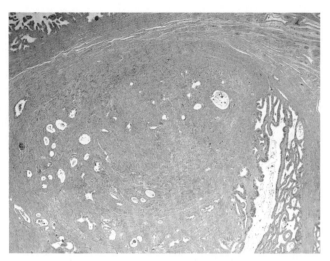

FIGURE 10-63 ■ Seminal vesicle adenofibroma.

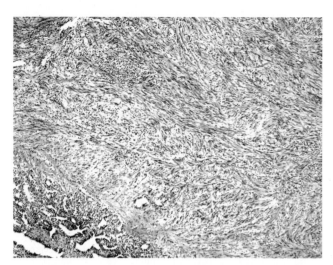

FIGURE 10-64 ■ Leiomyosarcoma primary in the seminal vesicle (*lower left*).

mucin (colloid carcinoma). The diagnosis requires exclusion of secondary involvement by carcinomas of the prostate, bladder, or rectum, based on clinical information and immunohistochemistry. Normal seminal vesicles and seminal vesicle adenocarcinomas are positive for CEA and CK7 and negative for PSA, PAP, and CK20.

Prognosis and Treatment

The prognosis of primary seminal vesicle adenocarcinoma is poor. Most patients present with metastases and in 95% of patients the survival is <3 years

Mixed Epithelial–Stromal Tumors

Mixed epithelial–stromal tumors are extremely rare neoplasms composed of both neoplastic epithelial and stromal elements.[154] Less than 25 cases have been reported and the mean age at presentation is 51 years. Presenting symptoms include obstructive urinary symptoms, abdominal pain, constipation, and painful ejaculation. They range in biologic behavior from benign, such as adenofibroma and adenomyoma, to low-grade and high-grade malignant mixed epithelial–stromal tumors, with the grade determined based on stromal cellularity, atypia, mitoses, and necrosis (Fig. 10-63).

Sarcomas

Sarcomas of the seminal vesicle are even rarer than carcinomas. As with carcinomas, many of the published cases are poorly documented in terms of both the origin of tumor and the histologic subtype. Well-documented cases of angiosarcoma and leiomyosarcoma of the seminal vesicles have been reported[155,156] (Fig. 10-64).

Miscellaneous

Rare primary germ cell tumors of the seminal vesicle such as seminoma and choriocarcinoma have been reported.[157,158] These probably arise from germ cells entrapped there during fetal development.

REFERENCES

1. Parwani AV, Kronz JD, Genega EM, et al. Prostate carcinoma with squamous differentiation: an analysis of 33 cases. *Am J Surg Pathol* 2004;28:651–657.
2. Bassler TJ Jr, Orozco R, Bassler IC, et al. Adenosquamous carcinoma of the prostate: case report with DNA analysis, immunohistochemistry, and literature review. *Urology* 1999;53:832–834.
3. Eble JN, Sauter G, Epstein JI, et al. *The World Health Organization Classification of Tumours of the Urinary System and Male Genital System*. Lyon, France: IARC Press, 2004:209–211.
4. Dundore PA, Cheville JC, Nascimento AG, et al. Carcinosarcoma of the prostate. Report of 21 cases. *Cancer* 1995;76:1035–1042.
5. Lauwers GY, Schevchuk M, Armenakas N, et al. Carcinosarcoma of the prostate. *Am J Surg Pathol* 1993;17:342–349.
6. Hansel DE, Epstein JI. Sarcomatoid carcinoma of the prostate: a study of 42 cases. *Am J Surg Pathol* 2006;30:1316–1321.
7. Shannon RL, Ro JY, Grignon DJ, et al. Sarcomatoid carcinoma of the prostate. A clinicopathologic study of 12 patients. *Cancer* 1992;69:2676–2682.
8. Abrahamsson PA. Neuroendocrine cells in tumour growth of the prostate. *Endocr Relat Cancer* 1999;6:503–519.
9. Abrahamsson PA, Falkmer S, Falt K, et al. The course of neuroendocrine differentiation in prostatic carcinomas. An immunohistochemical study testing chromogranin A as an "endocrine marker." *Pathol Res Pract* 1989;185:373–380.
10. Aprikian AG, Cordon-Cardo C, Fair WR, et al. Characterization of neuroendocrine differentiation in human benign prostate and prostatic adenocarcinoma. *Cancer* 1993;71:3952–3965.
11. Johnson DE, Chalbaud R, Ayala AG. Secondary tumors of the prostate. *J Urol* 1974;112:507–508.
12. Jongsma J, Oomen MH, Noordzij MA, et al. Different profiles of neuroendocrine cell differentiation evolve in the PC-310 human prostate cancer model during long-term androgen deprivation. *Prostate* 2002;50:203–215.
13. Jongsma J, Oomen MH, Noordzij MA, et al. Kinetics of neuroendocrine differentiation in an androgen-dependent human prostate xenograft model. *Am J Pathol* 1999;154:543–551.
14. Burchardt T, Burchardt M, Chen MW, et al. Transdifferentiation of prostate cancer cells to a neuroendocrine cell phenotype in vitro and in vivo. *J Urol* 1999;162:1800–1805.
15. Berruti A, Mosca A, Tucci M, et al. Independent prognostic role of circulating chromogranin A in prostate cancer patients with hormone-refractory disease. *Endocr Relat Cancer* 2005;12:109–117.

16. Bostwick DG, Qian J, Pacelli A, et al. Neuroendocrine expression in node positive prostate cancer: correlation with systemic progression and patient survival. *J Urol* 2002;168:1204–1211.

17. Cohen RJ, Glezerson G, Haffejee Z. Neuro-endocrine cells—a new prognostic parameter in prostate cancer. *Br J Urol* 1991;68:258–262.

18. Shariff AH, Ather MH. Neuroendocrine differentiation in prostate cancer. *Urology* 2006;68:2–8.

19. Bostwick DG, Grignon DJ, Hammond ME, et al. Prognostic factors in prostate cancer. College of American Pathologists Consensus Statement 1999. *Arch Pathol Lab Med* 2000;124:995–1000.

20. Weaver MG, Abdul-Karim FW, Srigley J, et al. Paneth cell-like change of the prostate gland. A histological, immunohistochemical, and electron microscopic study. *Am J Surg Pathol* 1992;16:62–68.

21. Tamas EF, Epstein JI. Prognostic significance of Paneth cell-like neuroendocrine differentiation in adenocarcinoma of the prostate. *Am J Surg Pathol* 2006;30:980–985.

22. Adlakha H, Bostwick DG. Paneth cell-like change in prostatic adenocarcinoma represents neuroendocrine differentiation: report of 30 cases. *Hum Pathol* 1994;25:135–139.

23. Freschi M, Colombo R, Naspro R, et al. Primary and pure neuroendocrine tumor of the prostate. *Eur Urol* 2004;45:166–169; discussion 169–170.

24. Goulet-Salmon B, Berthe E, Franc S, et al. Prostatic neuroendocrine tumor in multiple endocrine neoplasia type 2B. *J Endocrinol Invest* 2004;27:570–573.

25. Murali R, Kneale K, Lalak N, et al. Carcinoid tumors of the urinary tract and prostate. *Arch Pathol Lab Med* 2006;130:1693–1706.

26. Tash JA, Reuter V, Russo P. Metastatic carcinoid tumor of the prostate. *J Urol* 2002;167:2526–2527.

27. Whelan T, Gatfield CT, Robertson S, et al. Primary carcinoid of the prostate in conjunction with multiple endocrine neoplasia IIb in a child. *J Urol* 1995;153:1080–1082.

28. Wang W, Epstein JI. Small cell carcinoma of the prostate: a morphological and immunohistochemical study of 95 cases. *Am J Surg Pathol* 2008;32:65–71.

29. Brambilla E, Travis WD, Colby TV, et al. The new World Health Organization classification of lung tumours. *Eur Respir J* 2001;18:1059–1068.

30. Choi H, Byhardt RW, Clowry LJ, et al. The prognostic significance of histologic subtyping in small cell carcinoma of the lung. *Am J Clin Oncol* 1984;7:389–397.

31. The World Health Organization histological typing of lung tumours. Second edition. *Am J Clin Pathol* 1982;77:123–136.

32. Hirsch FR, Matthews MJ, Aisner S, et al. Histopathologic classification of small cell lung cancer. changing concepts and terminology. *Cancer* 1988;62:973–977.

33. Nomori H, Shimosato Y, Kodama T, et al. Subtypes of small cell carcinoma of the lung: morphometric, ultrastructural, and immunohistochemical analyses. *Hum Pathol* 1986;17:604–613.

34. Bepler G, Neumann K, Holle R, et al. Clinical relevance of histologic subtyping in small cell lung cancer. *Cancer* 1989;64:74–79.

35. Nicholson SA, Beasley MB, Brambilla E, et al. Small cell lung carcinoma (SCLC): a clinicopathologic study of 100 cases with surgical specimens. *Am J Surg Pathol* 2002;26:1184–1197.

36. Yashi M, Ishikawa S, Ochi M, et al. Small cell/neuroendocrine carcinoma may be a more common phenotype in advanced prostate cancer. *Urol Int* 2002;69:166–168.

37. Oesterling JE, Hauzeur CG, Farrow GM. Small cell anaplastic carcinoma of the prostate: a clinical, pathological and immunohistological study of 27 patients. *J Urol* 1992;147:804–807.

38. Mackey JR, Au HJ, Hugh J, et al. Genitourinary small cell carcinoma: determination of clinical and therapeutic factors associated with survival. *J Urol* 1998;159:1624–1629.

39. Amato RJ, Logothetis CJ, Hallinan R, et al. Chemotherapy for small cell carcinoma of prostatic origin. *J Urol* 1992;147:935–937.

40. Rubenstein JH, Katin MJ, Mangano MM, et al. Small cell anaplastic carcinoma of the prostate: seven new cases, review of the literature, and discussion of a therapeutic strategy. *Am J Clin Oncol* 1997;20:376–380.

41. Yao JL, Madeb R, Bourne P, et al. Small cell carcinoma of the prostate: an immunohistochemical study. *Am J Surg Pathol* 2006;30:705–712.

42. Evans AJ, Humphrey PA, Belani J, et al. Large cell neuroendocrine carcinoma of prostate: a clinicopathologic summary of 7 cases of a rare manifestation of advanced prostate cancer. *Am J Surg Pathol* 2006;30:684–693.

43. Lopez-Beltran A, Cheng L, Prieto R, et al. Lymphoepithelioma-like carcinoma of the prostate. *Hum Pathol* 2009;40:982–987.

44. Campodonico F, Bandelloni R, Maffezzini M. Paraganglioma of the prostate in a young adult. *Urology* 2005;66:657.

45. Dennis PJ, Lewandowski AE, Rohner TJ Jr, et al. Pheochromocytoma of the prostate: an unusual location. *J Urol* 1989;141:130–132.

46. Voges GE, Wippermann F, Duber C, et al. Pheochromocytoma in the pediatric age group: the prostate—an unusual location. *J Urol* 1990;144:1219–1221.

47. Mahadevia PS, Koss LG, Tar IJ. Prostatic involvement in bladder cancer. Prostate mapping in 20 cystoprostatectomy specimens. *Cancer* 1986;58:2096–2102.

48. Schellhammer PF, Bean MA, Whitmore WF Jr. Prostatic involvement by transitional cell carcinoma: pathogenesis, patterns and prognosis. *J Urol* 1977;118:399–403.

49. Esrig D, Freeman JA, Elmajian DA, et al. Transitional cell carcinoma involving the prostate with a proposed staging classification for stromal invasion. *J Urol* 1996;156:1071–1076.

50. Ellis DW, Leffers S, Davies JS, et al. Multiple immunoperoxidase markers in benign hyperplasia and adenocarcinoma of the prostate. *Am J Clin Pathol* 1984;81:279–284.

51. Ford TF, Butcher DN, Masters JR, et al. Immunocytochemical localisation of prostate-specific antigen: specificity and application to clinical practice. *Br J Urol* 1985;57:50–55.

52. Svanholm H. Evaluation of commercial immunoperoxidase kits for prostatic specific antigen and prostatic specific acid phosphatase. *Acta Pathol Microbiol Immunol Scand A* 1986;94:7–12.

53. Feiner HD, Gonzalez R. Carcinoma of the prostate with atypical immunohistological features. Clinical and histologic correlates. *Am J Surg Pathol* 1986;10:765–770.

54. Keillor JS, Aterman K. The response of poorly differentiated prostatic tumors to staining for prostate specific antigen and prostatic acid phosphatase: a comparative study. *J Urol* 1987;137:894–896.

55. Epstein JI. PSAP and PSA as immunohistochemical markers. *Urol Clin North Am* 1993;20:757–770.

56. Chuang AY, DeMarzo AM, Veltri RW, et al. Immunohistochemical differentiation of high-grade prostate carcinoma from urothelial carcinoma. *Am J Surg Pathol* 2007;31:1246–1255.

57. Heyderman E, Brown BM, Richardson TC. Epithelial markers in prostatic, bladder, and colorectal cancer: an immunoperoxidase study of epithelial membrane antigen, carcinoembryonic antigen, and prostatic acid phosphatase. *J Clin Pathol* 1984;37:1363–1369.

58. Nadji M, Tabei SZ, Castro A, et al. Prostatic-specific antigen: an immunohistologic marker for prostatic neoplasms. *Cancer* 1981;48:1229–1232.

59. Wood DP Jr, Montie JE, Pontes JE, et al. Transitional cell carcinoma of the prostate in cystoprostatectomy specimens removed for bladder cancer. *J Urol* 1989;141:346–349.

60. Genega EM, Hutchinson B, Reuter VE, et al. Immunophenotype of high-grade prostatic adenocarcinoma and urothelial carcinoma. *Mod Pathol* 2000;13:1186–1191.

61. Mhawech P, Uchida T, Pelte MF. Immunohistochemical profile of high-grade urothelial bladder carcinoma and prostate adenocarcinoma. *Hum Pathol* 2002;33:1136–1140.

62. Varma M, Morgan M, Amin MB, et al. High molecular weight cytokeratin antibody (clone 34betaE12): a sensitive marker for differentiation of high-grade invasive urothelial carcinoma from prostate cancer. *Histopathology* 2003;42:167–172.

63. Oliai BR, Kahane H, Epstein JI. A clinicopathologic analysis of urothelial carcinomas diagnosed on prostate needle biopsy. *Am J Surg Pathol* 2001;25:794–801.

64. Shen SS, Lerner SP, Muezzinoglu B, et al. Prostatic involvement by transitional cell carcinoma in patients with bladder cancer and its prognostic significance. *Hum Pathol* 2006;37:726–734.

65. Njinou Ngninkeu B, Lorge F, Moulin P, et al. Transitional cell carcinoma involving the prostate: a clinicopathological retrospective study of 76 cases. *J Urol* 2003;169:149–152.

66. Wishnow KI, Ro JY. Importance of early treatment of transitional cell carcinoma of prostatic ducts. *Urology* 1988;32:11–12.

67. Chibber PJ, McIntyre MA, Hindmarsh JR, et al. Transitional cell carcinoma involving the prostate. *Br J Urol* 1981;53:605–609.

68. Greene LF, O'Dea MJ, Dockerty MB. Primary transitional cell carcinoma of the prostate. *J Urol* 1976;116:761–763.

69. Goebbels R, Amberger L, Wernert N, et al. Urothelial carcinoma of the prostate. *Appl Pathol* 1985;3:242–254.

70. Nicolaisen GS, Williams RD. Primary transitional cell carcinoma of prostate. *Urology* 1984;24:544–549.

71. Rubenstein AB, Rubnitz ME. Transitional cell carcinoma of the prostate. *Cancer* 1969;24:543–546.

72. Sawczuk I, Tannenbaum M, Olsson CA, et al. Primary transitional cell carcinoma of prostatic periurethral ducts. *Urology* 1985;25:339–343.

73. Ullmann AS, Ross OA. Hyperplasia, atypism, and carcinoma in situ in prostatic periurethral glands. *Am J Clin Pathol* 1967;47:497–504.

74. McKenney JK, Amin MB, Srigley JR, et al. Basal cell proliferations of the prostate other than usual basal cell hyperplasia: a clinicopathologic study of 23 cases, including four carcinomas, with a proposed classification. *Am J Surg Pathol* 2004;28:1289–1298.

75. Iczkowski KA, Ferguson KL, Grier DD, et al. Adenoid cystic/basal cell carcinoma of the prostate: clinicopathologic findings in 19 cases. *Am J Surg Pathol* 2003;27:1523–1529.

76. Ali TZ, Epstein JI. Basal cell carcinoma of the prostate: a clinicopathologic study of 29 cases. *Am J Surg Pathol* 2007;31:697–705.

77. Hosler GA, Epstein JI. Basal cell hyperplasia: an unusual diagnostic dilemma on prostate needle biopsies. *Hum Pathol* 2005;36:480–485.

78. Yang XJ, McEntee M, Epstein JI. Distinction of basaloid carcinoma of the prostate from benign basal cell lesions by using immunohistochemistry for bcl-2 and Ki-67. *Hum Pathol* 1998;29:1447–1450.

79. Manrique JJ, Albores-Saavedra J, Orantes A, et al. Malignant mixed tumor of the salivary-gland type, primary in the prostate. *Am J Clin Pathol* 1978;70:932–937.

80. Schmid HP, Semjonow A, Eltze E, et al. Late recurrence of adenoid cystic carcinoma of the prostate. *Scand J Urol Nephrol* 2002;36:158–159.

81. Sarris A, Dimopoulos M, Pugh W, et al. Primary lymphoma of the prostate: good outcome with doxorubicin-based combination chemotherapy. *J Urol* 1995;153:1852–1854.

82. Iczkowski KA, Lopez-Beltran A, Sakr WA. Hematolymphoid tumors of prostate. In: Eble JN, Sauter G, Epstein JI, et al., eds. *Tumors of the Urinary System and Male Genital Organs*. Lyon, France: IAR Press, 2004:212.

83. Chu PG, Huang Q, Weiss LM. Incidental and concurrent malignant lymphomas discovered at the time of prostatectomy and prostate biopsy: a study of 29 cases. *Am J Surg Pathol* 2005;29:693–699.

84. Bostwick DG, Iczkowski KA, Amin MB, et al. Malignant lymphoma involving the prostate: report of 62 cases. *Cancer* 1998;83:732–738.

85. Steuter J, Weisenburger DD, Bociek RG, et al. Non-Hodgkin lymphoma of the prostate. *Am J Hematol* 2011;86:952–954.

86. Bostwick DG, Mann RB. Malignant lymphomas involving the prostate. A study of 13 cases. *Cancer* 1985;56:2932–2938.

87. Chim CS, Loong F, Yau T, et al. Common malignancies with uncommon sites of presentation: case 2. Mantle-cell lymphoma of the prostate. *J Clin Oncol* 2003;21:4456–4458.

88. Estrada PC, Scardino PL. Myeloma of the prostate: a case report. *J Urol* 1971;106:586–587.

89. Hollenberg GM. Extraosseous multiple myeloma simulating primary prostatic neoplasm. *J Urol* 1978;119:292–294.

90. Klotz LH, Herr HW. Hodgkin's disease of the prostate: a detailed case report. *J Urol* 1986;135:1261–1262.

91. Peison B, Benisch B, Nicora B, et al. Acute urinary obstruction secondary to pseudolymphoma of prostate. *Urology* 1977;10:478–479.

92. Quien ET, Wallach B, Sandhaus L, et al. Primary extramedullary leukemia of the prostate: case report and review of the literature. *Am J Hematol* 1996;53:267–271.

93. Dajani YF, Burke M. Leukemic infiltration of the prostate: a case study and clinicopathological review. *Cancer* 1976;38:2442–2446.

94. Spethmann S, Heuer R, Hopfer H, et al. Myeloid sarcoma of the prostate as first clinical manifestation of acute myeloid leukaemia. *Lancet Oncol* 2004;5:62–63.

95. Yasuda N, Ohmori S, Usui T. IgD myelomas involving the prostate. *Am J Hematol* 1994;47:65–66.

96. Tay HP, Bidair M, Shabaik A, et al. Primary yolk sac tumor of the prostate in a patient with Klinefelter's syndrome. *J Urol* 1995;153:1066–1069.

97. Hayman R, Patel A, Fisher C, et al. Primary seminoma of the prostate. *Br J Urol* 1995;76:273–274.

98. Han G, Miura K, Takayama T, et al. Primary prostatic endodermal sinus tumor (yolk sac tumor) combined with a small focal seminoma. *Am J Surg Pathol* 2003;27:554–559.

99. Michel F, Gattegno B, Roland J, et al. Primary nonseminomatous germ cell tumor of the prostate. *J Urol* 1986;135:597–599.

100. Namiki K, Tsuchiya A, Noda K, et al. Extragonadal germ cell tumor of the prostate associated with Klinefelter's syndrome. *Int J Urol* 1999;6:158–161.

101. Ekfors TO, Aho HJ, Kekomaki M. Malignant rhabdoid tumor of the prostatic region. Immunohistological and ultrastructural evidence for epithelial origin. *Virchows Arch A Pathol Anat Histopathol* 1985;406:381–388.

102. Kojima K, Uehara H, Naruo S, et al. Papillary cystadenocarcinoma of the prostate. *Int J Urol* 1996;3:511–513.

103. Pan CC, Chiang H, Chang YH, et al. Tubulocystic clear cell adenocarcinoma arising within the prostate. *Am J Surg Pathol* 2000;24:1433–1436.

104. Singh H, Flores-Sandoval N, Abrams J. Renal-type clear cell carcinoma occurring in the prostate. *Am J Surg Pathol* 2003;27:407–410.

105. Govender D, Hadley GP. Ectomesenchymoma of the prostate: histological diagnostic criteria. *Pediatr Surg Int* 1999;15:68–70.

106. Colecchia M, Dagrada G, Poliani PL, et al. Primary primitive peripheral neuroectodermal tumor of the prostate. Immunophenotypic and molecular study of a case. *Arch Pathol Lab Med* 2003;127:e190–e193.

107. Pan CC, Yang AH, Chiang H. Malignant perivascular epithelioid cell tumor involving the prostate. *Arch Pathol Lab Med* 2003;127:E96–E98.

108. Serizawa RR, Norgaard N, Horn T, et al. Hemangioma of the prostate—an unusual cause of lower urinary tract symptoms: case report. *BMC Urol* 2011;11:4.

109. Owens CL, Epstein JI, Netto GJ. Distinguishing prostatic from colorectal adenocarcinoma on biopsy samples: the role of morphology and immunohistochemistry. *Arch Pathol Lab Med* 2007;131:599–603.

110. Gaudin PB, Rosai J, Epstein JI. Sarcomas and related proliferative lesions of specialized prostatic stroma: a clinicopathologic study of 22 cases. *Am J Surg Pathol* 1998;22:148–162.

111. Bostwick DG, Hossain D, Qian J, et al. Phyllodes tumor of the prostate: long-term followup study of 23 cases. *J Urol* 2004;172:894–899.

112. Herawi M, Epstein JI. Specialized stromal tumors of the prostate: a clinicopathologic study of 50 cases. *Am J Surg Pathol* 2006;30:694–704.

113. Nagar M, Epstein JI. Epithelial proliferations in prostatic stromal tumors of uncertain malignant potential (STUMP). *Am J Surg Pathol* 2011;35:898–903.

114. Dailey VL, Hameed O. Blue nevus of the prostate. *Arch Pathol Lab Med* 2011;135:799–802.

115. Moore R. Benign hypertrophy of the prostate: a morphologic study. *J Urol* 1943;50:680–710.

116. Regan JB, Barrett DM, Wold LE. Giant leiomyoma of the prostate. *Arch Pathol Lab Med* 1987;111:381–382.

117. Michaels MM, Brown HE, Favino CJ. Leiomyoma of prostate. *Urology* 1974;3:617–620.

118. Herawi M, Epstein JI. Solitary fibrous tumor on needle biopsy and transurethral resection of the prostate: a clinicopathologic study of 13 cases. *Am J Surg Pathol* 2007;31:870–876.

119. Sexton WJ, Lance RE, Reyes AO, et al. Adult prostate sarcoma: the MD Anderson cancer center experience. *J Urol* 2001;166:521–525.

120. Cheville JC, Dundore PA, Nascimento AG, et al. Leiomyosarcoma of the prostate. Report of 23 cases. *Cancer* 1995;76:1422–1427.

121. Stenram U, Holby LE. A case of circumscribed myosarcoma of the prostate. *Cancer* 1969;24:803–806.

122. Kelley TW, Borden EC, Goldblum JR. Estrogen and progesterone receptor expression in uterine and extrauterine leiomyosarcomas: an immunohistochemical study. *Appl Immunohistochem Mol Morphol* 2004;12:338–341.

123. Herawi M, Montgomery EA, Epstein JI. Gastrointestinal stromal tumors (GISTs) on prostate needle biopsy: a clinicopathologic study of 8 cases. *Am J Surg Pathol* 2006;30:1389–1395.

124. Van der Aa F, Sciot R, Blyweert W, et al. Gastrointestinal stromal tumor of the prostate. *Urology* 2005;65:388.

125. Madden JF, Burchette JL, Raj GV, et al. Anterior rectal wall gastrointestinal stromal tumor presenting clinically as prostatic mass. *Urol Oncol* 2005;23:268–272.

126. Raney RB, Anderson JR, Barr FG, et al. Rhabdomyosarcoma and undifferentiated sarcoma in the first two decades of life: a selective review of intergroup rhabdomyosarcoma study group experience and rationale for intergroup rhabdomyosarcoma study V. *J Pediatr Hematol Oncol* 2001;23:215–220.

127. Lobe TE, Wiener E, Andrassy RJ, et al. The argument for conservative, delayed surgery in the management of prostatic rhabdomyosarcoma. *J Pediatr Surg* 1996;31:1084–1087.

128. Waring PM, Newland RC. Prostatic embryonal rhabdomyosarcoma in adults. a clinicopathologic review. *Cancer* 1992;69:755–762.

129. Nabi G, Dinda AK, Dogra PN. Primary embryonal rhabdomyosarcoma of prostate in adults: diagnosis and management. *Int Urol Nephrol* 2002;34:531–534.

130. Nuwal P, Solanki RL, Jain S, et al. Botryoid rhabdomyosarcoma of prostate—a case report. *Indian J Pathol Microbiol* 2001;44:65–66.

131. Sundarasivarao D, Banerjea S, Nageswararao A, et al. Hemangioma of the prostate: a case report. *J Urol* 1973;110:708–709.

132. Sloan SE, Rapoport JM. Prostatic chondroma. *Urology* 1985;25:319–321.

133. Bedrosian SA, Goldman RL, Sung MA. Heterotopic cartilage in prostate. *Urology* 1983;21:536–537.

134. Rames RA, Smith MT. Malignant peripheral nerve sheath tumor of the prostate: a rare manifestation of neurofibromatosis type 1. *J Urol* 1999;162:165–166.

135. Jiang R, Chen JH, Chen M, et al. Male genital schwannoma, review of 5 cases. *Asian J Androl* 2003;5:251–254.

136. Dogra PN, Aron M, Rajeev TP, et al. Primary chondrosarcoma of the prostate. *BJU Int* 1999;83:150–151.

137. Iwasaki H, Ishiguro M, Ohjimi Y, et al. Synovial sarcoma of the prostate with t(X;18)(p11.2;q11.2). *Am J Surg Pathol* 1999;23:220–226.

138. Pan CC, Chang YH. Primary synovial sarcoma of the prostate. *Histopathology* 2006;48:321–323.

139. Williams DH, Hua VN, Chowdhry AA, et al. Synovial sarcoma of the prostate. *J Urol* 2004;171:2376.

140. Furihata M, Sonobe H, Iwata J, et al. Granular cell tumor expressing myogenic markers in the prostate. *Pathol Int* 1996;46:298–300.

141. Chandan VS, Wolsh L. Postirradiation angiosarcoma of the prostate. *Arch Pathol Lab Med* 2003;127:876–878.

142. Chung AK, Michels V, Poland GA, et al. Neurofibromatosis with involvement of the prostate gland. *Urology* 1996;47:448–451.

143. Bain GO, Danyluk JM, Shnitka TK, et al. Malignant fibrous histiocytoma of prostate gland. *Urology* 1985;26:89–91.

144. Chin W, Fay R, Ortega P. Malignant fibrous histiocytoma of prostate. *Urology* 1986;27:363–365.

145. Kulmala RV, Seppanen JH, Vaajalahti PJ, et al. Malignant fibrous histiocytoma of the prostate. Case report. *Scand J Urol Nephrol* 1994;28:429–431.

146. Reyes JW, Shinozuka H, Garry P, et al. A light and electron microscopic study of a hemangiopericytoma of the prostate with local extension. *Cancer* 1977;40:1122–1126.

147. Nishiyama T, Ikarashi T, Terunuma M, et al. Osteogenic sarcoma of the prostate. *Int J Urol* 2001;8:199–201.

148. Maluf HM, King ME, DeLuca FR, et al. Giant multilocular prostatic cystadenoma: a distinctive lesion of the retroperitoneum in men. A report of two cases. *Am J Surg Pathol* 1991;15:131–135.

149. Patriarca C, Zucchini N, Corrada P. Giant multilocular prostate cystoadenoma: an entirely benign prostate neoplasm with some phenotypic features of malignancy. *Am J Surg Pathol* 2005;29:1252–1254.

150. Kirkland KL, Bale PM. A cystic adenoma of the prostate. *J Urol* 1967;97:324–327.

151. Damjanov I, Apic R. Cystadenoma of seminal vesicles. *J Urol* 1974;111:808–809.

152. Benson RC Jr, Clark WR, Farrow GM. Carcinoma of the seminal vesicle. *J Urol* 1984;132:483–485.

153. Zenklusen HR, Weymuth G, Rist M, et al. Carcinosarcoma of the prostate in combination with adenocarcinoma of the prostate and adenocarcinoma of the seminal vesicles. A case report with immunocytochemical analysis and review of the literature. *Cancer* 1990;66:998–1001.

154. Fain JS, Cosnow I, King BF, et al. Cystosarcoma phyllodes of the seminal vesicle. *Cancer* 1993;71:2055–2061.

155. Lamont JS, Hesketh PJ, de las Morenas A, et al. Primary angiosarcoma of the seminal vesicle. *J Urol* 1991;146:165–167.

156. Schned AR, Ledbetter JS, Selikowitz SM. Primary leiomyosarcoma of the seminal vesicle. *Cancer* 1986;57:2202–2206.

157. Adachi Y, Rokujyo M, Kojima H, et al. Primary seminoma of the seminal vesicle: report of a case. *J Urol* 1991;146:857–859.

158. Fairey AE, Mead GM, Murphy D, et al. Primary seminal vesicle choriocarcinoma. *Br J Urol* 1993;71:756–757.

CHAPTER 11

Nonneoplastic Lesions of the Testis

FERRAN ALGABA, MUKUL K. DIVATIA, ALBERTO G. AYALA, and JAE Y. RO

TESTICULAR EMBRYOLOGY

Genetic Mechanisms Regulating Testicular Development and Sex Determination

Although multiple genes play a role in testicular differentiation, the two genes of prime importance are NR5A1 and WT-1 (Wilms tumor gene). NR5A1 is located on chromosome 9q33.3 and comprises seven exons with a gene product known as SF-1 (steroidogenic factor 1). SF-1 is initially recovered from the Sertoli cells of the sex cords, but it is localized to the Leydig cells during later developmental stages.[1] It enhances the expression of anti-müllerian hormone (AMH) and plays a role in regulation of the AMH gene. A female phenotype is found in 46XY subjects with a heterozygous deletion of NR5A1 along with other features including adrenal failure in the first months after birth, persistence of normal müllerian structures and maldeveloped gonads comprising poorly differentiated tubules with abundant connective tissue stroma. The neonatal phenotype is not a reliable predictor of virilization at puberty. Male gender assignment in poorly virilized cases at birth may allow spontaneous puberty without signs of hypogonadotropic hypogonadism, and possibly fertility. Patients with SF-1 mutations are at increased risk for malignant germ cell tumors. Early orchidopexy and germ cell tumor screening are mandated in the presence of preserved gonads. In cases where premalignant and/or malignant changes are identified, gonadectomy with or without possible irradiation constitutes the modality of treatment.[2] Adrenal failure is the sole presenting feature in patients with 46XX since SF-1 does not influence ovarian development.[3] These disorders aid in highlighting the significant position of NR5A1 expressed in the primitive urogenital ridge, which differentiates into the gonads and adrenal glands.

WT1 is located on chromosome 11p13 and contains 10 exons with alternative splicing sites in introns 5 and 9. The splicing of intron 9 can result in KTS+ (three amino acids viz. lysine, threonine, and serine) or KTS− isoforms. Normal gene expression mandates a proper balance of both isoforms.

The WT1 gene is predominantly expressed in the kidneys and gonads. It is responsible for stromal–epithelial transition and inhibition of genes encoding proliferative factors for epithelial differentiation and simultaneous activation of genes enhancing the process. A host of phenotypic alterations are observed with WT1 gene anomalies.[4] Loss of the KTS+ isoform gives rise to Frasier syndrome characterized by 46XY gonadal dysgenesis, absence of Wilms tumor, and renal disease of late-onset type.[5] Missense heterozygous mutations are manifested as Denys-Drash syndrome with partial or complete 46XY gonadal dysgenesis, Wilms tumor, and early-onset renal disease with diffuse mesangial sclerosis.[6] WT1 deletions are linked to an increased propensity to develop Wilms tumor and variable genitourinary system manifestations. Other genes identified in the formation of kidneys and gonads are LIM1 and FGF-9 (fibroblast growth factor 9).

The signal for gonadal differentiation is initiated by the SRY gene on the sex-determining region of chromosome Y (Yp11.3) otherwise known as testis determining factor gene.[7] It is this gene that is responsible for production of the AMH, differentiation of Sertoli cell precursors and germ cells, and downstream gene regulation.[8] The pathway of testicular differentiation is complex and involves activation and inhibition of both autosomal and sex chromosomal genes. The SRY gene has been demonstrated in the nuclei of germ cells and Sertoli cells. It contains a single exon encoding a 204–amino acid protein of the central part that is responsible for encoding a DNA-binding domain referred to as high mobility group (HMG). SRY also regulates steroid hormonal expression and interacts with the AMH promoter gene.[9] Mutations of SRY give rise to pure gonadal dysgenesis (Swyer syndrome) or true hermaphroditism. Although all affected cases possess male external genitalia and testes, they have no müllerian structures and azoospermia. The karyotype of patients with the male phenotype without the Y chromosome is 46XX SRY+ in 80% cases and 46XX SRY− in 20% cases. SOX9 duplication may also be present in some instances.[10]

Several other genes encode associated transcription factors and play a role in gonadal differentiation including DAX-1, SOX-8, SOX-9, LHX-9, LIM-1, and DMRT-1. DAX-1 (dosage-sensitive sex reversal) gene is situated on X chromosome and is part of the pathway for development of ovaries, testes, and adrenal glands. It is inhibited by SRY during testicular differentiation and activated during ovarian differentiation. DAX mutations are associated with decreased levels of gene expression causing nondevelopment of the adrenal cortex and hypogonadotrophic hypogonadism with normal testicular development.[11] Human DAX1 duplications result in dosage-sensitive sex reversal (DSS) subsequent to which individuals with a chromosomal XY pattern can develop as females due to gonadal dysgenesis. The exact mechanism of DSS-adrenal hypoplasia congenita on X, gene 1 (DAX1) action in the fetal testis is albeit unknown. It has been demonstrated that in fetal testes from XY Dax1-overexpressing transgenic mice, the expression of the key testis-promoting gene sex-determining region on Y (SRY)-box-9 (Sox9) is reduced. Also, in XY Sox9 heterozygotes, in which testis development is usually normal, Dax1 overexpression results in ovotestes, thereby indicating a DAX1–SOX9 antagonism. The ovarian portion of the XY ovotestes in a recent study was characterized by expression of the granulosa cell marker, forkhead box-L2, with complete loss of the Sertoli cell markers, SOX9 and AMH, and the Leydig cell marker CYP17A1. However, the expression of SRY and SF-1, two key transcriptional regulators of Sox9, was retained in the ovarian portion of the XY ovotestes. Dax1 overexpression reduced activation of TES, the testis enhancer of Sox9, indicating that DAX1 might repress Sox9 expression via TES in reporter mice. Increasing levels of DAX1 antagonized SF-1-, SF-1/SRY−, and SF-1/SOX9-mediated activation of TES in cultured cells, as a result of reduced binding of SF-1 to TES, thus providing a possible mechanism for DSS.[12]

SOX-8 and SOX-9 (SRYY box 8 and 9) are linked to autosomal genes. SOX9 is located on chromosome 17q24.3q25.1 and is expressed after SRY expression in pre-Sertoli cells.[13] The protein encoded by this gene recognizes the sequence CCTTGAG along with other members of the HMG-box class DNA-binding proteins. It acts during chondrocyte differentiation and, with SF-1, regulates transcription of the AMH gene. Functional allelic losses lead to the skeletal malformation syndrome (campomelic dysplasia), frequently with 46XY constitution with female phenotype.[13] Duplication of SOX-9 results in 46XX patients with male phenotype.[14] SOX-8 is another gene involved in AMH regulation and interacts with SF-1 through protein–protein interactions. It has been demonstrated experimentally that SOX-9 dysfunction leads to SOX-8 expression as a replacement through a feedback process.[15]

Deletions in chromosome 9p[16] and 10q[17] result in expression of a female phenotype in 46XY genotype cases. Deletions of chromosome 9p are also associated with hydronephrosis, facial malformations, and delayed development.

In 46XY females, deletions of two genes (DMRT1 and DMRT2) are located on chromosome 9p24.3. Chromosome 10q deletions are associated with genital malformations, mental retardation, and other systemic manifestations.

Hormonal Control

Multiple hormones are involved in the development of the male genital system at various stages, including AMH, testosterone, dihydrotestosterone (DHT) and the pituitary gland hormones, follicle-stimulating hormone (FSH), and the luteinizing hormone (LH).

AMH (also known as müllerian inhibitory substance, MIS) is a glycoprotein consisting of two identical 72-kDa subunits linked by disulfide bonds that is secreted by Sertoli cells in males and granulosa cells in females.[18] Its expression is regulated by SF-1, which is a transcriptional regulator of many steroid genes.[19] AMH is a member of the TGF-β family encoded by a 2.75-kb gene situated on 19p13.2. The amount of AMH secreted is inversely proportional to degree of Sertoli cell maturation. It can be detected during the 8th to 9th week of gestation, and its concentration rises in the second trimester and decreases significantly in the third trimester.[20] Although its level rises upon birth and AMH is detectable during childhood, its levels decline to undetectable with the onset of puberty when it is negatively regulated by androgens.[21]

The target sites of AMH include the genital tract, testis, and surrounding structures with AMH causing involution of the ipsilateral müllerian duct beginning from the caudal pole with rapid progression upward. It regulates SRY expression being expressed around the same time frame. The tunica albuginea forms through mesenchymal insertion between primitive sex cords and coelomic epithelium and its development is promoted by AMH.[22] This hormone presents a barrier to spermatogonia entering meiosis.[23] Of note is the role played by AMH in the development of fetal lungs.[24]

Testosterone synthesis commences during the 8th week of gestation and is synthesized by Leydig cells, which appear during the 8th week of gestation and constitute approximately 50% of the testicular volume by the 16th week.[25] However, the secretion of testosterone is regulated by hCG and LH levels. hCG levels are at their peak during the 11th to 18th weeks and fall to significantly lower levels after this duration. This period of hCG-dependent testosterone secretion is crucial in terms of genital differentiation. Wolffian duct differentiation occurs when testosterone is secreted by the testis on each side and leads to differentiation of epididymis, ductus deferens, and seminal vesicle. Defects in androgen synthesis are evidenced as cryptorchidism and incomplete masculinization.

The enzyme 5α-reductase acts on testosterone to produce DHT, which in turn is responsible for differentiation of the prostate along with external genitalia, male urethra, scrotum, and penis. The midline fusion of labioscrotal folds (day 70) to form the scrotum with the midline raphe is induced by DHT.

The penile urethra is formed by fusion of the urethral folds (day 74), and the genital tubercle subsequently enlarges to form the glans penis. The terminal urethra develops from an invagination of the glans tip. The prostate, urinary bladder, and prostatic urethra are formed from the urogenital sinus.[26]

The roles played by FSH and LH gain importance toward the last weeks of gestation. LH levels start rising in fetal circulation during the 10th week and peak by the 18th week after which they decline gradually until birth. LH regulates fetal androgen production in the second and third trimesters. FSH is responsible for Sertoli cell mitogenic activity, which peaks at the time of delivery.[27]

NORMAL TESTICULAR STRUCTURE

Fetal Testis

In their initial stages, germ cells acquire diverse evolutionary morphologic appearances. Three types of germ cells have been identified, and some authors[28] have proposed that these should be known as gonocytes (OCT4 positive, c-kit positive), intermediate germ cells (OCT4 low expression/negative, c-kit negative), and prespermatogonia (OCT4 negative, c-kit negative). In the first trimester, most germ cells have a gonocyte phenotype; however, from the 18th week of gestation, prespermatogonia are the most abundant cell type (Fig. 11-1). These data provide evidence for the functional differentiation of human testicular germ cells during the second trimester of pregnancy and argue against these germ cells being considered a homogeneous population.

Prepubertal Testis

From birth until puberty, the testicles develop continuously, but some phenomena permit this period to be subdivided into the following three phases:

Testicle Development in Newborns and Perinatal Period

Testicular development in the newborn is characterized by solid tubules with Sertoli cells and gonocytes (centrally located). At 6 months after birth, there are no gonocytes because they have been transformed into spermatogonia by the testosterone from the Leydig cells.[29] The morphologic features of Leydig cells at this stage are similar to those in adults, without Reinke crystalloids.

Testicle Development in Infants

After the changes that occur in the testicle during the first 6 months following birth, the testicle remains at rest until age 3 years. After this time, margination of the cells can be observed, which provides a pseudoluminal appearance of the tubules; in addition, some meiosis can be seen, which rapidly stops in what appears to be cellular rests. The tubular cells are typically composed of Sertoli cells, undifferentiated cells, and some spermatogonia (Fig. 11-2). The Leydig cells have involuted and have decreased in number in this phase, with minimal levels of testosterone.

Testicle Development in Boys

From age 9 years onward and especially between ages 13 and 15 years, the interstitial mesenchymal cells are definitively transformed into adult Leydig cells that produce testosterone under the action of LH; in addition, LH stimulates the development of the germinal cells, growth of the tubule, and appearance of the central lumen.[29]

Pubertal and Adult Testis

When the testicle is totally developed, it has a supporting structure—the albuginea—that surrounds the testis like an external capsule. Between the thickened mediastinum testis

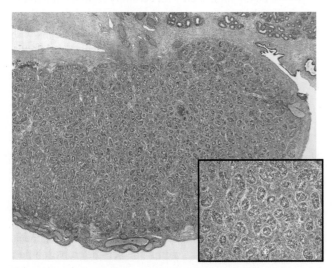

FIGURE 11-1 ■ Fetal testis. Solid seminiferous tubules with prespermatogonia and interstitial Leydig cells; 24th week of gestation (**Inset:** Higher magnification).

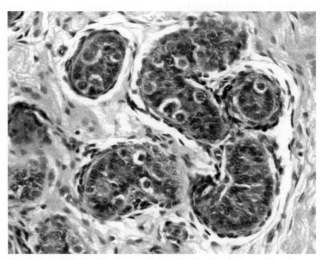

FIGURE 11-2 ■ Infantile testis. Small solid seminiferous tubules. Immature Sertoli cells with undifferentiated cells and some spermatogonias (cells with halo).

Table 11-1 ■ AVERAGE NUMBER OF CELLS PER TUBULE FOR VARIOUS CELLULAR SUBTYPES, PER TRANSVERSE TUBULAR SECTION

Cellular Subtype	Cells Per Tubule
Sertoli cells	10.2 ± 2
Spermatogonia	21.4 ± 4
Spermatocytes first order	31 ± 6
Immature spermatids	37 ± 7
Mature spermatids	25 ± 4
Leydig cells	5 ± 0.2

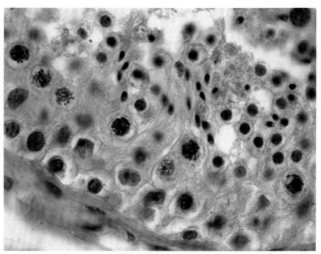

FIGURE 11-3 ■ Adult testis. Mature Sertoli cells (with triangular nuclei and prominent nucleoli). Normal spermatogenesis with spermatogonia (cells with perinuclear halo near the seminiferous wall), spermatocytes of first order (filamentous nuclei), spermatocytes of second order, and immature spermatids (cells with small nuclei). Mature spermatids (elongated nuclei, some with subnuclear vacuole).

area and the surface of the organ are fibrous septa that project toward the interior and divide the testicular parenchyma into about 250 segments or lobules. The albuginea has three layers; from outside to inside they include the external mesothelial layer (tunica vaginalis testicular); the medial, relatively acellular layer with fibroblasts, myocytes, and nerve fibers (tunica albuginea); and the internal vascular layer (tunica vasculosa).[30]

The seminiferous tubules occupy 70% to 75% of the testicular volume. Each seminiferous tubule has a closed-loop structure with intercommunication between the arms of the loop. The size varies according to the section angle. In the cross sections of the tubules in an adult, the average diameter is about 180 μm. Each seminiferous tubule is composed of a tubular wall, Sertoli cells, and germ cells (Table 11-1).

The tubular wall comprises five layers; they include the basement membrane (periodic acid–Schiff positive), the internal acellular layer, the internal myofibroblastic layer, the external acellular layer, and the external fibroblastic layer from the inner to the outer aspect. The innermost strata have contraction functions, apparently useful for intratubular motility, and thus mobilize the spermatozoids toward the rete testis or network of canals at the termination of the straight seminiferous tubules in the mediastinum testis.[31] The elastic fibers appear in puberty, are located more externally, and may be lacking in dysgenetic testicles.[32]

The Sertoli cells (10.2 ± 2 per tubule) have abundant cytoplasm with triangular nuclei and prominent nucleoli that extend from the basal membrane to the tubular lumen. Sertoli cells express vimentin and have the greatest metabolic activity of all cells in the entire tubule since they induce the process of differentiation and the maturation of spermatocytes, regulate the maturation of the Leydig cells, secrete inhibin, and produce tubular fluid.[33] These cells have strong desmosomal junctions in their lower portions and weak ones in their upper portions.[34] Sertoli cells synthesize and secrete a large variety of factors: proteins, cytokines, growth factors, opioids, steroids, prostaglandins that explain the presence of endoplasmic reticulum smooth and rough type and a prominent Golgi apparatus.

The germ cells progressively mature from spermatogonia to their final mature forms within 70 to 74 days. From the morphologic point of view, 13 distinct types of germ cells

can be identified, but at the typical light microscopic level, only the following principal levels of maturation are recognized (Fig. 11-3):

1. **Spermatogonia** (21.4 ± 4 per seminiferous tubule), located near the tubular wall, are placed in rows, with round nuclei, regular chromatin, and a perinuclear halo.

2. **Spermatocytes** (31 ± 6 per tubule) of the first order have nuclei with filamentous chromatin because of their involvement in meiosis. The spermatocytes of second order are not recognized because they have a very short average life (about 8 hours),[29] and since they are already haploid cells, they have very small nuclei that cannot be distinguished with certainty from the immature spermatids.

3. **Immature spermatids** (37 ± 7 per tubule) are cells with central nuclei with lymphoid characteristics and somewhat abundant and clear cytoplasm.

4. **Mature spermatids** (25 ± 4 per tubule), the last maturing phase that we can recognize, are located near the tubular lumens and have elongated nuclei with scanty cytoplasm.

The order of these germ cells in the tubule is apparently irregular, but for some time it has been recorded that there are six distinct stages,[35] a consequence of a helicoidal ordering throughout the tubule. These stages of spermatogenesis are defined as a characteristic association of germ cells representing several waves of spermatogenesis that occur simultaneously within the seminiferous tubules. Each stage has a specific duration, and the groups always occur in the same order, so that once the complete cycle is finalized it begins again.[36] During the maturation process,

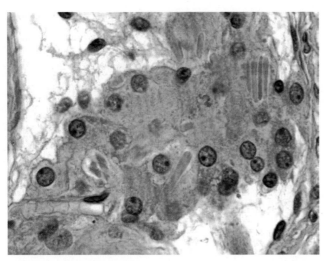

FIGURE 11-4 ■ Adult testis. Normal Leydig cells around capillary vessels with abundant eosinophilic cytoplasm and Reinke crystalloids.

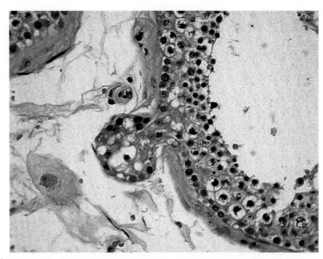

FIGURE 11-5 ■ Elderly testis. Seminiferous tubule with germ cell atrophy and parietal diverticulum.

from spermatogonium to mature spermatids, all the cells belonging to the same clone are interconnected.[37] Stage I is composed of spermatogonia, pachytene primary spermatocytes, and round and elongating spermatids. Stage II includes spermatogonia, pachytene primary spermatocytes, round and elongated spermatids, and residual bodies derived from spermatid cytoplasm within Sertoli cells. Stage III is characterized by the beginning of spermatid nuclear condensation and the entrance of type B spermatogonia into meiosis. Stages IV and V comprise pachytene primary spermatocytes, and can be differentiated by the presence of leptotene and zygotene primary spermatocytes. In Stage V, the secondary spermatocytes undergo a second meiotic division after a very short interphase.

In the interstitium, connective tissue collagen fibers with contractile capacity are present. The Leydig cells are the most important component, making up 5% to 12% of the testicular volume.[38] They are polygonal and have PAS-positive, eosinophilic cytoplasm with a central nucleus and prominent nucleolus, grouped in small nests (1 or 2 nest per tubule or 5 ± 0.2 cells per tubule) around the capillaries of the intertubular space. The fetal Leydig cells produce testosterone; immature Leydig cells produce 3α and 17β-diol and adult Leydig cells steroids. Characteristically, some eosinophilic crystalline structures can be found in the cytoplasm (Reinke crystalloids); these are probably subunits of globular proteins whose functional meaning is not known[39] (Fig. 11-4). Other cellular elements of the interstitium are the macrophages that secrete interleukin 1, which stimulates the proliferation of the germ cells, and the mast cells.

AGING TESTIS

The changes considered as age-related involution do not have a specific age at commencement, and the fact that we are able to see normal testicles in all age groups indicates

that there are marked individual variations.[40] The involution seems to be related more to hormonal levels than to age; however, after age 70 years, the changes of atrophy are frequent, and after age 80 years, the testicles of almost all men have a certain degree of fibrosis in the tubular wall, although they can preserve spermatogenesis.[40]

Several authors have observed foci of total tubular sclerosis, suggestive of a local ischemic phenomenon, as well as the appearance of tubular diverticula (Fig. 11-5) directly proportional to age, for possible weakening of the tubular wall together with obstructive phenomenon due to storage of fluid in the Sertoli cells.[41] The Sertoli cells store glycogen, ascorbic acid, and lipids, but it is difficult to interpret the significance of this accumulation because it starts at a very early age.[42] There can also be a decrease in the number of cells[40] in the aged testis and multinucleation in 4% of testicles.[43,44]

The loss of germ cells begins with the spermatids and progressively affects the predecessor cells,[45] with the pale spermatogonia disappearing in about the sixth decade and the dark ones in about the eighth decade.[46] A curious finding is the appearance of multinucleated spermatids (from 5 to 86 nuclei) that have been interpreted as an expression of active karyokinesis without cytokinesis, typical of aging.[47]

In the interstitium, one can observe an increase in the connective tissue earlier than in the tubule, and there are data indicating that this increase is regulated by differential expression of TGF-β proteins and decreased levels of TGF-β2.[48] As with the Leydig cells, there are contradictory observations; some authors have reported that their numbers decrease with age, especially in relation to the decrease of LH,[40] whereas others have found a certain compensatory increase.[49] Other changes that can be attributed to involution are intercellular fibrosis, cytoplasmic microvacuolization with accumulation of lipofuscin, and binucleation.[50]

ANATOMY OF THE ADULT TESTIS

Gross Anatomy and Microanatomy

The adult testis measures approximately 4 to 5 cm × 3.5 cm × 3 cm and weighs 15 to 19 g with the right usually being 10% heavier that the left. The external surface is covered by a capsule (tunica albuginea), which is a smooth and homogeneous layer measuring 400 to 459 µm in thickness in the adult. The tunica albuginea is composed of three layers. The outermost layer comprises of dense connective tissue and is lined by mesothelium. The middle layer represents less dense fibrous tissue. The inner most layer is rich vascular connective tissue. From this tunica albuginea layer, numerous fibrous septa emerge to divide the testicular parenchyma into approximately 250 lobules, and meet in a solid posterior area at the hilum of the testis, near the epididymis, which is called the mediastinum of the testis.

Each lobule of the testis contains one to four seminiferous tubules. Every tubule has a diameter of 180 µm and a total average length of 540 m. The tubules are a convoluted structure with numerous communications between the arms of the loop. Each arm of the loop empties into the mediastinum.

The mediastinum contains the rete testis, a connecting structure between the seminiferous tubules with the ductuli efferentes in the epididymis. There are around 1,500 units of seminiferous tubules to the rete. It is divided into three parts: the septal portion with the *tubulae reti*, which are short tubules 0.5 to 1.0 mm in length that connect the two ends of the seminiferous tubules to the mediastinal part with the *tunical rete*, which is a cavernous network of interconnecting channels between tubular reti and the extratesticular part with the *bullae retis*, which are vesicular channels measuring 3 mm in width that anastomose together to form the ductuli efferentes. In the mediastinal and external rete testis parts, fibrous columns or strands covered by epithelium called *chordae retis* are present to connect the different walls.

The rete testis epithelium is composed of flattened cells interspersed with small areas of columnar cells. Both cell types have single centrally located cilia and numerous microvilli on their free surfaces. These cells rest on a basal lamina surrounded by a layer of myofibroblasts and external layer of fibroblasts and collagen and elastic fibers.

Apart from the connection between the testis and the epididymis, the rete testis produces a pressure gradient internally for reabsorption of protein and potassium from tubular fluid.

Blood Supply and Lymphatics

The testis is supplied by the testicular *artery*, which arises from the abdominal aorta. In the spermatic cord, the testicular artery gives multiple branches that run along the interlobular septa of the testis. These centripetal arteries lead to the mediastinum testis and give off branches called centrifugal arteries.

The inner two-thirds of the testicular parenchyma are drained by *veins* that follow the interlobular septa to the mediastinum (centripetal veins). The outer third is drained by veins that lead to the tunica albuginea (centrifugal veins). Both centripetal and centrifugal veins join to form the pampiniform plexus, which drains the testis via the spermatic cord.

Lymphatic vessels are poorly developed in the testis and limited to the tunica vasculosa and interlobular septa where they accompany arterioles and venules.

Nerves

Efferent innervation of the testis is mainly supplied by neurons of the pelvic ganglia, where contralateral and bilateral neural connections occur. Postganglionic nerve fibers enter the testis via the pelvic nerves, extend throughout the tunica vasculosa, and follow the interlobular septa to reach the interstitium. The nerve fibers end in the wall of arterioles, the wall of seminiferous tubules, and the Leydig cells. Adrenergic nerve fibers innervate the tunica albuginea and the blood vessels of the tunica vasculosa. Peptidenergic nerve endings are uncommon. Afferent nerve endings from corpuscles similar to those of Meissner and Pacini are observed in the tunica albuginea.

CONGENITAL ANOMALIES

Disorders in Number and Size

Congenital disorders in number and size constitute one of the less frequently seen groups of testicular anomalies.

Monorchidism

Monorchidism is the congenital absence of one testicle. Its incidence is 1 in 5,000 masculine births, with a predominance of the left side (68.7%).[29] Among boys with monorchidism, 20% have other congenital genital malformations, and 30% have anomalies of the urinary tract. For a correct diagnosis, the possibility of any evidence of a testicle must be excluded; it is not sufficient to find blind seminal canals. All remnants found at exploration should be removed, and the absence of testicular parenchyma should be confirmed before diagnosing monorchidism. The finding of blindly ending spermatic vessels is the only accepted evidence of monorchidism.[16] The contralateral testicle can present a compensatory hypertrophy that can double the volume of the normal testicle; this is a consequence of the change in endocrine feedback that increases the FSH.[51] The increase in testis weight is correlated, in experimental models, with an increase in total seminiferous tubule length and a larger cross-sectional area, which is due in part to the greater number of germ cells per testis.[52]

Anorchidism

Although the term *anorchidism* strictly refers to the total absence of both testicles, a series of pathologic situations is usually included in this term that varies from the actual lack of gonads to extreme hypoplasia or very prolonged concealment of the testicles, for which reason the term *testicular regression syndrome*[53] has been created and includes the following disorders:

True Agonadism

True agonadism is a genuine absence of testicles in 46XY patients with ambiguous external genitals, and more rarely, in 46XX patients with external feminine genitals, with the possibility of there being a rudimentary uterine tube. The cause is unknown, although there are cases associated with heterozygote mutation of gene WT1.[54] This disorder can be associated with various syndromes of multiorganic malformations.[55]

Rudimentary Testes Syndrome

Rudimentary testes syndrome is the presence of cryptorchidic rests of testicles with occasional seminiferous tubules in which Sertoli cells and some spermatogonia are present. The external genitals are not ambiguous but are hypoplastic (micropenis).[56]

Congenital Bilateral Anorchidism

Congenital bilateral anorchidism is the strict bilateral absence of testicles with only wolffian elements and without müllerian rests. The phenotype is normal masculine or hypoplasia, and its incidence is 1 in 20,000 male births. The cause is unknown; there have been attempts to find mutations of the SRY gene, but convincing proof has not been found.[57]

Vanishing Testes Syndrome

Vanishing testes syndrome is the disappearance of the testicles from the last months of pregnancy until puberty; this disorder should be considered only as a prolonged concealment of the testicles, since they can be found in the inguinal canal or in the upper scrotum. The deep alterations of these testicles, represented only by occasional seminiferous tubules accompanied by epididymis, are more attributable to perinatal scrotal torsion than to genetic causes.[55]

Leydig-cell-only Syndrome

Leydig-cell-only syndrome is characterized by finding only clusters of functioning Leydig cells in the spermatic cords, with sufficient testosterone for male phenotype but insufficient for the complete development of secondary sex characteristics.

Sinorchidism

Sinorchidism is an extremely infrequent anomaly, characterized by the fusion of both testicles, each with their respective epididymis located in the midline. This fusion is usually associated with other fusions such as those of the adrenal glands and horseshoe kidney.[29]

Polyorchidism

Polyorchidism is the presence of more than two testicles, with three being the most frequent. This anomaly occurs infrequently, and the embryologic origin is not clear; the longitudinal division of all the structures of the genital ridges

and mesonephric ducts with only the longitudinal division of the genital ridges, and the high transverse division of the genital ridges and the low transverse division of the genital ridges have been proposed. The extra testicle is frequently intrascrotal and many times presents diverse alterations of spermatogenesis. There is no reason for a greater incidence of malignant transformation, although some cases have been reported with germ cell tumors.[58,59]

Macroorchidism

An increase in volume of testicular parenchyma can correspond to diverse pathologic situations. Some of them are consequences of other pathologic conditions, such as the loss of total testicular parenchyma (e.g., the aforementioned compensatory hypertrophy) or the secretion of androgens by Leydig cell tumors; but others are considered true intrinsic anomalies, such as the following:

Idiopathic Benign Macroorchidism

Idiopathic benign macroorchidism is characterized by an increase in the longitude of the tubules. It is caused perhaps by the greater sensitivity of hormonal receptors, which in the development of these testicular alterations are curiously found during spermatogenesis.[60]

Precocious Puberty

For practical purposes, this is considered to be before 8 years of age in girls and 9 years in boys. The incidence is estimated at between 1 in 5,000 and 1 in 10,000, with a female:male ratio higher than 20:1. In boys, the first symptom is rapid testicular enlargement followed by growth of pubic and axillary hair, enlargement of the penis, and acceleration of skeletal growth.

Precocious puberty results from the early differentiation of Leydig cells, with complete spermatogenesis and abnormal spermatids and, in the absence of stimulus, by pituitary gonadotropin (familial testotoxicosis)[61,62]; it can also result from alterations of the central nervous system such as those that occur in McCune-Albright or von Recklinghausen syndromes.[29] Other causes are the Leydig cell tumors and congenital adrenal hyperplasia.

Other Macroorchidisms

Other alterations such as *fragile X chromosome (Martin-Bell syndrome)*[63] or congenital Leydig cell hyperplasia can also be accompanied by macroorchidism because of the transfer of human chorionic gonadotropin from the mother to the fetus, similar to what occurs in diabetic mothers with hypertension.[64,65] In *bilateral megalotestes* with low gonadotropin, with excellent fertility parameters despite the unusually low hormone levels, no specific pathology underlying the large gonadal volume could be identified.[66]

Alterations of Location

Some congenital anomalies can be classified by their locations outside the normal path of testicular descent (ectopia) or in the path of descent (undescended testes). The location in the superficial inguinal pouch is considered to be ectopia by some researchers or to be cryptorchidism by others.

Ectopia

There are two types of ectopia: one that involves the complete testicle and the other that involves parts of the testicular parenchyma.

Complete Ectopia of the Testicle

Complete ectopia of the testicle occurs when the testicles complete the transinguinal migration and then divert to another location under the superficial inguinal ring. This anomaly is considered to be related to alterations in the gubernaculum testis and its branches since the ectopias that can be observed (suprapubic, superficial inguinal, femoral, transverse scrotal, and perineal)[67] correspond to the sites of these branches. These testicles have normal characteristics and are not associated with a greater incidence of neoplasia.[52]

Testicular Parenchymal Ectopia

Seminiferous tubule ectopia is characterized by the presence of seminiferous tubules in a normal albuginea, in contiguity with the tubules of the parenchyma, without evidence of ovarian stroma (fundamental to distinguish it from some testicular dysgenesis), and with clear delimitation between the tunica albuginea and the testicular parenchyma.[68]

Leydig cells ectopia can be located in the testicle (interlobular septa, rete testis, tunica albuginea, or complete fibrotic tubules) or in extratesticular structures such as the epididymis or spermatic cord (generally perineural). These cells seem to be less functional than do those with a normal location. Their origin is not clear, and cell migrations can be assumed since cells do not display ectopic differentiation.[69–71]

Undescended Testis (Cryptorchidism)

Undescended testes are the most common testicular anomaly. Scrotal testicular absence is seen in 30.3% of premature boys, and incomplete descent is seen in 3.2% of full-term boys. In most boys with incomplete descent, the testes will descend spontaneously within the first 3 months; by the end of the 1st year, the testes will not have descended in only 0.8%. Spontaneous resolution is rare after the 1st year.[72]

True Cryptorchidism

In boys with cryptorchidism, the testicle remains immovable along some areas of the testicular descent path; this occurs in 25% of cases of empty scrotum. It can be associated with complex syndromes (e.g., Klinefelter, Kallmann, or Noonan) or with other malformations such as omphalocele and myelomeningocele.

The mechanism for testicular descent involves participation by hormonal and mechanical factors and although it is not completely clear, the process involves three stages viz. nephric displacement (7th week), transabdominal descent (12th week), and inguinal descent (between 7th month and birth).[73]

The gubernaculum testis regulates testicular descent along with the formation of the inguinal canal and processus vaginalis.[74] It is a complex process involving a normally functioning hypothalamo-pituitary–gonadal axis, normal development of abdominal wall musculature, gubernaculum, and the processus vaginalis,[75] along with a normally functioning endocrine system of the testis.

The hormonal requisites for testicular descent are varied and not entirely elucidated. One of the most essential factors for testicular descent is insulin-like factor-3 (INSF-3), which is produced by Leydig cells and is independent of the androgen pathway. It stimulates gubernacular swelling, which is required for the initiation of testicular descent.[76] INSF-3 gene mutations or mutations of its receptors GREAT (G-protein-coupled receptor affecting testicular descent) or LGRB-8 (leucine-rich repeat-containing G-protein-coupled receptor-8) result in improper testicular descent and cryptorchidism.[77] Gubernaculum swelling also involves contributions from AMH and androgens.

Inguinoscrotal descent has not been fully explained; however, androgens and the genitofemoral nerve are two significant factors behind the process. Androgens act on the nucleus of the genitofemoral nerve in the spinal cord as opposed to direct action on the gubernaculums testis, effectively bringing about the masculinization of the neurons comprising the nucleus[78] accompanied by secretion of large amounts of calcitonin gene-related peptide (CGRP). In turn, CGRP acts on the cremasteric muscle that develops in the gubernaculum and is innervated by the genitofemoral nerve. This theory is supported by the fact that neurogenic atrophy of this muscle is seen in cryptorchid patients.[79]

A host of other factors are involved in testicular descent including epidermal growth factor (EGF) and estrogens. Experimental studies have demonstrated that estradiol decreases gubernacular swelling and plays a role in stabilizing müllerian ducts. One of the proposed hypotheses states that cell proliferation resulting in gubernacular swelling is inhibited by estradiol.[80] EGF is involved in testicular descent by its action at various sites along the entire gonadal–placental axis. EGF levels in maternal circulation rise immediately prior to fetal masculinization.[81] The placenta has an increased concentration of EGF receptors, and placental stimulation by EGF may cause hCG production. This chain of events may also stimulate androgen production by Leydig cells and a summation of these might bring about testicular descent.

The gubernaculum and processus vaginalis regress upon birth and the gubernaculum is replaced by fibrous tissue comprising the scrotal ligament. The processus vaginalis atrophies along its cephalic portion after testicular descent. If this process is exaggerated, a testis that descended normally may be caused to ascend and lead to a cryptorchid condition.[82]

The pathogenesis of testicular alteration is very controversial, and opinions vary from those who believe the alterations are based on immunologic changes (due to the alteration of the hemato-testicular barrier because of hyperthermia)[83] to those who believe that the alterations are a result of dysgenetic expression. Independent of the etiopathogenetic hypotheses, the important consideration is to know the morphologic variations, their chronology, and the possibility of preventing them.

We can systematize the testicular changes of cryptorchidism by age groups, as follows:

Changes in Prepubertal Cryptorchid Testes. In patients with prepubertal cryptorchid testes, 74% of the testes showed severe decrease in the average tubular diameter, marked decrease of the tubular fertility index, and hyperplasia of the Sertoli cells.[84] These findings, together with the frequent alteration of the contralateral testicle, reinforce the hypothesis that some cases represent authentic testicular dysgenesis. Other changes such as annular tubules and calcospherites (for probable cellular peeling and subsequent calcification)[85] are more difficult to explain.

Changes in Pubertal Cryptorchid Testes. During puberty in patients with pubertal cryptorchid testes, the lesions are very deep, and almost all patients experience some of the anomalies already described in the prepubertal cryptorchidic testes.[86] This disorder appears to be associated with progressive worsening of the structures until becoming terminal, typically at 13 years of age.[87]

Changes in the Adult Cryptorchid Testes. In adult men with cryptorchid testes, the entire testicle shows advanced atrophic changes[88] (Fig. 11-6). In a series by one of the authors (F.A.), changes in the cryptorchid testes that descended at prepubertal ages showed structural normality in only 7.7% of patients, and fibrotic changes in 46% of the cases.

Several foci of infantile (immature) seminiferous tubules can be present. Each group of tubules appears well delimited but unencapsulated. Nodule size varies from microscopic to 5 mm. On cut section, each nodule is distinguished by its

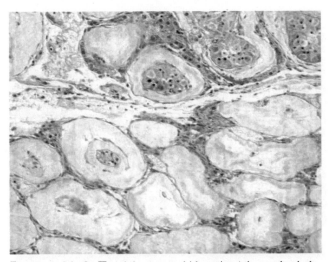

FIGURE 11-6 ■ Adult cryptorchid testis. Advanced tubular wall fibrosis with complete absence of tubular cells or only residual Sertoli cells.

whitish color. The seminiferous tubules have a prepubertal diameter and may be anastomotic. The epithelium is columnar or pseudostratified, devoid of lumina, and usually consists only of Sertoli cells. The cells have elongated hyperchromatic nuclei with one or several peripherally placed small nucleoli. The interstitium varies from scant to well collagenized. Leydig cells are usually absent in these areas and, if present, their numbers are low. Sertoli cell nodule is found in most adult cryptorchid testes, regardless of when the testes descended. It is also present in 22% of normal scrotal testes in some series and is an occasional finding in males with idiopathic infertility.

Much has been discussed on the use of orchiopexy in improving fertility, but its success has not been proven.[86] Also not proven is the justification for a systematic biopsy of the cryptorchid testis to predict its functional capacity or to detect an intratubular germ cell neoplasia. One of the most debated subjects is the incidence of a germ cell tumor in a cryptorchid testis since the risk of developing germ cell tumors is 4 to 10 times higher than in a normally descended testicle.[89] Seminoma is the most common histologic type. Orchiopexy does not decrease the incidence of neoplasia, which supports the hypothesis that changes of these testicles are dysgenetic.

Obstructed Testes

The testes are located superficially in the inguinal Denis-Browne pouch. Some authors consider them as ectopic and others as true cryptorchidism. The morphologic changes are similar to those in cryptorchidism.

Retractile Testes

The testicle may ascend to the scrotum at the time of exploration. Some alterations such as variable germ cell atrophy can be present from one lobule to the other.[90]

Gonadal/Testicular Dysgenesis

Gonadal dysgenesis is characterized by a feminine phenotype with amenorrhea and hypoplasia of the uterus and fallopian tubes. Dysgenesis is usually classified according to karyotype and therefore can be

(a) *46XY GONADAL DYSGENESIS* (Swyer syndrome) is characterized by a female phenotype without signs of the Turner syndrome with infantilism. It is possible to find fused labia majora, hypertrophic clitoris, and hypospadias. Some patients have mental retardation and chronic renal insufficiency. The typical gonads are the fibrous streak (see below).

(b) *46XX GONADAL DYSGENESIS* with normal genitals and ovarian hypoplasia (see below) rather than streak gonads.

(c) 45XO GONADAL DYSGENESIS with stigmata of the Turner syndrome; the external genitalia are female and infantile. The typical streak gonads are present.

(d) *MIXED DYSGENESIS* with streak gonads in some cases associated with testis.

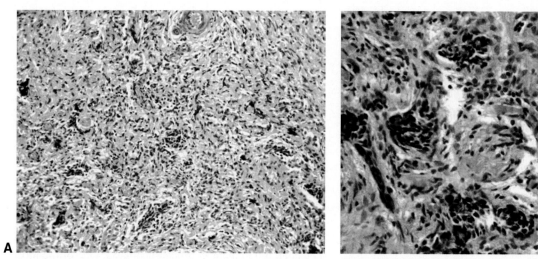

FIGURE 11-7 ■ Gonadal dysgenesis. Fibrous streak with ovarian-like stroma **(A)** and occasional rete testis like channels **(B).**

The streak gonads may consist only of ovarian stroma with a nodular pattern (typical of 46XY, and 45XO), fibrous tissue with occasional ovarian follicles (especially in 46XX/45XO), or fibrous tissue with tubules and channels resembling rete testis (in 46XY)[55,91] (Fig. 11-7).

The hypoplasic ovaries, in *46XX gonadal dysgenesis* are characterized by small ovaries that are more often hypoplastic and rarely streak gonads. The histologic picture of the ovaries consists of fibrous stroma without generative elements or with a small number of primary follicles, but sometimes also with a single growing graafian follicle.[92]

The incidence of tumors in gonadal dysgenesis is variable. Approximately 25% to 30% of patients with 46XY dysgenesis can develop gonadoblastomas, seminomas, or other germ cell tumors (Fig. 11-8), for which preventive extirpation is recommended.[93] In mixed dysgenesis, tumors develop in 25% of the cases[94]; in the other forms, the incidence of tumors is lower.[55]

In mixed dysgenesis, along with a fibrous streak, testicular dysgenesis can be found that is characterized by a central testicular area comprising of seminiferous tubules that are smaller than normal but identifiable, surrounded by ovarian stroma and branched tubules with an albuginea that may differ by the absence of tunica vasculosa.[55]

True Hermaphroditism

The term *hermaphroditism* should be applied only to patients who have both testicular and ovarian tissue (Fig. 11-9). It is a pathologic entity with a difficult clinical diagnosis. In patients with a masculine phenotype, hermaphroditism can often be recognized only in puberty by developing gynecomastia, which is present in nearly all of these patients[29]; in those who have a feminine phenotype, clitoromegaly or irregular menstruation can indicate this condition.

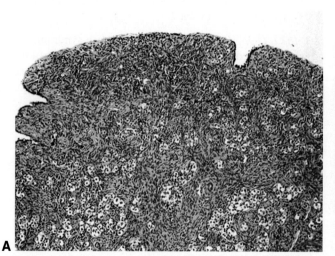

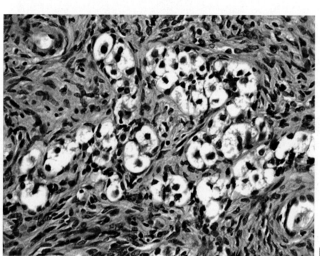

FIGURE 11-8 ■ Gonadoblastoma in gonadal dysgenesis. **(A)** Low power view; **(B)** high magnification. Large germ cells with clear cytoplasm (seminoma) surrounded by small cells resembling immature Sertoli cells and granulosa cells.

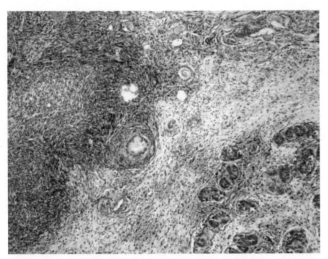

FIGURE 11-9 ■ True hermaphroditism. Ovotestis with ovarian tissue in *upper left* area and seminiferous tubules in *lower right* area, separated by nonspecific stromal tissue.

The gonads can be any type of combination of both tissues, but in 44.4% of cases it constitutes ovotestis. In about half of the cases, the location is intra-abdominal. In the rest of the cases, the location is inguinal, scrotal, or labial. Only 5% of patients with ovotestis are bilateral and the remainder are unilateral, with a predominance of the right side.[95] The ovotestis can be (a) bilobated, with one of the tissues having a pedicle and in each of the lobes, (b) ovoid, with the central testicular parenchyma and the ovarian tissue around it,[29] or (c) intermixed (occasionally), with both ovocytes and seminiferous tubules.[55] After puberty, seminiferous tubules remain small and often contain dysgenetic Sertoli cells similar to cryptorchid testis. Incomplete spermatogenesis has been reported, but complete spermatogenesis is very rare. The ovary is most frequently on the left side and usually hypoplastic with few primordial follicles. Occasionally, it is functionally and histologically normal.

About 4.6% of ovotestes develop germ cell tumors[96,97] and the most frequent lesions are gonadoblastoma and dysgerminoma/seminoma, followed by yolk sac tumors, mature teratoma, and carcinoid tumors. These tumors can grow to a large size. The testicle must be removed, and the residual gonad should be monitored by regular sonography explorations, particularly in patients with chromosomal mosaicisms.

Male Pseudohermaphroditism

Any process that alters any of the mechanisms for the correct expression of masculine differentiation can result in a state of male pseudohermaphroditism (Table 11-2). Situations inducing male pseudohermaphroditism include the following:

Alterations in Leydig Cell Activity
Alterations in Leydig cell activity are associated with *deficiencies in androgen synthesis* or with *deficient formation of pregnenolone, 3β-hydroxysteroid dehydrogenase,*

Table 11-2 ■ CAUSES OF MALE PSEUDOHERMAPHRODITISM

Deficiencies in androgen synthesis:
Alterations in Leydig cell activity
Androgen insensitivity syndromes:
Testicular feminization syndrome
Defective müllerian inhibiting substances:
Dysgenetic male pseudohermaphroditism
Persistent müllerian ducts syndrome

17α-hydroxylase, 17.20 desmolase, or 17β-hydroxysteroid dehydrogenase.[29]

Insufficient secretion of testosterone also can be motivated by *Leydig cell hypoplasia.* This defect can be due to an alteration of gonadotropin receptors, and their expression varies from hypogonadism to male pseudohermaphroditism according to the quantity or absence of Leydig cells.[98] The seminiferous tubules in the testicles are reduced in size, with moderate thickening of the tubular wall; Sertoli cells and occasional spermatogonia are typically present (Fig. 11-10).

In patients with defective functioning of the Leydig cells, the incidence of testicular tumors is very low.[55]

Androgen Insensitivity Syndromes
Androgen insensitivity syndromes are a spectrum of disorders characterized by peripheral resistance to the action of androgens. These syndromes are a consequence of a partial or complete absence of the response of target organs to the effect of androgens with the resultant phenotypes ranging from complete male[99] to prototypical complete testicular feminization.[100] These syndromes occur owing to an absence, decreased levels, or impairment of androgen receptors (ARs) or postreceptor anomaly.[102] As the AR is X-linked, only males are affected, and maternal carriers are phenotypically

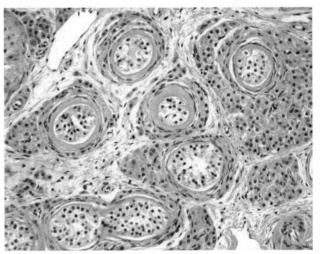

FIGURE 11-10 ■ Male pseudohermaphroditism. *Alteration in the Leydig cells activity* with reduced seminiferous tubules, wall fibrosis, and Leydig pseudohyperplasia for testicular parenchyma reduction but probable loss of function.

normal. The karyotype is usually 46XY but 47XXY and several mosaicisms have been reported.[103] These disorders affect 1:20,000 to 1:40,000 newborns.

These syndromes may be classified as follows:

1. Complete androgen insensitivity syndrome or complete testicular feminization syndrome (Morris syndrome)

2. Partial androgen insensitivity syndromes (including syndromes of Reifenstein, Gilbert-Dreyfus, Lubs, and Rosewater); mild androgen insensitivity syndrome

3. Kennedy disease

Complete Androgen Insensitivity Syndrome. Individuals with *complete AIS (formerly called testicular feminization syndrome)* have a female phenotype, normal breast development (due to aromatization of testosterone), a short vagina but no uterus (because MIS production is normal), scanty pubic and axillary hair, and female psychosexual orientation. Gonadotropins and testosterone levels can be low, normal, or elevated, depending on the degree of androgen resistance and the contribution of estradiol to feedback inhibition of the hypothalamic–pituitary gonadal axis. Most patients present with inguinal hernia (containing testes) in childhood or with primary amenorrhea in adulthood. The most prototypical is the *testicular feminization syndrome*, with a feminine phenotype, testicles with seminiferous tubules, and only Sertoli cells with occasional spermatogonia.

The testes may be in the inguinal canal, abdomen, or labia majora and may be normal upon histologic examination during the 1st year of life. Reduced germ cells are observed after the 1st year with few viable spermatogonia seen in seminiferous tubules.

In adults, the testes range in size from small to large, are tan-brown, and contain abluminal small seminiferous tubules with only Sertoli cells.[104] The accumulation of Leydig cells stands out, without Reinke crystalloids (Fig. 11-11). In 70%

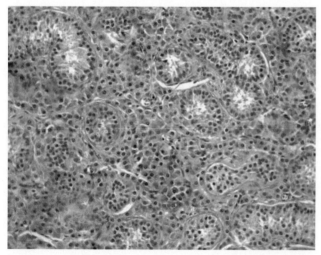

Figure 11-11 ■ Male pseudohermaphroditism. *Testicular feminization syndrome (Morris syndrome).* Seminiferous tubules with only Sertoli cells and Leydig cell accumulation without Reinke crystalloids.

of cases, yellowish nodal areas appear with the tubules and the large amount of Leydig cells, which has led some researchers to call them Sertoli-Leydig hamartomas.[29] About one-fourth have Sertoli cell adenoma comprising tubules resembling infantile testes but lacking germ cells and peritubular myoblasts. No Leydig cells are identified between the tubules.[105] Other associated tumors include large cell calcifying Sertoli cell tumor, sex cord tumor with annular tubules, Leydig cell tumor, fibroma, and leiomyoma.[101] Approximately two-thirds of cases have small cystic structures associated closely to the testes and about 80% of cases demonstrate thick smooth muscle bundles resembling myometrium near the testes. Ovarian stroma may be identified in the interstitial testicular tissue. Paratesticular cysts can also be found.[55]

Gonadectomy is usually performed immediately after puberty,[106] as there is a 10% risk of malignancy, and estrogen replacement is prescribed. The gonads can be left in situ until breast development is complete as malignancy is rarely seen before puberty. The tumors that can develop include intratubular germ cell neoplasia,[104] seminoma, nonseminomatous germ cell tumors of various types, and sex cord stromal tumors.

Partial Androgen Insensitivity Syndrome. This disorder includes the following four syndromes:

a) Reifenstein syndrome characterized by azoospermia, infertility, absent or weak virilization, hypospadias, testicular atrophy, and gynecomastia.[107]

b) Lubs syndrome with features including clitoromegaly, pubic and axillary hair, poor breast development, fusion of labioscrotal folds, and introitus formation.[108]

c) Gilbert-Dreyfus syndrome characterized by gynecomastia, hypospadias, small penis, and incomplete development of wolffian duct derivatives.[109]

d) Rosewater syndrome characterized by gynecomastia and infertility.[110]

The phenotype in the above syndromes ranges from normal male to normal female.

Mild Androgen Insensitivity Syndrome. Some patients with a male phenotype present with infertility due to a mild form of androgen insensitivity.[111] This is due to androgen resistance seen in these azoospermic or oligospermic males and is related to mutations in exons 6 or 7 or loss of exon 4.

Kennedy Disease. Spinal and bulbar muscular atrophy (Kennedy disease) is an X-linked recessive disorder usually affecting adult males.[112] Symptoms include muscle weakness, cramps, and fasciculations with onset around 20 years of age.[113] Progressive loss of motor neurons in the spinal cord and brain stem is associated with sensory neuron loss and denervation atrophy.[112]

Although testicular function and fertility may be unimpaired in the early stages of the disease, progression to secondary testicular atrophy and gynecomastia occurs with a fall in testosterone levels.

The pathologic basis behind this disease is mutations in the first exon of the AR gene. The SMBA gene located on Xq11-12 has expansion of a repetitive CAG sequence in exon A.

Defective Regression of Müllerian Ducts

Individual with anomalies in this category are typically characterized by the presence of müllerian derivatives and testicular dysgenesis (unilateral or bilateral). The expression of these anomalies can be traced back to AMH gene mutations and sensitivity of the target organs.[114]

AMH regulates inhibition of the ipsilateral müllerian ducts and collagenization of the tunica albuginea during development. Three variants of müllerian duct agenesis are described, viz. mixed gonadal dysgenesis, dysgenetic male pseudohermaphroditism, and persistent müllerian duct syndrome.

Mixed Gonadal Dysgenesis. This entity is characterized by the presence of a streak gonad on one side and a testis on the contralateral side.[115] In case of intra-abdominal gonads, the labioscrotal folds may appear as empty scrotal sacs or normal labia. The gonad is usually a testis if it is descended. If the labia appear normal, the entity cannot be detected in newborns unless an enlarged penis-like clitoris is also present. Fallopian tubes (a müllerian derivative) may be present with both a streak gonad and testis in a large percentage of cases. The testis is accompanied by an epididymis and vas deferens on the same side usually and the contralateral side usually contains a streak gonad with a fallopian tube. Other findings encountered commonly are a poorly developed vagina and a hypoplastic uterus.

Fifteen percent of intersex cases are accounted for by this condition. Patients may be reared as males as a consequence of ambiguous external genitalia subjected to virilizing effects. The penis is clitoriform with a perineal urethral meatus. However, most are considered like girls although they have cryptorchid testis and undergo virilization at puberty. Most patients report infertility as a symptom. Observed karyotypes include 45X0/46XY in >50% patients (especially those with Turner-like features), 45X0/47XYY, and 46XY. Most of the patients have one Y chromosome.

Morphologically, the testis may show two different patterns—streak testis and testicular dysgenesis. Testicular dysgenesis is typically described as having a tunica albuginea that varies in width and resembles ovarian stroma due to storiform distribution of cells and fibers. Maldeveloped seminiferous tubules with small size, absent lumina, and containing immature Sertoli cells only are also seen. Increased interstitial Leydig cells are noted with rare instances of spermatogenesis. Streak testes are complex gonads in which a fibrous streak area is seen along with testicular dysgenesis. Although the testis predominantly demonstrates features of testicular dysgenesis, a fibrous streak is identified at a gonadal pole or in continuity with the dysgenetic areas. These features may be also be encountered in some male pseudohermaphrodites. No ovocytes are identified in the streak in persistent müllerian duct syndrome. On microscopic examination, features include a spectrum of testicular lesions, ranging from true hermaphroditism to those resembling pure gonadal dysgenesis. A controversial debate herein involves the distinction between ovotestis and ovocyte-containing streak testis.[116,117]

The testis in this syndrome is unable to bring about regression of müllerian ducts and hence there is total differentiation of wolffian derivatives, virilization of external genitalia, and testicular descent in most of the cases. This syndrome is associated with a high risk of germ cell neoplasia (up to 50% in the third decade of life), especially gonadoblastoma. It is advised for patients to undergo orchiectomy after puberty.

Dysgenetic Male Pseudohermaphroditism. The above disorder of sexual differentiation is characterized by bilateral dysgenetic testes or streak testes, cryptorchidism, and persistent müllerian structures. This entity is also considered a variant of mixed gonadal dysgenesis.[118] Observed karyotypes include 45X0/46XY or 46XY with or without Turner-like features. The uterus and fallopian tubes are present and both are usually hypoplastic.[119] Lesions identified in the testes include characteristic features of testicular dysgenesis with germ cell hypoplasia. In adults, interstitial Leydig cell hyperplasia is seen along with poor or absent spermatogenesis. Gonadoblastoma arises in approximately a quarter of the patients with this syndrome.[120]

Persistent Müllerian Duct Syndrome. This syndrome is also referred to as persistent oviduct syndrome, male with uterus, tubular hermaphroditism, and hernia uteri inguinalis.[121] It is a rare form of pseudohermaphroditism wherein the müllerian derivatives persist in a phenotypically normal male. This syndrome represents the most typical form of isolated AMH deficiency.

The etiology behind the occurrence of this syndrome is multifactorial. Suggested hypotheses include the following theories: (a) defect in AMH synthesis owing to mutations in the AMH gene, (b) resistance of end organs to the effects of this hormone due to mutation in the receptor II for this hormone, and (c) failed action of this hormone just prior to the 8th week of pregnancy.[122]

One (25% cases) or both (75% cases) testes may be cryptorchid in spite of external genitalia being male. Other manifestations include inguinal hernia contralateral to the undescended testis, with a uterus and fallopian tubes situated within the hernia sac,[123] infertility,[124] and testicular tumor.[125] The testes in childhood have a decreased tubular diameter and a low fertility index. The tunica albuginea is variably thickened in adults with tissue resembling ovarian stroma and may contain rudimentary tubular structures. The seminiferous tubules are hyalinized and atrophic with decreased spermatogenesis or a mixed pattern with some tubules capable of spermatogenesis being seen. Interstitial Leydig cells are increased. Oligospermia and azoospermia are often seen.[122]

This syndrome is familial or sporadic with X-linked or autosomal inheritance.[126] All types of germ cell tumors have been reported in these patients who are at increased risk for testicular tumor.[127]

Table 11-3 ■ CHROMOSOMAL AND GENETIC ANOMALIES WITH TESTICULAR CHANGES

Name of Syndrome	Chromosomal Anomaly
Kallmann syndrome	Anomaly in the short arm of the X chromosome
Prader-Willi syndrome	Long arm of chromosome 15
Bardet-Biedl syndrome	Alteration in chromosome 16
Klinefelter syndrome	Extra X chromosome
Noonan syndrome	XYY, 46XX, and 4XY syndrome
Cystic fibrosis	q31.2 on the long (q) arm of chromosome 7
5α-reductase deficiency	SRD5A2 gene in chromosome 2p23
Down syndrome	Trisomy 21
Structural anomalies of the Y chromosome	Y chromosome abnormalities

Chromosomal and Genetic Anomalies (Table 11-3)

Genetic Anomalies that Induce Pretesticular Changes

In the group of genetic anomalies that induce pretesticular changes, we can include Kallmann syndrome (anomaly in the short arm of the X chromosome),[128] with anosmia, deafness, cryptorchidism, and testicular hypoplasia and anomalies of the palate, in which the testicle shows diverse degrees of hypoplasia and blockage in the maturation of the germ cells.[129]

Even rarer are Prader-Willi syndrome (obesity, mental retardation, and hypotonia of the hands and feet due to loss of genetic material in the long arm of chromosome 15)[130]; Bardet-Biedl syndrome (alteration in the chromosome 16); as well as congenital hypogonadotrophism due to sickle cell anemia and beta-thalassemia.[131]

Genetic Anomalies Associated with Testicular Alterations

Klinefelter syndrome is caused by an extra X chromosome due to nondysjunction in sex chromosome migration during the meiotic division of spermatocyte or ovule. In 73% of cases, the extra chromosome X belongs to the mother; for this reason advanced maternal age increases the incidence of Klinefelter syndrome.

Klinefelter syndrome is the most common genetic cause of human male infertility.[132]

In 80% of cases, the karyotype is 47XXY. The remaining 20% are mosaics with at least two X chromosomes in many different combinations: XY/XXY, XY/XXXY, XX/XXY, XY/X0/XXY, etc.

Clinically, an eunuchoid phenotype, increased stature, incomplete virilization, small testes, infertility (in 50%), gynecomastia, mental retardation, and low bone mineral density can be present; for that the incidence varies according to the population of reference (1:500 general male newborns, 1:100 among mental institutions, and 3.4:100 of infertile men).[133]

However, despite its relatively high frequency, the syndrome is often overlooked because it lacks many of these features.

Testicular biopsies of prepubertal Klinefelter syndrome have shown preservation of seminiferous tubules with reduced numbers of germ cells, but Sertoli and Leydig cells have appeared normal. During puberty, the testicle loses a large numbers of germ cells, and thus in the adult male they are characterized by extensive fibrosis and hyalinization of the seminiferous tubules (Fig. 11-12), loss of elastic fibers, and hyperplasia of the interstitium, but the tubules may show residual foci of spermatogenesis.[134] Treatment consists of testosterone replacement therapy to correct the androgen deficiency and to provide patients with appropriate virilization. This therapy also has positive effects on mood and self-esteem and has been shown to protect against osteoporosis, although it will not reverse infertility.[135] Early diagnosis and treatment can improve the quality of life and the overall health of men with Klinefelter syndrome.[133]

Testicular germ cell tumors are rare in Klinefelter syndrome, but extragonadal germ cell tumors (teratoma, and choriocarcinoma), especially in the mediastinum, are more frequent. Breast cancers also are more frequent. Both types probably are related to hormonal stimulation.[136]

The 46XX males have hypergonadotropic hypogonadism with elevated levels of FSH and elevated LH with normal testosterone. During childhood, the seminiferous tubules have a decreased number of germ cells. In the adults, the testes show a similar aspect as Klinefelter testicles with or without Sertoli cell–only tubules, and the Leydig cells demonstrate an absence of Reinke crystalloids.[29] The 47XYY syndrome men have a normal external genitalia, decreased fertility, and Sertoli cell–only tubules associated with normal spermatogenesis in tubules.[137]

Other chromosomal anomalies such as 46XY (Noonan) syndrome, 45X0, show different degrees of atrophy of the testicle.[131]

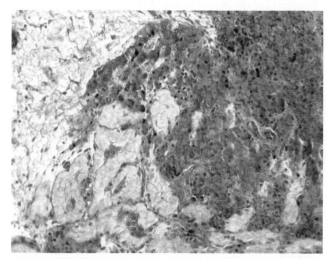

FIGURE 11-12 ■ Klinefelter syndrome. Tubular hyalinization with Leydig cell nodular pseudohyperplasia (Masson trichrome stain, low power.).

Genetic Anomalies Associated with Posttesticular Changes

In the group of genetic anomalies associated with post-testicular changes, very diverse pathologic features can be found, such as 5α-reductase deficiency (a variant of male pseudohermaphroditism that results in anomalous genitals in infancy, normal masculine development with libido and ejaculation, prostatic hypoplasia, and testicles with small seminiferous tubules without lumina and only immature Sertoli cells),[138] cystic fibrosis, or Kartagener syndrome with immobility of the cilia[131] and preserved spermatogenesis. Down syndrome and structural anomalies of the Y chromosome can also cause male pseudohermaphroditism.

Other Congenital Anomalies

Other testicular alterations can be found in addition to those described, which can be classified as follows:

Heterotopias and Rests of the Wolffian and Müllerian Ducts

In tunica albuginea and rete testis, *adrenal cortical rests* are found relatively frequently, with an incidence ranging from 2.5% to 15%.[139,140] They are made up of adrenal cortical tissue surrounded by a connective tissue band (Fig. 11-13). They are about 5 mm in diameter on average and are thus not clinically palpable.

Other heterotopic tissues involve the liver (*hepatic–gonadal fusion*, very infrequently)[141] and the spleen (*splenic–gonadal fusion*) (Fig. 11-14). The latter occurs more frequently on the left side and has been described in about 148 published cases.[142] The ectopic splenic tissue can be in close proximity to the head of the epididymis or to the upper pole of the testis, or it can be separated from them. Likewise, there may or may not be structural continuity between the normal spleen and the ectopic tissue.[143] In about 30% of cases, splenic–gonadal fusion has been associated with complex malformations such as micrognathia

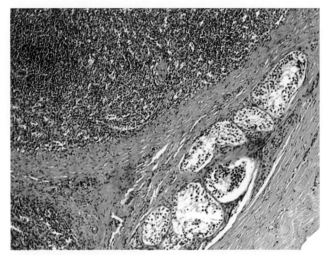

FIGURE 11-14 ■ Splenic–gonadal fusion. Splenic tissue in close relation with seminiferous tubules. Both tissues are separated by non-specific fibrous tissue.

(abnormal smallness of the jaws, especially of the lower jaw), peromelia (severe congenital malformations of extremities, including absence of the hand or foot), or phocomelia (absence of the upper portion of a limb).[143–145] In three of the reported cases, the fusion was associated with a germ cell tumor of the testis.[142]

The presence of rests of the wolffian duct, such as the paradidymis (*Giraldes organ*) and the *Haller organ*, are relatively frequent anomalies.[29] Much rarer is finding epithelial, solid, or cystic rests in albuginea, sometimes accompanied by an inflammatory reaction, known as *Walthard cellular rests*, probably of müllerian origin, since the epithelium has cilia.[146]

Cysts

Cysts occur in approximately 8% to 10% of patients with a lump in the testis, including those of the tunica albuginea or the parenchyma.[147]

Tunica Albuginea Cysts. Tunica albuginea cysts usually are small, asymptomatic, unilocular, or multilocular, probably mesothelial rests (with occasional squamous metaplasia)[148] or mesonephric rests.[149]

Parenchymal Testicular Cysts. Parenchymal testicular cysts are simple, very rare, and can be mesothelial rests or ectopic rete testis. The testicular *epidermoid cyst* deserves special consideration, which must only be covered with squamous epithelium (Fig. 11-15). It is recommended that the specimen be examined in toto to avoid underdiagnosis of any area of teratoma (especially among postpubertal patients) or intratubular germ cell neoplasia, since sonographically it is not possible to distinguish between epidermoid cyst and cystic teratoma.[150] Epidermoid cysts represent 1% of the masses of the testes. Recent genetic studies have shown that there is no chromosome 12p abnormality,[151] thus supporting its distinction from teratoma.

Cystic Dysplasia of the Rete Testis. Cystic dysplasia of the rete testis (Fig. 11-16) is a congenital lesion with complete testicular parenchymal substitution by the cyst.[152] The

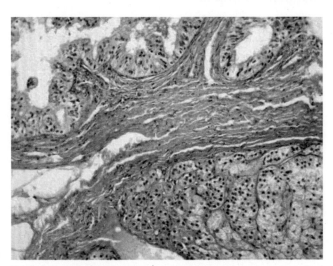

FIGURE 11-13 ■ Adrenal–gonadal fusion. Adrenal cortical cells (*bottom*) in close relation with epididymis (*top*).

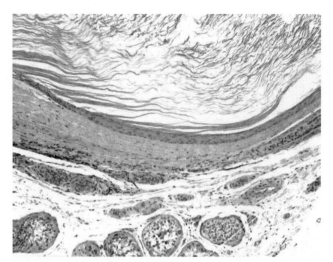

FIGURE 11-15 ■ Testicular epidermoid cyst. Intratesticular cyst covered by mature squamous cell epithelium with keratinization.

cysts of the rete testis are not always contiguous to it, and they are characterized by being covered by flat epithelium alternating with cuboidal epithelium. It is believed that they are a consequence of a defect in the connection between the efferent tubules and the rete testis, for which reason they can also be found in the literature under the term *testicular cystic dysplasia*,[153] especially when it substitutes nearly the entire parenchyma.

Congenital Testicular Lymphangiectasis. The disease is a congenital malformation consisting of an abnormal expansive development of lymphatic vessels in the parenchyma and the tunica vasculosa in both testes with absence of other lymphangiectasis.[154] It was described for the first time in a patient with bilateral inguinal cryptorchidism but also in Noonan syndrome, and cases without any other coexisting pathology have also been reported.[155] The testes show

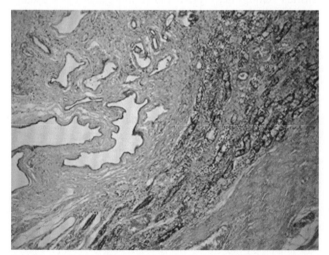

FIGURE 11-16 ■ Cystic dysplasia of rete testis. Testicular parenchyma is nearly completely replaced by the rete testis cysts (*upper left*) so that they are covered by flat epithelium alternating with cuboidal epithelium.

normal tubular development with normal germ cell numbers and also normal Leydig cell numbers or changes of cryptorchidism or Noonans syndrome.

Gonadoblastoid Testicular Dysplasia

Gonadoblastoid testicular dysplasia is a rare lesion with only seven published cases in the literature.[156] Several cases with this disorder have been reported in patients with *Walker-Warburg syndrome* (lethal genetic disease associated with a cobblestone-type lissencephaly, eye abnormalities, and a type of muscular dystrophy)[157] or with 46XY karyotype and multiple congenital anomalies.[158]

It consists of large tubular or nodular structures within a dense stroma, reminiscent of ovarian stroma. Each structure is composed of three cell types: cells with vesicular nuclei and vacuolated cytoplasm; cells with hyperchromatic nuclei; and germ cell–like cells. The former two types are arranged at the periphery, forming a pseudostratified epithelium. The third type resembles fetal spermatogonia and is smaller in number. These structures contain eosinophilic, periodic acid–Schiff–positive material, similar to Call-Exner bodies. The differential diagnosis is with testicular dysgenesis, but these are male pseudohermaphrodites with müllerian remnants, and gonadoblastoma usually appears in a streak gonad or dysgenetic gonad and the testes contain granulosa–Sertoli cells and germ cells that are similar to those of dysgerminoma or seminoma; these cells are absent in gonadoblastoid testicular dysplasia.

VASCULAR LESIONS

The testicle can present with various vascular lesions that lead to ischemia or hemorrhage. Among the causes of vascular lesions, traumas and torsions are the most common, although one must not overlook the states of hypercoagulability and vasculitis.

Testicular Infarction

Testicular infarctions related to vasculitis (see Testicular Vasculitis) and hematologic disorders have been described, but the most common cause is torsion.

Testicular Torsion

It can be intravaginal or extravaginal (infrequent and more common in prepubertal age). The two ages of highest incidence are perinatal and pubertal, but this pattern seems to change, and more cases, especially of the intravaginal variant, are beginning to be seen in young adults.[159]

The causes of torsion have not been sufficiently clarified, but anomalies of the tunica vaginalis seem to play a role. The testis is fixed to the scrotal wall by three structures. The reduction of these attachment surfaces facilitates intravaginal torsion. The hypercontractibility of the dartos and the spiral insertion of the muscular fibers of the cremaster with a high reflection of tunica vaginalis can explain the cord torsions by sudden body movements or by energic cremasteric contractions.[160] Other predisposing factors are a very long gubernaculum testis, a long or badly placed epididymis, and spermatic artery anomalies. The rate at which ischemia is established depends on the degree of vascular disturbance and whether it affects only the venous portion (great congestion and subsequent infarction) or both venous and arterial portions.

The morphologic appearance, both macroscopic and microscopic, depends on the degree of torsion (and consequently on the ischemia) and on the time of testis incarceration. Interruption of venous drainage causes edema, vascular congestion, rupture of venous wall, and interstitial bleeding. In the most evident cases, the testis turns dark red, has a greater solid consistency to the touch, and has a smooth external surface; the cut surface has an appearance similar to the external surface. Microscopically, hemorrhagic infarction with extravasated erythrocytes is seen; initially, there is conservation of germ cells, which later disappear (Fig. 11-17). Occasionally, a granulomatous reaction with macrophages, multinucleated giant cells, lymphocytes, plasma cells, and/or fibrous connective tissue at the periphery of the lesion has been reported. In the spermatic cord, lipomembranous fat necrosis with cystic cavities that are bounded by wavy hyaline membranes has been reported.[161]

The most important clinicopathologic questions include the following: (a) when should torsion be suspected? (b) how soon does the urologist have to untwist the testicle before irreversible changes take place? and (c) how does the torsion impact fertility? Testicular torsion produces acute pain, and that can induce inflammation of the scrotal skin. Therefore, torsion is clinically suspected if cord thickening and lateralization or anterior positioning of the epididymis is found.[162] The time required for irreversible changes is very difficult to estimate. Experience has shown that there will be severe alterations within 2 hours and necrosis within 6 hours,[163] but that

chronology is difficult to transfer into clinical practice since it depends on the intensity and type of obstructed vessels.

One of the most debated dilemmas is the influence of torsion on the contralateral testicle. Studies have shown that serious alterations in the untwisted contralateral testicle can develop via the twisted testicle through some type of immune reaction,[164] but more recent studies have shown that unilateral testicular and epididymal torsion had no effect on the contralateral testis.[165]

Segmental Infarction

An infrequent situation is focal testicular infarction; both its clinical picture and ultrasonographic image can be confused with a testicular tumor.[166] A venous rupture followed by thrombosis and infarction can be the origin of this focal infarction (for more information see the section on nonneoplastic tumorous conditions.).

Appendix Torsion

The testicular appendix (hydatid of Morgagni), seen in 80% to 92% of men, undergoes torsion and infarction more frequently than the epididymis appendix does. The clinical picture is identical to that of testicular infarction, and its appearance is that of a hemorrhagic infarction.[167] Its etiopathogenesis is unknown.

Other Infarction Causes

Many other causes of testicular infarction are refereed in the literature and amongst them trauma, orchitis, epididymitis, and cryptorchidism are the most important.[168–170]

Hematocele

The accumulation of hemorrhagic material in the vaginal space is known as hematocele. Many times it is distributed diffusely, although it occasionally acquires a more

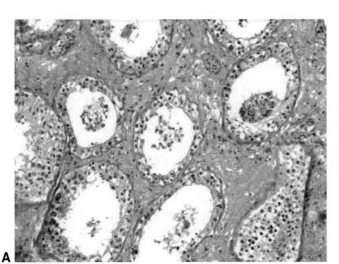
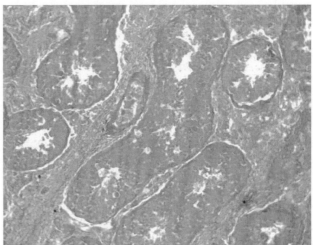

FIGURE 11-17 ■ Testicular infarction. **A:** Initial changes with interstitial hemorrhage, seminiferous tubules compression, and germ cell desquamation. **B:** Advanced changes with complete tubular necrosis (phantom contours).

pseudotumoral appearance. The long-standing hematocele can lead to fibrosis and calcification, with accumulation of hemosiderin[171] and cholesterol crystals associated with the formation of granulomas.[172]

Varicocele

Varicocele is characterized by dilation, elongation, and increase of the sinuosity of the vessels in the spermatic (pampiniform) plexus secondary to the increase in venous pressure that leads to anomalous blood flow to that venous system. The cause is unknown, but there is speculation that the cause is associated with conditions that damage venous drainage (venous valve anomalies, alterations of the muscles of the venous wall, extrinsic compressions, and pressure problems).

Varicoceles are found in 8% to 23% of the general population.[173] They occur more frequently in smokers and on the left side (probably because of the greater hydrostatic pressure secondary to its greater length or because its drainage in the renal vein occurs at a right angle). Although they can present at any age, they are more common in puberty.[174]

Alterations in the testicle are very diverse and difficult to attribute only to varicocele since many of these changes are nonspecific and common to many other processes. The usual changes with varicoceles include fibrosis of the wall in the veins of the albuginea, dilation of the interstitial veins, cytoplasmic vacuolization of the Sertoli cells, abnormal spermatogenesis, and germ cell sloughing; except for the venous ectasia in the testicular stroma, no specific feature is associated with the vascular origin of these changes, and their influence on infertility is still debated.[175]

Testicular Lesions in Arteriosclerosis and Hypertension

It is difficult to evaluate the changes that are secondary to generalized vascular pathologic changes because these pathologic changes are typically seen in advanced ages and cannot be easily distinguished from the changes caused by aging.[88]

Testicular Vasculitis

As seen in other organs, vasculitis can be isolated or can be in the context of a systemic form. Its morphologic features are not unique or pathognomonic toward one form of vasculitis or the other[176]; thus, the clinical history continues to be used for making these diagnoses. Many different types of vasculitis in the testicle have been described, including *Henoch-Schönlein purpura*,[177] *rheumatoid arthritis*,[178] and *dermatomyositis*[179]; however, the most frequent types of vasculitis seen in the testis are *polyarteritis nodosa* (PAN)[180] (Fig. 11-18), *giant cell vasculitis*,[181] and *Wegener granulomatosis*.[182,183]

Clinically, vasculitis of the reproductive system occurs in up to 18% of males with systemic PAN. At autopsy this

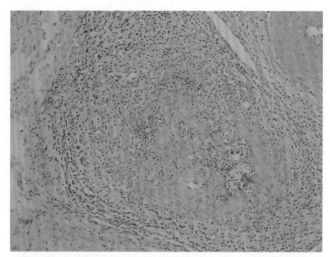

FIGURE 11-18 ■ Testicular vasculitis. Isolated vasculitis of PAN type.

system is involved in 60% to 86% of cases.[184] The testes usually show arterial lesions in different stages of evolution. The parenchyma has areas of infarction and scar lesions. PAN is the type of systemic vasculitis most frequently associated with testicular involvement. Testicular vasculitis occurs as isolated vasculitis in men usually presenting with a testicular mass in the absence of systemic symptoms and normal laboratory results. It is an unexpected finding in most isolated testicular vasculitis patients wherein a testicular neoplasm is initially suspected. Isolated testicular vasculitis does not require systemic therapy.[185]

LYSOSOMAL STORAGE DISEASES

Lysosomal storage diseases are a heterogeneous group of disorders caused by lysosomal enzyme dysfunction. Individually they are very rare, but this group as a whole has a prevalence of more than 1:8,000 live births. Musculoskeletal complaints are frequently the first reason for the patient to seek medical advice.[186]

Types A and B Niemann-Pick disease, lysosomal storage disorders resulting from the deficient activity of acid sphingomyelinase, in mice present characteristic lipid-filled vacuoles with storage vesicles within Sertoli cells of the seminiferous tubules. Lipid accumulation in the seminiferous tubules in the gonads results in regulatory volume decrease defects within the developing sperm with morphologic abnormalities such as kinks and bends at the midpiece–principle piece junction evident in spermatozoa.[187]

INFLAMMATORY DISEASES

A number of agents can produce a testicular inflammatory reaction (Table 11-4), but as in other organs, inflammatory lesions of the testicle can be classified as acute or chronic,

Table 11-4 ■ MOST FREQUENT AGENTS OF TESTICULAR INFLAMMATION

Bacterial:
- *Escherichia coli*
- *Klebsiella*
- *Pseudomonas*
- *Haemophilus influenzae*
- *Proteus mirabilis*
- *Neisseria meningitidis*
- *Salmonella*
- Pneumococci
- Streptococci
- Staphylococci
- *Mycobacterium tuberculosis*
- *Mycobacterium leprae*
- *Brucella melitensis*
- *Treponema pallidum*

Fungal:
- *Coccidioides immitis*
- *Blastomyces dermatitidis*
- *Cryptococcus neoformans*
- *Histoplasma capsulatum*

Parasites:
- *Schistosoma haematobium*
- *Wuchereria bancrofti* (filariasis)

Virus:
- Mumps
- Coxsackie B
- Echovirus
- Infectious mononucleosis
- Smallpox
- Varicella
- Rubella
- Adenovirus
- SARS

Special Tissular Reactions of Unknown Agent:
- Idiopathic granulomatous orchitis
- Malakoplakia
- Xantogranulomatous orchitis
- Sarcoidosis
- Lymphocytic orchitis
- Rosai-Dorfman disease

and in turn as bacterial, nonbacterial, or idiopathic with a peculiar tissue response. Moreover, inflammatory lesions of the testicle can be an expression of another infectious or generalized inflammatory process. Given that the greater part of the infectious processes, whether local or systemic, affects both the testicular parenchyma and the epididymis, it is a general rule to use the term *epididymo-orchitis*.

Acute Epididymo-orchitis

Acute epididymo-orchitis can be subdivided into *acute bacterial* and *acute nonbacterial (acute viral) epididymo-orchitis*.

Acute Bacterial Epididymo-orchitis

Acute bacterial epididymo-orchitis in young men is usually an infection of venereal origin. Men between 14 and 35 years of age are most often affected and *Chlamydia trachomatis* and *Neisseria gonorrhoeae* are the causative organisms, whereas in older adults, this condition is usually associated with a Gram-negative bacillary infection secondary to infections of the urinary system,[188] the most frequent being *Escherichia coli*, *Klebsiella*, *Pseudomonas*, *Haemophilus influenzae*, *Proteus mirabilis*, *Neisseria meningitidis*, *Salmonella*, pneumococci, streptococci, and staphylococci.

The clinical picture includes fever, pain, and increased size of the organ, a consequence of edema and the infiltration of neutrophils, lymphocytes, and plasma cells that, in a diffuse manner, start from the interstitium and expand into the seminiferous tubules with destroying germ cells (Fig. 11-19). Although not common, occasionally abscesses or infarctions can result, in which case one must search for anaerobic organisms and exclude the possibility of AIDS or diabetes.[189]

Acute Viral Epididymo-orchitis

Many viruses can affect the testicle. The mumps virus and Coxsackie virus are the most frequent,[190] but cases caused by the echovirus or by infectious mononucleosis, smallpox, varicella, rubella,[191] adenovirus and even severe acute respiratory syndrome (SARS) viruses have been reported.[192]

Mumps virus *epididymo-orchitis* occurs in 36% of patients with acute viral *epididymo-orchitis* and is bilateral in 15% of them. In the inflammatory exudate, the lymphocytes predominate over the neutrophils (Fig. 11-20). About the 3rd week after infection, fibrosis of the tubules is produced and is frequently the cause of sterility, either through direct destruction or through production of antisperm antibodies.[193]

In AIDS the testis shows many CD4+ lymphocytes, indicating the presence of abundant host cells (T-helper/-inducer

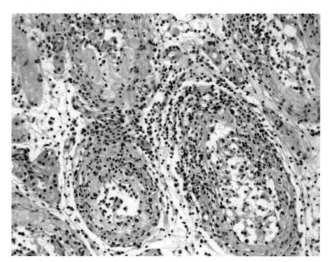

FIGURE 11-19 ■ Acute bacterial orchiepididymitis. Acute interstitial inflammation with tubular extension and germ cell destruction.

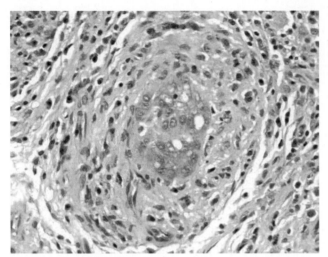

FIGURE 11-20 ■ Viral orchitis. Tubular fibrosis with scant lymphocytic infiltration and residual intratubular Sertoli cells.

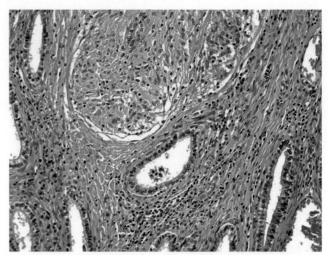

FIGURE 11-21 ■ Epididymal tuberculosis. Non-necrotizing granulomatous inflammation in the interstitium of epididymis.

lymphocytes and macrophages) for HIV-1. Furthermore, macrophages and cells of lymphocytic morphology were observed migrating across the boundary walls of hyalinized seminiferous in tubules to enter the lumen.[194]

Chronic Epididymo-orchitis

Chronic epididymo-orchitis can be subdivided into *nonspecific chronic epididymo-orchitis* and *granulomatous epididymo-orchitis*.

Nonspecific Chronic Epididymo-orchitis

Inadequate therapeutics or certain immunologic characteristics of the patient can cause acute inflammatory lesions to progress to a chronic form, focal or diffuse, with a predominance of scarring changes and lymphocytic infiltrate. If the patient does not seek medical attention until his or her disease is in advanced phases, it is impossible to determine the cause.

Granulomatous Epididymo-orchitis

A large percentage of chronic epididymo-orchitis cases are characterized microscopically by granulomatous inflammation. This is a very heterogeneous group with a common morphologic microscopic appearance of granuloma formation; these cases are often secondary to systemic infections or correspond to particular tissue responses.

Epididymo-orchitis in Systemic Infections

Practically all viral epididymo-orchitis belong in this group of epididymo-orchitis in systemic infections, and although it was described earlier, other variants will be discussed.

Bacterial Infection with Testicular Involvement

Tuberculosis

The incidence of tuberculosis has increased with the increased incidence of immunodeficiency diseases (such as HIV)[195]

and with intravesical treatment with bacille Calmette-Guérin (BCG).[196] Testicular involvement usually begins through the seminal duct system and within the context of renal tuberculosis (50% of the patients with renal or prostatic tuberculosis develop testicular tuberculosis). Testicular tuberculosis is more prominent and occurs earlier in the epididymis than in the testicle itself.

In orchiectomized cases, testicular tuberculosis is characterized by multiple, small (2 to 4 mm) white to yellow nodules with a uniform appearance, preferably located near the epididymis and corresponding to the initial granulomas (Fig. 11-21). In later phases, a broad substitution for the testicular parenchyma can be seen with characteristics similar to those seen in the epididymis. The typical microscopic features are necrotizing caseating granulomas with epithelioid histiocytes and Langhans giant cells[29] (Fig. 11-22). In children, dissemination to the testis appears to be more hematogenous than does dissemination to the seminal duct system.[197]

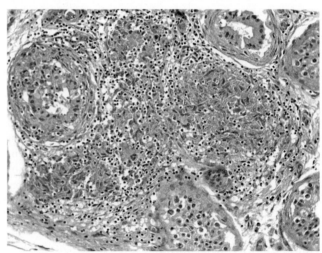

FIGURE 11-22 ■ **Testicular tuberculosis.** Well formed granulomata (with Langhans giant cells) without necrosis in testicular interstitium.

Brucellosis

Brucella melitensis in endemic areas can produce orchiepididymitis[198]: specifically, 6.8% of brucellosis patients have an orchiepididymitis and 6.5% of acute orchiepididymitis cases are etiologically related to brucellosis.[199] Microscopically, there is dense lymphohistiocytic infiltrate, often with nonnecrotizing granulomas.[29]

Syphilis

The typical lesion in syphilis is the gumma, a broad area of necrosis with "phantom" preservation of the tubule edges and inflammatory granulomatous reaction with lymphocytes and plasma cells. Endarteritis is also present.[200] In congenital syphilis, the testicular involvement can be bilateral. Recent reports cite the development of syphilitic testicular involvement in males with HIV 1 viral infection.[200]

Leprosy

Men with lepromatous or borderline leprosy can develop testicular and epididymal changes.[201] Semen analysis has revealed marked oligospermia or azoospermia in up to 10% of cases.[202] Very rarely, testicular involvement is the primary manifestation of the disease.[203] It is usually bilateral, although the degrees of involvement may differ. Classically, three morphologic phases are defined: the vascular phase (perivascular lymphocyte infiltrate), the interstitial phase (with lymphocytes and intertubular macrophages), and the obliterative phase (with tubular fibrosis, Leydig cell aggregates, and endarteritis obliterans). However, there is marked variation in histopathologic findings in testes; hence, it is difficult to categorize results into the vascular, interstitial, or obliterative phase.[201]

Fungal Infection with Testicular Involvement

Fungal infection with testicular involvement is rare. The most frequent fungal infections of this type include coccidioidomycosis,[204] blastomycosis, cryptococcosis, and histoplasmosis. These infections have been observed in immunosuppressed patients and usually cause abscesses or granulomas with characteristics similar to those of tuberculosis; therefore, only a demonstration of fungi (microscopically or through culture) permits a precise diagnosis. An isolated epidydimatis for histoplasma is referred in the literature.[205]

Parasitic Infection with Testicular Involvement

Parasitic infections can be found in the gonads, with filariasis[206] and schistosomiasis[207] being the most frequent. In both infections, there is a predominant spermatic cord and epididymal involvement, and the testicular lesions are usually secondary to the vascular manifestation by the parasites.

Special Inflammatory Testicular Reactions

This section includes inflammatory processes that are characterized by a particular tissue response; most are of unknown etiology.

Idiopathic Granulomatous Orchitis

This entity was identified in a group of patients with lesions that clinically mimic tuberculosis or neoplasia and had testicular enlargement associated with a noncaseating granulomatous inflammatory process without tuberculosis bacilli. An attempt was made to correlate this disorder with thrombotic phenomena of the pampiniform plexus[208]; however, most researchers support an autoimmune origin for this condition.[209] Patients are usually in the fifth or sixth decade of life.

The lesion typically affects the testicle, giving it a whitish and homogeneous appearance that is sometimes macroscopically indistinguishable from a seminoma or lymphoma. The albuginea can be thickened. The section surface is nodular with occasional necrotic areas.

Microscopically, the inflammatory involvement has two patterns: (i) *interstitial* when the granulomas predominate in the interstitium and (ii) *tubular* when the granulomas are predominantly in the seminiferous tubules. Epithelioid histiocytes and occasional giant cells, which give a distinct granulomatous appearance, are most commonly seen but polymorphonuclear cells can also be recognized. The germ cells are destroyed. Characteristically the granulomas in this lesion are intratubular (Fig. 11-23). Forty percent of the patients have spermatic granulomas in the epididymis. These two morphologic types correlate with two experimental animal models (injection of immune cells for interstitial and injection of the serum of affected animals) suggesting two different immunologic ways.[88]

It is mandatory to distinguish this entity from the granulomatous lesions in systemic infections, in which the granulomas are in general situated in the interstitium with secondary intratubular extension.[210] If the location of the granuloma is in doubt, staining with reticulin silver can be of help.

Malakoplakia

Malakoplakia is secondary to a decrease in cyclin–guanine monophosphate in mononuclear cells that impairs the killing

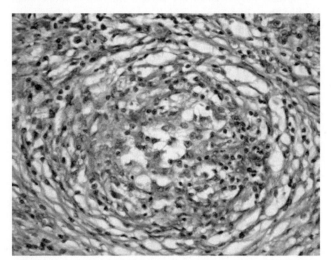

FIGURE 11-23 ■ Idiopathic granulomatous orchitis. Tubular granulomatous inflammation without necrosis. The interstitium is noninvolved or shows scanty inflammatory reaction.

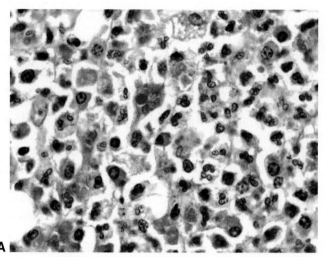
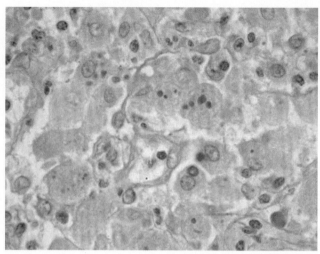

A   B

Figure 11-24 ■ Testicular malakoplakia. **A:** Plasma cells, lymphocytes, and macrophages with eosinophilic inclusion bodies (H&E). **B:** Macrophages/von Hansemann cells with inclusion bodies (Michaelis-Gutmann bodies) representing fusion of the phagolysosomes with bacterial rests (PAS).

of bacteria. Fusion of the phagolysosomes with bacterial rests produces the characteristic Michaelis-Gutmann bodies (granular basophilic periodic acid–Schiff–positive, diastase-resistant inclusions of 5 to 8 μm with calcification with a targetoid appearance with a dense central core) in the cytoplasm of the macrophages (von Hansemann cells)[211] (Fig. 11-24).

Testicular involvement is seen in only 12% of genital malakoplakia, with about 400 reported cases[212,213]; however, genital malakoplakia may affect only the epididymis.[214] Macroscopically yellowish-brown nodules are present, often with formation of abscesses. Microscopically, early in the disease, inflammatory cells mixed with histiocytes and scant Michaelis-Gutmann bodies, very difficult to appreciate with H&E, are seen. In the terminal phase, the characteristic von Hansemann cells are present with tubular destruction. Late in the disease, an extensive fibrosis can appear. Giant cells are occasionally seen or are absent. Immunohistochemical studies show histiocytes, which are positive for CD68 antibodies, lysosomes, and α-chymotrypsin. Gram stain may demonstrate Gram-negative bacteria. Ultrastructurally, there are curved membrane-bound phagolysosomes containing whorled and parallel lamellar phospholipids.

The differential diagnosis includes idiopathic granulomatous orchitis (but both conditions have been related in their pathogenesis to idiopathic granulomatous orchitis)[213,215] and Leydig cell tumors with eosinophilic cells containing Reinke crystalloids and without a significant inflammatory component.

Xanthogranulomatous Orchitis

Some cases of xanthogranulomatous orchitis in the testes[216,217] have been described as having a homogeneous appearance on cutting and the characteristic accumulations of foamy histiocytic cells (Fig. 11-25), which have been correlated with malakoplakia.[218] However, characteristic

Michaelis-Gutmann bodies cannot be demonstrated. Some cases of xanthogranulomatous periorchitis[219] have also been reported.

Sarcoidosis

Testicular involvement in systemic sarcoidosis[220] is exceedingly rare, and its presentation as the primary form is even rarer; in these cases, the epididymis is affected more, with the testicle being involved by contiguity.[221]

Lymphocytic Orchitis

Lymphocytic orchitis is also called *testicular pseudolymphoma*[222] and is characterized by a lymphocytic and plasmacytic cell reaction with germinal center formation and destruction of the testicular parenchyma (Fig. 11-26) that may be confused with a lymphoma; immunohistochemical

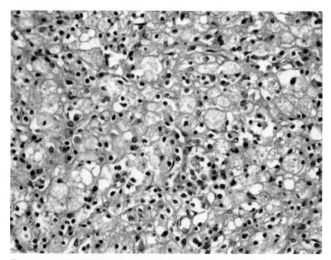

Figure 11-25 ■ Xanthogranulomatous orchitis. Accumulation of foamy histiocytes without Michaelis-Gutmann bodies.

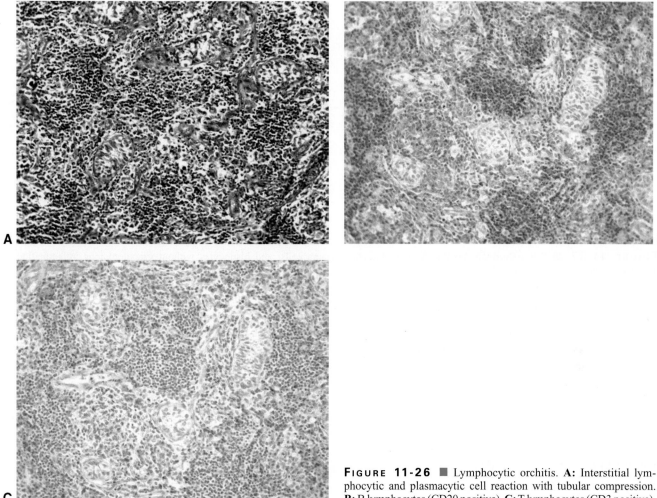

FIGURE 11-26 ■ Lymphocytic orchitis. **A:** Interstitial lymphocytic and plasmacytic cell reaction with tubular compression. **B:** B lymphocytes (CD20 positive). **C:** T lymphocytes (CD3 positive).

analysis, however, shows that the cellular infiltrate is polyclonal. The absence of endarterial lesion and of granulomas distinguishes lymphocytic orchitis from syphilis.[29]

Rosai-Dorfman Disease

Histologic examination of the testicular mass in Rosai-Dorfman disease reveals an inflammatory lesion comprising lymphocytes, plasma cells, and sheets of pale staining histiocytes, some containing lymphocytes within their ample cytoplasm, suggestive of emperipolesis (Fig. 11-27). The histiocytes characteristically stain positively for CD68 and S100 and negatively for CD1a by immunohistochemical analysis. Ultrastructural examination confirms that macrophages phagocyte intact lymphocytes (emperipolesis).[223]

INFERTILITY

There are many reasons why a male is infertile. Many of the pathologic conditions described up to now can cause it; thus, some of them are diagnosed in an infertility study. Infertility can also be secondary to pharmacologic treatments. Many

times, however, the cause of infertility is unknown. This has led to testicular biopsies being conducted to try to find the causes of infertility so that actions can be taken to resolve the problem. From the first biopsies performed in the 1940s[224,225] until now, however, biopsies have rarely disclosed the responsible etiologies or clinicopathologic entities, and if we add these disappointing attempts to the results from genetic (karyotyping) and endocrinologic studies, the clinical utility of these attempts is poorer than ever before. Nevertheless, the testicular biopsy in the assessment of male infertility continues to have its uses, and pathologists must therefore know about the interpretation of these biopsies for conveying optimal information to andrologists.

If we group male infertility by seminogram findings, the principal states are azoospermia, cryptozoospermia, and oligozoospermia with more or less asthenozoospermia. If we group types of male infertility by pathology we could subdivide them into pretesticular, testicular, and posttesticular.

The indications for testicular biopsy are for diagnosis and for testicular sperm extraction. According to these guidelines, the obstructive azoospermia and the normogonadotropic or hypergonadotropic azoospermia are the most common

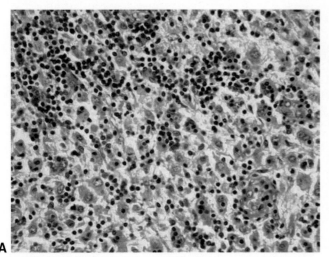
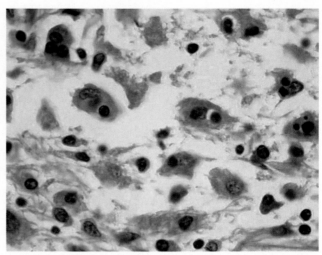

FIGURE 11-27 ■ Rosai-Dorfman disease. **A:** Lymphocytes, plasma cells, and histiocytes without granulomatous inflammation. **B:** Histiocytes with emperipolesis.

indications in infertility. Testicular biopsy is also indicated in case of azoospermic Klinefelter patients, because spermatogenesis, even at a very low rate, might occur.[226]

A diagnostic biopsy is also indicated to exclude intratubular germ cell neoplasia especially in cases of nonhomogeneous testicular ultrasonography and more controversially in the contralateral testis of a patient with a testicular germ cell tumor.

Handling of Testicular Biopsies

To correctly assess the testicular biopsy, careful handling of the sample is necessary to avoid artifacts of the cellular components of the seminiferous tubule.

The size of the biopsy specimen should not exceed 3 mm and should be bilateral. In these specimens, rapid and proper fixation is of utmost importance, for which reason it is recommended that they be preserved in Bouin liquid. This type of biopsy is typically prepared for various studies; for this reason, one must take into account that some portion of the specimen (or minimum parts of that sent to the pathologist) must be preserved for ancillary studies. The fresh tissue can be preserved about 5 hours in a wet chamber at 4°C. For each of the biopsies, three consecutive sections must be cut for each of the following recommended histochemical stains: hematoxylin–eosin, Masson trichrome, and orcein for elastic fibers.

Testicular biopsies for infertility are distinguished from other biopsies by the fact that most of the time, a diagnosis of a clinicopathologic entity is not reached, but rather an assessment is made of the functional state. This means that a "reading" of the findings must be made rather than an interpretation, and consequently one must be highly quantified to recognize the different parameters without omitting an assessment of the qualitative variations; from the integration of all these parameters, useful information can be provided in the assessment of male infertility. A diagnostic algorithm of testis biopsy for infertility interpretation is seen in Figure 11-28.

As in any pathologic study, the assessment must start at a low magnification to be able to assess whether it is a diffuse or focal lesion. After this observation, the state of the tubules, the characteristics of the intertubular cells, and finally the characteristics of the stroma must be evaluated. The morphologic evaluation is made with quantitative and qualitative criteria.

Evaluation of the Testis Biopsy

A quantitative study of the testis biopsy usually refers to the quantification of the different cell types and structural measures (tubular wall, vessels, interstitium). For counting of the cells, at least 10 tubules must be chosen from each side, which is possible if five or six sections are obtained; tubules must be selected with the most perpendicular section possible (avoiding tubules with elliptical sections).

Tubular Cells

The normal amount of Sertoli cells and of each of the germ cells is mentioned in the description of the normal adult testicle. There is a certain correlation between the number of mature spermatids and that of spermatozoids in the semen, so a possible obstruction should be suspected if more spermatids are counted than expected from the concentration of the semen.[227]

In the literature, correlation indices are also used between histologic structures such as the number of germ cells per Sertoli cells, the number of germ cells per length unit of the tubular perimeter (average of 31 μm), or the number of Sertoli cells per tubule (10.4 ± 2). Other indices are more generic such as Johnsen's, which varies from 0 (complete inactivity) to 10 (preserved spermatogenesis); the normal index is 9.1.[228] The Bergmann and Kliesch[229] score based on the percentage of tubules showing elongated spermatids is also used. These indices are usually used more to compare results in articles than for the daily assessment of patients.

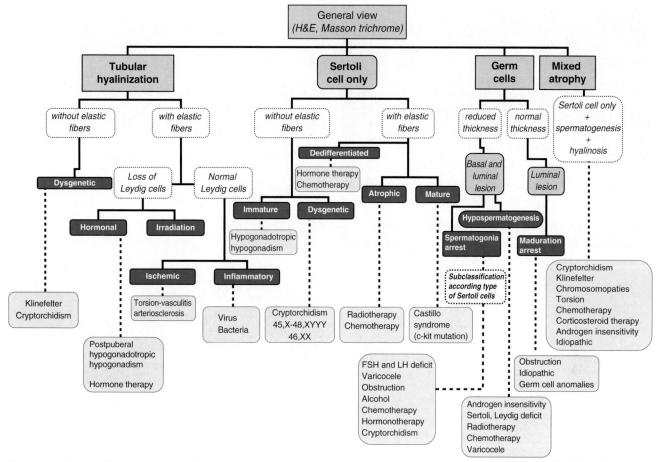

FIGURE 11-28 ■ Algorithm for assessment of infertility.

It is also necessary to describe the anomalies of germ cells, such as the presence of the following: *giant spermatogonia* that must be distinguished from intratubular neoplastic cells (with the latter expressing PLAP and OCT3/4)[230,231]; *multinucleated spermatogonia and spermatids* that appear with age and in cryptorchid testis; *megalospermatocytes*; and *abnormal spermatids*.[39]

Interstitial Cells

Quantifying interstitial cells in an isolated manner is more difficult; for this reason, the number of Leydig cells per tubule (5 ± 0.2) or per nest (1.2 ± 0.3) is evaluated.

One must bear in mind that interstitial cells such as Leydig cells tend to be grouped according to age; for this reason, in conditions in which tubules are reduced in diameter, the Leydig cells acquire a pseudohyperplastic appearance. To recognize true *Leydig cell hyperplasia,* one must take into account not only the increase in cell number but also the increased cell size, the increased number of nucleoli, and the absence of Reinke crystalloids.[232] This infrequent situation can be found in patients treated with nonsteroidal antiandrogens and in syndromes of insensitivity to androgens.[233] Any aggregate of inflammatory cells must be reported by the pathologist, with special reference to the mast cells.[234]

Tubular Wall

The thickness of the tubular wall is usually assessed subjectively, but it is worthwhile to remember that in the normal state, it usually has a thickness of 5.3 ± 1 μm.

Histologic evaluation additionally includes the consideration of cytologic alterations in Sertoli cells and germ cells. Bouin-fixed and paraffin blocks provide the opportunity for functional gene and protein expression studies.

Basic Testicular Lesions

Tubular Hyalinization

All of the pathologic conditions that profoundly damage the tubular germ cells can result in a total loss of these cells and in tubular hyalinization representing the end stage of several pathologies. According to the pathologic features of the tubular hyalinosis, it is possible to trace its etiology.

Dysgenetic Lesions

Dysgenetic lesions are usually observed in *Klinefelter syndrome.* The tubules lack elastic fibers, there is marked reduction of the tubular diameter, and tubules can have a homogeneous disc-like appearance (Fig. 11-29A). Occasionally, Sertoli cells persist and even some germ cells may be seen.[235]

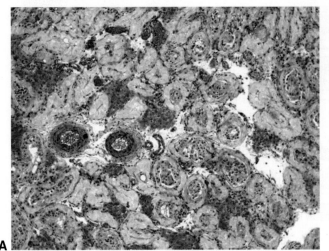

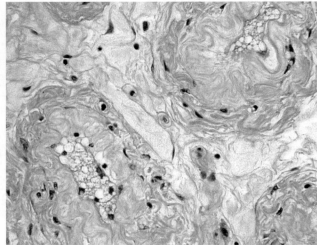

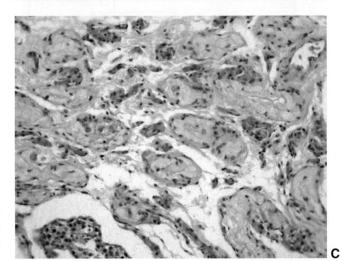

FIGURE 11-29 ■ Testicular tubular hyalinization. **A:** Dysgenetic type in a Klinefelter syndrome. **B:** Hormonal deprivation type in a prostate cancer patient treated with hormone therapy. **C:** Ischemic type post-testicular infarction.

Dysgenetic changes also are observed in the Leydig cells, which acquire an irregular appearance (from large-sized cells to very small ones); in addition, there is a decrease in Reinke crystalloids and an increase in paracrystalline structures. The general arrangement of the Leydig cells is pseudoadenomatous, although their total number is decreased. Functionally, the secretion of testosterone decreases.[39]

Hormonal Deprivation
Hormonal deprivation can be primary (lesions of the hypophysis or the sella turcica) or secondary to prolonged treatments with estrogens or antiandrogens.[236–238] The sclerosed tubules have preserved elastic fibers. The peritubular cells are seen around the tubules, and there is a loss of Leydig cells (Fig. 11-29B).

Ischemic Etiology
In cases with an ischemic etiology, the intratubular cells are more affected than the interstitial cells; for this reason, the Leydig cells are more preserved than in the other variants (Fig. 11-29C).[39]

Post-inflammation
Severe inflammation associated with bacterial infections usually produces generalized scar fibrosis, whereas viral infections preferentially affect the seminiferous tubules and usually show focal tubular sclerosis among areas of better preserved tubules.

Other Types of Tubular Hyalinization
Other types of tubular hyalinization can be found in obstructive etiologies, in endocrine diseases (Addison disease and diabetes), and surrounding germ cell tumors or in tubules with germ cell intratubular neoplasia.

Sertoli Cell–only Syndrome

The absence of germ cells with persistent Sertoli cells (Sertoli cell–only syndrome) was first called Del Castillo syndrome[239] and was attributed to a lack of migration of the germ cells from the wall of the yolk sac to the genital ridges. It has been proven that this type of azoospermia can be due to very different reasons, which is why the descriptive term of Sertoli cell–only syndrome is now used.

On the basis of the morphologic features of Sertoli cells and the characteristics of the tubules, five different types have been distinguished for their morphologic features, and these subtypes can correlate with the etiology of the syndrome (Table 11-5).[240]

Table 11-5 ■ MORPHOLOGIC FEATURES OF THE DIFFERENT SERTOLI CELLS IN SERTOLI CELL–ONLY SYNDROME

	Immature	Dysgenetic	Mature	Atrophic	Dedifferentiated
Nuclei	Oval	Spherical/oval	Triangular	Lobed	Round
Nucleolus	Absent/small	Normal	Normal	Normal	Small
Cytoplasm	Eosinophilic	Eosinophilic	Clear Big vacuoles	Clear apical Eosinophilic basal	Small vacuoles
Tubular features	No elastic fibers; no lumen; pseudostratified arrangement of Sertoli cells	Few elastic fibers; small lumen	Normal lumen	Fibrosis; normal lumen	Fibrosis; reduced lumen

Immature Sertoli Cell–only Syndrome

In patients with immature Sertoli cell–only syndrome, the Sertoli cells have a prepubertal appearance, distinguished by their pseudostratified distribution and oval nuclei without nucleolus (Fig. 11-30A). The number of Sertoli cells is increased. The elastic fibers of the tubular wall are usually lacking, and although occasional isolated spermatogonias can be found, it is usually the tubules that lack a central light. Immature Sertoli cell–only syndrome usually appears in patients with a deficiency of FSH or LH, which explains why the Leydig cells are also typically lacking.[240,241]

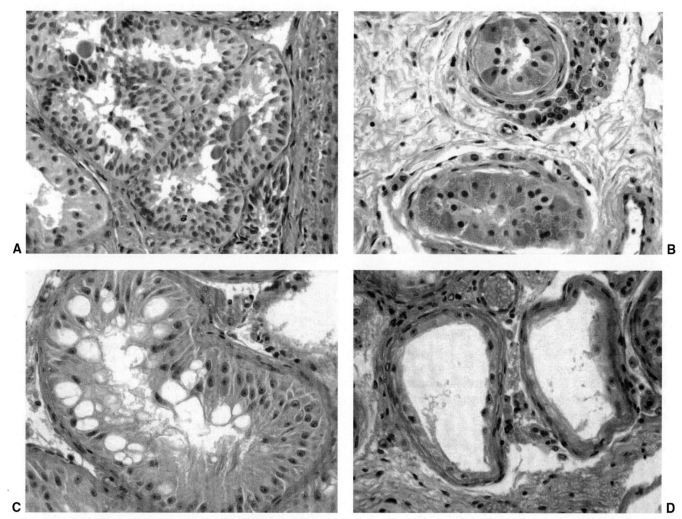

FIGURE 11-30 ■ Sertoli cell–only syndrome. **A:** Immature Sertoli cells with pseudostratified arrangement of elongated cells. **B:** Dysgenetic Sertoli cells with spherical nuclei and eosinophilic cytoplasm. **C:** Mature Sertoli cells with normal features and big "vacuoles." **D:** Atrophic Sertoli cells with flat cytoplasm, spherical nuclei.

Dysgenetic Sertoli Cell–only Syndrome

Dysgenetic Sertoli cell–only syndrome is considered dysgenetic because the Sertoli cells show different degrees of maturation in different tubules or in the same tubule (Fig. 11-30B). Sertoli cells can demonstrate focal immunohistochemical expression of AMH,[242] and the nucleus is spherical or oval. Tubular lesions are present, indicating dysgenesis (such as a reduction and even loss of the tubular lumen). Dysgenetic Sertoli cell–only syndrome is found in cryptorchid testicles and in Y chromosome anomalies.[243]

Mature Sertoli Cell–only Syndrome

In mature Sertoli cell–only syndrome, the Sertoli cells are normal morphologically, although they are present in greater amounts than in a normal testicle (14 ± 0.8) (Fig. 11-30C).[39] The tubules are reduced in size but larger than in other variants, the cells have cytoplasmic vacuoles, and some degree of fibrosis of the wall can be seen. This variant could be the same as described by Del Castillo et al.[239]

Atrophic Sertoli Cell–only Syndrome

Atrophic Sertoli cell–only syndrome is characterized by Sertoli cells with degenerative nuclear changes (lobed appearance with nucleolus) and cytoplasmic changes (apical vacuoles and fibrils of vimentin in the basal area) (Fig. 11-30D). There is a progressive loss of the germ cells, reduction of the tubular diameter, fibrosis, and tubular hyalinization. Disorders of Leydig cells can also be found.[244] The cause is usually unknown, except in case of prolonged chemotherapy or irradiation.

Dedifferentiated Sertoli Cell–only Syndrome

Dedifferentiated Sertoli cell–only syndrome occurs very infrequently and is observed in patients with previously normal testicles who are subjected to prolonged estrogen or antiandrogen treatments. The intensity of the changes is related to the dosage and is characterized by the loss of germ cells and dedifferentiated Sertoli cells with a round nuclei with small nucleolus.[245]

Germ Cell Changes

Most testicular biopsies for infertility are associated with germ cell alterations.

Many methods to evaluate changes in the germ cells have been described. Two different compartments, basal (spermatogonias) and luminal (spermatocytes and spermatids), can be considered. Logically, disorders of the basal compartment affect cells of the luminal compartment, and changes of the luminal compartment affect the spermatogonias.

Based on germ cell involvement, cell changes can be subdivided into two distinct categories—hypospermatogenesis and maturation arrest.

Hypospermatogenesis

Hypospermatogenesis involves disorders in both compartments and entails a global decrease of all the cell series, but preserves the proportion between spermatogonias and spermatocytes of first order. It can be accompanied by tubular hyalinization.[246] The pure form usually has from 10 to 17

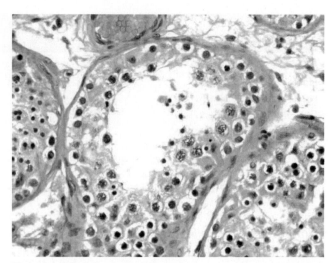

FIGURE 11-31 ■ Hyperspermatogenesis. All germ cell types are identified but in reduced numbers.

spermatogonia per tubule and a similar proportion of mature spermatids (Fig. 11-31). The cause has been ascribed to a primary defect in the stem cell population but recently Sertoli cell failure has been considered, but many other causes can be implicated such as hormonal, vascular, and chemical. Unfortunately, the morphologic features contribute little to the identification of the etiology.

Maturation Arrest

Maturation arrest is a block at a particular stage of spermatogenesis; and the precursor cells are normal in this category. The arrest can be subclassified as (i) *spermatogonia arrest*, in which there are fewer than 17 spermatogonias per tubule and a lower number of spermatocytes, and mature spermatids are almost always lacking (Fig. 11-32). The type of Sertoli cells, such as those identified in the Sertoli cell–only syndrome, can indicate the etiology of this lesion.[247] (ii) *Maturation arrest in spermatocyte of first order* (Fig. 11-33) is described as adequate maturation

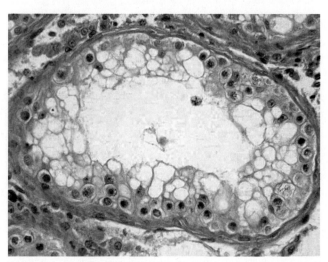

FIGURE 11-32 ■ Spermatogonia arrest. Vacuolated Sertoli cells with few spermatogonia and spermatocytes of first order without evidence of other germ cells.

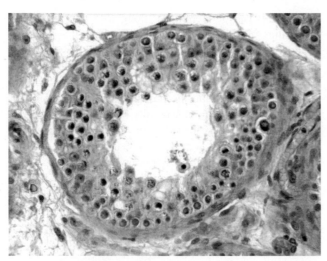

FIGURE 11-33 ■ Maturation arrest in spermatocytes of first order. Spermatogonia and spermatocytes of first order in normal quantity without evidence of spermatids.

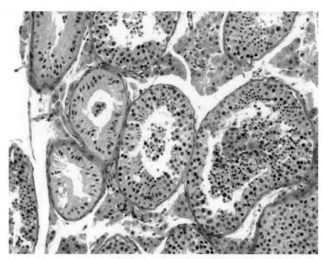

FIGURE 11-35 ■ Mixed atrophy. Seminiferous tubules with spermatogenesis intermixed with tubules with Sertoli cells only.

of spermatogonia and primary spermatocyte with a reduction in all types of spermatids; in addition, a notably low cell nuclear antigen proliferating index in the tubules has been shown when compared with the index in normal testicle (29.8% vs. 86.5%).[248] A similar finding has been observed with Ki67.[249] Some researchers call this condition late desquamation of spermatocytes of first order.[39] (iii) *Maturation arrest in spermatids* (Fig. 11-34) is the most common profile; for this condition, pathologists are obliged to count the mature spermatids to be able to correlate them with the concentration of spermatozoids in the semen. Some researchers call this condition desquamation of mature spermatids.[39]

Basal and luminal compartment changes are present in 44% of biopsy specimens for infertility.[39] Seventy percent of testicles with lesions in the luminal compartment have patching or mosaic of lesions and are often associated with obstruction phenomena.

Mixed Atrophy

When tubules are found without germinal epithelium (Sertoli cell only) and are intermixed with tubules in which there is either complete or incomplete spermatogenesis and even tubular hyalinization, the descriptive term of *tubular atrophic mosaicism* or *mixed atrophy*[250] (Fig. 11-35) can be used. The different tubules can correspond to the different lobes or can be tubules of the same lobe but with differences in their route.[39] This can be secondary to varicoceles or chemotherapy but is also very typical of cryptorchidism, chromosomal syndromes (e.g., Klinefelter), and pseudohermaphroditism. When the pathologist encounters one of these biopsy specimens, they must evaluate the percentage of tubules with spermatogenesis, as well as their quality.

Other changes are the presence of *giant spermatogonia* (Fig. 11-36) and true *Leydig cell hyperplasia* (Fig. 11-37) without Reinke crystalloids that can be present in patients

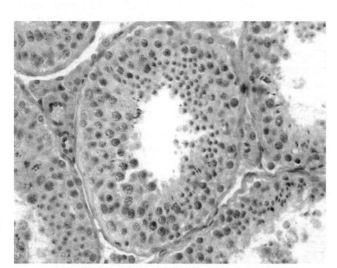

FIGURE 11-34 ■ Maturation arrest in spermatids. Spermatogonia, spermatocytes of first order, and immature spermatids in normal proportion but few mature spermatids.

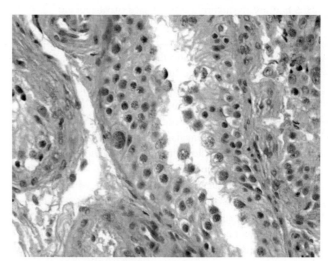

FIGURE 11-36 ■ Anomalies of germ cells. Giant spermatogonia without nuclear atypia.

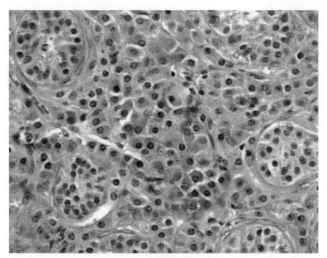

FIGURE 11-37 ■ Leydig cell hyperplasia. Increased number of Leydig cells without Reinke crystalloids.

treated with nonsteroidal antiandrogens and in insensitivity to androgens syndromes.

Changes in Obstructive Infertility

The seminiferous tubules are followed by straight tubules, which are concentrated in the rete testis (covered by cuboidal epithelium), and these continue forward as the efferent ductules in the head of the epididymis, which are covered by columnar epithelium. All these ductules come together in a single epididymal duct (with high columnar epithelium), constituting the body and tail of the epididymis, which is in continuity with the ductus deferens, reaching the area of the seminal vesicles; from this confluence emerges the ejaculatory duct, which feeds into the back portion of the prostatic urethra.[251] Obstruction of this long route can occur owing to many causes and at different levels. These can be divided into intratesticular and extratesticular obstructions.

Intratesticular obstructions can be tubular or of the rete testis. Tubular obstruction appears in cases of testicular dysgenesis or after epididymo-orchitis. Obstruction of the rete testis is more frequently seen in cases of varicocele.[252]

Extratesticular obstructions can be systematized as proximal, middle, or distal. *Proximal obstructions* occur between the seminiferous tubules and the ductus deferens; the most typical cause is pathologic lesions of the head and body of the epididymis resulting in lack of connection between the rete testis and the efferent ductules. *Middle obstructions* are due to ductus deferens obstruction near the testicle and can be secondary to the agenesis of the former. *Distal obstructions* appear between the distal portion of the deferent duct and the ejaculatory duct.

The changes induced by the obstruction of the seminal secretion depend on the location of the obstruction and when it occurred. The intratesticular obstructions produce tubular ectasias only in patches (affected areas next to other normal areas). The extratesticular proximal obstructions also induce changes similar to those of the intratesticular obstruction, with lobular tubular fibrosis (in which occasional remaining

Sertoli cells can be identified), along with normal testicular lobules.[253] Middle obstructions are those that have the greatest impact on the epididymal head, with ectasia of the tubules, and which even affect the rete testis. The congenital forms of obstruction usually produce fewer lesions than the acquired forms, and the obstructions after the level of the efferent ductules do not usually affect the seminiferous tubules since they absorb 90% of the tubular fluid and therefore protect the testicular parenchyma. The distal obstructions induce almost no testicular or epididymal changes.

Post-vasectomy testicles can show fibrosis of the tubular wall, stromal fibrosis, and loss of germ cells,[254] which could be partially responsible for the decrease in postseminal channel reconstruction for paternity, since it is decreased by 15% to 75%, according to various researchers.[255]

NONNEOPLASTIC TUMOROUS CONDITIONS

Many lesions can simulate a neoplasm in the testis. These pseudoneoplastic lesions can be divided into those that macroscopically imitate neoplasia and those that microscopically imitate neoplasia, regardless of whether they form a macroscopic mass.[256]

The frequently encountered lesions that can simulate a neoplasm in the testis are described below.

Macroscopic Mimickers of Testicular Neoplasia

Frequently, lesions that macroscopically mimic testicular neoplasia affect the testicle and paratesticular structures and look like a tumor with atypical clinical features. According to their etiology, the following lesions can mimic a tumor:

Segmental Testicular Infarction

Most vascular disorders of the male gonad, such as intratesticular hemorrhage and organizing testicular hematocele, are not confused with a tumor because, in addition to causing acute symptoms, they usually affect the entire gonad. However, in the rare situation in which the vascular lesion is segmental, it can simulate neoplasia. The *segmental testicular infarction* is a lesion clinically characterized by slight local pain unrelated to any acute episode[257]; it may be related to isolated or systemic vasculitis[258,259] and have the morphologic features of PAN,[260] giant cell vasculitis,[261] or Wegener granulomatosis.[262] Other cases are seen in the context of hematologic disease (sickle cell anemia)[263] or are associated with nonspecific perivascular fibrosis. Any of the phases of an infarction can be observed from an acute (with hemorrhage) to healing stage. Currently, a clinical diagnosis can be obtained with Doppler sonography,[264] avoiding orchiectomy.

Meconium Periorchitis

Meconium periorchitis is an infrequent inflammatory lesion (30 cases having been reported) that typically presents in the first months of life; typically, there is a clinical history of obstetric problems that caused meconium to be passed

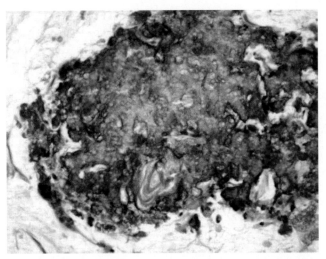

FIGURE 11-38 ■ Meconium periorchitis. Residual keratin from meconium with calcification in a background of myxoid fibrous tissue.

toward the testicular surrounding structures.[265] The macroscopic appearance is a myxoid material with calcification of the remains of squamous cells or lanugo hairs (Fig. 11-38).[266] Clinically, meconium periorchitis can simulate paratesticular rhabdomyosarcoma.

Sperm Granuloma

As the name indicates, this granulomatous lesion with few giant cells results from the extravasation of spermatozoa generally postvasectomy (40% of vasectomized men and 2.5% of general population) (Fig. 11-39).[267] When it produces a tumor-like lesion, it is usually located in the vas deferens or the epididymis with firm nodules of 0.7 to 4 cm with occasional cysts formation.[268]

Orchitis

Orchitis is characterized by nonspecific infectious inflammatory lesions with a tumor-like presentation, resulting frequently from chronic processes causing progressive

fibrosis that may clinically[269] or sonographically[270] simulate neoplasia. The specific infectious inflammatory lesions and chronic noninfectious inflammatory lesions most often confused with neoplasias include granulomatous inflammation in tuberculosis,[271] brucellosis,[272] syphilis,[273] fungal infections,[274] parasite diseases,[274] and malakoplakia.

Testicular Cysts

Parenchymal testicular cysts can be more difficult than other paratesticular cystic structures to distinguish from neoplasia, and if there is the slightest suspicion of intracystic content, one must suspect a malignant neoplasm.[256] Testicular cysts have been discussed previously under "Congenital Anomalies."

Ectopic Tissues

Only in cases of congenital adrenal hyperplasia or Cushing syndrome can ectopic adrenocortical tissue be prominent and appear as a tumor-like lesion.[275] Other ectopic tissues are encountered less frequently, and their pseudotumoral presentation is exceptionally rare.[256] Ectopic tissues have been discussed previously under "Congenital Anomalies."

Fibrous Pseudotumor

This entity refers to a phenomenon of fibrosis with paucicellular hyalinized collagen presenting as a nodular (single or multiple) or diffuse lesion in the testicular tunics (Fig. 11-40),[276,277] and sometimes a node can be free floating (scrotal mouse).[267] This broad spectrum of lesions has been labeled with a variety of names: chronic periorchitis, fibromatous periorchitis, nodular periorchitis, fibrous proliferation of the tunica, nonspecific paratesticular fibrosis, granulomatous periorchitis, nodular fibrous pseudotumor, fibrous pseudotumor, inflammatory pseudotumor, fibroma, reactive periorchitis, indicating its controversial pathogenesis. Some cases have been reported preceded by trauma or infection, and on occasion, an inflammatory component and

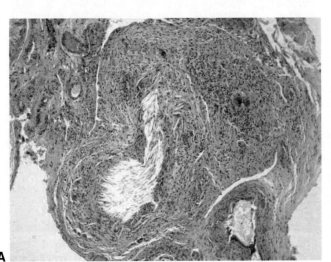

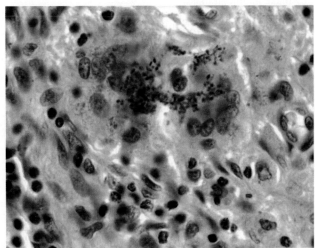

A ⎯ B

FIGURE 11-39 ■ Sperm granuloma. **A:** Seminal duct with crystalloid material in the lumen and granulomatous reaction in the wall. **B:** High power view of a sperm granuloma with giant cell reaction around residual spermatozoa.

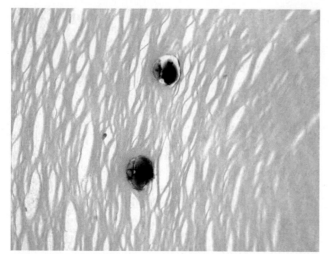

FIGURE 11-40 ■ Fibrous pseudotumor. Paucicellular hyalinized collagen with focal calcification.

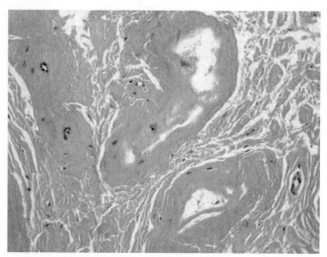

FIGURE 11-41 ■ Testicular amyloidosis. Seminiferous tubules replaced by amyloid deposition.

granulation tissue can be observed suggesting the possibility that there might be the healing of an inflammatory pseudotumor.[278] Recently it has been demonstrated that a subset of these cases have a high number of IgG4-positive plasma cells with an IgG4 to IgG ratio of 44% to 48%, indicating that paratesticular fibrous pseudotumor might belong to the spectrum of IgG4-related sclerosing disease.[279] Although it is not difficult to recognize radiologically, an intraoperative frozen section becomes necessary on occasion.

Amyloidosis

Amyloidosis is usually bilateral and presents in patients with a prior history of amyloidosis[280]; more rarely, if in cryptorchidic patients it presents in a primary form that simulates a testicular tumor (Fig. 11-41).[281]

Microscopic Mimickers of Testicular Neoplasia

Lesions or cellular changes that microscopically imitate a neoplasia are included under this category, whether or not they make a clinical mass.

Inflammatory Lesions

Some inflammatory lesions, such as xanthogranulomatous orchitis, idiopathic granulomatous orchitis, malakoplakia, lymphocytic orchitis (testicular pseudolymphoma), and Rosai-Dorfman disease (described previously), can microscopically imitate a neoplasm, but immunohistochemical studies can to serve to distinguish these entities and arrive at a diagnosis.

Sertoli Cell Hyperplasia

In a series of situations, nonencapsulated nodules of Sertoli cells known as Pick adenomas can be found, especially in cryptorchid testes[282] (Fig. 11-42). On account of their appearance, these should be distinguished from actual Sertoli cell tumors, which generally are larger and sometimes have

areas that mimic Call-Exner bodies. A differential diagnosis that includes a yolk sac tumor is not usually considered, but immunohistochemical stains with markers including α-fetoprotein, calretinin, α-inhibin, and CD99 can help to establish a correct diagnosis.

Of patients with androgen insensitivity syndrome or testicular feminization (male pseudohermaphroditism), 63% have tubular hamartomas (tubules lined by immature Sertoli cells)[283] that must be differentiated from Sertoli cell adenomas and sex cord tumors with annular tubules.[284]

Interstitial Cell Hyperplasia

Leydig cell hyperplasia, although usually diffuse, may form nodules mimicking a tumor; but this is an interstitial nondestructive process.

Nodules of Leydig cells are found in patients with adrenogenital syndrome[285,286] and Nelson syndrome (Fig. 11-43).

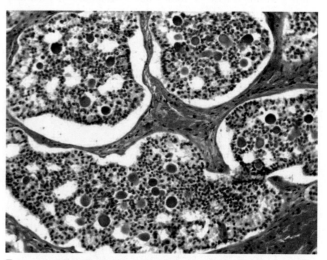

FIGURE 11-42 ■ Sertoli cell hyperplasia. Localized Sertoli cell proliferation in a nodular arrangement with hyaline material (Pick adenoma).

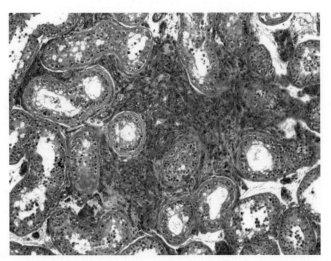

FIGURE 11-43 ■ Leydig cell hyperplasia. Localized Leydig cell accumulation with collagen fibers among the cells (Masson trichrome stain). In some cases it can acquire a nodular contour.

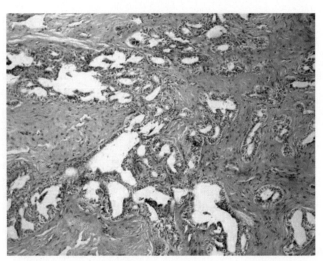

FIGURE 11-44 ■ Rete testis hyperplasia. Columnar cells with some small papillary projections.

These nodules are usually bilateral and large, with cellular pleomorphism and pigmentation. The clinical history and a complete endocrinologic profile can prevent an unnecessary orchiectomy[287] given the fact that only one case of aggressive behavior has been published.[212] Apparent Leydig cell hyperplasia can be present in many atrophic testicles such as in Klinefelter syndrome.

The distinction from a Leydig cell tumor can be made upon consideration of the multifocality and bilaterality of the nodules, the uniform absence of Reinke crystalloids, the prominent lipofucsin deposits[288] and correlation with clinical history.

Hyperplasia of Rete Testis

In some hyperestrogenic situations, the flat epithelium of the rete testis may become columnar, and rarely a micropapillary growth of bland cells can be observed. The diagnosis of rete testis hyperplasia is subjective, and adenomatous lesions are rarely seen (Fig. 11-44).[289,290] In some cases, there are intracytoplasmic hyaline eosinophilic globules resembling a yolk sac tumor, but the negative stains of AFP or PLAP help to rule this differential diagnosis.[291]

Mesothelial Hyperplasia

It is present as a reactive lesion in hydrocele or hernia but may also be found microscopically in older men.[292] The mesothelial proliferation has a predominantly epithelial appearance with papillary growth (Fig. 11-45), but rarely a spindle cell proliferation can be present. In the differential diagnosis with mesothelioma, the bland cytology, lack of true invasion, and presence of associated inflammatory elements can be useful.[293,294]

MISCELLANEOUS TESTICULAR LESIONS

Other testicular lesions of interest include the following:

Mechanical Lesions

Forces of <50 kg over the testicle cause *luxation* or *dislocation*, whereas greater forces can lead to *albugineal rupture* on exceeding tissue resistance.[295] *Testicular rupture* can produce hemorrhage in the vaginal space and seminiferous tubules protruding through the tear into the cavity, whereas *testicular dislocation* is the displacement of a testicle outside the scrotal bag; to date, 150 cases of dislocation have been reported.[296] Most dislocations are unilateral (90%), superficial (80%), and of superficial inguinal location (50% of cases).

Microlithiasis

In the testicle, it is possible to find hyaline bodies and microlithiasis on the wall of the tubules as well as in its lumen and in the interstitium (Fig. 11-46). It has been suggested that the origin of these microliths are desquamated and necrosed

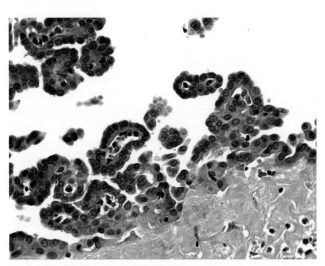

FIGURE 11-45 ■ Mesothelial hyperplasia. Mesothelial papillary proliferation without nuclear atypia and no invasion.

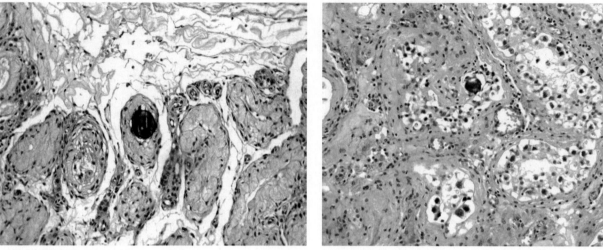

FIGURE 11-46 ■ Testicular microlithiasis. **A:** Intratubular microlithiasis with tubular hyalinization. **B:** Microlithiasis in intratubular germ cell neoplasia.

cells that have become calcified; although this mechanism is possible, it is not sufficient to explain all cases. Recent studies of the composition and the microlithiasis location have suggested that most testicular microliths are initiated in the wall of the tubule and that as they grow; they are surrounded by Sertoli cells and tunica propria and are able to end up in the lumen of the tubule or in the stroma.[297] This hypothesis can explain why microliths are found more frequently in cryptorchid testicles, in patients with Klinefelter syndrome, or in other situations in which there is a certain dysgenesis of the wall of the tubule; this also explains why more cases of testicular lithiasis are being found, detectable by sonography, in patients with testicular germ cell tumors, many of which are accompanied by intratubular germ cell tumors (that lead to disorders of the tubule wall).[298–300] Testicular microlithiasis is common (in 5.6% of the male population between 17 and 35 years of age and in 14.1% of African American males), and although microcalcifications do exist in approximately 50% of germ cell tumors, most men with testicular microlithiasis will not develop testicular neoplasms. Increased emphasis on testicular examination is the recommended follow-up for men identified with testicular microlithiasis.[301] The management of patients with testicular microlithiasis depends upon the specific requirements on an individual basis. A conservative approach involving testicular self-examination is recommended for asymptomatic patients with testicular microlithiasis. Early testicular biopsy should be considered in patients with testicular microlithiasis and associated features of testicular dysgenesis, including atrophic testes and cryptorchidism, considering the increased frequency of intratubular germ cell neoplasia and testicular germ cell tumor detection in this subset. Surveillance is a more suitable option than definitive treatment in individuals with bilateral testicular microlithiasis and intratubular germ cell neoplasia who desire to retain reproductive function, due to the long latency period of transformation of intratubular germ cell neoplasia. The clinical benefit of testicular

biopsy versus surveillance for these individuals is unclear as an aggressive approach to testicular biopsy is likely to be further associated with impaired fertility. The detection of testicular microlithiasis on radiologic studies should probably be investigated by performing a testicular biopsy at age 18 years in cases where individuals are at particularly increased risk of testicular germ cell tumor development, especially in cases with gonadal dysgenesis and/or cryptorchidism as the advantage of early detection and definitive treatment of intratubular germ cell neoplasia exceeds the potential risks.[302]

Testicular Arteriolar Hyalinosis

Testicular arteriolar hyalinosis is characterized by the accumulation of amorphous eosinophilic substance, which is PAS positive, negative on amyloid staining, and shows no necrosis or inflammatory reaction (Fig. 11-47). This is an age-related change, with maximum incidence at about 30

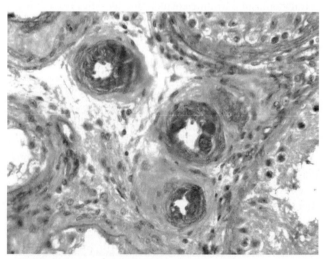

FIGURE 11-47 ■ Testicular arteriolar hyalinosis. Amorphous eosinophilic substance in the arteriolar wall (PAS).

years of age. Its origin is believed to be related to disorders of endothelial cell permeability since a large component of its material includes immunoglobulins, fibrin, and fibrinogen.[303] The effects depend on the intensity of vascular obliteration and the extent of the lesion, but on occasion it is difficult to determine whether the vascular lesion led to tubular fibrosis or if both lesions appeared at the same time for unknown causes, as occurs in Klinefelter syndrome.

Sclerosing Lipogranuloma

The term *sclerosing lipogranuloma* was introduced to describe a subcutaneous granulomatous reaction believed to result from a local reactive process after injury to adipose tissue from injection of foreign bodies, such as paraffin, mineral oil, or silicon. In patients without this history, the pathogenesis of the disease is controversial, whether endogenous or exogenous, and has not been resolved to date. In the testis, only one case of this entity has been reported.[304]

REFERENCES

1. Hanley NA, Ball SG, Clement-Jones M, et al. Expression of steroidogenic factor-1 and Wilms' tumour 1 during early human gonadal development and sex determination. *Mech Dev* 1999;87:175–180.
2. Cools M, Hoebeke P, Wolffenbuttel KP, et al. Pubertal androgenization and gonadal histology in two 46,XY adolescents with NR5A1 mutations and predominantly female phenotype at birth. *Eur J Endocrinol* 2012;166:341–349.
3. Biason-Lauber A, Schoenle EJ. Apparently normal ovarian differentiation in a prepubertal girl with transcriptionally inactive steroidogenic factor 1 (NR5A1/SF-1) and adrenal cortical insufficiency. *Am J Hum Genet* 2000;67:1563–1568.
4. Kreidberg JA, Sariola H, Loring JM, et al. WT-1 is required for early kidney development. *Cell* 1993;74:679–691.
5. Pelletier J, Bruening W, Kashtan CE, et al. Germline mutations in the Wilms; tumour suppressor gene are associated with abnormal urogenital development in Denys-Drash syndrome. *Cell* 1991;67:437–447.
6. Barbaux S, Niaudet P, Gubler MC, et al. Donor splice-site mutations in WT1 are responsible for Frasier syndrome. *Nat Genet* 1997;17:467–470.
7. Bishop CE, Guellaen G, Geloworth D, et al. Single copy DNA sequences specific for the human Y chromosome. *Nature* 1984;309:253–255.
8. McElreavery K, Fellous M. Sex determination and the Y chromosome. *Am J Med Genet* 1999;89:176–185.
9. Haqq CM, King CY, Ukiyama E, et al. Molecular basis of mammalian sexual determination: activation of Mullerian inhibiting substance gene expression by SRY. *Science* 1999;266:1494–1500.
10. Huang B, Wang S, Ning Y, et al. Autosomal XX sex reversal caused by duplication of SOX-9. *Am J Med Genet* 1999;87:349–353.
11. Lim HN, Hawkins JR. Genetic control of gonadal differentiation. *Baillieres Clin Endocrinol Metab* 1998;12:1–16.
12. Ludbrook LM, Bernard P, Bagheri-Fam S, et al. Excess DAX1 leads to XY ovotesticular disorder of sex development (DSD) in mice by inhibiting steroidogenic factor-1 (SF1) activation of the testis enhancer of SRY-box-9 (Sox9). *Endocrinology* 2012;153:1948–1958.
13. Foster JW, Dominguez-Steglich MA, Guioli S, et al. Campomelic dysplasia and autosomal sex reversal caused by mutations in an SRY-related gene. *Nature* 1994;372:525–530.
14. Zhou R, Liu L, Guo Y, et al. Similar gene structure of two Sox9a genes and their expression patterns during gonadal differentiation in a teleost fish, rice field eel (Monopterus albus). *Mol Reprod Dev* 2003;66:211–217.
15. Koopman P. Sex determination: a tale of two Sox genes. *Trends Genet* 2005;21:367–370.
16. Bennett CP, Docherty Z, Robb SA, et al. Deletion 9p and sex reversal. *J Med Genet* 1993;30:518–520.
17. Wilkie AOM, Campbell FM, Daubeney P. Complete and partial XY sex reversal associated with terminal deletion of 10q: report of two cases and literature review. *Am J Med Genet* 1993;46:597–600.
18. Behringer RR, Finegold MJ, Cate RL. Mullerian–inhibiting substance function during mammalian sexual development. *Cell* 1994;79:415–425.
19. Shen WH, Moore CC, Ikeda Y, et al. Nuclear receptor steroidogenic factor 1 regulates the mullerian inhibiting substance gene: a link to the sex determination cascade. *Cell* 1994;77:651–661.
20. Josso N, Cate RL, Picard JY, et al. Anti-Mullerian hormone, the Jost factor. *Recent Prog Horm Res* 1993;48:1–59.
21. Rey R, Josso N. Regulation of testicular anti-Mullerian hormone secretion. *Eur J Endocrinol* 1996;135:144–152.
22. Jirasek JE. *Development of the Genital System and Male Pseudohermaphroditism*. Baltimore, MD: Johns Hopkins; 1971.
23. Munsterberg A, Lovell-Badge R. Expression of the mouse anti-mullerian hormone gene suggests a role in both male and female sexual differentiation. *Development* 1991;113:613–624.
24. Catlin EA, Powell SM, Manganaro TF, et al. Sex-specific fetal lung development and Mullerian inhibiting substance. *Am Rev Respir Dis* 1990;141:466–470.
25. Cunha GR, Alarid ET, Turner T, et al. Normal and abnormal development of the male urogenital tract. Role of androgens, mesenchymal-epithelial interactions, and growth factors. *J Androl* 1992;13:465–475.
26. Larsen WJ. *Human Embryology*. London, UK: Churchill Livingstone; 1993:247.
27. Orth JM. The role of follicle-stimulating hormone in controlling Sertoli cell proliferation in testes of fetal rats. *Endocrinology* 1984;115:1248–1255.
28. Gaskell TL, Esnal A, Robinson LL, et al. Immunohistochemical profiling of germ cells within the human fetal testis: identification of three subpopulations. *Biol Reprod* 2004;71:2012–2021.
29. Nistal M, Paniagua R. Non-neoplastic disease of the testis. In: Bostwick DG, Eble JN, eds. *Urologic Surgical Pathology*. St. Louis, MO: Mosby; 1996:458.
30. Trainer TD. Histology of the normal testis. *Am J Surg Pathol* 1987;11:797–809.
31. Ross MH, Long IR. Contractile cells in human seminiferous tubules. *Science* 1966;153:1271–1273.
32. De Menezes AP. Elastic tissue in the limiting membrane of the human seminiferous tubule. *Am J Anat* 1977;150:349–373.
33. Nistal M, Abaurrea MA, Paniagua R. Morphological and histometric study on the human Sertoli cell from birth to the onset of puberty. *J Anat* 1982;134:351–363.
34. Hafez E. Testicular biopsy: fine structure. In: Bain J, Hafez EH, eds. *Diagnosis in Andrology*. Leiden, Netherlands: The Hagve Martinus Nijhoff Publishers; 1980:93.
35. Clermont Y. The cycle of the seminiferous epithelium in man. *Am J Anat* 1963;112:35–51.
36. Schulze W. Evidence of a wave of spermatogenesis in the human testis. *Andrologia* 1982;14:200–207.
37. Dym M, Fawcett DW. Further observations on the differentiation of spermatogonia, spermatocytes and spermatids connected by intercellular bridges in the mammalian testis. *Biol Reprod* 1971;4:195–215.
38. Mancini RE. Testicular biopsy evaluation. In: *International Congress of Andrology*. Barcelona, Spain; 1976:25.
39. Nistal M, Regadera J, González-Peramato P. Biopsia testicular e infertilidad. *Madrid Harcourt* 2001:4–15.
40. Paniagua R, Martín A, Nistal M, et al. Testicular involution in elderly men: comparison of histology quantitative studies with hormone patterns. *Fertil Steril* 1987;47:671–679.
41. Nistal M, Santamaria L, Regadera J, et al. Diverticula of human seminiferous tubules in the normal and pathologic testis. *J Androl* 1988;9:55–61.

42. Leathem JH. Aging and the testis. In: Johnson AD, Gomes WR, eds. *The Testis, p-547 Advances in Physiology, Biochemistry and Function.* New York: Academic Press; 1977.

43. Schulze W, Schulze C. Multinucleate Sertoli cells in aged human testes. *Cell Tissue Res* 1981;217:259–266.

44. Paniagua R, Amat P, Nistal M. Ultrastructural changes in Sertoli cells in ageing humans. *Int J Androl* 1985;8:295–312.

45. Paniagua R, Nistal M, Amat P, et al. Seminiferous tubule involution in elderly men. *Biol Reprod* 1987;36:939–947.

46. Nistal M, Codesal J, Paniagua R, et al. Decrease in the number of human Ap and Ad spermatogonia and in the Ap/Ad ratio with advancing age. New data on the spermatogonial stem cell. *J Androl* 1987;8:64–68.

47. Nistal M, Codesal J, Paniagua R. Multinucleated spermatids in aging human testes. *Arch Androl* 1986;16:125–129.

48. Jung JC, Park GT, Kim KH, et al. Differential expression of transforming growth factor-beta in the interstitial tissue of testis during aging. *J Cell Biochem* 2004;92:92–98.

49. Kothari LK, Gupta AS. Effect of ageing on the volume, structure and total Leydig cell content of the human testis. *Int J Fertil* 1974;19:140–146.

50. Paniagua R, Amat P, Nistal M et al. Ultrastructure of Leydig cells in human ageing testes. *J Anat* 1986;146:173–183.

51. Huff DS, Snyder HM, Hadziselimovic F, et al. An absent testis is associated with contralateral testicular hypertrophy. *J Urol* 1992;148;627–628.

52. Putra DK, Blackshaw AW. Morphometric studies of compensatory testicular hypertrophy in the rat after hemicastration. *Aust J Biol Sci* 1982;35:287–293.

53. Josso N, Briard ML. Embryonic testicular regression syndrome: variable phenotypic expression in siblings. *J Pediatr* 1980;97:200–204.

54. Devriendt K, Deloof E, Moerman P, et al. Diaphragmatic hernia in Denys-Drash syndrome. *Am J Med Genet* 1995;57:97–101.

55. Nistal M, García-Fernández E, Mariño-Enriquez A, et al. Diagnostic value of the gonadal biopsy in the disorders of sex development. *Actas Urol Esp* 2007;31:1056–1075.

56. Acquafredda A, Vassal J, Job JC. Rudimentary testes syndrome revisited. *Pediatrics* 1987;80:209–214.

57. Parigi GB, Bardoni B, Avoltini V, et al. Is bilateral congenital anorchia genetically determined? *Eur J Pediatr Surg* 1999;9:312–315.

58. Grechi G, Zampi GC, Selli C, et al. Polyorchidism and seminoma in a child. *J Urol* 1980;123:291–292.

59. Scott KW. A case of polyorchidism with testicular teratoma. *J Urol* 1980;124:930–932.

60. Nistal M, Martinez-Garcia F, Regadera J, et al. Macroorchidism: light and electron microscopic study of four cases. *Hum Pathol* 1992;23:1011–1018.

61. Gondos B, Egli CA, Rosenthal SM. Testicular changes in gonadotropin-independent familial male sexual precocity: familial testotoxicosis. *Arch Pathol Lab Med* 1985;109:990–995.

62. Egli CA, Rosenthal SM, Grumbach MM, et al. Pituitary gonadotropin-independent male-limited autosomal dominant sexual precocity in nine generations: familial testotoxicosis. *J Pediatr* 1985;106:33–40.

63. Sutherland GR, Judge CG, Wiener S. Familial X-linked mental retardation with an X chromosome abnormality and macro-orchidism. *J Med Genet* 1980;17:73–74.

64. Schedewie HK, Reiter EO, Beitins IZ. Testicular Leydig cell hyperplasia as a cause of familial sexual precocity. *J Clin Endocrinol Metab* 1981;52:271–278.

65. Leschek EW, Chan WY, Diamond DA, et al. Nodular Leydig cell hyperplasia in a boy with familial male-limited precocious puberty. *J Pediatr* 2001;138:949–951.

66. Meschede D, Behre HM, Nieschlag E. Endocrine and spermatological characteristics of 135 patients with bilateral megalotestis. *Andrologia* 1995;27:207–212.

67. Pillai SB, Besner GE. Pediatric testicular problems. *Pediatr Clin North Am* 1998;45:813–830.

68. Nistal M, Paniagua R, León L, et al. Ectopic seminiferous tubules in the tunica albuginea of normal and dysgenetic testes. *Appl Pathol* 1985;3:123–128.

69. Mori H, Tamai M, Fushimi H, et al. Leydig cells within the aspermatogenic seminiferous tubules. *Hum Pathol* 1987;18:1227–1231.

70. Mori H, Shiraishi T, Matsumoto K. Ectopic Leydig cells in seminiferous tubules of an infertile human male with a chromosomal aberration. *Andrologia* 1978;10:434–443.

71. Jun SY, Ro JY, Park YW, et al. Ectopic Leydig cells of testis: an immunohistochemical study on tissue microarray. *Ann Diagn Pathol* 2008;12:29–32.

72. Frey HL, Rajfer J. Incidence of cryptorchidism. *Urol Clin North Am* 1982;9:327–329.

73. Wensing CJ. The embryology of testicular descent. *Horm Res* 1988;30:144–152.

74. Heyns CF. The gubernaculum during testicular descent in the human fetus. *J Anat* 1987;153:93–112.

75. Backhouse KM. Mechanism of testicular descent. *Karger Prog Reprod Biol Med* 1984;10:16–23.

76. Baker LA, Nef S, Nguyen MT, et al. The insulin-3 gene: lack of a genetic basis for human cryptorchidism. *J Urol* 2002;167:2534–2537.

77. Foresta C, Bettella A, Vinanzi C, et al. A novel circulating hormone of testis origin in humans. *J Clin Endocrinol Metab* 2004;89:5952–5958.

78. Goh DW, Middlesworth W, Farmer PJ, et al. Prenatal androgen blockade with flutamide inhibits masculinization of the genitofemoral nerve and testicular descent. *J Pediatr Surg* 1994;29:836–838.

79. Tanyel FC, Erdem S, Buyukpamukcu N, et al. Cremaster muscles obtained from boys with an undescended testis show significant neurological changes. *BJU Int* 2000;85:116–119.

80. Spencer JR. The endocrinology of testicular descent. American Urological Association Update Series 1994;12:94–99.

81. Cain MP, Kramer SA, Tindall DJ, et al. Expression of androgen receptor protein within the lumbar spinal cord during ontologic development and following antiandrogen induced cryptorchidism. *J Urol* 1994;152:766–769.

82. Belman AB. Acquired undescended (ascended) testis: effects of human chorionic gonadotropin. *J Urol* 1988;140:1189–1190.

83. Mengel W, Zimmermann FA. Immunologic aspects of cryptorchidism. *Urol Clin North Am* 1982;9:349–352.

84. Nistal M, Paniagua R, Diez-Pardo J. Histologic classification of undescended testes. *Hum Pathol* 1980;11:666–674.

85. Lopez A, Vilches J, Castiñeiras J. Criptorquidia III B: Cambios cualitativos y cuantitativos en testículos criptorquídicos inducidos de forma experimental. *Actas Urol Esp* 1988;12:88–93.

86. Schilder AM, Díaz P, Cuendet A, et al. Follicle-stimulating hormone IV. Study of the histology of puberal cryptorchid and scrotal testes in relation to the secretion of gonadotropins. *Fertil Steril* 1982;37:828–836.

87. Hezmall HP, Lipshulz LI. Cryptorchidism and infertility. *Urol Clin North Am* 1982;9:361–369.

88. Nistal M, Paniagua R. *Testicular and epididymal pathology*. New York: Thieme-Stratton; 1984:120–139.

89. Abratt RP, Reddi VB, Sarembock LA. Testicular cancer and cryptorchidism. *Br J Urol* 1992;70:656–659.

90. Nistal M, Paniagua R. Infertility in adult males with retractile testes. *Fertil Steril* 1984;41:395–403.

91. Marrakchi A, Belhaj L, Boussouf H, et al. Pure gonadal dysgenesis XX and XY: observations in fifteen patients. *Ann Endocrinol* 2005;66:553–556.

92. Davis GH, McEwan JC, Fennessy PF, et al. Infertility due to bilateral ovarian hypoplasia in sheep homozygous (FecXI FecXI) for the Inverdale prolificacy gene located on the X chromosome. *Biol Reprod* 1992;46:636–640.

93. Słowikowska-Hilczer J, Romer TE, Kula K. Neoplastic potential of germ cells in relation to disturbances of gonadal organogenesis and changes in karyotype. *J Androl* 2003;24:270–278.

94. Haddad NG, Walvoord EC, Cain MP, et al. Seminoma and a gonadoblastoma in an infant with mixed gonadal dysgenesis. *J Pediatr* 2003;143:136–139.

95. Kropp BP, Keating MA, Moshang T, et al. True hermaphroditism and normal male genitalia: an unusual presentation. *Urology* 1995;46:736–739.

96. Malavaud B, Mazerolles C, Bieth E, et al. Pure seminoma in a male phenotype 46,XX true hermaphrodite. *J Urol* 2000;164:125–126.

97. Malik V, Gupta D, Gill M, et al. Seminoma in a male phenotype 46XX true hermaphrodite. *Asian J Surg* 2007;30:85–87.

98. Pals-Rylaarsdam R, Liu G, Brickman, et al. A novel double mutation in the luteinizing hormone receptor in a kindred with familial Leydig cell hypoplasia and male pseudohermaphroditism. *Endocr Res* 2005;31:307–323.

99. Brinkmann AO. Molecular basis of androgen insensitivity. *Mol Cell Endocrinol* 2001;179:105–109.

100. Morris JM. The syndrome of testicular feminization in male pseudo-hermaphrodites. *Am J Obstet Gynecol* 1953;65:1192–1211.

101. Rutgers JL, Scully RE. The androgen insensitivity syndrome (testicular feminization). A clinicopathologic study of 43 cases. *Int J Gynecol Pathol* 1991;10:126–145.

102. Griffin JE, Durrant JL. Quantitative receptor defects in families with androgen resistance; failure of stabilization of the fibroblast cytosol androgen receptor. *J Clin Endocrinol Metab* 1982;55:465–474.

103. Gerli M, Migliorini G, Bocchini V, et al. A case of complete testicular feminization and 47XXY karyotype. *J Med Genet* 1979;16:480–483.

104. Muller J. Morphometry and histology of gonads from twelve children and adolescents with the androgen insensitivity (testicular feminization) syndrome. *J Clin Endocrinol Metab* 1984;59:485–789.

105. Ko HM, Chung JH, Jung IS, et al. Androgen receptor gene mutation associated with complete androgen insensitivity syndrome and Sertoli cell adenoma. *Int J Gynecol Pathol* 2001;20:196–199.

106. Papadimitriou DT, Linglart A, Morel Y, et al. Puberty in subjects with complete androgen insensitivity syndrome. *Horm Res* 2006;65:126–131.

107. Reifenstein EC Jr. Hereditary familial hypogonadism. *Clin Res* 1947;3:86–89.

108. Lubs HA Jr, Vilar O, Bergenstal DM. Familial male psudohermaphroditism and partial feminization: endocrine studies and genetic aspects. *J Clin Endocrinol Metab* 1959;19:1110–1120.

109. Gilbert-Dreyfus S, Sebaoum CIA, Belaisch J. Etude d'un cas familial d'androgynoidisme avec hypospadias grave, gynecomastie et hyperestrogenie. *Ann Endocrinol* 1957;18:93–101.

110. Rosewater S, Gwinup G, Hamwi GJ. Familial gynecomastia. *Ann Intern Med* 1965;63:377–385.

111. Lombardo F, Sgro P, Salacone P, et al. Androgens and fertility. *J Endocrinol Invest* 2005;28:51–55.

112. Kennedy WR, Alter M, Sung JH. Progressive proximal spinal and bulbar atrophy of late onset. A sex-linked recessive trait. *Neurology* 1968;18:671–680.

113. La Spada AR, Wilson EM, Lubahn DB, et al. Androgen receptor gene mutations in X-linked spinal and bulbar muscular atrophy. *Nature* 1991;352:77–79.

114. Josso N, Picard JY, Imbeaud S, et al. The persistent mullerian duct syndrome: a rare cause of cryptorchidism. *Eur J Pediatr* 1993;152:S76–S78.

115. Sohval AR. Hermaphroditism with atypical or 'mixed' gonadal dysgenesis. Relationship to gonadal neoplasm. *Am J Med* 1964;36:281–292.

116. Robboy SJ, Miller T, Donahoe PK, et al. Dysgenesis of testicular and streak gonads in the syndrome of mixed gonadal dysgenesis. Perspective derived from a clinicopathologic analysis of twenty-one cases. *Hum Pathol* 1982;13:700–716.

117. Berkowitz GD, Fechner PY, Zacur HW, et al. Clinical and pathologic spectrum of 46,XY gonadal dysgenesis: its relevance to the understanding of sex differentiation. *Medicine (Baltimore)* 1991;70:375–383.

118. Rajfer J, Mendelsohn G, Arnheim J et al. Dysgenetic male pseudohermaphroditism. *J Urol* 1978;119:525–527.

119. Ribeiro-Scolfaro M, Aparecida-Cardinalli I, Gabas-Stuchi-Perez E, et al. Morphometry and histology of gonads from 13 children with dysgenetic male pseudohermaphroditism. *Arch Pathol Lab Med* 2001;125:652–656.

120. Slowikoska-Hilczer J, Szarras-Czapnik M, et al. Testicular pathology in 46,XY dysgenetic male pseudohermaphroditism: an approach to pathogenesis of testis cancer. *J Androl* 2001;22:781–792.

121. Nilson O. Hernia uteri inguinalis beim Manne. *Acta Chir Scand* 1939;83:231–240.

122. Belville C, Josso N, Picard JY. Persistence of mullerian derivatives in males. *Am J Med Genet* 1999;89:218–223.

123. Sheehan SJ, Tobbia IN, Ismail MA, et al. Persistent mullerian duct syndrome. Review and report of 3 cases. *Br J Urol* 1985;57:548–551.

124. Hershlag A, Spitz IM, Hochner-Celnikier D, et al. Persistent mullerian structures in infertile male. *Urology* 1986;28:138–141.

125. Malayaman D, Armiger G, D'Arcangues C, et al. Male pseudohermaphroditism with persistent mullerian and wolffian structures complicated by intraabdominal seminoma. *Urology* 1984;24:67–69.

126. Sloan WR, Walsh PC. Familial persistent mullerian duct syndrome. *J Urol* 1976;115:459–461.

127. Duenas A, Saldivar C, Castillero C, et al. A case of bilateral seminoma in the setting of persistent mullerian duct syndrome. *Rev Invest Clin* 2001;53:193–196.

128. Franco B, Guioli S, Pragliola A, et al. A gene deleted in Kallma's syndrome shares homology with neural cell adhesion and axonal pathfinding molecules. *Nature* 1991;353:529–536.

129. Males JL, Townsend JL, Schneider RA. Hypogonadotropic hypogonadism with anosmia-Kallmann's syndrome. A disorder of olfactory and hypothalamic function. *Arch Intern Med* 1973;131:501–507.

130. Smeets DF, Hamel BC, Nelen MR, et al. Prader-Willi syndrome and Angelman syndrome in cousins from a family with a translocation between chromosomes 6 and 15. *N Engl J Med* 1992;326:807–811.

131. Mak V, Jarvi KA. The genetics of male infertility. *J Urol* 1996;156:1245–1256.

132. Lanfranco F, Kamischke A, Zitzmann M, et al. Klinefelter's syndrome. *Lancet* 2004;364:273–283.

133. Paduch DA, Fine RG, Bolyakov A, et al. New concepts in Klinefelter syndrome. *Curr Opin Urol* 2008;18:621–627.

134. Wikström AM, Dunkel L. Testicular function in Klinefelter syndrome. *Horm Res* 2008;69:317–326.

135. Smyth CM, Bremner WJ. Klinefelter syndrome. *Arch Intern Med* 1998;158:1309–1314.

136. Mies R, Fischer H, Pfeiff B, et al. Klinefelter's syndrome and breast cancer. *Andrologia* 1982;14:317–321.

137. Speed RM, Faed MJ, Batstone PJ, et al. Persistence of two Y chromosomes through meiotic prophase and metaphase I in an XYY man. *Hum Genet* 1991;87:416–420.

138. Imperato-McGinley J, Peterson RE, Leshin M, et al. Steroid 5 alpha-reductase deficiency in a 65-year-old male pseudohermaphrodite: the natural history, ultrastructure of the testes, and evidence for inherited enzyme heterogeneity. *J Clin Endocrinol Metab* 1980;50:15–22.

139. Dahl EV, Bahn RC. Aberrant adrenal cortical tissue near the testis in human infants. *Am J Pathol* 1962;40:587–598.

140. Vaos G, Zavras N, Boukouvalea I. Ectopic adrenocortical tissue along the inguinoscrotal path of children *Int Surg* 2006;91:125–128.

141. Ferro F, Lais A, Boldrini R, et al. Hepatogonadal fusion. *J Pediatr Surg* 1996;31:435–436.

142. Imperial SL, Sidhu JS. Nonseminomatous germ cell tumor arising in splenogonadal fusion. *Arch Pathol Lab Med* 2002;126:1222–1225.

143. Gouw AS, Elema JD, Bink-Boelkens MT, et al. The spectrum of splenogonadal fusion. Case report and review of 82 reported cases. *Eur J Pediatr* 1985;144:316–323.

144. Murray RS, Keeling JW, Ellis PM, et al. Symmetrical upper limb peromelia and lower limb phocomelia associated with a de novo apparently balanced reciprocal translocation: XX (2; 12) (p25.1;q24.1). *Clin Dysmorphol* 2002;11:87–90.

145. Tank ES, Forsyth M. Splenic gonadal fusion. *J Urol* 1988;139:798–799.

146. Nistal M, Indigoes L, Paniagua R. Tubular embryonal remnants in the human spermatic cord. *Urol Int* 1987;42:260–264.

147. Hamm B, Fobbed F, Loy V. Testicular cysts: differentiation with US and clinical findings. *Radiology* 1988;168:19–23.

148. Nistal M, Indigoes L, Paniagua R. Cysts of testicular parenchyma and tunicas albuginea. *Arch Pathol Lab Med* 1989;113:902–906.

149. Bryant J. Efferent ductule cyst of tunica albuginea. *Urology* 1986;27:172–173.

150. Maizlin ZV, Belenky A, Baniel J, et al. Epidermoid cyst and teratoma of the testis: sonographic and histologic similarities. *J Ultrasound Med* 2005;24:1403–1409.

151. Cheng L, Zhang S, MacLennan GT, et al. Interphase fluorescence in situ hybridization analysis of chromosome 12p abnormalities is useful for distinguishing epidermoid cysts of the testis from pure mature teratoma. *Clin Cancer Res* 2006;12:5668–5672.

152. Jeyaratnam R, Bakalinova D. Cystic dysplasia of the rete testis: a case of spontaneous regression and review of published reports. *Urology* 2010;75:687–690.

153. Glantz L, Hansen K, Caldamone A, et al. Cystic dysplasia of the testis. *Hum Pathol* 1993;24:1142–1145.

154. Nistal M, Garcia-Rojo M, Paniagua R. Congenital testicular lymphangiectasis in children with otherwise normal testes. *Histopathol* 1990;17:335–338.

155. Nistal M, Paniagua R, Bravo MP. Testicular lymphangiectasis in Noonan's syndrome. *J Urol* 1984;131:759–761.

156. Nistal M, Rodríguez JI, García-Fernández E, et al. Fetal gonadoblastoid testicular dysplasia: a focal failure of testicular development. *Pediatr Dev Pathol* 2007;10:274–281.

157. Hung NA, Silver MM, Chitayat D, et al. Gonadoblastoid testicular dysplasia in Walker-Warburg syndrome. *Pediatr Dev Pathol* 1998;1:393–404.

158. Spear GS, Martin CG. Fetal gonadoblastoid testicular dysplasia. *Hum Pathol* 1986;17:531–533.

159. Lee LM, Wright JE, McLoughlin MG. Testicular torsion in the adult. *J Urol* 1983;130:93–94.

160. Muschat M. The pathological anatomy of testicular torsion: explanation of its mechanism. *Surg Gynecol Obstet* 1932;54:758–762.

161. Nistal M, González-Peramato P, Paniagua R. Lipomembranous fat necrosis in three cases of testicular torsion. *Histopathology* 2001;38:443–447.

162. Flanigan RC, DeKernion JB, Persky L. Acute scrotal pain and swelling in children: a surgical emergency. *Urology* 1981;17:51–53.

163. Burton JA. Atrophy following testicular torsion. *Br J Surg* 1972;59:422–426.

164. Cosentino MJ, Nishida M, Rabionowitz R, et al. Histological changes occurring in the contralateral testes of prepuberal rats subjected to various durations of unilateral spermatic cord torsion. *J Urol* 1985;133:906–911.

165. Turner TT. On unilateral testicular and epididymal torsion: no effect on the contralateral testis. *J Urol* 1987;138:1285–1290.

166. Arce Terroba Y, Algaba F, Villavicencio Maverich H. Segmental infarct of testicle: an infrequent pseudotumor. *Actas Urol Esp* 2010;34:194–200.

167. Skoglund RW, McRoberts JW, Ragde H. Torsion of testicular appendages: presentation on 43 new cases and collective review. *J Urol* 1970;104:598–600.

168. Lefort C, Thoumas D, Badachi Y, et al. Ischemic orchitis: review of 5 cases diagnosed by color Doppler ultrasonography. *J Radiol* 2001;82:839–842.

169. Vieras F. Evolution of acute epididymitis to testicular infarction. Scintigraphic demonstration. *Clin Nucl Med* 1986;11:158–160.

170. Ameur A, Zarzur J, Albouzidi A, et al. Testicular infarction without torsion in cryptorchidism. *Prog Urol* 2003;13:321–323.

171. Bostwick DG. Spermatic cord and testicular adnexa. In: Bostwick DG, Eble JN. eds. *Urologic Surgical Pathology*. St. Louis, MO: Mosby; 1996:653.

172. Nativ O, Mor Y, Nass D, et al. Cholesterol granuloma of the tunica vaginalis mimicking a neoplasm. *Isr J Med Sci* 1995;31:235–236.

173. Uehling DT. Fertility in men with varicocele. *Int J Fertil* 1968;13:58–60.

174. Hienz HA, Voggenthaler J, Weissbach L. Histological findings in testes with varicocele during childhood and their therapeutic consequences. *Eur J Pediatr* 1980;133:139–146.

175. Redondo E, Regadera J, Nistal M. Etiopatogenia e histopatologia del varicocele. *Med Clin (Barc)* 1989;92:309–315.

176. Levine TS. Testicular and epididymal vasculitides. Is morphology of help in classification and prognosis? *J Urol Pathol* 1994;2:81–88.

177. Hara Y, Tajiri T, Matsuura K, et al. Acute scrotum caused by Henoch-Schönlein purpura. *Int J Urol* 2004;11:578–580.

178. Mayer DF, Matteson EL. Testicular involvement in rheumatoid vasculitis. *Clin Exp Rheumatol* 2004;22:S62–S64.

179. Jalleh RP, Swift RI, Sundaresan M, et al. Necrotizing testicular vasculitis associated with dermatomyositis. *Br J Urol* 1990;66:660.

180. Dotan ZA, Laufer M, Heldenberg E, et al. Isolated testicular polyarteritis nodosa mimicking testicular neoplasm-long-term follow-up. *Urology* 2003;62:352.

181. Sundaram S, Smith DH. Giant cell arteritis mimicking a testicular tumour. *Rheumatol Int* 2001;20:215–216.

182. Kariv R, Sidi Y, Gur H. Systemic vasculitis presenting as a tumorlike lesion. Four case reports and an analysis of 77 reported cases. *Medicine (Baltimore)* 2000;79:349–359.

183. Davenport A, Downey SE, Goel S, et al. Wegener's granulomatosis involving the urogenital tract. *Br J Urol* 1996;78:354–357.

184. Shurbaji MS, Epstein JI. Testicular vasculitis: implications for systemic disease. *Hum Pathol* 1988;19:186–189.

185. Hernández-Rodríguez J, Tan CD, Koening CL, et al. Testicular vasculitis: findings differentiating isolated disease from systemic disease in 72 patients. *Medicine (Baltimore)* 2012;91:75–85.

186. Aldenhoven M, Sakkers RJ, Boelens J, et al. Musculoskeletal manifestations of lysosomal storage isorders. *Ann Rheum Dis* 2009;68:1659–1665.

187. Butler A, He X, Gordon RE, et al. Reproductive pathology and sperm physiology in acid sphingomyelinase-deficient mice. *Am J Pathol* 2002;161:1061–1075.

188. Berger RE, Alexander EF, Harnisch JP. Etiology, manifestations and therapy of acute epididymitis: prospective study of 50 cases. *J Urol* 1979;121:750–754.

189. Natarajan V, Burgess NA, Gaches CGC, et al. Emphysematous infarction of the testis following epididymo-orchitis. *Br J Urol* 1995;76:270–271.

190. Riggs S, Sanford JP. Viral orchitis. *N Engl J Med* 1962;266:990–993.

191. Preblud SR, Dobbs HI, Sedmak GV, et al. Testalgia associated with rubella infection. *South Med J* 1980;73:594–595.

192. Xu J, Qi L, Chi X, et al. Orchitis: a complication of severe acute respiratory syndrome (SARS). *Biol Reprod* 2006;74:410–416.

193. Jalal H, Bahadur G, Knowles W, et al. Mumps epididymo-orchitis with prolonged detection of virus in semen and the development of anti-sperm antibodies. *J Med Virol* 2004;73:147–150.

194. Pudney J, Anderson D. Orchitis and human immunodeficiency virus type 1nfected cells in reproductive tissues from men with the acquired immune deficiency syndrome. *Am J Pathol* 1991;139:149–160.

195. Anglada Curado FJ, Gómez Bermudo J, Carmona Campos E, et al. Tuberculous orchiepididymitis as clinical onset of human immunodeficiency virus (HIV) infection. *Actas Urol Esp* 1999;23:898–899.

196. Briceño-García EM, Gómez-Pardal A, Alvarez-Bustos G, et al. Tuberculous orchiepididymitis after BCG therapy for bladder cancer. *J Ultrasound Med* 2007;26:977–979.

197. Cabral DA, Johnson HW, Coleman GU, et al. Tuberculous epididymitis as a cause of testicular pseudomalignancy in two young children. *Pediatr Infect Dis* 1985;4:59–62.

198. Namiduru M, Gungor K, Dikensoy O, et al. Epidemiological, clinical and laboratory features of brucellosis: a prospective evaluation of 120 adult patients. *Int J Clin Pract* 2003;57:20–24.

199. Valdelvira Nadal P, Nicolás Torralba JA, Bañón Pérez VJ, et al. Brucellar orchiepididymitis. *Actas Urol Esp* 2001;25:140–142.

200. Varma R, Baithun S, Alexander S, et al. Acute syphilitic interstitial orchitis mimicking testicular malignancy in an HIV-1 infected man diagnosed by *Treponema pallidum* polymerase chain reaction. *Int J STD AIDS* 2009;20:65–66.

201. Nigam P, Mukhija RD, Kapoor KK, et al. Male gonads in leprosy—a clinico-pathological study. *Indian J Lepr* 1988;60:77–83.

202. El-Beheiry A, Abou Zeid S, El-Ghazzawi E, et al. The leprous testis. *Arch Androl* 1979;3:173–176.

203. Akhtar M, Ali MA, Mackey DM. Lepromatous leprosy presenting as orchitis. *Am J Clin Pathol* 1980;73:712–715.

204. Haddad FS. Coccidioidomycosis of the genitourinary tract with special emphasis on the epididymis and the prostate. Four case reports and review of the literature. *J Urol Pathol* 1996;4:205–211.

205. Kauffman CA, Slama TG, Wheat LJ. *Histoplasma capsulatum* epididymitis. *J Urol* 1981;125:434–435.

206. Williams PB, Henderson RJ, Sanusi ID, et al. Ultrasound diagnosis of filarial funiculoepididymitis. *Urology* 1996;48:644–646.

207. Mikhail NE, Tawfic MI, Hadi AA, et al. Schistosomal orchitis simulating malignancy. *J Urol* 1988;140:147–148.

208. Fajardo LF, Dueker GE, Kosek JC. Light and electron microscopic observations on granulomatous orchitis. *Invest Urol* 1968;6:158–169.

209. Capers TH. Granulomatous orchitis. *Am J Clin Pathol* 1960;34:139–145.

210. Osca Garcia JM, Alfaro Ferreres L, Ruiz Cerda JL, et al. Idiopathic granulomatous orchitis. *Actas Urol Esp* 1993;17:53–56.

211. Abdou NI, NaPombejara C, Sagawa A, et al. Malakoplakia: evidence for monocyte lysosomal abnormality correctable by cholinergic agonist in vitro and in vivo. *N Engl J Med* 1977;297:1413–1419.

212. Dieckmann KP, Henke RP, Zimmer-Krolzig G. Malacoplakia of the epididymis. Report of a case and review of the literature. *Urol Int* 1995;55:222–225.

213. McClure J. Malakoplakia of the testis and its relationship to granulomatous orchitis. *J Clin Pathol* 1980;33:670–678.

214. Green WO Jr. Malacoplakia of the epididymis (without testicular involvement). The first reported case. *Arch Pathol* 1968;86:438–441.

215. Mikuz G. Ultrastructural study of two cases of granulomatous orchitis. *Virchows Arch A Pathol Anat* 1973;360:223–234.

216. Al-Said S, Ali A, Alobaidy AK, et al. Xanthogranulomatous orchitis: review of the published work and report of one case. *Int J Urol* 2007;14:452–454.

217. Yap RL, Jang TL, Gupta R, et al. Xanthogranulomatous orchitis. *Urology* 2004;63:176–177.

218. Woodward PJ, Sohaey R, O'Donoghue MJ, et al. From the archives of the AFIP: tumors and tumorlike lesions of the testis: radiologic-pathologic correlation. *Radiographics* 2002;22:189–216.

219. Nishimura T, Akimoto M, Kawai H, et al. Peritesticular xanthogranuloma. *Urology* 1981;18:189–190.

220. Hurd DS, Olsen T. Cutaneous sarcoidosis presenting as a testicular mass. *Cutis* 2000;66:435–438.

221. Ryan DM, Lesser BA, Crumley LA, et al. Epididymal sarcoidosis. *J Urol* 1993;149:134–136.

222. Algaba F, Santaularia JM, Garat JM, et al. Testicular pseudolymphoma. *Eur Urol* 1986;12:362–363.

223. Fernandopulle SM, Hwang JS, Kuick CH, et al. Rosai-Dorfman disease of the testis: an unusual entity that mimics testicular malignancy. *J Clin Pathol* 2006;59:325–327.

224. Nelson WO. Testicular morphology in eunuchoidal and infertile men. *Fertil Steril* 1950;1:477–488.

225. McLachlan RI, Rajpert-De Meyts E, Hoei-Hansen CE, et al. Histological evaluation of the human testis-approaches to optimizing the clinical value of the assessment: mini review. *Hum Reprod* 2007;22:2–16.

226. Schiff JD, Palermo GD, Veeck LL, et al. Success of testicular sperm extraction [corrected] and intracytoplasmic sperm injection in men with Klinefelter syndrome. *J Clin Endocrinol Metab* 2005;90:6263–6267.

227. Silber SJ, Rodriguez-Rigau LJ. Quantitative analysis of testicular biopsy: determination of partial obstruction and prediction of sperm count after surgery for obstruction. *Fertil Steril* 1981;36:480–485.

228. Lennox B. The infertile testis. In: Anthony PP, MacSween RNM, eds. *Recent Advances in Histopathology*. Edinburgh, UK: Churchill Livingstone; 1981:135.

229. Bergmann M, Kliesch S. Testicular biopsy and histology. In: Nieschlag E, Behre HM, Niesschlag S, eds. *Andrology*. Chapter 11. Berlin, Germany: Springer Velag; 2010:155.

230. Loftus BM, Gilmartin LG, O'Brien MJ, et al. Intratubular germ cell neoplasia of the testis: identification by placental alkaline phosphatase immunostaining and argyrophilic nucleolar organizer region quantification. *Hum Pathol* 1990;21:941–948.

231. Cheng L, Sung MT, Cossu-Rocca P, et al. OCT4: biological functions and clinical applications as a marker of germ cell neoplasia. *J Pathol* 2007;211:1–9.

232. Söderström KO. Leydig cell hyperplasia. *Arch Androl* .1986;17:57–65.

233. Bjerklund Johansen TE, Majak M, Nesland JM. Testicular histology after treatment with the new antiandrogen Casodex for carcinoma of the prostate. A preliminary report. *Scand J Urol Nephrol* 1994;28:67–70.

234. Jezek D, Banek L, Hittmair A, et al. Mast cells in testicular biopsies of infertile men with 'mixed atrophy' of seminiferous tubules. *Andrologia* 1999;31:203–210.

235. Söderström KO. Tubular hyalinization in human testes. *Andrologia* 1986;18:97–103.

236. Hikim AP, Wang C, Leung A, et al. Involvement of apoptosis in the induction of germ cell degeneration in adult rats after gonadotropin-releasing hormone antagonist treatment. *Endocrinology* 1995;136:2770–2775.

237. Sinha Hikim AP, Rajavashisth TB, Sinha Hikim I, et al. Significance of apoptosis in the temporal and stage-specific loss of germ cells in the adult rat after gonadotropin deprivation. *Biol Reprod* 1997;57:1193–1201.

238. Atanassova N, McKinnell C, Walker M, et al. Permanent effects of neonatal estrogen exposure in rats on reproductive hormone levels, Sertoli cell number, and the efficiency of spermatogenesis in adulthood. *Endocrinology* 1999;140:5364–5373.

239. Del Castillo EB, Trabucco A, de la Balze FA. Syndrome produced by absence of germinal epithelium without impairment of Sertoli or Leydig cells. *J Clin Endocrinol Metab* 1947;7:493.

240. Nistal M, Jimenez F, Paniagua R. Sertoli cell types in the Sertoli-cell-only syndrome: relationships between Sertoli cell morphology and aetiology. *Histopathology* 1990;16:173–180.

241. DeKretser DM. The fine structure of the immature human testis in hypogonadotropic hypogonadism. *Virchows Arch B Cell Pathol* 1968;1:283–296.

242. Steger K, Rey R, Kliesch S, et al. Immunohistochemical detection of immature Sertoli cell markers in testicular tissue of infertile adult men: a preliminary study. *Int J Androl* 1996;19:122–128.

243. Mack WS, Scott LS, Ferguson-Smith MA. Ectopic testis and the undescended testis: a histological comparison. *J Pathol Bacteriol* 1961;82:439–443.

244. Rothman MC, Sims SA, Stotts CI. Sertoli cell only syndrome in 1982. *Fertil Steril* 1982;38:388–390.

245. Decensi AU, Guarneri D, Marroni P. Evidence for testicular impairment after long-term treatment with a luteinizing hormone-releasing agonist in elderly men. *J Urol* 1989;142:1235–1238.

246. Gulizia S, Vicari E, Aleffi A. Abnormal germ cell exfoliation in semen of hypogonadotrophic patients during a hCG treatment. *Andrologia* 1981;13:74–77.

247. Nistal M, De Mora JC, Paniagua R. Classification of several types of maturational arrest of spermatogonia according to Sertoli cell morphology: an approach to aetiology. *Int J Androl* 1998;21:317–326.

248. Zeng L, Kong XT, Su JW, et al. Evaluation of germ-cell kinetics in infertile patients with proliferating cell nuclear antigen proliferation index. *Asian J Androl* 2001;3:63–66.

249. Steger K, Aleithe I, Behre H, et al. The proliferation of spermatogonia in normal and pathological human seminiferous epithelium: an immunohistochemical study using monoclonal antibodies against Ki-67 protein and proliferating cell nuclear antigen. *Mol Hum Reprod* 1998;4:227–233.

250. Takizawa T, Hatakeyama S. Age-associated changes in microvasculature of human adult testis. *Acta Pathol Jpn* 1978;28:541–554.

251. Saitoh K, Terada T, Hatakeyama S. A morphological study of the efferent ducts of the human epididymis. *Int J Androl* 1990;13:369–376.

252. Nistal M, Paniagua R, Regadera J. Obstruction of the tubuli recti and ductuli efferentes by dilated veins in the testes of men with varicocele and its possible role in causing atrophy of the seminiferous tubules. *Int J Androl* 1984;7:309–323.

253. Santamaría L, Martín R, Nistal M, et al. The peritubular myoid cells in the testes from men with varicocele. An ultrastructural, immunohistochemical and quantitative study. *Histopathology* 1992;21:423–433.

254. Hirsch IH, Choi H. Quantitative testicular biopsy in congenital and acquired genital obstruction. *J Urol* 1990;143:311–312.

255. Urry RL, Heaton JB, Moore M. A fifteen-year study of alterations in semen quality occurring after vasectomy reversal. *Fertil Steril* 1990;53:341–345.

256. Algaba F, Mikuz G, Boccon-Gibod L, et al. Pseudoneoplastic lesions of the testis and paratesticular structures. *Virchows Arch* 2007;451:987–997.

257. McCabe J, Das S, Hamid B, et al. Localized traumatic infarction of the testicle. *Scand J Urol Nephrol* 2004;38:442–443.

258. Joudi FN, Austin JC, Vogelgesang SA, et al. Isolated testicular vasculitis presenting as a tumor-like lesion. *J Urol* 2004;171:799–803.

259. Warfield AT, Lee SJ, Phillips SM, et al. Isolated testicular vasculitis mimicking a testicular neoplasm. *J Clin Pathol* 1994;47:1121–1123.

260. Dotan ZA, Laufer M, Heldenberg E, et al. Isolated testicular polyarteritis nodosa mimicking testicular neoplasm-long-term follow-up. *Urology* 2003;62:352.

261. Sundaram S, Smith DH. Giant cell arteritis mimicking a testicular tumour. *Rheumatol Int* 2001;20:215–216.

262. Kariv R, Sidi Y, Gur H. Systemic vasculitis presenting as a tumorlike lesion. Four case reports and an analysis of 77 reported cases. *Medicine (Baltimore)* 2000;79:349–359.

263. Li M, Fogarty J, Whitney KD, et al. Repeated testicular infarction in a patient with sickle cell disease: a possible mechanism for testicular failure. *Urology* 2003;62:551.

264. Ruibal M, Quintana JL, Fernández G, et al. Segmental testicular infarction. *J Urol* 2003;170:187–188.

265. Garat JM, Algaba F, Parra L, et al. Meconium vaginalitis. *Br J Urol* 1991;68:430–431.

266. Williams HJ, Abernethy LJ, Losty PD, et al. Meconium periorchitis—a rare cause of a paratesticular mass. *Pediatr Radiol* 2004;34:421–423.

267. Woodward PJ, Schwab CM, Sesterhenn IA. From the archives of the AFIP: extratesticular scrotal masses: radiologic-pathologic correlation. *Radiographics* 2003;23:215–240.

268. Dunner PS, Lipsit ER, Nochomovitz L. Epididymal sperm granuloma simulating a testicular neoplasm. *J Clin Ultrasound* 1982;10:353–355.

269. Honore LH. Nonspecific peritesticular fibrosis manifested as testicular enlargement. Clinicopathological study of nine cases. *Arch Surg* 1978;113:814–816.

270. Einstein DM, Paushter DM, Singer AA, et al. Fibrotic lesions of the testicle: sonographic patterns mimicking malignancy. *Urol Radiol* 1992;14:205–210.

271. Kundu S, Sengupta A, Dey A, et al. Testicular tuberculosis mimicking testicular malignancy. *J Indian Med Assoc* 2003;101:204–205.

272. Kocak I, Dundar M, Culhaci N, et al. Relapse of brucellosis simulating testis tumor. *Int J Urol* 2004;11:683–685.

273. Archimbaud A, Bonvalet D, Levy-Klotz B, et al. Syphilitic orchiepididymitis. Apropos of a pseudotumoral case. *Ann Dermatol Venereol* 1984;111:169–171.

274. Jani AN, Casibang V, Mufarrij WA. Disseminated actinomycosis presenting as a testicular mass: a case report. *J Urol* 1990;143:1012–1014.

275. Shawker TH, Doppman JL, Choyke PL, et al. Intratesticular masses associated with abnormally functioning adrenal glands. *J Clin Ultrasound* 1992;20:51–58.

276. Thompson JE, van der Walt JD. Nodular fibrous proliferation (fibrous pseudotumour) of the tunica vaginalis testis. A light, electron microscopic and immunocytochemical study of a case and review of the literature. *Histopathology* 1986;10:741–748.

277. Parveen T, Fleischmann J, Petrelli M. Benign fibrous tumor of the tunica vaginalis testis. Report of a case with light, electron microscopic, and immunocytochemical study, and review of the literature. *Arch Pathol Lab Med* 1992;116:277–280.

278. Begin LR, Frail D, Brzezinski A. Myofibroblastoma of the tunica testis: evolving phase of so-called fibrous pseudotumor? *Hum Pathol* 1990;21:866–868.

279. Bösmüller H, von Weyhern CH, Adam P, et al. Paratesticular fibrous pseudotumor—an IgG4-related disorder? *Virchows Arch* 2011;458:109–113.

280. Handelsman DJ, Yue DK, Turtle JR. Hypogonadism and massive testicular infiltration due to amyloidosis. *J Urol* 1983;129:610–612.

281. Casella R, Nudell D, Cozzolino D, et al. Primary testicular amyloidosis mimicking tumor in a cryptorchid testis. *Urology* 2002;59:445.

282. Ricco R, Bufo P. Histologic study of 3 cases of so-called tubular adenoma of the testis. *Boll Soc Ital Biol Sper* 1980;56:2110–2115.

283. Rutgers JL, Scully RE. The androgen insensitivity syndrome (testicular feminization): a clinicopathologic study of 43 cases. *Int J Gynecol Pathol* 1991;10:126–144.

284. Ramaswamy G, Jagadha V, Tchertkoff V. A testicular tumor resembling the sex cord with annular tubules in a case of the androgen insensitivity syndrome. *Cancer* 1985;55:1607–1611.

285. Davis JM, Woodroof J, Sadasivan R, et al. Case report: congenital adrenal hyperplasia and malignant Leydig cell tumor. *Am J Med Sci* 1995;309:63–65.

286. Knudsen JL, Savage A, Mobb GE. The testicular 'tumour' of adrenogenital syndrome—a persistent diagnostic pitfall. *Histopathology* 1991;19:468–470.

287. Rich MA, Keating MA, Levin HS, et al. Tumors of the adrenogenital syndrome: an aggressive conservative approach. *J Urol* 1998;160:1838–1841.

288. Young RH, Talerman A. Testicular tumors other than germ cell tumors. *Semin Diagn Pathol* 1987;4:342–360.

289. Hartwick RW, Ro JY, Srigley JR, et al. Adenomatous hyperplasia of the rete testis. A clinicopathologic study of nine cases. *Am J Surg Pathol* 1991;15:350–357.

290. Nistal M, Castillo MC, Regadera J, et al. Adenomatous hyperplasia of the rete testis. A review and report of new cases. *Histol Histopathol* 2003;18:741–752.

291. Ulbright TM, Gersell DJ. Rete testis hyperplasia with hyaline globule formation. A lesion simulating yolk sac tumor. *Am J Surg Pathol* 1991;15:66–74.

292. Rosai J, Dehner LP. Nodular mesothelial hyperplasia in hernia sacs: a benign reactive condition simulating a neoplastic process. *Cancer* 1975;35:165–175.

293. Bolen JW, Hammar SP, McNutt MA. Reactive and neoplastic serosal tissue. A light-microscopic, ultrastructural, and immunocytochemical study. *Am J Surg Pathol* 1986;10:34–47.

294. Tyagi G, Munn CS, Kiser LC, et al. Malignant mesothelioma of tunica vaginalis testis. *Urology* 1989;34:102–104.

295. Perez-Arbej JA, Rosa Arias J, Aranda Lassa JM, et al. Testicular injury: presentation of 3 cases and review of the literature. *Arch Esp Urol* 1986;39:398–402.

296. Luján Marco S, Budía Alba A, Bango García V, et al. Traumatic testicular dislocation. *Actas Urol Esp* 2006;30:409–411.

297. Nistal M, Martínez-García C, Paniagua R. The origin of testicular microliths. *Int J Androl* 1995;18:221–229.

298. Yagci C, Zcan H, Ayta S, et al. Testicular microlithiasis associated with seminoma: gray-scale and color doppler ultrasound findings. *Urol Int* 1996;57:255–258.

299. Kaveggia FF, Strassman MJ, Apfelbach GL, et al. Diffuse testicular microlithiasis associated with intratubular germ cell neoplasia and seminoma. *Urology* 1996;48:794–796.

300. Parra BL, Venable DD, Gonzalez E, et al. Testicular microlithiasis as a predictor of intratubular germ cell neoplasia. *Urology* 1996;48:797–799.

301. Costabile RA. How worrisome is testicular microlithiasis? *Curr Opin Urol* 2007;17:419–423.

302. Tan MH, Eng C; Medscape. Testicular microlithiasis: recent advances in understanding and management. *Nat Rev Urol* 2011;8:153–163.

303. Hatakeyama S, Sengoku R, Takayama S. Histological and submicroscopic studies on arteriolar hyalinosis of the human testis. *Bull Tokyo Med Dent Univ* 1966;13:511–530.

304. Ricchiuti VS, Richman MB, Haas CA, et al. Sclerosing lipogranuloma of the testis. *Urology* 2002;60:515.

CHAPTER 12

Tumors of the Testis

VICTOR E. REUTER and SATISH K. TICKOO

ANATOMY OF THE TESTIS

The adult testes are suspended by the spermatic cord and located within the scrotum. The testis proper is surrounded by a thick connective tissue layer called the tunica albuginea that itself is lined by the visceral tunica vaginalis (Fig. 12-1). In the posterior aspect of the gonad is the mediastinum testis that contains blood vessels, lymphatics, nerves, and portions of the rete testis. The testis contains multiple fibrous septa that radiate from the mediastinum testis to the tunica albuginea, and these divide the organ into approximately 250 compartments that contain the seminiferous tubules.[1,2] Surrounding the seminiferous tubules is the interstitium, which contains Leydig cells, blood vessels, lymphatics, and nerves. Each compartment of the testis contains a maximum of four seminiferous tubules that are very convoluted and that usually empty into the straight portion of the rete (tubuli recti). Each seminiferous tubule is lined by a basement membrane and a thin lamina propria. Within the seminiferous tubule are Sertoli cells and germ cells at different stages of differentiation (Fig. 12-2).

Sertoli cells comprise 10% to 15% of cells within the tubule. They are columnar to pyramidal in shape with their long axis is perpendicular to the basement membrane. The cytoplasm is granular–eosinophilic and may contain fine vacuoles. The nuclei are round to oval with finely granular chromatin and are commonly located within a cell or two of the basement membrane. They contain a prominent nucleolus, the only normal cell within the tubule to do so. Intracytoplasmic Charcot-Böttcher crystalloids are best seen preferentially by electron microscopy.

Sertoli cells have phagocytic capacity but also play an important role in regulating spermatogenesis. By immunohistochemistry, they have been shown to express vimentin; cytokeratins 8, 18, and 19; as well as inhibin.[3,4] Cytokeratin positivity is routinely observed in immature but not mature Sertoli cells; however, expression of this intermediate filament may be seen in adults in association with various conditions including testicular atrophy, Sertoli cell tumors (SCTs) and

Sertoli cells adjacent to germ cell tumors (GCTs), orchitis, and infarct. In these settings, it is not unusual to see a gradient of immunoreactivity from positive to negative the farther away the tubules are located from the lesion.

Germ cells originate in the yolk sac and migrate to the genital ridge during the first 7 weeks of gestation.[5,6] They comprise 85% to 90% of cells within the seminiferous tubule and have the capacity to differentiate (mature). Spermatogonia are undifferentiated cells located adjacent to the basement membrane. They have clear or basophilic cytoplasm, distinct cytoplasmic membranes, small round nuclei with dark chromatin, and no nucleoli. They have the capacity to proliferate and give rise to primary spermatocytes. The latter cells are subclassified into preleptotene, leptotene, zygotene, pachytene, and diplotene spermatocytes based on their nuclear chromatin pattern. These subtle differences are difficult, if not impossible, to discern on routine histologic preparations and irrelevant when evaluating tumor-bearing gonads. In general, primary spermatocytes are larger than spermatogonia, have basophilic cytoplasm, indistinct nuclear borders, round nuclei with distinct chromatin patterns, and absent nucleoli. Completion of the first meiotic division gives rise to secondary spermatocytes, which have a short half-life and undergo a second meiotic division to form spermatids. Secondary spermatocytes are smaller than their progenitor cells and have denser chromatin. Spermatids are located toward the lumen of the tubule and have small nuclei with dense chromatin. They transform into spermatozoa through metamorphosis.

Leydig cells are present in the interstitium as single cells or in clusters. Interestingly, they may also be observed in the tunica albuginea, mediastinum testis, epididymis, and even along the spermatic cord, usually intimately associated to nerve bundles.[5,7] Leydig cells have abundant eosinophilic cytoplasm and round, regular nuclei with prominent nucleoli. Intracytoplasmic lipofuscin pigment may be seen, more commonly in older males. Intracytoplasmic Reinke crystals are characteristic of Leydig cells, rarely seen in normal cells, and more commonly observed by electron microscopy where they appear as a hexagonal prism.[8,9]

749

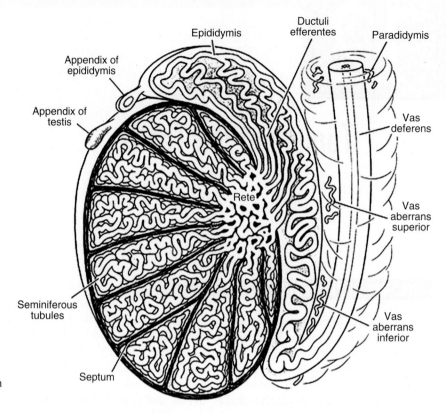

FIGURE 12-1 ■ Schematic representation of the testis and its adnexa.

Leydig cells have the capacity to produce testosterone and share an important paracrine function with Sertoli cells.[10] They express inhibin but not cytokeratins or vimentin by immunohistochemistry.[11]

The rete testis collects the effluent from the seminiferous tubules. It is located within the hilus of the testis and includes the tubuli recti, the mediastinal rete, and the extratesticular rete. The tubuli recti are short segments within the septa that connect the seminiferous tubules to the mediastinal rete. The mediastinum rete forms a series of epithelium-lined, interconnecting channels that lead to several dilated vesicular channels constituting the extratesticular rete, which anastomose to give rise to the efferent ducts or tubuli efferentia. The epithelium of the rete is low columnar and exhibits luminal microvilli. Every cell contains a flagellum that is not visible by routine light microscopy. The cells are immunoreactive for cytokeratins as well as vimentin.[12]

The efferent tubules have an irregular (undulating) luminal contour. They receive the luminal content from the rete testis and are responsible for resorption of fluid. The epithelial lining is a mixture of ciliated and nonciliated columnar pseudostratified cells that express cytokeratin and variably vimentin by immunohistochemistry. The epithelial cells are surrounded by a thick basement membrane, which in turn is surrounded by a layer of smooth muscle. These tubules lead into the epididymis, a convoluted tubular structure that plays a role in the transport, maturation, and storage of sperm.[7] Transport is aided by a thick smooth muscle layer that surrounds the epididymis. The epididymis is lined by a thick basement membrane and can be divided anatomically into three sections: head, body, and tail, the latter where sperm storage and maturation occurs. The epithelial lining of the epididymis is predominantly tall columnar cells (principal cells), many of which exhibit stereocilia, but basal cells, clear cells, and luminal cells are also present. The luminal contour of the epididymis is rigid rather than undulating.

The vas deferens arises from the caudal portion of the epididymis, which proximally joins the excretory duct of the seminal vesicles to form the ejaculatory duct. The vas deferens is lined by pseudostratified, columnar epithelium

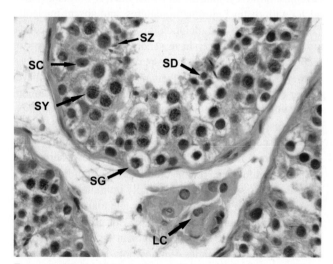

FIGURE 12-2 ■ Normal seminiferous tubules in an adult containing spermatogonia (SG), spermatocytes (SY), spermatids (SD), spermatozoa (SZ), and Sertoli cells (SC). A cluster of Leydig cells (LC) is present in the interstitium.

and basal cells, the former containing long stereocilia. The luminal contour of the vas is variably folded, and the epithelium is surrounded by loose connective tissue and a very thick smooth muscle layer.

Several appendages may be encountered on the testis, testicular adnexa, or spermatic cord, the most common being the appendix testis and appendix epididymis.[13,14] The appendix testis is a vestige of the müllerian duct attached to the tunica vaginalis along the anterosuperior surface of the testis adjacent to the head of the epididymis. It is a small pedunculated structure lined by columnar nonciliated epithelium. The epithelium covers richly vascular connective tissue. The appendix epididymis is a vestige of the mesonephric duct. It is a cystic, pedunculated structure attached to the head of the epididymis. The cyst is lined by low columnar epithelial cells, and the external surface is lined by mesothelium. Two other types of appendages are present as incidental findings and represent remnants of mesonephric tubules. They appear as epithelial-lined tubular or cystic structures, which are seen along the testicular adnexa or spermatic cord. Depending on their location, they are called vas aberrans or paradidymis.[7,14]

TUMORS OF THE TESTIS

Introduction

Primary testicular neoplasms are rare with <10,000 new cases reported each year in the United States. It is not unusual for there to be a delay in diagnosis since patients can present with testicular pain and be treated with antibiotics for a presumed orchitis or epididymitis. Metastases usually are first seen in retroperitoneal lymph nodes and then to lungs, consistent with the fact that metastases are usually through lymphatic spread except in the case of choriocarcinoma where dissemination is usually vascular. In more advanced cases, metastases are to the mediastinum and viscera, particularly the liver, and brain. The overwhelming majority of primary tumors are unilateral, whether of germ cell or sex cord–stromal origin. Because of the rarity of these tumors, it is prudent to always consider the possibility of secondary (metastatic) disease, even if the tumor is unilateral and particularly in older patients. However, as we discuss later, it is rare for a metastasis to the testis to be the first site of diagnosis since it is usually part of systemic disease. Primary lymphoma of the testis may present as unilateral disease and may mimic seminoma in its gross appearance as well as superficially at the microscopic level.

Gross Examination and Sampling of Testicular Tumors

In general, testicular neoplasms are managed surgically by a radical orchiectomy. This entails an inguinal incision and evacuation of the testis, surrounding tunica vaginalis, and extraperitoneal spermatic cord. Gross examination and proper prosecting of the orchiectomy specimen are crucial in establishing a proper diagnosis and pathologic staging of the tumor.[15] The tunica vaginalis should be opened and any adhesions to the tunica albuginea noted since these may be secondary to invasion by tumor. The tunica albuginea should be carefully examined for any areas of bulging, discoloration, or disruption. Palpation of the gonad will allow us to locate any mass within the testicular parenchyma and its relation to the overlying tunica albuginea, rete testis, mediastinum testis, and testicular adnexa. In general, it is best to incise the testis along its long axis from the lateral aspect of the gonad toward the mediastinum testis.

Sampling of the mass should include a minimum of one section per centimeter of lesional tissue unless the entire lesion can be submitted in 10 cassettes or less, in which case the entire tumor should be submitted. Tumors that have a variegated gross appearance should be sampled in a manner that will allow examination of these areas microscopically; this need may require more through sampling. In cases where the morphology of the tumor is not straightforward, for example, in cases of atypical-looking seminomas or undifferentiated sex cord–stromal tumors, it may be necessary to go back to the specimen to take additional sections. The importance of serum tumor markers cannot be overstated. In general, seminomas are associated with normal serum levels of alfa fetoprotein (AFP) and either normal or mildly elevated levels of beta-human chorionic gonadotropin (β-HCG). Sex cord–stromal tumors are not associated with elevation of either of these markers. Cases in which there is a discrepancy between the pathologic diagnosis and serum levels of these oncoproteins should be reexamined and, if needed, additional sections taken.

Staging and Morphologic Prognostic Factors in Testicular Tumors

It is important to note that proper sampling is required not only to classify the tumor but also to stage it pathologically and evaluate risk factors for clinical progression. In the case of GCTs, staging is quite complicated and takes into consideration pathologic factors, size and sites of metastases, and serum levels of oncofetal proteins (AFP and β-HCG) as well as lactic dehydrogenase [LDH]) (Tables 12-1A to 12-1C). In the case of GCTs, the percentage of the embryonal carcinoma (EC) component as well as the presence of lymphovascular invasion has been associated with the development of metastatic disease in clinical stage 1 tumors. Lymphovascular invasion is particularly important since it is included in the AJCC-UICC staging system (Table 12-1B). A tumor that is otherwise pathologic stage 1 but with lymphovascular invasion is classified as pathologic stage 2 (pT2). Since vascular invasion (VI) is commonly seen adjacent to the mass, sections must include the tumor–parenchymal interface; sections that only include tumor are of no utility other than to classify the tumor and are discouraged. As mentioned earlier, lymphatic drainage

Table 12-1A ■ TNM CLASSIFICATION OF GCTs OF THE TESTIS

pTNM Pathologic Classification of the Primary Tumor (pT)

pTX	Primary tumor cannot be assessed
pT0	No evidence of primary tumor (e.g., histologic scar in testis)
pTis	Intratubular germ cell neoplasia
pT1	Tumor limited to testis and epididymis without vascular/lymphatic invasion; tumor may invade the tunica albuginea but not the tunica vaginalis
pT2	Tumor limited to testis and epididymis with vascular/lymphatic invasion, or tumor extending through the tunica albuginea with involvement of the tunica vaginalis
pT3	Tumor invades spermatic cord with or without vascular/lymphatic invasion
pT4	Tumor invades scrotum with or without vascular/lymphatic invasion

pTNM Pathologic Classification of the Regional Lymph Nodes (pN)

pNX	Regional lymph nodes cannot be assessed
pN0	No regional lymph node metastasis
pN1	Metastasis with a lymph node mass 2 cm or less in greatest dimension; or multiple lymph nodes, none more than 2 cm in greatest dimension
pN2	Metastasis with a lymph node mass more than 2 cm but not more than 5 cm in greatest dimension; or multiple lymph nodes, any one mass >2 cm but not more than 5 cm in greatest dimension
pN3	Metastasis with a lymph node mass more than 5 cm in greatest dimension

From Edge SB, Byrd DR, Compton CC, et al., eds. *AJCC Cancer Staging Manual.* 7th ed. New York: Springer; 2010, with permission, Ref.[16]

Table 12-1B ■ CLINICAL STAGING OF GCTs OF THE TESTIS

Anatomic Stage/Prognostic Groups

Group	T	N	M	S*
Stage 0	pTis	N0	M0	S0
Stage I	pT1-4	N0	M0	SX
IA	pT1	N0	M0	S0
IB	pT2	N0	M0	S0
	pT3	N0	M0	S0
	pT4	N0	M0	S0
IS	Any pT/Tx	N0	M0	S1–3[†]
Stage II	Any pT/Tx	N1-3	M0	SX
IIA	Any pT/Tx	N1	M0	S0
	Any pT/Tx	N1	M0	S1
IIB	Any pT/Tx	N2	M0	S0
	Any pT/Tx	N2	M0	S1
IIC	Any pT/Tx	N3	M0	S0
	Any pT/Tx	N3	M0	S1
Stage III	Any pT/Tx	Any N	M1	SX
IIIA	Any pT/Tx	Any N	M1[‡]	S0
	Any pT/Tx	Any N	M1[‡]	S1
IIIB	Any pT/Tx	N1-3	M0	S2
	Any pT/Tx	Any N	M1[‡]	S2
IIIC	Any pT/Tx	N1-3	M0	S3
	Any pT/Tx	Any N	M1[‡]	S3
	Any pT/Tx	Any N	M1*	Any S

*Serum tumor markers.
[†]Measured after orchiectomy.
[‡]N indicates upper limit of normal for the LDH assay.
From Edge SB, Byrd DR, Compton CC, et al., eds. *AJCC Cancer Staging Manual.* 7th ed. New York: Springer; 2010, with permission, Ref.[16]

of the gonad flows toward the rete testis/mediastinum testis as well as toward the tunica albuginea (Figs. 12-3A and B). For this reason, sections that include tumor and overlying tunica as well as tumor with adjacent rete testis/mediastinum testis are particularly informative. Sections of the testicular adnexa (efferent tubules and epididymis) should be taken although involvement of these structures by tumor does not affect pathologic stage and does not seem to affect prognosis. This also applies to tumor involvement of soft tissue in the mediastinum, in the absence of lymphovascular invasion. A recent publication suggests that both rete testis involvement and hilar fat involvement are independently associated with advanced disease at presentation, but the study does not address the issue of association with relapse in clinical stage 1 disease[17] (Fig. 12-4). We suggest that at

Table 12-1C ■ SERUM TUMOR MARKERS IN TESTICULAR GCTs*

SX	Marker studies not available or not performed
S0	Marker study levels within normal limits
S1	LDH <1.5 × N[†] *and* hCG (mIU/mL) <5,000 *and* AFP (ng/mL) <1,000
S2	LDH 1.5–10 × N *or* hCG (mIU/mL) 5,000–50,000 *or* AFP (ng/mL) 1,000–10,000
S3	LDH >10 × N *or* hCG (mIU/mL) >50,000 *or* AFP (ng/mL) >10,000

*Measured after orchiectomy.
[†]N indicates the upper limit of normal for the LDH assay.
From Edge SB, Byrd DR, Compton CC, et al., eds. *AJCC Cancer Staging Manual.* 7th ed. New York: Springer; 2010, with permission, Ref. [16]

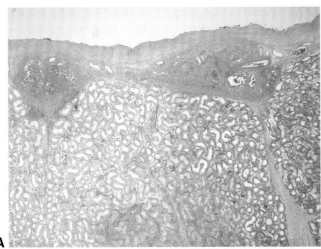
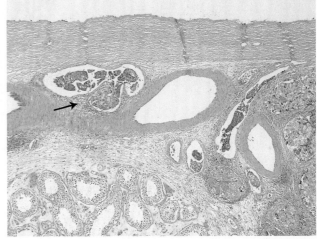

A **B**

FIGURE 12-3 ■ **A:** Extensive lymphovascular invasion by EC. Notice that the tumor involves lymphatics beneath the tunica albuginea, away from the main tumor mass. For this reason, sections should always include the interface between the tumor and the tunica albuginea. **B:** Lymphovascular invasion. The invasive tumor cells conform to the contours of the lymphatic channel and are focally attached to the vascular wall. Focal stromal response to the tumor emboli is present (*arrow*).

least three sections of the spermatic cord be taken: proximal (margin of resection), mid, and distal (near the adnexa). Involvement of the soft tissue of the spermatic cord is considered pathologic stage 3 and clinical stage 2 disease and is commonly associated with the presence of metastatic disease at the time of orchiectomy. Of note, intravascular or intralymphatic involvement within any part of the spermatic cord is still considered pT2 (Fig. 12-5).

Criteria for establishing VI are similar to those used in other organ systems but may present a greater challenge at this site due to the fact that the tumor cells are very discohesive and commonly contaminate the adjacent parenchyma and vascular structures at the time of sectioning. It is imperative to restrict the diagnosis of VI to vessels, usually

lymphatics, at the periphery of (not within) the tumor; in which the tumor cells conform to the shape of the vessel and preferably are attached to the wall with associated red blood cells or fibrin. While the use of immunohistochemistry is rarely necessary and not encouraged, we have recently found that ERG, a nuclear protein expressed in endothelial cells, may be of some utility when lymphovascular invasion is suspected but the presumed vascular space is entirely filled with tumor, as commonly happens with EC. In pure seminoma we should also mention if VI is present as it affects pathologic stage. However, its importance in establishing a higher risk of disease progression has not been proven. While most investigators suggest that tumor size (>4 cm) and rete testis involvement by seminoma predicts disease progression

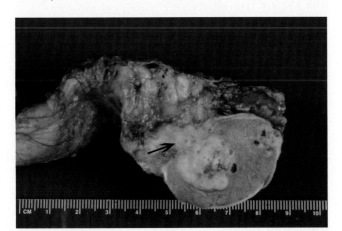

FIGURE 12-4 ■ Gross appearance of mixed GCT. The large lesion can be seen invading into the testicular hilum (mediastinum) and hilar soft tissue. The rete testis and hilum is the most common site where tumors extend outside the testicular parenchyma. It has also been associated with metastatic disease at presentation. The smaller lesion involves the overlying tunica albuginea.

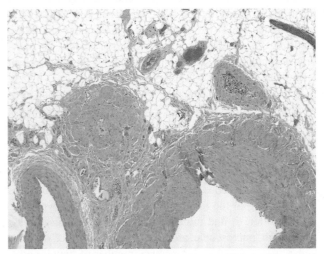

FIGURE 12-5 ■ VI in a blood vessel within the spermatic cord. This finding is commonly seen in patients with advanced disease at presentation. However, in the absence of stromal invasion at this site, it is still regarded as pT2 disease.

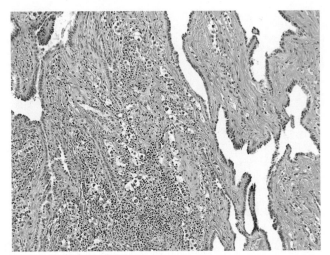

FIGURE 12-6 ■ Seminoma invading the rete testis. While this finding has been associated with tumor relapse on multivariate analysis, this finding has been recently challenged. However, rete testis involvement should be reported.

on multivariate analysis, at least one recent large study that included 687 stage 1 tumors puts this belief into question[18] (Fig. 12-6).

Sampling of primary (chemotherapy naïve) retroperitoneal resections requires a thorough gross examination of the sample and submission of all suspected lymph nodes for microscopic examination. When this surgical procedure is performed, it is in a setting of nonseminomatous primary tumor with a high risk for relapse or when imaging of the retroperitoneum is questionable. In other words, the presence of metastatic disease is likely to be minimal and microscopic. The average number of lymph nodes found at our institution in this setting is more than 50.[19] In fact, cases in which <40 lymph nodes are identified are submitted to regrossing of the residual tissue, with many additional lymph nodes identified. When reporting metastatic disease, the histologic type, number, and size of involved lymph nodes should be reported. Extranodal extension by tumor should be mentioned although the clinical significance of this finding has recently come into question.[20]

Great care should also be placed in sampling postchemotherapy resections. These resections should be carefully described grossly and sampled thoroughly, particularly those that are not obviously necrotic. A minimum of one section for each centimeter of lesional tissue should be submitted, making sure that all variegated areas are sampled. The sampling of an apparent mass does not mean that a thorough examination and sampling of the remaining soft tissue can be bypassed. It is common to find multiple lymph nodes in these areas, some with microscopic areas of treatment effect or even viable tumor. Once again, the size, number of lymph nodes involved, and the histology of the residual viable disease and the presence of extranodal extension should be reported.

In the case of sex cord–stromal tumors, similar care should be taken in the gross examination and prosecting

of the specimen. Sampling of the mass is similar to germ cells tumors, with special attention paid to variegated areas, tumor–parenchymal interface, rete testis, adnexa, and cord. While no single morphologic factor can predict disease progression, a combination of factors has been associated with the development of metastatic disease and should be included in the pathology report. The report should include size, presence or absence of infiltrative borders, coagulative necrosis, nuclear atypia, mitotic activity, and lymphovascular invasion; more details are provided in the subsequent sections of this chapter. Because there is no effective chemotherapy for these tumors, it is customary for patients with clinical stage 1 disease with multiple high-risk factors to undergo retroperitoneal lymph node dissection (RPLND) since surgery is their best chance for cure.

Clinical Management of Testicular Tumors

While all agree that radical orchiectomy is the treatment of choice for primary testicular GCTs, there is disagreement on how best to manage cases with a high risk of progression.[21-24] Many investigators advocate clinical surveillance since salvage chemotherapy at recurrence is associated with a high cure rate. Some advocate for a primary RPLND in this setting because the presence of minimal metastatic disease will allow the oncologist to give fewer cycles of chemotherapy. All agree that patients with bulky retroperitoneal disease or metastasis above the diaphragm should receive a full course of systemic chemotherapy although the exact regimen to follow will depend on the sites, the number of metastases, the levels of AFP, β-HCG, and LDH in serum.[25] Postchemotherapy retroperitoneal node dissection is controversial but advocated by some investigators as a means to diminish the incidence of late recurrences.

CLASSIFICATION

The 2004 World Health Organization classification of testicular tumors is presented in Table 12-2. This classification varies very little from the one described in the third edition of the Armed Forces Institute of Pathology Fascicle.[26] It builds upon previous classifications proposed by pioneers in this field, including Friedman and Moore,[27,28] Dixon and Moore,[29] Melicow,[30] and Mostofi and Price.[31] Practically speaking, these efforts at classifying testicular tumors are morphology based and reproducible. However, the present classification scheme described in Table 12-1A correlates with serum tumor marker abnormalities and has superior clinical application.

Germ Cell Tumors

Epidemiology and Pathogenesis

Testicular GCTs constitute approximately 98% of all testicular neoplasms and are the most common malignancy in males between the ages of 15 and 35 years.[32] They are relatively uncommon; approximately 7,920 new cases will have

Table 12-2 ■ WHO HISTOLOGIC CLASSIFICATION OF TESTIS TUMORS*

GCTs

Intratubular germ cell neoplasia, unclassified

Other types

Tumors of One Histologic Type (Pure Forms)

Seminoma

  Seminoma with syncytiotrophoblastic cells

Spermatocytic Seminoma (SS)

  SS with sarcoma

EC

YST

Trophoblastic tumors

  Choriocarcinoma

  Trophoblastic neoplasms other than choriocarcinoma

    Monophasic choriocarcinoma

    Placental site trophoblastic tumor

Teratoma

  Dermoid cyst

  Monodermal teratoma

  Teratoma with somatic-type malignancies

Tumors of More Than One Histologic Type (Mixed Forms)

Mixed EC and teratoma

Mixed teratoma and seminoma

Choriocarcinoma and teratoma/EC

Others

Sex Cord/Gonadal Stromal Tumors

Pure forms

LCT

SCT

  SCT lipid-rich variant

  Sclerosing SCT

  LCCSCT

Granulosa cell tumor

  Adult-type granulosa cell tumor

  Juvenile-type granulosa cell tumor

Tumors of the thecoma/fibroma group

  Fibroma

  Thecoma

Sex cord/gonadal stromal tumor, incompletely differentiated

Sex cord/gonadal stromal tumors, mixed forms

Tumors containing both germ cell and sex cord/gonadal stromal elements

  Gonadoblastoma

  Germ cell/sex cord/gonadal stromal tumor, unclassified

Miscellaneous Tumors

Carcinoid tumor

Nephroblastoma

Paraganglioma

Hematopoietic Tumors

Secondary Tumors of the Testis

*Modified from the World Health Organization Classification of Tumours, Pathology & Genetics: Tumours of the Urinary System and Male Genital Organs. In: Eble JN, Sauter G, Epstein JI, et al., eds. WHO Histological Classification of Testis Tumours. Lyon, France: IARC Press; 2004:218.

been diagnosed in the United States in 2013 with only 370 dying of disease[33] (Table 12-3). Because of their relative rarity, they present a diagnostic challenge to most practicing pathologist (Box 12-1).

Testicular GCTs can be divided into three groups (infantile/prepubertal, adolescent/young adult, and spermatocytic seminoma [SS]), each with its own constellation of clinical histology, molecular, and clinical features.[34,35] (Table 12-4) They originate from germ cells at different stages of development. Tumors arising in prepubertal gonads are either teratomas or yolk sac tumors (YSTs), tend to be diploid, and are not associated with i(12p) or intratubular germ cell neoplasia unclassified (IGCNU). The annual incidence is approximately 0.12 per 100,000. SS arises in older patients. These benign tumors may be either diploid or aneuploid and have losses of chromosome 9 rather than i(12p). Intratubular SS is commonly encountered but IGCNU is not. Their annual incidence is approximately 0.2 per 100,000. The pathogenesis of prepubertal GCT and SS is poorly understood.

The most common testicular cancers arise in postpubertal men; they are characterized genetically by the presence of excess genetic material of the short arm chromosome 12, usually due to one or more copies of i(12p), or other forms of 12p amplification and aneuploidy[36] (Fig. 12-7). The consistent gain of genetic material from chromosome 12 seen in these tumors suggests that it has a crucial role in their development. IGCNU is the precursor to these invasive tumors.

While IGCNU is considered to be the precursor of all GCTs, the stage in GC development at which transformation occurs is not known. One model proposed by Skakkebaek et al.[37] suggests that fetal gonocytes (primordial germ cells) undergo abnormal cell division (polyploidization) in utero, primarily due to environmental factors. These cells undergo abnormal cell division mediated by a kit receptor/kit ligand (stem cell factor) paracrine loop, leading to uncontrolled proliferation of gonocytes. Subsequent invasive growth may be mediated by postnatal and pubertal gonadotrophin stimulation. In this model 1(12p) is seen only after there is stromal invasion. A second model proposed by Chaganti et al. suggests that aberrant chromatid exchange events during meiotic crossing-over may lead to increased 12p copy number and overexpression of cyclin D2 (*CCND2*). In a cell containing unrepaired DNA breaks (recombination-associated), overexpressed cyclin D2 may block a p53-dependent apoptotic response and lead to reinitiation of cell cycle and genomic instability. This aberrant, genomically unstable cell is now able to escape the apoptotic effects of p53 and may reenter the cell cycle, now as a neoplastic cell. In this model, i(12p) is present in IGCNU.[38]

The incidence of adult-onset GCTs is approximately 6.0 per 100,000 per year with the majority being discovered between 15 and 40 years of age. The incidence of GCTs has increased over the last five decades while the death rate has decreased.[39,40] The increase in incidence is seen across all histologies but mostly in seminomas. While more effective therapy is responsible for the dramatic increase in the cure rate, it is less evident why the incidence continues to climb.

Table 12-3 ■ IMMUNOHISTOCHEMICAL PROFILE OF TESTICULAR TUMORS

Marker	IGCNU	Seminoma	Spermatocytic Seminoma	Embryonal Carcinoma	YST	Trophoblastic Tumors	Sex Cord/ Gonadal Stromal Tumors
PLAP	+ Diffuse cytoplasmic/ membranous	+ Diffuse cytoplasmic/ membranous	−	+ Diffuse cytoplasmic/ membranous	+/− Focal cytoplasmic/ membranous	−	−
CD117 (c-kit)	+ Diffuse membranous	+ Diffuse membranous	−/+ Focal weak	−	−	−	−
Oct3/4	+ Diffuse nuclear	+ Diffuse nuclear	−	+ Diffuse Nuclear	−	−	−
AFP	−	−	−	−	+ Variable cytoplasmic	−	−
SALL4	+ Diffuse nuclear	+ Diffuse nuclear	+/− Weak	+ Diffuse nuclear	+ Diffuse nuclear	+ Mononucleated trophoblastic cells	−
Glypican 3	−	−	−	−	+	+/−	−
Cytokeratin	−	− Focal dot-like	−	+ Membranous/ cytoplasmic, may be focal and weak	+	+	+/− SCTs
HCG	−	−	−	−	−	+ syncytiotro-phoblasts	−
Inhibin	−	−	−	−	−	−	+
Calretinin	−	−	−	−	−	−	+
SF-1	−	−	−	−	−	−	+
WT1	−	−	−	−	−	−	+

There appears to be a geographic and racial predisposition to the development of testicular GCTs with a twofold increase in Scandinavian countries as compared to the United States and a lower incidence in other countries such as Africa and some Latin American countries such as Puerto Rico.[39] Patients with prior testicular GCT are more likely to develop a contralateral tumor than does the general population.

The overwhelming majority of GCTs are sporadic with approximately 2% having a familial basis in which first-degree male relatives of patients with testicular GCTs will develop the disease.[41–44] Several other factors have been associated with their pathogenesis, including cryptorchidism, gonadal dysgenesis, and infertility. Testicular microlithiasis has been associated with the presence of GCT, but it may be seen in other conditions as well.

Cryptorchidism is one of the best-established risk factors,[43] with approximately 3.5 to 5 times elevated risk of development of a testicular GCT compared with control populations.[45–47] Testicular biopsies are commonly performed

Box 12-1 ● TESTICULAR GERM CELL TUMORS IN ADULTS

- Most common malignancy in males between the ages of 15 and 35
- Excess genetic material of chromosome 12p
- Mixed histologies are more common than pure forms
- Dissemination is commonly through lymphatics, initially to retroperitoneal lymph nodes

Table 12-4 ■ TESTICULAR GERM CELL TUMORS

Histology	Age	Ploidy	Chromosomes
Teratoma/ YST	Infantile	Diploid aneuploid	−1p, −6q
Seminoma/ NS	Postpubertal	CIS: hypertriploid	1(12p) or +12p
		SEM: hypertriploid	1(12p)
		NS: hypotriploid	1(12p)
SS	Older	Diploid or tetraploid	+9

Modified from Oosterhuis JW, Looijenga LH. Current views on the pathogenesis of testicular germ cell tumours and perspectives for future research: highlights of the 5th copenhagen workshop on carcinoma in situ and cancer of the testis. *APMIS* 2003;111:280–289.

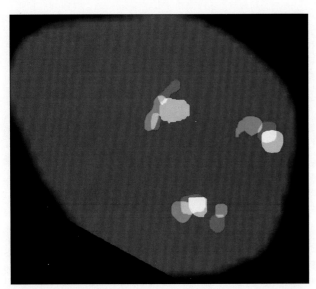

FIGURE 12-7 ■ Three color FISH probe demonstrating two copies of i(12p). The aqua is a cep12 probe while the red and green are ETV6(12p13). There is one normal chromosome (aqua adjacent to one red and one green signal) and two isochromosomes in which the cep12 signal is flanked by two red-green signals.

piece of evidence linking these tumors comes to us from genetics, since approximately 80% of tumors regardless of the primary site and histology will have at least one isochromosome of the short arm of chromosome 12, which is known as i(12p) (Fig. 12-3). This genetic abnormality is not absolutely pathognomonic of germ cell neoplasia, yet it is a very useful diagnostic tool in selected circumstances due to its rare occurrence in other solid tumors.[54–56]

Intratubular Germ Cell Neoplasia

This term refers to the lesion initially described by Skakkebaek as "carcinoma in situ" as well as to other "differentiated" forms of intratubular germ cell neoplasia.[57–60] Strictly speaking, the lesion originally described by Skakkebaek is now called "intratubular germ cell neoplasia, unclassified" by most, at least in the Western hemisphere; with increasing frequency in other parts of the world as well. It is the precursor lesion of all invasive GCTs with the exceptions of SS, prepubertal YST, and teratoma. It is found in virtually all cases in which residual seminiferous tubules are identified around an invasive GCT. It also is present in 5% to 8% of cases of cryptorchidism,[61] 5% of patients with an invasive GCT in the contralateral testis,[61] and frequently in dysgenetic gonads.

The story of testicular "carcinoma in situ" (intratubular germ cell neoplasia) is fascinating and serves as a paradigm for the concept of progression from incipient or preinvasive neoplasia to invasive disease.[59,62,63] In 1972, Skakkebaek reported "atypical spermatogonia" in two men undergoing testicular biopsies during a workup for infertility who subsequently developed invasive testicular GCTs. He hypothesized that these cells constituted "carcinoma in situ." Two subsequent seminal studies by his group proved that this was indeed the case. In 1978, he reported a series of 555 men who underwent testicular biopsies for infertility.[62,63] They identified six patients with evidence of "carcinoma in situ." With a median follow-up period of approximately 3 years, three of these patients developed evidence of an invasive GCT; one of them with bilateral disease. The remaining 449 patients were tumor free during the same follow-up period (Box 12-2).

In 1986, the Skakkebaek group reported their experience with contralateral biopsies in 500 patients with unilateral GCT.[64] Twenty-seven patients (5.4%) were found to have "CIS." Eight patients received systemic chemotherapy for advanced disease. Of the remaining 19 patients, 7 (37%)

in these high-risk patients to detect incipient neoplasia. In a large series, only one of more than 1,500 cryptorchid patients with testicular biopsy specimens negative for IGCNU developed testicular cancer over a follow-up period of 8 years,[48] in contrast to 50% of patients with IGCNU who developed invasive tumors over a 5-year period.[49]

There is an approximately 30% risk of GCTs observed in men with gonadal dysgenesis who carry a Y chromosome.[48] Gonadoblastoma is the most frequent tumor type arising in this setting, and its presence predisposes to the development of invasive GCTs, most commonly seminoma. Of patients with androgen insensitivity syndrome, 5% to 10% develop GCTs. These tumors generally are diagnosed after the complete development of female secondary sexual characteristics.[50,51]

The frequency of IGCNU in subfertile men has been reported to be 0.4% to 1.1%.[52,53] However, the relative risk of infertile men developing GCTs is not clear. Since many cases are associated with cryptorchidism or gonadal dysgenesis, it is difficult to judge whether infertility itself is an independent risk factor.

It is remarkable that GCTs, having such diverse morphology and clinical behavior, should be considered as variants of one entity. Nevertheless, there is circumstantial and laboratory evidence to support this practice. First, these tumors, in the postpubertal setting, tend to arise along the axial skeleton, be it the pineal gland, anterior mediastinum, retroperitoneum, or gonads. Second, mixed histologic patterns predominate over tumors with one histologic type. A third compelling piece of evidence relates to the so-called precursor lesion. When these tumors arise in the male gonad, irrespective of the morphology, one is likely to identify IGCNU in adjacent seminiferous tubules, originally described as in situ carcinoma by Neils Skakkebaek. A fourth important

Box 12-2 ● INTRATUBULAR GERM CELL NEOPLASIA

- Seen in adult-onset GCTs but not prepubertal tumors
- Associated with irregular hyalinization of tumor-bearing seminiferous tubules
- May be seen in association with microlithiasis
- Characterized cytoplasmic clearing, irregular nuclear contours, coarse chromatin, and prominent nucleoli
- Tumor cytology and immunophenotype are identical in seminoma and IGCNU

developed invasive GCT at this site within the follow-up period. Mathematical modeling suggested that 50% of biopsy-positive cases would develop disease within 5 years. Remarkably, not a single case of contralateral GCT developed in the remaining 463 biopsy-negative patients during the same follow-up period. In a subsequent report the authors revealed that at least two of the biopsy-positive cases that received systemic therapy subsequently developed contralateral tumors, suggesting that systemic therapy is not always effective against preinvasive disease.[65]

It is clear that the original lesion described by Skakkebaek is the precursor to all types of GCTs, at least for those that originate in postpubertal gonads other than SS. In early 1980, a group of distinguished pathologists including Drs. Robert Scully, Juan Rosai, F.K. Mostofi, and Robert Kurman met in Minnesota to discuss the nomenclature of incipient germ cell neoplasia. They agreed that "carcinoma in situ" was a poor choice to describe this lesion since it had no features of epithelial differentiation. They suggested the term "intratubular germ cell neoplasia, unclassified" (IGCNU) because it was associated with all morphologic types of GCT with the exception of SS. It also underscores the fact that differentiated forms of intratubular germ cell neoplasia may occur, including intratubular EC.

IGCNU can be seen adjacent to invasive GCTs in virtually all cases in which residual testicular parenchyma is present.[57,66] As previously mentioned, it is present in up to 4% of cryptorchid patients, up to 5% of contralateral gonads in patients with unilateral GCT, and up to 1% of patients biopsied for oligospermic infertility. Its association with testicular GCTs arising in prepubertal patients is still a source of controversy.[34,67,68] While some authors suggest that it does not occur, others state that it does. In either case, we can state with reasonable certainty that, if IGCNU does occur in childhood tumors, it is certainly less apparent.

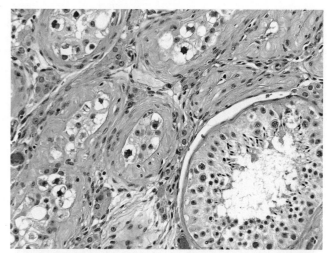

FIGURE 12-8 ■ Intratubular germ cell neoplasia. Notice the seminiferous tubules with irregular thickening of the basement membrane that contain cells with perinuclear clearing, irregular hyperchromatic nuclei with prominent nucleoli. An adjacent uninvolved tubule is present.

Microscopic Features

IGCNU is characterized morphologically by the presence of enlarged, atypical germ cells located adjacent to a usually irregularly thickened basement membrane (Figs. 12-8, 12-9A and B). The atypical cells are either isolated or form a single row along the basement membrane. They are typically larger than spermatogonia, the other cell that usually resides near the basement membrane. IGCNU cells have clear cytoplasm, irregular nuclear contours, coarse chromatin, and enlarged nucleoli, which may be single or multiple. Spermatogonia may also have clear cytoplasm but the cells are small, have round and regular nuclear contours, densely packed

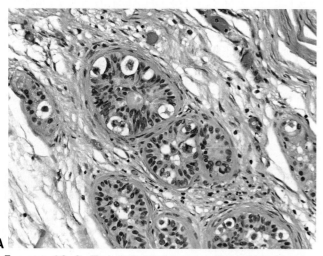
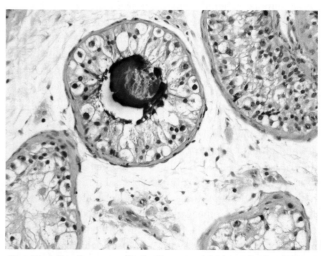

FIGURE 12-9 ■ **A:** Intratubular germ cell neoplasia. The surrounding Sertoli cells are small, fusiform, and lack nucleoli, similar to what is seen in prepubertal gonads. In adults the presence of seminiferous tubules with immature Sertoli cells is believed to be a sign of testicular dysgenesis. The combination of IGCNU and immature Sertoli cells is also a feature of gonadoblastoma. **B:** Testicular microlithiasis associated with IGCNU. While this finding can be associated with the presence of a germ cell neoplasm, it is in no way specific as it can be seen in many other conditions.

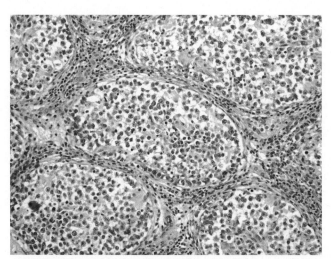

Figure 12-10 ■ Seminoma cells fill the lumen of a seminiferous tubule. This should not be called intratubular germ cell neoplasia.

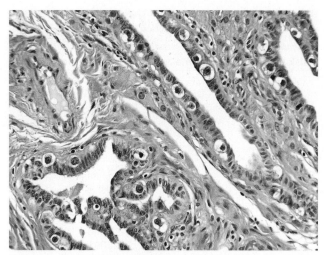

Figure 12-11 ■ Intratubular germ cell neoplasia extends into the rete testis in a pagetoid fashion.

chromatin, and absent nucleoli. In most cases, tumor-bearing tubules do not have active spermatogenesis and contain mostly Sertoli cells. Sertoli cells may be displaced toward the tubular lumen. Characteristically, they contain a single nucleolus that is small and regular. The nuclei are oval or round with regular borders and the chromatin is fine. The cytoplasm is amphophilic/eosinophilic and not vacuolated.

In essence, the cytologic features of classic IGCNU are those of seminoma. The relationship is supported by the coexpression of a host of histochemical and immunohistochemical markers among both cell types. Further evidence comes from electron microscopy, which has shown that both share common ultrastructural features: including the absence of well-developed cytoplasmic intermediate filaments, inconspicuous organelles, glycogen particles, lack of mature desmosomes and cell junctions, and nucleoli with ropy nucleolonema. Tubules whose lumens are filled with these cells may be regarded as "intratubular seminoma" (Fig. 12-10). The presence of i(12p) in IGCNU remains controversial with some investigators suggesting it is an early event and present in this stage of the disease while others suggest that it occurs only after the tumor cells invade into the parenchyma.[37] This debate is interesting in understanding the pathogenesis and progression of testicular GCTs but is of little or no clinical and diagnostic importance. Given the availability of excellent immunohistochemical markers, it is never necessary to resort to fluorescence in situ hybridization (FISH) or other molecular tests to document its presence. It is said that ICGNU is triploid or hypertetraploid. However, once again, this finding is of little diagnostic consequence.[38]

IGCNU may extend into the rete testis, usually undermining the epithelium in a "pagetoid" pattern (Fig. 12-11). At times, the epithelium of the rete may become hyperplastic, and in this setting, it is important not to confuse this finding with the presence of nonseminomatous GCT. At times, the rete testis epithelium adjacent to the tumor may contain

intracytoplasmic eosinophilic droplets that may be confused with YST (Fig. 12-12).[69]

Histochemistry and Immunohistochemistry

IGCNU cells contain glycogen and thus are PAS-positive, diastase-sensitive. Rarely will other intratubular cells, whether spermatogonia, spermatocytes, or Sertoli cells, show similar positivity. Placental-like alkaline phosphatase (PLAP) is one of the isoforms of alkaline phosphatase (Table 12-5). PLAP antibodies will stain IGCNU, the majority of seminomas and ECs, as well as a smaller percentage of YSTs. Immunoreactivity is seen in virtually all cases of IGCNU and the staining pattern is usually membranous or cytoplasmic. No other nonneoplastic intratubular cells are immunoreactive for PLAP, but immunoreactivity may be

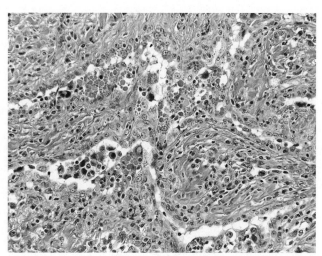

Figure 12-12 ■ Rete testis epithelium with reactive changes and intracytoplasmic eosinophilic globules, mimicking YST. This pitfall can be avoided by paying close attention to the location of the findings, since transition to more typical rete testis epithelium is usually seen.

Table 12-5 ■ GCTs RISK CLASSIFICATION: INTERNATIONAL CONSENSUS

Risk Group	Seminoma	Nonseminoma
Good	Any HCG Any LDH Nonpulmonary visceral metastases absent	AFP < 1,000 ng/mL HCG < 5,000 mIU/mL LDH < 1.5 × ULN
	Any primary site	Nonpulmonary visceral metastases absent Gonadal or retroperitoneal primary tumor
Intermediate	Nonpulmonary visceral metastases present	AFP 1,000–10,000 ng/mL
	Any HCG	HCG 5,000–50,000 mIU/mL
	Any LDH	LDH 1.5–10.0 × ULN
	Any primary site	Nonpulmonary visceral metastases absent Gonadal or retroperitoneal primary site
Poor	Does not exist	Mediastinal primary site Nonpulmonary visceral metastases present (e.g., bone, liver, brain) AFP 10,000 ng/mL HCG 50,000 mIU/mL LDH 10 × ULN

AFP, α-fetoprotein; HCG, human chorionic gonadotropin; LDH, lactate dehydrogenase; ULN, upper limit of normal.
Manivel JC, Jessurun J, Wick MR, et al. Placental alkaline phosphatase immunoreactivity in testicular germ-cell neoplasms. *Am J Surg Pathol* 1987;11:21–29.

seen in other types of non–germ cell malignancies.[70–73] C-kit (CD 117) is expressed in a large percentage of IGCNU as well as seminomas, but not in other GCTs.[74] Once again, the staining pattern is cytoplasmic/membranous (Fig. 12-13A). Despite the overexpression of this antigen, C-kit is rarely mutated in these tumors. Other antibodies that immunoreact with IGCNU but are rarely used in clinical practice include M2A and 43-F.[73,75,76] POU5F1 (Oct3/4) is a very interesting marker with great clinical utility.[77] The gene serves as a transcription factor and its product is expressed in pluripotent mouse and human embryonic stem cells and is downregulated during differentiation. Since the gene is also required for self-renewal of embryonic stem cells, knocking out the gene is lethal. This antigen is expressed solely in IGCNU, seminoma, and EC, suggesting that these are the types of GCT cells with pluripotency, that is, with the capacity to differentiate. As a transcription factor, staining is localized to the nucleus (Fig. 12-13B).

Another transcription factor expressed in IGCNU is SALL4; however, this nuclear marker is expressed in a wider spectrum of GCTs including seminoma, EC, yolk sac, tumor, and some glandular elements of teratoma.[78,79] As such, it is a useful marker in the characterization of GCTs but cannot be used in isolation. Podoplanin (clone D2-40) is an excellent cytoplasmic (membranous) marker with nuclear staining restricted to ICGNU and seminoma.[80,81]

Differential Diagnosis

When the tumor cells fill the seminiferous tubules, the term IGCNU is no longer used but rather intratubular seminoma, assuming that the cytomorphologic features of the tumor cells are identical to those described above. It is important to keep in mind that the presence of neoplastic cells within tubules does not always constitute IGCNU and that one

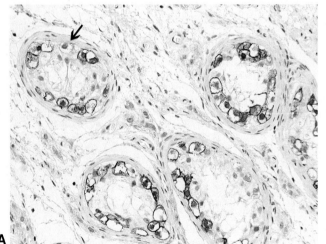 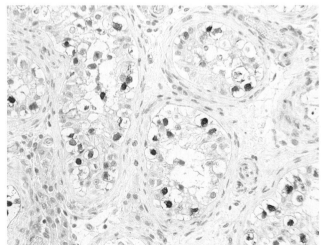

FIGURE 12-13 ■ **A:** Intratubular germ cell neoplasia. C-kit is positive in a membranous distribution. Notice that a few spermatogonia may be immunoreactive (*arrow*). **B:** Intratubular germ cell neoplasia. Oct3/4 is positive in a nuclear distribution.

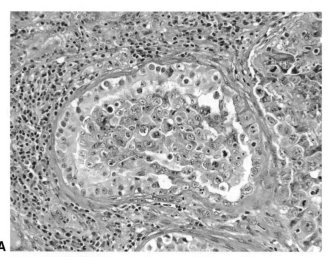 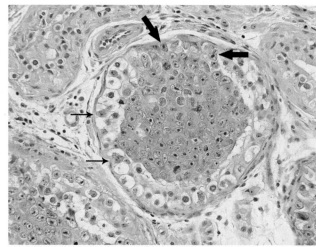

FIGURE 12-14 ■ **A:** Intratubular embryonal carcinoma. Tumor cells line a portion of the seminiferous tubule and fill the lumen. **B:** IGCNU and intratubular EC. IGCNU is characterized by atypical cells with irregular nuclear contours, prominent nucleoli, and cytoplasmic clearing (*thin arrows*) whereas the EC cells have larger, more irregular nuclei and nucleoli as well as amphophilic cytoplasm (*thick arrows*).

must adhere strictly to the established diagnostic criteria. On occasion spermatogonia may be enlarged and notably hyperchromatic, superficially mimicking ICGNU at low magnification. These changes are thought to be degenerative and are not associated with the development of tumor. These cells can be easily seen at intermediate to high magnification since they lack the characteristic coarse chromatin, nuclear contour irregularities, and prominent nucleoli seen in ICGNU. As you might expect, the immunoprofile of these cells is quite different, lacking expression of PLAP and OCT4. At times, spermatogonia can express C-kit and SALL4. Proper care must be taken to examine closely the cytologic features of the immunoreactive cells. While some investigators have reported PLAP immunoreactivity in rare spermatogonis, we have not encountered this problem. Besides intratubular seminoma, one can encounter intratubular EC (Fig. 12-14A and B), intratubular SS, and even metastatic disease such as melanoma and prostatic carcinoma. Intratubular lymphoma and even mesothelioma may also be confused with IGCNU.

ICGNU is commonly encountered adjacent to invasive germ cell tumors, more rarely during the workup of infertility, and in countries where patients with unilateral GCT undergo a diagnostic biopsy of the contralateral gonad. Biopsy of the contralateral side is rarely performed in this country but has been advocated in countries where the incidence of developing a contralateral tumor is high, such as in Scandinavia. In these settings, the cytologic features of ICGNU are identical to what we have described, but the diagnosis can be a bit more challenging because the number of neoplastic cells tends to be more limited. It is important to evaluate well-fixed, well-stained samples and to place close attention to the nuclear detains of the cells. In this setting prudent use of a limited panel of immunohistochemical markers, such as

Oct4 and podoplanin, may be very useful. PLAP and C-kit can also be used, with the caveats mentioned above.

Seminoma

Seminomas are the most common GCTs arising in the male gonad, whether they arise in a pure state or mixed with other morphologic types.[26,82–87] "Pure" seminoma account for 30% of testicular GCT and another 15% to 20% contain syncytiotrophoblasts without other germ cell components. Seminoma is extremely rare in children younger than 10 years of age, and uncommon in adolescents.[88] Approximately 1% to 2% are bilateral and bilaterality can occur synchronously or asynchronously. Seminomas reach a peak incidence between the fourth and fifth decades of life, which is approximately one decade later than nonseminomatous GCTs. Most patients present with self-identified testicular swelling, approximately 10% have acute groin pain, and fewer than 3% have symptoms secondary to metastatic disease, most commonly lumbar pain resulting from retroperitoneal involvement.[26,89] At the time of presentation, clinically about 75% of patients have disease limited to the testis, 20% have retroperitoneal involvement, and 5% have supradiaphragmatic or visceral metastases (Box 12-3).

A subset of seminomas, specifically those containing syncytiotrophoblastic cells, may have mildly elevated

---

Box 12-3 ● SEMINOMA

- Most common GCT presenting in its pure form
- Most common GCT in males above the age of 50
- Does not occur in prepubertal patients
- Only invasive GCT to consistently express D2-40 (podoplanin)

serum levels of β-HCG. Patients with metastases are more likely to have elevated levels of β-HCG; however, elevation of this marker does not appear to be an adverse prognostic marker but rather a marker of bulkier disease or advanced stage.[89] AFP levels generally are not elevated in pure seminoma, and any elevations require more thorough sampling of the tumor for a nonseminomatous component. LDH can be elevated in seminoma but this elevation is in no way specific to this disease but generally is a marker of the extent of disease; the larger the tumor burden, the high the serum levels.

Gross Features

Seminomas appear as a fleshy, well-circumscribed, bulging cream or light tan mass that, depending on size, may occupy a variable amount of testicular parenchyma or replace it entirely (Fig. 12-15). Tumor size can be quite variable with some measuring less than a centimeter while rare cases may reach a size of 10 cm or greater. Areas of necrosis may be observed grossly in up to 20% to 25% of cases, with this finding being more common in larger tumors. Some seminomas are associated with a granulomatous reaction, and in these cases the tumor takes on a fibrous and nodular gross appearance. Tumors with trophoblastic elements may be associated with punctate foci of hemorrhage. In general, one section per centimeter of tumor is sufficient sampling. However, tumors with a variegated appearance and those with nodularity must be sampled in a manner that all areas are sampled adequately. It is better to oversample in these cases since the management between pure seminomas and tumors with mixed histologies may be quite different. As previously mentioned, it is important to sample in a manner that allows the examination of the interface between the tumor–parenchyma, tumor–rete testis, tumor–mediastinum, and tumor–adnexa.[15] Sections of the spermatic cord should be taken as mentioned earlier in this chapter.

Microscopic Features

Seminoma usually grows in a sheet-like arrangement intersected by thin fibrous septa containing mature lymphocytes (Fig. 12-16). Occasionally, the fibrous septa are thicker, imparting a more nodular appearance to the tumor. Rarely seminomas may exhibit unusual patterns such as cribriform, pseudoglandular, and tubular growth[90] (Fig. 12-17A and B). These do not represent separate entities, but rather histologic variants of classic seminoma. Most tumors efface the underlying testicular parenchyma although an interstitial pattern of infiltration may be seen at the periphery in many cases. Rarely the pattern of growth is preferentially interstitial.[91] Interestingly, we have encountered a few cases of seminoma in which the component of the tumor with an interstitial pattern of growth took on micropapillary features due to retraction from the surrounding stroma (Fig. 12-18A and B). In two cases, the possibility of a metastatic carcinoma was entertained. The lymphocytes associated with the fibrous septa are mostly T cells, many with γ/δ phenotype.[92,93] Some tumors may contain lymphoid aggregates with germinal center formation. Up to 50% of tumors may exhibit a granulomatous reaction that may be so intense as to obscure the underlying neoplasm (Fig. 12-19). Some cases exhibit extensive fibrosis, particularly those associated with a granulomatous reaction or tumors that have undergone partial regression.

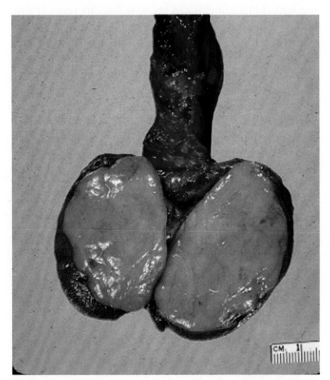

FIGURE 12-15 ■ Seminoma gross. A well-circumscribed fleshy tan mass occupies most of the testicular parenchyma.

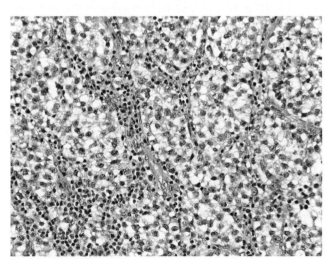

FIGURE 12-16 ■ Seminoma, classic type. Cells have squared-off nuclei, clear cytoplasm with little nuclear overlap. Mature lymphocytes are present in the septa.

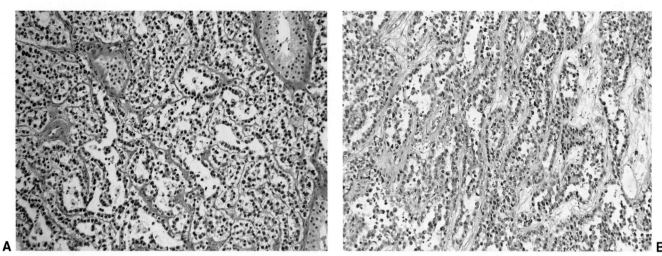

FIGURE 12-17 ■ **A:** Seminoma with a tubular pattern of growth. The cytologic features of the tumor cells are identical to those seen in classic seminoma. **B:** Seminoma with a tubular pattern of infiltration. At low power it is easy to understand why it might be confused with a SCT. It would be highly unusual for a seminoma to have this pattern of growth throughout the lesion.

Seminomas seen in association with a parenchymal scar should bring to mind the possibility of partial regression of the tumor, which may have been seminoma or possibly another GCT component other than teratoma. This phenomenon may be the explanation in some cases for nonseminomatous metastases in otherwise pure testicular seminomas. Whenever a parenchymal scar suggestive of partial regression is encountered, it is important to include it in the pathology report as a comment since this finding may account for the discrepancy between the pathology of the viable tumor and serum tumor markers.

Seminoma cells have a moderate amount of clear to pale eosinophilic cytoplasm with prominent cytoplasmic membranes and distinct cell borders (Fig. 12-16). The nuclei are large, round to rhomboid in shape and centrally located. The chromatin is evenly distributed and one or more prominent nucleoli are invariably present. In well-preserved specimens, one is unlikely to encounter nuclear overcrowding and overlap or syncytial growth. Mitotic activity is variable but may be quite brisk, a feature that has no bearing on prognosis. A significant proportion of seminomas contain syncytiotrophoblasts and their presence may be associated with focal areas of hemorrhage (Fig. 12-20). The absence of cytotrophoblast distinguishes these lesions from choriocarcinoma. Seminomas with syncytiotrophoblasts are generally accompanied by serum elevation of human chorionic gonadotropin (HCG), but levels will rarely reach levels above 500 IU/mL.[86]

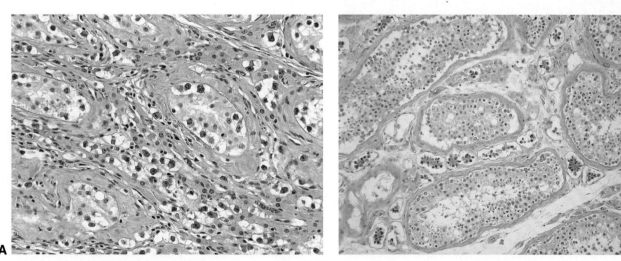

FIGURE 12-18 ■ Seminoma with an interstitial pattern of infiltration. IGCNU is present, and the walls of the seminiferous tubules are irregularly thickened. **A:** Seminoma with an interstitial pattern of infiltration. Tumor cells infiltrate among seminiferous tubules. **B:** Seminoma with an interstitial pattern of infiltration. Notice the retraction artifact, giving the tumor cell a "micropapillary" appearance.

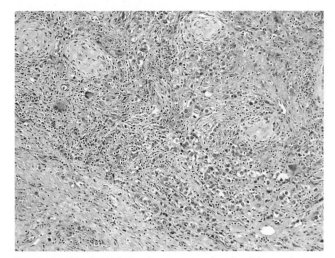

FIGURE 12-19 ■ Seminoma associated with an intense granulomatous reaction.

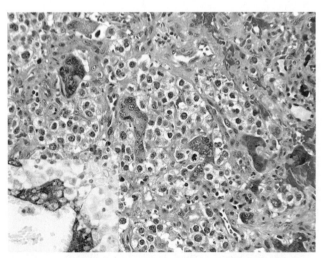

FIGURE 12-20 ■ Seminoma with syncytiotrophoblasts. Hematoxylin and eosin (H&E) stain reveals multinucleated syncytiotrophoblasts among classic seminoma cells, in the absence of cytotrophoblast. **Inset** demonstrates immunoreactivity for HCG in syncytiotrophoblastic cells.

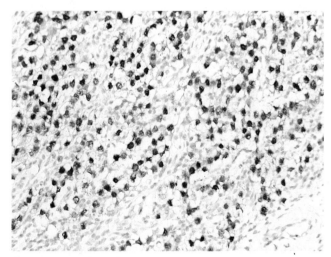

FIGURE 12-21 ■ Cytokeratin immunoreactivity in classic seminoma. Notice the dot-like cytoplasmic positivity in occasional cells.

Histochemistry and Immunohistochemistry

The expression profile of seminomas is detailed in Table 12-3. Briefly, tumor cells contain glycogen (PAS-positive) and express PLAP, C-kit (CD117), by immunohistochemistry[70,71,94–100] but not cytokeratins, CD30, or inhibin. In our practice, PAS and PLAP are rarely relied upon because of the availability of better discriminating markers. On occasion weak CD30 cytoplasmic immunoreactivity may be encountered in isolated seminoma cells, a finding that should not warrant a change in diagnosis. It is important to remember that CD30 may be expressed in some hematopoietic cells as well so attention to nuclear detail is warranted. A minority of seminoma cells may express focal and weak, dot-like or linear immunoreactivity for cytokeratin AE1/AE3 and CAM 5.2, however, never diffuse and strong staining throughout the cytoplasm (Fig. 12-21). Caution must be taken when interpreting cytokeratin markers since syncytiotrophoblasts are usually strongly immunoreactive, as are its mononuclear variants. If one relies on panels of markers this issue is resolved easily since syncytiotrophoblasts lack immunoreactivity to POU5F1 (OCT4), SALL4, podoplanin, and so on. Like IGCNU, seminoma cells express (OCT4) in a nuclear distribution[70,74,101,102] (Fig. 12-22). SALL4 is positive in a nuclear distribution while podoplanin (D2-40) is expressed in a cytoplasmic membranous distribution, once again similar to ICGNU.

Differential Diagnosis

Some seminomas exhibit a significant degree of cytologic atypia[103–111] and this fact led to the now abandoned concept

FIGURE 12-22 ■ OCT4 immunoreactivity in seminoma showing diffuse nuclear staining.

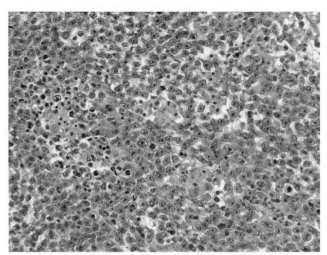

FIGURE 12-23 ■ Seminoma with atypia. While some tumors may lack a lymphocytic infiltrate and exhibit atypical cytologic features, one must consider other possibilities in the differential diagnosis.

of "anaplastic seminoma" as a discreet entity with a worse prognosis.[31,112] As described, this tumor was characterized by overall morphologic features of a seminoma but containing more pleomorphic cells with nonclear cytoplasm and abundant mitotic figures. Fibrovascular septa and lymphocytes were absent and focal necrosis was commonly seen. This concept did not withstand the test of time since many series later showed that stage for stage there was no difference in clinical outcome between classic and anaplastic seminomas.[26,103,113] In addition, it has become quite evident that mitotic activity in seminomas is quite variable and, in fact, may be quite high even in classical cases.[105] For the last decade or so, we have used the term "seminoma with atypia" not as a diagnostic entity but rather as a reminder to consider all possible explanations for the atypical morphologic findings (Fig. 12-23).

We need to emphasize that the "classic" growth and cytologic features of seminoma are not always present. This fact can bring problems in establishing the correct diagnosis. Poor fixation is a major culprit. In this setting the tumor cells are poorly preserved, the cytoplasm is condensed and eosinophilic, with the nuclei becoming irregular and hyperchromatic. In this setting, isolated necrotic nuclei may be present. In cases of poor tissue fixation, these changes are usually seen in a geographic distribution. The presence of a granulomatous and fibrous reaction mechanically distorts the diffuse growth pattern of the seminoma cells, which is now seen as aggregates or nests of cells with irregular cytoplasmic features. In extreme examples they can mimic neoplastic epithelial and even hematopoietic cells. If the seminoma is associated with an intense lymphocytic infiltrate, the tumor cells may be difficult to identify at low magnification, although the neoplastic component can be readily identified at high magnification, if necessary supplemented by immunohistochemistry. The problem associated with seminomas containing a tubular or interstitial growth

pattern has been mentioned and must be kept in mind. Attention to cytologic detail should lead us to the correct diagnosis since in these cases the classic nuclear cytology of seminoma is preserved. A myxoid stromal response is rarely encountered in seminoma, a feature more commonly associated with SS. Once again, nuclear cytology should solve the differential diagnosis, with immunohistochemistry limited to truly difficult cases.

Tumors thought to be seminoma but exhibiting atypical histology should trigger consideration of a differential diagnosis of seminoma, which includes (a) seminoma with "early carcinomatous differentiation," (b) solid variants of EC or YST, (c) lymphoma, (d) sex cord–gonadal stromal tumor (particularly SCT), (e) SS, (f) monophasic trophoblastic tumor (choriocarcinoma), and (g) metastatic disease, including poorly differentiated carcinoma and melanoma. Some examples are illustrated later in this chapter.

"Early carcinomatous differentiation" refers to areas of transition from seminoma to EC (Fig. 12-24). This concept suggests that seminoma cells are not terminally differentiated but rather, under certain poorly understood circumstances, may differentiate into other GCT types.[86,108,114] These tumors are characterized by either focal or diffuse nuclear atypia, nuclear overlapping, and on immunohistologic evaluation may show small clusters with intense membrane-predominant cytokeratin or CD30 (Ber-H2) positivity (Fig. 12-24). We would expect for OCT4 and SALL4 to be retained while C-kit and podoplanin expression would be lost in the EC component. The management of these tumors, whether as seminomas or as mixed GCTs, is controversial and is institution-dependent. Some investigators feel that these tumors should be approached clinically as mixed GCTs since the seminoma has already manifested its propensity to differentiate toward a more aggressive

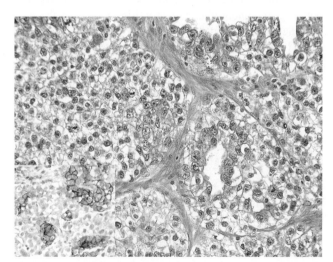

FIGURE 12-24 ■ Seminoma with early carcinomatous transformation. On the H&E stain you are able to notice subtle changes in cytology of the tumor cells with the EC cells having indistinct cells borders, nuclear overlap, and larger, more irregular nuclei. **Inset** demonstrates an AE1/AE3 cytokeratin stain in which strong cytoplasmic immunoreactivity is seen in the EC component.

phenotype. Others would not change management based on this finding alone since, in the absence of other adverse prognostic factors, the patient would likely be placed on surveillance either way. The fact of the matter is that decisions on how to treat these patients are at best empiric because of the rarity of the situation and the absence of clinical studies.

In contrast to a typical seminoma, EC has consistently a higher nuclear grade, irregular chromatin distribution, and syncytial arrangement of the cells (Fig. 12-18). The cytoplasm often is amphophilic to basophilic, the cell borders are poorly defined and glandular, or papillary areas may be present. The solid pattern in YSTs may also mimic seminoma. However, this pattern is usually accompanied by other diagnostic patterns of YST, making the distinction usually easy. YST cells generally have smaller nuclei without prominent nucleoli and may contain hyaline globules. Conversely, edema and microcysts in a seminoma may raise the possibility of a reticular or microcystic pattern of YST. The immunohistochemical profile of each of these tumors is distinct, as seen in Table 12-4. Lymphomas of the testis usually are bilateral tumors, occur in older men, have an interstitial growth pattern, and lack intratubular germ cell neoplasia. The nuclei are generally more convoluted and lack cytoplasmic clearing. Leukocyte common antigen and other lymphoid markers usually are positive, and PLAP is negative.

Rarely, seminomas with conspicuous tubular architecture may superficially resemble SCTs (Fig. 12-17B). The classic cytomorphology of seminoma cells is retained in tubular areas; however, invariably some areas of the tumor retain the typical sheet-like architecture. Conversely, because of a nested growth pattern, stromal fibrosis, and presence of lymphoid cells and intracytoplasmic glycogen, rare clear cell variants of sex cord–stromal tumors may be mistaken for a seminoma. The smaller, less pleomorphic nuclei, low mitotic count, and absence of IGCNU in the former, together with the immunoprofile, should aid in arriving at the correct diagnosis. SS may bear a superficial resemblance to typical seminoma, but on closer scrutiny the polymorphous cell population is invariably evident and IGCNU is absent. Rarely, metastatic tumors, including renal cell carcinomas, prostatic carcinomas, and malignant melanomas, may create differential diagnostic problems. Accurate clinical history, together with features such as angiolymphatic invasion and interstitial growth pattern, is important in arriving at the correct diagnosis, sometimes with the aid of immunohistochemistry. Finally, other causes of atypical histology in seminoma include poor fixation and faulty processing in the pathology laboratory.

Clinical Management of Seminoma

Primary testicular seminoma is managed by radical inguinal orchiectomy. Many clinicians no longer give adjuvant low-dose external beam radiation therapy to the retroperitoneum in clinical stage 1 disease but rather place them on surveillance; one important reason is the documented increased incidence of second malignancies.[115–118] Metastatic disease is treated with combination chemotherapy and postchemotherapy surgical resection is seldom, if ever, indicated. Cure rates for adequately treated seminoma are over 95% although chemotherapy-resistant tumors have been rarely described. As previously mentioned, the availability of adverse prognostic features in primary seminoma remains controversial.[18,21] Lymphovascular invasion places the tumor in the pT2 category but does not seem to be associated with disease progression. Involvement of the rete testis was thought to predict recurrence but a more recent study calls this issue into question. Involvement of the adnexa does not seem to influence progression while involvement of the soft tissue of the spermatic cord is classified as stage pT3 and is usually seen in patients with documented advanced disease.

SPERMATOCYTIC SEMINOMA

Etiology and Pathogenesis

SSs are rare, constituting <2% of testicular neoplasms.[86,119–121] In our institution, they account for significantly <1% of primary testicular tumors resected. They represent an entirely separate and distinct clinicopathologic entity from classic seminoma. The peak incidence is in the sixth decade of life[122] (median 54 years). Patients as old as 87 years and as young as 25 years of age have been affected. This tumor occurs only in the male gonad, is not associated with either cryptorchidism, other types of GCTs, i(12p), or nuclear expression of the stem cell marker OCT4. IGCNU is not present although tumor cells may fill seminiferous tubules (intratubular SS) and these neoplastic cells exhibit the identical level of cytologic heterogeneity seen in the invasive component. It was described as a distinct entity by Masson[123] in 1946 who considered it to mimic spermatogenesis, based on the polymorphous cell population and meiotic-like chromatin pattern in some cells. To date, no race or geographic predilection has been described although the rarity of the disease makes this type of analysis difficult.

Clinical Features

Men usually present with a unilateral painless testicular mass, although up to 9% are bilateral.[121] It is essentially a benign tumor with very few cases having metastasized[124]; possibly only one bona fide case with metastasis has been documented in the literature. When we make this diagnosis, our advice to the treating urologist is to treat is as a benign tumor with the possible exception of a postorchiectomy baseline CT scan of the abdomen. An exception to this rule is the rare case of "spermatocytic seminoma with sarcoma,"[125,126] which is commonly associated with metastatic disease at the time of initial diagnosis and poor prognosis. It is difficult to establish the rate of sarcomatous transformation since these cases are reported as small series, mostly based

- Peak incidence in the sixth decade of life
- Not associated with gains of chromosome 12p or i(12p)
- Not associated with serum elevation of oncofetal proteins
- Composed of three cell types; small (6 to 8 μm), medium (15 to 20 μm), and large (50 to 100 μm)
- Benign clinical course unless associated with sarcomatous transformation

on consultation cases, or isolated case reports. Suffice it to say that it is very rare. Outside of our consultation practice, we have collectively only seen a single primary case. One report introduced the concept of "anaplastic spermatocytic seminoma" as a variant of this disease.[127] SS is not associated with serum elevations of β-HCG, AFP, or any other oncofetal protein (Box 12-4).

Gross Features

SSs are well circumscribed and multilobulated or multinodular. Extension beyond the testis is rare. The cut surface typically is soft, with a fleshy, gelatinous, or mucoid consistency. Areas of hemorrhage and cystic change are common. Tumors tend to be large at presentation with a median size of 7.0 cm and a range of 2.0 to 20 cm.

Microscopic Features

The tumor cells are arranged in solid sheets or nests. Occasionally the tumor cells may be arranged in nests or pseudoglandular arrangements within an edematous or mucoid stroma (Fig. 12-25A and B). Cytologically, it is possible to identify three distinct cell types; small, medium and large although cells of medium size predominate (Fig. 12-26). The small cells have round, lymphocyte-like nuclei with dense chromatin and scant eosinophilic cytoplasm

and measure between 6 and 8 μm. The intermediate cells, measuring between 15 and 20 μm, have a small amount of eosinophilic or amphophilic cytoplasm. The nuclei are round and contain coarse chromatin, at times exhibiting a "spireme" (filamentous or string-like) pattern. The large cells, which can be multinucleated and measure between 50 and 100 μm, have round or oval nuclei and may exhibit spireme chromatic distribution. All three cell types may be present within seminiferous tubules (intratubular SS) but classic IGCNU is not seen (Fig. 12-27). Mitoses are frequent, including atypical forms (Fig. 12-25B). These tumors rarely contain a lymphocytic infiltrate and are not associated with a granulomatous reaction. When SS is associated with sarcoma, this component is usually undifferentiated or may exhibit rhabdomyosarcomatous differentiation.[125,126]

Tumor cells do not contain glycogen (negative PAS stain). Immunohistochemical stains for PLAP are negative, although occasional cells may be weakly immunoreactive. Cytokeratins are negative, although occasional cells may exhibit dot-like cytoplasmic staining. CD30, Oct3/4, and podoplanin are negative, while some investigators have reported variable immunoreactivity for CD117 (C-kit) and SALL4.[74,86,101,128,129]

EMBRYONAL CARCINOMA

Clinical Features

In its pure form, EC comprises up to 3% of GCT, although approximately 40% of all GCTs contain an EC component. Over 50% of tumors with either pure or predominant EC components will present with metastatic disease. Pure EC most commonly occurs in patients during the third or fourth decades of life, with an average age of 32 years,[130] and is extremely rare in prepubertal children.[131] Most patients present with a testicular mass that may be painful. Up to 10% of

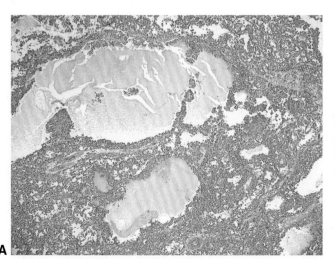

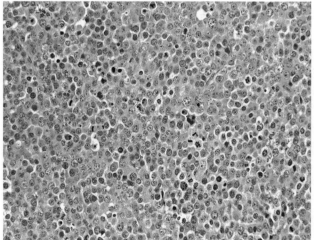

A   B

FIGURE 12-25 ■ **A:** Spermatocytic seminoma. Low-power magnification reveals densely packed tumor cells associated with pools of eosinophilic/basophilic fluid. **B:** Spermatocytic seminoma. The tumor cells are variable in size and mitotic activity is brisk.

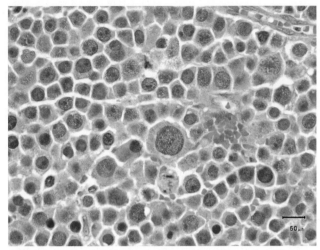

FIGURE 12-26 ■ Spermatocytic seminoma. High magnification clearly illustrates tumor cells of three sizes. The smaller lymphocyte-like cells measure 10 μm or less while the largest, with "spireme" chromatin, measure 50 μm or more.

patients present with symptoms related to metastatic disease. Metastases most commonly occur first to retroperitoneal lymph nodes, which in turn leads to back pain. Twenty percent of patients presenting with metastatic disease will also have supradiaphragmatic involvement.[132]

EC is not associated with elevation of serum β-HCG or AFP.[26,86] Earlier reports suggested an association with elevation of these markers were likely due to misclassification of the tumor, largely caused by not recognizing variants of YST. Similarly, EC cells should not express immunoreactivity for either of these markers, with earlier reports suggesting the contrary suffering from the same issues mentioned above. However, it is possible that focal AFP immunoreactivity in a tumor that otherwise fulfills the criteria for EC represents early transformation to YST. If this were the case, one would also expect absent or decreased expression

of CD30 and OCT4 while SALL4 expression is retained (Box 12-5).

Gross Features

ECs may vary in size, color, and texture, are commonly hemorrhagic, and exhibit areas of cystic degeneration and necrosis (Fig. 12-28). They may be poorly circumscribed and often extend into the mediastinum of the testis or adnexa. Color can vary from tan to dark brown, depending on the amount of hemorrhage and necrosis present. On average, pure ECs are smaller at diagnosis than other GCTs.

Microscopic Features

The pattern of growth is quite variable: gland-like, papillary, syncytial, and solid areas are commonly encountered[132] (Fig. 12-29A and B). A solid pattern with a sheet-like arrangement is present in almost all ECs but rarely predominates (Fig. 12-29C). It is usually associated with multiple microscopic foci of necrosis. In the solid areas, darkly staining, degenerate-looking cells with hyperchromatic, smudged nuclei often are present at the periphery of cell groups (so-called appliqué pattern) (Fig. 12-30). These cells may be confused with syncytiotrophoblastic cells, raising the possibility

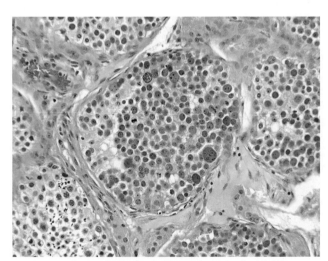

FIGURE 12-27 ■ Intratubular spermatocytic seminoma. The tumor cells tend to fill the lumen of the tubule and the same degree of variability in nuclear size is observed.

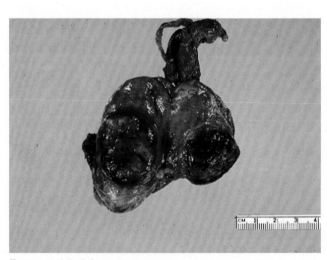

FIGURE 12-28 ■ Embryonal carcinoma gross. This tumor is extensively hemorrhagic but well circumscribed.

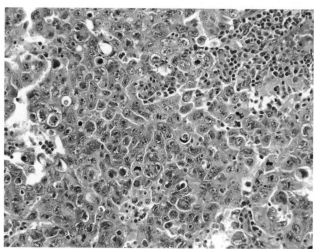

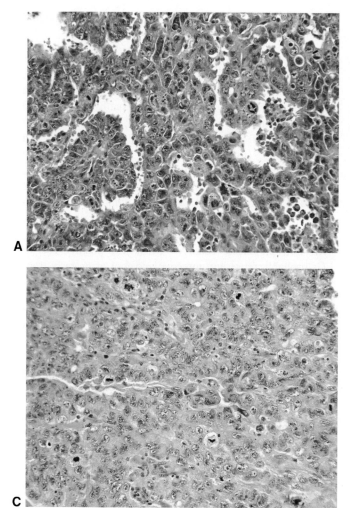

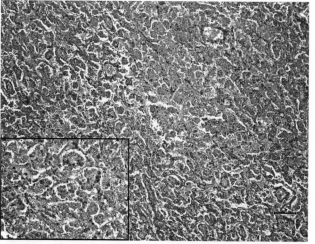

FIGURE 12-29 ■ **A:** Embryonal carcinoma. The tumor cells are arranged in a pseudoglandular/papillary pattern, likely due to cell drop-off. **B:** EC with a solid pattern of growth. The tumor cells have inconspicuous cell borders. The nuclei are irregular, hyperchromatic, and overlap with each other. Karyorrhectic debris is common. **C:** EC, solid variant. The tumor cells are very atypical with large irregular nuclei and pleomorphic nucleoli. The nuclear to cytoplasmic ratio is variable, and the cytoplasm is amphophilic. Notice the degree of karyorrhexis and mitotic activity, features that would not be seen in solid variants of YST.

of a choriocarcinoma. A tubular and tubulopapillary pattern is present in approximately 75% of tumors. In this pattern, tumor cells form true glandular or papillary structures, the latter organized around fibrovascular cores (Fig. 12-31). In many cases, a glandular or papillary appearance may be

present due to cell drop-off. Rarely a micropapillary pattern may be observed. Fibrous septations are rare, as are lymphocytic infiltrate and granulomatous reaction. Frequently, intratubular growth by EC is present at the periphery of the

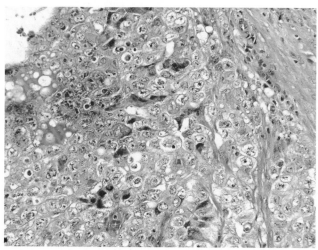

FIGURE 12-30 ■ Embryonal carcinoma. Notice the presence of degenerated cells with hyperchromatic, smudged nuclei intermingled with viable tumor cells (so-called appliqué pattern).

FIGURE 12-31 ■ EC with papillary growth. The papillary architecture suggests the possibility of YST, but close attention to the cytology of the tumor cells support a diagnosis of EC. **Inset** reveals very atypical pleomorphic nuclei, classic for EC.

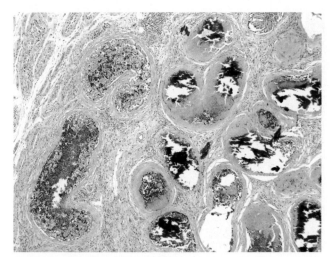

FIGURE 12-32 ■ Intratubular EC. Notice the distended tubules containing tumors cell, necrotic debris, and irregular calcifications. The surrounding stroma is inflamed and fibrotic.

tumor, and often the cells in these tubules show extensive necrosis and dystrophic calcification (Fig. 12-32). The presence of peritubular fibrosis helps distinguish intratubular growth from VI that frequently occurs in EC. An undifferentiated primitive-appearing spindle cell component may be seen in close association with the epithelial component of EC. Although a minor component of such stroma is accepted by some experts as EC,[132] many others, including us, believe this to indicate a teratomatous component, requiring careful evaluation for other teratomatous components.

The cells of EC are large, irregular, and epithelioid (Fig. 12-30). The cytoplasm is quite variable, ranging from abundant to minimal, although the nuclear to cytoplasmic ratio is invariably high. The cytoplasm is basophilic to amphophilic and rarely clear. Cell borders are characteristically indistinct. The nuclei are large and irregular with coarse chromatin and one or more irregular nucleoli. Common

findings include nuclear crowding and overlap, individual cell necrosis, and apoptotic bodies.[133]

Immunohistochemistry

The immunohistochemical features of EC are summarized in Table 12-4. Briefly, these tumors usually show intense and diffuse immunoreactivity for PLAP, cytokeratins (AE1/AE3 and CAM 5.2), CD30 (Ber-H2), OCT4, SOX-2, and SALL4[101,133,134] (Fig. 12-33A and B). Cytokeratin staining may be variable but is usually cytoplasmic; CD30 tends to be mostly membranous while OCT4, SOX2, and SALL4 are nuclear. Only about 2% of cases react with epithelial membrane antigen (EMA).[102] Staining for C-kit protein generally is negative, and β-HCG is demonstrable only in intermingled syncytiotrophoblastic cells.[74,129] Most AFP-positive foci in ECs probably represent unrecognized foci of or early transition to YST. Pertinent negatives include C-kit and podoplanin, remembering that C-kit can rarely stain isolated cells.

Differential Diagnosis

The solid variant of EC may be confused with "atypical" forms of seminoma, although the latter does not exhibit the same degree of cytologic anaplasia as EC. It is important to make this distinction because of the markedly different therapeutic implications and biologic behavior. The solid and papillary patterns of EC may be confused with similar patterns of YST. However, YST typically shows myriad patterns within the same tumor. The cells in EC have greater nuclear pleomorphism than in YSTs.[133] The presence of Schiller-Duval formations, hyaline globules, or basement membrane material favors YST. An immunopanel including CD30, OCT4, SALL-4 and AFP is further discriminatory.

Depending on the cell of origin, large cell lymphomas will be immunoreactive for B- or T-cell markers.[70,71,94–96,98–100] Large cell lymphoma (including Ki-1 lymphoma) sometimes

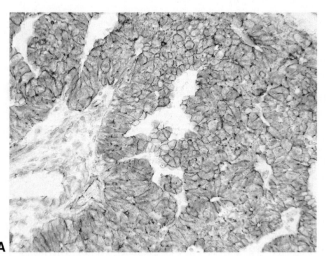
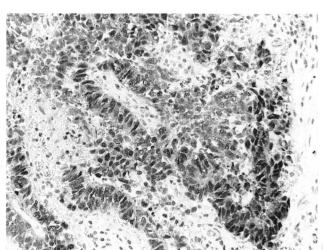

FIGURE 12-33 ■ **A:** Embryonal carcinoma. Diffuse cytoplasmic immunoreactivity for CD30 in a cytoplasmic membranous distribution. **B:** Embryonal carcinoma. Diffuse nuclear expression of OCT4 in a nuclear distribution.

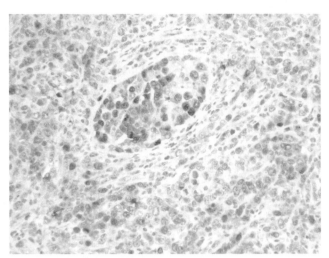

Figure 12-34 ■ Malignant lymphoma with nuclear immunoreactivity for OCT4. Admittedly, this finding is rare, but it is a good example of why it is better to use a panel of antibodies rather than a single marker to characterize a tumor. In this case, OCT4 led to an erroneous diagnosis of seminoma.

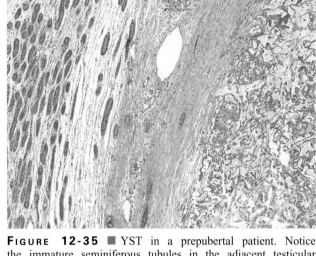

Figure 12-35 ■ YST in a prepubertal patient. Notice the immature seminiferous tubules in the adjacent testicular parenchyma.

may be confused with EC. However, patients with lymphoma generally are older and usually have bilateral and extragonadal disease. Lymphomas have an interstitial growth pattern, lack intratubular germ cell neoplasia (although lymphoma cells may be present within seminiferous tubules), and are negative for PLAP. Although Ki-1-positive lymphomas are positive for CD30, rare cases may show focal expression of cytokeratin, diffuse and strong coexpression of CD30, OCT4, and cytokeratins establishes the diagnosis of EC over a large cell anaplastic lymphoma. We have observed a single case of testicular large cell lymphoma with focal nuclear expression of OCT4, a finding that is not entirely surprising since OCT4 is a stem cell marker (Fig. 12-34). This fact may be a good reason to add SALL4 to the immunopanel when faced with this differential diagnosis.

One of the most difficult differential diagnoses is between EC in an extra testicular site and metastatic undifferentiated carcinoma. In such situations, judicious use of mucin stains (positive in some metastatic carcinomas), immunohistochemistry, particularly OCT4 and SALL4, and clinical correlation are helpful (see Table 12-4).

Clinical Management

In the introduction we discussed issues relating to prognostic factors and treatment. It is worth repeating that the extent of EC within a mixed GCT is associated with an increased risk of disease progression. This fact is amplified in the presence of pure EC. It is not surprising that lymphovascular invasion is the rule rather than the exception. In fact, in well-prosected cases of pure EC, lymphovascular invasion is almost always found microscopically. Management decisions are based on the stage at presentation but these patients are almost never offered surveillance, receiving either adjuvant chemotherapy or, more controversial, primary retroperitoneal node dissection followed by chemotherapy, if needed.[122,135-137]

YOLK SAC (ENDODERMAL SINUS) TUMOR

YSTs are characterized by multiple patterns of growth that recapitulate the yolk sac, allantois, and extra-embryonic mesenchyme. It has a bimodal age distribution: infants and young children and postpubertal males. In children, it commonly presents in its pure form, usually within the first 2 years of life (Fig. 12-35). They account for 75% of childhood testicular GCTs. In the postpubertal setting, it rarely presents in a pure form but is present in almost half of mixed GCTs.[26,138] The incidence of a YST component is higher in primary mediastinal GCT.

Patients at any age usually present with a painless testicular mass. Most childhood YSTs are stage I disease at presentation and radical orchiectomy is curative. Even in children with more advanced disease, the prognosis is better than in adults, suggesting a greater degree of chemosensitivity. There is some evidence that adults with a YST component in a mixed GCT have a higher frequency of stage I disease.[139-141] However, the presence of YST elements in metastatic testicular cancer has been associated with a poor prognosis, suggesting that YST has lower metastatic potential but less chemosensitivity than EC.[26,32] It is not uncommon for YST elements to be the sole or predominant component in patients with chemotherapy-refractory disease. It is important to keep in mind that residual yolk sac components after chemotherapy as well as those seen long after systemic therapy may exhibit unusual morphologies (Box 12-6).

Of patients with a YST component in their tumors, 95% to 100% have elevated serum AFP.[97,142] Serum levels below 15 ng/mL are considered normal, and its half-life is 5 to 7 days.

Box 12-6 ● YOLK SAC TUMOR

- Bimodal (prepubertal and adult) age distribution
- Multiple morphologic variants with microcystic being the most prevalent
- Unusual morphologies may be encountered post chemotherapy and in late recurrences
- Characterized by immunohistochemical coexpression of SALL4 and glypican 3 but not OCT4

Modest physiologic elevations above this value may occur in normal young children,[26] and it is important not to overinterpret such elevations. Additionally, low levels of serum AFP elevation may be encountered in patients with postchemotherapy residual teratoma, an issue that must be considered before concluding that the patient has residual chemotherapy-resistant YST.[122,143]

Gross Features

Most pediatric YSTs are nonencapsulated gray-tan to yellow homogeneous tumors usually with a myxoid and variably cystic quality. The gross appearance in adults is quite variable because YST components are usually closely admixed with other elements. A YST component is present in over 30% of mixed GCT. Pure YST in adults is rare, comprising <2% of tumors. If pure, they commonly appear gray-white with a myxoid or even mucoid appearance with areas of hemorrhage.

Microscopic Features

These tumors can have variable morphologic appearance due to the multiple subtypes, which are usually intermixed.[26,144–146]

- Reticular or microcystic: It is the most commonly encountered pattern, characterized by cells with prominent cytoplasmic vacuoles forming a meshwork of spaces as well as an irregular arrangement of interanastomosing cords of tumor cells and microcysts (Fig. 12-36).

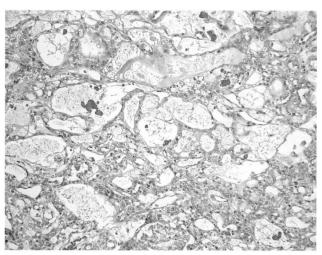

FIGURE 12-37 ■ YST, micro- and macrocystic.

These cysts vary in size and may contain an amorphous eosinophilic or basophilic fluid. Occasionally the epithelial cords attenuate and disperse into surrounding stroma as single spindle cells. The stroma frequently is myxoid.

- Macrocystic: This pattern is seen as a result of coalesced microcysts (Fig. 12-37).

- Endodermal sinus: This pattern is the most distinctive and widely recognized pattern. It is characterized by a papillary core of fibrous tissue containing a central blood vessel that is covered by a layer of cuboidal to columnar tumor cells (Fig. 12-38). The papillary structure is surrounded by a cystic space, which in turn is lined by flattened tumor cells. The entire structure is known as a Schiller-Duval body. When cut tangentially this structure may take on the appearance of elongated fibrous tissue cores draped (festooned) by malignant epithelium. While Schiller-Duval bodies are recognized by most pathologists, they are seen in only a minority of tumors.

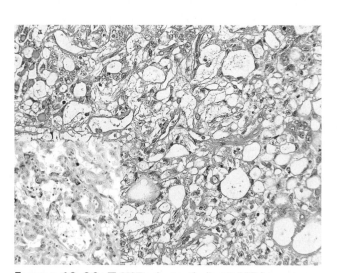

FIGURE 12-36 ■ YST, microcystic. **Inset:** AFP immunoreactivity in the tumor. We do not find this stain to be very dependable.

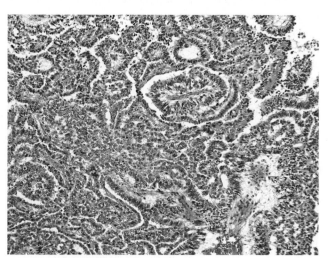

FIGURE 12-38 ■ YST, endodermal sinus type. Notice the presence of Schiller-Duval bodies.

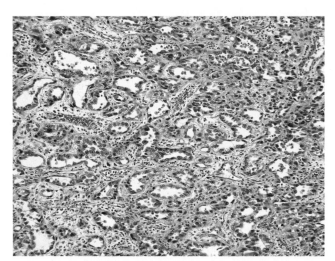

FIGURE 12-39 ■ YST with glandular/parietal features.

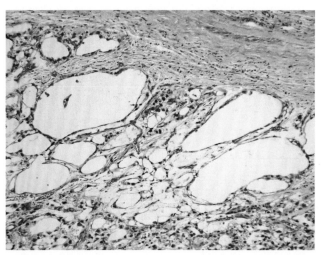

FIGURE 12-41 ■ YST with polyvesicular vitelline growth pattern. Variably sized cysts are lined by flattened tumor cells. The cysts have a central or eccentric constriction and are embedded in variably cellular mesenchyme.

- Papillary: This pattern is characterized by small irregular papillae, with or without fibrous cores, projecting into cystic spaces. If cut tangentially these may appear as detached papillae or cell clusters present within cystic spaces that often are lined by cuboidal to low columnar cells.

- Glandular–alveolar: Here glands and alveoli are lined by flattened epithelium or columnar, pseudostratified epithelium with brush borders (enteric features) (Fig. 12-39). Rarely, basal cytoplasmic vacuoles, reminiscent of early secretory endometrium, may be present, a feature more commonly seen in teratoma.

- Myxomatous: This pattern is quite common and characterized by cords or nests of neoplastic fusiform cells embedded in a myxoid stoma rich in hyaluronic acid. This pattern is most commonly seen adjacent to microcystic and reticular areas, the spindle cells appearing to emanate from them (Fig. 12-40).

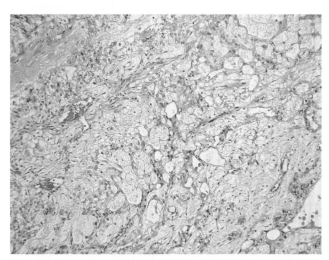

FIGURE 12-40 ■ YST with myxomatous pattern. Attenuated tumor cells line microcysts. Cords of neoplastic fusiform cells are embedded in a myxomatous stroma.

- Spindle cell: Rarely, YSTs have a cellular neoplastic (sarcomatoid) component. The spindle cells retain cytokeratin positivity, supporting their derivation from the epithelial component of microcystic/reticular YST.

- Parietal: This pattern is characterized by a variable amount of eosinophilic basement membrane material, which is present in the extracellular space between tumor cells.

- Polyvesicular vitelline: This pattern shows cysts often with an eccentric constriction, scattered in edematous to fibrous stroma. The cysts are lined by flattened to columnar epithelium, and the transition from the flattened to columnar epithelium usually occurs at the site of constriction (Fig. 12-41).

- Hepatoid: This pattern is not infrequent and presents itself as small clusters of cells with abundant eosinophilic cytoplasm and a large central nucleus with prominent nucleolus (Fig. 12-42). The cells may be arranged in nests, cords, or trabeculae and may show bile canalicular formation. These areas are diffusely and strongly AFP-positive and frequently show hyaline globules and positivity for hepatocyte immunostain, Hep Par-1.

- Solid: It consists of a sheet-like arrangement of polygonal cells, with eosinophilic to clear cytoplasm, well-defined cell borders, and relatively uniform nuclei (Figs. 12-43, 12-44, and 12-45A and B). This pattern may be confused with other GCTs, particularly seminoma. Occasionally it is possible to see eosinophilic droplets or hyaline bodies in the interstitium, a helpful feature in making a diagnosis of YST in this setting.

Tumor cells of YST are not as primitive or pleomorphic as those seen in EC. They have more abundant clear or weakly granular cytoplasm, which is often vacuolated. Individual cell necrosis and apoptotic bodies are not as conspicuous as

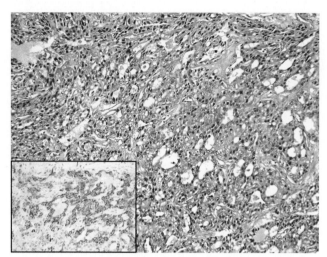

FIGURE 12-42 ■ YST, hepatoid variant. The tumor cells have large, regular nuclei with prominent nucleoli and abundant eosinophilic cytoplasm. **Inset** reveals strong granular cytoplasmic immunoreactivity for hepatocyte marker 1 (Hepar-1).

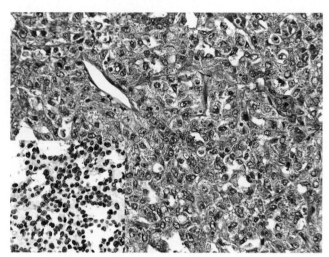

FIGURE 12-44 ■ YST, solid. The level of nuclear abnormalities is less than what is seen in EC. **Inset** shows diffuse nuclear immunoreactivity for SALL-4.

in EC; in the epithelial-looking areas the level of cytologic atypia lies somewhere between seminoma and EC. In the microcystic and spindle areas, the cells are usually more fusiform or stellate but lack marked cytologic atypia, as seen commonly in teratomatous mesenchyme. The cytoplasm may contain small, spherical, and densely eosinophilic intra-cytoplasmic droplets, which are PAS positive and diastase resistant. These represent either AFP or, more commonly, alpha-1-antytrypsin deposition.

Immunohistochemistry

Tumor cells of YST are usually immunoreactive for AFP and low-molecular-weight cytokeratins (Fig. 12-32). PLAP staining is variable and may be absent. CD117 (C-kit), CD30, and OCT4 are usually negative but SOX2, SALL4,

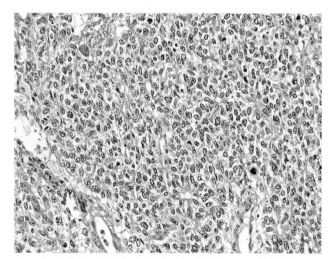

FIGURE 12-43 ■ YST, solid. Notice the deposition of eosinophilic, basement membrane–type material in the stroma as well as an occasional eosinophilic droplet, likely to be AFP.

and glypican 3 are positive[70,71,74,94–96,98–100,133,147,148] (Fig. 12-46) (Table 12-3). We have found that AFP immunohistochemistry can be difficult to interpret. Staining can be weak, patchy and it is often associated with a dirty background. While we admit that some of these findings could be laboratory-associated, the fact of the matter is that we never perform or interpret this assay in isolation. Because we now have better antibodies, we do not consider this assay to be absolutely necessary.

Differential Diagnosis

Differentiation of the solid pattern of YST from pure semi-noma is of great therapeutic and biologic importance and more crucial than its distinction from EC. Differentiation of YST from seminoma and EC has been discussed earlier.

Rare purely glandular YST may be confused with an immature teratoma. The enteric glands in YST often branch extensively, in contrast to the usually simple glands seen in teratoma, sometimes surrounded by a smooth muscle layer. A clinically major consideration is the distinction of juve-nile granulosa cell tumor from a YST in infants. Both tumors show solid and cystic areas. The cells in juvenile granulosa cell tumors do not appear as primitive as in YST, however. The presence of other YST patterns is helpful. Juvenile gran-ulosa cell tumor does not stain for AFP but stains for inhibin A. From a practical point of view, any testicular tumor seen in a neonate or within the first year of life is a juvenile granu-losa cell tumor until proven otherwise.

CHORIOCARCINOMA

Choriocarcinoma is composed of syncytiotrophoblastic, cytotrophoblastic, and other trophoblastic cells. It comprises <1% of testicular GCT in its pure form; however, it may be encountered as a component of a mixed GCT in up to 15% of

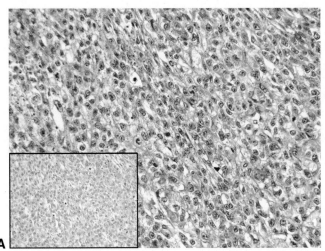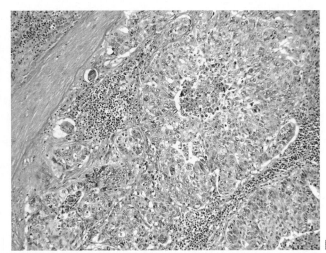

FIGURE 12-45 ■ **A:** YST, solid variant. In this microscopic field, the tumor is devoid of eosinophilic droplets or basement membrane–type stroma (see Fig. 12-43). In this setting, the tumor can be confused with seminoma. However, infiltrating lipocytes are absent, and the nuclei are a bit more irregular than in seminoma. **Inset** demonstrates lack of immunoreactivity for Oct4. **B:** YST after chemotherapy. This tumor recurred in the retoperitoneum 38 years after primary therapy and was confirmed genetically (i12p). While we classified it originally as secondary somatic malignancy (adenocarcinoma), it is likely to represent an unusual morphologic manifestation of YST. Unusual morphologies are not uncommon in the postchemotherapy setting.

cases.[26,86,130] In its pure form, these highly malignant tumors occur in the second and third decades of life, are commonly associated with very high levels of serum HCG (usually above 50,000 mIU/mL), and exhibit metastatic disease at the time of initial presentation. In this setting metastatic disease is found not only in the usual sites for other testicular tumors but also via hematogenous spread to viscera, including lungs, liver, gastrointestinal tract, spleen, brain, and adrenals. About 10% present with gynecomastia as a result of the marked elevation of serum β-HCG levels.[26] Because of the structural similarities between β-HCG and thyroid-stimulating hormone, thyrotoxicosis also may occur. Since pure choriocarcinoma usually presents with widespread hematogenous spread, nonpulmonary visceral metastases, and very high serum

levels of β-HCG, they usually fall into the poor risk category (Table 12-5). It is important to note, however that the choice of systemic therapy is based on risk category rather than histology. Small foci of choriocarcinoma within a mixed GCT are not uncommon and do not influence therapy or prognosis (Box 12-7).

Gross Features

These tumors usually present as a hemorrhagic, necrotic mass with areas of blood-filled cysts. The amount of residual viable tumor may be minimal, requiring thorough sampling. Similarly, identification in mixed GCTs requires proper sampling, paying close attention to areas of apparent hemorrhage. The mass may be small despite the presence of metastatic disease and lymphovascular invasion is common.

Microscopic Features

The majority of cases contain abundant necrotic tumor and hemorrhage and the amount of viable disease can be minimal. These tumors exhibit an admixture of trophoblastic

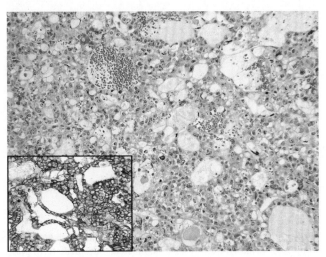

FIGURE 12-46 ■ YST with diffuse cytoplasmic immunoreactivity for glypican 3.

Box 12-7 ● CHORIOCARCINOMA

- Seen in up to 40% of testicular mixed GCTs
- Pure cases are rare but usually are associated with hematogenous metastases and very high serum levels of β-HCG (>50,000 mIU/mL)
- Admixture of syncytiotrophoblasts and cytotrophoblasts
- Monophasic, implantation site–like and cystic trophoblastic variants are rare but more commonly seen post chemotherapy

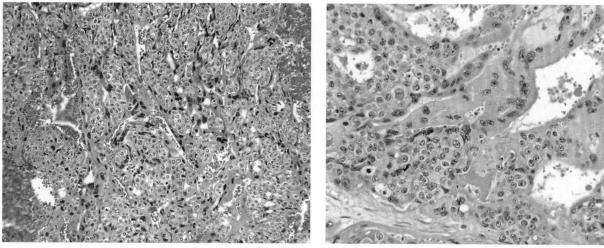

FIGURE 12-47 ■ **A:** Choriocarcinoma. Nests of cytotrophoblasts are surrounded by syncytiotrophoblasts. Hemorrhage and necrosis may be extensive. **B:** Choriocarcinoma. Syncytiotrophoblasts "cap" nests of cytotrophoblasts.

cells in varying proportions (Fig. 12-47A and B). Classic cases will have syncytiotrophoblasts, defined as multinucleated cells with smudged nuclear chromatin and abundant amphophilic cytoplasm and cytotrophoblast, which are mononuclear cells with clear to amphophilic cytoplasm and mild to moderate nuclear pleomorphism. In better-preserved areas, masses of cytotrophoblast are capped by syncytiotrophoblasts whereas in others the relationship between these components is more random. Very rare cases lack syncytiotrophoblasts and are composed predominantly of mononucleated cytotrophoblast and intermediate trophoblastic cells with abundant eosinophilic cytoplasm and squamoid appearance (Figs. 12-48 and 12-49). These tumors have been descriptively called "monophasic" variants of choriocarcinoma and have no association to a distinct clinical meaning except for the fact that they are more commonly encountered in the postchemotherapy setting.[149,150] Another recently described and even rarer variant of trophoblastic

disease is called implantation site trophoblastic tumor, a term taken from the morphologically analogous gestational tumor seen in women.[151] It is composed of intermediate trophoblasts exclusively (Fig. 12-50). These cells are mononuclear, pleomorphic, and exhibit eosinophilic cytoplasm. They are immunoreactive for human placental lactogen (HPL), EMA, and cytokeratins. Cystic trophoblastic tumor refers to cystic lesions rarely seen in the postchemotherapy setting, in association with residual teratoma (Fig. 12-51). These cysts are lined by epithelioid cells with abundant eosinophilic cytoplasm and a squamoid appearance. These cells are not mitotically active and should not be in continuity with other epithelial teratomatous elements within the same cyst. Its clinical meaning is unknown but should be regarded as a component of the teratoma rather than residual nonteratomatous GCT.[152,153]

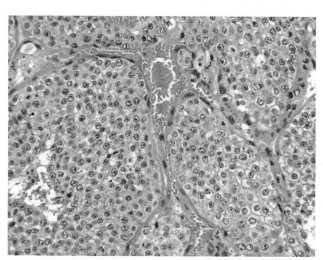

FIGURE 12-48 ■ Choriocarcinoma predominantly composed of cytotrophoblast. Flattened and deeply eosinophilic syncytiotrophoblasts are seen surrounding the nests of cytotrophoblasts.

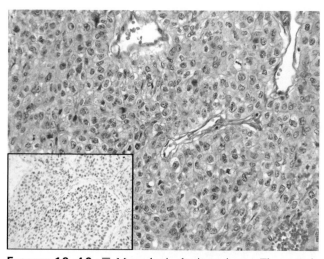

FIGURE 12-49 ■ Monophasic choriocarcinoma. The tumor is composed virtually entirely of mononuclear intermediate trophoblasts of the chorionic type. It was the sole histology seen in several lung metastases resected following systemic therapy **Inset** demonstrates nuclear immunoreactivity for p63 (clone 4A4).

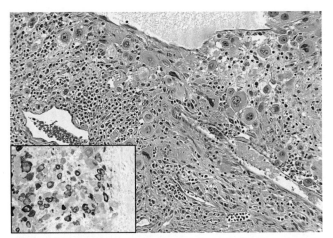

Figure 12-50 ■ Implantation site trophoblastic tumor. The lesion is characterized by epithelioid cells with abundant eosinophilic cytoplasm, similar to the similarly named gestation-related lesion seen in women. In males, it is very rare and seen exclusively in the postchemotherapy setting. **Inset** reveals immunoreactivity for EMA.

Syncytiotrophoblasts are immunoreactive for β-HCG as well as inhibin, EMA, and low molecular weight cytokeratins. PLAP may be positive, but staining is variable.[86] Cytotrophoblast are either negative or weakly positive for β-HCG. Pregnancy-specific β1-glycoprotein and HPL also are positive in syncytiotrophoblasts and intermediate-sized trophoblasts but are negative in cytotrophoblast.[26,154]

Differential Diagnosis

Choriocarcinoma with extensive hemorrhage and necrosis must be differentiated from testicular hemorrhagic infarction resulting from torsion or other causes. The onset of acute pain and swelling are commonly associated with infarction. It is important not to confuse seminomas with abundant syncytiotrophoblasts with choriocarcinoma. In both scenarios, the syncytiotrophoblasts may be associated with hemorrhage. However, in seminoma it is less likely to encounter necrosis and cytotrophoblast will be absent. These rules also hold true in the setting of other mixed GCTs.

TERATOMA

The term teratoma refers to neoplasms composed of tissues, which have differentiated along any of the three somatic pathways: ectoderm, mesoderm, or endoderm.[26,86,145] Tumors composed of only one of these components are regarded as monodermal teratomas. Teratomas may be composed of mature tissues, embryonal-type tissues, or a mixture of both. Historically, they were subclassified as immature and mature forms based on their degree of differentiation. The World Health Organization now recommends that these morphologies be considered as a single entity based on their overlapping genetic and clinical features.[155] Testicular teratomas occur in both prepubertal and adult patients with each having distinct biology. In prepubertal patients, they account for up to 20% of cases and are invariably benign. They usually appear in a pure form with the mean age at diagnosis being 20 months; rarely will they occur after 4 years of age. These tumors are not associated with intratubular germ cell neoplasia, are likely to be diploid, and will not exhibit i(12p). Teratomas in postpubertal patients are usually a component of a mixed GCT, tumors with a pure teratomatous histology being rare, <7%. These tumors, whether mature or immature, are considered malignant since both may be seen in primary and metastatic sites. They are commonly aneuploid and will exhibit i(12p). Whether mature teratomatous components are capable of metastasis or whether their presence in a metastatic site represents differentiation within a more primitive clone that has metastasized, such as EC or YST, is debatable. Teratomatous components may be the only remaining recognizable tumor after spontaneous regression or after systemic therapy. Pure teratomas are not usually associated with elevation of serum oncofetal markers. However, the fluid in cystic teratomas postchemotherapy has been shown to express high levels of these markers.[156] In this setting it is believed that these proteins may leach into the circulation, leading to low-level elevations of oncofetal proteins that clinically should not be interpreted as evidence of residual, chemotherapy-resistant, and/or nonteratomatous GCT (Box 12-8).

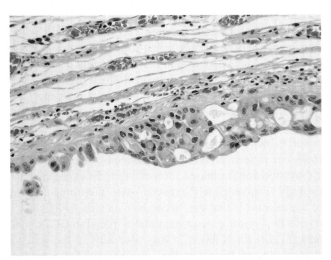

Figure 12-51 ■ Cystic trophoblastic tumor. Cystic spaces are lined by cells with abundant eosinophilic cytoplasm, some with a squamoid appearance. By definition, these cells do not merge with more typical epithelial teratomatous cells within the same cyst. This lesion is seen exclusively in metastatic sites post chemotherapy and should be regarded as a variant of teratoma.

Box 12-8 ● TERATOMA

- Subclassification into mature and immature categories is not recommended
- Pure cases are more common in prepubertal than in adult patients
- May be associated with secondary somatic malignancies, most commonly post chemotherapy and in late recurrences
- Best treated by surgery since all forms are chemoresistant

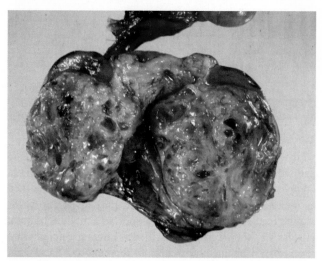

FIGURE 12-52 ■ Teratoma gross. Cystic and solid areas are evident.

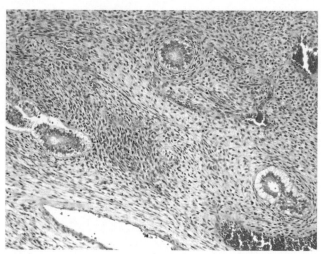

FIGURE 12-54 ■ Teratoma composed of fetal-type tissues.

Gross Features

Tumors are usually heterogeneous, firm or soft, nodular, and well circumscribed. They may be solid or cystic depending on histologic components (Fig. 12-52). The cysts may contain keratinaceous or viscous material or serous fluid. Cartilaginous elements may be grossly evident.

Microscopic Features

Mature elements ("mature" teratoma) resemble those seen in postnatal tissues from any or all three germ cell layers. Attempts at organ formation are common, particularly in children, but generally, the different components are intermixed but disorganized (Figs. 12-53 and 12-54). Skin and its adnexa are common ectodermal components whereas endoderm may be represented by any of a host of epithelia such as enteric, respiratory, or intestinal glands. Mesoderm may be represented by smooth and skeletal muscle, cartilage, and bone. Foci of adult-type neural tissue are common.

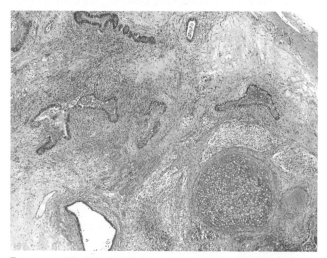

FIGURE 12-53 ■ Teratoma. Notice the intermingling of multiple cell types.

Fetal-type tissues ("immature" teratoma) are usually seen juxtaposed to mature elements and may derive from any of the germinal layers (Figs. 12-54, 12-55A and B). The immature elements are commonly represented by cellular, undifferentiated, primitive-appearing spindle cells (mesenchyme) that may surround fetal-type glands. Primitive, central-type neuroepithelium, embryonal skeletal muscle, and blastema may also be seen (Fig. 12-56).

When one of the teratomatous components, whether mesenchymal (skeletal muscle), neural (primitive neuroepithelium), or epithelial (glandular or squamous), predominates and forms an "expansile" mass, the term "teratoma with secondary somatic type malignancy" is used[86,157–161] (Fig. 12-57A–C). These tumors were originally called "teratoma with malignant transformation," a term no longer in use. The definition of what constitutes somatic-type malignancy is controversial, but most authors suggest that the expansile nodule should be equal or greater to the area viewed with a 4× objective (40× total magnification) (Figs. 12-58 and 12-59). The incidence of secondary somatic malignancy is approximately 3%. This phenomenon may be seen de novo in testicular GCT, more commonly in mediastinal primaries, and in retroperitoneal disease resected after chemotherapy.[158,159] It can also be seen in cases of late recurrence, many years after systemic chemotherapy was completed.[162] If limited to the gonad it is not associated with a worse prognosis. However, if seen in the retroperitoneum or mediastinum, progression and decreased survival are to be expected, particularly if incompletely excised.[156] An interesting feature of this disease is that the "secondary somatic malignancy" retains the typical genetic abnormality found in GCTs, that being i(12p). In addition, it may also acquire the genetic abnormality of the secondary malignancy, for example, primitive neuroepithelial component may exhibit an 11;22 translocation along with i(12p).[163,164] Rare cases of pure primitive central-type neuroectodermal tumors have been described.[145] Recently it has been shown that the majority

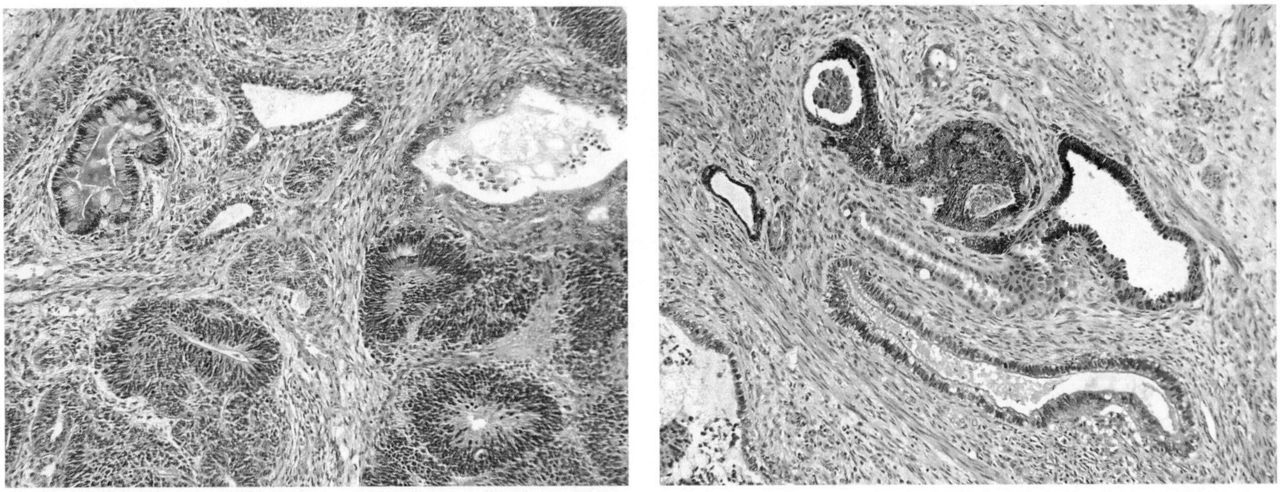

FIGURE 12-55 ■ **A:** Teratoma. In this image, more mature enteric-like glands are seen adjacent to a primitive neuroepithelial component. **B:** Teratoma. In this image, we can see immature, müllerian-type glands. The cells have subnuclear and supranuclear cytoplasmic vacuoles. An adjacent gland is partially lined retinal-type cells containing neuromelanin. Mesenchyme and smooth muscle cells are also present.

of neuroepithelial elements seen in this setting are central rather than peripheral type.[165] While some have regarded them as a form of monodermal teratoma, we consider them as examples of secondary somatic malignancy. These tumors are characterized by the presence of poorly differentiated cells arranged in sheets or forming primitive neural-type tubules, ependymal-type rosettes, or neuroblastic cells embedded in a fibrillary neuropil. This is a particularly ominous clinical finding in patients who have been previously treated with systemic chemotherapy.[156]

The immunohistochemical profile of teratomas will depend on the histologic component present. In addition, glandular elements are likely not to be immunoreactive for SALL4 and glypican 3 although focal staining may be evident for either marker; whether this represents early yolk sac differentiation is unknown (Fig. 12-60). AFP may also be focally positive in glandular elements, which may be associated with the elevation of AFP in the cystic fluid.[156]

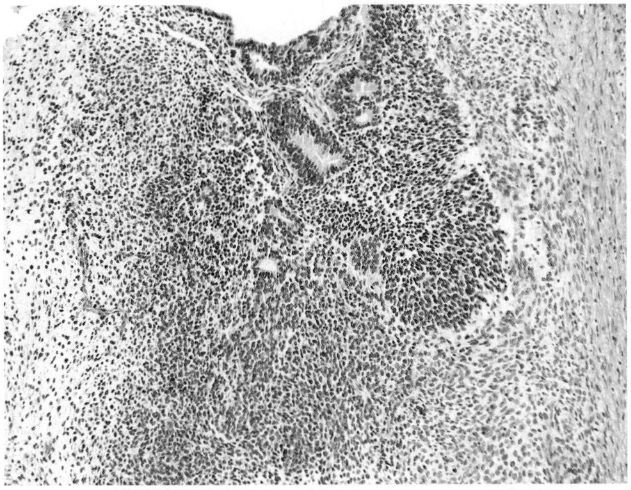

FIGURE 12-56 ■ Teratoma composed of primitive neuroepithelial elements surrounded by mesenchyme.

Differential Diagnosis

Rarely will teratomatous elements be confused with other entities although occasionally immature glands may mimic EC or YST. It is important to distinguish teratomas with mature elements from epidermoid and dermoid cysts, both of which are benign and will be discussed later in the chapter. Intratubular germ cell neoplasia is likely to be present in teratoma but is absent in epidermoid and dermoid cysts. The presence of scarring in the adjacent testicular parenchyma could be a sign of partial regression (partially burned-out lesion), and its presence should always be mentioned in the pathology report. This phenomenon is likely to account for some of the cases of divergent histology between the primary and metastatic sites, the nonteratomatous component having regressed in the primary but not before spreading and growing at a metastatic site.

If teratoma is present in a resected metastatic site, usually postchemotherapy, no additional therapy is required. An exception to this approach is in the presence of secondary somatic malignancy, in which case some investigators may choose to give systemic therapy geared toward histology of the secondary malignancy. However, this issue remains controversial, and clinical responses are anecdotal.

EPIDERMOID AND DERMOID CYSTS

Epidermoid cysts constitute 1% or less of all testicular neoplasms.[86,166,167] Their histogenesis is unclear, although most investigators suggest that they represent monodermally

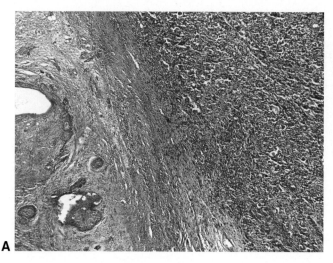

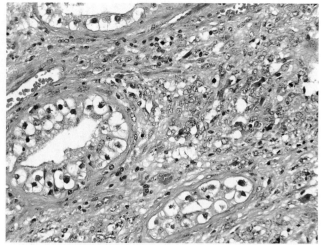

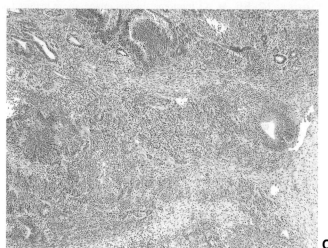

FIGURE 12-57 ■ **A:** Teratoma with an associated secondary somatic malignancy. Teratomatous components (**left**) adjacent to an expansile mass composed entirely of embryonal rhabdomyosarcoma. **B:** Secondary somatic malignancy. Embryonal rhabdomyosarcoma juxtaposed to intratubular germ cell neoplasia. **C:** Secondary somatic malignancy. Low-power magnification of a tumor composed exclusively of primitive neuroepithelial elements.

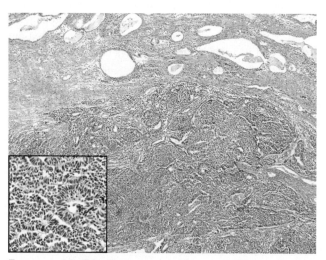

FIGURE 12-58 ■ Teratoma with an associated secondary somatic malignancy. A small amount of cystic teratomatous elements are present in the top portion of the image. But the majority of the tumor was composed of central-type primitive neuroepithelial tumor (PNET). The patient subsequently developed lung metastases entirely composed on PNET (**inset**).

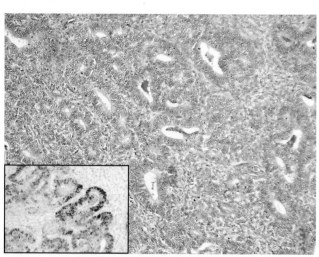

FIGURE 12-59 ■ Secondary somatic malignancy. This postchemotherapy metastatic tumor has the biphasic features of Wilms tumor. The **inset** demonstrates nuclear immunoreactivity for PAX8, mostly in the epithelial but not blastemal component. WT1 was also positive.

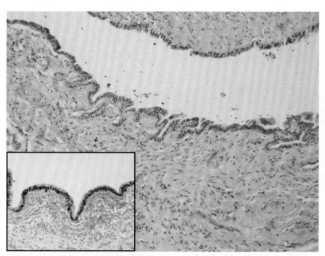

FIGURE 12-60 ■ Teratoma. Cystic space is lined by bland cuboidal epithelial cells. **Inset** shows nuclear immunoreactivity for SALL4. SALL4 is expressed in a wide spectrum of GCTs including IGCNU, seminoma, EC, and YST. It is important to remember that it can also be expressed in some elements of teratoma.

differentiated mature teratoma, supported by the fact that a recent case with adjacent IGCNU was identified.[168] Some have suggested that they arise from inclusion cysts, while others propose squamous metaplasia of seminiferous tubules or the rete testis (tumor-like condition). They are commonly discovered between the second and fourth decades of life and are often asymptomatic. These tumors may be as large as 10 cm although most measure <2 cm (Box 12-9).

Grossly they appear as well-circumscribed cystic masses filled with keratinized debris similar to an epidermal inclusion cyst (Fig. 12-61A). The cyst wall is composed of fibrous tissue surrounding flattened squamous epithelium (Fig. 12-61B). No dermal adnexal elements or other teratomatous elements are present in the cyst wall or surrounding testicular parenchyma. These tumors are not associated with a testicular scar; furthermore, IGCNU is not present except in the above-mentioned case.

These unusual neoplasms are invariably benign and should be managed conservatively. Nevertheless, the lesion should be thoroughly sampled and examined by the pathologist to rule out other elements or IGCNU. The treatment of choice for classic examples of this disease is enucleation,

---

Box 12-9 ● EPIDERMOID CYST

- Benign lesion that constitute <1% of resected testicular neoplasms
- Characteristic features on ultrasound that allows conservative enucleation of the lesion, which is the treatment of choice
- Keratin-filled cyst lined by squamous epithelium, classically without skin adnexal glands
- Not associated with IGCNU or parenchymal scar (regression)

---

which is made possible by the fact that the diagnosis can be suggested on testicular ultrasound.

Dermoid cysts have been described in the testis and are characterized by the presence of squamous epithelium overlying skin appendages, including hair follicles and sebaceous glands[86,169] (Figs. 12-62 and 12-63). They are extremely rare, and those described behave in a benign fashion. They differ from "usual" teratoma with mature elements by the absence of solid elements and IGCNU. Occasionally other teratomatous components may be present. Isolated cases with i(12p) have been described, an important fact to keep in mind when understanding the histogenesis of these lesions but an assay that is not required for proper classification. They are considered a benign variant of cystic teratoma analogous to what is seen in the ovary. From a practical point of view, we report such lesion as "teratoma" and include a comment stating that this lesion has the morphologic features of a dermoid cyst that we consider to be a benign monodermal variant of teratoma. Personally, we feel uncomfortable with these tumors being treated by simple enucleation although this issue remains controversial. Importantly, the presence of parenchymal scarring should raise the possibility of partial regression of other germ cell elements and should be mentioned in the pathology report.

Carcinoid Tumor

Primary carcinoid tumor of the testis is rare and is thought to represent a form of monodermal teratoma. Approximately 75% of cases are pure carcinoid tumors while the remainder present as a component of teratoma.[170–172] Mean age at presentation is in the fifth decade of life although they have a wide age distribution. The minority have symptoms associated with the carcinoid syndrome, and <10% will experience metastasis.[171,172] Features associated with metastasis include size larger than 7 cm, pure histology, and the presence of carcinoid syndrome.

Pure carcinoid tumors are pale yellow to dark tan, well-circumscribed, and firm. Size can be quite variable. If other teratomatous elements are present, the gross appearance will be more variegated. Microscopically, carcinoid tumors of the testis may have all the features seen in these tumors elsewhere, including insular, acinar, or trabecular patterns of growth (Figs. 12-64 and 12-65). The cytoplasm is abundant and the nuclei uniformly round with finely dispersed chromatin and inconspicuous nucleoli. The tumor cells will be immunoreactive for neuroendocrine markers and cytokeratin.

The principal differential diagnosis is with metastatic disease. In fact, one should first consider the possibility of a metastasis prior to making a diagnosis of a primary carcinoid tumor of the testis. Bilateral, multifocal diseases as well as prominent angiolymphatic invasion are features of metastatic rather than primary disease, whereas association with other teratomatous components or ICGNU is a sure sign of primary disease.

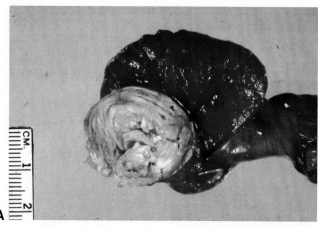
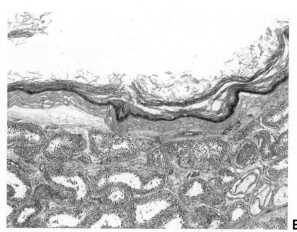

FIGURE 12-61 ■ **A:** Epidermoid cyst. Gross appearance shows a well-circumscribed mass containing keratin debris. The adjacent testicular parenchyma is grossly unremarkable. **B:** Epidermoid cyst. The cystic cavity is lined by keratinized squamous epithelium without evidence of skin adnexal structures. Intratubular germ cell neoplasia is absent.

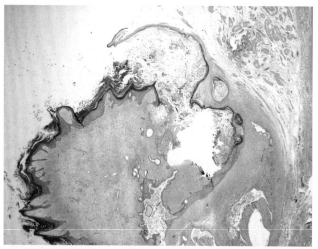

FIGURE 12-62 ■ Dermoid cyst. Skin adnexal structures and other teratomatous elements may be present. This lesion should be considered a variant of teratoma.

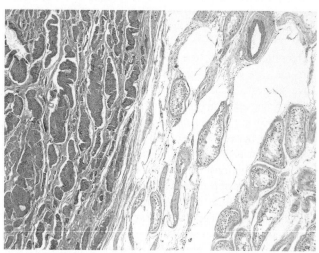

FIGURE 12-64 ■ Testicular carcinoid. When present in its pure form, the possibility of a metastasis must be entertained.

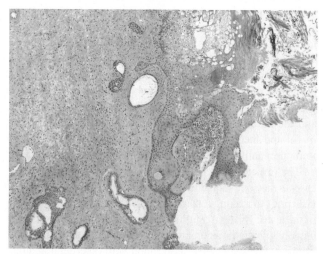

FIGURE 12-63 ■ Teratoma with dermoid-like areas. A central cystic space is lined by squamous epithelium, which is undermined by adnexal-type glands. Other teratomatous elements were present elsewhere, as was IGCNU.

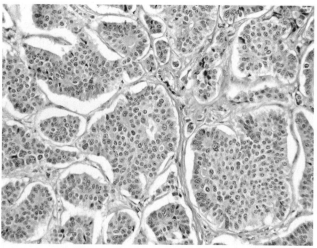

FIGURE 12-65 ■ Carcinoid tumor. Nests and cords of neoplastic cells with amphophilic cytoplasm. When cords predominate, this tumor could be confused with a sex cord–stromal tumor, particularly SCT.

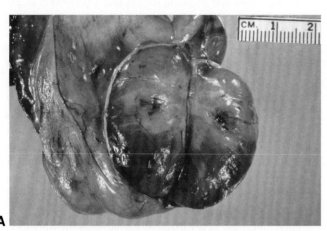
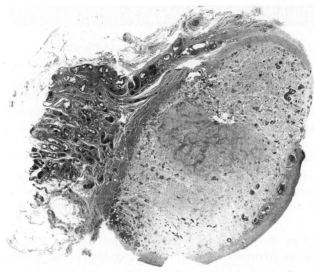

A   **B**

FIGURE 12-66 ■ **A:** Burned-out tumor (regression). Grossly, the testicular parenchyma exhibits an area of tan-white discoloration. The gross appearance of the surrounding testicular parenchyma is variable. **B:** Burned-out tumor (regression). Whole mount highlighting the area of scarring. These changes can also be seen after chemotherapy.

COMPLETELY OR PARTIALLY "BURNED-OUT" GERM CELL TUMOR

A possible explanation for most—if not all—presumed "primary" retroperitoneal GCT lies in the concept of partially or completely "burned-out" GCT (Fig. 12-66A and B). For many decades, pathologists have observed areas of regression within GCTs. These usually take the form of a well-defined stellate fibrous scar at the periphery where sclerosed seminiferous tubules are evident.[173–175] The scar may be accompanied by a sparse plasma cell infiltrate and aggregates of hemosiderin and macrophages may be present (Fig. 12-67). The scar is usually located well within the substance of the testis. It may abut the mediastinum testis

but is rarely located toward the poles or directly below the tunica albuginea. The latter location suggests the possibility of a posttraumatic scar. Another occasional feature seen in burned-out lesions is the presence of peculiar hematoxyphilic deposits having an amorphous or granular structure. These deposits appear to be located within hyalinized seminiferous tubules. Infrequently, these hematoxylin-staining bodies may be associated with scattered malignant germ cells (ICGNU). Variably hyalinized and atrophic seminiferous tubules, some containing microliths, dispersed within the testicular parenchyma, and seminiferous tubules with a Sertoli cell–only pattern are common findings associated with regression. However, testicular microlithiasis is in no way specific to testicular GCTs. A burned-out lesion without any viable GCT may be the only evidence of a regressed testicular primary. If viable germ cell components are present, they usually are in the form of teratoma, seminoma, or IGCNU. Burned-out lesions may be very small, rendering them nonpalpable; nevertheless, they are usually discernible by testicular ultrasound. Nonspecific testicular scars are commonly located near the tunica albuginea, and the seminiferous tubules away from the scar are normal in morphologic appearance with normal spermatogenesis (Box 12-10).

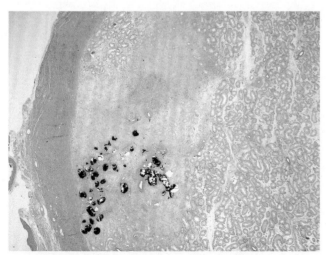

FIGURE 12-67 ■ Burned-out lesion. Low-power magnification shows parenchymal scarring as well as irregular dystrophic calcifications; the latter could signal the prior presence of intratubular EC.

Box 12-10 ● BURNED-OUT LESION

- Parenchymal fibrous scar with effacement of the normal cellular architecture
- Scar may contain macrophages, plasma cells, and/or calcifications
- Hyalinization of seminiferous tubules adjacent to and away from the area(s) of scarring
- May be associated with viable GCT at a metastatic site

TUMORS OF MORE THAN ONE HISTOLOGIC TYPE

Mixed GCTs constitute between 35% and 54% of GCT, exclusive of seminomas with trophoblastic cells and SS with sarcoma.[26,86] They are rarely seen in prepubertal gonads. All the morphologic variants previously described may be encountered with the exception of SS. The most common combinations are EC and teratoma (26%); EC and seminoma (16%); and EC, YST, and teratoma (11%)[82,112,130] (Fig. 12-68A–C). Cases containing a component of seminoma tend to occur later in life than those that do not. Elevation of serum oncofetal proteins will depend on the histologic components of the tumor (Fig. 12-69). As expected, the gross and microscopic features are quite variable and will depend on the histologic components encountered. In reporting this tumor,[176] we should mention each of the components present, giving the percentage of each. The term "teratocarcinoma" should be avoided since it lacks diagnostic specificity.

As previously mentioned, in reporting the pathology of mixed GCTs, it is important to mention the percentage of each of the histologic components, particularly the percentage of EC. Tumors with a predominance of EC (variably reported to be more than 55% to 80%) are four times more like to develop metastatic disease, usually to the retroperitoneum, via the lymphatics. Since these tumors are also more likely to be associated with lymphovascular invasion, the relative contribution of EC as a risk factor has been questioned by some. In our institution clinical stage 1 patients with a percentage of EC above 55% are rarely, if ever, managed by surveillance but rather undergo a primary RPLND. Admittedly, this remains a controversial topic. We do not recommend subclassifying the teratomatous components by their level of maturity, for reasons previously discussed. However, mentioning the presence of teratoma is important. The presence of teratoma in a primary tumor correlates with the presence of teratoma in a residual postchemotherapy mass. In this setting and in the absence of serum marker elevation, the presence of residual teratomatous elements can be inferred clinically. Although controversial, such residual masses, if small, are not resected but rather monitored.

Polyembryoma is a variant of mixed GCT in which EC and yolk sac components are arranged in a pattern resembling the embryo prior to day 18 of development.[57,61] It is characterized by the presence of scattered embryoid bodies, defined as a central plate of primitive cells exhibiting EC-like features, a "dorsal amnion–like cavity" lined by flat cells; and a "ventral yolk sac–like" vesicle composed of

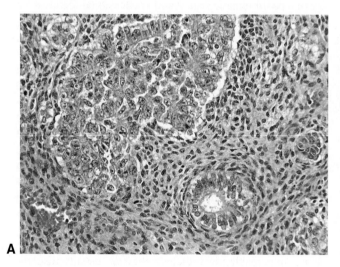

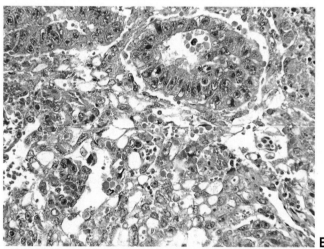

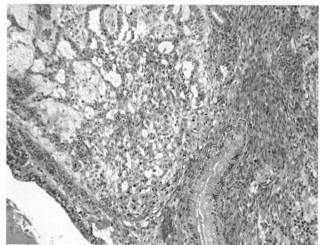

FIGURE 12-68 ■ A: Mixed GCT (EC and teratoma). A nest of EC with classic, highly atypical cytology is surrounded by teratomatous mesenchyme and a single gland with subnuclear vacuolization. **B:** Mixed GCT (EC and YST). **C:** Mixed GCT (YST and teratoma).

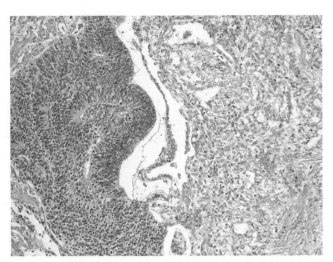

FIGURE 12-69 ■ Mixed GCT composed of YST and primitive neuroepithelium.

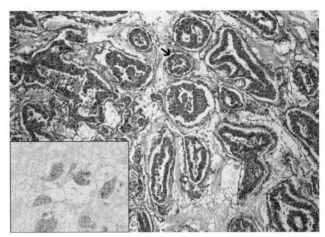

FIGURE 12-71 ■ Diffuse embryoma. Irregular gland-like structures lined by EC cells are surrounded by YST. **Inset** demonstrates membranous immunoreactivity for CD30 in the EC cells but not YST.

reticular and myxoid YST (Fig. 12-70). The bodies generally are surrounded by myxoid mesenchyme. Polyembryoma is invariably encountered in a setting of mixed GCT.

The term *diffuse embryoma* is used for tumors that exhibit an equal proportion of EC and YST where each of these elements encircles the other in a necklace or ribbon-like fashion (Fig. 12-71). The presence of polyembryoma or diffuse embryoma has no known clinical significance.

Pathologic Prognostic Factors in Stage I Nonseminomatous Germ Cell Tumors

Until recently, the treatment of choice for stage I nonseminomatous germ cell tumor was radical orchiectomy followed by RPLND. Given the advent of highly effective chemotherapy,

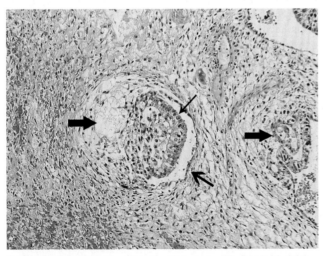

FIGURE 12-70 ■ Polyembryoma. This type of tumor is characterized by the presence of embryoid bodies embedded in a loose mesenchyme. An embryoid body is characterized by the presence of an "embryonic disc" composed of EC cells (*thin arrow*), an amniotic-like cavity (*intermediate-sized arrow*), and a yolk sac component (*thick arrow*). From a practical point of view, this lesion should be regarded as a mixed GCT.

the availability of sensitive serum tumor markers, as well as more precise staging techniques, orchiectomy alone followed by close surveillance is a viable option for some patients. Overall, 20% to 25% of patients treated in this manner will recur, usually in the retroperitoneum and within a year of the orchiectomy (Box 12-11).

Many studies have shown that the presence of VI in the primary tumor is the best predictor of recurrence. In fact, the importance of VI in the primary is reflected in the TMN classification. The impact of tumor histology on future relapse remains controversial, but most authors have suggested that a pure or predominant EC component also is more likely to metastasize.[139–141]

Large tumor size and rete testis invasion, but not lymphovascular invasion, have been considered pathologic risk factors for relapse in stage I seminoma by some, although the significance of rete testis invasion remains controversial.[18]

SEX CORD–STROMAL (GONADAL STROMAL) TUMORS OF THE TESTIS

Sex cord–stromal (gonadal stromal) tumors are rare, comprising approximately 4% of testicular neoplasms and almost 8% of tumors arising in prepubertal males.[26,86,177]

Box 12-11 ● STAGE 1 MIXED GERM CELL TUMORS

- Twenty-five percent will relapse
- Morphologic predictors of relapse include percent of embryonal carcinoma and vascular invasion (VI)
- The presence of VI defines the tumor as pathologic stage 2 (pT2) disease, even if organ-confined
- Tumor extension into rete testis, hilar soft tissue and/or adnexa do not influence pathologic stage or relapse rate

Similar tumors may arise in the female gonads. The term refers to neoplasms containing Leydig (interstitial) cells, Sertoli cells, granulosa cells, or theca cells (Box 12-12).

While tumors may be made up of one or a combination of these cell types in varying degrees of differentiation, mixed histologic types are common in the ovary but rarely occur in the male gonad. The terminology used to describe these tumors is confusing and controversial but it is best to adhere to the classification set forth by the World Health Organization (Table 12-2).

LEYDIG (INTERSTITIAL) CELL TUMOR

Leydig cell tumors (LCTs) are the most common pure testicular sex cord–stromal neoplasm and account for 1% to 3% of testicular neoplasms. They may occur at any age, though most common between the third and sixth decades of life.[26,86,178–180] Fifteen to twenty percent of cases will present in prepubertal children. Approximately 10% will metastasize with metastasis more commonly seen in older patients. LCTs usually arise in normally descended testes although they have been described in cryptorchid gonads as well as in testes that have undergone orchiopexy. Only three cases have been reported in patients with Klinefelter syndrome.

Most, if not all, children with LCT present with isosexual precocity, which is characterized by deepening of the voice, appearance of body hair, penile enlargement, and advanced bone age.[177] Often these physical changes are accompanied by excessive aggression or shyness. LCT must be considered in the differential diagnosis in all prepubertal patients with a testicular mass and precocious puberty. Painless testicular swelling is the most common manifestation in adults, followed by bilateral gynecomastia. It is not unusual for gynecomastia to precede the appearance of a testicular mass and in 15% of cases, the former being the only complaint at initial presentation. Approximately 25% of patients with gynecomastia experience a decrease in potency or libido. Given the low incidence of these tumors, endocrinologic studies are limited and incomplete. Prepubertal patients will usually have elevated serum testosterone as well as elevated urinary 17-ketosteroids. In adults, elevated estrogen levels

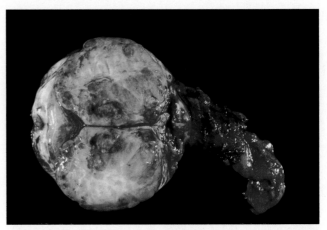

FIGURE 12-72 ■ LCT gross. The mass is heterogeneous and replaces most of the testicular parenchyma.

have been documented in patients with, as well as without, gynecomastia. Testosterone levels may be low or normal in patients with gynecomastia, associated with high levels of serum estradiol.

Gross Features

LCTs are well circumscribed and solid or lobulated in appearance (Fig. 12-72). They are yellow-tan or brown-gray with macroscopic evidence of hemorrhage or necrosis seen in up to 25% of cases. Extension outside the testicular parenchyma is rarely encountered.

Microscopic Features

LCTs usually exhibit a solid or nodular pattern of growth although fibrous septa may give them a pseudofollicular, tubular, or trabecular appearance (Fig. 12-73A and B). The cells are large and polyclonal with abundant eosinophilic cytoplasm. Less frequently, the cytoplasm may be clear or vacuolated due to the presence of lipid.[181,182] Nuclei are round or vesicular with delicate chromatin and a single prominent nucleolus. Spindle cells with abundant eosinophilic cytoplasm may predominate in some cases (Fig. 12-74). Rarely the tumor cells can take on a microcystic appearance, mimicking YST (Fig. 12-75). Crystalloids of Reinke are pathognomonic but seen in <40%, even with the assistance of electron microscopy. On light microscopy, they appear as densely eosinophilic needle-like or rhomboid structures within the cytoplasm.

Immunohistochemical Features

LCTs are immunoreactive for inhibin, melan A, calretinin, WT1 and vimentin (Fig. 12-73A). Cytokeratins and S-100 protein are either negative or only focally positive. CD30, CD117, Oct3/4, and PLAP are negative[86,134,183–187] (Table 12-3). Steriogenic factor 1 (SF-1) is a nuclear transcription factor expressed in testicular Sertoli cells as well as sex cord–stromal cells.[188] It is expressed in a high percentage of sex cord–stromal tumors of all types and is useful in the differential diagnosis of other tumor types.

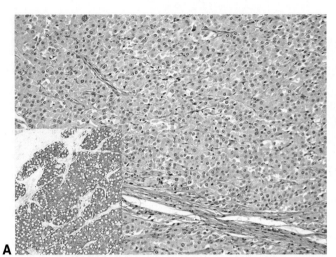
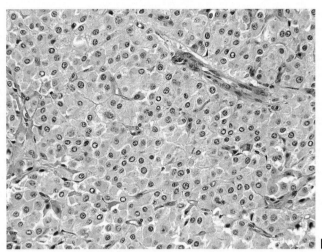

FIGURE 12-73 ■ **A:** Leydig cell tumor. In this tumor, the cells are arranged in solid sheets with abundant eosinophilic cytoplasm; round-to-oval nuclei with occasional prominent nucleoli. **Inset** shows diffuse cytoplasmic staining for inhibin. **B:** Leydig cell tumor. The cells are arranged in solid sheets interlaced by a delicate vascular network. Areas of fibrosis may be seen within and surrounding the tumor. At this magnification we can easily observe the classic cytology that includes abundant eosinophilic cytoplasm, round-to-oval nuclei with occasional prominent nucleoli.

It is difficult to determine histologically those tumors that will metastasize. Kim et al.[178] reported their experience with 40 cases as well as reviewed the literature and postulated that older age at presentation, tumors larger than 5 cm as well as those with infiltrative margins, VI, nuclear atypia, or increased mitotic rate were associated with aggressive behavior (Fig. 12-76). The presence of four or more of these features is strongly correlated with disease progression. Interestingly, none of the malignant cases presented with endocrine manifestations or occurred in prepubertal children. Cheville et al.[189] confirmed these findings but also found that malignant LCTs were more likely to have a high proliferation rate and to be nondiploid. Unless metastatic disease has been documented at the time of orchiectomy, we do not make a primary diagnosis of malignant LCT. Our

practice is to report all gross and microscopic features that have been found to be associated with a greater risk of progression. Based on the numbers of adverse features found, we add a statement stating whether the lesion is at high risk or low risk of malignant behavior.

Most series suggest that 90% of cases behave in a benign fashion with radical orchiectomy being curative. Once metastatic disease occurs the prognosis is poor. The most common metastatic sites are retroperitoneal and inguinal lymph nodes followed by the lungs and liver. Effective systemic

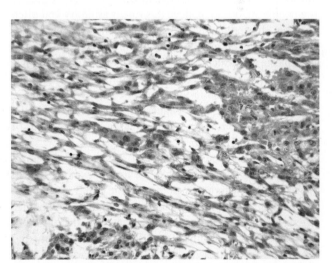

FIGURE 12-75 ■ LCT with microcystic features. In the microcystic areas, the tumor cells are elongated and flattened rather than round and associated with myxoid stroma. A tumor like this could be mistaken for YST. If necessary, immunohistochemistry could easily solve this diagnostic dilemma since LCT would be expected to be positive for inhibin, calretinin, and/or WT1 but negative for SALL4 and glypican 3.

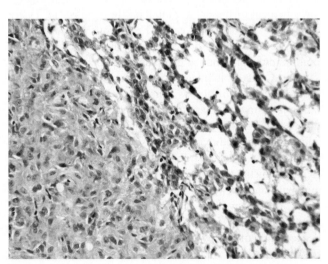

FIGURE 12-74 ■ LCT with spindle and microcystic features.

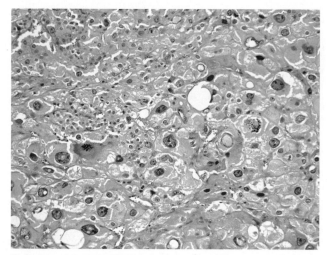

FIGURE 12-76 ■ Malignant LCT. Notice the degree of nuclear pleomorphism and mitotic activity. This patient presented with metastatic disease and subsequently died.

therapy for metastatic disease is lacking, so surgery remains the most effective treatment to achieve cure. Consequently, it is common for patients with increased risk for progression or with limited metastatic disease to the retroperitoneum to undergo a RPLND.

Differential Diagnosis

LCT must be distinguished from Leydig cell hyperplasia or nodular aggregates of Leydig cells that occur in atrophic testes (including patients with Klinefelter syndrome) and in testicular parenchyma adjacent to germ cell neoplasia. Here Leydig cells infiltrate between seminiferous tubules without displacing or obliterating them. It is common practice to consider any Leydig cell nodule measuring 5 mm or greater as a neoplasm, but we believe this rule is arbitrary and often incorrect, depending on other features. If the adjacent testicular parenchyma is atrophic and multiple foci of Leydig cell hyperplasia are evident, the presence of one or more nodules measuring 5 mm or slightly more should not trigger a diagnosis of "tumor." The lesion should be clearly described in the pathology report, and a suggestion should be made to the clinician for establishing a medical reason for the findings of Leydig cell hyperplasia.

LCT must also be distinguished from other sex cord–stromal tumors, especially when the former exhibits a cord-like or tubular pattern, which may mimic a SCT. Secondary lesions such as lymphoma, malignant melanoma, and poorly differentiated carcinoma may also enter in the differential diagnosis. LCT with microcystic features and myxoid stroma may be confused with YSTs.[181] Similarly, one must not confuse LCT with malakoplakia.

A lesion that must not be confused with LCT is that which occurs in association with congenital adrenal hyperplasia (CAH, *tumor of the adrenogenital syndrome*).[26,86,190] CAH is due to a defect of any one of five enzymatic steps involved in steroid synthesis (Box 12-13).

Box 12-13 ● TUMOR OF THE ADRENOGENITAL SYNDROME

- Autosomal dominant defect in steroid synthesis
- Lesion may be single or multiple and located within the testicular parenchyma, adnexa, or cord
- Tumor cytology may be confused with Leydig cell tumor
- Characterized by dense (keloid-like) bands of fibrous tissue

---

This disorder is an inborn error of metabolism, has an autosomal recessive mode of inheritance, and is the most common cause of ambiguous genitalia in infants. Ninety to ninety-five percent of cases are due to 21-hydroxylase deficiency. A small percentage may be due to 11-B-hydroxylase, 3-B-hydroxysteroid, 17-a-hydroxylase, or cholesterol desmolase deficiency.

Persistent stimulation of adrenal cortical tissue by ACTH may give rise not only to hyperplasia, but rarely to adrenal cortical neoplasia (both adenomas and carcinomas). Heterotopic or accessory adrenal cortical tissue can also become hyperplastic and enlarged. A testicular "tumor" of adrenal cortical type is defined as a tumefactive lesion of uncertain histogenesis in the setting of CAH, which histologically resembles hyperplastic adrenal cortical cells stimulated by ACTH and in which endocrinologic evaluation may reveal ACTH dependency. These tumors are thought to arise from primordial rests within the testicular hilum. These rests are a collection of cells morphologically resembling Leydig cells and found in a large proportion of cases of well-studied CAH. Nodules of these cells may be clinically undetectable or demonstrated only through testicular ultrasound. Larger "tumors" are usually associated to undiagnosed cases of CAH or with patients who have demonstrated poor compliance with their treatment.

Testicular "tumors" in CAH usually occur in early adult life (average age of 22.5 years). Smaller tumors are seen in younger patients, typically located in the hilum of the testis. In adults, the lesions may measure up to 10.0 cm. Eighty-three percent of tumors are bilateral. In contrast, LCTs are bilateral in 3% or less of cases. The lesions are unencapsulated and are light tan-brown in color due to the absence of lipids and the presence of cytoplasmic lipochrome pigment. They are usually lobulated as a result of the presence of prominent bands of fibrous connective tissue. Occasionally, multiple extra testicular nodules measuring up to 1.5 cm in diameter have been described along the spermatic cord or adjacent to the epididymis. Microscopically, there are sheets and nests of cells with abundant granular cytoplasm and relatively distinct cell borders. Nuclei are uniform, round to oval with one or two prominent small nucleoli (Figs. 12-77 and 12-78). Many of the tumor cells contain lipochrome pigment (lipofuscin). Mitoses are very uncommon. Invariably dense bands of deeply eosinophilic fibrous tissue intersect between the nests of tumor cells, a distinguishing feature that we have observed even on biopsy material (Fig. 12-77).

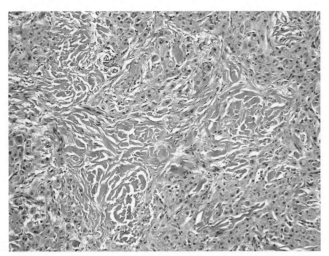

Figure 12-77 ■ Tumor of the adrenogenital syndrome. While the tumor cells may resemble those seen in LCT, the bands of densely eosinophilic (keloid-like) fibrous tissue are very characteristic.

As you might imagine from the microscopic description, there is great resemblance to Leydig cells. Indeed, LCT is the most common diagnosis made in these cases, a situation exacerbated by the fact that these tumors are also immunoreactive for inhibin and calretinin. Reinke crystals have not been described in tumors of CAH; however, are seen in up to 40% of LCT. Ultrastructurally, the cells have features of steroid producing cells with abundant smooth endoplasmic reticulum, numerous mitochondria, and accumulation of lipofuscin. The mitochondrial cristae may be lamellar or have a vesicular profile.

Another lesion that must be considered in the differential diagnosis is large cell calcifying Sertoli cell tumor (LCCSCT), an entity that is more thoroughly described in the section on SCT and its variants. Briefly, these tumors are usually <5 cm in size and microscopically are characterized by

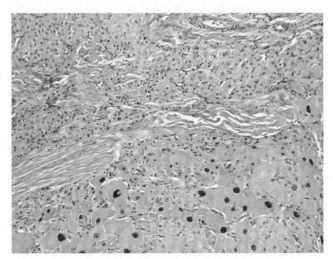

Figure 12-78 ■ Tumor of the adrenogenital syndrome. Tumor cells with endocrine-type atypia are present, as well as the characteristic densely eosinophilic (keloid-like) fibrous bands.

large polygonal cells with abundant eosinophilic cytoplasm, similar to Leydig cells, but arranged in sheets, nests, and cords embedded in a fibrous or myxoid stroma. Fifty percent of cases are associated with the presence of tumor cells within seminiferous. Variably sized stromal calcifications are a hallmark of this type of tumor, although they may be rare in selected cases. The tumor has a strong association with Carney syndrome, and up to a third of tumors are bilateral. These tumors cannot be distinguished from LCTs by immunohistochemistry. Additional details on LCCSCT are provided below.

Sertoli Cell Tumor, Not Otherwise Specified

SCTs are rare, comprising <1% of testicular neoplasms.[26,86,179,191,192] They were first described in the testis by Teilum who recognized their histologic similarity to SCTs of the canine testis. They may occur at any age and approximately 15% develop in children but rarely before the age of 10 years.[177] Patients characteristically present with a painless mass in a normally descended testis. Gynecomastia is evident in one-third of patients. Hormonal alterations in patients with SCT have been poorly documented; however, SCT should be in the differential diagnosis of prepubertal patients presenting with a testicular mass and gynecomastia. Three cases have been reported in boys with Peutz-Jeghers syndrome.[193] SCTs are usually benign, but about 10% behave in a malignant fashion.

Metastases will occur in approximately 10% of SCT.[192,194] Metastases are usually to inguinal or retroperitoneal lymph nodes, although skin and pulmonary involvement have been reported. Due to the rarity of this tumor, histologic criteria associated with malignant behavior may be unreliable. While the presence of metastasis remains as the best indicator of malignancy, large tumor size (>5 cm), VI, mitotic rate of >5/10 high-power fields, and solid and spindle cell architecture have been associated with disease progression.[192]

Gross Features

SCTs are well circumscribed, solid, and yellow-white or tan. The lesions may be lobulated and may contain small areas of hemorrhage. They are usually unilateral except in patients with Peutz-Jeghers syndrome.

Microscopic Features

Microscopic examination reveals mostly tubules but also cords, nests, and masses of tumor cells in a fibrous stroma (Fig. 12-79A and B). The tubules and cord-like structures vary in size and shape. The tubules may be round and hollow, solid, or elongated or may have a retiform pattern (Fig. 12-80). Some tumors may exhibit a predominant solid growth pattern (Fig. 12-81). A morphologic variant called sclerosing Sertoli cell tumor is characterized by the presence of prominent stromal sclerosis throughout the lesion although the growth pattern characteristics of

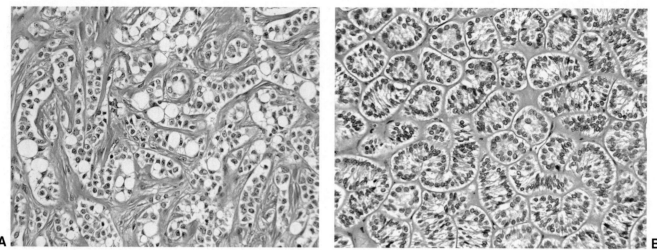

FIGURE 12-79 ■ **A:** Sertoli cell tumor. The tumor cells are arranged in tubules and cords. The tumor cells have scanty amphophilic cytoplasm. Many of the tumor cells are vacuolated, a feature that may be seen in this and other steroid-producing tumors. **B:** Sertoli cell tumor. A tubular pattern predominates. The tumor cells have finely stippled chromatin as well as occasional micronucleoli. The amount of cytoplasm is moderate, amphophilic, and reticulated.

the tumor cells remain the same[195] (Fig. 12-82). The clinical significance of this finding is uncertain. The sclerosing variant of SCT may be confused with adenomatoid tumor superficially although the former usually within the testicular parenchyma does not exhibit the degree of cytoplasmic vacuolization and sieve-like growth pattern seen in adenomatoid tumor, and is immunoreactive for sex cord rather than mesothelial markers.

The neoplastic cells usually have moderate amounts of pale or eosinophilic cytoplasm. Occasionally they contain abundant intracytoplasmic lipid giving them a clear or vacuolated appearance (Fig. 12-83). Most tumors have bland cytologic features with the cells exhibiting a vesicular nucleus

and a prominent central nucleolus. Pleomorphism may be evident in less differentiated tumors and a frankly malignant spindle cell component may be rarely encountered, even with heterologous differentiation. Electron microscopy may reveal Charcott-Böttcher filaments within the cytoplasm, which are characteristic of Sertoli cells.

Immunohistochemical Features

SCT are immunoreactive for vimentin, and staining for cytokeratin, inhibin and calretinin is variable[184–186,192] (Table 12-3). Cytokeratins and EMA are more likely to be expressed in LCT than in other types of sex cord–stromal

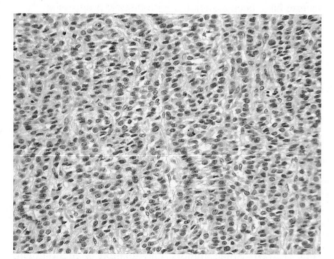

FIGURE 12-80 ■ Sertoli cell tumor. Tumor cells are arranged in cords. The intervening stroma is minimal. While there is some similarity to what can be seen in the tubular variant of seminoma (compare to image 17b), the nuclear features are quite different in these entities.

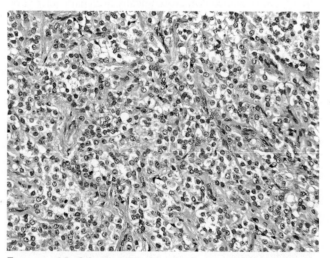

FIGURE 12-81 ■ SCT with a solid pattern of growth. Notice the presence of focal cytoplasmic clearing that could make a tumor such as this mistaken with seminoma. However, the presence of round-to-oval nuclei with finely stippled chromatin and micronucleoli seen in this image is not what is seen in seminoma.

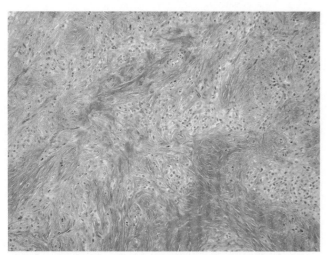

FIGURE 12-82 ■ SCT, sclerosing variant. Nests and cords of tumor cells with a moderate amount of clear to amphophilic cytoplasm are surrounded by abundant dense fibrous tissue.

tumors. Because they can coexpress calretinin, this marker cannot be used in isolation to differentiate them from adenomatoid tumor or mesothelioma. Markers typically seen in GCT are negative.[86]

Differential Diagnosis

The classification of SCT should be reserved for tumors composed entirely of Sertoli cells. Those neoplasms composed only partially of these cells should be classified as mixed or incompletely differentiated sex cord–stromal tumors. SCT must be distinguished from nonneoplastic, hyperplastic nodules of seminiferous tubules lined by Sertoli cells. These Sertoli cell nodules were previously mistakenly referred to as adenomas (Pick adenoma) (Fig. 12-84). They may contain central hyaline material resembling Call-Exner bodies or laminated calcifications. The nodules are usually small and are most frequently encountered in cryptorchid testes, in

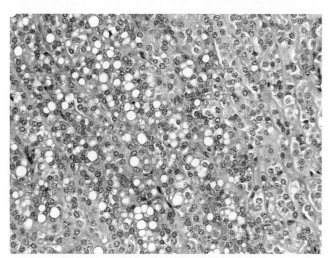

FIGURE 12-83 ■ SCT with cytoplasmic vacuolization. The classic nuclear features seen in SCT are retained.

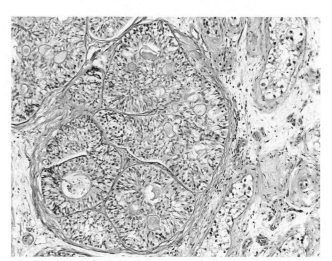

FIGURE 12-84 ■ Sertoli cell nodule. The Sertoli cells are immature and arranged around nodules of basement membrane–type material; similar to what is seen in gonadoblastoma. When seen adjacent to GCTs, this finding is thought to be evidence of dysgenesis. On occasion, it can be involved by IGCNU (see Fig. 12.9A). The adjacent tubules contain mature-appearing Sertoli cells.

atrophic scrotal testes, or adjacent to GCTs. In this setting, it is regarded by some as a sign of testicular dysgenesis, particularly when the Sertoli cells are immature (Fig. 12-9). SCT with a diffuse growth pattern and cytoplasmic eosinophilia may be confused with LCT. Immunohistochemistry may not aid in this differential diagnosis although Sertoli cell tumor is more likely to exhibit significant cytokeratin and EMA immunoreactivity. SCTs with clear cell features and diffuse growth pattern can easily be confused with seminoma (Fig. 12-81). The absence of intratubular germ cell neoplasia in the former and immunohistochemistry should help in arriving at the correct diagnosis.

Large Cell Calcifying Sertoli Cell Tumor

In 1980, Proppe and Scully described a subtype of SCT that they called large cell calcifying Sertoli cell tumor (LCCSCT).[196,197] It usually presents during the first three decades of life although cases in older males have been described. While patients may present exclusively with a testicular mass, given its strong association with Carney syndrome, their initial symptomatology could be related to other conditions such as pituitary adenomas, bilateral adrenocortical hyperplasia, cardiac myxomas, or other sex cord–stromal tumors. Besides gynecomastia and sexual precocity, other unusual associations have been described, including acromegaly, mucocutaneous pigmentation, sudden death, and Peutz-Jeghers syndrome. Approximately one-third of LCCSCTs are bilateral, and some will metastasize.[198] These tumors are usually <5 cm in size and microscopically are characterized by large polygonal cells with abundant eosinophilic cytoplasm arranged in sheets, nests and cords embedded in a fibrous or myxoid stroma (Fig. 12-85A and B). Tumor cells within seminiferous tubules are present in 50% of cases. Microcalcifications are usually abundant in the form of variably

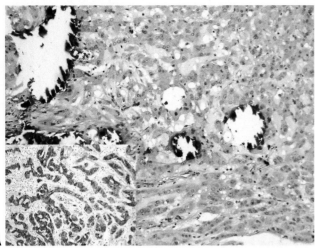 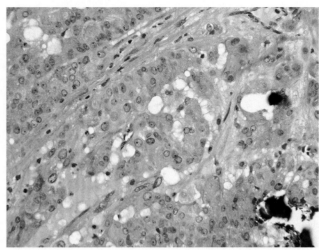

FIGURE 12-85 ■ **A:** Large cell calcifying SCT. **A:** The tumor cells are arranged in cords within a myxoid stroma containing calcifications. **Inset** reveals diffuse cytoplasmic immunoreactivity for inhibin. **B:** Large cell calcifying SCT. The tumor cells have abundant eosinophilic cytoplasm, round-to-vesicular nuclei with occasional nucleoli. Despite the cytologic similarity to LCT, notice the association with a myxoid stroma and microcalcifications.

sized basophilic, laminated calcific bodies. Ossification may also be present. A large series reported a metastatic rate of almost 20%, invariably in older and nonsyndromic patients.[197,199] LCCSCT has an immunophenotype that is virtually identical to other SCTs (Figs. 12-85A and 12-86). Aggressive tumors are more likely to be large (>4 cm) and have VI, cytologic atypia, and necrosis. LCCSCTs are often mistaken for LCT, but the abundant calcifications, frequent intratubular growth, absence of Reinke crystals, and unusual clinical associations should direct us toward the correct diagnosis (Box 12-14).

Granulosa Cell Tumor

There are two subtypes of granulosa cell tumor, adult and juvenile, similar to what is seen in the ovary. The adult variant of granulosa cell tumor very rarely develops in the testis

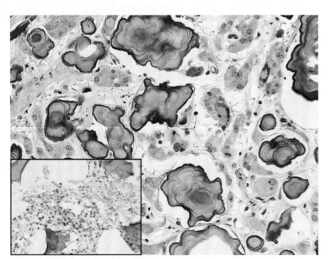

FIGURE 12-86 ■ Large cell calcifying Sertoli cell tumor. Abundant laminated calcifications are present while the tumor cells are less apparent. **Inset** demonstrates nuclear immunoreactivity for WT1.

with <30 bona fide cases reported in the literature.[179,180,200–202] They have been described in males between the ages of 21 and 73 years and usually present as a testicular mass that may have been present for several years. Up to 20% of cases may be associated with gynecomastia and, as such, urinary estrogen levels may be elevated. The tumors measure between 1 and 13 cm in greatest diameter. Grossly, the tumors are homogeneous or lobulated, yellow or yellow-tan and well circumscribed. Microscopically, the neoplastic cells are arranged in micro- or macrofollicular, solid, trabecular, insular, and gyriform patterns. Microfollicular pattern is the most common and is more likely to be associated with Call-Exner bodies (Fig. 12-87). The cells have scanty cytoplasm and pale, oval to elongated nuclei with longitudinal grooves. Metastases are rare.[202,203] Features associated with malignant behavior, as with other sex cord–stromal tumors, include, large size, mitotic activity above four per HPF, necrosis, and lymphovascular invasion. For this reason, these features must be included in the pathology report.

Juvenile granulosa cell tumors are the most common sex cord–stromal tumor of the infantile testis.[26,204,205] They are usually encountered in the first 6 months of life, with one isolated case reported in a 21-month-old and another in a 4-year-old.[206] Two cases developed in undescended testes. Juvenile granulosa cell tumors may arise in patients with an

---

Box 12-14 ● LARGE CELL CALCIFYING SERTOLI CELL TUMOR

- Up to 50% are associated with Carney syndrome
- Tumor cytology may be confused with Leydig cell tumor
- Tumor associated with myxoid stroma and calcifications
- Up to 50% of cases exhibit tumor cells within seminiferous tubules

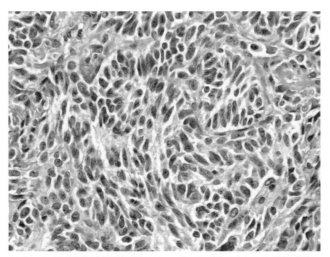

FIGURE 12-87 ■ Granulosa cell tumor, adult type. The tumor cells are elongated with inconspicuous nucleoli and occasional longitudinal nuclear grooves.

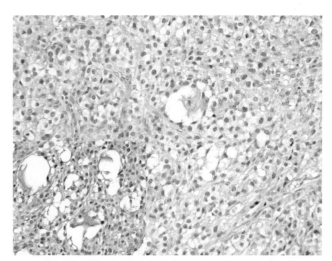

FIGURE 12-89 ■ Juvenile granulosa cell tumor. A solid area reveals the presence of microcysts containing basophilic or eosinophilic fluid. **Inset** shows the cyst fluid to be mucicarmine positive.

abnormal karyotype and ambiguous genitalia. Tumors may be solid, cystic, or both, and the cysts frequently contain a gelatinous material. Microscopically, the tumor exhibits either a follicular or solid pattern of growth (Fig. 12-88). The follicles vary greatly in size and typically contain eosinophilic fluid that is mucicarmine and PAS positive (Fig. 12-89). The cells lining the cysts are said to be follicular cells and have a modest amount of cytoplasm with round to oval nuclei. Grooves are not present. In the solid areas the cells are arranged in sheets, sometimes embedded in a loose, myxoid or hyalinizes stroma. These cells are characterized by a moderate to large amount of eosinophilic cytoplasm and round to irregular hyperchromatic nuclei. Although mitoses may be plentiful, no testicular tumor of this type has metastasized.[86,207]

Both subtypes of granulosa cell tumor are usually immunoreactive for inhibin. Cytokeratins may be focally positive in the adult type while the cells lining the follicles of juvenile granulosa cell tumors are likely to express cytokeratins.

Tumors of the Fibroma–Thecoma Group

These tumors very rarely occur in the testis, but, when they do, they resemble their ovarian counterparts[26,86,208] (Fig. 12-90). Mean age at presentation is 30 years, and, to this date, all cases have had a benign outcome. Similar to ovarian tumors, they are immunoreactive for estrogen/progesterone receptors as well as inhibin and calretinin. The lesion may be difficult to differentiate from an otherwise unclassified spindle cell sex cord–stromal tumor. The

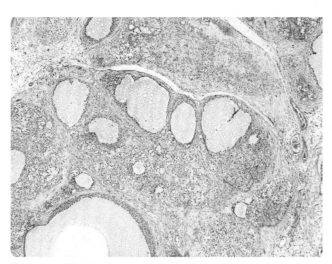

FIGURE 12-88 ■ Juvenile granulosa cell tumor. Low-power magnification shows solid and fluid-filled cystic components, the latter of variable size. A solid area reveals the presence of a microcyst containing basophilic or eosinophilic fluid.

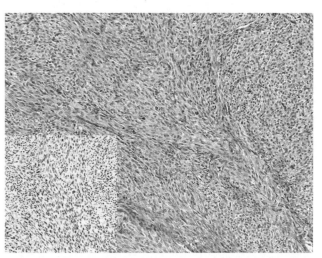

FIGURE 12-90 ■ Testicular fibroma. In this cellular variant, the plump fusiform cells are arranged in fascicles. **Inset** exhibits diffuse nuclear immunoreactivity for estrogen receptor. Immunoreactivity for steroid receptors (ER/PR) may be helpful in establishing the correct diagnosis.

morphologic criteria we have used in this setting include the presence of more sparse cellularity in the fibroma–thecoma tumors, together with zones of variable cellularity, typical fibrous-looking cells, and estrogen/progesterone expression. Obviously, transitions to more typical sex cord–stromal components are lacking.

Sex Cord–Gonadal Stromal Tumors, Mixed or Incompletely Differentiated (Undifferentiated) Forms

As you might expect, these two categories include tumors with more than one identifiable sex cord–stromal element as well as tumors in which the exact gonadal stromal cell of origin cannot be established with certainty.[86,88,209,210] Truly mixed sex cord–stromal cell tumors of the testis are rare, unlike what has been described in the ovary. The term unclassified sex cord–stromal tumor is used when the lesions lacks morphologic evidence of differentiation toward a specific type of differentiation but is deemed to belong to the gonadal stromal category (Fig. 12-91). However, there should be at least focal expression of one or more of the sex cord tumor–related antigens by immunohistochemistry (Table 12-3). We recently encountered a case that was composed predominantly of spindle cells and microcysts reminiscent of microcystic stromal tumor of the ovary, including strong and diffuse expression of β-catenin. They can exhibit a dominant spindle cell morphology or be associated with epithelial foci, either well or poorly differentiated. These neoplasms may occur at any age although more than half of the patients are either children or infants. Painless testicular enlargement is the most common presenting symptom, which is infrequently associated with gynecomastia. Approximately 30% of tumors presenting in patients older than 10 years of age are malignant while tumors presenting in younger patients follow a benign course.

Tumors Containing Both Sex Cord–Stromal and Germ Cell Elements

Gonadoblastoma

Gonadoblastomas are rare neoplasms composed of sex cord–stromal elements intimately admixed with germ cells.[86,209,211] These tumors generally arise in chromosomally abnormal individuals with dysgenetic gonads; 80% of cases occur in phenotypic females. Most patients are negative for sex chromatin associated with karyotypes 46, XY or mosaicism of 45, XO/46, XY.[212,213] Patients usually present with cryptorchidism, hypospadia, and internal female genitalia, although two cases have been reported arising in a scrotal testis. The gonads have features of mixed gonadal dysgenesis. Most patients are younger than 20 years of age and one third of cases are bilateral. Up to 60% of patients develop an invasive GCT, which is usually seminoma (50%) but may be YST or EC (10%). Metastasis from the associated GCT may occur.[214]

The tumors may be microscopic but, when visible, they are tan to yellow-brown. The microscopic appearance is distinctive and consists of tumor nests surrounded by connective tissue, which can exhibit features of ovarian-like stroma. The nests contain germ cells with clear cytoplasm, irregular nuclear contours, coarse chromatin, and prominent nucleoli, identical to intratubular germ cell neoplasia (Fig. 12-92). They are immunoreactive for CD117, PLAP, and Oct4.[215,216] The sex cord elements resemble immature Sertoli cells and are immunoreactive for inhibin. The nests may contain hyalinized eosinophilic deposits of basement membrane–like material, resembling Call-Exner bodies. Calcifications are common; the presence of an associated invasive GCT may efface the foci of gonadoblastoma. The prognosis of patients with gonadoblastoma is excellent with tumor-related morbidity usually dependent on the presence and extent of the associated GCT component.

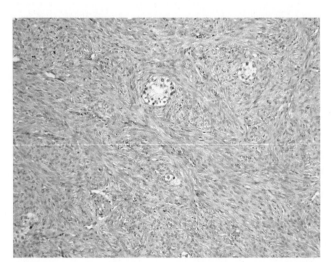

FIGURE 12-91 ■ Sex cord–stromal tumor, unclassified. The tumor cells are mostly spindled. Infiltration around seminiferous tubules is evident. The tumor cells were immunoreactive for inhibin.

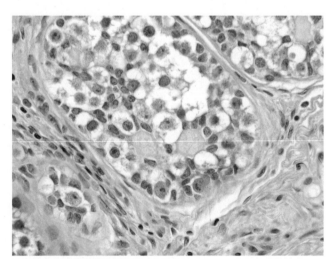

FIGURE 12-92 ■ Gonadoblastoma. The nests of tumor contain a mixture of immature Sertoli cells and germinal cells, including intratubular germ cell neoplasia.

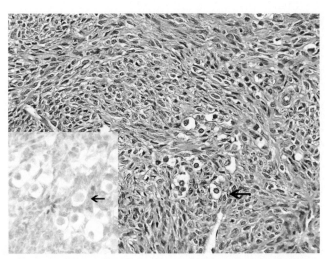

FIGURE 12-93 ■ Sex cord–stromal tumor with entrapped germ cells. The gonadal stromal component is undifferentiated while the entrapped germinal cells lack malignant features, bringing to mind spermatogonia. **Inset** demonstrates that both components lack immunoreactivity for Oct4. The lack of immunoreactivity for Oct4, SALL4, and podoplanin confirms that the germinal component is not seminoma (*arrows*).

Germ Cell/Sex Cord–Gonadal Stromal Tumor, Unclassified

This is a controversial entity that is also composed of an admixture of germ cells and sex cord–stromal elements but which occurs in phenotypically and genotypically normal males.[86,191,217,218] To date, there have been no endocrine abnormalities described with this lesion. The tumor may be large, measuring up to 12 cm in diameter. It is usually solid, gray-white, and well circumscribed. Microscopic examination reveals an admixture of germ cells and sex cord–stromal elements not arranged in nests, but instead, having a trabecular, tubular, or haphazard infiltrative pattern (Fig. 12-93). In our opinion, these tumors are likely to represent sex cord–stromal tumors with entrapped germ cells rather than true mixed tumors, an opinion that is supported by data showing that the germ cell component lacks immunoreactivity for PLAP and CD117.[210] Two cases we have seen recently also lack immunoreactivity for Oct4, further supporting this hypothesis. In fact, the cytologic features and immunophenotype is identical to spermatogonia.

Of course there is always the possibility of a true collision tumor.[180] We have seen a case of SCT associated with intratubular germ cell neoplasia and minimal invasive seminoma.

MISCELLANEOUS TUMORS

Lymphoma and Leukemia

Malignant lymphoma represents up to 5% of testicular neoplasms. It is the most common bilateral tumor (either synchronous or metachronous) and the most common testicular tumor

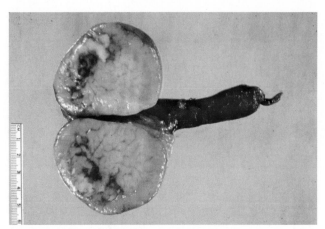

FIGURE 12-94 ■ Lymphoma gross. The tumor is fleshy, white-tan, and exhibits areas of hemorrhage and necrosis. Grossly this tumor is virtually impossible to differentiate from seminoma.

in men above the age of 60.[219,220] The majority of patients have localized disease but in a third of cases testicular involvement is part of either regional or systemic disease.[221,222] Survival is dependent on the type of lymphoma, associated sclerosis, and clinical stage, with recent publications reporting improving survival statistics, probably due to earlier diagnosis and better therapy. To accept a lymphoma as primary in the testis, imaging studies, peripheral blood, and bone marrow assessment must document that disease is limited to this site; even bilateral disease and/or limited retroperitoneal lymph node involvement (clinical stage II disease) should call testicular origin into question, even though it may be associated with better outcome that more advanced disease.

Grossly, the testicular parenchyma is replaced by a single or multiple fleshy, tan and homogeneous mass, which may extend into the adnexal structures (Fig. 12-94). Involvement of adnexal and peritesticular soft tissue is more common than in the cases of germ cell and sex cord–stromal tumors. On microscopy the tumor cells can efface the testicular parenchyma although an interstitial pattern of infiltration sparing the seminiferous tubules is common (Fig. 12-95A and B). It is important to note that tumor cells may be present within seminiferous tubules, superficially mimicking intratubular germ cell neoplasia (Fig. 12-95B).

The majority of lymphomas that involve the testis are of diffuse large cell type with most having a B-cell phenotype. Rare cases of anaplastic large cell, T cell, natural killer cell, MALT, and Hodgkin disease have been described.[223,224] Lymphoblastic T-cell lymphoma is more common in children and young adults (Fig. 12-96).

Lymphomas will express hematopoietic markers in accordance with its line of differentiation. They will not express cytokeratin or PLAP. We have seen a single large cell lymphoma with focal nuclear immunoreactivity for Oct4 (Fig. 12-34), but other GCT markers were negative while CD20 was positive. It is worth remembering that

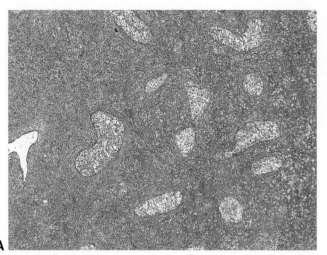
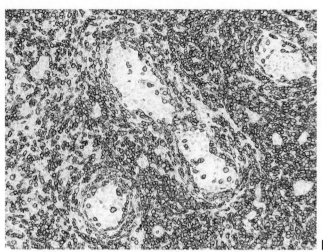

FIGURE 12-95 ■ **A:** Malignant lymphoma. At low-power magnification, there is a dense tumor infiltrate surrounding seminiferous tubules. **B:** Malignant lymphoma. An immunohistochemical stain for CD20 highlights the presence of tumor cells within the seminiferous tubules, which may mimic IGCNU (also see Fig. 12-34.)

anaplastic large cell lymphoma is likely to express CD30, similar to EC.

Primary leukemic tumors (granulocytic/myeloid sarcoma) of the testis are very rare.[225] Leukemic infiltration of the testis is most commonly seen on biopsy specimens in patents being evaluated for relapse after systemic therapy.[226–229] However, it may be seen at autopsy in up to 65% and 30% of patients with acute leukemia and chronic leukemia, respectively. Symptomatic enlargement of the gonad is encountered in 5% of cases. On microscopy, leukemic cells infiltrate between the seminiferous tubules and rarely extend into the seminiferous tubule itself. Marker expression will include MPO, lysozyme, CD68, and C-kit although the precise expression pattern will depend on the precise cell lineage. Common germ cell markers will be negative.

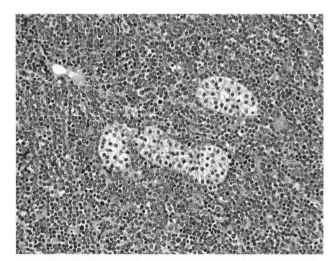

FIGURE 12-96 ■ Lymphoblastic lymphoma occupying the testis of a child. Tumor cells surround seminiferous tubules.

Plasma Cell Neoplasms

Involvement of the testis by multiple myeloma is rare and usually found at autopsy.[191] Rare cases of localized testicular plasmacytoma have been described but it is more likely to be an early manifestation of regional or systemic disease.[230] Mean age at presentation is in the sixth decade and up to a third of cases are bilateral. The tumor cells can involve the testis in an interstitial pattern of diffusely with effacement of the testicular parenchyma.

The differential diagnosis of testicular lymphoma, leukemia, and plasma cell neoplasms includes orchitis, seminoma, and SS. Lymphomas characteristically have a diffuse interstitial growth pattern but a similar pattern can be encountered in some seminoma. Peritumoral stromal sclerosis is also more common in association with hematopoietic neoplasms but can be occasionally in other primary tumors such as seminoma. While intratubular growth can be seen in lymphomas and many other primary and metastatic tumors, these cells are usually present free-floating in the lumen at all levels within the germinal epithelium. The classic perinuclear clearing seen in IGCNU is lacking. Rarely solid variants of EC and YST may enter the differential diagnosis since EC has nuclear cytology that is quite different to that seen in hematopoietic neoplasms and is rarely pure solid. Solid YSTs are also rarely pure; the nuclear and cytoplasmic features do not mimic what is seen in hematopoietic neoplasms. In cases of EC and YST, ICGNU should be present in adjacent seminiferous tubules. Seminoma is associated with cytoplasmic clearing, centrally located nuclei that are round to rhomboid with coarsely stippled but evenly distributed chromatin and prominent nucleolus. The margination of nuclear chromatin and irregular nuclear contours seen in lymphomas is characteristically absent in seminomas. Orchitis is characterized by a mixed inflammatory infiltrate which may include acute inflammatory cells, mature plasma cells, and lymphocytes.

Metastatic tumors such as melanoma may be mistaken for a hematopoietic neoplasm although these rarely present as a testicular primary but rather are encountered in the setting of disseminated disease. In these cases, the cytoplasm is usually more eosinophilic or spindled, and at least some nuclei contain large eosinophilic nucleoli. Lack of expression of any hematopoietic marker but rather expression markers documenting melanocytic differentiation may aid in the diagnosis, although a proper clinical history usually makes these stains unnecessary.

MESENCHYMAL TUMORS OF THE TESTIS

Primary mesenchymal tumors of the testis are rare since these neoplasms are unlikely to arise within the testicular parenchyma, but the parenchyma may be involved secondarily by tumors arising in the adjacent soft tissues. The possibility of a sex cord–stromal tumor with prominent spindle cell morphology should always be considered in the differential diagnosis, remembering that these tumors will express inhibin while other mesenchymal tumors will not. The possibility of metastatic disease should always enter in the differential diagnosis. If primary in the testis, these tumors may be derived from stromal cells of the testicular instertitium. Benign examples documented in the literature include leiomyomas,[231] neurofibromas,[232] hemangiomas,[233,234] and epithelioid hemangiomas.[235,236] Sarcomas reported in the literature include rhabdomyosarcoma,[237,238] leiomyosarcoma,[239] hemangioendothelioma,[240] Kaposi sarcoma,[241] osteosarcoma, and chondrosarcoma.[242] Care must be taken to search for the presence of intratubular germ cell neoplasia or other GCT components, particularly in young patients. We have observed several cases in which the dominant invasive tumor was sarcoma but other GCT components were present, thus fulfilling the criteria for GCT with secondary somatic malignancy, as described earlier in this chapter.

Box 12-15 ● METASTATIC TUMORS TO THE TESTIS

- Lymphoma and melanoma are the most common nonepithelial tumors
- Prostate, kidney, and colon are the most common epithelial tumors
- Usually seen in advanced disease although rarely may be the initial site of metastasis
- Tumor cells may be present within seminiferous tubules, mimicking IGCNU
- Differential diagnosis will drive the immunohistochemical workup

---

METASTATIC TUMORS

Metastasis to the testis from solid tumors is rare and usually presents in patients with known primary disease elsewhere and known metastatic disease.[243–245] It is typically encountered in patients beyond the age of 50 years (Box 12-15).

The most common primary sites include prostate (Fig. 12-97A and B) and lung, followed by melanoma (Fig. 12-98) of the skin, colon, and kidney[244] (Fig. 12-68A–C). In children the most common tumors to metastasize to the testis include neuroblastoma and rhabdomyosarcoma.[246–248] Metastatic tumors are commonly bilateral, multifocal, and frequently exhibit VI. Good clinical history, and sometimes immunohistochemistry, will aid at arriving at the correct diagnosis. Rarely will a metastatic tumor present as a testicular primary, and in these cases, it is important to remember that some of these tumors may mimic primary disease.[244,249–251] Metastatic melanoma with clear cell features may mimic either seminoma or a sex cord–stromal tumor while metastatic renal cell carcinoma may mimic a sex cord–stromal tumor as well. A poorly differentiated carcinoma may simulate an EC.

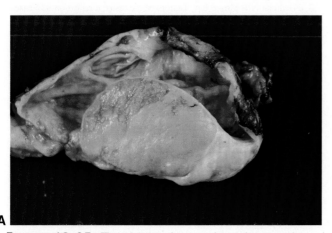

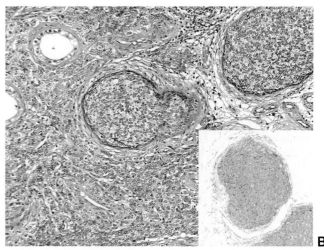

A   **B**

FIGURE 12-97 ■ **A:** Metastatic prostatic carcinoma to the testis. Grossly, the testicular parenchyma contains an ill-defined mass with no distinguishing features. **B:** Metastatic prostatic carcinoma to the testis. Tumor cells infiltrate the testicular parenchyma and are present within tubules. **Inset** demonstrates an immunohistochemical stain for PSA, which highlights the tumor cells within the seminiferous tubules.

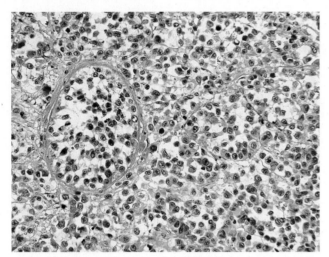

Figure 12-98 ■ Metastatic melanoma to the testis. This tumor was mistaken for seminoma, for obvious reasons. Notice that tumor cells are present within a seminiferous tubule.

We have seen two cases in which involvement of the testis by prostatic carcinoma was primarily intratubular and in both cases, a primary GCT was considered by the referring pathologist. In difficult cases an immunohistochemical panel that includes a broad spectrum of entities may be required, but there is no substitute for a detailed clinical history.[231]

REFERENCES

1. Trainer TD. Histology of the normal testis. *Am J Surg Pathol* 1987;11:797–809.
2. Vilar O. Histology of the human testis from the neonatal period to adolescence. In: Rosenberg E, Paulsen CA, eds. *Advances in Experimental and Medicine and Biology*. New York: Plenum Press; 1970:95–111.
3. Aumuller G, Schulze C, Viebahn C. Intermediate filaments in sertoli cells. *Microsc Res Tech* 1992;20:50–72.
4. Stosiek P, Kasper M, Karsten U. Expression of cytokeratins 8 and 18 in human sertoli cells of immature and atrophic seminiferous tubules. *Differentiation* 1990;43:66–70.
5. Moore K, Persaud TVN. *The Developing Human*. Philadelphia, PA: WB Saunders; 1993.
6. Moore KL, Persaud TVN. *The Developing Human: Clinically Oriented Embryology*. Philadelphia, PA: Saunders; 1998.
7. Trainer T. Testis and excretory duct system. In: Sternberg SS, ed. *Histology for Pathologists*. Philadelphia, PA: Lippincott-Raven Publishers; 1997:1019–1037.
8. Schulze C. Sertoli cells and leydig cells in man. *Adv Anat Embryol Cell Biol* 1984;88:1–104.
9. Nagano T, Otsuki I. Reinvestigation of the fine structure of reinke's crystal in the human testicular interstitial cell. *J Cell Biol* 1971;51:148–161.
10. Davidoff MS, Schulze W, Middendorff R, et al. The leydig cell of the human testis—a new member of the diffuse neuroendocrine system. *Cell Tissue Res* 1993;271:429–439.
11. Regadera J, Codesal J, Paniagua R, et al. Immunohistochemical and quantitative study of interstitial and intratubular leydig cells in normal men, cryptorchidism, and klinefelter's syndrome. *J Pathol* 1991;164:299–306.
12. Dinges HP, Zatloukal K, Schmid C, et al. Co-expression of cytokeratin and vimentin filaments in rete testis and epididymis. An immunohistochemical study. *Virchows Arch A Pathol Anat Histopathol* 1991;418:119–127.
13. Rolnick D, Kawanoue S, Szanto P, et al. Anatomical incidence of testicular appendages. *J Urol* 1968;100:755–756.
14. Srigley JR. The paratesticular region: histoanatomic and general considerations. *Semin Diagn Pathol* 2000;17:258–269.
15. Tickoo S, Reuter VE, Chang S, et al. College of American Pathologists (CAP) *Protocol for the Examination of Specimens from Patients with Malignant Germ Cell and Sex Cord-Stromal Tumors of the Testis*. 7th ed. 2008:1–17.
16. Edge SB, Byrd DR, Compton CC, et al., eds. *AJCC Cancer Staging Manual*. 7th ed. New York: Springer; 2010.
17. Yilmaz A, Cheng T, Zhang J, et al. Testicular hilum and vascular invasion predict advanced clinical stage in nonseminomatous germ cell tumors. *Mod Pathol* 2013;26:579–586.
18. Chung P, Daugaard G, Tyledesley S, et al. Prognostic factors for relapse in stage i seminoma managed with surveillance: a validation study [abstract]. *J Clin Oncol* 2010;28:7S.
19. Carver BS, Cronin AM, Eggener S, et al. The total number of retroperitoneal lymph nodes resected impacts clinical outcome after chemotherapy for metastatic testicular cancer. *Urology* 2010;75:1431–1435.
20. Beck SD, Cheng L, Bihrle R, et al. Does the presence of extranodal extension in pathological stage b1 nonseminomatous germ cell tumor necessitate adjuvant chemotherapy? *J Urol* 2007;177:944–946.
21. Warde P, Specht L, Horwich A, et al. Prognostic factors for relapse in stage i seminoma managed by surveillance: a pooled analysis. *J Clin Oncol* 2002;20:4448–4452.
22. van Dijk MR, Steyerberg EW, Habbema JD. Survival of non-seminomatous germ cell cancer patients according to the igcc classification: an update based on meta-analysis. *Eur J Cancer* 2006;42:820–826.
23. de Wit R, Stoter G, Kaye SB, et al. Importance of bleomycin in combination chemotherapy for good-prognosis testicular nonseminoma: a randomized study of the european organization for research and treatment of cancer genitourinary tract cancer cooperative group. *J Clin Oncol* 1997;15:1837–1843.
24. Bosl GJ, Reuter VE, Chaganti RS, et al. Cancer of the testis. In: Devita V, Lawrence T, Rosenberg S, eds. *Cancer: Principles and Practice of Oncology*. Philadelphia, PA: Lippincott Williams & Wilkins; 2011:1280–1301.
25. International Germ Cell Cancer Collaborative Group. International Germ Cell Consensus Classification: a prognostic factor-based staging system for metastatic germ cell cancers. *J Clin Oncol* 1997;15:594–603.
26. Ulbright TM, Amin MB, Young RH. Tumours of the testis, adnexa, spermatic cord, and scrotum. In: Rosai J, ed. *Atlas of Tumor Pathology*. Washington, DC: Armed Forces Institute of Pathology; 1999:59–181.
27. Friedman NB, Ash JE. Armed Forces Institute of Pathology (U.S.). *Atlas of Genitourinary Pathology*. Washington, DC: Army Institute of Pathology; 1946.
28. Friedman NB, Moore RA. Tumors of the testis; a report on 922 cases. *Mil Surg* 1946;99:573–593.
29. Dixon FJ, Moore RA. Tumors of the male sex organs. *Atlas of Tumor Pathology*, fascicles 31b and 32. Washington, DC: Army Institute of Pathology; 1952.
30. Melicow M. Classification of tumors of the testis. A clinical and pathological study based on 105 primary and 13 secondary cases in adults, adn 3 primary and 4 secondary cases in children. *J Urol* 1955;73:547–574.
31. Mostofi FK, Price EB. *Tumors of the Male Genital System*. Washington, DC: Armed Forces Institute of Pathology; 1973.
32. Bosl GJ, Motzer RJ. Testicular germ-cell cancer. *N Engl J Med* 1997;337:242–253.
33. Siegel R, Naishadham D, Jemal A. Cancer Statistics, 2013. *CA Cancer J Clin* 2013; 63:11-30
34. Looijenga LH, Oosterhuis JW. Pathogenesis of testicular germ cell tumours. *Rev Reprod* 1999;4:90–100.
35. Oosterhuis JW, Looijenga LH. Current views on the pathogenesis of testicular germ cell tumours and perspectives for future research: highlights of the 5th copenhagen workshop on carcinoma in situ and cancer of the testis. *APMIS* 2003;111:280–289.

36. Chaganti RS, Houldsworth J. Genetics and biology of adult human male germ cell tumors. *Cancer Res* 2000;60:1475–1482.

37. Skakkebaek NE, Rajpert-De Meyts E, Jorgensen N, et al. Germ cell cancer and disorders of spermatogenesis: an environmental connection? *APMIS* 1998;106:3–11; discussion 12.

38. Chaganti RS, Houldsworth J. The cytogenetic theory of the pathogenesis of human adult male germ cell tumors. Review article. *APMIS* 1998;106:80–83; discussion 83–84.

39. McGlynn KA, Cook MB. Etiologic factors in testicular germ-cell tumors. *Future Oncol* 2009;5:1389–1402.

40. Purdue MP, Devesa SS, Sigurdson AJ, et al. International patterns and trends in testis cancer incidence. *Int J Cancer* 2005;115:822–827.

41. Patel SR, Kvols LK, Richardson RL. Familial testicular cancer: report of six cases and review of the literature. *Mayo Clin Proc* 1990;65:804–808.

42. Forman D, Oliver RT, Brett AR, et al. Familial testicular cancer: a report of the uk family register, estimation of risk and an hla class 1 sib-pair analysis. *Br J Cancer* 1992;65:255–262.

43. Aetiology of testicular cancer: association with congenital abnormalities, age at puberty, infertility, and exercise. United Kingdom Testicular Cancer Study Group. *BMJ* 1994;308:1393–1399.

44. Manecksha RP, Fitzpatrick JM. Epidemiology of testicular cancer. *BJU Int* 2009;104:1329–1333.

45. Giwercman A, Grindsted J, Hansen B, et al. Testicular cancer risk in boys with maldescended testis: a cohort study. *J Urol* 1987;138:1214–1216.

46. Pottern LM, Brown LM, Hoover RN, et al. Testicular cancer risk among young men: role of cryptorchidism and inguinal hernia. *J Natl Cancer Inst* 1985;74:377–381.

47. Halme A, Kellokumpu-Lehtinen P, Lehtonen T, et al. Morphology of testicular germ cell tumours in treated and untreated cryptorchidism. *Br J Urol* 1989;64:78–83.

48. Giwercman A, Muller J, Skakkebaek NE. Carcinoma in situ of the undescended testis. *Semin Urol* 1988;6:110–119.

49. Sharpe RM, Skakkebaek NE. Are oestrogens involved in falling sperm counts and disorders of the male reproductive tract? *Lancet* 1993;341:1392–1395.

50. Manuel M, Katayama PK, Jones HW Jr. The age of occurrence of gonadal tumors in intersex patients with a y chromosome. *Am J Obstet Gynecol* 1976;124:293–300.

51. Rutgers JL, Scully RE. The androgen insensitivity syndrome (testicular feminization): a clinicopathologic study of 43 cases. *Int J Gynecol Pathol* 1991;10:126–144.

52. Skakkebaek NE, Berthelsen JG, Giwercman A, et al. Carcinoma-in-situ of the testis: possible origin from gonocytes and precursor of all types of germ cell tumours except spermatocytoma. *Int J Androl* 1987;10:19–28.

53. Gondos B, Migliozzi JA. Intratubular germ cell neoplasia. *Semin Diagn Pathol* 1987;4:292–303.

54. Bosl GJ, Dmitrovsky E, Reuter VE, et al. Isochromosome of the short arm of chromosome 12: clinically useful markers for male germ cell tumors. *J Natl Cancer Inst* 1989;81:1874–1878.

55. Motzer RJ, Rodriguez E, Reuter VE, et al. Genetic analysis as an aid in diagnosis for patients with midline carcinomas of uncertain histologies. *J Natl Cancer Inst* 1991;83:341–346.

56. Mukherjee AB, Murty VV, Rodriguez E, et al. Detection and analysis of origin of i(12p), a diagnostic marker of human male germ cell tumors, by fluorescence in situ hybridization. *Genes Chromosomes Cancer* 1991;3:300–307.

57. Dieckmann KP, Skakkebaek NE. Carcinoma in situ of the testis: review of biological and clinical features. *Int J Cancer* 1999;83:815–822.

58. Montironi R. Intratubular germ cell neoplasia of the testis: Testicular intraepithelial neoplasia. *Eur Urol* 2002;41:651–654.

59. Gondos B, Berthelsen JG, Skakkebaek NE. Intratubular germ cell neoplasia (carcinoma in situ): a preinvasive lesion of the testis. *Ann Clin Lab Sci* 1983;13:185–192.

60. Skakkebaek NE. Atypical germ cells in the adjacent "normal" tissue of testicular tumours. *Acta Pathol Microbiol Scand [A]* 1975;83:127–130.

61. Giwercman A, Brunn E, Frimodt-Moller C, et al. Prevalence of carcinoma in situ and other histopathologicl abnormalities in testis of men with a history of cryptorchidism. *J Urol* 1989;142:998–1001.

62. Skakkebaek NE. Carcinoma in situ of the testis: frequency and relationship to invasive germ cell tumours in infertile men. N. E. Skakkebaek. Histopathology 1978;2;157–170. *Histopathology* 2002;41:2.

63. Skakkebaek NE. Carcinoma in situ of the testis: frequency and relationship to invasive germ cell tumours in infertile men. *Histopathology* 1978;2:157–170.

64. von der Maase H, Rorth M, Walbom-Jorgensen S, et al. Carcinoma in situ of contralateral testis in patients with testicular germ cell cancer: study of 27 cases in 500 patients. *Br Med J (Clin Res Ed)* 1986;293:1398–1401.

65. von der Maase H, Meinecke B, Skakkebaek NE. Residual carcinoma-in-situ of contralateral testis after chemotherapy. *Lancet* 1988;1:477–478.

66. Jacobsen GK, Henriksen OB, von der Maase H. Carcinoma in situ of testicular tissue adjacent to malignant germ-cell tumors: a study of 105 cases. *Cancer* 1981;47:2660–2662.

67. Manivel JC, Simonton S, Wold LE, et al. Absence of intratubular germ cell neoplasia in testicular yolk sac tumors in children. A histochemical and immunohistochemical study. *Arch Pathol Lab Med* 1988;112:641–645.

68. Hu LM, Phillipson J, Barsky SH. Intratubular germ cell neoplasia in infantile yolk sac tumor. Verification by tandem repeat sequence in situ hybridization. *Diagn Mol Pathol* 1992;1:118–128.

69. Ulbright TM, Gersell DJ. Rete testis hyperplasia with hyaline globule formation. A lesion simulating yolk sac tumor. *Am J Surg Pathol* 1991;15:66–74.

70. Manivel JC, Jessurun J, Wick MR, et al. Placental alkaline phosphatase immunoreactivity in testicular germ-cell neoplasms. *Am J Surg Pathol* 1987;11:21–29.

71. Wick MR, Swanson PE, Manivel JC. Placental-like alkaline phosphatase reactivity in human tumors: an immunohistochemical study of 520 cases. *Hum Pathol* 1987;18:946–954.

72. Burke AP, Mostofi FK. Intratubular malignant germ cells in testicular biopsies: clinical course and identification by staining for placental alkaline phosphatase. *Mod Pathol* 1988;1:475–479.

73. Giwercman A, Cantell L, Marks A. Placental-like alkaline phosphatase as a marker of carcinoma-in-situ of the testis. Comparison with monoclonal antibodies m2a and 43-9f. *APMIS* 1991;99:586–594.

74. Leroy X, Augusto D, Leteurtre E, et al. Cd30 and cd117 (c-kit) used in combination are useful for distinguishing embryonal carcinoma from seminoma. *J Histochem Cytochem* 2002;50:283–285.

75. Giwercman A, Lindenberg S, Kimber SJ, et al. Monoclonal antibody 43-9f as a sensitive immunohistochemical marker of carcinoma in situ of human testis. *Cancer* 1990;65:1135–1142.

76. Marks A, Sutherland DR, Bailey D, et al. Characterization and distribution of an oncofetal antigen (m2a antigen) expressed on testicular germ cell tumours. *Br J Cancer* 1999;80:569–578.

77. Looijenga LH, Stoop H, de Leeuw HP, et al. Pou5f1 (oct3/4) identifies cells with pluripotent potential in human germ cell tumors. *Cancer Res* 2003;63:2244–2250.

78. Cao D, Guo S, Allan RW, et al. Sall4 is a novel sensitive and specific marker of ovarian primitive germ cell tumors and is particularly useful in distinguishing yolk sac tumor from clear cell carcinoma. *Am J Surg Pathol* 2009;33:894–904.

79. Cao D, Li J, Guo CC, et al. SALL4 is a novel diagnostic marker for testicular germ cell tumors. *Am J Surg Pathol* 2009;33:1065–1077.

80. Sonne SB, Herlihy AS, Hoei-Hansen CE, et al. Identity of m2a (d2-40) antigen and gp36 (aggrus, t1a-2, podoplanin) in human developing testis, testicular carcinoma in situ and germ-cell tumours. *Virchows Arch* 2006;449:200–206.

81. Lau SK, Weiss LM, Chu PG. D2-40 immunohistochemistry in the differential diagnosis of seminoma and embryonal carcinoma: a comparative immunohistochemical study with kit (cd117) and cd30. *Mod Pathol* 2007;20:320–325.

82. Mostofi FK, Sesterhenn I, Sobin LH. *Histological Typing of Testis Tumours*. Berlin, Germany: Springer; 1998.

83. Ulbright TM. Germ cell neoplasms of the testis. *Am J Surg Pathol* 1993;17:1075–1091.

84. Jacobsen GK, von der Maase H, Specht L, et al. Histopathological features in stage I seminoma treated with orchiectomy only. *J Urol Pathol* 1995;3:85–94.

85. Babaian RJ, Zagars GK. Testicular seminoma: the M. D. Anderson experience. An analysis of pathological and patient characteristics, and treatment recommendations. *J Urol* 1988;139:311–314.

86. Eble J, Sauter G, Epstein J, et al. *Pathology and Genetics of Tumours of the Urinary System and Male Genital Organs*. Lyon, France: IARC Press; 2004.

87. Ulbright T, Berney DM. Testicular and paratesticular tumors. In: Mills SE, ed. *Diagnostic Surgical Pathology*. Philadelphia, PA: Lippincott Williams & Wilkins; 2010:1944–2004.

88. Kay R. Prepubertal testicular tumor registry. *J Urol* 1993;150:671–674.

89. Hori K, Uematsu K, Yasoshima H, et al. Testicular seminoma with human chorionic gonadotropin production. *Pathol Int* 1997;47:592–599.

90. Ulbright TM. Morphologic variation in seminoma. *Am J Clin Pathol* 1994;102:395–396.

91. Henley JD, Young RH, Wade CL, et al. Seminomas with exclusive intertubular growth: a report of 12 clinically and grossly inconspicuous tumors. *Am J Surg Pathol* 2004;28:1163–1168.

92. Wilkins BS, Williamson JM, O'Brien CJ. Morphological and immunohistological study of testicular lymphomas. *Histopathology* 1989;15:147–156.

93. Zhao X, Wei YQ, Kariya Y, et al. Accumulation of gamma/delta t cells in human dysgerminoma and seminoma: roles in autologous tumor killing and granuloma formation. *Immunol Invest* 1995;24:607–618.

94. Jacobsen GK, Jacobsen M, Clausen PP. Distribution of tumor-associated antigens in the various histologic components of germ cell tumors of the testis. *Am J Surg Pathol* 1981;5:257–266.

95. Battifora H, Sheibani K, Tubbs RR, et al. Antikeratin antibodies in tumor diagnosis. Distinction between seminoma and embryonal carcinoma. *Cancer* 1984;54:843–848.

96. Jacobsen GK, Norgaard-Pedersen B. Placental alkaline phosphatase in testicular germ cell tumours and in carcinoma-in-situ of the testis. An immunohistochemical study. *Acta Pathol Microbiol Immunol Scand A* 1984;92:323–329.

97. Jacobsen GK, Jacobsen M. Alpha-fetoprotein (afp) and human chorionic gonadotropin (HCG) in testicular germ cell tumours. A prospective immunohistochemical study. *Acta Pathol Microbiol Immunol Scand A* 1983;91:165–176.

98. Mostofi FK, Sesterhenn IA, Davis CJ Jr. Immunopathology of germ cell tumors of the testis. *Semin Diagn Pathol* 1987;4:320–341.

99. Jacobsen GK. Histogenetic considerations concerning germ cell tumours. Morphological and immunohistochemical comparative investigation of the human embryo and testicular germ cell tumours. *Virchows Arch A Pathol Anat Histopathol* 1986;408:509–525.

100. Eglen DE, Ulbright TM. The differential diagnosis of yolk sac tumor and seminoma. Usefulness of cytokeratin, alpha-fetoprotein, and alpha-1-antitrypsin immunoperoxidase reactions. *Am J Clin Pathol* 1987;88:328–332.

101. Jones TD, Ulbright TM, Eble JN, et al. Oct4 staining in testicular tumors: a sensitive and specific marker for seminoma and embryonal carcinoma. *Am J Surg Pathol* 2004;28:935–940.

102. Niehans GA, Manivel JC, Copland GT, et al. Immunohistochemistry of germ cell and trophoblastic neoplasms. *Cancer* 1988;62:1113–1123.

103. Cockburn AG, Vugrin D, Batata M, et al. Poorly differentiated (anaplastic) seminoma of the testis. *Cancer* 1984;53:1991–1994.

104. Johnson DE, Gomez JJ, Ayala AG. Anaplastic seminoma. *J Urol* 1975;114:80–82.

105. von Hochstetter AR. Mitotic count in seminomas—an unreliable criterion for distinguishing between classical and anaplastic types. *Virchows Arch A Pathol Anat Histol* 1981;390:63–69.

106. Zuckman MH, Williams G, Levin HS. Mitosis counting in seminoma: an exercise of questionable significance. *Hum Pathol* 1988;19:329–335.

107. Denk H, Moll R, Weybora W, et al. Intermediate filaments and desmosomal plaque proteins in testicular seminomas and non-seminomatous germ cell tumours as revealed by immunohistochemistry. *Virchows Arch A Pathol Anat Histopathol* 1987;410:295–307.

108. Motzer RJ, Reuter VE, Cordon-Cardo C, et al. Blood group-related antigens in human germ cell tumors. *Cancer Res* 1988;48:5342–5347.

109. Srigley JR, Mackay B, Toth P, et al. The ultrastructure and histogenesis of male germ neoplasia with emphasis on seminoma with early carcinomatous features. *Ultrastruct Pathol* 1988;12:67–86.

110. Raghavan D, Heyderman E, Monaghan P, et al. Hypothesis: when is a seminoma not a seminoma? *J Clin Pathol* 1981;34:123–128.

111. Walt H, Arrenbrecht S, DeLozier-Blanchet CD, et al. A human testicular germ cell tumor with borderline histology between seminoma and embryonal carcinoma secreted beta-human chorionic gonadotropin and alpha-fetoprotein only as a xenograft. *Cancer* 1986;58:139–146.

112. Mostofi FK. Pathology of germ cell tumors of testis: a progress report. *Cancer* 1980;45:1735–1754.

113. Tickoo SK, Hutchinson B, Bacik J, et al. Testicular seminoma: a clinicopathologic and immunohistochemical study of 105 cases with special reference to seminomas with atypical features. *Int J Surg Pathol* 2002;10:23–32.

114. Czaja JT, Ulbright TM. Evidence for the transformation of seminoma to yolk sac tumor, with histogenetic considerations. *Am J Clin Pathol* 1992;97:468–477.

115. Travis LB, Fossa SD, Schonfeld SJ, et al. Second cancers among 40,576 testicular cancer patients: focus on long-term survivors. *J Natl Cancer Inst* 2005;97:1354–1365.

116. Feldman DR, Bosl GJ. Treatment of stage i seminoma: is it time to change your practice? *J Hematol Oncol* 2008;1:22.

117. Aparicio J, Germa JR, Garcia del Muro X, et al. Risk-adapted management for patients with clinical stage I seminoma: the second spanish germ cell cancer cooperative group study. *J Clin Oncol* 2005;23:8717–8723.

118. Warde P, Gospodarowicz M. Evolving concepts in stage I seminoma. *BJU Int* 2009;104:1357–1361.

119. Talerman A. Spermatocytic seminoma: clinicopathological study of 22 cases. *Cancer* 1980;45:2169–2176.

120. Eble JN. Spermatocytic seminoma. *Hum Pathol* 1994;25:1035–1042.

121. Burke AP, Mostofi FK. Spermatocytic seminoma. *J Urol Pathol* 1993;1:21–32.

122. Dash A, Carver BS, Stasi J, et al. The indication for postchemotherapy lymph node dissection in clinical stage is nonseminomatous germ cell tumor. *Cancer* 2008;112:800–805.

123. Masson P. Etude sur le seminoma. *Rev Cancer Biol* 1946;5:361–387.

124. Steiner H, Gozzi C, Verdorfer I, et al. Metastatic spermatocytic seminoma—an extremely rare disease: part 2. *Eur Urol* 2006;49:408–409.

125. Floyd C, Ayala AG, Logothetis CJ, et al. Spermatocytic seminoma with associated sarcoma of the testis. *Cancer* 1988;61:409–414.

126. True LD, Otis CN, Rosai J, et al. Spermatocytic seminoma of testis with sarcomatous transformation. *Am J Surg Pathol* 1988;12:806.

127. Albores-Saavedra J, Huffman H, Alvarado-Cabrero I, et al. Anaplastic variant of spermatocytic seminoma. *Hum Pathol* 1996;27:650–655.

128. Kraggerud SM, Berner A, Bryne M, et al. Spermatocytic seminoma as compared to classical seminoma: an immunohistochemical and DNA flow cytometric study. *APMIS* 1999;107:297–302.

129. Latza U, Foss HD, Durkop H, et al. Cd30 antigen in embryonal carcinoma and embryogenesis and release of the soluble molecule. *Am J Pathol* 1995;146:463–471.

130. Krag Jacobsen G, Barlebo H, Olsen J, et al. Testicular germ cell tumours in denmark 1976-1980. Pathology of 1058 consecutive cases. *Acta Radiol Oncol* 1984;23:239–247.

131. Hawkins EP, Finegold MJ, Hawkins HK, et al. Nongerminomatous malignant germ cell tumors in children. A review of 89 cases from the pediatric oncology group, 1971-1984. *Cancer* 1986;58:2579–2584.

132. Ulbright T, Amin M, Young RH. Tumors of the testis, adnexa, spermatic cord, and scrotum. In: *Atlas of Tumor Pathology, Third Series Fascicle.* Washington, DC: Armed Forces Institute of Pathology; 1999.

133. Gopalan A, Dhall D, Olgac S, et al. Testicular mixed germ cell tumors: a morphological and immunohistochemical study using stem cell markers, oct3/4, sox2 and gdf3, with emphasis on morphologically difficult-to-classify areas. *Mod Pathol* 2009;22:1066–1074.

134. Emerson RE, Ulbright TM. The use of immunohistochemistry in the differential diagnosis of tumors of the testis and paratestis. *Semin Diagn Pathol* 2005;22:33–50.

135. Donohue JP, Thornhill JA, Foster RS, et al. Retroperitoneal lymphadenectomy for clinical stage a testis cancer (1965 to 1989): modifications of technique and impact on ejaculation. *J Urol* 1993;149:237–243.

136. Stephenson AJ, Bosl GJ, Motzer RJ, et al. Nonrandomized comparison of primary chemotherapy and retroperitoneal lymph node dissection for clinical stage iia and iib nonseminomatous germ cell testicular cancer. *J Clin Oncol* 2007;25:5597–5602.

137. Scheinfeld J, Bartsch G, Bosl GJ. *Surgery of Testicular Neoplasams.* Philadelphia, PA: WB Saunders Co.; 2010.

138. Talerman A. Endodermal sinus (yolk sac) tumor elements in testicular germ-cell tumors in adults: comparison of prospective and retrospective studies. *Cancer* 1980;46:1213–1217.

139. Sogani PC, Perrotti M, Herr HW, et al. Clinical stage i testis cancer: long-term outcome of patients on surveillance. *J Urol* 1998;159: 855–858.

140. Sesterhenn IA, Weiss RB, Mostofi FK, et al. Prognosis and other clinical correlates of pathologic review in stage i and ii testicular carcinoma: a report from the testicular cancer intergroup study. *J Clin Oncol* 1992;10:69–78.

141. Albers P, Siener R, Kliesch S, et al. Risk factors for relapse in clinical stage i nonseminomatous testicular germ cell tumors: results of the German Testicular Cancer Study Group Trial. *J Clin Oncol* 2003;21:1505–1512.

142. Talerman A, Haije WG, Baggerman L. Serum alphafetoprotein (afp) in patients with germ cell tumors of the gonads and extragonadal sites: correlation between endodermal sinus (yolk sac) tumor and raised serum afp. *Cancer* 1980;46:380–385.

143. Carver BS, Bianco FJ Jr, Shayegan B, et al. Predicting teratoma in the retroperitoneum in men undergoing post-chemotherapy retroperitoneal lymph node dissection. *J Urol* 2006;176:100–104.

144. Ulbright TM, Roth LM, Brodhecker CA. Yolk sac differentiation in germ cell tumors. A morphologic study of 50 cases with emphasis on hepatic, enteric, and parietal yolk sac features. *Am J Surg Pathol* 1986;10:151–164.

145. Ulbright TM. Testicular and paratesticular tumors. In: Sternberg SS, ed. *Diagnostic Surgical Pathology.* Philadelphia, PA: Lippincott Williams & Wilkins; 1999:1973–2004.

146. Talerman A. Germ cell tumors. In: Talerman A, Roth LM, eds. *Pathology of the Testis and Its Adnexa.* New York: Churchill Livingstone; 1986:60.

147. Emerson RE, Ulbright TM. Intratubular germ cell neoplasia of the testis and its associated cancers: the use of novel biomarkers. *Pathology* 2010;42:344–355.

148. Wang F, Liu A, Peng Y, et al. Diagnostic utility of SALL4 in extragonadal yolk sac tumors: an immunohistochemical study of 59 cases with comparison to placental-like alkaline phosphatase, alpha-fetoprotein, and glypican-3. *Am J Surg Pathol* 2009;33:1529–1539.

149. Ulbright TM, Loehrer PJ. Choriocarcinoma-like lesions in patients with testicular germ cell tumors. Two histologic variants. *Am J Surg Pathol* 1988;12:531–541.

150. Ulbright TM, Roth LM. A pathologic analysis of lesions following modern chemotherapy for metastatic germ-cell tumors. *Pathol Annu* 1990;25 Pt 1:313–340.

151. Ulbright TM, Young RH, Scully RE. Trophoblastic tumors of the testis other than classic choriocarcinoma: "monophasic" choriocarcinoma and placental site trophoblastic tumor: a report of two cases. *Am J Surg Pathol* 1997;21:282–288.

152. Little JS Jr, Foster RS, Ulbright TM, et al. Unusual neoplasms detected in testicular cancer patients undergoing postchemotherapy retroperitoneal lymphadenectomy. *World J Urol* 1994;12:200–206.

153. Ulbright TM, Henley JD, Cummings OW, et al. Cystic trophoblastic tumor: a nonaggressive lesion in postchemotherapy resections of patients with testicular germ cell tumors. *Am J Surg Pathol* 2004;28:1212–1216.

154. Manivel JC, Niehans G, Wick MR, et al. Intermediate trophoblast in germ cell neoplasms. *Am J Surg Pathol* 1987;11:693–701.

155. World Health Organization Classification of Tumours. *Pathology and Genetics of Tumours of the Urinary System and Male Genital Organs.* Lyon, France: IARC press; 2004.

156. Beck SD, Patel MI, Sheinfeld J. Tumor marker levels in postchemotherapy cystic masses: clinical implications for patients with germ cell tumors. *J Urol* 2004;171:168–171.

157. Ulbright TM, Loehrer PJ, Roth LM, et al. The development of nongerm cell malignancies within germ cell tumors. A clinicopathologic study of 11 cases. *Cancer* 1984;54:1824–1833.

158. Motzer RJ, Amsterdam A, Prieto V, et al. Teratoma with malignant transformation: diverse malignant histologies arising in men with germ cell tumors. *J Urol* 1998;159:133–138.

159. Ahlgren AD, Simrell CR, Triche TJ, et al. Sarcoma arising in a residual testicular teratoma after cytoreductive chemotherapy. *Cancer* 1984;54:2015–2018.

160. Ahmed T, Bosl GJ, Hajdu SI. Teratoma with malignant transformation in germ cell tumors in men. *Cancer* 1985;56:860–863.

161. Michael H, Ulbright TM, Brodhecker CA. The pluripotential nature of the mesenchyme-like component of yolk sac tumor. *Arch Pathol Lab Med* 1989;113:1115–1119.

162. Michael H, Lucia J, Foster RS, et al. The pathology of late recurrence of testicular germ cell tumors. *Am J Surg Pathol* 2000;24: 257–273.

163. Dmitrovsky E, Rodriguez E, Samaniego F, et al. Analysis of chromosome 12 abnormalities in male germ cell cancers. *Recent Results Cancer Res* 1991;123:119–123.

164. Ladanyi M, Samaniego F, Reuter VE, et al. Cytogenetic and immunohistochemical evidence for the germ cell origin of a subset of acute leukemias associated with mediastinal germ cell tumors. *J Natl Cancer Inst* 1990;82:221–227.

165. Ulbright TM, Hattab EM, Zhang S, et al. Primitive neuroectodermal tumors in patients with testicular germ cell tumors usually resemble pediatric-type central nervous system embryonal neoplasms and lack chromosome 22 rearrangements. *Mod Pathol* 2010;23:972–980.

166. Malek RS, Rosen JS, Farrow GM. Epidermoid cyst of the testis: a critical analysis. *Br J Urol* 1986;58:55–59.

167. Price EB Jr. Epidermoid cysts of the testis: a clinical and pathologic analysis of 69 cases from the testicular tumor registry. *J Urol* 1969;102:708–713.

168. Younger C, Ulbright TM, Zhang S, et al. Molecular evidence supporting the neoplastic nature of some epidermoid cysts of the testis. *Arch Pathol Lab Med* 2003;127:858–860.

169. Ulbright TM, Srigley JR. Dermoid cyst of the testis: a study of five postpubertal cases, including a pilomatrixoma-like variant, with evidence supporting its separate classification from mature testicular teratoma. *Am J Surg Pathol* 2001;25:788–793.

170. Berdjis CC, Mostofi FK. Carcinoid tumors of the testis. *J Urol* 1977;118:777–782.

171. Zavala-Pompa A, Ro JY, el-Naggar A, et al. Primary carcinoid tumor of testis. Immunohistochemical, ultrastructural, and DNA flow cytometric study of three cases with a review of the literature. *Cancer* 1993;72:1726–1732.

172. Ordonez NG, Ayala AG. Primary malignant carcinoid of the testis. *Arch Pathol Lab Med* 1982;106:539.

173. Azzopardi JG, Mostofi FK, Theiss EA. Lesions of testes observed in certain patients with widespread choriocarcinoma and related tumors. The significance and genesis of hematoxylin-staining bodies in the human testis. *Am J Pathol* 1961;38:207–225.

174. Azzopardi JG, Hoffbrand AV. Retrogression in testicular seminoma with viable metastases. *J Clin Pathol* 1965;18:135–141.

175. Meares EM Jr, Briggs EM. Occult seminoma of the testis masquerading as primary extragonadal germinal neoplasms. *Cancer* 1972;30:300–306.

176. Evans RW. Developmental stages of embryo-like bodies in teratoma testis. *J Clin Pathol* 1957;10:31–39.

177. Kaplan GW, Cromie WJ, Kelalis PP, et al. Gonadal stromal tumors: a report of the prepubertal testicular tumor registry. *J Urol* 1986;136:300–302.

178. Kim I, Young RH, Scully RE. Leydig cell tumors of the testis. A clinicopathological analysis of 40 cases and review of the literature. *Am J Surg Pathol* 1985;9:177–192.

179. Lawrence WD, Young RH, Scully RE. Sex cord-stromal tumors. In: Talerman A, Roth LM, eds. *Pathology of the Testis and Its Adnexa.* New York: Churchill Livingstone; 1986:67.

180. Cheville JC. Classification and pathology of testicular germ cell and sex cord-stromal tumors. *Urol Clin North Am* 1999;26:595–609.

181. Billings SD, Roth LM, Ulbright TM. Microcystic leydig cell tumors mimicking yolk sac tumor: a report of four cases. *Am J Surg Pathol* 1999;23:546–551.

182. Ulbright TM, Srigley JR, Hatzianastassiou DK, et al. Leydig cell tumors of the testis with unusual features: adipose differentiation, calcification with ossification, and spindle-shaped tumor cells. *Am J Surg Pathol* 2002;26:1424–1433.

183. Augusto D, Leteurtre E, De La Taille A, et al. Calretinin: a valuable marker of normal and neoplastic leydig cells of the testis. *Appl Immunohistochem Mol Morphol* 2002;10:159–162.

184. Zheng W, Senturk BZ, Parkash V. Inhibin immunohistochemical staining: a practical approach for the surgical pathologist in the diagnoses of ovarian sex cord-stromal tumors. *Adv Anat Pathol* 2003;10:27–38.

185. Cobellis L, Cataldi P, Reis FM, et al. Gonadal malignant germ cell tumors express immunoreactive inhibin/activin subunits. *Eur J Endocrinol* 2001;145:779–784.

186. Iczkowski KA, Bostwick DG, Roche PC, et al. Inhibin a is a sensitive and specific marker for testicular sex cord-stromal tumors. *Mod Pathol* 1998;11:774–779.

187. Busam KJ, Iversen K, Coplan KA, et al. Immunoreactivity for a 103, an antibody to melan-a (mart-1), in adrenocortical and other steroid tumors. *Am J Surg Pathol* 1998;22:57–63.

188. Zhao C, Barner R, Vinh TN, et al. Sf-1 is a diagnostically useful immunohistochemical marker and comparable to other sex cord-stromal tumor markers for the differential diagnosis of ovarian sertoli cell tumor. *Int J Gynecol Pathol* 2008;27:507–514.

189. Cheville JC, Sebo TJ, Lager DJ, et al. Leydig cell tumor of the testis: a clinicopathologic, DNA content, and mib-1 comparison of nonmetastasizing and metastasizing tumors. *Am J Surg Pathol* 1998;22:1361–1367.

190. Rutgers JL, Young RH, Scully RE. The testicular "tumor" of the adrenogenital syndrome. A report of six cases and review of the literature on testicular masses in patients with adrenocortical disorders. *Am J Surg Pathol* 1988;12:503–513.

191. Young RH, Talerman A. Testicular tumors other than germ cell tumors. *Semin Diagn Pathol* 1987;4:342–360.

192. Young RH, Koelliker DD, Scully RE. Sertoli cell tumors of the testis, not otherwise specified: a clinicopathologic analysis of 60 cases. *Am J Surg Pathol* 1998;22:709–721.

193. Cantu JM, Rivera H, Ocampo-Campos R, et al. Peutz-jeghers syndrome with feminizing sertoli cell tumor. *Cancer* 1980;46:223–228.

194. Krag Jacobsen G. Malignant sertolic cell tumors of the testis. *J Urol Pathol* 1993;1:233–255.

195. Zukerberg LR, Young RH, Scully RE. Sclerosing sertoli cell tumor of the testis. A report of 10 cases. *Am J Surg Pathol* 1991;15:829–834.

196. Proppe KH, Scully RE. Large-cell calcifying sertoli cell tumor of the testis. *Am J Clin Pathol* 1980;74:607–619.

197. Proppe KH, Dickersin GR. Large-cell calcifying sertoli cell tumor of the testis: light microscopic and ultrastructural study. *Hum Pathol* 1982;13:1109–1114.

198. Kratzer SS, Ulbright TM, Talerman A, et al. Large cell calcifying sertoli cell tumor of the testis: contrasting features of six malignant and six benign tumors and a review of the literature. *Am J Surg Pathol* 1997;21:1271–1280.

199. De Raeve H, Schoonooghe P, Wibowo R, et al. Malignant large cell calcifying sertoli cell tumor of the testis. *Pathol Res Pract* 2003;199:113–117.

200. Wang BY, Rabinowitz DS, Granato RC Sr, et al. Gonadal tumor with granulosa cell tumor features in an adult testis. *Ann Diagn Pathol* 2002;6:56–60.

201. Mostofi FK, Theiss EA, Ashley DJ. Tumors of specialized gonadal stroma in human male patients. Androblastoma, sertoli cell tumor, granulosa-theca cell tumor of the testis, and gonadal stromal tumor. *Cancer* 1959;12:944–957.

202. Jimenez-Quintero LP, Ro JY, Zavala-Pompa A, et al. Granulosa cell tumor of the adult testis: a clinicopathologic study of seven cases and a review of the literature. *Hum Pathol* 1993;24:1120–1125.

203. Suppiah A, Musa MM, Morgan DR, et al. Adult granulosa cell tumour of the testis and bony metastasis. A report of the first case of granulosa cell tumour of the testicle metastasising to bone. *Urol Int* 2005;75:91–93.

204. Lawrence WD, Young RH, Scully RE. Juvenile granulosa cell tumor of the infantile testis. A report of 14 cases. *Am J Surg Pathol* 1985;9:87–94.

205. Young RH, Lawrence WD, Scully RE. Juvenile granulosa cell tumor—another neoplasm associated with abnormal chromosomes and ambiguous genitalia. A report of three cases. *Am J Surg Pathol* 1985;9:737–743.

206. Fidda N, Weeks DA. Juvenile granulosa cell tumor of the testis: a case presenting as a small round cell tumor of childhood. *Ultrastruct Pathol* 2003;27:451–455.

207. Fagin R, Berbescu E, Landis S, et al. Juvenile granulosa cell tumor of the testis. *Urology* 2003;62:351.

208. Jones MA, Young RH, Scully RE. Benign fibromatous tumors of the testis and paratesticular region: a report of 9 cases with a proposed classification of fibromatous tumors and tumor-like lesions. *Am J Surg Pathol* 1997;21:296–305.

209. Scully RE. Gonadoblastoma. A review of 74 cases. *Cancer* 1970;25:1340–1356.

210. Ulbright TM, Srigley JR, Reuter VE, et al. Sex cord-stromal tumors of the testis with entrapped germ cells: a lesion mimicking unclassified mixed germ cell sex cord-stromal tumors. *Am J Surg Pathol* 2000;24:535–542.

211. Talerman A. The pathology of gonadal neoplasms composed of germ cells and sex cord stroma derivatives. *Pathol Res Pract* 1980;170:24–38.

212. Rutgers JL. Advances in the pathology of intersex conditions. *Hum Pathol* 1991;22:884–891.

213. Iezzoni JC, Von Kap-Herr C, Golden WL, et al. Gonadoblastomas in 45,x/46,xy mosaicism: analysis of y chromosome distribution by fluorescence in situ hybridization. *Am J Clin Pathol* 1997;108:197–201.

214. Hart WR, Burkons DM. Germ cell neoplasms arising in gonadoblastomas. *Cancer* 1979;43:669–678.

215. Jorgensen N, Muller J, Jaubert F, et al. Heterogeneity of gonadoblastoma germ cells: similarities with immature germ cells, spermatogonia and testicular carcinoma in situ cells. *Histopathology* 1997;30:177–186.

216. Kersemaekers AM, Honecker F, Stoop H, et al. Identification of germ cells at risk for neoplastic transformation in gonadoblastoma: an immunohistochemical study for oct3/4 and tspy. *Hum Pathol* 2005;36:512–521.

217. Talerman A. A distinctive gonadal neoplasm related to gonadoblastoma. *Cancer* 1972;30:1219–1224.

218. Bolen JW. Mixed germ cell-sex cord stromal tumor. A gonadal tumor distinct from gonadoblastoma. *Am J Clin Pathol* 1981;75:565–573.

219. Ferry JA, Harris NL, Young RH, et al. Malignant lymphoma of the testis, epididymis, and spermatic cord. A clinicopathologic study of 69 cases with immunophenotypic analysis. *Am J Surg Pathol* 1994;18:376–390.

220. Sussman EB, Hajdu SI, Lieberman PH, et al. Malignant lymphoma of the testis: a clinicopathologic study of 37 cases. *J Urol* 1977;118:1004–1007.

221. Lagrange JL, Ramaioli A, Theodore CH, et al. Non-hodgkin's lymphoma of the testis: a retrospective study of 84 patients treated in the french anticancer centres. *Ann Oncol* 2001;12:1313–1319.

222. Zouhair A, Weber D, Belkacemi Y, et al. Outcome and patterns of failure in testicular lymphoma: a multicenter rare cancer network study. *Int J Radiat Oncol Biol Phys* 2002;52:652–656.

223. Ferry J, Ulbright T, Young R. Anaplastic large-cell lymphoma presenting in the testis: a lesion that may be confused with embryonal carcinoma. *J Urol Pathol* 1996;5:139–148.

224. Chan JK, Tsang WY, Lau WH, et al. Aggressive t/natural killer cell lymphoma presenting as testicular tumor. *Cancer* 1996;77:1198–1205.

225. Valbuena JR, Admirand JH, Lin P, et al. Myeloid sarcoma involving the testis. *Am J Clin Pathol* 2005;124:445–452.

226. Givler RL. Testicular involvement in leukemia and lymphoma. *Cancer* 1969;23:1290–1295.

227. Reid H, Marsden HB. Gonadal infiltration in children with leukaemia and lymphoma. *J Clin Pathol* 1980;33:722–729.

228. Askin FB, Land VJ, Sullivan MP, et al. Occult testicular leukemia: testicular biopsy at three years continuous complete remission of childhood leukemia: a southwest oncology group study. *Cancer* 1981;47:470–475.

229. Nesbit ME Jr, Robison LL, Ortega JA, et al. Testicular relapse in childhood acute lymphoblastic leukemia: association with pretreatment patient characteristics and treatment. A report for childrens cancer study group. *Cancer* 1980;45:2009–2016.

230. Ferry JA, Young RH, Scully RE. Testicular and epididymal plasmacytoma: a report of 7 cases, including three that were the initial manifestation of plasma cell myeloma. *Am J Surg Pathol* 1997;21:590–598.

231. Honore LH, Sullivan LD. Intratesticulr leiomyoma: a case report with discussion of differential diagnosis and histogenesis. *J Urol* 1975;114:631–635.

232. Livolsi VA, Schiff M. Myxoid neurofibroma of the testis. *J Urol* 1977;118:341–342.

233. Nistal M, Paniagua R, Regadera J, et al. Testicular capillary haemangioma. *Br J Urol* 1982;54:433.

234. Mazal PR, Kratzik C, Kain R, et al. Capillary haemangioma of the testis. *J Clin Pathol* 2000;53:641–642.

235. Banks ER, Mills SE. Histiocytoid (epithelioid) hemangioma of the testis. The so-called vascular variant of "adenomatoid tumor". *Am J Surg Pathol* 1990;14:584–589.

236. Mazzella FM, Sieber SC, Lopez V. Histiocytoid hemangioma of the testis: a case report. *J Urol* 1995;153:743–744.

237. Kumar PV, Khezri AA. Pure testicular rhabdomyosarcoma. *Br J Urol* 1987;59:282.

238. Alexander F. Pure testicular rhabdomyosarcoma. *Br J Cancer* 1968;22:498–501.

239. Yachia D, Auslaender L. Primary leiomyosarcoma of the testis. *J Urol* 1989;141:955–956.

240. Tsolos C, Polychronidis A, Sivridis E, et al. Epithelioid hemangioendothelioma of the testis. *J Urol* 2001;166:1834.

241. Kneale BJ, Bishop NL, Britton JP. Kaposi's sarcoma of the testis. *Br J Urol* 1993;72:116–117.

242. Washecka RM, Mariani AJ, Zuna RE, et al. Primary intratesticular sarcoma. Immunohistochemical ultrastructural and DNA flow cytometric study of three cases with a review of the literature. *Cancer* 1996;77:1524–1528.

243. Amin MB. Selected other problematic testicular and paratesticular lesions: rete testis neoplasms and pseudotumors, mesothelial lesions and secondary tumors. *Mod Pathol* 2005;18(suppl 2):S131–S145.

244. Haupt HM, Mann RB, Trump DL, et al. Metastatic carcinoma involving the testis. Clinical and pathologic distinction from primary testicular neoplasms. *Cancer* 1984;54:709–714.

245. Tiltman AJ. Metastatic tumours in the testis. *Histopathology* 1979;3:31–37.

246. Dutt N, Bates AW, Baithun SI. Secondary neoplasms of the male genital tract with different patterns of involvement in adults and children. *Histopathology* 2000;37:323–331.

247. Backhaus BO, Kaefer M, Engum SA, et al. Contralateral testicular metastasis in paratesticular rhabdomyosarcoma. *J Urol* 2000;164:1709–1710.

248. Simon T, Hero B, Berthold F. Testicular and paratesticular involvement by metastatic neuroblastoma. *Cancer* 2000;88:2636–2641.

249. Datta MW, Ulbright TM, Young RH. Renal cell carcinoma metastatic to the testis and its adnexa: a report of five cases including three that accounted for the initial clinical presentation. *Int J Surg Pathol* 2001;9:49–56.

250. Richardson PG, Millward MJ, Shrimankar JJ, et al. Metastatic melanoma to the testis simulating primary seminoma. *Br J Urol* 1992;69:663–665.

251. Datta MW, Young RH. Malignant melanoma metastatic to the testis: a report of three cases with clinically significant manifestations. *Int J Surg Pathol* 2000;8:49–57.

Pathology of the Paratesticular Region

HELEN MICHAEL and JOHN R. SRIGLEY

INTRODUCTION

The paratesticular region is a relatively small anatomical compartment containing a disproportionately large number of anatomic structures. In addition to the testicular collecting system there are mesothelial and mesenchymal components representing extensions of the abdominal cavity and retroperitoneum. The epithelial, mesothelial, and connective tissue elements give rise to a wide variety of pathologic conditions including an interesting array of neoplasms and tumor-like lesions.

EMBRYOLOGY, ANATOMY, AND HISTOLOGY

Embryology

The embryology of the testis and paratesticular region is complex and has been the topic of various monographs.[1–5] The gonads are first evident as paired mesenchymal ridges between the dorsal mesentery and the mesonephric ridge at about 4 weeks' gestation (Fig. 13-1). The coelomic epithelium that covers these mesenchymal ridges extends into the underlying mesenchyme to form the primitive sex cords. Germ cells are first seen in the embryonic yolk sac. They then migrate along the wall of the hindgut and the dorsal mesenteric root into the developing gonads by the 6th week of gestation (Fig. 13-2). The sex cords proliferate under the influence of the germ cells. Testicular tissue with primitive seminiferous tubules is detectable by the 7th week of gestation. At about the same time, the primitive tunica albuginea forms as a layer of flattened cells around the gonad, and the primitive testis becomes separated from the overlying coelomic epithelium.

In the hilum of the developing testis, the sex cords form a network of cellular strands that admix with mesonephric cells from the degenerating mesonephric tubule (Fig. 13-3). Both sex cords and the mesonephros are thought to contribute to the formation of the rete testis. Hormones from the embryonic testis are thought to stimulate the mesonephric duct to develop into the male genital tract collecting system and, at the same time, to suppress development of the paramesonephric duct. By the end of the 4th month of gestation, the rete cords have merged with the epigenital tubules of the mesonephros, which form the efferent ductules and head of the epididymis (Fig. 13-4). The mesonephric duct develops into the epididymal body and tail and the vas deferens. The caudal portion of the vas deferens joins with the seminal vesicles, which are also derived from the mesonephric duct. The enlarging testis becomes separated from the degenerating mesonephros.

The descent of the testis into the scrotum through the inguinal canal is complex and not totally understood.[2] At the same time that the mesonephros degenerates, a ligament called a gubernaculum descends from the lower pole of each gonad along each side of the abdomen, passing through the abdominal wall at the site of the future inguinal canal, and it attaches to the scrotal swelling. A peritoneal sac called the processus vaginalis develops bilaterally, ventral to the gubernaculum, and herniates through the abdominal wall along the pathway formed by the gubernaculum. The processus vaginalis carries with it extensions of the abdominal wall layers, thus forming the wall of the inguinal canal. The opening formed in the external oblique aponeurosis forms the superficial inguinal ring, and the defect in the transversalis fascia forms a deep inguinal ring. The external spermatic fascia is a thin membrane derived from the aponeurosis of the external oblique muscle at the outer abdominal ring. The cremasteric fascia originates from the lower border of the internal oblique muscle. The internal spermatic fascia is derived from the transversalis fascia.[6] These layers become part of the spermatic cord and the wall of the scrotum.

By about 7 months' gestation, the testes are located distal to the deep inguinal ring, a change in position that is attributed to growth of the trunk and pelvis of the embryo.[2] The gubernaculum does not grow after it is formed, and the exact process of testicular descent into the scrotum is not well understood. The gubernaculum serves as an anchor that aids

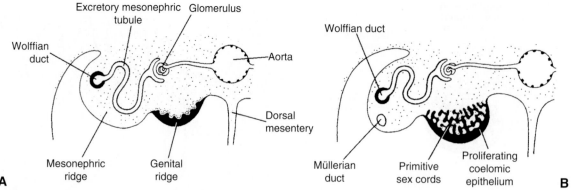

Figure 13-1 ■ Embryology of the testis and paratestis. **A:** At 4 weeks, the genital ridges are apparent as mesenchymal condensations with a covering of coelomic epithelium that has proliferated. **B:** At 6 weeks, there is ingrowth of the coelomic epithelium with extension into the mesenchyme to form the primitive sex cords. (Reprinted from Langman J. *Medical Embryology and Human Development—Normal and Abnormal.* 2nd ed. Baltimore, MD: Williams & Wilkins; 1972, Fig. 11-13, with permission.)

in testicular descent, but it does not pull the testis caudally. Increasing abdominal pressure due to developing organs may have a role in the process. Androgenic and gonadotrophic hormones are also thought to be important in the descent of the testes into the scrotum.[2] The testis is positioned posterior to the processus vaginalis, and it is located in the scrotum by about the 8th month of gestation. The layers of the inguinal canal then contract around the spermatic cord.

The vas deferens crosses anterior to the ureter as a result of the pathway of testicular descent into the scrotum.[2,6] The blood vessels that supply the testis follow a pathway along the dorsal abdominal wall. The cranial part of the processus vaginalis is obliterated in the perinatal period. The tunica vaginalis is then an isolated sac lined by mesothelium.

Anatomy and Histology

The rete testis, efferent ductules, and epididymis represent a continuous conduit for seminiferous fluid to be transported from the seminiferous tubules to the vas deferens.

Rete Testis

The rete testis represents a group of anastomotic channels in the hilum of the testis (Fig. 13-5). These channels receive the contents of the seminiferous tubules. The rete also serves as a chamber for mixing the seminiferous tubule contents, a possible source of seminal fluid, a site of resorption of protein, and the site of a pressure gradient between the testis and the epididymis.[7] There are intratesticular and

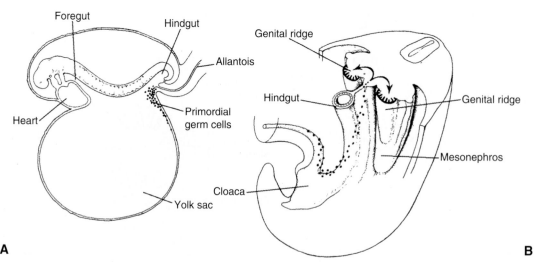

Figure 13-2 ■ Embryology of the testis and paratestis. **A:** At 3 weeks, the primordial germ cells form in the wall of the yolk sac. **B:** At 6 weeks, the primordial germ cells migrate to the wall of the hindgut, along the dorsal mesenteric root, and into the genital ridges. (Reprinted from Langman J. *Medical Embryology and Human Development—Normal and Abnormal.* 2nd ed. Baltimore, MD: Williams & Wilkins; 1972, Fig. 11-14, with permission.)

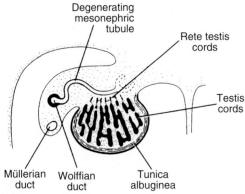

FIGURE 13-3 ■ Embryology of the testis and paratestis. At 8 weeks of gestation, the tunical albuginea surrounds the developing testis, and the rete testis cords intermingle with mesonephric tubules at the hilum. (Reprinted from Langman J. *Medical Embryology and Human Development—Normal and Abnormal.* 2nd ed. Baltimore, MD: Williams & Wilkins; 1972, Fig. 11-15A, with permission.)

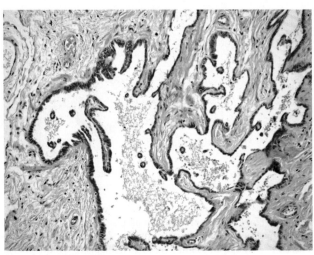

FIGURE 13-5 ■ Complex anastomosing channels are present in the rete testis. The channels are lined by low columnar epithelium.

extratesticular portions of the rete testis. The tubulae rete are located in testicular interlobular septa, and they connect the two ends of each seminiferous tubule. They also connect to the mediastinal rete, which exit the testis as the extratesticular bullae retis. The latter structures anastomose to form the efferent ductules.

The rete testis is lined by low columnar, cuboidal, or simple squamous epithelium that rests on basal lamina surrounded by fibroblasts, myoid cells, collagen, and elastin. These connective tissue components constitute the wall of

the rete testis. Microvilli are present on the luminal surfaces of the epithelial cells. Each cell also contains a single flagellum that can be seen by electron microscopy.[8]

Efferent Ductules

Twelve to fifteen efferent ductules connect with the extratesticular rete testis. They make up most of the head of the epididymis and resorb seminal fluid components. The efferent ductule epithelium is composed of two layers, including columnar epithelial cells and flattened, cuboidal basal

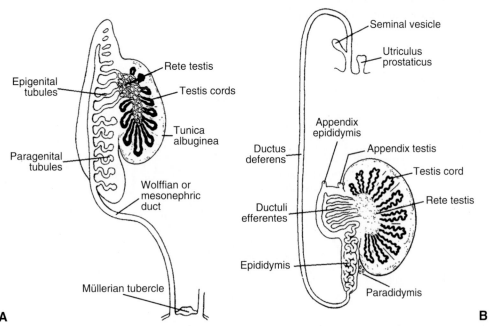

A   **B**

FIGURE 13-4 ■ Embryology of the testis and paratestis. **A:** By 4 months of gestation, the rete testis cords have merged with the epigenital tubules of the mesonephros. **B:** Diagram of the mature testis after descent showing the relationships of various structures. (Reprinted from Langman J. *Medical Embryology and Human Development—Normal and Abnormal.* 2nd ed. Baltimore, MD: Williams & Wilkins; 1972, Fig. 11-18, with permission.)

cells. The luminal surface of the tubules is undulating. Sometimes, the epithelial cells may display nuclear atypia and cytoplasmic pigment reminiscent of that in the seminal vesicles.[9] The epithelium is surrounded by basement membrane, smooth muscle, and some fibroblasts.[8]

Epididymis

Most of the head of the epididymis contains the efferent ductules. The body and tail contain a coiled, 4- to 5-m-long duct.[7,10] The epididymis is involved with sperm storage, sperm transfer, sperm maturation, and sperm concentration.[7] Sperm matures, develops motility, and is stored in the tail of the epididymis.[11] The well-developed smooth muscle wall surrounding the epididymal tubules assists in transportation of sperm through the epididymis.

Unlike the wavy luminal surface of the efferent ductules, the epididymal ducts have a smooth luminal contour (Fig. 13-6). The epididymal epithelium contains tall columnar cells, dark columnar cells, clear cells, and basal cells. The columnar cells are ciliated, and the cilia decrease in length from the head to the tail of the organ. The duct lumen of the tail of the epididymis contains abundant spermatozoa, and clear cells are more prominent in the epithelium in this area. Periodic acid–Schiff–positive diastase-resistant intranuclear inclusions are often present in the columnar cells of the epididymal epithelium,[12] most commonly in the distal portion. Electron-dense, membrane-enclosed bodies are identified by ultrastructural examination, but no viral features have been seen.[12] Cytoplasmic lipochrome pigment may also be present. The epididymal epithelium is surrounded by both basement membrane and smooth muscle; the latter is important for sperm transport. The epithelium may have a cribriform pattern that should not be mistaken for hyperplasia.[13–15]

Vas Deferens (Ductus Deferens)

The tail of the epididymis connects with the vas deferens, a 30- to 40-cm-long tubular structure that merges with the seminal vesicle to form the ejaculatory duct.[7] The vas deferens epithelium contains pseudostratified columnar epithelial cells and cuboidal to flattened basal cells. Electron microscopic examination has shown principal cells, peg cells, mitochondria-rich cells, and basal cells in the epithelium.[16] The luminal side of the epithelium is ciliated, and the cilia become shorter and less abundant as the seminal vesicle is approached. The epithelium is surrounded by a basement membrane. In adults, there is a layer of connective tissue containing elastic fibers between the basement membrane and the muscular wall of the vas deferens. The muscularis contains inner and outer longitudinal layers and a middle circular or oblique layer. Like the epididymis, the vas deferens epithelium may display cribriform architecture, intranuclear inclusions,[12] and lipochrome pigment. The epithelium of the vas is thrown into folds, and some of these complex infoldings and outpouchings may reach into the muscularis layer.

Testicular Tunics

The tunica albuginea is internal to the tunica vaginalis. It is composed of thick fibrous tissue that contains smooth muscle cells and nerve fibers and surrounds the testis except at the testicular hilus. The myocytes may contract and lead to an increase in intratesticular pressure. Tumor-like lesions and rare neoplasms may arise from the tunica albuginea.

The tunica vaginalis is a layer of mesothelium and associated basement membrane that represents the inner lining of the intrascrotal structures. The visceral tunica vaginalis forms a serosal lining over the tunica albuginea, covering the testis and most of the epididymal head. It reflects

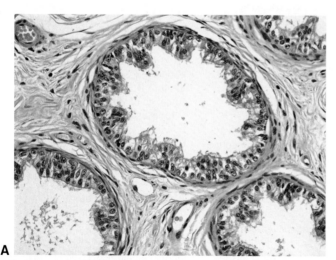 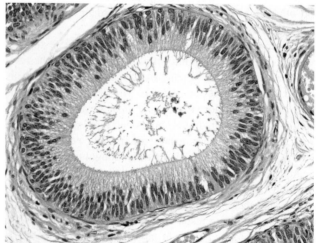

FIGURE 13-6 ■ Normal epididymis. **A:** The head of epididymis is composed of efferent ductules. They contain pseudostratified epithelium with ciliated cells. The luminal border is undulating. **B:** Ductus epididymis. Cilia are prominent, and the pseudostratified lining cells have a smooth luminal border. Smooth muscle surrounds the duct.

back on itself superiorly and posteriorly at the mediastinum testis to become the parietal tunica vaginalis. Urothelial metaplasia may occur in the tunica vaginalis,[17] with formation of von Brunn nest–like structures.[8] Squamous metaplasia may also occur, and after cystic transformation, it may account for some epidermoid cysts in the testis and paratestis.[18,19]

While the cranial part of the tunica vaginalis normally becomes obliterated in the perinatal period, sometimes residual mesothelium present in the spermatic cord may result in cysts or other lesions of mesothelial origin.

Spermatic Cord

During its descent into the scrotum, the testis brings with it the elements of the spermatic cord, including the vas deferens, blood vessels, and nerves.[1,2,4,5] The cord is covered by the spermatic and cremasteric fascia that accompany the processus vaginalis through the abdominal wall into the inguinal canal.[2,6] The cremasteric muscle is composed of skeletal muscle bundles present along the outer part of the spermatic cord and in the wall of the scrotal sac. The loose connective tissue matrix of the spermatic cord contains scattered bundles of smooth muscle.

The arteries present in the spermatic cord supply blood to the testis and paratesticular structures. They include the testicular (spermatic) artery, the artery of the vas deferens, and the cremasteric artery.[6] The testicular artery originates from the aorta inferior to the renal artery and penetrates the tunica albuginea to provide the main blood supply to the testis and the epididymis. The anterior and posterior epididymal arteries arise from the testicular artery and supply the head of the epididymis and the epididymal body and tail, respectively. The artery of the vas deferens is a branch of the superior vesicle artery that accompanies the vas deferens and anastomoses with the main testicular artery or the posterior epididymal artery. The cremasteric artery is a branch of the deep epigastric artery. It supplies the cremasteric muscle and other coverings of the spermatic cord. It anastomoses with branches of the testicular artery.

The epididymal veins anastomose with the testicular veins[6] to form the pampiniform plexus that invests the testicular artery.[8] Further venous anastomoses eventually lead to the right and left testicular veins. The right testicular vein opens into the inferior vena cava at an acute angle, whereas the left testicular vein drains into the left renal vein at a right angle. Increased hydrostatic pressure from the perpendicular venous anastomosis on the left side is thought to account for the greater incidence of varicoceles on that side.

The lymphatic channels of the testis and epididymis arise from a superficial plexus beneath the tunica vaginalis and a deep plexus in the testis and epididymis.[6] These vessels anastomose into four to eight larger channels that accompany the main testicular blood vessels through the spermatic cord to drain into the lateral paraaortic and preaortic lymph node groups.[8]

The spermatic cord nerves include the genital branch of the genitofemoral nerve, which innervates the cremasteric muscle and sends branches to the scrotal skin.[6] The testicular plexus of sympathetic nerve fibers is derived from branches of renal and aortic nerve plexuses with contributions from the superior and inferior hypogastric plexuses. These nerves travel with the testicular artery as well as give off branches to the epididymis and the vas deferens. Nerves from the pelvic plexus may accompany the artery of the vas deferens.[8]

Congenital Abnormalities and Ectopia

Rete Testis

The term "dysgenesis of the rete testis" refers to the underdeveloped rete testis associated with cryptorchidism[20] (Table 13-1).

Testicular abnormalities reported in cryptorchidism include Sertoli cell–only syndrome (23 cases), diffuse tubular hyalinization (8 cases), mixed tubular atrophy (3 cases), and maturation arrest of spermatogonia (4 cases).[20]

The rete has been described as diffusely hypoplastic in 37.5%, hypoplastic and cystic in 50%, and hyperplastic in 12.5% of 40 cryptorchid testes.[20] The latter pattern is identical to the lesion described as (idiopathic) rete testis hyperplasia, characterized by tubular, papillary, and cribriform intratubular epithelial proliferations. Cystic change in the rete testis associated with cryptorchidism is manifested by dilated epithelial structures measuring up to 500 μm lined

Table 13-1 ■ CONGENITAL ABNORMALITIES AND ASSOCIATED CONDITIONS

Type	Associated Conditions
Rete testis	
Dysgenesis	Cryptorchid testis, epididymal abnormalities
Cystic dysplasia	Renal agenesis or cystic dysplasia of kidney
Epididymis	
Anomalies of attachment to testis	
Cysts	Von Hippel-Lindau syndrome In utero DES exposure
Agenesis	Absence of vas deferens and renal anomalies
Vas deferens	
Congenital absence	Cystic fibrosis Absent epididymis Renal anomalies
Ectopic	Imperforate anus, hypospadias
Splenic–gonadal fusion (continuous form)	Peromelia, micrognathia, gastrointestinal abnormalities
Ectopic adrenal tissue	TTAGS Nelson syndrome in some
Ectopic renal tissue	Undescended testis; rarely associated with extrarenal Wilms' tumor

by large cuboidal epithelial cells. The epithelium stains for both cytokeratin and vimentin in the same manner as the normal rete epithelium. Some cases have been associated with efferent duct atrophy, with small duct diameters and more space than usual between the ducts. Other associated findings included epididymal duct ectasia (21 cases), an underdeveloped muscular layer in the epididymis (11 cases), and fat and dilated veins in the mediastinum testis (3 cases each).

Cryptorchidism is also associated with anomalies of mesonephric structures, including luminal dilation of the spermatic duct system, immature muscle layers, and malformations of the epididymis. These multiple abnormalities associated with cryptorchidism suggest a primary developmental disorder of the mesonephros.[21]

Epididymis

Congenital anomalies of the epididymis include anomalies of the attachment to the testes, epididymal cysts, agenesis or accessory epididymis, ectopic epididymis, and duplication of the epididymis.

Anomalies of fusion, with detachment of the head of the epididymis from the testis, and anomalies of suspension have been reported in children who have had surgery for cryptorchidism.[22–24] Fusion anomalies are more commonly associated with abdominal testes, and suspension anomalies are more often seen when the cryptorchid testis is located more distally. Some epididymal anomalies are associated with an absent testis. Anomalies of attachment of the epididymis to the testis include attachment of the caput and cauda with a detached corpus, attachment of the epididymal head only, attachment of the cauda only, and complete separation of the testes and epididymis.[23] Epididymal anomalies may also be seen in about one-third of boys with hernias and hydroceles without cryptorchidism, especially if there is a patent processus vaginalis. Detachment of the head of the epididymis bilaterally results in infertility.

Epididymal cysts are usually asymptomatic lesions that are discovered incidentally on physical examination or ultrasound. Epididymal cysts may be acquired, but some authors believe that they have a congenital basis,[25] perhaps related to maturation of the mesonephric ductal system. They are seen in patients with von Hippel-Lindau syndrome and in some patients exposed to diethylstilbestrol in utero[26] (Table 13-1). The cysts may represent efferent ducts that did not fuse with the mesonephric duct during embryogenesis.

Epididymal agenesis is almost always associated with unilateral or bilateral absence of the vas deferens (Table 13-1). The epididymal head is usually present because it is composed of efferent ducts derived from the genital ridge, whereas the epididymal body and tail are of mesonephric derivation.[25] A high frequency of renal anomalies is present in these patients.

Aberrant epididymal tissue is rare. It may be associated with an undescended testis. One case of ectopic epididymal tissue

in the appendix testis has been reported.[27] Ectopic epididymal tissue has also been associated with an inguinal hernia sac.[28]

Epididymal duplication is rare. It is characterized by a small accessory epididymis branching from the main epididymis. These patients are asymptomatic, and the lesions are discovered incidentally.

Vas Deferens

Congenital bilateral absence of the vas deferens is a well-studied abnormality of the wolffian ducts that represents a primary genital form of cystic fibrosis[29] (Table 13-1). Mutations in the cystic fibrosis transmembrane conductance gene are associated with wolffian duct abnormalities, including unilateral and bilateral congenital absence of the vas deferens and idiopathic epididymal obstruction.[29] The body and tail of the epididymis are also often absent, so the epididymal head may be prominent and distended with sperm. In some cases, there may be complete absence of the epididymis. Renal anomalies may be present due to the associated embryologic origins of these structures.[25]

Unilateral absence of the vas deferens occurs in <1% of healthy men. It represents the most frequent congenital anomaly of the vas deferens and involves the left side more often than the right side.[25] It is often detected at the time of vasectomy. It is not a common cause of infertility if the contralateral vas is normal. The epididymis associated with the absent vas may be of variable length. Ipsilateral renal agenesis may be associated with this condition (Table 13-1).

Only a few cases of duplicated vas deferens have been reported.[25] This term is restricted to cases where a second vas deferens is identified within the spermatic cord. The condition needs to be recognized at the time of vasectomy.

Ectopic vas deferens (persisting mesonephric duct) is a condition wherein the ureter enters the vas deferens.[25] A triad of ectopic vas deferens, imperforate anus, and hypospadias has been described[30] (Table 13-1); it has been present in about one-fourth of patients with ectopic vas deferens. The diagnosis of persisting mesonephric duct should be considered in male children with imperforate anus and recurring urinary tract infections.

One case of a large diverticulum of the vas deferens has been reported.[31] A thickened scrotal vas deferens and azoospermia were present. Another rare congenital anomaly is crossed dystopia of the vas deferens, a condition in which the vas deferens crosses the midline and communicates with the contralateral seminal vesicles.[31] Infertility is not associated with that lesion unless additional abnormalities are present. The diagnosis is made by vasography. Segmental aplasia of the vas deferens (skip vas) may be unilateral or bilateral; bilateral lesions result in infertility. Segments of vas deferens may also be hypoplastic. These conditions represent abnormal mesonephric duct development and may be associated with abnormalities of the epididymis and seminal vesicles.

Ectopic Splenic Tissue and Splenic–Gonadal Fusion

Splenic and gonadal tissue may fuse during embryogenesis.[32] The left gonad is most frequently involved.[33] There is a continuous form of this lesion in which a cord connects the spleen to the testis; many of those patients have marked defects of the extremities (peromelia), as well as micrognathia and gastrointestinal abnormalities (Table 13-1). Those patients may have a scrotal or inguinal mass that becomes apparent during an inguinal hernia operation or during surgery for an undescended testis. Small aggregates of splenic tissue may be found in the spermatic cord, or the cord may be composed entirely of splenic tissue.[34]

The discontinuous form of splenic–gonadal fusion is manifested by accessory splenic tissue in the paratestis region rather than continuity between the spleen and testis. Accessory splenic tissue has been reported in the epididymis, in the spermatic cord, and between the scrotal skin and the spermatic cord.[33] The splenic tissue has the gross and microscopic characteristics of normal spleen.

Ectopic Adrenal Tissue

Ectopic adrenal cortical tissue is seen in the paratestis of 1.6% to 15% of male patients.[35,36] It typically appears as yellow-orange nodules in the spermatic cord, epididymis, rete testis, tunica albuginea, and between the epididymis and the testis. It is most often seen in infants, but it may occur in adults. Nodules of ectopic adrenal tissue may measure 2 to 6 mm in diameter.[37] They display three well-defined layers of adrenal cortex. The zona fasciculata is the predominant tissue. Adrenal medulla is not present in ectopic adrenal tissue. The characteristic zonation seen in the adrenal cortex is an important factor in distinguishing ectopic adrenal tissue from other steroid cell proliferations in this region.

Ectopic adrenal cortex may be the source for neoplasms such as the testicular tumor of the adrenal genital syndrome (TTAGS) that may be seen in the spermatic cord.[38] Similar tumors are seen in patients with Nelson syndrome[39] (Table 13-1). These lesions actually represent reversible hyperplasia of steroid-producing cells in response to high circulating levels of ACTH.[40] Reduction of the ACTH levels causes regression of the lesion. TTAGS displays nests of cells with eosinophilic cytoplasm; the cell nests are separated by fibrous stoma. Intracytoplasmic lipofuscin may be present. Some authors have suggested that TTAGS arise from pluripotential cells in the testicular hilus rather than adrenal rests.[38]

Ectopic Renal Tissue

Ectopic renal tissue in the paratesticular region is rare and usually occurs in association with an undescended testis.[41–43] One case occurred in a 36-year-old man with a painful inguinal swelling.[41] An undescended testis was present with an adjacent ectopic kidney that measured 3 cm in diameter and contained renal cortex and medulla as well as some immature mesenchyme. An additional patient had heterotopic renal tissue that was discovered in association with an intrascrotal Wilms tumor[44] (Table 13-1). The renal heterotopia consisted of renal tubules and immature glomeruli that may have arisen from caudal mesonephric elements present in the paratesticular area. Primary extrarenal nephrogenic rests occur rarely in the paratesticular region.[45] They display blastema and immature glomeruli and tubules.

Extraparenchymal Leydig Cells

Clusters of Leydig cells are often present in the paratesticular region (Fig. 13-7). They have been reported in the tunica albuginea and rete testis,[46,47] the adventitial tissue between the tunica albuginea and epididymis, the epididymis, the vas deferens, and the spermatic cord.[36,48] A recent study found Leydig cells outside the testis in 90 of 97 orchiectomy specimens reviewed.[49] The testicular tunics were involved in 50% of cases, and 14.4% of spermatic cords contained Leydig cells. These cells were associated with nerves in 25.5% of cases and with vascular spaces in 7.8% of orchiectomy specimens, but some aggregates of Leydig cells were not associated with either nerves or blood vessels.[49] Leydig cells sometimes contain lipochrome pigment, Reinke crystals, and multiple nuclei.[47] Large aggregates of extratesticular Leydig cells may be misinterpreted as a primary paratesticular Leydig cell neoplasm, spread from a testicular Leydig cell tumor or other rare neoplasms or metastatic disease. Extratesticular Leydig cells may form small nodules, but the location along nerves and vessels combined with the lack of an expansile paratesticular mass or testicular neoplasm distinguishes testicular adnexal Leydig cells from Leydig cell tumor of paratesticular or testis origin. In contrast to metastatic deposits, no atypia, mitosis, or stromal reaction is associated with extratesticular Leydig cell aggregate.

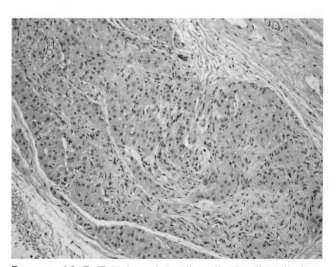

FIGURE 13-7 ■ Perineural Leydig cells. Leydig cells have abundant eosinophilic cytoplasm and are often associated with nerve bundles in the paratesticular region.

Remnants of Wolffian and Müllerian Ducts

Remnants of the embryonic müllerian and wolffian ducts give rise to the appendix testis and the appendix epididymis, respectively. These structures may be subject to various pathologic processes, including cysts, infarcts, and tumors. Cysts usually occur in the retroperitoneum, mesentery, pelvis, or paratesticular region. However, one cyst thought to be derived from a wolffian duct remnant occurred in the liver of an infant boy. It was connected by a stalk to the head of the epididymis adjacent to his right abdominal undescended testis.[50]

Appendix Testis

The appendix testis is a remnant of the paramesonephric (müllerian) duct that is usually found on the anterosuperior aspect of the testis in the groove between the testis and the head of the epididymis.[5,7] It is most commonly attached to the tunica vaginalis of the testis, but it may also be attached to the epididymis. The appendix testis can be identified in 80% to 90% of men, and it has been found bilaterally in 60% of patients.[7] A thickened area of the tunica vaginalis or focal calcification may be the only evidence of this structure in some men. However, it is generally an ovoid structure that measures 0.5 to 2.5 cm in length.[51] It is covered by cuboidal to columnar epithelium that may be stratified (Fig. 13-8). The connective tissue core contains blood vessels and, sometimes, smooth muscle cells. Stroma resembling ovarian stroma may also be present. Torsion and infarction of the appendix testis is usually seen in children or adolescents, and it is associated with scrotal pain[52] that may be mistaken for processes involving other intrascrotal areas. Chronic torsion may cause detachment of the appendix testis.

Appendix Epididymis

The appendix epididymis is derived from the cranial aspect of the mesonephric (wolffian) duct. It is identifiable in only about 25% of specimens.[53] It is a cystic structure that

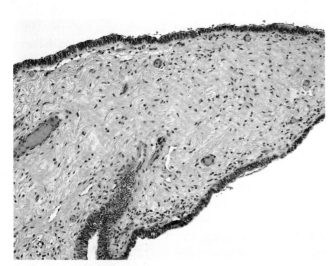

FIGURE 13-8 ■ Appendix testis. The oblong structure has a fibrovascular core and is covered by columnar cells.

may contain eosinophilic fluid and is lined by cuboidal to columnar epithelium. The epithelium is surrounded by a basement membrane, with a small amount of connective tissue and mesothelial cells on the external aspect. The appendix epididymis may be pedunculated, or it may be adherent to the head of the epididymis. It may be involved by torsion and infarction causing scrotal pain, and sometimes it may become enlarged and suggest a mass lesion.

Aberrant Ductules and Paradidymis

The superior and inferior aberrant ductules (organ of Haller) and paradidymis (organ of Giraldes) are mesonephric duct (wolffian) remnants.[8] They are near the head or body of the epididymis in the case of the superior aberrant ductule or the junction of the tail of the epididymis and the vas deferens in the case of the inferior aberrant ductule.[7] Both are small tubules or cysts with low columnar epithelium surrounded by smooth muscle. They may be the source of some epididymal cysts, although epididymal cysts are also encountered in patients with the von Hippel-Lindau syndrome and in some patients who were exposed to diethyl-stilbestrol in utero.[7,26,54]

The paradidymis is usually located adjacent to the vas deferens in the area of the head of the epididymis. It is a small tubular structure similar to the aberrant ductules, and it may result in a spermatic cord cyst.[28] It is important not to mistake the paradidymis for vas deferens in inguinal hernia specimens.[55] The well-developed, three-layered muscular wall of the vas deferens aids in the distinction.

Hernia Sac Inclusions

Hernia sacs from young boys contain glandular or ductal structures in 1.5% to 6% of cases[55–57] (Box 13-1). These embryonal rests must be distinguished from transected vas deferens and epididymal tissue because gland inclusions do not affect reproductive function.

The three types of embryonal rests seen in inguinal hernia sacs include vas deferens–like, epididymis-like and müllerian-like inclusions.[56] The diameter of the remnants,

Box 13-1 ● GLANDULAR INCLUSIONS IN INGUINAL HERNIA SACS

Type of Inclusion	Diagnostic Features
Vas deferens–like	CD10 negative, smooth muscle actin positive, diameter ≤0.8 mm
Epididymis-like	7/13 CD10 positive, others negative
Müllerian-like	CD10 negative
Normal Anatomic Structures	
Normal vas deferens	At least focal CD10 positive, smooth muscle actin positive, diameter ≥1 mm
Normal epididymis	At least focal CD10 positive

correlated with patient age, may aid in distinguishing them from normal vas deferens.[56] Trichrome and immunohistochemical stains for smooth muscle actin are useful because they distinguish periglandular mesenchymal condensations in the inclusions from the subepithelial muscle layer seen in the vas deferens and epididymis. Vas deferens–like and müllerian-like inclusions do not display the luminal CD10 staining that is seen in normal vas deferens. Two types of epididymis-like inclusions have been reported.[56] One group displays luminal decoration by CD10 and may represent aberrant wolffian ductules. The other group does not stain with this antibody and may represent müllerian remnants.

Congenital Hydrocele

Congenital hydroceles result from a persistent communication between the tunica vaginalis and the peritoneal cavity. This communication is normally obliterated after descent of the testis into the scrotum and usually before the age of 2 years.

Cystic Dysplasia

Cystic testicular dysplasia is rare, and it is an entity seen in infants and young children.[58] It is usually a unilateral lesion that is associated with an ipsilateral urogenital lesion such as renal agenesis or cystic dysplasia of the kidney[59] (Table 13-1). The lesion is usually manifested by painless testicular enlargement, although one recently reported patient complained of scrotal pain.[60] Involvement of the rete may be segmental or diffuse. The rete testis in patients with this disorder displays cystically dilated channels (Fig. 13-9) that maintain the normal branching pattern of the rete and do not display epithelial proliferation.[21] The rete spaces are lined by cuboidal to flattened epithelial cells that are surrounded by fibrous stroma. The cysts range in size from 1 to 5 mm in diameter and are visible on gross examination. Seminiferous tubules are normal. Cystic dysplasia of the rete testis does not appear to be caused by obstruction of the duct system, which causes extensive dilation of the rete channels

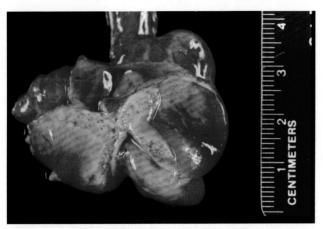

FIGURE 13-9 ■ Cystic dysplasia. This gross photograph displays distorted rete testis architecture due to multilocular cystic dilation of the rete channels.

as well as dilation of seminiferous tubules in young children. It is more likely related to an embryologic defect. During embryogenesis, the rete testis is formed from sex cord stromal tissue; the connection with epididymis (of wolffian duct origin) may be defective in this disorder, leading to dilated, blind-ended rete channels.[21] Abnormal sodium metabolism has also been proposed as a cause for this disorder.[26] Cystic dysplasia has also been reported in the epididymis.[61]

Inflammation and Infection

Inflammatory conditions of infectious or noninfectious origin may principally affect epididymis, tumor, or spermatic cord or may involve more than one of those structures. Furthermore, paratesticular inflammation may be secondary to orchitis. In this section the entities are discussed under headers of nonspecific and granulomatous inflammation, realizing that both may have active (acute) and chronic components. Diverse etiologic agents are associated with these conditions, and in some instances no identifiable agent is found.

Nonspecific Acute and Chronic Inflammations

Epididymitis represents the most common intrascrotal inflammation.[62,63] Chronic infection and inflammation are associated with reactive changes and fibrosis that may simulate a neoplasm. Acute epididymitis is the most common cause of an acutely painful scrotum. Bacterial infection may be caused by a variety of organisms. It is often associated with anatomic abnormalities, and it is the most common type of epididymitis seen in older men.[34] Sexually transmitted *Chlamydia trachomatis* or *Neisseria gonorrhoeae* epididymitis represent the most common cause of acute scrotal swelling in men under the age of 35 years.[34] Sexually transmitted epididymitis is associated with underlying urologic abnormalities.[64] *Chlamydia trachomatis* epididymitis is minimally destructive, with periductal and intraepithelial inflammation, epithelial proliferation, and, sometimes, squamous metaplasia.[65] On the other hand, pyogenic infections such as *N. gonorrhoeae* are associated with destructive abscess formation and may create masses that mimic neoplasia. Low-risk and high-risk types of human papillomavirus have been detected in epididymal and ductus deferens tissue from some patients with epididymitis, although neither koilocytotic atypia nor dysplasia was identified.[66] The male urogenital tract may therefore serve as a reservoir of HPV infection. Older men who develop bacterial epididymitis are more often infected with *Escherichia coli*.

Whereas epididymitis is rare in childhood, an increasing frequency has been reported in children admitted with the diagnosis of acute scrotum.[67] In some cases, *E. coli* has been cultured from children with epididymo-orchitis who had no underlying urinary tract abnormalities.[68]

Chemical epididymitis occurs when sterile urine refluxes into the vas deferens, sometimes after heavy lifting or blunt abdominal trauma that increases the intra-abdominal pressure.[69] The vas deferens and the tail of the epididymis become inflamed, but no organisms are identified.

Schistosomal funiculitis has been reported in a patient with chronic schistosomal infection of long duration.[70] Dirofilaria conjunctivae infection has been seen in the spermatic cord, where it has simulated a neoplasm.[71]

Granulomatous Inflammation

The most common cause of granulomatous epididymitis is tuberculosis (Fig. 13-10). The incidence of this disease has increased because of human immunodeficiency virus infection and intravesical bacille Calmette-Guerin therapy for superficial bladder tumors.[72] There is an association between renal and genital tuberculosis, with frequent involvement of the epididymis.[73] Painful or painless scrotal enlargement is a common presenting symptom. Epididymal tuberculosis may present as a mass lesion in patients that have widespread disease. Secondary hydroceles may be associated with epididymal tuberculosis. Extensive infection can result in sinuses that communicate with the scrotum.[72]

Gross examination of tuberculous epididymitis reveals multiple small white to yellow nodules that typically contain caseous necrosis. Microscopic examination displays necrotizing granulomatous inflammation with palisading histiocytes and Langhans giant cells. Granulomas originate in the epididymal stroma and then enlarge, become confluent, and spread to and secondarily involve the tubules.[74]

Brucella[75,76] and blastomycosis[77] have also been implicated in granulomatous epididymitis clinically simulating neoplasia. Some cases of granulomatous epididymitis have

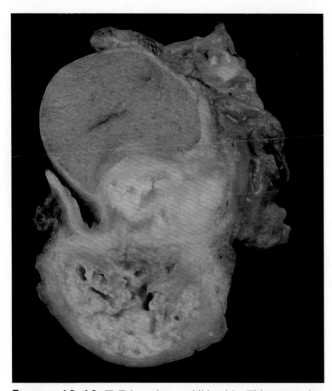

FIGURE 13-10 ■ Tuberculous epididymitis. This gross photograph shows partially necrotic tumor-like lesion involving epididymis and paratesticular soft tissue.

not been associated with any detectable infectious agent.[78] One such case occurred in a 41-year-old man who presented with a scrotal mass and had a 2.3-cm firm lesion in the tail of the epididymis.[34] Epididymal tubules had necrotic walls, and there was a significant histiocytic infiltrate associated with squamous metaplasia.[34] No necrosis or Langhans-type giant cells were seen, and no organisms could be identified on special stains.

Granulomatous epididymitis may also be caused by fungal organisms. However, fungal epididymitis is very rare and usually associated with orchitis. Demonstration of the organisms with special histologic stains or culture is necessary if this diagnosis is a consideration.

Some cases of granulomatous epididymitis with no apparent infectious agent may have an ischemic etiology.[79] In cases thought to be ischemic, granulomatous lesions display predominantly histiocytic infiltrates and typically involve tubular walls rather than the epididymal stroma.[79] Areas of necrosis and squamous metaplasia may be present. Ischemic lesions are more frequently located in the head of the epididymis, where the blood supply is more easily compromised than in the body and tail.[34] The vascular supply for the head of the epididymis consists of only the superior epididymal artery. The vascular supply for the body and tail of the epididymis includes numerous anastomoses between the inferior epididymal and vas deferens arteries, thereby protecting these areas against ischemia.

Xanthogranulomatous epididymitis is associated with Gram-negative bacteria and usually requires surgical excision.[34,80] These lesions display prominent aggregates of foamy histiocytes in addition to plasma cells, lymphocytes, and neutrophils. One reported case[80] was bilateral and so severe that it was difficult to distinguish the epididymis from the adjacent testis. Xanthogranulomatous funiculitis and epididymitis have been described in a quadriplegic patient with unsuccessful voiding.[81] Other rare cases of xanthogranulomatous funiculitis have been reported.[82] The lesion presents with spermatic cord enlargement, and the histologic features are identical to those of xanthogranulomatous epididymitis.

Sarcoidosis

Genitourinary involvement by sarcoidosis is very uncommon. The average age at onset of genital sarcoidosis is 33 years (range 2 to 67).[83] Epididymal sarcoidosis has been reported mainly in black men, some of whom also had testicular sarcoidosis.[84] The spermatic cord may also be involved. These lesions are often asymptomatic and unilateral, although they may be bilateral.[85,86] Firm nodules may replace the entire epididymis. Nonnecrotizing granulomas may cause nodules that measure up to 2.5 cm in diameter and mimic a tumor.[84,87,88] Special stains for acid-fast bacilli and fungi show no organisms. Diffuse involvement of the epididymis may also be present. Most patients have hilar adenopathy or reticulonodular lung infiltrates on chest radiographs. However, genitourinary sarcoidosis has been reported in the absence of radiographically detectable lung or mediastinal disease.[83]

Sclerosing Lipogranuloma

Injection of lipids to increase the size of the genitalia has resulted in granulomatous lesions in the scrotum, the spermatic cord, or the epididymis.[89,90] Some have presented as mass lesions requiring surgical excision.[91,92] Most cases have been associated with a history of exogenous lipid injection or a history of trauma, but some may have been idiopathic.[93] Most patients have presented with localized masses measuring from a few to several centimeters in size.[5]

Gross examination of resected sclerosing lipogranulomas reveals fragmented or intact specimens that are gray to yellow and solid or solid with small cysts on gross examination.[5] Microscopic examination displays patchy fibrous tissue containing empty vacuoles of varying size without epithelial lining cells. Foreign body giant cells may be present. Areas of hyalinization may be seen, and inflammatory cells include histiocytes, lymphocytes, plasma cells, and eosinophils. This lesion is typically patchy in the involved area of the epididymis or spermatic cord. The differential diagnosis of sclerosing lipogranuloma in the epididymis includes adenomatoid tumor, sclerosing lipogranuloma, and signet ring carcinoma. None of those neoplasms contains the empty vacuoles devoid of lining cells that are characteristic of sclerosing lipogranuloma. Mesothelial-lined tubular structures typical of adenomatoid tumor are not seen in sclerosing lipogranulomas. Sclerosing liposarcoma displays atypical nuclei and rare lipoblasts in fibrous tissue alternating with "lipoma-like" areas. Neither atypical nuclei nor lipoblasts are seen in sclerosing lipogranuloma. Signet ring carcinomas contain mucinous cytoplasmic vacuoles that are not present in sclerosing lipogranuloma.

Other Rare Granulomas

Granulomas of paratesticular structures have been reported due to powder from surgical gloves.[94] This was the etiology in the case of a 2-cm hard mass in the head of the epididymis and tunica albuginea in one patient.[94] Microscopic examination of the mass showed fibrous tissue and epithelioid histiocytes intermingled with foreign body–type giant cells that contained crystalline material. Radiopaque contrast dye containing lipid has also been reported as a cause of granulomas of the vas deferens in a 35-year-old infertile man who underwent vesiculoepididymography.[95] Partial resection of the vas deferens revealed a small nodule that showed acute, chronic, and granulomatous inflammation on microscopic examination. The granulomas contained refractile foreign material.

Cholesterol granulomas (also called cholesteatoma) of the tunica vaginalis simulating neoplasm have also been reported.[96,97] One such lesion was described in a 52-year-old man who had a 7-cm mass that had been present since an episode of trauma 25 years earlier.[97] Excision of the mass showed thickening of the tunica vaginalis. Microscopic examination showed granulomas and fibrosis with foreign body–type giant cells containing cytoplasmic cholesterol clefts.

Malakoplakia

About one-third of reported cases of testicular and paratesticular malakoplakia involve the epididymis. The testis is usually involved also,[98,99] although sometimes only the epididymis is affected.[100] Rare cases of epididymal malakoplakia present as masses in patients with remote histories of vasectomy or associated with a hydrocele, and they have occasionally required surgical excision.[101] Other examples of this lesion have been detected incidentally in orchiectomy specimens from men with prostate cancer.[100] Some patients have histories of urinary tract infections, especially with *E. coli*. On microscopic examination, malakoplakia displays aggregates of histiocytes and inflammatory cells with the characteristic targetoid Michaelis-Gutmann bodies. The inflammatory infiltrate may overshadow the population of histiocytes in some cases. Stains for iron (Prussian blue), calcium (von Kossa), and the periodic acid–Schiff stain may help identify these structures if they are not seen on routine H&E stains.

Meconium Periorchitis (Also Called Meconium Vaginalitis)

This lesion usually becomes evident in infants <1 month of age. Rare infants with this condition have had cystic fibrosis.[102] However, several cases have been reported in black infants, a group that is rarely affected by cystic fibrosis. Meconium periorchitis is the result of perforation of the wall of the intestine in utero with subsequent extravasation of meconium into the tunica vaginalis. It is sometimes present as a firm, nontender scrotal mass that is separate from the testis and simulates a neoplasm.[102] On gross examination, the tunica vaginalis and/or spermatic cord typically displays numerous nodules composed of yellow-green material. However, masses measuring up to 3 cm in diameter have been reported.[102] The presence of numerous greenish-yellow small nodules on the tunica vaginalis or spermatic cord in young infants argues against a neoplasm. Microscopic examination shows myxoid tissue and spindle cells, macrophages, squamous cells with and without nuclei, rare lanugo hairs, and mesothelial hyperplasia.[34] The lesion typically does not have much inflammatory infiltrate.

Sperm Granulomas

Sperm granulomas occur at the superior pole of the epididymis or in the vas deferens.[103,104] They are more common in the vas deferens. They sometimes simulate neoplasms and have resulted in orchiectomies.[62,103–107] One patient with an epididymal sperm granuloma had clinical features of an intratesticular tumor.[107] The lesion was associated with testicular swelling and pain 2 years after trauma, and ultrasound studies revealed a solid, hypoechoic mass consistent with an intratesticular tumor. The possibility of a sperm granuloma should be considered when there is a firm, discrete, tender, persistent nodule in the epididymis or vas deferens, especially if the patient has a history of a vasectomy.[104]

More than 40% of sperm granulomas are related to a previous vasectomy,[34] and 1% to 10% of men who have vasectomies develop sperm granulomas.[104,108,109] Trauma, infection, obstruction, and previous surgery are also associated with this lesion. It may also be a complication of secondary oxalosis in patients with chronic renal failure.[108] Most patients are younger than 40 years of age.[103]

The average size of sperm granulomas is 7 mm, although they may be as large as 4 cm, and they are sometimes multiple.[104,106–110] They are firm, yellow-white lesions that contain sperm surrounded by neutrophils, histiocytes, and giant cells. Cystic spaces may be present due to obstruction and dilation of epididymal tubules, which may display squamous metaplasia.[34] Dystrophic calcification may occur. The lesion eventually becomes replaced by fibrous tissue that may contain lipochrome pigment. Vasitis nodosa accompanies one-third of sperm granulomas present in the vas deferens.[34]

Vasitis Nodosa and Epididymitis Nodosa

Vasitis nodosa and epididymitis nodosa are usually postvasectomy changes. Vasitis nodosa is usually identified during a vasovasostomy from 1 to 15 years after vasectomy.[111] The lesions occur in as many as half of men who have had vasectomies, and they may be bilateral. However, vasitis nodosa and epididymitis nodosa may also follow trauma, herniorrhaphy, and prostatectomy.[112] They have been described in patients with primary infertility, chronic severe cystitis, and bladder diverticula.[112] Most cases are asymptomatic, possibly because the lesions are small (<1 cm). Some patients have scrotal swelling, pain, and nodularity. Patients with vasitis nodosa usually have a firm nodule in the scrotal part of the vas. Both lesions display a proliferation of small ducts and gland-like structures in the walls of the vas deferens and epididymis in response to mechanical obstruction and increased intraluminal pressure. The glands may be located in a perineural location, resulting in confusion with adenocarcinoma.[113–115] The gland proliferation seen in vasitis and epididymitis nodosa does not display mitotic figures or epithelial atypia, and the presence of sperm in gland lumina is evidence against a neoplasm. Extravasation of sperm leads to sperm granulomas and subsequent inflammation and fibrosis. Sperm granulomas coexist with vasitis and epididymitis nodosa in 70% of patients.[34]

Vascular Abnormalities and Ischemia

Arterial Venous Malformations

Arterial venous malformations are rare in the paratesticular region. A case of an intrascrotal, extratesticular lesion was detected after a bicycle accident resulted in a scrotal hematoma.[116] A case has also been described in the spermatic cord.[117] Some other arterial venous malformations have been reported in the "scrotum" without specification of exact locations.

There has been one reported case of a spermatic artery aneurysm.[118] It presented as a round, firm, nonpulsating tender mass in the left spermatic cord of a 50-year-old man. It was attached to a segment of a muscular artery, and the cut surface showed aneurysmal dilation of the artery with blood clot. There was a transition from the wall of the artery to the aneurysm.[118]

Varicocele

Varicoceles represent abnormal venous dilation in the pampiniform vascular plexus. They occur in about 15% of men.[119] They may be detected during investigation of infertility, or they may present with scrotal pain and swelling. They occur most commonly on the left side due to increased hydrostatic pressure from the left spermatic vein entering the left renal vein perpendicularly. The pampiniform plexus becomes dilated and tortuous. More unusual causes of varicoceles include compression of the renal vein, an aberrant renal vein, or an obstructed renal vein.[119] Varicoceles that occur on the right side and those with recent onset in older men should prompt evaluation of a possible abdominal mass compressing veins downstream from the scrotum. Gross and microscopic examination of the rete testis in patients with varicoceles often reveals dilated rete testis veins that compress and obstruct the rete tubules, although some patients have dilated efferent ductule veins that result in dilated rete testis channels.[120]

Torsion

Testicular torsion has been diagnosed in one-third of patients under the age of 40 who present with acute scrotal pain and undergo emergency scrotal exploration.[121] Torsion of the spermatic cord results in hemorrhagic infarction of the testis. The next most common entity in the patients with acute scrotal pain followed by emergency surgery is torsion of the appendix testis. Torsion of the appendix testis has been reported to be the most common cause of acute scrotum in children.[122] Torsion of the epididymis has been described in a 11-year-old boy who presented with an acute scrotum and was found to have an abnormal attachment of the epididymis to the testis.[123] Torsion of the testicular or epididymal appendages may simulate the clinical symptoms of testicular torsion. Gross and microscopic features of the structures affected by torsion are those of hemorrhagic infarction. Dark red, hemorrhagic tissue is present. Extravasated blood often overshadows any residual parenchymal architecture, and ischemic changes may obliterate normal histology.

Vasculitis

Polyarteritis nodosa is the most common vasculitis seen in the paratesticular region.[34] Unilateral or bilateral epididymal enlargement and tenderness may be either the presenting symptom of the disease or a component of systemic disease.[124–126] A review of autopsy tissue from patients with known polyarteritis nodosa showed epididymal vasculitis in two-thirds of cases.[127] Isolated arteritis of the epididymis has also been reported, and it may be either an incidental finding or associated with a mass.[128] A case of limited Wegener granulomatosis involving the epididymis has been described in a 32-year-old man.[129]

Other types of vasculitis seen in the paratestis include Henoch-Schoenlein purpura,[130] thromboangiitis obliterans, and granulomatous vasculitis. One 6-year-old boy with Henoch-Schoenlein purpura developed a swollen, painful right scrotum 24 hours after an appendectomy.[130] The tunica albuginea, epididymis, spermatic cord, and testis displayed vascular necrosis, red blood cell extravasation, and vascular infiltration by neutrophils.[130] There was hemorrhagic infarction of the testis and spermatic cord. Microscopic examination displayed necrotic vessel walls with areas of acute inflammation and extravasated red blood cells in the testis, tunica albuginea, epididymis, and spermatic cord.

Thromboangiitis obliterans has been reported in the epididymis and spermatic cord.[34] The patients reported have been in the third or fourth decades of life, and they have presented with firm, tender scrotal masses.[131–133] Gross examination of the lesions revealed enlarged, thickened vasa deferentia or epididymal nodules. Microscopic examination displayed arterial and venous thrombi and focal aggregates of mononuclear inflammatory cells and giant cells in the vessel walls.

Granulomatous vasculitis (Fig. 13-11) has been reported in the epididymis or spermatic cord in five patients, either with or without involvement of the adjacent testis.[134–136] These lesions have been unilateral or bilateral and synchronous or metachronous. One 70-year-old patient had a painless paratesticular mass that was clinically suspicious for a neoplasm. He had no signs or symptoms of vasculitis before resection of the mass. Microscopic examination of the mass displayed a nonnecrotizing granulomatous vasculitis containing giant cells in arteries and veins of the spermatic cord.[136]

Two reported patients developed hemorrhagic infarction of the testis as a result of intimal fibroplasia of the spermatic artery.[137] Both patients had orchiectomies because clinical features were suspicious for neoplasms. Microscopic

examination of both lesions showed moderate or marked luminal obstruction of branches of the spermatic artery under the tunica albuginea and in the testis. The arterial wall intima contained a proliferation of loose connective tissue, but there were no abnormalities of the elastic lamina. These lesions resemble intimal fibroplasia of the renal artery seen in patients with arterial hypertension.[34]

Miscellaneous Cysts, Celes and Pseudotumorous Conditions

Cystic Transformation of the Rete Testis (Synonym: Also Called Giant Cystic Degeneration of the Rete Testis)

Nistal et al.[138] studied 1,798 autopsy and 518 surgical specimens from the testis and epididymis, and identified cystic transformation of the rete testis in 20 autopsy and 18 surgical pathology specimens.[138] The cystic transformation was thought to be due to several different etiologies. One cause of this lesion is mechanical compression of the extratesticular excretory ducts, resulting from neoplasia or other masses such as hematoceles. Cystic transformation may also follow postvasectomy inflammation or it may be related to infection such as epididymitis. An ischemic etiology has also been proposed in elderly men who have atherosclerosis in the epididymal branch of the testicular artery with associated atrophy of the head of the epididymis. Hormonal abnormalities may cause cystic transformation of the rete testis in patients with cirrhosis; these patients have increased peripheral conversion of androgen to estrogen and develop bilateral epididymal atrophy and columnar transformation of the rete testis epithelium. One case of giant cystic degeneration of the rete testis has been reported recently in an elderly adult man treated with LHRH for prostate adenocarcinoma.[139] The patient age, the postulated effect to antiandrogen therapy, and the 10-cm size of the lesion are all unusual for this lesion. Malformations, such as cryptorchidism, that have dissociation between the rete testis (derived from the sex cords) and the epididymis (derived from the mesonephric duct) may also result in cystic transformation of the rete testis (Box 13-2).

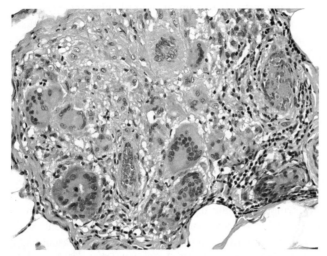

FIGURE 13-11 ■ Granulomatous vasculitis involving the spermatic cord. Small blood vessels are surrounded by giant cells.

Box 13-2 ● CELES/CYSTS OF THE PARATESTIS: ETIOLOGY AND ASSOCIATED LESIONS	
Cystic transformation of the rete testis	Mechanical compression, postvasectomy, ischemia, hormonal factors, cryptorchidism
Acquired cysts of the rete testis	Hemodialysis
Cysts of the epididymis	Polycystic kidney disease, von Hippel-Lindau (rare), renal cell carcinoma (rare), in utero DES exposure
Hydrocele (acquired)	Idiopathic or may be secondary to infection or neoplasm
Hematocele	Trauma, torsion, tumor, surgery

Acquired Cysts of the Rete Testis

Acquired cysts of the rete testis have been reported in patients on hemodialysis, who may have oxalate crystals in the cyst lumens[140] (Box 13-2). Benign rete testis cysts are lined by a single layer of flat or columnar epithelial cells.

Mesothelial Cysts

Mesothelial-lined cysts of the paratesticular area are rare and may involve the tunica albuginea, tunica vaginalis, epididymis, or spermatic cord.[18,141–144] They usually occur in men over 40 years of age. They may either be asymptomatic or patients may present with a painful mass simulating testicular tumors. These cysts may be single or multiple, but they are usually unilateral and located on the anterolateral surface of the testis.[144] They measure from 0.3 to 0.4 cm in diameter and contain serous or blood-tinged fluid. The cysts are lined by single-layered, non-atypical, flattened, or cuboidal mesothelial cells. The epithelium is surrounded by hyalinized connective tissue. Squamous metaplasia may be present. The cysts are surrounded by fibrous tissue. They are benign lesions that should be treated conservatively.

Cysts of the Epididymis

Small benign cysts of the epididymis are common. They measure 1 to 2 cm in diameter. Pain and torsion may occur with larger cysts.[145] Polycystic kidney disease has been associated with multiple epididymal cysts.[146] Bilateral epididymal cysts have been described in a patient with von Hippel–Lindau disease and early-onset renal cell carcinoma.[147] Epididymal cysts have also been reported in 10% of men exposed to DES in utero[148] (Box 13-2).

Epididymal cysts usually occur in the head of the epididymis. They are thought to arise from efferent ductules.[21] They may be unilocular or multilocular, and they are lined by a single layer of flat to cuboidal epithelial cells that may display variable numbers of cilia (Fig. 13-12). Cytologic

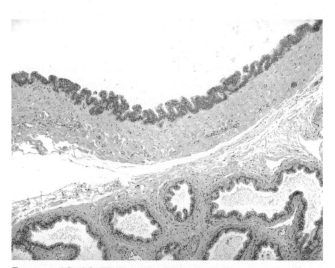

FIGURE 13-12 ■ Cyst of epididymis. A dilated, cystic efferent duct is present adjacent to normal ducts.

atypia is not a feature of epididymal cysts. If spermatozoa are present in the cysts, the lesions are called spermatoceles. Small papillary structures containing connective tissue cores lined by a single layer of bland epithelium may protrude into the cysts.[149]

Spermatocele

Spermatoceles result from cystic dilation of the efferent ductules, the tubules of the rete testis, or the aberrant ducts. Cysts may become large, with thin walls. Cloudy fluid present in spermatoceles is a result of sperm present in the cystic spaces. The fibromuscular walls are lined by cuboidal to columnar, sometimes ciliated, epithelium. The epithelial lining of long-standing spermatocele may be quite attenuated and may resemble a mesothelial or simple squamous layer.[18] Sometimes they contain papillary proliferations lined by benign epithelial cells.[149] Calcification may occur.[150] Clusters of small blue cells have been reported in spermatocele and hydrocele specimens. They may represent sloughed rete testis epithelium and they may mimic the appearance of small cell carcinoma.[151] Bland nuclei, lack of mitotic figures, and lack of staining with neuroendocrine markers are features indicative of benign epithelium.

Dermoid and Epidermoid Cysts

Epidermoid cysts are rare in the paratestis.[152] They present either incidentally during hernia repair procedures or as painless enlarging masses located in the spermatic cord. They are lined by keratinizing squamous epithelium and contain intracystic keratinous debris. Dermoid cysts have also been reported in the spermatic cord.[153,154] They contain skin appendage structures in addition to squamous epithelium.

Most epidermoid and dermoid cysts are considered benign neoplasms, in contrast to teratomas. Some epidermoid cysts may represent a metaplastic process derived from mesothelium. The possibility of extension or metastasis from a tumor in the testis should be excluded before making this diagnosis.

Hydrocele (Acquired)

A hydrocele is a fluid accumulation between the visceral and parietal layers of the tunica vaginalis. Congenital hydroceles have been discussed above (congenital abnormalities). Acquired hydroceles may be idiopathic or secondary to infections or neoplasms (Box 13-2). They represent the most common cause of painless scrotal swelling. They form over time, and neoplasm should be excluded in the case of a rapid formation of a hydrocele. Hydroceles usually transilluminate, except in cases where the tunica vaginalis is thickened. Ultrasound shows an anechoic fluid collection. The pathogenesis of acquired hydroceles reflects an imbalance between fluid secretion and resorption in the tunica vaginalis.[155] Defective lymphatic drainage has been suggested as a cause of hydroceles.[156]

Chronic hydroceles may become inflamed, with a proliferation of fibrous tissue. The testis may become adherent to the parietal tunica vaginalis. These features may mimic neoplasms clinically.[34,62,63] The resulting mass-like lesions may be more than twice the normal size of the normal testis, but they are diffuse and symmetrical.[34] Patients in one series of nine patients ranged from 22 to 88 years of age.[63] Most patients had hydroceles that were excised because of the clinical similarity to neoplasms.[63] Microscopic examination showed features typical of a reactive process, including mesothelial hyperplasia with fibrosis and some chronic inflammation.[63] Organizing hemorrhage in a hydrocele may also simulate a neoplasm until it is examined microscopically.

Hematocele

Hematoceles represent collections of blood in the tunica vaginalis. They may be acute or chronic, and they may have a mass effect. Causes include trauma, torsion, tumor, and surgery (Box 13-2). Varicoceles may be present, and minor trauma may cause rupture of one of the dilated blood vessels.[69] Patients present with a mass and scrotal pain. Most hematoceles resolve spontaneously with conservative therapy, but some may become fibrotic and calcified.[157]

Endometriosis

Endometriosis has been reported in an elderly man who presented with a mass in the tail of the epididymis on a follow-up examination after taking diethylstilbestrol for 3 years for prostate carcinoma. On gross examination, a 5-cm mass was present between the vas deferens and the tail of the epididymis. Microscopic examination showed tubular glands lined by columnar to cuboidal epithelium without atypia. The glands were surrounded by stroma typical of that normally seen in the endometrium.

Prostatic-Type Glands

Prostatic-type glands have been found rarely in the epididymis.[158] One example was found incidentally in a grossly normal epididymis in a 30-year-old man.[158] The glands displayed the two cell layers normally seen in prostate glands. While these glands were different from the epididymal gland epithelium, there was a focal transition from epididymal ducts to the prostatic epithelium. The prostate glands stained positively for prostatic acid phosphatase (PAP) and prostate-specific antigen (PSA), but some epididymal duct tissue was also positive with these markers. The lesion probably represents prostatic metaplasia in the epididymis rather than true ectopic prostate glands.[158,159]

Metanephric Dysplastic Hamartoma

There is one report of metanephric dysplastic hamartoma presenting as an epididymal mass in an 18-month-old boy. Blastema associated with papillae, glomeruloid structures, and dysplastic tubules were seen on microscopic examination.[5] This lesion must be distinguished from the rare Wilms tumors that have been reported in the paratesticular region.

Rosai-Dorfman Disease

A few cases of Rosai-Dorfman disease (sinus histiocytosis with massive lymphadenopathy) have been described in the epididymis.[160] Patients may be either children or adults, and lymph nodes are also often involved.[5] This process may result in nodules, or it may diffusely involve the epididymis. Microscopic examination shows sheets of histiocytes that contain oval nuclei and abundant pale cytoplasm with poorly defined cell borders. The histiocytes may contain phagocytosed lymphocytes, plasma cells, neutrophils, and erythrocytes.

Calcification, Bone, and Cartilage

An autopsy study of testes and associated rete testes showed a rare lesion called "nodular proliferation of calcifying connective tissue in the rete testis"[161] in three men with histories of myocardial infarction. Polypoid projections in the rete spaces had connective tissue cores with calcification and were covered by benign, flattened epithelial cells.

Calcification may cause firm nodules in the epididymis, usually associated with sperm granuloma, filarial infection, or tuberculosis.[162] Calcification of the epididymis may also be seen in patients on hemodialysis.[163] Two cases of heterotopic bone trabeculae in the epididymis have been reported.[18,164] Cartilage has also been seen in the epididymis of infants.[165]

Calcification of the seminal vesicles and vasa deferentia may indicate systemic disease.[166] This lesion may be associated with diabetes, uremia with secondary hyperparathyroidism, prostatitis, infections (tuberculosis, schistosomiasis, gonorrhoea), and congenital abnormalities. Bilateral calcification of the vas deferens has been reported in a hemodialysis patient[167] and, rarely, the condition is idiopathic.

Amyloidosis

One histochemical and ultrastructural study of six men with secondary amyloidosis showed amyloid deposits in the walls of the blood vessels of the epididymis and spermatic cord.[168] Localized amyloidosis involving vasa deferentia has been described in two patients with prostate carcinoma.[169]

Inflammatory Myofibroblastic Tumor (Synonyms: Also Called Inflammatory Pseudotumor, Pseudosarcomatous Myofibroblastic Proliferation, and Proliferative Funiculitis)

Inflammatory myofibroblastic tumor and related lesions in the paratestis occur most often in the spermatic cord,[62,170–176] but isolated cases have also been reported in the rete testis

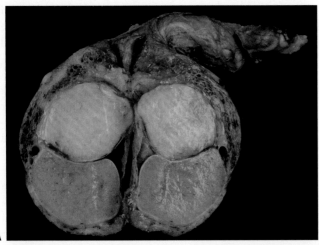

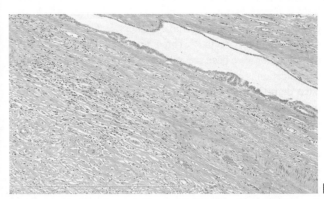

FIGURE 13-13 ■ Inflammatory myofibroblastic tumor. **A:** Gross photograph showing circumscribed paratesticular tan tumor-like nodule; **B:** Note dense fibroblastic connective tissue and chronic inflammation adjacent to mesothelial lined space. Sclerosis is often present in long-standing cases.

and epididymis.[171,172] They may present as mass lesions, or they may be incidental findings in inguinal hernia specimens. Some of these lesions in the epididymis may be a reaction to torsion and chronic ischemia.[170,176]

These lesions are usually gray or tan, firm nodules that are <3 cm in size, although an occasional lesion has measured 7 cm.[5] Some are well circumscribed (Fig. 13-13), but many are poorly demarcated. Areas of hemorrhage or cystic change may occur rarely. Inflammatory myofibroblastic tumors are composed of tapering spindle to stellate-shaped cells with vesicular nuclei and eosinophilic cytoplasm. The stroma is fibrous or myxoid. Cellularity varies in different parts of the lesions and may be greater in the central portion of the lesion. Inflammatory and giant cells may cause the lesion to resemble fasciitis seen elsewhere in the body.[5] Hyalinized fibrous tissue characteristically surrounds blood vessels. The mitotic rate is usually low, although torsion has been associated with greater numbers of mitotic figures.[176] Atypical mitotic figures are not present. It is possible that these lesions may progress to the densely collagenous and hyalinized "fibrous pseudotumors."[5] Immunohistochemical stains performed on inflammatory myofibroblastic tumors show cells will be of myofibroblastic phenotype; stains may be positive for actins, vimentin, desmin, and sometimes keratin,[34] although these stains are not usually necessary for diagnosis of this lesion.

The differential diagnosis of inflammatory pseudotumors includes rhabdomyosarcoma, leiomyosarcoma, sclerosing liposarcoma, malignant fibrous histiocytoma, and spindle cell mesothelioma. The bland cytologic features, low mitotic rate, lack of atypical mitoses, and overall resemblance to fasciitis are features that are helpful in recognizing the reactive nature of this lesion and distinguishing it from malignant neoplasms.

Fibrous Pseudotumor (Synonyms: Called Fibromatous Periorchitis, Nodular Periorchitis Additional Synonyms: Chronic Periorchitis, Proliferative Funiculitis, Fibrous Proliferation of Tunics, Fibroma, Nonspecific Testicular Fibrosis, Nodular Fibrous Periorchitis, Nodular Fibrous Pseudotumor, Inflammatory Pseudotumor, Reactive Periorchitis, Pseudofibromatous Periorchitis)

Paratesticular fibrous pseudotumors present as mass lesions. They are most often seen in the third decade of life,[177,178] but one case has been reported in a 5-year-old boy.[179] One patient had retroperitoneal fibrosis, one had Gorlin syndrome,[180] and one lesion was associated with testicular infarction.[181] After adenomatoid tumors, these lesions represent the most common cause of masses in the paratestis. Patients have single or multiple nodules or plaques in the tunica vaginalis,[182,183] epididymis,[184,185] or spermatic cord, and the nodules range from 0.5 to

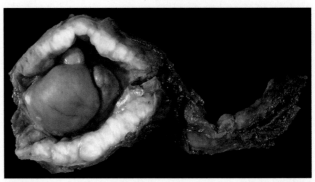

FIGURE 13-14 ■ Fibroma of the tunica vaginalis. Gross photograph showing extensive involvement of tunica vaginalis by white nodular fibrous tissue.

8 cm[177] (Fig. 13-14). In a diffuse form, dense fibrous tissue involves the tunica vaginalis.

Microscopically, this lesion is characterized by dense, hyalinized, fibrous tissue often containing lymphocytes and plasma cells with occasional germinal centers.[186] Calcification and ossification may occur.[187] Three histologic types of fibrous pseudotumor have been recently described,[188] although this subclassification is mainly of academic interest. Plaque-like lesions have dense fibrous stroma without significant inflammation, inflammatory sclerotic pseudotumors contain dense fibrous tissue with significant inflammation and myofibroblastic lesions have reactive appearing cells with numerous capillaries and sparse chronic inflammation.[188] Paratesticular fibrous pseudotumor does not display significant nuclear atypia, mitotic activity, or necrosis. The differential diagnosis of paratesticular fibrous pseudotumor includes solitary fibrous tumor, leiomyoma, fibromatosis, spindle cell mesothelioma, and neurofibroma.[188]

Immunohistochemical stains performed on paratesticular fibrous pseudotumors display positive staining for smooth muscle actin in more than 80% of cases.[188] Surprisingly, stains for cytokeratin, calretinin, and CD34 are positive in about half of the cases.[188] All cases in a recent study were negative for B-catenin and ALK-1, and these lesions have a very low proliferation index as measured by Ki-67 staining.[188]

Potential cells of origin include myofibroblasts and submesothelial stromal cells, but paratesticular fibrous pseudotumors may be a nonspecific pattern resulting from a variety of pathogenetic processes.[188] Past histories of trauma, surgery, infection, and inflamed hydroceles in some patients suggest a reactive etiology,[63,189] although some patients have no such prior events. Some fibrous pseudotumors are thought to represent an advanced stage of inflammatory pseudotumors.[149,177,190] Paratesticular fibrous pseudotumors are benign lesions, and local excision is curative.

"Tumor" of the Adrenogenital Syndrome and Related Lesions

This lesion develops in the paratesticular region of men with the adrenogenital syndrome who are not adequately treated, especially men with the salt-losing form of the syndrome. Nodules of steroid-type cells may occur in the epididymis, the spermatic cord, or the tunica albuginea.[38,191–193] The paratesticular lesions may either extend from testicular nodules or be separate dark brown nodules measuring up to 1.5 cm in diameter.[38] Sometimes, fibrous septa are present in the nodules. The microscopic appearance of these lesions is quite characteristic. Paratesticular nodules of steroid type cells are present. Bands of fibrous tissue and focal nuclear atypia are also seen.

Five cases of rete testis–associated nodular steroid cell nests associated with the rete testis have recently been reported.[194] They are discrete conspicuous, unencapsulated nodules with vascular sinusoids between nests or cords of cells. They display strong melan A immunostaining, absent-to-weak inhibin staining and absent-to-moderate calretinin

expression, in contrast to interstitial Leydig cells and testicular adnexal Leydig cells (TTAGS). The cells in rete testis–associated nodular steroid nests have been postulated to represent the precursor of testicular tumors of the adrenogenital syndrome.[194]

Patients with Nelson syndrome have ACTH-secreting pituitary adenomas following bilateral adrenalectomy for Cushing syndrome. These patients may also develop paratesticular steroid cell nodules.[39,195,196] All reported cases have been bilateral, with nodules ranging up to 5.5 cm in diameter.[195,196] They may produce cortisol and result in recurrence of Cushing syndrome. Gross and microscopic features are similar to those seen in patients with the adrenogenital syndrome. Bilateral small steroid cell nodules have also been described in children with Cushing syndrome and nodular hyperplasia of the adrenal cortex.[38,197] They also have the same morphologic characteristics as the nodules associated with the adrenogenital syndrome.

Some masses of paratesticular steroid cells may also develop by stimulation of ectopic adrenocortical tissue found in about 10% of infants and some older patients.[5,34,35,198,199]

Hyperplasias

Hyperplasia of the Rete Testis (Synonym: Also Called Adenomatous Hyperplasia)

Hyperplasia of the rete testis includes both epithelial hyperplasia and smooth muscle hyperplasia. Epithelial hyperplasia may be real or apparent, so-called rete testis prominence.[200]

The cause of rete testis hyperplasia is not clear, but it may reflect hormonal factors including estrogen effect.[201,202] Mice exposed in utero to DES have developed rete hyperplasia.[203] Cryptorchidism, thought to be related to abnormalities of the hypothalamic–pituitary–testicular hormonal axis, is associated with both testicular atrophy and rete testis hyperplasia.[204] One reported patient had been treated with DES for 15 months and androgen blockade for 19 months before diagnosis of rete testis hyperplasia.[201] Increased numbers and stratification of rete epithelial cells has also been described after estrogen therapy in male-to-female transsexual patients.[202] Columnar change of the rete epithelium has been associated with chronic liver failure,[202] further supporting a hormonal basis for hyperplasia of the rete testis. Rete testis hyperplasia may also be associated with testicular atrophy and hypospermatogenesis.[13,18,201,205,206] There is no clear dividing line between prominent rete testis associated with testicular atrophy and true rete hyperplasia. Rete hyperplasia may also be associated with epididymal cribriform change.[13] It has also been described in a child with bilateral renal dysplasia[207] and in patients with carcinoma of the prostate[208] and breast.[205]

Some authors have proposed separating hyperplasia of the rete testis into two types: congenital and acquired.[209] Lesions associated with cryptorchid testes, as well as some that are associated with testicular germ cell tumors, are included in the congenital group. Cases related to chemical

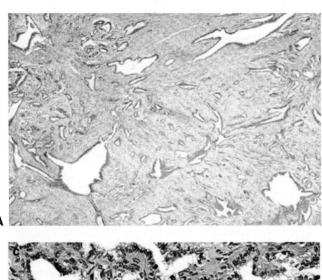

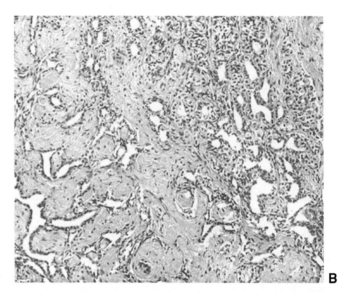

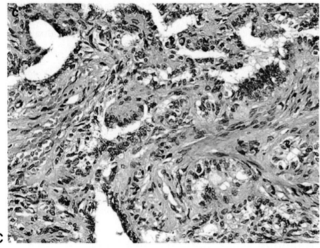

FIGURE 13-15 ■ Adenomatous hyperplasia of rete testis. Complex, interconnecting proliferation of tubular channels with and without cystic dilation, low power (**A, B**). The lining cells are cuboidal to low columnar with innocuous cytology (**C**). (Reprinted from Amin MB. Selected other problematic testicular and paratesticular lesions: rete testis neoplasms and pseudotumors, mesothelial lesions and secondary tumors. *Mod Pathol* 2005;18:S131–S145, with permission.)

agents, some hormonal changes such as androgen blockage, and most lesions related to testicular germ cell tumors are considered acquired hyperplasias.

Nine patients in one study of rete testis hyperplasia[201] ranged in age from 30 to 74 years of age (mean 59 years). Three patients presented with a clinically identifiable solid or cystic testicular hilar mass; however, the lesion is more likely to be an incidental finding. Rete testis hyperplasia may be multinodular and/or bilateral.

Two histologic types of rete testis hyperplasia have been described. Adenomatous hyperplasia (Fig. 13-15) displays a complex focal or diffuse interconnecting labyrinth of tubulopapillary channels that may be cystically dilated.[200] Gland lumina may be empty or they may contain either sperm or eosinophilic secretions. A second type of rete testis hyperplasia represents an incidental finding in patients with testicular germ cell tumors. This lesion is characterized by a focal or diffuse epithelial proliferation within dilated rete testis spaces (Fig. 13-16). Hyaline globules within the hyperplastic rete epithelium may simulate the appearance of yolk sac tumor. Cells of rete hyperplasia are

cuboidal, with pale, eosinophilic cytoplasm and round to oval, uniform nuclei. There is no cytologic atypia, necrosis, or mitotic activity. Epithelial cells stain positively for cytokeratin and epithelial membrane antigen, and the mesenchyme between the hyperplastic tubules displays variable staining for vimentin, muscle-specific actin, desmin, and S-100 protein.[201] Ultrastructural examination of the epithelial cells shows intracellular junctions and complex interdigitation of cell membranes.[201] Important indicators of the benign, reactive nature of this lesion are overall conformation to the normal branching tubular architecture of the rete testis and its continuity with nonhyperplastic rete testicular tubules.

Rete testis hyperplasia may resemble a primary or metastatic carcinoma.[5,18,21,201,205,208] PSA and PAP stains may be useful in distinguishing rete hyperplasia from prostatic carcinoma.[206] Testicular germ cell tumors may be associated with papillary, squamous, or vacuolated rete testis epithelium.[210] Furthermore, there may be invasive or intraepithelial pagetoid spread of the germ cell tumor in the rete testis.[210–213] Immunohistochemical stains for

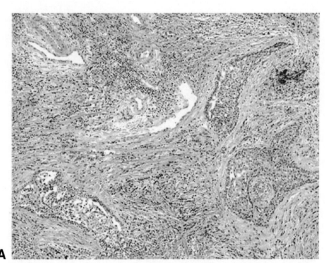
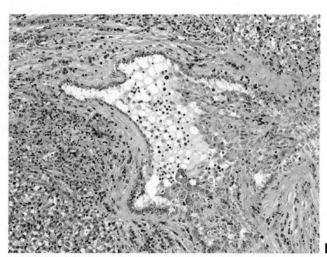

FIGURE 13-16 ■ Rete testis hyperplasia associated with germ cell tumor. Hyperplastic rete epithelium fills expanded channels (low power) **(A)**. Seminoma associated with rete testis hyperplasia **(B)**. Hyperplastic rete epithelium shows intracytoplasmic and extracellular hyaline globules that result in an appearance simulating yolk sac tumor. If misinterpreted as such, this would lead a pure seminoma to be diagnosed as a mixed germ cell tumor with seminoma and yolk sac tumor components. (Reprinted from Amin MB. Selected other problematic testicular and paratesticular lesions: rete testis neoplasms and pseudotumor, mesothelial lesions and secondary tumors. *Mod Pathol* 2005;18:S131–S145, with permission.)

germ cell tumors can resolve any diagnostic confusion.[214] Rete testis hyperplasia may contain eosinophilic hyaline globules that are PAS-positive and may stain for alpha-1-anti-trypsin, but they are alpha-fetoprotein negative. They may contain proteins absorbed from the rete lumen by lining epithelial cells.[210] Rete hyperplasia with hyaline globules needs to be distinguished from the many and various morphologic patterns of yolk sac tumor.[210,215] One case of rete testis hyperplasia with hyaline globules also had eosinophilic basement membrane material between the hyperplastic rete epithelial cells, simulating the parietal type of yolk sac tumor.[210,215] Papillary adenoma of the rete testis, a small lesion that is usually identified incidentally in the testicular hilum at the time of microscopic examination, also needs to be distinguished from rete testis hyperplasia.

Cribriform Hyperplasia and Atypical Nuclei in the Epididymis

The normal epididymis, which usually has a simple columnar epithelium, may display a cribriform epithelial pattern (Fig. 13-17).[15,216] The cribriform change is usually focal but can sometimes be more extensive raising the possibility of hyperplasia, although the latter has not been well defined in the epididymis. The incidence of this histologic finding has ranged from 8% to 50% in the literature.[13–15] Intratubular confinement of the cribriform epithelium and lack of mitotic activity or cytologic atypia are features that are helpful in distinguishing this architectural variant from epididymal carcinoma.

Enlarged and atypical nuclei similar to those seen in the seminal vesicles may also occur in the efferent ductules, ductus epididymis,[9] and vas deferens. This cytologic

atypia has been attributed to fusion of epithelial cells into multinucleated giant cells that then form large pyknotic nuclei.[34] These atypical nuclei are more frequently encountered in older patients and are not associated with any systemic disease, but the association with age supports a hormonal or degenerative process.[34] This is a focal or spotty process, and the atypical nuclei may contain cytoplasmic pseudoinclusions, but there are no mitotic figures.

Reactive Mesothelial Hyperplasia

Reactive mesothelial hyperplasia is an uncommon lesion that may be associated with hydrocele, hematocele, hernia sacs, and paratesticular fibrous pseudotumors.[18,149,217] It is

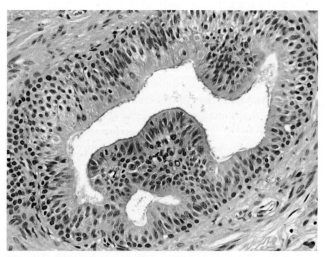

FIGURE 13-17 ■ Cribriform architecture in the epididymis. The cells are cuboidal or columnar. There are no mitotic figures.

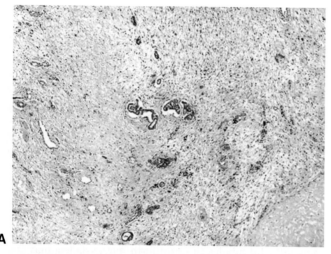

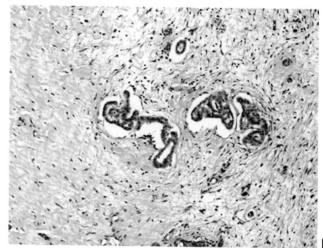

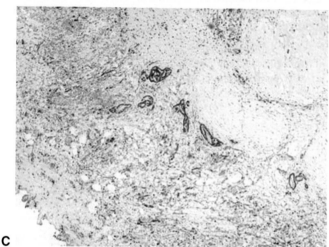

FIGURE 13-18 ■ Reactive mesothelial hyperplasia with mesothelial entrapment occurring in a background of organizing hematocele. Low-power observation of linear disposition of tubules rather than a haphazard infiltrative growth is an important feature to recognize (**A**). Higher power shows small reactive tubulopapillary mesothelial clusters with retraction artifact that may mimic vascular invasion (**B**). Immunohistochemical stain for WT1 confirms the mesothelial nature of the proliferation (**C**). (Reprinted from Amin MB. Selected other problematic testicular and paratesticular lesions: rete testis neoplasms and pseudotumors, mesothelial lesions and secondary tumors. *Mod Pathol* 2005;18:S131–S145, with permission.)

usually an incidental histologic finding in those lesions, and it appears to be a response to serosal injury.[200] Mesothelial hyperplasia usually displays submesothelial aggregates of mesothelial cells that are well circumscribed and surrounded by fibrous tissue.[218] Small papillary structures and solid nodules of mesothelial cells may also protrude into the lumen of the involved structure. Most cases show no cytologic atypia, but nuclear atypia and rare mitoses[217] are present in some cases. The combination of the mesothelial proliferation and submesothelial fibrosis may result in clusters of mesothelial cells or small glands being trapped in fibrous tissue in a pseudoinvasive pattern. The overall proliferation, however, has a linear distribution without destructive invasion of the underlying tissue (Fig. 13-18).

Reactive mesothelial hyperplasia must be distinguished from well-differentiated papillary mesothelioma, malignant mesothelioma, paratesticular serous tumors, and metastatic adenocarcinoma. Reactive mesothelial hyperplasia lacks the significant cytologic atypia and invasive or complex destructive tubulopapillary pattern seen in malignant tumors,[144] and it often contains inflammatory cells. It does not form a mass lesion. A desmin immunohistochemical stain may be useful in differential diagnosis because it stains reactive

mesothelial cells but not malignant mesothelial proliferations.[219] The presence of mesothelial immunohistochemical markers[220] and the lack of an invasive pattern are useful in excluding adenocarcinoma.

Smooth Muscle Hyperplasia

Smooth muscle hyperplasia of the testicular adnexa represents an idiopathic overgrowth of muscle normally present in the paratesticular region. It proliferates around or between normal structures.[221] The largest series of these unusual lesions reported 16 cases that involved the epididymis, the spermatic cord, the tunica vaginalis, and the tunica albuginea.[221]

Smooth muscle hyperplasia in the paratestis has been seen in adults between 46 and 81 years of age.[221] All patients presented with palpable intrascrotal mass lesions ranging from a few millimeters to several centimeters in diameter. The average size was 2.5 cm, but some of these masses measured up to 7 cm in diameter. Some were nodular or fusiform masses, whereas others were more poorly defined thickenings of paratesticular structures. Gross examination showed firm gray to white cut surfaces.[34] Microscopic examination revealed a diffuse or nodular increase in smooth muscle that displayed a perivascular, periductal or interstitial location.[221] No inflammatory infiltrate or mitotic figures were seen in the smooth muscle hyperplasia. The well-circumscribed architecture seen in leiomyomas was not present. Proliferations of smooth muscle surrounded the vas deferens and epididymal ducts. This lesion was associated with vasitis nodosa, interstitial fibrosis, calcium deposition, and duct ectasia in some cases. One case of simultaneous leiomyoma and contralateral smooth muscle hyperplasia of the epididymis has been reported.[222] A complex cystic mass of the rete testis associated with smooth muscle hyperplasia and myxoid stroma containing Leydig cells has also been described in a 26-year-old man.[223] Smooth muscle hyperplasia of paratesticular structures is a benign lesion that does not recur after excision.

Multicystic Mass of Probable Wolffian Origin

A multicystic mass of presumed wolffian origin in the paratestis displayed multiple cysts lined by cuboidal to columnar epithelium and surrounded by strands of smooth muscle and was considered to represent cystic hyperplasia of wolffian duct remnants.[224]

NEOPLASMS OF THE PARATESTICULAR REGION

Epithelial Tumors

Rete Testis and Epididymis — General Considerations

Primary tumors of the rete testis are rare. Pagetoid or direct stromal extension of tumors from the testis and metastatic tumor from other sites are seen more commonly than primary rete testis tumors. Primary tumors are seen in the hilar aspect of the testis and are continuous with the branching channels of the normal rete. The hilar location is apparent in small tumors. The site of origin of larger neoplasms may not be apparent on gross examination.

Only 5% of intrascrotal neoplasms arise in the epididymis.[225] One large series of epididymal tumors found that 75% were benign and 25% were malignant.[226] The most common tumor seen in the epididymis is adenomatoid tumor. Papillary cystadenomas, leiomyomas, and lipomas also occur at this site.[149] Most primary malignant tumors of the epididymis are sarcomas, but carcinomas, primary germ cell tumors and metastatic tumors may be encountered.[227,228]

Benign Tumors of the Rete Testis

Benign epithelial tumors of the rete testis are rare. They have been called adenomas,[229] benign papillary tumors,[230] cystadenomas,[231] papillary cystadenomas,[232] and adenofibromas.[233] These neoplasms have occurred in patients between 12 and 51 years of age; the average age has been 26 years. Patients with these tumors have unilateral scrotal masses.

These tumors are well-circumscribed, usually solid masses of the rete testis. Cystic and mixed cystic and solid masses also occur.[231] Tumors range from 1.5 to 3.6 cm in diameter.[21] Smaller tumors may be incidentally found during microscopic examination of the rete testis. Microscopic examination shows cysts and intracystic papillary structures lined by cuboidal cells without atypia or mitotic figures. A transition with normal rete channels is helpful in making the diagnosis. A rare adenofibroma has been reported.[233] It displayed a fibrous tissue component in addition to short tubules and longer slit-like spaces lined by cells similar to those of the normal rete testis.

Five cases of sertoliform rete cystadenoma[21,231,234] have all contained solid tubules resembling those seen in testicular Sertoli cell tumors (Fig. 13-19). The similar appearance of solid tubules in sertoliform rete cystadenomas and Sertoli cell tumors of the testis reflects the common sex cord embryogenesis of the rete testis and testicular sex cord elements.[235] One sertoliform rete cystadenoma showed small areas of tumor at the junction of the rete with the seminiferous tubules.[21] Some authors[21] have suggested that the origin of sertoliform cystadenomas is from the "transition zone" between rete and seminiferous tubules. Since both anatomic structures develop from gonadal sex cord tissue, cells in the rete testis near the seminiferous tubules may have the capacity to differentiate toward Sertoli cells. The presence of inhibin positivity in one tumor[21] further supports this hypothesis. It is important to distinguish primary rete testis tumors from secondary rete involvement by adjacent Sertoli cell tumors of the testis.[236] Location of the tumor in the rete testis only, not accompanied by a coexisting testicular Sertoli cell tumor, a noninvasive growth pattern, and lack of nodular aggregates of cells are features supportive of a primary rete testis tumor.[21] Inhibin staining is not helpful in distinguishing between rete testis cystadenomas and testicular Sertoli cell tumors, since it stains both tumors.[21]

Benign Tumors of the Epididymis

Papillary cystadenomas[237–239] and cystadenofibromas[240] are benign tumors that occur in men from 16 to 65 years of age (mean 36 years). They usually present as palpable, nonpainful masses in the head of the epididymis.[238,239] About one-third of epididymal tumors are papillary cystadenomas, and about two-third of these occur in patients with von Hippel-Lindau syndrome.[238,239,241–243] More than half of patients with this syndrome develop unilateral or bilateral epididymal cystadenomas,[239] and the cystadenoma may be the initial sign of the syndrome.[238] Most bilateral tumors are associated with von Hippel-Lindau syndrome[238,239,241–243] but some bilateral tumors are nonsyndromic.[238,244] Most patients developing epididymal cystadenomas in the absence of von Hippel-Lindau syndrome have unilateral tumors.[238,241,245] A molecular pathology analysis of epididymal cystadenomas collected from von Hippel-Lindau patients at autopsy demonstrated that these lesions are true neoplasms that arise following a

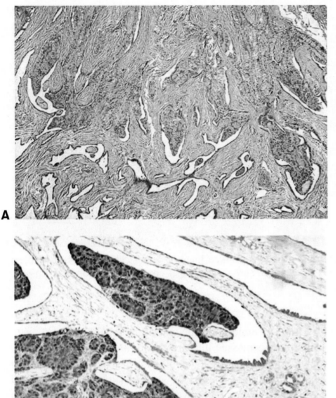

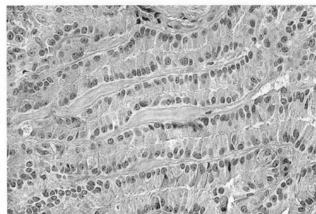

FIGURE 13-19 ■ Sertoliform cystadenoma of the rete testis. The neoplasm expands the native rete. Low power (**A**). Elongated trabeculae and solid tubules of tumor resembling a Sertoli cell tumor (**B**). Inhibin positivity (**C**). Note the nonneoplastic rete epithelium is also positive for inhibin. (Reprinted from Amin MB. Selected other problematic testicular and paratesticular lesions: rete testis neoplasms and pseudotumors, mesothelial lesions and secondary tumors. *Mod Pathol* 2005;18:S131–S145, with permission.)

sequence of inactivation of the wild-type copy of the von Hippel-Lindau gene, and activation of hypoxia-inducible factor.[246] The epididymal cystadenomas in von Hippel-Lindau patients are thought by some authors to evolve from a subset of microscopic epithelial tumorlets in the efferent ductular system.[246] Sporadic tumors do show a mutation in the von Hippel-Lindau gene,[247] and some authors have suggested that unilateral, sporadic epididymal cystadenomas represent a forme fruste of this disease.[21] Epididymal cystadenomas may cause infertility and obstructive azoospermia.[242,248,249]

On gross examination, epididymal cystadenomas are well-circumscribed masses in the head of the epididymis. Most are relatively small, but sizes as large as 5 cm have been reported.[238] These tumors may be solid, cystic, or partially cystic, and they are usually gray-tan in color.[238,245] Small, fluid filled cysts may be seen on cut sections.[238]

Microscopic examination reveals tubules, cysts, and papillary structures lined by one or two layers of bland, cuboidal to columnar epithelial cells that may be ciliated (Fig. 13-20).[237,238,242] Cystic fluid or an eosinophilic colloid material may be present. The cells lining this lesion have vacuolated or clear cytoplasm that contains glycogen.[242] Efferent ductules may be ecstatic.[242] Solid cores of clear cells may be present in the cyst walls.[21] While the epithelium of this tumor contains glycogen[238,245] and fat,[245] mucin is not present.[238] Cytokeratin, epithelial membrane antigen, and carcinoembryonic antigen all are positive in the tumor cells.[244]

The papillary cystadenomas of the epididymis generally have a characteristic appearance, and the diagnosis is usually straightforward. However, it is important not to confuse papillary cystadenoma composed of cells with clear cytoplasm with clear cell carcinoma of the epididymis. Cystadenomas lack the invasive pattern, nuclear atypia, and mitoses seen in clear cell carcinoma. Metastatic renal cell carcinoma may metastasize to the paratesticular region, but the prominent thin-walled blood vessels characteristically situated between nests of clear cell carcinoma of the kidney are not seen in epididymal cystadenomas. Immunohistochemical stains performed on epididymal cystadenomas are negative for RCC antigen and CD10, in contrast to renal cell carcinomas.[250]

Benign Ovarian-Type Epithelial Tumors

Ovarian-type epithelial tumors occur infrequently in the paratesticular region, and they are identical to their more frequent counterparts in the ovary. Benign ovarian-type epithelial tumors include serous cystadenoma, mucinous cystadenoma,

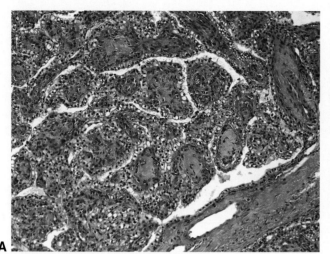
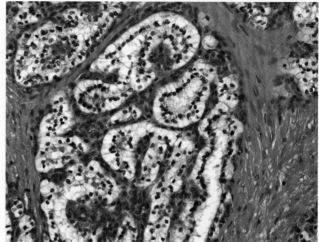

Figure 13-20 ■ Papillary cystadenoma of epididymis. **A:** Note tightly packed papillae lined by small cuboidal cells with clear cytoplasm; **(B)** cuboidal epithelial cells with small uniform nuclei and clear cytoplasm are seen. (Images courtesy of Dr Jonathan Epstein, Baltimore, MD.)

and Brenner tumor. Ovarian-type epithelial tumors are usually seen in adults, and they typically present as mass lesions.[5]

Two serous cystadenomas of ovarian type have been reported in the epididymis.[251,252] These are cystic lesions that may be surrounded by ovarian-type stroma. These cysts are often translucent and thin-walled. They typically have smooth linings, but a few blunt, club-shaped papillary processes may occur. Microscopically, the cysts are lined by a single layer of ciliated cells that suggest derivation from müllerian duct remnants. There is no epithelial stratification, tufting, or atypia in these lesions. Immunohistochemical stains are not necessary for the diagnosis of serous cystadenomas, and the ciliated lining distinguishes serous lesions from mesothelial cysts. The presence of ovarian stroma associated with benign serous tumors is not seen in epididymal cysts, which also may contain ciliated epithelium.

Paratesticular mucinous cystadenomas have been reported adjacent to the testis and in the spermatic cord.[253] Mucinous cystadenomas are cystic lesions that are usually translucent on gross examination. They may be multilocular, but they do not contain solid or necrotic areas. They are usually lined by a single layer of endocervical-type mucinous epithelium that does not display tufting, stratification, atypia, or mitoses, but one paratesticular mucinous cystadenoma has been lined by intestinal-type mucinous epithelium.[254] One reported case had smooth muscle in its wall and had ruptured, with mucin extravasation.[253] The diagnosis is straightforward if one remembers that ovarian type lesion can arise in the paratesticular region. Immunohistochemical stains are not of much use. The etiology of benign mucinous tumors of the paratesticular region has been a topic of debate. Origin of a mucinous cystadenoma from the ovarian component of a dysgenetic gonad has been considered,[255] but these lesions may also arise from metaplastic mesothelium, from müllerian remnants,[254] or from the mucinous components of teratomas.[253]

Brenner tumors of the paratesticular region are firm, white or tan masses that are predominantly solid, but they may contain scattered small cystic spaces. Microscopic examination reveals fibrous stroma surrounding nests of urothelial-type epithelium that often contain longitudinal nuclear grooves (Fig. 13-21). Cystic spaces lined by columnar or cuboidal mucinous epithelial cells may be present within the epithelial nests. The diagnosis is straightforward, and no ancillary studies are necessary. Brenner tumors most likely arise from metaplastic mesothelium, where Walthard cell nests also occur.[51,256] It is not unusual to find Walthard cell nests in the mesothelium at the junction of the testis and epididymis. A Brenner tumor associated with an adenomatoid tumor has been reported, further supporting derivation of Brenner tumors from mesothelium.[257]

Malignant Epithelial Neoplasms

Carcinoma of the Rete Testis

Primary carcinomas of the rete testis are rare tumors, although they are more common than benign rete testis tumors.[258,259] They have been reported only in Caucasian men. While patients have ranged from 8 to 91 years of age, 70% of reported cases have been in men over the age of 60 years.[21,259,260] Both rete testes are involved with equal frequency. Most patients present with scrotal pain or swelling.[200] Some have clinical features suggesting inflammatory disorders such as epididymitis rather than a mass lesion,[260,261] and a clinical presentation that does not suggest neoplasm may delay the correct diagnosis. One quarter of reported cases have been associated with a hydrocele[259,262] that may mask the underlying tumor and delay detection of the neoplasm.[263,264] Since the tumor is most often located on the posterior aspect of the testis, it may be difficult to palpate. Patients with advanced neoplasm may have tumor nodules occur on the scrotal skin, penis, or the perineum,[260]

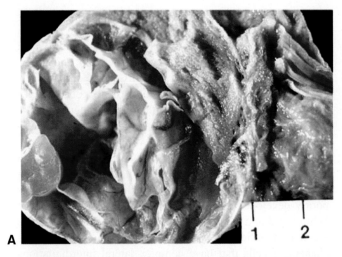

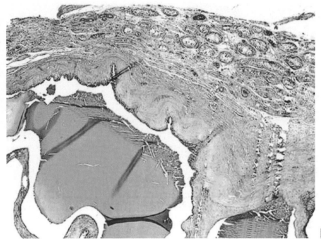

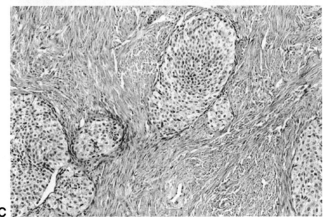

FIGURE 13-21 ■ Brenner tumor of testis. Gross appearance of multiloculated cystic tumor that replaces the testis **(A)**. Low power of cystic component of tumor **(B)**. Solid area shows more characteristic histology of Brenner tumor **(C)**. (Reprinted from Amin MB. Selected other problematic testicular and paratesticular lesions: rete testis neoplasms and pseudotumors, mesothelial lesions and secondary tumors. *Mod Pathol* 2005;18:S131–S145, with permission.)

and draining sinuses may occur[265] in some patients. The prognosis for patients with adenocarcinoma of the rete testis is very poor. The average survival is 8 months, although survival of over 4 years has been reported.[200] The etiology of these neoplasms is not clear. Carcinomas do not arise from cystadenomas, although there is one report of a patient with a history of rete testis hyperplasia who subsequently developed a rete adenocarcinoma.[266] Some younger patients have had a history of testicular maldescent,[267] and one case has been associated with asbestos exposure.[262]

It is likely that some tumors formerly diagnosed as rete testis carcinomas actually represent other entities such as serous neoplasms. Nochomovitz and Orenstein[259] listed five criteria for the diagnosis of rete testis tumors: (1) absence of tumor with similar histologic features outside the scrotum, (2) tumor centered in the testicular hilus, (3) morphologic features not consistent with another testicular or paratesticular tumor type, (4) a transition exists between the tumor and the normal rete testis, and (5) a predominantly solid architecture. More recently, Amin[200] added the additional requirement for immunohistochemical exclusion of other paratesticular malignancies, such as malignant mesothelioma and papillary serous carcinoma. The requirement for a predominantly solid architecture is not absolute. We now recognize that rete testis carcinomas can have cystic areas,

and that not all cystic rete tumors are of serous derivation, although it is likely that some cases reported in the earlier literature, especially those with longer survivals, actually represent serous tumors.[21] It may be difficult to see the transition between the rete carcinoma and the uninvolved rete testis. The first three criteria of Nochomovitz and Orenstein and the additional criterion proposed by Amin should be met for a diagnosis of rete testis adenocarcinoma.[21,200]

Careful attention should be given to the location of the tumor in the hilar region of the testis on gross examination of the specimen; this location suggests a rete testis origin for the neoplasm. Rete testis carcinomas are most often large solid tan masses that range from 6 to up to 12 cm in size.[21,263] Rare tumors may have cystic areas[5,259–261,268] that contain fluid. Areas of hemorrhage and necrosis may be present.[269] Satellite tumor nodules may be seen in the tunica albuginea. About one-third of tumors extend into other paratesticular structures, including the spermatic cord,[259,260] but spermatic cord involvement may be apparent only on microscopic examination.[260,269,270]

Microscopic examination of these neoplasms shows solid, glandular, and papillary nodules of tumor (Fig. 13-22). Papillary structures may project into cysts.[235,260–263,267–270] Tubular and glandular structures often have elongated, slit-like shapes, or even a sertoliform appearance.[235] A retiform

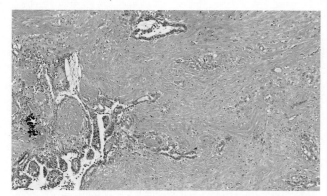

FIGURE 13-22 ■ Adenocarcinoma of rete testis. Note infiltrating adenocarcinoma with a tubulopapillary growth pattern associated with fibrous stroma.

pattern displays elongated and compressed branching tubules.[200] Many neoplasms display confluent growth of tumor cells.[235,259,263,269,270] A Kaposiform pattern has been described and is mainly solid with scattered very small, slit-like channels.[200] Tumor cells have enlarged, hyperchromatic nuclei, but marked pleomorphism is not usually seen. The mitotic rate is variable, and areas of necrosis may be present. Tumors with a cellular spindle-cell component have been reported.[269,270] Transition between benign rete testis epithelium, atypical epithelium, and the carcinoma is helpful in establishing the diagnosis, but it may be difficult to identify.[259,260,271]

Special stains and immunohistochemical stains are not specific for carcinomas of the rete testis, but they are very useful in excluding other lesions such as mesothelioma or papillary serous carcinoma (Box 13-3). Carcinomas of the rete testis do not usually contain mucin. They are diffusely reactive for cytokeratin and EMA,[269,270] even when a spindle cell component is present in the tumor. CEA has been detected in these tumors by some investigators, but not by others.[208,239,240] These tumors do not stain for hCG, AFP, S-100 protein, Leu-M1, placental alkaline phosphatase, or PSA.[235,269] Stains for malignant mesothelioma and serous

carcinoma should be performed to exclude those possibilities before a diagnosis of rete testis adenocarcinoma is made. Malignant mesotheliomas are positive for calretinin, WT-1, CK5/6, and negative for CEA, Leu-M1, Ber EP4, and B72.3. Serous carcinoma stains positively for CA-125 and WT-1.

Electron microscopic examination of adenocarcinomas of the rete testis shows cells with oval to irregular nuclei and sometimes deep nuclear indentations. One or two nucleoli are present, and microvilli are variable in number.[260,269] Cytoplasm contains variable amounts of smooth and rough endoplasmic reticulum, rod-shaped mitochondria, and occasional clusters of tonofilaments, but the Golgi apparatus is poorly developed and microvilli lack core rootlets.[260,269–271] While lipid and glycogen may be present, mucin vacuoles are not identified.[260,270] A basement membrane surrounds clusters of cells that have complex lateral interdigitations with numerous desmosomes.[260,270]

The differential diagnosis of high-grade tubulopapillary carcinoma histology in the testicular mediastinum includes rete testis carcinoma, papillary serous carcinoma, malignant mesothelioma, metastatic adenocarcinoma, and epididymal carcinoma (Box 13-4). Nochomovitz and Orenstein concluded that many cystic tumors reported as rete carcinomas actually represented serous tumors of low malignant potential or serous carcinomas.[259,260,272–274] The site of origin is different for the two tumor types, with serous tumors arising in the groove between the testis and epididymis and rete carcinomas arising in the testicular hilus.[259,260,275] Both the clinical presentation and the histologic features of mesothelioma may mimic rete testis carcinoma.[259,260] The tumor location is helpful in making the diagnosis. Mesotheliomas typically involve the tunica vaginalis and do not involve or replace the rete testis. The use of immunohistochemistry in the differential diagnosis has been described above. Metastatic carcinoma should especially be considered if tumors are bilateral, multinodular, or have lymphatic/vascular space invasion or an interstitial growth pattern. Sex cord stromal tumors of the testis can rarely mimic rete testis carcinomas.[259,260,276,277]

Carcinomas of the rete testis have a poor prognosis. Only 37% of patients have been free of disease at last clinical follow-up,[259] and the mean survival is 8 months after diagnosis of the tumor.[260] A few patients have experienced longer

---

Box 13-3 ● LIKELY IMMUNOHISTOCHEMICAL REACTIONS IN TUBULOGLANDULAR NEOPLASMS*

Malignant mesothelioma	WT1+, calretinin+, thrombomodulin±, Leu M1−, CEA−, CK7+, CK20−
Papillary serous carcinoma	WT1+, CA 125+, Leu M1±, CEA±, calretinin±, thrombomodulin±, CD10±
Rete/epididymal carcinoma	CD10+, calretinin±, Leu M1±, CEA±, WT1−, Thrombomodulin±
Metastatic carcinoma	Lung (CK7+, CK20−, TTF1+, Leu M1+), colorectal (CK7−, CK20+, CDX2+, CEA+) Prostate (CK7−, CK20−, PSA+, PLAP+)

*Redrawn from Amin MB. Selected other problematic testicular and paratesticular lesions: rete testis neoplasms and pseudotumors, mesothelial lesions and secondary tumors. *Mod Pathol* 2005;18: S131–S145, with permission.

Box 13-4 ● DIFFERENTIAL DIAGNOSIS OF TUBULOPAPILLARY NEOPLASMS OF THE PARATESTIS*

Rete testis adenocarcinoma
Epididymal carcinoma
Malignant mesothelioma arising from the tunica vaginalis
Ovarian-type (serous, endometrioid or clear cell) carcinomas
Metastatic adenocarcinoma

*Redrawn and modified from Amin MB. Selected other problematic testicular and paratesticular lesions: rete testis neoplasms and pseudotumors, mesothelial lesions and secondary tumors. *Mod Pathol* 2005;18:S131–S145, with permission.

survival, but those patients had cystic tumors that may have actually represented serous tumors of low malignant potential.[259] Rete testis carcinomas typically spread locally and metastasize to the para-aortic and iliac lymph nodes as well as hematogenously to the lungs.[278] The inguinal lymph nodes may also be affected. Early diagnosis offers the best chance for favorable outcome. Most patients who die of disease have advanced-stage disease at the time of diagnosis. Treatment is primarily surgical; chemotherapy and radiation have been of limited value in the therapy of these tumors.[259]

Carcinoma of the Epididymis

Epididymal carcinoma is a rare tumor. It has occurred in adults between 22 and 82 years of age; the average patient age has been 47 years.[227,279,280] Patients have presented with scrotal masses either with or without pain. Approximately half of the patients have had associated hydroceles.[280] None have been associated with von Hippel-Lindau disease.

Gross examination of epididymal carcinomas shows solid and cystic gray-white tumor with areas of hemorrhage and necrosis.[280] Tumors have ranged from <1 cm[281] to 14 cm in diameter.[280,282] The tumor typically obliterates part or all of the epididymis with at most limited involvement of the testis.[280] The spermatic cord and tunica vaginalis may be involved by tumor.

Microscopic examination reveals adenocarcinoma containing invasive glands, tubules, and papillary aggregates of tumor cells that have clear cytoplasm containing glycogen, at least focally (Fig. 13-23).[279,280] Moderate nuclear atypia is present, although more anaplastic, pleomorphic nuclei may also occur. Cysts and intracystic papillary structures may be present. In some cases, the appearance is reminiscent of endometrioid carcinoma.[21,280] Squamous differentiation may be admixed with the adenocarcinoma, and pure squamous carcinoma of the epididymis has been reported.[280]

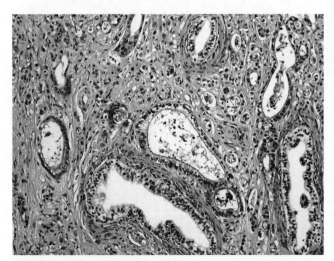

FIGURE 13-23 ■ Adenocarcinoma of epididymis. Note infiltrating adenocarcinoma between epididymal tubules. (Image courtesy of Dr Steven Shen, Houston, TX.)

PAS stains highlight the glycogen present in tumor cells. Mucin stains are negative.[280] Immunohistochemical stains are positive for cytokeratin and EMA; the latter stains the luminal surface of the cytoplasm.[280] Studies have yielded conflicting results regarding CEA staining.[280] Electron microscopy shows characteristics of adenocarcinoma.[280]

The differential diagnosis of epididymal carcinoma includes clear cell papillary cystadenoma. In contrast to benign neoplasms, adenocarcinomas are infiltrating and destructive tumors that display hemorrhage, necrosis, nuclear atypia, and mitotic activity. Adenomatoid tumors are smaller and more circumscribed tumors that are composed of tubules lined by flattened cells. Adenomas of the rete testis enter the differential diagnosis, but they do not involve the epididymis proper and they do not display nuclear atypia and mitotic figures. Epididymal adenocarcinoma also needs to be distinguished from mesothelioma of the tunica vaginalis,[283] papillary serous carcinoma,[274] and adenocarcinoma of the rete testis.[259,260] Clear cytoplasm, seen in epididymal adenocarcinoma, is not a typical feature of rete carcinomas. Serous carcinomas display more epithelial budding, papillary structures surrounded by desmoplastic stroma, and psammoma bodies than epididymal carcinoma. Mesothelioma is a more diffuse process than epididymal carcinoma and often is associated with hydrocele and tumor nucleolus along the tunica vaginalis.

The number of reported cases of primary epididymal adenocarcinoma has been small, but it appears that about 50% of patients with this neoplasm eventually die with metastatic disease.[21,280,284] This tumor usually metastasizes via lymphatic channels to the retroperitoneal lymph nodes,[280] but inguinal lymph nodes may also be involved by tumor. Metastatic disease has also been reported in the right para-ureteral area and the lung.[280]

Borderline and Malignant Ovarian-Type Epithelial Tumors

Borderline and malignant ovarian-type epithelial tumors occur infrequently in the paratesticular region, and they are identical to their more frequent counterparts in the ovary. Most of these tumors in the paratesticular region are serous tumors of low malignant potential,[18,285–289] but serous carcinomas,[274] Brenner tumors,[257,290,291] mucinous tumors,[253,292,293] endometrioid tumors,[288] and clear cell carcinomas[294] have also been reported in this location (Box 13-5).

These neoplasms may arise from müllerian metaplasia of the peritoneal surface of the tunica vaginalis in a process similar to that of primary peritoneal serous tumors in women. Many of these tumors are centered in the epididymal–testicular groove.[274,291,292] That location suggests origin from the appendix testis.[286] It is a müllerian remnant, and other müllerian remnants also exist in the paratesticular region.[51,273,295] Some ovarian-type epithelial tumors have been located in the spermatic cord.[296]

Serous tumors of low malignant potential typically occur in midlife. The median age for borderline serous tumors in the paratestis is 54 years, with an average age of 49 years.[272,273,285,286,288,295,297] Paratesticular serous carcinomas occur mainly in younger adults with a mean age of 31 years.[274] One case of paratesticular papillary serous cystadenocarcinoma has been reported in a child,[298] and one was recently reported in an 87-year-old man.[299] Two cases of malignant ovarian-type epithelial tumor have been reported in men who received hormonal therapy for prostate carcinoma; they included an endometrioid carcinoma and a mixed endometrioid and smooth muscle tumor.[5,286,288]

Presenting symptoms include scrotal enlargement and palpable masses that may be painless or associated with discomfort. There may be an associated hydrocele.[293]

Serous and mucinous tumors of low malignant potential have pink-tan, smooth outer surfaces. Cut sections reveal variable numbers of cysts[255] that contain watery or thick, mucoid material[300] and papillary excrescences.[292] In contrast to borderline tumors, carcinomas have a solid gray-tan tissue component that is not well demarcated from surrounding structures.[274]

Histologic features of ovarian-type epithelial tumors are identical to tumors of the same type seen more commonly in the ovaries. Borderline serous tumors typically display papillary connective tissue fronds with a hierarchical branching architecture. The lining epithelium shows stratification, tufting, nuclear atypia, and mitotic figures. Borderline tumors do not display invasion into the surrounding stroma, in contrast to serous carcinomas. Stromal invasion is the characteristic that defines serous carcinoma and separates carcinoma from borderline tumors. Stromal invasion may be recognized by a desmoplastic stromal response, a solid growth pattern, or isolated papillary structures surrounded by clear spaces (Fig. 13-24). Some tumors may be predominantly borderline serous tumors with only small foci of invasive tumor.[274,287]

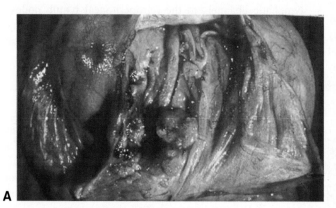
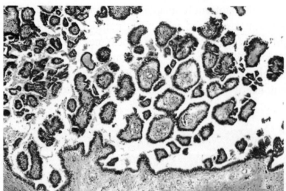
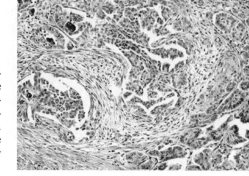

FIGURE 13-24 ■ Ovarian-type serous papillary tumor of paratestis. Gross appearance of a serous papillary cystic tumor of borderline malignancy (**A**). Intracystic growth with papillae demonstrating hierarchical branching (**B**). Serous carcinoma with tubulopapillary architecture and psammomatous calcification (**C**). (Reprinted from Amin MB. Selected other problematic testicular and paratesticular lesions: rete testis neoplasms and pseudotumors, mesothelial lesions and secondary tumors. *Mod Pathol* 2005;18:S131–S145, with permission.)

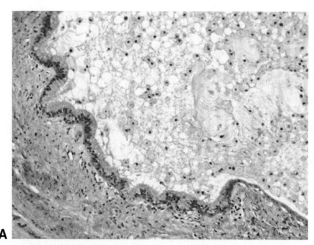
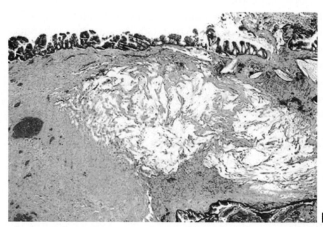

FIGURE 13-25 ■ Ovarian-type paratesticular/testicular mucinous tumor. Cystadenoma histology with lining by endocervical-like cells **(A)**. Testicular mucinous tumor of borderline malignancy with mucin extravasation **(B)**. (Case courtesy of Dr Thomas Ulbright, Indianapolis, IN, USA; Reprinted from Amin MB. Selected other problematic testicular and paratesticular lesions: rete testis neoplasms and pseudotumors, mesothelial lesions and secondary tumors. *Mod Pathol* 2005;18:S131–S145, with permission.)

In contrast to the single layer of bland epithelium seen in mucinous cystadenomas, the presence of endocervical or enteric-type epithelium with stratification, tufting, atypia and mitotic figures is diagnostic of a borderline mucinous tumor (Fig. 13-25). Borderline mucinous tumors do not display destructive stromal invasion. Two mucinous borderline tumors and one mucinous carcinoma have been recently reported in the paratesticular region.[253] The paratesticular mucinous carcinoma appeared as a thickening of the tunica vaginalis on gross examination. Destructive stromal invasion in mucinous tumors is indicative of carcinoma.

Endometrioid and clear cell tumors have been reported rarely in the paratesticular region.[40] Endometrioid tumors are reminiscent of endometrial carcinoma. Clear cell carcinomas display solid, glandular or papillary architecture. One malignant Brenner tumor was associated with areas of squamous and transitional cell carcinoma.[291]

Immunohistochemistry is useful in the diagnosis of ovarian-type epithelial tumors. Tumors of müllerian derivation stain positively with antibodies to WT1. They are cytokeratin positive, and most ovarian-type epithelial tumors display a predominance of cytokeratin 7 staining, with less cytokeratin 20 positivity. CEA[274,285,287] and CA-125 may also be positive. Serous tumors stain positively for B72.3.

Serous tumors need to be distinguished from carcinoma of the rete testis and malignant mesothelioma. Location of a tumor in the testicular hilus and the rete testis is typical of rete testis carcinomas. Rete carcinomas also typically display a greater degree of cytologic atypia and a more solid growth pattern than the well-defined papillary fronds seen in serous tumors. Psammoma bodies may occur in both serous tumors and carcinoma of the rete testis.[269] Both serous tumors and malignant mesotheliomas display papillary architecture. Serous carcinoma displays more tufting and stratification than is typically seen in mesotheliomas.

Immunohistochemistry is quite useful in distinguishing the two neoplasms (Box 13-3). Papillary serous tumors are positive for Leu M1, B72.3, and WT1. Mesotheliomas are positive for WT1, CK5/6 and calretinin and negative for Leu M1 and B72.3. The possibility of metastatic carcinoma should be excluded when considering a diagnosis of endometrioid, mucinous, or clear cell tumors of the paratesticular region. Bilateral tumors and prominent lymphatic or vascular space involvement supports a metastatic lesion. The majority of paratesticular ovarian-type epithelial tumors present with disease limited to the paratestis, in contrast to advanced-stage disease associated with tumors metastatic to the paratesticular region.

There is very limited experience with müllerian-type tumors of the paratesticular region. Completely excised borderline tumors have a good prognosis; no case has recurred or metastasized after radical orchiectomy.[289] Nistal reported that mucinous tumors of the paratestis are locally aggressive tumors with little metastatic potential.[293] Two patients reported to have mucinous cystadenocarcinomas[292,293] were alive without disease after 2 years, but other authors do not think these tumors were actually invasive.[40] The single patient reported to have a malignant Brenner tumor had a metastasis to retroperitoneal lymph nodes at the time of diagnosis, but he was alive without disease 1 year later.[291] Complete surgical excision of ovarian-type epithelial tumors of the paratestis is recommended.[40] Adjuvant therapy should only be considered for patients whose tumors represent carcinoma.[40]

Ovarian serous borderline tumors with microscopic foci of invasion have a prognosis similar to that of tumors of low malignant potential, but the significance of very small foci of invasive tumor in the paratesticular region has not been determined. One man with a serous borderline tumor with "focal" invasion was disease-free 1 year after surgical excision.[287] A different patient reported to have focal invasion had diffuse abdominal recurrent disease 7 years after surgery.[274] Some authors[40] believe that microinvasion measuring <3 mm is associated with a good prognosis, but no actual data from paratesticular tumors exist to confirm this impression. At least one reported case of a testicular borderline serous tumor with microinvasion by criteria used for ovarian tumors has been clinically malignant, indicating that additional experience with these lesions is necessary before drawing conclusions about the prognostic significance of microinvasive foci.[200] Thorough sampling of borderline tumors should be performed. Patients with larger amounts of invasive serous carcinoma are at risk for recurrent or metastatic disease.[274] The role of retroperitoneal lymph node dissection in this context is unclear.

Mesothelial Neoplasms

Benign Mesothelial Tumors

Adenomatoid Tumor

Adenomatoid tumors are the most common mesothelial tumors of the paratesticular region. Srigley and Hartwick reported 23 cases,[18] and Mostofi and Price[149] found that these tumors represent about one-third of all tumors in the paratesticular region. While most paratesticular adenomatoid tumors occur in the head of the epididymis,[301,302] some are seen in the tunica albuginea, spermatic cord, and tunica vaginalis.[284,301,303–307] Patients range in age from 18 to 79 years, but the lesion is seen most commonly in the fourth decade of life. Adenomatoid tumors are usually asymptomatic lesions that are discovered during physical examinations or in the course of other procedures. However, if infarction occurs due to torsion, patients may present with pain.[308]

Adenomatoid tumors are well-circumscribed, firm tan, gray or white nodules that may be as large as 5 cm, although most measure <2 cm (Fig. 13-26A). Microscopic

examination displays a plexiform pattern of nests, cords, and tubules composed of cells with moderate to abundant eosinophilic cytoplasm containing vacuoles (Fig. 13-26B). The cytoplasmic vacuoles represent an important clue to the diagnosis. Coalescence of the vacuoles gives rise to tubular spaces. Attenuated extensions of cytoplasm called "thread-like bridging strands" are often seen crossing these tubular spaces.[309] Nuclei are round and uniform. Mitoses are rare. The tubules are surrounded by fibrous stroma that may contain smooth muscle cells. Occasionally, smooth muscle cells may be admixed with the larger, epithelioid cells to form an adenomatoid leiomyoma.[310,311] Rarely, the tumor may infiltrate the testis[312,313] and it may masquerade as a testicular neoplasm. Brenner tumors occasionally occur in association with adenomatoid tumors of the paratesticular region.[257] Necrosis is a rare occurrence in adenomatoid tumors and is presumably due to infarction.[308] Some cases have been associated with rete testis hyperplasia.[308]

While the typical pattern of adenomatoid tumor results in a straightforward "pattern recognition" diagnosis, there are variants of this tumor that may be more challenging to pathologists[200,314] (Box 13-6). Adenoid, angiomatoid, cystic, glandular, solid, tubular, oncocytic, and ischemic patterns may be seen.[314] Signet ring cells resulting from cytoplasmic vacuoles may mimic the appearance of metastatic adenocarcinoma. Vacuolated cells may suggest liposarcoma or vascular neoplasms, and the combination of vacuolated cells with gland-like tubules can mimic yolk sac tumor or Sertoli cell tumor. Nests or solid areas of eosinophilic cells can suggest variants of Leydig cell tumor. Awareness that smooth muscle cells may be admixed with the tubules of adenomatoid tumor will prevent an erroneous diagnosis of leiomyoma. Although adenomatoid tumors are grossly well-circumscribed, some infiltration of surrounding muscle may be seen at the edges of the lesion. Muscle infiltration and any atypia resulting from reaction to infarction need to be

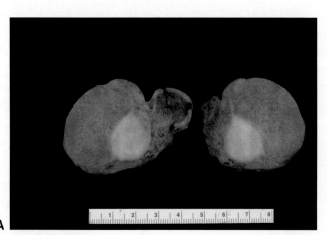

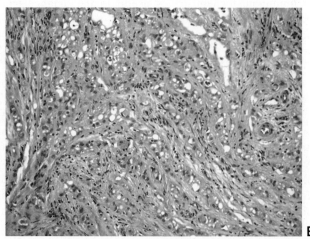

FIGURE 13-26 ■ Adenomatoid tumor. **A:** Gross photograph of bisected testis. Note circumscribed white-yellow nodule with a hilar epicenter. **B:** Microscopically, these tumors display cords and tubules composed of cells with moderate to abundant eosinophilic cytoplasm containing vacuoles.

Histologic Pattern	Differential Diagnosis
Signet ring cells	Metastatic carcinoma
Vacuolated cells	Liposarcoma
	Vascular neoplasm
Vacuolated cells and gland-like tubules	Yolk sac tumor
	Metastatic carcinoma
	Sertoli cell tumor
Nests/solid areas of eosinophilic cells	Leydig cell tumor
	Large cell calcifying Sertoli cell tumor
Prominent smooth muscle component	Leiomyoma
Infiltration of testicular parenchyma	Mesothelioma
Infarction with atypia	Mesothelioma

*Redrawn and modified from Amin MB. Selected other problematic testicular and paratesticular lesions: rete testis neoplasms and pseudotumors, mesothelial lesions and secondary tumors. *Mod Pathol* 2005;18:S131–S145, with permission.

carefully evaluated in view of the low-power architecture and gross appearance of the tumor because they can be suggestive of mesothelioma to observers not familiar with their occurrence.

Frozen section diagnosis of adenomatoid tumor may be crucial in steering therapy toward a conservative resection. The gross appearance of a white circumscribed nodule is helpful in achieving the correct intraoperative diagnosis. Appreciation of the pattern of anastomosing tubules and cytoplasmic vacuolation are important diagnostic factors, even if some solid areas, signet ring cells, or admixed smooth muscle are identified microscopically. The absence of nuclear atypia or mitotic activity is helpful at the time of frozen section, but the gross appearance of the lesion and the low-power pattern of tubules and vacuolated cells are keys to the correct diagnosis.

Immunohistochemical stains are useful in diagnosing adenomatoid tumors. These neoplasms are positive for cytokeratin and epithelial membrane antigen and negative for vimentin, carcinoembryonic antigen, and vascular markers. A recent study emphasized the value of a positive D2-40 stain for adenomatoid tumors of the genital tract.[314] Electron microscopy demonstrates the long, slender microvilli seen in mesothelial lesions.[315,316]

Adenomatoid tumors are benign lesions that should be conservatively excised. The differential diagnosis includes vascular lesions and malignant mesothelioma (Box 13-6). Immunohistochemical stains and electron microscopy[315,317,318] confirm the mesothelial nature of the tumor. Adenomatoid tumors may be infiltrative, but they do not show the papillary architecture and cytologic atypia characteristic of malignant mesotheliomas. Furthermore, the cytoplasmic vacuoles characteristic of adenomatoid tumors are not a feature of malignant mesotheliomas.

Well-Differentiated Papillary Mesothelioma and Mesothelial Tumors of Uncertain Malignant Potential

Well-differentiated papillary mesotheliomas are usually seen in the peritoneum of young women,[319] but a few cases have been reported in the tunica vaginalis of men.[149,320–322] They are rare paratesticular tumors.[322] Most occur in the second or third decade of life in men who present with unilateral or recurrent hydroceles.[149,321,322] This tumor has not been shown to be associated with asbestos exposure.

Gross examination of these lesions shows single or multiple nodules of tumor studding a hydrocele sac. Microscopic examination reveals papillae and tubules that are lined by a single layer of flattened to cuboidal mesothelial cells that do not contain glycogen or mucin.[320,322] Solid aggregates of mesothelial cells with luminal spaces may also be present. Mitoses are rare or absent, and cytologic atypia is not a feature of this neoplasm. Psammoma bodies may be seen. Fibrosis can cause some irregular architecture that should not be mistaken for invasive tumor.[321] Immunohistochemical stains performed in a small number of cases have shown cytokeratin and epithelial membrane antigen positivity in these neoplasms.[321] Electron microscopy displays epithelial cells containing mitochondria and rough endoplasmic reticulum; an adjacent basement membrane is present. Luminal spaces contain short microvilli. Nuclear p53 protein accumulation was demonstrated in one case that had benign histology and an uneventful 3-year follow-up.[323]

The differential diagnosis of well-differentiated papillary mesothelioma includes reactive mesothelial hyperplasia, malignant mesothelioma, and papillary carcinoma of the paratesticular region. Well-differentiated papillary mesothelioma is a larger and more complex lesion than papillary mesothelial hyperplasia. Malignant mesotheliomas and carcinomas of the paratestis characteristically have significant cytologic atypia, mitotic activity, and invasive patterns that are not seen in well-differentiated papillary mesotheliomas. Malignant mesotheliomas may contain noninvasive areas that are indistinguishable from well-differentiated papillary mesothelioma, so it is essential that the lesion be thoroughly sampled. Well-differentiated papillary mesothelioma may represent a noninvasive stage of malignant mesothelioma, and complete excision is necessary. Recurrent disease has not been reported, but most cases reported do not have long follow-up,[320–322,324] so careful follow-up of patients is essential.

Eight cases of mesothelioma of the tunica vaginalis of uncertain malignant potential have been recently reported.[325] These neoplasms had papillary and tubulopapillary architecture similar to well-differentiated papillary mesotheliomas, but they also displayed more complex cribriform and condensed architecture. None of the neoplasms demonstrated any areas of invasive tumor. An average of 2.1 mitotic figures/50 HPF was seen in most of the neoplasms. Only rare cells stained for Ki-67 and p53, and only one case stained positively for GLUT-1. Five patients had follow-up data. Three were alive 2, 3, and 9 years after diagnosis, and two other patients died of unknown causes. Survival was much better than that associated with malignant mesotheliomas, although additional studies of these neoplasms are needed to define their biologic behavior.

Malignant Mesothelial Neoplasms

Malignant Mesothelioma

Malignant mesothelioma is the most common malignant neoplasm of the paratesticular region that displays an epithelial growth pattern. Individual case reports and small series of these tumors have been reported. Most arise in the tunica vaginalis testis, but they may also be seen in the epididymis and spermatic cord. Patients have ranged in age from 6 to 91 years. The highest incidence of this tumor has been in men between 55 and 75 years of age. A recent study reported a mean age of 60 years for this neoplasm.[326] However, 10% of cases reported have been in patients younger than 25 years of age,[283,327] so these neoplasms need to be considered in the diagnosis of paratesticular masses and hydroceles, even in pediatric patients. The only known risk factor for malignant mesothelioma of the paratesticular region is asbestos exposure. Up to one-third of patients with this lesion have a history of asbestos exposure, but the prevalence of asbestos exposure is probably higher than reported due to a lack of clinical information in many reported cases.

Most men present with either unilateral testicular enlargement, a hydrocele that develops over the period of several months, or a recurrent hydrocele. Rare patients have presented with metastatic disease.[328,329] Malignant mesothelioma involves the left and right paratesticular regions with equal frequency. Rare patients may present with symptoms of advanced disease such as scrotal nodules[329] or spinal metastases.[328]

Ultrasound or CT scans with or without cytology may suggest a preoperative diagnosis of malignant mesothelioma.[330]

Ultrasound shows a hypoechoic hydrocele with hyperechoic peripheral masses ranging from 2 to 20 mm in size.[331] These studies are very useful in determining surgical therapy because there is a high rate of recurrence if a local resection is performed instead of the indicated inguinal orchiectomy.

Malignant mesothelioma most characteristically consists of multiple firm, white nodules with papillary excrescences on the surface of a hydrocele sac.[144,283,332] The nodules or papillary areas may range from very small to 2 cm. The fluid in the hydrocele may be clear or hemorrhagic. The tunica vaginalis may also be thickened and studded with firm, white, plaque-like lesions. A few tumors consist of single well-circumscribed masses between 2.5 and 7.8 cm in diameter.[333]

Paratesticular malignant mesotheliomas may display epithelial (60% to 70%) (Fig. 13-27A), sarcomatous (rare), or biphasic (30% to 40%) patterns.[144] No desmoplastic mesotheliomas have been reported in this site. Some well-differentiated, epithelial paratesticular mesotheliomas display papillary structures containing fibrous tissue cores covered with cuboidal mesothelial cells with little nuclear atypia. The presence of slight atypia, a low mitotic rate, and tubules invading the wall of the hydrocele sac are clues to the malignant nature in these well-differentiated neoplasms. More commonly, malignant mesothelioma displays a tubulopapillary pattern that includes both exophytic papillary structures and invasive tubules and papillae. The arborizing papillae are covered by multiple layers of atypical mesothelial cells with moderate amounts of cytoplasm and large, vesicular nuclei that contain moderate-sized nucleoli. Solid areas of highly atypical cells and foci of necrosis may be present, especially in high-grade tumors. Tubulopapillary and solid mesotheliomas have mitotic rates varying from low to very high, with higher mitotic rates occurring in more poorly differentiated tumors. Areas of mesothelioma in situ may sometimes be present in the tunica adjacent to the invasive

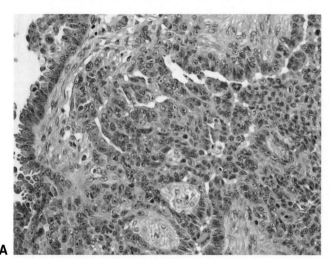
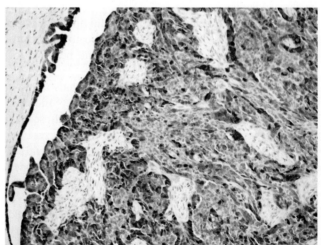

FIGURE 13-27 ■ Malignant mesothelioma. **A:** This tumor displays a tubular, papillary and solid pattern. Atypical rete tubule epithelium **(left)** is associated with the invasive neoplasm. **B:** A calretinin stain is positive. This stain is useful in distinguishing mesothelioma from serous carcinoma in the paratesticular region.

mesothelioma. A transition from benign mesothelium to mesothelioma in situ to invasive malignant mesothelioma may be demonstrable.

Biphasic malignant mesothelioma consists of an admixture of tubulopapillary elements with a spindle cell sarcomatous stroma arranged in fascicles or a storiform pattern resembling malignant fibrous histiocytoma. The degree of atypia in the stroma is variable. Some tumors contain uniform, mildly atypical spindle cells, whereas others display a great deal of nuclear pleomorphism, numerous mitoses, and areas of necrosis. One case had metaplastic osseous and chondroid differentiation of the stroma, and these stromal elements were attributed to metaplasia of the stromal cells.[334]

The only reported case of a sarcomatous mesothelioma of the paratesticular region occurred in a 32-year-old man with no history of asbestos exposure.[335] The tumor displayed spindle and polygonal cells containing ample eosinophilic cytoplasm and oval, vesicular nuclei with prominent nucleoli and numerous mitotic figures. Some cells at the edge of the tumor had cytoplasmic vacuoles that contained hyaluronidase-sensitive Alcian blue material. No microvilli were identified on ultrastructural examination of this sarcomatous mesothelioma.

Immunohistochemical studies of malignant mesothelioma have shown positive staining for CK5/6, WT-1, and calretinin (Fig. 13-27B).[336,337] Negative stains include CEA, Leu-M1, Ber EP4, B72.3, and E-cadherin. Some biphasic mesotheliomas have displayed cytokeratin staining of the spindle cell component of the neoplasms.[144] Some authors have reported that a negative E-cadherin stain coupled with a positive calretinin stain is helpful in the diagnosis of mesothelioma.[337] Some mesothelioma markers may overlap with immunohistochemical markers of other tumors in the differential diagnosis of mesothelioma. WT-1 is positive in both mesothelioma and papillary serous carcinoma. Calretinin is positive in mesothelioma, carcinoma of the rete testis, and epididymal carcinoma. Therefore, a panel of immunostains is useful in eliminating other neoplasms from the differential diagnosis of malignant mesothelioma (Table 13-2).

Ultrastructural study of mesothelioma[326,338–340] displays long, branching microvilli, abundant cytoplasmic fibrils, desmosomes, and sparse intracellular organelles. These features are the same as those seen in malignant mesotheliomas at other sites.

The differential diagnosis of malignant mesothelioma of the paratesticular region includes mesothelial hyperplasia, well-differentiated papillary mesothelioma, paratesticular müllerian-type tumors, adenocarcinoma of the rete testis, adenocarcinoma of the epididymis, adenomatoid tumor, and metastatic carcinoma. The differential diagnoses of malignant mesothelioma compared to mesothelial hyperplasia, adenomatoid tumor, well-differentiated papillary mesothelioma, and paratesticular serous carcinomas have been discussed. Distinction of paratesticular malignant mesothelioma from rete testis adenocarcinoma may be difficult. The latter tumor is located at the testicular hilum and displays

Table 13-2 ■ DIFFERENTIAL DIAGNOSIS OF HIGH-GRADE TUBULOPAPILLARY NEOPLASMS IN THE RETE TESTIS*

Malignant mesothelioma	WT-1 and other Mesothelial markers (calretinin, CK56) positive Adenocarcinoma related markers negative (BerEP4, B72.3, E-cadherin)
Papillary serous carcinoma	Adenocarcinoma-related markers positive Mesothelioma markers negative WT-1 and CA 125 positive Psammoma bodies may be present
Other	Adenocarcinoma markers positive Mesothelioma markers negative WT-1 positive CA 125 negative
Rete testis or epididymal carcinoma	No primary tumor elsewhere Areas of transition from normal structures CD10 positive Calretinin ±
Metastatic carcinoma	History of primary tumor in other location Bilateral tumor Vascular and lymphatic space invasion Interstitial growth between normal glandular structures Perform immunostains for unknown primary tumor

*Modified from Amin MB. Selected other problematic testicular and paratesticular lesions: rete testis neoplasms and pseudotumors, mesothelial lesions and secondary tumors. *Mod Pathol* 2005;18: S131–S145, with permission.

a transition from rete adenocarcinoma in situ to invasive neoplasm.[341] Epididymal adenocarcinomas are centered in the epididymis and not usually associated with a hydrocele.[280] Furthermore, they are often composed of epithelial cells that display clear cytoplasm, at least focally. A history of prior neoplasms is helpful in distinguishing malignant mesothelioma from metastatic carcinoma in the paratesticular region.

Malignant mesotheliomas are aggressive tumors with high recurrence rates. The median time to tumor recurrence is 10.5 months.[332] More than half of the patients reported developed recurrences and/or metastatic tumor. Thirty-nine percent have had local recurrences, 56% have had inguinal, retroperitoneal, or cervical lymph node metastases, and 65% developed lung, mediastinal, bone,[328] or brain[307] metastases. Only one-third of reported patients were alive without disease at last follow-up. Univariate analysis showed that patients younger than age 60 and those with organ-confined disease[332] have longer survival than other patients.

The optimal treatment for paratesticular malignant mesothelioma is radical inguinal orchiectomy.[332] Limited local resection should be avoided due to the high frequency of local recurrence.[332] Some investigators have recommended that retroperitoneal lymph node dissection or postoperative radiation therapy should be performed.[342] The value of adjuvant chemotherapy and radiation therapy is not clear at this time, although recent randomized trials have shown significant improvement in time to progression and survival with chemotherapy for malignant mesothelioma.[343]

Mesenchymal Neoplasms

The incidence of paratesticular soft tissue tumors is difficult to determine.[284,344–346] Benign and malignant soft tissue tumors represented 52% of all paratesticular tumors in the Canadian Reference Center for Cancer Pathology cases.[18] About 70% of paratesticular tumors reported have been benign (Box 13-7) and 30% have been malignant (Box 13-8).[347] The proportion of benign mesenchymal tumors, especially lipomas, may be considerably >30% since most of these tumors are not referred for consultation.

Benign Mesenchymal Tumors

The most common soft tissue tumors of the paratesticular region are lipomas and leiomyomas. Lipomas account for 90% of the soft tissue tumors in this area. Some paratesticular

lipomas may actually represent lipomatous hyperplasia rather than true neoplasms. Variants of lipoma, including angiolipoma, vascular myxolipoma, and myolipoma also occur in the paratestis.[284,348] These lipoma variants are distinguished from liposarcomas by the lack of cytologic atypia, lipoblasts, or a plexiform capillary network in the lipomas. Leiomyomas may have epithelioid or myxoid patterns.[349] Other benign mesenchymal tumors of the paratesticular region include schwannoma, neurofibroma, hemangioma, rhabdomyoma, and granular cell tumor.

Aggressive Angiomyxoma

Aggressive angiomyxoma was originally described in the pelvic soft tissue of women,[350] but it is now known to occur in the spermatic cord in both adults and children.[351–353] These tumors are locally infiltrative and therefore characterized by disease recurrences, but they do not metastasize. They are often large at the time of diagnosis. They typically appear to be well-circumscribed and myxoid on gross examination. Aggressive angiomyxomas are not encapsulated, and microscopic examination shows small nests and tongues of the lesion extend beyond the grossly apparent edge of the neoplasm. Microscopically, these lesions have a background of hypocellular stroma containing blood vessels of variable size. Prominent large dilated blood vessel walls usually contain smooth muscle. Some vessel walls are typically hyalinized. Cellularity may be increased around blood vessels. Foci of hemorrhage may be present. The tumor stroma is myxoid and contains collagen as well as bland spindle and stellate cells with oval round to oval nuclei, no nuclear atypia and no more than a very rare mitotic figure. Some angiomyxomas have microscopic features that overlap with angiomyofibroblastomas.

The rate of recurrence of aggressive angiomyxoma in the paratestis (20%) is lower than that seen in women[354] because lesions of the paratestis are easier to completely resect. The recommended therapy is wide resection with careful follow-up.[354]

Angiomyofibroblastoma (Synonym: Also Called Angiomyofibroblastoma-Like Lesions; Cellular Angiofibroma)

Like angiomyxoma, angiomyofibroblastoma is most commonly seen in the soft tissue of the female pelvis, especially vulva.[355] Some cases do occur in the inguinal region and scrotum of men.[356] These lesions are small, rubbery, well-circumscribed tumors. They are more cellular than angiomyxomas, and they may contain both hypercellular and hypocellular areas (Fig. 13-28). They display a network of blood vessels that are smaller, less dilated, and less hyalinized than those seen in angiomyxomas. Stromal cells are stellate or spindle-shaped without atypia or significant mitotic activity. They may aggregate and whorl around blood vessels.[354] Multinucleated stromal cells are often present. Enlarged nuclei that display degenerative changes characterized by smudged nuclei may be seen. Fat may be present in the stroma. Cellular angiofibroma[357] and "angiomyofibroblastoma-like tumor of the male

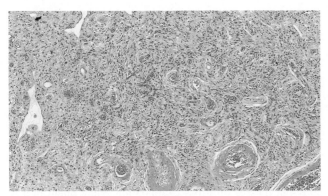

FIGURE 13-28 ■ Angiomyofibroblastoma. Note proliferation of bland small spindle cells with a vaguely storiform growth pattern on a background of abundant small blood vessels, some of which have hyalinized walls.

genital tract"[356] represent variants of angiomyofibroblastoma. Angiomyofibroblastomas are benign neoplasms that should be treated by local resection,[354] although very rare angiomyofibroblastomas have had malignant histologic features, with sarcomatous transformation.[358]

Some tumors may show features of both angiomyxoma and angiomyofibroblastoma. Immunohistochemical stains have been proposed as a way to separate the two entities, but more recent studies show great overlap of the two lesions. Both stain positively for smooth muscle actin, desmin, CD34, and sex hormone receptors.[359,360] Tumors with criteria suggestive of both angiomyxoma and angiomyofibroblastoma should be completely resected with subsequent follow-up clinical examinations.[354]

Malignant Mesenchymal Tumors

Leiomyosarcoma, rhabdomyosarcoma, liposarcoma, malignant fibrous histiocytoma, and fibrosarcoma are the most frequent malignant mesenchymal tumors that occur in the paratestis.[344,345,354,361–363] A recent study of adult spermatic cord sarcomas showed that 51% were liposarcomas, 19% were leiomyosarcomas, 13% were embryonal rhabdomyosarcomas, and 11% represented malignant fibrous histiocytomas,[364] and 62% of patients had high-grade sarcomas in that study. Between 7% and 10% of pediatric rhabdomyosarcomas occur in the paratestis.[365] A rare example of a primary spermatic cord osteosarcoma has been reported.[366] One malignant mesenchymoma composed of distinct areas of liposarcoma and leiomyosarcoma[367] and one mixed liposarcoma and osteosarcoma of the spermatic cord[368] have been reported. We have seen a malignant mesenchymoma composed of ganglioneuroblastoma and rhabdomyosarcoma. A rare case of epithelioid sarcoma arising from the vas deferens has also been reported.[369] Other paratesticular sarcomas include synovial sarcoma and extraskeletal myxoid chondrosarcoma.[354] With the exception of embryonal rhabdomyosarcoma, soft tissue sarcomas of the paratesticular region are tumors of the adult population. Almost all patients with paratesticular sarcomas come to attention because of a palpable mass in the scrotum or inguinal area.

Rhabdomyosarcoma

The most common site for rhabdomyosarcomas is the paratesticular region (Fig. 13-29A).[354] The median age is 15 years, with a range from 7 years of age to adults. Half of all paratesticular rhabdomyosarcomas occur in pediatric patients. On gross examination, paratesticular rhabdomyosarcomas are infiltrating, firm, gray-white neoplasms that may demonstrate areas of necrosis.

Embryonal rhabdomyosarcoma is the most common type of rhabdomyosarcoma in the paratestis, although any type may occur in this region.[370] Embryonal rhabdomyosarcomas are very cellular small round blue cell tumors. There are also variable numbers of rhabdomyoblasts that have abundant eosinophilic cytoplasm (Fig. 13-29B). Strap cells with

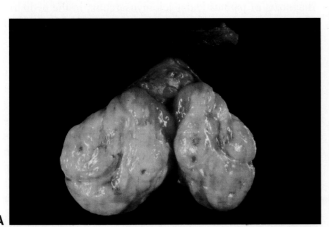

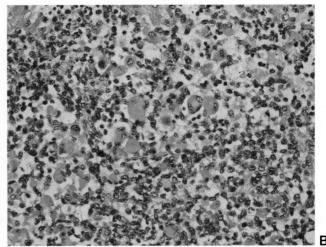

A **B**

FIGURE 13-29 ■ Rhabdomyosarcoma. **A:** This paratesticular rhabdomyosarcoma is a multilobular, fleshy white mass adjacent to the testis. **B:** Embryonal rhabdomyosarcoma displays a proliferation of small, round, blue cells. Cells with more abundant, eosinophilic cytoplasm are rhabdomyoblasts.

cross-striations may be present. They often display partial monosomy of chromosome 11.[371]

Sixty percent of tumors classified as the spindle cell variant of embryonal rhabdomyosarcomas occur in the paratesticular region.[370] Spindle cell rhabdomyosarcomas display elongated fusiform cells that may resemble the cells of leiomyosarcoma, a tumor rarely seen in the paratesticular region in children. Careful examination of spindle cell rhabdomyosarcomas reveals cross-striations, and immunostains are also helpful in this differential diagnosis. The spindle cell variant has a better prognosis than other embryonal rhabdomyosarcomas,[354] and pediatric rhabdomyosarcomas have a better prognosis than adult rhabdomyosarcomas in the paratesticular region.

Alveolar rhabdomyosarcoma is an uncommon type of rhabdomyosarcoma seen in the paratesticular region, but these are very aggressive tumors. Fibrous trabeculae separate the tumor cells into "alveolar" nests of primitive tumor cells with poor cell cohesion, so that the peripheral cells appear to adhere to the fibrous stroma. Tumor nests may therefore appear to be solid or alveolar, with peripheral cells lining the fibrous stroma separating tumor cell nests. Multinucleated giant cells may be present, and cells may display clear cytoplasm. Any amount of alveolar pattern is sufficient to classify the tumor as an alveolar rhabdomyosarcoma for prognostic and therapeutic purposes, because this tumor has a worse prognosis than other types of rhabdomyosarcoma. A solid variant of alveolar rhabdomyosarcoma has been reported in this location.[372] These tumors have a specific chromosome translocation t(2;13) or t(1;13) resulting in formation of PAX-FKHR fusion genes.[373] Genetic studies may be useful in establishing the diagnosis.

The least common type of rhabdomyosarcoma to occur in the paratesticular region is pleomorphic rhabdomyosarcoma, which is usually seen only in adult patients. The incidence of this tumor type has probably been overestimated. Pleomorphic rhabdomyosarcoma displays a patternless proliferation of spindle and polygonal cells with abundant brightly eosinophilic cytoplasm, highly atypical nuclei, and mitotic figures. Although strap-shaped cells may be present, cross-striations are difficult to identify.[374]

Immunohistochemical staining of these tumors is recommended because many of the tumors formerly thought to represent pleomorphic rhabdomyosarcoma would probably be classified today as malignant fibrous histiocytomas.[354] Antibodies to desmin are the most sensitive marker of striated muscle differentiation,[375] but these antibodies are not specific and may stain other types of sarcomas. Antibodies to MyoD1 and myogenin are the most specific markers for rhabdomyosarcoma.[376,377] Actin stains, including those using antibodies to smooth muscle actin, may be positive in some rhabdomyosarcomas[374,378]; these stains alone do not distinguish between leiomyosarcoma and rhabdomyosarcoma.

Leiomyosarcoma

Nearly one-third of paratesticular sarcomas in adults represent leiomyosarcomas.[344,345,354,361,362] Paratesticular leiomyosarcomas are typically painless scrotal masses that occur in

men between 34 and 86 years of age, with an average age of 62 years and a median age of 64 years.[379] They are tumors of the adult population; they are very rare in childhood. Most of these neoplasms involve the spermatic cord or testicular tunics, but the epididymis may also be affected.[379] A recent review of 24 primary paratesticular leiomyosarcomas found 11 tumors in the testicular tunics, 10 in the spermatic cord, 1 in the scrotal subcutis, 1 in the dartos muscle, and 1 in the epididymis.[379]

Leiomyosarcomas are often well circumscribed, but some have an infiltrative growth pattern. These tumors are firm, gray-tan masses on gross examination. They range in size from 2 to 9 cm. Microscopic examination of these tumors displays features of smooth muscle differentiation, including interlacing bundles of spindle-shaped cells with blunt-ended nuclei. Leiomyosarcomas may resemble leiomyomas with abnormal mitotic activity, or they may display marked cellular and nuclear pleomorphism and areas of necrosis. Even highly pleomorphic tumors that may resemble malignant fibrous histiocytomas usually contain some areas that are typical of smooth muscle neoplasms. Epithelioid areas are present in some tumors, and one paratesticular leiomyosarcoma recently studied also displayed vascular invasion.[379] Necrosis is present in less than half of paratesticular leiomyosarcomas. Scattered lymphocytes, lymphoid aggregates, and foamy macrophages are seen in some tumors.[379] Myxoid stromal tissue may be present. A few sarcomas in the paratesticular area have had components of both leiomyosarcoma and liposarcoma.[380] Mitotic figures are present in all paratesticular leiomyosarcomas; the number of mitotic figures has ranged from <1 MF per 10 high power fields to >70 MF/10 HPF.[379] Any mitotic activity in a paratesticular smooth muscle tumor is an indicator of a leiomyosarcoma.[354]

Immunohistochemistry is helpful in confirming smooth muscle differentiation.[381] Most cases stain strongly with antibodies to muscle-specific actin, smooth muscle actin, and desmin. Some also display CD34 positivity. Focal cytokeratin and S-100 protein positivity may occur, but myogenin stains have been negative.[379] Some spindle cell rhabdomyosarcomas in children may resemble leiomyosarcomas. The diagnosis of paratesticular leiomyosarcoma in the pediatric age group should not be made unless immunohistochemical stains for MyoD1 and myogenin are negative.[354]

The differential diagnosis of paratesticular leiomyosarcomas includes inflammatory myofibroblastic tumor. The latter lesion may have mitotic figures, but cells have nuclei with tapered rather than blunt ends. An inflammatory element is often seen and cytologic atypia is not a feature of inflammatory myofibroblastic tumor. Aggressive fibromatosis occurs in the paratestis,[382] and it has a more infiltrative pattern than seen in leiomyosarcoma. Solitary fibrous tumors[383] have been reported in the spermatic cord. They often have a hemangiopericytomatous pattern, and they lack the desmin positivity that is characteristic of leiomyosarcomas. Careful examination and thorough sectioning of pleomorphic leiomyosarcomas in order to identify areas typical of smooth muscle tumor is helpful in excluding other pleomorphic sarcomas such as dedifferentiated liposarcoma and malignant fibrous histiocytoma.

Most low-grade leiomyosarcomas of the paratestis are indolent neoplasms, but high-grade tumors behave aggressively. Fisher et al.[379] recently showed that the grade of the tumor correlates with clinical outcome when necrosis, mitotic activity, and nuclear pleomorphism are considered together. Grade 1 tumors lack necrosis, have <6 MF/10 HPF, and have only occasional pleomorphic nuclei. Grade 2 tumors have focal necrosis (<15%) and/or >6 MF/10 HPF or prominent nuclear pleomorphism. Grade 3 tumors have >15% necrosis with any degree of nuclear pleomorphism and mitotic count. These authors found that all seven patients with grade 1 tumors (some of whom had had tumor recurrences) and all three patients with grade 2 tumors were alive without disease at last follow-up. However, all four patients with grade 3 tumors died of their disease. Complete, and even radical, resection of these tumors is necessary for optimal results. Literature addressing adjuvant therapy after radical orchiectomy is limited and inconclusive because these neoplasms are uncommon.

Liposarcoma

Liposarcoma is the most common malignant tumor of the paratesticular region.[354,384] Twelve percent of liposarcomas in one study were seen in inguinal or paratesticular areas.[384] Paratesticular liposarcomas are usually well-differentiated tumors that have a prolonged clinical course. Myxoid, round cell, and pleomorphic liposarcomas also occur in this location.[354]

Paratesticular liposarcomas are detected as painless mass lesions.[385] Some are found during repair of hernias. The age range is 41 to 87 years, with a mean age of 63 years.[385] In a recent study of paratesticular liposarcomas, tumors involved the spermatic cord, testicular tunica, and epididymis.[385]

Liposarcomas often resemble fat on gross examination, although some are firm due to fibrous tissue components

(Fig. 13-30A) and others are more myxoid than fatty. These neoplasms range from 3 to 30 cm in diameter, with a mean size of 11.7 cm.[385] Well-differentiated liposarcomas resemble fat on gross examination, although the sclerosing variant displays areas of dense fibrotic tissue. Any firm or solid areas evident in a grossly fatty tumor should be carefully sectioned in an attempt to identify foci of dedifferentiation. Myxoid liposarcomas have a gelatinous appearance. Any firmer or whiter nodules in the gelatinous tissue should be sectioned because they may represent focal round cell differentiation. Pleomorphic liposarcomas typically display areas of necrosis. While liposarcomas may appear lobulated and well circumscribed, they typically infiltrate the surrounding tissue.

All types of liposarcomas may occur in this area, but well-differentiated sclerosing or lipoma-like liposarcomas are the most common. Well-differentiated sclerosing liposarcoma contains a significant component of fibrous tissue admixed with adipocytes (Fig. 13-30B). Atypical nuclei are present in the fat or fibrous tissue or both, but lipoblasts are rare and do not need to be identified for the diagnosis of this subtype of well-differentiated liposarcoma. A chronic inflammatory infiltrate may obscure part of the lesion.[384] Lipoma-like well-differentiated liposarcomas resemble mature fat, but they contain cells with enlarged, hyperchromatic nuclei as well as scatted lipoblasts. The term "atypical lipoma" should not be used for these neoplasms in the paratestis because they are associated with both a high (79%) risk of recurrence and the possibility of dedifferentiation.[386] Myxoid change may occur in well-differentiated liposarcoma, but it lacks the plexiform vascular component seen in myxoid liposarcoma. Dedifferentiated liposarcoma is defined as a high-grade sarcoma arising in the setting of a well-differentiated liposarcoma.[387–389] The dedifferentiated component of the tumor displays features of malignant fibrous histiocytoma, high-grade fibrosarcoma,[387] or other types of mesenchymal neoplasms. Dedifferentiated liposarcoma

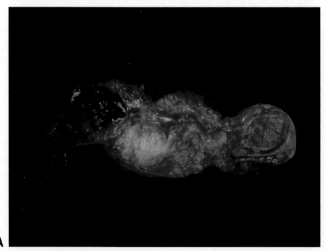

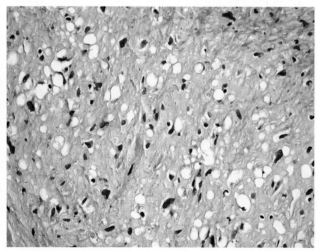

A **B**

FIGURE 13-30 ■ Liposarcoma. **A:** The ill-demarcated white mass represents a dedifferentiated liposarcoma. **B:** Well-differentiated sclerosing liposarcoma has atypical nuclei in a collagenous background. Lipoblasts and mitotic figures are not often identified in this type of liposarcoma.

must be distinguished from other types of high-grade sarcoma by the presence of coexisting well-differentiated liposarcoma. The high-grade sarcomatous component has a different gross appearance, with firmer fibrous-appearing tissue, than the juxtaposed well differentiated liposarcoma. Approximately 8% of dedifferentiated liposarcomas have occurred in the paratesticular region.[387]

More than half of the well-differentiated liposarcomas in a recent study[385] recurred and dedifferentiation was noted in some of the recurrences, but there were no metastases of well-differentiated liposarcoma in that series except in a case with dedifferentiation. Recurrences may occur many years after the original tumor is excised. The prognosis of tumors with dedifferentiation is more guarded.

Myxoid liposarcoma is less common in the paratesticular region than well-differentiated liposarcoma.[390] Patients with these tumors have soft, gelatinous tumor masses. Microscopically, these tumors display myxoid, lobulated tissue with a prominent network of branching thin-walled blood vessels. Lipoblasts are present and easily identified. Increased cellularity is seen at the edge of tumor nodules. Round cell liposarcoma may arise in the setting of myxoid liposarcoma. Round cell liposarcoma is very cellular, and contains crowded, enlarged, atypical nuclei. It lacks any prominent vascular pattern. Both of these liposarcoma variants display the same chromosomal abnormality, t(12;16), resulting in fusion of the CHOP gene on chromosome 12q13 with the FUS (TLS) gene on chromosome 16p11.[391] Round cell liposarcoma is diagnosed when it either exceeds 25% of the area of the original myxoid liposarcoma or produces a nodule in the myxoid liposarcoma.[392] About 20% of patients with paratesticular myxoid liposarcoma develop metastatic disease,[393,394] but a round cell component is predictive of an adverse outcome.[393,394]

Pleomorphic liposarcoma, a variant not commonly seen in the paratesticular region, presents as a mass that often has necrotic areas. This tumor is very cellular, with highly atypical, pleomorphic nuclei and numerous mitotic figures. Pleomorphic liposarcoma may resemble malignant fibrous histiocytoma with intermingled lipoblasts, or it may be composed of sheets of epithelioid, pleomorphic, lipoblast-like cells.[395] These are high-grade sarcomas, and associated mortality exceeds 40%.[394]

The differential diagnosis of well-differentiated liposarcoma of the paratestis is with benign lipomas. Cytologic characteristics are important in the assessment of these lesions because well-differentiated lipoma-like liposarcomas have nuclear atypia that is not seen in benign lesions of fat. The appearance of sclerosing liposarcomas is sufficiently characteristic that is should not be confused with other lesions. Dedifferentiated liposarcomas must be distinguished from other sarcomas by the presence of a well-differentiated liposarcoma component. The possibility of extension of metastasis from retroperitoneal liposarcomas must be excluded before classifying a liposarcoma as a primary paratesticular liposarcoma.

Malignant Fibrous Histiocytoma

Malignant fibrous histiocytoma occurs rarely in the paratesticular area.[396–398] Fewer than 20 cases have been reported in the English literature. Most paratesticular malignant fibrous histiocytomas occur in men over the age of 50.[399] They occur as solitary mass lesions that range in size from <1 cm to more than 20 cm.[399] Nine patients in one recent series[399] had satellite tumor nodules at presentation. These tumors are grayish-tan masses that may contain necrosis. Microscopic examination shows intermediate- to high-grade sarcomas that usually display a storiform pattern of spindle-shaped cells. Myxoid, giant cell, and inflammatory variants of malignant fibrous histiocytomas are less common that the storiform type. Lin et al.[399] recently reported that 83% of paratesticular malignant fibroma histiocytomas are of the storiform–pleomorphic type, with only a few giant cells, inflammatory and myxoid variants. Cells are pleomorphic, with atypical hyperchromatic nuclei, variable numbers of mitotic figures, and sometimes an associated inflammatory infiltrate. Tumors with a prominent inflammatory infiltrate may be misdiagnosed as inflammatory myofibroblastic tumor.

The differential diagnosis of malignant fibrous histiocytoma includes other pleomorphic sarcomas, metastatic carcinoma, and metastatic melanoma. Immunohistochemical stains are useful in confirming the diagnosis. Tumor cells stain positively for vimentin and CD68. Stains for cytokeratin, S-100 protein, desmin, smooth muscle actin, muscle-specific actin, CD34, epithelial membrane antigen, and CD117 are negative. Stains for cytokeratin and melanoma markers are useful in excluding the possibility of metastatic carcinoma or melanoma.

Malignant fibrous histiocytoma may be diagnosed earlier in the paratesticular region than at other sites and may therefore be associated with a better prognosis than the same tumor at other locations,[398] although retroperitoneal and mediastinal adenopathy has been reported in some cases.[400] Lin et al.[399] found that tumor size does not predict clinical progression, but satellite nodules at the time of disease presentation are an indication of early local metastasis; progression of disease was commonly associated with these satellite nodules. Recurrence and metastasis is common for paratesticular malignant fibrous histiocytomas. The overall prognosis is poor despite adjuvant therapy.

Grading and Staging of Paratesticular Sarcomas

The American Joint Committee on Cancer staging system is currently used in the United States.[401] Paratesticular sarcomas are classified as either low-grade or high-grade sarcomas. Low-grade tumors include those classified as grade 1 in a three-tier system and those classified as grades 1 and 2 in a four-tier grading system. High-grade sarcomas are those classified as grades 2 and 3 in a three-tier grading system and those classified as grades 3 and 4 in a four-tier system. All paratesticular sarcomas should be considered deep neoplasms. The TNM stage grouping takes into account the size of the primary tumor, presence or absence of lymph node and distant metastases, and tumor grade.

Treatment of Paratesticular Sarcomas

All paratesticular sarcomas should be managed by complete resection with high ligation of the spermatic cord.[402–404] Inadequately resected tumors should be treated with wide inguinal reresection, including completion orchiectomy or removal of the cord remnant to the level of the internal inguinal ring with surrounding soft tissue and scar excision, all with negative surgical margins.[364] Large tumors, those with an inguinal location, prior transection of the tumor, and involved or close margins are associated with increased risk of local recurrence[403] that may be decreased with adjuvant radiotherapy.[402–404] The question of whether a retroperitoneal lymph node dissection should be performed is controversial,[362,402–404] but no study has shown that a prophylactic lymph node dissection is beneficial in general. Retroperitoneal lymph node dissection has been recommended for patients with rhabdomyosarcoma and radiographically suspicious lymph nodes.[346,365,405] Adjuvant chemotherapy has been very effective in children with paratesticular rhabdomyosarcoma,[346,365] but there has not been a controlled study of its benefit in adult patients. In other anatomic sites, it has been shown to increase time to recurrence or metastasis at other sites[406] and to increase overall survival in patients with high-grade sarcomas.[407]

Hematopoietic and Lymphoid Neoplasms

Malignant Lymphoma

Paratesticular lymphoma is usually the result of spread to the epididymis or spermatic cord from a primary lymphoma in the testis,[408,409] although lymphoma may also spread from other primary sites. There are only a few reported cases of lymphoma presenting as an epididymal mass, and patient ages have ranged the third decade to the eighth decade of life.[408,410]

Types of lymphoma presenting as paratesticular masses are variable. One young patient had an extranodal marginal zone B-cell lymphoma of the mucosa-associated lymphoid tissue type confined to the epididymis; this patient was disease-free 36 months after surgical excision.[411] Three other patients in the third and fourth decades of life had sclerosing lymphomas that were either partially or totally follicular and either mixed small and large cell type or a large cell lymphoma.[408,411,412] While one of these three tumors was bilateral, none had spread beyond the epididymis. Two patients were not initially treated because they were not recognized as lymphoma, and both recurred.[408,413] One older patient had an Epstein-Barr virus–positive intravascular lymphoma of T-cell lineage. Although the tumor initially presented as an epididymal tumor, disseminated tumor was later discovered. It resulted in patient death in spite of chemotherapy.[410] Two elderly patients had stage I diffuse large cell lymphomas that were treated with radiation in one case and chemotherapy in the other case.[414,415] Follow-up was short in both cases, but one patient had developed widespread disease and died within a year of diagnosis. While the number of epididymal lymphomas has been quite limited, some authors[40] have suggested that epididymal lymphomas in young men are more likely to be low- to intermediate-grade tumors with indolent behavior, in contrast to more aggressive lymphomas seen in older patients.

Spermatic cord lymphoma usually represents spread from testicular lymphoma.[408] Only 13 cases of primary spermatic cord lymphoma have been reported.[408,416,417] Those patients ranged in age from 21 to 89 years and presented with hard, painless masses in the upper scrotum or inguinal canal. The tumors were usually diffuse large cell lymphomas. Most patients were treated surgically, either with or without radiation, and most developed widespread or central nervous system relapses shortly after diagnosis. Lymphomas involving the spermatic cord behave in a manner similar to those in the testis, and local therapy alone is not adequate treatment. One reported case of paratesticular lymphoma involved the tunica albuginea bilaterally.[408] One adult patient presented with right inguinoscrotal pain and swelling 7 years after a renal transplant and died despite chemotherapy for his aggressive posttransplant epididymal lymphoma.[418]

Most lymphomas of the paratesticular area have been B-cell lymphomas, but an epididymal T-cell lymphoma[410] and a case of secondary mycosis fungoides[419] have been reported in the epididymis.

Plasmacytoma

Plasmacytoma has been reported in the epididymis of middle-aged to elderly patients, some of whom have had multiple myeloma.[420] These tumors are composed of aggregates of plasma cells that may be atypical or immature and express either monotypic immunoglobulins of IgG or IgA type or light chains without heavy chains. They do not usually stain with the B-cell marker CD20 or leukocyte common antigen, but they usually do express CD79a and (often) epithelial membrane antigen.[40] Poorly differentiated tumors may stain for epithelial membrane antigen and/or CD138 without CD20 or CD45 staining, causing a mistaken consideration of an epithelial tumor.[40] Attention to the cytologic features and clinical history are helpful in achieving the correct diagnosis.

Granulocytic Sarcoma

Granulocytic sarcoma is very rare in the paratesticular region, and it usually represents disease spread from the testis.[421] One 73-year-old man who presented with granulocytic sarcoma of the epididymis with extension to the spermatic cord later developed acute myeloid leukemia.[40] This tumor may be mistaken for lymphoma. The presence of eosinophils in the infiltrate may be helpful in establishing the correct diagnosis. Patients may have circulating blasts and acute myeloid leukemia. Neoplastic myeloid cells usually stain positively by histochemical stains for chloroacetate esterase and by immunohistochemical stains for myeloperoxidase and lysozyme, but not for the B- and T-cell markers seen in lymphomas.[40]

Other Rare Neoplasms

Melanotic Neuroectodermal Tumor of Infancy (Synonyms: Retinal Anlage Tumor, Melanotic Hamartoma, Melanotic Progonoma)

Melanotic neuroectodermal tumor of infancy is also known as melanotic progonoma and retinal anlage tumor. It is rare and is seen in children <1 year of age. Most of these tumors occur in the head and neck.[422] Several cases have been reported in the paratesticular region, especially in the epididymis.[423–425] Some authors believe that melanotic neuroectodermal tumors are dysembryogenetic neoplasms that are always congenital.[425] These tumors are of neuroectodermal origin. They occur in young children, although one paratesticular tumor was reported in an 8-year-old child.[425]

The typical clinical presentation of melanotic neuroectodermal tumors is a scrotal firm mass, sometimes associated with a hydrocele, in an infant. Urinary vanillylmandelic acid/homovanillic acid levels are elevated in some patients and are potentially useful in detecting recurrent disease.[426]

Melanotic neuroectodermal tumors of infancy typically involve the epididymis. They are well-circumscribed, blue-gray rubbery masses that measure <4 cm in diameter. Microscopically, these tumors display two cell populations. Cellular aggregates of tumor cells are separated by fibrous stroma. Large, melanin-containing, columnar to cuboidal epithelioid cells are located peripherally around nests of smaller neuroblastic cells with scant cytoplasm and a neurofibrillary background (Fig. 13-31). Mitoses are usually rare,

but they may be seen in the small cell component. Necrosis is rare in these tumors. Tumor cells may surround tubules of the epididymis in an infiltrative pattern. Metastatic lesions may contain either the larger, pigmented cells or the neuroblast-like cells, and ganglion cell differentiation has been described in metastatic lesions.[423,427]

Melanotic neuroectodermal tumor of infancy expresses epithelial, neural, and melanocytic immunohistochemical markers. The pigmented cells stain for both cytokeratin and HMB.45; they may also be EMA-positive. Both cell populations often stain positively with antibodies to neuron-specific enolase and Leu7. The cells resembling neuroblasts stain positively for glial fibrillary acidic protein, neurofilament protein, and synaptophysin.[428] Negative staining for desmin excludes rhabdomyosarcoma and desmoplastic round cell tumor from the differential diagnosis, but occasional melanotic tumors of infancy do display desmin positivity.[425]

Ultrastructural analysis shows both epithelial and melanocytic differentiation in the large cells, which contain desmosomes as well as melanosomes and pre-melanosomes. The smaller, neuroblast-like cells contain dense-core granules and microtubules; they also form dendritic processes.[425] Rare cells may contain both dense-core granules and melanosomes.[40]

Recognition of the dual cell population in a paratesticular tumor in a young infant is the key to the correct diagnosis. If pigmented cells are scant or only one cell population is seen, the differential diagnosis includes other small round blue cell tumors. Thorough sampling to reveal both cell populations is

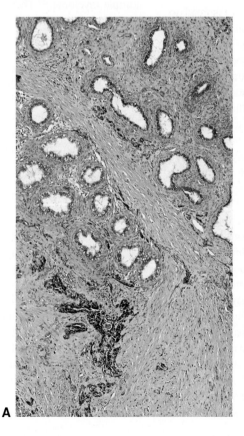 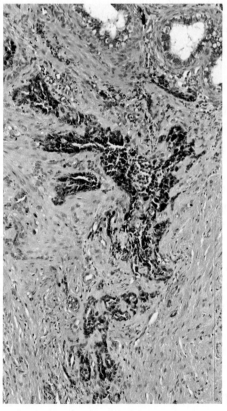

FIGURE 13-31 ■ Melanotic neuroectodermal tumor of infancy. **A:** Low-power photograph showing infiltrating melanocytic lesion involving epididymis. **B:** Note nests and cords of epithelioid cells with abundant melanin pigment.

A

B

essential. Positivity of the large cells for HMB45 excludes the possibility of either rhabdomyosarcoma or desmoplastic small round cell tumor. Homer-Wright rosettes characteristic of neuroblastoma are not seen in melanotic neuroectodermal tumor of infancy. A panel of immunostains is useful, but the fact that melanotic neuroectodermal tumor of infancy may be desmin-positive should be borne in mind.

Behavior of melanotic neuroectodermal tumors of infancy is unpredictable. Recurrences may be seen in about half of patients when all primary disease sites are considered, with metastatic disease occurring in 5% to 10% of cases.[427,428] Two of twenty-four patients with paratesticular tumors have had local or regional lymph node metastases. One patient was treated with chemotherapy and the other with lymph node dissection; both were disease free after 24 and 48 months.[423,427] There are no histologic criteria to predict which tumors may recur or metastasize.

Desmoplastic Small Round Cell Tumor

Desmoplastic small round cell tumors are highly aggressive small round blue cell tumors that arise in association with mesothelial surfaces. They are much more common in males than in females. They have a distinctive immunophenotype and they are associated with a specific chromosomal abnormality. They metastasize and also spread by serosal seeding. Paratesticular desmoplastic small round cell tumors are associated with the tunica vaginalis. They may be primary or secondary. Several of these tumors have been reported in patients who presented with symptoms in the paratesticular region.[429–433]

These neoplasms occur in young patients between the ages 17 and 35 years. Patients typically present with a painless scrotal mass that may be accompanied by swelling of the scrotum and leg. Some patients have had symptoms for only 1 month, whereas others report symptoms for 2 years before diagnosis.[432]

Desmoplastic small round cell tumors are firm, gray-white neoplasms that may display areas of necrosis or myxoid change on gross examination. In the paratestis, these tumors usually consist of a dominant nodule that measures between 2.5 and 5.5 cm in diameter, with surrounding satellite nodules studding the testicular tunics and involving the epididymis.[40]

Microscopic examination (Fig. 13-32) typically shows fibrous stroma surrounding nests of tumor cells with enlarged, hyperchromatic round nuclei, little cytoplasm, numerous mitotic figures, and areas of necrosis. Cell borders are indistinct. Lymphovascular space invasion is often present. However, atypical histologic features may complicate the diagnosis. Glands, pseudorosettes, signet ring cells, and rhabdoid features may be present.[434,435] Some tumors have abundant eosinophilic cytoplasm that produces a rhabdoid appearance to the cells, some contain glycogen, and some tumors have mucin-negative cytoplasmic vacuoles that produce a signet ring appearance in the neoplastic cell

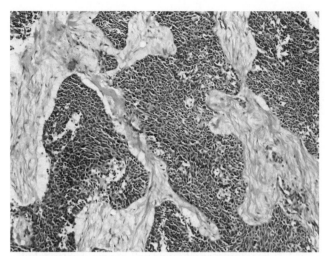

FIGURE 13-32 ■ Desmoplastic small round cell tumor. Note sheets and broad trabeculae of poorly differentiated cohesive cells separated by abundant fibrous stroma. (Image courtesy of Dr Steven Shen, Houston, TX.)

nests.[434–436] Pseudorosettes and tubular formations mimic the appearance of primitive neuroectodermal tumor in some cases of desmoplastic small round cell tumor. Psammoma bodies have been reported in one case of paratesticular desmoplastic small round cell tumor.[430]

Desmoplastic small round cell tumors have a very distinct, polyphenotypic immunohistochemical profile. These neoplasms express three different intermediate filaments, including cytokeratin, desmin, and vimentin. Immunohistochemical stains are useful in distinguishing these tumors from other round cell sarcomas including rhabdomyosarcoma and primitive neuroectodermal tumors.[436] Desmoplastic round cell tumors show positive staining for desmin, cytokeratin (often with a dot-like pattern), epithelial membrane antigen, neuron-specific enolase, vimentin, and often WT1. Some tumors stain for MIC2.[436] Stains for actin and chromogranin are generally negative. Rare tumors with the characteristic chromosomal translocation seen in desmoplastic small round cell tumors have failed to express cytokeratin or epithelial membrane antigen.[437]

Electron microscopy reveals nonspecific features that include primitive cells with a few poorly developed cell junctions, aggregates of intermediate filaments, some glycogen, and rare dense-core granules.[437]

Desmoplastic small round cell tumors display a unique chromosomal abnormality, t(11;22) (p13,q12) that results in the fusion of the EWS gene on chromosome 22 to the Wilms tumor suppressor gene (WT1) on chromosome 11. The EWS-WT1 transcript can be detected by reverse transcriptase–polymerase chain reaction or by immunohistochemistry.[437]

The differential diagnosis of paratesticular desmoplastic small round cell tumor includes embryonal rhabdomyosarcoma, lymphoma, primitive neuroectodermal tumor, and melanotic neuroectodermal tumor of infancy. Paratesticular rhabdomyosarcoma most commonly occurs in children, whereas desmoplastic small round cell tumor is usually seen in young adults. Rhabdomyosarcomas stain with antibodies to muscle-specific actin (HHF35), in contrast to desmoplastic small round cell tumor, which is negative for actin markers. Both tumors stain for desmin. Only desmoplastic small round cell tumor is polyimmunophenotypic, with positive staining to cytokeratin, epithelial membrane antigen, and neuron-specific enolase in addition to desmin and vimentin.

Malignant lymphoma also displays a small round blue cell population, but the cells are not arranged in the nested aggregates seen in desmoplastic small round cell tumor. Immunohistochemical profiles of these two neoplasms are completely different and will resolve any diagnostic problems between the two tumors. As mentioned above, occasional desmoplastic small round cell tumors display tubules and rosettes, leading to potential confusion with primitive neuroectodermal tumor.[430] Cytokeratin and desmin positivity are characteristic of desmoplastic small round cell tumor, in contrast to the MIC2 (HBA71) positivity that is seen in primitive neuroectodermal tumors. However, MIC2 may be seen in some desmoplastic small round cell tumors, and we have seen some desmin staining in primitive neuroectodermal tumors. Cytokeratin staining is not seen in primitive neuroectodermal tumors. Cytogenetic testing should resolve the dilemma in difficult cases.

Desmoplastic small round cell tumors are very aggressive malignant neoplasms; most patients do not survive more than 2 years. Paratesticular tumors may be detected at an earlier stage than abdominal tumors and therefore have a slightly better prognosis. A few patients have been alive without disease 2.5 to 3 years after diagnosis.[432] Treatment includes aggressive surgery and intensive multidrug chemotherapy.[438]

Extratesticular Germ Cell Tumors

Primary paratesticular germ cell tumors have been rarely described.[439,440] Concurrent or regressed testicular germ cell tumors should be excluded before diagnosing a primary germ cell tumor in the paratestis. Significant scarring and/or the presence of intratubular germ cell neoplasia provide evidence for a regressed testicular germ cell tumor. The possibility of undescended testes should also be excluded because they may be a source of inguinal germ cell tumors.

Extratesticular Sex Cord–Stromal Tumors

Extratesticular sex cord–stromal tumors have been described in the paratestis,[441,442] but they are very rare. Some may arise from Leydig cells present in the spermatic cord or from incidental Sertoli cell nodules in the epididymis or rete testis.[40] Fibromas of gonadal stromal origin occur in the testis, but some are adjacent to the tunica albuginea and may be confused with fibromas originating from the testicular tunics. Fibromas of gonadal stromal origin have stroma resembling ovarian fibromas, in contrast to the more collagenous and less cellular fibromas originating from the testicular tunics.

Neuroblastoma

The paratestis has been a presenting location for neuroblastoma in some young infants.[443–445] Some neuroblastomas represent metastases from primary tumors in the adrenal gland,[443] but one paratesticular neuroblastoma associated with ectopic adrenal cortical tissue was considered to represent multifocal origin of the tumor.[444] These tumors are small round blue cell tumors with a neurofibrillary background, often a high mitotic rate, and variable numbers of Homer-Wright pseudorosettes.

Paraganglioma

Six cases of paraganglioma have been reported in the spermatic cord.[446] These lesions usually present as mass lesions without neuropeptide production. These tumors display the typical "zellballen" surrounded by a delicate vascular network as seen in paragangliomas in more typical locations. Immunohistochemical markers such as CD56, chromogranin, and synaptophysin are useful in confirming a diagnosis of paraganglioma. All cases reported in the paratesticular region have been benign tumors.[40]

Carcinoid Tumor

One case of primary carcinoid tumor of the epididymis has been reported.[447] Other rare carcinoid tumors of the paratesticular region have been metastatic, rarely as the first manifestation of carcinoid tumors of the small intestine.[448]

Wilms Tumor

Fifteen cases of inguinal and scrotal Wilms tumor have been reported.[449] Primary extrarenal Wilms tumor has been reported in the paratestis in two young children[44,450] and a 23-year-old man.[40] These tumors present as mass lesions and have the epithelial, blastema, and stromal components characteristic of Wilms tumor. The possibility of metastatic tumor from the kidney should be excluded, although metanephric rests in the paratesticular region could represent a precursor lesion. Primary extrarenal nephrogenic rests also occur rarely in this anatomic region[45] and must be distinguished from Wilms tumor.

Squamous Cell Carcinoma

There is a single report of paratesticular squamous cell carcinoma in a hydrocele sac of an 85-year-old man.[451] The hydrocele sac displayed squamous metaplasia, dysplasia, and invasive squamous carcinoma.

Secondary Neoplasms

Metastatic tumors may be seen in the epididymis, testicular tunics, and the spermatic cord. In one review of 112 paratesticular tumors, 5 neoplasms represented tumor metastatic to the paratesticular region.[441] A different study found that

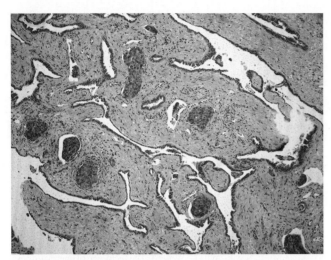

FIGURE 13-33 ■ Metastatic prostatic carcinoma in rete testis. Tumor present in lymphatic and vascular spaces is characteristic of metastatic carcinoma.

metastatic tumors accounted for only 8.1% of all malignant tumors of the epididymis and/or spermatic cord.[452] Most cancers that metastasize to the paratestis are known carcinomas in men over the age of 50 with high-stage disease, but paratesticular metastases may rarely be the presenting finding. Metastatic tumors in the paratestis may present as fixed inguinal hernias, intrascrotal masses, or areas of thickening of the spermatic cord. Some metastatic tumors are discovered incidentally.

Stomach cancer has been the most frequent type of metastatic tumor in the spermatic cord and epididymis; it accounts for 42.8% of metastases to these sites.[452] Prostate cancer accounts for 28.5% of metastases (Fig. 13-33).[452] Other primary tumor sites include the testis, kidney,[453] lung, intestine, and appendix,[454,455] liver and biliary tract,[456,457] pancreas,[458] skin (melanoma),[459] and brain medulloblastoma.[460] Prostate carcinoma may spread through the vas deferens. Other neoplasms metastasize by way of lymphatic and vascular channels. There may be a tendency for left-sided renal cell carcinoma to metastasize to the paratesticular region because the left gonadal vein enters the left renal vein.[461]

Tumors that are metastatic to the paratestis may mimic the appearance of primary paratesticular neoplasms. The differential diagnosis of metastatic carcinoma in the paratesticular region includes adenocarcinoma of the epididymis, rete testis adenocarcinoma, primary serous carcinoma of the paratesticular region, and malignant mesothelioma. Evaluation of the medical history, the location of the tumor, the histologic pattern, and judicious use of immunohistochemical are very useful in distinguishing metastatic carcinoma from primary tubulopapillary tumors of the paratesticular region.

Papillary cystadenoma of the epididymis and metastatic renal cell carcinoma both occur in patients with von Hippel-Lindau syndrome, but the bland cytologic features and cystic spaces seen in cystadenoma are helpful for that diagnosis. In general, the presence of bilateral tumors, multiple masses, prominent lymphatic or vascular space invasion by tumor, signet ring cells, or architecture not typical of known tumors of the paratesticular region should prompt consideration of a metastatic lesion.

Since metastases in the paratesticular region are usually associated with advanced disease, patients have a very poor prognosis. The average survival after discovery of the metastatic tumor was 9.1 months in one series.[452]

REFERENCES

1. Langman J. *Medical Embryology and Human Development—Normal and Abnormal.* 2nd ed. Baltimore, MD: Williams & Wilkins; 1969.
2. Moore KL. *The Developing Human. Clinically Oriented Embryology.* Philadelphia, PA: Saunders; 1973.
3. Neville AM, Grigor KM. Structure, function, and development of the human testis. In: Pugh R, ed. *Pathology of the Testis.* Oxford, UK: Blackwell Scientific; 1976:1–37.
4. Carlson BM. *Patten's Foundations of Embryology.* New York: McGraw-Hill; 1988:567–580.
5. Ulbright TM, Amin MB, Young RH. *Tumors of the Testis, Adnexa, Spermatic Cord and Scrotum: Atlas of Tumor Pathology, Third Series, Fascicle 25.* Washington, DC: Armed Forces Institute of Pathology; 1999.
6. Warwick R, Williams BL. *Gray's Anatomy.* 35th ed. London, UK: Longman; 1973:1336–1351.
7. Trainer TD. Testis and excretory duct system. In: Sternberg SS, ed. *Histology for Pathologists.* New York: Raven Press; 1992:731–747.
8. Srigley JR. The paratesticular region: histoanatomic and general considerations. *Semin Diagn Pathol* 2000;17:258–269.
9. Kuo T, Gomez LC. Monstrous epithelial cells in human epididymis and seminal vesicles. A pseudomalignant change. *Am J Surg Pathol* 1981;5:483–490.
10. Manely RE. Epididymal structure and function. A historical and critical review. *Acta Zool* 1959;40:1–21.
11. Hinrichsen MJ. Evidence supporting the existence of sperm maturation in the human epididymis. *J Reprod Fertil* 1980;60:291–294.
12. Madara JL, Haggitt RC, Federman M. Intranuclear inclusions of the human vas deferens. *Arch Pathol Lab Med* 1978;102:648–650.
13. Butterworth DM, Bisset DL. Cribriform intra-tubular epididymal change and adenomatous hyperplasia of the rete testis—a consequence of testicular atrophy? *Histopathology* 1992;21:435–438.
14. Calder CJ, Aluwihare N, Graham CT. Cribriform intra-tubular epididymal change. *Histopathology* 1993;22:406.
15. Sharp SC, Batt MA, Lennington WJ. Epididymal cribriform hyperplasia. A variant of normal epididymal histology. *Arch Pathol Lab Med* 1994;118:1020–1022.
16. Paniagua R, Regadera J, Nistal M, et al. Histological, histochemical and ultrastructural variations along the length of the human vas deferens before and after puberty. *Acta Anat* 1981;111:190–203.
17. Brennan MB, Srigley JR. Brenner tumors of testis and paratestis: case report and literature review. *J Urol Pathol* 1999;10:219–228.
18. Srigley J, Hartwick RW. Tumors and cysts of the paratesticular region. *Pathol Ann* 1990;25:51–108.
19. Shah KH, Maxted WC, Chun B. Epidermoid cysts of the testis: a report of three cases and analysis of 141 cases from the world literature. *Cancer* 1981;47:577–582.
20. Nistal M, Jimenez-Heffernan J. Rete testis dysgenesis. A characteristic lesion of undescended testes. *Arch Pathol Lab Med* 1997;121:1259–1264.
21. Jones EC, Murray SK, Young RH. Cysts and epithelial proliferations of the testicular collecting system (including rete testis). *Semin Diagn Pathol* 2000;17:270–293.
22. Gill B, Kogan S, Starr S, et al. Significance of epididymal and ductal anomalies associated with testicular maldescent. *J Urol* 1989;142:556–558.

23. Heath AL, Mann DW, Eckstein HB. Epididymal abnormalities associated with maldescent of the testis. *J Ped Surg* 1984;19:47.

24. Elder JS. Epididymal anomalies associated with hydrocele/hernia and cryptorchidism: implications regarding testicular descent. *J Urol* 1992;148:624.

25. Vohra S, Morgentaler A. Congenital anomalies of the vas deferens, epididymis, and seminal vesicles. *Urology* 1997;49:313–321.

26. Whitehead ED, Leiter E. Genital abnormalities and abnormal semen analysis in male patients exposed to diethylstilbestrol in utero. *J Urol* 1981;125:47–51.

27. Val-Bernal JF, Val D, Garijo MF. Ectopic epididymal tissue in appendix testis. *Virchows Arch* 2006;449:373–375.

28. Wollin M, Marshall F, Fink M, et al. Aberrant epididymal tissue: a significant clinical entity. *J Urol* 1987;138:1247–1250.

29. Daudin M, Bieth E, Bujan L, et al. Congenital bilateral absence of the vas deferens: clinical characteristics, biological parameters, cystic fibrosis transmembrane conductance regulator gene mutations, and implications for genetic counseling. *Fertil Steril* 2000;74:1164–1174.

30. Hicks CM, Skoog SJ, Done S. Ectopic vas deferens, imperforate anus and hypospadias. *J Urol* 1989;141:586.

31. Malatinsky E, Labady F, Lepies P. Congenital anomalies of the seminal ducts. *Int Urol Nephrol* 1987;19:189.

32. Putschar W. Die Entwicklungsstorungen der Milz. In: Schwalbe E, Gruber GB, eds. *Die Morphologie der Missbildungen des menschen und der Tiere*. Jena, Germany: G Fisher; 1934:760–856.

33. Putschar WG, Manion WC. Splenic-gonadal fusion. *Am J Pathol* 1956;32:15–33.

34. Oliva E, Young RH. Paratesticular tumor-like lesions. *Semin Diagn Pathol* 2000;17:340–358.

35. Dahl EV, Bahn RC. Aberrant adrenal cortical tissue near the testis in human infants. *Am J Pathol* 1962;40:587–598.

36. McDonald J, Calams J. A histological study of extraparenchymal Leydig-like cells. *J Urol* 1958;79:850–858.

37. Ketata S, Ketata H, Sahnoun A, et al. Ectopic adrenal cortex tissue: an incidental finding during inguinoscrotal operations in pediatric patients. *Urol Int* 2008;81:316–319.

38. Rutgers J, Young RH, Scully RE. The testicular "tumor" of the adrenogenital syndrome. A report of six cases and review of the literature on testicular masses in patients with adrenocortical disorders. *Am J Surg Pathol* 1988;12:503–513.

39. Ntalles K, Kostoglou-Athanassiou I, Geogiou E, et al. Paratesticular tumours in a patient with Nelson's syndrome. *Horm Res* 1996;45:291–294.

40. Henley JD, Ferry J, Ulbright TM. Miscellaneous rare paratesticular tumors. *Semin Diagn Pathol* 2000;17:319–339.

41. Kusuma V, Hemalata B, Suguna BV. Ectopic supernumerary kidney presenting as inguinal hernia. *J Clin Pathol* 2005;58:446–448.

42. McDougall EM, Mikhail BR, Carpenter B. Ectopic renal tissue associated with an undescended testis: a case report. *J Urol* 1986;135:1018–1019.

43. Shono T, Kai H, Suita S. Ectopic renal tissue in the gubernaculum associated with undescended testis. *BJU Int* 2002;89:320–321.

44. Orlowski J, Levin H, Dyment P, et al. Intrascrotal Wilms' tumor developing in a heterotopic renal anlage of probable mesonephric origin. *J Pediatr Surg* 1980;15:679–682.

45. Bennett S, Defoor W, Minevich E. Primary extrarenal nephrogenic rest. *J Urol* 2002;168:1529.

46. Berger L. Coexistence de cellulares sympathicotropes et de cellules pheocromes dans un testicule de noveau-ne. *Arch d'anat micr* 1935;31:101–109.

47. Nelson A. Giant interstitial cells and extraparenchymal interstitial cells of the human testis. *Am J Pathol* 1938;14:831–841.

48. Halley J. The infiltrative activity of Leydig cells. *J Pathol Bacteriol* 1961;81:347–353.

49. Park YW, Ro JY, Kim C, et al. Location, distribution, pattern, and quantity of testicular adnexal Leydig cells (TALC) [abstract]. *Mod Pathol* 1998;11:92A.

50. Ceccanti S, Mele E, Masselli G, et al. Intrahepatic paratesticular cyst: unique presentation of vestigial remnants of Wolffian duct. *Urology* 2012;79:212–214.

51. Sundarasivarao D. The mullerian vestiges and benign epithelial tumours of the epididymis. *J Pathol Bacteriol* 1953;LXVI:417–432.

52. Skoglund RW, McRoberts JW, Radge H. Torsion of testicular appendages. Presentation of 43 new cases and a collective review. *J Urol* 1970;104:598–600.

53. Rolnick D, Kawanoue S, Szanto P, et al. Anatomical incidence of testicular appendages. *J Urol* 1988;100:755–756.

54. Bernstein J, Gardner KD Jr. Renal cystic disease and renal dysplasia. In: Walsh PC, Gittes RF, Permutter AD, et al., eds. *Campbell's Urology*. vol. 2. Philadelphia, PA: Saunders; 1986:1760–1803.

55. Popek EJ. Embryonal remnants in inguinal hernia sacs. *Hum Pathol* 1990;21:339–349.

56. Cerilli LA, Sotelo-Avila C, Mills SE. Glandular inclusions in inguinal hernia sacs: morphologic and immunohistochemcal distinction from epididymis and vas deferens. *Am J Surg Pathol* 2003;27:469–476.

57. Steigman C, Sotelo-Avila C, Weber T. The incidence of spermatic cord structures in inguinal hernia sacs from male children. *Am J Surg Pathol* 1999;23:880–885.

58. Nistal M, Regadera J, Paniagua R. Cystic dysplasia of the testis. Light and electron microscopic study of three cases. *Arch Pathol Lab Med* 1984;108:579–583.

59. Bouron-Dal Soglio D, Harvey I, Jovanovic M, et al. Bilateral cystic dysplasia of the rete testis with renal adysplasia. *Ped Devel Pathol* 2006;9:157–160.

60. Smith PJ, DeSouza R, Roth DR. Cystic dysplasia of the rete testis. *Urology* 2008;72:230e7–230e10.

61. Nistal M. Cystic dysplasia of the epididymis: a disorder of mesonephric differentiation associated with renal maldevelopment. *Virchows Archiv* 2010;456:695–702.

62. Morgan A. Inflammatory lesions simulating malignancy. *Br J Urol* 1964;36(suppl):95–102.

63. Honore L. Nonspecific peritesticular fibrosis manifested as testicular enlargement. *Arch Surg* 1978;113:814–816.

64. Krieger J. Epididymitis, orchitis, and related conditions. *Sex Transm Dis* 1984;11:173–181.

65. Hori S, Tsutsumi Y. Histological differentiation between chlamydial and bacterial epididymitis: nondestructive and proliferative versus destructive and abscess forming: immunohistochemical and clinico-pathological findings. *Hum Pathol* 1995;26:402–407.

66. Svec A, Mikyskova I, Hes O, et al. Human papillomavirus infection of the epididymis and ductus deferens: an evaluation by nested polymerase chain reaction. *Arch Pathol Lab Med* 2003;127:1471–1474.

67. Klin B, Zlotkevich L, Horne T, et al. Epididymitis in childhood: a clinical retrospective study over 5 years. *Israel Med Assoc J* 2001;3:833–835.

68. McAndrew HF, Pemberton R, Kikiros CS, et al. The incidence and investigation of acute scrotal problems in children. *Ped Surg Int* 2002;18:435–437.

69. Woodward PJ, Schwab CM, Sesterhenn IA. Extratesticular scrotal masses: radiologic–pathologic correlation. *Radiographics* 2003;23:215–240.

70. Durand F, Brion JP, Terrier N, et al. Funiculitis due to *Schistosoma haematobium*: uncommon diagnosis using parasitologic analysis of semen. *Am J Trop Med Hygiene* 2004;70:46–47.

71. Munichor M, Gold D, Lengy J, et al. An unusual case of Dirofilaria conjunctivae infection suspected to be malignancy of the spermatic cord. *Isr Med Assoc J* 2001;3:860–861.

72. Lai AY-H, Lu S-H, Yu H-J, et al. Tuberculous epididymitis presenting as huge scrotal tumor. *Urology* 2009;73:1163.e5–1163.e37.

73. Ross J, Gow J, St. Hill C. Tuberculous epididymitis. A review of 170 patients. *Br J Surg* 1961;48:663–666.

74. Jaffar A, Hehta J, Godfrey J. Tuberculous epididymoorchitis and granulomatous prostatitis mimicking neoplasia. *J Tenn Med Assoc* 1990;83:605–606.

75. Afsar H, Baydar I, Sirmatel F. Epididymo-orchitis due to brucellosis. *Br J Urol* 1993;72:104–105.

76. Gonzalez Sanchez F, Encinas Gaspar M, Napal Lecumberri S, et al. Brucellar orchiepididymitis with abscess. *Arch Esp Urol* 1997;50:289–292.

77. Eickenberg H, Amin M, Lich R Jr. Blastomycosis of the genitourinary tract. *J Urol* 1975;113:650–652.

78. Yantiss R, Young RH. Idiopathic granulomatous epididymitis: report of a case and review of the literature. *J Urol Pathol* 1998;8:171–179.

79. Nistal M, Mate A, Paniagua R. Granulomatous epididymal lesion of possible ischemic origin. *Am J Surg Pathol* 1997;21:951–956.

80. Wiener L, Riehl P, Baum N. Xanthogranulomatous epididymitis: a case report. *J Urol* 1987;138:621–622.

81. Vaidyanathan S, Mansour P, Parsons KF, et al. Xanthogranulomatous funiculitis and epididymo-orchitis in a tetraplegic patient. *Spinal Cord* 2000;38:769–772.

82. Nistal M, Gonzales-Peramato P, Serrano A, et al. Xanthogranulomatous funiculitis and orchiepididymitis: report of 2 cases with immuno-histochemical study and literature review. [Review]. *Arch Pathol Lab Med* 2004;128:911–914.

83. Kodama K, Hasegawa T, Egawa M, et al. Bilateral epididymal sarcoidosis presenting without radiographic evidence of intrathoracic lesion: review of sarcoidosis involving the male reproductive tract. *Int J Urol* 2004;11:345–348.

84. Ryan D, Lesser B, Crumley L, et al. Epididymal sarcoidosis. *J Urol* 1993;149:134–136.

85. Ritchie A, Hindmarsh J. Bilateral epididymal sarcoid. *Br J Urol* 1983;55:240–241.

86. McWilliams W, Abramowitz L, Tiamson E. Epididymal sarcoidosis: case report and review. *J Urol* 1983;130:1201–1203.

87. Gazaigne J, Mozzionacci J, Mornet M, et al. Epididymal and renal sarcoidosis. *Br J Urol* 1995;75:413–414.

88. Gross A, Heinzer H, Loy V, et al. Unusual differential diagnosis of testis tumor: intrascrotal sarcoidosis. *J Urol* 1992;147:1112–1114.

89. Oertel YC, Johnson FB. Sclerosing lipogranuloma of male genitalia. Review of 23 cases. *Arch Pathol Lab Med* 1977;101:321–326.

90. Smetana HF, Bernhard W. Sclerosing lipogranuloma of male genitalia. *J Urol* 1950;50:296–325.

91. Arduino LJ. Sclerosing lipogranuloma of male genitalia. *J Urol* 1959;82:155–161.

92. Matsushima M, Tajima M, Maki A, et al. Primary lipogranuloma of male genitalia. *Urology* 1988;31:75–77.

93. Vargas J, Arguelles M, Prada I, et al. Lipogranuloma esclerosante paratesticular. *Patologia* 1992;25:57–58.

94. Pugh JI, Stringer P. Glove-powder granuloma of the testis after surgery. *Br J Surg* 1973;60:240–242.

95. Talerman A. Granulomatous lesions in the vas deferens caused by injection of radiopaque contrast medium. *J Urol* 1972;107:818–820.

96. Lin JI, Tseng CH, Marsidi PJ, et al. Cholesterol granuloma of right testis. *Urology* 1979;14:522–523.

97. Lowenthal SB, Goldstein AM, Terry R. Cholesterol granuloma of tunica vaginalis simulating testicular tumor. *Urology* 1981;18:89–90.

98. McClure J. Malakoplakia. *J Pathol* 1983;140:275–330.

99. McClure J. Malakoplakia of the testis and its relationship to granulomatous orchitis. *J Clin Pathol* 1980;33:670–678.

100. Green W Jr. Malacoplakia of the epididymis (without testicular involvement). The first reported case. *Arch Pathol* 1968;86:438–441.

101. Povysil C. Extravesical malakoplakia. *Arch Pathol* 1974;97:273–276.

102. Dehner LP, Scott D, Stocker JT. Meconium periorchitis: a clinicopathologic study of four cases with a review of the literature. *Hum Pathol* 1986;17:807–812.

103. Glassy FJ, Mostofi FK. Spermatic granulomas of the epididymis. *Am J Clin Pathol* 1956;26:1303–1313.

104. Schmidt SS, Morris RR. Spermatic granuloma: the complication of vasectomy. *Fertil Steril* 1973;24:941–947.

105. Cullen TH, Voss HJ. Sperm granulomata of the testis and epididymis. *Br J Urol* 1966;38:202–207.

106. Friedman N, Garske GL. Inflammatory reactions involving sperm and the seminiferous tubules. Extravasation, spermatic granulomas and granulomatous orchitis. *J Urol* 1949;62:363–374.

107. Dunner PS, Lipsit ER, Nochomovitz LE. Epididymal sperm granuloma simulating a testicular neoplasm. *J Clin Ultrasound* 1982;10:353–355.

108. Leader AJ, Axelrad SD, Frankowski R, et al. Complications of 2,711 vasectomies. *J Urol* 1974;111:365–369.

109. Schmidt SS. Technics and complications of elective vasectomy. The role of spermatic granuloma in spontaneous recanalization. *Fertil Steril* 1966;17:467–482.

110. Coyne J, al-Nakib L, Goldsmith D, et al. Secondary oxalosis and sperm granuloma of the epididymis. *J Clin Pathol* 1994;47:470–471.

111. Kiser GC, Fuchs EF, Kessler S. The significance of vasitis nodosa. *J Urol* 1986;136:42–44.

112. Easley S, MacLennan GT. Vasitis and epididymitis nodosa. *J Urol* 2006;175:1502.

113. Goldman RL, Azzopardi JG. Benign neural invasion in vasitis nodosa. *Histopathology* 1982;6:309–315.

114. Kovi J, Agbata A. Benign neural invasion in vasitis nodosa. *JAMA* 1974;228:1519.

115. Balogh K, Travis WD. The frequency of perineurial ductules in vasitis nodosa. *Am J Clin Pathol* 1984;82:710–713.

116. Kang TW, Choi YD, Jeong YY, et al. Intrascrotal extratesticular arteriovenous malformation. *Urology* 2004;64:590.e26–590.e27.

117. Guz BV, Ziegelbaum M, Pontes JE. Arteriovenous malformation of spermatic cord. *Urology* 1989;33:427–428.

118. Bush IM, Bauer S, Rosenbeld LJ. Aneurysm of the spermatic artery. *J Urol* 1964;92:47–50.

119. Beddy P, Geoghegan T, Browne RF, et al. Testicular varicoceles. *Clin Radiol* 2005;60:1248–1255.

120. Nistal M, Paniagua R, Regadera J, et al. Obstruction of the tubuli recti and ductuli efferentes by dilated veins in the testes of men with varicocele and its possible role in causing atrophy of the seminiferous tubules. *Int J Androl* 1984;7:309–323.

121. Hegarty PK, Walsch E, Corcoran MO. Exploration of the acute scrotum: a retrospective analysis of 100 consecutive cases. *Irish J Med Science* 2001;170:181–182.

122. Rakha E, Puls F, Saidul I, et al. Torsion of the testicular appendix: importance of associated acute inflammation. *J Clin Pathol* 2006;59:831–834.

123. Brisson P, Feins N, Patel H. Torsion of the epididymis. *J Ped Surg* 2005;40:1795–1797.

124. Wright L, Bicknell S. Systemic necrotizing vasculitis presenting as epididymitis. *J Urol* 1986;136:1094.

125. Shurbaji MS, Epstein JI. Testicular vasculitis: implications for systemic disease. *Hum Pathol* 1998;19:186–189.

126. Levine TS. Testicular and epididymal vasculitides. Is morphology of help in classification and prognosis? *J Urol Pathol* 1994;2:81–88.

127. Dahl EV, Bagenstoss AH, DeWeerd JH. Testicular lesion of periarteritis nodosa, with special reference to diagnosis. *Am J Med* 1960;28:222–228.

128. Womack C, Ansell ID. Isolated arteritis of the epididymis. *J Clin Pathol* 1985;38:797–800.

129. Al-Arfaj A. Limited Wegener's granulomatosis of the epididymis. *Int J Urol* 2001;8:333–335.

130. Mikuz G, Hofstadter F, Hager J. Testis involvement in Schoenlein–Henoch purpura. *Pathol Res Pract* 1979;165:323–329.

131. Nesbit RM, Hodges NB. Thrombo-angiitis obliterans of the spermatic cord. *J Urol* 1960;83:445.

132. Abercrombie G. Thrombo-angiitis obliterans of the spermatic cord. *Br J Surg* 1965;52:632.

133. Tartakoff J, Hazard JB. Thromboangiitis obliterans of the spermatic cord. *N Engl J Med* 1938;218:173–175.

134. Halim A, Neild GH, Levine T, et al. Isolated necrotizing granulomatous vasculitis of the epididymis and spermatic cords. *World J Urol* 1994;12:357–358.

135. Karnauchow PN, Steele AA. Isolated necrotizing granulomatous vasculitis of the spermatic cords. *J Urol* 1989;141:379–381.

136. Corless CL, Daut D, Burke R. Localized giant cell vasculitis of the spermatic cord presenting as a mass lesion. *J Urol Pathol* 1997;6: 235–242.

137. Brehmer-Anderson E, Anderson L, Johansson JE. Hemorrhagic infarctions of testis due to intimal fibroplasia of spermatic artery. *Urology* 1985;25:379–382.

138. Nistal M, Mate A, Paniagua R. Cystic transformation of the rete testis. *Am J Surg Pathol* 1996;20:1231–1239.

139. Busto Martin LA, Lopez Garcia D, Barghoutti I, et al. Giant cystic degeneration of the rete testis. *Arch Esp Urol* 2009;62:592–595.

140. Nistal M, Santaaria L, Paniagua R. Acquired cystic transformation of the rete testis secondary to renal failure. *Hum Pathol* 1989;20: 1065–1070.

141. Warner KE, Noyes DT, Ross JS. Cysts of the tunica albuginea. Report of 4 cases and review of the literature. *J Urol* 1984;132:131–132.

142. Mancilla-Jiminez R, Matsuda GT. Cysts of the tunica albuginea. Report of 4 cases and review of the literature. *J Urol* 1975;114: 730–733.

143. Tammela TL, Karttunen TJ, Mattila SI, et al. Cysts of the tunica albuginea—more common testicular masses than previously thought? *Br J Urol* 1991;68:280–284.

144. Perez-Ordonez B, Srigley JR. Mesothelial lesions of the paratesticular region. *Semin Diagn Pathol* 2000;17:294–306.

145. Jassie M, Mahmood P. Torsion of spermatocele: a newly described entity with 2 cases. *J Urol* 1985;133:683–684.

146. Engelbrecht K, Bornman M, du Plessis D. Multicystic epididymis and seminal vesicles in a patient with polycystic kidney disease. *Br J Urol* 1995;75:554–555.

147. Kroes H, Sijmons R, Van Den Berg A, et al. Early-onset renal cell cancer and bilateral epididymal cysts as presenting symptoms of von Hippel-Lindau disease. *Br J Urol* 1998;81:915.

148. Bibbo M, Al-Naqeeb M, Baccarini S, et al. Follow-up study of male and female offspring of DES-treated mothers a preliminary report. *J Reprod Med* 1975;15:29–32.

149. Mostofi FK, Price EB. Tumors and tumor-like conditions of testicular adnexal structures. In: Hartman WH, Sobin LH, eds. *Tumors of the Male Genital System, Atlas of Tumor Pathology*, 2nd series. Washington, DC: Armed Forces Institute of Pathology; 1973.

150. Medina Perez M, Sanchez Gonzalez M, Valero Puerta J, et al. Calcified spermatocele simulating a neoplasm. *Arch Esp Urol* 1998;51: 725–726.

151. Lane Z, Epstein JI. Small blue cells mimicking small cell carcinoma in spermatocele and hydrocele specimens: a report of 5 cases. *Hum Pathol* 2010;41:88–93.

152. Katergiannakis V, Lagoudianakis EE, Markogiannakis H, et al. Huge epidermoid cyst of the spermatic cord in an adult patient. *Int J Urol* 2006;13:95–97.

153. Ford J Jr, Singh S. Paratesticular dermoid cyst in a 6-month old infant. *J Urol* 1988;139:89–90.

154. Wegner H, Herbst H, Dieckmann KP. Paratesticular epidermoid cyst and ipsilateral spermatic cord dermoid cyst: case report and discussion of pathogenesis, diagnosis and treatment. *J Urol* 1994;152: 2101–2103.

155. Ozdilek S. The pathogenesis of idiopathic hydrocele and a simple operative technique. *J Urol* 1957;77:282.

156. Rinker JR, Allen L. Lymphatic defect in hydrocele. *Am Surg* 1951;17:681.

157. Bostwick D. Spermatic cord and testicular adnexa. In: Bostwick D, Eble JN, eds. *Urologic Surgical Pathology*. St. Louis, MO: Mosby; 1997:647–674.

158. Bromberg WE, Kozlowski JM, Oyasu R. Prostate-type gland in the epididymis. *J Urol* 1991;145:1273–1274.

159. Lee L, Tzeng J, Grosman M, et al. Prostate gland-like epithelium in the epididymis: a case report and review of the literature [review]. *Arch Pathol Lab Med* 2004;128:e60–e62.

160. Foucar E, Rosai J, Dorfman R. Sinus histiocytosis with massive lymphadenopathy (Rosai–Dorfman disease): review of the entity. *Semin Diagn Pathol* 1990;7:19–73.

161. Nistal M, Paniagua R. Nodular proliferation of calcifying connective tissue in the rete testis: a study of three cases. *Hum Pathol* 1989;20:58–61.

162. Raghavaiah NV. Epididymal calcification in genital filariasis. *Urology* 1981;18:78–79.

163. Guvel S, Pourbagher MA, Torun D, et al. Calcification of the epididymis and the tunica albuginea of the corpora cavernosa in patients on maintenance hemodialysis. *J Androl* 2004;25:752–756.

164. Demirci D, Ekmekciolu O, Inci M, et al. Heterotopic ossification of the spermatic cord. *Int Urol Nephrol* 2003;35:513–514.

165. Nistal M, Paniagua R. Congenital anomalies of the testis and epididymis. In: *Testicular and Epididymal Pathology*. New York: Thieme-Stratton, Inc.; 1984.

166. Patel HTH, Arya M, O'Donoghue EPN. Calcified seminal vesicles and vasa deferentia: "beware or be aware". *Scand J Urol Nephrol* 2001;35:79–80.

167. Lin C-J, Wu C-J. Unusual metastatic soft tissue calcification in a hemodialysis patient. *South Med J* 2008;101:851–852.

168. Nistal M, Santamaria L, Codesal J, et al. Secondary amyloidosis of the testis: an electron microscopic and histochemical study. *Applied Pathol* 1989;7:2–7.

169. Jun SY, Kim KR, Cho KS, et al. Localized amyloidosis of seminal vesicle and vas deferens: report of two cases [review]. *J Korean Med Sci* 2003;18:447–451.

170. Hollowood K, Fletcher CD. Pseudosarcomatous myofibroblastic proliferations of the spermatic cord ("proliferative funiculitis"). Histologic and immunohistochemical analysis of a distinctive entity. *Am J Surg Pathol* 1992;16:448–454.

171. Khalil KH, Ball RY, Eardley I, et al. Inflammatory pseudotumor of the epididymis. *J Urol Pathol* 1996;5:39–43.

172. Lam KY, Chan KW, Ho MH. Inflammatory pseudotumour of the epididymis. *Br J Urol* 1995;75:255–257.

173. Donnellan R, Bramdev A, Chetty R. A paratesticular pseudosarcomatous myofibroblastic proliferation. A case report. *Int J Surg Pathol* 1998;6:235–238.

174. Nishimura T, Akimoto M, Kawai H, et al. Peritesticular xanthogranuloma. *Urology* 1981;18:189–190.

175. Piscioli F, Polla E, Pusiol T, et al. Pseudomalignant cytologic presentation of spermatic hydrocele fluid. *Acta Cytol* 1983;27:666–670.

176. Yamashina M, Honma T, Uchijima Y. Myofibroblastic pseudotumor mimicking epididymal sarcoma. A clinicopathological study of three cases. *Pathol Res Pract* 1992;188:1054–1059.

177. Sen S, Patterson DE, Sandoval O Jr, et al. Testicular adnexal fibrous pseudotumors. *Urology* 1984;23:594–597.

178. Vates TS, Ruemmler-Fisch C, Smilow PC, et al. Benign fibrous testicular pseudotumors in children. *J Urol* 1993;150:1886–1888.

179. Bajwa RPS, Skinner R, Barrett AM. Fibrous pseudotumor of the tunica vaginalis testis. *Med Pediatr Oncol* 2001;36:665–666.

180. Watson RA, Harper BN. Paratesticular fibrous pseudotumor in a patient with Gorlin's syndrome: nevoid basal cell carcinoma syndrome. *J Urol* 1992;148:1254–1255.

181. Sonmez K, Turkyilmaz Z, Boyaciolu M, et al. Diffuse fibrous proliferation of tunica vaginalis associated with testicular infarction: a case report. *J Ped Surg* 2001;36:1057–1058.

182. Meyer AW. Corpora libera in the tunica vaginalis testis. *Am J Pathol* 1928;4:445–455.

183. Goodwin WE. Multiple, benign, fibrous tumors of tunica vaginalis testis. 1946;56:438–447.

184. Perez Herms S, Cosme MA, Pellice C Jr, et al. Fibrous pseudotumor of the epididymis. *Actas Urol Esp* 1995;19:322–324.

185. Gogus O, Bulay O, Yurdakul T, et al. A rare scrotal mass: fibrous pseudotumor of epididymis. *Urol Int* 1990;45:63–64.

186. Thompson JE, van der Walt JD. Nodular fibrous proliferation (fibrous pseudotumour) of the tunica vaginalis testis. A light, electron

microscopic and immunocytochemical study of a case and review of the literature. *Histopathology* 1986;10:741–748.

187. Parveen T, Fleischmann J, Petrelli M. Benign fibrous tumor of the tunica vaginalis testis. Report of a case with light, electron microscopic, and immunocytochemical study of a case and review of the literature. *Arch Pathol Lab Med* 1992;116:277–280.

188. Miyamoto H, Montgomery EA, Epstein JI. Paratesticular fibrous pseudotumor: a morphologic and immunohistochemical study of 13 cases. *Am J Surg Pathol* 2010;34:569–574.

189. Elem B, Patil PS, Lambert TK. Giant fibrous pseudotumor of the testicular tunics in association with schistosoma haematobium infection. *J Urol* 1988;141:376–377.

190. Begin LR, Frail D, Brzezinski A. Myofibroblastoma of the tunica testis: evolving phase of co-called fibrous pseudotumor? *Hum Pathol* 1990;21:866–868.

191. Garvey FK, Daniel TB. Bilateral interstitial cell tumor of the testicle. *J Urol* 1951;66:713–719.

192. Cutfield RG, Bateman JM, Odell WD. Infertility caused by bilateral testicular masses secondary to congenital adrenal hyperplasia (21-hydroxylase deficiency). *Fertil Steril* 1983;20:809–814.

193. Rich MA, Keating MA, Levin HS, et al. Tumors of the adrenogenital syndrome: an aggressive conservative approach. *J Urol* 1998;160:1838–1841.

194. Paner GP, Kristiansen G, McKenney JK, et al. Rete testis-associated nodular steroid cell nests: description of putative pluripotential testicular hilus steroid cells. *Am J Surg Pathol* 2011;35:505–511.

195. Krieger DT, Samojlik E, Bardin CW. Cortisol and androgen secretion in a case of Nelson's syndrome with paratesticular tumors: response to cyproheptadine therapy. *J Clin Endocrinol Metab* 1978;47:837–844.

196. Johnson RE, Scheithauer BW. Massive hyperplasia of testicular adrenal rests in a patient with Nelson's syndrome. *Am J Clin Pathol* 1982;77:501–507.

197. Rose IK, Enterline HT, Rhoads JE, et al. Adrenal cortical hyperfunction in childhood. Report of a case with adrenocortical hyperplasia and testicular adrenal rests. *Pediatrics* 1951;9:475–484.

198. Delmas V, Dauge MC. Accessory adrenals in the spermatic cord. A propos of 2 cases. *Ann Urol* 1986;20:261–264.

199. Nelson A. Accessory adrenal cortical tissue. *Arch Pathol* 1939;27:955–965.

200. Amin MB. Selected other problematic testicular and paratesticular lesions: rete testis neoplasms and pseudotumors, mesothelial lesions and secondary tumors. *Mod Pathol* 2005;18:S131–S145.

201. Hartwick RW, Ro J, Srigley J, et al. Adenomatous hyperplasia of the rete testis. A clinicopathologic study of nine cases. *Am J Surg Pathol* 1991;15:350–357.

202. Sapino A, Pagani A, Godano A, et al. Effects of estrogens on the testis of transsexuals. A pathological and immunocytochemical study. *Virchows Arch [A] Pathol Anat Histopathol* 1987;411:409–414.

203. Newbold R, Bullock B, McLachlan J. Adenocarcinoma of the rete testis. Diethylstilbestrol-induced lesions of the mouse rete testis. *Am J Pathol* 1986;125:625–628.

204. Job J, Gendrel D, Safar A, et al. Pituitary LH and FSH and testosterone sectetion in infants with undescended testes. *Acta Endocrinol* 1977;85:644–649.

205. Nistal M, Paniagua R. Adenomatous hyperplasia of the rete testis. *J Pathol* 1988;20:343–346.

206. Cooper K, Govender D. Adenomatous hyperplasia of the rete testis in the undescended testis. *J Pathol* 1990;162:333–334.

207. Nistal M, Garcia Vilanueva M, Sanchez J. Displasia quistica del testiculo: anomalia en la defferenciacion del parenchquima testicular por probable fallo de la connexion entre los conductos de origen mesonefrico y os cordones testiculares (Abstract in English). *Arch Exp Urol* 1976;29:431–444.

208. Channer J, MacIver A. Glandular changes in the rete testis: metastatic tumor or adenomatous hyperplasia? (letter). *J Pathol* 1989;157:81–83.

209. Nistal M, Castillo M, Regedera J, et al. Adenomatous hyperplasia of the rete testis. A review and report of new cases. *Histol Histopathol* 2003;18:741–752.

210. Ulbright TM, Gersell D. Rete testis hyperplasia with hyaline globule formation. A lesion simulating yolk sac tumor. *Am J Surg Pathol* 1991;15:66–74.

211. Lee H, Theaker J. Pagetoid spread into the rete testis by testicular tumours. *Histopathology* 1994;24:385–389.

212. Ulbright TM. Germ cell neoplasms of the testis. *Am J Surg Pathol* 1993;17:1075–1091.

213. Hasan N, Shareef D, Al-Jafari M. Pagetoid spread into the rete testis by intratubular germ cell neoplasia in an undescended testis. *Histopathology* 1995;27:391–392.

214. Perry A, Wiley E, Albores-Saavedra J. Pagetoid spread of intratubular germ cell neoplasia into rete testis: a morphologic and histochemical study of 100 orchiectomy specimens with invasive germ cell tumors. *Hum Pathol* 1994;25:235–239.

215. Ulbright TM, Roth L. Recent developments in the pathology of germ cell tumors. *Semin Diagn Pathol* 1987;4:304–319.

216. Shah V, Ro J, Amin MB, et al. Histologic variations in the epididymis. Findings in 167 orchiectomy specimens. *Am J Surg Pathol* 1998;22:990–996.

217. Rosai J, Dehner LP. Nodular mesothelial hyperplasia in hernia sacs. A benign reactive condition simulating a neoplastic process. *Cancer* 1975;35:165–175.

218. Churg A, Colby TV, Cagle P, et al. The sepration of benign and malignant mesothelial proliferations. *Am J Surg Pathol* 2000;24:1183–1200.

219. Attanoos RL, Griffin A, Gibbs AR. The use of immunohistochemistry in distinguishing reactive from neoplastic mesothelium. A novel use for desmin and comparative evaluation with epithelial membrane antigen, p53, platelet-derived growth factor-receptor, P-glycoprotein and Bcl-2. *Histopathology* 2003;43:231–238.

220. Amin MB, Ulbright TM, Mendrinos SE, et al. Utility of a comprehensive immunohistochemical panel in the differential diagnosis of paratesticular neoplasms with tubulopapillary/glandular architecture. *Mod Pathol* 2004;17:137A.

221. Barton JH, Davis CJ Jr, Sesterhenn IA, et al. Smooth muscle hyperplasia of the testicular adnexa clinically mimicking neoplasia: clinicopathologic study of sixteen cases. *Am J Surg Pathol* 1999;23:903–909.

222. Lanzafame S, Leonardi R, Caltabiano R. Simultaneous leiomyoma and contralateral smooth muscle hyperplasia of the epididymis: a case report. *Pathologica* 2009;101:119–122.

223. Friedman E, Skarda J, Ofek-Moravsky E, et al. Complex multilocular cystic lesion of rete testis, accompanied by smooth muscle hyperplasia, mimicking intratesticular Leydig cell neoplasm. *Virchows Arch* 2005;447:768–771.

224. Schned AR, Seremetis G, Rous S. Paratesticular multi-cystic mass of Wolffian, probably paradidymal, origin. *Am J Clin Pathol* 1994;101:543–546.

225. Elsasser E. Tumors of the epididymis. Recent results. *Cancer Res* 1977;60:163.

226. Beccia D, Drane R, Olsson C. Clinical management of non-testicular intrascrotal tumors. *J Urol* 1976;116:476–479.

227. Salm R. Papillary cystadenoma of the epididymis. A clinicopathologic analysis of 20 cases. *Arch Pathol* 1971;91:456–470.

228. Powell B, Craig J, Muss H. Secondary malignancies of the penis and epididymis: a case report and review of the literature. *J Clin Oncol* 1985;3:110–116.

229. Altaffer L, Fufour D, Castleberry G, et al. Co-existing rete testis adenoma and gonadoblastoma. *J Urol* 1982;127:332–335.

230. Gupta R. Benign papillary tumor of the rete testis. *Indian J Cancer* 1974;11:480–481.

231. Jones MA, Young RH. Sertoliform rete cystadenoma: a report of two cases. *J Urol Pathol* 1997;7:47–53.

232. Yadav S, Patel P, Karkhanis R. Primary tumours of spermatic cord, epididymis and rete testis. *J Postgrad Med* 1969;15:49–52.

233. Murao T, Tanahashi T. Adenofibroma of the rete testis. A case report with electron microscopy findings. *Acta Pathol Jpn* 1988;38:105–112.

234. Sinclair AM, Gunendran T, Napier-Hemy RD, et al. Sertoliform cystadenoma of the rete testis. *Pathol Int* 2006;56:568–569.

235. Watson P, Jacob V. Adenocarcinoma of the rete testis with sertoliform differentiation. *Arch Pathol Lab Med* 1989;113:1169–1171.

236. Young R, Koelliker D, Scully RE. Sertoli cell tumors of the testis, not otherwise specified. A clinicopathologic analysis of 60 cases. *Am J Surg Pathol* 1998;22:709–721.

237. Witten F, O'Brien D, Sewell C, et al. Bilateral clear cell papillary cystadenoma of the epididymides. *J Urol* 1985;133:1062–1064.

238. Price E. Papillary cystadenoma of the epididymis. A clinicopathologic analysis of 20 cases. *Arch Pathol* 1971;91:456–470.

239. Choyke P, Glenn G, Wagner J, et al. Epididymal cystadenomas in von Hippel-Lindau disease. *Urology* 1997;49:926–931.

240. Iczkowski KA, Pantazis CG. Papillary cystadenofibroma of epididymis: a case report. *Int J Clin Exp Pathol* 2011;4:629–631.

241. Billesbolle P, Nielsen K. Papillary cystadenoma of the epididymis. *J Urol* 1988;239:1062.

242. De Souza A, Bambirra E, Bicalho O, et al. Bilateral papillary cystadenoma of the epididymis as a component of von Hippel–Lindau's syndrome: report of a case presenting as infertility. *J Urol* 1985;133:288–289.

243. Tsuda S, Fukushima S, Takahashi M, et al. Familial bilateral papillary cystadenoma of the epididymis. *Cancer* 1976;37:1831–1839.

244. Calder C, Gregory J. Papillary cystadenoma of the epididymis: a report of two cases with an immunohistochemical study. *Histopathology* 1993;23:89–91.

245. Greka H, Morley A, Evans D. Papillary cystadenoma of the epididymis. *Br J Urol* 1985;57:356–357.

246. Glasker S, Tran MG, Shively SB, et al. Epididymal cystadenomas and epithelial tumourlets: effects of VHL deficiency on the human epididymis. *J Pathol* 2006;210:32–41.

247. Gilcrease M, Schmidt L, Abar B, et al. Somatic von Hippel-Lindau mutation in clear cell papillary cystadenoma of the epididymis. *Hum Pathol* 1995;26:1341–1346.

248. Pozza D, Masci P, Amodeo S, et al. Papillary cystadenoma of the epididymis as a cause of obstructive azoospermia. *Urol Int* 1994;53:222–224.

249. Crisp J, Roberts P. A case of bilateral cystadenoma of the epididymides presenting as infertility. *Br J Urol* 1975;47:682.

250. Aydin H, Young RH, Ronnett BM, et al. Clear cell papillary cystadenoma of the epididymis and mesosalpinx: immunohistochemical differentiation from metastatic clear cell renal cell carcinoma. *Am J Surg Pathol* 2005;29:520–523.

251. Klimis T, Vlahos P, Kokotas N. Serous cystadenoma of the epididymis of common epithelial ovarian type: case report with an immunohistochemical study. *J Balk Union Oncol* 2006;11:237–240.

252. Talmon G, Johnaason S. Serous cystadenoma of the epididymis. *Urology* 2007;70:372.e7–372.e8.

253. Ulbright TM, Young RH. Primary mucinous tumors of the testis and paratestis. A report of nine cases. *Am J Surg Pathol* 2003;27:1221–1228.

254. Uschuplich V, Hilsenbeck JR, Velasco CR. Paratesticular mucinous cystadenoma arising from an oviduct-like müllerian remnant. *Arch Pathol Lab Med* 2006;130:1715–1717.

255. Kellert E. An ovarian type pseudomucinous cystadenoma in the scrotum. *Cancer* 1959;12:187–190.

256. Hartz PH. Occurrence of Walthard cell rests of Brenner-like epithelium in the serosa of the epididymis. *Am J Clin Pathol* 1947;17:654–656.

257. Nogales FF Jr, Matilla A, Ortega I, et al. Mixed Brenner and adenomatoid tumor of the testis: an ultrastructural study and histogenetic considerations. *Cancer* 1979;43:539–543.

258. Toklu C, Ozen H, Ergen A, et al. Rete testis adenocarcinoma recurring in the inguinal lymph nodes. A case report. *Int Urol Nephrol* 1997;29:581–586.

259. Nochomovitz LE, Orenstein JM. Adenocarcinoma of the rete testis. Review and regrouping of reported cases and a consideration of miscellaneous entities. *J Urogenit Pathol* 1991;1:11–40.

260. Nochomovitz LE, Orenstein JM. Adenocarcinoma of the rete testis. Case report, ultrastructural observations, and clinicopathologic correlates. *Am J Surg Pathol* 1984;8:625–634.

261. Erlandson R, Lieberman P. Paratesticular tumor in a 44 year-old male. *Ultrastruct Pathol* 1985;8:107–113.

262. Gisser S, Nayak S, Kaneko M, et al. Adenocarcinoma of the rete testis: a review of the literature and report of a case with associated asbestosis. *Hum Pathol* 1977;1977:219–224.

263. Schoen S, Rush B. Adenocarcinoma of the rete testis. *J Urol* 1959;82:356–363.

264. Turner R, Williamson J. Adenocarcinoma of the rete testis. *J Urol* 1973;109:850–851.

265. Roy J, Baumann W, Lewis T, et al. Adenocarcinoma of the rete testis. *Urology* 1979;14:270–272.

266. Gruber H, Ratschek M, Pummer K, et al. Adenocarcinoma of the rete testis: report of a case with surgical history of adenomatous hyperplasia of the rete testis. *J Urol* 1997;158:1525–1526.

267. Jacobellis U, Ricco R, Ruotolo G. Adenocarcinoma of the rete testis 21 years after orchiopexy. A case report and review of the literature. *J Urol* 1981;125:429–431.

268. Whitehead E, Valensi Q, Brown J. Adenocarcinoma of the rete testis. *J Urol* 1972;107:992–999.

269. Crisp-Lindgren N, Travers H, Wells MM, et al. Papillary adenocarcinoma of rete testis. Autopsy findings, histochemistry, immunohistochemistry, ultrastructure, and clinical correlation. *Am J Surg Pathol* 1988;12:492–501.

270. Visscher D, Talerman A, Rivera I, et al. Adenocarcinoma of the rete testis with a spindle cell component. A possible metaplastic carcinoma. *Cancer* 1989;64:770–775.

271. Fukunaga M, Aizawa S, Fursusato M, et al. Papillary adenocarcinoma of the rete testis. *Cancer* 1982;50:134–138.

272. Brito CG, Bloch T, Foster RS, et al. Testicular papillary cystadenomatous tumor of low malignant potential. A case report and discussion of the literature. *J Urol* 1988;139:378–379.

273. Herschman BR, Ross MM. Papillary cystadenoma within the testis. *Am J Clin Pathol* 1974;61:724–729.

274. Jones MA, Young RH, Srigley JR, et al. Paratesticular serous papillary carcinoma. A report of six cases. *Am J Surg Pathol* 1995;19:1359–1365.

275. Jones M, Young RH, Srigley JR, et al. Paratesticular serous papillary carcinoma. A report of 6 cases. *Am J Surg Pathol* 1995;19:1359–1366.

276. Jacobsen G. Malignant Sertoli cell tumors of the testis. *J urol Pathol* 1993;1:233–255.

277. Zukerberg L, Young RH, Scully RE. Sclerosing Sertoli cell tumor of the testis: a report of 10 cases. *Am J Surg Pathol* 1991;15:829–834.

278. Burns M, Chandler W, Kreiger J. Adenocarcinoma of the rete testis. Role of inguinal orchiectomy plus retroperitoneal lymph node dissection. *Urology* 1991;37:571–573.

279. Kurihara K, Oka A, Mannami M, et al. Papillary adenocarcinoma of the epididymis. *Acta Pathol Jpn* 1993;43:440–443.

280. Jones MA, Young RH, Scully RE. Adenocarcinoma of the epididymis: a report of four cases and review of the literature. *Am J Surg Pathol* 1997;21:1474–1480.

281. Ganem J, Jhaveri F, Marroum M. Primary adenocarcinoma of the epididymis: case report and review of the literature. *Urology* 1998;52:904–908.

282. Yu C, Huang J, Chiang H, et al. Papillary cystadenocarcinoma of the epididymis: a case report and review of the literature. *J Urol* 1992;147:162–165.

283. Jones MA, Young RH, Scully RE. Malignant mesothelioma of the tunica vaginalis. A clinicopathologic analysis of 11 cases with review of the literature. *Am J Surg Pathol* 1995;19:815–825.

284. Srigley JR, Hartwick RW. Tumors and cysts of the paratesticular region. *Pathol Ann* 1990;25:51–108.

285. De Nictolis M, Tommasoni S, Fabris G, et al. Intratesticular serous cystadenoma of borderline malignancy. A pathological, histochemical and DNA content study of a case with long-term follow-up. *Virchows Arch A Pathol Anat Histopathol* 1993;423:221–225.

286. Kernohan NM, Coutts AG, Best PV. Cystadenocarcinoma of the appendix testis. *Histopathology* 1990;17:147–154.

287. Remmele W, Kaiserling E, Zerban U, et al. Serous papillary cystic tumor of borderline malignancy with focal carcinoma: a case report with immunohistochemical and ultrastructural observations. *Hum Pathol* 1992;23:75–79.

288. Young RH, Scully RE. Testicular and paratesticular tumors and tumor-like lesions of ovarian common epithelial and mullerian types. A report of four cases and review of the literature. *Am J Clin Pathol* 1986;86:146–152.

289. McClure RF, Keeney GL, Sebo TJ, et al. Serous borderline tumor of the paratestis: a report of seven cases. *Am J Surg Pathol* 2001;25:373–378.

290. Goldman RL. A Brenner tumor of the testis. *Cancer* 1970;26:853–856.

291. Caccamo D, Socias M, Truchet C. Malignant Brenner tumor of the testis and epididymis. *Arch Pathol Lab Med* 1991;115:280–284.

292. Elbadawi A, Batchvarov MM, Linke CA. Intratesticular papillary mucinous cystadenocarcinoma. *Urology* 1979;14:280–284.

293. Nistal M, Revistido R, Paniagua R. Bilateral mucinous cystadenocarcinoma of the testis and epididymis. *Arch Pathol Lab Med* 1992;116:1360–1363.

294. Teilum G. Histogenesis and classification of mesonephric tumors of the female and male genital system and relationship to benign so-called adenomatoid tumors (mesotheliomas). A comparative histological study. *Acta Pathol Microbiol Scand* 1954;34:431–481.

295. Axiotis CA. Intratesticular serous papillary cystadenoma of low malignant potential: an ultrastructural and immunohistochemical study suggesting mullerian differentiation. *Am J Surg Pathol* 1988;12:56–63.

296. Walker AN, Mills SE. Glandular inclusions in inguinal hernial sacs and spermatic cords. Müllerian-like remnants confused with functional reproductive structures. *Am J Clin Pathol* 1984;82:85–89.

297. Meister P, Keiditsch E, Stampfl B. Intratesticular papillary cystadenoma. A rare analogue of serous papillary cystadenoma of the ovary. *Pathologe* 1990;11:183–187.

298. Kurian RR, Prema NS, Belthazar A. Paratesticular papillary serous cystadenocarcinoma—a case report. *Ind J Pathol Microbiol* 2006;49:36–37.

299. Anchala PR, Dhir R, Parwani AV, et al. Immunohistochemical profile of paratesticular serous papillary adenocarcinoma and tunica vaginalis facilitates distinction from malignant mesothelioma. *Int J Surg Pathol* 2011;19:692–698.

300. Mai KT, Carlier M, Lajeunesse C. Paratesticular composite tumour of epididymal-like and mucinous cells of low malignant potential. *Histopathology* 1998;33:193–194.

301. Aubert J, Touchard G, Mazet B, et al. Adenomatoid tumor of the tunica vaginalis testis. Apropos of 5 cases. *J Urol* 1983;89:677–682.

302. Zanollo A, Jerano A. Para-epididymal adenomatoid tumor infiltrating the tunica vaginalis testis. *Minerva Urol* 1967;19:204–209.

303. Estebanez Zarranz MJ, Lobo MC, Sanz Jaka JP, et al. Adenomatoid tumor of the albuginea testis. *Actas Urol Esp* 1989;13:391–392.

304. Horstman WG, Sands JP, Hooper DG. Adenomatoid tumor of testicle. *Urology* 1992;40:359–361.

305. Samad AA, Pereiro B, Badiola A, et al. Adenomatoid tumor of intratesticular localization. *Eur Urol* 1996;30:127–128.

306. Nistal M, Paniagua R, Fuentes E, et al. Histogenesis of adenomatoid tumor associated to pseudofibromatous periorchitis in an infant with hydrocele. *J Pathol Bacteriol* 1984;144:275–280.

307. Silberblatt JM, Gellman SZ. Mesotheliomas of spermatic cord, epididymis, and tunica vaginalis. *Urology* 1974;3:235–237.

308. Skinnider BF, Young RH. Infarcted adenomatoid tumor: a report of five cases of a facet of a benign neoplasm that may cause diagnostic difficulty. *Am J Surg Pathol* 2004;28:77–83.

309. Hes O, Perez-Montiel DM, Alvarado Cabrero I, et al. Thread-like bridging strands: a morphologic feature present in all adenomatoid tumors. *Ann Diagn Pathol* 2003;7:273–277.

310. Romanelli R, Sanna A. Adenomatoid leiomyoma and papillary cystadenoma of the epididymis. *Pathologica* 1985;77:445–448.

311. Kausch I, Galle J, Buettner H, et al. Leiomy-adenomatoid tumor of the epididymis. *J Urol* 2002;168:636.

312. Manson AL. Adenomatoid tumor of the testicular tunica albuginea mimicking testicular carcinoma. *J Urol* 1988;139:819–820.

313. Evans K. Rapidly growing adenomatoid tumor extending into testicular parenchyma mimics testicular carcinoma. *Urology* 2004;64:589.

314. Sangoi AR, McKenney JK, Schwartz EJ, et al. Adenomatoid tumors of the female and male genital tracts: a clinicopathological and immunohistochemical study of 44 cases. *Mod Pathol* 2009;22:1228–1235.

315. Macay B, Bennington JL, Skoglund RW. The adenomatoid tumor. Fine structural evidence for a mesothelial origin. *Cancer* 1971;27:109–115.

316. Ferenczy A, Fenoglio J, Richart RM. Observations on benign mesothelioma of the genital tract (adenomatoid tumor). A comparative ultrastructural study. *Cancer* 1972;30:244–260.

317. Lehto VP, Miettinen M, Virtanen I. Adenomatoid tumor: immunohistological features suggesting a mesothelial origin. *Virchows Arch B Cell Pathol Mol Pathol* 1983;42:153–159.

318. Moch H, Ohnacker H, Epper R, et al. A new case of malignant mesothelioma of the tunica vaginalis testis. Immunohistochemistry in comparison with an adenomatoid tumor of the testis. *Pathol Res Pract* 1994;190:400–404.

319. Daya D, McCaughey WTE. Well-differentiated papillary mesothelioma of the peritoneum. A clinicopathologic study of 22 cases. *Cancer* 1990;65:292–296.

320. Barbera V, Rubine M. Papillary mesothelioma of the tunica vaginalis. *Cancer* 1957;10:183–189.

321. Chetty R. Well differentiated (benign) papillary mesothelioma of the tunica vaginalis. *J Clin Pathol* 1992;45:1029–1030.

322. Mikuz G, Hopftel-Kreiner I. Papillary mesothelioma of the tunica vaginalis propia. Case report and ultrastructural study. *Virchows Arch A Pathol Anat Histol* 1982;396:231–238.

323. Xiao SY, Rizzo P, Carbone M. Benign papillary mesothelioma of the tunica vaginalis testis. *Arch Pathol Lab Med* 2000;124:143–147.

324. Johnson DE, Fuerst DE. Mesothelioma of tunica vaginalis. *South Med J* 1973;66:1295–1297.

325. Brimo F, Illei PB, Epstein JI. Mesothelioma of the tunica vaginalis: a series of eight cases with uncertain malignant potential. *Mod Pathol* 2010;23:1165–1172.

326. Winstanley AM, Landon G, Berney D, et al. The immunohistochemical profile of malignant mesotheliomas of the tunica vaginalis: a study of 20 cases. *Am J Surg Pathol* 2006;30:1–6.

327. Khan MA, Ruri P, Devaney D. Mesothelioma of tunica vaginalis testis in a child. *J Urol* 1997;158:198–199.

328. Mathew BS, Jyothirmayi R, Mair MK. Case report: malignant mesothelioma of tunica vaginalis testis presenting with spinal metastasis—report of two cases. *Br J Radiol* 1996;69:1067–1068.

329. Lopez JI, Angulo JC, Ibanez T. Combined therapy in a case of malignant mesothelioma of the tunica vaginalis testis. *Scand J Urol Nephrol* 1995;29:361–364.

330. Gupta SC, Gupta AK, Misra V, et al. Pre-operative diagnosis of malignant mesothelioma of tunica vaginalis testis by hydrocele fluid cytology. *Eur J Surg Oncol* 1998;24:153–154.

331. Pfister M, Saez D, Celeste F. Sonographic appearance of malignant mesothelioma of the tunica vaginalis testis in a child. *J Clin Ultrasound* 1992;20:129–131.

332. Plas E, Riedl DR, Pfluger H. Malignant mesothelioma of the tunica vaginalis testis. Review of the literature and assessment of prognostic parameters. *Cancer* 1998;83:1437–2446.

333. Kossow AS, McCann LS. Malignant mesothelioma of the testicular tunic. *J Urol* 1981;126:272–274.

334. Saw KC, Barker TH, Khalil KH, et al. Biphasic malignant mesothelioma of the tunica vaginalis testis. *Br J Urol* 1994;74:381–382.

335. Eimoto T, Inoue I. Malignant fibrous mesothelioma of the tunica vaginalis: a histologic and ultrastructural study. *Cancer* 1977;39:1059–1066.

336. Ordonez NG. The immunohistochemical diagnosis of mesothelioma: a comparative study of epithelioid mesothelioma and lung adenocarcinoma. *Am J Surg Pathol* 2003;27:1031–1051.

337. Ordonez NG. The immunohistochemical diagnosis of epithelial mesothelioma. *Hum Pathol* 1999;30:313–323.

338. Agapitos E, Pavlopoulos PM, Marinos E, et al. Malignant mesothelioma of the tunica vaginalis testis: an immunohistochemical and ultrastructural study of two cases. *Br J Urol* 1997;80:345–346.

339. Berti E, Schiaffino E, Minervini MS, et al. Primary malignant mesothelioma of the tunica vaginalis of the testis. Immunohistochemistry and electron microscopy. *Pathology* 1997;29:96–99.

340. Chekol SS, Sun C-C. Malignant mesothelioma of the tunica vaginalis testis. Diagnostic studies and differential diagnosis. *Arch Pathol Lab Med* 2012;136:113–117.

341. Nochomovitz LE, Orenstein JM. Adenocarcinoma of the rete testis. Consolidation and analysis of 31 reported cases with a review of miscellaneous entities. *J Urol Pathol* 1994;2:1–37.

342. Smith JJ III, Malone MJ, Geffin J, et al. Retroperitoneal lymph node dissection in malignant mesothelioma of tunica vaginalis testis. *J Urol* 1990;144:1242–1243.

343. Antman K, Hassan R, Eisner M, et al. Update on malignant mesothelioma. *Oncology (Williston Park)* 2005;19:1301–1309.

344. Soosay GN, Parkinson MC, Paradinas J, et al. Paratesticular sarcomas revisited. A review of cases in the British Testicular Tumour Panel and Registry. *Br J Urol* 1996;77:143–146.

345. Russo P, Prady MS, Conlon K, et al. Adult urological sarcoma. *J Urol* 1992;147:1032–1037.

346. Raney RB Jr, Tefft M, Lawrence W Jr, et al. Paratesticular sarcoma in childhood and adolescence. A report from the Intergroup Rhabdomyosarcoma Studies I and II, 1973–1983. *Cancer* 1987;60: 2337–2343.

347. Banik S, Guha PK. Paratesticular rhabdomyosarcomas and leiomyosarcomas: a clinicopathological review. *J Urol* 1979;121:823–826.

348. Mai KT, Yazdi HM, Collins JP. Vascular myxolipoma ("angiomyxolipoma") of the spermatic cord. *Am J Surg Pathol* 1996;20: 1145–1148.

349. Satyanarayana S, Jawed KZ, Sirki V, et al. Myxoid leiomyoma of the tunica vaginalis testis. *Ind J Pathol Microbiol* 2001;44:373–374.

350. Steeper TA, Rosai J. Aggressive angiomyxoma of the female pelvis and perineum. Report of nine cases of a distinctive type of gynecologic soft-tissue neoplasm. *Am J Surg Pathol* 1983;7:462–475.

351. Durdov MG, Tomic S, Pisac V, et al. Aggressive angiomyxoma of scrotum. *Scand J Urol Nephrol* 1998;32:299–302.

352. Iezzoni JC, Fechner RE, Wong LS, et al Aggressive angiomyxoma in males. A report of four cases. *Am J Clin Pathol* 1995;104: 391–396.

353. Calinfante G, De Marco L, Mori M, et al. Aggressive angiomyxoma of the spermatic cord. Two unusual cases occurring in childhood. *Path Res Pract* 2001;197:139–144.

354. Folpe AL, Weiss SW. Paratesticular soft tissue neoplasms. *Semin Diagn Pathol* 2000;17:307–318.

355. Fletcher CD, Tsang WY, Fisher C, et al. Angiomyofibrolastoma of the vulva. A benign neoplasm distinct from aggressive angiomyxoma. *Am J Surg Pathol* 1992;16:373–382.

356. Laskin WB, Fetsch JF, Mostofi FK. Angiomyofibroblastomalike tumor of the male genital tract: analysis of 11 cases with comparison to female angiomyofibroblastoma and spindle cell lipoma. *Am J Surg Pathol* 1998;22:6–16.

357. Nucci MR, Grantner SR, Fletcher CD. Cellular angiofibroma; A benign neoplasm distinct from angiomyofibroblastoma and spindle cell lipoma. *Am J Surg Pathol* 1997;21:636–644.

358. Nielsen GP, Young RH, Dickersin GR, et al. Angiomyofibroblastoma of the vulva with sarcomatous transformation ("angiomyofibrosarcoma"). *Am J Surg Pathol* 1997;21:1104–1108.

359. Silverman JS, Albukerk J, Tamsen A. Comparison of angiomyofibroblastoma and aggressive angiomyxoma in both sexes: four cases composed of bimodal CD34 and factor XIIIa positive dendritic cell subsets. *Pathol Res Practice* 1997;193:673–682.

360. Granter SR, Nucci MR, Fletcher CD. Aggressive angiomyxoma: reappraisal of its relationship to angiomyofibroblastoma in a series of 16 cases. *Histopathology* 1997;30:3–10.

361. Rao CR, Srinivasulu M, Naresh KN, et al. Adult paratesticular sarcomas: a report of eight cases. *J Surg Oncol* 1994;56:89–93.

362. Catton CN, Cummings BJ, Founasier V, et al. Adult paratesticular sarcomas: a review of 21 cases. *J Urol* 1991;146:342–345.

363. Sugita Y, Clarnette TD, Cooke-Yarborough C, et al. Testicular and paratesticular tumours in children: 30 years' experience. *Aust N Z J Surg* 1999;69:505–508.

364. Coleman J, Brennan M, Alektiar K, et al. Adult spermatic cord sarcomas: management and results. *Ann Surg Oncol* 2003;10:669–675.

365. De Vries JD. Paratesticular rhabdomyosarcoma. *World J Urol* 1995;13:219–225.

366. Stella M, Di Somma C, Sorari N, et al. Primary osteosarcoma of the spermatic cord: case report and literature review. *Anticancer Res* 2007;27:1605–1608.

367. Paul R, Leyh H, Hillemanns M, et al. Giant malignant mesenchymoma of the spermatic cord with bidirectional differentiation. *Onkologie* 2001;24:73–75.

368. Ugidos L, Suarez A, Cubillo A, et al. Mixed paratesticular liposarcoma with osteosarcoma elements. *Clin Transl Oncol* 2010;12:148–149.

369. Bajaj P, Aiyer H, Sinha BK, et al. Pitfalls in the diagnosis of epithelioid sarcoma presenting in an unusual site: a case report. *Diagn Cytopathol* 2001;24:36–38.

370. Cavazzana AO, Schmidt D, Ninfo V, et al. Spindle cell rhabdomyosarcoma. A prognostically favorable variant of rhabdomyosarcoma. *Am J Surg Pathol* 1992;16:229–235.

371. Scrable H, Witte D, Shimada H, et al. Molecular differential pathology of rhabdomyosarcoma. *Genes Chromosomes Cancer* 1989;1:23–35.

372. Zamolo G, Cocklo M, Stifter S, et al. Solid variant of alveolar rhabdomyosarcoma of the spermatic cord. *Wien Klin Wochenschr* 2005;117:323.

373. Parham DM. The molecular biology of childhood rhabdomyosarcoma. *Semin Diagn Pathol* 1994;11:39–46.

374. Gaffney EF, Dervan PA, Fletcher CD. Pleomorphic rhabdomyosarcoma in adulthood. Analysis of 11 cases with definition of diagnostic criteria. *Am J Surg Pathol* 1993;17:601–609.

375. Rangdaeng S, Truong LD. Comparative immunohistochemical staining for desmin and muscle-specific actin. A study of 576 cases. *Am J Clin Pathol* 1991;96:32–45.

376. Folpe AL, Patterson K, Gown AM. Antibodies to desmin identify the blastemal component of nephroblastoma. *Mod Pathol* 1997;10: 895–900.

377. Wang NP, Marx J, McNutt MA, et al. Expression of myogenic regulatory proteins (myogenin and MyoD1) in small blue round cell tumors of childhood. *Am J Pathol* 1995;147:1799–1810.

378. Rubin BP, Hasserjian RP, Singer S, et al. Spindle cell rhabdomyosarcoma (so-called) in adults: report of two cases with emphasis on differential diagnosis. *Am J Surg Pathol* 1998;22:459–464.

379. Fisher C, Goldblum JR, Epstein J, et al. Leiomyosarcoma of the paratesticular region: a clinicopathologic study. *Am J Surg Pathol* 2001;25:1143–1149.

380. Suster S, Wong TY, Moran CA. Sarcomas with combined features of liposarcoma and leiomyosarcoma. Study of two cases of an unusual soft-tissue tumor showing dual lineage differentiation. *Am J Surg Pathol* 1993;17:905–911.

381. Alberghini M, Zanella L, Bacchini P, et al. Leiomyosarcoma of the spermatic cord: a light and ultrastructural description of one case. *Path Res Pract* 2004;200:487–491.

382. Lai FM, Allen PW, Chan LW, et al. Aggressive fibromatosis of the spermatic cord: a typical lesion in a 'new' location. *Am J Clin Pathol* 1995;104:403–407.

383. Fisher C, Bisceglia M. Solitary fibrous tumour of the spermatic cord. *Br J Urol* 1994;74:798–799.

384. Kraus MD, Guillou L, Fletcher CD. Well-differentiated inflammatory liposarcoma: an uncommon and easily overlooked variant of a common sarcoma. *Am J Surg Pathol* 1997;21:518–527.

385. Montgomery E, Fisher C. Paratesticular liposarcoma: a clinicopathologic study. *Am J Surg Pathol* 2003;27:40–47.

386. Weiss SW, Rao VK. Well-differentiated liposarcoma (atypical lipoma) of deep soft tissue of the extremities, retroperitoneum, and miscellaneous sites. A follow-up study of 92 cases with analysis of the incidence of "dedifferentiation". *Am J Surg Pathol* 1997;21:271–281.

387. Henricks WH, Chu YC, Goldblum JR, et al. Dedifferentiated liposarcoma: a clinicopathological analysis of 155 cases with a proposal for an expanded definition of dedifferentiation. *Am J Surg Pathol* 1997;21:271–281.

388. Fanburg-Smith JC, Miettinen M. Liposarcoma with meningothelial-like whorls: a study of 17 cases of a distinctive histological pattern associated with dedifferentiated liposarcoma. *Histopathology* 1998;33:414–424.

389. Nasciemento AG, Kurtin PJ, Gillou L, et al. Dedifferentiated liposarcoma: a report of nine cases with a peculiar neurallike whorling pattern associated with metaplastic bone formation. *Am J Surg Pathol* 1998;22:945–955.

390. Panagis A, Karydas G, Vasilakakis J, et al. Myxoid liposarcoma of the spermatic cord: a case report and review of the literature. *Int Urol Nephrol* 2003;35:369–372.

391. Tallini G, Akerman M, Dal Cin P, et al. Combined morphologic and karyotypic study of 28 myxoid liposarcomas. Implications for a revised morphologic typing (a report from the CHAMP Group). *Am J Surg Pathol* 1996;20:1047–1055.

392. Smith TA, Easley KA, Goldblum JR. Myxoid/round cell liposarcoma of the extremities. A clinicopathologic study of 29 cases with particular attention to extent of round cell liposarcoma. *Am J Surg Pathol* 1996;20:171–180.

393. Kilpatrick SE, Doyon J, Choong PF, et al. The clinicopathologic spectrum of myxoid and round cell liposarcoma. A study of 95 cases. *Cancer* 1996;77:1450–1458.

394. Zagars GK, Goswitz MS, Pollack A. Liposarcoma: outcome and prognostic factors following conservation surgery and radiation therapy. *Int J Radiat Oncol Biol Phys* 1996;36:311–319.

395. Miettinen M, Enzinger FM. Epithelioid variant of pleomorphic liposarcoma: a study of 12 cases of a distinctive variant of high-grade liposarcoma. *Mod Pathol* 1999;12:722–728.

396. Weiss SW, Enzinger FM. Malignant fibrous histiocytoma: an analysis of 200 cases. *Cancer* 1978;41:2250–2266.

397. Weiss SW. Malignant fibrous histiocytoma. A reaffirmation. *Am J Surg Pathol* 1982;6:773–784.

398. Sethi S, Ashok S. Malignant fibrous histiocytoma of the spermatic cord. *J Indian Med Assoc* 2003;101:599–600.

399. Lin BTY, Harvey DA, Medeiros J. Malignant fibrous histiocytoma of the spermatic cord: report of two cases and review of the literature. *Mod Pathol* 2002;15:59–65.

400. Shoja MM. Malignant fibrous histiocytoma of the spermatic cord: a case report and review of the literature. *Folia Morphologica* 2006;65:390–395.

401. Edge SB, Byrd DR, Compton CC, et al. *AJCC Cancer Staging Manual.* 7th ed. New York: Springer; 2010.

402. Merimsky O, Terrier P, Bonvalot S, et al. Spermatic cord sarcoma in adults. *Acta Oncol* 1999;38:635–638.

403. Catton C, Jewett M, O'Sullivan B, et al. Paratesticular sarcoma. Failure patterns after definitive local therapy. *J Urol* 1999;161:1844–1847.

404. Fagundes MA, Zeitman AL, Althausen AF, et al. The management of spermatic cord sarcoma. *Cancer* 1996;77:1873–1876.

405. Goldfarb B, Khoury AE, Greenberg ML, et al. The role of retroperitoneal lymphadenectomy in localized paratesticular rhabdomyosarcoma. *J Urol* 1994;152:785–787.

406. Anonymous. Adjuvant chemotherapy for localized resectable soft-tissue sarcoma of adults: meta-analysis of individual data. Sarcoma meta-analysis collaboration. *Lancet* 1997;350:1647–1654.

407. Coindre JM, Terrier P, Bui NB, et al. Prognostic factors in adult patients with locally controlled soft tissue sarcoma. A study of 546 patients from the French Federation of Cancer Centers Sarcoma Group. *J Clin Oncol* 1996;14:869–877.

408. Ferry JA, Harris NL, Young RH, et al. Malignant lymphoma of the testis, epididymis and spermatic cord. A clinicopathologic study of 69 cases with immunophenotypic analysis. *Am J Surg Pathol* 1994;18:376–390.

409. Al-Abbadi MA, Hattab EM, Tarawneh M, et al. Primary testicular and paratesticular lymphoma. A retrospective clinicopathologic study of 34 cases with emphasis on differential diagnosis. *Arch Pathol Lab Med* 2007;131:1040–1046.

410. Au WY, Shek WH, Nicholls J, et al. T-cell intravascular lymphomatosis (angiotropic large cell lymphoma): association with Epstein-Barr viral infection. *Histopathology* 1997;31:563–567.

411. Kausch I, Doehn C, Buttner H, et al. Primary lymphoma of the epididymis. *J Urol* 1998;160:1801–1802.

412. Schned AR, Variakojis D, Straus FH, et al. Primary histiocytic lymphoma of the epididymis. *Cancer* 1979;43:1156–1163.

413. McDermott MB, O'Briain DS, Shiels OM, et al. Malignant lymphoma of the epididymis. A case report of bilateral involvement by a follicular large cell lymphoma. *Cancer* 1995;75:2174–2179.

414. Ginaldi L, De Pasquale A, De Martinis M, et al. Epididymal lymphoma. A case report. *Tumori* 1993;79:147–149.

415. Heaton JP, Morales A. Epididymal lymphoma: an unusual scrotal mass. *J Urol* 1984;131:353–354.

416. Lands RH. Non-Hodgkin's lymphoma originating in the spermatic cord. *South Med J* 1996;89:352–356.

417. Moller MB. Non-Hodgkin's lymphoma of the spermatic cord. *Acta Haematol* 1994;91:70–72.

418. Maniyur R, Anant K, Aneesh S, et al. Posttransplant epididymal lymphoma: an aggressive variant (Letter to the Editor). *Transplantation* 2003;75:246–247.

419. Tykocinski M, Schinella R, Greco MA. The pleomorphic cells of advanced mycosis fungoides. An ultrastructural study. *Arch Pathol Lab Med* 1984;108:387–391.

420. Ferry JA, Young RH, Scully RE. Testicular and epididymal plasmacytoma: a report of 7 cases, including 3 that were the initial manifestation of plasma cell myeloma. *Am J Surg Pathol* 1997;21:590–598.

421. Ferry JA, Srigley JR, Young RH. Granulocytic sarcoma of the testis: a report of two cases of a neoplasm prone to misinterpretation. *Mod Pathol* 1997;10:320–325.

422. Diamond DA, Breitfeld PP, Bur M, et al. Melantoic neuroecodermal tumor of infancy: an important mimicker of paratesticular rhabdomyosarcoma. *J Urol* 1992;147:673–675.

423. De Chiara A, Van Tornout JM, Hachitanda Y, et al. Melanotic neuroectodermal tumor of infancy. A case report of paratesticular primary with lymph node involvement. *Am J Pediatr Hematol Oncol* 1992;14:356–360.

424. Calabrese F, Danieli D, Valente M. Melanotic neuroectodermal tumor of the epididymis in infancy: case report and review of the literature. *Urology* 1995;46:415–418.

425. Pettinato G, Manviel JC, d'Amore ES, et al. Melanotic neuroectodermal tumor of infancy. A reexamination of a histogenetic problem based on immunohistochemical, flow cytometric, and ultrastructural study of 10 cases. *Am J Surg Pathol* 1991;15:233–245.

426. Dehner LP, Sibley RK, Sauk JJ Jr, et al. Malignant melanotic neuroectodermal tumor of infancy: a clinical, pathologic, ultrastructural and tissue culture study. *Cancer* 1979;43:1389–1410.

427. Johnson RE, Scheithauer BW, Dahlin DC. Melanotic neuroectodermal tumor of infancy. A review of seven cases. *Cancer* 1983;52:661–666.

428. Kapadia SB, Frisman DM, Hitchcock CL, et al. Melanotic neuroectodermal tumor of infancy. Clinicopathological, immunohistochemical, and flow cytometric study. *Am J Surg Pathol* 1993;17:566–573.

429. Prat J, Matias-Guiu X, Algaba F. Desmoplastic small round cell tumor. *Am J Surg Pathol* 1992;16:306–307.

430. Cummings OW, Ulbright TM, Young RH, et al. Desmoplastic small round cell tumors of the paratesticular region. A report of six cases. *Am J Surg Pathol* 1997;21:219–225.

431. Furman J, Murphy WM, Wajasman Z, et al. Urogenital involvement by desmoplastic small round-cell tumor. *J Urol* 1997;158:1506–1507.

432. Roganovich J, Bisogno G, Cecchetto G, et al. Paratesticular desmoplastic small round cell tumor: case report and review of the literature. *J Surg Oncol* 1999;71:269–272.

433. Kawano N, Inayama Y, Nagashima Y, et al. Desmoplastic small round-cell tumor of the paratesticular region: report of an adult case with demonstration of EWS and WTI gene fusion using paraffin-embedded tissue. *Mod Pathol* 1999;12:729–734.

434. Ordonez NG. Desmoplastic small round cell tumor I: a histopathologic study of 39 cases with emphasis on unusual histological patterns. *Am J Surg Pathol* 1998;22:1303–1313.

435. Gerald WL, Rosai J. Desmoplastic small cell tumor with divergent differentiation. *Pediatr Pathol* 1989;9:177–183.

436. Ordonez NG. Desmoplastic small round cell tumor: II: an ultrastructural and immunohistochemical study with emphasis on new immunohistochemical markers. *Am J Surg Pathol* 1998;22: 1314–1327.

437. Gerald WL, Ladanyi M, de Alava E, et al. Clinical, pathologic, and molecular spectrum of tumors associated with t(11;22)(p13;q12). Desmoplastic small round-cell tumor and its variants. *J Clin Oncol* 1998;16:3028–3036.

438. Schwarz RE, Gerald WL, Kushner BH, et al. Desmoplastic small round cell tumors; Prognostic indicators and results of surgical management. *Ann Surg Oncol* 1998;5:416–422.

439. Leaf D, Tucker G, Harrison L. Embryonal cell carcinoma originating in the spermatic cord: case report. *J Urol* 1974;112:285–286.

440. Dichmann O, Engel U, Jensen D, et al. Juxtatesticular seminoma. *Br J Urol* 1990;66:324–325.

441. Hartwick RWJ, Srigley JR, Burns B, et al. A clinicopathologic review of 112 paratesticular tumors [abstract]. *Lab Invest* 1987;56:30A.

442. Maurer R, Taylor C, Schmucki O, et al. Extratesticular gonadal stromal tumor in the pelvis. A case report with immunoperoxidase findings. *Cancer* 1980;45:985–990.

443. Yamashina M, Kayan H, Katayama I, et al. Congenital neuroblastoma presenting as a paratesticular tumor. *J Urol* 1988;139:796–797.

444. Matsunaga T, Takahashi H, Ohnuma N, et al. Paratesticular neuroblastoma with N-myc activation. *J Pediatr Surg* 1993;28:1612–1614.

445. Krieger JN, Chasko S, Keuhnelian J. Paratesticular neuroblastoma associated with subependymal giant cell astrocytoma. *J Urol* 1980;124:736–738.

446. Calonge WM, Heitor F, Castro LP, et al. Neonatal paratesticular neuroblastoma misdiagnosed as in utero torsion of testis. *J Pediatr Hematol Oncol* 2004;26:693–695.

447. Zeng L, Xia T, Kong X, et al. Primary carcinoid tumor of the epididymis. *Chin Med J* 2001;114:544–545.

448. Lodato RF, Zentner GJ, Gomez CA, et al. Scrotal carcinoid. Presenting manifestation of multiple lesions in the small intestine. *Cancer* 1991;96:664–668.

449. Arkovitz MS, Ginsburg HB, Eidelman J, et al. Primary extrarenal Wilms' tumor in the inguinal canal: case report and review of the literature. *J Pediatr Surg* 1996;31:957–959.

450. Taylor W, Myers M, Taylor W. Extrarenal Wilms' tumor in an infant exposed to intrauterine phenytoin. *Lancet* 1980;2:481–482.

451. Bryan RL, Liu S, Newman J, et al. Squamous carcinoma arising in a chronic hydrocoele. *Histopathology* 1990;17:178–180.

452. Algaba F, Santauiaria J, Villavicencio H. Metastatic tumor of the epididymis and spermatic cord. *Eur Urol* 1983;9:56–59.

453. Datta MW, Ulbright TM, Young RH. Renal cell carcinoma metastatic to the testis and its adnexa: a report of five cases including three that accounted for the initial clinical presentation. *Int J Surg Pathol* 2001;9:49–56.

454. Parra R, Boulleir J, Mehan D. Malignant tumor of the colon metastatic to the epididymis a first sign of recurrence of colon cancer. *Mo Med* 1992;89:298–300.

455. Patel S, Richardson R, Kvols L. Metastatic cancer to the testes: a report of 20 cases and review of the literature. *J Urol* 1989;142:1003–1005.

456. Tozawa K, Akita H, Kusada S, et al. Testicular metastases from carcinoma of the bile duct: a case report. *Int J Urol* 1998;5:106–107.

457. Young RH, van Patter H, Scully RE. Hepatocellular carcinoma metastatic to the testis. *Am J Clin Pathol* 1987;87:117–120.

458. Kandmata N, Eble JN. Adenocarcinoma of the pancreas presenting as an epididymal mass. *J Urol Pathol* 1997;6:159–170.

459. Hammad FA. Metastatic malignant melanoma of the epididymis. *Br J Urol* 1992;69:661.

460. Thamba dorai CR, Azmi A, Rahman AJ, et al. Spermatic cord metastasis from a medulloblastoma. *Pediatr Surg Int* 2001;17:654–656.

461. Ribalta T, Ro J, Sahin A, et al. Intrascrotally metastatic renal cell carcinoma. Report of two cases and review of the literature. *J Urol Pathol* 1993;1:201–209.

Penis and Scrotum

ELSA F. VELAZQUEZ, MAHUL B. AMIN, and ANTONIO L. CUBILLA

THE PENIS

Embryology

The genital eminence, an external mound arising between the umbilicus and the tail, is made up of the genital tubercle and the genital swellings.[1] The urogenital sinus opens at the base of the genital tubercle, between the genital swellings. These structures form identically in male and female embryos up to 7 weeks' gestational age. Development of the male external genitalia is dependent upon dihydrotestosterone, which is produced by the testes. At 9 weeks of gestational age, and under the influence of testosterone, the genital tubercle starts to lengthen. In addition, the genital swellings (also called the labioscrotal folds) enlarge and rotate posteriorly. As they meet, they begin to fuse from posterior to anterior. As the genital tubercle becomes longer, two sets of tissue folds develop on its ventral surface on either side of a developing trough, the urethral groove. The more medial endodermal folds will fuse in the ventral midline to form the male urethra. The more lateral ectodermal folds will fuse over the developing urethra to form the penile shaft skin and the prepuce. As these two layers fuse from posterior to anterior, they leave behind a skin line: the median raphe. By 13 weeks, the urethra is almost complete. A ring of ectoderm forms just proximal to the developing glans penis. This skin advances over the corona glandis and eventually covers the glans entirely as the prepuce or foreskin. The tip of the penis, which is now called the glans, then begins to form a cord of ectoderm that grows toward the spongy urethra. This cord is known as the urethral plate and when it canalizes, the end of the urethra (external urethral orifice) is at the tip of the penis.

The foreskin is formed in the 12th week of development. A septum of ectoderm moves inward around the edges of the penis and then breaks down, leaving a thin layer of skin surrounding the penis. During this time, the penis is also developing its corpora cavernosa and spongiosa from proliferating mesenchyme within the genital tubercle.

Anatomical Features

The complexity of the penis is partially related to the characteristics of the surface epithelium, which includes both skin and mucous membrane. The penis is composed of three portions: the distal part (glans or head), mid part (corpus or shaft), and proximal part (root) (Figs. 14-1 and 14-2).[2,3] The head consists of the glans, coronal sulcus, and foreskin. The cutaneous portions of the penis include the root, shaft, and outer foreskin. The mucosal portions are the glans, coronal sulcus, and inner surface of the foreskin. The mucosal (distal) portion of the penis is particularly important from the surgical pathology viewpoint because it is from this portion that most squamous cell carcinomas (the most frequent malignancy at this site) arise. The foreskin or prepuce is a virtual sac that encases the head of the penis and distally reflects over the preputial orifice (Figs. 14-2 and 14-3). The inner (mucosal) surface of the prepuce is smooth and pink and the outer (cutaneous) surface is wrinkled and dark.[3]

The rubbery and conical glans contains the meatus urethralis, corona, and frenulum (Fig. 14-1). The meatus is vertical and is located at the apex, from which the frenulum arises, traversing the ventral portion of the glans to its insertion at the base where the glans is attached to the foreskin. The glans corona is a circumferential elevated rim at the base of the glans (Fig. 14-1). Grossly, the cut surface of the glans reveals four anatomical layers that from the surface to deep portions are a thin and white epithelium, lamina propria, corpus spongiosum, and corpora cavernosa (Figs. 14-2 and 14-3). The tunica albuginea is seen as a thick white sheath encasing the corpora cavernosa (Figs. 14-2 and 14-3). The coronal sulcus (balanopreputial sulcus) is a cul-de-sac located between the glans corona and foreskin. The preputial length is variable. In short foreskins, the preputial orifice is located proximally to the corona; in intermediate foreskins, the preputial orifice is located between the meatus and corona. Long foreskins entirely cover the glans. There is a significant association between long and phimotic foreskins and penile cancer.[3]

The main components of the shaft are the erectile tissues of the corpora cavernosa. A transverse cut section of the shaft

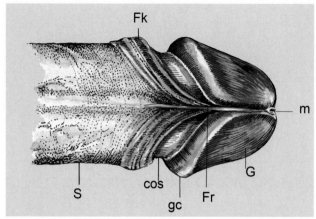

FIGURE 14-1 ■ Diagram illustrating the distal and mid portions of the penis. The distal part corresponds to the glans or head (G) and the mid part corresponds to the corpus or shaft (S). The distal portion consists of the glans, coronal sulcus (cos), and foreskin (Fk). The foreskin was retracted to better illustrate the other structures. In the glans, there is the glans corona (gc), meatus (m), and frenulum (Fr).

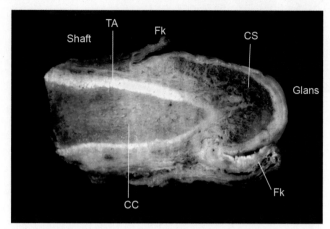

FIGURE 14-3 ■ Cut surface of a partial penectomy specimen. Fk, foreskin; CS, corpus spongiosum; TA, tunica albuginea; CC, corpus cavernosum. (Reprinted from Mills, SE, ed. *Histology for Pathologists*. 4th ed. Philadelphia: Lippincott Williams & Wilkins; 2012, with permission.)

reveals, from outside to inside, the skin, dartos, penile fascia (Buck fascia), albuginea, erectile tissue (corpus spongiosum and corpora cavernosa), and urethra (Fig. 14-4).[3] The penile or pendulous urethra is ventrally located in the corpus and head and runs surrounded by the corpus spongiosum (Fig. 14-4).

Microscopic Features

The glans is covered by a nonkeratinizing to slightly keratinized squamous epithelium without adnexal structures. The lamina propria, which measures 2 to 3 mm in thickness, is

composed of loose connective tissue containing small blood and lymphatic vessels and nerves (Fig. 14-5). The corpus spongiosum is a complex erectile tissue predominantly composed of interanastomosed vascular channels separated by fibrous trabeculae. The thickness of the glans corpus spongiosum varies from 6 to 13 mm.[3,8] The corpora cavernosa slightly protrudes into the glans in more than two-thirds of the specimens (Fig. 14-2).[8] The penile shaft is predominantly formed by the erectile tissues of the thick corpora cavernosa and the thinner corpus spongiosum, the latter surrounding the urethra (Figs. 14-6 and 14-7).[8] The corpora cavernosa are predominantly composed of thick and interanastomosing erectile vascular structures separated by a complex tridimensional

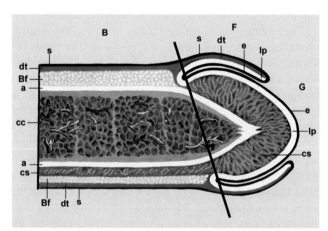

FIGURE 14-2 ■ Diagram to illustrate the different parts of the penis. The *blue line* passing through the coronal sulcus separates the glans (G) from the shaft or body (B). The anatomical levels in the glans are the epithelium (e), lamina propria (lp), corpus spongiosum (cs), and, in two-thirds of the cases, the distal portion of the corpus cavernosum (cc) and tunica albuginea (a). Anatomical levels of the foreskin (F) include the epithelium (e), lamina propria (dt), and skin (s). The levels of the coronal sulcus are epithelium, lamina propria, dartos, and Buck fascia (Bf). In some cases, there is no dartos between lamina propria and Buck fascia at this level.

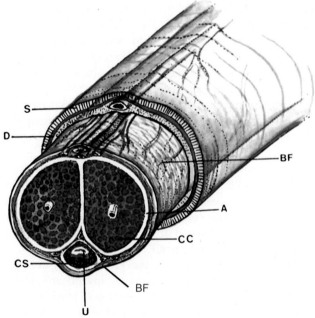

FIGURE 14-4 ■ Diagram of a cross section passing through the mid shaft of a partial penectomy specimen. S, skin; D, dartos; BF, Buck fascia; A, tunica albuginea; CC, corpus cavernosum; CS, corpus spongiosum; U, urethra.

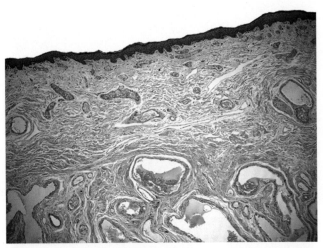

FIGURE 14-5 ■ Glans anatomical layers: squamous epithelium, lamina propria, and corpus spongiosum.

network of trabecula (Fig. 14-7). The vascular structures of the corpora cavernosa are thicker and more complex, and the connective tissue of the trabecula contains more smooth muscle bundles when compared with the corpus spongiosum.[3] There are also thin nutritional vessels within the matrix

of the corpora cavernosa. The tunica albuginea is a hyaline fibrous sheath measuring approximately 1 to 3 mm in thickness that surrounds and separates the corpus spongiosum and corpora cavernosa (Figs. 14-4, 14-6C, and 14-7). The Buck fascia surrounds the tunica albuginea and erectile tissues of the shaft and extends distally to the coronal sulcus where it is continuous imperceptibly with the connective tissue of the dartos or with the lamina propria (Figs. 14-4 and 14-6C). The Buck fascia is an important pathway of tumor progression and is composed of loose fibroadipose tissue with numerous blood vessels and nerves (Fig. 14-6C). It is surrounded by the dartos of the shaft that is present underneath the skin surface (Fig. 14-4).

The foreskin shows five histologic layers that, from the inner to the outer surface, are the mucosal squamous epithelium, lamina propria, dartos, dermis, and epidermis (Fig. 14-8). The mucosal epithelium is nonkeratinizing to slightly keranized squamous, similar to that of the glans. Skin adnexa are absent; however, scarce, small sebaceous glands not associated with hair follicles may be rarely identified, especially near the cutaneous transition. The preputial lamina propria is thin and composed of loose fibrous tissue containing small vessels and nerves. Numerous genital corpuscles

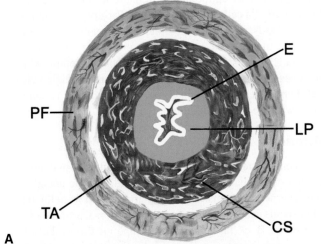

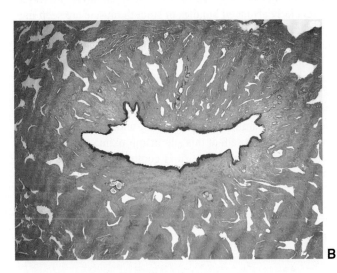

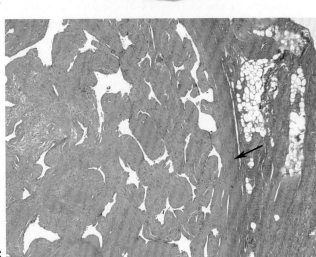

FIGURE 14-6 ■ **A–C:** Urethra and periurethral cylinder. **A:** Diagram to illustrate the anatomical layers at this level—from inside to outside: urethral epithelium (E), lamina propria (LP), corpus spongiosum (CS), tunica albuginea (TA), and Buck fascia (PF). (Reprinted from Mills, SE, ed. *Histology for Pathologists*. 4th ed. Philadelphia: Lippincott Williams & Wilkins; 2012, with permission.) **B:** Microscopic section showing the urethra surrounded by the corpus spongiosum. **C:** Periurethral corpus spongiosum (**left**) surrounded by a thin tunica albuginea (*marked with the arrow*) and Buck fascia (**right**). The urethra and periurethral cylinder represent an important pathway of tumor progression and an important margin to be evaluated in partial penectomies.

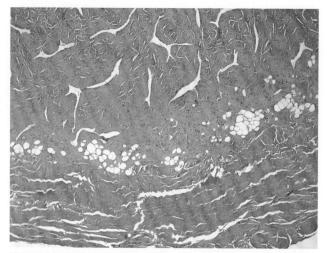

FIGURE 14-7 ■ Histologic features of the corpus cavernosum surrounded by the tunica albuginea. There are irregular and interanastomosing thick-walled vessels separated by a fibromuscular stroma. This erectile tissue is surrounded by the thick dense connective tissue of the albuginea. A few adipose cells may be seen in the tunica albuginea and corpus cavernosum.

are present in the superficial lamina propria just underneath the epithelium.[6] The dartos is a muscular layer, in which irregularly arranged bundles of smooth muscle are seen in a background of loose connective tissue associated with vascular structures, nerves, and pacinian corpuscles.[3] The skin is composed of the epidermis with a slightly hyperpigmented basal layer and a few small adnexal structures in the dermis.

The anatomical levels in the coronal sulcus vary from three to four and from top to bottom include the squamous epithelium, lamina propria, dartos, and Buck fascia.[3] The dartos is not present at this site in approximately half of the specimens. When present, it is continuous with the corporal and preputial dartos. The squamous epithelium is often

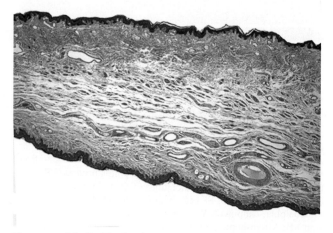

FIGURE 14-8 ■ Histology of the foreskin to show its five anatomical layers. From top to bottom: epidermis, dermis, dartos, lamina propria, and squamous epithelium of the mucosal surface. Most squamous cell carcinomas arise from the mucosal surface of the foreskin.

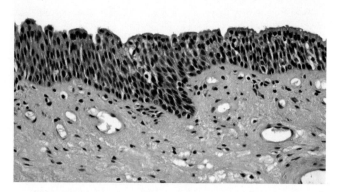

FIGURE 14-9 ■ Histologic features of the penile urethral epithelium composed of stratified basaloid cells with a columnar cell layer at the surface.

keratinized but not associated with adnexal structures. The lamina propria is identical to that seen in the glans.

The penile urethral epithelium is composed of stratified basaloid cells with a columnar cell layer at the surface (Fig. 14-9). This epithelium differs from classical urothelium; umbrella cells are not present.[4,9] Periurethral mucinous Littre glands as well as prostate-specific antigen–positive prostatic-like glands and ducts are associated with the urethra.[10] The distal 5 to 6 mm of the penile urethra, which includes the fossa navicularis, shows a nonkeratinizing clear cell/hyperglycogenated squamous epithelium that is continuous with the glans epithelium.

Arteries

The penile arteries are branches of the internal pudenda, a branch of the iliac artery. They are divided in the dorsal and the cavernous systems. The dorsal arteries run from the base of the penis near and on both sides of the dorsal profunda vein within the Buck fascia and in the superior groove between the corpora cavernosa (Fig. 14-4). Smaller branches, the circumflex arteries, irrigate the corpora cavernosa and the periurethral corpus spongiosum. Terminal branches irrigate the glans, and collateral branches irrigate the skin. The cavernous arteries penetrate the corpora cavernosa at the site where the corpora join, and they run longitudinally near the central septum, which divides the corpora. The vasa vasorum, small arteries that irrigate the erectile tissues and the helicine branches, responsible for filling the vascular spaces during erection, originate from the cavernous arteries.[13]

Veins

The superficial dorsal vein drains the prepuce and skin and runs straight from the foreskin to the base of the penis located in the space between the dermis and Buck fascia. It opens into the superficial external pudendal vein. The deep dorsal vein runs along the superficial dorsal vein but in a deeper plane beneath the Buck fascia. It receives the blood from the glans and corpora cavernosa and courses backward in the middle line between the dorsal arteries. The deep dorsal vein divides into two branches that drain into the pudendal plexus. It is noteworthy that the cavernous venous system delays venous drainage and in doing so assists in maintaining erections.[14] The deep dorsal vein of the penis has a connection with the vertebral veins; hence it is possible for metastases to make their way to the vertebrae or even to the skull and brain without going through the heart and lungs. Pyogenic organisms may be transported by the same route.[2]

Nerves

The nerves originate in the sacral and lumbar plexuses. Peripheral nerves run along the arteries. Dorsal nerves are located external to the arteries, giving circumflex branches to the corpora cavernosa. The terminal branches end in the glans and foreskin.[2,15]

Lymphatics

The lymphatics of the foreskin spring from a network that covers its internal and external surfaces; they arise from the lateral aspect and converge dorsally with the skin of the shaft lymphatics to form 4 to 10 vessels that run toward the pubis; here they diverge to drain into the right and left superficial inguinal lymph nodes. The lymphatics draining the glans form a rich network that, beginning in the lamina propria, course toward the frenulum where they coalesce with two or three trunks from the distal urethra to form several collecting trunks following the coronal sulcus. A collar of lymphatics entirely surrounds the corona, forming two or three trunks that run along the dorsal surface of the penis deep to the fascia together with the deep dorsal vein. At the presymphyseal region they form a rich anastomosing plexus draining into superficial and deep inguinal lymph nodes. The male urethra has a dense plexus in the mucosa. The lymphatic capillaries are especially abundant around the fossa navicularis.[2] The lymphatics of the urethra, corpus spongiosum, and corpora cavernosa run toward the ventral surface of the body of the penis, reaching the raphe and the dorsum, where they run with the dorsal vein ending in the superficial and deep inguinal lymph nodes.[11,12]

Regional Lymph Nodes

Inguinal nodes are the first and most frequent site of metastasis in penile carcinomas. The inguinal lymph nodes can be divided into superficial and deep. A horizontal line crossing the point where the saphenous vein enters the femoral vein marks the division of these two compartments. The superficial nodes (approximately 10 to 13) are located above the cribriform fascia.[2,9,11] The sentinel node is usually part of the superficial group of nodes located at the superior inner quadrant.[11] Deep nodes are few, and their lymphatic vessels

drain into the pelvic (iliac) lymph nodes, located externally or medially along the major iliac vessels.[11,12]

CONGENITAL ANOMALIES

Penile Agenesis

Congenital absence of the penis (aphallia) is caused by developmental failure of the genital tubercle.[16-18] This rare anomaly has an incidence of approximately 1 in 30 million population. The phallus is completely absent, including the corpora cavernosa and corpus spongiosum. It is usually associated with normal scrotum and undescended testes. The urethra opens at any point of the perineal midline from over the pubis to the anus or anterior wall of the rectum. These patients often have other associated genitourinary anomalies.

Microphallus (Penile Hypoplasia)

The terms microphallus or micropenis refers to a penis with a stretched length more than 2.5 standard deviations less than the mean for age. It is usually associated with a normal scrotum and small, undescended testes. Micropenis should be differentiated from other types of pseudomicropenis, particularly the buried penis in the obese infant and the penis concealed by an abnormal skin attachment. Micropenis may be associated with endocrine and nonendocrine conditions.[17,18]

Penile Duplication

Duplication of the penis (diphallia) is another rare anomaly that results from incomplete fusion of the genital tubercle.[17,18] It may present in two distinct forms. In the most common form, the patient exhibits a bifid penis, which consists of two separated corpora cavernosa that are associated with two independent hemiglans. The second form, or true diphallia, is extremely rare and varies from duplication of the glans alone to duplication of the entire lower genitourinary tract. The urethral opening can be in its normal position or in a hypospadiac or epispadiac position. Associated anomalies of the gastrointestinal, genitourinary, and musculoskeletal systems are frequently present.

Webbed and Buried Penis

Webbed penis is a common congenital abnormality in which a web or fold of scrotal skin obscures the penoscrotal angle. In the buried (concealed) penis, the penile shaft is hidden below the surface of the prepubic skin (Fig. 14-10A). This condition usually occurs in obese children in whom the abundant prepubic fat covers the penis.[17,18]

Penile Torsion

In penile torsion, there is a rotational defect of the penile shaft. The rotation usually is to the left in a counterclockwise fashion. The urethral meatus is placed in an oblique position, and the median raphe makes a spiral curve from the base of

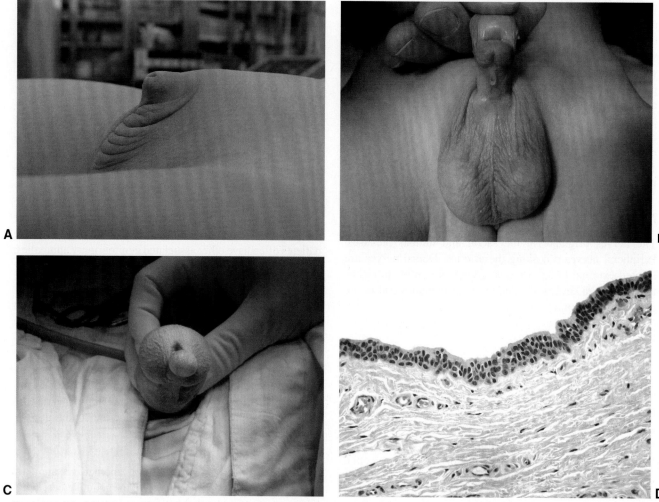

FIGURE 14-10 ■ Congenital anomalies. **A:** Buried (concealed) penis in which the penile shaft is hidden below the surface of the prepubic skin. **B:** Second-degree hypospadias with the urethral meatus opening on the shaft. **C:** Clinical appearance of a median raphe (parameatal) cyst. **D:** Median raphe cysts. Histologically, the epithelial lining is stratified columnar reminiscent of the penile urethral epithelium. (Courtesy of Professor Jae Ro, Methodist Hospital, Houston, Texas.)

the penis to the meatus. The embryologic abnormality often is an isolated skin and dartos defect. Penile torsion may also be associated with hypospadias or hooded prepuce.[17,18]

Lateral Penile Curvature

Congenital penile curvature is a rare deformity secondary to asymmetry of corpora cavernosa length. Hemihypertrophy of a corpus cavernosum and its accompanying thickened tunica albuginea, with or without contralateral concomitant hypoplasia (rudimentary corpus), are responsible for the lateral deviation in congenital curvature of the penis.[17,18]

Penoscrotal Transposition

Complete penoscrotal transposition is an uncommon condition in which the scrotum is located in a cephalad position with respect to the penis. A less severe form is a bifid scrotum, in which the two halves of the scrotum meet above the penis. It is a heterogeneous anomaly, and detection warrants careful clinical evaluation to rule out other major and

life-threatening anomalies, especially of the urinary system, gastrointestinal tract, upper limbs, craniofacial region, and central nervous system.[17,18]

Epispadias

Epispadias is a rare type of malformation in which the urethra ends in an opening on the dorsal aspect of the penis.[17,18] It is the partial form of a spectrum of failures of abdominal and pelvic fusion in the first months of embryogenesis. The opening of the urethra may occur on the dorsal aspect of the glans (glandular epispadias), between the pubic symphysis and the coronal sulcus (penile epispadias) and at the penopubic junction (penopubic hypospadias).[17,18]

Hypospadias

Hypospadias is a birth defect in which the urethral meatus is abnormally placed on the ventral aspect of the shaft.[17–18] The urethral opening may be seen at any point along the urethral groove from the glans to the perineum. The urethral meatus

First degree: urethra opens on the glans
Second degree: urethra opens on the shaft
Third degree: urethra opens on the perineum

opens on the glans (first degree hypospadias) in about 50% to 75% of cases. Second degree (when the urethra opens on the shaft) (Fig. 14-10B) and third degree (when the urethra opens on the perineum) occur in up to 20% and 30% of cases, respectively (Box 14-1). The more severe degrees are more likely to be associated with other malformations. Hypospadias is among the most common birth defects of the male genitalia.[17,18]

Chordee

This anomaly is ventral or rotational curvature of the penis, which is most apparent with erection and is caused by fibrous tissue along the usual course of the corpus spongiosum. It is often associated with hypospadias.

Urethral Meatal Stenosis

Most commonly acquired after newborn circumcision in boys, urethral meatal stenosis is occasionally congenital and associated with hypospadias. Meatotomy is needed for a significantly deflected stream or for a pinpoint stream.

Median Raphe Cysts (Genitoperineal Raphe)

Median raphe cysts are unusual lesions that result from anomalies in the development of the urethral groove (ectopia of urethral and periurethral mucosa).[18,19] They occur in the midline and ventral aspect of the penis, most frequently near the glans or prepuce, although they may be found anywhere from the urethral meatus (Fig. 14-10C) to the anus. They appear as a solitary, usually asymptomatic papule or nodule. Histologically, the epithelial lining has been described as squamous, pseudostratified columnar, stratified columnar, mucus-producing, ciliated, and apocrine (Fig. 14-10D).[19,20]

INFECTIONS

Balanitis is defined as inflammation of the glans penis, often involving the prepuce (balanoposthitis).

Bacterial Infections

Balanoposthitis is more frequently seen in uncircumcised men due to the greater propensity of pathogenetic bacteria to adhere to and colonize the mucosal surface of the foreskin.[21–23] Several common Gram-positive bacteria may affect the genital skin; however, they are rarely biopsied. Balanoposthitis caused by *Gardnerella vaginalis*[24] has rarely been reported. These infections usually are sexually transmitted. Histologically, a nonspecific inflammatory infiltrate is found.

Gonococcal infections are typically sexually transmitted, but they more frequently produce urethritis. Gonococcal infections have been reported to infect penile median raphe as well.[25]

Cellulitis can result as a complication of localized infections especially in newborns and immunosuppressed patients. It is usually caused by group A streptococcus and less frequently by group B streptococcus and commonly involves the scrotum.[26] Cellulitis is characterized by marked dermal edema with perivascular and interstitial predominantly neutrophilic infiltrate. This diagnosis needs confirmation by culture.

Trichomycosis pubis is an often asymptomatic colonization of the hair by various corynebacteria (especially *Corynebacterium tenuis*). It is characterized by a yellow, red, or black coating around pubic and/or scrotal hairs that under the microscope correspond to aggregates of Gram-positive bacteria adhering to the hair shaft (Fig. 14-70A and B).[27,28] This condition is discussed in more detail in the scrotal section.

Fournier gangrene is a necrotizing fasciitis of the genitalia, perianal, and perineal regions that when affecting the penis (and scrotal skin) usually involves the dartos and Buck fascia.[29,30] This condition particularly affects the scrotum and is discussed in more detail in the scrotal section.

Gangrenous balanitis (Corbus disease) is a rapidly progressing necrotizing infection, frequently caused by anaerobic organisms; it usually affects the glans penis, which sometimes may suffer complete necrosis.[31] Necrotizing gangrene is an exceptional condition that may be seen in diabetic patients and associated with penile prosthesis.

Ecthyma gangrenosum (Pseudomonal cellulitis) is usually a complication of pseudomonal sepsis, and it is characterized by necrotizing bacterial vasculitis with thrombosis and secondary tissular necrosis and ulceration. Gram-negative bacteria can be found surrounding the blood vessels. This condition has been reported in drug abusers and neutropenic patients.[21]

Mycobacterial Infections

Penile mycobacterial infections are exceptionally rare with *Mycobacterium tuberculosis* being the most frequent species. Tuberculosis of the penis can present as a primary focus, a direct spread from nearby areas, or by hematogenous spread in generalized tuberculosis.[32] Histologic features do not differ from tuberculous granulomas of other sites. BCG balanitis as a complication of intravesical BCG immunotherapy is extremely rare.[33] A case of penile infection caused by *Mycobacterium celatum* in a man with acquired immunodeficiency syndrome has been reported.[34]

Syphilis

This sexually transmitted disease caused by the *Treponema pallidum* can manifest by anogenital lesions during the primary, secondary, tertiary, and congenital stages of the infection.[21,35] The primary syphilis chancre occurs at the inoculation site 3 weeks after exposure to the spirochete; it usually starts as a painless papule that enlarges and ulcerates centrally. This ulcerated lesion that has an indurated base is known as the hard chancre. Chancres are most often solitary and in the penis commonly affect the inner prepuce, coronal sulcus, penile shaft, and penile base.[21] Secondary syphilis results from hematogenous dissemination of organisms. *Condyloma lata*, the characteristic anogenital lesions of secondary syphilis, are large verruciform papules, nodules, or plaques, which may become confluent.[35] Gummas are characteristic of tertiary syphilis. Histologic hallmark of the lesions is obliterative endarteritis surrounded by a plasma cell–rich infiltrate (Fig. 14-11A and B). In primary syphilis the endarteritis can be found at the base of the ulcer. Secondary syphilis is usually associated with psoriasiform epidermal hyperplasia with a superficial lichenoid and deep perivascular plasma cell–rich infiltrate; the endarteritis can be superficial or deep.[36–38] Spongiform pustular lesions can also be seen. The causative agent can be identified in primary and secondary lesions using Steiner or Warthin-Starry stains (Fig. 14-11C). The presence of *T. pallidum* in the tissues can also be detected by immunohistochemistry and by PCR. Condyloma latum is usually characterized by

prominent epidermal hyperplasia and numerous neutrophils in the epidermis and cornified layer.[36–38] When intraepidermal/intracorneal neutrophils are prominent, spirochetes tend to be easily identified within the epidermis (Fig. 14-11C). Gummas of tertiary syphilis are necrotizing granulomatous lesions associated with obliterative endarteritis. Treponema organisms usually cannot be demonstrated in these lesions by special stains. Reactivation of syphilis in patients infected with human immunodeficiency virus (HIV) is becoming more frequent[39,40] and the affected patients may present with an atypical course.

Chancroid

Chancroid or soft chancre is a sexually transmitted disease caused by a Gram-negative, facultative anaerobic bacterium, *Haemophilus ducreyi*.[21,41,42] It is clinically characterized by a soft-based painful ulcer with yellow-gray base and sharp undermined border usually located in the coronal sulcus or glans. The ulcerated lesion can be small (dwarf chancroid) or rapidly enlarging and associated with ruptured inguinal abscess (giant chancroid). The combination of a painful

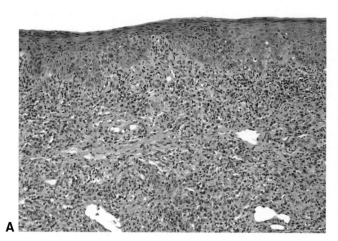

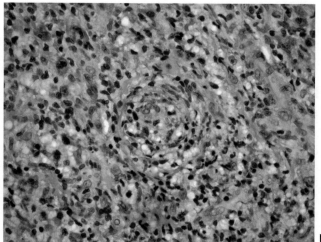

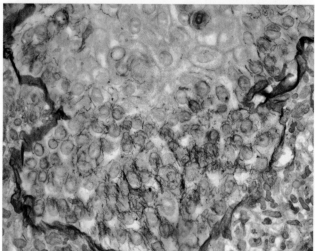

FIGURE 14-11 ■ Primary syphilis. **A:** Histopathologic features seen at the peripheral border of the hard chancre. There is a superficial and deep plasma cell–rich inflammatory infiltrate. **B:** Higher-power view to illustrate the so-called obliterative endarteritis that is characteristic of syphilis. **C:** Steiner stain highlights numerous slender spirochetes.

ulcer with tender adenopathy is suggestive of chancroid. Phagedenic chancroids are widely necrotic and destructive lesions usually secondary to superimposed infection by *Fusobacterium* organisms. Histologically, the soft chancre is characterized by a zonation phenomenon. The upper layer shows necrosis, fibrin, and numerous neutrophils; the middle layer shows abundant granulation tissue with prominent blood vessels, some with partial thrombosis; the deepest layer shows an intense plasma and lymphoid cell infiltrate.[37,38,42] Diagnosis is made isolating *H. ducreyi* on special culture media.

Granuloma Inguinale (Donovanosis)

Granuloma inguinale is a sexually transmitted disease caused by the Gram-negative bacillus *Calymmatobacterium granulomatis*.[21,43] The first clinical manifestation is a small, relatively painless nodule, occurring on the prepuce, glans, penile shaft, or scrotum that later ulcerates and may show large size. The ulcer has a red beefy base and hyperplastic borders. Histologically, the base of the ulcer shows exuberant granulation tissue with pseudoepitheliomatous hyperplasia at the borders (Fig. 14-12A). Numerous plasma cells and

neutrophils are seen in the granulation tissue (Fig. 14-12B). A characteristic feature is the presence of large mononuclear foamy histiocytes with intracytoplasmic Donovan bodies representing the microorganisms (Fig. 14-12B). The organisms are difficult to see with hematoxylin and eosin stain and can be highlighted with Warthin-Starry and Giemsa stains as short bacilli, either singly or in clumps (Fig. 14-12C).[37,38,43] Electron microscopy reveals that the bacteria reside in phagosomes.[43] Long-standing cases may be associated with elephantiasis of the penis and scrotum. Subcutaneous satellite lesions (pseudobuboes) can be seen. Lymph node involvement is rare.

Lymphogranuloma Venereum (Inguinale)

Lymphogranuloma venereum is a sexually transmitted disease caused by an obligate intracellular bacterium, *Chlamydia trachomatis*.[21,37,38] Clinically, a painless papule or ulcer appears at the site of inoculation and then rapidly disappears. Within 1 to 2 weeks after the appearance of the primary lesion, enlargement of the inguinal lymph nodes begins (bubo formation). Histologically, the primary penile lesion shows nonspecific changes consisting of ulceration

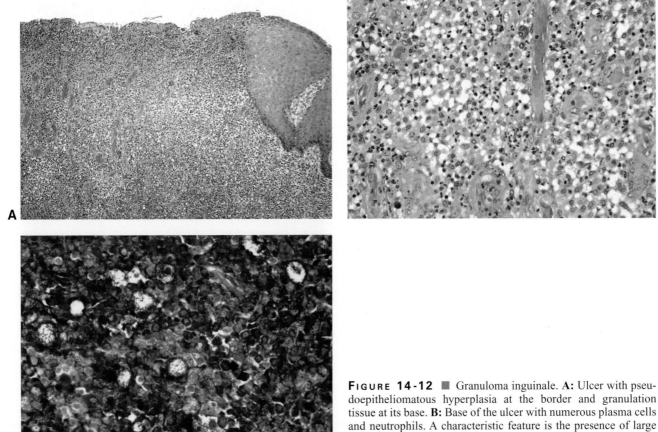

FIGURE 14-12 ■ Granuloma inguinale. **A:** Ulcer with pseudoepitheliomatous hyperplasia at the border and granulation tissue at its base. **B:** Base of the ulcer with numerous plasma cells and neutrophils. A characteristic feature is the presence of large mononuclear foamy histiocytes containing the microorganisms. **C:** Giemsa stain highlights the intracytoplasmic microorganisms also known as Donovan bodies.

and a nonspecific granulation tissue with plasma cells and lymphocytes. Nonnecrotizing granulomas composed of epithelioid histiocytes and a few giant cells surrounded by plasma cells also can be seen.[37,44] The lymph nodes show focal aggregates of neutrophils in necrotic foci followed by follicular hyperplasia with massive plasma cell infiltration. The small suppurative foci eventually coalesce to form the classical stellate abscesses with surrounding epithelioid cells and multinucleated giant cells.[45] Sinuses and tracts can develop. Old lesions are characterized by extensively fibrotic lymph nodes. The microorganisms cannot be seen by ordinary histologic stains. The diagnosis can be confirmed by cultures. Serology may be useful.[44]

Viral Infections

Human Papillomaviruses: Condyloma Acuminatum

Human papillomaviruses (HPVs) are epitheliotropic DNA viruses that infect epithelial cells of the skin and anogenital and oropharyngeal mucosa. More than 100 genotypes have been described, several of which cause specific types of cancers and benign warts.[45–56] Genital wart (condyloma acuminatum) is one of the most common sexually transmitted diseases, affecting approximately 20 million people in the United States. HPV-6 and HPV-11, considered as low-risk types, are the ones most often associated with condyloma acuminatum.[50] Condyloma acuminata tend to affect young adults and are often multiple. They may occur sporadically (usually associated with other genital infections) or in the setting of immunosuppression.[51] They usually affect the glans, corona, frenulum, prepuce, and shaft and may extend into the meatus.[21] They appear as soft, fleshy plaques with cobblestone or filiform appearance. Microscopically, classical lesions of condylomata acuminata are exophytic, branching, arborescent proliferations with acanthosis, hyperparakeratosis, and a fairly regular pushing, rounded base (Fig. 14-13A). The papillae frequently show a tree-like pattern with prominent central fibrovascular cores (Fig. 14-13A and B). The hallmark of the lesion is the presence of koilocytosis secondary to cytopathic viral effect (Fig. 14-13C).[37,38] Koilocytes have enlarged, wrinkled nuclei surrounded by a perinuclear halo. Binucleated and multinucleated forms and dyskeratotic cells may be seen (Fig. 14-13C). These changes tend to be more prominent on the upper levels of the epithelium. The koilocytic changes are more difficult to detect in old lesions

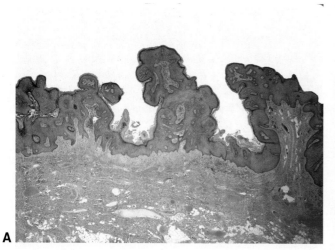

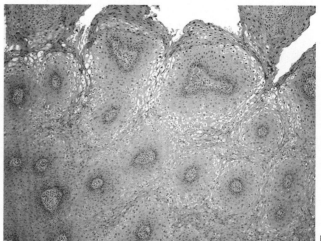

FIGURE 14-13 ■ Condyloma acuminatum. **A:** Branching, arborescent papillae and fairly regular pushing, rounded base. The papillae show a tree-like pattern with prominent central fibrovascular cores. **B:** Higher-power view of the papillae with prominent koilocytosis. **C:** Koilocytes have enlarged, wrinkled nuclei surrounded by a perinuclear halo. Binucleated and multinucleated forms and dyskeratotic cells may be seen.

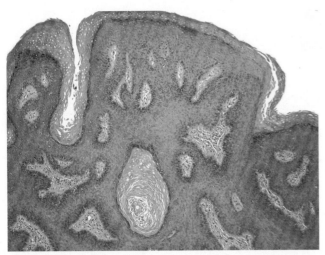

Figure 14-14 ■ Old lesion of condyoma acuminatum mimicking a seborrheic keratosis. The koilocytic changes are more difficult to detect in such old lesions.

that can look like fibroepithelial papillomas. Less frequently, condylomata may closely resemble seborrheic keratoses with basaloid cells, horn pseudocysts, and inconspicuous viral cytopathic changes (Fig. 14-14). Flat condylomata may also be seen (Fig. 14-15). Condyloma acuminatum is a benign lesion showing normal maturation with no atypias except for the koilocytosis that is usually restricted to the upper levels of the epithelium. Interestingly, it has been demonstrated that in genital locations lesions with features of fibroepithelial polyps and seborrheic keratosis without koilocytosis are often associated with HPV.[57,58] Methods of virus identification include immunohistochemistry, in situ hybridization, and polymerase chain reaction.[55,56,59,60]

It is important to differentiate condylomata previously treated with podophyllin from carcinoma. Treated condylomata may display prominent degenerative changes such as pallor of the epithelium, nuclear enlargement, necrotic keratinocytes, and increase in the number of mitotic figures

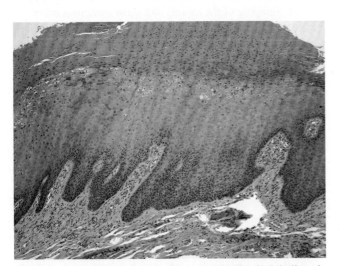

Figure 14-15 ■ Flat condyloma with classical koilocytic changes on the surface.

(metaphase arrest).[61] These degenerative changes tend to be focal and atypical mitoses should not be seen. Clinical correlation is necessary to make the correct diagnosis. True koilocytes should also be distinguished from the normal glycogenated keratinocytes of mucosal epithelia. Normal glycogenated keratinocytes appear vacuolated; however, they don't show enlarged nuclei with irregular contours and are not binucleated.

Penile condylomata may reach large sizes (usually more than 8 cm), and after many years of neglect may become locally destructive (giant or atypical condyloma) or may harbor foci of evolving carcinoma.[62] Due to the frequent association with squamous cell carcinoma, giant condylomata are discussed in the sections on squamous neoplasia. High-risk types of HPV are discussed in the section on squamous cell carcinoma.

Herpes

Herpes infection is caused by a DNA virus, the herpes simplex virus (HSV). Sexually transmitted genital herpes is primarily caused by HSV-2.[21,63] Clinically, primary lesions present as multiple millimeter-sized fragile vesicles that rupture to form painful erosions and tend to be accompanied by lymphadenopathy. Recurrences tend to be less extensive. Penile lesions may affect the prepuce, shaft, and/or glans. Immunosuppressed patients may present with chronic herpetic ulcers. Histologically, lesions are characterized by intraepithelial vesicles containing prominent round acantholytic keratinocytes showing viral cytopathic changes. The latter consist of multinucleation, nuclear ground-glass appearance, and molding (Fig. 14-16A).[37,38] Well-defined acidophilic inclusions can also be seen. The diagnosis can be made on Tzanck preparations. Herpes zoster can also affect the anogenital area and usually appears as grouped vesicles in a dermatomal distribution. Immunohistochemical analysis to identify HSV-1, HSV-2, and herpes zoster in paraffin-embedded sections is now available (Fig. 14-16B).

Molluscum Contagiosum

This cutaneous DNA pox virus infection can be sexually transmitted. Lesions involving the anogenital region may also be secondary to autoinoculation, especially in children. Clinically, the lesions present as clustered, 3- to 6-mm dome-shaped papules with central umbilication.[21] Histologically, there are endophytic lobules of squamous epithelium separated by compressed dermis. Infected keratinocytes show the characteristic intracytoplasmic eosinophilic inclusions called Henderson bodies (Fig. 14-17).[37,38] These inclusions are usually identified in the stratum spinosum and granulosum.

Penile Lesion in AIDS

HIV is a retrovirus of which two types, 1 and 2, are recognized. HIV-1 is the causative agent of AIDS in the United States and Europe. Immunodeficiency in AIDS is secondary to the depletion of T-helper cells as a result of HIV replication

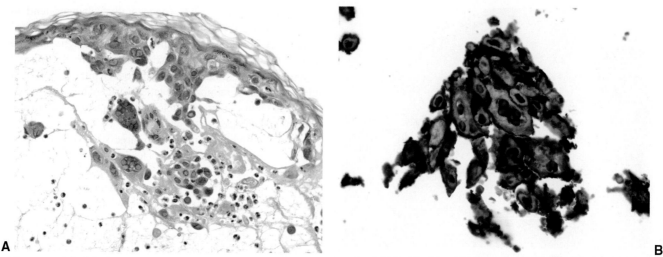

A   **B**

FIGURE 14-16 ■ Herpes simplex viral infection. **A:** Classical appearance of the viral cytopathic changes. The infected keratinocytes show multinucleation, nuclear ground-glass appearance, and molding. Well-defined acidophilic inclusions can also be seen. **B:** Immunohistochemistry for HSV-2 is positive in the infected keratinocytes.

selectively within those cells.[21,37,38] The result of T helper cell depletion is a severe defect in cell-mediated immunity making the affected individuals particularly susceptible to infections. AIDS patients are often concomitantly infected with several different types of microorganisms. Skin diseases (including genital lesions) are common manifestations of HIV infection and they can be classified as noninfective dermatosis, infective disorders, and neoplasms.[38,64–67] These conditions are discussed in other parts of this chapter; however, they can be more frequent or severe in patients with AIDS. Immunosuppression often results in an atypical presentation, increased severity, and aggressive course of a dermatosis. Such lesions may also fail to respond to standard treatment regimens. A high index of suspicion is important to make the diagnosis.

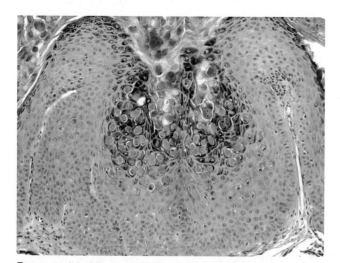

FIGURE 14-17 ■ Molluscum contagiosum. There are endophytic lobules of squamous epithelium separated by compressed dermis. Infected keratinocytes show the characteristic intracytoplasmic Henderson bodies.

Noninfective dermatosis includes seborrheic dermatitis-like eruption, psoriasis, genital (aphthous ulcers), atopic dermatitis, and drug reactions. These conditions tend to be more widespread and severe in patients with AIDS. Histologically, the findings are similar (although they may be more florid) to those seen in patients without AIDS. A common finding in patients with AIDS is the presence of numerous plasma cells in the infiltrate.

Infective dermatosis includes a variety of bacterial, viral, and fungal disorders. Particularly common in AIDS patients are HPV-related lesions such as verruca vulgaris and condyloma accuminata that may be widespread and often associated with preneoplastic and neoplastic HPV-related tumors. Other common genital infections in AIDS patients include herpes viral infection (herpes simplex and herpes zoster), molluscum contagiosum, syphilis, Candida, and tinea cruris. Infestations such as scabies can be seen and often present as the Norwegian variant. Scraping of the lesions will show numerous mites.

Neoplastic conditions are also increased in AIDS patients. The most common tumors in such population include Kaposi sarcoma and HPV-related squamous cell carcinomas.[66,67] Precursor lesions of squamous cell carcinoma (such as bowenoid papulosis and penile intraepithelial neoplasia [PeIN]) are also more frequently encountered.

Fungal Infections

Superficial Fungal Infections

Dermatophytosis

Dermatophytosis (tinea) is a superficial fungal infection caused by *Trichophyton, Epidermophyton,* and *Microsporum* species. *Trichophyton rubrum* and *Trichophyton mentagrophytes* are the most common agents.[21,22] The fungus may infect the penis through local spread from more commonly affected areas such as the groin (tinea cruris). Patients may

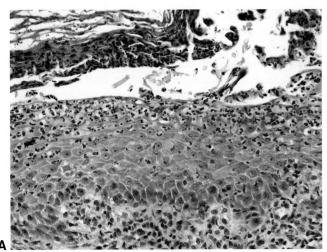
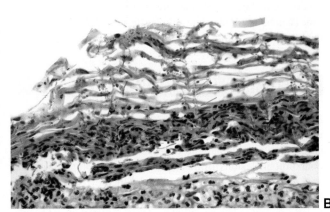

FIGURE 14-18 ■ Candidiasis. **A:** There are acanthosis and numerous neutrophils in the superficial layers of the epithelium. **B:** Numerous pseudohyphae and yeast-like forms are seen even on hematoxylin and eosin stain.

also transfer the fungus from the feet or other areas by hand. Clinically, the lesion presents as an erythematous, often annular plaque with scaling. Histologically, the fungus may be difficult to identify on H&E-stained sections. Superficial fungal infections should be especially suspected when neutrophils are present in the squamous epithelium and keratin (often parakeratotic) layer. Special stains such as diastase–PAS and silver stains will highlight the presence of septate hyphae, frequently admixed with globose hyphal segments and chains of arthroconidia within the stratum corneum.[22,37,38]

Pytiriasis Versicolor (Tinea Versicolor)

This condition caused by the fungus *Malassezia globosa* may affect the penile shaft as hypo- or hyperpigmented macules.[21,22,37,38] Unlike dermatophytes, the causative agent of pityriasis versicolor is usually easily identified on H&E-stained sections as thin and basophilic septate hyphae and round yeasts (spaghetti and meatballs appearance). The fungus will also stain with PAS and silver stains. There is usually only a very mild inflammatory response within the dermis.

Candidiasis

Candidal balanoposthitis is the most common fungal infection of the penis. It is usually associated with a predisposing factor such as immunosuppression or diabetes mellitus. It may be sexually transmitted; however, approximately 15% to 20% of men may be asymptomatic carriers and this could explain some recurrent lesions. Primary lesions are characterized by papules and pustules that expand to form erosive plaques with small satellite pustules. Histologically, within the cornified layer and extending to the upper levels of the epithelium, there are long pseudohyphae and budding yeasts that stain with diastase–PAS and silver stains (Fig. 14-18A and B).[21,22,37,38]

Deep Mycotic Infections

Deep fungal infections of the penis such as cryptococcosis and histoplasmosis have been described, but they are

extremely rare. They usually represent hematogenous spread from other primary sites.[68,69]

Parasitic Infections

Several parasitic infestations including cutaneous larva migrans, schistosomiasis, amebiasis, and trichomoniasis have been described in the penis but are rare.[21,70] The most common is scabies. This itchy infection is caused by the mite *Sarcoptes scabiei*, hominis variety, an obligate human parasite.[21,37,38] The penis is commonly affected in the setting of a generalized infestation. The hallmark lesion is the burrow, which presents as a short, waxy, dark line. The lesions tend to be secondarily excoriated, eczematized, and impetiginized. Definitive diagnosis rests on microscopic identification of the mites, eggs, or pellets (*scyballa*). This is usually done by direct examination following scraping of the lesions or in shave or punch biopsies. On direct exam the mite measures about 400 µm in length and has a round to oval body (Fig. 14-19). On

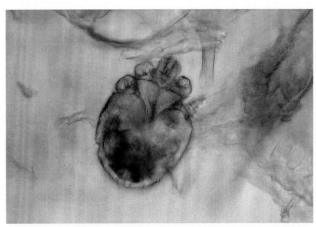

FIGURE 14-19 ■ Scabies. Direct examination following scraping of the lesions reveals the mite *S. scabiei*, which is round to oval and has four pairs of limbs.

histologic examination, there is usually a dermal lymphoid infiltrate with variable numbers of eosinophils. Several serial sections may need to be examined before identifying the burrow (which is almost entirely located within the cornified layer) and its contents (e.g., mite, eggs or fecal deposits).

NONINFECTIOUS INFLAMMATORY CONDITIONS

A variety of noninfectious dermatoses can preferentially or incidentally involve the penis and, especially in the latter case, can be problematic to diagnose.[21,22,37,38] Examination of concomitant lesions from other sites (e.g., nongenital skin, oral mucosa, nails) can help to make the correct diagnosis. Dermatoses with a preferential and often exclusive genital location will be discussed below. Dermatoses that only incidentally affect the penis are too numerous; therefore, only the most frequent entities will be discussed.

Eczematous Dermatitis

Seborrheic dermatitis is the commonest form of eczema affecting this area and may be especially exuberant in patients with AIDS.[21,22,64-44] Other eczematous processes such as irritant contact dermatitis, allergic contact dermatitis, nummular dermatitis, and atopic dermatitis may all affect the penis. Allergic contact dermatitis may result from latex, lubricants, deodorant spray, and spermicides. More often, contact dermatitis is an irritant, resulting from persistent moisture and maceration. Clinically, the lesions may be prominent and atypical due to the highly vascularized and usually occluded nature of this area. Histologically, eczematous dermatitides are characterized by variable degree of epithelial hyperplasia, spongiosis, parakeratosis, and a superficial predominantly lymphoid infiltrate.[37,38] Eosinophils may be numerous, especially in allergic contact dermatitis (Fig. 14-20). Seborrheic dermatitis, irritant contact dermatitis, and in general any of these dermatitides may

be associated with neutrophils in the cornified layer and this is sometimes related to secondary impetiginization. In cases where aggregates of neutrophils are seen in the parakeratotic layer, one should consider the possibility of psoriasis and superficial fungal infection. A diastase–PAS stain is necessary to rule out the latter possibility.

Lichen Simplex Chronicus and Prurigo Nodularis

Lichen simplex chronicus (also known as circumscribed neurodermatitis) is characterized by the development of localized thickened scaly patches or plaques secondary to persistent scratching in patients who usually do not have an underlying dermatologic condition.[21,38] Patients with atopic dermatitis and other eczematous processes may develop lesions of lichen simplex chronicus.

Lichen simplex chronicus preferentially affects the scrotum but the penis may also be involved. Histologically, there is epidermal hyperplasia with elongated rete ridges, ortho-hyperkeratosis often with patchy parakeratosis, a prominent granular layer, and variable but usually mild spongiosis.[37] There is also papillary dermal fibrosis associated with a mild predominantly lymphoid infiltrate (Fig. 14-71). In some cases, nerve hyperplasia may be seen. The differential diagnosis includes psoriasis. Distinguishing features include irregularly thickened and long rete ridges associated with prominent granular layer and orthokeratosis in lichen simplex chronicus compared with the more uniform rete ridges and parakeratosis with diminished to absent granular layer in psoriasis. The characteristically fibrotic papillary dermis of lichen simplex chronicus is not a feature seen in psoriasis where usually there is a more edematous papillary dermis with prominent blood vessels.

Prurigo nodularis is characterized by intensely pruritic, chronic, lichenified nodules that are often excoriated. It shows a significant overlap and may be associated with lichen simplex chronicus. The histologic findings are similar to those seen in lichen simplex chronicus but usually the lesions are better circumscribed and the epidermal hyperplasia more prominent.

Prurigo nodule (Picker nodule) represents a solitary variant of prurigo nodularis.

Psoriasis

Psoriasis is a chronic relapsing and remitting common skin condition that may affect any site. It is one of the commonest of all skin diseases affecting approximately 2% of the US population.[22,38] The classical cutaneous lesions are described as raised, sharply demarcated plaques with scaly surface. The clinical features, however, show regional variation. Lesions located on the penis may not show the classical features, and scaling may be minimal and moist and erosion-prominent.[71] The clinical features may be mistaken by an eczematous process or even a preneoplastic condition (PeIN). Classical histopathologic features of well-established lesions of psoriasis include acanthosis showing evenly elongated rete ridges with club-shaped bases and characteristic

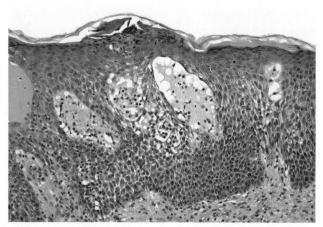

FIGURE 14-20 ■ Allergic contact dermatitis. Acanthosis, parakeratosis, spondylosis with intraepidermal vesicles, and a superficial lymphoid infiltrate with eosinophils.

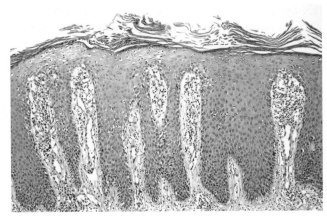

FIGURE 14-21 ■ Psoriasis. Note the evenly elongated rete ridges with club-shaped bases. Prominent blood vessels are seen within an edematous papillary dermis. There is confluent parakeratosis containing aggregates of neutrophils.

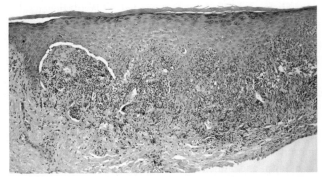

FIGURE 14-22 ■ Lichen planus showing an acanthotic epithelium with saw-toothed appearance associated with a dense, band-like lymphohistiocytic infiltrate obscuring the dermal–epidermal junction where there are numerous cytoid (Civatte) bodies. Because this lesion was located on the cutaneous surface, there is hyperorthokeratosis and typically wedge-shaped hypergranulosis. Note the subepidermal cleft formation.

thinning of the suprapapillary plates. The papillary dermis appears edematous with prominent blood vessels.[37,38] There is confluent parakeratosis containing neutrophilic aggregates and diminution to loss of granular layer (Fig. 14-21). Lesions in the genital location, however, may show more prominent spongiosis and even erosion. Therefore, often, the histologic features are not typical and the diagnosis is supported by the presence of classical psoriasis at other sites (scalp, nails, extensor surface, etc.). When dealing with a psoriasiform dermatitis containing neutrophils in the parakeratotic layer, a PAS stain to rule out superficial fungal infection is mandatory.

Reiter Syndrome

Reiter syndrome represents a triad of polyarthritis, urethritis, and nongonococcal conjunctivitis most commonly affecting males between 20 and 30 years of age.[37,38,72] The pathogenesis is poorly understood but it appears that the condition develops in predisposed individuals usually following enteric or urogenital infections. Cutaneous and mucosal manifestations of the disease may be seen including a form of circinate balanitis presenting as a moist erosion affecting the glans and urethral meatus. Histologically, the lesions show a psoriasiform morphology with uniform elongation of rete ridges, parakeratosis, and edematous papillary dermis with prominent blood vessels. Neutrophils are numerous in the parakeratotic layer as well as in the epidermis, similar to what is seen in the pustular variant of psoriasis. A PAS stain should always be performed to rule out a fungal infection.

Lichen Planus

Lichen planus is a common, usually pruritic, and symmetrical papulosquamous dermatosis that affects the genital area in up to 40% of the patients with generalized lesions.[21,38] Cases predominantly affecting the mucosal surface need to be distinguished from mucous membrane pemphigoid. The rare cases showing an exclusive genital or mucosal location may

be difficult to diagnose. The classical lesions are violaceous, flat-topped shiny papules sometimes showing delicate white lines on the surface, namely, Wickham striae. Penile lesions tend to be associated with erosions. Histologically, lichen planus is characterized by a thickened or effaced epidermis often showing a saw-toothed appearance associated with a dense, band-like lymphohistiocytic infiltrate obscuring the dermal–epidermal junction where there is basal cell liquefactive degeneration and a variable number of cytoid (Civatte) bodies. When the lesions are located on the cutaneous surface, there is hyperorthokeratosis and typically wedge-shaped hypergranulosis (Fig. 14-22). Mucosal lesions tend to be associated with patchy hypergranulosis, parakeratosis, and a plasma cell–rich inflammatory infiltrate. Old lesions of lichen planus with only subtle interface changes and numerous plasma cells may be misdiagnosed as Zoon balanitis. Eosinophils are not a feature of lichen planus and when numerous, one should think of a lichenoid drug reaction. The features of lichen planus may overlap with lichen sclerosus and in some patients the two disorders may coexist.

Direct immunofluorescence studies in lichen planus may show fibrinogen and IgM along the basement membrane zone. Civatte bodies may also be highlighted, especially with IgM. Immunofluorescence helps to distinguish lichen planus from cicatricial pemphigoid.

Long-standing anogenital lichen planus appears to carry a small increased risk of squamous cell carcinoma.[73,74]

Lichen Sclerosus (Et atrophicus) (Balanitis Xerotica Obliterans)

Lichen sclerosus is a chronic and atrophic mucocutaneous condition preferentially affecting anogenital areas of men and women. Extragenital location is less common. This condition was described in the penis as balanitis xerotica obliterans by Stuhmer in 1928; however, because some authors prefer to use the term balanitis xerotica obliterans for the end-stage condition and to unify gynecologic and urologic terminology, the use of lichen sclerosus is recommended.[75,76] Penile lichen sclerosus tends to affect middle-aged adults. Grossly, the lesions appear as white gray, irregular geographic and atrophic areas most commonly compromising the inner aspect of the foreskin, glans, and perimeatal region. Erosion, ulceration, and elevated hyperkeratotic foci may also be seen. In advanced cases, the preputial mucosal folds may disappear resulting in acquired phimosis or paraphimosis.[21] Histologically, the lesions are characterized by an atrophic epithelium frequently intermixed with hyperplastic areas, vacuolar alteration of the basal layer, and a thickened lamina propria with the classical hyalinization/sclerosis (Fig. 14-23A).[37,38] A variable amount of band-like lymphoid infiltrate is usually seen underneath the area of hyalinization. Because of marked basal cell vacuolar alteration, some cases may show dermal–epidermal clefting. Marked edema of the lamina propria may precede or coexist with the classical sclerotic changes.[37,38] Lichen sclerosus is a superficial mucosal disorder preferentially affecting the epithelium and lamina propria and typically sparing the preputial dartos and corpus spongiosum of the glans. The lesions, however, tend to be broad and multifocal and may affect more than one epithelial compartment, and even extend to the epithelium and lamina propria of the distal urethra.[76] While extragenital lichen sclerosus appears to carry no risk for malignant transformation, the relationship of anogenital lichen sclerosus and squamous cell carcinoma is well-documented.[76–82] In a prospective study, the incidence of carcinoma arising in the setting of long-standing lichen sclerosus of the penis was 9.3%.[80,81] In a retrospective review of 200 penectomy specimens with penile invasive carcinoma, 33% of the cases were associated with lichen sclerosus[76] and

this figure was much higher (69%) when considering carcinomas affecting the foreskin exclusively.[82] When present adjacent to invasive carcinomas, lichen sclerosus is almost always associated with areas of epithelial hyperplasia and frequently shows squamous cell atypias (Fig. 14-23B).[76,82] A significant association of lichen sclerosus with special (usually HPV-unrelated) variants of carcinoma such as usual, pseudohyperplastic, verrucous, and papillary carcinoma has been demonstrated. There is also a distinct association of lichen sclerosus with differentiated (simplex) PeIN.[83] These findings suggest that lichen sclerosus may represent a precancerous condition for a subset of penile squamous cell carcinoma, especially the HPV-unrelated variants.

Balanitis Circumscripta Plasmacellularis (Zoon Balanitis)

This is an inflammatory condition of unknown etiology preferentially occurring in uncircumcised men.[21,38,84,85] The classical clinical presentation is that of a solitary, reddish plaque with speckled and hemorrhagic surface usually affecting the glans. The clinical appearance usually raises the concern of a carcinoma in situ. Histologically, there is a thinned epidermis with no granular layer and a very thin to absent parakeratotic layer. There is some epidermal spongiosis and the keratinocytes are sometimes described as lozenge or diamond shaped.[21] The classical (although nonspecific) feature that gave name to this entity is the presence of a dense, band-like, plasma cell–rich dermal inflammatory infiltrate, usually associated with lymphocytes, extravasated erythrocytes, and siderophages. The blood vessels are prominent. The papillary dermal edema usually seen in early stage is replaced by fibrosis in long-standing lesions. The diagnosis of Zoon balanitis is largely one of exclusion. One must consider other specific entities such as lichen planus, syphilis, and pemphigoid

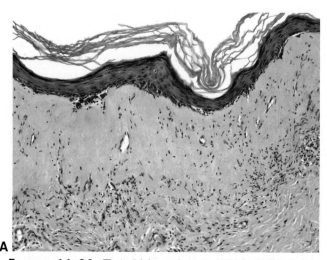

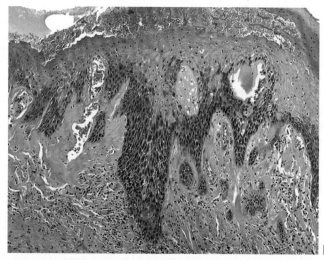

A   B

FIGURE 14-23 ■ **A:** Lichen sclerosus. Histologically, the lesion is characterized by an atrophic epithelium with vacuolar alteration of the basal layer and a thickened lamina propria with the classical hyalinization/sclerosis. **B:** Lichen sclerosus with epithelial hyperplasia showing keratinocytic atypia. Such changes are frequently found adjacent to invasive carcinomas.

before making this diagnosis. Based on the nonspecific findings in Zoon balanitis and the similarities with other plasma cell–rich dermatitis and mucositis, the more generic term idiopathic lymphoplasmacellular mucositis-dermatitis was suggested by some authors to encompass etiologically uncertain lymphoplasmacellular infiltrates in the skin and mucosal surfaces.[86]

Fixed Drug Reaction

Fixed drug eruptions present as a one or more circumscribed erythematous to violaceous or brown plaques that show predilection for the extremities and external genitalia.[21,38] Vesiculation and blister formation are common. Resolution is characterized by postinflammatory hyperpigmentation. The lesions classically recur at the same site each time that the patient is exposed to the same drug. The most common penile locations include the glans and distal shaft.[21] Histopathologically, there is an interface dermatitis with prominent vacuolar degeneration of the basal layer, lymphocyte tagging of basal keratinocytes, and scattered apoptotic keratinocytes.[37,38] These epidermal changes are associated with a superficial and midperivascular and interstitial mixed cell dermal infiltrate with lymphoid cells, eosinophils, and melanophages (Fig. 14-24). Old lesions may only show pigment incontinence. Fixed drug reactions can be distinguished from erythema multiforme by the deeper dermal infiltrate and presence of eosinophils.

Aphthous Ulcer and Behçet Disease

Aphthous ulcers may involve the scrotum and penis and they may or may not be associated with Behçet disease. Lesions are usually painful, solitary, and sharply marginated with necrotic gray fibrinoid base.[21] Histologically, the changes are nonspecific and similar to those seen in oral aphthous lesions. At the center of the ulcer, there is necrosis with a dense neutrophilic infiltrate. At the periphery, there is a predominantly lymphoid infiltrate with exocytosis. Aphthous ulcer is a diagnosis of exclusion and should only be made after other causes (especially infection) have been ruled out. When chronic aphthous ulcers occur, the diagnosis of Behçet syndrome should be considered. Behçet disease is a poorly understand, chronic condition likely due to disturbances in the immune system. The presence of oral (apthtous) ulcers, along with any two out of the four additional signs: genital ulcers, skin lesions (e.g., pustules, erythema nodosum), eye lesions (e.g., iritis, uveitis) and pathergy reaction is necessary for the diagnosis.[37]

Bullous Pemphigoid

It is the most frequent autoimmune blistering disorder and usually affects the elderly.[21,37] There are several variants that can variably affect the skin and mucosal surface. The characteristic lesion is a tense blister with an erythematous border. Approximately 7% of the patients have genital lesions. Histologically, well-established lesions show a subepithelial blister associated with edema of the underlying dermis or lamina propria and a mixed cell infiltrate containing numerous eosinophils. Direct immunofluorescence shows linear deposition of IgG and C3 at the basement zone. Two main bullous pemphigoid antigens are recognized: one is the intracellular protein 230 kD (BPAG1) and the other is the transmembrane protein 180 kD (BPSG2); both of them are located in the hemidesmosomal area of the basal keratinocyte.[38]

Cicatricial Pemphigoid (Mucous Membrane Pemphigoid)

Cicatricial pemphigoid is an autoimmune bullous disease that has a predilection for mucous membranes and often results in scarring. Oral and ocular lesions predominate; however, the genital area may also be involved. In males, genital lesions usually affect the foreskin and glans.[38] Long-standing lesions may lead to urethral stricture formation and

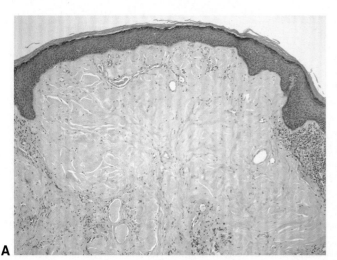 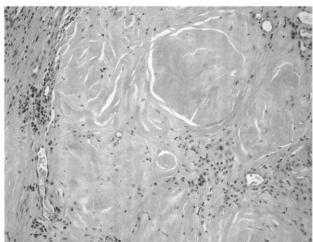

FIGURE 14-24 ■ **A,B:** Amyloidosis. There are nodular amorphous aggregates of eosinophilic material in the lamina propria.

phimosis.[38,87] Histologically, there is a subepithelial blister associated with a mixed inflammatory infiltrate containing lymphoid cells, eosinophils, neutrophils, and plasma cells. The lamina propria may be edematous or fibrotic. Apart from scarring fibrosis in old lesions, these changes are identical to those seen in bullous pemphigoid. The mucosal lesions are often eroded and ulcerated showing fibrosing–granulation tissue with no specific acute and chronic inflammation. Direct immunofluorescence findings on perilesional mucosa (the site of choice) are similar to those seen in bullous pemphigoid.

Pemphigus

Pemphigus refers to a group of chronic blistering conditions that develop as a consequence of autoantibodies against a variety of desmosomal proteins.[21,37] Several variants exist, including pemphigus vulgaris, vegetans, erythematosus, and foliaceous. Penile involvement is rare but may be observed.[88,89] The hallmark of pemphigus is the presence of acantholysis, which is located at different levels of the epidermis in the different variants. Pemphigus vulgaris, the most common variant, is characterized by suprabasilar acantholysis with intraepidermal blister formation. In pemphigus vegetans, there is also suprabasilar acantholysis but this is more subtle and associated with a hyperplastic epidermis with scattered neutrophilic and eosinophilic abscesses.[38] Pemphigus foliaceous and erythematosus are characterized by superficial acantholysis involving the upper levels of the epidermis. Direct immunofluorescence shows intercellular deposition of IgG and often C3.

Paraneoplastic pemphigus is a distinct variant of pemphigus that may be associated with a variety of malignancies. The penis may rarely be affected.[38,90] The pathologic features are variable and often consist of a combination of suprabasal acantholysis and interface changes.[38] Direct immunofluorescence may be negative in a fourth of the cases.

Acantholytic Dermatosis of the Genitocrural Area

This condition appears to represent a distinct acantholytic eruption of the genital/perineal area that should be distinguished from other generalized blistering acantholytic and dyskeratotic disorders that may also involve the genitalia. Originally reported as a localized form of acantholysis and dyskeratosis affecting the vulvocrural region in females, this rare condition was more recently described confined to the genital and perineal areas in male patients.[38,91] The etiopathogenesis is unknown and perhaps somehow related to the moist environment of this area. Clinically, the lesions are characterized by multiple discrete papules or macerated patches involving the penis, scrotum, inner thighs, and perineum. Histologically, the acantholytic dermatosis had features resembling both Hailey-Hailey disease and Darier disease. The lesions show hyperkeratosis, parakeratosis, acanthosis, and acantholysis sometimes associated with dyskeratosis. Warty dyskeratoma–like features and follicular

involvement may also be seen. Typically, inflammation is minimal or absent.

MISCELLANEOUS CONDITIONS

Amyloidosis

Penile amyloidosis is a rare disease that has been occasionally reported.[92,93] It usually affects middle-aged men and presents as nodules or papules most commonly involving the glans. Coronal and shaft lesions may occur. Because of the nodular presentation, they may raise the clinical concern of a tumor. Penile amyloidosis is a localized disorder with excellent prognosis. It is usually limited to the skin/mucosa with rare systemic involvement. Histopathologically, nodular amorphous aggregates of eosinophilic material are identified in the dermis or lamina propria (Fig. 14-25). These deposits are positive with Congo red, crystal violet, and thioflavin T stain. Penile amyloidosis involving the skin or mucosa should be distinguished from urethral amyloidosis. Patients with urethral amyloid deposition most frequently present with hematuria, and the lesions are identified endoscopically.

Tancho Nodules and Paraffinomas

Tancho nodules refer to an unusual custom among some Asian populations to implant foreign material under the skin of the penis to improve sexual pleasure.[94] Paraffinomas (also known as sclerosing lipogranulomas) result from the injection of mineral oil in the penis usually done with the purpose of penile enlargement. Histologically, these materials may cause foreign body reaction that may need surgical resection. Such foreign substances that are injected or inserted into the penis include paraffin, silicone, or wax. A characteristic foreign body reaction called paraffinoma similar to

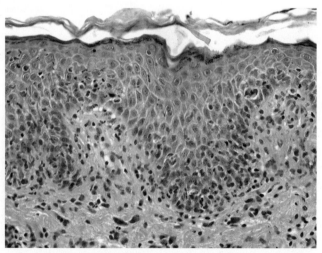

FIGURE 14-25 ■ Fixed drug reaction. There is an interface dermatitis with necrotic keratinocytes and a dermal mixed cell dermal infiltrate with lymphoid cells, eosinophils, and melanophages.

the one seen in the scrotum is produced (Fig. 14-74).[95] This reaction may occur several years after the injection.[96]

Peyronie Disease

Peyronie disease is a relatively common condition (recent studies suggest that it may occur in up to 9% of the male population) that affects men in the third to seventh decade. It is characterized by dense fibrosis with formation of a plaque-like lesion affecting the tunica albuginea and penile fascia and sometimes extending to the dermis. This fibrotic plaque causes an abnormal penile curvature and very often pain and erectile dysfunction. In some cases, there are several firm nodules over the middorsal line. The histologic appearance varies with the duration of the disease. Early lesions are characterized by a loose proliferation of plum fibroblasts/myofibroblasta admixed with some inflammatory cells (similar to an early scar). Older lesions are more fibrotic and less cellular. Finally, large hypocellular nodules of hyalinized fibrotic tissue are the prominent finding. The changes in Peyronie disease recapitulate the sequence of events that characterize the development of tissue fibrosis in general. These are essentially an initial tissue insult (trauma, microtrauma, or local toxicity), followed by acute and then chronic inflammation that leads to deposition of excessive collagen and other extracellular matrix, fragmentation of elastin, and persistence of myofibroblasts. Fibrosis may then progress to partial ectopic calcification or ossification.[97] An important experimental finding is increased levels of transforming growth factor β1 (*TGFβ1*), in the fibrotic plaques. Injury to the erect penis is thought to trigger the disease by inducing extravasation of fibrin and subsequent synthesis of *TGFβ1*. Some studies demonstrate a role for oxidative stress and cytokine release primarily TGFβ1 in the development of the fibrotic plaques.[98,99] There is evidence indicating that these profibrotic factors interact with antifibrotic defense mechanisms, such as decrease of myofibroblast accumulation and elimination of reactive oxygen species by inducible nitric oxide synthase and neutralization of TGFβ1 by decorin, suggesting that some plaques are in dynamic turnover. Treatment is mainly surgical, as pharmacologic therapy has limited efficacy.[98,99] The development of animal and cell culture models has advanced the understanding of this disease and uncovered several promising molecular targets for antifibrotic treatments.

Sclerosing Lymphangitis of the Penis

This unusual and usually self-limited condition preferentially affecting young adults is characterized by firm subcutaneous cord-like structures located along the dorsal shaft of the penis or around the coronal sulcus.[100,101] The pathogenesis is poorly understood but it may be associated with trauma and vigorous sexual activity. Concurrent infections including herpes simplex infection have been described, but most likely they are not the cause of the disease. Because of the difficulty in distinguishing between large lymphatic vessels

and veins in this location there is controversy as to whether this condition preferentially affects large lymphatic vessels or veins and perhaps either could be affected in different patients. This condition may show overlapping features with Mondor phlebitis. Histologically, one or more vessels of the superficial plexus show thickening of the wall, sometimes associated with thrombosis and various stages of recanalization. Inflammation is not prominent.

Vascular Disorders

Penile involvement by vascular disorders is rare. A few case reports of polyarteritis nodosa involving the penis can be found in the literature.[102] Wegener granulomatosis affecting the penis has also been reported. Most reported patients developed penile lesions in the clinical context of upper respiratory tract, pulmonary, and/or renal involvement by the disorder.[103]

Crohn Disease

Anogenital lesions occur in about 30% of the patients with intestinal Crohn disease, either by direct extension of active intestinal disease or as noncontiguous lesions, or so-called metastatic disease. Skin involvement is more common in patients with colonic disorder. Importantly, skin lesions may be the first manifestation of the disease. Genital lesions in patients with Crohn disease include edema, ulcers, abscesses, sinus, and fistulas.[37,38,104,105] Histopathologically, the findings are nonspecific and vary from edema and lymphangietasis to noncaseating granulomas that may have a perivascular distribution. Clinical correlation is important to confirm the diagnosis.

Papillomatosis of Glans Corona (Penile Pearly Papules)

This is an HPV-unrelated, asymptomatic, and benign condition occurring in 20% to 30% of normal men characterized by multiple pearly gray-white fibroepithelial papules located in the dorsal aspect of the glans corona.[106] These minute papillomas are characteristically arranged in two to three rows. Each lesion is dome shaped or filiform and arises on a solitary base. Histologically, there is a normal or slightly thickened squamous epithelium overlying a central fibrovascular core (Fig. 14-26).

Penile Cutaneous Horn (Cornu Cutaneoum)

This is a clinical term based on the appearance of the lesion that presents as a keratotic protuberance mimicking a horn. Nonneoplastic and neoplastic conditions may present clinically as a cutaneous horn. The diagnosis rests upon histologic examination of the viable epithelium underneath the thick cornified layer. Cutaneous horns may correspond to viral warts, seborrheic keratosis, or squamous cell carcinoma among other possibilities.[37,38,107]

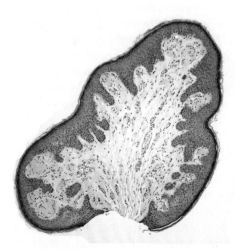

FIGURE 14-26 ■ Penile pearly papules. There is a small fibroepithelial polyp characterized by slightly thickened squamous epithelium overlying a central fibrovascular core.

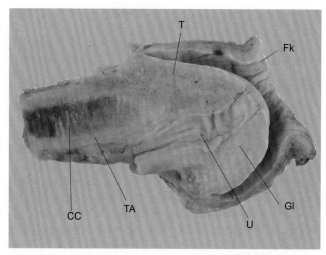

FIGURE 14-27 ■ Phimosis and cancer. Cut section of a partial penectomy specimen with a long phimotic foreskin and glans carcinoma. Fk, foreskin; T, tumor; Gl, glans; U, urethra; TA, albuginea; CC, corpus cavernosum.

Verruciform Xanthoma

The vast majority of these lesions affect the oral cavity (70%) followed by the anogenital region.[21,38,108] Verruciform xanthoma usually affects adults and presents as a yellowish to red plaque. Most patients do not have associated lipid disorders. Histologically, most lesions shows acanthosis, papillomatosis, and a thick parakeratotic layer exhibiting a bright orange hue. Within the connective tissue core of the papillae and between rete ridges, there are numerous large, foamy, lipid-laden macrophages (Fig. 14-76). Multinucleated cells are usually not seen. Lymphocytes and neutrophils may be present. These lesions are nonrelated to HPV and should be differentiated from condylomata.

Phimosis

This is a condition in which the prepuce cannot be retracted, usually as a consequence of nonspecific chronic bacterial infections, lichen sclerosus, or congenitally abnormally long foreskin.[21,109–110] Phimosis may also be seen secondary to graft versus host disease. The accumulation of smegma induces a diffuse inflammation of all mucosal epithelial compartments of the glans and foreskin. The treatment of choice is the surgical removal of the foreskin. Histologically, there is usually fibrosis of the lamina propria associated with a nonspecific lymphoid and plasmacytic infiltrate.[110] It is important for the surgical pathologist to liberally sample phimotic foreskin specimens from adults to rule out dysplasia, carcinoma in situ, or occult early invasive carcinoma. Special attention is advised to hyperkeratotic, thick, and slightly elevated or irregular foci. Penile cancer has been reported to occur more frequently in patients with long phimotic foreskins (Fig. 14-27).[7] In paraphimosis, the prepuce cannot be advanced over the glans and becomes trapped in the space located between the coronal sulcus and the glans corona. Unusual cases of

penile infarct secondary to arterial obstruction resulting from edema have been described.

Squamous Hyperplasia

Squamous hyperplasia is characterized by an acanthotic thickening of the squamous epithelium without atypia[3,11,111,112] that may involve any of the penile anatomical compartments. It represents a reaction pattern more than a specific entity and it may be seen associated to a rather broad spectrum of conditions from inflammatory dermatitis (i.e., lichen sclerosus) to squamous cell carcinoma. Squamous hyperplasia is usually seen in the epithelium adjacent to special subtypes of carcinomas, particularly usual (keratinizing), verrucous, and low-grade papillary variants. Grossly, lesions appear flat, smooth, and pearly white with occasional slightly elevated to papillary configuration. Microscopically, squamous hyperplasia shows acanthosis, hyper-/orthokeratosis, and normal maturation of squamous cells (Fig. 14-28). Patchy parakeratosis may occasionally be seen. Koilocytosis, deep keratin whorls, and cytologic atypia are not present. Pseudoepitheliomatous hyperplasia may be confused with squamous cell carcinoma (SCC) because the florid complex downward proliferation of squamous rete ridges may appear as detached from the epithelium in cut sections. Important features that may be helpful to differentiate pseudoepitheliomatous hyperplasia from carcinoma include the superficial nature of the lesion, absence of atypia, absence of deep keratin whorls (keratin pearls), and lack of stromal reaction or desmoplasia. Another pattern is that of verrucous hyperplasia, typically found adjacent to verrucous carcinomas (Fig. 14-28). The frequent association of squamous hyperplasia with differentiated PeIN and invasive carcinomas, especially low-grade variants and the usual continuity with the invasive tumor, suggests that squamous hyperplasia with or without lichen sclerosus may be a precancerous lesion of the penis.[76] Its role as a potential precursor remains controversial.

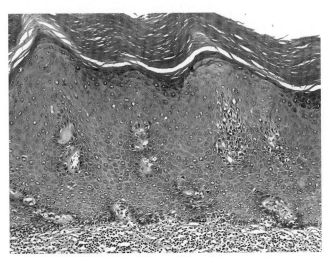

Figure 14-28 ■ Squamous hyperplasia, verrucous. There is acanthosis with hyperorthokeratosis. The lesion has a spiky (slightly verrucous surface). The epithelium shows normal maturation without atypia.

SQUAMOUS NEOPLASIA

Penile Intraepithelial Neoplasia

Invasive squamous cell carcinomas are thought to be preceded by precursor lesions, namely, PeIN. In keeping with the notion of a bimodal pathway of carcinogenesis in penile carcinoma, precursor lesions can be broadly classified into two main groups: HPV-related and HPV-unrelated variants.[83,111–118] Taking into consideration the striking similarities in morphology and pathogenesis between vulvar and penile carcinomas,[119–121] and in an attempt to have a simplified and more uniform terminology, we have recently proposed a slightly modified nomenclature for penile preinvasive lesions.[83] The term PeIN is preferred over old terms such as squamous intraepithelial lesion (SIL), erythroplasia of Queyrat, and Bowen disease. These latter two terms are synonymous with carcinoma in situ and have been used for lesions in the glans (erythroplasia of Queyrat) and skin of the shaft (Bowen disease).[122–124] PeIN can be classified as differentiated/simplex (HPV-unrelated) and undifferentiated (HPV-related) variants (Box 14-2). The latter can be subclassified as warty, basaloid, and mixed warty/basaloid.[83] PeIN may be solitary or multifocal, and tends to be associated with infiltrating SCCs in about two-thirds of cases. In our experience of these cases, approximately 65% are associated with differentiated PeIN and 35% with warty/basaloid PeIN. Differentiated PeIN affects older patients, it usually arises in the setting of a chronic scarring inflammatory dermatosis, and it is more frequently located in the foreskin when compared with HPV-related variants. The latter affect younger patients and are usually more centrally located in the glans and perimeatal region. The gross appearance of PeIN is heterogeneous and does not allow one to distinguish between the two main types. Lesions vary from flat to slightly elevated, pearly white or moist erythematous, dark

Box 14-2 ● PENILE INTRAEPITHELIAL NEOPLASIA

1. Differentiated
   - HPV unrelated
   - Well differentiated (pink cell predominates)
   - Precursor of HPV-unrelated SCC
   - Associated with LSA
2. Undifferentiated
   Basaloid
   - HPV-related
   - Blue cell predominates
   - Precursor of HPV-related SCC
   Warty
   - HPV-related
   - Blue cells and koilocytes
   - Precursor of HPV-related SCC
   Mixed warty–basaloid
   - HPV-related
   - Mixed basaloid and warty features (Blue cells and koilocytes)
   - Precursor of HPV-related SCC

brown or black, macules, papules, or plaques. The contours may be sharp or subtle and irregular. Occasionally, a granular or low papillary appearance may be noted. Microscopically, differentiated (simplex) PeIN is characterized by a thickened epithelium, usually associated with elongated and anastomosing rete ridges, subtle abnormal maturation (enlarged keratinocytes with abundant eosinophilic cytoplasm), whorling and keratin pearl formation (usually in deep rete ridges), prominent intercellular bridges (spongiosis and sometimes acantholysis), and atypical basal cells with hyperchromatic nuclei.[83,118,119] Parakeratosis is frequent (Fig. 14-29). At low power, the atypia seems to be present only in lower levels of the epidermis; however, at higher power, it is more clear that

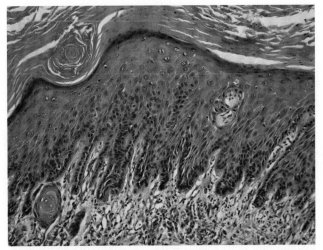

Figure 14-29 ■ Differentiated penile intraepithelial neoplasia (PeIN). There is a thickened epithelium, associated with elongated and anastomosing rete ridges, basilar atypia, enlarged keratinocytes with abundant eosinophilic cytoplasm, and keratin pearl formation. There is also spongiosis with acantholysis and parakeratosis.

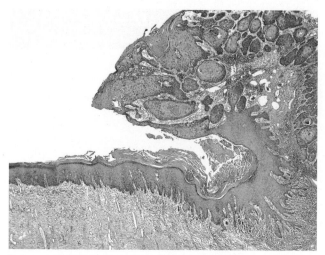

FIGURE 14-30 ■ Differentiated PeIN **(left)** is seen adjacent to a well-differentiated invasive carcinoma **(right)**.

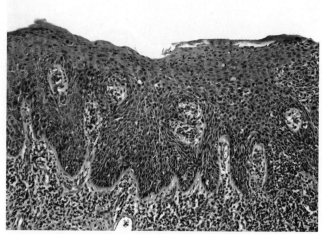

FIGURE 14-31 ■ Undifferentiated PeIN, basaloid type. There is replacement of the epithelium by a monotonous proliferation of small round cells with high nuclear/cytoplasmic ratio.

there is subtle but abnormal maturation in all levels of the epithelium. Despite the subtle changes, we believe that differentiated PeIN represents a high-grade (although differentiated) lesion that may evolve to frank invasive carcinoma without showing more significant atypia (Fig. 14-30).[83,118,119,121]

It is not surprising that the precursor lesions of well-differentiated invasive tumors show such a high degree of differentiation. It is important to recognize this lesion because it appears to be the most frequent precursor lesion of penile carcinomas, especially the keratinizing and well-differentiated variants. Unfortunately, most studies on simplex PeIN are retrospective and have been done in penectomies for invasive carcinoma. It is also important to acknowledge the difficulty of this diagnosis and the need of molecular or immunohistochemical markers to more easily prospectively identify differentiated PeIN. p53 expression is more frequently seen in differentiated PeIN when compared with warty/basaloid variants[112]; however, p53 expression is also seen in benign condylomata and other inflammatory or reactive conditions and therefore cannot be considered a specific marker of differentiated PeIN. A preferential association was seen between lichen sclerosus and differentiated PeIN when compared with warty/basaloid variants.[76,82,83] It is therefore important to keep a high level of suspicion when dealing with hyperkeratotic and hyperplastic lesions with subtle keratinocytic atypia arising in the setting of long-standing lichen sclerosus.

The second major type of PeIN (the undifferentiated, HPV-related type) shows distinctive morphologic changes. It is subclassified as warty, basaloid, and mixed PeIN. In the basaloid variant, the epithelium is replaced by a monotonous population of small immature cells with a high nuclear/cytoplasmic ratio (Fig. 14-31).[83,118] Apoptosis and mitotic figures are numerous. Basaloid PeIN should be distinguished from transitional cell urethral carcinoma in situ, which may secondarily involve the penile meatal region.[125] In the warty pattern, the involved epithelium has an undulating or spiking

surface with atypical parakeratosis. There is striking cellular pleomorphism and koilocytosis (multinucleation, nuclei with irregular contours, perinuclear halo, and dyskeratosis) (Fig. 14-32). Mitotic figures tend to be numerous. Frequently, lesions show overlapping features of both, namely, mixed warty and basaloid PeIN. These mixed lesions tend to have a spiking surface with koilocytic changes while the lower half of the epithelium is predominantly composed of small basaloid cells (Fig. 14-33). Basaloid and warty PeIN can be divided into low-grade and high-grade lesions when the atypical cells occupy less than half and more than half of the epithelial thickness, respectively. Most of the warty and basaloid PeIN will fall within the high-grade category. Full-thickness atypia of the epithelium equals carcinoma in situ. Low-grade lesions are exceptional and should be distinguished from

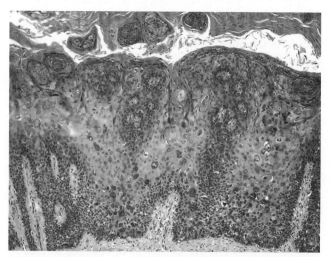

FIGURE 14-32 ■ Undifferentiated PeIN, warty type. The involved epithelium has an undulating/spiking surface with atypical parakeratosis. There is marked cellular pleomorphism and koilocytosis (multinucleation, nuclei with irregular contours, perinuclear halo, and dyskeratosis).

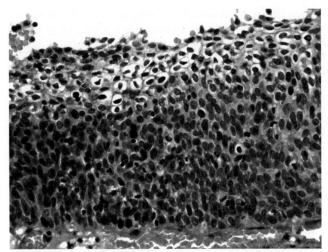

FIGURE 14-33 ■ Undifferentiated PeIN, mixed, warty–basaloid type. The lower part of the lesion shows classical features of basaloid PeIN. The top part shows atypical koilocytic changes characteristic of warty PeIN. This example has a flat surface; most cases have a slightly undulating surface.

benign condyloma, with the latter not being considered a preneoplastic condition. p16 is usually overexpressed in undifferentiated PeIN (Fig. 14-34) and negative in differentiated PeIN, further supporting the association of undifferentiated PeIN with high-risk variants of HPV.[112] Other rare morphologic patterns of precursor lesions include pleomorphic, pagetoid, clear, spindle, and small cell; all of these are more likely to represent variants of the HPV-related group. A recent study found a distinctive geographical distribution of penile precursor lesions. PeIN with warty and/or basaloid features predominated in low-incidence areas, whereas differentiated PeIN was more prevalent in endemic regions for penile cancer. With few exceptions there is a good correlation between the microscopic appearance of the preinvasive process and the associated invasive carcinoma, further supporting the concept of a dual pathway of penile tumorigenesis.

Some authors still use the old terminology of mild (PeIN 1), moderate (PeIN 2), and severe dysplasia (PeIN 3 or carcinoma in situ) based on the degree, in thirds, that the epithelium is atypical.[37,38,113–116] Because of the overlapping features between moderate and severe dysplasia, PeIN 2 and 3 are combined in one category in some systems. Such systems divide PeIN into only two grades: low and high. These systems mainly apply to the HPV-related group of lesions.

It has been suggested that the use of a triple p16/p53/Ki-67 immunohistochemical panel may be helpful in the classification, differential diagnosis, and morphologic standardization of penile intraepithelial lesions.[112]

Bowenoid Papulosis

Bowenoid papulosis is a multifocal HPV-related condition affecting the anogenital region of young adults.[126–129] Clinically, penile bowenoid papulosis is characterized by multiple soft papules or macules mostly affecting the skin of the shaft, and less frequently the epithelium of the glans, sulcus, or foreskin. Despite the clinical benign-looking appearance of these papular lesions, histopathologic findings reveal features of a squamous cell carcinoma in situ.[37,38] There is a proliferation of atypical cells with a high nuclear/cytoplasmic ratio that tend to have a more patchy and less continuous disposition when compared with carcinoma in situ (Fig. 14-35). There may be a variable increased pigmentation of the basal layer.[127] Definitive histologic distinction between carcinoma in situ and bowenoid papulosis is not possible; therefore, clinical correlation is necessary to confirm this diagnosis. Immunosuppression, including HIV infection, greatly increases the risk for bowenoid papulosis, with the lesions in this setting tending to be more widespread. Lesions of bowenoid papulosis may regress spontaneously or (especially in immunocompromised patients) may evolve to invasive carcinoma.[128] High-risk HPVs, mainly HPV-16, are regularly found in the lesions.[129]

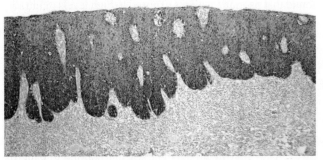

FIGURE 14-34 ■ Basaloid PeIN. Note the overexpression of p16 by the BC in situ.

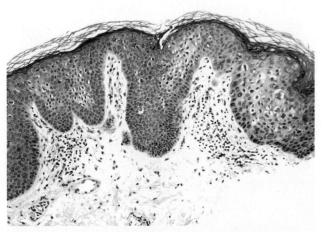

FIGURE 14-35 ■ Bowenoid papulosis. There is a proliferation of atypical cells with high nuclear/cytoplasmic ratio that tend to have a more patchy and less continuous disposition when compared with carcinoma in situ.

Squamous Cell Carcinoma

The majority of penile carcinomas are squamous cell carcinomas that arise on the mucosal squamous epithelium of the distal portion of the organ including glans, coronal sulcus, and foreskin (Fig. 14-36).[3,9] Primary squamous cell carcinomas arising from the cutaneous surface of the foreskin and shaft are extremely rare. Squamous cell carcinoma of the penis is relatively infrequent in the United States and Europe, where it accounts for <1% of all malignancies in males. However, it is still common in some parts of Asia, Africa, and Latin America, accounting for over 10% of all carcinomas in males.[130–136] Penile cancer most frequently affects elderly men, but age variations are seen with certain histologic subtypes (i.e., basaloid and warty carcinomas affect slightly younger patients than the other variants). There is no racial preference.[137] Familial cases also have been noted.[130] Cancer of the penis is relatively common in Africa, being the most common form of cancer in males in Uganda.[132] There is wide variation in prevalence in India.[136] Regional differences in the prevalence of penile carcinoma are noted, even in the same country. It is the second most common urologic cancer after prostate cancer in males in the rural population of Paraguay; interestingly, it is extremely rare in the urban population of the same country.

Etiopathogenesis

Circumcision has a protective effect against carcinoma, especially when performed shortly after birth.[138–142] Late circumcision does not seem to have the same preventive effect. Carcinoma of the penis is exceptional in the Jewish population. Penile carcinomas arising on circumcision scars in cases of adult circumcision have been described.[143,144] It is likely that carcinoma is related to personal hygiene and possibly the carcinogenic effect of smegma, factors that may be enhanced by lack of circumcision. In keeping with this notion, it has been shown that long phimotic foreskins are associated with penile carcinoma.[7] It has also been shown that male circumcision is associated with a reduced risk of penile HPV infection and, in the case of men with a history of multiple sexual partners, a reduced risk of cervical cancer in their current female partners.[139,145] The etiology of a subset of cancer of the penis has been linked to HPVs, with a high preponderance of HPV-16.[45–48,145–150] In a combined study of cases from the United States and Paraguay, HPV DNA was detected in 42% of penile carcinomas.[55] HPV is more frequently associated with basaloid or warty carcinoma variants (85%). The majority of usual/keratinizing and verrucous carcinomas are not related to HPV. There appears to be strong evidence that at least HPV-16 is involved in penile carcinogenesis; the role of other HPV types remains controversial.[45–47] In the majority of cases HPV-16 is integrated into the genome (host cell chromosomes)[148] and it has been shown that both primary and metastatic tumors contain the same integrated HPV subtype with identical cleavage patterns, suggesting that it is a stable component of cancer progression.[150] Molecular studies have shown E6 transcriptional activity and a high viral load in HPV-16 DNA–positive squamous cell carcinomas. Additionally, HPV-16 molecular findings were strongly associated with HPV-16 L1-, E6-, and E7-antibody seropositivity.[47] For additional discussion on HPV, please review the section on molecular studies. Although an association of Epstein-Barr virus (EBV) with penile carcinomas has been reported, a possible carcinogenic role of EBV in penile tumors has not been proved and remains controversial.[151,152] Numerous reports have linked lichen sclerosus to penile cancer.[76,78–83,153–155] It is possible that lichen sclerosus is a precancerous condition for a subset of squamous cell carcinomas, mainly the HPV-unrelated variants.[76,83] The relation between lichen planus and penile cancer remains controversial.[73,74] A significant association was reported among smoking, chewing tobacco, and the use of snuff in patients with penile cancer, with a dose–response relationship for the first two.[156] Daling found that the adjusted odds ratio for penis cancer associated with current smoking was 2.8 times that of men who never smoked,[157] and it was dose dependent. Radiation-induced carcinoma of the penis has been reported.[158] They usually are more aggressive than the original tumor. Radiation-induced transformation of verrucous to anaplastic carcinoma has been noted.[159] It has been found that psoriatic patients exposed to high levels of ultraviolet B radiation have a higher risk of genital tumors (including penile carcinoma). Psoralens and ultraviolet A radiation (PUVA) were found to have a strong dose-dependent correlation with penile cancer.[160] Squamous cell carcinoma may be associated with scars (e.g., secondary to a burn).[161]

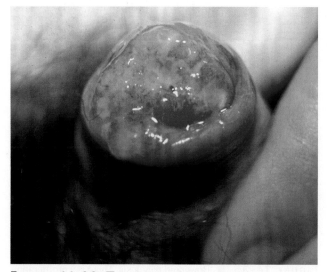

FIGURE 14-36 ■ Invasive squamous cell carcinoma arising from the mucosal surface of the glans. The surface of the lesion appears flat and ulcerated. On cut sections, such flat lesions may be deeply invasive tumors.

Classification

The vast majority of malignant neoplasms of the penis are SCCs. They may be broadly classified according to patterns of growth and more specifically classified according to histologic variant.

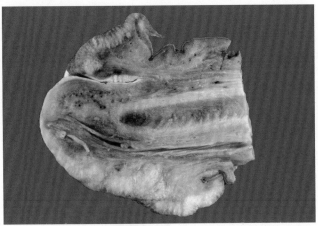

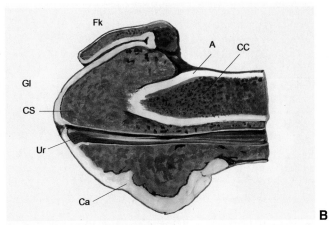

FIGURE 14-37 ■ Superficial spreading pattern of growth. Gross picture **(A)** and diagram **(B)** illustrating the cut section of a superficially spreading carcinoma composed of an extensive intraepithelial component (horizontal growth), associated with a superficially invasive cancer. Gl, glans; Fk, foreskin; CS, corpus spongiosum; CC, corpus cavernosum; A, albuginea; Ur, urethra; Ca, carcinoma.

Patterns of Growth

SCCs of the penis can be classified in three major growth patterns with different prognostic implications.[3,9,162–166] Superficial spreading corresponds to slowly growing neoplasms widely involving the superficial anatomic layers of glans, sulcus, and/or foreskin. Neoplasms showing this pattern tend to have a long and initially horizontal phase (mainly involving the epithelium and sometimes lamina propria) followed by a more advanced phase with focal vertical growth pattern with invasion of corpus spongiosum and cavernosum. Grossly, the lesions appear as slightly raised white-gray granular firm neoplasms usually affecting more than one anatomical compartment (i.e., glans, foreskin, and coronal sulcus). A cut section of the specimen will show a wide, band-like thickening of the surface extensively limited to the lamina propria; focally, deeper infiltration may be seen (Fig. 14-37A and B). Microscopically, these lesions show an extensive in situ component with focal (and less often multifocal) infiltration of lamina propria or deeper anatomical layers. The most common histologic variant associated with the superficial spreading pattern is SCC of the usual type. It is important to keep in mind when dealing with such tumors that because of the characteristic centrifugal growth, they can extend to the urethral or cutaneous surgical margins of resection. If a foreskin specimen is evaluated, the entire circumferential margin near the coronal sulcus should be submitted for histologic evaluation to avoid recurrences in the glans. Vertical growth pattern is seen in large, endophytic, deeply infiltrative tumors. These lesions often show a fungating and ulcerated surface. Cut sections show a solid, deeply invasive neoplasm with nodular appearance (Fig. 14-38A and B). Rounded satellite nodules separated from the main tumor and usually deeply located in the corpus spongiosum or cavernosum may be

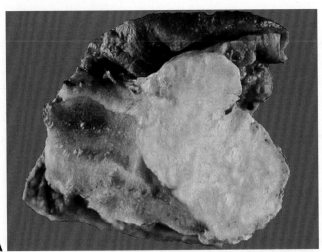

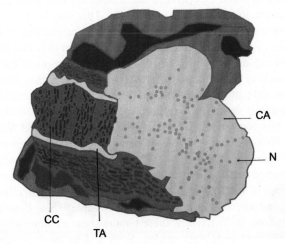

FIGURE 14-38 ■ Vertical pattern of growth. Gross **(A)** and diagram **(B)** of the cut surface of a deeply invasive squamous cell carcinoma. Such tumors are associated with a high rate of regional metastasis. On microscopic examination, this case corresponded to a BC. CA, carcinoma; N, foci of comedonecrosis; TA, albuginea; CC, corpus cavernosum.

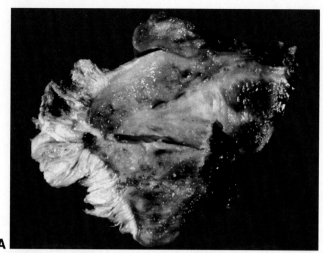

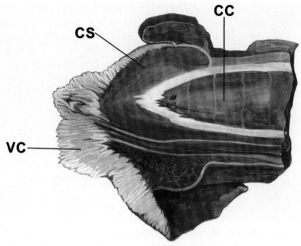

A   **B**

FIGURE 14-39 ■ Verruciform growth pattern. **A:** Cut sections of a partial penectomy specimen illustrating a verrucous carcinoma replacing the distal glans. Note papillomatous (verruciform) surface of the tumor. **B:** Diagram of the same lesion. VC, verrucous carcinoma; CS, corpus spongiosum; CC, corpus cavernosum.

seen. The tumors tend to show high histologic grade and lymphovascular invasion. The histologic types most commonly associated with this pattern of growth are basaloid, sarcomatoid, and usual SCC.[167] The vertical pattern of growth is associated with a high risk of regional metastasis and poor outcome. The verruciform growth pattern is seen in approximately 25% of penile tumors and corresponds to slowly growing, exophytic, well-differentiated neoplasms with papillary surfaces (Fig. 14-39A and B).[3,9,22] They are usually confined to the lamina propria or superficial corpus spongiosum or more rarely may invade deeper structures. This pattern of growth is usually seen in histologic variants such as verrucous carcinoma, condylomatous (warty) carcinoma, papillary carcinoma, and carcinoma cuniculatum.[168] Benign conditions such as verruciform xanthomas and common and giant condylomata may show a similar pattern of growth. Multicentric carcinoma refers to the presence of two or more independent carcinomatous foci separated by nonneoplastic tissue (Fig. 14-40). This may be a clinical or a microscopic finding. Multicentric carcinomas may affect different anatomical compartments and may be synchronous or metachronous. The pattern of growth of each tumor may be similar or different (i.e., one tumor may show a vertical pattern of growth and the other may be superficial spreading) and they may correspond to similar or different histologic types. The prognosis would be related with the tumor showing histologic parameters of more aggressive behavior. The margins of resection should be carefully evaluated in these multicentric lesions. Mixed patterns may be seen in about a third of penile tumors, especially in clinically advanced stages. A classical example is the hybrid/verrucous SCC. Usually, these tumors show a combination of different histologic grades. Such lesions may also be multicentric. It is important to recognize growth patterns because they can determine the best therapeutic approach.

Large tumors of the penis may be treated conservatively if they are verruciform or superficially spreading, whereas small vertical growth tumors often require radical surgery and lymphadenectomy.

Histologic Subtypes

The majority of penile carcinomas show a conventional nonverruciform keratinizing squamous cell appearance (SCC of usual type). Other histologic variants included in the WHO histologic classification of penile SCCs are basaloid carcinoma (BC), warty (condylomatous) carcinoma, verrucous carcinoma, papillary carcinoma, sarcomatoid carcinoma, mixed carcinomas, and adenosquamous carcinomas.[9,162,166–169] Additional histologic variants such as pseudohyperplastic SCC, mixed warty–basaloid, papillary basaloid, carcinoma cuniculatum, acantholytic SCC, and clear cell SCC have also been described[3,9,170–174] (Box 14-3).

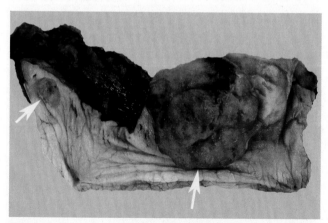

FIGURE 14-40 ■ Multicentric squamous cell carcinoma of the foreskin. There are two separate neoplasms, each of which is indicated by an *arrow*. The smaller tumor was a well-differentiated SCC, and the larger one was a sarcomatoid.

Box 14-3 ● SQUAMOUS CELL CARCINOMA OF PENIS: HISTOLOGIC VARIANTS

SCC, usual type
Basaloid carcinoma
Warty carcinoma
Verrucous carcinoma
Carcinoma cuniculatum
Papillary SCC (NOS)
Sarcomatoid carcinoma
Acantholytic/adenoid SCC
Adenosquamous SCC
Pseudohyperplastic SCC
Mixed SCC (warty–basaloid; hybrid verrucous/usual type SCC)

Squamous Cell Carcinoma, Usual Type

Invasive keratinizing carcinoma without any special features is similar to squamous carcinomas of other sites.[175–183] It is the most common type of penile cancer, accounting for 60% to 70% of all cases. The most frequent clinical presentation is that of an irregular mass in the glans penis with or without palpable inguinal lymph nodes. Enlarged metastatic inguinal lymph nodes associated with an occult primary penile cancer owing to severe phimosis is a less likely but possible presentation.

The median age is about 58 years. Grossly, it appears as an irregular granular mass with variably, flat, exophytic, or even polypoid surface. Large lesions tend to be ulcerated. The cut surface shows a white to tan solid irregular tumor with either superficial or deep penetration into the various penile anatomical layers. Microscopically, SCC of the usual type is an infiltrating keratinizing squamous carcinoma that can be classified based on a three-grade system.[3,9,164] Well-differentiated (grade 1) tumors are characterized by squamous cells with almost normal to slightly enlarged nuclei and abundant eosinophilic cytoplasm. Intercellular bridges are easily identified and keratinization is prominent. There is minimal pleomorphism, usually seen near the basal layer (Fig. 14-41A). Moderately differentiated (grade 2) carcinomas show a more disorganized growth compared to grade 1 lesions, higher nuclear cytoplasmic ratio, evident mitoses, and, although present, less prominent keratinization (Fig. 14-41B). The majority of the SCC of usual type show moderate degree of differentiation. Poorly differentiated (grade 3) neoplasms show little to no keratinization. In such lesions, the tumoral cells are arranged as solid sheets or irregular aggregates, nests or cords. The atypical cells

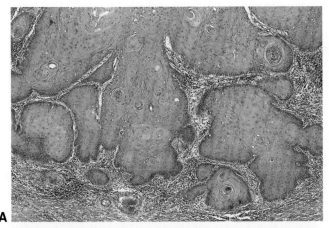

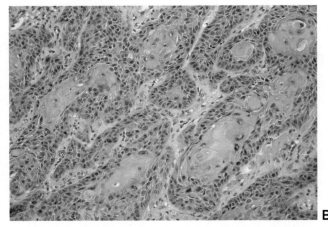

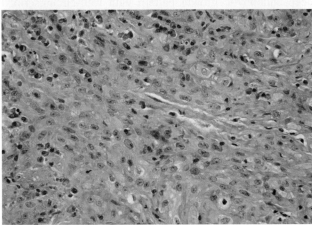

FIGURE 14-41 ■ Squamous cell carcinoma, usual type. **A:** Well-differentiated tumor composed of neoplastic cells with ample eosinophilic cytoplasm and relatively uniform nuclei; **(B)** moderately differentiated neoplasm showing more pleomorphic nuclei compared with well-differentiated lesions; **(C)** poorly differentiated SCC showing sheets and cords of neoplastic cells with high nuclear/cytoplasmic ratio and scant or no keratinization.

show marked nuclear pleomorphism, high nuclear cytoplasmic ratio, prominent nucleoli, and numerous mitosis figures (Fig. 14-41C). A tumor should be graded on the least differentiated element even if this constitutes only a minor component of the neoplasm. Any proportion of grade 3 should be reported.[184,185] Poorly differentiated areas may be focal. When they are the predominant component, it may be difficult to establish the true nature of the neoplasm. In these cases, immunohistochemical studies may be necessary to achieve the diagnosis and to differentiate these tumors from other less common malignancies such as melanoma and sarcoma. Urothelial urethral carcinomas can also be confused with poorly differentiated solid variants of SCC. Urethral neoplasms usually affect the ventral portion of the penis and show no evidence of squamous intraepithelial atypia; the identification of urothelial carcinoma in situ in urethral epithelium or the history of a previous bladder cancer facilitates the diagnosis. Unusual patterns such as pseudohyperplastic, acantholytic, spindle cell, lymphoepithelioma-like, trabecular, giant cell/pleomorphic, small cell, rhabdoid, and clear cell may be focally seen. The stroma shows a mild to severe inflammatory lymphoplasmacytic infiltrate. Eosinophils are occasionally prominent. Foreign body–type giant cell reaction to the keratin may be noted, especially in highly keratinized tumors. Desmoplasia is unusual. The adjacent epidermis usually shows squamous hyperplasia. Associated PeIN is present in two-thirds of the cases. Lichen sclerosus can be seen in the adjacent mucosa, especially associated with low-grade carcinomas of the foreskin.

Basaloid Carcinoma

Basaloid carcinoma is an aggressive, high-grade, and deeply invasive penile neoplasm, usually associated with HPV.[167] It accounts for 5% to 10% of all penile cancers; the median age is 52. More than half the patients show enlarged inguinal nodes owing to metastasis at the time of diagnosis. The glans is the main location. Grossly, there is a rather flat, ulcerated irregular mass. The cut surface shows a solid, tan tissue usually replacing corpus spongiosum, with involvement of albuginea and corpora cavernosa. Minute dot-like necrotic foci within the tumor are frequently seen (Fig. 14-38A and B). Microscopically, characteristic solid infiltrative nests composed of monotonous blue round small tumor cells are noted (Fig. 14-42A and B). These tumoral aggregates may show peripheral palisading surrounded by peripheral clefts and central foci of comedonecrosis (Fig. 14-42C). The cells are small, with a high nuclear/cytoplasmic ratio, similar to basal cells, and show inconspicuous nucleoli. Numerous mitoses are characteristic of this lesion. A starry-sky appearance may be noted because of prominent apoptosis (Fig. 14-42B). Occasionally, the central areas of the neoplastic aggregates show pleomorphic cells with larger size. Focal and abrupt keratinization in the central portion of the nests can be seen in some cases. The adjacent epidermis usually shows atypical

basal cell hyperplasia, basaloid or mixed basaloid/warty PeIN (Figs. 14-31 and 14-33), and, less often, warty carcinoma in situ (Fig. 14-32). The stroma may show chronic inflammatory cells or hyalinization. Lymphovascular invasion tends to be prominent (Fig. 14-42D). The mortality rate of patients with BC is near 60%.[167] Most BCs have a flat and often ulcerated surface. A rare papillary variant of BC has been recently described. These tumors have a better prognosis than the classical type of BC; however, deeply invasive tumors were associated with regional nodal metastasis indicating a potential for tumor-related death.[171]

Warty (Condylomatous) Carcinoma

Warty carcinomas are unusual, low- to intermediate-grade, slowly growing malignant tumors with a verruciform pattern, identical to their counterpart in the vulva.[168,186] Because of their prominent HPV-related changes, they have some morphologic features that may be confused with condyloma.[3,9,22,168] Grossly, the tumors are exo-endophytic, cauliflower-like measuring 5 cm in average diameter. The surface of the tumor may show a cobblestone appearance. The cut surface reveals a papillomatous growth, with frequent deep penetration into corpus spongiosum or cavernosum (Fig. 14-43A). The deep border varies from irregular to broad and pushing. Microscopically, an arborescent papillary pattern is noted (Fig. 14-43B and D). The papillae are long, undulating, rounded, or spiky, with prominent fibrovascular cores (Fig. 14-43B and D). The neoplastic cells are pleomorphic with prominent koilocytic changes (enlarged nuclei with irregular contours, binucleation, clear perinuclear halo, and dyskeratosis are prominent) (Fig. 14-43C and F). Compared to benign condylomata, these HPV-related changes are not restricted to the surface but are present throughout the tumor, including in its deep portion (Fig. 14-43E). The boundary between the neoplasm and stroma is infiltrative (jagged) in the majority of cases; however, some cases may show a predominantly pushing border. Intraepithelial abscesses may be prominent, especially in the basal areas. Hyperkeratosis and atypical parakeratosis are prominent. In some cases a deep endophytic growth pattern with well-circumscribed deep pseudocystic nodular aggregates can be seen. Some warty carcinomas may show prominent clear cell features (Fig. 14-43F). These clear cell squamous cell carcinomas should be differentiated from sweat gland carcinomas and metastatic renal clear cell carcinomas to the penis. Warty carcinomas should be distinguished from giant condylomata (Box 14-4), which are benign tumors with koilocytosis restricted to the surface and pushing deep borders. Benign condylomata lacks the cellular pleomorphism seen in warty carcinomas. Verrucous and papillary carcinomas show no HPV-related changes. Warty carcinomas may be associated with regional lymph node metastasis and this appears to be more frequent in deeply invasive and high-grade tumors. Warty carcinomas have an intermediate biologic behavior, between

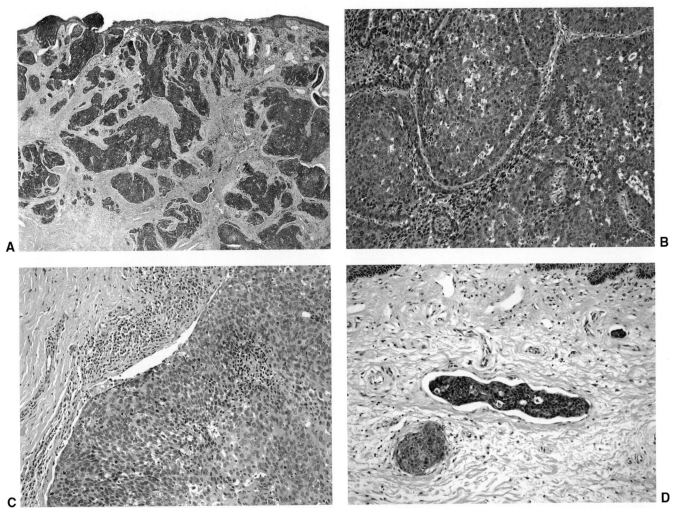

FIGURE 14-42 ■ Basaloid carcinoma. **A:** Solid and confluent infiltrative nests composed of small blue round cells with scant cytoplasm. **B:** Higher-power view of the infiltrating nests composed of a monotonous population of small basaloid cells with high mitotic rate. Note the starry-sky appearance due to prominent apoptosis. **C:** Cleft formation between the tumor aggregate and the stroma. **D:** Lymphovascular invasion is commonly identified in BCs.

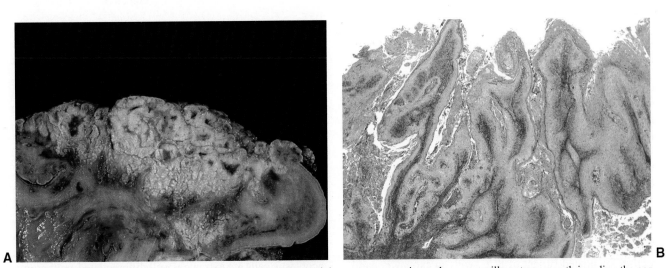

FIGURE 14-43 ■ Warty carcinoma. **A:** Cut surface of a partial penectomy specimen shows a papillomatous growth invading the corpus spongiosum. The epithelium of the papillae is white, and the vascular core appears dark in this picture. **B:** Low-power view of a warty carcinoma showing long undulating papillae and deep jagged borders.

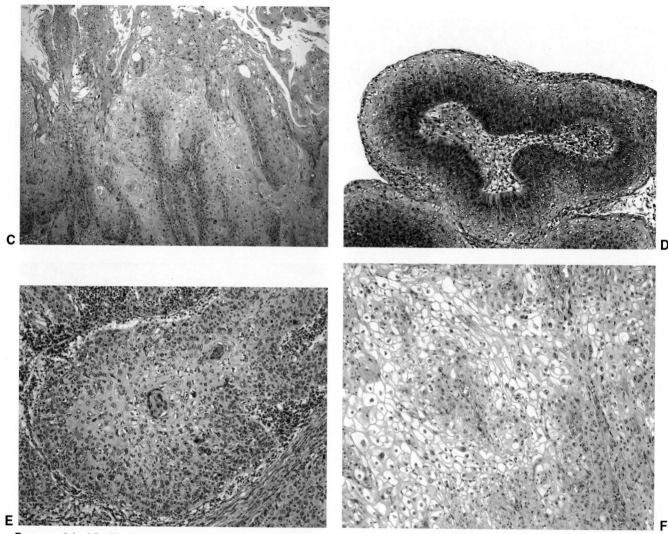

FIGURE 14-43 ■ *(Continued)* **C:** Higher-power view of the papillae-prominent koilocytosis. **D:** The papillae of warty carcinoma vary from long and spiky to round. This picture illustrates a round papilla similar to those seen in condylomata. **E:** Koilocytosis is not restricted to the surface but also present in deep invasive portions of the tumor. **F:** Warty carcinoma with prominent clear cell features.

other types of low-grade verruciform tumors (verrucous, papillary) and the usual SCC of the penis.

Warty carcinoma is the most frequent variant of penile carcinoma seen in immunosuppressed patients. It has been shown that p16 overexpression is strongly associated with high-risk HPV (16 and 18)-related carcinomas in different locations including the penis.[187,188] The majority of BCs, warty carcinomas, and warty/BCs (high-risk HPV-related tumors) show diffuse p16 expression while the majority of the non–HPV-related tumors do not overexpress p16.[188]

Verrucous Carcinoma

Verrucous carcinoma is an unusual, slowly growing, extremely well-differentiated variant of SCC, with an exophytic papillary appearance and characteristic broadly based boundary between tumor and stroma (Figs. 14-39A and B, 14-44A)

(Box 14-4).[3,166,189–191] Grossly, they are exophytic white-gray neoplasms measuring from 1 to 3 cm in diameter; larger destructive lesions can be seen but they usually harbor hybrid/higher-grade areas. Verrucous carcinomas commonly affect the glans or the foreskin. Microscopically, the lesions are characterized by thick acanthotic papillae with thin and generally inconspicuous fibrovascular cores. There is prominent piling up of keratin between the papillae sometimes forming keratin craters (Figs. 14-44B and 14-45B). Orthokeratosis, with presence of keratohyaline granules, is frequently present, but parakeratosis may also be seen. Koilocytosis is not a feature of verrucous carcinoma; however, occasional vacuolated clear cells (likely not true koilocytes) may be seen at the surface. In any case, these changes are nonprominent. The neoplastic cells are extremely well differentiated, with prominent intercellular bridges (Fig. 14-44C). There is minimal atypia at the base of the nests as well as rare mitosis. The

Verrucous carcinoma
    Papillary surface without koilocytosis
    Broad pushing base
    HPV-unrelated
Carcinoma cuniculatum
    Variant of verrucous carcinoma
    Deep invaginations
Papillary carcinoma (NOS)
    Papillary surface without koilocytosis
    Irregular/ infiltrative base
    HPV-unrelated
Warty carcinoma
    Papillary surface with prominent koilocytosis
    Irregular/infiltrative base
    Koilocytosis throughout the tumor
    HPV-related (High-risk HPV-16 and -18)
Condyloma acuminatum/giant condyloma
    Benign lesion
    Papillary surface with koilocytosis
    Koilocytosis limited to the surface
    Broad/pushing base
    HPV-related (Low-risk HPV-6 and -11)

base of the tumor is broad and pushing and sometimes shows a characteristic club-shaped pattern (Fig. 14-44B and C). A dense inflammatory cell infiltrate may obscure the boundaries between tumor and stroma. Most verrucous carcinomas are limited to the lamina propria; deeper invasion is unusual but may occur. The majority of large and deep verrucous carcinomas harbor smaller foci of invasive carcinoma of the usual type.[195] These mixed or hybrid variants should be distinguished from pure verrucous carcinomas. In our experience, pure verrucous carcinomas have an excellent prognosis while hybrid verrucous carcinomas are associated with regional metastasis in approximately 25% of the cases.[166,191] The presence of regional metastasis in verrucous carcinomas is related to higher-grade areas and deeper infiltration. Verrucous carcinomas can be associated with local recurrence (up to a third of the cases in different series), and this may be related to insufficient surgery or due to multicentricity. Multicentric carcinomas are usually seen in the setting of long-standing lichen sclerosus (Fig. 14-44A). The absence of koilocytosis helps to distinguished verrucous carcinoma from giant condyloma and warty carcinoma. Verrucous carcinoma does not

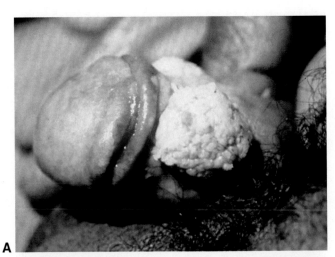

A

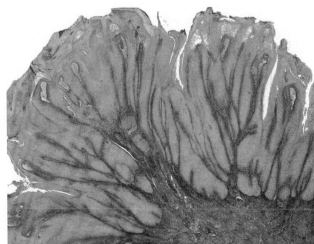

B

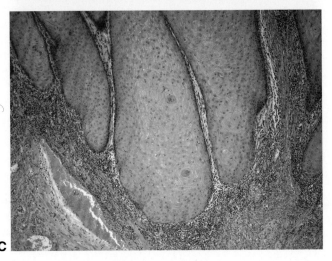

C

FIGURE 14-44 ■ Verrucous carcinoma. **A:** Two separate preputial verrucous carcinomas arising in a background of lichen sclerosus. **B, C:** Low-power view illustrating the verrucous surface and bulbous and club-shaped deep borders. The papillae show thick acanthotic epithelium and thin fibrovascular cores. Note the characteristic piling up of orange keratin among the papillae. Higher-power view to illustrate the high degree of differentiation and bulbous, pushing deep borders.

show the pleomorphic features and jagged borders that are seen in warty carcinoma. Papillary carcinomas can be very similar to verrucous, but they are more atypical and show infiltrative, jagged deep borders.

Carcinoma Cuniculatum

This unusual tumor was originally described by Ayrd et al.[192] in the plantar skin as a peculiar variant of verrucous carcinoma characterized by a deep burrowing growth pattern mimicking rabbit burrows (cuniculum) (Box 14-4). Rare cases have been reported in the penis.[173] The patients' mean age is 77 years. Grossly, the tumors are large, papillomatous lesions with cobblestone appearance, usually affecting the glans and extending to the coronal sulcus and foreskin. Cut surfaces show the hallmark of the lesion represented by deep and narrow, complex tumor invaginations that connect to the surface through sinus tracts (Fig. 14-45A). Microscopically, the bulk of the lesion has features of a verrucous carcinoma (extremely well differentiated with bulbous deep borders) (Fig. 14-45B) usually associated with a minor component that is more infiltrative and less differentiated. In most cases, therefore, it represents a hybrid verrucous/usual SCC with a peculiar growth pattern. The deep invaginations form interanastomosing channels and pseudocystic structures that are lined by well-differentiated carcinoma and filled with keratin material (Fig. 14-45C). Carcinoma cuniculatum appears to have a good prognosis. None of the reported cases metastasized.[173]

Papillary Carcinoma

Papillary carcinoma is an exophytic, slowly growing, low-grade squamous cell carcinoma without HPV-related changes that usually shows an irregular infiltrating base (Box 14-4).[9,193] The diagnosis is made by exclusion of the other more specific types of verruciform tumors. It is usually located in the glans, although other compartments also may be involved. Inguinal lymph node metastasis is unusual. Grossly, they are white-gray exophytic destructive lesions. The cut surface usually shows a pearly white tumor with a serrated papillomatous surface and ill-defined deep borders. Microscopically, the appearance is that of a well-differentiated papillary squamous neoplasm. Hyperkeratosis and acanthosis are prominent. The papillae are variable, short or long, usually with prominent

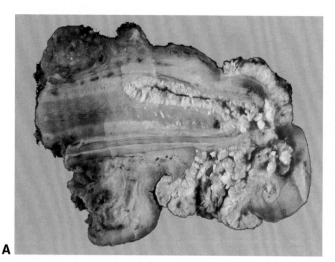

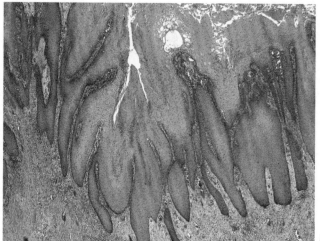

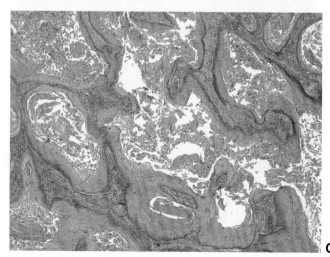

FIGURE 14-45 ■ Carcinoma cuniculatum. **A:** Cut section of a partial penectomy specimen illustrating the characteristic deep burrowing pattern. **B:** Microscopically, most of the tumor looks like a verrucous carcinoma. Note the club-shaped deep borders and piling up of keratin among the acanthotic papillae. **C:** Interanastomosing sinus-like structures lined by a well-differentiated squamous cell carcinoma and filled with keratin.

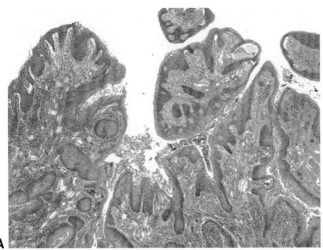

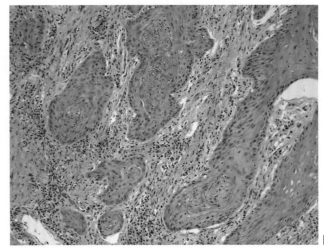

FIGURE 14-46 ■ Papillary carcinoma. **A:** Complex arborescent papillae with prominent fibrovascular cores. The tumor is well to moderately differentiated. **B:** The interface between the tumor and stroma is infiltrative.

fibrovascular cores (Fig. 14-46A). Keratin cysts or intraepithelial abscesses can be noted. Koilocytotic-like changes may be present focally but are never prominent. The base of the lesion is irregular and infiltrative (Fig. 14-46B). Verrucous carcinomas share some architectural (papillary surface) and cytologic (degree of differentiation and lack of koilocytosis) features with papillary carcinoma; however, the deep border of verrucous carcinoma is classically broad and pushing compared to the jagged borders of papillary carcinoma. In addition, papillary carcinoma tends to be slightly less differentiated that verrucous carcinoma, especially in deeper portions of the neoplasm. Warty carcinomas can be distinguished from papillary carcinomas by the marked pleomorphism and koilocytosis.

Sarcomatoid Carcinoma

Sarcomatoid carcinomas are uncommon (representing approximately 4% of penile carcinomas), high-grade tumors, predominantly composed of spindle cells.[194–196] The patients' mean age is 60 years. Grossly, tumors are large, polypoid, and ulcerated masses frequently affecting the glans and deeply invading corpora spongiosa and cavernosa (Fig. 14-47A and B). Microscopically, the neoplasms are predominantly composed of atypical spindle cells disposed in interlacing fascicles, resembling fibrosarcoma or leiomyosarcoma (Fig. 14-48A), sometimes admixed with pleomorphic giant cells mimicking malignant fibrous histiocytoma. Myxoid changes may be prominent. Lesions showing a prominent pseudovascular pattern

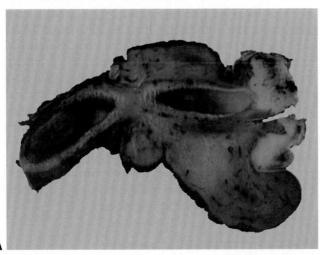

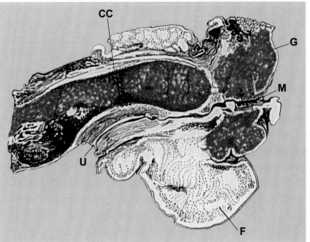

FIGURE 14-47 ■ Sarcomatoid carcinoma. **A, B:** Cut surface and diagram of a penectomy specimen with an ulcerated and large tumor deeply invading into the corpus spongiosum of the glans and extending into the coronal sulcus and foreskin. There are satellite nodules in the corpus cavernosum; this last feature is frequent in this highly aggressive neoplasm. The primary tumor and satellite nodules are shown in red in the diagram. F, foreskin; G, glans; CC, corpus cavernosum; U, urethra; M, meatus.

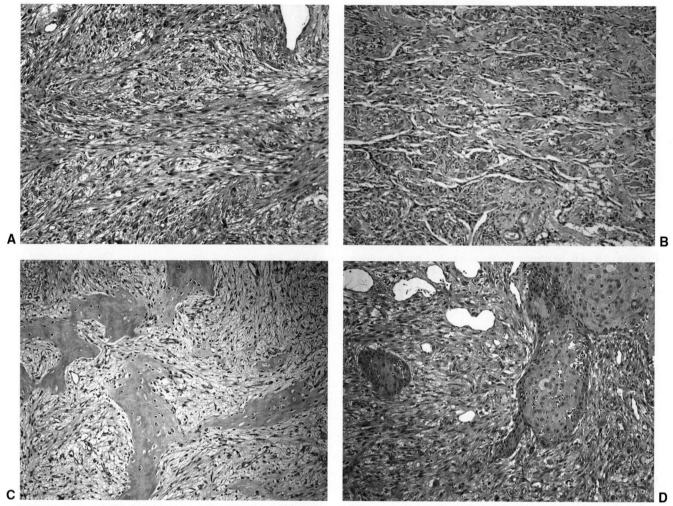

FIGURE 14-48 ■ Sarcomatoid carcinoma. **A:** Microscopically, these tumors are predominantly composed of interlacing fascicles of spindle cells simulating a sarcoma. **B:** Sarcomatoid carcinoma with angiosarcomatoid features. **C:** Sarcomatoid carcinoma with bone formation. **D:** Foci of clear-cut squamous differentiation may be present and are usually a minor component.

mimicking angiosarcoma have been described (Fig. 14-48B).[195] Mitotic figures are numerous, and necrosis is prominent. Foci of bone and cartilaginous heterologous differentiation (osteosarcomatous and chondrosarcomatous components) may be observed (Fig. 14-48C). Because foci of carcinoma in situ and a clear-cut keratinizing invasive component may be very focal (Fig. 14-48D), multiple sections and immunohistochemical studies may be necessary to make a correct diagnosis. The spindle cells are usually positive for vimentin, different cytokeratins, and p63. In our experience, cytokeratin 34betaE12 and p63 appear to be the more specific and sensitive markers to categorize these tumors as epithelial (Fig. 14-49A and B).[195] AE1/AE3 and Cam 5.2 tend to be more variably and focally positive, sometimes highlighting only scattered single cells. Smooth muscle actin may be focally positive; however, desmin and S-100 are negative. Penile sarcomatoid carcinomas are aggressive tumors usually associated with lymph node metastasis and poor outcome.[198,199] Differential diagnoses include different sarcomas and melanoma. Penile sarcomas are exceedingly rare tumors, usually arising in deep tissues (such as the corpora

cavernosa). A poorly differentiated spindle cell neoplasm arising from the epithelium of the distal penis most likely represents a sarcomatoid carcinoma. In advanced ulcerated lesions, the connection to the overlying epithelium may be difficult to prove and occasionally they may be mostly (or even entirely) composed of spindle cells. A large tumor involving and ulcerating the distal penis most likely represents a sarcomatoid carcinoma, despite lack of clear-cut connection to the epithelium. When present, identification of PeIN in the adjacent epithelium and foci showing clear-cut squamous differentiation are helpful in making the diagnosis of carcinoma. When these features are not present and the tumor is entirely composed of spindle cells (monophasic sarcomatoid carcinomas), immunohistochemical analysis is crucial in making the diagnosis.

Pseudohyperplastic Carcinomas

Pseudohyperplastic squamous cell carcinomas are nonverruciform low-grade tumors preferentially affecting the foreskin of older patients (eighth decade) and strongly

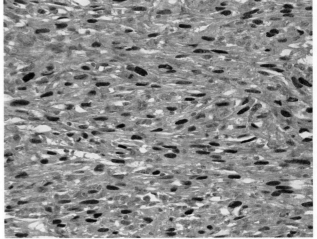

FIGURE 14-49 ■ Sarcomatoid carcinoma, immunohistochemistry. **A:** The expression of cytokeratin 34BetaE12 by the spindle cells supports the epithelial nature of the neoplasm. **B:** Immunohistochemical stain for p63 shows diffuse nuclear expression.

associated with lichen sclerosus.[79,172] There is extreme differentiation and in small biopsies the tumors mimic pseudoepitheliomatous hyperplasia. They are often multicentric and the second or third independent tumor may show some verrucous features. Grossly, they are flat or slightly elevated lesions measuring about 2 cm. Characteristic microscopic features are keratinizing nests of squamous cells with no or minimal atypia surrounded by a reactive stroma (Fig. 14-50A and B). This degree of differentiation is noted only in low-grade verruciform tumors such as verrucous or papillary cancers. The consistent association with lichen sclerosus suggests that this inflammatory condition may play a precancerous role. In a series of 10 cases, recurrence was noted in the glans of 1 patient who was circumcised for a multicentric carcinoma of the foreskin 2 years after diagnosis. No metastases were found in any of these cases.[79,172]

Acantholytic (Pseudoglandular or Adenoid) SCC

The unusual variant of SCC is characterized by the presence of pseudoglandular spaces secondary to acantholysis (Fig. 14-51).[174] The patient's median age is 54 years. Tumors tend to be large, involve multiple penile anatomical compartments, and deeply invade into erectile corpora. The pseudoglandular spaces contain acantholytic neoplastic keratinocytes sometimes admixed with keratin material and necrotic debris. Carcinoembryonic antigen (CEA) and mucin stains are negative. Acantholytic squamous cell carcinomas usually harbor high-grade foci, invade deep anatomical structures, and therefore tend to be associated with a high incidence of regional metastasis and mortality. The differential diagnosis includes gland forming penile tumors (surface adenosquamous, mucoepidermoid, and urethral adenocarcinomas) and angiosarcoma.

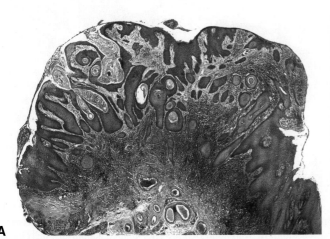

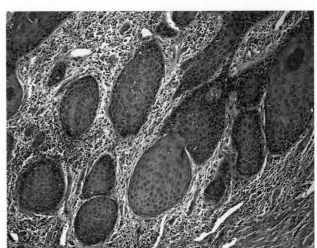

FIGURE 14-50 ■ **A, B:** Pseudohyperplastic squamous cell carcinoma. Low-power and high-power views of this extremely well-differentiated carcinoma that may be confused with pseudoepitheliomatous hyperplasia.

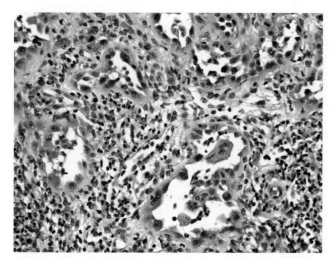

FIGURE 14-51 ■ Squamous cell carcinoma with acantholytic features. Note the presence of acantholytic neoplastic cells within the pseudoglandular spaces.

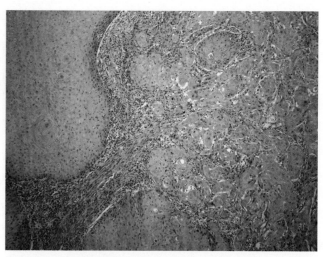

FIGURE 14-52 ■ Hybrid carcinoma, mixed verrucous and usual type. This tumor shows, in addition to areas of verrucous carcinoma (**left**), other less differentiated foci of squamous cell carcinoma of the usual type (**right**). These mixed tumors have a worse prognosis when compared with pure verrucous carcinoma.

Mixed Squamous Cell Carcinomas

Squamous cell carcinomas of the usual type can be found in association with any other subtypes of penile cancer. Mixed carcinomas account for about 25% of penile SCCs. The classical example is that of a verrucous carcinoma with higher-grade foci consisting of usual SCC, so-called *hybrid carcinoma* (Fig. 14-52).[191] The metastatic potential of these hybrid tumors is related to the grade and depth of invasion of the nonverrucous component. Another interesting tumor is the *warty basaloid*, where an exophytic warty tumor is associated with a deeply invasive BC[170] (Fig. 14-53). The clinical behavior is related to the basaloid component, with a high rate of regional metastasis. As warty and BCs, the mixed variant also overexpresses p16. Another rare mixed tumor is the SCC, usual type, admixed with neuroendocrine areas.[9]

Adenosquamous Carcinoma

Adenosquamous carcinoma is an exceedingly rare form of mixed carcinoma probably originating from misplaced glandular cells in the perimeatal region of the penis.[169] Grossly, the lesions are large and indistinguishable from the usual variant of SCC. Cut sections show a firm and granular tumor deeply invading the corpus spongiosum or cavernosum. Microscopically, these are biphasic tumors showing squamous cell and glandular differentiation (Fig. 14-54). The squamous component predominates in most cases. The glands are mucin producing and stain for CEA and with mucicarmine. PeIN is usually present in the adjacent epithelium. Adenosquamous carcinomas of the penis should be

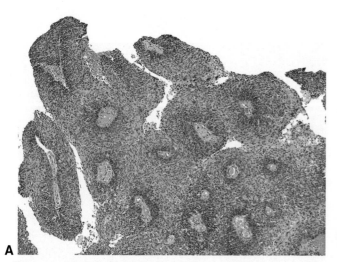

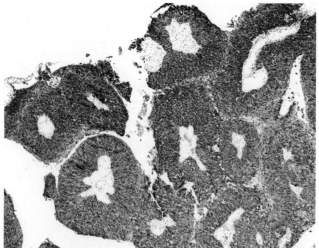

A   **B**

FIGURE 14-53 ■ Warty–basaloid (mixed) carcinoma. **A:** The upper portion of the lesion is predominantly composed of neoplastic cells with marked koilocytic changes; the lower portion is predominantly basaloid. **B:** Warty and BCs are HPV-related neoplasms; therefore immunohistochemical stain for p16 usually shows diffuse expression in warty, basaloid, and warty/basaloid tumors. The latter is illustrated in this picture.

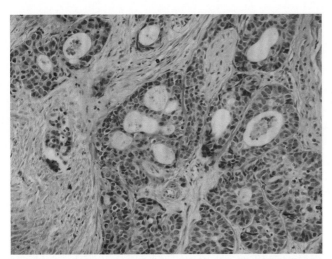

FIGURE 14-54 ■ Adenosquamous carcinoma. Biphasic squamous and glandular infiltrating carcinoma. Note the presence of perineural invasion.

distinguished from the acantholytic SCC, adenosquamous (mucoepidermoid) carcinomas of the urethra,[9] and adenocarcinoma arising in Littre glands.

Molecular Changes in Penile Carcinomas

Molecular, immunohistochemical, and genetic studies support the notion that penile cancer occurs through mechanisms both dependent and independent of HPV.[197–218] The overall prevalence of HPV DNA detection in penile cancers is approximately 40% to 45%, and this figure is very similar to that detected in vulvar carcinomas.[55] No significant differences in HPV prevalence were seen when comparing cases from the United States and Paraguay.[55] Although HPV reveals a remarkable plurality of different genotypes, only a limited number are associated with penile carcinomas. High-risk HPV-16 is by far the most frequent type associated with penile cancer, followed by HPV-18. Tumor types that are significantly related to HPV include the warty and basaloid variants. It is believed that HPV infection by itself is insufficient to induce malignant transformation so that additional cellular changes are necessary in the tumorigenic process. Two viral oncoproteins, E6 and E7, appear crucial in the process of carcinogenesis. The HPV oncogenic product E6 interferes with the p53 pathway causing suppression of the p53 normal inhibitory function of the cell cycle.[45–47] The retinoblastoma protein (pRB) is a target of the viral oncoprotein E7; thus its inactivation appears to contribute to carcinogenic events interfering with the p16INK4a/cyclinD/retinoblastoma pathway. Although E6 and E7 proteins may immortalize various types of human cells independently, their cooperative interaction leads to a substantial enhancement in immortalization efficiency. Several studies in cervix, vulvar, and penile cancers support the hypothesis that p16INK4a is a specific marker for cells that express the viral E6-E7 oncogenes.[187,188] Since expression of p16INK4a underlies a negative feedback control through pRB, the enhanced expression of p16 is probably due to reduced or lost pRB function. Binding of HPV-E7 oncoprotein to pRb causes degradation of pRb with consequent loss of Rb-tumor suppressor function and p16 overexpression, which can be demonstrated immunohistochemically. Basaloid, warty, and warty–BCs show a significant overexpression of p16 when compared with HPV-unrelated variants (Fig. 14-53B).[188] Interestingly, the precursor lesions of HPV-related tumors (basaloid, warty, and warty/basaloid PeIN) are also strongly positive for p16 (Fig. 14-34) while the majority of precursor lesions of HPV-unrelated tumors (differentiated PeIN and lichen sclerosus) do not express p16, further supporting the concept of a bimodal pathway of tumor progression.

It is important to recognize that the majority (approximately 55% to 60%) of penile cancers appear to be HPV-unrelated. There are data indicating that both HPV-related and -unrelated modes of p16INK4a cyclin D/Rb inactivation exist in penile carcinoma. The tumor suppressor gene Tp53 and its functional protein product p53 are believed to be involved in the HPV-unrelated pathway of carcinogenesis as well. Taking into consideration that mutant p53 accumulates in the cells, several studies analyzing the expression of p53 in invasive penile carcinoma have been done. The overall expression of the proteins varies between 40% and 89%.[202,203] The evidence linking p53 expression and presence of HPV DNA in penile cancer is contradictory. Lam and Chan[204] studied 42 penile carcinomas for HPV and p53 protein status and found that all HPV-positive cases showed p53 immunostaining. However, several other reports have shown an inverse or negative relation between these two factors. In a recent study on verruciform tumors, we found p53 expression to be independent from p16 expression (therefore independent from high-risk HPV infection) and its expression was preferentially seen in less differentiated areas supporting the concept that p53 expression is a marker of worse prognosis. Lopes et al.[206] showed that p53 expression was an independent predictor of lymph node metastasis on multivariate analysis. Patients with p53-negative tumors had a significantly better overall survival. Overall outcome was significantly worse if tumors were positive for p53 and HPV DNA. In this study, patients who were HPV positive but p53 negative had the best survival rates. Patients who died of disease also expressed higher levels of p53. p53-negative tumors were associated with higher overall survival. It is important to keep in mind that overexpression of p53 does not necessarily indicate a p53 mutation. Castren et al. found absence of p53 mutations in benign and premalignant lesions that overexpressed p53 by immunohistochemistry. These findings suggest that overexpression of p53 does not indicate a p53 mutation in these lesions and that p53 mutations are not important, or at least not early, events in male genital carcinogenesis.[200]

Many other molecular markers have been investigated. Considering that p21 and p53 interplay in the regulation of the cell cycle, Lam and Chan analyzed the expression of both markers in penile carcinomas. p21 was found in 40% of invasive carcinomas and its expression was also seen in the adjacent dysplastic epithelium. An inverse relationship between p21 and p53 was seen in 50% of the squamous cell carcinomas.[206] Telomerase activity was found in 85% of invasive penile carcinomas, but also in over 80% of normal epithelium and corpus cavernosum.[208] Cytogenetic changes have been described, but none are characteristic.[209,210] Missense mutation in the c-RasHa codon 61was found only in the second metastasis of a penile carcinoma with HPV-18. This suggests that changes in *ras* may be associated with late progression.[211] Up-regulation of COX-2 and prostaglandin synthase 1 was shown in a small cohort of patients with penile cancer.[212] The use of DNA ploidy in penile cancer is controversial. Some studies found no prognostic significance and others found that diploid cancers had a better prognosis than aneuploid tumors.[213,214] With the aim to explore the disease progression, Campos et al. analyzed E-cadherin (involved in intercellular adhesion) and matrix metalloproteinases (MMP-2 and MMP-9; involved in breakdown of extracellular matrix) in 125 patients with penile cancer. They demonstrated that low E-cadherin immunoreactivity is associated with greater risk of lymph node metastasis and high MMP-9 expression appears to be an independent risk factor for disease recurrence.[215]

A study of the MYC cytogenetic profile by fluorescence in situ hybridization found that MYC gains progressively increased during penile squamous cell carcinoma progression from in situ samples to metastases.[216] A recent study suggests that SOX2 amplification and consequent SOX2 protein overexpression may represent important mechanisms of tumor initiation and progression in a considerable subset of SCCs, including penile carcinomas.[217]

A clearer picture is slowly emerging from these reports, with most cases of penile SCCs following a different and yet-to-be-determined pathway involving p53,[218] whereas HPV is involved in the tumorigenesis of only a subset of penile carcinomas, preferentially basaloid and warty carcinomas.

Pathologic Factors Related to Prognosis

Pathologic factors related to the presence of lymph node metastasis and prognosis in penile cancer are tumor location, tumor size, growth pattern, histologic type, histologic grade, depth of invasion, vascular invasion, and perineural invasion.[219–236] Tumors exclusively of the foreskin (Figs. 14-48 to 14-70) carry a better prognosis than those of the glans because low-grade and superficially invasive variants of SCC more frequently arise in the foreskin.[82,172,224] There is a correlation between tumor pattern of growth and the presence of regional metastasis and survival.[164,225,229] The incidence of metastasis in verruciform tumors is minimal. Mortality in patients with superficially spreading carcinomas is 10%, compared with 67% for patients with vertical growth pattern.[225] If we exclude verruciform neoplasms (that tend to be large but well differentiated), there is a correlation between larger tumor size and metastasis. There is also a correlation between histologic type and regional metastasis and

outcome.[235] Metastasis and mortality in verrucous, papillary, and warty (condylomatous) carcinomas are rare. Basaloid and sarcomatoid carcinomas show a high rate of metastasis and mortality.[225] In a recent study of 333 patients with homogeneous surgical treatment we found that higher histologic grade, deeper anatomical infiltration, and vascular and perineural invasion were common findings in sarcomatoid, basaloid, and adenosquamous carcinoma cases, correlating with a higher rate of nodal metastasis and mortality. These features were unusual in verrucous, papillary, and warty carcinoma cases.[224] Taking into consideration the presence of nodal metastasis and mortality, we found that SCC can be divided into low-, intermediate-, and high-risk groups. Verrucous, papillary, and warty carcinomas are in the low-risk group for nodal metastasis, usual and mixed SCC fall in the intermediate-risk group, and sarcomatoid, basaloid, and adenosquamous belong to the high-risk group.[224] The prognostic influence of HPV infection in patients with penile cancer is controversial and the evidence contradictory. A large series found that high-risk HPV-related cancers were associated with an overall better survival.[237] The histologic grade correlates with prognosis. A major study found an incidence of regional metastasis in 24%, 46%, and 82% of patients with well, moderate, and poorly differentiated tumors, respectively.[229] We have found that any proportion of grade 3 adversely affects prognosis.[184] There is also a correlation between depth of tumor infiltration and presence of inguinal metastasis in penile SCC. Measurement of depth of tumor invasion in millimeters may be performed from the basement membrane of adjacent squamous epithelium to the deepest point of invasion.[221] In cases of large destructive and bulky exophytic tumors, it may be more practical to measure the thickness from the nonkeratinizing surface of the tumor to the deepest point of invasion. The evaluation of the anatomic levels of tumor invasion is valid for all cancers. The stage of the primary lesion in the current TNM system is based on anatomical levels of invasion (Tables 14-1 and 14-2).[238] Superficial neoplasms, especially those infiltrating only the lamina propria (<5 mm), have minimal to almost no risk of regional spread. The risk for metastasis increases in tumors infiltrating more than 5 mm and it is especially high when corpora cavernosa (glans) and dermis (foreskin) are affected. The limitation of this method is that corpus spongiosum measures approximately 8 to 13 mm in depth and that the threshold for penile carcinoma metastasis is approximately 4 to 6 mm in the corpus spongiosum, suggesting a necessary subdivision in superficial or deep corpus spongiosum. The three statistically more important pathologic factors related to regional metastasis are histologic grade, depth of invasion, and vascular invasion. Because the combination of histologic grade and depth of invasion is thought to better predict metastasis and mortality,[222,223] the use of a prognostic index has been proposed.[239] The prognostic index is measured from 1 to 6 and it results from the addition of the numerical values given to the histologic grade and anatomical level of invasion. The numerical values that are

Table 14-1 ■ TNM CLASSIFICATION OF CARCINOMAS OF THE PENIS

T—primary tumor

TX primary tumor cannot be assessed

T0 No evidence of primary tumor

Tis carcinoma in situ

Ta Noninvasive verrucous carcinoma

T1 Tumor invades subepithelial connective tissue (lamina propria)

T2 Tumor invades corpus spongiosum or cavernosum

T3 Tumor invades urethra or prostate

T4 Tumor invades other adjacent structures

N—Regional lymph nodes

Regional lymph nodes cannot be assessed

N0 No regional lymph metastasis

N1 Metastasis in a single superficial inguinal lymph node

N2 Metastasis in multiple or bilateral superficial inguinal lymph nodes

N3 Metastasis in deep inguinal or pelvic lymph nodes (s), unilateral or bilateral

M—Distant metastasis

MX Distant metastasis cannot be assessed

M0 No distant metastasis

M1 Distant metastasis

given to histologic grades are 1, 2, and 3 (for well, moderately, and poorly differentiated tumors) and anatomic level of invasion (1, 2, and 3; corresponding to lamina propria, corpus spongiosum, and corpus cavernosum in the glans and lamina propria, dartos and skin in the foreskin). When the sum of the two values is <3 (low index), tumors are usually associated with no mortality. Metastatic and mortality rates are high in patients with indexes of 5 and 6.[239] The behavior of tumors with intermediate prognostic indexes is more difficult to predict. We have recently demonstrated that perineural invasion is an independent parameter associated with regional metastasis.[185] The single most important prognostic factor for overall outcome in penile carcinomas is nodal status.[183,227,229,234] Patients with clinically node-negative disease have cancer-specific survival probabilities between 75% and

Table 14-2 ■ TNM STAGE GROUPING FOR PENILE CARCINOMAS

Stage 0	Tis	N0	M0
	Ta	N0	M0
Stage I	T1	N0	M0
Stage II	T1	N1	M0
	T2	N0, N1	M0
Stage III	T1, T2	N2	M0
	T3	N0, N1, N2	M0
Stage IV	T4	Any N	M0
	Any T	N3	M0
	Any T	Any N	M1

93% and those with pathologically proven negative nodes have 5-year cancer-specific survival probabilities ranging from 85% to 100%. While patients with a single positive superficial lymph node on pathology have very good cancer-related outcomes, patients with multiple involved lymph nodes have significantly less favorable outcomes.[227]

An evaluation of clinical and pathologic variables using a nomogram was developed.[240] The selected factors were clinical stage of lymph nodes, microscopic growth pattern, grade, vascular invasion, and invasion of corpora spongiosa and cavernosa and urethra. The probability of nodal metastasis as predicted by the nomogram was close to the real incidence of metastasis observed at follow-up. A second nomogram to estimate predictions of survival at 5 years using the same clinical and pathologic factors gave similar results.[241] More recently, a nomogram using perineural invasion and histologic grade as predictors of mortality in penile tumors 5 to 10 mm thick was developed.[185] In a recent study of a large number of cases, the overall metastasis rate was 24% and the 10-year survival rate was 82%. The highest mortality rate was observed within the first 3 years of follow-up.[224]

Local Spread

Pathways of local tumor spread may be grossly or microscopically detected (Fig. 14-55). Penile tumors may spread from one mucosal compartment to the other. Typically, foreskin carcinomas spread to skin of the shaft, coronal sulcus, or glans; carcinomas originating in the glans may spread to the coronal sulcus and foreskin. Penile SCC may spread horizontally and externally to skin of the shaft and internally to the proximal urethral margin of resection (Fig. 14-55). This centrifugal mode of spread is observed in superficially spreading carcinomas. The vertical spread may sequentially involve from surface to deep areas: (a) in the glans, lamina propria to corpus spongiosum, albuginea, and corpus cavernosum; (b) in the foreskin, lamina propria to dartos and outer skin; and (c) in the sulcus, lamina propria to fascia. This is the pattern of spread of vertical growth carcinoma. An important and underrecognized route of spread of penile

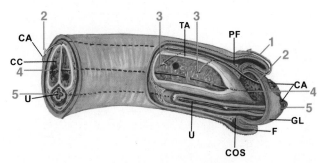

FIGURE 14-55 ■ Local spread of squamous cell carcinoma. Diagram showing possible routes of local spread, from distal penis to shaft and urethral resection margins. The arrows and the green numbers indicate the different pathways. Abbreviations: CA, carcinoma; GL, glans; F, foreskin; COS, coronal sulcus; TA, tunica albuginea; PF, penile fascia; U, urethra; CC, corpus cavernosum.

carcinomas is the penile fascia, a common site of positive surgical margin of resection.[5] The fascial involvement in glans tumors is usually through the coronal sulcus. Tumor compromising fascia may secondarily penetrate into the corpora cavernosa via nutritional vessels and adipose tissue traversing the tunical albuginea (Fig. 14-7). It is not unusual to find rounded nodules of carcinoma separated from the main invasive tumor ("satellite" nodules) in penectomy or circumcision specimens of advanced tumors (Fig. 14-55). These are strong indicators of regional metastasis and poor outcome. Macroscopic evaluation and inclusion of the entire urethral resection margin for microscopic evaluation is crucial. In a series of partial penectomies for penile cancer, urethral and periurethral tissues were found to be the second-most frequent sites of margin involvement.[5] In this area corresponding to the urethra and periurethral cylinder (Fig. 14-6A–C), the tumor may compromise the urethral epithelium, lamina propria, periurethral corpus spongiosum, and fascia (Fig. 14-56). Lymphatic or perineural invasion may also be seen (Fig. 14-57). A pagetoid intraepithelial spread simulating Paget disease may be observed. In clinically more advanced cases, penile carcinomas may spread directly to inguinal, pubic, or scrotal skin and soft tissues. These cases are usually associated with poor prognosis. However, it is important to determine the tumor histologic type because occasionally, giant condylomata and verrucous or low-grade warty carcinomas (which are less aggressive, albeit locally destructive lesions) may spread in this pattern and yet have a good outcome.

Regional and Systemic Spread

Regionally, penile carcinoma disseminates to inguinal lymph nodes bilaterally. Rarely, skip metastases directly to deep inguinal or to pelvic nodes are found. The first site of metastasis is in the "sentinel" lymph node(s). Although originally thought to be in a constant anatomical location associated with the superficial epigastric vein in the superomedial quadrant of the inguinal field,[11] later studies

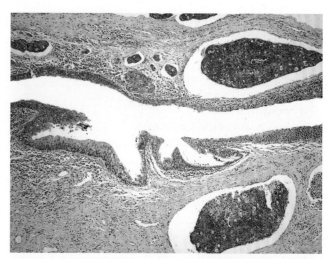

FIGURE 14-57 ■ Squamous cell carcinoma of the penis showing massive lymphovascular invasion at the urethral resection margin. Note the tumor emboli within lymphovascular spaces in urethral lamina propria.

found that anatomical variations exist in the position of the sentinel node(s).[242] Superficial inguinal lymph node dissection remains the most common practice for ascertaining inguinal node status for select patients at high risk among most urologists.[242] Results from preoperative lymphoscintigraphy and dynamic sentinel node biopsy appear promising.[242–245] There are studies suggesting that early detection of lymph node metastases by dynamic sentinel node biopsy and subsequent resection in clinically node-negative T2-3 penile carcinoma improves survival compared with a policy of surveillance.[246] These techniques, however, are still in evolution and require further optimization at high-volume centers.[242] Systemic dissemination of penile cancer may involve retroperitoneal nodes, the heart, lungs, bone, and liver.

Handling of the Specimen with Penile Carcinoma

Circumcision specimen: Describe the specimen and take measurements. Identify and describe the tumor. It is important to identify and ink the mucosal and cutaneous margins with different colors. Most SCCs arise from the mucosal surface of the foreskin; therefore, the coronal sulcus (mucosal) margin is especially important.[9] Lightly stretch and pin the specimen to a cardboard. Fix for several hours in formalin. Cut vertically the whole specimen labeling from 1 to 12, clockwise.[247]

Penectomy specimen: Take measurements, describe specimen, and identify and describe tumor. Most SCCs of the penis arise from the epithelium of the distal portion of the organ (glans, coronal sulcus, and mucosal surface of the prepuce; the tumor may involve one or more of these anatomical compartments).[9,247] If present, classify the foreskin as short, medium, long, and/or phimotic.[7] Cut the proximal

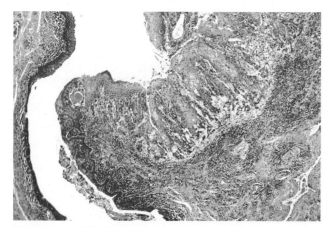

FIGURE 14-56 ■ Involvement of the urethral resection margin by squamous cell carcinoma. The epithelium is totally replaced by squamous cell carcinoma that infiltrates into the periurethral tissues.

margin of resection en face, making sure to include the entire circumference of the urethra (Figs. 14-4, 14-6A and B). If the urethra has retracted, it is important to identify its resection margin and submit it entirely. The resection margin can be divided in three important areas that need to be analyzed: the skin of the shaft with underlying dartos and penile fascia; corpora cavernosa with albuginea; and urethra with periurethral cylinder that includes the lamina propria, corpus spongiosum, albuginea, and penile fascia (Figs. 14-4 and 14-6A–C). The urethra and periurethral cylinder can be placed in one cassette. The skin of the shaft with dartos and fascia can be included together with the corpora cavernosa. Because this is a large specimen, it may need to be included in several cassettes to include the entire resection margin. Fix the rest of the specimen overnight. Then, in the fixed state and if the tumor is large and involves most of the glans, cut longitudinally and centrally using the meatus and the proximal urethra as reference points (Fig. 14-3). Do not probe the urethra. Separate the specimen in two halves: left and right. Then cut two to six serial sections of each half. If the tumor is small and asymmetrically located in the dorsal or ventral area, the central portion of the tumor may be used as the axis of sectioning. If the tumor is large involving multiple sites (glans, sulcus, and foreskin), it is important not to remove the foreskin leaving the entire specimen intact for sectioning.

In cases of small carcinomas exclusively located in the glans with no foreskin involvement, one may choose to remove the foreskin leaving a 3-mm redundant edge around the sulcus. Proceed cutting the foreskin as indicated for circumcision specimens. Even if the primary tumor is located in the glans, submit the foreskin serially and in an orderly fashion labeled from 1 to 12 clockwise. The rest of the penectomy specimen should be handled as described above.

OTHER RARE EPITHELIAL TUMORS

Giant Condyloma Acuminatum

Giant condylomata are rare, benign, exuberant exophytic condylomata that reach large sizes after many years of neglect (Box 14-4). Like common condylomata, they are preferentially associated with HPV-6 and -11. They tend to affect patients slightly older than those with common condylomata. Giant condylomata frequently affect the coronal sulcus and the foreskin, but the glans can also be involved. Grossly, they are large (usually more than 5 cm), unicentric, cauliflower-like, verruciform tumors with cobblestone surfaces. The cut surface shows a papillomatous surface and bulbous deep borders with a sharp separation from the underlying stroma. The tumor tends to show deeper penetration into subjacent structures than common condyloma. Microscopic features are identical to the common condyloma acuminatum, with arborescent papillae showing prominent fibrovascular cores with surface koilocytosis (Fig. 14-58). Giant condylomata, however, tend to show a more exuberant growth and the

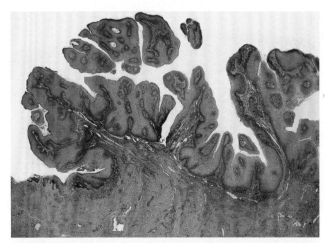

FIGURE 14-58 ■ Giant condyloma. Microscopic features are identical to the common condyloma acuminatum, with arborescent papillae showing prominent fibrovascular cores with surface koilocytosis.

base with bulbous expansion into underlying tissues, often with a burrowing pattern. No atypia is seen in these deep areas. The differential diagnosis includes other verruciform tumors such as warty (condylomatous) carcinoma, verrucous carcinoma, and papillary carcinoma. Warty carcinoma is a clearly malignant neoplasm showing pleomorphic cytologic features and often infiltrative deep borders. Verrucous carcinoma is characterized by acanthotic papillae with thin fibrovascular cores and no evidence of koilocytosis. HPV studies are negative in most cases of verrucous carcinoma. Papillary carcinoma is a non–HPV-related tumor; therefore koilocytosis is not present and the deep borders tend to be jagged and irregular.

In our experience, small foci of frank SCC can be found in at least a fourth of these giant condylomata; therefore, extensive sampling and a high level of suspicion is advised when dealing with large and deep lesions. We avoid the term Buschke-Löwenstein tumor because it has been used for several different verruciform tumors, including benign and malignant ones.[248]

Basal Cell Carcinoma

Basal cell carcinomas arise on the skin of the shaft and in general show no metastatic potential.[249,250] They are identical to basal cell carcinomas of the skin elsewhere (Fig. 14-59) and should be distinguished from BCs, a high-grade deeply invasive squamous cell carcinoma arising from the mucosal surfaces. Basal cell carcinomas arise from the skin surface of the penis, are not associated with HPV, and have locally aggressive potential.

Merkel Cell Carcinoma

Merkel cell carcinoma of the penis is exceptional but has been described. The histopathologic and immunohistochemical features are similar to those seen in other locations.[251]

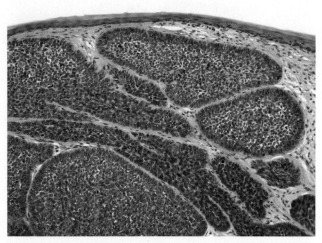

FIGURE 14-59 ■ Basal cell carcinoma from the skin of the shaft. The lesion shows identical features to cutaneous basal cell carcinoma in nongenital locations.

CYSTS

Benign epidermoid and dermoid cysts have been described in the literature. The histopathologic features are similar to those seen in other locations.[252–254]

ADNEXAL CYSTS AND TUMORS

Benign adnexal cysts and tumors such as hidrocystomas and syringomas have been reported.[255,256] Syringomas are appendageal tumors exhibiting features of eccrine differentiation that may be single or multiple. Histologically, they are characterized by a proliferation of small comma-shaped ducts, the walls of which are lined by two rows of epithelial cells, embedded in a fibrous stroma (Fig. 14-60).[256,257] Sebaceous gland hyperplasia and a

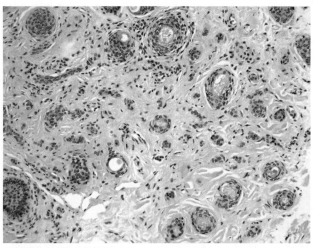

FIGURE 14-60 ■ Syringoma. Histologically, the lesion is characterized by a proliferation of small comma-shaped ducts, the walls of which are lined by two rows of epithelial cells, embedded in a fibrous stroma.

rare adnexal tumor with composite ductal and follicular differentiation have also been described.[258,259]

Paget Disease

Extramammary Paget disease affecting the penis can be classified as primary and secondary. Primary Paget disease can be confined to the epidermis or may be associated with an underlying sweat gland adenocarcinoma.[260–262] Dermal invasion from a predominantly epidermal lesion can also be seen. Secondary Paget disease usually represents an extension from a urethral or bladder carcinoma.[263–265] Primary Paget disease may rarely show an exclusively penile location. Most frequently, however, it involves the skin of the shaft as part of a more extensive scrotal, inguinal, perineal, or perianal lesion. Secondary Paget disease tends to affect the glans and especially the perimeatal region.[263–265]

Typically, patients are in the sixth or seventh decade and present with thickened red, pale plaques with scaling or oozing. Microscopically, there is an intraepithelial proliferation of large atypical cells with abundant pale cytoplasm (Fig. 14-61A). Nuclei are vesicular and nucleoli prominent. These cells may extend to the epithelium of adnexal structures. Such in situ lesions have a favorable prognosis when completely excised. The prognosis is more serious in cases in which Paget cells invade the dermis from the epidermis or from an underlying sweat gland carcinoma.[262] Primary Paget disease should be distinguished from squamous cell carcinoma in situ with pagetoid pattern, pagetoid extension at the periphery of an invasive squamous cell carcinoma, secondary extension from urothelial and anal/rectal carcinomas, and melanoma in situ. Clear cell papulosis,[266] pagetoid dyskeratosis,[267] and mucinous metaplasia[268] should also be ruled out. Primary Paget disease is usually positive for mucins (Fig. 14-61B).[269] Immunohistochemically, primary Paget disease characteristically expresses CEA, low molecular weight cytokeratins, especially cytokeratin 7 (Fig. 14-79B), and CAM 5.2, EMA, MUC1, and GCDFP15 and is negative for CK20.[270,271] Secondary Paget disease associated with urothelial carcinoma usually expresses both cytokeratin 20 and cytokeratin 7 and is negative for CEA.[272] The expression of uroplakin III would support Paget disease secondary to urothelial carcinoma.[273] A recent publication in the vulvar literature suggests that p63 is positive in Paget disease secondary to urothelial carcinoma and negative in primary Paget disease of the vulva.[274] Similar analysis in penile lesions and in a larger series would be necessary to confirm the utility of this marker. Another possible scenario would be the extension to the penis from a perianal lesion of Paget disease. Such lesions may be primary (having the same immunohistochemical profile described in primary penile lesions) or associated with an anal/rectal adenocarcinoma. Paget disease secondary to anal/rectal carcinomas usually expresses CK20 and CEA and shows a variable (most frequently negative) expression of CK7. GCDFP15 is negative in such cases. Some studies suggest that the expression of CDX-2 by Paget cells would be another strong indicator

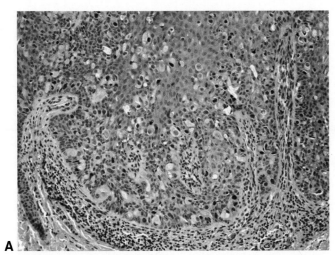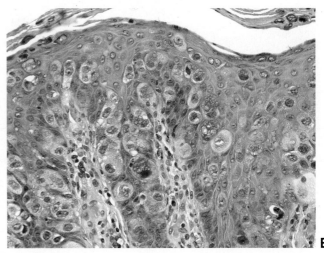

FIGURE 14-61 ■ Paget disease. **A:** Intraepithelial proliferation of large atypical (pagetoid) cells with pale cytoplasm. **B:** The neoplastic cells are positive with mucicarmine stain.

of an associated synchronous or metachronous anal/rectal malignancy.[272,275] Squamous cell carcinoma in situ is usually negative for mucicarmine, CEA, GCDFP15, CK 7, and CK20 and positive for high molecular weight keratins and p63. The lack of expression of melanocytic markers (such as S100 and Melan-A) in Paget disease (primary and secondary) will allow the distinction from melanoma in situ.

Clear Cell Carcinoma

A series of five penile clear cell carcinomas likely of sweat gland origin was recently described.[276] The reported cases affected the inner side of the foreskin of middle-aged men. They were large, exophytic, partly ulcerated, and widely invasive tumors with sharp demarcation from the surrounding normal tissues. Histologically, they were composed of large clear cells with intracytoplasmic PAS-D-positive material and showed extensive lymphatic and blood vessel invasion (Fig. 14-62). The neoplastic

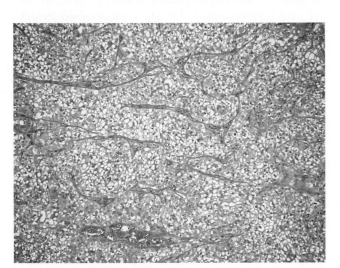

FIGURE 14-62 ■ Clear cell carcinoma of the penis. Solid tumor composed of clear cells arranged in large nests and trabecular structures. (Courtesy of S. Regauer, Medical University Graz.)

cells were positive for cytokeratins, MUC-1, EMA, and CEA. All patients had extensive inguinal lymph node metastases. One of the patients died of metastatic disease. The histologic and immunohistochemical features as well as the occasional presence of an in situ component in the eccrine ducts support a sweat gland differentiation. Distinction of sweat gland clear cell carcinomas from ordinary SCC of the penis is important because of a potentially more aggressive course of sweat gland clear cell carcinomas. It is important to keep in mind that SCCs can show prominent clear cell changes. We have seen more than a few cases mainly composed of clear cells. These clear cell features are usually associated with warty carcinomas. The differential diagnosis of penile clear cell carcinomas includes metastatic renal cell carcinoma and extension of a urothelial clear cell carcinoma.

PIGMENTARY AND MELANOCYTIC DISORDERS

Penile Melanosis

Also called melanotic macules or genital lentiginosis, this condition is clinically characterized by large and pigmented macules that may be multifocal and show irregular borders. They may affect the glans and foreskin.[277,278] Histologically, there are basal layer hyperpigmentation, slight melanocytic hyperplasia, epithelial hyperplasia, and stromal melanophages.[277] No cytologic atypia of melanocytes should be detectable. It is considered a benign condition; however, the available information is insufficient to predict the natural history of genital lentiginosis or its relation to mucocutaneous melanoma.[278]

Malignant Melanoma

Penile malignant melanoma is rare and mainly localized in the glans (Fig. 14-63).[279–281] Although classically associated with a poor prognosis, there is a recent study suggesting that

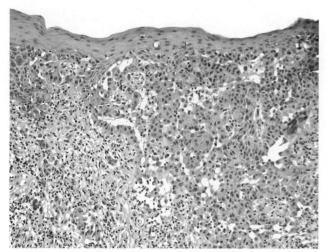

Figure 14-63 ■ Invasive malignant melanoma of the glans.

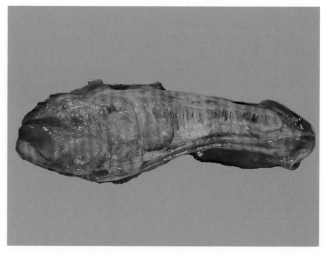

Figure 14-64 ■ Leiomyosarcoma. Total penectomy specimen with a large and deeply located mass in the proximal portion of penile shaft. The tumor replaces the corpora cavernosa.

the prognosis of primary mucosal penile melanoma is not worse than that for cutaneous melanoma with comparable tumor thickness.[285] Presence of ulceration, tumor depth of 3.5 mm or more, and tumor diameter >15 mm had a significantly adverse effect on prognosis.[281] In two separate studies, all patients with nodal and/or distant metastases at presentation died of the disease.[280,281] Melanoma in situ can mimic Paget disease; the demonstration of immunohistochemical expression of melanocytic markers (i.e., S100, HMB-45, Melan-A) may be necessary to make the correct diagnosis in such difficult cases.

SOFT TISSUE TUMORS

Although rare, there are a great variety of benign and malignant penile soft tissue tumors that can be broadly classified as superficial and deep according to their location.[282,283] The most common benign soft tissue tumors that affect the penis are vascular neoplasms such as hemangiomas (including epithelioid hemangiomas), angiokeratomas (Fig. 14-80), and lymphangiomas.[282–287] Glomus tumors and vascular malformations have also been described.[288,289] The histopathologic appearance of these lesions is similar to that seen at any other location. Multiple angiokeratomas may be seen associated with Fabry disease and other more rare genetic enzymatic deficiencies. Myointimoma is an unusual but distinct vascular/myointimal benign tumor characteristically affecting the corpus spongiosum of the glans. Histologically, the lesion shows a peculiar myointimal proliferation of the preexisting vascular spaces of the corpus spongiosum, creating a multinodular/plexiform architecture.[290,291] Benign tumors of neural (e.g., neurofibromas, granular cell tumors),[292–294] myoid (e.g., leiomyomas),[295] and fibrous (e.g., dermatofibromas)[296] origin can also be seen. The most frequent malignant penile soft tissue tumors are leiomyosarcoma and vascular

neoplasms.[283,297–301] Leiomyosarcomas can be classified as superficial and deep.[301] The latter, usually affecting deep structures of the penile shaft, are associated with a worse prognosis (Fig. 14-64). Superficial lesions tend to be indolent and cured by complete wide excision. Tumors with a deep-seated component may require more aggressive intervention to ensure complete removal. Leiomyosarcomas are composed of smooth muscle cells with both cytologic atypia and mitotic activity. Immunoreactivity for smooth muscle action, desmin, and calponin is characteristic. The best predictors of outcome are tumor depth and tumor size.[301] The most commonly found vascular sarcomas include Kaposi sarcoma, epithelioid hemangioendothelioma, and angiosarcoma.[283,297,302–307] Kaposi sarcoma may affect the penis in the setting of multiple disseminated lesions, especially in AIDS patients.[302–304] Cases limited to the penis or affecting immunocompetent patients are rare but have been described.[306,307] The most common location appears to be the glans. Histologically, Kaposi sarcoma shows features similar to those described in other locations. Early lesions may be subtle and mimic benign angiomas. Well-established lesions show the characteristic spindle cell proliferation admixed with slit-like vascular spaces, extravasated erythrocytes, and hemosiderin deposition (Fig. 14-65A). Immunohistochemistry for human herpes virus-8 (HHV-8) is now available and is helpful in confirming the diagnosis (Fig. 14-65B). Epithelioid hemangioendothelioma is considered a low-grade malignant tumor that rarely may affect the penis and can recur or even metastasize.[308,309] Epithelioid hemangioendothelioma is often multifocal and shows a lobulated pattern of growth. Histologically, the neoplastic cells have abundant eosinophilic cytoplasm with frequent intracytoplasmic vacuoles (Fig. 14-66A). The neoplastic cells are often arranged in cords that may be seen embedded in a hyalinized or chondroid stroma.

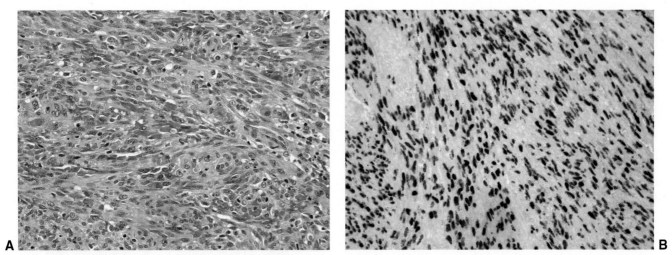

FIGURE 14-65 ■ Kaposi sarcoma. **A:** There is a spindle cell proliferation admixed with slit-like vascular spaces, extravasated erythrocytes, and hemosiderin deposition. **B:** Immunohistochemistry for HHV-8 is helpful to confirm the diagnosis.

An angiocentric pattern that may be occlusive has been described.[310] Immunohistochemically, the neoplastic cells express vascular markers such as CD31, CD34, and factor VIII (Fig. 14-66B). Occasionally, they may express keratins and smooth muscle actin.[310] Epithelioid hemangioendotheliomas should be distinguished from another sarcoma with epithelioid features that may also affect the penis, the epithelioid sarcoma.[311,312] Lesions in this more proximal location tend to have a different morphology from conventional epithelioid sarcomas and are especially aggressive.[312] Proximal type of epithelioid sarcomas show a more sheet-like growth and large, epithelioid tumor cells with large vesicular nuclei and rhabdoid features (Fig. 14-67). Areas of necrosis are frequent.[312] The conventional form of

epithelioid sarcoma, which is composed of a monotonous population of eosinophilic cells with epithelioid or spindle shapes often surrounding geographic foci of necrosis, may also be seen in this location. Immunohistochemically, epithelioid sarcoma shows consistent positivity for keratin, vimentin, and EMA. Around half of the cases also express CD34.[312] Other malignant soft tissue neoplasms reported are rhabdomyosarcoma,[313,314] malignant fibrohistiocytoma,[315] clear cell sarcoma,[316] dermatofibrosarcoma protuberans,[317] and fibrosarcoma.[318] Correctly diagnosing penile soft tissue tumors is important, because the biologic behavior and the clinical management of these neoplasms vary considerably.[283] Distinguishing sarcomas from sarcomatoid carcinoma and melanoma is particularly important.[283]

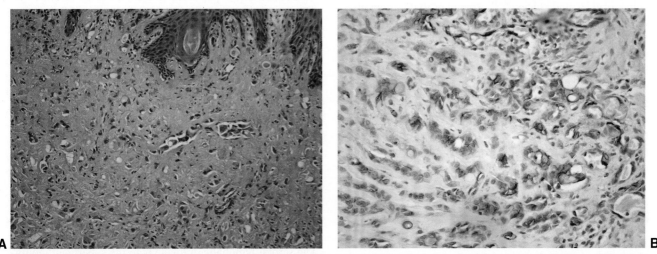

FIGURE 14-66 ■ Epithelioid hemangioendothelioma. This was a multicentric lesion. **A:** Microscopic appearance of one of the tumors affecting the foreskin. The neoplastic cells are arranged in cords that are embedded in a hyalinized stroma. Note the abundant eosinophilic cytoplasm with frequent intracytoplasmic vacuoles. **B:** Immunohistochemically, the neoplastic cells express CD34. (Courtesy of Dr. CD Fletcher, Brigham and Women's Hospital and Harvard Medical School, Boston, USA.)

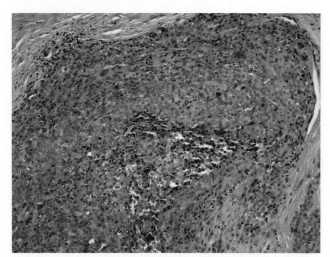

FIGURE 14-67 ■ Epithelioid sarcoma, proximal type. There are sheet-like aggregates of large, epithelioid tumor cells with large vesicular nuclei and foci of necrosis. (Courtesy of Dr. CD Fletcher, Brigham and Women's Hospital and Harvard Medical School, Boston, USA.)

LYMPHOPROLIFERATIVE AND OTHER HEMATOPOIETIC DISORDERS

Lymphomas of the penis are very rare and may be observed as a primary lesion or a secondary involvement of the organ in the setting of a systemic disease.[319–326] Priapism, a urologic emergency, may be seen in leukemic patients.[326] Histiocytic disorders have been reported, but they are rare.[327–329]

METASTATIC TUMORS TO THE PENIS

Although the penis is a highly vascularized organ, metastatic lesions to the penis are rare.[297,330–339] When encountered, the primary site is most frequently of pelvic origin; the most common primary site is the prostate, followed by the rectosigmoid colon, bladder, and kidney.[330–336] Among prostate carcinomas, the ductal–endometrioid variant appears to be the more prone to develop penile metastasis.[335] Less common primary sites include the testis, ureter, and other nonpelvic organs such as lung, stomach, pancreas, nasopharynx, and bone.[297,337,338]

The most common location of the metastatic lesions is the corpus cavernosum.[297] The clinical presentation is that of multiple, palpable nodules that may ulcerate. A prominent clinical feature of metastatic carcinoma is the so-called malignant priapism, caused by massive replacement of the corpora cavernosa by the neoplasm.[339]

THE SCROTUM

Normal Anatomy and Histology

The scrotum originates from the genital swellings that meet ventral to the anus and unite to form the two scrotal sacs. A median raphe of fibrovascular connective tissue separates both

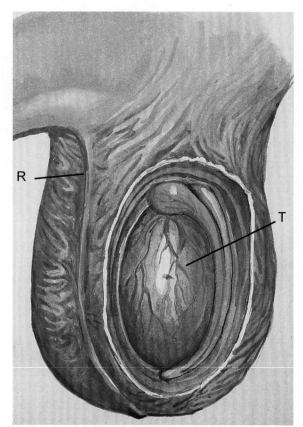

FIGURE 14-68 ■ The surface of the scrotum is divided into right and left halves by a cutaneous raphe (R) that continues ventrally to the inferior penile surface and dorsally along the midline of the perineum to the anus. The scrotum contains the testes (T) and the lower parts of the spermatic cords.

halves.[1] The scrotum contains the testes and the lower parts of the spermatic cords.[2] The surface of the scrotum is divided into right and left halves by a cutaneous raphe that continues ventrally to the inferior penile surface and dorsally along the midline of the perineum to the anus (Fig. 14-68).[340] The left side of the scrotum is usually lower because of the greater length of the left spermatic cord. The anatomical layers of the scrotum are the skin, dartos muscle, and external spermatic, cremasteric, and internal spermatic fascia (Fig. 14-69A). The internal fascia is loosely attached to the parietal layer of the tunica vaginalis. The skin is composed of the epidermis and dermis. The dermis contains hair follicles and sebaceous, eccrine, and apocrine glands. There is not well-formed subcutaneous tissue at this level; however, scattered adipocytes may be seen in the deep dermis. The dermis merges imperceptibly with the dartos tunic where there are numerous smooth muscle bundles embedded in loose connective tissue (Fig. 14-69B).[2]

The vascular supply of the scrotum derives from the external and internal pudendal arteries. Additional blood comes to the scrotum from the cremasteric and testicular arteries. The scrotal lymphatic drainage is to the superficial inguinal lymph nodes.[340] There is free communication between the superficial lymphatic network on both sides of the scrotum and the median raphe does not act as a barrier.[341,342]

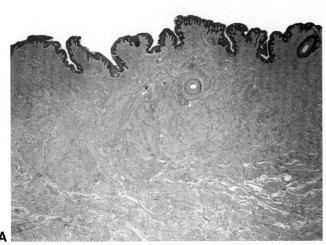
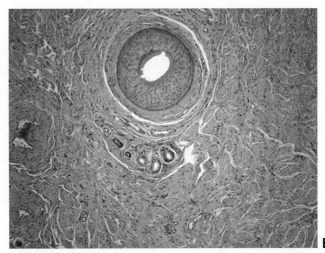

FIGURE 14-69 ■ **A:** The skin covering the scrotum is composed of epidermis and dermis. The dermis merges imperceptibly with the dartos. **B:** The dartos tunic is composed of numerous smooth muscle bundles embedded in loose connective tissue.

Congenital Anomalies

Penoscrotal transposition is an anomaly frequently associated with other congenital abnormalities especially hypospadias. It results from incomplete migration of the inferomedial labioscrotal swelling. This condition has been termed *bifid scrotum*, *doughnut scrotum*, *prepenile scrotum*, and *shawl scrotum*. In complete transposition, the penis lies entirely behind the scrotum. In less severe forms, the penis may appear to arise from the center of the scrotum or be enveloped by the scrotum.[17,18]

Ectopic scrotum is very uncommon and usually occurs in the presence of severe colloquial exstrophy. Occasionally ectopic scrotal tissue can be found in a child with otherwise normal genitalia. The ectopic scrotal tissue is usually located in the inner thigh or near the external inguinal ring. Typically the ipsilateral testicle lies within the ectopic scrotum.[17,18]

NONNEOPLASTIC CONDITIONS

Scabies

Scabies is the infestation with the itch mite, *S. scabiei* var *humanus* (Fig. 14-19).[21,37,38] The disease is found worldwide, in all races and in all age groups.[21] It is transmitted by close skin-to-skin contact. The penis and scrotum are commonly affected in addition to web spaces, fingers, wrists, elbows, and axillary folds. The characteristics of the parasite as well as histologic findings were described in the penile section.

Trichomycosis

Despite its name, trichomycosis is a superficial bacterial colonization of the hair shafts in sweat gland–bearing areas such as the axillae, pubis, and scrotum.[21,27,28,37,38,343] It is caused by the genus Corynebacteria (mostly *C. tenuis*). The condition typically is asymptomatic; however, patients may complain of malodorous sweat. Clinically, there are 1- to 2-mm

yellow, red (and less often black) granular concretions (minute nodules) that adhere firmly to the hair shaft. The exact origin of the cement substance that creates the grossly visible nodules is debated. Some studies favor origin from the causative agents, while others have favored elaboration from apocrine sweat.[21,38,344] The actual nidus may be through the modification of apocrine sweat by elaborated cement substance to create the insoluble material that holds bacteria to the hair shaft. Under the microscope, an amorphous thick material can be appreciated surrounding and attached to the hair shaft (Fig. 14-70A). Admixed with this amorphous material are long, slender Gram-positive rods (Fig. 14-70B). The bacteria may invade and destroy the cuticle of the hair shaft (Fig. 14-70A). Differential diagnosis includes pediculosis (the minute nodules of Corynebacteria may be confused with nits), black piedra, and white piedra. Black piedra is a fungal infection of the hair shaft caused by *Piedraia hortae*, an ascomycetous fungus forming hard black nodules on the shafts of the scalp, beard, moustache, and pubic hair. White piedra (or tinea blanca) is a mycosis of the hair associated with *Trichosporon beigelii* and it is characterized by nodules composed of hyphae that encircle the hair shaft. Distinction from white piedra may be more difficult and some cases appear to be the result of a synergistic interaction between *Corynebacteria* and *T. beigelii*.[345]

Fournier Gangrene

Fournier gangrene is a necrotizing fasciitis of the genitals and perineum that particularly affects the scrotum.[29,30] It tends to be a polymicrobial infection caused by a mixture of aerobic and anaerobic organisms. The source of the infection may be colorectal, urologic, and cutaneous. It begins as painful reddish plaques with necrosis and is accompanied by systemic symptoms including fever. The scrotum becomes edematous and the lesions progress to form blisters. Scrotal emphysema and frank gangrenous necrosis follow. The key pathophysiologic event is thought to be thrombosis of the small vessels, known

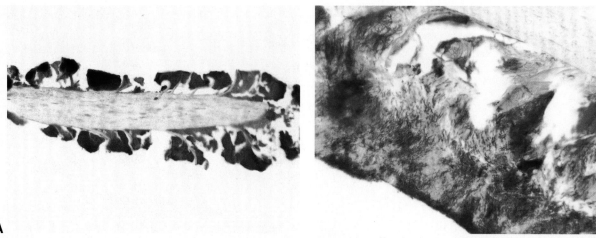

A   **B**

Figure 14-70 ■ Trichomycosis; Gram stain **(A)** Under the microscope, an amorphous thick material can be seen surrounding and attached to the hair shaft. Note how the bacteria invaded and destroyed the cuticle of the hair shaft. **B:** Higher-power view to illustrate the slender Gram-positive rods admixed with the amorphous material.

as obliterative endarteritis.[29,30] Fournier gangrene is a serious and life-threatening condition.[29] Predisposing factors include diabetes mellitus, immunosuppression, contaminated genitourinary trauma, lower urinary tract instrumentation, and septic injection into the penile vein.

Lichen Simplex Chronicus/Prurigo Nodularis

Lichen simplex chronicus is characterized by the development of localized thickened scaly patches or plaques secondary to persistent scratching in patients who usually do not have an underlying dermatologic condition.[37,38] The clinicopathologic features are similar in the penis and scrotum and were described in the penile section (Fig. 14-71).

Acantholytic Dermatosis of the Genitocrural Area

This distinct acantholytic eruption of the genital/perineal area including the scrotum has been described in the penile section.[38,91]

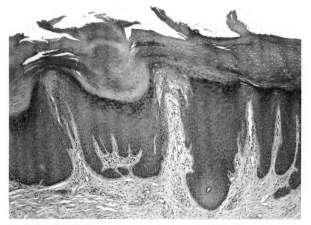

Figure 14-71 ■ Lichen simplex chronicus/prurigo nodularis of the scrotum. There is irregular epidermal hyperplasia with hypergranulosis, hyperkeratosis, and minimal dermal inflammatory infiltrate associated with dermal fibrosis.

Hidradenitis Suppurativa

Hidradenitis suppurativa is a chronic relapsing suppurative inflammatory process.[346,347] The precise pathogenesis is not well understood, but it seems likely that in most cases, follicular occlusion with formation of acne-like lesions is the primary event.[37,38] The preferential anatomic distribution of the lesions in areas containing apocrine glands supports the concept of an underlying apocrine gland defect. Clinically, the lesion starts as a firm painful nodule that may discharge foul-smelling pus and slowly involute. The lesions tend to recur and may progress to form indurated plaques and nodules associated with marked scarring and numerous sinus tracts. Secondary bacterial infection perpetuates the process. Histologically, keratin plugging of dilated hair follicles is regularly seen. This may be accompanied by acute inflammation of the associated apocrine glands in early lesions. Well-established lesions show sinus tracts with marked suppuration and abscess formation, lined by a mixture of squamous epithelium and granulation tissue (Fig. 14-72). The squamous epithelium lining the sinuses extends from adjacent follicular structures. These sinuses contain keratin and sometimes hair shafts. They are surrounded by marked fibrosis and acute and chronic inflammation including giant cell reaction to the keratin material. At this stage, apocrine glands are no longer identified in the scarred and inflamed area.[38]

Scrotal Calcinosis

Scrotal calcinosis is an uncommon condition characterized by single or multiple hard nodules that vary in size from a few millimeters to few centimeters.[37,38,348–351] These nodules may break down to discharge a chalky material.[38] Rarely lesions may be polypoid. It usually affects young adults, but it may also be seen in children and elderly patients.

Although originally considered an idiopathic condition, it is now accepted that the vast majority of cases develop from dystrophic calcification of cysts' contents (including epidermoid cysts, adnexal cysts, and cystically dilated eccrine

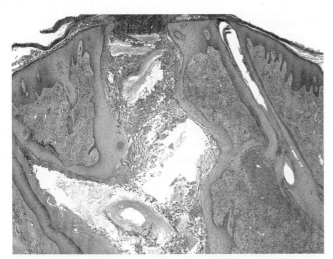

FIGURE 14-72 ■ Hidradenitis suppurativa. Dilated hair follicles forming sinus tracts containing keratin material and inflammatory debris. Within the dermis, there is fibrosis and chronic and acute inflammation with abscess formation.

ducts).[38,348–351] Histologically, the epidermis is usually intact or less frequently ulcerated. The process is located within the dermis and may extend to the dartos. It is characterized by granular and globular deposition of hematoxylinophilic purple calcified material. A giant cell granulomatous inflammatory response may be associated with the deposits (Fig. 14-73). Sometimes, histologic remnants of the preexisting epidermoid cyst or even more rarely a partially cystic adnexal tumor (e.g., syringoma) may be identified.

Sclerosing Lipogranuloma

Sclerosing lipogranuloma, also known as paraffinoma, may involve the penis or scrotum.[95,297,352] It is usually secondary to the injection or less frequently topical application of oil-based substances such as paraffin, silicone, oil, or wax for cosmetic or therapeutic purposes. Rarely, they may also

be related to cold weather or trauma. Most cases are seen in patients younger than 40 years who present with an indurated and sometimes tender plaque or mass that varies in size from a few centimeters to massive replacement of the scrotum. Biopsy is necessary to exclude a neoplasm, especially if there is no history of injection or exogenous material. Grossly, the specimen consists of firm yellow to gray/white pieces of tissue with a solid or multicystic appearance. Microscopically, sclerosing lipogranulomas are characterized by numerous lipid vacuoles of variable size embedded in a sclerotic stroma (Fig. 14-74). There is also an infiltrate of foamy histiocytes and a variable amount of multinucleated giant cells, lymphoid cells, and eosinophils. The inflammatory infiltrate may be nodular or interspersed in the sclerotic stroma. The diagnosis is usually not difficult especially when there is a good clinical history. If necessary, sections from frozen tissue showing a positive staining with oil red O can be helpful. Immunohistochemical studies have shown expression of lysozyme, alpha-1-antitrypsin, alpha-1-antichymotrypsin, KP-1, and CD68 by multinucleated giant cells and epithelioid histiocytes.[353,354] Most of the lymphocytes infiltrating the lesions are T cells associated with some S-100-positive dendritic cells. T-cell-mediated immune reaction appears to be important in the histogenesis of sclerosing lipogranuloma.[353] The differential diagnosis includes liposarcoma (Fig. 14-83A and B), metastatic carcinoma, adenomatoid tumor, and lymphangioma. The presence of a foreign body giant cell reaction and foamy histiocytes helps to distinguish this condition from liposarcoma. Immunohistochemistry for epithelial and vascular markers may be helpful to distinguish it from carcinomas and lymphangiomas, respectively.

Fat Necrosis

Fat necrosis of the scrotum presents as firm nodules in the lower portion of the scrotal wall.[355] Most cases affect children and adolescents, and the lesions are often bilateral. The lesion

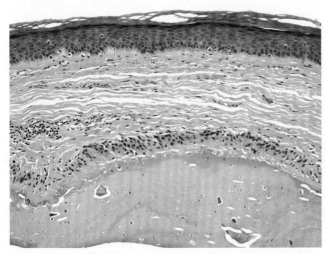

FIGURE 14-73 ■ Scrotal calcinosis. Underneath an intact epidermis, there is granular deposition of an amorphous purple calcified material. These calcified deposits are surrounded by a palisading histiocytic reaction.

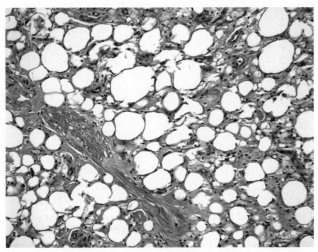

FIGURE 14-74 ■ Sclerosing lipogranuloma. There are numerous lipid vacuoles of variable size embedded in a sclerotic stroma where there are foamy histiocytes.

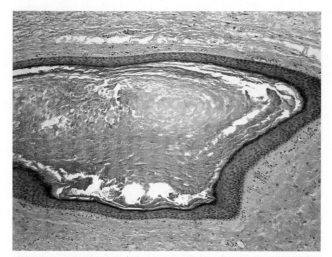

FIGURE 14-75 ■ Epidermal inclusion cyst. Microscopically, the lesion is lined by a keratinizing squamous epithelium with granular layer and contains abundant keratin material.

may develop when scrotal fat crystallizes following exposure to cold. Biopsies are exceptional since the lesion has specific imaging features and the ultrasound appearance combined with the characteristic clinical presentation can confirm the diagnosis.[356]

Epidermal Inclusion Cyst

Epidermal inclusion cysts are common in the scrotum and they present as single or multiple firm rubbery intradermal or subdermal nodules. Grossly, they contain a characteristic gray-white cheesy material.[297] Microscopically, they are lined by a keratinizing squamous epithelium with granular layer and contain abundant keratin (Fig. 14-75).

Verruciform Xanthoma

Verruciform xanthomas occur most commonly in the oral mucosa followed by genital areas (scrotum and penis).[37,38,357] Trauma is probably the triggering event. The importance of verruciform xanthoma is that it may be clinically confused with condyloma. Microscopically, the low-power view is also similar to that of a wart (Fig. 14-76A), and this may be misleading. There is marked acanthosis with a papillomatous surface and marked elongation and thinning of the dermal papillae. The clue to the diagnosis is the presence of the characteristic foamy to granular xanthomatous histiocytes within the dermal papillae (Fig. 14-76B). The blood vessels at the base of the lesion appear prominent. Another helpful feature is the presence of prominent (usually orange) parakeratosis and superficial keratinocytic necrosis admixed with neutrophils (Fig. 14-76B). Candidal hyphae and bacteria may be found in this thick parakeratotic layer. An unusual scrotal case associated with HPV-6 has been described.[358]

Condyloma Acuminatum

Condyloma acuminatum may affect the scrotum showing identical gross and microscopic features as penile condylomata and it was discussed in the penile section (Figs. 14-13 to 14-15).[50,60] Giant condylomata acuminata may also affect the scrotum.[359]

EPITHELIAL NEOPLASMS

Neoplastic lesions of the scrotum including benign and malignant are rare.

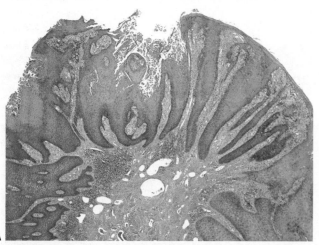
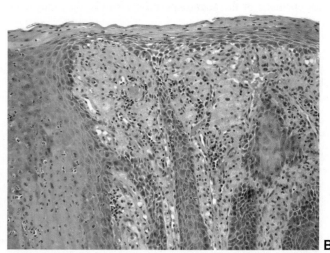

FIGURE 14-76 ■ Verruciform xanthoma. **A:** At low power, the lesion can be confused with a viral wart or a condyloma. There is marked acanthosis with a papillomatous surface and marked elongation and thinning of the dermal papillae. **B:** The diagnostic features are appreciated at higher power. Note the presence of characteristic xanthomatous histiocytes within the dermal papillae. There is prominent parakeratosis and superficial keratinocytic necrosis admixed with neutrophils.

Squamous Cell Carcinoma

Epidemiology and Etiopathogenesis

Squamous cell carcinoma of the scrotum is the most common malignant tumor in this location, and yet it is extremely infrequent.[360–369] The incidence of squamous cell carcinoma of the scrotum is much lower than that of penile carcinoma.[297,361,362,364] In 1976, the incidence in the United States was reported to be <10 cases per year.[364] The reported incidence from large cancer centers is one case every 2 or 3 years.[362,363,364]

This tumor is of great historical interest because it was the first cancer to be directly linked to exposure to occupational carcinogens. In the eighteen century, Sir Percival Pott noted a high incidence of this tumor in chimney sweeps.[362,364] Since then, an increased incidence of scrotal cancer has been noted in tar workers, paraffin and shale oil workers, and cotton factory workers.[362,364] Scrotal cancer is more frequent in the lower social class and rural populations when compared with the higher social class and urban population, and this may be related to hygienic measures.[364] Occupation-related scrotal carcinomas are much less frequent now because of better hygiene, protective clothing, and awareness. HPV infection is another risk factor in the development of scrotal cancer.[363,364,366] From a series of 14 cases of scrotal cancer from the Mayo Clinic files, 45% had documented HPV infection.[363] The combination of PUVA has been shown to increase the incidence of both penile and scrotal carcinomas. Squamous cell carcinomas arising in the setting of scars have also been described.[370,371]

Clinical Presentation and Gross Appearance

Carcinoma of the scrotum usually affects patients in the sixth decade of life and most frequently presents as a solitary lesion. Tumors start as pimple and wart-like lesions or nodules that slowly grow for several months and then ulcerate. The ulcerated lesions have an indurated base and raised rolled borders. Invasion of the scrotal contents or the penis may eventually occur. The median time before seeking medical assistance is approximately 8 months.[361,362,364] Nearly 40% to 50% of patients with scrotal cancer have inguinal lymphadenopathy at the time of presentation, and half of these men (25% overall) will have metastasis in the surgical specimens.[364] Less frequent presentations include that of an exophytic papillomatous lesion such as in cases of verrucous carcinoma.[372]

Microscopic Features

The majority of scrotal cancers are keratinizing well or moderately differentiated squamous cell carcinomas of the usual type (Fig. 14-77) similar to those seen in the penis.[297,340,364] Tumors can be graded as well, moderately, and poorly differentiated lesions following the same guidelines that were discussed in the penile section. Even more rarely, other variants such as verrucous, sarcomatoid, warty, and basaloid carcinomas may be seen (Fig. 14-78A).[372]

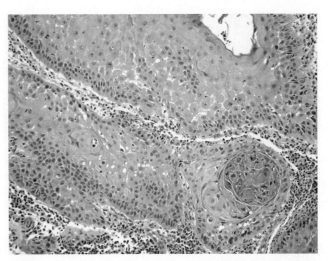

FIGURE 14-77 ■ Invasive squamous cell carcinoma of the scrotum. Keratinizing squamous cell carcinoma of the usual type as the one depicted in this picture is the most commonly found variant.

The epidermis adjacent to the invasive tumors may show dysplastic changes (Fig. 14-78B). Although there are not enough data published on scrotal precancerous conditions to make definitive statements, it is our experience that the precancerous lesions appear similar to those seen in the penis. Differentiated SILs appear more frequently adjacent to the usual type of squamous cell carcinomas, and warty and basaloid type of precancerous lesions are seen more frequently adjacent to HPV-related variant (e.g., warty and basaloid) invasive carcinomas (Fig. 14-78B).

Prognosis and Treatment

The significance of the histologic grade is uncertain because of the scarcity of published data. The most commonly used staging system is the Lowe's modification of the system proposed by Ray and Whitmore (Table 14-3).[364] Data regarding survival are also limited, but overall outcome is poor for invasive carcinoma. Survival appears to correlate with stage; approximately 75% of patients with stage A1 and 44% of patients with stage A2 have a chance for long-term survival.[360–362,364] Patients with stage C or stage D disease have little chance for long-term survival. Surgery is the preferred treatment of scrotal carcinoma.

Basal Cell Carcinoma

Basal cell carcinoma is a rare scrotal neoplasm with clinical, histopathologic, and behavioral features similar to those seen in nongenital skin locations[297,373–376] (Fig. 14-59). Clinically, the most common presentation is that of a pearly papule with telangiectases, but ulcerative, infiltrative, cicatricial, and superficial multicentric variants also occur.[21] It is usually an indolent tumor; however, metastasis has been documented in some cases. Complete local excision with negative margins is the preferred treatment for basal cell carcinomas. Small tumors with classical features of basal

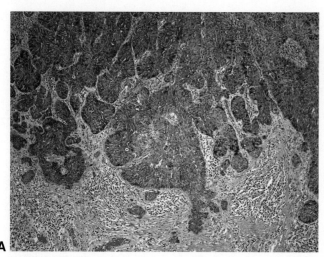
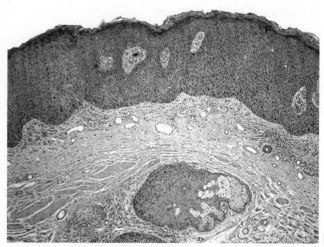

FIGURE 14-78 ■ **A:** Invasive BC of the scrotum. Note the invasive aggregates of small uniform basaloid cells. **B:** The adjacent epithelium shows carcinoma in situ with warty–basaloid features. Note the extension of dysplastic keratinocytes to the underlying adnexal structure; this should not be confused with true invasion. (Courtesy of John Hopkins Medical Center, Department of Pathology, USA.)

cell carcinomas (without foci of necrosis or squamous differentiation) have an excellent prognosis in most cases. It is important to distinguish basal cell carcinoma from BC (Figs. 14-42A–D and 14-78A); the latter is a highly aggressive HPV-related variant of squamous cell carcinoma. BC usually presents as a highly aggressive tumor frequently associated with lymphovascular invasion and poor outcome. For a more detailed description of the basaloid variant of squamous cell carcinoma, please review the penile section. It is possible that some of the reported cases of metastasizing basal cell carcinomas of the scrotum corresponded to basaloid squamous cell carcinomas.

Extramammary Paget Disease

Extramammary Paget disease of the scrotum can be classified as primary and secondary.[377,378] Primary Paget disease may be confined to the epidermis or may invade the dermis. They may also be associated with an underlying sweat gland

carcinoma. Secondary Paget disease results from an epidermotropic spread from a colorectal or urogenital carcinoma. Clinical, histopathologic, and immunohistochemical features are similar to those described in penile location (Figs. 14-61A and B, 14-79A and B).

Other Epithelial Tumors

Practically, any tumor that may affect the skin rarely affects the scrotum. Benign adnexal tumors include syringomas and hidrocystomas. Malignant adnexal neoplasms such as eccrine porocarcinoma have also been reported.[379]

MELANOCYTIC NEOPLASMS

Benign nevi may affect the scrotum. Scrotal malignant melanoma is rare; therefore the data available are scarce. In a recent series from a large institution, the authors reported six cases of scrotal melanoma.[280] The outcome of this series was poor; the 5-year actuarial disease-specific and recurrence-free survival rates were 33.3% and 33.3%, respectively, at a median follow-up of 36 months. Melanoma in situ can mimic Paget disease; the demonstration of immunohistochemical expression of melanocytic markers (i.e., S100, HMB-45, Melan-A) may be necessary to make the correct diagnosis in such difficult cases.

SOFT TISSUE TUMORS

Benign mesenchymal tumors such as hemangiomas, angiokeratomas (Fig. 14-80), leiomyomas (Fig. 14-81), lipomas, granular cell tumor, schwannomas, and solitary fibrous tumor may rarely affect the scrotum.[298,380–382] A rare angiomyofibroblastoma-like tumor with features similar to female

Table 14-3 ■ STAGING SYSTEM FOR SCROTAL CARCINOMA

Stage	Description
A1	Localized to the scrotal wall
A2	Locally extensive tumor invading adjacent structures (testis, spermatic cord, penis, pubis, perineum)
B	Metastatic disease involving inguinal lymph nodes only
C	Metastatic disease involving pelvic lymph nodes without evidence of distant spread
D	Metastasis beyond the pelvic lymph nodes, to involve distant organs.

From Lowe FC. Squamous cell carcinoma of the scrotum. *J Urol* 1983;130:423–427.

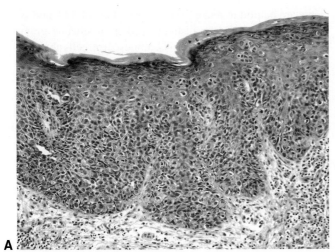
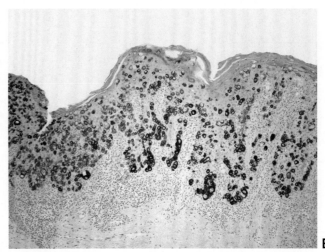

FIGURE 14-79 ■ Paget disease of the scrotum. **A:** Intraepithelial proliferation of large atypical (pagetoid) cells with pale cytoplasm. **B:** Immunohistochemistry for cytokeratin 7 highlights the neoplastic pagetoid cells.

angiomyofibroblastoma and spindle cell lipoma was also described in this location.[383] Rare cases of fibrous hamartoma of infancy have been reported in the scrotum.[37,38,384] The affected patients are usually younger than 2 years. Grossly, the lesion is firm and gray-white with admixed yellow foci. The tumor has ill-defined borders on gross and microscopic examination. Histologically, the lesion is composed of lobules of mature adipose tissue separated by intervening dense fibrous tissue. There are admixed foci of primitive myxoid mesenchymal tissue. Immunohistochemical analysis shows positivity with vimentin, smooth muscle actin, and desmin.

Some cases of aggressive angiomyxoma, a distinctive, locally aggressive but nonmetastasizing soft tissue tumor of the pelvic soft tissues and perineum classically affecting adult women, were also reported in the scrotum.[385,386] These tumors are infiltrative and composed of a fibromyxoid matrix sparsely populated by bland-looking spindled and stellate cells with delicate cytoplasmic processes. There are haphazardly scattered small and large blood vessels, some of which exhibit hypertrophy or hyalinization of the wall. Immunohistochemically, the stromal cells stain for vimentin and variably for muscle-specific actin, but not alpha-smooth muscle actin, desmin, and S-100 protein.[385] This uncommon tumor occurring around the genital region in men merits wider recognition because of its potential for recurrence. It should be distinguished from benign myxoid tumors with a low risk of local recurrence and fully malignant myxoid tumors with distant metastatic potential.[385,386]

Sarcoma of the scrotum, excluding extension from the spermatic cord or other adjacent areas, is extremely rare. The most common malignant soft tissue tumor is

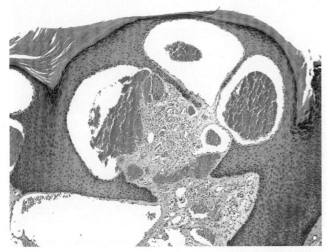

FIGURE 14-80 ■ Angiokeratoma of the scrotum. Underneath a hyperplastic epidermis, there is a proliferation of dilated blood vessels.

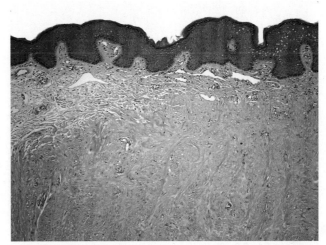

FIGURE 14-81 ■ Leiomyoma of the scrotum. Within the dartos and dermis, there is a proliferation of bland-looking smooth muscle bundles. (Courtesy of John Hopkins Medical Center, Department of Pathology, USA.)

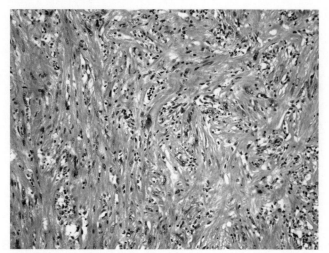

FIGURE 14-82 ■ Leiomyosarcoma of the scrotum. Histologically, the tumor is composed of sweeping fascicles of cells with blunt-end nuclei and perinuclear halos. Nuclear pleomorphism and mitosis are present. (Courtesy of John Hopkins Medical Center, Department of Pathology, USA.)

leiomyosarcoma,[387–390] which usually arises within the dartos. Clinically, it presents as a rapidly growing, painless mass. Histologically, the tumor is composed of sweeping fascicles of cells with blunt-end nuclei and perinuclear halos. Nuclear pleomorphism and mitosis are present (Fig. 14-82).

Liposarcoma may also affect the scrotum. Well-differentiated (including the dedifferentiated variant), myxoid (including the round cell variant), and pleomorphic forms have been described.[390–393] Identification of the classical lipoblasts and, in the well-differentiated variants, the presence of hyperchromatic spindle and bizarre cells in the fibrous

septa are helpful to make the diagnosis (Fig. 14-83A and B). Liposarcoma should be distinguished from silicone granuloma or paraffinoma, which is composed of cells that may really mimic lipoblasts. The presence of multinucleated giant cell reaction and too many multivacuolated "lipoblast-like" cells in silicone granuloma compared with a well-differentiated liposarcoma are helpful to make the distinction. S100 immunostain may be helpful to highlight lipoblasts in liposarcoma. An unusual scrotal sarcoma characterized histologically by the intimate admixture of areas displaying the features of liposarcoma and leiomyosarcoma has been described.[394]

Epithelioid sarcoma (especially the proximal variant) (Fig. 14-67), rhabdomyosarcoma, and other sarcomas exceptionally affect the scrotum.[297,395,396] Scrotal posttraumatic spindle cell nodules may mimic a sarcoma.[397]

LYMPHOPROLIFERATIVE AND OTHER HEMATOPOIETIC DISORDERS

Lymphomas and leukemic infiltration of the scrotum are exceptional but may be seen as primary or secondary events[398–403] (Fig. 14-84A and B).

METASTATIC TUMORS TO THE SCROTUM

Metastasis to the scrotum is very rare.[404–408] The primary site is most frequently a pelvic organ such as the prostate, rectosigmoid colon, bladder, and penis.[404–406] Metastasis from kidney tumors has also been described.[407] Exceptional cases such as desmoplastic small round cell tumor of the abdomen with scrotal metastases[408] and an unusual case of gastrointestinal stromal tumor extending through the inguinal canal to present as a scrotal mass have been reported.[409]

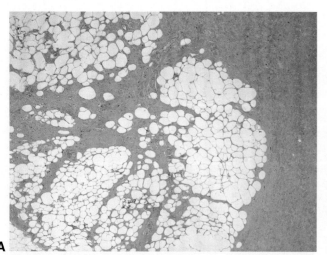
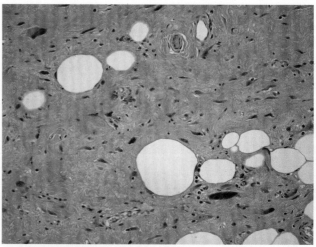

A   **B**

FIGURE 14-83 ■ Well-differentiated liposarcoma of the scrotum. **A:** Low-power view illustrating the adipocytic nature of the lesion. **B:** Higher-power view to show the characteristic bizarre stromal cell within the fibrous septa.

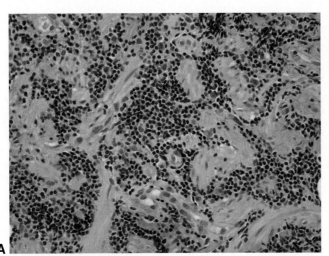
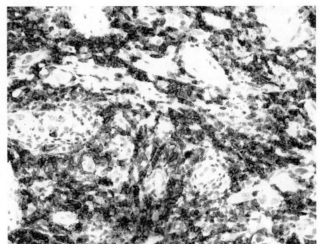

FIGURE 14-84 ■ Chronic lymphocytic leukemia involving the scrotum. **A:** There is a diffuse infiltrate composed of small lymphoid cells. **B:** Immunohistochemistry for the B-cell marker CD20 highlights the neoplastic cells.

REFERENCES

1. Sadler TW. *Langman's Medical Embryology*. 11th ed. Philadelphia, PA: Lippincott Williams & Wilkins; 2009.

2. Clemente C. *Gray's Anatomy of the Human Body*. 30th ed. Philadelphia, PA: Lea & Febiger; 1985.

3. Velazquez EF, Barreto JE, Ayala G, et al. The penis. In: Mills SE, ed. *Sternberg's Diagnostic Surgical Pathology*. 5th ed. Lippincott Williams & Wilkins; 2009.

4. Velazquez EF, Soskin A, Bock A, et al. Epithelial abnormalities and precancerous lesions of anterior urethra in patients with penile carcinoma: a report of 89 cases. *Mod Pathol* 2005;18:917–923.

5. Velazquez EF, Soskin A, Bock A, et al. Positive resection margins in partial penectomies: sites of involvement and proposal of local routes of spread of penile squamous cell carcinoma. *Am J Surg Pathol* 2004;28:384–389.

6. Cold CJ, Taylor JR. The prepuce. *BJU Int* 1999;83:34–44.

7. Velazquez EF, Bock A, Soskin A, et al. Preputial variability and preferential association of long phimotic foreskins with penile cancer. An anatomic comparative study of types of foreskin in a general population and cancer patients. *Am J Surg Pathol* 2003;27:994–998.

8. Cubilla AL, Piris A, Pfannl R, et al. Anatomic levels: important landmarks in penectomy specimens: a detailed anatomic and histologic study based on examination of 44 cases. *Am J Surg Pathol* 2001;25:1091–1094.

9. Young RH, Srigley JR, Amin MB. *Tumors of the Prostate Gland, Seminal Vesicles, Male Urethra and Penis*. 3rd ed. Washington, DC: Armed Forces Institute of Pathology; 2000.

10. Cohen RJ, Garrett K, Golding JL, et al. Epithelial differentiation of the lower urinary tract with recognition of the minor prostatic glands. *Hum Pathol* 2002;33:905–909.

11. Cabanas RM. Anatomy and biopsy of sentinel lymph nodes. *Urol Clin North Am* 1992;19:267–276.

12. Crawford ED, Daneshgari F. Management of regional lymphatic drainage in carcinoma of the penis. *Urol Clin North Am* 1992;19:305–317.

13. Breza J, Aboseif SR, Owis BR, et al. Detailed anatomy of penile neurovascular structures: surgical significance. *J Urol* 1989;141:437–443.

14. Fitzpatrick T. The corpus cavernosum intercommunicating venous drainage system. *J Urol* 1975;113:494–496.

15. Leport H, Gregerman M, Ranice C, et al. Precise localization of the autonomic nerves from the pelvic plexus to the corpora cavernosa: a detailed study of the adult male pelvis. *J Urol* 1985;133:207–212.

16. Oesch IL, Pinter A, Ransley PG. Penile agenesis: a report of six cases. *J Pediatr Surg* 1987;22:172–174.

17. Elder J. *Congenital Anomalies of the Genitalia*. Philadelphia, PA: WB Saunders; 1982.

18. Chesney T, Murphy WM. Diseases of the penis and scrotum. In: *Urologic Pathology*. Philadelphia, PA: WB Saunders; 1989:380–408.

19. Nagore E, Sanchez-Motilla JM, Febrer MI, et al. Median raphe cysts of the penis: a report of five cases. *Pediatr Dermatol* 1998;15:191–193.

20. Romani J, Barnadas MA, Miralles J, et al. Median raphe cyst of the penis with ciliated cells. *J Cutan Pathol* 1995;22:378–381.

21. Johnson RA. Diseases and disorders of the anogenitalia of males. In: *Fitzpatrick's Dermatology in General Medicine*. 6th ed. New York: McGraw-Hill; 2003:1091–1107.

22. Tannenbaum M, Madden, JF, eds. *Diagnostic Atlas of Genitourinary Pathology*. Philadelphia, PA: Churchill Livingstone; 2006.

23. Fussell EN, Kaack MB, Cherry R, et al. Adherence of bacteria to human foreskins. *J Urol* 1988;140:997–1001.

24. Burdge DR, Bowie WR, Chow AW. *Gardnerella vaginalis*-associated balanoposthitis. *Sex Transm Dis* 1986;13:159–162.

25. Ramon Quiles D, Betlloch Mas I, Jimenez Martinez A, et al. Gonococcal infection of the penile median raphe. *Int J Dermatol* 1987;26:242–243.

26. Brady MT. Cellulitis of the penis and scrotum due to group B streptococcus. *J Urol* 1987;137:736–737.

27. White SW, Smith J. Trichomycosis pubis. *Arch Dermatol* 1979;115:444–445.

28. Bargman H. Trichomycosis of the scrotal hair. *Arch Dermatol* 1984;120:299.

29. Kuo CF, Wang WS, Lee CM, et al. Fournier's gangrene: ten-year experience in a medical center in northern Taiwan. *J Microbiol Immunol Infect* 2007;40:500–506.

30. Adams JR Jr, Mata JA, Venable DD, et al. Fournier's gangrene in children. *Urology* 1990;35:439–441.

31. Corbus BC. Erosive and gangrenous balanitis. The fourth venereal disease. *JAMA* 1909;52:1474.

32. Jeyakumar W, Ganesh R, Mohanram MS, et al. Papulonecrotic tuberculids of the glans penis: case report. *Genitourin Med* 1988;64:130–132.

33. Erol A, Ozgür S, Tahtali N, et al. Bacillus Calmette-Guerin (BCG) balanitis as a complication of intravesical BCG immunotherapy: a case report. *Int Urol Nephrol* 1995;27:307–310.

34. Dahl DM, Klein D, Morgentaler A. Penile mass caused by the newly described organism *Mycobacterium celatum*. *Urology* 1996;47:266–268.

35. Abell E, Marks R, Jones EW. Secondary syphilis: a clinico-pathological review. *Br J Dermatol* 1975;93:53–61.

36. Jeerapaet P, Ackerman AB. Histologic patterns of secondary syphilis. *Arch Dermatol* 1973;107:373–377.

37. David EE, ed. *Lever's Histopathology of the Skin*. 10th ed. Philadelphia, PA: Lippincott Williams & Wilkins; 2008.

38. Mc Kee PH, Calonje E, Brenn TL, eds. *Pathology of the Skin*. 4th ed. Philadelphia, PA: Elsevier Saunders; 2011:297.

39. Bari MM, Shulkin DJ, Abell E. Ulcerative syphilis in acquired immunodeficiency syndrome: a case of precocious tertiary syphilis in a patient infected with human immunodeficiency virus. *J Am Acad Dermatol* 1989;21:1310–1312.

40. Hay PE, Tam FW, Kitchen VS, et al. Gummatous lesions in men infected with human immunodeficiency virus and syphilis. *Genitourin Med* 1990;66:374–379.

41. Sheldon WH. Studies on chancroid: observations of the histology with an evaluation of biopsy as a diagnostic procedure. *Am J Pathol* 1946;22:415–425.

42. Freinkel AL. Histological aspects of sexually transmitted genital lesions. *Histopathology* 1987;11:819–831.

43. Davis CM. Granuloma inguinale. A clinical, histological and ultrastructural study. *JAMA* 1970;211:632–636.

44. Smith E. The histopathology of lymphogranuloma venerum. *J Urol* 1950;63:546–563.

45. zur Hausen H. Papillomaviruses causing cancer: evasion from host-cell control in early events in carcinogenesis. *J Natl Cancer Inst.* 2000;92:690–698.

46. zur Hausen H. Papillomaviruses in the causation of human cancers—a brief historical account. *Virology* 2009;384:260–265.

47. Heideman DA, Waterboer T, Pawlita M, et al. Human papillomavirus-16 is the predominant type etiologically involved in penile squamous cell carcinoma. *Clin Oncol* 2007;25:4550–4556.

48. Pascual A, Pariente M, Godínez JM, et al. High prevalence of human papillomavirus 16 in penile carcinoma. *Histol Histopathol* 2007;22:177–183.

49. Woodworth CD, Waggoner S, Barnes W, et al. Human cervical and foreskin epithelial cells immortalized by human papillomavirus DNAs exhibit dysplastic differentiation in vivo. *Cancer Res* 1990;50:3709–3715.

50. O'Brien WM, Jenson AB, Lancaster WD, et al. Human papillomavirus typing of penile condyloma. *J Urol* 1989;141:863–865.

51. Milburn PB, Brandsma JL, Goldsman CI, et al. Disseminated warts and evolving squamous cell carcinoma in a patient with acquired immunodeficiency syndrome. *J Am Acad Dermatol* 1988;19:401–405.

52. Barrasso R, De Brux J, Croissant O, et al. High prevalence of papillomavirus-associated penile intraepithelial neoplasia in sexual partners of women with cervical intraepithelial neoplasia. *N Engl J Med* 1987;317:916–923.

53. Campion MJ, McCance DJ, Mitchell HS, et al. Subclinical penile human papillomavirus infection and dysplasia in consorts of women with cervical neoplasia. *Genitourin Med* 1988;64:90–99.

54. Campion MJ, Singer A, Clarkson PK, et al. Increased risk of cervical neoplasia in consorts of men with penile condylomata acuminata. *Lancet* 1985;1:943–946.

55. Rubin MA, Kleter B, Zhou M, et al. Detection and typing of human papillomavirus DNA in penile carcinoma: evidence for multiple independent pathways of penile carcinogenesis. *Am J Pathol* 2001;159:1211–1218.

56. Gregoire L, Cubilla AL, Reuter VE, et al. Preferential association of human papillomavirus with high-grade histologic variants of penile-invasive squamous cell carcinoma. *J Natl Cancer Inst* 1995;87:1705–1709.

57. Li J, Ackerman AB. "Seborrheic keratoses" that contain human papillomavirus are condylomata acuminata. *Am J Dermatopathol* 1994;16:398–405.

58. Bai H, Cviko A, Granter S, et al. Immunophenotypic and viral (human papillomavirus) correlates of vulvar seborrheic keratosis. *Hum Pathol* 2003;34:559–564.

59. Nuovo GJ, Hochman HA, Eliezri YD, et al. Detection of human papillomavirus DNA in penile lesions histologically negative for condylomata. Analysis by in situ hybridization and the polymerase chain reaction. *Am J Surg Pathol* 1990;14:829–836.

60. Syrjanen SM, von Krogh G, Syrjanen KJ. Detection of human papillomavirus DNA in anogenital condylomata in men using in situ DNA hybridization applied to paraffin sections. *Genitourin Med* 1987;63:32–39.

61. Wade TR, Ackerman AB. The effects of resin of podophyllin on condylomas acuminatum. *Am J Dermatopathol* 1984;6:109–122.

62. Adanali G, Hacilar A, Verdi M, et al. Epidermoid carcinoma arising in a giant condyloma acuminata of 20 years' duration. *Ann Plast Surg* 2002;48:333–334.

63. Gupta R, Warren T, Wald A. Genital herpes. *Lancet* 2007;370:2127–2137.

64. Cedeno-Laurent F, Gómez-Flores M, Mendez N, et al. New insights into HIV-1-primary skin disorders. *J Int AIDS Soc* 2011;14:5.

65. Cockerell CJ. Cutaneous manifestations of HIV infection other than Kaposi's sarcoma: clinical and histologic aspects. *J Am Acad Dermatol* 1990;22:1260–1269.

66. Gormley RH, Kovarik CL. Dermatologic manifestations of HPV in HIV-infected individuals. *Curr HIV/AIDS Rep* 2009;6:130–138.

67. Woldrich JM, Silberstein JL, Saltzstein SL, et al. Penile Kaposis sarcoma in the state of California. *Can J Urol* 2012;19:6178–6182.

68. Perfect JR, Seaworth BA. Penile cryptococcosis with review of mycotic infections of penis. *Urology* 1985;25:528–531.

69. Ariyanayagam-Baksh SM, Baksh FK, Cartun RW, et al. Histoplasma phimosis: an uncommon presentation of a not uncommon pathogen. *Am J Dermatopathol* 2007;29:300–302.

70. Soendjojo A, Pindha S. *Trichomonas vaginalis* infection of the median raphe of the penis. *Sex Transm Dis* 1981;8:255–257.

71. Buechner SA. Common skin disorders of the penis. *BJU Int* 2002;90:498–506.

72. Schneider JM, Matthews JH, Graham BS. Reiter's syndrome. *Cutis* 2003;71:198–200.

73. Bain L, Geronemus R. The association of lichen planus of the penis with squamous cell carcinoma in situ and with verrucous squamous carcinoma. *J Dermatol Surg Oncol* 1989;15:413–417.

74. Hoshi A, Usui Y, Terachi T. Penile carcinoma originating from lichen planus on glans penis. *Urology* 2008;71:816–817.

75. Stühmer A. Balanitis xerotica obliterans (post operationem) und ihre Beziehungen zur 'Kraurosis glandis et praeputii penis.' *Arch Dermatol Syphilis* 1928;156:613–623.

76. Velazquez EF, Cubilla AL. Lichen sclerosus in 68 patients with squamous cell carcinoma of the penis: frequent atypias and correlation with special carcinoma variants suggests a precancerous role. *Am J Surg Pathol* 2003;27:1448–1453.

77. Carlson JA, Ambros R, Malfetano J, et al. Vulvar lichen sclerosus and squamous cell carcinoma: a cohort, case control, and investigational study with historical perspective; implications for chronic inflammation and sclerosis in the development of neoplasia. *Hum Pathol* 1998;29:932–948.

78. Powell J, Robson A, Cranston D, et al. High incidence of lichen sclerosus in patients with squamous cell carcinoma of the penis. *Br J Dermatol* 2001;145:85–89.

79. Cubilla AL, Velazquez EF, Young RH. Pseudohyperplastic squamous cell carcinoma of the penis associated with lichen sclerosus. An extremely well-differentiated, nonverruciform neoplasm that preferentially affects the foreskin and is frequently misdiagnosed: a report of 10 cases of a distinctive clinicopathologic entity. *Am J Surg Pathol* 2004;28:895–900.

80. Nasca MR, Innocenzi D, Micali G. Penile cancer among patients with genital lichen sclerosus. *J Am Acad Dermatol* 1999;41:911–914.

81. Micali G, Nasca MR, Innocenzi D. Lichen sclerosus of the glans is significantly associated with penile carcinoma. *Sex Transm Infect* 2001;77:226.

82. Oertell J, Caballero C, Iglesias M, et al. Differentiated precursor lesions and low-grade variants of squamous cell carcinomas are frequent findings in foreskins of patients from a region of high penile cancer incidence. *Histopathology* 2011;58:925–933.

83. Chaux A, Velazquez EF, Amin A, et al. Distribution and characterization of subtypes of penile intraepithelial neoplasia and their association with invasive carcinomas: a pathological study of 139 lesions in 121 patients. *Hum Pathol* 2012;43:1020–1027.

84. Zoon JI. Balanopostithe Chronique Circonscrite Benigne a Plasmocytes. *Dermatologica* 1952;105:1–7.

85. Souteyrand P, Wong E, MacDonald DM. Zoon's balanitis (balanitis circumscripta plasmacellularis). *Br J Dermatol* 1981;105:195–199.

86. Brix WK, Nassau SR, Patterson JW, et al. Idiopathic lymphoplasma-cellular mucositis-dermatitis. *J Cutan Pathol* 2010;37:426–431.

87. Fueston JC, Adams BB, Mutasim DF. Cicatricial pemphigoid-induced phimosis. *J Am Acad Dermatol* 2002;46:S128–S129.

88. Sami N, Ahmed AR. Penile pemphigus. *Arch Dermatol* 2001;137:756–758.

89. Palleschi GM, Giomi B, Giacomelli A. Juvenile pemphigus vegetans of the glans penis. *Acta Derm Venereol* 2004;84:316–317.

90. Anhalt GJ. Paraneoplastic pemphigus. *Investig Dermatol Symp Proc* 2004;9:29–33.

91. Wong TY, Mihm MC Jr. Acantholytic dermatosis localized to genitalia and crural areas of male patients: a report of three cases. *J Cutan Pathol* 1994;21:27–32.

92. Muneer A, Ali I, Blick C, et al. An unusual solitary lesion on the glans penis. *Clin Exp Dermatol* 2009;34:929–930.

93. Domínguez Domínguez M, Valero Puerta JA, Jiménez Leiro JF, et al. [Primary localized amyloidosis of glans penis. A new case and review of the literature (Review)]. *Actas Urol Esp* 2007;31:168–171.

94. Gilmore WA, Weigand DA, Burgdorf WH. Penile nodules in Southeast Asian men. *Arch Dermatol* 1983;119:446–447.

95. Oertel YC, Johnson FB. Sclerosing lipogranuloma of male genitalia. Review of 23 cases. *Arch Pathol Lab Med* 1977;101:321–326.

96. Eandi JA, Yao AP, Javidan J. Penile paraffinoma: the delayed presentation. *Int Urol Nephrol* 2007;39:553–555.

97. Gelbard MK. Dystrophic penile calcification in Peyronie's disease. *J Urol* 1988;139:738–740.

98. Abdel-Hamid IA, Anis T. Peyronie's disease: perspectives on therapeutic targets. *Expert Opin Ther Targets* 2011;15:913–929.

99. Gonzalez-Cadavid NF, Rajfer J. Experimental models of Peyronie's disease. Implications for new therapies. *J Sex Med* 2009;6:303–313.

100. Gharpuray MB, Tolat SN. Nonvenereal sclerosing lymphangitis of the penis. *Cutis* 1991;47:421–422.

101. Rosen T, Hwong H. Sclerosing lymphangitis of the penis. *Am Acad Dermatol* 2003;49:916–918.

102. Karademir K, Senkul T, Atasoyu E, et al. Ulcerative necrosis of the glans penis resulting from polyarteritis nodosa. *J Clin Rheumatol* 2005;11:167–169.

103. Dufour JF, Le Gallou T, Cordier JF, et al. Urogenital manifestations in Wegener granulomatosis: a study of 11 cases and review of the literature. *Medicine (Baltimore)* 2012;91:67–74.

104. Reitsma W, Wiegman MJ, Damstra RJ. Penile and scrotal lymphedema as an unusual presentation of Crohn's disease: case report and review of the literature. *Lymphology* 2012;45:37–41.

105. Cockburn AG, Krolikowski J, Balogh K, et al. Crohn disease of penile and scrotal skin. *Urology* 1980;15:596–598.

106. Tannenbaum M. Papillae of the corona of the glans penis. *J Urol* 1965;93:391–395.

107. Manchanda Y, Sethuraman G, Paderwani PP, et al. Molluscum contagiosum presenting as penile horn in an HIV positive patient. *Sex Transm Infect* 2005;81:183–184.

108. George WM, Azadeh B. Verruciform xanthoma of the penis. *Cutis* 1989;44:167–170.

109. Chalmers RJ, Burton PA, Bennett RF, et al. Lichen sclerosus et atrophicus. A common and distinctive cause of phimosis in boys. *Arch Dermatol* 1984;120:1025–1027.

110. Clemmensen OJ, Krogh J, Petri M. The histologic spectrum of prepuces from patients with phimosis. *Am J Dermatopathol* 1988;10:104–108.

111. Chaux A, Pfannl R, Lloveras B, et al. Distinctive association of p16INK4a overexpression with penile intraepithelial neoplasia depicting warty and/or basaloid features: a study of 141 cases evaluating a new nomenclature. *Am J Surg Pathol* 2010;34:385–392.

112. Chaux A, Pfannl R, Rodríguez IM, et al. Distinctive immunohistochemical profile of penile intraepithelial lesions: a study of 74 cases. *Am J Surg Pathol* 2011;35:553–562.

113. Cubilla AL, Meijer CJ, Young RH. Morphological features of epithelial abnormalities and precancerous lesions of the penis. *Scand J Urol Nephrol Suppl* 2000;205:215–219.

114. Cubilla AL, Velazquez EF, Young RH. Epithelial lesions associated with invasive penile squamous cell carcinoma: a pathologic study of 288 cases. *Int J Surg Pathol* 2004;12:351–364.

115. Horenblas S, von Krogh G, Cubilla AL, et al. Squamous cell carcinoma of the penis: premalignant lesions. *Scand J Urol Nephrol Suppl* 2000;205:187–188.

116. Porter WM, Francis N, Hawkins D, et al. Penile intraepithelial neoplasia: clinical spectrum and treatment of 35 cases. *Br J Dermatol* 2002;147:1159–1165.

117. Soskin A, Vieillefond A, Carlotti A, et al. Warty/basaloid penile intraepithelial neoplasia is more prevalent than differentiated penile intraepithelial neoplasia in nonendemic regions for penile cancer when compared with endemic areas: a comparative study between pathologic series from Paris and Paraguay. *Hum Pathol* 2012;43:190–196.

118. Velazquez EF, Chaux A, Cubilla AL. Histologic classification of penile intraepithelial neoplasia. *Semin Diagn Pathol* 2012;29:96–102.

119. Hart WR. Vulvar intraepithelial neoplasia: historical aspects and current status. *Int J Gynecol Pathol* 2001;20:16–30.

120. Kurman RJ, Norris HJ, Wilkinson E. Tumors of the cervix, vagina and vulva. In: *Atlas of Tumor Pathology*. 3rd series ed. Washington, DC: Armed Forces Institute of Pathology; 1992:202–203.

121. Sideri M, Jones RW, Wilkinson EJ, et al. Squamous vulvar intraepithelial neoplasia: 2004 modified terminology, ISSVD Vulvar Oncology Subcommittee. *J Reprod Med* 2005;50:807–810.

122. Graham JH, Helwig EB. Erythroplasia of Queyrat. A clinicopathologic and histochemical study. *Cancer* 1973;32:1396–1414.

123. Kaye V, Zhang G, Dehner LP, et al. Carcinoma in situ of penis. Is distinction between erythroplasia of Queyrat and Bowen's disease relevant? *Urology* 1990;36:479–482.

124. Queyrat L. Erythroplasie Du Gland. *Bull Soc Fr Dermatol Syphiligr* 1911;22:378–382.

125. Metcalf JS, Lee RE, Maize JC. Epidermotropic urothelial carcinoma involving the glans penis. *Arch Dermatol* 1985;121:532–534.

126. Wade TR, Kopf AW, Ackerman AB. Bowenoid papulosis of the penis. *Cancer* 1978;42:1890–1903.

127. Patterson JW, Kao GF, Graham JH, et al. Bowenoid papulosis. A clinicopathologic study with ultrastructural observations. *Cancer* 1986;57:823–836.

128. Eisen RF, Bhawan J, Cahn TH. Spontaneous regression of bowenoid papulosis of the penis. *Cutis* 1983;32:269–272.

129. Hauser B, Gross G, Schneider A, et al. HPV-16-related Bowenoid papulosis. *Lancet* 1985;2:106.

130. Chaux A, Netto GJ, Rodríguez IM, et al. Epidemiologic profile, sexual history, pathologic features, and human papillomavirus status of 103 patients with penile carcinoma. *World J Urol* 2011. Nov 25. [Epub ahead of print].

131. Chiu TY, Huang HS, Lai MK, et al. Penile cancer in Taiwan—20 years' experience at National Taiwan University Hospital. *J Formos Med Assoc* 1998;97:673–678.

132. Dodge OG, Linsell CA. Carcinoma of the penis in Ugandan and Kenyan Africans. *Cancer* 1963;16:1255–1263.

133. Lebron RF, Riveros M. Geographical pathology of cancer of the penis. *Cancer* 1963;15:798–810.

134. Maiche AG. Epidemiological aspects of cancer of the penis in Finland. *Eur J Cancer Prev* 1992;1:153–158.

135. Persky L. Epidemiology of cancer of the penis. Recent results. *Cancer Res* 1977;60:97–109.

136. Reddy CR, Raghavaiah NV, Mouli KC. Prevalence of carcinoma of the penis with special reference to India. *Int Surg* 1975;60:474–476.

137. Hubbell CR, Rabin VR, Mora RG. Cancer of the skin in blacks. V. A review of 175 black patients with squamous cell carcinoma of the penis. *J Am Acad Dermatol* 1988;18:292–298.

138. Boczko S, Freed S. Penile carcinoma in circumcised males. *NY State J Med* 1979;79:1903–1904.

139. Castellsagué X, Bosch FX, Muñoz N, et al. Male circumcision, penile human papillomavirus infection, and cervical cancer in female partners. *N Engl J Med* 2002;346:1105–1112.

140. Maden C, Sherman KJ, Beckmann AM, et al. History of circumcision, medical conditions, and sexual activity and risk of penile cancer. *J Natl Cancer Inst* 1993;85:19–24.

141. Moses S, Bailey RC, Ronald AR. Male circumcision: assessment of health benefits and risks. *Sex Transm Infect* 1998;74:368–373.

142. Schoen EJ, Oehrli M, Colby C, et al. The highly protective effect of newborn circumcision against invasive penile cancer. *Pediatrics* 2000;105:E36.

143. Bissada NK, Morcos RR, el-Senoussi M. Post-circumcision carcinoma of the penis. I. Clinical aspects. *J Urol* 1986;135:283–285.

144. Bissada NK. Post-circumcision carcinoma of the penis: II. Surgical management. *J Surg Oncol* 1988;37:80–83.

145. Aynaud O, Piron D, Bijaoui G, et al. Developmental factors of urethral human papillomavirus lesions: correlation with circumcision. *BJU Int* 1999;84:57–60.

146. Chaux A, Cubilla AL. The role of human papillomavirus infection in the pathogenesis of penile squamous cell carcinomas. *Semin Diagn Pathol* 2012;29:67–71.

147. Malek RS, Goellner JR, Smith TF, et al. Human papillomavirus infection and intraepithelial, in situ, and invasive carcinoma of penis. *Urology* 1993;42:159–170.

148. Scinicariello F, Rady P, Saltzstein D, et al. Human papillomavirus 16 exhibits a similar integration pattern in primary squamous cell carcinoma of the penis and in its metastasis. *Cancer* 1992;70:2143–2148.

149. Villa LL, Lopes A. Human papillomavirus DNA sequences in penile carcinomas in Brazil. *Int J Cancer* 1986;37:853–855.

150. Wiener JS, Effert PJ, Humphrey PA, et al. Prevalence of human papillomavirus types 16 and 18 in squamous-cell carcinoma of the penis: a retrospective analysis of primary and metastatic lesions by differential polymerase chain reaction. *Int J Cancer* 1992;50:694–701.

151. Lam KY, Chan AC, Chan KW, et al. Absence of Epstein-Barr virus in penile carcinoma. A study of 42 cases using in situ hybridization. *Cancer* 1995;76:658–660.

152. Alves G, Macrini CM, de Souza Nascimento P, et al. Detection and expression of Epstein-Barr virus (EBV) DNA in tissues from penile tumors in Brazil. *Cancer Lett* 2004;215:79–82.

153. Bouyssou-Gauthier ML, Boulinguez S, Dumas JP, et al. [Penile lichen sclerosus: follow-up study]. *Ann Dermatol Venereol* 1999;126:804–807.

154. Campus GV, Alia F, Bosincu L. Squamous cell carcinoma and lichen sclerosus et atrophicus of the prepuce. *Plast Reconstr Surg* 1992;89:962–964.

155. Pride HB, Miller OF III, Tyler WB. Penile squamous cell carcinoma arising from balanitis xerotica obliterans. *J Am Acad Dermatol* 1993;29:469–473.

156. Harish K, Ravi R. The role of tobacco in penile carcinoma. *Br J Urol* 1995;75:375–377.

157. Daling JR, Sherman KJ, Hislop TG, et al. Cigarette smoking and the risk of anogenital cancer. *Am J Epidemiol* 1992;135:180–189.

158. Ravi R. Radiation-induced carcinoma of the penis. *Urol Int* 1995;54:147–149.

159. Fukunaga M, Yokoi K, Miyazawa Y, et al. Penile verrucous carcinoma with anaplastic transformation following radiotherapy. A case report with human papillomavirus typing and flow cytometric DNA studies. *Am J Surg Pathol* 1994;18:501–505.

160. Stern RS. Genital tumors among men with psoriasis exposed to psoralens and ultraviolet A radiation (PUVA) and ultraviolet B radiation. The Photochemotherapy Follow-up Study. *N Engl J Med* 1990;322:1093–1097.

161. Selli C, Scott CA, De Antoni P, et al. Squamous cell carcinoma arising at the base of the penis in a burn scar. *Urology* 1999;54:923.

162. Chaux A, Velazquez EF, Barreto JE, et al. New pathologic entities in penile carcinomas: an update of the 2004 world health organization classification. *Semin Diagn Pathol* 2012;29:59–66.

163. Cubilla AL. Carcinoma of the penis. *Mod Pathol* 1995;8:116–118.

164. Cubilla AL, Barreto J, Caballero C, et al. Pathologic features of epidermoid carcinoma of the penis. A prospective study of 66 cases. *Am J Surg Pathol* 1993;17:753–763.

165. Cubilla AL, Dillner J, Schellhammer PF, et al. Malignant epithelial tumors. In: *Tumors of the penis. Pathology and Genetics. Tumors of the Urinary System and Male Genital Organs, WHO*. Lyon, France: IARC Press; 2003.

166. Velazquez EF, Cubilla AL. Penile squamous cell carcinoma: anatomic, pathologic and viral studies in Paraguay (1993–2007). *Anal Quant Cytol Histol* 2007;29:185–98.

167. Cubilla AL, Reuter VE, Gregoire L, et al. Basaloid squamous cell carcinoma: a distinctive human papilloma virus-related penile neoplasm: a report of 20 cases. *Am J Surg Pathol* 1998;22:755–761.

168. Cubilla AL, Velazques EF, Reuter VE, et al. Warty (condylomatous) squamous cell carcinoma of the penis: a report of 11 cases and proposed classification of 'verruciform' penile tumors. *Am J Surg Pathol* 2000;24:505–512.

169. Cubilla AL, Ayala MT, Barreto JE, et al. Surface adenosquamous carcinoma of the penis. A report of three cases. *Am J Surg Pathol* 1996;20:156–160.

170. Chaux A, Tamboli P, Ayala A, et al. Warty-basaloid carcinoma: clinicopathological features of a distinctive penileneoplasm. Report of 45 cases. *Mod Pathol* 2010;23:896–904.

171. Cubilla AL, Lloveras B, Alemany L, et al. Basaloid squamous cell carcinoma of the penis with papillary features: a clinicopathologic study of 12 cases. *Am J Surg Pathol* 2012;36:869–875.

172. Velazquez EF, Cubilla AL. Pseudohyperplastic squamous cell carcinoma of the penis associated with lichen sclerosus. *Pathol Case Rev* 2005;10:21–26.

173. Barreto JE, Velazquez EF, Ayala E, et al. Carcinoma cuniculatum: a distinctive variant of penile squamous cell carcinoma: report of 7 cases. *Am J Surg Pathol* 2007;31:71–75.

174. Cunha IW, Guimaraes GC, Soares F, et al. Pseudoglandular (adenoid, acantholytic) penile squamous cell carcinoma: a clinicopathologic and outcome study of 7 patients. *Am J Surg Pathol* 2008;33:551–555.

175. Derrick FC Jr, Lynch KM Jr, Kretkowski RC, et al. Epidermoid carcinoma of the penis: computer analysis of 87 cases. *J Urol* 1973;110:303–305.

176. Jones WG, Fossa SD, Hamers H, et al. Penis cancer: a review by the Joint Radiotherapy Committee of the European Organization for Research and Treatment of Cancer (EORTC) Genitourinary and Radiotherapy Groups. *J Surg Oncol* 1989;40:227–331.

177. Hanash KA, Furlow WL, Utz DC, et al. Carcinoma of the penis: a clinicopathologic study. *J Urol* 1970;104:291–297.

178. Hoppmann HJ, Fraley EE. Squamous cell carcinoma of the penis. *J Urol* 1978;120:393–338.

179. Merrin CE. Cancer of the penis. *Cancer* 1980;45:1973–1979.

180. Narayana AS, Olney LE, Loening SA, et al. Carcinoma of the penis: analysis of 219 cases. *Cancer* 1982;49:2185–2191.

181. Ornellas AA, Seixas AL, Marota A, et al. Surgical treatment of invasive squamous cell carcinoma of the penis: retrospective analysis of 350 cases. *J Urol* 1994;151:1244–1249.

182. Ornellas AA, Seixas AL, de Moraes JR. Analyses of 200 lymphadenectomies in patients with penile carcinoma. *J Urol* 1991;146:330–332.

183. Srinivas V, Morse MJ, Herr HW, et al. Penile cancer: relation of extent of nodal metastasis to survival. *J Urol* 1987;137:880–882.

184. Chaux A, Torres J, Pfannl R, et al. Histologic grade in penile squamous cell carcinoma: visual estimation versus digital measurement of proportions of grades, adverse prognosis with any proportion of grade 3 and correlation of a Gleason-like system with nodal metastasis. *Am J Surg Pathol* 2009;33:1042–1048.

185. Velazquez EF, Ayala G, Liu H, et al. Histologic grade and perineural invasion are more important than tumor thickness as predictor of nodal metastasis in penile squamous cell carcinoma invading 5-10 mm. *Am J Surg Pathol* 2008;32:974–979.

186. Downey GO, Okagaki T, Ostrow RS, et al. Condylomatous carcinoma of the vulva with special reference to human papillomavirus DNA. *Obstet Gynecol* 1988;72:68–73.

187. Riethdorf S, Neffen EF, Cviko A, et al. p16INK4A expression as biomarker for HPV 16-related vulvar neoplasias. *Hum Pathol* 2004;35:1477–1483.

188. Cubilla AL, Lloveras B, Alejo M, et al. Value of p16(INK)⁴(a) in the pathology of invasive penile squamous cell carcinomas: a report of 202 cases. *Am J Surg Pathol* 2011;35:253–261.

189. Johnson DE, Lo RK, Srigley J, et al. Verrucous carcinoma of the penis. *J Urol* 1985;133:216–218.

190. McKee PH, Lowe D, Haigh RJ. Penile verrucous carcinoma. *Histopathology* 1983;7:897–906.

191. Kato N, Onozuka T, Yasukawa K, et al. Penile hybrid verrucous-squamous carcinoma associated with a superficial inguinal lymph node metastasis. *Am J Dermatopathol* 2000;22:339–343.

192. Ayrd I, Johnson HD, Lennox B, et al. Epithelioma cuniculatum: a variety of squamous carcinoma peculiar to the foot. *Br J Surg* 1954;42:245–250.

193. Chaux A, Soares F, Rodríguez I, et al. Papillary squamous cell carcinoma, not otherwise specified (NOS) ofthe penis: clinicopathologic features, differential diagnosis, and outcome of 35 cases. *Am J Surg Pathol* 2010;34:223–230.

194. Lont AP, Gallee MP, Snijders P, et al. Sarcomatoid squamous cell carcinoma of the penis: a clinical and pathological study of 5 cases. *J Urol* 2004;172:932–935.

195. Velazquez EF, Melamed J, Barreto JE, et al. Sarcomatoid carcinoma of the penis: a clinicopathologic study of 15 cases. *Am J Surg Pathol* 2005;29:1152–1158.

196. Manglani KS, Manaligod JR, Ray B. Spindle cell carcinoma of the glans penis: a light and electron microscopic study. *Cancer* 1980;46:2266–2272.

197. Kayes O, Ahmed HU, Arya M, et al. Molecular and genetic pathways in penile cancer. *Lancet Oncol* 2007;8:420–429.

198. Muneer A, Kayes O, Ahmed HU, et al. Molecular prognostic factors in penile cancer. *World J Urol* 2009;27:161–167.

199. Ferreux E, Lont AP, Horenblas S, et al. Evidence for at least three alternative mechanisms targeting the p16INK4A/cyclin D/Rb pathway in penile carcinoma, one of which is mediated by high-risk human papillomavirus. *J Pathol* 2003;201:109–118.

200. Castren K, Vahakangas K, Heikkinen E, et al. Absence of p53 mutations in benign and pre-malignant male genital lesions with overexpressed p53 protein. *Int J Cancer* 1998;77:674–678.

201. Ayala G, Cubilla AL. p53 and histologic subtypes of penile carcinomas. *J Surg Pathol* 1998;3:33–38.

202. Lam KY, Chan AC, Chan KW, et al. Expression of p53 and its relationship with human papillomavirus in penile carcinomas. *Eur J Surg Oncol* 1995;21:613–616.

203. Walts AE, Koeffler HP, Said JW. Localization of p53 protein and human papillomavirus in anogenital squamous lesions: immunohistochemical and in situ hybridization studies in benign, dysplastic, and malignant epithelia. *Hum Pathol* 1993;24:1238–1242.

204. Lam KY, Chan KW. Molecular pathology and clinicopathologic features of penile tumors: with special reference to analyses of p21 and p53 expression and unusual histologic features. *Arch Pathol Lab Med* 1999;123:895–904.

205. Schmidt-Grimminger DC, Wu X, Jian Y, et al. Post-transcriptional induction of p21cip1 protein in condylomata and dysplasias is inversely related to human papillomavirus activities. *Am J Pathol* 1998;152:1015–1024.

206. Lopes A, Bezerra AL, Pinto CA, et al. p53 as a new prognostic factor for lymph node metastasis in penile carcinoma: analysis of 82 patients treated with amputation and bilateral lymphadenectomy. *J Urol* 2002;168:81–86.

207. Ranki A, Lassus J, Niemi KM. Relation of p53 tumor suppressor protein expression to human papillomavirus (HPV) DNA and to cellular atypia in male genital warts and in premalignant lesions. *Acta Derm Venereol* 1995;75:180–186.

208. Alves G, Fiedler W, Guenther E, et al. Determination of telomerase activity in squamous cell carcinoma of the penis. *Int J Oncol* 2001; 18:67–70.

209. Ornellas AA, Ornellas MH, Simoes F, et al. Cytogenetic analysis of an invasive, poorly differentiated squamous cell carcinoma of the penis. *Cancer Genet Cytogenet* 1998;101:78–79.

210. Xiao S, Feng XL, Shi YH, et al. Cytogenetic abnormalities in a squamous cell carcinoma of the penis. *Cancer Genet Cytogenet* 1992;64:139–141.

211. Leis PF, Stevens KR, Baer SC, et al. A c-rasHa mutation in the metastasis of a human papillomavirus (HPV)-18 positive penile squamous cell carcinoma suggests a cooperative effect between HPV-18 and c-rasHa activation in malignant progression. *Cancer* 1998;83:122–129.

212. Golijanin D, Tan JY, Kazior A, et al. Cyclooxygenase-2 and microsomal prostaglandin E synthase-1 are overexpressed in squamous cell carcinoma of the penis. *Clin Cancer Res* 2004;10:1024–1031.

213. Hall MC, Sanders JS, Vuitch F, et al. Deoxyribonucleic acid flow cytometry and traditional pathologic variables in invasive penile carcinoma: assessment of prognostic significance. *Urology* 1998;52:111–116.

214. Yu DS, Chang SY, Ma CP. DNA ploidy, S-phase fraction and cytomorphometry in relation to survival of human penile cancer. *Urol Int* 1992;48:265–269.

215. Campos RS, Lopes A, Guimarães GC, et al. E-cadherin, MMP-2, and MMP-9 as prognostic markers in penile cancer: analysis of 125 patients. *Urology* 2006;67:797–802.

216. Masferrer E, Ferrándiz-Pulido C, Lloveras B, et al. MYC copy number gains are associated with poor outcome in penile squamous cell carcinoma. *J Urol* 2012;188:1965–1971.

217. Maier S, Wilbertz T, Braun M, et al. SOX2 amplification is a common event in squamous cell carcinomas of different organ sites. *Hum Pathol* 2011;42:1078–1088.

218. Rocha RM, Ignácio JA, Jordán J, et al. A clinical, pathologic, and molecular study of p53 and murine double minute 2 in penile carcinogénesis and its relation to prognosis. *Hum Pathol* 2012;43:481–488.

219. Cubilla AL. The role of pathologic prognostic factors in squamous cell carcinoma of the penis. *World J Urol* 2009;27:169–177.

220. Slaton JW, Morgenstern N, Levy DA, et al. Tumor stage, vascular invasion and the percentage of poorly differentiated cancer: independent prognosticators for inguinal lymph node metastasis in penile squamous cancer. *J Urol* 2001;165:1138–1142.

221. Emerson RE, Ulbright TM, Eble JN, et al. Predicting cancer progression in patients with penile squamous cell carcinoma: the importance of depth of invasion and vascular invasion. *Mod Pathol* 2001;14: 963–968.

222. McDougal WS. Carcinoma of the penis: improved survival by early regional lymphadenectomy based on the histological grade and depth of invasion of the primary lesion. *J Urol* 1995;154:1364–1366.

223. Solsona E, Iborra I, Rubio J, et al. Prospective validation of the association of local tumor stage and grade as a predictive factor for occult lymph node micrometastasis in patients with penile carcinoma and clinically negative inguinal lymph nodes. *J Urol* 2001;16:1506–1509.

224. Guimarães GC, Cunha IW, Soares FA, et al. Penile squamous cell carcinoma clinicopathological features, nodal metastasis andoutcome in 333 cases. *J Urol* 2009;182:528–534.

225. Cubilla AL, Reuter V, Velazquez E. Histologic classification of penile carcinoma and its relation to outcome in 61 patients with primary resection. *Int J Surg Pathol* 2001;9:111–120.

226. Ficarra V, Zattoni F, Cunisco SC, et al. Lymphatic and vascular embolizations are independent predictive variables of inguinal node involvement in patients with squamous cell carcinoma of the penis. *Cancer* 2005;103:2507–2516.

227. Novara G, Galfano A, De Marco V, et al. Prognostic factors in squamous cell carcinoma of the penis. *Nat Clin Pract Urol* 2007;4: 140–146.

228. Horenblas S, van Tinteren H, Delemarre JF, et al. Squamous cell carcinoma of the penis. III. Treatment of regional lymph nodes. *J Urol* 1993;149:492–497.

229. Horenblas S, van Tinteren H. Squamous cell carcinoma of the penis. IV. Prognostic factors of survival: analysis of tumor, nodes and metastasis classification system. *J Urol* 1994;151:1239–1243.

230. Maiche AG, Pyrhonen S, Karkinen M. Histological grading of squamous cell carcinoma of the penis: a new scoring system. *Br J Urol* 1991;67: 522–526.

231. Velazquez EF, Barreto JE, Rodriguez I, et al. Limitations in the interpretation of biopsies in patients with penile squamous cell carcinoma. *Int J Surg Pathol* 2004;12:139–146.

232. Korets R, Koppie TM, Snyder ME, et al. Partial penectomy for patients with squamous cell carcinoma of the penis: the Memorial Sloan-Kettering experience. *Ann Surg Oncol* 2007;14:3614–3619.

233. Mistry T, Jones RW, Dannatt E, et al. A 10-year retrospective audit of penile cancer management in the UK. *BJU Int* 2007;100:1277–1281.

234. Lont AP, Kroon BK, Gallee MP, et al. Pelvic lymph node dissection for penile carcinoma: extent of inguinal lymph node involvement as an indicator for pelvic lymph node involvement and survival. *J Urol* 2007;177:947–952.

235. Dai B, Ye DW, Kong YY, et al. Predicting regional lymph node metastasis in Chinese patients with penile squamous cell carcinoma: the role of histopathological classification, tumor stage and depth of invasion. *J Urol* 2006;176:1431–1435.

236. Hegarty PK, Kayes O, Freeman A, et al. A prospective study of 100 cases of penile cancer managed according to European Association of Urology guidelines. *BJU Int* 2006;98:526–531.

237. Lont AP, Kroon BK, Horenblas S, et al. Presence of high-risk human papillomavirus DNA in penile carcinoma predicts favorable outcome in survival. *Int J Cancer* 2006;119:1078–1081.

238. UICC. *TNM Classification of Malignant Tumors*. 6th ed. New York: Wiley & Sons; 2002.

239. Chaux A, Caballero C, Soares F, et al. The prognostic index: a useful pathologic guide for prediction of nodal metastases and survival in penile squamous cell carcinoma. *Am J Surg Pathol* 2009;33: 1049–1057.

240. Ficarra V, Zattoni F, Artibani W, et al. Penile Cancer Project Members. Nomogram predictive of pathological inguinal lymph node involvement in patients with squamous cell carcinoma of the penis. *J Urol* 2006;175:1700–1705.

241. Kattan MW, Ficarra V, Artibani W, et al. Nomogram predictive of cancer specific survival in patients undergoing partial or total amputation for squamous cell carcinoma of the penis. *J Urol* 2006;175:2103–2108.

242. Spiess PE, Izawa JI, Bassett R, et al. Preoperative lymphoscintigraphy and dynamic sentinel node biopsy for staging penile cancer: results with pathological correlation. *J Urol* 2007;177:2157–2161.

243. Tanis PJ, Lont AP, Meinhardt W, et al. Dynamic sentinel node biopsy for penile cancer: reliability of a staging technique. *J Urol* 2002;168:76.

244. Perdona S, Autorino R, De Sio M, et al. Dynamic sentinel node biopsy in clinically node-negative penile cancer versus radical inguinal lymphadenectomy: a comparative study. *Urology* 2005;66:1282.

245. Hadway P, Smith Y, Corbishley C, et al. Evaluation of dynamic lymphoscintigraphy and sentinel lymph-node biopsy for detecting occult metastases in patients with penile squamous cell carcinoma. *BJU Int* 2007;100:561–565.

246. Lont AP, Horenblas S, Tanis PJ, et al. Management of clinically node negative penile carcinoma: improved survival after the introduction of dynamic sentinel node biopsy. *J Urol* 2003;170:783–786.

247. Velazquez EF, Amin MB, Epstein JI, et al. Members of the Cancer Committee, College of American Pathologists. Protocol for the examination of specimens from patients with carcinoma of the penis. *Arch Pathol Lab Med* 2010;134:923–929.

248. Lowenstein LW. Carcinoma-like condylomata acuminata of the penis. *Med Clin North Am* 1939;23:789–795.

249. Gibson GE, Ahmed I. Perianal and genital basal cell carcinoma: a clinicopathologic review of 51 cases *J Am Acad Dermatol* 2001;45:68–71.

250. Peison B, Benisch B, Nicora B. Multicentric basal cell carcinoma of penile skin. *Urology* 1985;25:322–323.

251. Tomic S, Warner TF, Messing E, et al. Penile Merkel cell carcinoma. *Urology* 1995;45:1062–1065.

252. Suwa M, Takeda M, Bilim V et al. Epidermoid cyst of the penis: a case report and review of the literature. *Int J Urol* 2000;7:431–433.

253. Park HJ, Park NC, Park SW, et al. Penile epidermal inclusion cyst: a late complication of penile girth enhancement surgery. *J Sex Med* 2008;5:2238–2240.

254. Tomasini C, Aloi F, Puiatti P, et al. Dermoid cyst of the penis. *Dermatology* 1997;194:188–190.

255. Mataix J, Bañuls J, Blanes M, et al. Translucent nodular lesion of the penis. Apocrine hidrocystoma of the penis. *Arch Dermatol* 2006;142:1221–1226.

256. Lo JS, Dijkstra JW, Bergfeld WF. Syringomas on the penis. *Int J Dermatol* 1990;29:309–310.

257. Olson JM, Robles DT, Argenyi ZB, et al. Multiple penile syringomas. *Am Acad Dermatol* 2008;59:S46–S47.

258. Vergara G, Belinchón I, Silvestre JF, et al. Linear sebaceous gland hyperplasia of the penis: a case report. *J Am Acad Dermatol* 2003;48: 149–150.

259. Obaidat NA, Ghazarian DM. A proliferating composite adnexal tumour of the penis: report of the first case. *J Clin Pathol* 2007;60: 567–569.

260. Helwig EB, Graham JH. Anogenital extramammary Paget's disease. A clinicopathologic study. *Cancer* 1963;16:387–403.

261. Macedo A Jr, Fichtner J, Hohenfellner R. Extramammary Paget's disease of the penis. *Eur Urol* 1997;31:382–384.

262. Mitsudo S, Nakanishi I, Koss LG. Paget's disease of the penis and adjacent skin: its association with fatal sweat gland carcinoma. *Arch Pathol Lab Med* 1981;105:518–520.

263. Metcalf JS, Lee RE, Maize JC. Epidermotropic urothelial carcinoma involving the glans penis. *Arch Dermatol* 1985;121:532–534.

264. Tomaszewski JE, Korat OC, LiVolsi VA, et al. Paget's disease of the urethral meatus following transitional cell carcinoma of the bladder. *J Urol* 1986;135:368–370.

265. Salamanca J, Benito A, García-Peñalver C, et al. Paget's disease of the glans penis secondary to transitional cell carcinoma of the bladder: a report of two cases and review of the literature. *J Cutan Pathol* 2004;31:341–345.

266. Chen YH, Wong TW, Lee JY. Depigmented genital extramammary Paget's disease: a possible histogenetic link to Toker's clear cells and clear cell papulosis. *J Cutan Pathol* 2001;28:105–108.

267. Val-Bernal JF, Garijo MF. Pagetoid dyskeratosis of the prepuce. An incidental histologic finding resembling extramammary Paget's disease. *J Cutan Pathol* 2000;27:387–391.

268. Val-Bernal JF, Hernandez-Nieto E. Benign mucinous metaplasia of the penis. A lesion resembling extramammary Paget's disease. *J Cutan Pathol* 2000;27:76–79.

269. Kuan SF, Montag AG, Hart J, et al. Differential expression of mucin genes in mammary and extramammary Paget's disease. *Am J Surg Pathol* 2001;25:1469–1477.

270. Liegl B, Leibl S, Gogg-Kamerer M, et al. Mammary and extramammary Paget's disease: an immunohistochemical study of 83 cases. *Histopathology* 2007;50:439–447.

271. Smith KJ, Tuur S, Corvette D, et al. Cytokeratin 7 staining in mammary and extramammary Paget's disease. *Mod Pathol* 1997;10:1069–1074.

272. De Nisi MC, D'Amuri A, Toscano M, et al. Usefulness of CDX2 in the diagnosis of extramammary Paget disease associated with malignancies of intestinal type. *Br J Dermatol* 2005;153:677–679.

273. Brown HM, Wilkinson EJ. Uroplakin-III to distinguish primary vulvar Paget disease from Paget disease secondary to urothelial carcinoma. *Hum Pathol* 2002;33:545–548.

274. Yanai H, Takahashi N, Omori M, et al. Immunohistochemistry of p63 in primary and secondary vulvar Paget's disease. *Pathol Int* 2008;58: 648–651.

275. Zeng HA, Cartun R, Ricci A Jr. Potential diagnostic utility of CDX-2 immunophenotyping in extramammary Paget's disease. *Appl Immunohistochem Mol Morphol* 2005;13:342–346.

276. Liegl B, Regauer S. Penile clear cell carcinoma: a report of 5 cases of a distinct entity. *Am J Surg Pathol* 2004;28:1513–1517.

277. Revuz J, Clerici T. Penile melanosis. *J Am Acad Dermatol* 1989;20: 567–570.

278. Barnhill RL, Albert LS, Shama SK, et al. Genital lentiginosis: a clinical and histopathologic study. *J Am Acad Dermatol* 1990;22:453–460.

279. Das Gupta T, Grabstald H. Melanoma of the genitourinary tract. *J Urol* 1965;93:607–614.

280. Sánchez-Ortiz R, Huang SF, Tamboli P et al. Melanoma of the penis, scrotum and male urethra: a 40-year single institution experience. *J Urol* 2005;173:1958–1965.

281. van Geel AN, den Bakker MA, Kirkels W, et al. Prognosis of primary mucosal penile melanoma: a series of 19 Dutch patients and 47 patients from the literature. *Urology* 2007;70:143–147.

282. Dehner LP, Smith BH. Soft tissue tumors of the penis. A clinicopathologic study of 46 cases. *Cancer* 1970;25:1431–1447.

283. Katona TM, Lopez-Beltran A, MacLennan GT, et al. Soft tissue tumors of the penis: a review. *Anal Quant Cytol Histol* 2006;28:193–206.

284. Senoh K, Miyazaki T, Kikuchi I, et al. Angiomatous lesions of glans penis. *Urology* 1981;17:194–196.

285. Hemal AK, Goswami AK, Sharma SK, et al. Penile venous haemangioma. *Aust N Z J Surg* 1989;59:814–886.

286. Fetsch JF, Sesterhenn IA, Miettinen M, et al. Epithelioid hemangioma of the penis: a clinicopathologic and immunohistochemical analysis of 19 cases, with special reference to exuberant examples often confused with epithelioid hemangioendothelioma and epithelioid angiosarcoma. *Am J Surg Pathol* 2004;28:523–533.

287. Solsona E, Ricos J, Monros J, et al. [Cavernous lymphangioma of the penis]. *Acta Urol Esp* 1986;10:73–76.

288. Mortesenn H, Murphy L. Angiomatous malformations of the glans penis. *J Urol* 1950;64:396–399.

289. Macaluso JN Jr, Sullivan JW, Tomberlin S. Glomus tumor of glans penis. *Urology* 1985;25:409–410.

290. Fetsch JF, Brinsko RW, Davis CJ Jr, et al. A distinctive myointimal proliferation ('myointimoma') involving the corpus spongiosum of the glans penis: a clinicopathologic and immunohistochemical analysis of 10 cases. *Am J Surg Pathol* 2000;24:1524–1530.

291. McKenney JK, Collins MH, Carretero AP, et al. Penile myointimoma in children and adolescents: a clinicopathologic study of 5 cases supporting a distinct entity. *Am J Surg Pathol* 2007;31:1622–1626.

292. Ogawa A, Watanabe K. Genitourinary neurofibromatosis in a child presenting with an enlarged penis and scrotum. *J Urol* 1986;135:755–757.

293. Maher JD, Thompson GM, Loening S, et al. Penile plexiform neurofibroma: case report and review of the literature. *J Urol* 1988;139:1310–1312.

294. Bryant J. Granular cell tumor of penis and scrotum. *Urology* 1995;45:332–334.

295. Liu SP, Shun CT, Chang SJ, et al. Leiomyoma of the corpus cavernosum of the penis. *Int J Urol* 2007;14:257–258.

296. Fletcher CD, Lowe D. Inflammatory fibrous histiocytoma of the penis. *Histopathology* 1984;8:1079–1084.

297. Ro JY, Amin MB, Ayala AG. Penis and scrotum. In: Fletcher CDM, ed. *Diagnostic Histopathology of Tumors.* 3rd ed. Churchill Livingstone, Elsevier; 2007:861–879.

298. Pack GT, Trinidad SS, Humphreys JA. Primary leiomyosarcoma of the penis: report of a case. *J Urol* 1963;89:839–841.

299. Greenwood N, Fox H, Edwards EC. Leiomyosarcoma of the penis. *Cancer* 1972;29:481–483.

300. McDonald MW, O'Connell JR, Manning JT, et al. Leiomyosarcoma of the penis. *J Urol* 1983;130:788–789.

301. Fetsch JF, Davis Jr CJ, Miettinen M, et al. Leiomyosarcoma of the penis: a clinicopathologic study of 14 cases with review of the literature and discussion of the differential diagnosis. *Am J Surg Pathol* 2004;28:115–125.

302. Kagu MB, Nggada HA, Garandawa HI, et al. AIDS-associated Kaposi's sarcoma in Northeastern Nigeria. *Singapore Med J* 2006;47:1069–1074.

303. Hymes KB, Cheung T, Greene JB, et al. Kaposi's sarcoma in homosexual men-a report of eight cases. *Lancet* 1981;2:598–600.

304. Lowe FC, Lattimer DG, Metroka CE. Kaposi's sarcoma of the penis in patients with acquired immunodeficiency syndrome. *J Urol* 1989;142:1475–1477.

305. Zambolin T, Simeone C, Baronchelli C, et al. Kaposi's sarcoma of the penis. *Br J Urol* 1989;63:645–646.

306. Conger K, Sporer A. Kaposi's sarcoma limited to glans penis. *Urology* 1985;26:173–175.

307. Pacifico A, Piccolo D, Fargnoli MC, et al. Kaposi's sarcoma of the glans penis in an immunocompetent patient. *Eur J Dermatol* 2003;13:582–583.

308. Elhosseiny AA, Ramaswamy G, Healy RO. Epithelioid hemangioendothelioma of penis. *Urology* 1986;28:243–245.

309. Zastrow S, Baretton GB, Wirth MP. Multifocal recurring epithelioid hemangioendothelioma of the penis. *Urology* 2008;71:351.e9–e10.

310. Mentzel T, Beham A, Calonje E, et al. Epithelioid hemangioendothelioma of skin and soft tissues: clinicopathologic and immunohistochemical study of 30 cases. *Am J Surg Pathol* 1997;21:363–374.

311. Moore SW, Wheeler JE, Hefter LG. Epithelioid sarcoma masquerading as Peyronie's disease. *Cancer* 1975;35:1706–1710.

312. Guillou L, Wadden C, Coindre JM, et al. "Proximal-type" epithelioid sarcoma, a distinctive aggressive neoplasm showing rhabdoid features. Clinicopathologic, immunohistochemical, and ultrastructural study of a series. *Am J Surg Pathol* 1997;21:130–146.

313. Antoneli CB, Novaes PE, Alves AC, et al. Rhabdomyosarcoma of the penis in a 15-month-old boy. *J Urol* 1998;160:2200–2201.

314. Ramos JZ, Pack GT. Primary embryonal rhabdomyosarcoma of the penis in a 2-year-old child. *J Urol* 1966;96:928–932.

315. Moran CA, Kaneko M. Malignant fibrous histiocytoma of the glans penis. *Am J Dermatopathol* 1990;12:182–187.

316. Saw D, Tse CH, Chan J, et al. Clear cell sarcoma of the penis. *Hum Pathol* 1986;17:423–425.

317. Charuwichitratana S, Polnikorn N, Timpatanapong P. Dermatofibrosarcoma protuberans of the penis: a case report. *J Med Assoc Thai* 1981;64:148–151.

318. Lue TF, Macchia RJ, Vuletin JC, et al. Fibrosarcoma of penis. *Urology* 1980;15:498–500.

319. Arena F, di Stefano C, Peracchia G, et al. Primary lymphoma of the penis: diagnosis and treatment. *Eur Urol* 2001;39:232–235.

320. Gonzalez-Campora R, Nogales FF Jr, Lerma E, et al. Lymphoma of the penis. *J Urol* 1981;126:270–271.

321. Haque S, Noble J, Wotherspoon A, et al. MALT lymphoma of the foreskin. *Leuk Lymphoma* 2004;45:1699–1701.

322. Tomb RR, Stephan F, Klein-Tomb L, et al. Recurrent primary CD30+ lymphoma of the penis. *Br J Dermatol* 2003;149:903–905.

323. Thorns C, Urban H, Remmler K, et al. Primary cutaneous T-cell lymphoma of the penis. *Histopathology* 2003;42:513–514.

324. Lanesky JR, Law DW, Roth SJ, et al. Burkitt lymphoma metastatic to penis. *Urology* 1980;15:610–612.

325. Gallardo F, Pujol RM, Barranco C, et al. Progressive painless swelling of glans penis: uncommon clinical manifestation of systemic non-Hodgkin's lymphoma. *Urology* 2008;73:929.e3–929.e5.

326. Ponniah A, Brown CT, Taylor P. Priapism secondary to leukemia: effective management with prompt leukapheresis. *Int J Urol* 2004;11:809–810.

327. Myers DA, Strandjord SE, Marcus RB Jr, et al. Histiocytosis X presenting as a primary penile lesion. *J Urol* 1981;126:268–269.

328. Miettinen M, Fetsch JF. Reticulohistiocytoma (solitary epithelioid histiocytoma): a clinicopathologic and immunohistochemical study of 44 cases. *Am J Surg Pathol* 2006;30:521–528.

329. Hautmann RE, Bachor R. Juvenile xanthogranuloma of the penis. *J Urol* 1993;150:456–457.

330. Chaux A, Amin M, Cubilla AL, et al. Metastatic tumors to the penis: a report of 17 cases and review of the literature. *Int J Surg Pathol* 2011;19:597–606.

331. Powell BL, Craig JB, Muss HB. Secondary malignancies of the penis and epididymis: a case report and review of the literature. *J Clin Oncol* 1985;3:110–116.

332. Perez-Mesa C, Oxenhandler R. Metastatic tumors of the penis. *J Surg Oncol* 1989;42:11–15.

333. Hizli F, Berkmen F. Penile metastasis from other malignancies. A study of ten cases and review of the literature. *Urol Int* 2006;76:118–121.

334. Wang SQ, Mecca PS, Myskowski PL, et al. Scrotal and penile papules and plaques as the initial manifestation of a cutaneous metastasis of adenocarcinoma of the prostate: case report and review of the literature. *J Cutan Pathol* 2008;35:681–684.

335. Tu SM, Reyes A, Maa A, et al. Prostate carcinoma with testicular or penile metastases. Clinical, pathologic, and immunohistochemical features. *Cancer* 2002;94:2610–2617.

336. Ketata S, Boulaire JL, Soulimane B, et al. Metachronous metastasis to the penis from a rectal adenocarcinoma. *Clin Colorectal Cancer* 2007;6:657–659.

337. Zheng FF, Zhang ZY, Dai YP, et al. Metastasis to the penis in a patient with adenocarcinoma of lung, case report and literature review. *Med Oncol* 2009;26:228–232.

338. Karanjia ND, King H, Schweitzer FA. Metastases to the penis from carcinoma of the stomach. *Br J Urol* 1987;60:368.

339. Celma Doménech A, Planas Morin J, et al. [Priapism secondary to penis infiltration of bladder cancer]. *Actas Urol Esp* 2008;32:749–751.

340. Ulbright TM, Amin MB, Young RH. *Tumors of the testis, adnexa, spermatic cord and scrotum. Atlas of Tumor Pathology. Armed Forces Institute of Pathology.* 3rd Series. Washington, DC; 1999.

341. Morley J. The lymphatics of the scrotum. In relation to the radial operation for scrotal epithelioma. *Lancet* 1911;2:1545.

342. Lowe FC. Squamous cell carcinoma of the scrotum. *J Urol* 1983;130: 423–427.

343. Noble WC, Savin JA. Trichomycosis of the scrotal hair. *Arch Dermatol* 1985;121:25.

344. Shelley WB, Miller MA. Electron microscopy, histochemistry, and microbiology of bacterial adhesion in trichomycosis axillaris. *J Am Acad Dermatol* 1984;10:1005–1014.

345. Ellner KM, McBride ME, Kalter DC, et al. White piedra: evidence for a synergistic infection. *Br J Dermatol* 1990;123:355–363.

346. Anderson BB, Cadogan CA, Gangadharam D. Hidradenitis suppurativa of the perineum, scrotum, and gluteal area: presentation, complications, and treatment. *J Natl Med Assoc* 1982;74:999–1003.

347. Ray B. Hidradenitis suppurativa of the scrotum. *J Urol* 1977;118: 686–687.

348. Shah V, Shet T. Scrotal calcinosis results from calcification of cysts derived from hair follicles: a series of 20 cases evaluating the spectrum of changes resulting in scrotal calcinosis. *Am J Dermatopathol* 2007;29:172–175.

349. Bhawan J, Malhotra R, Franks S. The so-called idiopathic scrotal calcinosis. *Arch Dermatol* 1983;119:709.

350. Dare AJ, Axelsen RA. Scrotal calcinosis: origin from dystrophic calcification of eccrine duct milia. *J Cutan Pathol* 1988;15:142–149.

351. Ito A, Sakamoto F, Ito M. Dystrophic scrotal calcinosis originating from benign eccrine epithelial cysts. *Br J Dermatol* 2001;144: 146–150.

352. Jung SE, Lee JM, Kang CS, et al. Sclerosing lipogranuloma of the scrotum: sonographic findings and pathologic correlation. *J Ultrasound Med* 2007;26:1231–1233.

353. Ohtsuki Y, Miyazaki J, Kamei Y, et al. Three cases of sclerosing lipogranuloma: an immunohistochemical study. *Med Mol Morphol* 2007;40:108–111.

354. Watanabe K, Hoshi N, Baba K, et al. Immunohistochemical profile of primary sclerosing lipogranuloma of the scrotum: report of five cases. *Pathol Int* 1995;45:854–859.

355. Hollander JB, Begun FP, Lee RD. Scrotal fat necrosis. *J Urol* 1985;134:150–151.

356. Harkness G, Meikle G, Craw S, et al. Ultrasound appearance of scrotal fat necrosis in prepubertal boys. *Pediatr Radiol* 2007;37:370–373.

357. Mohsin SK, Lee MW, Amin MB, et al. Cutaneous verruciform xanthoma: a report of five cases investigating the etiology and nature of xanthomatous cells. *Am J Surg Pathol* 1998;22:479–487.

358. Khaskhely NM, Uezato H, Kamiyama T, et al. Association of human papillomavirus type 6 with a verruciform xanthoma. *Am J Dermatopathol* 2000;22:447–452.

359. Rabii R, Joual A, Bellabidia B, et al. [Giant scrotal condyloma acuminata: a case report]. *Ann Urol (Paris)* 2001;35:67–70.

360. Ray B, Whitmore WF Jr. Experience with carcinoma of the scrotum. *J Urol* 1977;117:741–745.

361. Lowe FC. Squamous cell carcinoma of the scrotum. *J Urol* 1983;130: 423–427.

362. Lowe FC. Squamous cell carcinoma of scrotum. *Urology* 1985;25:63–65.

363. Andrews PE, Farrow GM, Oesterling JE. Squamous cell carcinoma of the scrotum: long-term followup of 14 patients. *J Urol* 1991;146:1299–1304.

364. Lowe FC. Squamous-cell carcinoma of the scrotum. *Urol Clin North Am* 1992;19:397–405.

365. Taniguchi S, Furukawa M, Kutsuna H, et al. Squamous cell carcinoma of the scrotum. *Dermatology* 1996;193:253–254.

366. Orihuela E, Tyring SK, Pow-Sang M, et al. Development of human papillomavirus type 16 associated squamous cell carcinoma of the scrotum in a patient with Darier's disease treated with systemic isotretinoin. *J Urol* 1995;153:1940–1943.

367. Arias Fúnez F, Fernández Fernández E, Perales Cabanas L, et al. [Epidermoid carcinoma of the scrotum]. *Arch Esp Urol* 2000;53:937–940.

368. Shifrin DA, Lange MK, Kahnoski RJ, et al. Squamous cell carcinoma of the scrotum in a radiation technologist and the use of sentinel lymph node biopsy in recurrent disease. *Am Surg* 2007;73:302–303.

369. Peng W, Feng G, Lu H, et al. A case report of scrotal carcinoma and review of the literature. *Case Rep Oncol* 2012;5:434–438.

370. Chintamani, Shankar M, Singhal V, et al. Squamous cell carcinoma developing in the scar of Fournier's gangrene-case report. *BMC Cancer* 2004;4:16.

371. Kotwal S, Madaan S, Prescott S, et al. Unusual squamous cell carcinoma of the scrotum arising from a well healed, innocuous scar of an infertility procedure: a case report. *Ann R Coll Surg Engl* 2007;89: W17–W19.

372. Foroudi F, Turner S. Verrucous scrotal carcinoma: a radioresponsive tumor. *J Urol* 1999;162:1694–1695.

373. Schleicher SM, Milstein HJ, Ilowite R. Basal cell carcinoma of the scrotum. *Cutis* 1997;59:116.

374. Gibson GE, Ahmed I. Perianal and genital basal cell carcinoma: a clinicopathologic review of 51 cases. *J Am Acad Dermatol* 2001;45: 68–71.

375. Handa Y, Kato Y, Ishikawa H, et al. Giant superficial basal cell carcinoma of the scrotum. *Eur J Dermatol* 2005;15:186–188.

376. Dai B, Kong YY, Ye DW, et al. Basal cell carcinoma of the scrotum: clinicopathologic analysis of 10 cases. *Dermatol Surg* 2012;38:783–790.

377. Wang Z, Lu M, Dong GQ, et al. Penile and scrotal Paget's disease: 130 Chinese patients with long-term follow-up. *BJU Int* 2008;102: 485–488.

378. Parada D, Moreira O, López C, et al. Extramammary Paget's disease of scrotum. A case with local lymph node metastasis. *Arch Esp Urol* 2005;58:85–89.

379. Evans J, Datta MW, Goolsby M, et al. Eccrine porocarcinoma of the scrotum. *Can J Urol* 2005;12:2722–2723.

380. Braun-Falco M, Eberlein-König B, Ring J, et al. [Scrotal leiomyoma]. *Hautarzt* 2002;3:258–260.

381. Ameur A, Touiti D, Jira H, et al. [Multiple leiomyoma of the scrotum. A case report]. *Ann Urol (Paris)* 2002;36:154–156.

382. Popek EJ, Montgomery EA, Fourcroy JL. Fibrous hamartoma of infancy in the genital region: findings of 15 cases. *J Urol* 1994;152: 990–993.

383. Godoy G, Mufarrij PW, Tsou HC, et al. Granular cell tumor of scrotum: a rare tumor of the male external genitalia. *Urology* 2008;72:716.

384. Laskin WB, Fetsch JF, Mostofi FK. Angiomyofibroblastomalike tumor of the male genital tract: analysis of 11 cases with comparison to female angiomyofibroblastoma and spindle cell lipoma. *Am J Surg Pathol* 1998;22:6–16.

385. Tsang WY, Chan JK, Lee KC, et al. Aggressive angiomyxoma. A report of four cases occurring in men. *Am J Surg Pathol* 1992;16:1059–1065.

386. Iezzoni JC, Fechner RE, Wong LS, et al. Aggressive angiomyxoma in males. A report of four cases. *Am J Clin Pathol* 1995;104:391–396.

387. Fisher C, Goldblum JR, Epstein JI, et al. Leiomyosarcoma of the paratesticular region: a clinicopathologic study. *Am J Surg Pathol* 2001;25:1143–1149.

388. Jeddy TA, Vowles RH, Southam JA. Leiomyosarcoma of the dartos muscle. *Br J Urol* 1994;74:129–130.

389. Newman PL, Fletcher CD. Smooth muscle tumours of the external genitalia: clinicopathological analysis of a series. *Histopathology* 1991;18:523–529.

390. Lucas DR, Nascimento AG, Sanjay BK, et al. Well-differentiated liposarcoma. The Mayo Clinic experience with 58 cases. *Am J Clin Pathol* 1994;102:677–683.

391. Bauer JJ, Sesterhenn IA, Costabile RA. Myxoid liposarcoma of the scrotal wall. *J Urol* 1995;153:1938–1939.

392. Henricks WH, Chu YC, Goldblum JR, et al. Dedifferentiated liposarcoma: a clinicopathological analysis of 155 cases with a proposal for an expanded definition of dedifferentiation. *Am J Surg Pathol* 1997;21:271–281.

393. Thanakit V, Nelson SD, Udomsawaengsup S. Round cell liposarcoma of scrotum with indolent course in young adult. *J Med Assoc Thai* 2005;88:1302–1307.

394. Suster S, Wong TY, Moran CA. Sarcomas with combined features of liposarcoma and leiomyosarcoma. Study of two cases of an unusual soft-tissue tumor showing dual lineage differentiation. *Am J Surg Pathol* 1993;17:905–911.

395. Armah HB, Palekar A, Rao UN, et al. Proximal-type epithelioid sarcoma of the scrotum: a difficult diagnosis in an unusual location and review of the literature. *Pathology* 2008;40:326–330.

396. Yokozeki H, Inai T, Kagawa S, et al. [A case of intrascrotal rhabdomyosarcoma]. *Hinyokika Kiyo* 1987;33:625–628.

397. Papadimitriou JC, Drachenberg CB. Posttraumatic spindle cell nodules. Immunohistochemical and ultrastructural study of two scrotal lesions. *Arch Pathol Lab Med* 1994;118:709–711.

398. Nakamura Y, Tajima F, Omura H, et al. Primary effusion lymphoma of the left scrotum. *Intern Med* 2003;42:351–353.

399. Lan CC, Yu HS, Cheng ST, et al. Relapsing ulcerative papules over bilateral hands and scrotum in an Asian man: an atypical manifestation of primary cutaneous CD30-positive lymphoma. *J Dermatol* 2003;30:230–235.

400. McLellan RA, Norman RW. Primary extranodal lymphoma of the scrotum. *Can J Urol* 2000;7:949–951.

401. Da Silva E, Pesqueira D, Ferreira EL, et al. [Urology images. Cutaneous lymphoma in the perineal scrotum]. *Actas Urol Esp* 1999;23:287.

402. Allen DC, Walsh MY. Malignant lymphoma of the scrotum and Wegener's granulomatosis of the penis—genital presentation of systemic disease. *Ulster Med J* 1996;65:169–172.

403. Doll DC, Diaz-Arias AA. Peripheral T-cell lymphoma of the scrotum. *Acta Haematol* 1994;91:77–79.

404. Wang SQ, Mecca PS, Myskowski PL, et al. Scrotal and penile papules and plaques as the initial manifestation of a cutaneous metastasis of adenocarcinoma of the prostate: case report and review of the literature. *J Cutan Pathol* 2008;35:681–684.

405. Hayashi H, Shimizu T, Shimizu H. Scrotal metastases originating from colorectal carcinoma. *Clin Exp Dermatol* 2003;28:226–227.

406. Peng W, Feng G, Lu H, et al. A case report of scrotalcarcinoma and review of the literature. *Case Rep Oncol* 2012;5:434–438.

407. Aridogan IA, Satar N, Doran E, et al. Scrotal skin metastases of renal cell carcinoma: a case report. *Acta Chir Belg* 2004;104:599–600.

408. Takhtani D, Saleeb SF, Teplick SK. General case of the day. Desmoplastic small round cell tumor of the abdomen with scrotal metastases. *Radiographics* 1999;19:252–254.

409. Froehner M, Ockert D, Aust DE, et al. Gastrointestinal stromal tumor presenting as a scrotal mass. *Int J Urol* 2004;11:445–447.

Index

(Note: Page numbers in italics indicates figures and those followed by "t" indicates tables and those followed by "b" indicates boxes.)